Understanding Medical-Surgical Nursing

Understanding Medical-Surgical Nursing

Linda S. Williams, MSN, RN, C, CS

Associate Professor of Nursing
Jackson Community College
Registered Nurse Care Coordinator
W.A. Foote Memorial Hospital
Jackson, Michigan

Paula D. Hopper, MSN, RN

Associate Professor of Nursing
Jackson Community College
Registered Nurse Care Coordinator
W.A. Foote Memorial Hospital
Jackson, Michigan

 F. A. DAVIS COMPANY • Philadelphia

F. A. Davis Company
1915 Arch Street
Philadelphia, PA 19103

Printed in the United States of America

Last digit indicates print number: 10 9 8 7 6 5 4 3

Acquisitions Editor: Alan Sorkowitz
Developmental Editor: Peg Waltner
Production Editor: Samuel A. Rondinelli
Designer: Bill Donnelly
Cover Designer: Louis Forgione
Cover Photograph: Doug Rickards

As new scientific information becomes available through basic and clinical research, recommended treatments and drug therapies undergo changes. The author(s) and publisher have done everything possible to make this book accurate, up to date, and in accord with accepted standards at the time of publication. The authors, editors, and publisher are not responsible for errors or omissions or for consequences from application of the book, and make no warranty, expressed or implied, in regard to the contents of the book. Any practice described in this book should be applied by the reader in accordance with professional standards of care used in regard to the unique circumstances that may apply in each situation. The reader is advised always to check product information (package inserts) for changes and new information regarding dose and contraindications before administering any drug. Caution is especially urged when using new or infrequently ordered drugs.

Library of Congress Cataloging in Publication Data

Williams, Linda S. (Linda Sue), 1954-
    Understanding medical-surgical nursing / Linda S. Williams, Paula
D. Hopper
      p.   cm.
    Includes bibliographical references and index.
    ISBN 0-8036-0331-2
    1. Nursing.   2. Surgical nursing.   I. Hopper, Paula D.
II. Title.
    [DNLM: 1. Nursing Care.   2. Nursing.   WY 100 W724u 1998]
RT41.W576   1998
610.73--dc21
DNLM/DLC   98-50588
for Library of Congress   CIP

Dedication

To our students, who provide us with inspiration, motivation, and the joy of being a part of their learning experience.

To Garland for his continual loving support and encouragement; to Jami, Jacqueline, and Richard for their support and assistance; to MaryAnne Pietraniec-Shannon for friendship, humor, and encouragement when it was needed most; in memoriam Jeanine Stewart-Zelnis.

Linda Williams

With love, to my husband, Dave, who encouraged me, read many first drafts, and cooked a lot while I was writing. To my children, Dan and Libby, who were patient when I tied up the computer for days at a time. And to my parents, who raised me to believe I could do anything I set my mind to.

Paula Hopper

Preface

Understanding Medical Surgical Nursing is a comprehensive medical-surgical text intended for licensed practical and vocational nursing students. It resulted from our search for an excellent LPN/LVN–level text that would help students *understand* material rather than just memorize it. Many of the existing textbooks provided a lot of information but not enough rationale for the increasingly complex nursing care being provided by LPNs and LVNs. We requested such a book from the F.A. Davis representative for our college, who in turn said, "Why don't you write one?" So we did.

Features of the Textbook

Included in the textbook are items our students and we have found useful in our own LPN classrooms. These include:

- Chapter objectives
- Review of anatomy and physiology at the beginning of each unit
- New word pronunciation section at the beginning of each chapter
- Information on the effects of aging on body systems and on the nursing care of older adults
- Learning tips throughout the chapters
- Word-building techniques
- Comprehensive glossary of new words
- Nursing care plans with geriatric considerations highlighted
- Common laboratory and diagnostic tests
- Brief pathophysiology for each illness
- Boxed presentations on gerontological issues, therapeutic nutrition, ethical considerations, and cultural considerations
- Hints for home health care providers
- Critical thinking exercises throughout the chapters
- Review questions at the end of each chapter

Focus of the Textbook

We use the nursing process to provide a unifying framework for the book. Within this framework, we emphasize understanding, critical thinking, and application.

We believe that the student who learns to think critically will be better able to apply information to new situations. Case studies appear throughout the chapters to foster critical thinking. These are followed by questions that require more than simple recall of material. Answers to these questions are included in the textbook to provide immediate feedback and to reinforce learning.

Since illustrations enhance the understanding and readability of the text, we have included over 430 figures. Most of the artwork and photographs are original and specifically designed to support the text. Additional figures, tables, and boxed materials are used to clarify complex material.

How to Use This Textbook

Each chapter begins with a list of new words and their pronunciations. These words are then presented in bold type as they first appear in the textbook, indicating that they also appear in the glossary at the end of the text. Students are encouraged to learn the meanings of these words as they are encountered to enhance understanding of the material.

Chapter objectives help students focus on what is important in each chapter. After reading each chapter, students are encouraged to go back to the objectives and write out the answer for each objective.

Mnemonics, acrostics, and other learning tips are used within the text to enhance understanding and retention of material. Students may want to develop their own memory techniques in addition to those provided. Many of the learning tips have been developed and used in our own classrooms. We find them helpful in fostering understanding of complex concepts or as memory aids. However, we want to stress that memorization is not the primary focus of the text but rather a foundation for developing critical thinking skills. Understanding and application will serve the student far better than memorization will when dealing with new situations.

Each chapter includes one or more case studies designed to help students apply material that has been presented. A series of questions related to the case study helps students integrate the material into their thinking. These questions emphasize critical thinking, which is based on a foundation of recall and understanding of material. Students are encouraged to answer the questions before looking up the answers at the end of the chapter to enhance their learning.

Review questions appear at the end of each chapter. These are written in a multiple-choice format to help students prepare for the NCLEX-PN. Students are encouraged to answer the questions before looking up the answers at the end of the textbook to assess their understanding.

A bibliography at the end of each chapter provides students with sources for additional reading material. Web sites have been included in some chapters. We believe it is important for students to interact with current technology to expand their informational resources.

Appendices are included for easy reference. They cover nursing diagnoses, lab values, abbreviations, and common prefixes and suffixes to assist in learning word-building techniques.

Supplements to the Textbook

A *Study Guide* is available to provide the student additional contact and practice with the material. Each chapter includes vocabulary practice, objective exercises using a variety of question types (including figure labeling), a case study or other critical thinking exercise, and review questions written in NCLEX-PN format. Answers are provided so students can solidify their understanding and learning with immediate feedback. Rationales are provided for review question answers.

An *Instructor's Guide* provides materials for use in the classroom. Each chapter has a chapter outline with suggested classroom activities. Also included are student activities suitable for duplicating and using for individual practice or for collaborative learning activities. These activities help the student to interact with the material, understand it, and apply it. We have used many of these activities with our own practical nursing students, and their feedback has helped to refine them. Students have demonstrated increased retention of material, improved understanding, and enjoyment of these exercises. Another benefit is the sense of community the students develop as a result of working in groups. A brief introduction and guidelines for using collaborative learning techniques are included. We believe the use of collaborative learning has greatly enhanced our students' success in achieving their educational and licensure goals.

When we first began using collaborative learning exercises extensively, our students commented, "It hurts to think!" Over time, as they gained experience and practice in thinking critically, they enjoyed the challenge and became skilled in responding to new situations. If collaborative learning is a new concept to students, as with any skill, time needs to be allowed for students to learn to use it. However, it is rewarding to see the growth that occurs when students learn how to use this technique.

A computerized *Test Bank*, available free to instructors who adopt the textbook, provides test questions that assist students to prepare for state board examinations. These questions have been prepared according to test item writing protocols. Many of the questions have been critiqued by a testing expert to enhance their quality. These questions are in multiple-choice format and test recall and application of material. We have developed, used, and refined many of the test questions in our own medical-surgical course for practical nursing students. The test bank program allows instructors to choose and modify the questions that best suit their classroom needs.

A complimentary transparency package with 100 transparencies has been prepared for use by instructors who adopt the textbook. They include figures and tables from the textbook to facilitate classroom instruction.

Feedback

We plan to continually improve and develop future editions of this textbook. We welcome feedback from both students and faculty: let us know what works well for you, your suggestions for changes, and new ideas for future editions. Please contact us through F.A. Davis Company, 1915 Arch Street, Philadelphia, PA 19103, or by e-mail at www.fadavis.com with your comments and ideas.

Linda Williams

Paula Hopper

Acknowledgments

Many people have helped to make this book a reality. First and foremost are our students, who provided us with the inspiration to undertake this project. We hope they find this text worth reading.

The F.A. Davis Company has been an exceptional publishing company with which to work. We feel fortunate to have had their enthusiasm and confidence in our book. The staff at F.A. Davis has guided us through this project from its inception to publication to help us create a student-friendly book that truly promotes understanding of medical-surgical nursing.

F.A. Davis nursing editor Alan Sorkowitz has been our most ardent supporter and cheerleader. His humor and coaching abilities helped to keep us going. His efforts on this project were numerous and included being a wonderful historian and tour guide of the city of Philadelphia. We are indebted to his guidance and enthusiasm for this project, which allowed us to realize our dream of providing a tool to foster understanding for LPN/LVN students.

Director of production Herbert J. Powell, Jr., was endlessly patient as he guided us through the production process. Samuel Rondinelli concluded the process and kept us on schedule during the last months.

Developmental editor Peg Waltner helped us format the book, ensured that details were accurate, coordinated our photo shoot, and gave us encouragement.

We wish to thank the staff of Thomas Jefferson University Medical Center, in Philadelphia, and especially Ann Reynolds, for assisting us in a successful photo shoot. Thanks also to Nanine Hartzenbusch, our photographer, who provided a wonderful human touch to the photography.

Graphic World Publishing Services production editor Carol U. O'Connell did an outstanding job of coordinating the development of our manuscript into a book. Graphic World Illustration Studio's John Denk created wonderful art to enhance the students' understanding of concepts.

Contributors from across the United States and Canada, including many well-known experts in their fields, brought expertise, diversity, and regional perspectives to the content. Their hard work is much appreciated. Donna Ignatavicius was especially helpful in providing material at the last minute, offering much-needed expertise and encouraging us when we were feeling overwhelmed. Reviewers from throughout the United States provided valuable insights that enhanced the quality of the text. Kara Schmitt, Director, Testing Services Division, Michigan Department of Consumer and Industry Services, provided expertise in writing multiple-choice test questions. Cheryl White, LPN, gave us additional perspective about the role of the LPN in the current health care environment.

Many of our coworkers have contributed to this book and given us ongoing encouragement and validation of the worthiness of this project. Betty Ackley and Carroll Lutz were especially helpful in providing material, advice, and encouragement. Linda Nabozny assisted with pedagogical aids. Debbie, Anna, Deanna, Dollie, Kathy, Lynn, Stephanie, and Suzanne provided ongoing encouragement and insight.

We wish to thank everyone who played a role, however large or small, in helping us to provide a tool to help students realize their dreams of becoming LPN/LVNs. We hope this book will help train nurses who can provide safe and expert care because they are able to think critically.

Contributors

Jeanette Acker, RN, BSN
Manager, Stepdown Unit
W.A. Foote Memorial Hospital
Jackson, Michigan

Betty J. Ackley, RN, MSN, EdS
Professor of Nursing
Jackson Community College
Jackson, Michigan

Debra Aucoin-Ratcliff, RN, BSN, MN
Nursing Program Director
Western Career College
Sacramento, California

Joseph T. Catalano, RN, PhD
Professor of Nursing
East Central University
Ada, Oklahoma

Elizabeth Chapman, RN, MS, CCRN
Nursing Faculty
Mississippi Gulf Coast Community College
Gulfport, Mississippi
ICU Staff Nurse
Hancock Medical Center
Bay St. Louis, Mississippi

Linda Hopper Cook, RN, MN
University of Alberta
Grant MacEwan Community College
Collaborative Nursing Program
Edmonton, Alberta

Kathleen R. Culliton, APRN, MS, GNP
Assistant Professor
Weber State University
Ogden, Utah

Constance Monlezun Darbonne, RN, MPH, CFNP
Family Nurse Practitioner
Clinical Instructor, Community Health
McNeese State University
Lake Charles, Louisiana

Vera Dutro, RN, BS, OCN
Infusion Nurse
Zanesville Infusion Therapy
Zanesville, Ohio

Sharon Ivy Gordon, RN, MSN, CNOR
Instructor, Medical/Surgical Nursing
Associate Degree Nursing Program
Coordinator, LPN-to-RN Transition Program
Mississippi Gulf Coast Community College
Gulfport, Mississippi
Staff Nurse
Gulf Coast Medical Center
Biloxi, Mississippi

Paula D. Hopper, MSN, RN
Associate Professor of Nursing
Jackson Community College
Registered Nurse Care Coordinator
W.A. Foote Memorial Hospital
Jackson, Michigan

Donna D. Ignatavicius, MS, RN, CM
Clinical Nurse Specialist in
    Medical/Surgical/Gerontological Nursing
Calvert Memorial Hospital
Owner/Consultant, DI Associates
Prince Frederick, Maryland

Cheryl L. Ivey, RN, MSN, CS
Nurse Manager
Inpatient Oncology
Memorial Hospital at Gulfport
Gulfport, Mississippi

Josephine Whitney Johns, RN, OCN, CRNI
South Mississippi Home Health
Oncology Specialty Nurse
Board of Director, Mississippi Cancer Pain Initiative
Cofounder, Mississippi Gulf Coast Chapter
Oncology Nurse Association
Gulfport, Mississippi

Elaine Bishop Kennedy, RN, BSN, MS, EdD
Associate Professor, Nursing
Wor-Wie Community College
Salisbury, Maryland

Karen P. Kettelman, RN, BA
Pain Management Coordinator
Doctors Medical Center
Modesto, California

Gail Ladwig, RN, MSN, CHTP
Associate Professor of Nursing
Coordinator JCC/UM BSN Transfer Program
Jackson Community College
Jackson, Michigan

Diane Lewis, RN, MS
Hospice of Grant/Riverside Methodist Hospitals
Westerville, Ohio

Gary S. Lott, RN, MS
Instructor of Nursing
Mississippi Gulf Coast Community College
Gulfport, Mississippi

Carroll A. Lutz, RN, MA
Professor Emerita of Nursing
Jackson Community College
Jackson, Michigan

Deborah J. Mauffray, RN, MSN, CNS, CDE, CWOCN
Clinical Nurse Specialist in Wound, Ostomy, and
    Incontinence
Memorial Hospital at Gulfport
Gulfport, Mississippi

Cindy Meredith, RN, MSN
Adjunct Lecturer in Nursing
University of Michigan–Flint
Flint, Michigan

Marsha A. Miles, RN, MSN, CCRN
Instructor
Valdosta State University
College of Nursing
Valdosta, Georgia

Kathy Neeb, RN, BA
Training Designer
Health Risk Management
Former Instructor, Practical Nursing
Minneapolis Community and Technical College
Minneapolis, Minnesota

Sharon M. Nowak, RN, BSN, CCRN
Assistant Professor of Nursing
Jackson Community College
Jackson, Michigan

Lazette Nowicki, RN, MSN
Nursing Program Assistant Director
Western Career College
Sacramento, California

MaryAnne Pietraniec-Shannon, RN, MSN, CS
Associate Professor of Nursing
Lake Superior State University
Sault Ste. Marie, Michigan

Larry Purnell, RN, PhD
Associate Professor
College of Health and Nursing Sciences
University of Delaware
Newark, Delaware

Deborah L. Roush, RN, MSN
Assistant Professor
Valdosta State University
College of Nursing
Valdosta, Georgia

Valerie C. Scanlon, PhD
College of Mount St. Vincent
Riverdale, New York

Kate Schmitz, RN, MS
Clinical Nurse, Emergency Department
St. Joseph Hospital
Creighton University Medical Center
Omaha, Nebraska

Sally Schnell, RN, MSN, CNRN
Professional Education Coordinator
Regional Organ Bank of Illinois
Chicago, Illinois

Jill F. Secord, RN, BSN, CRNI
University of Michigan Health System—M-CARE
Jackson, Michigan

Patrick M. Shannon, JD, MPH
Chippewa County Prosecuting Attorney
Assistant Professor
Lake Superior State University
Sault Ste. Marie, Michigan

Martha Spray, RN, BSN, MS
Adult PN Instructor
Mid East Ohio Vocational School
Zanesville, Ohio

Rita Bolek Trofino, RN, MNEd
Nurse Educator
Former Assistant Professor
Nursing Department
St. Francis College
Loretto, Pennsylvania
Former Staff Development Instructor
Burn Unit
Western Pennsylvania Hospital
Pittsburgh, Pennsylvania

Kathleen Kelley Walsh, RN, MS
Professor of Nursing
Jackson Community College
Jackson, Michigan

JoAnn Widner, RN, MS
Health Educator
Central North Alabama Health Services, Inc.
Huntsville, Alabama

Linda S. Williams, MSN, RN, C, CS
Associate Professor of Nursing
Jackson Community College
Registered Nurse Care Coordinator
W.A. Foote Memorial Hospital
Jackson, Michigan

Reviewers

Ethel Jones Avery, RN, MSN, EDS
H. Councill Trenholm State Technical College
Montgomery, Alabama

Paula Barnaby, RN, BSN
T.H. Pickens Tech Center
Aurora, Colorado

Cheryl Brown, RN, MEd
Hillsborough County-Erwin Vocational-Technical Center
Tampa, Florida

Mollie Brown, RN, BSN
Maric College of Medical Careers
San Diego, California

Donna J. Burleson, RN, MS
Cisco Junior College
Abilene, Texas

Mary Ann Cosgarea, RN, BSN
Portage Lakes Career Center
W. Howard Nichol School of Practical Nursing
Green, Ohio

Phyllis Crownover, RN, BSN, MA
Maric College of Medical Careers
San Diego, California

Sandra S. Dawes, RN, MS
Louisiana Technical College–Jefferson Campus
Metarie, Louisiana

Gloria Ferritto, RN, BSN
Maric College of Medical Careers
Vista, California

Chris Herdlick, RN, BA
Marshalltown Community College
Marshalltown, Iowa

Nancy Jo Kastor, RN, BSN
Portage Lakes Career Center
W. Howard Nichol School of Practical Nursing
Green, Ohio

Margaret Maben, RN
Otsego Area School of Practical Nursing BOCES
Fox Hospital
Oneonta, New York

Robert G. McGee, AAS, BS, MSEd
Walters State Community College
Greeneville, Tennessee

Carol Mehrani, RN, ADN
Hillsborough County-Erwin Vocational-Technical Center
Tampa, Florida

Mary Frances Moorhouse, RN, CRRN, CLNC
TNT RN Enterprises
Colorado Springs, Colorado

M. Christine Neff, RN, BSN
Mid-East Ohio Vocational School
Zanesville, Ohio

Janine O'Buchon, BSN, MSNc
North Orange County ROP
Anaheim, California

Lynn Phillips, RN, MSN, CRNI
Butte Community College
Oroville, California

Donna N. Roddy, RN, MSN
Chattanooga State Technical Community College
Chattanooga, Tennessee

Judith S. Schell, RN, BSN
Clearfield County Area Vocational-Technical School
Clearfield, Pennsylvania

Kara Schmitt, PhD
Director, Testing Services Division
Michigan Department of Consumer and Industry Services
Lansing, Michigan

Martha Spray, RN, BSN, MS
Mid-East Ohio Vocational School
Zanesville, Ohio

Judith L. Stauder, MSN, RN
Practical Nursing Program of Canton City Schools
Canton, Ohio

Susan Corwin Stolz, RN, BSEd
Cincinnati Public School of Practical Nursing
Cincinnati, Ohio

Marie Thieleman, RN, BSN
West Kentucky Technical College
Paducah, Kentucky

Darlyn DeHart Weikel, MSN, RN, C
North Central Technical College
Mansfield, Ohio

Cheryl White, LPN
W.A. Foote Memorial Hospital
Jackson, Michigan

Rose Anne Wilcox, RN, BSN, MEd
Columbus Public Schools
School of Practical Nursing
Columbus, Ohio

Contents

UNIT 7
Understanding the Gastrointestinal System 553

COLOR PLATES 1–16 FOLLOW PAGE 384

COLOR PLATES 17–32 FOLLOW PAGE 1168

Understanding Health Care

The Nurse and the Health Care System

Linda S. Williams, Patrick Shannon, and Joseph Catalano

Learning Objectives

Upon completion of this chapter, the student will be able to:

1. Describe three factors influencing changes in the health care delivery system.
2. Define health and the health-illness continuum.
3. Explain three economic issues facing the health care industry and methods for controlling health care costs.
4. Describe members of the health care team and their roles.
5. Describe the concept of continuous quality improvement.
6. Explain two future trends in health care.
7. Define three legal concepts that relate to nursing practice.
8. Discuss the importance of ethical decisions in health care.
9. Define the important ethical principles that underlie ethical dilemmas.
10. Apply the steps of the ethical decision-making model in resolving ethical dilemmas.
11. Discuss values and how they relate to individuals and the nursing profession.
12. Explain two components in a professional relationship.
13. Define three leadership styles and the licensed practical nurse's and licensed vocational nurse's role in leadership.
14. Describe two caring behaviors.

Key Words

administrative laws (ad-MIN-i-**STRAY**-tive LAWZ)

autocratic leadership (AW-tuh-**KRAT**-ik **LEE**-der-ship)

beneficence (buh-**NEF**-i-sens)

caring (**KARE**-ring)

civil law (**SIV**-il LAW)

code of ethics (KOHD OF **ETH**-icks)

confidentiality (KON-fi-den-she-**AL**-i-tee)

criminal law (**KRIM**-i-nuhl LAW)

democratic leadership (DEM-ah-**KRAT**-ik **LEE**-der-ship)

diagnosis-related groups (DYE-ag-**NOH**-sis ree-**LAY**-ted GROOPS)

distributive justice (dis-**TRIB**-yoo-tiv **JUS**-tiss)

empathy (**EM**-puh-thee)

ethical rights (**ETH**-i-kuhl RIGHTS)

fidelity (fi-**DEL**-i-tee)

health (HELLTH)

health-illness continuum (HELLTH **ILL**-ness kon-**TIN**-u-um)

illness (**ILL**-ness)

laissez-faire leadership (LAYS-ay-**FAIR LEE**-der-ship)

law (LAW)

leadership (**LEE**-der-ship)

liability (LYE-uh-**BIL**-i-tee)

limitation of liability (LIM-i-**TAY**-shun OF LYE-uh-**BIL**-i-tee)

malpractice (mal-**PRAK**-tiss)

morality (muh-**RAL**-i-tee)

negligence (**NEG**-li-jense)

nonmaleficence (NON-muh-**LEF**-i-sens)

option rights (**OP**-shun RIGHTS)

paternalism (puh-**TER**-nuhl-izm)

respondeat superior (res-**POND**-ee-et sue-**PEER**-ee-or)

standard of best interest (**STAND**-erd OF BEST **IN**-ter-est)

summons (**SUM**-muns)

torts (TORTS)

values (**VAL**-use)

veracity (vuh-**RAS**-i-tee)

welfare rights (**WELL**-fare RIGHTS)

New concerns are facing the health care industry, which is in the midst of health care reform. Changes that are forcing policy makers, health care providers, and the public to look carefully at the way health care is provided include a dramatically increasing number of elderly people, increasing cultural diversity in our society, challenging new diseases, the emergence of disease strains that are resistant to common treatments, and the escalating costs of health care. Who will pay for health care and who will receive health care services are questions that society has to answer.

Health Care Delivery

The health care delivery system is undergoing rapid and dramatic change. Nursing is being greatly affected by the shifting focus in health care from acute care to outpatient and community settings. Hospitals are downsizing and redesigning delivery methods to respond to this shift in where care is being provided. An emphasis on prevention and wellness is also structuring how care is being delivered.

HEALTH-ILLNESS CONTINUUM

Individuals define **health** in different ways. The World Health Organization in the preamble of its constitution defines health as a "state of complete physical, mental and social well-being and not merely the absence of disease and infirmity." This definition provides a narrow view of health that does not provide for chronic **illness** effects or fluctuating levels of wellness. The **health-illness continuum** in contrast, addresses various levels of health that are continually shifting for an individual (Fig. 1–1). One end of the continuum represents high-level health and the other end poor health with impending death. Individuals continually move along the continuum throughout their lives. This continuum provides a broader definition of health that includes those with chronic illnesses. On this continuum, those with chronic illnesses can achieve wellness goals within the limitations of their illnesses.

HEALTH PROMOTION

Health care is shifting from a disease-focused model to one of wellness and prevention. The public is recognizing that personal responsibility for health is important to individuals and society. Consumers are requesting information with which to make choices and informed decisions about their

health. Increased nutritional labeling of food and restaurant menus that provide information and healthy options are examples of this.

Wellness services are being offered by companies to their employees. These services may include (1) health screening, such as blood pressure measurement, cholesterol levels, weight and body fat measurement, and safety in the areas of proper body mechanics and seat belt use; (2) education on a variety of health topics; and (3) cardiopulmonary resuscitation training and certification. Employers are motivated to offer these wellness services in an effort to contain health care costs. Employees want to participate in these activities to improve their health.

HEALTH CARE DELIVERY SYSTEMS

Today's health care system is a highly specialized industry that provides a network of services for clients. Instead of being treated by one health care provider for a lifetime as was common several decades ago, clients see health care members that specialize in one area of treatment. Some believe that specialization and fragmentation of health care have contributed to the rising costs of health care. Current efforts to keep costs down by the health care industry include the redesign of systems to integrate health care services. A focus on prevention and providing services from birth to death under one integrated system is an approach being used in some systems. Hospital consolidations and mergers are resulting in the development of health care systems that may cover large geographic areas. These systems are then purchasing or starting community agencies to deliver services not included under acute care, such as home health care and medical equipment sales. The hospital and these agencies provide the integrated care delivery network for the system (Fig. 1–2).

FACTORS INFLUENCING HEALTH CARE CHANGE

The health care needs of society are changing in response to several changes in society. Changing characteristics of the U.S. population is one important factor that includes the size of the population, the number of elderly, the birth rate decline, the homeless, and increasing cultural diversity. (See Gerontological Issues Box 1–1.) The size of the American population is increasing, with 300 million people projected for the year 2000. The population includes an increasing number of people over age 65, with those over 85 increasing the fastest. The health care needs of the elderly can be complex and chronic, which places increased demands on the health care system. The declining birth rate means there are fewer school-age children and fewer people to care for the elderly. The homeless population is increasing and includes whole families. The homeless have limited or no access to health care. The in-

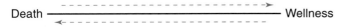

Figure 1–1. Health-illness continuum.

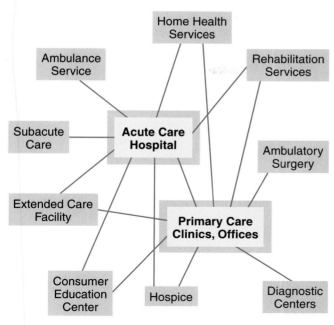

Figure 1–2. An integrated health care system.

crease in cultural diversity affects how health care is delivered.

The change in diseases being treated today greatly influences health care delivery. Chronic diseases are the most commonly treated conditions. During this century, advances in medicine, such as vaccines and antibiotics, have eradicated or controlled many infectious diseases. Other infectious diseases, such as acquired immunodeficiency syndrome (AIDS) and tuberculosis, are increasing. Superstrains of organisms are developing that are resistant to current treatments. This may be occurring because of the misuse of antibiotics when treating infections. Methods of treating these superorganisms need to be developed to prevent epidemics from occurring.

The development of new technology for communicating information and designing medical equipment for testing and treatment is rapidly changing the health care industry. New technology is continually being introduced that quickly outdates equipment in use. This means change and relearning are constant in today's health care environment.

GERONTOLOGICAL ISSUES BOX 1–1

Gerontological nursing, which is the support and care of older adults, is an emerging specialty in nursing. As the population of older adults increases, more nurses will be needed who recognize, support, and understand the unique health and illness care needs of this population.

Economic Issues

The health care system is mainly funded by the government and private insurers. Costs have risen dramatically in recent years, causing a movement for health care reform. Access to care is not available to everyone and is often linked to availability of resources. The number of uninsured or underinsured individuals is growing. Preventive care is not an option for many of these people with few resources. Care is often sought in the costly emergency room when a medical problem has become complex. Developing systems to deliver care to these individuals in a less costly manner is one area of health care reform.

Public opinion continues to shift toward the belief that health care is a right for all. However, to ensure this right is an enormous economic burden, and policy makers have not embraced the belief that health care is a right. Methods to deliver cost-effective care began in 1983 with **diagnosis-related groups** (DRGs) and continue today as part of the national health care reform debate.

MEDICARE AND DIAGNOSIS-RELATED GROUPS

Medicare was created in 1966 to provide health insurance as part of the Social Security Act. It is run by the U.S. government and covers all individuals age 65 and over and disabled people under 65 who are eligible for Social Security. It is funded by a deduction from every person's paycheck that is matched by the federal government. The DRG payment system was created by Congress in 1983 to help control costs in the Medicare program, which previously had no reimbursement limits. This payment system set fixed payment rates for 470 diagnostic categories. Hospitals everywhere are paid the same for clients in the same diagnostic category regardless of length of stay and supply costs. Hospitals lose money if the client's costs exceed the DRG payment but make money if the costs are less than the payment. The incentive to deliver more cost-effective care within the DRG payment system lies with the hospital. Effective discharge planning and nursing involvement in maintaining quality but cost-effective care are essential in this payment system.

MEDICAID

The Medicaid payment system was also created in 1966 to provide health insurance as part of the Social Security Act for low-income or disabled persons under 65 and their dependent children. Some low-income people over 65 may also qualify. Medicaid funding comes from federal, state, and local taxes. It is run by both the federal and state governments, causing benefits to vary from state to state.

text continues on page 10

Clinical Pathway for Acute Asthma

ICD-9 Code 097   ELOS 3 days

Nursing Diagnosis/ Collaborative Problem	Expected Outcome (The Patient Is Expected to...)	Met/ Not Met	Reason	Date/ Initials
Ineffective breathing pattern	Resume baseline breathing pattern and respiratory rate with a peak flow >70% of baseline			
Ineffective airway clearance	Clear airway without difficulty			
Activity intolerance	Resume activities of daily living with good exercise tolerance			
Ineffective individual and family coping	Identify successful coping strategies and participate in plan of care			

Aspect of Care	Date ____ Day 1	Date ____ Day 2	Date ____ Day 3
Assessment	Systems assessment q shift with focus on respiratory • Adventitious breath sounds and accessory muscle utilization VS q 4 h Sputum for color, tenacity, and amount Skin assessment for color, temp, diaphoresis Anxiety, fear, and fatigue levels; family support and resources	Same as Day 1	Same as Day 2 VS q 8 h

Figure 1–3. A sample clinical pathway. (From Ignatavicius and Hausman: Clinical Pathways for Collaborative Practice. WB Saunders, Philadelphia, 1995, pp 78–81, with permission.)

	Assess response to therapy Assess need for mechanical ventilation Monitor for complications • Hypoxemia • Pneumonia • Respiratory acidosis		
Teaching	Orient to hospital and unit Prepare for diagnostic tests Instruct on use of peak expiratory flow meter, nebulizer and MDI (metered dose inhaler) Provide information regarding diagnosis and medications Involve family in care of patient as appropriate Review plan of care/clinical pathway with patient and family	Stress reduction techniques, need for adequate rest and sleep How to recognize and prevent respiratory infection, irritants Adaptive breathing techniques (pursed lips, pushing/pulling during exhalation) and energy conserving measures	What to do during acute asthma attack and when to seek emergency care Medication administration and use of MDI Importance of diet and fluids Assess knowledge about factors that trigger asthma and how to pretreat before exposure to trigger Provide information concerning medications that may trigger asthma
Consults	Respiratory therapy Pulmonologist Social worker	N/A	N/A
Lab Tests	CBC with differential, lytes ABGs Theophylline level Total IgE Sputum culture	Theophylline level (while on IV or if dosage changes)	Same as Day 2

Continued

Figure 1–3. Continued

Clinical Pathway for Acute Asthma *Continued*

Aspect of Care (Cont'd)	Date ____ Day 1	Date ____ Day 2	Date ____ Day 3
Other Tests	Chest x-ray ECG (if >40 years of age) Pulmonary function tests	N/A	N/A
Meds	Bronchodilator or beta$_2$ agonist metaproterenol, albuterol via nebulizer q 4 h or IV bronchodilator (aminophylline) via continuous drip Corticosteroids IV q 6 h	Nebulizer q 4 h Consider changing to PO if patient stable Taper dosage and change to PO	Discontinue nebulizer and place on MDI Theo-Dur PO Prednisone PO BID
Treatments/Interventions	O$_2$ per NC or Ventimask at 2 L to maintain SaO$_2$ >90% Pulse oximeter Peak flow before and after nebulizer treatment Bronchodilator via nebulizer or MDI q 4 h Position to facilitate breathing Elevate HOB 45–90° Allergen-free pillow Frequent oral care Provide periods of uninterrupted sleep and rest Daily wts	Same as Day 1	Discontinue O$_2$ Pulse oximeter Peak expiratory flow q 8 h Incentive spirometer TID Aerosol inhalation QID Position to facilitate breathing Oral care as needed

Figure 1–3. Continued

Nutrition	DAT (low Na$^+$ if steroid dependent) Encourage fluids to 2000 mL/day (restrict if on steroids)	Same as Day 1	Same as Day 2
Lines/Tubes/Monitors	IV fluids for hydration and medications	Discontinue IV fluids; change to saline lock	Same as Day 2 D/C saline lock
Mobility/Self-Care	Bed rest with BRPs Sit on side of bed or up in bed leaning on overbed table	OOB and ambulate as tolerated	Same as Day 2
Discharge Planning	Assess need for home respiratory equipment	Refer to support group Continue as Day 1 with attention to home needs, modification of environment to reduce allergens	Arrange for follow-up visit with physician

Figure 1–3. Continued

MANAGED HEALTH CARE

The early movement to contain health care costs led to the formation of health maintenance organizations (HMOs) and then preferred provider organizations (PPOs). The HMO delivers holistic health care to individuals who enroll in this prepaid group practice health program. The purpose of the HMO is to reduce overlapping services and provide quality and cost-effective care. The HMO collects a yearly fee from clients, and then services are usually free. Healthy clients require fewer services, so preventive care is promoted. The PPOs are a method of reducing costs to businesses that insure employees. Hospitals and physicians develop a contract with employers to provide services at a negotiated fee. The employer saves money by negotiating a discounted fee, and the care providers expand their market base.

Managed care is currently being implemented in various stages across the country. Managed care's purpose is to control costs. To do this, the government, insurers, and businesses have taken more control over the funding of the health care system. The components of managed care, which are a blending of some of the features of HMOs and PPOs, include precertification requirements, prearranged payment rates, utilization review, provider choice limitations, and fixed-rate reimbursement. Managed care covers acute, long-term, home care, ambulatory, and diagnostic and therapeutic services.

LEARNING TIP

To understand what the term *managed care* means, think of it as: *care management.*

As managed care is implemented, trends are emerging. The need for hospital beds is decreasing. Skill cross-training that produces a multiskilled health care worker is occurring. Shorter lengths of stay for more acutely ill clients are being seen. Discharged clients are requiring more home care for more complex needs. Home care is rapidly expanding to meet this need. Nurses are leaving the acute care setting as downsizing occurs to go into community and home care. Competition and a for-profit environment is emerging in health care that was not previously evident. The challenge to the health care industry is to provide cost-effective care while maintaining quality health care that meets the needs of the client.

Case management is a model for providing client care designed to ensure that the best outcome is achieved while controlling costs. It is a strategy used in managed care. Case management uses clinical pathways, which are interdisciplinary care plans that are used to standardize care to a specific group of clients. A clinical pathway is usually developed for an illness or surgery that has a routine or predictable sequence of events. In the clinical pathway, timelines for interventions are given that promote quality outcomes (Fig. 1–3). Although the concept of clinical pathways is not new, the widespread development and use of them in health care is. There are many versions of clinical pathways and several settings in which they are used. The most common setting is the hospital, but some variations have been developed to include long-term care, subacute care, home care, or care from the hospital to the long-term care facility or home care.

Nursing and the Health Care Team

Nursing is an integral part of the health care network. Nurses work as licensed practical nurses (LPNs) or licensed vocational nurses (LVNs); registered nurses (RNs); and RNs with advanced practice skills that include nurse practitioners (NPs), clinical nurse specialists (CNSs), certified nurse midwives, and certified registered nurse anesthetists (CRNAs). The LPN/LVN works under the direct supervision of a registered nurse, physician, or dentist while giving direct client care. Certified nursing assistants are trained to assist nurses in providing health care to clients.

There are many other members of the health care team network. Nurses work in collaboration with these team members to meet client health care needs. Educational requirements, titles, and duties are described for some health care team members. Licensed physicians provide medical care to clients after graduating from a college of medical or osteopathic medicine. Physician assistants, after graduating from a physician's assistant program, work under the supervision of a physician and perform certain physician duties, such as history taking, injections, and suturing of wounds. Licensed pharmacists complete 5 or 6 years of college and dispense medications from prescriptions, consult with physicians, and provide medication information to clients. Social workers usually have a master's degree in social work and treat psychosocial problems of clients and their families. Dietitians provide nutrition information, analyze nutritional needs, and calculate special dietary needs. Licensed physical therapists complete a college physical therapy program and assist clients in reducing physical disability, bodily malfunction, movement dysfunction, and pain through evaluation, education, and treatment. Physical therapy assistants, whose educational requirements vary, may complete 2 years of education and be licensed and then work under the supervision of a physical therapist. Respiratory therapists have a 2-year college degree, may be registered (registered respiratory therapist, RRT), and work with clients who have respiratory problems. Respiratory therapy technicians have 1 year of education, may be certified (certified respiratory therapy technician, CRTT), and work under the supervision of a respiratory therapist to provide respiratory care. Occupational therapists complete a bachelor's or master's program, may be registered (occupational therapist, registered, OTR), and assist clients in restoring self-care, work, and leisure skills from developmental deficits or injury. Health unit secretaries manage the clerical work at a nursing station. Student nurses are enrolled in a nursing program and work under the supervision of nursing faculty in the clinical setting.

Continuous Quality Improvement

Society expects quality health care. To ensure the accountability of health care organizations for the care that they provide, assessment and improvement of health care quality are required for financial reimbursement and accreditation. Continuous quality improvement is a method used to increase the quality of health care. It is included in the Joint Commission on Accreditation of Healthcare Organizations (JCAHO) standards. The JCAHO standards recommend health care organizations implement continuous quality improvement to improve performance.

Continuous quality improvement assesses the processes of providing health care. Isolated problems are not analyzed in continuous quality improvement. Problem trends are examined, and methods to improve the quality of outcomes and client satisfaction are explored. Areas that are focused on include clinical client care, operating procedures, and financial issues. For example, if client satisfaction is found to be low regarding wait times for transport to other areas of the hospital for tests, surgery, or discharge, a focused study of factors contributing to transport delays will be conducted. Analysis of data will show areas for improvement, which might include decreasing elevator usage

and wait times, peak transport usage times, and staffing patterns or delays in client readiness for transport. Interventions to improve the interfering factors can then be designed and implemented. After the interventions have been implemented for a period of time, reassessment of transport wait times should be done to ensure that wait times have been reduced and client satisfaction has increased. If not, further assessment and analysis are required. Continuous quality improvement is an ongoing process that requires evaluation and reevaluation of outcomes (Fig. 1–4).

All nurses need to understand continuous quality improvement to improve client care outcomes. Nurse managers develop continuous quality improvement plans. Nurses providing client care collect and analyze data to implement changes for improved outcomes.

Future Trends

Health care is currently in a state of redesign. At this time it is uncertain what the final evolution of health care will be. Trends that are emerging today in health care delivery include managed care; case management; critical pathways; increased home health care; community-based health care; subacute care units, which can be freestanding or associated with a hospital; increased independent nursing practices and prescriptive authority for advanced practice registered nurses; hospital redesign and mergers of hospitals; specialized freestanding facilities for ambulatory surgery, dialysis, or childbirth; increased for-profit health care organizations; increased use of multiskilled and unlicensed health care workers; a shift in the job market from acute care settings to home and community care settings; and increased use of computers at the bedside and throughout health care. Employment trends for LPN/LVNs include employment in subacute care units and increased use of LPN/LVNs as primary caregivers with a registered nurse team leader in skilled nursing units of long-term care facilities.

Trends in society include increased population, rising number of elderly, increasing cultural diversity, rising number of uninsured or underinsured individuals, and an uncertain future for Social Security and Medicare. These trends have made health care inaccessible to some individuals. The U.S. Public Health Service has published a plan to improve health care in this country by the year 2000.[1] The goals of this plan are to (1) increase the healthy life span for Americans, (2) decrease health disparities among Americans, and (3) attain access to preventive services for all Americans.

Concern over health care is evident in all areas of today's society. Health care redesign is being driven by several forces. The primary forces include a society that is demanding improved quality and lower costs, employers that are seeking lowered insurance premiums, and insurers and health care providers that are seeking to lower operating

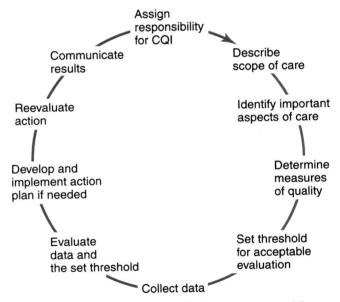

Figure 1–4. A continuous quality improvement model.

costs and increase utilization efficiency. The emerging trends are in response to these forces.

Leadership in Nursing Practice

Leadership skills are necessary for the LPN/LVN to effectively guide client care and achieve goals. Leadership involves decision making, communicating, and motivating and guiding others. The success of the entire leadership process depends on effective communication. The leadership process seeks to change behaviors in others in order to accomplish goals.

A leader is not just someone with a title. Anyone who influences others to achieve goals is a leader. Leaders must be respected by those with whom they work. They must be knowledgeable in the management process and able to make decisions. They should be role models and an inspiration to others. Positive thinking and the use of humor are valuable assets of good leaders.

LEADERSHIP STYLES

There are three basic leadership styles: autocratic, democratic, and laissez-faire. These styles differ according to the amount of control the leader exerts over the group, the amount of involvement the leader has with the group, and the level of decision making the leader assumes for the group.

Autocratic Leadership

An autocratic leader has a high degree of control. Almost no control is given to others. In **autocratic leadership,** the leader determines the goals and plans for achieving the goals. Others are instructed what to do but are not asked to provide input. The leader takes complete charge and re-sponsibility. The group usually achieves high-quality outcomes under this style of leadership. This is an efficient leadership style for situations in which decisions must be made quickly, as in an emergency such as evacuation of a building or a code for cardiac arrest.

Democratic Leadership

A democratic leader has a moderate degree of control. Others are given some control and freedom. In **democratic leadership,** participation is encouraged in determining goals and plans for achieving the goals (Fig. 1–5). Decisions are made within the group. The leader assists the group by steering and teaching rather than dominating. The leader shares responsibility with the group. The group usually achieves high-quality outcomes and is more creative under this style of leadership. This is an efficient leadership style for most situations. Group members are more satisfied and motivated to achieve goals because they are active participants.

Laissez-Faire Leadership

A laissez-faire leader exerts no control over the group. Others are given complete freedom under this leadership style. With **laissez-faire leadership,** no one is responsible for determining goals and plans for achieving the goals. This produces a feeling of chaos. If decisions are made, the group makes them. Little is accomplished under this type of leadership, and the quality of outcomes is poor.

MANAGEMENT FUNCTIONS

There are five major components in the management process: planning, organizing, directing, coordinating, and controlling. An effective leader understands each of these functions.

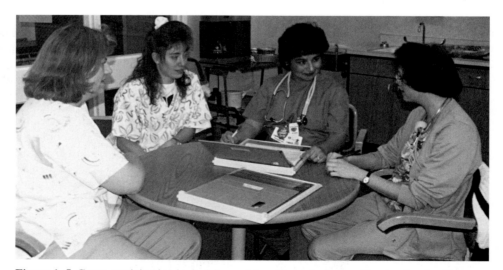

Figure 1–5. Group participation in decision making. (From Anderson: Nursing Leadership, Management, and Professional Practice for the LPN/LVN. FA Davis, Philadelphia, 1997, p 98, with permission.)

Planning

The first step of the management process is planning. A plan must be developed to ensure that desired client care outcomes are achieved. To formulate the plan, desired outcomes or problems are identified and data are collected about them. Alternatives or solutions are considered using the collected data and input from others. A decision is then made about the best option or course of action. The leader should ensure that the choice is realistic and can be implemented. Before implementation, the wise leader will determine how to communicate the action to be implemented so that it will be supported by others. Change can be upsetting and resisted by those not involved in the decision-making process. Involving others in the planning and decision-making process from beginning to end can assist in greater acceptance at time of implementation. After implementation, an evaluation must be done to determine the effects of the implemented action. If the evaluation indicates that the action is not satisfactory, the decision-making process to select another option begins.

Organizing

The purpose of organizing, the second step in the management process, is to provide an orderly environment that promotes cooperation and goal achievement. Providing a framework for goals and the activities that accomplish them is the initial step in organization. Policies and procedures provide this framework, as well as guidance for those carrying out tasks designed to accomplish the organization's goals. Assigning personnel to tasks that they are trained and qualified to complete also aids organization.

Directing

Making assignments is the primary function of directing. Nurses make assignments for patient care. One person, usually the nurse in charge or the team leader, makes the assignments. State nursing practice acts define who can make assignments and delegate care. The registered nurse is given this authority and responsibility, but LPN/LVNs are not usually given this authority under state nursing practice acts.

Communication is important in directing. Assignments must be clearly and specifically stated. Clarification should be sought by the individual making assignments to be sure that they are correctly understood. Effective directing can be accomplished by providing verbal and written assignment information, making requests rather than giving orders, and giving instructions as needed.

Coordinating

Coordination is the process of looking at a situation to ensure that it is being handled in the most effective way for the organization. The nurse may assess a particular activity or issues related to client care assignments. In a long-term care facility, for example, the nurse may want to review skin assessment and care throughout the facility to see whether it is being done consistently and uniformly. If a concern is found, problem-solving techniques are noted to ensure that protocols are followed for positive client outcomes.

Controlling

The final phase of the management process is controlling, which evaluates the accomplishment of the organization's goals. Continuous quality improvement is linked with controlling. If the organization's efficiency or ability to reach its goals is impaired, the use of the continuous quality improvement model can facilitate correction of the concern.

LEADERSHIP ROLE OF THE LPN/LVN

The LPN/LVN is a leader and manager for the care of the clients to whom they are assigned. Beyond this application of a leader and manager role for the LPN/LVN, the state nurse practice act specifies whether the LPN/LVN can assume other leader or manager roles. The LPN/LVN always practices under the supervision of a registered nurse, physician, or dentist.

The LPN/LVN in some cases may function as a team leader in the long-term care setting. When the LPN/LVN acts as a team leader, a registered nurse provides supervision. Team leaders are responsible for the coordination and delivery of client care to each of the clients assigned to the team. They collect data on all of the clients assigned to the team to plan appropriate care and update nursing care plans. Delivered care is evaluated and documented by the team leader. Team leaders receive information from team members and communicate clients' needs to appropriate individuals.

Because team leaders guide client care provided by the team, they must be knowledgeable about safety, clients' rights, and the accountability of being a team leader. Regulations related to safety apply to all health organizations and must be followed by all team members for the client's and their own safety. The team leader oversees the implementation of these regulations by team members. All clients are entitled to quality care and treatment with dignity and respect. A Patient's Bill of Rights was drafted in 1973 by the American Hospital Association (Table 1–1). It outlines the type of treatment and care a client has the right to expect. Knocking before entering a client's room and caregivers introducing themselves are examples of a client's rights. The team leader and team members should be aware of a client's rights and ensure them during client care. The team leader is accountable for all care provided by the team. Documentation must be accurate and complete. Institutional policy is followed regarding the taking

Table 1–1. **American Hospital Association's Patient's Bill of Rights**

The patient has the right to
1. Considerate and respectful care.
2. Obtain from physicians and other direct caregivers relevant, current, understandable information concerning diagnosis, treatment risks, benefits, alternatives, prognosis, financial implications, and identity of caregivers, including students, residents, and trainees.
3. Make decisions about the plan of care, be informed, and refuse treatment or a plan of care.
4. Have an advance directive (living will, health care proxy, or durable power of attorney) concerning treatment or designating a surrogate decision maker.
5. Every consideration of privacy.
6. Expect that all communications and records pertaining to his or her care will be treated as confidential.
7. Review the records pertaining to his or her medical care and have the information explained.
8. Expect reasonable response to care and service requests by the hospital.
9. Ask and be informed of the existence of business relationships among the hospital, educational institutions, or other health care providers or payers that may influence the patient's treatment and care.
10. Consent to or decline to participate in research studies and still receive the most effective care that the hospital can provide.
11. Expect reasonable continuity of care and be informed of care options when hospital care is no longer appropriate.
12. Be informed of hospital policies and practices that relate to patient care, treatment, responsibilities, charges for services, and payment methods.

Reprinted with permission of the American Hospital Association, copyright 1992.

of verbal physician orders and noting orders. At the end of the team's work shift, team leaders are responsible for transferring client care to the oncoming team. This transfer of care is accomplished by reporting the client's condition, status, and needs to the oncoming team leader (Fig. 1–6).

Institutional policy specifies whether the RN or LPN/LVN communicates the report.

Nurse-Client Relationship

HOLISTIC CARE

Nursing has a holistic approach to client care. Individuals are composed of many different parts. The sum of these parts creates a whole person. The interaction of these parts forms a complex person. Holistic care considers the needs of the entire person.

Every individual has a mind, body, and spirit. Each one of these components is affected by the others. The effects of illness must be considered on all of these components. A wound that heals but leaves a visible scar can affect the body image and self-esteem of the individual. When nurses provide care, they must care for the body as well as the mind and spirit. Nursing's uniqueness lies in providing holistic care for clients.

Nursing provides care for clients' responses to illness and other situations. These responses can be physical, physiological, psychological, cultural, spiritual, or sociological. Every individual has unique responses to illness. A holistic nursing plan of care is individualized to reflect the unique responses of individuals.

COMMUNICATION

The process of communication consists of a sender, a message, and a receiver (Fig. 1–7). The sender conveys a message to the receiver. The receiver listens, interprets the received message, and provides feedback indicating how the message was interpreted. Feedback allows the sender to verify that the intent of the message was correctly conveyed.

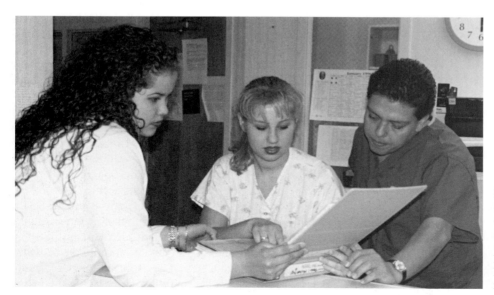

Figure 1-6. Communication of the client's status when transferring the client's care to another team leader. (From Anderson: Nursing Leadership, Management and Professional Practice for the LPN/LVN. FA Davis, Philadelphia, 1997, p 128, with permission.)

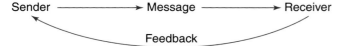

Sender ⟶ Message ⟶ Receiver

Feedback

Figure 1–7. Components of communication.

Communication may be verbal or nonverbal. Nonverbal communication is conveyed by body language and expressions of emotion. Examples of body language include gestures, body positioning, and body movements. Expressions of emotions include laughing, crying, grimacing, moaning, smiling, frowning, and facial affect.

Clear communication is essential in providing client care. Nurses must send clear, easily understood messages to clients and be attentive listeners and observers. When the nurse is sending a message to the client, complex medical terminology should be avoided. Words should be used that are easily understood by the client. When the nurse is receiving a message, being a good listener is important. The nurse should face the client, eliminate distractions, and focus on what the client is saying to enhance the listening process. Whenever the nurse interacts with clients, nonverbal messages should be noted. Conflicting messages can be sent by clients. The nurse must learn to interpret these messages to meet the client's needs. For example, clients who state they are not in pain but are grimacing and guarding their movements are sending a mixed message. The nurse must develop the skill of exploring the meaning of these messages to meet the comfort needs of these clients.

INTERACTION WITH CLIENTS

The nurse is entrusted with providing professional, competent care to clients. Nursing care should be provided using the following principles: ensuring dignity and respect, maintaining **confidentiality,** including the client and family in care explanations and decisions, respecting the client's right to make care choices, and maintaining a professional relationship with the client.

ENSURING DIGNITY AND RESPECT

All clients have the right to be treated with dignity and respect. Ensuring that clients are treated with dignity is done by recognizing that each person is a unique individual. As unique individuals, people have differences that should be appreciated. To acknowledge these differences, care should be individualized and nonjudgmental.

Showing respect for clients includes treating them with courtesy; asking their name preference; avoiding the use of endearment terms, such as "honey," "sweetie," or "dear"; and providing privacy. Courtesy is extended to clients when nurses use please and thank you and ask clients their time preferences for care. For older clients, Mr. or Mrs. is appropriate unless the client indicates a different preference. Endearment terms should be avoided, especially for the elderly. They are demeaning and convey a closer relationship than is present in professional interactions.

The nurse must always provide privacy when it is indicated for the client. Closing doors and privacy curtains, exposing only necessary areas of the client's body for care, and asking visitors to step out of the room while care is given are examples of providing privacy (Fig. 1–8). Clients often depend on the nurse for their needs. Showing that the client's need for privacy is recognized conveys dignity and respect. Clients value care that maintains their dignity and respect.

CONFIDENTIALITY

The nurse must maintain client confidentiality at all times. Client care should be discussed only in the professional setting with those involved in the client's care on a need to know basis. Discussions should not take place in a public area where others may hear them. Access to client records should also be safeguarded. Only care providers actually caring for the client have the right to access client records. Caregivers do not have the right to read the records of clients who are not assigned to them. This includes clients who are friends or acquaintances of the caregiver. The client or family may only have access to the client's records according to institutional policy. A written request is usually required to begin the process. Families do not automatically have the right to information about the

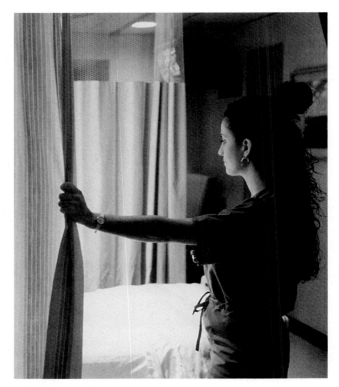

Figure 1–8. Maintaining privacy is a client right and conveys caring to the client.

client. If the client is able, consent must be given for the nurse to share information with specific family members. Some client information is private and should remain private. Institutional policy is followed for sharing information with those inquiring about the client's status. Breaching confidentiality can have serious consequences.

CARE EXPLANATIONS AND DECISIONS

Clients have the right to expect that all of their care will be explained to them (Fig. 1–9). Clients cannot make informed decisions without care explanations. When clients are informed they are able to make better decisions for their care and are in control of their lives. This feeling of control can reduce anxiety and make an illness less stressful for the client. Clients who are less anxious are more cooperative and appreciative of their care. The LPN/LVN should allow the team leader to provide initial information and instructions to clients. Then the LPN/LVN can assist the team leader in reinforcing the explanations as needed and referring further client questions to the team leader.

Families should be included in explanations if the client gives permission (Fig. 1–10). Families provide support to the client and are better able to do this if they are knowledgeable about the client's care. They can assist the client in making better care choices. Including families in explanations is an important way nurses can provide emotional support to them in stressful situations, such as emergency surgeries and after accidents.

CARE CHOICES

Clients have the right to make care choices. After they have made an informed choice the nurse should respect their choice and provide appropriate care. Many clients want to be active in guiding their care. Today's clients are better informed about health care. The nurse must respect clients' level of participation in care and enable clients to be as active in their care planning as they wish to be.

PROFESSIONAL RELATIONSHIP

The nurse in a professional relationship has entered that relationship to provide assistance to the client. Within this relationship there should be trust and security. The nurse can promote trust and security for the client by appearing confident, being skilled, and meeting commitments made to the client. The nurse should not divulge personal information or relate similar personal health experiences in a professional relationship.

A caring approach to client care is necessary in a professional role. The practice of nursing combines the science of medical knowledge with the art of nursing, which consists of **caring,** ethics, aesthetics, and beauty.[2] Caring involves having a deep concern for other individuals. A caring nursing behavior is providing care in which the client participates in care decisions. The nurse does not assume a "boss" role but instead works with the client. A caring moment is described by Watson[2] as the personal sharing of moments when the nurse is able to completely focus knowledge and attention on the client. Entering every client interaction with the intention of providing personalized, holistic care

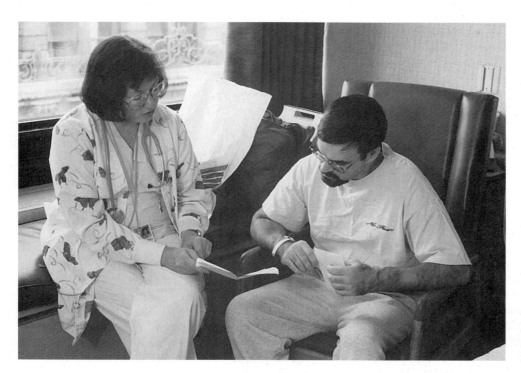

Figure 1–9. The nurse explains the client's care to reduce anxiety and allow the client to make informed decisions.

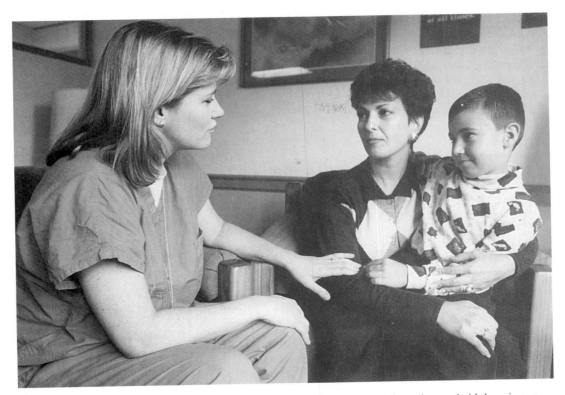

Figure 1–10. Families may be included in care explanations to reduce their anxiety and aid them in supporting the client.

is another caring behavior. The nurse should be kind and honest while providing care and able to set limits when needed. If clients need rest but are hesitant to limit visitors the nurse should assume that responsibility as the client's advocate. Being empathetic is an important part of caring. **Empathy** is the ability to remain objective while understanding a client's experience and responses. It is helpful to the client because the nurse is not immersed in the situation and can provide a calm and objective view of the situation.

Legal Concepts

All of us are members of society. To promote harmony, safety, and productivity, members of society create rules. The rules of society can be informal or formal. An informal social rule, for example, would be opening a door for someone. A criminal statute (**law**) would be an example of a formal rule of society. Social rules or codes promote our social well-being. It would be unsafe to live in a community that existed without rules.

Morality is a social barometer that dictates what is good or bad in a society. Moral teachings are an important adhesive for any society. Morality influences social rules or codes. The word ethics comes from the Greek word *ethos,* which means custom. Ethics can be thought of as a social

formalization of moral teachings. Ethics are those ideal standards that must be met if people are to behave with honor in their communities and professions. Health professionals are expected to behave in accordance with rules established by their professional organizations. Professional ethics establish the minimum requirements for honorable behavior within a profession. Ethics establish integrity. A member of a social or professional organization has a duty to adhere to the organization's ethics as a matter of personal and social integrity.

Law is the further formalization of moral considerations. It is necessary in all societies to require minimum standards of conduct for all its members. Laws require all social beings to behave in a manner that protects the individual and society as a whole. Many times these duties are enacted as codes, statutes, or laws by the government. Moral and ethical concerns can bleed into these laws. The government regulates behavior through these laws. Laws define individuals' duties to themselves, their neighbors, and the government. The failure to adhere to laws can result in punishment that can include imprisonment.

Morals establish what is good or bad for society. Ethics follow moral teachings and describe honorable behavior for a community or a profession. Laws are the governmental mandates of a society. As members of a social community, individuals are expected to behave in ways that will promote themselves and other members of society. The failure to follow social rules can result in informal social ostracism or formal legal punishment.

REGULATION OF THE PRACTICE OF NURSING

Nursing is a licensed health care profession. Nurses must be licensed by their state to practice nursing. The rationale for state licensure is to improve the quality of health care services and protect the public. As such, state governments have created licensing boards to establish the entry level requirements for nurses. These licensing boards also establish regulations that define the scope of appropriate nursing practice for licensed nurses. These licensing regulations are found in state nursing practice laws and within regulations that are made by the licensing agency.

The state nursing practice laws and the attendant nursing regulations establish the parameters within which nurses must practice in order to obtain and maintain their state license. These regulations are law and are referred to as **administrative laws.** Sometimes these regulations reflect the moral and ethical concerns of the society, community, and the state. Once these beliefs are codified in a written rule form, they are then enforceable by the licensing agency. These considerations and mandates can be the basis for disciplinary actions by the licensing body. The failure to adhere to the regulatory mandates of the nursing licensing body can result in the loss of the privilege to practice nursing. Unprofessional conduct and the conviction of a crime are examples of potential violations of nursing regulations.

A **code of ethics** is traditionally a compilation of ideal behaviors of a professional group. This list of ideals is intended to assist the professional in daily practice. Most professional organizations maintain these codes of ethics, and nursing associations have established ethical codes for their members. The codes are usually created by these private professional associations to reflect the ideals of that profession and the association. All LPN/LVNs must follow the ethical requirements found in the NAPNES Code of Ethics, which is the LPN/LVN professional code of ethics (Table 1–2).[3]

NURSING LIABILITY AND THE LAW

Liability refers to the level of responsibility that society places on individuals for their actions. In recent years, this responsibility has been interpreted to mean the financial responsibility owed to those who are injured by wrongful actions. Laws establish the minimum standards of behavior within society and communities. Laws also establish the liability or responsibility for the wrongs that are caused from the failure to adhere to these standards of behavior. The law is a major part of the practice of nursing.

Table 1–2. **NAPNES *Code of Ethics for LPN/LVNs***

The LPN/LVN shall:
1. Consider as a basic obligation the conservation of life and the prevention of disease.
2. Promote and protect the physical, mental, emotional and spiritual health of the patient and his family.
3. Fulfill all duties faithfully and efficiently.
4. Function within established legal guidelines.
5. Accept personal responsibility (for his/her acts) and seek to merit the respect and confidence of all members of the health care team.
6. Hold in confidence all matters coming to his/her knowledge in the practice of his profession, and in no way at no time violate this confidence.
7. Give conscientious service and charge just remuneration.
8. Learn and respect the religious and cultural beliefs of his/her patient and of all people.
9. Meet his/her obligation to the patient by keeping abreast of current trends in healthcare through reading and continuing education.
10. As a citizen of the United States of America, uphold the laws of the land and seek to promote legislation which shall meet the health needs of its people.

From The National Association for Practical Nurse Education and Service. Author, Silver Spring, Md, 1988, with permission.

Administrative laws establish the licensing authority of the state to create, license, and regulate the practice of nursing. **Criminal law** regulates behaviors for citizens within this country. **Civil law** provides the rules by which individuals seek to protect their personal and property rights.

CRIMINAL AND CIVIL LAW

All individuals, regardless of their occupations, are required to obey the criminal laws of the government. Criminal laws establish the rules of social behavior and provide the punishment for the breaking of those rules, which can result in the loss of freedom by imprisonment.

Criminal law is different from civil law by the nature of remedies that are used for punishment. A crime is viewed as an action taken by an individual against society that the government will prosecute and punish. The breaking of a criminal law may result in criminal punishment and civil liability. For instance, an intoxicated driver may go to jail for a crime and also be held civilly liable for any personal injury that resulted. Examples of criminal acts are assault, battery, rape, murder, and larceny.

Civil laws dictate how disputes are settled among individuals and how liability will be assigned for wrongful actions. For health care workers, civil liability is an everyday concern. The potential for civil liability is reflected by an increased use of health care procedures such as diagnostic testing, which results in higher health care costs. Civil liability is a method by which a client can seek financial recovery for injuries and losses caused by the wrongful action of a health care worker.

A civil liability suit begins with the filing of a complaint with a court. A copy of the complaint must be given or served by the plaintiff to the defendant. A **summons,** which is a notice to defendants that they are being sued, is attached to the complaint. The complaint will describe the claim being made by the plaintiff, and the summons will instruct the defendant that the complaint must be answered within a specified period of time, usually 20 to 30 days. Nurses served with a summons relating to work should notify their employer. These documents are important and must be taken seriously. The nurse must make sure that the summons is answered. If the employer does not answer the summons, the nurse must seek legal counsel to answer the summons within the specified time. If the nurse fails to answer the summons and complaint, it may result in a default judgment, which is acknowledgment of liability.

Civil wrongs caused by the act or omission of a health care worker can be physical, emotional, and financial in nature. The person claiming a civil cause of action and injury is the plaintiff, and the person alleged to have caused the injuries is the defendant. Lawsuits involving civil wrongs are called **torts.** The institution that employs the worker may also become liable for the acts or omissions of its employees. This theory of law is called **respondeat superior.** It is important for employees to understand that their work may result in civil liability for their employers.

Civil or tort liability for health care workers can be based on intentional actions, unintentional actions, and even the omission to act. **Malpractice** may be defined as a breach of the duty that arises out of the relationship that exists between the patient and the health care worker. This term includes liability that may arise from intentional torts and unintentional torts. Intentional torts are lawsuits wherein the defendant is accused of intentionally causing injury to the plaintiff. Examples of intentional torts are assault, battery, defamation, false imprisonment, outrage, invasion of privacy, and wrongful disclosure of confidential information (Table 1–3).

Negligence

An unintentional tort is known as **negligence.** Negligence occurs when injury results from the failure of the wrongdoer to exercise care. This failure to follow due care in the protection of the person injured is referred to as a breach of duty. Professionals owe a higher duty of care to their patients. The failure of a professional in health care to follow a prescribed duty of care is called malpractice. Professional negligence, therefore, is referred to as malpractice (Table 1–4). All professionals, including LPN/LVNs, are responsible for their own actions whether they are intentional or negligent in nature. Although the employing agency is also responsible for the actions of its employees, employees always remain responsible as well for their own actions.

All professions are concerned with the **limitation of liability.** This means that health care professionals can do some things to limit their individual and institutional liability. Some examples of liability limitations are accurate documentation of procedures, following institutional policies, acquiring individual malpractice or liability insurance, pursuing continuing education, and practicing in accordance with the current standards of the nursing profession. To limit liability the LPN/LVN should question directions that are controversial, are given verbally, or concern situations of high liability or when there is any discrepancy between the direction and standard policy. The LPN/LVN should document the individual giving a verbal direction.

It is important to understand that some employers do not provide malpractice insurance for their nursing employees. Nurses must always ask their employer whether they are covered under the employer's liability insurance. An employer's insurance will provide coverage from liability only as long as the nurse is in compliance with the employer's work policies. A nursing employee's failure to follow work policies and procedures may result in no liability insurance coverage for the employee. For this reason employer-provided liability insurance is not personal liability insurance. Nurses often carry personal liability insurance because of this.

Table 1-3. Intentional Torts

Assault	Unlawful conduct that places another in immediate fear of an unlawful touching or battery; real threat of bodily harm
Battery	Unlawful touching of another
Defamation	Wrongful injury to another's reputation or standing in a community; may be written (libel) or spoken (slander)
False Imprisonment	Unlawful restriction of a person's freedom
Outrage	Extreme and outrageous conduct by a defendant in the care of the client or the body of a deceased individual
Invasion of Privacy and Wrongful Disclosure of Confidential Information	Liability when a client's privacy is invaded physically or when records are released without authority

Table 1-4. Components Necessary for a Finding of Negligence

1. A duty of care owed to patients
2. A breach of duty to exercise care
3. Injury and damages occurring from this breach of duty

All LPN/LVNs must document their actions according to the orders that they are following in writing. This becomes a record of the LPN/LVN's work. The documentation must be clear, honest, and accurate.

Ethics and Values

Although many health care providers still think of ethics as an abstract exercise in thinking that is far removed from their daily practice, the simple truth is that every time a therapeutic relationship is established with a client, an ethical situation exists. In today's rapidly changing health care system, these situations are more common than they were a few years ago. Rapid advances in technology, changes in health care delivery systems, decreased personalization of health care, and increasing health care costs are all contributing to the ethical dilemmas seen today.

There are several different ways to approach ethical dilemmas. Some nurses may decide to do nothing at all, with the hope that the problem will resolve itself or that someone else will solve it. If that fails, these nurses may use the "it just feels right" technique: they choose the solution that produces the lowest degree of internal discomfort for them.[4]

However, ethical decision making is a skill that can be learned, much like inserting a catheter, changing a dressing, or assisting in data collection for care planning. Ethical decision making, like any learned skill, becomes easier the more it is practiced.

ETHICAL PRINCIPLES

Every ethical dilemma is different. However, when ethical dilemmas are carefully analyzed, there are several basic ethical principles that reoccur in each dilemma. These basic principles serve as the cause for various ethical problems. At the heart of many ethical dilemmas is a conflict between one or more of these basic principles. Understanding what the principle is and how it relates to the client's situation is necessary to resolve the dilemma. Some of the more important principles are discussed next.

Autonomy

Autonomy is the right of self-determination, independence, and freedom. Autonomy refers to clients' right to make health care decisions for themselves, even if health care providers do not agree with those decisions.

Autonomy, as with most rights, is not an absolute right, and under certain conditions, limitations can be imposed on it. Generally these limitations occur when an individual's autonomy interferes with the rights, health, or well-being of others. For example, clients generally can use their right to autonomy by refusing any or all treatments. However, in the case of contagious diseases that affect so-

ciety, such as tuberculosis (TB), an individual can be forced by the health care and legal systems to take medications to cure the disease. The individual can also be forced into isolation to prevent the spread of the disease.

Justice

Justice is the obligation to be fair to all people. The concept is often expanded into what is called **distributive justice,** which states that individuals have the right to be treated equally regardless of race, sex, marital status, sexual preference, medical diagnosis, social standing, economic level, or religious belief.[5] The principle of justice underlies the eighth statement in the NAPNES Code of Ethics for LPN/LVNs: "Learn and respect the religious and cultural beliefs of [the] patient and of all people" (Table 1–2). Distributive justice sometimes includes ideas such as equal access to health care by all citizens. As with other rights, limits can be placed on justice when it interferes with the rights of others.

Fidelity

Fidelity is the obligation to be faithful to commitments made to self and others. In health care, fidelity includes faithfulness or loyalty to agreements and responsibilities accepted as part of the practice of nursing. Fidelity is the main support for the concept of accountability, although conflicts in fidelity might arise because of obligations owed to different individuals or groups. For example, nurses have an obligation of fidelity to the clients they care for to provide the highest quality care possible, as well as an obligation of fidelity to their employing institution to follow its rules and policies. Nurses can be in an ethical dilemma when a hospital's policy on staffing creates a situation that does not allow the nurses to provide the quality of care they feel they should be providing.

Beneficence

Beneficence is one of the oldest requirements for health care providers. It views the primary goal of health care as doing good for clients under their care. In general, the term *good* includes more than just technically competent care for clients. Good care requires a holistic approach to clients, including their beliefs, feelings, and wishes, as well as those of their family and significant others. A problem sometimes encountered in implementing the principle of beneficence is in determining what exactly is good for another and who can best make the decision about this.

Nonmaleficence

Nonmaleficence is the requirement that health care providers do no harm to their clients, either intentionally or unintentionally. In a sense, it is the opposite side of the coin of beneficence, and it is difficult to speak of one term without mentioning the other. In current health care practice, the principle of nonmaleficence is often violated in the short run to produce a greater good in the long-term treatment of the client. For example, a client may undergo a painful and debilitating surgery to remove a cancerous growth in order to avoid death and prolong life.

By extension, the principle of nonmaleficence also requires the nurse to protect from harm those who cannot protect themselves. This protection from harm includes such groups as children, the mentally incompetent, the unconscious, and those who are too weak or debilitated to protect themselves.

Veracity

Veracity is the principle of truthfulness. It requires health care providers to tell the truth and not intentionally deceive or mislead clients. As with other rights and obligations, there are limitations to this principle. The primary limitation is when telling the client the truth would seriously harm (principle of nonmaleficence) his or her ability to recover, or produce greater illness. Although giving diagnostic information is the responsibility of the RN or physician and not an LPN/LVN role, LPN/LVNs sometimes find themselves caught in situations in which they must deal with clients' questions. If LPN/LVNs feel uncomfortable about reinforcing RN or physician explanations about unpleasant information, they may avoid answering clients' questions directly by using half-truths or claiming ignorance. However, clients have a right to know this information.

Standard of Best Interest

Standard of best interest is a type of decision made about clients' health care when they are unable to make an informed decision about their own care. The standard of best interest is based on what the health care providers or the family decide is best for that individual. It is important to consider the individual's expressed wishes, either formally in a written declaration, such as a living will, which states clients' wishes if they are unable to speak for themselves, or informally in what may have been said to family members.

The standard of best interest should be based on the principle of beneficence. Unfortunately, in situations in which clients are unable to make decisions for themselves, the resolution of the dilemma cannot be a unilateral decision made by health care providers. Although it is not an LPN/LVN role to determine what the standard of best interest is for clients, all nurses need to be aware that ignoring client wishes expressed in written documents can and has resulted in lawsuits against those providing care. A unilateral decision by health care providers that disregards a client's wishes implies that they alone know what is best and is called **paternalism.**

Obligations

Obligations are demands made on individuals, professions, society, or government to fulfill and honor the rights of others. Obligations are often divided into two categories:

1. Legal obligations are those which have become formal statements of law and are enforceable under the law. For example, nurses have a legal obligation to provide safe and adequate care for clients to whom they are assigned.
2. Moral obligations are those based on moral or ethical principles but are *not* enforceable under the law. For example, if a nurse is on vacation and comes on an automobile accident, in most states there is no legal obligation for the nurse to stop and help the victims. Most nurses would, however, feel a strong moral obligation to help.

Rights

Rights are generally defined as something due an individual according to just claims, legal guarantees, or moral and ethical principles. Although the term *right* is frequently used in both the legal and ethical systems, its meaning is often blurred in everyday usage. Individuals tend to claim things as rights that are really privileges, concessions, or freedoms. There are several classification systems for rights in which different types of rights are delineated. The following three types of rights are included in most of these systems:

1. **Welfare rights,** also called legal rights, are rights that are based on a legal entitlement to some good or benefit. These rights are guaranteed by laws such as the Bill of Rights and, if violated, can come under the powers of the legal system. For example, citizens of the United States have a right to equal access to employment regardless of race, sex, or religion.
2. **Ethical rights,** also called moral rights, are rights that are based on a moral or ethical principle. Ethical rights usually do not have the power of a law for enforcement. Ethical rights are, in reality, often privileges allotted to certain individuals or groups of individuals. Over time, popular acceptance of ethical rights can give them the appearance of a legal right. For example, the statements in the American Hospital Association's Patient's Bill of Rights are actually well-accepted privileges and are not legally binding on health care workers (Table 1–1).
3. **Option rights** are rights that are based on a fundamental belief in the dignity and freedom of human beings. Option rights are particularly evident in free and democratic countries such as the United States and are much less evident in totalitarian and restrictive societies. Option rights give individuals freedom of choice and the right to live their lives as they choose within a set of prescribed boundaries.

DECISION-MAKING MODEL IN ETHICS

Nurses, by definition, are problem solvers, and one of the important tools that is used regularly in problem solving is the nursing process. The nursing process is a systematic, step-by-step approach to resolving problems that deal with a client's health and well-being.

An ethical decision-making model provides a method for nurses to answer key questions about ethical dilemmas and to organize their thinking in a more logical and sequential manner, which is critical thinking. The chief goal of the ethical decision-making model is determining right from wrong in situations in which clear demarcations do not exist or are not readily apparent.

The following five-step ethical decision-making model is presented as a tool for resolving ethical dilemmas.

Step 1: Collect, Analyze, and Interpret the Data

Obtain as much information as possible concerning the ethical dilemma. Some important information to obtain includes the client's wishes, the family's wishes, the extent of the physical or emotional problems causing the dilemma, the physician's beliefs about health care, and the nurse's personal orientation to life-and-death issues.

For example, nurses often must deal with the question of whether to initiate resuscitation efforts when a terminally ill client is admitted to the hospital. Many states and hospitals now have requirements for written "no code" orders. In some areas, however, physicians may indicate verbally that the client should not be resuscitated but that the nurses should go through the motions of a code to make the family feel better. The dilemma for the nurse becomes whether to seriously attempt to revive the client or let the client die.

Important information that would help the nurse make the best decision might include the mental competency of the client to make a no resuscitation decision, the client's desires, the family's feelings, whether the physician sought input from the client and the family before giving orders, and the institution's policies concerning no resuscitation orders.

Step 2: State the Dilemma

After collecting and analyzing as much of the information as is available, the dilemma needs to be stated as clearly and briefly as possible. Recognizing the key aspects of the dilemma helps focus attention on the important ethical principles. Most of the time, the dilemma can be reduced to a statement or two that revolves around key ethical principles. These ethical principles often involve a question of conflicting rights, obligations, or basic ethical principles.

In the situation of slow resuscitation or no resuscitation, the statement of the dilemma might be, "The client's right to self-determination and death with dignity versus the nurse's obligation to preserve life and do no harm." In general, the principle that the competent client's wishes must be followed takes precedent. If the client has become unresponsive before expressing his or her wishes, the input of family members must be given serious consideration. Additional questions can arise if the family's wishes conflict with those of the client.

Step 3: Consider the Choices of Action

After having stated the dilemma as clearly as possible, the nurse should list all the possible courses of action that can be taken to resolve the dilemma without consideration of their consequences at this time. This brainstorming activity considers all possible courses of action and may require input from outside sources such as colleagues, supervisors, or even experts in the ethical field. The consequences of these different actions are considered later.

Some of the possible courses of action the nurse might consider for the slow resuscitation or no resuscitation question include the following: (1) resuscitating the client to the fullest ability despite what the physician has requested; (2) not resuscitating the client at all; (3) just going through the motions without any real attempt to revive the client; (4) seeking another assignment to avoid dealing with the situation; (5) reporting the problem to the supervisor; (6) attempting to clarify the question with the client; (7) attempting to clarify the question with the family; and (8) confronting the physician about the question.

Step 4: Analyze the Advantages and Disadvantages of Each Course of Action

Some of the courses of action listed during the previous step in the process are more realistic than other courses of action. The unrealistic actions become readily evident during this step in the decision-making process, when the nurse considers the advantages and the disadvantages of each action in detail. Along with each option, the consequences of taking each course of action must be evaluated as to their advantages and disadvantages.

For example, initiating discussion about the order might anger the physician or cause him or her to distrust the nurse in the future. Either of these responses might make practicing at that institution difficult. The same result might occur if the client is successfully resuscitated despite orders to the contrary. Not resuscitating the client has the potential to develop into a lawsuit if there is no clear order for no resuscitation. Presenting the situation to a supervisor may, if the supervisor supported the physician, cause the nurse to be labeled a troublemaker. The same process can be applied to the other courses of action listed in step 3.

By thoroughly considering the advantages and disadvantages of each possible action, it should be easier to reduce the choices to the most realistic ones. An important factor to include in the evaluation of the actions would be the NAPNES Code of Ethics (Table 1–2).

Step 5: Make the Decision

The most difficult part of the process is actually making the decision and living with the consequences. By their nature, ethical dilemmas produce differences of opinion, and not everyone will be pleased with the decision.

The client's wishes almost always supersede independent decisions on the nurse's part. Collaborative decision making among the client, physician, nurses, and family about resuscitation is the ideal solution and tends to produce fewer complications in the long-term resolution of such questions.

Nursing Code of Ethics

A code of ethics states the principles that govern a particular profession. Codes of ethics are presented in general statements and do not give specific answers to every possible ethical dilemma that might arise. However, these codes do offer guidance in making ethical decisions.

Ideally, codes of ethics should undergo periodic revision to reflect changes in the profession and society as a whole. Although codes of ethics are not legally enforceable as laws, if a nurse consistently violates the code of ethics, it is taken as an indication of an unwillingness to act in a professional manner and often results in disciplinary actions ranging from reprimands and fines to suspension and revocation of licensure.

The NAPNES Code of Ethics used by LPN/LVNs contains a set of clearly stated principles that must be applied to actual clinical situations. For example, nurses involved in the resuscitation dilemma described previously will not find any specific mention of no resuscitation orders in the NAPNES Code of Ethics. Instead, general statements such as the LPN/LVN shall "consider as a basic obligation the conservation of life and the prevention of disease," and the LPN/LVN "fulfills all duties faithfully and efficiently" are found in the NAPNES Code of Ethics and must be applied to a particular situation.

> **CRITICAL THINKING: Ethical Decisions**
>
> 1. Identify a health care–related ethical dilemma you have encountered as a student. How did you deal with it?
> 2. Apply the ethical decision-making model to the ethical dilemma. Would your decision or actions be any different?

Values

Values are ideals or concepts that give meaning to an individual's life. Values are most commonly derived from societal norms, religion, and family orientation. They serve as the framework for making decisions and taking certain actions in everyday life. Values are not usually written down, but it may be important for nurses at some time in their careers to make a list of their values and attempt to rank them by priority. Value conflicts often occur in everyday life and can force an individual to select a higher-priority value over a lower-priority value. For example, a nurse who values both her career and her family may be forced to decide between going to work or staying home with a sick child.

Values exist on many different levels. Individuals have personal values that govern their lives and actions. Many groups and organizations have values that may or may not be identical to personal values. When a person becomes a member of a group or organization, he or she agrees to accept the values of the group. Common groups include clubs, churches and church organizations, and professions. The values of a profession are best outlined in a code of ethics. Failure to adhere to a code of ethics of a profession may be an indication that the individual really does not want to belong to that group. Society as a whole has values. As a member of a society or country, the individual accepts the values of that culture.

Ethical issues and ethics are a part of the everyday practice of a nurse. In today's world, with rapidly advancing technology and unusual health care situations, ethical dilemmas are increasing. Nurses can prepare themselves to deal with most of these dilemmas if they keep current with the issues and are able to use a systematic process for making ethical decisions. One of the most difficult elements of ethical decision making is that it is unlikely that everyone will be pleased with the decision. But if decisions are made after thoughtful analysis of the situation and are based on ethical principles, nurses will be able to defend their decisions.

Review Questions

1. Factors influencing health care changes include which of the following?
   a. Increasing elderly population
   b. Increasing birth rate
   c. Decreasing cultural diversity
   d. Decreasing population in America

2. Where are licensing laws for nurses found?
   a. Office policies
   b. Association ethics codes
   c. State nursing practice laws
   d. National nursing standards

3. The law of negligence requires which of the following to create liability?
   a. A crime
   b. Assault
   c. A breach of duty
   d. Ethical violations

4. An ethical code can best be described as
   a. The "ball and chain" of the profession
   b. A collection of rules that are static
   c. A group of values legally binding
   d. A framework for decision making

5. A nurse believes that the most important consideration in client care is to do good for the client. This attitude represents support for the concept of
   a. Fidelity
   b. Beneficence
   c. Justice
   d. Nonmaleficence

6. The authoritarian leader makes decisions by
   a. Seeking information from all staff members
   b. Using own knowledge to decide
   c. Forming focus groups to gather information
   d. Forming a staff committee to provide input

7. Which of the following is a caring behavior of the art of nursing?
   a. A deep concern for other individuals.
   b. The nurse determines client care decisions.
   c. The nurse assumes a "boss" role for client care.
   d. Focusing on all assigned clients with every client interaction.

REFERENCES

1. United States Department of Health and Human Services, Public Health Service: Healthy People 2000: National Health Promotion and Disease Prevention Objectives. U.S. Government Printing Office, Washington, DC, 1992.
2. Watson, J: Nursing: Human Science and Human Care. National League of Nursing, New York, 1988.
3. NAPNES Code of Ethics. National Association for Practical Nurse Education and Service, Silver Spring, Md, 1988.
4. Catalano, JT: Ethical and Legal Aspects of Nursing, ed 2. Springhouse, Philadelphia, 1995.
5. Thompson, JE, and Thompson, HO: Teaching ethics to nursing students. Nurs Outlook 37:84, 1989.

BIBLIOGRAPHY

Aiken, TD, and Catalano, JT: Legal, Ethical, and Political Issues in Nursing. FA Davis, Philadelphia, 1995.
Anderson, M: Nursing Leadership, Management and Professional Practice for the LPN/LVN. FA Davis, Philadelphia, 1997.
Aroskar, MA: Nurses and unlicensed assistive personnel: Ethical perspectives. ANA Center for Ethics and Human Rights 4:2, 1995.
Catalano, JT: Contemporary Professional Nursing. FA Davis, Philadelphia, 1996.
Catalano, JT: Treatments not specifically listed in the living will: The ethical dilemmas. Dimens Crit Care Nurs 13:142, 1994.
Curtin, LH: How much is enough? Nurs Manage 25:30, 1994.
Reeves, DL: A licenced practical nurse/licensed vocational nurse's (LPN/LVN) guide to the changing healthcare system. Gastroenterol Nurs 20:54, 1997.

Critical Thinking and the Nursing Process

Paula D. Hopper and Linda S. Williams

2

Learning Objectives

Upon completion of this chapter, the student will be able to:

1. Identify the steps of the nursing process.
2. Define critical thinking.
3. Describe the role of the licensed practical nurse and licensed vocational nurse in using the nursing process.
4. Describe the process of collecting client data.
5. Use data clusters to select nursing diagnoses from a list of accepted North American Nursing Diagnosis Association diagnoses.
6. Prioritize client care based on Maslow's hierarchy of human needs.
7. Identify measurable client outcomes based on nursing diagnoses.
8. Collaborate in developing interventions to meet identified client outcomes.
9. Identify evaluation criteria for interventions and outcomes.
10. Explain how critical thinking enhances the implementation of the nursing process.

Key Words

auscultation (AWS-kul-**TAY**-shun)
assessment (ah-**SESS**-ment)
critical thinking (**KRIT**-i-kuhl **THING**-king)
data (**DAY**-tuh)
evaluation (e-VAL-yoo-**AY**-shun)
inspection (in-**SPEK**-shun)
intervention (in-ter-**VEN**-shun)
nursing diagnosis (**NUR**-sing DYE-ag-**NOH**-sis)
nursing process (**NUR**-sing **PRAH**-sess)
objective data (ob-**JEK**-tiv **DAY**-tuh)
palpation (pal-**PAY**-shun)
percussion (per-**KUSH**-un)
subjective data (sub-**JEK**-tiv **DAY**-tuh)

Excellence in nursing care delivery requires good thinking. Each day nurses make many decisions that affect the care of their clients. For the decisions to be effective, the thought processes behind them must be sound.

Critical Thinking

Nurses must learn to think critically. This means they use their knowledge and skills to make the best decisions possible in client care situations. Halpern[1] says that "**critical thinking** is the use of those cognitive (knowledge) skills or strategies that increase the probability of a desirable outcome." Critical thinking is sometimes termed *directed thinking,* because it focuses on a goal. Other terms used when talking about critical thinking include *reasoning, common sense, analysis,* and *inquiry.*

Problem Solving

Problem solving is a type of critical thinking. Nurses solve problems on a daily basis. However, a problem can be solved in a way that may or may not help the client.

For instance, consider the client who is in pain and requests pain medication. The nurse checks the medication record and finds that his analgesic medication is not due for another 40 minutes. The nurse can solve this problem in a variety of ways. One obvious solution is to return to the client and say that it is not time for the pain medication and the client will have to wait. The problem has been solved, but not in the best way for the client.

Another way to solve the problem is to do the following:

1. Gather **data.** You return to the client and make a further **assessment** of his pain. He states that his pain is in his back, and rates it as an 8 on a scale of 1 to 10. He is lying stiffly in bed and has a strained expression. You know from his history that he has compression fractures of his spine. You return to the medica-

25

tion record and find that he has no alternative pain medications ordered.

2. Formulate the problem. The client is in pain, and with the resources you currently have, you cannot provide pain relief.

3. Decide what outcome (sometimes called a goal) is desirable. The outcome should be determined by the nurse and the client. The client is intimately involved in this situation and deserves to be consulted. In this case, you talk to the client and determine that the client needs his pain controlled now; he cannot wait until the next scheduled dose of medication. He states that he will be satisfied if his pain rating is at 2 or less on a scale of 1 to 10.

4. Plan what to do about it. Formulate and evaluate some alternative solutions. For example, you can decide to tell the client that he has to wait 40 minutes. However, this will not help the client reach his desired outcome of pain control. Giving the medication early might relieve the client's pain, but this would not be following the physician's orders and could have harmful effects for the client. You could decide to try some alternative pain control methods, such as relaxation, distraction, or imagery. These might be helpful, but with a pain rating of 8, the client may also need medication. Another alternative is to inform the physician that the current pain control regimen is not working, and obtain new pain relief orders.

   Once you have several alternatives, it is time to choose the best options. Which ones will best help the client? Which ones will not harm the client? You confer with the registered nurse and decide the best thing to do is to have the registered nurse contact the physician while you work with the client on relaxation exercises. You tell the client that the physician is being contacted. This assures him that you understand his need and that his pain will be controlled soon.

5. Implement the plan of care. The registered nurse enters the room and informs you and the client that the physician has changed the analgesic orders, then hands you the first dose. The registered nurse also informs the client that the physician has ordered a consultation with the institution's pain clinic.

6. Evaluate the plan of care. Did the plan work? You think back to the desired outcome and compare it with the current assessment. As you reassess the client 30 minutes later, he rates his pain level at 2, and thanks you for your prompt and compassionate attention to his pain relief need.

Can you see how using the problem-solving process led to a better outcome than simply choosing the first obvious solution? You now have a satisfied client whose pain is controlled.

Nursing Process

You have just used the **nursing process** to solve a real problem. The nursing process is an organizing framework that links the process of thinking with actions in nursing practice. Nurses use the nursing process to assess client needs; formulate nursing diagnoses; and plan, implement, and evaluate care. The beginning nurse consciously uses the nursing process with each client problem. The experienced nurse has internalized the nursing process and can use it without as much conscious effort.

ROLE OF THE LICENSED PRACTICAL NURSE AND LICENSED VOCATIONAL NURSE

The licensed practical nurse (LPN) or licensed vocational nurse (LVN) carries out a specific role in the nursing process, as described in Table 2–1. The LPN/LVN collects data, assists in formulating nursing diagnoses, assists in determining outcomes and planning care to meet client needs, implements client care **intervention,** and assists in evaluating the effectiveness of nursing interventions in achieving the client's outcomes. Often the LPN/LVN spends more direct care time with the client than the registered nurse (RN) does and develops a relationship that aids in collecting valuable data. The LPN/LVN and the RN work as a team to analyze data and develop, implement, and evaluate the plan of care (Fig. 2–1).

DATA COLLECTION

The first step in the nursing process is data collection. The LPN/LVN assists the registered nurse in collecting data from a variety of sources. Information that is provided verbally by the client is called **subjective data.** Symptoms are subjective data. Subjective data are often placed in quotes, such as "I have a headache" or "I feel short of breath." The nurse must listen carefully to the client and understand that only the client truly knows how he or she feels.

Table 2–1. **Role of the LPN/LVN in the Nursing Process**

Steps of the Process	Role of the LPN/LVN
Assessment	Assists in collecting data
Nursing Diagnosis	Assists in choosing appropriate nursing diagnoses
Plan of Care	Assists in developing outcomes and planning care to meet outcomes
Implementation	Carries out those portions of the plan of care that are within the LPN/LVN's scope of practice
Evaluation	Assists in evaluation and revision of the plan of care

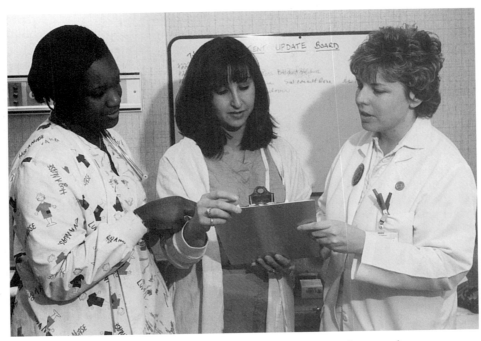

Figure 2–1. An LPN and an RN collaborating on a nursing care plan.

Objective data are factual data obtained through physical assessment and diagnostic tests, and are observable or knowable through the five senses. Objective data are sometimes called signs. Examples of objective data include the following: 3 cm red lesion, respiratory rate 36, blood glucose 326 mg/dL, and client moaning and holding abdomen. Note that these are all observable or measurable by the nurse and do not require explanation by the client.

Subjective Data

The nurse first assesses the chief complaint. Here the nurse focuses on the reason the client is seeking health care. The question "What brings you here?" can be helpful.

Once the client has identified the main concern, the nurse can use further questioning to gain more pertinent information. The WHAT'S UP questioning format can be helpful. The nurse can use the letters of WHAT'S UP to remember questions to ask the client (Table 2–2).

LEARNING TIP

Practice assessing a symptom on a classmate. Ask the WHAT'S UP questions.

Next the nurse obtains a client history. This is done by asking the client and family questions about the client's past and present health problems, specific questions about each body system, family health problems, and risk factors for health problems. The client's medical record may also be consulted for background history information.

In addition to assessment related to physiological functioning, the nurse asks the client about personal habits that relate to health, such as exercise, diet, and the presence of stressors. Finally, the client's family role, support systems, and cultural and spiritual beliefs or influences are assessed.

Objective Data

After the history is complete a physical assessment is done. During the physical assessment the nurse inspects, palpates, percusses, and auscultates (IPPA) to collect objective data. This is called the IPPA format. Special attention is given to those areas that the client has identified as problem areas.

Inspection

During the **inspection** phase of physical assessment the nurse uses observation skills to systematically gather data

Table 2–2. **WHAT'S UP Guide to Symptom Assessment**

W—Where is it?
H—How does it feel? Describe the quality.
A—Aggravating and alleviating factors. What makes it worse? What makes it better?
T—Timing. When did it start? How long does it last?
S—Severity. How bad is it? This can often be rated on a scale of 1 to 10.
U—Useful other data. What are other symptoms that are present that might be related?
P—Patient's perception of the problem. The patient (or client) often has an idea about what the problem is, or the cause, but may not believe that his or her thoughts are worth sharing unless specifically asked.

that can be seen. This may include noting the client's respiratory effort, observing skin color, or measuring a wound. This phase continues throughout the assessment.

Palpation

Palpation involves use of the fingers or hands to feel something. The nurse might palpate the abdomen for firmness or use the back of the hand to palpate a forehead for fever. Physicians and advanced practice nurses also use deep palpation to assess abdominal organs.

Percussion

Percussion is a technique used by physicians and advanced practice nurses to determine the consistency of underlying tissues. The examiner taps on the client to elicit a sound. Generally the middle finger of the nondominant hand is placed on the area to be percussed, and the middle finger of the dominant hand taps on the nondominant one (Fig. 2–2). This prevents client discomfort. A dull sound is heard over a fluid-filled area, such as the liver. A flat sound is heard over a solid area, such as muscle. Tympany is a drumlike sound heard over air, such as gas in the stomach. Resonance is a hollow sound heard over air-filled lung tissue. Although this technique is not generally used by LPN/LVNs, it is helpful to understand what it is when assisting someone performing it during a physical examination.

Auscultation

Auscultation is usually done with a stethoscope. The abdomen is auscultated for bowel sounds. The chest is auscultated for normal and adventitious lung sounds or for heart sounds. Major vessels may be auscultated for turbulent blood flow by a physician or registered nurse.

During physical assessment, the IPPA format is followed in the given order, except in the case of the abdomen. The order

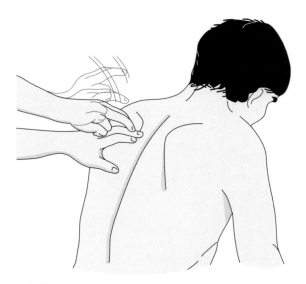

Figure 2–2. Percussion. (Modified from Morton: Health Assessment in Nursing, ed 2. FA Davis, Philadelphia, 1993, p 85, with permission.)

for the abdomen is IAPP, because percussion and palpation of the abdomen can alter the auscultation findings.

Data collection related to each body system is covered in individual chapters throughout the book. Specific ways to use the IPPA format will be discussed.

DOCUMENTATION OF DATA

Once the data have been collected, it is documented in the client's medical record. The recorded data should be accurate and concise. The nurse documents exactly what was observed or stated. Interpretation of the data and the use of words that have vague meanings should be avoided in documentation. For example, "nailbed color is pink" gives clearer information than "nailbed color is normal." "Capillary refill is two seconds" gives precise data when compared with "capillary refill is good." The statement "the wound looks better" is not meaningful unless the wound has been previously observed by the reader. Stating "the wound is one by two inches, red in color, with no drainage or odor" provides data with which to compare the future status of the wound and determine whether it is improving. When documenting subjective data, direct quotations from the client are desirable. Quotes accurately represent the client's view and are least open to interpretation. Meaningful documentation promotes continuity of client care.

LEARNING TIP

Documenting exactly what is observed is appropriate, easier, and less time-consuming than seeking other words or ways to state observations. Nursing students and novices often search for elaborate phrases or words when simple, direct words are best. State exactly what you see, and it should be appropriate.

NURSING DIAGNOSIS

Once data have been collected, the LPN/LVN assists the RN to compare the findings with what is considered "normal." Data are then grouped, or clustered, into sets of related information that can lead the nurse to the conclusion that a problem exists.

A **nursing diagnosis** is a standardized label placed on a client's problem to make it understandable to all nurses. It helps guide the development of the plan of care. A diagnosis is considered "nursing" instead of "medical" if the interventions necessary to treat the problem are primarily independent nursing functions. In other words, nurses can decide what to do about the problem without a physician's order. Of course, nurses commonly do consult with physicians about plans of care, and it is helpful to do so. If, however, the physician directs most of the care related to a particular problem, it is probably a medical, rather than a nursing diagnosis.

One commonly used nursing diagnosis is pain. In the previous example, the nurse assessed the pain, determined that it was a problem, and developed a brief plan of care to help resolve the pain. Although the physician was consulted for an analgesic order, the nurse also used relaxation and distraction to help the client. These do not require a physician's order.

Another nursing diagnosis is altered skin integrity. The nurse can assess the client's skin condition and provide care for many skin problems without specific physician orders. See the inside cover of this book for a complete list of nursing diagnoses recommended for use by the North American Nursing Diagnosis Association (NANDA).

Some client problems require more collaboration with a physician. For example, a client with pneumonia has many needs that depend on physician orders, such as respiratory treatments and antibiotics. The nurse, however, can provide important assessment findings related to the problem, and provide nursing measures such as increased fluid intake and encouragement to cough and deep breathe. When the physician and nurse work closely together on a client problem, it is called a collaborative problem. In reality, most problems are collaborative, if they are treated appropriately.

CRITICAL THINKING: Nursing Diagnosis

Which of the following is a nursing diagnosis? Medical? Collaborative?

1. Pain
2. Ineffective coping
3. Herniated disk
4. Fractured femur
5. Diabetes
6. Impaired gas exchange
7. Heart failure
8. Health-seeking behaviors

Answers at end of chapter.

A well-written nursing diagnosis is helpful in guiding development of a plan of care. There are three parts to a diagnosis:

1. *Problem*—the nursing diagnosis label
2. *Etiology*—the cause or related factor (often preceded by the words "related to")
3. *Signs and symptoms*—the evidence that this is indeed a valid diagnosis (often preceded by the words "as evidenced by")

This is called the PES format. Look again at the case study of the client with pain. A diagnosis using this format might read as follows: "Acute pain (related to) muscle spasms and nerve compression (as evidenced by) client pain rating of 8 and strained facial expression." Note how the complete diagnosis gives the nurse more helpful information than simply the label "pain." This additional information helps determine an appropriate outcome and directs interventions.

PLAN OF CARE

Once nurse diagnoses are identified, the nurse develops an individualized plan of care to help the client meet his or her care needs. It is important for the nurse to include the client in the development of the plan of care. The client should be in agreement with the plan for it to be successful in meeting the desired outcomes. The first step in planning care after diagnoses are selected is to prioritize the diagnoses and develop outcomes, or goals, for each. Actions can then be determined that will help the client meet the desired outcomes.

LEARNING TIP

If you are developing a plan of care for a complex client and are not sure where to start, go back to the assessment phase. Often additional information can help you better understand the client's needs and develop a plan of care that is individualized to the client's specific problem areas.

Prioritizing Care

The nurse and client decide which problems take priority. Maslow's hierarchy of human needs can be used as a basis for determining priorities (Fig. 2–3). According to Maslow, humans must meet their most basic needs first. They can then move up the hierarchy to meet higher-level needs.

Physiological needs are the most basic needs. Once physiological needs are met, the client can concentrate on meeting safety and security needs. Love, belonging, and self-esteem needs are next, and self-actualization needs are met last.

Throughout life, clients move up and down Maslow's hierarchy in response to life events. If a need occurs on a level below where the client currently is, the client will move down to the level of that need. Once the need is fulfilled, the client can move upward again on the hierarchy.

In a nursing plan of care, the client's most urgent problem is listed first. According to Maslow's hierarchy of human needs this usually involves a physiological need such as oxygen or water, because these are life-sustaining needs. Once physiological needs are met, needs related to the next level of the hierarchy, safety and security, can be addressed. Remaining diagnoses are listed in order of urgency as they relate to the hierarchy. Needs can occur simultaneously on different levels and must be addressed in a holistic manner with prioritization guiding the care provided.

CRITICAL THINKING: Prioritizing Care

Based on Maslow's hierarchy of needs, list the following nursing diagnoses in order from highest (1) to lowest (5) priority. Give rationale for your decisions.

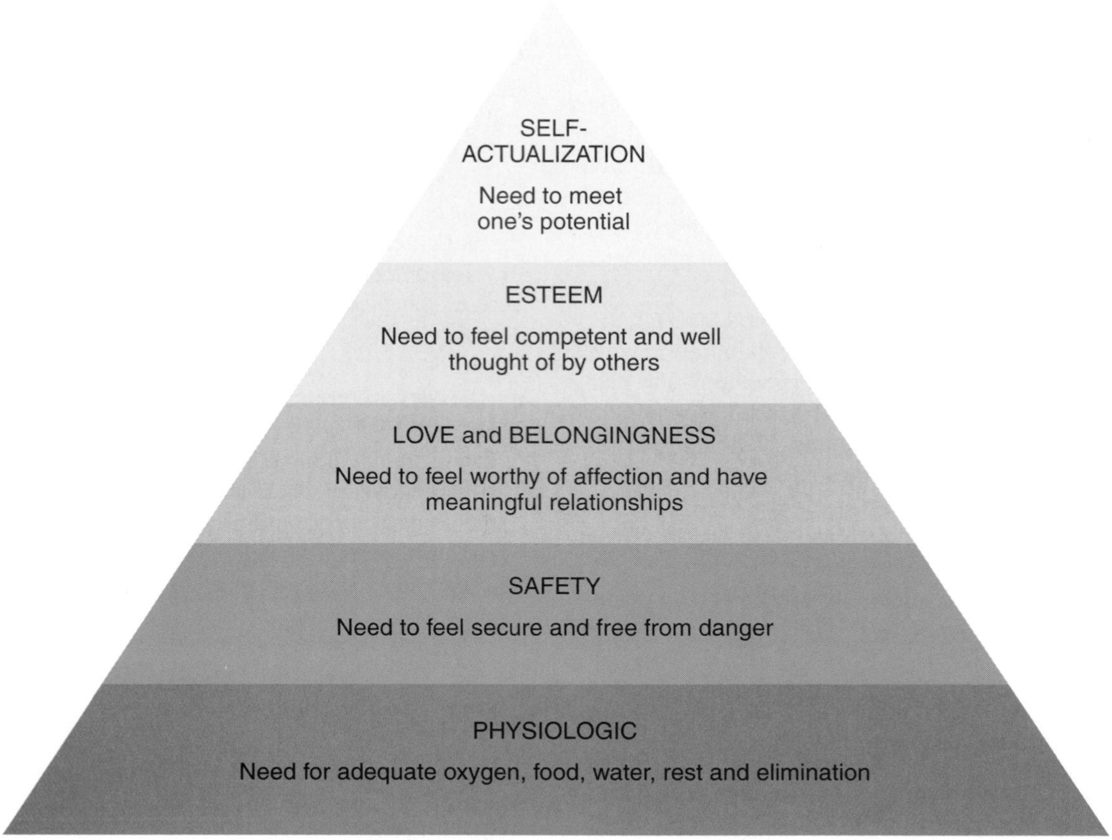

Figure 2–3. Maslow's hierarchy of human needs.

1. Knowledge deficit
2. Constipation
3. Ineffective family coping
4. Anxiety
5. Ineffective airway clearance.
   Answers at end of chapter.

Developing Outcomes

An outcome is a statement that describes the client's desired goal for a problem area. It should be measurable, be realistic for the client, and have an appropriate time frame for achievement. Measurable means that the outcome can be observed, or is objective. It should not be vague or open to interpretation with the use of subjective words such as normal, large, small, or moderate. Consider, for example, two outcomes:

1. The client's shortness of breath will improve.
2. The client will be less short of breath within 15 minutes as evidenced by client rating the shortness of breath less than 3 on a scale of 1 to 10, respiratory rate between 16 and 20, and relaxed appearance.

Although the first outcome seems appropriate, in reality it will be difficult for the nurse to know when it has been met. There is nothing to objectively indicate when the

problem has been resolved. The second outcome, however, is objective. It is easy to see that when the client rates his or her shortness of breath less than 3, is breathing at a rate of 16 to 20, and appears relaxed, the desired outcome will have been met. The outcome is realistic, and the 15-minute time frame ensures that the client will not suffer shortness of breath for longer than necessary. If the plan of care does not achieve the desired outcome in the given time frame, it should be evaluated and revised as needed.

When determining criteria for a measurable outcome, look at the signs and symptoms portion of the nursing diagnosis. The signs and symptoms that are evidence that the problem exists are the same criteria that need to be resolved. Look at another outcome example to see how criteria are used for measurement:

Nursing diagnosis: Ineffective airway clearance related to excess secretions *as evidenced by coarse crackles and nonproductive cough.*
Outcome: Improved airway clearance within 8 hours *as evidenced by clear lung sounds and productive cough.*

Identifying Interventions

Interventions are the actions the nurse takes to help the client meet the desired outcome. Interventions are therefore considered to be goal directed. Any intervention that does not contribute to meeting the outcome should not be part of the plan of care.

One way to create a plan is to include interventions that can be categorized as "take, treat, and teach." In the first intervention category, take, the nurse takes or identifies data that should be routinely collected related to the problem. Next, the nurse treats the problem by identifying deliberate actions to help reach the outcome. Last, the nurse identifies what to teach the client and family in order for the client to learn to care for himself or herself.

Look again at the nursing diagnosis of impaired airway clearance. A plan of care for this problem using the take, treat, and teach method might look like this:

Take: Auscultate lung sounds every 4 hours and prn.
          Assess respiratory rate every 4 hours and prn.
Treat: Provide 2 L of fluids every 24 hours.
          Offer expectorant as ordered.
          Provide cool mist vaporizer in room.
Teach: Teach the client the importance of fluid intake.
          Teach the client to cough and deep breathe every 1 to 2 hours.

In addition to identifying interventions, it is important for the nurse to understand how and why they will work. This is called identifying rationale. For example, the nurse will assess lung sounds and respiratory rate every 4 hours *because increased crackles and respiratory rate indicate retained secretions.* The nurse provides fluids *in order to help liquefy secretions and ease their removal.* Sound rationale should guide each intervention identified.

IMPLEMENTATION

Once the plan of care has been identified, it must be communicated to the client, family, and health team members, and then implemented. One way a plan of care is communicated is by writing it as a nursing care plan. The nursing care plan is documented on the client's medical record and lets other nurses know the client's priority problems, the desired outcomes, and the plan for meeting the outcomes. In this way, all nurses can be consistent in providing care for the client.

When implementing the plan of care the actions listed as interventions are performed. The client's response to each intervention is noted and documented. This documentation provides the basis for **evaluation** and revision of the plan of care.

EVALUATION

The last step of the process is evaluation. Evaluation examines both outcomes and interventions. The nurse continuously evaluates the client's progress toward the desired outcomes and the effectiveness of each intervention. If the outcomes are not reached within the given time frame, or if the interventions are ineffective, the plan of care is revised. Any part of the plan of care can be revised, from the diagnosis or desired outcome to the interventions. Acute care institutions require review and updating of the plan of care every 24 hours. See the Nursing Care Plan Box 2–1 for the Client with Pain.

NURSING CARE PLAN BOX 2–1 FOR THE CLIENT WITH PAIN*

Acute pain related to muscle spasms and nerve compression as evidenced by client pain rating of 8 on a scale of 1 to 10 and strained facial expression

Client Outcome
Pain level improved as evidenced by client pain rating of less than 3, relaxed facial expression, and statement that pain level is acceptable.

Evaluation of Outcomes
Is pain rating less than 3? Is facial expression relaxed? Does client state that pain level is acceptable?

Interventions	Rationale	Evaluation
• Assess pain level on a scale of 1 to 10 every 4 hours and as required (prn).	The client's report is the most reliable indicator of pain.	Is the client able to report pain level? Is it less than 3?
• Offer analgesic per order every 4 hours.	The client may not ask for analgesic medication.	Is the client using analgesic medication appropriately?
• Encourage client to take analgesic before pain becomes severe.	Pain is more easily relieved when it is less intense.	Is pain controlled, and is severe pain prevented?
• Assist client to comfortable position every 1 to 2 hours and prn.	Some positions may be more comfortable than others. Pain may prevent the client from moving.	Do position changes help the client's pain? Does the client need assistance to change position?
• Teach the client distraction and relaxation techniques.	These strategies may alter the sensation of pain. They also give the client control over the situation.	Does the client demonstrate use of distraction and relaxation techniques?

*Note: This is an example only. A more complete care plan for pain is found in Chapter 9.

Summary

Although the nursing process is presented in discrete steps in this chapter, in reality it is a continuous process. The nurse is constantly assessing, evaluating, and revising the plan of care to meet the client's current needs.

In most chapters throughout this book, sample nursing care plans are provided. These are guidelines for client care. Any plan of care must be individualized based on a client's unique characteristics and needs.

Review Questions

1. Which of the following *best* defines the nursing process?
   a. The process that nurses use to write nursing care plans.
   b. The process used by nurses to evaluate nursing care.
   c. A framework that links the process of thinking with nursing actions.
   d. A framework that promotes collaboration with other members of the health team.

2. Which of the following parts of the nursing process can be carried out by the LPN?
   a. implementation of interventions
   b. nursing diagnosis
   c. analysis of data
   d. evaluation of outcomes

3. Which of the following pieces of information would be considered objective data?
   a. Client is short of breath.
   b. Client states, "I feel short of breath."
   c. Client's respiratory rate is 28.
   d. Client is feeling panicky.

4. An LPN is collecting data on a newly admitted client. He has an ulcerated area on his left hip that is 2 inches in diameter, 1 inch deep, and has yellow exudate. Which of the following statements should be documented in the client's data base?
   a. Wound on left hip 2 inches in diameter, 1 inch deep, yellow exudate
   b. Left hip wound is large, deep, and has yellow drainage
   c. Pressure ulcer on left hip, yellow drainage
   d. Wound on left hip, 2 inches diameter, 1 inch deep, infected

5. A 34-year-old mother of three children is admitted to a respiratory unit with pneumonia. Based on Maslow's hierarchy of needs, which of the following client problems should the nurse address *first*?
   a. Frontal headache from stress of hospital admission
   b. Shortness of breath from newly diagnosed pneumonia
   c. Anxiety related to concern about leaving children
   d. Lack of knowledge about treatment plan

6. Which of the following is a nursing diagnosis?
   a. Stroke
   b. Renal failure
   c. Fracture
   d. Pain

ANSWERS TO CRITICAL THINKING

Critical Thinking: Nursing Diagnosis

1. Pain = nursing
2. Ineffective coping = nursing
3. Herniated disk = medical
4. Fractured femur = medical
5. Diabetes = collaborative
6. Impaired gas exchange = nursing
7. Heart failure = collaborative
8. Health-seeking behaviors = nursing

Critical Thinking: Prioritizing Care

1. Knowledge deficit, safety and security need—4
2. Constipation, physiological need—2
3. Ineffective family coping, love and belonging need—5
4. Anxiety, safety and security need—3
5. Ineffective airway clearance, physiological need—1

REFERENCE

1. Halpern, D: Thought and Knowledge: An Introduction to Critical Thinking, ed 3. Lawrence Erlbaum Associates, NJ, 1996, p 5.

BIBLIOGRAPHY

Ackley, BJ, and Ladwig, GB: Nursing Diagnosis Handbook: A Guide to Planning Care. Mosby, St Louis, 1995.

Baker, C: Reflective learning: A teaching strategy for critical thinking. J Nurs Educ 35(1):19, 1996.

Case, B: Walking around the elephant: A critical thinking strategy for decision making. J Contin Educ Nurs 25(3):101, 1994.

Dobrzykowski, T: Teaching strategies to promote critical thinking skills in nursing staff. J Contin Educ Nurs 25(6):272, 1994.

Maynard, C: Relationship of critical thinking ability to professional nursing competence. J Nurs Educ 35(1):13, 1996.

Morton, PG: Health Assessment in Nursing, ed 2. FA Davis, Philadelphia, 1993.

Rane-Szostak, D, and Fisher Robertson, J: Issues in measuring critical thinking: Meeting the challenge. J Nurs Educ 35(1):5, 1996.

Rubenfeld, MG, and Scheffer, BK: Critical Thinking in Nursing: An Interactive Approach. JB Lippincott, Philadelphia, 1995.

Cultural Influences on Nursing Care

Larry Purnell

Learning Objectives

Upon completion of this chapter, the student will be able to:

1. Define basic terms and concepts common to culture and ethnicity.
2. Identify his or her cultural characteristics, values, beliefs, and practices.
3. Discuss attributes of culturally diverse clients and their families as they influence nursing care.
4. Collect data from culturally diverse clients and their families.
5. Provide a holistic approach to client care according to cultural characteristics and attributes.

Key Words

beliefs (bee-**LEEFS**)
culture (**KUL**-chur)
cultural (**KUL**-chur-uhl)
cultural awareness (**KUL**-chur-uhl a-**WARE**-ness)
cultural competence (**KUL**-chur-uhl **KOM**-pe-tens)
cultural diversity (**KUL**-chur-uhl di-**VER**-si-tee)
cultural sensitivity (**KUL**-chur-uhl SEN-si-**TIV**-i-tee)
customs (**KUS**-tums)
ethnic (**ETH**-nick)
ethnocentrism (ETH-noh-**SEN**-trizm)
generalizations (JEN-er-al-i-**ZAY**-shuns)
stereotype (**STER**-ee-oh-TIGHP)
traditions (tra-**DISH**-uns)
values (**VAL**-use)
worldview (**WERLD**-vyoo)

Cultural diversity in the United States is increasing. As a result, **cultural** and **ethnic** differences between nurses and their clients are becoming more evident and must be recognized. Thus there is a need for nurses to become knowledgeable about cultures other than their own. This chapter provides the student with the basics of culture and its impact on health promotion and wellness.

Culture Defined

Culture refers to the socially transmitted behavior patterns, arts, **beliefs, values, customs,** and all other characteristics of people that guide their **worldview.**

Cultural beliefs, values, customs, and **traditions** are primarily learned within the family on an unconscious level. They are also learned from the community in which one lives, in religious organizations, and in schools. All individuals and groups have the right to maintain their cultural practices as they deem appropriate. Because culture has powerful influences on a client's interpretation of health and responses to nursing care, valuing diversity in nursing practice enhances the delivery and effectiveness of care (Fig. 3–1). As nurses accumulate knowledge about specific ethnic and cultural groups, they are challenged to look at the differences and similarities across cultures.

The terms **cultural sensitivity, cultural awareness,** and **cultural competence** are different. Cultural sensitivity is knowing politically correct language and not making statements that may be offensive to another person's cultural beliefs. Cultural awareness focuses on history and ancestry and emphasizes an appreciation and attention for arts, music, crafts, celebrations, foods, and traditional clothing. Cultural competence includes the skills and knowledge required to provide nursing care and has at least four components. The first component is having an awareness of one's own culture and not letting it have an undue influence on the client. The second is having specific knowledge about the client's culture. The third is accepting and respecting cultural differences. The fourth is adapting nursing care to the client's culture.

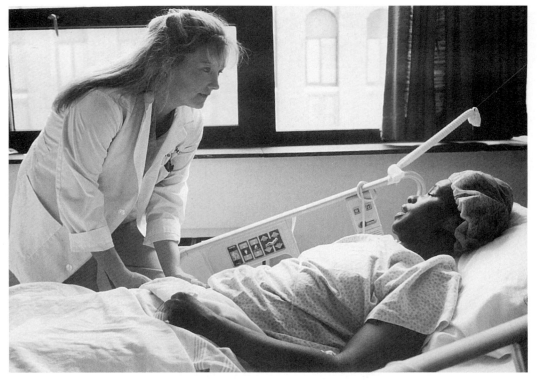

Figure 3–1. The nurse must assess clients' special needs related to their cultural backgrounds.

Even though one may have knowledge about another culture, **ethnocentrism** may still pervade one's attitudes and behavior. Ethnocentrism is the universal tendency for human beings to think that their ways of thinking, acting, and believing are the only right, proper, and natural ways. Ethnocentrism perpetrates an attitude that beliefs that differ greatly are strange or bizarre and therefore wrong. Ethnocentrism can be a major barrier to providing culturally competent care. Additionally, the nurse must be careful not to **stereotype** a client. A stereotype is an opinion or belief ascribed to an individual. For example, the statement "all Chinese people prefer traditional Chinese medicine" is a stereotype. This stereotype is not true. Although most Chinese people may prefer traditional Chinese medicine for some health conditions, not all Chinese people prefer traditional Chinese medicine. Some Chinese people prefer the Western medicine that is practiced in the United States.

However, one can still make **generalizations** about an ethnic individual without stereotyping. Whereas a generalization, an assumption, may be true for the group, it does not necessarily fit the individual. Therefore the nurse must seek additional information to determine whether the generalization fits the individual. The challenge for the nurse is to understand the client's cultural perspective. Nurses who have specific cultural knowledge improve therapeutic interventions by becoming co-participants with clients and their families. To do this, the nurse must develop a personal, open style of communication and be receptive to learning from multicultural clients.

Characteristics of Diversity

Primary and secondary characteristics of diversity affect how people view their culture. The primary characteristics of diversity include nationality, race, color, gender, age, and religious affiliation. Secondary characteristics include socioeconomic status, education, occupation, military experience, political beliefs, length of time away from the country of origin, urban versus rural residence, marital status, parental status, physical characteristics, sexual orientation, and gender issues.

CULTURAL GROUPS IN THE UNITED STATES

This chapter describes selected attributes of some of the cultural groups in the United States. These groups are European-Americans, Native-Americans, African-Ameri-

---

CULTURAL SELF-ASSESSMENT EXERCISE

• Identify your primary and secondary cultural characteristics. How do they affect your worldview?

• Share these views with others in your class.

ETHICAL CONSIDERATIONS BOX 3-1

Facing Cultural Diversity in Nursing

When dealing with patients from cultural backgrounds that are different, nurses sometimes try to impose their own values and standards in situations that they do not fully understand. The following is an example of that tendency.

A woman of Iranian cultural background delivered a stillborn baby. After the delivery, she was transferred to the medical-surgical unit for postpartum care, a practice commonly followed when stillbirths occur. Sharon, an experienced licensed practical nurse (LPN), was assigned to care for this patient. While reading through her chart, Sharon noticed that the woman's husband refused to let his wife see the baby. The chart also contained a photograph of the dead baby, an ultrasound picture, and the footprints and handprints that had been taken after the birth.

As expected, the woman was very depressed, and Sharon felt a great deal of sympathy for her. While caring for this lady, Sharon mentioned that there was a photograph and other mementos of the child and asked if she would like to see them. The woman's husband, who was visiting at the time, called Sharon out of the room and indicated very strongly his displeasure at letting his wife know that these pictures existed without first asking him. He expressed his desire to see them, but refused to let his wife see them. He also admonished Sharon to stop talking with his wife, and emphasized the fact that Sharon had no understanding at all of their culture.

Sharon completed the shift without additional communication with the woman, who was discharged before Sharon returned the next day for her shift. Sharon was plagued by a feeling that she had made a major error in caring for this woman and had failed to meet the client's emotional needs.

It becomes evident from this story that the American conception of what composes the ideal marital relationship is not the same for the Iranian culture. It would be easy to judge the husband as a domineering chauvinist who had no feelings for his wife's distress or emotions. But instead of judging, nurses must respect each patient's cultural origins and be sensitive to their differences. Obviously, the woman's role in the Iranian culture is much different from that in the American culture. Connecting with the family's culture and strengths increases the nurse's ability to communicate and help that family.

GERONTOLOGICAL ISSUES BOX 3-2

Aging, Ethnicity, Health, and Illness

In the United States, ethnic minority elders have serious health and well-being issues. Compared with white or European-American elders, ethnic minority elders are more likely to

Live in poverty.

Have a shorter life expectancy.

Experience debilitating disease processes or functional disability at a higher rate and at an earlier age.

Have difficulty accessing health care services.

Remember that older adults need to be assessed within their personal cultural context. Avoid generalizing cultural practices to individuals or families without first assessing whether this practice or belief is true for them. For example, it would be wrong to assume that an older Mexican-American woman who lives with her extended family will get the family's support for assistance with bathing and other activities of daily living. If an older Chinese woman uses herbs and folk treatments for common complaints, it does not mean that she will not use the services, treatments, or medications of Western medicine.

and ethnic biological variations, susceptibility to disease, and genetic diseases are covered elsewhere in this textbook. (See Ethical Considerations Box 3–1 and Gerontological Issues Box 3–2.)

CULTURAL SELF-ASSESSMENT EXERCISE

Whether we realize it or not, everyone has a cultural or ethnic background. This exercise is to help identify your personal beliefs and values, which are largely passed on to you through your family.

- How do you identify yourself in terms of racial, cultural, or ethnic background? From what country did your ancestors originate? Were your parents from the same or similar ethnic backgrounds?
- What stories do you remember that your parents, grandparents, or other relatives told about relocating in the United States? Do you know why they originally came to America?
- How do these stories compare with those of others from similar backgrounds?
- How do these stories compare with those of others from different backgrounds?

Remember, one's values and beliefs are not better than another's—they are just different.

cans, Hispanic-Americans, Asian/Pacific Islander–Americans, Arab-Americans, and Appalachians. Attributes presented for each group include communication styles, family organization, nutrition practices, death and dying issues, health care beliefs, and traditional health care practitioners. Traditional health care practitioners are those practitioners from the client's native culture such as shamans, herbalists, and other traditional healers. Racial

Communication Styles

Communication styles include verbal and nonverbal variations. Verbal communication includes spoken language, dialects, and voice volume. Dialects are variations in grammar, word meanings, and pronunciation of spoken language. Nonverbal communication includes the use and degree of eye contact, the perception of time, and physical closeness when talking with peers and perceived superiors.

In some societies, people are expected to maintain eye contact without staring, which denotes that they are listening and can be trusted. However, in other societies, as a sign of respect, people should not maintain eye contact with superiors such as teachers and those in positions of higher status.

The perception of time has two dimensions. The first dimension is related to clock versus social time. For example, some cultures have a flexible orientation to time and events, and appointments take place when the person arrives. An event scheduled for 2 P.M. may not begin until 2:30 or when a majority of the people arrive. For others, time is less flexible, and appointments and social events are expected to start at the agreed-on time. For many, social events may be flexible, whereas medical appointments and business engagements start on time.

The second dimension of time relates to whether the culture is predominantly concerned with the past, present, or future. Past-oriented individuals maintain traditions that were meaningful in the past and may worship ancestors. Present-oriented people accept the day as it comes with little regard for the past; the future is unpredictable. Future-oriented people anticipate a bigger and better future and place a high value on change. However, some individuals balance all three views—they respect the past, enjoy living in the present, and plan for the future.

NURSING ASSESSMENT AND STRATEGIES

Ask the following questions:

- By what name do you prefer to be called?
- What language do you speak at home?
- Are you normally on time for appointments?

Be sure to do the following:

- Take cues from the client for voice volume.
- Be an active listener, and become comfortable with silence.
- Avoid appearing rushed.
- Take greeting cues from the client.
- Speak slowly and clearly. Do not speak loudly or with exaggerated mouthing.
- Explain why you are asking specific questions.
- Give reasons for treatments.
- Repeat questions if necessary.
- Provide written instructions in the client's preferred language.
- Obtain an interpreter if necessary.

CULTURAL SELF-ENRICHMENT EXERCISE

- How many languages do you speak? Do you speak a dialect of your dominant language? Does it interfere with communication with your clients?
- Do you speak in a soft, medium, or loud tone of voice? Does this tone change in different situations? How close do you stand when you speak with close friends? Does this distance change when you converse with your teacher, your religious leader, or a politician?
- Identify characteristics from your worldview in terms of being present, past, and future oriented.
- By what name do you prefer to be called? Why? Does this change in different situations?

Family Organization

Family organization includes the perceived head of the household, gender roles, and roles of the elderly and extended family members. The head of the household may be patriarchal (male dominated), matriarchal (female dominated), or egalitarian (shared equally between men and women). An awareness of the family dominance pattern is important for determining which family member to speak with when health care decisions have to be made.

In some cultures, specific roles are outlined for men and women. Men are expected to protect and provide for the family, manage finances, and deal with the outside world. Women are expected to maintain the home environment, including child care and household tasks. The nurse must accept that not all societies share or even desire an egalitarian family structure.[1]

Roles for the elderly and extended family vary among culturally diverse groups. In some cultures, the elderly are seen as being wise, are deferred to for decision making, and are held in high esteem. Their children are expected to provide for them when they are no longer able to care for themselves. In other cultures, although the elderly may be loved by family members, they may not be given such high regard and may be cared for outside the home when self-care becomes a concern.

The extended family is very important in some groups, and a single household may include several generations living together out of desire rather than out of necessity. The extended family may include both blood-related and non-blood-related individuals who are provided with family status. For others, each generation lives separately and has its own living space.

CULTURAL SELF-ENRICHMENT EXERCISE

- Who is considered the head of the household in your family?
- Are there specified gender roles for family members?
- What are the roles of the elderly in your family?
- Do you identify with an extended family? Are they all blood relatives? What roles do they play?

NUTRITION NOTES BOX 3–3

Nutritional Considerations Related to Culture

Sometimes native eating patterns are better than modern ones. Adopting the dominant culture's dietary practices has been implicated in declining health of native populations or less healthful practices among immigrants. Examples include nursing bottle dental caries among Native-Americans; non-insulin-dependent diabetes mellitus among Native-Americans, Hawaiians, and native populations of Canada and Australia; and lower rates of breast feeding among Hispanic-American immigrants.

Foods that often are restricted by various groups include the following:

Pork by Orthodox Jews, Muslims, Hindus, and Seventh-Day Adventists

All meat by Buddhists

Coffee and tea by Muslims and Seventh-Day Adventists

Alcohol by Muslims, Seventh-Day Adventists, and some Catholics

Groups that seldom consume milk include Hispanics, Italians, and Asians, possibly because of a high incidence of lactose intolerance. Some Seventh-Day Adventists also restrict milk consumption.

Orthodox Jews may keep separate dishes and utensils for meat and dairy meals. To be kosher, certain meats must be obtained from ritually slaughtered animals and must be prepared in specific ways.

Although modern health care may be mysterious to many clients, they are experts in their own food preferences. Providing familiar meals is comforting to the client and demonstrates caring on the part of the health care provider.

NURSING ASSESSMENT AND STRATEGIES

Ask the following questions:

- Who makes the decisions in your household?
- Who takes care of money matters, does the cooking, is responsible for child care, and so forth?
- Who decides when it is time to see a health care provider?
- Who lives in your household? Are they all blood related?

Be sure to do the following:

- Observe the use of touch between family members.
- Allow family members to decide where they want to stand or sit for comfort.

Nutrition Practices

Nutrition practices include the meaning of food to individuals, food choices and rituals, food taboos, and how food and food substances are used for health promotion and wellness. Cultural beliefs influence what people eat or avoid. Food (1) offers security and acceptance; (2) is necessary as a means of survival and relief from hunger; (3) plays a significant role in socialization; (4) has symbolic meaning for peaceful coexistence; (5) is used to promote healing; (6) denotes caring, closeness, and kinship; and (7) may be used as an expression of love or anger.[2]

Culturally congruent dietary counseling such as changing amounts and preparation practices and including ethnic food choices can reduce health risks. Whenever possible, the nurse should determine a client's dietary practices during the intake interview. Culturally diverse clients may refuse to eat on a schedule of American mealtimes or eat American foods. Counseling about food group requirements, intake restrictions, and exercise that respects cultural behaviors is essential.

Most cultures have their own nutritional practices for health promotion and disease prevention. For many, a balance of different types of foods is important for maintaining health and preventing illness. Common folk practices recommend specific foods during illness and for prevention of illness or disease. Therefore a thorough history and assessment of dietary practices can be an important diagnostic tool to guide health promotion. (See Nutrition Notes Box 3–3.)

CULTURAL SELF-ENRICHMENT EXERCISE

- What is the meaning of food in your culture?
- Are there any dietary deficiencies or limitations in food for you?
- What cultural or ethnic foods do you prepare at home?
- When you eat out for lunch or dinner, what are your favorite ethnic foods? Which ethnic foods do you not like? Why?
- What are some of the dietary practices you engage in when you are ill?
- What kinds of foods do you eat to stay healthy?
- Are there any taboo or restricted foods in your culture or personal belief system?

NURSING ASSESSMENT AND STRATEGIES

Ask the following questions:

- What do you eat to stay healthy?
- What do you eat when you are ill?
- Are there certain foods that you do not eat? Why?
- Do certain foods cause you to become ill?
- Who prepares the food in your household?
- Who purchases the food in your household?

Death and Dying Issues

Death rituals of cultural groups are the least likely to change over time. To avoid cultural taboos, nurses must become knowledgeable about rituals surrounding death and bereavement. For some, the body should be buried whole. Thus an amputated limb may be buried in a future grave site. Cremation may be preferred for some, whereas for others it is taboo and burial is the preferred practice. Views toward autopsy vary accordingly. Some cultural groups have elaborate ceremonies that last for days in commemoration of the dead. To some individuals these rituals look like a celebration, and in a sense they are—a celebration of the person's life rather than a mourning of the person's death.

The expression of grief in response to death varies within and among cultural and ethnic groups. For example, in some cultures, loved ones are expected to suffer the grief of death in silence with little display of emotion. In other cultures, loved ones are expected to demonstrate an elaborate display of emotions to show that they cared for the individual. These variations in the grieving process may cause confusion for nurses who perceive some individuals as overreacting and others as not caring. The nurse must accept culturally diverse behaviors associated with the grieving process. Bereavement support strategies include (1) being physically present, (2) encouraging reality orientation, (3) openly acknowledging the family's right to grieve, (4) assisting the family to express their feelings, (5) encouraging interpersonal relationships, (6) promoting interest in a new life, and (7) making referrals to other staff and clergy as appropriate.

NURSING ASSESSMENT AND STRATEGIES

Ask the following questions:

- What are the usual burial practices in your family?
- Do you believe in autopsy?

Be sure to do the following:

- Observe expressions of grief. Support the family in their expression of grief.
- Observe for differences in the expression of grief among family members.
- Offer to obtain a religious counselor if the family wishes.

CULTURAL SELF-ENRICHMENT EXERCISE

- What are the usual burial practices in your family?
- What is expected of family members and friends after a loved one dies?
- How is grief expressed in your family? Are there different expectations for men and women?
- Are any specific rituals associated with death?

Health Care Beliefs

The focus of health care includes prevention versus acute care practices and traditional, religious, and biomedical beliefs. Additionally, individual responsibility for health, self-medicating practices, views toward mental illness, and the client's response to pain and the sick role are shaped by one's culture.

Most societies combine biomedical health care with traditional, folk, and religious practices, such as praying for good health and wearing amulets to ward off diseases and illnesses. The health care system abounds with individual and family folklore practices for curing or treating specific illnesses. Many times folk therapies are handed down from family members and may have their roots in religious beliefs. Examples of folk medicines include covering a boil with axle grease, wearing copper bracelets for arthritic pain, mixing wild turnip root and honey for a sore throat, and drinking herbal teas. As an adjunct to biomedical treatments, many people use complementary therapies such as acupressure, acumassage, reflexology, and other traditional therapies specific to the cultural group.

Often, folk practices are not harmful and should be incorporated into the client's plan of care. However, some may conflict with prescription medications, intensify the treatment regimen, or cause an overdose. It is essential to inquire about the full range of therapies being used, such as food items, teas, herbal remedies, nonfood substances, over-the-counter medications, medications prescribed by others, and medications borrowed from others. If clients perceive that the nurse does not accept their beliefs and practices, they may be less compliant with prescriptive treatment.

Mental illness may be seen by many as not being as important as physical illness. Mental illness is culture bound, and what may be perceived as a mental illness in one society may not be considered a mental illness in another society. Among some cultures, having a mental illness or an emotional difficulty is considered a disgrace and is taboo. As a result, the family is likely to keep the mentally ill or handicapped person at home as long as possible.[3]

CULTURAL SELF-ENRICHMENT EXERCISE

- How do you define health for yourself?
- How do you define illness for yourself?
- Identify preventive health care practices that you use.
- When you see a health care provider for a minor illness, what do you expect the health care provider to do for you?
- Identify your self-medicating behaviors.
- What home remedies do you use when you are ill?
- What meaning does pain have to you? What measures do you use when you are in pain?
- What are your personal views toward autopsy, organ donation, organ transplantation, and receiving blood or blood products?

Cultural responses to pain and the sick role vary among cultures. For example, some individuals are expected to openly express their pain. Others are expected to suffer their pain in silence. For some, the sick role is readily accepted, and any excuse is accepted for not fulfilling one's daily obligations. Others minimize their illness and make extended efforts to fulfill their obligations.

NURSING ASSESSMENT AND STRATEGIES

Ask the following questions:

- What do you usually do to maintain your health?
- What do you usually do when you are sick?
- What kind of home treatments do you use when you are sick?
- Who is the first person you see when you are sick?
- What do you do when you have pain?
- Do you wear charms or bracelets to ward off illness?
- Do you take herbs or drink special teas when you are sick?
- Do you recite special prayers to maintain your health?

Health Care Practitioners

Health care practitioners include the client's perceived status and use of traditional, religious, and biomedical health care providers. Individual perceptions of selected practitioners may be closely associated with previous contact and experiences with health care providers. In Western societies, educated health care providers are treated with great respect (Fig. 3-2). However, some people prefer tra-

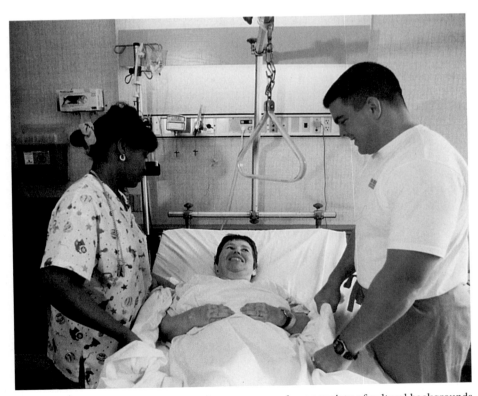

Figure 3–2. Clients and health care workers may come from a variety of cultural backgrounds.

CULTURAL SELF-ENRICHMENT EXERCISE

- What complementary health care practitioners have you used? Were they successful?
- Identify complementary health care practitioners used by your friends. Were they successful?
- When you are ill and need to see a health care provider, do you prefer a same-gender provider? Why or why not?

---

ditional healers because they are known to the individual, family, and community.[4]

Because some clients may be especially modest, the nurse should respect differences in gender relationships when providing care. Some people, because of their religion, may be especially modest, seeking out same-gender nurses and physicians for intimate care. Nurses need to respect these clients' modesty by providing privacy and assigning a same-gender care provider when possible.

NURSING ASSESSMENT AND STRATEGIES

Ask the following questions:

- Do you see any health care providers besides physicians and nurses when you are ill?
- Do you object to male or female health care providers giving physical care to you?

Be sure to do the following:

- Observe for alternative care providers who may visit the client in the health care facility.

Ethnic and Cultural Groups

NATIVE-AMERICANS

There are more than 400 Native-American and Alaskan Eskimo tribes in the United States, with a population of 257,906.[5] Although there are similarities among Native-Americans, each tribe has its own unique perspective on health and illness. Many traditional Native-Americans live on reservations; others live in urban areas and practice few of their traditions. Many Native-Americans have a strong belief that illness is caused by an imbalance with nature and the universe. Tribal identity is maintained through powwows, ceremonial events, and arts and crafts that are taught to children at a young age. Communicating with nature is important for maintaining life forces.[6] Native-Americans are the original inhabitants of North America.

Native-Americans are underrepresented in all the health professions. They are consistently identified as the most underrepresented minority group in institutions of higher

learning.[7] See Cultural Considerations Box 3–4 for cultural attributes of Native-Americans.

EUROPEAN-AMERICANS

European-American is the term used to describe people living in the United States whose heritage is from the countries of England, Scotland, Wales, Ireland, Norway, Switzerland, Sweden, the Netherlands, and other northern European countries. European-American groups include the white ethnic groups. Many of the descendants of these original European immigrants practice the unique attributes of the subcultures from which they originate. There is much diversity in this cultural group according to the primary and secondary characteristics of diversity.

Many European-Americans maintain the value of individualism, which is paramount over group norms, and are activity oriented. Most European-Americans practice Western medicine that uses high technology and scientific discovery.[4] See the Cultural Considerations box for common cultural attributes of European-Americans.

AFRICAN-AMERICANS

African-Americans are the largest ethnic group in the United States and represent more than 100 racial strains.[8] They make up 12 percent of the population and number over 29,000,000. Although African-Americans live in all 50 states, more than half live in the South. It is important to understand that not all people with black skin identify themselves as African-American. Many black-skinned people from the Caribbean prefer terms more personal to their identity, such as Haitian, Jamaican, or West Indian.

African-Americans have been called by many names. Their ancient African name is *Nehesu* or *Nubian.* During slavery days in America, they were called *Negro,* a Spanish-Portuguese word meaning black. After emancipation in 1863, they were called *colored,* a term adopted by the First Colored Men's Convention in the United States in 1831. The United States Bureau of the Census adopted the word *Negro* in 1880. During the Civil Rights movements in the 1960s, the term *black* was used to signify a philosophy of life instead of color. In the 1970s these ethnic peoples referred to themselves as African-Americans because they were proud of both their African and American heritages. In 1988 the term *African-American* was widely adopted in the United States by individuals whose ancestry originated from Africa. These terms continue to cause confusion when people attempt to use the "politically correct" term for this group in the United States. Some individuals prefer terms more appropriate to their individual heritage instead of the term *African-American.* Additionally, one still sees titles such as the National Black Nurses Association and the National Association for the Advancement of Colored People.[8]

text continues on page 47

CULTURAL CONSIDERATIONS BOX 3-4

Cultural Group	Communication Styles	Family Organization	Nutrition
Native-Americans	Each tribe has its own language. Many speak English, Spanish, or both. Talking loudly may be considered rude. Touch is not acceptable from strangers. Pointing with the finger may be considered rude. Direct eye contact may be considered rude, even with friends. Appointments may not be kept. Most are present oriented.	Most tribes are matriarchal, but some are egalitarian. Gender roles are usually flexible. Elderly are highly respected. Family bonds are strong. Extended family members are very important.	Herbs are used to cleanse the body of evil spirits and poison. Nontraditional diets tend to be high in fat. Diet commonly lacks fruits and vegetables on reservations.
European-Americans	Primary language is English. Dialects vary by region of the country but are mutually understandable. May also speak language of native country. Loud voice tone is the norm. Maintain eye contact without staring. Value change, are future oriented, and emphasize accomplishments. Punctual in social and business situations. Many concerned with status. Touch infrequently.	Goal is egalitarian family relationships, but some are nominally patriarchal or matriarchal. Goal is gender role flexibility. Impersonal relationships with outsiders. Elderly are loved but may not be respected for wisdom or sought for advice. Extended family not usually important on a daily basis. Stress individualism over the group.	Diets tend to be high in fat and sodium. The only group that uses the food pyramid. Believe a balanced diet promotes a healthy body. Eating and drinking may be social rituals.
African-Americans	Primary language is English. Many speak "Black English" some, depending on the situation. Usually loud voice volume. Punctuality is flexible. Many present oriented, believe there is little control over their destiny. Place emphasis on nonverbal behaviors. Direct eye contact may be interpreted as aggression.	Usually matriarchal or egalitarian household. Flexible gender roles. Augmented families with non–blood relatives sharing space. Group goals more important than individual goals. Strong family ties. Extended family assists in crisis. Elderly respected, especially maternal grandmothers.	Diet commonly high in fat and sodium. Many have a lactose intolerance. Food selections may vary according to socioeconomic class and rural versus urban residence. Being overweight is seen as positive. Food is a symbol of health and wealth.

continued

CULTURAL CONSIDERATIONS BOX 3–4 *(continued)*

Cultural Group	Communication Styles	Family Organization	Nutrition
	Are comfortable with close personal space. Touch frequently with friends, less so with strangers.	Church commonly plays a central role, and church members may be seen as family.	
Hispanic-Americans	Primary language either English or Spanish. Numerous Spanish dialects, which are regionally specific and may not be mutually understandable. Present oriented, cannot control destiny. Flexible with time and appointments. Some believe that direct eye contact can cause illness ("evil eye"). Touch with close same-gender friends but not with opposite-gender friends or strangers.	Usually patriarchal households with women taking a more active role in health care decisions. Usually strict gender roles. Children are highly valued and taken everywhere, rarely left with babysitters. Elderly are highly respected. Extended family members, including godparents, are important.	Important for food to be served warm—not too hot or too cold. Many subscribe to the hot-and-cold theory, the concept that illness is caused when the body is exposed to an imbalance of hot and cold substances. Foods are classified as hot and cold, and their consumption must be balanced or illness will occur. Food choices vary by country of origin. Many adults have a lactose intolerance.
Asian-Americans	Language specific to each country. Many dialects, with 55 in China alone. Loud talking is considered rude. Much communication is nonverbal. May be reluctant to maintain eye contact with elders or superiors. Touch acceptable only between members of the same gender. Present oriented. Flexible with social engagements, punctual in business appointments. "Yes" may not mean "I agree" or "I understand." It may mean "I hear you." Reluctant to disclose personal information.	Patriarchal households. Gender roles are well defined. Children are extremely important. Elderly are seen as wise and are respected. A child's bad behavior is reflected on the entire family. Multigenerational and extended family important and may share the same living space. Responsibility of the family is to care for elderly, handicapped, and mentally ill at home. Group takes priority over the individual.	Foods are balanced between the yin and yang. Foods are used for health maintenance and treatment of illness. Diet is high in salt. Many have a lactose intolerance. Food is a fundamental form of socialization. Food choices and preparation vary by specific country.

continued

CULTURAL CONSIDERATIONS BOX 3–4 *(continued)*

Cultural Group	Communication Styles	Family Organization	Nutrition
Arab-Americans	Primary language is Arabic. Most speak some English. Exaggerated, spirited, and loud voice. May be reluctant to disclose personal information. Maintain intense eye contact. Stand very close when talking. Touch only between the same gender. Flexible time schedules socially and for appointments. Present to future oriented according to socioeconomic status.	Patriarchal household. Well-defined gender roles. Overly protective of children. Physical punishment is common. Loyalty to family over self. Elders are respected. Family obligated to care for elders. Extended family members important, freely offer advice. Extended family live in close proximity.	Food is a symbol of love, friendship, and generosity. Food preparation takes a long time; only fresh meats and vegetables are used when possible. Lunch is the main meal. Some do not eat pork or drink alcohol (Islam). Fast to cure disease. Believe in the hot-and-cold theory of foods. Many fast from sunrise to sunset during the holy month of Ramadan.
Appalachians	English language spoken with dialectal variations—"ing" endings become "in," some plurals formed by adding "es" instead of "s" (e.g., "Breastes"). Individualism and self-reliance idealized. May deny anger and do not complain. Direct eye contact from strangers may be perceived as aggression or hostility. Comfortable with silence. Relaxed, enjoying body rhythms instead of strong adherence to clock time.	Traditional home was patriarchal but is currently changing to egalitarian. Women are providers of emotional strength. Women marry earlier than in many other cultures. Have larger families than the rest of the white American groups. Most believe in physical punishment as a form of discipline. Elders are respected. Usually care for elderly in the home.	Wealth means having plenty of food. High-cholesterol organ meats are commonly used. Use lard for frying and baking. Diet commonly deficient in iron, calcium, and vitamin A.

Cultural Attributes

Cultural Group	Death and Dying Issues	Health Care Beliefs	Health Care Practitioners
Native-Americans	Body should go into the afterlife whole. Some engage in a cleansing ceremony after touching a dead body.	Many practice acute care only. Use herbs, corn, dances, and prayers to cure and balance life forces with nature.	Traditional healers include shamans, singers, diviners, crystal gazers, hand tremblers. Elderly may request same-gender direct care provider.

continued

CULTURAL CONSIDERATIONS BOX 3–4 *(continued)*

Cultural Group	Death and Dying Issues	Health Care Beliefs	Health Care Practitioners
	Home has to be cleaned if person dies at home. Taboo to talk directly about death or a grave diagnosis. Open expression of grief. Tribal laws may dictate cremation versus burial.	Combine Western medicine with traditional practices. Have a fear of witchcraft. Inanimate objects are believed to ward off evil. Theology and medicine are interwoven. Promote harmony with nature. Pain is something to be endured. Sick role is not usually supported.	
European-Americans	Autopsy and burial or cremation usually connected with religious practices or are individual decisions. Varied expression of grief. Men are expected to be in more control of grief than women.	Believe humans can control nature. Strong belief and value in technology. Primary acute care practices, but recent trend is moving toward prevention. Value individual responsibility for health. May use folk remedies or over-the-counter medicines before seeing a health care practitioner. Use prayers and religious symbols for good health. Controlled expression of pain. Need little encouragement for pain relief. Sick role not well accepted unless a major illness.	Primarily use Western-educated health care providers. Recent trend is to use complementary therapists, such as chiropractors, reflexologists, and acumassage. Most accept physical care from either gender.
African-Americans	Death does not end connection between people. Body is kept intact after death; prefer no autopsy. Relatives may communicate with the dead person. Eulogy at burial with religious songs. Usually burial, rarely cremation. Express grief openly with emotional catharsis.	Diseases may be natural, caused by cold or bad air, food, or water. Diseases may be unnatural, caused by voodoo, witchcraft, or a hex. Serious illness may be sent from God. May resist preventive care because illness is God's will.	A respected elderly female community member commonly sought for initial health care. Spiritualists who receive their gift from God. Voodoo priest or priestess. Root doctor uses herbs, oils, candles, and ointments.

continued

CULTURAL CONSIDERATIONS BOX 3-4 (continued)

Cultural Group	Death and Dying Issues	Health Care Beliefs	Health Care Practitioners
		Folk medicine prevalent with herbs.	
		Use prayers for prevention and health recovery.	
		Pain is seen as a sign of illness.	
		Sick role not seen as a burden.	
Hispanic-Americans	Burial is the usual practice, rarely cremation.	Health beliefs strongly affected by religion.	Santero in Cuba practices Santeria, a religion with animal sacrifice and worship of many gods.
	May resist autopsy; body should be buried whole.	Health and illness largely God's will.	Curandero uses herbs.
	May have elaborate ceremonial burial.	May have shrines or statues in the home to pray for good health.	Espirituista uses prayers and amulets.
	Women very expressive with grief; men are expected to maintain control of their grief.	Frequent use of over-the-counter medicines and medicines brought from home country.	Sobador manipulates muscles and performs massage.
		Theory of hot and cold foods used for health maintenance and treatment of disease.	High degree of modesty, so may prefer same-gender provider for intimate care.
		Many are fearful and suspicious of hospitals.	
		Expressive with pain.	
		Easy to enter the sick role.	
		Primarily acute care practice with little prevention.	
		Children and women are more susceptible to the evil eye.	
Asian-Americans	Autopsy not understood by many.	Good health is a gift from ancestors.	Acupuncturist uses needle insertions at specific points to control pain.
	Cremation acceptable, but burial is also common depending on the specific population.	Imbalances in the yin and yang cause illness.	Acumassage: deep tissue and muscle massage.
	Extended grieving time (7 to 30 days) for the more traditional.	Believe blood is the source of life and is not replenished.	Moxibustion therapy uses heat instead of needles or massage.
	Expression of grief is highly varied between men and women and among specific countries.	Amulets are worn to ward off disease.	Coining: heated coin is rubbed over body surfaces, causing dermabrasion.
		Cleanliness is highly valued.	
		Prayers are used for healing.	

continued

CULTURAL CONSIDERATIONS BOX 3-4 (continued)

Cultural Group	Death and Dying Issues	Health Care Beliefs	Health Care Practitioners
		Over-the-counter medicine use is common.	Cupping: heated cups are applied over the body, which causes suction, leaving large ecchymotic areas.
		Use of herbal teas and medicine is common.	
		Commonly stoical with pain.	
		Many delay seeking help until very ill.	
Arab-Americans	Death is God's will.	Acute care primarily with little prevention.	Accept and prefer Western practitioners.
	At the time of death the bed should face the holy city of Mecca.	Little responsibility for self-care.	May use cupping and phlebotomy.
	Ritual washing of the body after death.	Pray five times each day for health.	Primarily same-gender care only, especially among elderly.
	No cremation or autopsy.	Combine prayers with meditation.	
	May weep with grief, but limited.	Freely use over-the-counter medication.	
		Illness is a punishment for sins.	
		Considered rude and cruel to communicate a grave diagnosis.	
		Organs may be purchased for transplantation.	
		Overt expression of pain.	
		Sick dependency role readily accepted.	
		Injections preferred over pills.	
		Able to enter the sick role easily.	
Appalachians	Funerals are plain and an important social function.	Prayer is a primary source of strength.	Physicians are commonly seen as outsiders.
	Family and friends remain at bedside when a death is expected.	Good health is largely a result of God's will.	Family folk practitioners used as a primary source of health care.
	Deceased usually buried in his or her best clothes.	Biomedical care may be used as a last resort.	Nurses are highly respected in the culture.
	Elaborate meals are served after the funeral.	Many folk remedies, primarily passed on by "granny" practitioners who use poultices, herbs, and teas.	Practitioner must ask the client what he or she thinks is the problem to be effective.
	Funeral services are accompanied by singing.	Self-medicate first before seeking a biomedical practitioner.	
	Clergy are good at helping family through the grieving process.	A major health concern is the state of the blood.	

African-Americans are underrepresented in colleges and universities, managerial and administrative positions, and the health care professions. They are overrepresented in high-risk, hazardous occupations such as the steel and tire industry, construction industries, and high-pollution factories. See Cultural Considerations Box 3–4 for cultural attributes of African-Americans.

HISPANIC-AMERICANS

The term *Hispanic* is used to describe people whose cultural heritage has a strong Spanish influence. Other names Hispanics use to identify themselves include *Latino, Chicano,* and terms that provide a country of origin such as *Mexican, Peruvian, Puerto Rican,* and *Cuban.*[9] The largest Hispanic populations in the United States are Mexican-Americans (64%), Puerto Ricans (11%), Central Americans (7%), South Americans (7%), Cubans (4%), Caribbean (3%), and other (4%). Additionally, Hispanics come from Venezuela, Colombia, Ecuador, Peru, Bolivia, Paraguay, Chile, Argentina, Uruguay, Dominican Republic, Guatemala, El Salvador, Costa Rica, Honduras, Nicaragua, and Panama. Thus there is much diversity in the Hispanic population in the United States.[10]

Some Hispanics speak only Spanish, some speak only English, some speak both Spanish and English, and some speak neither Spanish nor English but rather an Indian dialect, depending on individual circumstances and the length of time in the United States. Spanish is the second most common spoken language in the United States.

Hispanics total 27,000,000 and live in all 50 states. More than 90 percent live in cities. Four out of every five Hispanics are born and raised in the United States and are expected to become the largest ethnic group in the United States by the year 2000, with over 31,000,000.[10]

The majority of Hispanics practice adaptations from the Roman Catholic religion. Their close relationship with God makes it acceptable for people to experience visions and dreams in which God or the saints speak directly to them. Thus one must be careful not to attribute these culture-bound visions to hallucinations that indicate a need for psychiatric services.[9] See Cultural Considerations Box 3–4 for cultural attributes of Hispanics.

ASIAN-AMERICANS

This large group, with over 5,575,000 people, is far from homogeneous. The term *Asian,* as used in most references, includes 32 different groups (Fig. 3–3). These groups include Asians, Pacific Islanders, Indochinese, and other Asian groups. Asians include people from Korea, Japan, and 54 ethnic groups from China. Pacific Islanders include Hawaiians, Polynesians, Filipinos, Malaysians, and Guamanians. Indochinese populations include Cambodian, Vietnamese, Hmong, and Laotian. Other Asian groups include Asian Indian, Pakistani, and Thai.

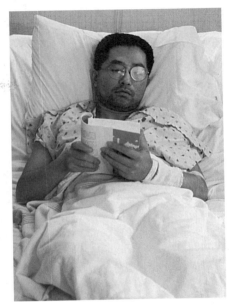

Figure 3–3. This Asian-American passes time reading a book in his native language.

Although it is difficult to determine exact numbers of Asians from specific countries because of the method of keeping population statistics, they are a significant and fast-growing population in the United States. Nurses must realize that it is important for many Asian clients to "save face." Individual shame is shared with the family and community. Most Asians see the nurse as an authority figure. Although known by different names, most Asian cultures practice the yin and yang balance of forces for illness prevention and maintaining health. Yin is considered female and represents cold and weakness. Yang is considered male and represents strength and warmth. Foods and all forces are classified as yin or yang and must be balanced, or illness occurs. Yin and yang forces are major components of traditional Chinese medicine, which includes acupressure, acumassage, cupping, and moxibustion.[11] See Cultural Considerations Box 3–4 for cultural attributes of Asian-Americans.

ARAB-AMERICANS

Arab-Americans are a large and diverse population, with over 3,000,000 in the United States. Some common bonds include the Arabic language and the Islamic religion. Arab-Americans include people from Morocco, Algeria, Tunisia, Libya, Sudan, and Egypt and the western Asian countries of Lebanon, occupied Palestine, Syria, Jordan, Iraq, Iran, Kuwait, Bahrain, Qatar, United Arab Emirates, Saudi Arabia, Oman, and Yemen. Many early Arab immigrants are Christians from Lebanon and Syria.

Although many Arab-Americans favor professional occupations, many are underemployed, have their own businesses, and work in a variety of other occupations. Arab-

Americans, whether born in the United States or in Arab countries, are more educated than the average American.[12,13] They are more likely to be in managerial and professional specialty occupations than any other ethnic group in America.[13] However, a significant number of primarily foreign-born Arab-Americans are unemployed and live in poverty.

APPALACHIANS

The term *Appalachian* is derived from the Apalache Indians, who inhabited what is today known as the Appalachian Mountain region. This chapter uses the term *Appalachian* to describe people born in this region and their descendants. Most Appalachians trace their heritage to Scotland, Wales, Ireland, England, or Germany. This large mountainous region consists of part or all of the states of Georgia, Alabama, Mississippi, Virginia, West Virginia, North Carolina, South Carolina, Kentucky, Tennessee, Ohio, Maryland, Pennsylvania, and New York. Parts of Appalachia have insufficient roads, public transportation systems, and airports, creating a disparity in educational and health care facilities.

Appalachians are loyal, caring, family oriented, religious, hardy, independent, honest, patriotic, and resourceful. They value home, which is a connectedness to the land rather than a physical structure. Additional characteristics ascribed to Appalachians are (1) avoiding aggression and assertiveness, (2) not interfering with others' lives, (3) avoiding dominance over others, and (4) avoiding arguments and seeking agreement. They are private people who want to offend no one and may not easily trust outsiders.[14]

Summary

Rarely do practicing nurses have the luxury to assess each client comprehensively on a first encounter. The essentials for culturally competent interventions are obtained as needed. The client data base can be added to as time permits. Astute observations, an openness to diversity, and a willingness to learn from clients are requirements for effective cross-cultural competence in clinical practice. Through these avenues, nurses can provide culturally competent nursing care. Cultural competence is not a luxury; it is a necessity.

  CRITICAL THINKING: Mr. Bautista

Mustafa Bautista, age 62, and his wife, Mina, age 60, immigrated to the United States three years ago from Saudia Arabia. During a celebration of Ramadan, Mustafa collapsed and was taken to the nearest emergency room. He was admitted to the observation unit for diagnostic testing. He does not speak or understand English well, and when the nurse asks him a question, he stares at her, does elaborate hand gesturing, and speaks in a very loud voice. Mustafa is a devoted adherent of Islam, and his wife brings him the Koran, from which he reads several times each day.

Even though Mustafa is prescribed bed rest, he gets out of bed several times each day, kneels on a small carpet, and prays. He refuses to let the female nurses bathe him. Yesterday, he refused his breakfast and lunch. Today, he refused his dinner, and insisted on keeping the tray at his bedside. At 8:00 P.M., he took the pork chops from his tray and placed them in the hall. Additionally, he refuses his oral medicines and insists on injections instead.

1. What nonverbal communication characteristics does this client display that are common among people of Arabic descent?
2. Does his loud voice mean that he is angry?
3. What might you do when Mr. Bautista gets out of bed to pray?
4. Why do you think Mr. Bautista refused his breakfast and lunch?
5. Why did Mr. Bautista remove the pork chops from his tray and leave them in the hall?
6. What might you do to improve Mr. Bautista's nutrition while he is in the hospital?
7. What is Ramadan?
8. Why does Mr. Bautista insist on injections rather than oral medication?
9. What might you do to get Mr. Bautista to take oral medications rather than injections?

Answers at end of chapter.

Review Questions

1. As the nurse, you are explaining the medication schedule to Mrs. Bing Bing, a 45-year-old Chinese woman with minimal English language skills. Which of the following will best help ensure compliance?
   a. Provide written instructions in English.
   b. Speak slowly and clearly using the same phrase each time.
   c. Speak loudly to make sure she understands you.
   d. Speak slowly and exaggerate the words.

2. A 12-year-old Mexican child needs an appendectomy. Who should sign the informed consent for the operation?
   a. The mother.
   b. The father.
   c. Both parents.
   d. Let the parents decide.

3. Your 42-year-old male Islamic client in a long-term care facility needs to have a urinary catheter inserted to ob-

tain a specimen. Who is the best person to do the procedure?
   a. A female registered nurse
   b. A male nurse
   c. An orderly
   d. The client's wife

4. A 22-year-old Osage Native-American woman is slow at giving responses and does not maintain eye contact with you when you are doing her intake interview. Which of the following interpretations of her behavior is most likely accurate?
   a. Direct eye contact may be interpreted as rude in her culture
   b. She does not want to answer personal questions.
   c. She does not understand you.
   d. She does not want to talk with a nurse and prefers a physician.

5. An 82-year-old African-American woman is in the coronary care unit to rule out a myocardial infarction. Several church members come to visit her on a daily basis. Which of the following actions by the nurse is correct?
   a. Carefully explain to them that only family members are allowed to visit in the coronary care unit.
   b. Allow two church members to visit and have them represent the entire group.
   c. Set up a specific time during which several of them can visit for brief periods.
   d. Report the situation to her physician.

6. A 42-year-old Puerto Rican man has been admitted for reconstructive orthopedic surgery on his knee. His wife brings jars of special blends of spices that he wants to put on his food because the hospital food is too bland. He is on a general diet. You would
   a. Allow him to use them.
   b. Carefully explain that family cannot bring food items to the hospital.
   c. Have the dietitian speak with the family.
   d. Report the situation to the physician.

7. The mother of a 6-year-old Vietnamese child admitted with pneumonia is rubbing a coin on the child's back. The coin leaves red marks. As the nurse caring for this child you would
   a. Not allow the mother to be alone with her child.
   b. Explain to the mother that she cannot do this in the hospital.
   c. Add a statement to the care plan that the family practices coining.
   d. Report the possibility of child abuse.

8. A 72-year-old Arab-American man has just been diagnosed with cancer of the colon. His family does not want him to be told about the diagnosis. You would
   a. Tell him anyway because he has a right to know.
   b. Call a religious counselor.
   c. Insist that his family tell him about his diagnosis.
   d. Respect the family's wishes.

9. Rebecca Lewis, age 35 years, manages a convenience store in a remote mountainous region of Kentucky. It is 35 miles to the closest health clinic, and she does not own an automobile. On this occasion, she accompanies her neighbor, Mary Kapp, to the clinic for her monthly diabetes checkup. You discover that Mrs. Lewis has never had a Papanicolaou test because of lack of time and transportation. She is agreeable to the examination. As the intake clinic nurse, you would
   a. Schedule the test for next month.
   b. Encourage the gynecological clinic to perform the test today.
   c. Give her the telephone number of the clinic and have her make an appointment.
   d. Refer her to the community health nurse practitioner.

10. William O'Donnell, age 66 years, is scheduled for surgery to remove a cyst from his perineum. While you are helping him onto the transport cart, he asks you to go slowly because his arthritis is bothering him today. Because he was NPO (nothing by mouth) for the surgery today, he was not able to take his home-brew medication for his arthritis. Four times a day he takes a tablespoon of a mixture of whiskey, wild honey, and vinegar. You explain to him that
    a. He should stop the home brew because it is dangerous.
    b. This is a very effective treatment and that he should continue it.
    c. He should have seen a physician for his arthritis before now.
    d. He can continue with his home brew, but he should also see the clinic nurse practitioner, who might be able to provide more relief from his arthritis pain.

ANSWERS TO CRITICAL THINKING

Critical Thinking: Mr. Bautista

1. Culture-bound communication patterns that Mr. Bautista displays include speaking in a loud voice, liberal use of hand gesturing, and maintaining intense eye contact.
2. A loud voice does not necessarily mean that Mr. Bautista is angry.
3. The nurse should instruct Mr. Bautista to call someone to help him get out of bed when he is ready to pray and when he is ready to return to bed. The danger of injury to himself while praying is minimal once he is out of bed and kneeling on his prayer rug.
4. During Ramadan, Islamic people fast from sunup to sundown. Breakfast and lunch are served dur-

ing daylight hours. Therefore Mr. Bautista refused his meals.

5. Because Islamic people do not eat pork, Mr. Bautista removed the pork chops from his room.

6. Because Islamics fast from sunup until sundown during Ramadan, serve Mr. Bautista breakfast before sunup and hold his dinner until sundown. Provide snacks between dinner and breakfast as necessary.

7. Ramadan is a holy month for adherents of Islam. It involves special religious observances.

8. Many Arab-Americans prefer injection over oral medications because it is believed that injections are stronger than oral medicine. Additionally, fasting may include not taking medications.

9. Administering medications after sundown may improve compliance. Explaining to Mr. Bautista that fasting is not required during times of illness may also improve compliance.

REFERENCES

1. Lipson, J, and Haifizi, H: Iranians. In Purnell, L, and Paulanka, B (eds): Transcultural Health Care: A Culturally Competent Approach. FA Davis, Philadelphia, 1998.
2. Leininger, ME: Transcultural eating patterns and nutrition: Transcultural nursing and anthropological perspectives. Holistic Nurs Pract 3(1):16, 1988.
3. Louie, KB: Providing health care to Chinese clients. Topics in Clinical Nursing 7(3):18, 1985.
4. Purnell, L: Purnell's model for cultural competence. In Purnell, L, and Paulanka, B (eds): Transcultural Health Care: A Culturally Competent Approach. FA Davis, Philadelphia, 1998.
5. Information Please: Almanac 1995. Houghton Mifflin, Boston, 1995.
6. Still, O, and Hodgins, D: Navajo Indians. In Purnell, L, and Paulanka, B (eds): Transcultural Health Care: A Culturally Competent Approach. FA Davis, Philadelphia, 1998.
7. Preito, D: American Indians in medicine: The need for Indian healers. Acad Med 64:388, 1989.
8. Campinha-Bacote, J: African-Americans. In Purnell, L, and Paulanka, B (eds): Transcultural Health Care: A Culturally Competent Approach. FA Davis, Philadelphia, 1998.
9. Purnell, L: Mexican-Americans. In Purnell, L, and Paulanka, B (eds): Transcultural Health Care: A Culturally Competent Approach. FA Davis, Philadelphia, 1998.
10. Hudson, T: Cutting of care. Hosp Health Netw 69(2):36,1995.
11. Matocha, L: Chinese-Americans. In Purnell, L, and Paulanka, B (eds): Transcultural Health Care: A Culturally Competent Approach. FA Davis, Philadelphia, 1998.
12. Meleis, A, and Meleis, M: Egyptian-Americans. In Purnell, L, and Paulanka, B (eds): Transcultural Health Care: A Culturally Competent Approach. FA Davis, Philadelphia, 1998.
13. Zogby, J: Arab American Today: A Demographic Profile of Arab-Americans. Arab American Institute, Washington, DC, 1990.
14. Purnell, L: Appalachians. In Purnell, L, and Paulanka, B (eds): Transcultural Health Care: A Culturally Competent Approach. FA Davis, Philadelphia, 1998.

BIBLIOGRAPHY

Nowak, T: Vietnamese-Americans. In Purnell, L, and Paulanka, B (eds): Transcultural Health Care: A Culturally Competent Approach. FA Davis, Philadelphia, 1998.

Trends in Health Care

4

Kathleen Kelley Walsh and Gail Ladwig

Learning Objectives

Upon completion of this chapter, the student will be able to:

1. Discuss changes that have occurred in the acute care setting in the past 20 years.
2. Identify distinguishing features of the various settings in which health care is delivered.
3. Explain how recent trends have affected the settings for health care delivery.
4. Define alternative therapies.
5. Demonstrate the use of focused breathing as an alternative therapy.

Key Words

alternative therapy (all-**TURN**-a-tive **THAIR**-a-pee)

diagnosis-related groups (DRGs) (DYE-ag-**NOH**-sis ree-**LAY**-ted GROOPS)

health care delivery systems (HELLTH KAIR dee-**LIV**-er-ee **SIS**-tems)

primary care (**PRY**-mer-ee KAIR)

Health care is delivered in a wide variety of settings in the United States and Canada. Specific health care needs of individuals vary widely from person to person and fluctuate over time for the same individual or family. Infants and children need frequent assessments, and their parents require a great deal of information to promote and maintain growth and development. Chronically ill clients may need ongoing management of their disease states and in-depth teaching for themselves and their family. Health care needs can be simple or complex; require infrequent or frequent contact; involve few or many different categories of health care workers, or consume many or few resources. This tremendous variability of need means that communities need to have a wide variety of services available.

An agency or institution may be highly specialized or provide many different services. A recent trend in health care delivery is the merger of several agencies into **health care delivery systems.** These systems attempt to develop a range of programs and services. They consist of both inpatient and outpatient care services and meet health needs from birth to death. This trend is due primarily to financial pressures, including the onset of managed care. Attracting or retaining business from insurance companies and others who purchase services necessitates marketing groups of services at discounted rates. There is also fierce competition between health care delivery systems to attract business and keep it.

An increasing emphasis on delivering care in the community such as in clinics or in the home is another trend that continues to grow. This change is being caused by economic, technological, and social factors, which are important to understand.

It is much less expensive to provide care in the home or in a facility with fewer built-in overhead costs. The most expensive setting in which to deliver care is the hospital. Hospitals have tried many strategies to decrease the resources consumed during a hospital stay. They have also focused on shortening the length of stay, or average time that a person spends as an inpatient. These strategies have included earlier and more focused discharge planning and providing incentives for physicians to use fewer resources such as laboratory tests or x-rays. These strategies have been successful in decreasing the length of stay. The average inpatient stay has been greatly reduced from previous levels.

In addition to financial pressures, there have been tremendous technological advances that have contributed to massive change. Managing information through computer systems has decreased the need for the client to go to a specific health care site. Today's diagnostic and treatment tools are more portable and user-friendly than they were in the past. Technology has also become less invasive, which means fewer complications occur and recuperation time is shortened. For example, laser surgery greatly decreases the length of time the client spends under anesthesia and decreases both recovery time and the incidence of side effects, such as hemorrhage, pain, and infection. Because of the smoother recovery, less time or even no time is required as an inpatient in the hospital. There is also pressure from consumers to make services more accessible and efficient.

As a result of all of these influences, health care needs that previously required lengthy hospital stays are now managed in the client's home or community settings. For example, clients with systemic infections or advanced cardiac conditions that require intravenous medications may now be treated at home. As more quality outpatient programs are developed, hospitals are mainly becoming places for treating the acutely ill in need of intensive services and technologies.

Hospitals

There are multiple ways of classifying hospitals. One way is according to size (Fig. 4–1). Rural hospitals may be very small with only a few beds. City hospitals may be very large with up to 1500 beds. Hospitals are also categorized as governmental, or public, and nongovernmental, or private. In the United States, public hospitals may be city, county, state, or federal operations; in Canada they are either federal or provincial. Military hospitals provide care to military personnel and their families. Many private hospitals are run by religious organizations or other charitable groups. Private hospitals can be operated for profit or as not for profit. Until recently, only a small number of hospitals operated for profit. There are now for-profit hospital chains that are growing rapidly. Fewer hospitals exist as stand-alone institutions.

Another way to categorize a hospital is by the population it serves. Many hospitals are general, which means that they provide a broad range of services. This often includes medical, surgical, obstetrical, pediatric, and sometimes psychiatric care. Other hospitals may serve only a

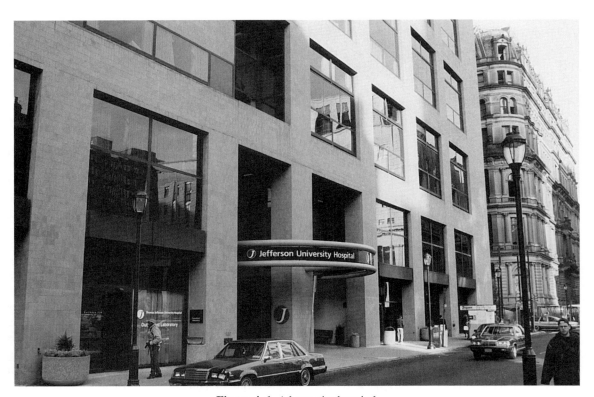

Figure 4–1. A large city hospital.

particular population, such as pediatric, rehabilitation, or psychiatric clients. The largest hospitals, usually in urban areas, may offer highly specialized care in units organized for the specialty. Examples of specialty units include burn units, transplant units, oncology units, spinal cord injury units, and neonatal intensive care units.

Hospitals provide services beyond the obvious care to inpatients. They serve as training facilities for nurses, physicians, and other disciplines. Many research studies are conducted to answer clinical questions. Hospitals also are adding more programs to promote health and cope with illness, disease, and death. Examples include support groups, exercise classes, and community health libraries.

Many hospitals are expanding into health care delivery systems or developing partnerships with other hospitals or systems in order to survive and remain competitive. In the past, hospitals were able to pass along costs to insurance companies and the various government agencies who paid for the services rendered. Now, however, hospitals have to operate like other businesses and carefully monitor and control costs.

This change in reimbursement began in 1983 with the onset of **diagnosis-related groups (DRGs).** Before this change, hospitals were paid for all costs associated with caring for a client who had Medicare coverage. The new system paid hospitals a set amount calculated to cover the average cost of caring for a Medicare client with a particu-

lar diagnosis. If the cost of caring for an individual client was more, hospitals had to absorb the cost, but if it was less, they were able to keep the money. For the first time, hospitals had an incentive to control costs. These incentives were developed over time by insurance companies and other government programs to control costs. The effects of these changes in reimbursement have been varied. Hospitals now need to carefully manage information and documentation. It is crucial to their operation that they learn which types of diagnoses they manage well and which ones they have problems managing. They have discovered that spending more money may or may not be associated with improvements in quality. They have had to learn how to analyze their operations and make adjustments on a continual basis.

Clients and physicians have had to recognize that admission to a hospital for acute care is now reserved for individuals requiring a high level of nursing care and technological support (Fig. 4–2). The majority of clients requiring this level of care are elderly, often chronically ill with multiple health problems. The hospital is increasingly becoming an intensive care center. All of these changes have many implications for those working in hospitals, for those using the services of a hospital, and for the development of services to meet the needs of clients who would have been hospitalized in the past.

The growing acuity of the clients and intensity of services provided means that hospital care continues to be-

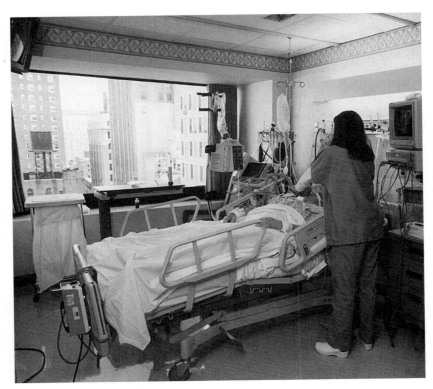

Figure 4–2. A client in an intensive care unit.

come more expensive. The business world, government, and insurance companies are all pressuring hospitals to contain their rapidly growing costs. As a result of this economic pressure, hospitals are rethinking how client care is provided. Many are making profound changes in the roles and responsibilities of the health care team members. Hospitals vary widely in how they are redesigning their care delivery. As a result, hospitals may change their system of care delivery and the role of the licensed practical nurse (LPN) and licensed vocational nurse (LVN). In some settings, these changes have expanded employment opportunities for LPN/LVNs. Multiskilled workers are in demand. A key point is that all nurses must understand their roles well in order to thoughtfully participate in redesign efforts and adapt to frequent changes in the environment of health care delivery.

CRITICAL THINKING: Health Care Trends

1. How are DRGs influencing client care today?
2. How are recent trends in health care affecting the role of the LPN/LVN?

Answers at end of chapter.

Rehabilitation Centers and Subacute Care Units

Rehabilitation centers can be separate facilities or special units of hospitals. Using a team approach, a variety of health care professionals, including nurses, work on maximizing the potential of the individual. Rehabilitation can refer to a place where concentrated efforts are made to optimize recovery from a disease or event. Rehabilitation may also refer to a concept as opposed to a place. The concept of rehabilitation includes planning for discharge beginning with admission, regardless of whether the setting is inpatient or outpatient. The concept is also applied to all types of physical and mental illnesses, including heart disease, respiratory illness, recovery from addiction, and other situations.

There are other concepts or settings evolving in response to the changes in health care reimbursement. For example, when independent self-care is projected to take a longer period of time than the stay in the acute care setting allows, subacute care may be an appropriate option. Subacute care may take place in a special unit of a hospital or in a separate, freestanding facility. In subacute care, the degree of intensity of services falls between acute care and long-term care. The individual receiving services has entered a more stable phase of recovery from illness or surgery, yet still requires frequent monitoring and a range of therapies provided by nursing and other professional staff.

Skilled Nursing Facilities

There are several different terms used to describe facilities that provide skilled nursing services for individuals with chronic health problems and self-care deficits. Commonly used titles include long-term care (LTC) or extended care (EC) facilities. In the past, LTC or EC facilities were referred to as nursing homes. The newer terms more accurately reflect the variety of services available today. Depending on the facility, care may range from providing personal services such as assistance with bathing and dressing to skilled nursing services such as wound care. Many people live months or years in these facilities, which in effect become their homes. Because of this, the term *resident* is used in place of client. Since the majority of residents in an EC facility are elderly, the physical environment, activities, and programs are designed accordingly. (See Gerontological Issues Box 4–1.)

Since hospitals began focusing on treating the acute phase of an illness and shortening lengths of stay, EC facil-

GERONTOLOGICAL ISSUES BOX 4–1

Nursing facilities (long-term care or nursing homes) are often thought to be the most common place to see and care for older adults. Statistics repeatedly demonstrate that no more than 5 percent of all adults over the age of 65 reside in a nursing facility at any one time. This has important implications for the nurse who is interested in caring for older people. Most older people live in the community. They live in their own homes, apartments, condominiums, and retirement centers. Some older adults live with family members, or members of their family live with them.

Admission to a nursing facility is often preceded by a life-altering event, such as debilitating illness, a fall or accident, cognitive impairment, or death of a spouse or caregiver. Usually, admission is not planned in advance and is more of a last resort or a crisis intervention. Older adults live in nursing facilities when they are no longer able to care for themselves in the community and they are unwilling or unable to live with family members.

Nursing facilities have changed over the years to accept a variety of care missions in the community. With shortened approved hospital stays, older adults that have had surgery or need rehabilitative services may be admitted to the nursing facility for a short time to take advantage of the support and care while they are recuperating. As these people get stronger and are able to assume self-care they are discharged back to their homes in the community. Another service area is hospice. Some nursing facilities have designated beds for providing hospice services. The resident and families are supported through the dying process.

ity usage has been affected. People who in the past would have had ample time to recover in the hospital and go home independently are now often discharged before independence is achieved. Extended care facilities can bridge this gap by offering nursing care and extended opportunities for recovering self-care skills. If residents have complex care needs, extended care may be necessary for a few weeks or months after hospitalization for illness or surgery. Extended care facilities employ a wide variety of professionals, including registered nurses (RNs), LPN/LVNs, nursing assistants, physical therapists, occupational therapists, speech therapists, activity specialists, social workers, and dietitians.

Beginning in 1987, the Omnibus Budget Reconciliation Act (OBRA) mandated that specific quality initiatives be undertaken by EC facilities. These initiatives include standards for training and competency evaluation of nursing assistants and increased recognition of residents' rights. This industry is considered one of the most highly regulated businesses in the country. Extended care facilities employ large numbers of LPN/LVNs, often placing a relatively high degree of responsibility in their hands. Although this setting often is less technically focused than the hospital setting, there is a high degree of complexity in the nursing care that is planned and implemented. Many residents have multiple chronic illnesses, sensory or motor impairments, and alterations in cognition.

Home Health Care Agencies

Home health care is not a new entity and has a long, productive history. It is, however, undergoing profound changes and is another rapidly growing segment of the health care industry. The early home health nursing movement was fueled by concerns over public health and well-being in the late 19th century and early 20th century. Threats to public health were recognized in the squalor of urban areas as well as in isolated regions with few facilities or health care professionals. Visits to the home by public health nurses often focused on teaching hygiene, recognition and treatment of common illness, and promotion of health via good nutrition. Although there have been many changes in home health since then, the emphasis on teaching persons how to better care for themselves remains a key feature of this service.

Earlier discharge from hospitals and the emphasis on managing illness from the home whenever possible has fueled tremendous growth in this setting. Home care aims to promote, maintain, or restore health and self-care abilities. Nurses and other health care professionals may provide either acute, short-term care or long-term monitoring of chronic illnesses by assessing, planning, delivering, and evaluating care in the client's home. Home health requires in-depth assessment of clients' functional status and needs across a wide spectrum. With this information the home

health nurse can develop a plan of care that meets the individualized learning needs of clients and families. The nurse has the advantage of working with clients in their natural environment where the client is usually most comfortable. The nurse can gather firsthand data about the opportunities and limitations afforded by the physical, social, and emotional environment of the client. Using this detailed information base the nurse can assist clients to build knowledge, skills, and abilities critical to their recovery or adaptation.

Registered nurses assess clients' needs for other services and then coordinate them. For example, a client recovering from a fractured hip may require in-home physical therapy and an aide to assist with activities of daily living. Recovery from a stroke may necessitate the services of a speech and occupational therapist. The services of a social worker may also be needed in some situations.

Home health care agencies may also specialize. Some provide maternal and child care, provide intravenous therapy, or coordinate services for brain-injured clients who are returning to a home setting.

Many agencies employ LPN/LVNs, who work under the direction of an RN. The RN delegates to the LPN/LVNs specific aspects of nursing care to be implemented from the overall plan of care. For example, an LPN/LVN may be asked to visit a stable, chronically ill diabetic client who requires insulin injections or other medications. The LPN/LVN can collect data, reinforce teaching, and administer the medications as ordered.

**CRITICAL THINKING:
Home Health Care Agencies**

1. What are some of the benefits of delivering care in the home for the client?
2. What are some of the benefits of delivering care in the home for the nurse?

Answers at end of chapter.

Hospice Services

The provision of hospice services began in England. The term *hospice* means shelter for those on a difficult journey. These services can occur in a client's home or in special facilities for the terminally ill. The hospice movement has grown tremendously in the last 20 years. There is increasing recognition by the public that terminally ill clients have special needs for comfort care, also known as palliative care. These needs are addressed well with the hospice focus on pain and other symptom management. Caring, humanity, and attention to the client's definition of quality of life are hallmarks of hospice. This unhurried and very personal approach to the care of the dying allows for richer dimensions of experience for dying clients and their families.

Hospice provides care to the client and support for the client's family and caregivers. Clients are admitted to hospice care when they are expected to live 6 months or less. Hospice accepts clients with a variety of diagnoses, such as cancer, end-stage heart failure, and end-stage pulmonary disease. Aggressive treatment for an illness is not the purpose of hospice care. The focus is on comfort care, maintaining quality of life, and providing death with dignity.

Public Health

Public health services can originate at the federal, state, or local level. At the federal level, the Public Health Service conducts research, assists communities in planning efforts around health, and provides training in the public health field. There are also federally funded research institutions that focus on health. One example is the National Institutes of Health (NIH) in Bethesda, Maryland. It has several divisions that investigate different illness, such as human immunodeficiency virus (HIV) and heart and lung disease. There is a separate division devoted to nursing research. Another government agency, Centers for Disease Control and Prevention, is located in Atlanta, Georgia. It has many programs and divisions related to surveying diseases and preventing infections. The federal government also operates the Veteran's Administration (VA) system of health care.

State health departments develop statewide plans for improving health and assist local health departments in executing the plans. Local health departments deliver the programs to their county or group of counties. These services vary but may include health screenings, immunizations, outpatient clinics, and health education. LPN/LVNs may be employed in public health clinics. Some health departments also have divisions that provide nursing services in the home for new mothers and infants, the chronically ill, the handicapped, the mentally ill, or other persons with special needs.

In Canada, the Canadian Department of Health and Welfare (CDHW) administers federal health programs, although provincial governments bear much of the responsibility for delivering health care in their region.

Office Settings

Nurse practitioners, physicians, and other health care professionals provide **primary care** in independent or group practice settings (Fig. 4–3). This setting provides diagnosis and care for illnesses and services that promote health and prevent disease. Nurses may function as the providers of primary care as nurse practitioners with advanced educational degrees or as providers of client care who register clients, perform vital sign measurements, and assist with procedures, treatments, or health education. A significant number of LPN/LVNs are employed in the office setting.

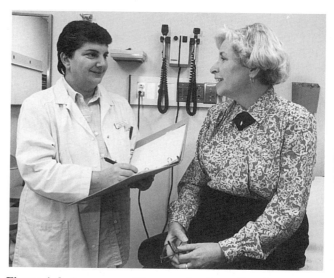

Figure 4–3. A nurse practitioner caring for a client in a primary care office setting.

Ambulatory Care Centers

Some office settings have broadened to include diagnostic and treatment facilities, such as laboratories, radiological services, and sometimes surgery. These settings are called ambulatory care centers. They are often operated by larger health care delivery systems, such as corporations who have hospitals and other facilities. When such a setting includes a center where surgery is performed on outpatients it is called an ambulatory surgical center or outpatient surgery center. This type of setting is growing in popularity because surgeries performed here are not burdened with the high built-in costs associated with a hospital setting. These settings also tend to offer more convenience to the client.

Clinic Settings

There are a wide variety of services in clinics. Many are located in public hospitals and offer everything from family practice to reproductive counseling to indigent medical care. In other clinics, the degree of specialization is expanded on. In a pain clinic, for instance, neurologists, neurosurgeons, nurses, psychologists, and other professionals may function as a team to recommend and carry out treatment plans for people with chronic pain syndromes. The variety of professionals who compose the team varies with the specialty area and the unique needs of the client.

Managed Care

There are a variety of organizations that consist of groups of health care providers who together attempt to provide all or most of the health care required for a group of people.

The types of organizations who meet this description continue to evolve as health care changes rapidly. Providers, insurance companies, and industries are struggling to control costs, meet customer expectations, and remain competitive. As a result, new organizational structures are developing to manage client care economically.

Health maintenance organizations (HMOs) were begun in the 1930s but did not flourish until the 1970s. Their emphasis is on wellness, health promotion, and illness prevention. Preferred provider organizations (PPOs) are much newer. A PPO is a network of providers who provide care to plan members at set discounted rates. Individual practice associations (IPAs) are physician-owned organizations that contract their services to HMOs and PPOs. Each of these organizations can be classified as managed care, which aims to control costs for medical care.

CRITICAL THINKING: Managed Care

1. What effect does managed care have on client care today?
Answer at end of chapter.

Alternative/Complementary Therapies

There is a current demand from the general public to receive health care treatment that is sometimes referred to as **alternative therapy** or complementary therapy. Sometimes clients are not satisfied with conventional medicine or simply want something that they view as more natural or less invasive. They may also have tried conventional medicine without achieving desired results.

Complementary or alternative medicine is defined as a practice used for the prevention and treatment of disease that is not taught widely in medical schools or is not generally available inside hospitals. According to the World Health Organization, between 65 and 80 percent of the world's health care services are classified as traditional medicine. These traditional medicine services become complementary, alternative, or unconventional when used in Western countries.

In the United States, one out of three Americans saw an alternative health care practitioner in 1990. This was more visits than were made to conventional primary care physicians. As a result, over 13 billion dollars were paid for these services. According to Jonas,[1] 10 billion dollars of this expense was out-of-pocket and not reimbursed.

Alternative medicine offers a wide variety of treatment options. Chiropractic, craniosacral therapy, and various systems of bodywork address structural imbalances within the body. Diet, nutritional supplements, herbal medicine, and enzyme therapy focus on maintaining the body's biochemical balance. Mind-body medicine, biofeedback train-

ing, meditation, hypnotherapy, guided imagery, and neurolinguistic programming seek to restore mental and emotional balance. Acupuncture, homeopathy, energy medicine, magnetic field therapy, and neural therapy address the energetic levels of the body.

Alternative therapies have been around for hundreds and even thousands of years in some cultures. Conventional medicine on the other hand is rather new. It is the predominant type of health care in Western civilization.

The LPN/LVN needs to be aware of these therapies and should ask clients whether they are using them. The primary caregiver should be aware of their use. Some clients use them alone, but many clients also use them with conventional medicine. It is helpful for caregivers to know everything that their clients are using so that comprehensive care may be delivered.

A common philosophy in alternative medicine is that alternative medicine treats the individual instead of just the symptoms. Nurses have been involved in delivering what is being called alternative medicine since nursing began. Nurses have always treated the whole person: body, mind, and spirit. Florence Nightingale[2] stated, "Nursing is putting the client in the best condition for nature to act upon him."

Many treatments that nurses do are noninvasive and do not require a physician's order. The following interventions might be considered alternative therapies: back massage and the use of music to promote relaxation; the use of visualization or imagery for pain control; and the use of presence of self when giving care.

A simple exercise that may be taught to clients that is used as part of many alternative therapies is called focused breathing (Table 4–1). There are many ways to teach focused breathing, but the following is an effective tool that the nurse can teach clients to use for a variety of problems. It can be used for pain control, to promote sleep, to relieve stress, or for general overall relaxation. It is also an easy

Table 4–1. *Steps for Focused Breathing*

1. Instruct client to be as comfortable as possible.
2. Depending on the setting and the client's comfort level, the nurse may suggest that the client close his or her eyes.
3. Instruct client to be aware of his or her breathing.
4. Instruct client that after the client is aware of his or her breathing to slowly breathe in and out and to notice both inspiration and expiration.
5. Have client concentrate on his or her breathing for a few minutes.
6. Have client notice any area of his or her body that is tense and consciously let that part of the body relax.
7. Have client continue to slowly breathe in and out for 20 seconds to 10 minutes.
8. To conclude the exercise, if the client had his or her eyes closed, either the nurse or the client can slowly count backward from 5, saying: "Five—get ready to come back; four—get ready to open the eyes; three—slowly open the eyes; two—open the eyes; one—feel comfortable and relaxed and ready to enjoy the rest of the day."

exercise for nurses to use for themselves to relieve their own stress and promote relaxation. This exercise may last from 2 to 10 minutes. It takes about 10 minutes to teach and practice this with clients. Clients can be instructed to use this exercise when they are in pain or stressed. They should be encouraged to practice this exercise at times when they are not in pain or stressed. Then, as situations arise in which the exercise will be helpful, it is second nature to use it.

Review Questions

1. Which of the following is a feature of integrated health care delivery systems?
   a. The health care services are delivered primarily from the hospital setting.
   b. Partnerships between different types of health care agencies create the system.
   c. They are stable organizations with long histories of service.
   d. Most integrated delivery systems specialize in one segment of health care.

2. Which of the following is a method HMOs use to control costs?
   a. Wellness and health promotion are emphasized.
   b. Their focus is the treatment of illnesses.
   c. Payment is made for the client's actual length of stay.
   d. A group of physicians sets a fixed fee schedule.

3. Working with clients in their home is of greatest benefit to the nurse in which phase of the nursing process?
   a. Assessment
   b. Planning
   c. Implementation
   d. Evaluation

4. A 53-year-old client with end-stage breast cancer that has spread to the lungs, bones, and brain asks the physician about entering a hospice program. The client's husband is unclear about hospice and states, "My wife will just be left to die." Which of the following is the best response by the nurse?
   a. "You can seek experimental treatment for your wife if you are not ready to let go."
   b. "Hospice is the best option for your wife at this time."
   c. "If you choose hospice, they will aggressively treat the cancer."
   d. "You seem to have questions that the doctor can answer for you."

5. Which of the following is most likely to contribute to the complexity of nursing care provided to residents of long-term care facilities?
   a. Cognitive, sensory, or motor impairments of residents
   b. Lack of health care insurance coverage for many of the residents
   c. The provision of many skilled technological services
   d. The frequent admissions and discharges of facility residents

6. A client admitted for abdominal surgery is taught focused breathing by the nurse to help control postoperative pain. Which of the following instructions regarding the use of focused breathing should the client be given?
   a. Begin the focused breathing after the pain is intense.
   b. Begin the focused breathing before pain is experienced.
   c. Use focused breathing on arising in the morning to be most alert.
   d. Use focused breathing up to four times a day.

7. A client asks the nurse if it will be all right to use herbal therapy at home for pain relief. Which of the following would be the best response for the nurse based on the understanding that alternative therapy has been practiced for many years in most cultures?
   a. "Herbs are natural and can always be used."
   b. "I would never recommend herbs, they taste awful."
   c. "It is a good idea to discuss this with your physician, so your medications can be reviewed for compatibility with the herbs."
   d. "I always use herbs and would recommend them to anyone."

ANSWERS TO CRITICAL THINKING

Critical Thinking: Health Care Trends

1. Acute care length of stays for clients have been shortened, resulting in reduced time for discharge planning and client teaching. Health care services such as home care are more in demand as a result.

2. The LPN/LVN may be learning a variety of skills, such as phlebotomy and running 12-lead electrocardiograms, that were not traditionally taught to LPN/LVNs. New or growing practice settings, including LTC, clinics, or home health care, are available for employment opportunities. The LPN/LVN is faced with continual adjustment to ongoing change in the workplace as health care is redesigned. Also, LPN/LVNs may work with new categories of workers such as unlicensed assistive personnel.

Critical Thinking: Home Health Care Agencies

1. Clients are able to recover in a setting that is familiar and comfortable to them. They are usually more motivated to increase their self-care abilities in settings where they have control. Clients' roles and social activities are more normal with their families around them. Family support is readily available. Home care is less expensive for clients and society.

2. The nurse can perform a well-rounded assessment of clients' functioning in their natural environment and adapt teaching to specific needs of a client's lifestyle and home setting. During a home care visit, the nurse's attention is focused on only one client at a time.

Critical Thinking: Managed Care

1. Institutions have incentives to control costs under managed care. The goal is to be more efficient. As a result, for example, clients may have fewer diagnostic tests ordered. Care is often coordinated by a case manager. The case manager oversees the client's case to ensure that care is timely and efficient.

REFERENCES

1. Jonas, W: Remarks by Wayne Jonas, M.D. Office of Alternative Medicine, National Institutes of Health, Eighth International Conference, The Psychology of Health, Immunity, and Disease, The National Institute for the Clinical Application of Behavioral Medicine, Hilton Head, SC, December 1996.
2. Nightingale, F: Notes on Nursing: What It Is and What It Is Not (fascimile ed.). JB Lippincott, Philadelphia, 1966. (Originally published by Harrison, London, 1859.)

BIBLIOGRAPHY

Burton Goldberg Group, James Strohecker, Executive Editor: Alternative Medicine: The Definitive Guide. Future Medicine, Puyallup, Wash, 1994.

Donahue, MP: Nursing: The Finest Art. Mosby, St Louis, 1985.

Dossey, B: Using imagery to help your patient heal. Am J Nurs 95(6):41, 1995.

Dossey, BM: Complementary and alternative therapies for our aging society. J of Gerontological Nursing 23:45, 1997.

Dunham-Taylor, J, Marquettee, P, and Pinczuk, J: Surviving Capitation. Am J Nurs 96(3):26, 1996.

Hunt, BH, and James, MK: Tomorrow's LPN: Understanding the role. Nursing 27(3):52, 1997.

Joel, LA: Restructuring: Under what conditions? Am J Nurs 94(3):7, 1994.

The health care revolution: Health care enterprise. Nurs Adm Q 21(2):vi, 1997.

Understanding Health and Illness

5

Fluid, Electrolyte, and Acid-Base Balance and Imbalance

Donna D. Ignatavicius

Learning Objectives

Upon completion of this chapter, the student will be able to:

1. Identify the purpose of fluids and electrolytes in the body.
2. Differentiate between the signs and symptoms of common fluid imbalances.
3. Identify clients who are at the highest risk for dehydration and fluid overload.
4. Describe the assessment that the nurse performs for clients with fluid imbalances.
5. Discuss the treatment plan for dehydration and fluid overload.
6. Identify patient education needs for clients with fluid imbalances.
7. Discuss the common causes, signs and symptoms, and treatment for sodium, potassium, calcium, and magnesium imbalances.
8. Identify foods that have high sodium, potassium, and calcium content.
9. Describe the common causes of acidosis and alkalosis.
10. Explain the changes in arterial blood gases for each type of acid-base imbalance.

Key Words

acidosis (ass-i-**DOH**-sis)
alkalosis (al-ka-**LOH**-sis)
anion (**AN**-eye-on)
antidiuretic (AN-ti-DYE-yoo-**RET**-ik)
baroreceptors (BA-roh-ree-**SEP**-turs)
cation (**KAT**-eye-on)
dehydration (DEE-high-**DRAY**-shun)
diffusion (di-**FEW**-zhun)
dysrhythmia (dis-**RITH**-mee-yah)
electrolytes (ee-**LEK**-troh-lites)
extracellular (EX-trah-**SELL**-yoo-ler)
filtration (fill-**TRAY**-shun)
homeostasis (HOH-mee-oh-**STAY**-sis)
hydrostatic (HIGH-droh-**STAT**-ik)

hypercalcemia (HIGH-per-kal-**SEE**-mee-ah)
hyperkalemia (HIGH-per-kuh-**LEE**-mee-ah)
hypermagnesemia (HIGH-per-MAG-nuh-**ZEE**-mee-ah)
hypernatremia (HIGH-per-nuh-**TREE**-mee-ah)
hypertonic (HIGH-per-**TAHN**-ik)
hyperventilation (HIGH-per-VEN-ti-**LAY**-shun)
hypervolemia (HIGH-poh-voh-**LEE**-mee-ah)
hypocalcemia (HIGH-poh-kal-**SEE**-mee-ah)
hypokalemia (HIGH-poh-kuh-**LEE**-mee-ah)
hypomagnesemia (HIGH-poh-MAG-nuh-**ZEE**-mee-ah)
hyponatremia (HIGH-poh-nuh-**TREE**-mee-ah)
hypotonic (HIGH-poh-**TAHN**-ik)
hypovolemia (HIGH-poh-voh-**LEE**-mee-ah)
interstitial (IN-ter-**STISH**-uhl)
intracellular (IN-trah-**SELL**-yoo-ler)
intracranial (IN-trah-**KRAY**-nee-uhl)
intravascular (IN-trah-**VAS**-kyoo-lar)
isotonic (EYE-so-**TAHN**-ik)
osmosis (ahs-**MOH**-sis)
osteoporosis (AHS-tee-oh-por-**OH**-sis)
semipermeable (SEM-ee-**PER**-mee-uh-buhl)
transcellular (trans-**SELL**-yoo-lar)

Fluids (primarily water) are found throughout the body and are needed for all cells to function. Approximately 60 percent of a young adult's body weight is water. The elderly have less than 50 percent. Women also have less body water because they have more fat than men. Fat cells do not contain water.

In addition to water, body fluids also contain solid substances that dissolve, called solutes. Some solutes are electrolytes and some are nonelectrolytes. **Electrolytes** are chemicals that when dissolved in water can conduct electricity. Examples of electrolytes are sodium, potassium, calcium, and magnesium, discussed later in this chapter. Nonelectrolytes do not conduct electricity. Examples are glucose and urea.

Fluid Balance

Fluids are located in two major areas of the body—within the cells (**intracellular** fluid [ICF]) and outside the cells (**extracellular** fluid [ECF]). As seen in Figure 5–1, ECF can be further divided into three types: **interstitial** fluid, **intravascular** fluid, and **transcellular** fluid.

Interstitial fluid is the water that surrounds the body's cells and includes the lymph. Fluids and electrolytes move freely between the interstitial fluid and the intravascular fluid, which is the plasma of the blood. Examples of transcellular fluid are cerebrospinal fluid, digestive juices, and synovial fluid in joints.

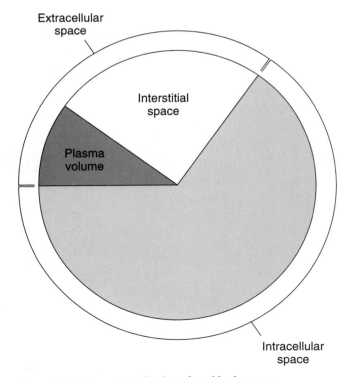

Figure 5–1. Normal distribution of total body water.

CONTROL OF FLUID BALANCE

The body works hard to keep the proper fluid balance. This balance is sometimes referred to as **homeostasis.** Four major processes help control the amount of extracellular fluid volume in the body. They are **baroreceptors,** volume receptors, the **antidiuretic** hormone, and the renin-angiotensin-aldosterone system.

Baroreceptors are special cells located in the heart and large vessels. When the body does not have enough fluid, the baroreceptors signal the kidneys to decrease their urinary output. This action conserves water in the body.

The volume receptors, also located in the heart, work just the opposite from the baroreceptors. They are special cells that respond to too much fluid in the body by signaling the kidneys to increase output. This action gets rid of extra water in the body.

The antidiuretic hormone (ADH) is an important substance produced by the pituitary gland located at the base of the brain. When the body has too much fluid, the pituitary gland decreases the amount of ADH so that the kidneys will rid the body of extra water. When the body has too little fluid, the pituitary gland increases the amount of ADH to conserve water by the kidneys.

The last process, the renin-angiotensin-aldosterone system, is much more complex. Renin is an enzyme secreted by the kidneys when body fluid is decreased. Renin helps form a substance in the body called angiotensin I. Angiotensin I is then converted in the lungs by the angiotensin-converting enzyme (ACE) to angiotensin II. Angiotensin II constricts blood vessels to raise blood pressure. It also signals the adrenal cortex to secrete aldosterone, a hormone that helps hold sodium in the body. When sodium is held in the body, water also stays in the body.

The response of hormones, such as aldosterone and antidiuretic hormone, to changes in body fluid level is called a negative feedback system. In a negative feedback system, the hormones are secreted only when needed by the body.

MOVEMENT OF FLUIDS AND ELECTROLYTES IN THE BODY

Fluids and electrolytes move within the body by passive and active transport systems. In passive transport, no en-

---

electrolyte: electro—electricity + lyte—dissolve
intracellular: intra—within + cellular—cell
extracellular: extra—outside of + cellular—cell
interstitial: inter—between + stitial—tissue
intravascular: intra—within + vascular—blood vessel
transcellular: trans—across + cellular—cell
homeostasis: homeo—likeness + stasis—a standing
baroreceptor: baro—heaviness + receptor—receiver
antidiuretic: anti—against + diuretic—urination

ergy is expended. The three passive transport systems are **diffusion, filtration,** and **osmosis.**

Diffusion is a process in which the solute moves across a biological membrane from an area of higher solute concentration to an area of lower concentration. The biological membrane is selectively **semipermeable,** meaning that only certain solutes can cross the membrane from one area to another. In the body, gases (oxygen and carbon dioxide) and electrolytes move across the capillary wall or across the cell membrane.

In some cases, the solute diffuses with the assistance of another substance. For example, insulin promotes the movement of glucose and potassium into the cells. This process is helpful in the treatment of clients who have excess glucose and potassium in their blood. By administering insulin, the extra glucose and potassium move from the blood, where they are life-threatening, into the cells of the body.

Filtration is the movement of both the solute and water caused by **hydrostatic** pressure differences between areas. Hydrostatic pressure is the force that water exerts, sometimes called water pushing pressure. In the body, filtration is important for the movement of water, nutrients, and waste products in the capillaries.

Osmosis is the movement of water from an area of lower solute concentration to an area of higher concentration. The solutes exert an osmotic pressure, sometimes called water pulling pressure. The term *osmolarity* refers to the concentration of the solutes in body fluids. The normal osmolarity of the blood is between 270 and 300 milliosmoles per liter (mOsm/L). Sodium, an important body electrolyte, is the primary solute in extracellular fluid and therefore helps hold water in the blood.

Another term for osmolarity is *tonicity.* Fluids or solutions can be classified as **isotonic, hypotonic,** or **hypertonic.** A fluid that has the same osmolarity as the blood is called isotonic. For example, a 0.9 percent saline solution (normal saline) is isotonic to the blood and is often used as a solution for intravenous therapy.

A solution that has a lower osmolarity than blood is called hypotonic, such as a 0.20 percent saline solution. When a hypotonic solution is given to a client, water leaves the blood and other extracellular fluid areas and enters the cells.

Hypertonic solutions, such as 3 percent saline, exert greater osmotic pressure than blood. When a hypertonic solution is given to a client, water leaves the cells and enters the bloodstream and other extracellular fluid spaces. Table 5–1 lists commonly used isotonic, hypotonic, and hypertonic intravenous solutions.

The other major way that fluids and electrolytes move in the body is by active transport. This process allows movement in the opposite direction from diffusion and depends on the presence of adequate cellular adenosine triphosphate (ATP) for energy. The principle of active transport is that solutes can be moved from an area of lower solute concentration to an area of higher concentration. The most common example of active transport is the sodium-potassium pump. This pump, located in the cell membrane, allows the movement of sodium out of the cell and potassium into the cell when needed.

FLUID GAINS AND FLUID LOSSES

Water is very important to the body for cellular metabolism, blood volume, body temperature regulation, and solute transport. Although an individual can survive without food for several weeks, he or she can survive only a few days without water.

Water is gained and lost from the body every day. When too much fluid is lost, the brain's thirst mechanism tells the individual that more fluid intake is needed. Older adults have a diminished thirst reflex, which makes them prone to fluid deficit. In addition to liquid intake, some fluid is obtained from solid foods.

An adult loses as much as 2500 mL of sensible and insensible fluid each day. Sensible losses are those of which the individual is aware, such as urination. Insensible losses

Table 5–1. **Commonly Used Intravenous Fluids**

Solution	Osmolarity (mOsm/L)	Tonicity
0.9%	308	Isotonic
0.45% saline	154	Hypotonic
5% dextrose in water (D_5W)	272	Isotonic*
10% dextrose in water ($D_{10}W$)	500	Hypertonic*
5% dextrose in 0.9% saline	560	Hypertonic*
5% dextrose in 0.45% saline	406	Hypertonic*
5% dextrose in 0.225% saline	321	Isotonic*
Ringer's lactate	273	Isotonic
5% dextrose in Ringer's lactate	525	Hypertonic*

*Solution tonicity at the time of administration. Within a short time after administration, the dextrose is metabolized and the tonicity of the infused solution decreases in proportion to the osmolarity or tonicity of the nondextrose components (electrolytes) within the water.
Source: Ignatavicius, DD, Workman, ML, and Mishler, MS: Medical-Surgical Nursing: A Nursing Process Approach, ed 2. WB Saunders, Philadelphia, 1995, with permission. (Data from Trissel, L: *Handbook on Injectable Drugs,* ed 7. American Society of Hospital Pharmacists, Bethesda, Md, 1992.)

diffusion: diffuse—spread, scattered
filtration: filter—strain through
osmosis: osmo—impulse + osis—condition
semipermeable: semi—half or part + permeable—passing through
hydrostatic: hydro—water + static—standing
isotonic: iso—equal + tonic—strength
hypotonic: hypo—less than + tonic—strength
hypertonic: hyper—more than + tonic—strength

may occur without the individual recognizing the loss. Perspiration and water lost through feces are examples of insensible losses.

Fluid Imbalances

Fluid imbalances are common in any clinical setting. The elderly are at the highest risk for life-threatening complications that can result from either fluid deficit, more commonly called **dehydration,** or fluid overload.

DEHYDRATION

Although there are several types of dehydration, only the most common type will be discussed in this chapter. Dehydration occurs when there is not enough fluid in the body, especially in the blood (intravascular area).

Pathophysiology and Etiology

The most common form of dehydration results from loss of fluid from the body resulting in decreased blood volume. This decrease is referred to as **hypovolemia.** Hypovolemia occurs when the client is hemorrhaging or when fluids from other parts of the body are lost. For example, severe vomiting and diarrhea, severely draining wounds, and profuse diaphoresis can cause dehydration.

Hypovolemia may also occur when fluid from the intravascular space moves into the interstitial fluid space. This process is called third spacing. Examples of conditions in which third spacing is common include burns, liver cirrhosis, and extensive trauma. Table 5–2 lists the common causes of dehydration.

As described earlier in this chapter, the body initially attempts to compensate for fluid loss by a number of mechanisms. If the cause of dehydration is not resolved or the client is not able to replace the fluid, a state of dehydration occurs.

Table 5–2. **Common Causes of Dehydration**

Long-term nothing by mouth (NPO)
Hemorrhage
Profuse diaphoresis (sweating)
Diuretic therapy
Diarrhea
Vomiting
Gastrointestinal suction
Draining fistulas
Draining abscesses
Severely draining wounds
Systemic infection
Fever
Frequent enemas
Ileostomy
Cecostomy
Diabetes insipidus

Prevention

The nurse can help prevent dehydration by identifying those clients at the highest risk for developing this condition. High-risk clients include the elderly and any client who has one of the conditions listed in Table 5–2.

Adequate hydration is another important intervention to help prevent dehydration. The nursing staff should encourage clients to increase fluid intake. If the client is unable to take fluids by mouth, the nurse checks with the physician for an order for intravenous therapy to replace fluid in the body.

Signs and Symptoms

The earliest symptom of dehydration in an elderly client is disorientation, confusion, or increased confusion. The brain needs oxygen supplied by the blood to function properly. In the client with hypovolemia, there is inadequate blood supply to the brain, which causes mental status changes, especially among elderly clients.

Other signs and symptoms include increased, weak pulse; low blood pressure; elevated temperature; dry skin and mouth; poor skin turgor ("tenting"); thirst; decreased urinary output; dark, concentrated urine; weight loss; and constipation. As mentioned earlier, the elderly client may not experience thirst. In addition, temperature may not appear elevated because an elder's normal body temperature is often several degrees lower than a younger person's.

Complications

If dehydration is not treated, lack of sufficient blood volume will cause multiple organ failure. The brain, kidneys, and heart must be adequately supplied with blood (perfused) to function properly. Multiple organ failure then results in death.

Diagnostic Tests

The client with dehydration usually has an elevated blood urea nitrogen (BUN) and elevated hematocrit. Both values are increased because there is less water in proportion to the solid substances being measured. The specific gravity of the urine also increases as the kidneys attempt to conserve water, resulting in a more concentrated urine.

Medical Treatment

The goals of medical treatment are to replace fluids and resolve the cause of dehydration. In the client with moderate or severe dehydration, intravenous therapy is used. Isotonic fluids that have the same osmolarity as blood are typically administered.

---

dehydration: de—down + hydration—water

hypovolemia: hypo—less than + vol—volume + emia—blood

Nursing Process

The nurse plays a major role in identifying clients who are dehydrated.

Assessment

The nurse assesses the client for signs and symptoms of dehydration. All of the classic signs and symptoms may not be present.

When assessing an elderly client for skin turgor, the skin over the forehead or sternum should be assessed. The skin over these areas usually retains elasticity and is therefore a more reliable indicator of skin turgor.

Weight is the most reliable indicator of fluid loss or gain. A loss of 1 to 2 pounds or more per day suggests water loss rather than fat loss. The client in the hospital setting should be weighed every day. The client in the nursing home or home setting should be weighed three times a week if the client is at risk for fluid imbalance. The nursing staff should weigh the client before breakfast using the same scale. The scale should be periodically evaluated by the manufacturer for accuracy.

Nursing Diagnosis

The primary nursing diagnoses for the client with dehydration are as follows:

- Fluid volume deficit related to fluid loss or inadequate fluid intake
- Decreased cardiac output related to insufficient blood volume
- Altered oral mucous membrane related to inadequate oral secretions
- Decreased tissue (cerebral) perfusion related to insufficient blood volume
- Constipation related to decreased body fluids

Planning

The health care team works together to restore fluids for the client. The expected outcome is that the client will be adequately hydrated and not experience further episodes of dehydration.

Implementation

Clients can become dehydrated in any setting. For the client who is mildly dehydrated, interventions can be implemented in the home or nursing home setting. For moderate or severe dehydration, the client may require hospitalization to treat the underlying cause and replace fluid losses. The nurse monitors the client to ensure that he or she does not receive too much fluid replacement and cause fluid overload, discussed in the next section of this chapter. Fluid intake and output should be carefully measured. (See Cultural Considerations Box 5–1.)

---

hypervolemia: hyper—more than + vol—volume + emia—blood

Evaluation

As part of evaluation, the nurse determines whether the client has been adequately rehydrated, using the assessment techniques described earlier.

Client Education

The client, family, and significant others need to be taught about the importance of reporting early signs and symptoms of dehydration to the physician or other health care provider. At home or in the nursing home, infections often cause fever and sepsis, a serious condition in which the infection invades the bloodstream. The client becomes dehydrated as a result and can become seriously ill.

 CRITICAL THINKING: Mrs. Levitt

Mrs. Levitt is a 92-year-old widow who has been in a nursing home for 4 years. Today she complains that her urine smells bad and that her heart feels like it is beating faster than usual. You suspect that she is becoming dehydrated.

1. When taking the client's vital signs, what changes would you expect and why?
2. What interventions should you provide at this time?

Answers at end of chapter.

FLUID OVERLOAD

Fluid overload, sometimes called overhydration, is a condition in which a client has too much fluid in the body. Most of the problems related to fluid overload result from too much fluid in the bloodstream or from dilution of electrolytes and red blood cells.

Pathophysiology and Etiology

The most common result of fluid overload is **hypervolemia,** in which there is excess fluid in the intravascular space. The healthy adult kidneys can compensate for mild to moderate hypervolemia. The kidneys increase urinary output to rid the body of the extra fluid.

The causes of fluid overload are related to excessive intake of fluids or inadequate excretion of fluids. Conditions that can cause excessive fluid intake are poorly controlled intravenous therapy, excessive irrigation of wounds or body cavities, and excessive ingestion of water. Conditions that can result in inadequate excretion of fluid include renal failure, heart failure, and syndrome of inappropriate antidiuretic hormone (SIADH). These conditions are discussed elsewhere in this textbook.

Prevention

One of the best ways to prevent fluid overload is to avoid excessive fluid intake. For example, the nurse monitors the client receiving intravenous therapy for signs and symptoms of fluid overload. The prescribed rate of infusion should be controlled by an electronic infusion pump.

The nurse also monitors the amount of fluid used for irrigations. For instance, continuous bladder irrigation after a transurethral resection of the prostate (TURP) procedure is typically ordered to infuse at a rate high enough to keep the urine clear. However, the irrigation may infuse too quickly and cause fluid overload.

Signs and Symptoms

The vital sign changes seen in the client with fluid overload are the opposite of those found in clients with dehydration. The blood pressure is elevated, pulse is bounding, and respirations are increased and shallow. The neck veins may become distended, and pitting edema in the feet and legs may be present. The skin is pale and cool. The kidneys increase their urinary output and the urine appears diluted, almost like water. The client rapidly gains weight. In severe fluid overload, the client has moist crackles in the lungs, dyspnea, and ascites (excess peritoneal fluid).

Complications

Acute fluid overload typically results in congestive heart failure. As the fluid builds up in the heart, the heart is not able to properly function as a pump. The fluid then backs up into the lungs, causing a condition known as pulmonary edema. Other major organs of the body cannot receive adequate oxygen, and organ failure can lead to death.

Diagnostic Tests

In the client experiencing fluid overload, the BUN and hematocrit tend to decrease as a consequence of hemodilution. The plasma content of the blood is proportionately increased when compared with the solid substances. The specific gravity of the urine also diminishes as the urinary output increases.

Medical Treatment

Once the client's breathing has been supported, the goal of treatment is to rid the body of excessive fluid and resolve the underlying cause of the overload. Drug therapy and diet therapy are commonly used to decrease fluid retention.

Positioning

To facilitate ease in breathing, the head of the client's bed should be in semi-Fowler's or high Fowler's position. These positions allow greater lung expansion and thus aid in respiratory effort. Once the client has been properly positioned, oxygen therapy may be necessary (Fig. 5–2).

Oxygen Therapy

To ensure adequate perfusion of major organs and minimize dyspnea, oxygen therapy is typically used. If the client has a history of chronic obstructive pulmonary disease (COPD), such as emphysema or chronic bronchitis, do *not* administer more than 2 L/min of oxygen. At higher oxygen doses, the client may lose his or her stimulus for breathing and will suffer respiratory arrest.

Drug Therapy

The drug of choice for fluid overload when the client has adequately functioning kidneys is usually furosemide (Lasix). Furosemide is a loop (high-ceiling) diuretic that causes the kidneys to excrete sodium, and thus water. Sodium (Na^+) and water tend to move together in the body. Potassium (K^+), another electrolyte, is also lost, which can lead to a potassium deficit, discussed later in this chapter.

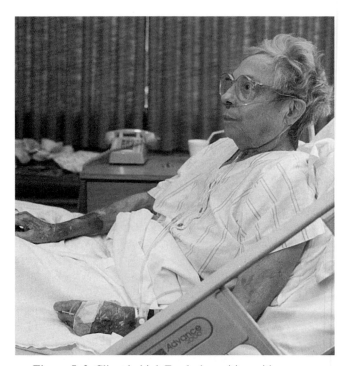

Figure 5–2. Client in high Fowler's position with oxygen.

Furosemide may be given by the oral, intramuscular, or intravenous route. The oral route is used most commonly for mild fluid overload. Intravenous (IV) furosemide is administered by a registered nurse or physician for severe overload. The client should begin diuresis in 30 minutes after IV furosemide. If not, another dose is given.

Diet Therapy

Mild to moderate fluid restriction may be necessary, as well as a sodium-restricted diet. In collaboration with the dietitian, the physician prescribes the specific restriction necessary, usually a 1 to 2 g Na restriction for severe overload.

Nursing Process

The nurse plays a pivotal role in the care of the client with fluid overload. Prompt action is needed to prevent life-threatening complications.

Assessment

The nurse observes the client who is at high risk for fluid overload and monitors fluid intake and output carefully. If the client is drinking adequate amounts of fluid (1500 mL/day or more) but is voiding in small amounts, the fluid is being retained by the body.

The nurse assesses for edema, which is fluid that accumulates in the interstitial tissues. (See Gerontological Issues Box 5–2.) If the edema is pitting, a finger pressed against the skin leaves a temporary indentation. For clients in bed, the nurse checks the sacrum for edema. For clients in the sitting position, the nurse checks the feet and legs.

As mentioned earlier, weight is the most reliable indicator of fluid gain. A gain of 1 to 2 pounds or more a day indicates fluid retention, even though other signs and symptoms may not be present.

Nursing Diagnoses

The common nursing diagnoses for the client experiencing fluid overload are as follows:

- Fluid volume excess related to excessive fluid intake or inadequate excretion of body fluid

GERONTOLOGICAL ISSUES BOX 5-2

Peripheral Fluid Retention in Older Adults

Older adults often comment or complain about retaining fluid in their feet and ankles. This is uncomfortable and is related to compromised peripheral circulation. Often, the symptoms can be decreased by elevation of the feet and legs. Peripheral fluid retention is not an accurate indicator of hydration for older adults. An older adult can have a serious fluid volume deficit and still have peripheral edema.

- Decreased cardiac output related to excess work on the heart from fluid retention
- Altered tissue perfusion related to dependent edema
- Risk for impaired gas exchange related to fluid in the lungs

Planning

The expected outcome for the client is that fluid balance is achieved and that the client does not experience life-threatening cardiac or pulmonary failure.

Implementation

The client at risk for fluid overload may be in the hospital, nursing home, or home. Severe overload requires hospitalization, possibly to a critical care unit on a ventilator if the client has severe pulmonary edema. Mild or moderate overload may be treated outside the hospital, but the client must follow the treatment plan carefully to avoid a worsening condition.

Evaluation

During treatment, the nurse evaluates whether the expected outcomes are achieved. Many clients must remain on drug and diet therapy after hospital discharge to prevent the problem from occurring again.

Client Education

In collaboration with the dietitian, the client, family, or other caregiver needs to be instructed about the fluid and sodium restrictions to prevent further problems. High-sodium foods to avoid are listed in Table 5–3. (See Nutrition Notes Box 5–3.)

Table 5–3. **Common Food Sources of Sodium***

Food Source	Amount (mg)
Table salt (1 tsp)	2000
Cheddar cheese (1 oz)	176
Cottage cheese (4 oz)	457
American cheese (1 oz)	439
Whole milk (8 oz)	120
Skim milk (8 oz)	126
Butter (1 tsp)	123
White bread (1 slice)	123
Whole-wheat bread (1 slice)	159
Soy sauce (1 tbsp)	1029
Ketchup (1 tbsp)	156
Mustard (1 tbsp)	188
Beef, lean (4 oz)	60
Pork, lean, fresh (4 oz)	60
Pork, cured (4 oz)	850
Chicken, light meat (4 oz)	70
Chicken, dark meat (4 oz)	70

*U.S. Department of Agriculture recommended daily allowance for adults: 1100–3300 mg.
Source: Ignativicius, DD, Workman, ML, and Mishler, MS: Medical-Surgical Nursing: A Nursing Process Approach, ed 2. WB Saunders, Philadelphia, 1995, with permission. (Data from Pennington, J: Bowe's and Church's Food Values of Portions Commonly Used, ed 16. JB Lippincott, Philadelphia, 1992.)

NUTRITION NOTES BOX 5–3

Sodium labeling definitions (serving size is an important variable):
Salt or sodium free—<5 mg sodium per serving
Very low sodium—<35 mg sodium per serving
Low sodium—<140 mg sodium per serving (per 100 g if main dish)

Teaching the caregivers about diuretic therapy is essential to prevent electrolyte imbalances. If a potassium-losing diuretic is prescribed, the nurse teaches which foods are high in potassium, such as oranges and other citrus fruits, melons, bananas, and potatoes. The client's serum potassium level needs to be periodically monitored by the physician or home care nurse. If it becomes too low, an oral potassium supplement is needed.

The family or other caregiver also needs to be taught the common signs and symptoms of fluid overload that should be reported to the physician or other health care provider. Of special importance is a weight gain. The client should be weighed at least three times a week in the home or nursing home if he or she is at high risk for fluid overload.

 CRITICAL THINKING: Mr. Peters

Mr. Peters is a 32-year-old man with a congenital heart problem. He has been recovering from congestive heart failure and fluid overload. Today his blood pressure is higher than usual, and his pulse is bounding. He is having trouble breathing and presses the call light for your assistance.

1. What should you do *first* when you assess Mr. Peters' condition?
2. What questions should you ask him?
3. What other assessments should you perform?

Answers at end of chapter.

Electrolyte Balance

Natural minerals in food become electrolytes or ions in the body through digestion and metabolism. Electrolytes are usually measured in milliequivalents per liter (mEq/L) or in milligrams per deciliter (mg/dL).

Electrolytes are one of two types: **cations,** which carry a positive electrical charge, and **anions,** which carry a negative electrical charge. Although there are many electrolytes in the body, this chapter discusses the most important ones, including sodium (Na^+), potassium (K^+), calcium (Ca^{++}), and magnesium (Mg^{++}).

Like fluid, electrolytes are essential substances in the body. Each electrolyte has specific functions. When there is a deficit or excess of any electrolyte, the client is at risk for potentially serious complications.

Electrolyte Imbalances

The two types of electrolyte imbalances are deficit and excess. A number of conditions and illnesses cause imbalances. In general, if a client experiences a deficit of an electrolyte, the electrolyte is replaced either orally or intravenously. If the client experiences an excess of the electrolyte, treatment focuses on getting rid of the excess, often via the kidneys. The underlying cause of the imbalance must also be treated.

The most important aspect of nursing care is preventing and assessing electrolyte imbalances. High-risk clients should be identified and monitored carefully. Patient education is another important nursing role for clients with electrolyte imbalances.

SODIUM IMBALANCES

The normal value for serum sodium is 135 to 145 mEg/L. Because sodium is the major cation in the blood, it helps maintain serum osmolarity. Therefore sodium imbalances are often associated with fluid imbalances, described earlier in this chapter. Sodium is also important for cell function, especially the central nervous system. The two sodium imbalances are **hyponatremia** (sodium deficit) and **hypernatremia** (sodium excess).

Hyponatremia

Hyponatremia occurs when the serum sodium level is less than 135 mEq/L.

Pathophysiology and Etiology

Many conditions can lead to either an actual or a relative decrease in sodium. In an actual decrease, the client has inadequate intake of sodium or excessive sodium loss from the body. In a relative decrease, the sodium is not lost from the body but leaves the intravascular space and moves into the interstitial tissues (third spacing). Another cause of a relative decrease occurs when the plasma volume increases (fluid overload) causing a dilutional effect of the sodium. The percentage of sodium compared with the fluid is diminished.

---

cation: cat—descending + ion—carrying
anion: an—without + ion—carrying
hyponatremia: hypo—less than + natr—sodium + emia—blood
hypernatremia: hyper—more than + natr—sodium + emia—blood

Table 5–4. *Clients at High Risk for Hyponatremia*

Nothing by mouth (NPO)
Excessive diaphoresis (sweating)
Diuretics
Gastrointestinal suction
Syndrome of inappropriate antidiuretic hormone
Excessive ingestion of hypotonic fluids
Freshwater near-drowning
Decreased aldosterone

Prevention

For clients at high risk for hyponatremia (Table 5–4), additional sodium is often administered, usually by the intravenous route to prevent a sodium deficit. Individuals who engage in strenuous exercise or physical labor, especially in the heat, need to replace sodium and water with drinks such as Gatorade that supply these vital substances. Water alone is not sufficient for electrolyte replacement.

Hyponatremia is especially dangerous for the elderly client. The client may not have specific signs and symptoms. The laboratory values for high-risk clients need to be monitored carefully.

Signs and Symptoms

Unfortunately, the signs and symptoms of hyponatremia are vague and depend somewhat on whether a fluid imbalance accompanies the hyponatremia. The client with sodium and fluid deficits has signs and symptoms of dehydration discussed earlier. The client with a sodium deficit and fluid overload has signs and symptoms associated with fluid overload.

In addition, the client experiences mental status changes, including disorientation, confusion, and personality changes, caused by cerebral edema (fluid around the brain). Weakness, nausea, and diarrhea may also occur.

Complications

In severe hyponatremia, respiratory arrest or coma can lead to death. The client who also has fluid overload may develop pulmonary edema, another life-threatening complication.

Diagnostic Tests

The primary diagnostic test is serum sodium, which is lower than the normal value. The serum osmolarity also decreases in clients with hyponatremia. Other laboratory tests may be affected if the client experiences an accompanying fluid imbalance. Serum chloride (Cl), an anion, is often depleted when sodium decreases because these two electrolytes commonly combine as NaCl (salt in solution, or saline).

Medical Treatment

The medical treatment focuses on resolving the underlying cause of hyponatremia and replacing the lost sodium. The physician orders intravenous saline for clients who have hyponatremia without fluid overload. The saline solution given may be isotonic (0.9%) or hypertonic (3%), depending on the severity of the problem.

For clients who have a fluid overload, a fluid restriction is often ordered. Diuretics that rid the body of fluid but do not cause sodium loss may also be needed. For clients with cerebral edema, dexamethasone (Decadron) may be prescribed to reduce the **intracranial** fluid. Intake and output are carefully monitored, as well as weights.

Hypernatremia

Hypernatremia occurs when the serum sodium level is above 145 mEq/L.

Pathophysiology and Etiology

Serum sodium increase may be an actual increase or a relative increase. In an actual increase, the client receives too much sodium or is unable to excrete sodium, as seen in renal failure. In a relative increase, the amount of sodium does not change but the amount of fluid in the intravascular space decreases. The percentage of sodium (solid) is increased in relationship to the amount of plasma (water).

In mild hypernatremia, most excitable tissues, such as muscle and neurons of the brain, become more stimulated. In severe cases, these tissues fail to respond.

Prevention

Prevention of hypernatremia is not as simple as prevention of hyponatremia. Most clients have a sodium excess as a result of an acute or chronic illness.

For clients receiving intravenous saline solutions, the nurse carefully regulates the flow rate as prescribed. Most IV solutions are controlled by an electronic infusion pump.

Signs and Symptoms

The signs and symptoms of hypernatremia are vague and nonspecific until severe excess is present. Like the client with a sodium deficit, the client experiencing sodium excess has mental status changes, such as agitation, confusion, and personality changes. Seizures may also occur.

At first, muscle twitches and unusual contractions may be present. Later, skeletal muscle weakness occurs that can lead to respiratory failure.

If fluid deficit or fluid overload accompanies the hypernatremic state, the client will have signs and symptoms associated with these imbalances as well.

Complications

The client experiencing severe hypernatremia may become comatose or have respiratory arrest as skeletal muscle weakness worsens.

---

intracranial: intra—within + cranial—cranium (skull)

Diagnostic Tests

The most reliable diagnostic test is serum sodium, which indicates an increase above the normal level. Serum osmolarity may also increase. If the client has a fluid imbalance, other laboratory values, such as BUN, hematocrit, and urine specific gravity, are affected (see earlier discussion in chapter).

Medical Treatment

If a fluid imbalance accompanies hypernatremia, it is treated first. For example, fluid replacement without sodium in a client with dehydration should correct a relative sodium excess. If the kidneys are not excreting adequate amounts of sodium, diuretics may help if the kidneys are functional. Intake and output is monitored, as well as weights.

The cause of hypernatremia is also treated in an attempt to prevent further episodes of this imbalance. For some clients, a sodium-restricted diet is prescribed.

POTASSIUM IMBALANCES

Potassium is the most common electrolyte in the intracellular fluid compartment. Therefore only a small amount, 3.5 to 5.0 mEq/L, is found in the bloodstream. Minimal changes in this laboratory value cause major changes in the body.

Potassium is especially important for muscle function—cardiac, skeletal, and smooth muscle. As the serum potassium level falls, the body attempts to compensate by moving intracellular potassium into the bloodstream.

The two potassium imbalances are **hypokalemia** (potassium deficit) and **hyperkalemia** (potassium excess). Hypokalemia is the most commonly occurring imbalance.

Hypokalemia

Hypokalemia occurs when the serum potassium level falls below 3.5 mEq/L.

Pathophysiology and Etiology

Most cases of hypokalemia result from inadequate intake of potassium or excessive loss of potassium by the kidneys. Hypokalemia most often occurs as a result of drug use. Potassium-losing diuretics (e.g., Lasix), digitalis preparations (e.g., Lanoxin), and corticosteroids (e.g., prednisone) are examples of drugs that cause excessive excretion of potassium from the body. Potassium may also be lost through the gastrointestinal (GI) tract, which is rich in potassium and other electrolytes. Severe vomiting, diarrhea, and prolonged GI suction cause hypokalemia. Major surgery and hemorrhage can also lead to potassium deficit.

Prevention

Most clients having major surgery receive potassium supplements in their intravenous fluids to prevent hypokale-

Table 5–5. *Common Food Sources of Potassium**

Food Source	Amount (mg)
Corn flakes (1¼ c)	26
Cooked oatmeal (¾ c)	99
Egg (1 large)	66
Codfish, raw (4 oz)	400
Salmon, pink, raw (3½ oz)	306
Tuna fish (4 oz)	375
Apple, raw with skin (1 medium)	159
Banana (1 medium)	451
Cantaloupe (1 c pieces)	494
Grapefruit (½ medium)	175
Orange (1 medium)	250
Raisins (½ c)	700
Strawberries, raw (1 c)	247
Watermelon (1 c pieces)	186
White bread (1 slice)	27
Whole-wheat bread (1 slice)	44
Beef (4 oz)	480
Beef liver (3½ oz)	281
Pork, fresh (4 oz)	525
Pork, cured (4 oz)	325
Chicken (4 oz)	225
Veal cutlet (3½ oz)	448
Whole milk (8 oz)	370
Skim milk (8 oz)	406
Avocado (1 medium)	1097
Carrot (1 large)	341
Corn (4-inch ear)	196
Cauliflower (1 c pieces)	295
Celery (1 stalk)	170
Green beans (1 c)	189
Mushrooms (10 small)	410
Onion (1 medium)	157
Peas (¾ c)	316
Potato, white (1 medium)	407
Spinach, raw (3½ oz)	470
Tomato (1 medium)	366

*U.S. Department of Agriculture recommended daily allowance for adults: 1875–5625 mg.
Sources: Pennington, J: Bowe's and Church's Food Values of Portions Commonly Used, ed 16. JB Lippincott, Philadelphia, 1992. Ignatavicius, DD, et al: Medical-Surgical Nursing: A Nursing Process Approach, ed 2. WB Saunders, Philadelphia, 1995, with permission.

mia. For clients receiving drugs known to cause hypokalemia, foods high in potassium may prevent a deficit (Table 5–5). Clients receiving digitalis must be closely monitored because hypokalemia can enhance the action of digitalis and cause digitalis toxicity.

Signs and Symptoms

Many body systems are affected when potassium imbalance occurs. Vital signs change because the respiratory and cardiovascular systems need potassium to function prop-

hypokalemia: hypo—less than + kal—potassium + emia—blood
hyperkalemia: hyper—more than + kal—potassium + emia—blood

erly. Skeletal muscle activity diminishes, resulting in shallow, ineffective respirations. The pulse rate is typically weak, irregular, and thready because the heart muscle is depleted of potassium. Orthostatic (postural) hypotension may also be present.

The nervous system is usually affected as well. The client experiences changes in mental status, followed by lethargy. The motility of the GI system is slowed, causing nausea, vomiting, abdominal distention, and constipation. These symptoms further increase potassium loss.

Complications

If not corrected, hypokalemia can result in death from **dysrhythmia,** respiratory failure and arrest, or coma. The client must be treated promptly before these complications occur.

Diagnostic Tests

In addition to a decrease in serum potassium, the client may have an acid-base imbalance known as metabolic alkalosis, which commonly accompanies hypokalemia. In metabolic alkalosis, the serum pH of the blood increases (above 7.45) such that the blood is more alkaline than usual. Acid-base imbalances are discussed later in this chapter.

The client's electrocardiogram (ECG) shows cardiac dysrhythmias associated with potassium deficit.

Medical Treatment

The goal of treatment is to replace potassium in the body and resolve the underlying cause of the imbalance. For mild to moderate hypokalemia, oral potassium supplements are given. For severe hypokalemia, intravenous potassium supplements are given. Potassium is a potentially dangerous drug, especially when administered by the IV route. The client's laboratory values must be monitored carefully to prevent giving too much potassium, another potentially life-threatening imbalance.

The nurse teaches the client about the side effects of oral potassium and precautions associated with potassium administration. Table 5–6 summarizes the precautions the nurse needs to be aware of when giving oral potassium supplements.

Hyperkalemia

Hyperkalemia is a condition in which the serum potassium is greater than 5.0 mEq/L. It is rare in an individual with healthy kidneys.

Pathophysiology and Etiology

Hyperkalemia may result from an actual increase in the amount of total body potassium or from the movement of

---

Table 5–6. _Patient Education Tips for Patients Receiving Oral Potassium Supplements_

- Do not substitute one potassium supplement for another.
- Dilute powders and liquids in juice or other desired liquid to improve taste and to prevent gastrointestinal irritation. Follow manufacturer's recommendations for the amount of fluid to use for dilution, most commonly 4 oz per 20 mEq of potassium.
- Do not drink diluted solutions until mixed thoroughly.
- Do not crush potassium tablets, such as Slow-K or K-tab tablets. Read manufacturer's directions regarding which tablets can be crushed.
- Administer slow-release tablets with 8 oz of water to help them dissolve.
- Do not take potassium supplements if taking potassium-sparing diuretics such as spironolactone or triamterene.
- Do not use salt substitutes containing potassium unless prescribed by the physician.
- Take potassium supplements with meals.
- Report adverse effects, such as nausea, vomiting, diarrhea, and abdominal cramping, to the physician.
- Have frequent laboratory testing for potassium levels as recommended by the physician.

Source: Adapted from Lee, CA, Barrett, CA, and Ignatavicius, DD: Fluids and Electrolytes: A Practical Approach, ed 4. FA Davis, Philadelphia, 1996.

---

intracellular potassium into the blood. Excessive potassium intake can be caused by overuse of potassium-based salt substitutes or potassium-sparing diuretics (e.g., Aldactone), or by excessive intake of oral or intravenous potassium supplements. Excessive serum potassium can also occur in clients with renal failure because the kidneys cannot excrete it.

Movement of potassium from the cells into the blood and other extracellular fluid is common in massive tissue trauma and metabolic acidosis. Metabolic acidosis is an acid-base imbalance commonly seen in clients with diabetes mellitus. Acid-base imbalances are discussed later in this chapter.

Prevention

For clients receiving potassium supplements, hyperkalemia can be prevented by monitoring laboratory values and client signs and symptoms.

Signs and Symptoms

Most cases of hyperkalemia occur in hospitalized clients or those undergoing medical treatment for a chronic condition. The classic manifestations are muscle twitches and cramps, later followed by profound muscular weakness; increased GI motility (diarrhea); slow, irregular heart rate; and decreased blood pressure.

Complications

Cardiac dysrhythmias and respiratory failure can occur in severe hyperkalemia, causing death.

---

dysrhythmia: dys—bad or disordered + rhythmia—measured motion

Diagnostic Tests

In addition to an elevated serum potassium, the client has an irregular ECG associated with hyperkalemia. If the client also has metabolic acidosis, the serum pH falls below 7.35.

Medical Treatment

For mild, chronic hyperkalemia, dietary limitation of potassium-rich foods may be helpful. (See Table 5–5.) Potassium supplements are discontinued, and potassium-losing diuretics are given to clients with healthy kidneys. For clients with renal problems, a cation exchange resin, such as sodium polystyrene sulfonate (Kayexalate), is administered either orally or rectally. This drug releases sodium and absorbs potassium for excretion through the feces and out of the body.

In cases in which cellular potassium has moved into the bloodstream, the administration of glucose and insulin can facilitate the movement of potassium back into the cells. During treatment of moderate to severe hyperkalemia, the client should be in a cardiac-monitored bed in the hospital.

CALCIUM IMBALANCES

Calcium is a mineral that is primarily stored in bones and teeth. A small amount is found in extracellular fluid. The normal value for serum calcium is 9 to 11 mg/dL, or 4.5 to 5.5 mEq/L. Minimal changes in serum calcium levels can have major negative effects in the body.

Calcium is needed for the proper function of excitable tissues, especially cardiac muscle. It is also needed for adequate blood clotting. The two calcium imbalances are **hypocalcemia** and **hypercalcemia.**

Hypocalcemia

Hypocalcemia occurs when the serum calcium falls below 9 mg/dL or 4.5 mEq/L.

Pathophysiology and Etiology

Although calcium deficit can be acute or chronic, most clients develop hypocalcemia slowly as a result of chronic disease or poor intake. The postmenopausal client is most at risk for hypocalcemia. As a woman ages, calcium intake typically declines. The parathyroid glands recognize this decrease and stimulate bone to release some of its stored calcium into the blood for replacement. The result is a condition known as **osteoporosis,** in which bones become porous and brittle and fracture easily. The postmenopausal woman has a decreased level of estrogens, hormones that help prevent bone loss in the younger woman. Immobility or decreased mobility also contributes to bone loss in many clients. The highest-risk clients for osteoporosis are thin, petite, Caucasian women.

Hypocalcemia may also result from inadequate absorption of calcium from the intestines, as seen in clients with Crohn's disease—a chronic inflammatory bowel disease. An insufficient intake of vitamin D prevents calcium absorption as well. Conditions that interfere with the production of parathyroid hormone can also cause hypocalcemia, such as partial or complete thyroid or parathyroid surgical removal.

Finally, clients with hyperphosphatemia (usually those with renal failure) often experience hypocalcemia. Calcium and phosphate have an inverse relationship. When one of these electrolytes increases, the other decreases, and vice versa.

Prevention

In the United States, the typical daily calcium intake is less than 550 mg. The recommended daily allowance of calcium is 800 mg, and many researchers believe that it should be twice that amount.

Hypocalcemia can be prevented in premenopausal and postmenopausal women by consuming calcium-rich foods and by taking calcium supplements. These supplements can be purchased over the counter in any pharmacy or large food store. An inexpensive source of calcium is Tums (calcium carbonate), which provides 240 mg of elemental calcium in each tablet.

Vitamin D supplementation may also be required for homebound or institutionalized clients who have no exposure to the sun, the best source of vitamin D.

Signs and Symptoms

Chronic hypocalcemia is usually not diagnosed until the client breaks a bone, usually a hip. Acute hypocalcemia, which can occur following surgery or in clients with acute pancreatitis, has several signs and symptoms. These signs and symptoms include increased and irregular heart rate, mental status changes, hyperactive deep tendon reflexes, and increased GI motility, including diarrhea and abdominal cramping. Two classic signs that can be used to assess for hypocalcemia are Trousseau's sign and Chvostek's sign.

To test for Trousseau's sign, a blood pressure cuff is inflated around the client's upper arm for 1 to 4 minutes. In a client with hypocalcemia, the hand and fingers become spastic and go into palmar flexion (Fig. 5–3). A positive Chvostek's sign also indicates calcium deficit. To test for this sign, the face just below and in front of the ear is tapped. Facial twitching on that side of the face results in a positive test (Fig. 5–4).

Complications

In severe hypocalcemia, seizures, respiratory failure, or cardiac failure can occur and lead to death if not aggressively treated.

---

hypocalcemia: hypo—less than + calc—calcium + emia—blood
hypercalcemia: hyper—more than + calc—calcium + emia—blood
osteoporosis: osteo—bone + porosis—porous

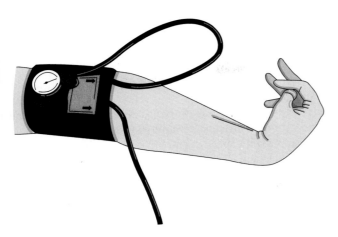

Figure 5–3. Trousseau's sign. (Modified from Morton: Health Assessment in Nursing, ed 2. FA Davis, Philadelphia, 1993, p 601, with permission.)

Diagnostic Tests

The client with hypocalcemia has a lowered serum calcium and an abnormal ECG. The parathyroid hormone level may be increased because it stimulates bone to release more calcium for the blood.

Medical Treatment

In addition to treating the cause of hypocalcemia, calcium is replaced. For mild or chronic hypocalcemia, oral calcium supplements with or without vitamin D are given. Calcium supplements should be administered 1 to 2 hours after meals to increase intestinal absorption.

For acute or severe hypocalcemia, intravenous calcium gluconate or calcium chloride is given. When a client has thyroid or parathyroid surgery, the medication must be readily available for emergency use.

For clients with hyperphosphatemia, usually those with renal failure, aluminum hydroxide is used to bind the excess phosphate for elimination via the GI tract. As the phosphate decreases, the serum calcium begins to increase closer to normal levels.

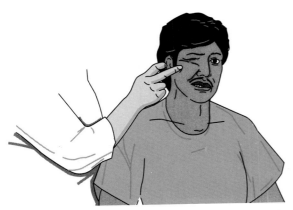

Figure 5–4. Chvostek's sign. (Modified from Morton: Health Assessment in Nursing, ed 2. FA Davis, Philadelphia, 1993, p 601, with permission.)

Diet therapy is an important part of treatment. The nurse teaches the client, family, or other caregiver which foods are high in calcium (Table 5–7). Many foods today are fortified with calcium. Vitamin D foods are also encouraged, especially milk and other dairy products.

CRITICAL THINKING: Mrs. Wright

Mrs. Wright is a 77-year-old petite Caucasian woman who lives alone at home. She is on a fixed income and rarely eats high-calcium foods. She recently fell and broke her hip. After surgery she returned to home under the care of a home health agency.

1. What made the client at high risk for a fracture?
2. What would you expect her serum calcium level to have been before the fall?
3. What client teaching related to diet and calcium supplements should the home health care nurse include during his or her home visits?

Answers at end of chapter.

Hypercalcemia

Hypercalcemia occurs when the serum calcium is above 11 mg/dL or 5.5 mEq/L.

Pathophysiology and Etiology

Chronic hypercalcemia can result from excessive intake of calcium or vitamin D, renal failure, hyperparathyroidism, and overuse or prolonged use of thiazide diuretics, such as hydrochlorothiazide (HydroDiuril). Acute hypercalcemia can occur as an oncologic emergency in clients with invasive or metastatic cancers.

Table 5–7. Quantities of Food Containing Calcium Equal to 1 Cup of Milk in Order of Energy Content

Food	Amount	Kilocalories
Skim milk	1 c	86
Grated Parmesan cheese	4.3 tbs	99
Plain low-fat yogurt	0.7 c	101
Swiss cheese	1.1 oz	118
2% milk	1 c	121
Whole milk	1 c	150
Cheddar cheese	1.5 oz	171
Processed American cheese	1.7 oz	180
Low-fat yogurt with fruit	0.9 c	199
Blue cheese	2 oz	200
Vanilla milkshake	0.9 c	273
2% low-fat cottage cheese	2 c	410
Hard ice cream, vanilla	1.7 c	459
Soft ice cream	1.3 c	479
Cottage cheese, creamed, large curd	2.25 c	529
Sherbet	2.9 c	786

Source: Adapted from Lutz, CA, and Przytulski, KR: Nutrition and Diet Therapy, ed 2. FA Davis, Philadelphia, 1997, p 172.

Prevention

Although many causes of increased calcium cannot be prevented, an individual receiving calcium supplements should be monitored carefully. Some women believe that if 2 or 3 tablets a day is helpful, they will consume twice that much. The result can be serum calcium excess. Educating the public about the proper amount of calcium needed each day and the danger of too much calcium is very important.

Signs and Symptoms

Clients who have mild hypercalcemia or a slowly progressing calcium increase may have no obvious signs and symptoms. However, acute hypercalcemia is associated with increased heart rate and blood pressure, skeletal muscle weakness, and decreased GI motility. The client also has a decreased ability for blood clotting.

Complications

In some cases, the client may experience renal or urinary calculi (stones) resulting from the buildup of calcium. In more severe cases of acute hypercalcemia, the client may experience respiratory failure caused by profound muscle weakness or heart failure caused by dysrhythmias.

Medical Treatment

Clients with severe hypercalcemia should be hospitalized and placed on a cardiac monitor. To prevent calculi formation and help the kidneys excrete some of the excess calcium, intravenous therapy is prescribed. Saline infusions are the most useful solutions to promote renal excretion of calcium.

The physician also discontinues thiazide diuretics if the client was receiving them and prescribes diuretics that promote calcium excretion, such as furosemide (Lasix). Other drugs that bind with calcium to lower calcium levels may also be used, such as plicamycin (mithramycin, Mithracin) and D-penicillamine (Cuprimine).

If hypercalcemia is so severe that cardiac problems are present, hemodialysis (artificial kidney), peritoneal dialysis, or ultrafiltration may be necessary. (See Chapter 35 for discussion of these procedures.)

MAGNESIUM IMBALANCES

Magnesium and calcium work together for the proper functioning of excitable cells, such as cardiac muscle and nerve cells. Therefore an imbalance of magnesium is usually accompanied by an imbalance of calcium.

The normal value for serum magnesium is 1.5 to 2.5 mEq/L. The magnesium imbalances are called **hypomagnesemia** and **hypermagnesemia.**

Hypomagnesemia

Hypomagnesemia occurs when the serum magnesium level falls below 1.5 mEq/L. It results from either a decreased

intake or an excessive loss of magnesium. Causes of inadequate intake include malnutrition and starvation diets. Clients with severe diarrhea and Crohn's disease are unable to absorb magnesium in the intestines.

One of the major causes of hypomagnesemia is alcoholism, from both a decreased intake and an increased renal excretion. Certain drugs, such as loop (high-ceiling) and osmotic diuretics, aminoglycosides (e.g., gentamicin), and some anticancer agents (e.g., cisplatin), can increase renal excretion of magnesium.

The signs and symptoms of hypomagnesemia are similar to those for hypocalcemia, including a positive Trousseau's and Chvostek's sign, described earlier in the chapter.

The goal of management is to treat the underlying cause and replace magnesium in the body. Magnesium sulfate is administered intravenously. If the serum calcium is also low, calcium replacement is prescribed. The client is placed on a cardiac monitor because of magnesium's effect on the heart. Life-threatening dysrhythmias can lead to cardiac failure and arrest.

Hypermagnesemia

Hypermagnesemia results when the serum magnesium level increases above 2.5 mEq/L. The most common cause of hypermagnesemia is increased intake coupled with decreased renal excretion caused by renal failure.

Signs and symptoms are usually not apparent until the serum level is greater than 4 mEq/L. Then the signs and symptoms include bradycardia and other dysrhythmias, hypotension, lethargy or drowsiness, and skeletal muscle weakness. If not treated, the client will experience coma, respiratory failure, or cardiac failure.

When kidneys are functioning properly, loop diuretics such as Lasix and intravenous fluids can help increase magnesium excretion. For clients with renal failure, dialysis may be the only option.

Acid-Base Balance

The cells of the body function best when the body fluids and electrolytes are within a very narrow range. Hydrogen (H+) is another ion that must stay within its normal limits. The amount of hydrogen determines whether a fluid is an acid or base.

An acid is a substance that releases hydrogen when dissolved in water. The stronger the acid, the more hydrogen ions are released. A common acid in the body is hydrochloric acid (HCl), which is found in the stomach. A base is a substance that binds hydrogen when dissolved

hypomagnesemia: hypo—less than + magnes—magnesium + emia—blood
hypermagnesemia: hyper—more than + magnes—magnesium + emia—blood

in water. A common base in the body is bicarbonate (HCO_3).

SOURCES OF ACIDS AND BASES

Acids and bases are formed in the body as part of normal metabolic processes. Acids are formed as end products of glucose, fat, and protein metabolism. These acids are called fixed acids because they do not change once they are formed. A weak acid, carbonic acid, can be formed when the carbon dioxide resulting from cellular metabolism combines with water. This acid can again change to bicarbonate (a base) and hydrogen and therefore is not a fixed acid.

The extracellular fluid maintains a delicate balance between acids and bases. The strength of the acids and bases can be measured by pH (potential of hydrogen). The pH of a solution can vary from 1 to 14, with 7 being neutral, 1 to 6.99 being acid, and 7.01 to 14 being base, also called alkaline. The serum pH is 7.35 to 7.45, or slightly alkaline. It must remain in this extremely narrow range to sustain life.

CONTROL OF ACID-BASE BALANCE

As discussed for fluid and electrolyte balance, the body has several ways in which it tries to compensate for changes in the serum pH. A pH below 6.9 or above 7.8 is usually fatal. Three major mechanisms may be used—cellular buffers, the lungs, and the kidneys.

Cellular buffers are the first to attempt a return of the pH to its normal range. Examples of cellular buffers are proteins, hemoglobin, bicarbonate, and phosphates. These buffers act as a type of "sponge" to "soak up" extra hydrogen ions if there are too many (too acidic) or release hydrogen ions if there are not enough (too alkaline).

The lungs are the second line of defense to restore normal pH. When the blood is too acidic (pH is decreased), the lungs "blow off" additional carbon dioxide, which would otherwise make more carbonic acid in the body, through rapid, deep breathing. If the blood is too alkaline (pH is increased), the lungs try to conserve carbon dioxide through shallow respirations.

The kidneys are the last to respond to changes in serum pH, taking as long as 24 to 48 hours to assist with compensation. The kidneys help in a number of ways, including regulating the amount of bicarbonate (base) that is kept in the body. If the serum pH lowers and becomes too acidic, the kidneys reabsorb additional bicarbonate rather than excreting it so that it can help neutralize the acid. If the serum pH increases and becomes too alkaline, the kidneys excrete additional bicarbonate to get rid of the extra base. The kidneys also buffer pH by forming acids and ammonium (a base).

Acid-Base Imbalances

Most acid-base imbalances are caused by a number of acute and chronic illnesses or conditions. The primary treatment for each of the imbalances is to manage the underlying cause, which corrects the imbalance. The role of the nurse is to identify clients at risk and monitor laboratory test values for significant changes.

LEARNING TIP

To remember the types and causes of acid-base imbalances:

> Lungs = Carbon Dioxide (CO_2) = acid
>
> Kidneys = Bicarbonate = Base

The laboratory tests that are used are called arterial blood gases (ABGs). As the name implies, the blood sample that is analyzed must be from an artery, rather than a vein. The femoral, brachial, and radial arteries are most often used to obtain the sample. Table 5–8 lists these major tests and normal values. The partial pressure of oxygen is not as helpful in determining the type of imbalance when compared with the serum pH, partial pressure of carbon dioxide, and bicarbonate levels.

The two broad types of acid-base imbalance are **acidosis** and **alkalosis.** Each of these types can occur suddenly, called an acute imbalance, or develop over a long period of time, referred to as a chronic imbalance.

When the serum pH falls below 7.35, the client has acidosis because the blood becomes more acidic than normal. Acidosis is caused by too much acid in the body or too little base. It can be divided into two types: respiratory acidosis and metabolic acidosis.

When the serum pH increases above 7.45, the client has alkalosis because the blood becomes more alkaline or basic. Alkalosis is caused by too little acid in the body or too much base. It can also be divided into two types: respiratory alkalosis and metabolic alkalosis.

Table 5–8. **Normal Values for Arterial Blood Gases**

Test	Normal Range
pH	7.35–7.45
PaO_2	>80 mm Hg
$PaCO_2$	32–45 mm Hg
HCO_3	20–26 mEq/L

---

acidosis: acid—acidic + osis—condition

alkalosis: alka—alkaline + (l)osis)—condition

RESPIRATORY ACIDOSIS

As the name indicates, the primary etiology of this type of acidosis is respiratory problems. Carbon dioxide is not adequately "blown off" during expiration, causing a buildup of carbon dioxide in the blood. As mentioned earlier, carbon dioxide mixes with water to create a weak acid in the body, thus increasing the acidity of the blood.

Acute respiratory acidosis occurs in clients with respiratory depression, caused by drugs and neurologic problems, such as strokes, and inadequate chest expansion, caused by muscle weakness, ascites (excess peritoneal fluid), hemothorax (blood in the thoracic cavity), or pneumothorax (air in the thoracic cavity).

More commonly seen is clients with chronic respiratory acidosis. Many clients with COPD are not able to exhale completely because of overinflated alveoli (emphysema) or obstructed bronchi (chronic bronchitis). The PaO_2 decreases and the $PaCO_2$ level increases (Table 5–9). As the kidneys try to conserve bicarbonate as a compensation mechanism, the bicarbonate value may also increase slightly.

The signs and symptoms of respiratory acidosis involve the central nervous system and the musculoskeletal system. As carbon dioxide increases, mental status changes become more profound, progressing from confusion and lethargy to stupor and coma, if not treated. The lungs are not able to get rid of excess carbon dioxide. Instead respirations become more depressed and shallow as muscle weakness worsens.

The treatment of respiratory acidosis is aggressive management of the underlying respiratory problem, discussed in the respiratory unit of this text.

METABOLIC ACIDOSIS

Metabolic acidosis can result from too much acid in the body (usually fixed acids) or too little bicarbonate in the body. Uncontrolled diabetes mellitus and end-stage renal failure are the two most common causes of metabolic acidosis resulting from increased fixed acids.

The GI tract is rich in bicarbonate. Clients experiencing severe diarrhea or prolonged nasointestinal suction are at high risk for metabolic acidosis as a result of bicarbonate (base) loss.

As seen in Table 5–9, the serum pH decreases and the bicarbonate level decreases. As mentioned earlier under the discussion on hyperkalemia, serum potassium tends to increase in the presence of metabolic acidosis. Excess hydrogen in the extracellular fluid moves into the cells in exchange for potassium, which leaves the cells and enters the blood. In a sense, this is a way of compensating for the acidotic state.

The signs and symptoms are similar to those associated with respiratory acidosis with the exception of the respiratory pattern. To help compensate for the acidotic state, the lungs get rid of extra carbon dioxide through Kussmaul's respirations. These respirations are deep and rapid and can occur only in clients with healthy lungs.

The treatment for the client with metabolic acidosis is management of the underlying disease or condition. Information about disease management, such as diabetes, is found elsewhere in this book.

RESPIRATORY ALKALOSIS

Respiratory alkalosis is probably the least common acid-base imbalance. It occurs when there is excessive loss of carbon dioxide through **hyperventilation.** Clients may hyperventilate when they are severely anxious or fearful. Mechanical ventilation can also cause respiratory alkalosis, as well as high altitudes.

Clients who hyperventilate have rapid shallow respirations, are light-headed, and may become confused. The heart rate increases and the pulse becomes weak and thready. The serum pH is increased and the $PaCO_2$ is very low.

The treatment for respiratory alkalosis is the administration of additional carbon dioxide through either a rebreathing oxygen mask or a plain paper bag.

METABOLIC ALKALOSIS

Metabolic alkalosis results from excessive ingestion of bicarbonate or other bases or loss of acids from the body. Overuse or abuse of antacids or baking soda (sodium bicarbonate) can lead to metabolic alkalosis. Because the stomach contains hydrochloric acid, prolonged vomiting or nasogastric suction can cause loss of acid and also lead to metabolic alkalosis.

The serum pH is increased and bicarbonate is also increased. As discussed under potassium imbalances, the serum potassium also decreases. Hydrogen from the intracellular fluid moves into the blood in exchange for

---

Table 5–9. **Arterial Blood Gas Value Changes in Acid-Base Imbalances**

Acid-Base Imbalance	pH	$PaCO_2$	HCO_3
Respiratory acidosis	Decreased	Increased	Unchanged
Metabolic acidosis	Decreased	Unchanged	Decreased
Respiratory alkalosis	Increased	Decreased	Unchanged
Metabolic alkalosis	Increased	Unchanged	Increased

---

hyperventilation: hyper—more than + ventilation—air

potassium, which moves from the blood into the cells. This is one way that the body works to keep an acid-base balance. Hypocalcemia may also accompany hypokalemia.

The signs and symptoms of metabolic alkalosis are related to hypokalemia and hypocalcemia rather than the alkalotic state itself. Treatment involves identifying the underlying cause and managing it as quickly as possible.

Review Questions

1. Mrs. Rodriguez is a 93-year-old client admitted to the hospital from an extended care facility with diarrhea and dehydration. Which of the following symptoms of dehydration do you expect to see?
   a. Pale-colored urine, bradycardia
   b. Disorientation, tenting
   c. Decreased hematocrit, hypothermia
   d. Lung congestion, abdominal discomfort

2. Which of the following is the *most* reliable way to monitor Mrs. Rodriguez's fluid status?
   a. Intake and output (I&O)
   b. Skin turgor
   c. Daily weights
   d. Lung sounds

3. When caring for a client with fluid overload, which of the following interventions will help relieve respiratory distress?
   a. Elevate the head of the bed.
   b. Encourage the client to cough and deep breathe.
   c. Increase fluids to promote urine output.
   d. Perform percussion and postural drainage.

4. Mr. Janes is being treated for hypokalemia. When evaluating his response to potassium replacement therapy, the nurse observes for which of the following changes in his assessment?
   a. Improving visual acuity
   b. Worsening constipation
   c. Decreasing serum glucose
   d. Increasing muscle strength

5. Which of the following organ systems is most at risk for life-threatening complications when a client has hyperkalemia?
   a. Cardiovascular
   b. Renal
   c. Nervous
   d. Musculoskeletal

6. When instructing a client to follow a high-potassium diet, the nurse includes the importance of eating which of the following foods?
   a. Fish and fruit
   b. Breads and cereals
   c. Pasta and cream soups
   d. Eggs and broth

7. David has respiratory acidosis. Which of the following conditions most likely predisposed him to this condition?
   a. Diabetes
   b. Anxiety
   c. Kidney failure
   d. Chronic lung disease

8. Which of the following adaptive responses occurs when a client is in metabolic acidosis?
   a. Respiratory depression
   b. Kussmaul's respirations
   c. Increased urine output
   d. Highly concentrated urine

 ANSWERS TO CRITICAL THINKING

Critical Thinking: Mrs. Levitt

1. Expect increased, weak, and thready pulse; decreased blood pressure; and possibly increased temperature caused by hypovolemia.
2. Encourage increased fluid intake; monitor fluid intake and output; recheck vital signs.

Critical Thinking: Mr. Peters

1. Place the head of the bed up to assist with breathing.
2. Questions to ask might include the following: When did your symptoms begin? Have you had these symptoms before? (If the client is too dyspneic to answer, do not ask many questions.)
3. Check breath sounds for crackles, observe for dependent edema and ascites, observe for distended neck veins, assess skin for color and temperature, and monitor intake and output.

Critical Thinking: Mrs. Wright

1. Osteoporosis because she is an elderly, petite, Caucasian woman.
2. Lower than normal.
3. Teach her about consuming foods high in calcium, teach her about the need to be compliant with taking her calcium supplements, and teach her to take them 1 to 2 hours after meals for best absorption by the body.

BIBLIOGRAPHY

Booker, MF, and Ignatavicius, DD: Infusion Therapy: Techniques and Medications. WB Saunders, Philadelphia, 1996.
Dennison, R, and Blevins, B: Myths and facts about fluid imbalance. Nursing 22(3):22, 1992.

Dennison, R, and Blevins, B: Myths and facts about electrolyte imbalances. Nursing 22(2):26, 1992.

Ignatavicius, DD, Workman, ML, and Mishler, MA: Medical-Surgical Nursing: A Nursing Process Approach. WB Saunders, Philadelphia, 1995.

Kokko, J, and Tannen, R: Fluids and Electrolytes, ed 3. WB Saunders, Philadelphia, 1995.

Lee, CA, Barrett, A, and Ignatavicius, DD: Fluids and Electrolytes: A Practical Approach, ed 4. FA Davis, Philadelphia, 1996.

Lipson, J, and Haifizi, H: Iranians. In Purnell, L, and Paulanka, B (eds): Transcultural Health Care: A Culturally Competent Approach. FA Davis, Philadelphia, 1997.

Lutz, CA, and Przytulski, KR: Nutrition and Diet Therapy. FA Davis, Philadelphia, 1994.

Metheney, N: Fluid and Electrolyte Balance: Nursing Considerations. JB Lippincott, Philadelphia, 1992.

Norris, MK: Evaluating sodium levels. Nursing 22(7):20, 1992.

Tasota, F, and Wesmiller, S: Assessing ABGs: Maintaining the delicate balance. Nursing 24(5):34, 1994.

Terry, J: The major electrolytes: Sodium, potassium, and chloride. J Intravenous Nurs 17(5):240, 1994.

Towle, C: Turkish Americans. In Purnell, L, and Paulanka, B (eds): Transcultural Health Care: A Culturally Competent Approach. FA Davis, Philadelphia, 1997.

Nursing Care of Clients Receiving Intravenous Therapy

Jill Secord

6

Learning Objectives

Upon completion of this chapter, the student will be able to:

1. Define intravenous therapy.
2. Explain how the practice of intravenous therapy is regulated.
3. Identify rationale for the use of intravenous therapy.
4. Identify the preferred sites for the initiation of intravenous therapy.
5. Discuss factors that influence the condition, size, and long-term use of veins.
6. Describe the technique for insertion of an intravenous catheter.
7. Identify and describe nursing interventions for complications of intravenous therapy.
8. Calculate a drip rate for a client receiving a parenteral solution.
9. Identify the difference between isotonic, hypertonic, and hypotonic solutions.
10. Develop beginning knowledge of midline catheters, subcutaneous infusions, and implanted pumps.

Key Words

bolus (**BOH**-lus)
cannula (**KAN**-yoo-lah)
hypertonic (HIGH-per-**TAHN**-ik)
hypotonic (HIGH-poh-**TAHN**-ik)
intravenous (IN-trah-**VEE**-nus)
isotonic (EYE-so-**TAHN**-ik)

Intravenous (IV) therapy is the administration of fluids or medication via a needle or catheter (**cannula**) directly into the bloodstream. The practice of IV therapy is regulated by the Intravenous Nursing Society and is guided by the Intravenous Standards of Practice. These standards define the nurse's scope of practice and educational requirements. The Centers for Disease Control (CDC) provide guidelines for prevention of infection. The Occupational Safety and Health Administration (OSHA) provides regulations to maintain health care worker safety. State licensing and institution policy determines who can administer IV therapy. Some states now include IV therapy within the licensed practical nurse (LPN) and licensed vocational nurse (LVN) job role.

Rationale for Intravenous Therapy

Clients receive IV therapy for a variety of purposes, including administration of fluids, electrolytes, nutrients, medications, and blood products. Clients can receive life-sustaining fluids, electrolytes, and nutrition when they are unable to eat or drink adequate amounts. The IV route provides rapid access for medication in an emergency. Many medications are faster acting and more effective when given via this route. Other medications can be administered continuously in order to maintain a therapeutic blood level. Clients with anemia or blood loss receive lifesaving IV transfusions. Clients who are unable to eat for an extended period of time can have their nutritional needs met with total parenteral nutrition (TPN). Clients may have an IV catheter inserted and capped with a needle access port, to provide access to the bloodstream for intermittent or emergency medications.

Intravenous Access

Intravenous therapy can be administered into either peripheral or central veins. Peripheral veins lie near the surface of

81

the skin. They are usually an easy way to gain access to the venous system. Central veins are close to the heart. Special catheters that end in a large vessel near the heart are called central lines. This chapter will primarily discuss peripheral catheters. Central catheters are explained briefly at the end of the chapter.

Administering Peripheral Intravenous Therapy

STARTING THE INTRAVENOUS NEEDLE

Gather Equipment

The nurse obtains an assortment of cannulas, a tourniquet, tape, antimicrobial solution (such as alcohol), clean gloves, and IV solution and tubing set or injection cap, depending on whether a fluid infusion is planned. An arm board, IV pole, adhesive bandages, syringes, sterile sponges, filter, and antiseptic swabs may also be used based on intended therapy, nurse preference, and institution policy. Note that OSHA guidelines allow the tourniquet to be kept and reused for the same client, but it cannot be used on another client. Some institutions carry IV start kits, which contain a tourniquet, gloves, alcohol, bandage, and antimicrobial solution.

Wash Hands

Before beginning the procedure, hands should be washed for 15 to 20 seconds. Gloves are worn when inserting the needle.

Choose the Cannula

Needles have been largely replaced with flexible plastic catheters, or cannulas, that are inserted over a needle (Fig. 6–1). The needle is removed after the catheter is in place. These are available in a variety of sizes (gauges) and lengths. For client comfort, the nurse chooses the smallest-gauge catheter that will work for the intended purpose. Smaller-gauge needles (20 to 24 gauge) are used for fluids and slow infusion rates. Larger needles (18 gauge) are used for rapid fluid administration and viscous solutions such as blood. The nurse also considers vein size when choosing a catheter gauge. The nurse should refer to institution policy and equipment stock for specific recommendations.

Explain the Procedure

The nurse briefly explains the procedure to the client. The client should be told to expect some discomfort. Use of distraction such as music or television can be helpful.

Choose the Vein

Proper vein selection is important in order to accommodate the prescribed therapy and to minimize potential complications (Tables 6–1 and 6–2). The nurse avoids use of an arm on the side where the client has had a mastectomy, has a dialysis access site, or is scheduled for a surgical procedure. The nurse should also be careful to avoid a vessel that is pulsating, because accidental arterial puncture could cause serious bleeding. The client's condition and diagnosis, age, vein condition, size, location, and type and duration of therapy are considered. The vein should be able to accommodate the gauge and length of catheter used. (See Cultural Considerations Box 6–1.)

Hand veins are used first if intravenous therapy will be prolonged. This allows for each successive **venipuncture** to be made proximal to the site of the previous one. This eliminates irritating fluids passing through a previously injured vein and discourages leaking through old puncture sites. Hand veins can be used successfully for most hydrating solutions, but they are best avoided when irritating solutions of potassium or antibiotics are anticipated.

Vein size must also be considered. Small veins do not tolerate large volumes of fluid, high infusion rates, or irritating solutions. Large veins should be used for these purposes. See Figure 6–2 for peripheral veins that may be used for IV therapy.

LEARNING TIP

As you insert the IV needle, try to visualize the veins in your mind even if they are not readily visible on the client.

Factors That Influence Vein Condition

Multiple needle sticks and caustic medications can render a vein unusable for life. Care should be used during the needle insertion to minimize trauma.

If veins are constricted, venipuncture is more difficult. Fever, anxiety, and cold temperatures can cause veins to constrict. Smoking before the insertion of an IV will also cause veins to constrict. The home care client is instructed to refrain from smoking for at least one-half hour before the IV insertion to ensure successful venipuncture.

Dilate the Vein

A tourniquet helps dilate and stabilize the vein, easing venipuncture and threading of the catheter. The tourniquet is placed 6 to 8 in above the insertion site. If the tourniquet is too close to the insertion site it will create too much pres-

---

venipuncture: veni—vein + puncture—to prick

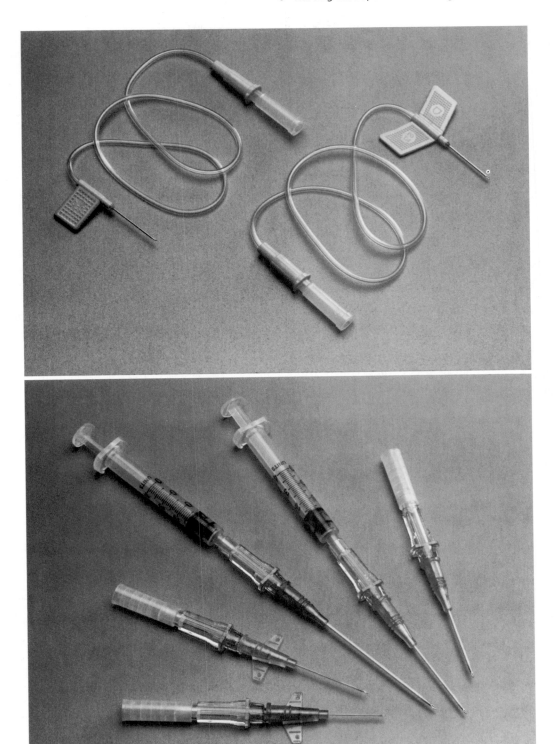

Figure 6–1. Types of gauges of IV cannulas and needles. (From Phillips, L: Manual of IV Therapeutics, ed 2. FA Davis, Philadelphia, 1997, pp 195, 197, with permission.)

sure and cause the vein to burst. It should be tight enough to impede venous flow while maintaining arterial flow. A tourniquet should be at least 1 in wide and should not be left on for more than 3 minutes, to prevent impaired blood flow to the extremity.

Occasionally additional techniques are necessary to distend the vein. Placing the arm in a dependent position or using a warm towel over the site for several minutes before applying the tourniquet will help dilate a vein. The whole extremity must be warmed to improve blood flow to the

Table 6–1. **Considerations for Vein Selection**

- Availability of the site
- Size of the needle to be used
- Type of fluid to be infused
- Volume, rate, and length of infusion
- Degree of mobility desired
- Skill of nurse initiating therapy

Among the Vietnamese, the head is considered sacred. Thus the practice of starting IV lines in scalp veins may cause a Vietnamese client significant anxiety.[1]

area. Opening and closing the fist will "pump" blood to the extremity and increase blood flow in order to dilate the vein. A blood pressure cuff inflated to the midpoint between the systolic and diastolic pressures (e.g., if the blood pressure is 130/90, pump the cuff to 110) is another good method.

Clean the Site

The peripheral insertion site is cleaned with an antimicrobial solution before cannula placement. If the skin is dirty it should be washed with soap and water before the application of an antimicrobial solution. The nurse follows institution policy when choosing a solution. Most institutions use an alcohol- or iodine-based product. Alcohol is avoided after an iodine prep because the alcohol negates the effect of iodine. The solution is applied in a circular motion, starting at the intended site and working outward to clean an area 2 to 3 in in diameter. If alcohol is used, it should be applied with friction for a minimum of 30 seconds or until the final applicator is visually clean. Blotting of the excess solution at the insertion site is not recommended. The solution is allowed to completely air dry. If the client has excess hair it can be clipped with scissors.

Insert the Cannula

The catheter is held with the bevel (slanted opening) of the needle facing upward during insertion. With the tourniquet

Table 6–2. **General Considerations When Initiating Intravenous Therapy**

1. Use veins in the upper part of the body.
2. When multiple sticks are anticipated, make the first venipuncture distally and work proximal with subsequent punctures.
3. If therapy will be prescribed for longer than 3 weeks, a long-term access device should be considered.
4. Avoid using venipunctures in affected arms of clients with radical mastectomies or a dialysis access site.
5. If possible, avoid taking a blood pressure on the arm receiving an infusion because the cuff interferes with blood flow and forces blood back into the needle. This may cause a clot or cause the vein or catheter to rupture.
6. No more than two attempts should be made at venipuncture before getting help.
7. Immobilizers should not be placed on or above an infusion site.

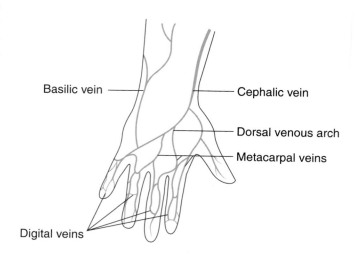

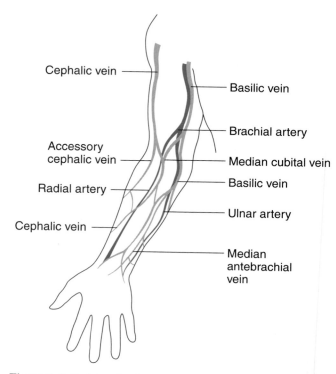

Figure 6–2. Peripheral veins used for IV therapy. (Modified from Phillips, L: Manual of IV Therapeutics, ed 2. FA Davis, Philadelphia, 1997, pp 237, 238.)

in place, the vein is entered either from the side (indirect entry) or from above (direct entry). When using the direct entry approach, the needle is held at an angle of 30 to 45 degrees. When using some newer catheters the angle of insertion is minimal. The lateral approach may help decrease vein collapse. The skin is pierced with the needle and the vein is entered. Depending on the type of device used, a small flash of blood may be seen in the tubing or at the hub of the catheter when the needle is in the vein. The angle of the needle is then lowered so that it is parallel with the skin as it is threaded into the lumen of the vein. If a catheter-over-needle device is used, the needle is advanced one-fourth of an inch, and then the catheter is advanced for its remaining length as the metal needle is withdrawn. The tourniquet is released, and the IV solution or injection cap is connected to the hub of the catheter. Blood may ooze from the hub at this time. If it does not, the needle may not be in the vein. If an injection cap is being used, the catheter is flushed with 0.9 percent sodium chloride solution to check for patency. If a bubble develops at the insertion site, the line is not patent and should be removed. A smooth easy flush and no signs of infiltration indicate that the catheter is patent and that the prescribed solution can be administered.

LEARNING TIP

Inserting an intravenous needle is like flying a plane. Come in at a low angle and level off immediately when you hit the ground.

Stabilize the Cannula

A common problem in IV therapy is dislodging of the cannula. Secure taping will keep the catheter patent and stable. A transparent dressing is a good way to stabilize the cannula and monitor for redness or swelling. Some institutions use plastic bandages (Band-Aid bandages) at the insertion site as a sterile dressing. It is wise to allow some slack in the tubing for movement. Arm boards are used to restrict movement in clients who have a cannula placed in an area of flexion. The extremity can be immobilized with a physician order as a last resort if a confused client is unable to protect the IV site. Care is taken to apply a dressing in a manner that does not constrict blood flow to the extremity.

Dispose of Equipment

All needles and blood-contaminated equipment should be disposed of according to institution policy.

Label and Document

Once the procedure is completed, the nurse labels the IV dressing with the date, time, catheter type and size, and nurse's initials. Documentation is done in the medical record according to institution policy.

CRITICAL THINKING:
Insertion of Peripheral Line

You are assisting Dr. Louis in the insertion of a peripheral line on a client with poor venous access. Because of the difficulty of the venipuncture, Dr. Louis is using the antecubital area. Suddenly blood begins to pulsate out of the insertion site.

1. What has happened?
2. What should you do?

Answers at end of chapter.

INITIATING THE SOLUTION

Before starting IV therapy the nurse first validates the physician's order. The order should include solution, volume, rate, and route. If medication is ordered, the order also includes the medication, dosage, and frequency.

The expiration dates of solutions and medications should be checked before administration. Medications packaged as individual doses are best because multiple-dose containers increase the risk for infection. If multiple dose vials are used, they are labeled with the date and time that the vial is initially entered.

Before starting the IV solution, the nurse should inspect the fluid for particles or discoloration and the container for cracks, leaks, or punctures. If the appearance of the fluid is in question, it should not be given. After medication is added to a solution, it must be infused or discarded within 24 hours. Solutions mixed in a container specific for home therapy or an infusion device may have an extended expiration date based on drug stability.

Once the solution is verified, the nurse uses the tubing spike to puncture the solution bag or bottle, taking care to keep the spike and the bag opening sterile. Solution is flushed through the tubing to remove air and is then attached to the IV cannula. The flow rate is set according to the physician's order.

All IV solutions are labeled with the solution (usually done by the manufacturer or pharmacist), client's name, date and time initiated, and flow rate. In addition, the nurse uses a strip of tape or a premade strip along the length of the solution container to mark the expected level of fluid each hour. This allows the nurse to see at a glance whether the infusion is running too slow or too fast. The IV tubing is labeled with the date and time initiated and the nurse's initials. Tubing should be changed every 24 to 72 hours, depending on the solution and according to institution policy, to prevent infection. All IV solutions are also documented on the medication administration record in the medical record.

Types of Infusion

CONTINUOUS

A continuous solution is kept running constantly until discontinued by the physician. An IV controller or roller clamp allows the solution to infuse at a constant rate. The physician orders the infusion in milliliters to be delivered over a specific amount of time.

BOLUS

A **bolus** drug (sometimes called an IV push drug, or IVP drug) is injected slowly via a syringe into the IV site or tubing port. It provides a rapid effect because it is delivered directly into the client's bloodstream. The IV push drugs can be dangerous if they are not given correctly, and the nurse should check a drug reference to determine the safe amount of time over which the drug can be injected. The IV push drugs are administered by the registered nurse (RN) and are not within the scope of practice of the LPN/LVN. The LPN/LVN should be aware of the drug being given and assist with observing for desired or adverse effects.

INTERMITTENT

Intermittent IV therapy is administered at prescribed intervals. Intermittent intravenous lines are any lines that are "capped off" with an injection port and used periodically. Patency must be ensured before an intermittent site is used to inject a drug or solution. The nurse checks for backflow of blood in the syringe before injection.

Sites that are capped with an injection cap are termed *saline* or *heparin locks*. A diluted solution of heparin, an anticoagulant, is used to flush the needle after each use and every 8 hours or according to institution policy. Many institutions are changing this practice, however, and are now using saline for flushes, which is believed to be safer and less costly. Regular flushing ensures cannula patency. Flushing also prevents the mixing of medications and solutions that are incompatible with one another. Positive pressure within the lumen of the catheter must be maintained during the administration of the flush solution to prevent a backflow of blood into the cannula lumen. This is accomplished by continuing to slowly inject the saline or heparin even as the needle is withdrawn from the cap. Intermittent cannulas should be flushed after IV medication administration, after blood sampling, and after the conversion from continuous IV therapy to intermittent IV therapy. If resistance is met while a cannula is being flushed, a clot may be occluding the cannula. Pressure should not be exerted in the attempt to restore patency, because it may result in the dislodgment of a clot into the vascular system or rupture of the catheter.

Some medications that are given intermittently are not compatible with heparin and therefore are given by the SASH method:

1. Flush with **S**aline.
2. **A**dminister medication
3. Flush with **S**aline
4. Flush with **H**eparin

Methods of Infusion

GRAVITY DRIP

Gravity is often used to drip the solution into the vein (Fig. 6–3). The solution is positioned about 3 ft above the infusion site. If it is positioned too high above the client, the in-

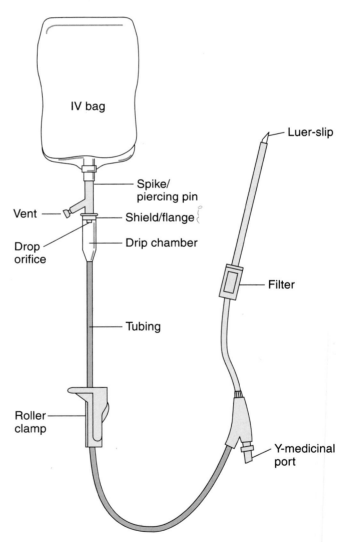

Figure 6–3. Gravity drip setup, including detailed drawing of tubing. (Modified from Phillips, L: Manual of IV Therapeutics, ed 2. FA Davis, Philadelphia, 1997, p 191.)

fusion may run too fast. A solution positioned too low may run too slowly. Flow is controlled with a roller, screw, or slide clamp. A manual flow device can achieve accurate delivery of fluid with minimal deviation.

It is recommended by the Intravenous Nursing Standards of Practice that filters be used routinely for the delivery of IV therapy. Filters fit onto the IV tubing between the solution and the insertion site and remove contaminants from the IV fluid. A 0.22 μm filter removes bacteria and fungi from IV fluids. The nurse should check institution policy and manufacturers' guidelines for use of filters.

Calculating Drip Rates

When a gravity set is used, the nurse must calculate the drops per minute required to deliver fluid at the rate ordered. Commercial parenteral administration sets vary in the number of drops delivering 1 mL. Sets generally deliver 10, 15, 20, or 60 drops per milliliter of fluid. For example, to deliver 5 mL per minute using a set with 10 drops per milliliter, a flow rate of 50 drops per minute would be necessary. To administer the same amount using a set with 15 drops per milliliter, a flow rate of 75 drops per minute would be necessary. The nurse checks the manufacturer's instructions on the administration set to determine how many drops per milliliter (drop factor) are delivered by the set. Sets delivering 60 drops per milliliter are called minidrip or microdrip sets and are used for solutions that need to be infused slowly.

To determine drops per minute of an IV solution, the nurse needs to know the amount of fluid to be given in a specified time interval and the drop factor of the administration set to be used. The formula for determining drops per minute is as follows:

$$\text{mL/Total number of hours} \times \text{Drops/mL} \times \text{1 hour/60 min} = \text{Drops per min}$$

Sample Problem: Dr. Elizabeth orders 1000 mL of 5 percent dextrose in water to be infused over 8 hours. You have on hand an administration set that delivers 10 drops per 1 mL.

Total volume: 1000 mL

Drops/mL (drop factor):   10/1

Total time of infusion: 8 hours

$$\frac{1000 \text{ mL}}{8 \text{ hours}} \times \frac{10 \text{ gtts}}{1 \text{ mL}} \times \frac{1 \text{ hour}}{60 \text{ min}} = \frac{1000}{480} = \sim 21 \text{ gtts/min}$$

If the IV is ordered as milliliters per hour, the following formula can be used:

$$\text{mL/60 min} \times \text{Drops/mL} = \text{Drops/min}$$

Sample Problem: The order reads 75 mL of 0.9 percent saline per hour. You have on hand an administration set that delivers 15 drops per 1 mL.

Volume per hour: 75 mL

Drops/mL: 15/1

Total time of infusion: 60 min

$$\frac{75 \text{ mL}}{60 \text{ min}} \times \frac{15 \text{ gtts}}{1 \text{ mL}} = \frac{75}{4} = 19 \text{ drops/min}$$

Factors Affecting Flow Rates (Troubleshooting Problems)

Change in Catheter Position

A change in the catheter's position may push the bevel either against the venous wall, which will obstruct blood flow, or away from the venous wall, which can increase the flow. Careful taping and avoidance of joint flexion areas will minimize this problem.

Height of the Solution

Because infusions flow by gravity, a change in the height of the infusion bottle or a change in the level of the bed can increase or decrease the flow rate. The flow rate increases as the distance between the solution and the client increases. A client may alter the flow rate greatly simply by standing up. The ideal height for a solution is 3 ft above the level of the heart.

Patency of the Catheter

A small clot or fibrin sheath may occlude the needle lumen and decrease or stop the flow rate. Clot formation can occur from irritation, increase in venous pressure, or backup of blood into the line. Use of a blood pressure cuff on the affected extremity is avoided because of the resulting transient increase in venous pressure. A regular flush schedule helps maintain patency.

ELECTRONIC CONTROL DEVICES

Electronic pumps and controllers regulate the rate of infusion (Fig. 6–4). Controllers measure the amount of solution delivered and depend on gravity to deliver the infusion. Pumps use positive pressure to deliver the solution. Pumps are often used for central lines to help overcome the high pressure of the central circulation.

Pumps and controllers are used for the infusion of precise volumes of solution. Institution policy often dictates use of controllers for infusion of potent medications such as heparin, concentrated morphine, and chemotherapy solutions and for very fast or slow rates. Some electronic in-

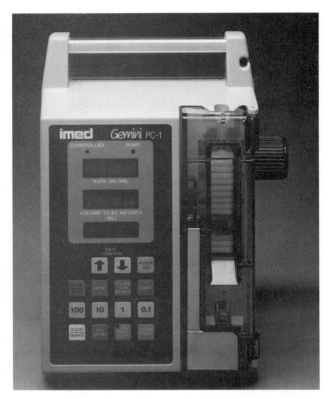

Figure 6–4. Electronic control device.

fusion devices are portable and are designed to be worn on the body. These are called ambulatory infusion devices. It is important for the nurse to know the type of pump being used and its manufacturer's guidelines.

Types of Fluids

Fluids and electrolytes administered intravenously pass directly into the plasma space of the extracellular fluid compartment. They are then absorbed based on the characteristics of the fluid and the hydration status of the client. The most commonly infused fluids are dextrose and sodium solutions. These are called crystalloid solutions.

DEXTROSE SOLUTIONS

Dextrose in water is available in many concentrations and provides carbohydrates in a readily usable form. Solutions of 2.5 percent, 5 percent, and 10 percent dextrose in water are used for peripheral infusions. Concentrations of 20 percent and above must be given into a large vein and are infused via a central line access. These high concentrations can be used for treatment of hypoglycemia or for TPN because they supply a large number of calories in a minimal amount of solution.

SODIUM CHLORIDE SOLUTIONS

Sodium chloride solutions are available in concentrations of 0.225 percent, 0.3 percent, 0.45 percent, 0.9 percent, 3 percent, and 5 percent. Combination dextrose and sodium chloride solutions, such as 5 percent dextrose with 0.45 percent sodium chloride (often referred to as "D5 and a half"), are commonly used.

TONICITY

Intravenous fluids may be classified as isotonic, hypotonic, or hypertonic. (See Chapter 5 to review these concepts.) **Isotonic** fluids have the same concentration of solutes to water as body fluids. **Hypertonic** solutions have more solutes (i.e., are more concentrated) than body fluids. **Hypotonic** solutions have fewer solutes (i.e., are less concentrated) than body fluids. Water moves from areas of lesser concentration to areas of greater concentration. Therefore hypotonic solutions send water into areas of greater concentration (cells), and hypertonic solutions pull water from the more highly concentrated cells.

Isotonic Solutions

Normal saline (0.9% sodium chloride) is an isotonic solution that has the same tonicity as body fluid. When administered to a client requiring water it neither enters cells nor pulls water from cells; it therefore expands the extracellular fluid volume. A solution of 5 percent dextrose in water (D_5W) is also isotonic when infused, but the dextrose is quickly metabolized, making the solution hypotonic.

Hypotonic Solutions

Hypotonic fluids are used when fluid is needed to enter the cells, as in the client with cellular dehydration. They are also used as fluid maintenance therapy. An example of a hypotonic solution is 0.45 percent sodium chloride.

Hypertonic Solutions

Examples of hypertonic solutions include 5 percent dextrose in 0.45 percent sodium chloride, 5 percent dextrose in 0.9 percent sodium chloride, and 5 percent dextrose in lactated Ringer's solution. Hypertonic solutions are used to expand the plasma volume, as in the hypovolemic client. They are also used to replace electrolytes.

---

isotonic: iso—equal + tonic—tension or tone
hypotonic: hypo—deficient + tonic—tension or tone
hypertonic: hyper—excessive + tonic—tension or tone

ELECTROLYTE SOLUTIONS

Electrolyte solutions are used to replace fluid and electrolyte loss. Lactated Ringer's solution is an example of a premixed electrolyte solution. Potassium is an electrolyte that is commonly added to a solution to replace deficits. High concentrations of potassium in the bloodstream can cause cardiac arrest. No more than 10 to 20 mEq of potassium should be infused in 1 hour. Potassium is *never* administered in an IV bolus.

Nursing Process for the Client Receiving IV Therapy

ASSESSMENT

The nurse routinely assesses the client receiving IV therapy. Some institution policies require assessment as often as every hour. Assessment should be systematic and thorough. One method is to start at the site and work toward the solution. The nurse first assesses the client for signs of fluid imbalance. This is especially important when caring for an older patient (see Gerontological Box 6-2). Daily weights and intake and output help determine whether the client is retaining too much fluid. Skin turgor, mucous membrane moisture, vital signs, and level of consciousness also indicate hydration status. New onset of fine crackles in the lungs indicates fluid retention. See Table 6–3 for other symptoms of complications.

Next, the nurse inspects the site for redness or swelling. The dressing should be intact and the date on the dressing within institution policy for change interval. The tubing is inspected to ensure tight connections and the absence of kinks or defects. Last, the fluid is inspected and compared with the physician's order for type, amount, and rate. Complications are reported to the RN or physician.

The nurse should be aware of the purpose of the individual client's IV therapy. This allows appropriate attention to prevention of complications that are most likely to occur. Because IV therapy is a medical intervention, the nurse is responsible primarily for appropriate monitoring, documenting, and reporting related to the therapeutic goals.

NURSING DIAGNOSIS, PLANNING, AND IMPLEMENTATION

The nurse is responsible for safe administration of IV therapy. All clients receiving IV therapy have a risk for complications. The LPN/LVN monitors carefully for the onset of complications (Table 6–3) and reports them promptly to the RN. Clients may also experience some anxiety related to IV therapy. The nurse explains all actions and rationale for therapy.

EVALUATION

The nurse monitors the client for evidence that the goals of therapy are being met. For example, if antibiotic therapy is administered, the nurse monitors temperature and other signs of resolution of infection. If IV therapy is ordered to correct dehydration, the nurse monitors skin turgor, vital signs, and other appropriate signs of improved fluid balance. All findings are documented.

In addition to meeting therapeutic goals, complications should be prevented or recognized and reported immediately.

CRITICAL THINKING: Blood in IV Tubing

You have walked into the room of a client whose IV has blood backed up in the tubing. When you open the clamp to increase the flow, nothing happens. What do you do?

Answer at end of chapter.

GERONTOLOGICAL BOX 6-2

Care of the Patient with Intravenous Therapy

When an older patient is receiving fluids intravenously (IV) the nurse must regularly assess the patient for potential fluid volume excess. Symptoms of fluid volume excess include:

Elevated blood pressure

Full bounding pulse

Shallow but rapid respirations

Jugular-venous distention

Increased urine output

Lung sounds—moist crackles related to pulmonary edema

If these signs are present:

Immediately turn down IV to a minimum drip rate (1 mL per minute); do not discontinue or shut IV off as the doctor may want to administer IV diuretics

Position the patient to maximize lung expansion

Check peripheral oxygen perfusion with an oximeter

Start emergency oxygen per mask or nasal cannula if indicated

Closely monitor patient's vital signs, level of consciousness, and oxygen perfusion along with fluid output

Assist the physician or registered nurse with IV, push administration of diuretic medication like furosemide, if ordered.

Table 6–3. **Complications of Intravenous Therapy**

Local Complications	Symptoms	Prevention	Treatment
Phlebitis (inflammation of vein)	Pain and erythema at insertion site	Anchor cannula well. Avoid insertion near joint. Dilute medication. Use large veins. Use an in-line filter.	Remove cannula. Restart in new site.
Infiltration (solution leaks out of the vein into tissues)	Insertion site puffy and cool	Monitor patency of intravenous line. Check for blood return if unsure.	Stop the infusion. Apply warm compresses. Elevate extremity. Restart in new site.
Infection	Redness, edema, exudate at site	Strict aseptic technique during insertion and site care. Inspect fluid before hanging.	Discontinue infusion. Replace in new site.
Extravasation—infiltration of a vesicant (drug that causes tissue necrosis)	Serious local tissue necrosis or death of the surrounding tissue; pain	Check that IV line is patent with blood return before and during vesicant drug infusion.	Stop infusion immediately. Follow institution policy. Many have extravasation kits. Pharmacist can provide information related to specific drug.
Pain (can occur with some medications even if IV is patent)	Complaint of discomfort at or above infusion site	Check manufacturer recommendations for specific drugs.	Obtain physician order to slow infusion, dilute medication, or add lidocaine.

Systemic Complications	Symptoms	Prevention	Treatment
Circulatory overload (fluid administered too fast or too much)	Dyspnea, new-onset crackles, bounding pulse, intake greater than output	Monitor flow rate, lung sounds, and intake and output. Use controller in elderly clients.	Raise head of bed. Reduce flow rate and contact physician.
Infection (septicemia)	Fever, chills, thready pulse, tachycardia	Strict aseptic technique at all times. Inspect all fluids and equipment before infusion.	Discontinue infusion. Be prepared to send catheter and tubing to laboratory for culture. Culture IV site if ordered by physician.
Pulmonary embolism (clot or particle in pulmonary artery)	Shortness of breath, feeling of panic, chest pain, bloody sputum	Never irrigate a plugged cannula. Inspect all fluids for particles.	Notify physician for emergency treatment. Administer IV anticoagulants per order.
Air embolism (air in bloodstream)	Cyanosis; hypotension; weak, rapid pulse; loss of consciousness	Inspect tubing for cracks, poor connections, other places where air could enter. Highest risk in central lines.	Clamp tubing. Administer oxygen. Place client on left side with head down to allow air to rise into the right atrium and be excreted via pulmonary circulation.
Speed shock (shock symptoms from infusing drug too rapidly)	Syncope, flushing, headache, chest pain, hypotension, respiratory distress, cardiac arrest	Check drug manufacturer recommendations for proper dilution and rate of administration. Use IV controllers.	Discontinue infusion. Contact physician or pharmacist for treatment for specific drug.
Incompatibility (two drugs do not dissolve together)	Symptoms of embolism	Check drug reference or pharmacist before mixing medications or infusing via same IV tubing. If a precipitate is noted in tubing, do not infuse.	Notify physician and pharmacist for drug-specific remedy.

Complications of IV Therapy

Any complication or unusual incident should be reported to the physician, and an incident report should be prepared according to institution policy. This applies to the hospital and the home situation. See Table 6–3 for complications, prevention, and treatment.

CRITICAL THINKING:
Complications of IV Therapy

Mr. Lyn is receiving 5 percent dextrose in water at 83 mL per hour. One hour after the infusion starts the client complains of pain at the site. The site is puffy.

1. What might be happening?
2. How do you further assess the client?

3. What action steps do you take?

Answers at end of chapter.

Alternative Access Routes

CENTRAL VENOUS CATHETERS

Central catheter devices include subclavian or jugular lines, ports, peripherally inserted central catheter (PICC) lines, and tunneled catheters. Central catheters terminate in the superior vena cava near the heart (Fig. 6–5). They are used when peripheral sites are inadequate or when large amounts of fluid or irritating medication must be given. These devices can have one, two, or three lumens in the catheter, or one or more port chambers. Each lumen exits the site in a separate line, called a tail. Multilumen catheters allow for the administration of incompatible solutions at the same time.

Central Lines

Central lines are inserted by the physician into the jugular or subclavian vein. Hickman, Broviac, and Groshong implanted central catheters are examples of radiopaque central catheters that are surgically tunneled under the skin before entering the vein. After insertion by a physician, correct placement is determined by x-ray before use.

Central lines have sterile dressings to protect the site. Sterile gloves and mask should be worn during the dressing change. Whenever tubing is disconnected for changing, the client is instructed to perform a Valsalva maneuver if able, to increase thoracic pressure and prevent air from entering the central line. Institution policy directs specific dressing and tubing change procedure.

Ports

A port is a reservoir that is surgically implanted into a pocket created under the skin, usually in the upper chest (Fig. 6–6). An attached catheter is tunneled under the skin into a central vein. An advantage of a port is that when not in use it can be flushed and left unused for long periods of time. Because the port is under the skin, the client can swim and shower without risk of contaminating the site.

Ports come in a variety of sizes and styles and are now being used in many areas of the body. Ports can be used for the administration of chemotherapy, for the administration of antibiotics that are toxic to tissues, or as a choice for long-term therapy.

Ports should only be accessed by a specially trained technician. Aseptic technique is used. Most ports require the use of needles that are specially designed for this use. Confirmation of correct needle placement is essential and should be established before the administration of any medication.

Peripherally Inserted Central Catheters and Midline Catheters

A peripherally inserted central catheter (PICC) is a long catheter that is inserted in the arm and terminates in the central circulation. A midline catheter tip rests at or before the axilla. These lines are used when therapy will be over 2 weeks in duration or the medication is too caustic for peripheral administration. Specially trained RNs insert PICC lines and midline catheters. They can be left in place for long periods of time, minimizing the trauma of frequent IV insertions. The nurse should consult with the physician if long-term therapy is anticipated.

When flushing a PICC line, a 5 mL or larger syringe is used because of the high pressures generated by small syringes and the possibility of catheter rupture. Heparin solution rather than saline is used to flush a PICC line. It is important to follow the manufacturer's recommended guidelines for flushing the catheter and to be aware of institutional policy.

The RN removes the PICC or midline catheter when therapy is terminated. The LPN/LVN may assist with this procedure. Caution is taken during removal, especially if it has remained in place for an extended period of time. Precautions should be made for air embolism, because a catheter that has been in place for 2 weeks or more will create a hole in the vein that can allow air to enter the internal circulation. The arm should be abducted for removal of these catheters. If resistance is encountered when attempting to remove the catheter, warm moist heat over the extremity and attempting to have the client relax may help relax the vein. If this technique does not work, the physician should be notified. After catheter removal, the nurse applies pressure, antiseptic ointment, and a sterile dressing to the site.

IMPLANTED PUMPS

An implanted pump is a catheter and an internal pump that are surgically placed into a vessel, body cavity, or organ and attached to a reservoir that contains a mechanism for continuous medication administration. The medication reservoir is placed under the skin. Implantable infusion pumps are used in clients who need continuous IV therapy with medication delivered into the central blood system. These pumps were originally used for the administration of insulin for individuals with diabetes who wanted to avoid the discomfort of daily injections. Pumps are now used to administer chemotherapy directly into tumor sites and to infuse intrathecal muscle relaxants to manage severe spasticity caused by neurological disorders such as multiple sclerosis, among other purposes.

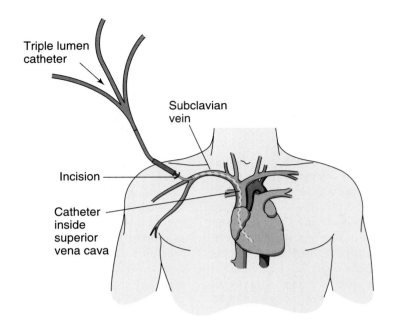

A

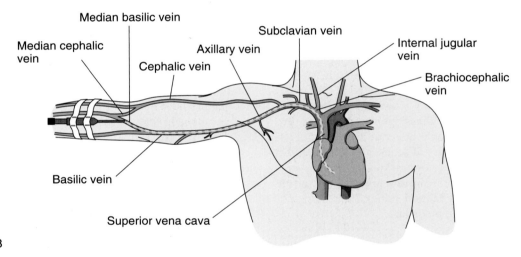

B

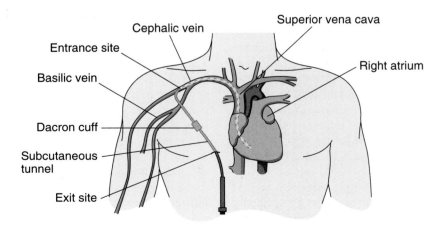

C

Figure 6–5. Central lines. *(A)* Triple-lumen subclavian catheter. *(B)* PICC line. *(C)* Tunneled catheter. *(B and C modified from Phillips, L: Manual of IV Therapeutics, ed 2. FA Davis, Philadelphia, 1997, pp 404, 412.)*

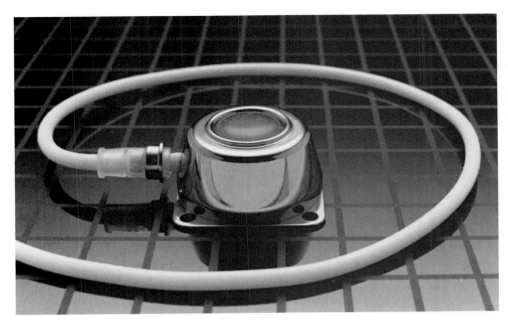

Figure 6–6. Port. (From Phillips, L: Manual of IV Therapeutics, ed 2. FA Davis, Philadelphia, 1997, p 203.)

Nutrition Support

Total parenteral nutrition is complete IV nutrition that is administered to clients who are unable to take adequate nutrients via the enteral route (mouth or tube feeding). It may be used to promote wound healing, to promote optimal weight in preparation for surgery, or to avoid malnutrition from chronic disease or surgery. Clients with ulcerative colitis, trauma, or cancer cachexia are candidates for TPN. Every effort should be made to return a client on TPN to oral or tube feedings as soon as possible.

Total parenteral nutrition provides and maintains the essential nutrients required by the body. Solutions contain carbohydrates, amino acids, lipid emulsions, electrolytes, trace elements, and vitamins in varied amounts according to the client's needs. Parenteral nutrition requires filtration and an electronic infusion device for administration. In the home setting, an ambulatory infusion device is used to allow the client more mobility. (See Nutrition Notes Box 6–3.)

The nurse is responsible for assessment of the client's height, daily weight, nutritional status, and current laboratory values. Because of the high glucose concentration of TPN, the client is at risk for infection and blood sugar disturbances. Insulin therapy may be necessary during TPN administration. The nurse assesses blood glucose levels according to institution policy and monitors for signs and symptoms of infection, hyperglycemia, and hypoglycemia. On initiation of TPN, the rate is increased gradually to the prescribed rate to help prevent hyperglycemia. On termination, the rate is gradually decreased to prevent hypoglycemia.

When nutritional solutions contain final concentrations exceeding 10 percent dextrose or 5 percent protein, they must be administered via a central catheter. When final concentrations are 10 percent dextrose or lower or 5 percent protein, they may be administered through a peripheral vein. Peripheral therapy is a short-term intervention, because it does not provide adequate nutrition over an extended period of time.

Because TPN is total replacement for food, it is essential that the entire health care team be involved. The

---

NUTRITION NOTES BOX 6–3

Nutritional Implications of Total Parenteral Nutrition

Serious metabolic complications of total parenteral nutrition (TPN) can occur quickly. Rapid shifts in potassium, magnesium, phosphorus, and glucose among the fluid compartments of the body can become life threatening. Glucose in excess of body needs can produce carbon dioxide retention, hyperlipoproteinemia, and fatty deposits in the liver. Therefore administration of TPN requires careful monitoring. The goal is to provide sufficient nutrients, but not excessive amounts that create physiological stress.

To this end, TPN infusions are started slowly at low concentrations. Adjustments in therapy are made cautiously, changing one component (amount, concentration, or rate) at a time and observing the client's reaction.

The client whose only nutrition is obtained from TPN suffers atrophy of the gastrointestinal cells. Consequently, weaning from parenteral to enteral feeding is necessary. Oral or tube feedings are introduced slowly. As gastrointestinal intake increases, TPN is decreased.[2]

pharmacist, dietitian, physician, and nurse communicate in a team conference to discuss the assessment, plan, and outcome criteria. Many institutions have nutrition teams that assess the appropriateness of TPN for individual clients.

Home Intravenous Therapy

As health care costs continue to escalate, clients are using more alternatives to hospitalization. Subacute care, skilled nursing care in nursing homes, and home health care are growing by leaps and bounds. Home IV therapy allows many clients the benefit of early discharge and the ability to accomplish health care in the privacy and comfort of their own home (Fig. 6–7). Some home health agencies employ nurses to instruct clients and their families in the administration of home IV therapy.

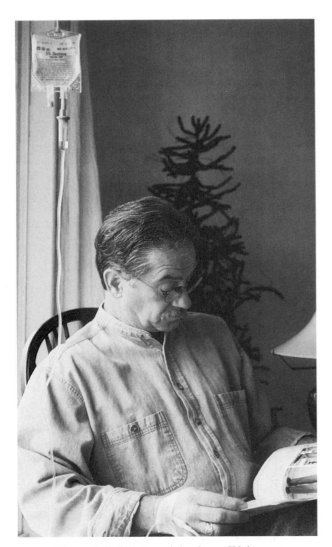

Figure 6–7. Client receiving home IV therapy.

Home IV antibiotic therapy is becoming the method of choice in the long-term treatment of a number of infections, including bacterial endocarditis, osteomyelitis, and septic arthritis. Other clients with chronic diseases choose to receive TPN at home. The health team can assess clients and their families for their ability to manage home IV therapy.

CRITICAL THINKING:
Home Intravenous Therapy

Mrs. Karas is an 86-year-old hospitalized client who is receiving TPN for malnutrition. Her daughter wants to take care of her at home. What criteria would you look for in determining whether your client is a candidate for home intravenous therapy?
Answers at end of chapter.

Review Questions

1. Which of the following is the *best* resource for the nurse who has a question about implementation of IV therapy at a specific institution?
   a. An experienced nurse
   b. Institution policy
   c. The physician
   d. The pharmacist

2. Which of the following sites is the best choice for initiating an IV needle?
   a. In the antecubital fossa
   b. In a lower extremity
   c. In the hand or arm
   d. Distal to previous insertion sites

3. Which of the following actions will help dilate a vein for IV catheter insertion?
   a. Apply a warm, moist compress.
   b. Elevate the extremity.
   c. Apply an ice pack.
   d. Loosen the tourniquet.

4. The drop factor for minidrip tubing is
   a. 10
   b. 15
   c. 30
   d. 60

5. The client is to receive 1000 mL of 5 percent dextrose in water over 12 hours. The tubing has a drop factor of 10. The nurse adjusts the drip rate to how many drops per minute?
   a. 10
   b. 14
   c. 28
   d. 50

6. Which of the following factors can slow the flow rate of a gravity solution?
   a. Raising the level of the solution container.
   b. Opening the roller clamp.
   c. Flexing the extremity above the insertion site.
   d. Flushing the cannula with saline solution.

7. A hypertonic IV solution will draw fluid from the
   a. Venous circulation into the interstitial space
   b. Interstitial space into the venous circulation
   c. Arterial circulation into the venous circulation
   d. Plasma into the cells

8. The nurse assesses a client receiving IV therapy and suspects fluid overload. Which of the following assessments is most important?
   a. Inspect insertion site for infiltration.
   b. Assess lung sounds for crackles.
   c. Question the client about pain at the site.
   d. Monitor the client's temperature.

ANSWERS TO CRITICAL THINKING

Critical Thinking: Insertion of Peripheral Line

1. Dr. Louis has probably entered the artery rather than the vein.
2. Apply pressure by using a 4 × 4 in gauze pad or other dressing and apply a firm, steady pressure over the artery, pushing against the bone to ensure that the bleeding is stopped and to discourage hematoma formation. This steady pressure should be maintained for 5 full minutes or until the bleeding stops.

Critical Thinking: Blood in IV Tubing

Your client's IV is clotted. If the IV is clotted and has been so for a period of time it will not be salvageable. *Do not flush,* because this can dislodge the clot into the circulation. Discontinue the IV and insert a new catheter.

Critical Thinking: Complications of IV Therapy

1. The IV fluid may be leaking at the insertion site under the skin. This causes the IV site to become puffy.
2. The pain can be caused by the buildup of fluid under the skin.
3. Take another look at the site. Feel the site to see if it is cool to touch. Compare it with the opposite extremity. If it is infiltrated, stop the infusion and restart the needle in a new site.

Critical Thinking: Home Intravenous Therapy

The client has good venous access; the client is motivated to care for himself or herself at home, or has a caregiver who is capable; and the solution can be given safely at home.

REFERENCES

1. Anderson, JN: Health and illness in Philippino immigrants. West J Med 139(6):811, 1983.
2. Lutz, CA, and Przytulski, KR: Nutrition and Diet Therapy, ed 2. FA Davis, Philadelphia, 1997.

BIBLIOGRAPHY

Intravenous Nursing Society: Intravenous Nursing Standards of Practice. Author, Belmont, Mass, 1990.

Metheny, N: Fluid and Electrolyte Balance: Nursing Considerations, ed 3. JB Lippincott, Philadelphia, 1996.

Phillips, D: Teaching intravenous therapy using innovative strategies. J Intravenous Nurs 17:40, 1994.

Phillips, L: Manual of IV Therapeutics, ed 2. FA Davis, Philadelphia, 1997.

Robathan, G, Woodger, S, and Merante, D: A prospective study evaluating the effects of extending total parenteral nutrition line changes to 72 hours. J Intravenous Nurs 18:84, 1995.

Robertson, Kathryn: The role of the IV specialist in health care reform. J Intravenous Nurs 18:130, 1995.

Weinstein, SM: Plumer's Principles and Practice of IV Therapy, ed 6. JB Lippincott, Philadelphia, 1996.

Nursing Care of Clients with Infections

Elizabeth Chapman

Learning Objectives

Upon completion of this chapter, the student will be able to:

1. Identify microorganisms that cause infectious diseases.
2. Identify the route of transmission of an infectious disease.
3. Identify the body's defense mechanisms against agents that cause disease.
4. Describe differences between localized and generalized infections.
5. List the methods used to diagnose an infectious disease.
6. Explain the difference between active and passive immunity.
7. Describe the differences between community-acquired and nosocomial infections.
8. Explain medical and surgical asepsis.
9. Explain types of isolation techniques.
10. Discuss treatments for infectious diseases.
11. Develop a plan of care for a client with an infectious disease.

Key Words

active immunity (**AK**-tiv im-**YOO**-ni-tee)

antibodies (**AN**-ti-bod-es)

antigen (**AN**-ti-jen)

asepsis (ah-**SEP**-sis)

bacteria (back-**TEAR**-e-ah)

fungi (**FUNG**-guy)

histoplasmosis (HISS-toh-plaz-**MOH**-sis)

nosocomial infection (no-zoh-**KOH**-mee-uhl in-**FECK**-shun)

passive immunity (**PASS**-iv im-**YOO**-ni-tee)

pathogen (**PATH**-o-jen)

phagocytosis (fay-go-sigh-**TOH**-sis)

protozoa (pro-tow-**ZOH**-ah)

rickettsia (ra-**KET**-see-ah)

sepsis (**SEP**-sis)

standard precautions (**STAN**-derd pre-**KAW**-shuns)

staphylococcus (STAFF-il-oh-**KOCK**-uss)

streptococcus (STREP-toh-**KOCK**-uss)

universal precautions (yoo-ni-**VER**-sel pre-**KAW**-shuns)

virus (**VI**-rus)

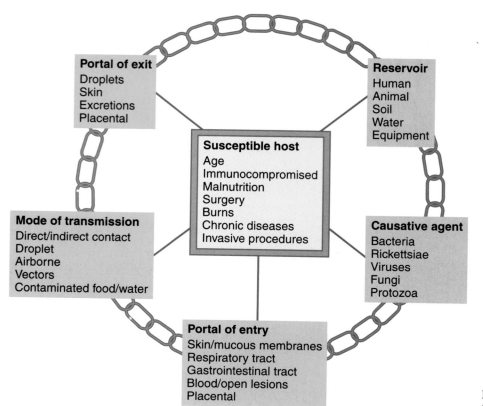

Portal of exit
Droplets
Skin
Excretions
Placental

Reservoir
Human
Animal
Soil
Water
Equipment

Susceptible host
Age
Immunocompromised
Malnutrition
Surgery
Burns
Chronic diseases
Invasive procedures

Mode of transmission
Direct/indirect contact
Droplet
Airborne
Vectors
Contaminated food/water

Causative agent
Bacteria
Rickettsiae
Viruses
Fungi
Protozoa

Portal of entry
Skin/mucous membranes
Respiratory tract
Gastrointestinal tract
Blood/open lesions
Placental

Figure 7–1. Chain of events in the infectious process.

An infection is a condition in which the body is invaded by microorganisms that can produce injurious effects. There are many reasons that infections occur. A large number of microorganisms invading the body can lower the resistance of the host. If the host's immune system is impaired and the infection is severe, the body's defense mechanisms may be unable to guard against the invasion of the microorganisms, and infectious disease results. In addition, more complex reasons may contribute to the inability to control some infections. Microorganisms may become resistant to antibiotics, limiting treatment options. Vaccination can be difficult because many microorganisms have several types of strains. Also, some infections occur in areas of the body where treatment is difficult, such as within a bone.

The Infectious Process

Many factors play a role in the development of an infectious disease (Fig. 7–1). The events in the chain of infection include the following:

1. Causative agents
2. Reservoir
3. Portal of exit
4. Mode of transmission
5. Portal of entry
6. Susceptible host

To prevent the development of an infection, the progression or chain of infection must be broken. Many factors play a role in the chain of infection. Treatment is geared at breaking the chain to prevent the spread of infectious disease. (See Cultural Considerations Box 7–1.)

CAUSATIVE AGENTS

Throughout life, many microorganisms are found in and on the body. Microorganisms that occur naturally in or on a particular body part are known as normal flora. They are harmless, or nonpathogenic, because they do not usually produce disease in their normal environment and can even be helpful to the host. For example, intestinal normal flora assist in vitamin K production, which is useful to the host. However, if these microorganisms gain access to an area of the body where they are not considered normal flora, they may produce disease and are referred to as **pathogens.**

Several factors must be present for a microorganism to be pathogenic, or disease producing. The microorganism must be able to live and multiply outside of the host and the resistance of the host must be impaired, thereby increasing the susceptibility of the host to the microorganism's invasion. Microorganisms that can become causative agents for infection include **bacteria, viruses, fungi,** and **protozoa.**

---

protozoa: proto—first + zoon—animal

CULTURAL CONSIDERATIONS BOX 7-1

An immediate concern with refugees and some newer immigrants is treating infectious conditions that jeopardize both the client and the resident population. Some immigrant Vietnamese, Mexicans, Guatemalans, Asian Indians, Turks, Brazilians, and Egyptians suffer from malaria, dengue fever, gastrointestinal parasites, tuberculosis, hepatitis A and B, and other infectious diseases associated with the tropics and crowded and substandard living conditions. Positive tuberculin tests are particularly prevalent among some immigrant and refugee populations. The hepatitis B virus is hyperendemic in Vietnam, Cambodia, and Laos. Most people are infected during childhood and then bring it with them when they immigrate to the United States. Given the high incidence of infectious diseases among migrant workers, immigrants, and refugees, the nurse must be careful to use standard precautions when working with these populations.

Among the Navajo, infectious health problems include the plague, tick fever, and the Muerto Canyon Hantavirus.

Many of these illnesses are due to the reservation's rodent population, which includes prairie dogs and deer mice.[1] Symptoms of the plague, tick fever, and Muerto Canyon Hantavirus include high fever, restlessness, mental confusion, delirium, confusion, shock, and coma.

Many Appalachians live in rural areas that lack electricity, plumbing, and running water. Thus they are at an increased susceptibility to parasitic and bacterial infections. The nurse needs to teach clients to thoroughly wash their hands after coming in contact with contaminated food and water and after toileting.

The drug isoniazid (INH), used in the treatment of tuberculosis, may be metabolized differently by some ethnic and racial groups. Half of European-Americans and a smaller percentage of Asians are slow eliminators of isoniazid. These individuals may have high blood concentrations of this medicine leading to harmful reactions.[2] The nurse needs to carefully monitor these clients for reactions to isoniazid.

Bacteria

Bacteria are single-celled microorganisms that contain both deoxyribonucleic acid (DNA) and ribonucleic acid (RNA). They usually reproduce by simple cellular division. They depend on a host to supply food and a supportive living environment. Most bacteria produce cell walls that are susceptible to antibiotics. However, bacteria can mutate to survive lethal agents such as antibiotics.

Bacteria have three shapes: spherical, rod, and spiral (Fig. 7–2). Spherical bacteria can reproduce into formations of micrococci, which are single bacteria; diplococci, which are paired bacteria; **staphylococci,** which are irregular clusters; and **streptococci,** which are chains. Rod-shaped bacteria are called bacilli. Spiral bacteria can be rigid (spirilla), flexible (spirochetes), or curved (vibrios).

To study bacteria, staining methods, including Gram's method and acid-fast staining, are used. Bacteria respond to the stains in one of three ways and are classified by their response. Gram-positive bacteria stain purple when a basic dye is applied; gram-negative bacteria lose the purple stain when exposed to alcohol but stain red with a second dye; and acid-fast bacteria retain the purple stain even when an acid is applied.

Bacteria are named according to their shape and classified according to their staining properties. For example, *Mycobacterium tuberculosis,* the organism causing tuberculosis, is an acid-fast, rod-shaped organism, and *Legionella pneumophila,* the bacteria causing legionnaires' disease, is a

gram-negative rod. Table 7–1 gives examples of other bacteria and the common bacterial infections they cause.

Bacterial growth requirements relate to oxygen, nutrition, light, temperature, and humidity. Aerobic bacteria rely on the presence of free or atmospheric oxygen to grow and multiply. Anaerobic bacteria, such as bacteria in the gastrointestinal (GI) tract, live in environments without oxygen. Most bacteria require moderate temperatures of 98.6°F (37°C) for growth. The various types of bacteria have many different growth requirements that range from being highly adaptable to very strict. The bacteria *Neisseria gonorrhoeae,* which causes gonorrhea, has strict growth requirements and cannot survive very long outside of the environment of the body.

Bacteria reproduce independently. Rod-shaped bacteria form spores that are thick walled and in a resting state, which acts as a defense mechanism in unfavorable environments. These spores remain in a resting state until favorable conditions exist that allow the organism to resume normal function. These spores are difficult to kill because they are resistant to heat, drying, and disinfectant action. Prolonged exposure to high temperature is required to destroy them.

Rickettsiae

Rickettsiae are a type of bacteria. They are parasites that must be inside living cells to reproduce. They contain DNA and RNA, reproduce by cellular division, and produce a rigid cell wall. They are the causative agents of many diseases. Their vectors are infected fleas, ticks, mites, and lice, which bite humans to transmit disease. Several diseases are caused by rickettsia. Rocky Mountain spotted fever, caused by *Rickettsia rickettsii* whose reser-

---

staphylococcus: staphyte—a bunch of grapes + kokkos—berry
streptococcus: streptos—twisted + kokkos—berry

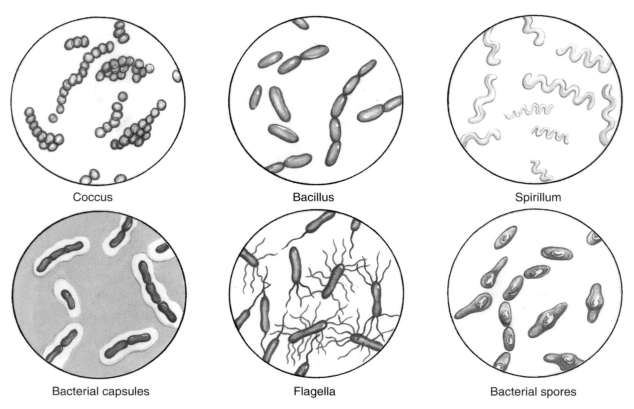

Coccus   Bacillus   Spirillum

Bacterial capsules   Flagella   Bacterial spores

Figure 7–2. Types of bacteria shapes (×1000). (From Scanlon, VC, and Sanders, T: Essentials of Anatomy and Physiology, ed 2. FA Davis, Philadelphia, 1995, p 514, with permission.)

voirs are rodents and dogs, is transmitted by ticks. Rickettsialpox, epidemic typhus, endemic typhus, and trench fever are other diseases caused by rickettsiae. Some of these diseases may be severe and fatal. Antibiotic therapy can be used for treatment.

Table 7–1. **Common Bacterial Infections**

Organisms	Type or Site of Infection
Gram-Positive Bacteria	
Staphylococcus aureus	Pneumonia, cellulitis, peritonitis, and toxic shock
Staphylococcus epidermidis	Postoperative bone/joints, IV line–related phlebitis
Streptococcus pneumoniae	Pneumonia, meningitis, otitis media, sinusitis, septicemia
Gram-Negative Bacteria	
Escherichia coli	Urinary tract, pyelonephritis, septicemia, and gastroenteritis
Klebsiella pneumoniae	Pneumonia and wounds
Legionella pneumophila	Pneumonia
Neisseria gonorrhoeae	Gonorrhea
Pseudomonas aeruginosa	Wounds, urinary tract, pneumonia, and IV lines
Salmonella enteritidis	Gastroenteritis, food poisoning

Viruses

Viruses are minute organisms that contain either a strand of DNA or RNA. They are classified according to their origin, mode of transportation, size, and manifestations produced in their host. They depend on nutrients inside host cells for their metabolic and reproductive needs. Host cells are damaged because viruses block the host cell's normal protein synthesis. Viruses cannot reproduce outside of living cells. They must use the host cell's structures to replicate. Then, after replication, new virus particles are released either by destroying the host cell or by forming small buds that break away to infect other cells.

When a virus enters a cell, it may immediately trigger a disease process or remain dormant for years without causing illness. An example of this is the herpes virus, which after being latent for years can start replicating, causing chickenpox or shingles. Viruses, such as the herpes virus, can also change host cells into malignant cells. Table 7–2 shows examples of infections caused by viruses. Antibiotics are not effective against viruses.

Fungi

Fungi are a group of plantlike organisms that includes yeast, molds, and mushrooms. They grow as single cells, as in yeast, or as multicellular colonies, as in molds and mushrooms. They can produce highly resistant spores. They do not contain chlorophyll, so they must obtain food

Table 7–2. *Common Viral Infections*

Virus	Type or Site of Infection
Herpes virus group	Cold sores/fever blisters; genital herpes
Epstein-Barr	Infectious mononucleosis
Varicella zoster	Skin (chickenpox) and shingles
Hepatitis (A, B, C, D, E)	Liver
Human immunodeficiency virus	Acquired immunodeficiency syndrome
Influenza (A, B, C)	Bronciolitis, pneumonia
Rubella	German measles
Rubeola	Measles

Table 7–3. *Protozoal Infections*

Protozoa	Type or Site of Infection
Giardia lamblia	Gastroenteritis
Trichomonas vaginalis	Trichomoniasis
Dientamoeba fragilis	Diarrhea, fever
Entamoeba histolytica	Amebic dysentery
Toxoplasma gondii	Toxoplasmosis
Plasmodium malariae	Quartan malaria

from dead organic matter or from living organisms. Fungi produce a rigid cell wall layer that is not destroyed by antibiotics, so fungi are not susceptible to antibiotic therapy as bacteria are.

The body's normal flora of the mouth, skin, vagina, and intestinal tract include many fungi. Most fungi are not pathogenic, and serious fungal infections are rare. Fungi that cause disease come from a group of fungi called Fungi Imperfecti. Diseases that result from fungi are called a mycosis, such as dermatomycosis, a fungus infection of the skin.

In people with competent immune systems, fungi can cause minor infections of the hair, nails, mucous membranes, or skin. In people with compromised immune systems due to acquired immunodeficiency syndrome (AIDS) or immunosuppressive drug therapy, fungi are a source of opportunistic infections that can be severe and overwhelm the immune system, causing death. (See chapter 53.) Examples of fungal infections include **histoplasmosis,** which is a systemic, fungal, respiratory disease that can be mild or fatal; ringworm, which is a dermatomycosis that can affect the scalp (tinea capitis), the body (tinea corporis), the nails (tinea unguium), or the foot (athlete's foot); and candidiasis, a yeast, which is an infection of the skin causing a red rash or of the mucous membranes that produces painless, white lesions in the mouth.

Protozoa

Protozoa are single-celled parasitic organisms with flexible membranes and usually the ability to move. They live in the soil and obtain nourishment from dead or decaying organic material. Most protozoa infect only humans without adequate immunological defenses. Infections are spread by the fecal-oral route through ingestion of food or water contaminated with cysts or spores, through host-to-host contact, or by the bite of a mosquito or other insect

that has previously bitten an infected person. Common protozoan infections include malaria, gastroenteritis, sleeping sickness, and vaginal infections (Table 7–3).

Helminths

Helminths are wormlike parasitic animals. They include roundworms, flatworms, tapeworms, pinworms, hookworms, flukes, and *Trichinella*. These helminths mate and reproduce in the host. Disease transmission occurs through skin penetration of larva or ingestion of helminth eggs. Trichinosis is a disease caused by eating raw or undercooked meat, such as pork, that contains *Trichinella*.

RESERVOIR

A reservoir is where infectious agents live, multiply, and reproduce, in order to be transmitted to a susceptible host. A reservoir can be animate, such as people, insect, animals, and plants, or inanimate, such as equipment or soil.

PORTAL OF EXIT

The portal of exit is the route by which the infectious agent leaves the reservoir or source host. This route may be the same as the portal of entry. The respiratory tract, skin, mucous membranes, gastrointestinal tract, genitourinary tract, blood, open lesions, and placenta are points of exit for the infectious agent.

MODE OF TRANSMISSION

Once the causative agent exits the reservoir or source host, a means of transfer to a susceptible host is needed. Transmission methods for microorganisms include contact, airborne, droplet, common vehicle, or vector-borne transmission.

Contact transmission occurs by direct or indirect contact. Direct contact occurs person to person. It involves body surface–to–body surface contact. Examples of activities of direct contact include hand contact, performance of client care activities, and sexual contact. Indirect contact is the spreading of an infectious microorganism by

histoplasmosis: histo—web + plasm—plasma + osis—condition

contact with a contaminated object. Examples of inanimate objects include gloves not changed between clients, used needles, and used dressings. Illnesses that can be spread via contact include impetigo, scabies, viral conjunctivitis, pediculosis, *Clostridium difficile,* and herpes simplex virus.

Airborne transmission is the spreading of small particles of infectious material in dust particles or in evaporated droplets that can remain suspended in the air for a long time and travel large distances. These microorganisms can be inhaled or deposited on a susceptible host. Measles and tuberculosis are transmitted by airborne droplet nuclei.

Droplet transmission occurs during talking, coughing, sneezing, or suctioning when large infectious particles are propelled through the air and come in contact with the mucous membranes of the nose and mouth or conjunctivae of the susceptible host. Droplet transmission is different from airborne transmission because the droplets do not stay suspended in the air. Diphtheria, influenza, mumps, streptococcal pharyngitis, and rubella are transmitted in this manner.

Common vehicle transmission of microorganisms occurs by consumption of contaminated food or water that can lead to salmonella, gastroenteritis, or typhoid and equipment that has been contaminated by the source host and then touched by the susceptible host.

Vector-borne transmission occurs when a vector bites a person or animal and transmits an infectious agent. Vectors such as the tick can transmit Rocky Mountain spotted fever. The mosquito transmits malaria and yellow fever.

PORTAL OF ENTRY

To produce disease, microorganisms must gain entry into a susceptible host. Routes of entry into a susceptible host include the respiratory tract, skin, mucous membranes, gastrointestinal tract, genitourinary tract, and placenta. Once the organism enters the host, it may be able to begin the process that will lead to illness or disease.

SUSCEPTIBLE HOST

Many factors influence the susceptibility of a person in acquiring infections. The body uses many defense mechanisms, such as intact skin and mucous membranes, white blood cells, and the immune system, in an attempt to prevent infection. A breakdown in these defenses increases the possibility of developing an infection. Factors that contribute to people being more susceptible as hosts to microorganisms are very young age, old age, malnourishment, being immunocompromised, having a chronic disease, being under stress, or undergoing an invasive procedure. (See Gerontological Issues Box 7–2.)

GERONTOLOGICAL ISSUES BOX 7–2

Infection and Older Clients

Often an older client may not have typical symptoms of an infection. This can cause a significant delay in providing appropriate treatment and care. The nurse should be alert for the following in the elderly client, which may indicate an infection:

One of the first signs of an infection in an older client may be a behavior change, such as pacing or irritability.

A chronic disease process may make it difficult for the older client to recognize the symptoms of infection as different from the symptoms of the chronic disease. For example, the inflammation and pain of degenerative joint disease may make it difficult for a client to recognize an infection in an afflicted joint.

An older adult may have a serious bacterial infection with no elevation in temperature. A fever is not a common complaint or sign of infection for an older adult.

The Human Body's Defense Mechanisms

The human body's defense mechanisms are designed to prevent the invasion of microorganisms. When any of these defense mechanisms are weakened or fail, an individual is more susceptible to the entry of microorganisms, thereby increasing the risk of infectious disease. Some of the major defense mechanisms are discussed.

SKIN AND MUCOUS MEMBRANES

Intact skin and mucous membranes are the body's first line of defense against infection. In addition, skin and mucous membranes have other defense characteristics. Oral mucous membranes have many layers that make it difficult for microorganisms to gain entrance into the body. The skin has acidic (pH < 7.0) properties that render some microorganisms unable to produce disease because many bacteria prefer an alkaline (pH > 7.0) environment for multiplication or reproduction. There is also an abundance of normal flora that impairs the growth of pathogens both on the skin and in the GI tract.

MUCOCILIARY MEMBRANES

Cilia are hairlike structures that line the mucous membranes of the upper respiratory tract. They are responsible for trapping mucus, pus, dust, and foreign particles to prevent them from entering the lungs. After these particles are trapped, the cilia push them up to the pharynx with wavelike movements so they can be expectorated. This protects the lungs from infection.

GASTRIC JUICES

Gastric juices within the stomach are very acidic (pH 1.0 to 5.0). This acidic environment destroys most microorganisms that enter the GI tract and travel through the stomach.

LEUKOCYTES AND MACROPHAGES

Leukocytes, or white blood cells, are the primary cells that protect against infection and tissue damage. There are five types of leukocytes: neutrophils, which are phagocytic cells focusing on bacteria and small particles; monocytes, which become macrophages and are mainly phagocytic on tissue debris and large particles; lymphocytes, whose several functions include **antigen** recognition and antibody production; basophils that respond to inflammation from injury; and eosinophils that destroy parasites and respond in allergic reactions.

After recognizing a foreign antigen, neutrophils and macrophages engulf it and digest it. This is referred to as **phagocytosis** (Fig. 7–3). Macrophages then move the antigen fragments to the cell surface to be recognized by T lymphocytes to further stimulate the action of the immune system. Phagocytes ingest and destroy bacteria, damaged or dead cells, cellular debris, and foreign substances. They play a major role in the immune response.

LYSOZYMES

Lysozymes are bactericidal enzymes present in white blood cells and most body fluids such as tears, saliva, and sweat. These enzymes dissolve the walls of the bacteria, which destroys them.

IMMUNOGLOBULINS

Immunoglobulins are proteins found in serum and body fluids that may act as **antibodies** to destroy invading microorganisms and prevent the development of an infectious disease. Antibodies are proteins that are produced by B lymphocytes when foreign antigens of invading cells are detected. Antigens are markers on the surface of cells that identify cells as being the body's own cells (autoantigens) or as being foreign cells (foreign antigens). Antibodies combine with specific foreign antigens on the surface of the invading microorganisms, such as bacteria or viruses,

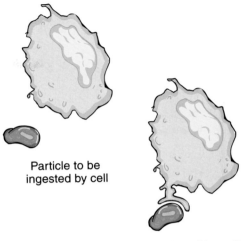

Particle to be ingested by cell

Beginning of ingestion

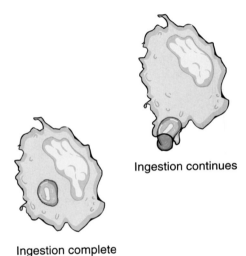

Ingestion continues

Ingestion complete

Figure 7–3. Phagocytosis.

to control or destroy them. Antigens are neutralized or destroyed by antibodies in several ways. Antibodies can initiate lysis of the antigen, neutralize toxins released by bacteria, promote antigen clumping with the antibody, or prevent the antigen from adhering to host cells. This defense mechanism helps provide protection against most common infections.

INTERFERON

If an invading organism is a virus, white blood cells and fibroblasts release a group of antiviral proteins called interferon. These proteins aid in the destruction of infected cells and inhibit production of the virus within infected cells. This prevents the spread of the virus to other cells. The growth of some tumor cells may also be inhibited by interferon.

---

antigen: anti—against + gennan—to produce
phagocytosis: phagein—to eat + dytos—cell + osis—condition

INFLAMMATORY RESPONSE

The inflammatory response occurs as a result of any bodily injury. It can be caused by pathogens, trauma, or other events leading to injury to body tissues. Infection may or may not be present. Regardless of the cause, the inflammatory process is always the same.

Vascular Response

The first step of the inflammatory process is local vasodilation that increases blood flow to the injured area. This increased blood flow creates redness and heat production at the injured site. An invasion of pathogenic microorganisms can trigger the first step of the inflammatory process.

Inflammatory Exudate

Following the vascular response, there is increased permeability of the blood vessels that allows plasma to move out of the capillaries and into the tissues. As a result, swelling of the tissues and pain from pressure on the nearby nerve endings is produced. The exudation of fluid helps dilute toxic agents.

Phagocytosis and Purulent Exudate

The final step of the inflammatory process involves the destruction by leukocytes of pathogenic microorganisms and their toxins at the injury site. During this process, a purulent exudate may form that contains protein, cellular debris, and dead leukocytes.

IMMUNE SYSTEM

The immune system is the body's final line of defense against infection. It is composed of immune cells and lymphoid tissue that work with the body's other defense mechanisms. Immune cells include the lymphocyte classes of T cells, B cells, and natural killer cells, which have protective functions related to specific antigens. Macrophages are accessory cells for the functioning of T cells and B cells.

The lymphoid organs are the thymus, which is vital to the development of the immune system, and the bone marrow, which produces leukocytes. Other lymphoid structures include the spleen, tonsils, intestinal lymphoid tissue, and lymph nodes where immune cells grow and whose filtering of foreign materials prevents them from entering the bloodstream. The spleen destroys old or damaged red blood cells and contains large amounts of lymphocytes.

The immune system is a finely tuned network of structures that function together to protect the body from invasion by pathogenic microorganisms. When this network breaks down, infectious disease and illness can result.

Infectious Disease

GENERAL CLINICAL MANIFESTATIONS OF INFECTIONS

Localized Infection

A localized infection is caused by the lodging and multiplication of a microorganism in one area of a tissue, which activates the inflammatory response. Classic manifestations of a local infection include pain, redness, swelling, and warmth at the site. Pain is especially prominent when the infection is confined within closed cavities and is proportional to the pathogen's virulence, or ability to cause disease, and the extent of the infection. Redness and swelling become prominent when superficial structures are involved but is not evident if the infection is within a rigid tissue or deep in a cavity. Warmth may be felt at the site, and there might be an elevation in body temperature even with only minor infections.

Generalized Infection

Generalized infections occur when there is systemic or whole body involvement. The symptoms for generalized infections are sometimes nonspecific and vague, but may include headache, malaise, muscle aches, fever, and anorexia. As the infection progresses and becomes more severe, there can be a marked increase in fever, elevated white blood cell count, decreased blood pressure, mental confusion, tachycardia, and shock. **Sepsis** is the term used when an infection has spread to the bloodstream. It can be a very severe condition.

LABORATORY ASSESSMENT

To determine the presence of an infectious disease, the microorganism present in the host must be identified. Several methods can be used to identify the pathogen. One method is performing a microscopic examination such as Gram's method of staining. Bacteria retaining the purple stain are gram-positive, such as *Staphylococcus aureus*. Bacteria that are gram-negative take on a red counterstain, such as *Escherichia coli*. Another method is the culture examination, in which a growth medium is used to identify the causative agent within 24 to 48 hours. A sensitivity examination is then done, which exposes the specimen to a number of antibiotics to determine which ones the pathogen is sensitive to and which ones it is resistant to. A culture and sensitivity helps guide treatment.

A serology test can be performed to look for the host's level of serum antibodies that react with a certain antigen. A positive or high result on this test does not always mean an active infection is present. It can simply mean there has been an exposure to the antigen, so it is not as accurate a test as a culture.

A complete blood count with differential is usually performed on a client suspected of having an infectious disease. It identifies the five different types of leukocytes and their levels. Elevations in specific leukocytes occur based on the type and severity of the pathogen.

Erythrocyte sedimentation rate (ESR, sed rate) is an early screening test for inflammation. It is not a definitive test for infection. During the inflammatory process, red blood cells become heavier and during the test settle to the bottom of a tube. The ESR measures in millimeters per hour the speed at which the red blood cells settle in the tube. The faster the settling, the greater the inflammation.

Other tests such as x-rays, computed tomography (CT), and magnetic resonance imagery (MRI) are helpful in identifying abscesses, which are walled-off areas of infection. Skin tests can also be used to diagnose infections, such as the tine test or intradermal purified protein derivative test, which both screen for tuberculosis. (See Chapter 28.)

IMMUNITY

Immunity is the ability of the body to protect itself from disease. There are several types of immunity. Natural immunity occurs in species and prevents one species from contracting illnesses found in another species. Innate immunity is genetic, hereditary immunity that a person is born with. Acquired immunity is obtained either actively or passively. It is usually the result of having been exposed to a microorganism and recovering or having had a vaccine to provide protection from a microorganism. It can also be the result of immunity passed on from mother to baby or an injection of immunoglobulins (antibodies) to give immediate immunity to a certain disease.

Active Immunity

Active immunity is a cellular (T lymphocyte) and humoral (B cell antibody production) immune response. The cellular response involves sensitized T cells that destroy the infectious agent. With humoral immunity, antibodies are produced by B cells, which are formed from lymphocytes. Active immunity is longer lasting, because it is the individual's own body forming the immunity.

Active immunity results from the body's natural response to an invading pathogen. This natural response, leading to active immunity, may also be triggered by a vaccination. Vaccines contain foreign antigens that trigger the immune response when they enter the body. Vaccines are used to prevent infection if an individual can be at risk of exposure to an infectious disease.

An antibody titer can be drawn to determine if there is immunity to a specific microorganism or toxin. A positive titer means a person has active immunity. Examples include the immunity a person has after recovering from the flu or after receiving a vaccine.

Passive Immunity

Passive immunity is acquired when preformed antibodies are introduced into an unprotected individual. In this case, the body is not required to form an immune response because the immunity is transferred directly into the individual via the antibodies. Preformed antibodies can come directly from someone else, as in mother-to-baby transfer through the placenta or in breast milk, or in a prepared antitoxin or serum such as an immune globulin preparation. Examples for use include a rattlesnake bite or exposure to hepatitis A within the previous 2 weeks and without illness development.

Antibodies are given to remove toxins and pathogens before damage or disease can occur. Passive immunity is given to people who are unable to form antibodies or who do not have sufficient time to form antibodies to prevent illness. This type of immunity is temporary and short term.

CRITICAL THINKING: Charles

Charles has acquired immunodeficiency syndrome (AIDS). Why should Charles not be given a live virus vaccine?
Answer at end of chapter.

Infection Control in the Community

A communicable disease is one that can be transmitted, directly or indirectly, from one individual to another. It results from an infectious agent or toxic products produced by the agent that gain entry into a susceptible host.

Many communicable diseases have been eradicated through worldwide efforts. Diseases such as smallpox and rubella have been successfully controlled. Many organizations, such as the World Health Organization (WHO) and the Centers for Disease Control and Prevention (CDC), work closely together. These organizations monitor disease outbreaks and teach standards to use to prevent and control diseases. Local health departments also teach how to prevent and control the spread of disease. The community health nurse role is vital in the collection of health data, in setting up immunization programs within the community, and in educating the public about health and illness.

Education is of great importance in preventing the spread of disease. Education programs are set up in schools and homes to teach the public the importance of preventing the spread of infectious disease. Physicians and health agencies are responsible for reporting communicable diseases to public health departments.

INFECTION PREVENTION AND CONTROL METHODS

Immunization programs established in communities have helped reduce infectious diseases. In the past, elementary schools required proof of immunization; now many colleges also require proof of immunization to help control the outbreak of diseases such as measles. Vaccination has played a major role in preventing many infectious diseases and controlling the spread of an existing disease outbreak. Educating the public to understand the importance of hand washing and immunization in preventing the spread of disease cannot be overemphasized.

HOME CARE

The hospital nurse has a responsibility to provide discharge teaching for the client and family in the care for and prevention of the spread of infection. The home care nurse teaches family members and friends how to care for the client with an infectious disease. Many of the same principles used in the hospital can be modified for home use. The client and family should be taught not to share personal items such as drinking cups or towels. Separate beds and bathrooms should be used if possible when an infection is present. Disposable dishes and utensils can be used for meals to help eliminate transmission of infection via these items. Disposable gloves, which can be purchased at many stores, should be used when providing personal care to clients or handling body fluids or feces. Teaching family members how to dispose of contaminated items properly will help limit the exposure and spread of infectious diseases in the home.

Infection Control in Health Care Agencies

On admission to a hospital or health care agency, some clients may already have an infectious process started. This is referred to as a community-acquired infection because it is present or incubating at the time of admission to the health care facility. An infection that develops after the client is admitted to the hospital or health care agency is called a **nosocomial infection** and is a major concern for health care facilities.

During the infectious process, the host's resistance to infection plays a major role in whether or not an infection is acquired. Clients in the hospital are commonly debilitated, malnourished, or immunocompromised. Multiple antibiotic therapy also increases susceptibility to other types of infection and promotes the resistance of the pathogens to the antibiotics. Therefore the risk of developing a nosocomial infection is very high. Some areas within an institution tend to have an increased number of nosocomial infections. They include intensive care, neonatal, dialysis, oncology, and burn units. Clients in these areas tend to un-

dergo invasive procedures and are very ill and debilitated. These factors increase the client's susceptibility to infection.

Several pathogens are commonly responsible for causing nosocomial infections. *E. coli* is the most common pathogen causing nosocomial urinary tract infections. *E. coli* normally lives in the intestinal tract. It can be spread by the client, unwashed hands of a health care worker, or contaminated food and water. *S. aureus* is the most common pathogen causing nosocomial surgical wound infections and nosocomial bacteremia. *S. aureus* lives in the respiratory tract in the anterior nares and on the skin. Many individuals are carriers of this organism and transmit it from person to person. *P. aeruginosa* is the most common pathogen in nosocomial pneumonia. This organism is present in the environment, especially around sinks, water, and irrigating solutions and nebulizers on respiratory equipment.

ANTIBIOTIC-RESISTANT INFECTIONS

Antibiotic-resistant infections are on the rise and are creating significant treatment problems. These infections result in increased health care costs, morbidity, and mortality. Preventive measures to reduce the occurrence of antibiotic-resistant infections are important to implement. Two infections that are on the rise include methicillin-resistant *S. aureus* (MRSA) and vancomycin-resistant enterococci (VRE).

A serious antibiotic-resistant infection is caused by MRSA.[3] This infection is very difficult to treat and mortality can be high. It affects mainly the elderly and those who are chronically ill. Vancomycin hydrochloride, an antibiotic, can be used to treat MRSA. It is a very potent and expensive antibiotic that is only administered intravenously.

Vancomycin-resistant enterococci infections are becoming more common.[3] Enterococci are normal flora in the GI and female genital tracts. These organisms can be transmitted via direct or indirect contact. Populations at increased risk for VRE infections include those with indwelling urinary or central venous catheters, immunocompromised and critically ill clients, clients receiving multiple antibiotics or vancomycin therapy, surgical clients, or those with extended hospital stays. Preventive measures focus on proper hand-washing technique, prudent use of vancomycin for defined situations, continuing education for health care workers on the need for high standards, and aggressive infection-control methods to prevent this serious infection. Clients with VRE infections should be isolated, and current CDC and institutional isolation policies should be implemented and strictly followed (Fig. 7–4). Treatment is difficult. It may involve combination antibiotic therapy, but VRE infections are often also resistant to these antibiotics.

INFECTION PREVENTION AND CONTROL

The single most effective way to prevent and control the spread of infection is by hand washing. Most organisms are

Antibiotic-Resistant Organism Precautions

Visitors: Report to the Nurses' Station before entering the room.

1. **Private Room** required.
2. **Gloves** <u>must</u> be worn by <u>all hospital personnel</u> entering the room.
3. **Wash Hands** on entering and leaving the room.
4. **Gowns:** required **IF** contamination of clothing is likely.
5. **Decontaminate All Equipment** used in the room before removal from the room.

Form #: 0204-01   Revised 8/97

Figure 7–4. Antibiotic-resistant organism precautions for Vancomycin resistant enterococci (VRE).

transmitted via the hands of health care workers. Health care workers must wash their hands before and after every client contact to prevent the transmission of microorganisms (Fig. 7–5). Clients may also transmit microorganisms with improper hand-washing methods. Instructing clients on the importance of hand washing after handling their own secretions helps reduce pathogen transmission and client reinfection. The use of gloves also decreases the transmission of microorganisms but still requires hand washing before and after their use.

▼ **CRITICAL THINKING: Mrs. Sampson**

Mrs. Sampson has neutropenia from chemotherapy treatments.

1. Why is hand washing the most important intervention the nurse can do to help prevent infection development in Mrs. Sampson?
2. What would be a priority nursing diagnosis for Mrs. Sampson?
3. What type of isolation could be beneficial to Mrs. Sampson?

Answers at end of chapter.

Asepsis

The concept of **asepsis,** which is freedom from microorganisms, should be stressed to all health care workers who come in direct or indirect contact with clients. Aseptic technique reduces the spread of microorganisms and thereby reduces infection. There are two kinds of asepsis: medical and surgical. In hospitals, the most common sites for infectious diseases are the genitourinary tract, respiratory tract, bloodstream, and surgical wounds. The nurse must be aware of clients at risk of developing these infec-

tions and help protect them from acquiring an infection. Using aseptic techniques can help prevent these infections from occurring.

Medical Asepsis

Medical asepsis is commonly referred to as clean technique. The goal is to reduce the number of pathogens or prevent and reduce the transmission of pathogens from one person to an-

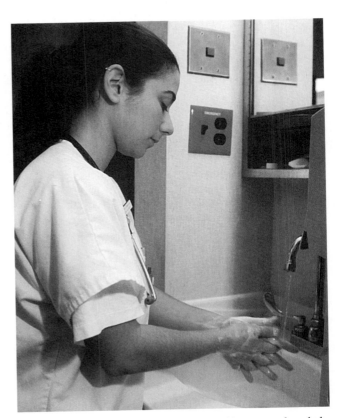

Figure 7–5. Frequent hand washing by health care workers helps reduce the spread of microorganisms.

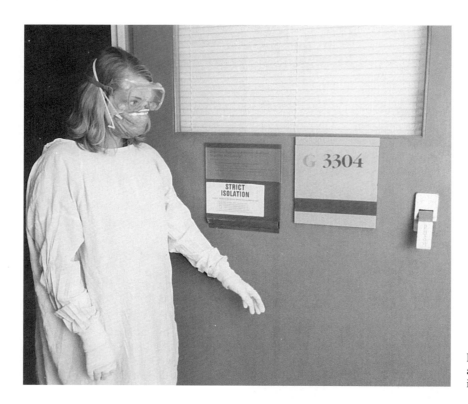

Figure 7–6. Gloves, gowns, masks, goggles, and face shields help prevent the spread of infection to health care workers and clients.

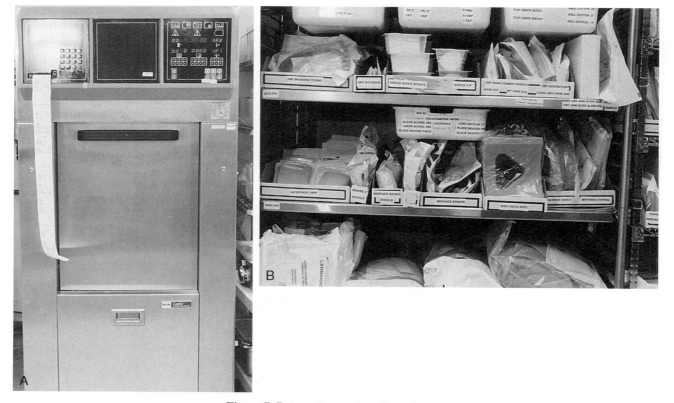

Figure 7–7. Autoclave and sterile packages.

other. This is accomplished by frequent, proper hand washing; use of gowns, gloves, masks, and protective eyewear; use of rooms with special ventilation; use of disinfectants; and standard precautions as defined by the CDC (Fig. 7–6).

Surgical Asepsis

Surgical asepsis refers to an item or area that is free of all microorganisms and spores and is also referred to as sterile technique. Surgical asepsis is used in surgery and to sterilize equipment. It can be accomplished by several different methods. Articles can be subjected to intense heat or chemical disinfectants to destroy all microorganisms. The use of pressurized steam sterilizers, known as autoclaves, will kill even the most powerful microorganisms (Fig. 7–7). Some equipment cannot be exposed to moist heat, so gas sterilizers are used instead. Once these articles are sterilized, they are dated, packaged, and sealed. Once a package is opened or outdated, it is no longer considered sterile.

Signs of Infections

Symptoms of localized and generalized infections were discussed earlier. Following are site-specific symptoms associated with infections.

RESPIRATORY TRACT INFECTIONS

Clients with respiratory tract infections may have a cough, a congested or runny nose, a sore throat, chest congestion, or chest pain. The throat may be reddened or there may be white patches in the back of the throat. Lung sounds can include crackles, rhonchi, or wheezing. The nurse should ask clients if they have a productive cough and the amount, frequency, and color of the sputum. Usually a sputum culture will be ordered by the physician and obtained by the nurse to identify the presence of microorganisms and the appropriate treatment.

GASTROINTESTINAL TRACT INFECTIONS

The symptoms of GI tract infections may include nausea, vomiting, diarrhea, cramping, and anorexia. Clients may have frequent episodes of emesis and diarrhea and need to be monitored closely for signs of dehydration. Dehydration can result from the loss of fluid in emesis or diarrhea. Stool cultures may be ordered by the physician.

GENITOURINARY TRACT INFECTION

The symptoms for a urinary tract infection can include voiding urgency, frequency, and burning; flank pain; change in color of urine; foul odor; and discharge. The nurse should monitor frequency, amount, color, and odor of the urine. Urinalysis and urine cultures are ordered to determine if a microorganism is present. Urine cultures must be collected using sterile technique. Urinary tract infections need to be treated because those left untreated can lead to serious kidney problems.

Infection Prevention

PREVENTION OF RESPIRATORY TRACT INFECTIONS

Nosocomial pneumonia has been linked with the highest infection mortality rate in hospitalized clients. Clients who are at highest risk for pneumonia are those with endotracheal, nasotracheal, or tracheostomy tubes because these invasive tubes bypass the normal defenses of the upper respiratory tract. To prevent infection in these clients, care of these tubes requires sterile technique. When suctioning a client through these tubes, the equipment and solutions used are sterile. If clients are on ventilators or receiving respiratory treatments, the tubing and equipment are usually changed every 48 hours. Institution policy regarding this should be followed. Protecting debilitated clients or those with an ineffective cough from aspirating can also help prevent pneumonia from occurring.

PREVENTION OF GENITOURINARY TRACT INFECTIONS

The most common hospital-acquired infection is a urinary tract infection. Clients with urinary catheters have the greatest risk of developing an infection. The urinary tract is a sterile tract. Introduction of a catheter into the bladder may allow bacteria to enter the bladder along the catheter. Many institutions have policies on appropriate use of Foley catheters and their removal. Catheters should be used only when necessary because of the morbidity and mortality associated with infections that develop from them. Appropriate uses of catheters include clients with urinary obstructions, clients with neurogenic bladder, and clients in shock.

Indwelling urinary catheters should be removed as soon as possible. For clients requiring long-term use of urinary catheters, intermittent catheterization is preferred because it has been shown to significantly reduce the risk of infection. Using strict aseptic technique while inserting and caring for the catheter in the health care agency is imperative regardless of which type of catheterization is used. The catheter tubing must be securely anchored to the client's leg, according to agency protocol, so it does not move in and out of the urethra because this movement can encourage bacteria to enter the urinary tract.

The closed urinary drainage system seal should never be opened. If intermittent irrigation is ordered, sterile technique must be used to protect both ends from contamination. The drainage bag should be positioned so that it is never higher than the level of the bladder to prevent backflow of urine into the bladder, which could contaminate the sterile urinary tract. If an indwelling urinary catheter and drainage system is used long term, the catheter and the entire system should be changed regularly using sterile technique.

PREVENTION OF SURGICAL WOUND INFECTIONS

The initial dressing for surgical wounds is applied in the operating room using sterile aseptic technique. Institutions have policies and procedures on the frequency of dressing changes. Many surgeons prefer to remove the first dressing themselves. Others leave postoperative orders indicating when to change the dressing. Dressing changes should be done using sterile technique. The nurse must monitor the wound with every dressing change for signs of infection. The institution's policy and physician's orders on wound care and dressing changes should be followed.

PROTECTION FROM BACTEREMIA

Bacteremia means bacteria in the bloodstream. It is referred to as sepsis or blood poisoning and has a variety of causes. Bacteremias commonly occur secondary to an infection from another site in the body. Prevention for bacteremia from another infection would be to aggressively treat the underlying infection to prevent its spread. Another common cause of bacteremia is the use of invasive catheters, such as central lines, arterial lines, and pulmonary artery catheters. Insertion and care of these catheters requires sterile technique and careful observation for infection signs. Institutional policy on care of invasive catheters should be followed. Solutions, such as those used intravenously, in suctioning, for irrigating, in tube feedings, or in medications, can also be a source of contamination. The nurse must examine all solutions for expiration date, signs of contamination, cloudiness, particles, or discoloration before using them.

Indications of bacteremia such as fever, tachypnea, tachycardia, hypotension, and elevated white blood cell count should be reported promptly to the physician for immediate treatment. Blood cultures may be ordered when fever occurs to detect the presence of the pathogen that is triggering the fever. Antibiotics are used to treat the bacteremia.

INFECTION PREVENTION GUIDELINES

The Centers for Disease Control and Prevention publishes guidelines for isolation precautions in hospitals and health care agencies and infection control in health care personnel. Health care agencies then use these guidelines to establish their own policies. CDC and agency guidelines are continuously updated, and their current guidelines should always be followed. In 1998 the CDC guidelines for infection control in health care personnel were updated for release.

The 1996 CDC guidelines for isolation precautions in hospitals established two tiers of precautions.[4] The first tier of precautions consider that all clients are presumed infec-

tious regardless of their diagnosis. The use of these **standard precautions** is the best method for prevention of nosocomial infections. The second tier establishes precautions for clients with a specific diagnosis. These precautions include transmission-based precautions along with the standard precautions. Transmission-based precautions are used for clients with known or suspected infections from pathogens that can be transmitted by airborne or droplet transmission, or by contact with dry skin or contaminated surfaces.

No specific guidelines are written by CDC pertaining directly to the client who has an immune system incapable of responding to pathogens. Disease or immunosuppressant agents, such as corticosteroids, can affect the functioning of the immune system. Immunocompromised clients are at an increased risk for bacterial, parasitic, fungal, and viral infections. The use of standard precautions and transmission-based precautions helps reduce the risk of infection for these clients also. Each institution may establish additional guidelines for these clients, which should be reviewed by health care workers interacting with these clients.

Standard Precautions

Standard precautions combine universal precautions and body substance isolation techniques. **Universal precautions** focus on reducing the spread of blood-borne pathogens found in blood and body fluids. Universal precautions are used in some agencies such as child care centers where hospital guidelines would not be appropriate. The aim of body substance isolation is to decrease transmission of moist body substance pathogens. The purpose of both these precautions is to decrease the spread of pathogens in recognized and unrecognized client infections. Standard precautions apply to blood, secretions, excretions, open skin, mucous membranes, and all body fluids excluding sweat. All clients with draining wounds or secretions of body fluids are considered infectious until an infection is confirmed or ruled out.

Most institutions have adopted standard precautions. Using gloves, gowns, masks, goggles, face shields, and, most important, hand washing helps prevent the spread of infection to health care workers and other clients (see Fig. 7–6). Standard precautions are used whenever there is a risk of spreading an infectious disease, when a client needs to be protected against cross-infection, and for any client with signs of infection until it is confirmed or ruled out. Institutions have policies and procedures on the detailed use of standard precautions, and every health care worker should read and follow them.

Transmission-based Precautions

Infections transmitted through the air, such as tuberculosis (TB), varicella (chickenpox), and rubella (German measles), require transmission-based precautions. A special type of filter respirator mask, individually fitted for each health care worker, is required for those likely to come in contact with the client with this type of diagnosis. Also required for the TB client is a room equipped with a negative pressure ventilation system to prevent the spread of TB in the air.

Treatment of Infectious Diseases

Treatment is begun once an infectious organism and the affected body system is identified. Many factors play a part in determining the drug to be used. The type of organism is very important in selecting an appropriate medication. Antibiotics treat bacterial infections. Antiviral medications treat viral infections, but their use is relatively new and limited. Antifungal drugs are used for fungal infections. The drug of choice must be able to destroy the pathogen while preserving the client's healthy cells. Cost-effectiveness is another concern when selecting a medication. For example, newer antibiotics can be very expensive and therefore are not available to everyone.

Numerous antibiotics are available on the market today to treat bacterial infections. When choosing an antibiotic, several things must first be considered. First, any allergies the client may have to a particular group or class of antibiotics prevents the use of that drug. The client must have good kidney and liver function. Many antibiotics are metabolized by the liver and excreted by the kidneys. Diseases of these organs may require a lower dose to be given. Antibiotic peak and trough levels need to be monitored to prevent toxicity and damage to the kidneys. Site of infection is another factor and will determine what the route of the antibiotic will be. Possible routes include oral, parenteral, intravenous, or instillation into a body cavity.

Antibiotics can be classified as either bactericidal or bacteriostatic. Bactericidal agents destroy bacteria without the help of the infected host's immune system. Bacteriostatic agents inhibit or retard bacterial growth and usually leave the final destruction of the bacteria up to the infected host's immune system. Bacteriostatic agents therefore would not be helpful for the client who is immunocompromised.

A sampling of medications and important information related to their administration follows. The nurse should consult drug references for further information on anti-infective medications. The nurse is responsible for administering medications correctly and for teaching the client the importance of taking these medications properly.

BACTERICIDAL ANTIBIOTICS

Penicillin

Penicillin is the most widely used antibiotic. Examples of penicillin include amoxicillin (Amoxil), ticarcillin (Ticar), penicillin G, and ampicillin (Omnipen). Penicillin is most effective in treating gram-positive organisms.

Nursing Responsibilities

1. Allergies to penicillins are noted.
2. If the client is receiving penicillin for the first time, the nurse should remain with the client for the first 30 minutes to watch for signs of an allergic reaction and anaphylactic shock. Ventilatory support and epinephrine must be available.
3. Side effect occurrences are monitored.
   a. Rash, hives, and itching
   b. Fever and chills
   c. Allergic reaction and anaphylactic shock
4. If any signs of an allergic reaction occur, the parenteral dose is stopped and the physician is notified immediately.
5. Signs of a superinfection are noted.

Client Education

1. The importance of completing the entire course of antibiotic therapy is stressed.
2. The client and family are told to stop the drug and call the physician if any signs of allergic reaction occur.
3. The physician should be notified of white patches in the mouth or vaginal irritation for treatment.

Cephalosporins

Cephalosporins are similar to the penicillins. They are classified in three groups: first, second, and third generations. The first-generation cephalosporins are most effective against gram-positive organisms. The second and third generations are more effective against gram-negative organisms. Examples are cephalothin (Keflin), cefazolin (Ancef), cefaclor (Ceclor), and ceftriaxone (Rocephin).

Nursing Responsibilities

1. Allergies to cephalosporins or penicillins are noted.
2. Side effect occurrences are monitored and reported to the physician.
   a. Gastrointestinal disturbances (most common side effect)
   b. Phlebitis or localized pain at site of injection
   c. Rashes and urticaria
   d. Anaphylaxis
   e. Nephrotoxicity
   f. Hepatotoxicity
   g. Superinfection
3. Lab work is monitored—blood urea nitrogen (BUN), creatinine, lactic dehydrogenase (LDH), aspartate aminotransferase (AST), and alanine aminotransferase (ALT).

Client Teaching

1. The importance of completing the entire course of antibiotic therapy is stressed.

2. The client and family are taught when to report adverse signs.
3. Instructions include taking the medication on an empty stomach, 1 hour before or 2 hours after meals.
4. Dosages are taken at specified intervals to cover a 24-hour period.

Aminoglycosides

The aminoglycosides were the first antibiotics to treat gram-negative organisms effectively. These drugs are usually given parenterally, because they are not well absorbed in the gastrointestinal tract. Examples are amikacin (Amikin), gentamicin (Garamycin), and tobramycin (Nebcin).

Nursing Responsibilities

1. If any signs of an allergic reaction occur, the medication is stopped and the physician is notified immediately.
2. Side effects:
   a. Nephrotoxicity
   b. Ototoxicity
3. This type of medication should not be mixed or infused with any other drug.

Client Teaching

1. Teach the client to report signs of allergy, tinnitus, vertigo, or hearing loss.
2. The client should obtain daily weights because weight gain can be an indication of kidney problems.

BACTERIOSTATIC ANTIBIOTICS

Tetracyclines

Tetracyclines were the first broad-spectrum antibiotics developed that were effective against most gram-positive and gram-negative organisms. Examples are tetracycline HCl, doxycycline (Vibramycin), and minocycline HCl (Minocin). Tetracycline HCl is available only in oral preparations. The other tetracyclines are given parenterally. The intravenous route is preferred because intramuscular routes are poorly absorbed.

Nursing Responsibilities

1. Medications are given 1 hour before or 2 hours after meals. They are not given with milk, milk products, or antacids because absorption is affected.
2. Signs of superinfection are noted.
3. Gastrointestinal disturbances are the most common side effect.
4. Tetracyclines increase the activity of anticoagulants. If the client is on anticoagulant therapy, prothrombin times, international normalized ratios, and partial prothrombin times are monitored as appropriate. Signs of bleeding are also monitored.

Client Teaching

1. Explain that eating crackers with tetracyclines and drinking juice can alleviate gastrointestinal upset.
2. Teach that prolonged exposure to the sun can cause photosensitivity reactions to occur.

Erythromycin

Erythromycin is a broad-spectrum antibiotic. It is effective against gram-negative and gram-positive organisms. It is also the medication primarily used for clients allergic to penicillins. Examples are E-Mycin, E.E.S., and Erythrocin.

Nursing Responsibilities

1. Erythromycin is given on an empty stomach 1 hour before meals or 2 hours after meals.
2. The medication should be taken with a full glass of water. It should not be given with acidic fruit juices, such as orange juice or grapefruit juice.
3. When giving medication intravenously, it should be administered slowly to decrease vein irritation.

Client Teaching

1. The client is instructed to take the medication around the clock and complete the entire treatment.
2. Gastric distress is a common side effect and is not an indication to stop the medication. If symptoms persist and are not tolerable, the client is told to contact the physician.
3. The client should contact the physician if signs of superinfection appear.

Sulfonamides

Developed in the 1930s, sulfonamides were the first effective systemic antibiotics. They were effective against most gram-positive and many gram-negative organisms. Sulfonamides are commonly used in urinary tract infections, *Pneumocystis carinii* pneumonia, and otitis media. Examples include sulfamethoxazole (Gantanol), sulfasalazine (Azulfidine), sulfisoxazole (Gantrisin), and trimethoprim-sulfamethoxazole (Bactrim, Septra).

Nursing Responsibilities

1. Side effects are monitored.
   a. Rashes and pruritis (most common)
   b. Nausea and vomiting
   c. Phlebitis
   d. Signs of bleeding
2. The intravenous route should be infused over 1 hour.
3. Intake and output are monitored.
4. Fluid intake should be at least 1500 mL per day.
5. Bleeding time can be increased, so caution is used with anticoagulants.
6. The toxicity of phenytoin (Dilantin) can be increased.
7. The risk of hypoglycemia can be increased.

Client Teaching

1. The client is instructed to take the medication on an empty stomach 1 hour before or 2 hours after meals.
2. The medication is taken with a full glass of water. Fluids are encouraged.
3. Teach that prolonged exposure to the sun can cause photosensitivity reactions to occur.
4. Tell client to stop medication and call physician if signs of allergic reaction or bleeding occur.

ANTIFUNGAL AGENTS

Antifungal agents are available in systemic and topical form. Antifungal agents interfere with the cell wall structure of the fungus, causing it to die.

Amphotericin B

Amphotericin B is given parenterally only. It is reserved for treating life-threatening fungal infections.

Nursing Responsibilities

1. The client is closely monitored during first hour of drug infusion for signs of febrile reactions.
2. The injection site is monitored frequently because this drug is very irritating to the tissues.
3. Side effects are monitored.
   a. Nausea, vomiting, and diarrhea
   b. Nephrotoxic
4. Nursing implications:
   a. Intake and output are monitored.
   b. Daily weight is obtained.
   c. Fluid intake of 2000 to 3000 mL per day is encouraged.
   d. BUN and creatinine levels are monitored.

Client Education

1. The purpose of the treatment and use of long-term intravenous therapy is explained.
2. The client is instructed on side effects and possible discomfort at intravenous site.

Fluconazole (Diflucan)

Fluconazole (Diflucan) is used to treat candidal and urinary tract infections, as well as cryptococcal meningitis. It can be given either parenterally or orally.

Nursing Responsibilities

1. Cultures are obtained before administering the medication.
2. BUN and creatinine are monitored. The medication must be used with caution in clients with renal impairment.
3. Liver function tests are monitored.
4. Side effects are monitored.
   a. Hepatotoxicity
   b. Nausea, vomiting, diarrhea, and abdominal discomfort

Client Education

1. The client is taught the importance of completing the medication therapy.
2. The client is taught to take the medication the same time each day.
3. The client is instructed not to double a dose, if a dose is missed.
4. The client is taught to notify the physician at the first sign of yellow skin, dark urine, or pale stools.

Nursing Process

ASSESSMENT

The ability of the nurse to recognize the signs and symptoms of infection is extremely important. Early detection can help prevent major complications and provide early treatment. The nurse must be aware of body systems that can commonly be affected by infections and clients who are at risk for development of infections.

NURSING DIAGNOSIS

Nursing diagnoses are made by the registered nurse. These diagnoses are made based on assessment data gathered by the registered nurse and consideration of data collected by the LPN/LVN. (See Nursing Care Plan Box 7–3 for the Client with an Infection.) The diagnoses may include but are not limited to the following:

1. Increased risk for infection related to external factors
2. Alteration of comfort related to the infectious process
3. Knowledge deficit related to disease process and treatment

PLANNING

Diligence in carrying out the plan of care is extremely important. Ensuring that the appropriate medication is given on time and understanding how to care for clients with infections can help the client recover quickly. All members of the health care team must be aware of the client's infection and their role in helping the client recover.

IMPLEMENTATION

Diligence in following infection control procedures can help prevent the development of infections. Understanding

NURSING CARE PLAN BOX 7–3 FOR THE CLIENT WITH AN INFECTION

Risk for infection related to external factors

Client Outcomes
Client will remain afebrile. White blood cell count (WBC) remains within normal limits.

Evaluation of Outcomes
Is client's temperature within normal range? Is client's WBC normal?

Interventions	Rationale	Evaluation
Assess client for signs/symptoms of infection.	Detection of infection allows treatment to begin.	Are signs/symptoms of infection present?
Monitor temperature every 4 hours and record.	Elevated temperature can indicate presence of infection.	Is temperature within normal limits?
Monitor WBC as ordered.	Elevated WBC can indicate infection.	Is WBC normal?
Use standard precautions.	Standard precautions protect clients from transmission of microorganisms.	Are standard precautions used?
Obtain cultures as ordered.	Cultures allow detection and identification of microorganisms.	Are cultures negative?
Teach client infection prevention techniques.	Understanding prevention techniques can help reduce infection risk.	Does client state understanding of prevention techniques?

GERIATRIC

Assist client with activities of daily living as needed.	Proper hygiene can reduce infection risk.	Are client's activities of daily living done?

Alteration in comfort related to infection and hyperthermia

Client Outcomes
Client reports satisfactory comfort level.

Evaluation of Outcomes
Does client report comfort?

Interventions	Rationale	Evaluation
Assess pain levels using a scale of 1 to 10, pain location, duration, and intensity.	Determines severity and location of pain consistently.	Does client report pain level on scale of 1 to 10, location, duration, and intensity?
Administer analgesics or antipyretics as ordered.	Analgesics and antipyretics promote comfort by relieving pain and fever.	Does client report that pain and fever are relieved?
Perform comfort measures to promote relaxation.	Comfort measures help reduce pain.	Do comfort measures relieve pain?

GERIATRIC

Assess pain levels and provide pain relief for elderly clients.	Pain is not a normal aging change and requires treatment.	Does client report that pain is relieved?

Knowledge deficit related to lack of knowledge about disorder and treatment

Client Outcomes
Verbalizes knowledge of disorder and willingness to comply with therapeutic regimen.

continued

NURSING CARE PLAN BOX 7–3 (continued)

Evaluation of Outcomes
Does client report understanding and willingness to comply?

Interventions	Rationale	Evaluation
Explain condition, symptoms, and complications. Explain medications and therapies ordered, including teaching client importance of following treatment regimen.	Client must have basic knowledge to comply with therapy. Compliance and safe use of medications are promoted with an adequate knowledge base.	Is client able to verbalize knowledge taught? Can client explain medications and therapies?
GERIATRIC		
Allow elderly clients more time to learn.	Reaction times in elderly clients are slower, but learning can take place.	Does elderly client state understanding within time provided for teaching sessions?

of how infections are contracted and spread will help in controlling infectious diseases.

EVALUATION

Evaluating laboratory data helps determine that the infection is controlled and the client is recovering. Absence of signs and symptoms helps evaluate the effectiveness of treatment. The client's compliance with treatment evaluates the effectiveness of client teaching.

Client Education

Clients, families, and all members of the health care team must be aware of the events that cause the infectious process and treatment plans when an infection occurs. Education should be directed toward prevention and spread of infectious diseases. Teaching clients how to participate in their care and assisting in the development of their plan of care promotes compliance with treatment. Clients' understanding of how infections occur helps them in controlling their risk for developing an infection.

Review Questions

1. Which of the following are disease-producing microorganisms?
   a. Normal flora
   b. Antibodies
   c. Pathogens
   d. Antigens

2. As the nurse plans client care, defense mechanisms against infections are considered. Which of the following is the body's first line of defense against infection?
   a. Phagocytosis
   b. Immune response
   c. Intact skin and mucous membranes
   d. Inflammatory response

3. Which one of the following is a common sign or symptom of a localized infection?
   a. Fever
   b. Site warmth
   c. Malaise
   d. Headache

4. Which of the following is the purpose of a sensitivity test?
   a. Identifying pathogens
   b. Assessing the client's response to a medication
   c. Identifying an antibiotic's effect on a pathogen
   d. Determining the appropriate medication dosage

5. A client has been exposed to hepatitis A. Treatment to provide passive immunity is recommended. Which of the following provides passive immunity?
   a. Administration of immune globulin
   b. Administration of a vaccine
   c. Antibodies produced by client's own B cells
   d. Stimulation of the client's immune system by the pathogen

6. Which of the following is the most important nursing action to prevent a nosocomial urinary tract infection in a client with an indwelling urinary catheter?
   a. Ensure an adequate intake of IV and oral fluids.
   b. Use clean technique for catheter insertion.

c. Review urine culture and sensitivity results.

d. Maintain a closed urinary drainage system.

7. Which of the following is the purpose of medical asepsis?
   a. Eliminating any microorganisms from coming in contact with a client.
   b. Preventing the spread of infection from one person to another.
   c. Preventing the spread of infection during a surgical procedure.
   d. Removing bacteria from objects that come in contact with an open wound.

8. Before administering a newly ordered antibiotic to a client with a wound infection, which of the following should the nurse do first?
   a. Ensure that a culture of the wound is done.
   b. Check the client's temperature.
   c. Change the dressing and note the wound's appearance.
   d. Wait until meal time to give the antibiotic.

9. Which one of the following standard precautions is most important for the nurse to use during client care when the possibility of body secretions being sprayed in the air exists?
   a. Gloves
   b. Gown
   c. Face shield
   d. Mask

ANSWERS TO CRITICAL THINKING

CRITICAL THINKING: Charles

Charles should not be given a live virus to develop active immunity because his immune system is not functioning properly. If his immune system is not able to develop antibodies against the live virus, Charles could become ill and even die from the virus.

CRITICAL THINKING: Mrs. Sampson

1. Hand washing reduces the microorganisms on the nurse's hands to help reduce their transmission from client to client. This helps prevent exposure to pathogens and infection.
2. Risk for infection.
3. Reverse isolation, the goal of which is to protect the client from exposure to microorganisms rather than to protect others from exposure to the client.

REFERENCES

1. Still, O, and Hodgins, D: Navajo Indians. In Purnell, L, and Paulanka, B (eds): Transcultural Health Care: A Culturally Competent Approach. FA Davis, Philadelphia, 1998.
2. Levy, RA: Ethnic and racial differences in response to medicines: Preserving individualized therapy in managed pharmaceutical programmes. Pharmaceutical Medicine 7:139, 1993.
3. Humphreys, H, and Keane, C: Methicillin-resistant *Staphylococcus aureus* and vancomycin-resistant enterococci. Lancet 350(9079):737, 1997.
4. The Hospital Infection Control Practices Advisory Committee, Centers for Disease Control and Prevention: CDC Guideline for Isolation Precautions in Hospitals. American Journal Infection Contol 24(1):32, 1996.

BIBLIOGRAPHY

Boyce, JM: Vancomycin-resistant enterococcus. Detection, epidemiology, and control measures. Infect Dis Clin North Am 11(2):367, 1997.
Catianno, C: Nosocomial pneumonia: Repelling a deadly invader. Nursing 26:5, 1996.
Corwin, EJ: Handbook of Pathophysiology. JB Lippincott, Philadelphia, 1996.
Deglin, J, and Vallerand, A: Davis's Drug Guide for Nurses. FA Davis, Philadelphia, 1997.
Edmond, MB, et al: Vancomyin-resistant enterococcus bacteremia: natural history and attributable mortality. Clin Infect Dis 23(6):1234, 1996.
Garna, J: Guidelines for isolation precautions in hospitals. Infect Control Hosp Epidemiol 17(1):53, 1996.
Guyton, AC, and Hall, JE: Textbook of Medical Physiology, ed 9. WB Saunders, Philadelphia, 1996.
Horland, WA: Defending your client against nosocomial pneumonia. Nursing 25:8, 1995.
Lee, YL, et al: Surveillance of colonization and infection with *Staphylococcus aureus* susceptible or resistant to methicillin in a community skilled-nursing facility. Am J Infect Control 25(4):312, 1997.
Jaffe, MS: Medical-Surgical Nursing Care Plans: Nursing Diagnosis and Interventions, ed 3. Appleton & Lange, Norwalk, Conn, 1996.
Jaffe, M, and McVan, B: Davis's Laboratory and Diagnostic Test Handbook. FA Davis, Philadelphia, 1997.
McDonald, LC, et al: Vancomycin-resistant enterococcus outside the health-care setting: Prevalence, sources and public health implications. Emerg Infect Dis 3(3):311, 1997.
Polaski, AL, and Tatro, SE: Luckmann's Core Principles and Practice of Medical-Surgical Nursing. WB Saunders, Philadelphia, 1996.
Reiss, P: Battling the super bugs. RN 59:3, 1996.
Shlaes, DM, et al: Society for Healthcare Epidemiology of America and Infectious Diseases Society of America Joint Committee on the prevention of antimicrobial resistance: Guidelines for the prevention of antimicrobial resistance in hospitals. Clin Infect Dis 25(3):584, 1997.
Stein, A, et al: Infection control: For our clients and ourselves. Journal of Emergency Medical Services 20:6, 1995.
Thomas, CL (ed): Taber's Cyclopedic Medical Dictionary, ed 18. FA Davis, Philadelphia, 1997.
Washio, M: Risk factors for methicillin-resistant *Staphylococcus aureus* (MRSA) infection in a Japanese elderly care nursing home. Epidemiol Infect 119(2):285, 1997.

Care of Clients in Shock

JoAnn Widner

8

Learning Objectives

Upon completion of this chapter, the student will be able to:

1. Define shock.
2. Explain the causes and pathophysiology of shock.
3. Explain how the body compensates for shock.
4. Explain how shock affects the organ systems of the body.
5. Differentiate between the four categories of shock.
6. Identify the signs and symptoms of shock.
7. Describe comprehensive assessment of the client in shock.
8. Apply the nursing process to the care of the client in shock.

Key Words

acidosis (ass-i-**DOH**-sis)

acute pulmonary hypertension (ah-**KEWT PULL**-muh-NER-ee HIGH-per-**TEN**-shun)

anaerobic (AN-air-**ROH**-bik)

anaphylaxis (AN-uh-fi-**LAK**-sis)

antiarrhythmic (an-ti-a-**RITH**-mik)

bronchospasm (**BRONG**-koh-spazm)

cardiac output (**KAR**-dee-yak **OWT**-put)

cardiogenic (KAR-dee-oh-**JEN**-ik)

cyanosis (SIGH-uh-**NOH**-sis)

distributive (dis-**TRIB**-yoo-tiv)

dysrhythmia (dis-**RITH**-mee-yah)

epinephrine (EP-i-**NEFF**-rin)

extracardiac (EX-trah-**KAR**-dee-yak)

hypotension (HIGH-poh-**TEN**-shun)

hypovolemic (HIGH-poh-voh-**LEEM**-ick)

ischemia (iss-**KEY**-me-ah)

lactic acid (LAK-tik **ASS**-id)

laryngeal edema (lah-**RIN**-jee-uhl uh-**DEE**-muh)

myocardium (MY-oh-**KAR**-dee-um)

myocarditis (MY-oh-kar-**DYE**-tis)

neurogenic (NEW-roh-**JEN**-ik)

norepinephrine (NOR-ep-i-**NEFF**-rin)

oliguria (AH-li-**GYOO**-ree-ah)

perfusion (per-**FEW**-zhun)

pericardial tamponade (PER-ee-**KAR**-dee-uhl TAM-pon-**AYD**)

sepsis (**SEP**-sis)

tachycardia (TAK-ee-**KAR**-dee-yah)

tachypnea (TAK-ip-**NEE**-ah)

tension pneumothorax (**TEN**-shun NEW-moh-**THAW**-raks)

thrombi (**THROM**-bye)

toxemia (tock-**SEE**-me-ah)

transmural myocardial infarction (trans-**MYOOR**-uhl MY-oh-**KAR**dee-uhl in-**FARK**-shun)

trauma (**TRAW**-mah)

trendelenburg (Tren-**DELL**-en-berg)

urticaria (UR-ti-**KAIR**-ee-ah)

Table 8–1. **Signs and Symptoms of Shock Phases**

Signs and Symptoms	Mild/Compensating	Moderate/Progressive	Severe/Irreversible
		Phases	
Heart Rate	Elevated	Tachycardia	Slowing
Pulses	Bounding	Weaker, thready	Absent
Blood Pressure			
Systolic	Normal	Below 90 mm Hg In hypertensive 25% below baseline	Below 60 mm Hg
Diastolic	Normal	Decreased	Decreasing to 0
Respirations	Elevated	Tachypnea	Slowing
Depth	Deep	Shallow	Irregular, shallow
Temperature	Varies	Decreased May elevate in septic shock	Decreasing
Level of Consciousness	Anxious, restless, irritable, alert, oriented	Confused, lethargy	Unconscious, comatose
Skin and Mucous Membranes	Cool, pale	Cold, moist, clammy, pale	Cyanosis, mottled, cold, clammy
Urine Output	Normal	Decreasing to less than 20 mL/h	15 mL/h decreasing to anuria
Bowel Sounds	Normal	Decreasing	Absent

The client in shock is in a state of severe circulatory collapse that will result in death without immediate treatment. Massive bleeding, overwhelming infection, severe allergic reactions, and cardiac failure are examples of conditions that may lead to shock. No matter what its source, shock is a medical emergency requiring rapid nursing assessment and intervention.

Whenever shock occurs, there is insufficient delivery of oxygen and nutrients to the body's tissues and inadequate removal of waste products from the tissues. When oxygen delivery is insufficient, cellular metabolism becomes abnormal. All body systems are affected at both the organ and cellular level. The resulting injury to the body is treatable in early stages, but when prolonged, it leads to irreversible cell damage and death.

Pathophysiology of Shock

Shock occurs when the cardiovascular system is unable to meet the oxygen and nutritional needs of the body's cells and is usually reflected by a sudden drop in blood pressure. Insufficient blood pressure may be due to a variety of factors. Common causes include inadequate **cardiac output** due to heart failure, a sudden loss of blood volume due to hemorrhage, or a sudden decrease in peripheral vascular resistance due to **anaphylaxis.**

METABOLIC AND HEMODYNAMIC CHANGES

When blood pressure falls below a critical level, the body responds by activating the sympathetic nervous system (SNS). The SNS secretes epinephrine and norepinephrine to increase cardiac output by causing the heart to beat faster and stronger. Blood is shunted away from the skin, kidneys, and intestines to preserve blood flow to the brain, liver, and heart. Epinephrine, cortisol, and glucagon raise blood glucose levels to supply cells with fuel. Stimulation of the renin-angiotensin-aldosterone system from decreased cardiac output causes vasoconstriction and sodium and water to be retained to decrease further fluid loss. Respiratory rate increases to deliver more oxygen to the tissues. Together, these compensatory responses produce the classic signs and symptoms of shock seen in the initial phase of shock: **tachycardia; tachypnea; oliguria;** and cool, clammy skin with pallor. If oxygen delivery remains inadequate, signs and symptoms of moderate and irreversible shock phases are seen (Table 8–1).

---

anaphylaxis: an—without + phylaxis—protection
tachycardia: tachy—fast + cardia—heart condition
tachypnea: tachy—fast + pnea—breathing
oliguria: olig—few + uria—urine condition

LEARNING TIP

Tachycardia is a compensatory mechanism that is usually the first sign of shock. When a client develops sustained tachycardia it is a signal that the client's condition is changing. Be aware that elderly clients cannot tolerate tachycardia very long because their reserves for adapting to stress are reduced.

Consider what the cause of the tachycardia could be for the client. For example, a surgical client who develops tachycardia may be hemorrhaging and should be assessed for bleeding. With internal hemorrhaging there may not be any visible signs of bleeding.

Provide prompt intervention, such as applying direct pressure to an area of hemorrhage, and implement the physician's orders immediately.

Inadequate tissue blood flow causes an important change in cellular metabolism. When cells are deprived of oxygen, they shift to **anaerobic** metabolism to provide nutrition and energy for the cell. Anaerobic metabolism, however, can only supply the energy needs of the cell for a period of a few minutes, and then metabolic rate and body temperature fall. Anaerobic metabolism also results in the production of **lactic acid,** and unless the lactic acid can be circulated to the liver and removed from the bloodstream, the blood will become increasingly acidic. Metabolic **acidosis** and a fall in blood pH, below 7.35, are the hallmarks of shock.

 CRITICAL THINKING:
Anaerobic Metabolism

Why is anaerobic metabolism necessary and helpful when it produces the complication of metabolic acidosis?

Answer at end of chapter.

EFFECT ON ORGANS AND ORGAN SYSTEMS

Prolonged shock causes extensive damage to the organs and organ systems (Table 8–2). Inadequate blood flow results in tissue **ischemia** and injury. Because blood is shunted away from the kidneys early in shock, they are often injured first. The kidneys can tolerate low blood flow for approximately 1 hour before sustaining permanent damage. Renal failure resulting from inadequate blood

---

anaerobic: an—without + aerobic—presence of oxygen
acidosis: acid—sour + osis—condition
dysrhythmia: dys—difficult or abnormal + rhythm—rhythm

Table 8–2. *Effect of Shock on Organs and Organ Systems*

Lungs	Acute respiratory failure Adult respiratory distress syndrome
Renal	Pre–renal failure, intrinsic renal failure, complete renal failure
Heart	Dysrhythmias, myocardial ischemia, and myocardial depression
Liver	Abnormal clotting; decreased production of plasma proteins; elevated serum levels of ammonia, bilirubin, and liver enzymes
Immune System	Depletion of defense components
Gastrointestinal System	Mucosal injury, paralytic ileus, pancreatitis, absorption of endotoxins and bacteria
Central Nervous System	Ischemic damage, necrosis, brain death

flow to the kidneys can be prevented or treated by replacing lost fluids. Cells within the kidneys die when there is a lack of oxygen and nutrients. If there is widespread damage to the kidneys, complete renal failure is likely.

Several organs of the gastrointestinal system may be injured early in shock. Inadequate circulation to the intestines may result in injury of the mucosa and even cause paralytic ileus. **Toxemia** may result when the body absorbs into the circulation normally occurring bacteria and endotoxins from inside the bowel. The liver may be injured both by ischemia and by toxins created by the shock state as blood is circulated through it for cleansing. Signs and symptoms of liver injury include abnormal clotting, decreased production of plasma proteins, and elevated serum levels of ammonia, bilirubin, and liver enzymes.

The immune system is also affected by shock. Many of the body's defense components become depleted from shock, leaving the body vulnerable to infection. Also, if the liver has been damaged, it will be unable to assist the immune system in providing defense.

The body attempts to preserve blood supply to the heart and brain because these are vital organs that require a continuous supply of oxygen. Shock places extra demands on the heart itself, creating a situation in which the heart is in extra need of oxygen at a time when oxygen supplies are already low. When the **myocardium** itself does not receive adequate oxygenation, cardiac output decreases and shock worsens. The pumping ability of the heart may further be depressed by toxins released into the blood from ischemic tissues and by ischemia-induced **dysrhythmia.** If the brain is deprived of circulation for more than 4 minutes, brain cells will die from a lack of oxygen and glucose. Lengthy shock may eventually cause brain death.

COMPLICATIONS FROM SHOCK

Adult respiratory distress syndrome (ARDS), disseminated intravascular coagulation (DIC), and multisystem organ failure (MSOF) are three especially grave conditions that may follow a prolonged episode of shock. Clients with ARDS will usually develop pulmonary failure despite high levels of supplemental oxygen and mechanical ventilation. Disseminated intravascular coagulation results from ischemic damage to the endothelial lining of blood vessels. The formation of multiple tiny **thrombi,** microscopic debris, and depletion of tissue clotting factors causes abnormal bleeding and additional tissue damage, and DIC itself may precipitate shock and death. Multisystem organ failure is a major cause of mortality following shock. It usually begins with respiratory failure, followed by failure of the kidneys, heart, liver, and finally cerebral and gastrointestinal functioning.

LEARNING TIP

To understand what disseminated intravascular coagulation means, define each of the words and then put the definitions together:

Disseminated: scattered or widespread
Intravascular: intra—inside + vascular—vessels
Coagulation: clotting

When these definitions are put together it means that DIC is scattered, widespread clotting inside vessels.

In response to stressors, many clots with no useful purpose form throughout the body, leaving few clotting factors available to form clots necessary to prevent hemorrhage. As a result, hemorrhage may be seen in DIC.

Classification of Shock

Different forms of shock are categorized and named by the cardiovascular characteristics that occur. The four shock categories are (1) **hypovolemic** shock caused by a decrease in the circulating blood volume; (2) **cardiogenic** shock caused by cardiac failure; (3) **extracardiac** obstructive shock caused by a blockage of blood flow in the cardiovascular circuit outside the heart; and (4) **distributive** shock caused by excessive dilation of the venules and arterioles (Table 8–3). Most cases of clinical shock show some components of each of these categories. However, this classification system is helpful in understanding shock. The hallmark characteristic that all forms of shock exhibit is a decrease in blood pressure. The blood pressure usually falls below the level required to provide an adequate supply of blood to the tissues.

HYPOVOLEMIC SHOCK

Any severe loss of body fluid may lead to hypovolemic shock. Hypovolemic shock can be caused by dehydration; internal or external hemorrhage; fluid loss from burns, vomiting, or diarrhea; or loss of intravascular fluid into the interstitium due to **sepsis** or **trauma.** Clinical signs and symptoms include pale, cool, clammy skin; tachycardia; tachypnea; flat, nondistended peripheral veins; decreased jugular vein circumference; decreased urine output; and altered mental status. With a 10 percent loss of blood volume, tachycardia is the only obvious sign. At 20 to 25 percent blood loss, tachycardia and mild to moderate **hypotension** are present. With a loss of 40 percent or greater, all clinical signs and symptoms of shock are present.

CARDIOGENIC SHOCK

Cardiogenic shock results when the heart fails as a pump. It is a common cause of death among clients who have suffered a **transmural** (full thickness of the heart wall) **myocardial infarction** (MI). In most cases, approximately 40 percent of the myocardium must be lost to produce cardiogenic shock. Clients with cardiogenic shock will have signs and symptoms similar to hypovolemic shock, except that they may display distended jugular and peripheral veins, as well as other symptoms of heart failure, such as pulmonary edema. Other causes of cardiogenic shock include rupture of heart valves, acute **myocarditis,** end-stage heart disease, severe dysrhythmias, or traumatic injury to the heart.

OBSTRUCTIVE SHOCK

Extracardiac obstructive shock occurs when there is a blockage in the flow of blood within the cardiovascular circuit outside of the heart. Several conditions may cause obstructive shock. **Pericardial tamponade,** which is the filling of the pericardial sac with blood, compresses the heart and limits its filling capacity. **Tension pneumothorax** compresses the heart from an abnormal collection of air in the pleural space and interferes with normal cardiac functioning. **Acute pulmonary hypertension,** a sudden abnormal elevated pressure in the pulmonary artery, increases resistance for blood flowing out of the right side of the heart. All of these conditions cause a decrease in cardiac output, which can lead to shock. Tumors or large emboli may also cause shock. Obstructive shock signs and symptoms are similar to those of hypovolemic shock, except that jugular veins are usually distended.

DISTRIBUTIVE SHOCK

Distributive shock occurs when peripheral vascular resistance is lost because of massive vasodilation of the periph-

Table 8–3. **Categories of Shock**

Category	Causes	Signs and Symptoms
Hypovolemic Shock	Any severe loss of body fluid. Dehydration, internal or external hemorrhage, fluid loss from burns or from vomiting or diarrhea, or loss of intravascular fluid into the interstitium.	Tachycardia, tachypnea, hypotension, cyanosis, oliguria, flat nondistended peripheral veins, decreased jugular veins, and altered mental status.
Cardiogenic Shock	Myocardial infarction, myocarditis, end-stage cardiomyopathy, severe dysrhythmias, valvular disease, severe electrolyte imbalance, and drug overdoses.	Dysrhythmias, labored respirations, hypotension, cyanosis, oliguria, altered mental status, possibly distended jugular and peripheral veins, and symptoms of congestive heart failure.
Obstructive Shock	Any block to the cardiovascular flow. Pericardial tamponade, tension pneumothorax, intrathoracic tumors, massive pulmonary emboli, and large systemic emboli.	Tachycardia, tachypnea, hypotension, cyanosis, oliguria, and altered mental status. Jugular veins may be distended.
Distributive Shock	Any condition causing massive vasodilation of the peripheral circulation. Subcategories include anaphylactic, septic, and neurogenic shock.	See subcategories below.
Anaphylactic shock	Insect stings, antibiotics, anesthetics, dye contrast, and blood products are typical allergens.	Tachycardia, tachypnea, hypotension, cyanosis, oliguria, and altered mental status. May also have urticaria, laryngeal edema, and severe bronchospasm. If conscious, may be extremely apprehensive and complain of a metallic taste.
Septic shock	Massive release of chemical mediators and endotoxins causes loss of vascular autoregulatory control and loss of fluid into the interstitium. Bacteria, especially gram-negative strains, protozoans, and viruses.	Early or warm phase: blood pressure, urine output, and neck veins may be normal. Skin warm and flushed with full veins. Fever usually present, although temperature may be subnormal. Late phase: tachycardia, tachypnea, hypotension, oliguria, flat jugular and peripheral veins, and cool clammy skin. Normal or subnormal temperature.
Neurogenic shock	Dysfunction or injury to the nervous system. Spinal cord injury, general anesthesia, fever, metabolic disturbances, and brain injuries.	Early phase: hypotension and altered mental status, bradycardia, and skin that is warm and dry. Late phase: tachycardia, tachypnea, and cool clammy skin.

eral circulation. Distributive shock includes anaphylactic, septic, and **neurogenic** shock.

Anaphylactic Shock

Anaphylactic shock occurs when the body has an extreme hypersensitivity reaction. It occurs most commonly from insect stings, antibiotics, anesthetics, dye contrast, and blood products. The signs and symptoms are similar to those seen in hypovolemic shock. Additionally, clients may have symptoms specific to allergic reactions, including **urticaria,** wheezing, **laryngeal edema,** and severe **bronchospasm.** If conscious, they may be extremely apprehensive and short of breath and may complain of a metallic taste.

Septic Shock

Septic shock is caused by systemic infection and inflammation. Extensive release of chemical mediators and endotoxins causes dilation of blood vessels and loss of fluid into

the interstitial space. Most cases of sepsis are caused by gram-negative bacteria, although other bacteria, protozoans, and viruses may be the cause. Septic shock is the leading cause of death among critical care clients. Predisposing conditions include trauma, diabetes mellitus, corticosteroid therapy, acquired immunodeficiency syndrome (AIDS), poor nutrition, and radiation therapy.

During the early or warm phase of septic shock, blood pressure, urine output, and neck vein size may be normal, but the skin is warm and flushed. Fever is present in the majority of clients, although some may have a subnormal temperature. Untreated, septic shock progresses to a second phase with signs and symptoms similar to hypovolemic shock: hypotension, oliguria, tachycardia, tachypnea, flat jugular and peripheral veins, and cold, clammy skin. Body temperature may be normal or subnormal.

Neurogenic Shock

Neurogenic shock occurs when dysfunction or injury to the nervous system causes extensive dilation of peripheral blood vessels. It is a rarer form of shock. It occurs most commonly with injury to the spinal cord, which is referred to as spinal shock. Other causes include general anesthesia, fever, metabolic disturbances, and brain contusions and concussions. Signs and symptoms include hypotension and altered mental status, and during the early phases, bradycardia and skin that is warm and dry. As shock progresses, however, tachycardia and cool, clammy skin develop.

Medical-Surgical Management

Because of the emergency nature of shock, life-threatening symptoms must be treated immediately (Table 8–4). Assessment of the exact nature of the shock must be done as interventions such as ventilatory and circulatory support are being implemented (Table 8–5). The order of interventions and testing is guided by the stability of the client. Intervention priorities are as follows: (1) respiratory support; (2) cardiovascular support; (3) adequate circulatory volume; (4) control of bleeding if present; (5) treatment of life-

Table 8–4. Medical-Surgical Management of Shock

Intervention Priorities	Respiratory support Cardiovascular support Adequate circulatory volume Control of bleeding Assess neurological status Treat life-threatening injuries Determine and treat cause of shock
Immediate Goals	Systolic BP > 90 mm Hg MVo_2 > 60 mm Hg with O_2 saturation > 92% Urine output > 30 mL/h Hemoglobin > 10 g/dL Serum lactate < 2.2 mM/L Restore normal level of consciousness
Fluid Resuscitation	1–3 L of IV fluids for hemorrhagic and septic shock IV fluids: lactated Ringer's solution, normal saline, and plasmalyte Blood products: whole blood, packed red blood cells, albumin, and plasma protein fraction
Medications	Morphine sulfate Dopamine Norepinephrine, epinephrine Isoproterenol, dobutamine Digoxin, nitroglycerin, nitroprusside, isosorbide
Antiarrhythmics	Tachycardias: verapamil, digoxin Bradycardias: atropine, Isuprel Ventricular dysrhythmias: lidocaine, procainamide, bretylium Atrial dysrhythmias: digoxin, quinidine, propranolol

Table 8–5. Assessment of the Client in Shock

Signs and Symptoms	Tachycardia, tachypnea, hypotension, oliguria, cyanosis, and altered mental status
Laboratory Tests	Complete blood count, serum osmolarity, blood chemistries, prothrombin time, partial thromboplastin time, blood typing and crossmatch, serum lactate, arterial blood gases, cardiac isoenzymes, urinalysis
Imaging	Chest x-ray, spinal films, computed tomography, echocardiogram
Monitoring	Electrocardiogram, arterial pressure monitor, central venous pressure monitor, pulmonary artery catheter, gastric pH

threatening injuries; and (6) determination and treatment of the cause of shock. Immediate goals include (1) stabilization of blood pressure; (2) adequate tissue oxygenation; (3) adequate renal **perfusion;** and (4) resolution of acidosis.

FLUID RESUSCITATION

Most clients in circulatory shock receive a fluid bolus with intravenous (IV) fluids. The exception would be clients who are in cardiogenic shock and marked pulmonary edema. The volume of the fluid bolus varies according to the client's needs. Commonly used IV fluids include normal saline, lactated Ringer's solution, and plasmalyte. Blood products such as whole blood, packed red blood cells, albumin, and plasma protein fraction are often given, particularly in the case of hemorrhage shock. Clients receiving blood products are monitored closely for signs of transfusion reaction.

MEDICATIONS

For the conscious client in pain, morphine sulfate may be given, provided there has not been a closed head injury and blood pressure is high enough to offset the vasodilation caused by analgesics. Respirations should be carefully monitored. Morphine is particularly helpful in the case of myocardial infarction because it reduces anxiety, pain, and myocardial oxygen consumption.

If the client continues to be unstable despite adequate hydration, vasoactive drugs may be needed for adequate tissue perfusion. Dopamine (Intropin) IV may be used to treat shock because it causes vasoconstriction, which raises blood pressure. **Norepinephrine** (Levophed) and **epinephrine** also act by causing systemic vasoconstriction. Epinephrine acts by increasing myocardial contractility, as does isoproterenol and dobutamine. Digoxin (Lanoxin) may be used if the heart rate needs to be slowed and contractility increased. Perfusion of the myocardium itself can be increased with drugs such as nitroglycerin (Nitro-Bid), nitroprusside (Nipride), and isosorbide (Isordil).

Clients suffering from cardiogenic shock secondary to acute myocardial infarction may have underlying cardiac dysrhythmias requiring treatment. Commonly used **antiarrhythmic** agents include verapamil (Calan) and digoxin (Lanoxin) for tachycardias, atropine (Atropair) and isoproterenol (Isuprel) for bradycardias, lidocaine (Xylocaine), procainamide (Pronestyl), and bretylium (Bretylol) for ventricular dysrhythmias, and digoxin (Lanoxin), quinidine (Quinaglute), and propanolol (Inderal) for atrial dysrhythmias.

MANAGEMENT OF ACIDOSIS

Acidosis occurs when serum pH falls below 7.35. Symptoms of metabolic acidosis include fatigue, nausea, vomiting, hyperventilation, and decreased level of consciousness (LOC). Acidosis is treated by improving systemic and hepatic perfusion, thus decreasing the body's production of lactate and increasing its removal by the liver. Nursing measures such as providing comfort and decreasing anxiety help decrease metabolic demands. Serial arterial blood gases (ABGs) and blood lactate levels are drawn to evaluate client progress. Sodium bicarbonate, once standard therapy, is now rarely given and only if based on ABG results indicating that it is needed.

SURGICAL INTERVENTION

Surgical intervention may be necessary to treat the underlying cause of shock. Examples of corrective surgical procedures include vascular and surgical repair of major wounds and fractures, repair of bleeding ulcers and esophageal varicosities, removal of obstructions, repair of ruptured heart valves, and skull decompression to relieve elevated intracranial pressure from closed head injuries.

Nursing Process

ASSESSMENT

Assessment of the client in shock must be carried out quickly. A "head to toe" approach can be used, starting with LOC. Client responsiveness and ability to move all extremities is checked. Respiratory status is assessed. The airway is checked for patency. The cardiovascular system is assessed. Vital signs are taken. A rapid scan of the entire body for evidence of bleeding or other injuries is done. The condition of the jugular veins is noted. Are they collapsed or full? The peripheral pulses are palpated. The skin is palpated to note whether it is warm or cold, wet or dry, reddened, pale, cyanotic, or mottled. The skin around the

mouth and the mucous membranes is closely observed because **cyanosis** is often evident in these areas first. The presence, severity, and location of pain or nausea and vomiting is assessed. Chest expansion is noted for symmetry. Respirations are assessed for depth and ease. Breath sounds are ascultated to see whether they are normal, diminished, absent, or abnormal. The abdomen is inspected for normal contour and softness or firmness and distention. Bowel sounds are ascultated to determine whether they are normal, absent, hyperactive, or hypoactive. When an indwelling urinary catheter has been placed, the color of the urine and the rate of urine output are noted.

CRITICAL THINKING: Classic Signs of Shock

What is the cause and compensatory purpose of each of the classic signs of shock: tachycardia, tachypnea, oliguria, pallor, and cool, clammy skin?
Answer at end of chapter.

NURSING DIAGNOSIS

The major nursing diagnoses for shock include but are not limited to the following:

- Decreased cardiac output related to reduced circulating blood volume
- Fear related to severity of condition and unknown outcome
- Knowledge deficit related to unfamiliar condition

See Nursing Care Plan Box 8–1 for the Client in Shock.

PLANNING

The client's goals are to (1) maintain vital signs and oxygen saturation within normal range, (2) verbalize reduced fear, and (3) understand the condition and its treatment.

NURSING INTERVENTIONS

Decreased Cardiac Output

Heart rhythm and pumping ability may fail if tissue perfusion decreases to the point that vital organs are receiving an insufficient supply of oxygen. In addition to cardiogenic shock, other categories of shock may lead to cardiac instability. The cardiovascular status of clients in shock must be carefully monitored based on their stability. Intravenous fluids, medications, and oxygen are given as ordered.

Trendelenburg or modified Trendelenburg positioning has been used in the past to position clients in shock, but research has not shown these positions to be beneficial in improving tissue oxygenation. Using the Trendelenburg position may be harmful for some clients by increasing intracranial pressure, stimulating cardiac reflexes, compress-

---

antiarrhythmic: anti—against + a—not + rhythmic—rhythm

NURSING CARE PLAN BOX 8–1 FOR THE CLIENT IN SHOCK

Decreased cardiac output related to reduced circulating blood volume

Client Outcome
Client has adequate cardiac output as evidenced by vital signs and cardiac rhythm within normal limits (WNL).

Evaluation of Outcomes
Are blood pressure, heart rate, and cardiac rhythm within normal limits? Are nailbeds or mucous membranes pink? Is skin warm and dry?

Interventions	Rationale	Evaluation
Monitor heart rate and cardiac rhythm with ECG and report abnormalities.	Changes in heart rate and cardiac rhythm can be detected immediately and treated appropriately.	Are heart rate and rhythm normal?
Assess skin/nailbed color, capillary refill, and peripheral pulses and report abnormalities.	Inadequate perfusion is first evident in skin/nailbeds and peripheral pulses.	What color and temperature are the skin/nailbeds? Is capillary refill normal? Are peripheral pulses present?
Give cardiovascular medications and oxygen as ordered.	Cardiac function can be supported with medications. Supplemental oxygen increases oxygenation of heart and tissues.	Are heart rate and rhythm normal?
Reduce myocardial oxygen demand by utilizing comfort measures to alleviate pain and anxiety and by keeping the body at an appropriate temperature.	Pain, anxiety, and cold all increase tissue demands for blood and oxygen, which places increased workload on the heart to supply it.	Is body temperature within normal limits? Is the client free of pain and anxiety?

Fear related to severity of condition and unknown outcome

Client Outcome
Client states fear is reduced.

Evaluation of Outcomes
Does client state fear is decreased?

Interventions	Rationale	Evaluation
Provide explanations for procedures, the condition, and its treatment.	Knowledge allows a feeling of control and reduces fear.	Does client state fear is reduced?

Knowledge deficit related to unfamiliar condition of shock

Client Outcome
Client explains shock and its treatment.

Evaluation of Outcomes
Can client explain shock and how it is treated?

Interventions	Rationale	Evaluation
Assess client's ability to learn and identify barriers to learning.	For learning, the client must be ready to learn. Barriers such as lifestyle changes or the shock of the diagnosis may decrease learning.	Is client alert and stable? Does client indicate willingness to learn? Does client express concerns about condition?
Provide information that is most relevant to client first.	Giving necessary information first meets client's immediate needs.	Does client state understanding of important information?
Allow time for questions and clarification.	Clarification ensures that accurate information is learned.	Does client state accurate information?

ing coronary arteries, and causing the abdominal organs to press against the diaphragm, which restricts ventilations.

Fear

Reducing fear is important in controlling shock and preventing complications. It can be accomplished by providing explanations for procedures and educating the client about the condition and its treatment. The client should be allowed to express fears and ask questions. Family members should be allowed to provide support to the client.

Knowledge Deficit

Teaching the client and family about the condition and its treatment is important for compliance with treatment and to reduce anxiety. Simple explanations should be given in the critical stages of shock. As the client recovers, educational sessions can be expanded.

EVALUATION

The ultimate goal of nursing care for the client in shock is to restore normal tissue perfusion quickly enough to ensure recovery without complications. Short-term goals include the following: (1) reduce blood and fluid loss; (2) maintain adequate cardiac output; (3) restore adequate circulating volume; (4) reduce fear; (5) maintain optimal body temperature; and (6) maintain normal baseline LOC. Once these goals have been met, discharge planning for home care or rehabilitation can begin based on the client's individualized needs.

CLIENT EDUCATION

The client's participation in teaching sessions depends on the client's LOC. Family members should be included in the sessions. Initially, the client will need reorientation to person, place, and time. The client is unlikely to remember events immediately preceding and following the onset of shock. Simple explanations of what has occurred and what is happening at the present time can be followed by more complete explanations as the client's condition improves. Interventions should include explanation of all diagnostic and treatment procedures, rationales, and outcome goals. The cause of shock needs to be explained to both the family and the client once the client has stabilized. If the client has suffered complications from shock, these also need to be addressed and desired outcomes explained.

CRITICAL THINKING: Mr. Hall

Mr. Hall, 55 years old, has suffered a large transmural myocardial infarction (MI). He is complaining of chest pain and difficulty breathing. Crackles are heard on auscultation of breath sounds. The electrocardiogram shows an irregular and rapid heartbeat.

He is restless and apprehensive. Mr. Hall is given morphine sulfate IV for pain relief.

1. Name three nursing priorities for Mr. Hall's care.
2. Why is morphine sulfate useful in treating an MI?
3. What are possible side effects of morphine?
4. What signs and symptoms would indicate a worsening of Mr. Hall's shock?

Answers at end of chapter.

CRITICAL THINKING: Mrs. Neal

Mrs. Neal, 45 years old, is admitted to the emergency room in severe hypovolemic shock after sustaining several bleeding wounds in an automobile accident. Her shock is resolving after receiving several transfusions and surgical repair of her injuries. She has just been admitted to the surgical unit for postoperative care.

1. What postoperative nursing assessments are performed first?
2. Mrs. Neal's family is very alarmed by her condition. What interventions could you provide to decrease their anxiety?
3. What postoperative complications may develop in Mrs. Neal?

Answers at end of chapter.

Review Questions

1. Which one of the following mechanisms does the body use to compensate for shock?
   a. Bradycardia
   b. Bradypnea
   c. Sympathetic nervous system stimulation
   d. Parasympathetic nervous system stimulation

2. The metabolic acidosis of shock is caused by which of the following?
   a. Tachypnea
   b. Release of cortisol and glucagon
   c. Excessive aerobic metabolism
   d. Excessive anaerobic metabolism

3. Anaphylactic, septic, and neurogenic shock are all examples of which of the following type of shock?
   a. Hypovolemic
   b. Cardiogenic
   c. Obstructive
   d. Distributive

4. Which one of the following is a serious complication commonly associated with shock?
   a. Malnutrition
   b. Adult respiratory distress syndrome

c. Diabetes mellitus
d. Cerebral vascular accident

5. Which one of the following can be a serious complication for clients receiving blood products?
   a. Transfusion reaction
   b. Inadequate oxygenation
   c. Nausea and vomiting
   d. Infection

6. Which one of the following findings would be seen specifically with anaphylactic shock?
   a. Tachycardia
   b. Hypotension
   c. Laryngeal edema
   d. Oliguria

7. Which one of the following causes the decrease in level of consciousness commonly found in clients experiencing shock?
   a. Severe pain
   b. Endotoxins
   c. Cerebral anoxia
   d. Cerebral edema

8. Which one of the following knowledge deficit outcomes would be appropriate for the client recovering from shock?
   a. Accepts responsibility
   b. States understanding
   c. Interacts with others
   d. Verbalizes fears

 ANSWERS TO CRITICAL THINKING

CRITICAL THINKING: Anaerobic Metabolism

It is the source of nutrition and energy for the cell to prevent cellular death when oxygen is not available. It is a short-term compensatory mechanism to save the cell until oxygen becomes available again.

CRITICAL THINKING: Classic Signs of Shock

Tachycardia is caused by decreased cardiac output and reduced tissue oxygenation. Its purpose is to increase cardiac output and oxygen delivery by causing more heartbeats to pump out blood from the heart.

Tachypnea is caused by decreased tissue oxygenation. Its purpose is to increase respirations so more oxygen is available for delivery to tissues.

Oliguria is caused by a reduced blood flow to the kidneys. Its purpose as a compensatory mechanism is to conserve as much fluid as possible to help maintain a normal blood pressure.

Pallor is caused by reduced blood volume or flow. When pallor results from compensation it is due to peripheral vasoconstriction that occurs to shunt blood volume to the vital organs.

Cool, clammy skin is the result of decreased blood flow to the skin and the release of moisture (sweat) from the skin. The sympathetic nervous system causes these compensatory mechanisms of peripheral vasoconstriction to shunt blood volume to the vital organs and sweating to cool the body in anticipation of the fight or flight response, which would generate body heat if it occurred.

CRITICAL THINKING: Mr. Hall

1. Relief of chest pain and anxiety. Stabilization of cardiac rhythm and vital signs. Adequate tissue oxygenation.
2. It relieves pain and anxiety. Myocardial oxygen consumption is reduced because resistance in the blood vessels is reduced, so the heart does not have to work as hard in pumping out blood.
3. A decrease in systolic blood pressure below 90 mm Hg, depressed respirations, and signs and symptoms of allergic reaction.
4. A decrease in blood pressure, increase in heart and respiratory rate, cyanosis, a decrease in urine output, and a decrease in mental status.

CRITICAL THINKING: Mrs. Neal

1. Assessment of respiratory status, cardiovascular status, inspection of surgical wounds for bleeding, assessment of mental status and need for pain relief.
2. Explain the cause of shock and all interventions, rationales, and desired outcomes. Keep environment calm, provide for privacy, and answer all questions in a matter-of-fact and reassuring manner. Allow them to visit.
3. Unrelieved pain, bleeding, infection, or respiratory complications.

BIBLIOGRAPHY

Brown, K: Critical intervention in septic shock. Am J Nurs 94(10):20, 1994.
Harwood, S: Anaphylaxis. Nursing 27(2):33, 1997.
Huston, C: Emergency! Hemolytic transfusion reaction. Am J Nurs 94(3):47, 1996.
Kumar, A, and Parrillo, JE: Shock: Classification, pathophysiology, and approach to management. In Parrillo, JE, and Bone, RC (eds): Critical Care Medicine: Principles of Diagnosis and Management. Mosby, St. Louis, 1995.
O'Neal, P: How to spot early signs of cardiogenic shock. Am J Nurs 94(5):36, 1994.
Ostrow, CL: Use of the Trendelenberg position by critical care nurses: Trendelenberg survey. Am J Crit Care 6(3):172, 1997.
Sing, R, et al: Trendelenberg position and oxygen transport in hypovolemic adults. Ann Emerg Med 23(3):564, 1994.
Tierney, LM, Jr., McPhee, SJ, and Papadakis, MA (eds): Current Medical Diagnosis and Treatment, ed 35. Appleton and Lange, Stamford, Conn, 1996.

Nursing Care of Clients in Pain

9

*Josephine Whitney Johns and
Karen P. Kettelman*

Learning Objectives

Upon completion of this chapter, the student will be able to:

1. Define pain.
2. Identify myths and barriers to the effective management of pain.
3. Explain the differences between addiction, physical dependence, and tolerance.
4. Explain current knowledge of the physiology of the pain response.
5. Define acute, chronic nonmalignant, and cancer pain.
6. Discuss the components of pain assessment.
7. Describe the use of the World Health Organization analgesic ladder.
8. List three categories of analgesics and their uses.
9. Identify various pain treatment modalities and when they might be used.
10. Describe the use of nondrug pain management techniques.
11. Explain how ethical decision making plays a role in the care of the client in pain.

Key Words

addiction (uh-**DIK**-shun)

adjuvant (ad-**JOO**-vant)

agonist (**AG**-on-ist)

analgesic (AN-uhl-**JEE**-zik)

antagonist (an-**TAG**-on-ist)

ceiling effect (**SEE**-ling e-**FEKT**)

endorphins (en-**DOR**-fins)

enkephalins (en-**KEF**-e-lins)

equianalgesic (EE-kwee-AN-uhl-**JEE**-zik)

neuropathic pain (NEW-roh-**PATH**-ik PAYN)

nociceptive (NOH-see-**SEP**-tiv)

opioid (**O**-pe-OYD)

pain (PAYN)

patient-controlled analgesia (**PAY**-shent kon-**TROHLD** an-uhl-**JEE**-zee-ah)

physical dependence (**FIZ**-ik-uhl dee-**PEN**-dens)

prostaglandins (PRAHS-tah-**GLAND**-ins)

pseudoaddiction (soo-doh-ad-**DICK**-shun)

psychological dependence (SY-ko-**LOJ**-ick-al dee-**PEN**-dens)

serotonin (SER-ah-**TOH**-nin)

suffering (**SUFF**-er-ing)

titration (tigh-**TRAY**-shun)

tolerance (**TALL**-er-ens)

transdermal (trans-**DER**-mal)

The Pain Puzzle

Pain is the most common reason for which medical advice is sought. However, even as widespread as the problem is, pain continues to be left untreated or undertreated much of the time. The care of clients with pain is challenging and requires a systematic approach to assessment and treatment.

Decisions about pain management require careful assessment and attention to ethical principles that influence the care of the client. Providing information and giving the client choices help maintain autonomy and provide opportunities for informed consent. When clients are not involved in the process of choosing their own pain management options, they cannot be autonomous. Just as risks and benefits related to surgery and anesthesia are discussed with the client, so should pain management options be discussed in the process of obtaining informed consent. Nurses often worry about overmedicating clients, thinking that they are "doing good" (beneficence) or "doing no harm" (nonmaleficence) by withholding medication from a client who they do not believe is having pain. (See Ethical Considerations Box 9–1.) It is important that nurses learn as much as they can about pain and pain management, so they can effectively advocate for their clients, assist with client education, and provide appropriate resources.

Cultural and ethnic differences must be considered when planning care for the client in pain. People from various cultures have different ways of expressing pain. Some may be dramatic and emotional; others tend to be stoic and quiet. Widely accepted information about different ethnic and cultural groups can be useful in understanding a client's experience and what care might be considered acceptable. It is important, however, to assess a client's pain care needs individually and not make assumptions based on culture or ethnicity alone. See Cultural Considerations Box 9–2 for more information about how clients from different cultures may express pain.

Because of the importance of controlling health care costs, the entire health team must provide care in the most cost-effective manner possible while continuing to provide the best quality of care. Effective pain management can help reach those goals by enhancing comfort, minimizing side effects and complications related to poor pain control, and reducing the lengths of hospital stays.

It is not possible to record a client's pain on a machine or measure it with a blood or urine sample. It is difficult to gauge the effect of a nursing intervention or treatment of pain, whether the intervention is medication or a nondrug therapy. Pain can be likened to a difficult puzzle that requires many pieces to solve.

In this chapter, the many challenges of pain assessment and treatment will be discussed. Some of the tools needed to effectively deal with these challenges will also be pre-

---

ETHICAL CONSIDERATIONS BOX 9-1

Case Study—Controlling Pain

A client was admitted to the medical unit 2 days after his 83rd birthday with a diagnosis of metastatic cancer of the pancreas. He had several full-course treatments of chemotherapy and radiation during the previous year with only temporary remissions of the disease. His condition deteriorated rapidly during the previous month, and his family was no longer able to care for him at home. The client's physician expected him to die within a few weeks, if not sooner, and admitted him to the hospital primarily for pain control. On admission, the physician ordered morphine sulfate (MS) 5 mg IV to be given every 2 hours around the clock.

Although this seemed like a relatively large dose of a strong narcotic medication to be given this frequently, the client tolerated the treatment for the first 36 hours, and reported a significant reduction in his pain. On the third morning after his admission, he was difficult to arouse for his morning vital signs and breakfast. When his nurse, Kathy P., LPN, finally did manage to awaken the client, he was confused, his blood pressure was 82/50 with shallow respirations at 10/min. He still complained of severe generalized pain and asked for "more of that medication that helped so much the day before."

Kathy did not give the client his scheduled 0800 dose of MS. She phoned the physician and reported her assessment of the client, expressing her belief that continuing the medication at the previously prescribed dose and frequency would be fatal to this patient. The physician, who had been up most of the night with an emergency patient, stated sarcastically, ". . . and your client has such a productive life to look forward to—give the #$@& medication like I ordered it! And don't call me any more about this—I'll be in after lunch!" and slammed down the phone.

What should Kathy do? If she continues to give the medication at the prescribed dose and frequency, and the client does die, could she be held liable for his death? What about her ethical obligations as a nurse to reduce pain and suffering, and also to follow the physician's orders? Use the ethical decision-making model to resolve this ethical dilemma.

---

sented. Common myths and barriers that continue to affect nursing practice will be clarified.

Definitions of Pain

According to Margo McCaffery, a consultant in the care of clients with pain, "Pain is whatever the experiencing person says it is, existing whenever the experiencing person

CULTURAL CONSIDERATIONS BOX 9-2

The pain experience may differ between and among ethnocultural individuals. Remember that individuals within groups will vary, and not all will fit the general descriptions and previous experience with pain. (See Chapter 2.)

Culture	Expression and Meaning of Pain	Client Preferences	Assessment	Interventions
Native-American	Frequently do not request pain medicine and are undertreated. May not realize that they can ask for pain medicine. Many believe pain is something that must be endured. May describe pain in general terms such as "not feeling right" or "not feeling good." The word for pain varies according to the tribal language.	Many prefer traditional herbal medicines. May complain to family member or visitor, who relays message to caregiver.	Frequently ask client and family members or visitors if client has pain. Observe for nonverbal clues of pain.	Explain that the control of pain can promote healing. Offer pain medicine as needed. Allow adequate time for response; silence is valued. Maintain a calm, relaxing environment. Incorporate traditional practices for pain relief if not harmful.
European-American	Strong sense of stoicism, especially men. Fear of being dependent may decrease use of pain medicine. Many have fear of addiction. May continue to work and carry out daily activities and minimize pain.	Prefer relaxation and distraction as means of pain control.	Observe for nonverbal signs of pain. Use visual analog or numerical pain scales to assess severity of pain.	Encourage use of pain medicine as needed. Incorporate distraction and relaxation techniques.
African-American	Usually openly and publicly display pain, but this is highly variable. Many, especially the elderly, fear that medication may be addictive. Pain is seen as a sign of illness or disease. Many believe that suffering and pain are inevitable and should be endured.	May focus on spirituality and religious beliefs to endure pain. Prayers and the laying on of hands are thought to relieve pain if the client has enough faith.	Observe for verbal and nonverbal expressions of pain. Use of pain scales is helpful.	Offer pain medication as needed. Allow meditation and prayer along with pain medication.

continued

CULTURAL CONSIDERATIONS BOX 9–2 (continued)

Culture	Expression and Meaning of Pain	Client Preferences	Assessment	Interventions
Hispanic-American	Puerto Ricans tend to be expressive of pain and discomfort. Moaning, groaning, and crying are culturally accepted ways of dealing with and reducing pain. Mexicans may bear pain stoically because it is "God's will." Many feel that pain and suffering are a consequence of immoral behavior. For men, expressing pain shows weakness and a possible loss of respect. The Spanish word for pain is *dolor*.	Prefer oral or intravenous medication for pain. Heat, herbal teas, and prayer are used to manage pain.	Visual analog and numerical scales may be helpful. Observe and compare verbal and nonverbal behaviors indicating pain.	Do not censor verbal expression of pain. Incorporate traditional practices as permitted. For individuals who are stoical with pain, encourage pain medicine frequently. Explain that pain control can hasten healing.
Asian-American	Chinese and Koreans tend to be stoical, although there is a wide variation, and describe pain in terms of diverse body symptoms instead of locally. Filipinos may view pain as a part of living an honorable life. Some view this as an opportunity to reach a fuller life and to atone for past transgressions. Frequently stoic and tolerate pain to a high degree. Some moan as an expression of pain.	Prefer oral or intravenous pain medications. Like warm compresses. For Koreans, intramuscular injections may be seen as an invasion of privacy.	Observe for nonverbal signs of pain. Vietnamese may not understand numerical scale of rating pain. Observing facial expression may be a good indicator of pain.	Incorporate traditional healing methods as much as possible. Offer and encourage pain medicines to promote healing.

continued

CULTURAL CONSIDERATIONS BOX 9–2 (continued)

Culture	Expression and Meaning of Pain	Client Preferences	Assessment	Interventions
	For the Japanese, bearing pain is a virtue and a matter of family honor. Some, especially older individuals, may fear addiction.			
	For Vietnamese, enduring pain is an indication of strong character. Family may be very attentive and request pain medication for the client.	Vietnamese maintain self-control as a means of pain relief.		
Arab-American	See pain as something to be controlled. May express pain openly to family with elaborate verbal expressions, less so with caregivers. Expect prompt interventions for pain control. Tend to describe pain as diffuse rather than locally. May use terms such as fire, hot, and cold.	Intramuscular or intravenous usually preferred over oral medications.	Compare verbal and nonverbal characteristics of pain to determine degree of pain.	Engage family to help with distraction and relaxation techniques. Administer medication promptly.
Appalachian	Pain is something to be endured, and many respond stoically, especially men. May continue activities until pain forces cessation of work.	Some may place a knife or axe under the bed or mattress to "cut pain."	Observe for verbal and nonverbal signs of pain. Many do not like visual analog or numerical pain scales.	Offer pain medication frequently. Encourage relaxation techniques and distraction. Talking about the pain may have pain-relieving results.

says it does."[1] This is a reminder to nurses to remember to believe the client when pain is reported.

In 1979, pain was defined as "an unpleasant sensory and emotional experience associated with actual or potential tissue damage or described in terms of such damage" by the International Association for the Study of Pain (IASP).[2] This indicates that pain is complex and not only has a physical component but an emotional one as well.

What is pain for, and why does it exist? Pain is a protective mechanism, or a warning. It may take place before serious injury, allowing further injury to be prevented, such as when a bone is fractured and the client holds it still to prevent further damage or a child touches a hot burner on a stove and pulls back before a serious burn occurs.

Why is untreated or undertreated pain a bad thing? There are basic complications that occur when pain is experienced. The body experiences a stress response in the presence of pain during which harmful substances are released from injured tissue. Reactions include breakdown of tissue, increased metabolic rate, impaired immune function, and negative emotions. In addition, pain prevents the client from participating in self-care activities such as walking, deep breathing, and coughing. Think of the client who had a chest surgery and now has to cough and deep breathe. It hurts! If it hurts the client tries not to cough, turn, or even move. Retained pulmonary secretions and pneumonia can develop. If the client does not walk and move about, return of bowel function is delayed, and an ileus can result. When pain is well controlled the client is able to do what he or she needs to do to get well and out of the hospital.

Suffering often accompanies pain, but not all pain has the element of suffering. Suffering refers to a sense of threat to one's self-image or life. According to the Agency for Health Care Policy and Research Management of Cancer Pain Guideline, suffering is defined as "the state of severe distress associated with events that threaten the intactness of the person."[3] Suffering can often be relieved if clients believe that their pain can be relieved. Pain can be a constant reminder for the client with cancer that he or she has a life-threatening illness.

Myths and Barriers to Effective Pain Management

The way clients in pain are treated is influenced by a number of factors, including the way the nurse was treated when in pain growing up in his or her own home. Why is the client often disbelieved when he or she reports pain? Why do nurses and other health care team members insist that clients behave a certain way before they can be believed? Various myths about pain impair the nurse's ability to be objective about pain and create barriers to effective treatment. Because there is no objective measuring device for pain, nurses tend to rely on what is comfortable rather than what has been proven to be effective.

Myth: A person who is laughing and talking is not in pain.

Fact: A person in pain is likely to use laughing and talking as a form of distraction, which can be very useful in the management of pain when used in conjunction with appropriate drug therapies.

Myth: If morphine is given too early to the client with cancer pain, it will not work when the client really needs it, toward the end, when the pain is worse.

Fact: Morphine is an **opioid** agonist. Opioid doses can be escalated (titrated upward) indefinitely as needed as the client's pain increases. There is no **ceiling effect,** or dose that is limited by side effects. Side effects such as sedation or clinically significant respiratory depression may temporarily limit the dose or the rate at which the dose can be increased.

Myth: Respiratory depression is common in clients receiving opioid pain medications.

Fact: Respiratory depression is uncommon in clients receiving opioid pain medications. If clients are monitored carefully when they are at risk, such as with the first dose of an opioid or when a dose is increased, respiratory depression is preventable. A client's respiratory status and level of sedation (LOS) should be routinely monitored using an LOS scale.

Myth: Pain medication is more effective when given by injection.

Fact: Intramuscular (IM) injections are not recommended by experts because they are painful, have unreliable absorption from the muscle, and have a lag time to peak effect and rapid falloff compared with oral administration. Oral administration is the first choice if possible; the intravenous (IV) route has the most rapid onset of action and is the preferred route for postoperative administration.

Myth: Teenagers are more likely to become addicted than older clients.

Fact: Addiction to opioids is very uncommon in all age groups when taken for pain in clients without a prior drug abuse history.

CRITICAL THINKING: Smithers and Barnett

Mrs. Smithers had an abdominal hysterectomy yesterday and is sitting up in bed putting on her makeup the morning after surgery. On morning rounds she is smiling but reports that her pain is at 6 on a scale of 0 to 10. Mr. Barnett has just been transferred from the surgical intensive care unit the day after surgery for multiple injuries. He is moaning and reports his pain at 6 on a scale of 0 to 10. Which of these clients is really having as much pain as they say they are? How is that judgment made?

Answers at end of chapter.

Some More Definitions

Nurses often complain about clients who require large amounts of pain medication or know exactly when their next dose of pain medication is due. Nurses may say that such clients are addicted, or that they are "clock watchers," but do nurses really know what that means? Clients are expected to be informed about their medications and involved in their care, but when they know when their medications are due, nurses become suspicious. If a client is watching the clock the most likely reason is because he or she is in pain. The most common reason that clients ask for more pain medicine is because they have increased pain. It is important to understand the differences between addiction, physical dependence, and tolerance. When talking with clients and teaching them about their medications it is important to help them understand these differences as well. It is something many clients worry about. **Tolerance** simply means that it takes a larger dose to provide the same level of pain relief. **Physical dependence** is a physiological phenomenon that any person would experience after continuous opioid use for a few weeks, such as following a traumatic injury. If the opioid is abruptly discontinued the client would experience a withdrawal or abstinence syndrome demonstrated by symptoms such as sweating, tearing, runny nose, restlessness, irritability, tremors, dilated pupils, sleeplessness, nausea and vomiting, and diarrhea. These symptoms can be prevented by slowly weaning a client from an opioid, rather than quick discontinuation. **Psychological dependence** or **addiction** is defined as a pattern of compulsive drug use characterized by a continued craving for an opioid and the need to use the opioid for effects other than pain relief. **Pseudoaddiction** has been described in clients who are prescribed opioid doses that are too low or spaced too far apart to relieve their pain and certain behavioral characteristics resembling psychological dependence, such as drug-seeking behaviors, have developed.[4]

Educating clients and families about these concerns will help alleviate their fears and increase their satisfaction with the pain relief measures that are employed.

Mechanisms of Pain Transmission

Many theories of how pain is transmitted are in the literature. The specificity theory, developed by Descartes in 1644, proposed that body trauma sends a message directly to the brain, causing a sort of "bell" to ring, prompting a response from the brain. In 1965 Melzack and Wall proposed the gate control theory, which describes the dorsal horn of the spinal cord as a gate, allowing impulses to go through when there is a pain stimulus and closing the gate when

those impulses are inhibited. The gate control theory stimulated massive research on the physiology of pain.

We know much more about the transmission of pain today than these and other theories demonstrate. **Endorphins** are endogenous chemicals that act similar to opioids to inhibit pain impulses in the spinal cord and brain. Unfortunately they degrade too quickly to be considered effective analgesics. These are the chemicals that stimulate the long-distance runner's "high." **Enkephalins** are one type of endorphin.

Pain is transmitted through the dorsal horn of the spinal cord and other points in the central nervous system to higher centers of the brain with the influence of chemicals known as neurotransmitters, which are released during pain or trauma. These chemicals include **serotonin, prostaglandins,** and others. Many treatments and analgesics are designed based on known principles to inhibit the release of these chemicals.

Mechanisms of pain transmission are **nociceptive** and **neuropathic.** Nociception refers to the body's reaction to noxious stimuli, such as tissue damage, with the release of pain-producing substances. Nociceptive pain in the visceral organs may be referred to other parts of the body. See Figure 9–1 for sites of referred pain. Neuropathic pain is pain associated with injury to either the peripheral or central nervous system. Unlike nociceptive pain, neuropathic pain is not usually localized, and it may spread to involve other areas along the nerve pathway.

Types of Pain

Pain is often categorized according to whether it is acute, related to cancer, or chronic nonmalignant. *Acute pain* is described as pain that follows injury to the body and subsides when healing takes place. It is often, although not always, associated with objective physical signs such as increased heart rate and elevated blood pressure. Examples of acute pain include pain related to fractures, burns, or other trauma. *Cancer pain* may be acute, chronic, or intermittent and often has a definable cause such as tumor pressure or a neuropathy caused by the cancer treatment. *Chronic nonmalignant pain* is described as pain that persists beyond the time when healing usually takes place. Conditions considered chronic nonmalignant pain include low back pain, arthritic pain, and phantom limb pain. Chronic nonmalignant pain may have nociceptive as well as neuropathic components and may require a variety of medications and nondrug treatments to manage. Clients with chronic nonmalignant pain or chronic cancer pain may not appear to be in pain because the body adapts very quickly. The physiological responses that accompany acute pain, such as elevated heart rate and blood pressure, cannot be sustained without harm to the body, so the body adapts.

---

pseudoaddiction: pseudo—false + addiction—psychological dependence

nociceptive: noci—pain + ceptive—reception

neuropathic: neuro—nerves + pathy—disease, suffering

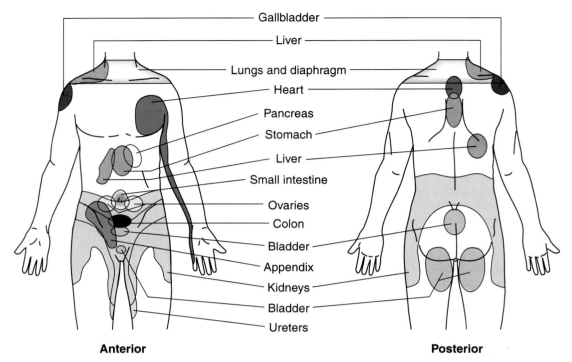

Figure 9–1. Sites of referred pain. (Modified from Ignatavicius, Workman, and Mishler: Medical-Surgical Nursing: A Nursing Process Approach. WB Saunders, Philadelphia, 1995, p 122, with permission.)

Options for Treatment of Pain

ANALGESICS

Medications that relieve pain are called **analgesics.** Analgesics are the biggest pieces of the pain management puzzle. There are three main categories of analgesics: opioids, nonopioids, and **adjuvants.** Opioids are classified by their affinity or ability to attach or bind to opioid receptors in the brain and spinal cord, as well as other areas of the body, inhibiting the perception of pain. Nonopioids include nonsteroidal anti-inflammatory drugs (NSAIDs) and acetaminophen (Tylenol). Adjuvants include classes of drugs that were originally developed for a different purpose but have been found to have pain-relieving properties of their own in some painful conditions.

Nonopioids

Nonopioids are generally the first class of drugs used for treatment of pain. They can be useful for acute and chronic pain from a variety of causes, such as surgery, trauma, arthritis, and cancer. These medications are limited in their use because they have a ceiling effect to analgesia. A ceiling effect indicates that there is a dose beyond which there is no improvement in the analgesic effect, and there may be an increase in side effects. When used in combination with opioids, care must be taken to ensure that the dose of the nonopioid drug does not exceed the maximum safe dose for a 24-hour period. For example, if a client receiving two aspirin with codeine tablets every 4 hours continues to ex-perience pain, the dose cannot be increased because of the potential toxic effects of the aspirin (Table 9–1).

Nonopioids do not produce tolerance or physical or psychological dependence. They do have antipyretic (fever-reducing) effects. This class of drugs works primarily at the site of injury, or peripherally, rather than in the central nervous system as with opioids. In general, it is helpful to include a nonopioid in any analgesic regimen, even if the pain is severe enough to require the addition of an opioid.

Opioids

Opioids are added to nonopioids to manage pain that cannot be managed effectively by nonopioids alone. Opioids are classified as full agonists, partial agonists, or mixed agonists and **antagonists.** Full agonists have a complete re-

Table 9–1. **Side Effects of Nonopioids**

Drug	Side Effects
NSAIDs (including aspirin)	Gastrointestinal (GI) irritation and bleeding Inhibition of platelet aggregation, increasing risk of GI bleeding Renal insufficiency in some clients, especially the elderly Clients with asthma at risk for hypersensitive reactions
Acetaminophen	Necrosis of the liver with overdose

sponse on the opioid receptor; the partial agonist has a lesser response. The mixed agonist and antagonist activates one type of opioid receptor while blocking another.

Opioids alone have no ceiling effect to analgesia. Doses can safely be increased to treat increasing pain if the client's respiratory status and level of sedation are stable. See Table 9–2 for side effects of opioids.

Sustained-release opioids such as oxycodone (Oxycontin) and sustained-release morphine (MS Contin) are effective for prolonged periods of time. Sustained- or time-release medication should never be crushed, but always taken whole. Whenever a sustained-release preparation is used it is important to have an immediate-release medication available for breakthrough pain, such as oral morphine solution (OMS).

Morphine is the drug of choice for the treatment of moderate to severe pain. It is the drug used as a standard against which all other analgesics are compared. (See Table 9–3 for **equianalgesic** doses of medications.) Morphine is long acting (4 to 5 hours) and available in many forms, making it convenient for the client, as well as inexpensive. It has a slower onset than the other opioid agonists.

Hydromorphone (Dilaudid) is commonly used for moderate to severe pain as well. It is shorter acting than morphine and has a somewhat faster onset. It is a good choice for pain management in most clients.

Meperidine (Demerol), also an opioid agonist, should be reserved for healthy clients requiring opioids for a short period of time or for those who have unusual reactions or allergic response to other opioids. When broken down in the body it produces a toxic metabolite called normeperidine. Normeperidine is a cerebral irritant that can cause side effects ranging from dysphoria and irritable mood to seizures. It has a long half-life even in healthy clients, so clients with impaired renal function are at increased risk. The use of meperidine (Demerol) should be avoided in clients with impaired renal function or those receiving medications from the monoamine oxidase (MAO) inhibitor class of antidepressants. Additionally, the effective dose of oral meperidine (Demerol) is three to four times the parenteral dose, which is toxic and not recommended.

Fentanyl (Sublimaze, Duragesic) can be administered parenterally, intraspinally, or by **transdermal** patch (Duragesic patch). It is about 10 times more potent than morphine. Fentanyl is commonly used intravenously with anesthesia for surgery and is also commonly used for relief of postoperative pain via the epidural route. Administration can also be effective via IV patient-controlled analgesia (see later in chapter) for postoperative pain management, but other drugs may be preferred. Fentanyl is very short acting, so it must be administered frequently. The fentanyl patch is useful for the client with stable cancer pain and requires dosing only every 3 days.

equianalgesic: equi—equal + analgesic—relieving pain
transdermal: trans—across + dermal—the skin

Table 9–2. Common Side Effects of Opioids

Sedation
Respiratory depression*
Constipation
Nausea, vomiting
Itching
Constricted pupils*

*These effects are not common, but they alert the nurse to possible overdose.

Methadone (Dolophine) is a potent analgesic that has a longer duration of action than morphine. It has a very long half-life and accumulates in the body with continued dosing. Dosing intervals should be lengthened after pain relief has been achieved. Methadone is well absorbed from the gastrointestinal tract and is very effective when given orally at doses similar to the parenteral dose. Methadone is also used in drug treatment programs during detoxification from heroin and other opioids. Clients on methadone maintenance can present a unique problem for the nurse when admitted to the hospital. It is important to continue the maintenance dose even if other medications for pain are given after surgery or trauma.

LEARNING TIP

It is important to monitor level of sedation and respiratory status whenever administering opioids. Increased sedation, decreased respiratory effort, and constricted pupils can be signs of opioid overdose. Careful monitoring and **titration** of opioids can prevent opioid-induced respiratory depression.

CRITICAL THINKING: Mrs. Shepard

Mrs. Shepard is 92 years old and has undergone an open cholecystectomy. Her continuous epidural infusion has been discontinued. She has oral hydrocodone with acetaminophen (Vicodin) ordered every 3 to 4 hours as required for pain. This is her second postoperative day, and she refuses to get out of bed because her pain is 7 on a scale of 0 to 10.

The medication record shows that Mrs. Shepard has not received any pain medication since the continuous epidural infusion was stopped 3 hours ago.

1. Why is Mrs. Shepard in so much pain?
2. What complications can occur as a result of her pain?
3. What can be done to relieve her pain and better prevent her pain in the future?

Answers at end of chapter.

Table 9–3. **Equianalgesic Chart**

Approximate doses of medications in milligrams to equal same amount of pain relief.

Drug	Parenteral (IM/IV/SQ)	Oral Dose	Conversion Factor (Parenteral to PO)
Morphine	10 mg	30 mg	3
Codeine	130 mg	200 mg NR	1.5
Hydromorphone (Dilaudid)	1.5 mg	7.5 mg	5
Methadone (Dolophine)	10 mg	20 mg	2
Meperidine (Demerol)	75 mg	300 mg NR	4

Source: Adapted from McCaffery, M: Pain: Assessment and Use of Analgesics (conference handouts). Fall 1996. NR—not recommended at that dose.

Opioid Antagonists

Naloxone (Narcan) is a pure opioid antagonist. It is used to counteract or antagonize the effect of opioids. It is often used in the emergency department setting for treatment of opioid overdose. Caution must be used when naloxone is given to the client receiving opioids for the treatment of pain. If too much naloxone is given too fast it can reverse not only the respiratory depression and sedation but the analgesia as well.

Antagonists are generally shorter acting than the opioid that is being used. If the antagonist is given because of respiratory depression the dose may need to be repeated because its effect will wear off before that of the opioid.

As previously mentioned, some analgesics are classified as combined agonist and antagonist. These drugs bind with some opioid receptors and block others. The most commonly used agonist-antagonist drugs are pentazocine (Talwin), butorphanol (Stadol), and nalbuphine (Nubain).

How does this information translate into nursing practice? Consider, for example, a client who is taking sustained-release morphine every 12 hours to control metastatic bone pain and is experiencing breakthrough pain between doses. The nurse observes that Stadol has been ordered for pain by another doctor and administers it. The Stadol will antagonize or counteract the effects of the morphine, and the client may develop acute pain. It is important to be informed about the actions of all drugs that are administered and to be aware of possible drug-drug interactions that may interfere with client care.

Agonist-antagonist drugs are also used sometimes to counteract other opioid side effects. Nalbuphine (Nubain) is often used to counteract itching and nausea that can accompany the administration of opioids. A smaller than therapeutic dose is given so that the analgesia is not reversed completely along with the reversal of the side effect.

Analgesic Adjuvants

Adjuvants are classes of medications that may either potentiate the effects of opioids or nonopioids, have analgesic activity themselves in certain situations, or counteract unwanted effects of other analgesics. Adjuvants are especially important when treating pain that does not respond well to traditional analgesics alone.

Steroids can be used to treat a variety of pain conditions, including acute and chronic cancer-related pain. They may be used as part of actual cancer treatment because of their toxicity to some cancer cells, or they may reduce pain by reducing inflammation and resulting compression of healthy tissues. Their use is standard emergency practice in the treatment of suspected spinal cord compression. Clients with pain caused by malignant lesions pressing on nerves such as brachial or lumbosacral plexus may receive large doses of steroids.

Benzodiazepines such as midazolam (Versed) or diazepam (Valium) are effective for the treatment of anxiety or muscle spasms associated with pain. These drugs are not analgesic except in the treatment of muscle spasms. They cause sedation, which may limit the amount of opioid that may be given safely.

Tricyclic antidepressants such as amitriptyline, imipramine, desipramine, and doxepin have been shown to relieve pain related to neuropathy and other nerve-related painful conditions. These medications must be taken for a period of time before they are effective, and clients must be instructed about this so that they do not stop taking the medication after a few days. Benefits of this class of medications may include mood-elevating and sleep-aid effects.

Anticonvulsants such as phenytoin (Dilantin) and carbamazepine (Tegretol) may relieve the sharp or cutting pain caused by peripheral nerve syndromes. Again, these medications must be taken regularly before full benefit may be realized.

Amphetamines such as methylphenidate hydrochloride (Ritalin) may be used to counteract the sedating effects of opioids in some clients.

Other Interventions

Other pain treatments include the use of radiation therapy or antineoplastic chemotherapy to help shrink tumors that are causing pain for a client with cancer. Chemotherapy is also used for treating pain associated with connective tissue disorders such as rheumatoid arthritis or systemic lupus erythematosus. Bowel regimens, laxatives, enemas, or antigas medication to decrease abdominal fullness may be considered pain management if it is the primary source of discomfort for the client. Drugs that result in calcium uptake by the bones in osteoporosis can also aid in relief of pain. This may include hormonal agents and medications that decrease calcium resorption from bone such as etidronate (Didronel).

The IV administration of strontium-89 chloride (Metastron) by a qualified physician helps ease the bone pain of some clients with metastatic bone cancer. It is most effective for clients who have hormone-related cancers such as cancer of the breast or prostate.

Lidocaine/prilocaine (EMLA, eutectic mixture of local anesthetics) cream is a topical local anesthetic that decreases pain associated with procedures such as venipunctures and lumbar punctures. It is most effective if left in place for 1 hour before the procedure and covered with a semipermeable membrane dressing such as Tegaderm or Opsite before the needle stick.

Placebos

Use of placebos involves the administration of nonmedication such as normal saline in place of a real medication. Placebos have been given in an attempt to determine whether a client's pain is "real." Placebos are also given in drug-testing studies (clinical trials) to compare a new drug with an inactive substance. There is no research to justify the use of placebos to treat pain, unless the client has agreed to be a part of a research study and has consented to the possibility that he or she may be receiving a placebo. Clients may actually experience pain relief after the administration of a placebo even if they have an organic basis for pain. The use of placebos is unethical and deceptive and should not be practiced. It is contrary to all that is taught about believing clients when they say that they have pain. If a placebo is ordered for a client, the nurse should discuss his or her concerns with the physician and nurse supervisor. Except in a research setting, it is *never* appropriate to administer placebos to clients experiencing pain.

Routes for Medication Administration

Oral

Medication administration by the oral (PO) route is preferred whenever possible. It is convenient, flexible, and inexpensive and provides consistent blood level when given around the clock (ATC).

Rectal

When the client is not able to take medications by the oral route, rectal administration is a good alternative. Many medications may be given by the rectal route. Often oral preparations (tablets or capsules) can be administered rectally, as well as intrastomally, intravaginally, or buccally.

Inhalation

Butorphanol (Stadol) can be administered via the nasal route and is sometimes used for treatment of migraine headaches. It is an agonist-antagonist, and caution must be used if the client is also taking opioids, as discussed earlier.

There is ongoing research about the use of aerosolized morphine in clients with diseased lungs.

Transdermal

Fentanyl (Duragesic) patches are used in the treatment of chronic pain and are dosed in micrograms (μg) per hour. It may seem easy enough to apply a patch, but there are some special considerations when using this route.

- There is about a 12-hour delay until peak effectiveness is reached, and the client may require an immediate-release form of pain medication until that time.
- The patches may not be as effective in clients who smoke.
- Absorption may be reduced if the patch is placed in an area with little or no fatty tissue.
- Absorption may be increased in clients with body temperatures of 101°F or greater. Increased or erratic absorption may require patches to be replaced more frequently.
- When applying the patch, the nurse must use caution to prevent contact with the membrane covering the medication to prevent exposure. If contact occurs, rinse with plain water.
- Patches should not be used with other sustained-release analgesics.
- Multiple patches may be used.
- When the patch is discontinued, the residual medication in the skin continues to be absorbed for about 17 hours. During this time the client must be monitored for pain control and overdose if another pain medication has been administered.

Intramuscular

The IM route is appropriate only if the medication cannot be delivered by another route. IM injections are not recommended in the treatment of chronic pain because injections are painful and inconvenient and absorption is unpredictable.

Intravenous

The IV route is the preferred route of opioid administration for postoperative pain and when the client is unable to tolerate oral medications. IV infusions of opioids are preferred for chronic cancer pain over intermittent doses of IM or subcutaneous medication. Continuous infusion of an opioid will provide a steady blood level, which tends to provide the most effective analgesia with the fewest side effects. Routes other than IV require lag time for absorption of the drug into the circulation. Self-administration of an opioid by the client is called **patient-controlled analgesia** (PCA). In most cases we think of PCA as an IV route, but it is a concept rather than a modality and can mean oral, subcutaneous, epidural, or other routes. This chapter will focus on IV PCA.

IV PCA is a safe method for postoperative pain management that many clients prefer over intermittent injections. A special pump designed for the purpose of delivering medication by the use of a client-controlled button is used. The pump can be programmed to administer the prescribed dose of opioid at the press of the button. A lockout interval is also programmed into the pump, which regulates the frequency with which the client can receive a dose of medication, to protect against overdose. A typical dose of morphine is 1 mg (hydromorphone 0.2 mg) with a lockout interval of 5 to 10 minutes. Most PCA pumps can also deliver a continuous, or basal, infusion in addition to the client-controlled dose. The purpose of the basal, or continuous, infusion is to allow the client to have intervals of uninterrupted sleep. An hourly limit is also prescribed by the physician and programmed into the pump. The pump keeps track of the number of doses a client uses (doses actually received by the client) and the number of attempts made (times the button was pushed). This helps the nurse know how much medication the client is using and if the use of the pump is understood. If the client has a record of many attempts and very few injections, the client may not be waiting the full interval between doses. This occurs because the client is in severe pain and cannot wait or because he or she does not understand the instructions. Client education should include information about the medication that is being administered, safety features and the use of the pump, potential side effects, and what to report to the nurse. The nurse should consult with institution policy for safe PCA administration guidelines. It is important that clients, families, and caregivers understand that no one should push the button except the client. This modality is safe if it is client controlled. Family members can help by reminding their loved one to use the PCA if they think the person is in pain.

Subcutaneous

This is the route of administration into subcutaneous tissue. It can be used as an alternative to IV infusion, if IV access is problematic, for opioid therapy in clients with chronic cancer pain. A needle is placed into the subcutaneous tissue and a small volume of a high concentration of opioid can be infused for effective pain management.

Intraspinal

The intraspinal (epidural or subarachnoid) route is an appropriate pain relief modality for some clients. Clients with traumatic injuries, including rib fractures or orthopedic injuries of the pelvis and lower extremities, or clients undergoing chest, abdominal, or lower extremity orthopedic sur-

gical procedures may benefit from the epidural route of opioid administration. Advantages to the intraspinal route of administration include the ability to provide superior pain relief while administering overall lower doses of opioid. There is less systemic effect of the opioid because it is administered close to the site of the nerves serving the area of injury or surgical incision and not into the systemic circulation. Intraspinal opioids can be safely administered in a variety of hospital and home care settings if protocols for the care and monitoring of the client are in place and enforced. Nurses must have appropriate education to prepare for the care of these clients.

NONDRUG THERAPIES

Nondrug treatments are usually classified as cognitive-behavioral interventions or physical agents. The goals of these two groups of treatments are different. Cognitive-behavioral interventions can help clients understand and cope with pain and take an active part in its assessment and control. The goals of physical agents may include providing comfort, correcting physical dysfunction, altering physiological response, and reducing fear that might be associated with immobility.

Cognitive-Behavioral Interventions

Included in this group are interventions such as educational information, relaxation exercises, guided imagery, distraction (e.g., music, television), and biofeedback. These treatments require extra time for detailed instruction and demonstration.

Providing the client with educational information related to what to expect and how the client can participate in his or her own care has been shown to decrease the client's report of postoperative pain and analgesic use. Relaxation can be accomplished through the use of a variety of methods. The client may prefer a relaxation exercise with a script that can be practiced and used the same way each time or simply the use of a favorite piece of music that will allow a state of muscle relaxation and freedom from anxiety. Guided imagery uses the client's imagination to take the client away from the pain to a favorite place, such as the beach on Tahiti. The success of guided imagery does not mean that the pain is in any way imaginary. The use of distraction is something that many of us do without thinking about it. We focus our attention on something other than the pain. Clients watch a favorite television program or laugh with visitors when they are in pain. When the program is over or the visitors leave the client may ask for a dose of pain medication. Biofeedback is commonly used in behavioral chronic pain programs to teach clients how to teach their body to respond to different signals. Biofeedback has been very useful in clients with migraine headaches. When clients experience the aura that many migraine sufferers experience, they begin the exercise that relaxes them and prevents the migraine from coming on.

Physical Agents

Physical agents may be more commonly used because they contribute directly to the client's comfort. Applications of heat or cold, massage, exercise and immobilization, and transcutaneous electrical nerve stimulation (TENS) are commonly used physical agents.

The application of heat to sore muscles and joints is effective for pain relief. Heat works to increase circulation, induce muscle relaxation, and decrease inflammation when applied to a painful area. Heat can be applied using dry or moist packs or wraps, as well as in a bath or whirlpool. Heat is contraindicated in conditions that would be worsened by the use of heat, such as an area of trauma, because of the possibility of increased swelling due to vasodilation. Heat should not be applied over areas of decreased sensation, to prevent burns. Cold can be used to reduce swelling, bleeding, and pain when applied to a new injury. Cold can be applied by a variety of methods such as cold wraps and cold packs, as well as a localized ice massage. Clients often chose heat over cold if they have the choice. Cold is better tolerated over a small area. Heat and cold are most effective when alternated if not contraindicated. Massage and exercise are used to stretch and regain muscle and tendon length and probably work by relaxing the muscles. Massage can be superficial or deep pressure as with acupressure techniques. It is important that massage is acceptable and not offensive to the client. Immobilization is used following a variety of orthopedic procedures, as well as fractures and other injuries worsened by movement.

Physical agents are readily available, are inexpensive, and require little preparation or instruction. It is important to use nondrug treatments to enhance appropriate drug treatments, not as a substitute for them.

Nursing Process

ASSESSMENT

Accurate assessment of pain is the key to effective treatment. Without appropriate assessment it is not possible to intervene in a way that will meet the client's needs. Use of the WHAT'S UP? format found in chapter 2 assists the nurse in performing a complete and effective assessment (Table 9–4). Following are some additional key points for assessing pain and putting together more pieces of the pain puzzle.

Believe the Client

Pain is what the client says it is, *not* what the nurse or physician thinks it should be. When a member of the health care team distrusts the client's report of pain, the client can

Table 9–4. *WHAT'S UP?* Format for Assessment of Pain

W—Where is the pain? Be specific. Use drawing of body if necessary.
H—How does the pain feel? Is it shooting, burning, dull, sharp?
A—Aggravating and alleviating factors. What makes the pain better? Worse?
T—Timing. When did the pain start? Is it intermittent? Continuous?
S—Severity. How bad is the pain on a 0 to 10 (0 to 5; faces) scale?
U—Useful other data. Are you experiencing any other symptoms associated with the pain or pain treatment? Itching, nausea, sedation, constipation?
P—Perception. What is the client's perception of what caused the pain?

usually sense that he or she is not believed. The client may compensate by either underreporting pain or, less commonly, anxiously overreporting.

Take a Pain History

History is information obtained from the client about the pain that he or she is experiencing. Allowing and encouraging the client to describe the pain in his or her own terms helps establish a trust relationship between the nurse and the client and also helps discover the effects the pain is having on the client's lifestyle. Is the pain keeping the client from eating, sleeping, or participating in work or family activities? The client's emotional and spiritual distress and coping abilities should be assessed to individualize the interventions to the client's needs. The client can tell the nurse how he or she has coped with pain previously and what treatment measures have been effective in the past.

A variety of tools are available to assist in accurate and complete pain assessment. The tools vary in size, content, and questions asked. The nurse should become familiar with the tool used in his or her setting and use it consistently. It is of utmost importance that all health care personnel caring for the client use the same pain rating scale, whether it is a numerical scale (0 to 5; 0 to 10), a visual analog scale (a 10 cm line on which the level is marked and then measured from the beginning of the line to indicate the amount of pain), or the Wong-Baker faces scale (Figs. 9–2 and 9–3). Whichever scale is used, it must be one that has been validated with research. Some scales are cute and

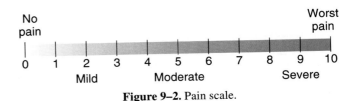

Figure 9–2. Pain scale.

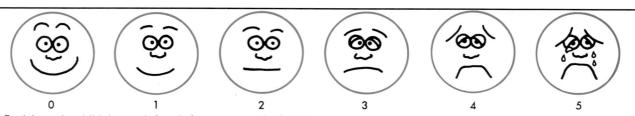

0   1   2   3   4   5

1) Explain to the child that each face is for a person who feels happy because he or she has no pain (hurt, or whatever word the child uses) or feels sad because he or she has some or a lot of pain.
2) Point to the appropriate face and state, "This face is . . .":
   0—"very happy because he doesn't hurt at all."
   1—"hurts just a little bit."
   2—"hurts a little more."
   3—"hurts even more."
   4—"hurts a whole lot."
   5—"hurts as much as you can imagine, although you don't have to be crying to feel this bad."
3) Ask the child to choose the face that best describes how he or she feels. Be specific about which pain (e.g., "shot" or incision) and what time (e.g., now? earlier before lunch?).

Figure 9–3. Wong-Baker faces. (From Wong, DL: Whaley & Wong's Essentials of Pediatric Nursing, ed 5. Mosby, St Louis, 1997, with permission.)

interesting but may not be accurate or even useful. The best tools are simple and easy to use. Longer questionnaires require more time and may cause distress for the client in acute pain but may be helpful when doing a complete pain history (Fig. 9–4). A scale should be used also to monitor the client's level of sedation following opioid administration. A scale such as S for normal sleep, 1 for awake and alert, 2 for occasionally drowsy, 3 for frequently drowsy (falls asleep in midsentence), and 4 for unable to arouse should be used (Fig. 9–5). Any unexpected decrease in the client's level of consciousness should be reported promptly to the RN or physician.

It is important to use the client's own descriptions and words when taking the pain history, such as aching, knifelike, or throbbing. This is also true when the client is experiencing neuropathic pain. Neuropathic pain is often more difficult to define. Commonly used terms when describing neuropathic pain include *burning, shocklike,* and *tingling.*

Do a Complete Physical Assessment

A good physical assessment is necessary to assess the effect of the pain and pain treatments on the body. It helps identify all of the pain sites and helps the nurse prioritize the seemingly overwhelming task of helping the client achieve acceptable pain management and good qualify of life. As discussed before, the client with acute pain may exhibit signs such as grimacing and moaning or elevated pulse and blood pressure, but these signs cannot be relied on to "prove" that the client is in pain. The *only* reliable source of pain assessment is the client's self-report. See also Gerontological Issues Box 9–3.

CRITICAL THINKING: Mr. Sebastian

Mr. Sebastian is a 75-year-old gentleman who has been diagnosed with lung cancer and is anxious about leaving the hospital to return home following a thoracotomy. The nursing assessment reveals the need for home health care for dressing changes and teaching about the medications he will need at home. While in the hospital, Mr. Sebastian has required morphine 5 mg IV every 4 hours around the clock.

What discharge instructions must be given to Mr. Sebastian and his wife before sending him home? How might his pain be managed at home to prevent unnecessary readmissions to the hospital?

Answers at end of chapter.

PLANNING AND IMPLEMENTATION

During the planning phase a pain control goal should be established. The client must be asked to determine an acceptable level of pain if complete freedom from pain is not possible. It is also important to identify what the client's goals are for activity. After surgery goals may include the ability to ambulate and to sleep without pain. For clients with chronic pain the goals may be different. For example, if a client with terminal cancer wants to be able to attend her granddaughter's wedding, the nurse should assist the client in reaching that goal. She can be taught to reserve energy that day for the activity that is most important to her. Instructing her for optimal timing of her pain medication will assist her in reaching a good level of comfort for the activity.

Pain Assessment Chart (For Admission and/or Follow-up)

1. Patient _____   2. DX _____

Assessment on Admission

Date _____ / _____ / _____   Pain ☐   No Pain ☐   Date of Pain Onset _____ / _____ / _____

1. Location of Pain (indicate on drawing)

2. Description of Predominant Pain (in patient's words) _____
_____
_____
_____

3. Intensity [Scale 0 (no pain) — 10 (most intense)] _____   Right   Left   Left   Right
_____

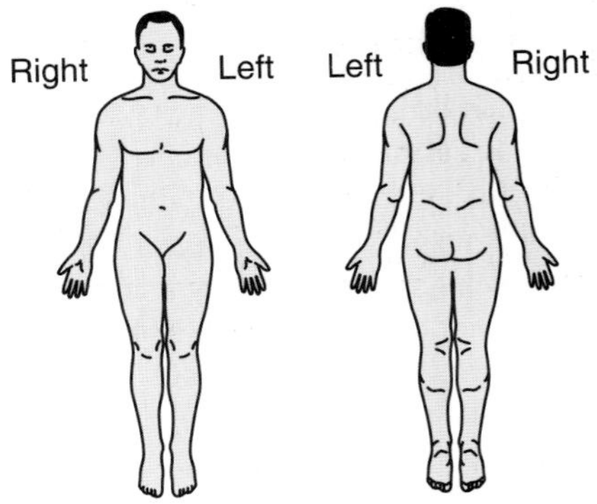

4. Duration and when occurs _____
_____

5. Precipitating Factors _____
_____

6. Alleviating Factors _____
_____

7. Accompanying Symptoms

   GI: Nausea ☐   Emesis ☐   Constipation ☐   Anorexia ☐

   CNS: Drowsiness ☐   Confusion ☐   Hallucinations ☐

   Psychosocial: Mood _____   Anger _____

   Anxiety _____   Depression _____

   Relationships _____

8. Other Symptoms

   Sleep _____   Fatigue _____

   Activity _____   Other _____

9. Present Medications _____
_____
_____

   Doses and times medicated last 48 hours _____
_____

10. Breakthrough Pain _____
_____

Signature: _____

Figure 9–4. Pain assessment chart. (Modified from The Purdue Frederick Company, Norwalk, Conn, with permission.)

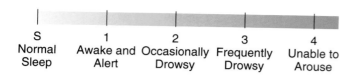

Figure 9–5. LOS scale.

Some additional principles to consider during the planning phase follow.

Client Should Maintain As Much Control As Possible

Pain can bring forth feelings of helplessness and hopelessness. By giving the client choices of pain management options he or she can maintain some control. It is also the nurse's responsibility to teach the client about the goals of pain management and why it is an important part of care. If clients understand that the health care provider's goals and theirs are the same, they are likely to cooperate with and contribute to the pain management plan.

Pain Affects the Whole Family

It is important to include the whole family in the plan. Understanding family dynamics helps the nurse in implementing an effective pain management plan. Cultural influences are important to consider when planning pain treatment. It is difficult for family members to see loved ones in pain. Including them in the planning helps them feel that they may be helping to make the client more comfortable.

GERONTOLOGICAL ISSUES BOX 9–3

The older client may have different manifestations of pain than a younger client. Older clients who are confused may be unable to tell the nurse that they are feeling pain. The nurse should consider incidents of restlessness and confusion as possible signs of pain. Pulling at dressings, tugging at IV sites, and trying to climb over the side rails to get out of bed can also be symptoms of discomfort.

The nurse can anticipate pain and provide relief measures to prevent severe pain. Pain medications and basic comfort care can be administered routinely if pain is likely. Nagging achiness in hands and feet is often noted as a reason for decreased activity, inability to sleep, and altered functional ability. A hand or foot massage using lotion and gentle massage strokes is often a very relaxing comfort measure.

Pain Is Exhausting

Pain may keep the client from sleeping. This cycle of sleeplessness and pain must be interrupted in order to help the client. The need for adequate rest must not be ignored. This is more often an ongoing problem for the client with chronic nonmalignant pain or chronic cancer pain, and it is perhaps more difficult to manage. The client needs to get at least 4 to 6 hours of uninterrupted sleep to be relaxed enough to break the cycle. Sustained-release pain medications may help maintain pain relief, allowing the client to sleep. If sustained-release medications are not used, it may be necessary to wake a client to administer pain medication so that the pain does not get out of control. The addition of a sedative may be necessary to allow the client to sleep. Pain medications are not designed to make the client sleep.

A Team Approach to Pain Management Is Best

A plan must be developed using an interdisciplinary approach, including the client and family, the nurse, and the physician. Others such as occupational and physical therapists, the chaplain, social worker, and pharmacist should be included as appropriate. Communication is the important link for this team to be effective in creating a plan that will work for the client. Plans must be individualized to meet the special needs of each client and will vary greatly for the client with acute pain as compared with cancer pain and chronic nonmalignant pain.

In 1990 the World Health Organization (WHO) developed the WHO analgesic ladder, which involves choosing among three levels of treatments based on intensity of pain (Fig. 9–6). The ladder was developed for the treatment of cancer pain but can be used when treating other types of pain as well. The ladder helps direct the interventions required when using medications to treat pain.

When treating mild pain (level I on the WHO ladder) the client can usually sleep, perform activities of daily living, and even work. The first level of the ladder primarily recommends the use of nonopioid analgesics. When pain is unrelieved by maximum ATC dosing, the treatment moves up the ladder to level II (mild to moderate pain) and adds an opioid analgesic. The client with mild to moderate pain may not be able to sleep or may have trouble working and staying focused. If pain increases beyond that which is controlled by the level II analgesics, it is time to move on to level III. At this level the pain is moderate to severe and is affecting the quality of the client's life, and he or she may not be able to perform activities of daily living. At level III an adjuvant analgesic may be added.

Analgesics should be given on an ATC basis to prevent the pain from breaking through, especially for cancer and

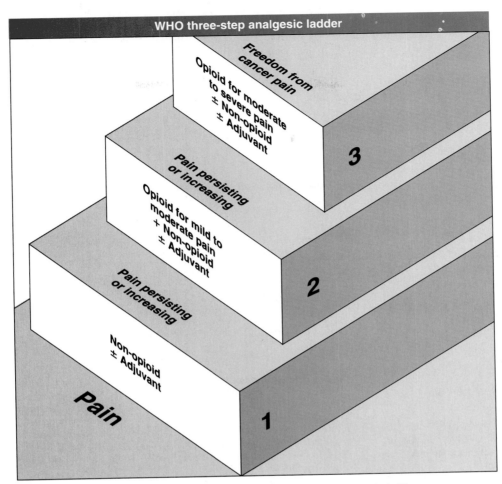

Figure 9–6. World Health Organization three-step analgesic ladder.

chronic benign pain. For clients experiencing surgical or traumatic pain, analgesics should be given ATC until the pain decreases to a level that allows medications to be given as required (prn). When using the WHO ladder it is important to keep in mind that it may not be necessary to start at level I if the client is having severe pain. Analgesics from level III on the WHO ladder may be the starting point in some cases.

 CRITICAL THINKING: Mrs. Zales

A 32-year-old woman was admitted for a hysterectomy after being treated for painful endometriosis for 12 months. After her surgery she had a PCA pump with hydomorphone (Dilaudid), which was effective in relieving her pain. Forty-eight hours postoperatively, the surgeon discontinued the PCA pump and ordered oral hydrocodone with acetaminophen (Lortab) for her. It was ineffective, so an order for hydomorphone (Dilaudid) 2 to 4 mg orally every 3 to 4 hours as needed was added. The nurses gave only one dose of the hydromorphone, then, thinking that her pain should be lessening, switched her back to the hydrocodone with acetaminophen. By the next morning she was in severe pain, and the on-call physician ordered IM meperidine (Demerol) and promethazine (Phenergan). Mrs. Zales' discharge was delayed until her pain could be controlled.

What do you think happened? How could the delayed discharge have been avoided?

Answers at end of chapter.

CLIENT EDUCATION

Clients must be informed about the medications that they are taking for pain management so they can take an active role in their care. Clients informed about the goals of pain management will be more likely to report unrelieved pain so that they can receive prompt and effective treatment. Goals include a satisfactory comfort level with minimal side effects and complications of pain and its treatment, as well as an appropriate length of hospital stay.

It is important for the nurse to provide the client with information about the drug's common side effects, the frequency of the dose and its duration of action, and potential drug-drug interactions if indicated. Education must be pre-sented at a level that the client can understand. Clients who are informed will use their medications more effectively and safely.

CRITICAL THINKING: Ms. Jackson

Ms. Jackson had abdominal surgery 2 days ago. She has been receiving morphine via IV PCA at an aver-

---

NURSING CARE PLAN BOX 9–4 FOR THE CLIENT IN PAIN

Pain

Client Outcomes

Pain is at a level that is acceptable to the client. Client is able to participate in activities that are important to him or her.

Evaluation of Outcomes

Is pain at a level that is acceptable to the client? Is the client able to participate in activities that he or she has identified as important?

Interventions	*Rationale*	*Evaluation*
Assess pain based on client report. Use the WHAT'S UP format.	Client's pain is defined as what the client says it is, when the client says it is occurring.	Does the client verbalize his or her pain? Does the client use verbal or nonverbal messages that imply trust in nurse's belief of pain report?
Teach the client to use a pain rating scale. Use the same scale consistently.	A rating scale is the most reliable method for assessing pain severity.	Does the client understand the use of the scale and use it to report pain?
Determine with client what is an acceptable pain level.	Only the client can decide what pain level is tolerable.	Is the client's pain at an acceptable level?
Assess whether pain is acute, chronic, or both.	Acute and chronic pain may present differently and may require different interventions.	Has acute versus chronic pain been identified? Are treatments appropriate?
Assess need for and offer emotional and spiritual support for the experience of pain and suffering.	Pain, as well as disease processes, can be accompanied by feelings of powerlessness and distress.	Does the client appear emotional, angry, or withdrawn? Does the client have difficulty making decisions? Is the client-nurse relationship therapeutic?
Give analgesics before pain becomes severe. For moderate to severe pain, give analgesic ATC.	Severe pain is more difficult to relieve.	Is analgesic schedule effective?
Observe for anticipated side effects of pain medication.	Many pain medications cause nausea and constipation. The nausea usually subsides after several days, but the constipation does not.	Are side effects occurring? Can they be managed? Does medication regimen need to be adjusted?
If opioids are being used, assess for respiratory depression and reduced level of consciousness at regular intervals.	High doses or sudden increases in dose of an opioid can result in respiratory depression and reduced level of consciousness.	Is the client's respiratory rate greater than 8 per minute or above the parameter ordered by the physician? Is the client alert and oriented?
Institute measures to prevent constipation: 8 to 10 glasses of fluid daily (unless contraindicated), fiber in meals, fiber or bulk laxatives, exercise as tolerated.	Opioids cause constipation.	Are the client's bowels moving according to his or her usual pattern?
Teach client alternative pain relief interventions, such as relaxation and distraction, to be used with medication.	Alternative interventions can help the client feel in control and may help reduce the perception of pain.	Does the client use alternative interventions effectively?
Assess whether client is taking pain medications appropriately, and if not, assess reasons. Instruct in how to manage pain interventions.	Pain medications must be taken appropriately in order to be effective.	Is the client able to manage the pain control regimen? Are adjustments necessary?

age of 2.5 mg per hour for the last 6 hours. She rates her pain at 3 on a scale of 0 to 10. She is to be discharged today. Her physician has ordered codeine 30 mg with acetaminophen (Tylenol with Codeine No. 3), 1 or 2 tablets every 4 hours as needed for pain at home.

Will Ms. Jackson be comfortable at home? Why or why not?

Answers at end of chapter.

LEARNING TIP

Many medication interventions are available for the treatment of pain. Whenever possible, the nurse should administer analgesics by the mouth, by the WHO ladder, and by the clock.

EVALUATION

The final phase of the nursing process is evaluation. Once the plan of care has been implemented, the nurse must evaluate whether the client's goals have been met. Evaluation is an ongoing process as the plan of care is carried out to be sure that pain management is effective and changes are made as needs are identified. Has the client's identified goal for an acceptable level of pain been met? How well were the pain treatments tolerated? Were there any adverse effects to the medications that were given? Were the side effects managed appropriately? Poorly managed side effects can be as problematic as poorly managed pain. When nausea is a problem that the client has identified as something that is always a problem for him or her after surgery, it is imperative that we include in our plan how it will be addressed. Was monitoring appropriate at each point in the pain management plan for the prevention of uncontrolled pain and clinically significant respiratory depression? Was the client able to participate in activities that he or she identified as important? The plan was effective if all of these questions can be answered positively.

See also Nursing Care Plan Box 9–4 for the Client in Pain.

Review Questions

1. Mr. White is walking up and down the hall and visiting with other clients. He is laughing and joking. He approaches the nurse's station and asks for his pain shot, and reports that his pain is 6 on a scale of 0 to 10. Based on McCaffery's definition, which of the following assumptions by the nurse is correct?
   a. Mr. White is not really in pain but just wants his medication.
   b. Mr. White is having pain at 6 on a scale of 0 to 10.
   c. Mr. White is in minimal pain and should receive a pill instead of a shot.
   d. Mr. White is in pain but does not need his pain medication now.

2. Mrs. Yates has chronic cancer pain. She is receiving 120 mg of MS Contin every 12 hours orally. She recently required an increase in her dose because of increased pain. Mrs. Yates is most likely experiencing which of the following?
   a. Addiction
   b. Tolerance
   c. Psychological dependence
   d. Ceiling effect

3. Ms. Williams has incisional pain following total hip replacement surgery. Which of the following types of pain is she experiencing?
   a. Nociceptive
   b. Neuropathic
   c. Both of the above

4. Which of the following assessment methods is the most reliable way to objectively assess a client's pain?
   a. Obtain a pain history from the client.
   b. Observe the client for signs of pain.
   c. Ask the client to rate his or her pain on a validated assessment scale.
   d. Ask a family member to rate the client's pain.

5. Jim is hospitalized following a motor vehicle accident. He has multiple orthopedic injuries and is in acute pain. He has an order for morphine 6 mg IV every 2 to 3 hours as needed. Assuming his respiratory rate and level of sedation are acceptable and his pain is controlled, which of the following analgesic schedules will be most effective for relieving his pain?
   a. Offer the analgesic every 2 to 3 hours.
   b. Tell him to put on his light when he feels pain, and give it immediately when he requests it.
   c. Give the IV analgesic every 2 to 3 hours ATC.
   d. Alternate the IV analgesic with an oral analgesic.

6. Which of the following classes of medications is likely to be most effective for the treatment of pain with a neuropathic component?
   a. Tricyclic antidepressants
   b. Opioids
   c. NSAIDs
   d. All of the above

7. Mrs. Edwards has terminal cancer and has been requiring 5 mg of IV morphine every 1 to 2 hours to control her pain, yet she is laughing and enjoying her visitors. Which of the following explanations of her behavior is most likely correct?
   a. Denial of pain is common in clients with cancer.
   b. Mrs. Edwards' cancer is improving.

c. Mrs. Edwards is hiding her pain when visitors are present.

d. Distraction can be an effective treatment for pain when used with appropriate drug treatments.

ANSWERS TO CRITICAL THINKING

CRITICAL THINKING: *Smithers and Barnett*

It is important to believe both clients' pain reports. Assessment should be based on what the client says rather than what is observed. Each client copes with his or her pain in a unique way, and the nurse cannot judge whether one is in more pain than the other.

CRITICAL THINKING: *Mrs. Shepard*

1. Pain medication is most effective when given on a routine schedule around the clock so that the pain is not allowed to break through. Mrs. Shepard's epidural infusion will continue to relieve her pain for several hours after it is discontinued, depending on the medication used. The oral medication is most effective when given at the time the epidural is stopped so that it is taking effect as the epidural effects wear off.

2. Pain prevents clients from moving freely. Postoperative complications such as retained pulmonary secretions and ileus can occur when clients are immobile. Effective pain management can help prevent these complications.

3. Mrs. Shepard should be instructed what her role will be when her pain management regimen is altered. Does she have to ask for the pain medication or will it just be brought to her? Client and family education is vital to success in management of a client's pain.

CRITICAL THINKING: *Mr. Sebastian*

Home instruction regarding ATC administration of pain medication is indicated. MS Contin, a long-acting form of morphine, may be an option for him with an immediate-release preparation for breakthrough pain. Also, information about what to do and who to contact if pain becomes unmanageable is necessary to help prevent readmissions to the hospital.

CRITICAL THINKING: *Mrs. Zales*

Mrs. Zales was probably tolerant to opioids because of her need for medication for chronic pain over the last year. For this reason, she needed more medication than a nontolerant, opioid-naive person to relieve her pain. Also, the belief that promethazine and other phenothiazines potentiate opioids is a myth. It does cause increased levels of sedation and may limit the amount of opioid that can be safely given. IM injections are not recommended because they are painful, absorption is not predictable, and there is a delay between injection and relief. Nurses often base the treatment of a client's pain on what they usually do or what they think *should* be effective rather than on sound pain management practices and principles. A more rational approach to Mrs. Zales would have been regular pain assessment with ATC treatment until pain began to subside. If her pain level had been better controlled, she could have been discharged on oral analgesics without the delay.

CRITICAL THINKING: *Ms. Jackson*

Using an equianalgesic conversion we can determine whether she is likely to have good pain relief based on her requirement with the PCA. Her current pain level of 3 shows that the morphine has been effective. Remember that the pump keeps a history of what the client uses, which is the best indicator of what the client needs. Ms. Jackson has used 15 mg of morphine during the past 6 hours. An equianalgesic dose of Tylenol with Codeine No. 3 would be almost 200 mg of codeine, but she has only 30 to 60 mg ordered. In addition, if Ms. Jackson takes enough Tylenol with Codeine No. 3 to get 200 mg of codeine, she will receive a dangerous dose of both the codeine and the acetaminophen. The physician needs to be contacted for different analgesic orders.

REFERENCES

1. McCaffery, M, and Beebe, A: Pain: Clinical Manual for Nursing Practice. Mosby, St Louis, 1989.
2. Principles of Analgesic Use in the Treatment of Acute Pain and Cancer Pain, ed 3. American Pain Society, Skokie, Ill, 1992, p 2.
3. AHCPR Clinical Practice Guideline: Management of Cancer Pain. US Department of Health and Human Services, Rockville, Md, 1994.
4. Principles of Analgesic Use in the Treatment of Acute Pain and Cancer Pain. American Pain Society, Skokie, Ill, 1993.

BIBLIOGRAPHY

Acute Pain Management Guideline Panel. Acute Pain Management: Operative or Medical Procedures and Trauma. Clincal Practice Guideline. AHCPR Pub No 92-0032. Agency for Health Care Policy and Research, Public Health Service, US Department of Health and Human Services, Rockville, Md, 1992.

Altman, GB, and Lee, CA: Strontium-89 for treatment of painful bone metastasis from prostate cancer. Oncol Nurs Forum 23(3):523, 1997.

American Nurses' Association Position Paper on Promotion of Comfort and Relief of Pain in Dying Patients. American Nurses' Association, Kansas City, Mo, 1990.

Gahart, B, and Nazareno, A: Intravenous Medications. Mosby, St Louis, 1996.

Guidelines for the Treatment of Cancer Pain. Final Report of the Texas Cancer Council's Workgroup on Pain Control in Cancer Patients. Austin, Tx, 1991.

Mackey, R: Discover the Healing Power of Therapeutic Touch. Am J Nurs 95:26, April 1995.

McCaffery, M: Analgesic administration via rectum or stoma. ET Nurs 19:114, 1992.

McCaffery, M, and Beebe, A: Pain: Clinical Manual for Nursing Practice. Mosby, St Louis, 1989.

O'Brien, S, et al: The knowledge and attitudes of experienced oncology nurses regarding the management of cancer-related pain. Oncol Nurs Forum 23:3, 515, 1996.

Paice, J, and Buck, M: Intraspinal devices for pain management. Nurs Clin North Am 18:46, December 1994.

Pain management as a legal responsibility. Nursing October 1992.

Pharmacy Formulary and Therapeutic Index. University of Texas, MD Anderson (ed), Houston, Tex, 1994-1995.

Principles of Analgesic Use in the Treatment of Acute Pain and Cancer Pain. American Pain Society, Skokie, Ill, 1993.

Roberts, M: Basic Pain Management. South Mississippi Home Health, Hattiesburg, Miss, 1997.

Spross, J: Cancer pain relief: An international perspective. Caring February 1993.

Zenz, M, Strumpf, M, and Tryba, M: Long term oral opioid therapy in patients with chronic nonmalignant pain. J Pain Symptom Manage 22, July 1992.

Nursing Care of Clients with Cancer

Martha Spray and Vera Dutro

10

Learning Objectives

Upon completion of this chapter, the student will be able to:

1. Review normal anatomy and physiology of the cell.
2. Relate the changes that occur in the cell when it becomes malignant.
3. Describe the special nursing needs of the client receiving chemotherapy or radiation therapy.
4. Identify medications commonly used as chemotherapy agents.
5. Discuss the appropriate nursing assessment and interventions for common oncological emergencies.
6. Use the nursing process as a framework to provide care for clients with cancer.
7. Describe the concept of hospice in providing care for clients with advanced cancer.

Key Words

alopecia (AL-oh-**PEE**-she-ah)
anemia (uh-**NEE**-mee-yah)
anorexia (AN-oh-**REK**-see-ah)
benign (bee-**NIGHN**)
biopsy (**BY**-ahp-see)
cancer (**KAN**-sir)
carcinogen (kar-**SIN**-oh-jen)
chemotherapy (KEE-moh-**THER**-uh-pee)
cytotoxic (SIGH-toh-**TOCK**-sick)
leukopenia (LOO-koh-**PEE**-nee-yah)
malignant (muh-**LIG**-nunt)
metastasis (muh-**TASS**-tuh-sis)
mucositis (MYOO-koh-**SIGH**-tis)
neoplasm (**NEE**-oh-PLAZ-uhm)
oncology (on-**KAH**-luh-jee)
oncovirus (**ONK**-oh-VIGH-russ)
palliation (pal-ee-**AY**-shun)
radiation therapy (RAY-dee-**AY**-shun **THER**-uh-pee)
stomatitis (STOH-mah-**TIGH**-tis)

thrombocytopenia (THROM-boh-SIGH-toh-**PEE**-nee-ah)
tumor (**TOO**-mur)
vesicant (**VESS**-i-kant)
xerostomia (ZEE-roh-**STOH**-mee-ah)

149

Review of Normal Anatomy and Physiology of Cells

Cells are the smallest living structural and functional sub-units of the body. Although human cells vary in size, shape, and certain metabolic activities, they have many characteristics in common.

CELL STRUCTURE

Human cells, with the exception of mature red blood cells, have a cell membrane, cytoplasm, cell organelles, and a nucleus. In the mature red blood cell the nucleus has been lost. In either case, the cell structures have a specific and vital function. The cell membrane forms the outer boundary of the cell and is made up of protein, phospholipids, and cholesterol. Proteins serve three different purposes: (1) they can act as pores or enzymes to permit transport of certain materials, (2) they can act as receptor sites for hormones to trigger a cell's activity, or (3) they can act as antigens to identify the cell as belonging in the body.

Materials may enter or leave a cell in one of several ways. These transport mechanisms are summarized in Table 10–1, with examples of their importance in the body. A cell membrane is selectively permeable, meaning that not all substances will pass through. The lipids permit the diffusion of lipid-soluble materials into or out of the cell.

CYTOPLASM AND CELL ORGANELLES

Cytoplasm is a watery solution of minerals, gases, and organic molecules that is found between the cell membrane and the nucleus. Chemical reactions (such as the synthesis of adenosine triphosphate [ATP]) take place within the cytoplasm. Many cell organelles are found within the cyto-

plasm. Cell organelles are subcellular structures with specific functions; these are summarized in Table 10–2 and shown in Figure 10–1.

NUCLEUS

The nucleus of a cell is surrounded by a double-layered nuclear membrane with many pores. Within the nucleus are one or more nucleoli and the chromosomes of the cell.

A nucleolus is a small sphere made of deoxyribonucleic acid (DNA), ribonucleic acid (RNA), and protein. The nucleoli together form a type of RNA called ribosomal RNA.

Table 10–2. **Functions of Cell Organelles**

Organelle	Function(s)
Endoplasmic Reticulum	Passageway for transport of materials within the cell Synthesis of lipids
Ribosomes	Site of protein synthesis
Golgi Apparatus	Synthesis of carbohydrates Packaging of materials for secretion from the cell
Mitochondria	Site of aerobic cell respiration, synthesis of ATP
Lysosomes	Contain enzymes to digest ingested material or damaged tissue
Centrioles	Organize the spindle fibers during cell division
Cilia	Sweep materials across the cell surface, as in the respiratory passages
Flagellum	Enables a sperm cell to move

Table 10–1. **Cellular Transport Mechanisms**

Mechanism	Definition	Example in the Body
Diffusion	Movement of molecules from an area of greater concentration to an area of lesser concentration	Exchange of gases in the lungs or body tissues
Osmosis	The diffusion of water	Absorption of water by the intestines or kidneys
Facilitated Diffusion	Carrier enzymes move molecules across cell membranes	Intake of glucose by most cells
Active Transport	The use of ATP to move molecules from an area of lesser concentration to an area of greater concentration	Absorption of glucose and amino acids by the small intestine
Filtration	Movement of water and dissolved materials from an area of higher pressure to an area of lower pressure (blood pressure)	Formation of tissue fluid; the first step in the formation of urine
Phagocytosis	A moving cell engulfs something	White blood cells engulf bacteria
Pinocytosis	A stationary cell engulfs something	Cells of the kidney tubules reabsorb small proteins

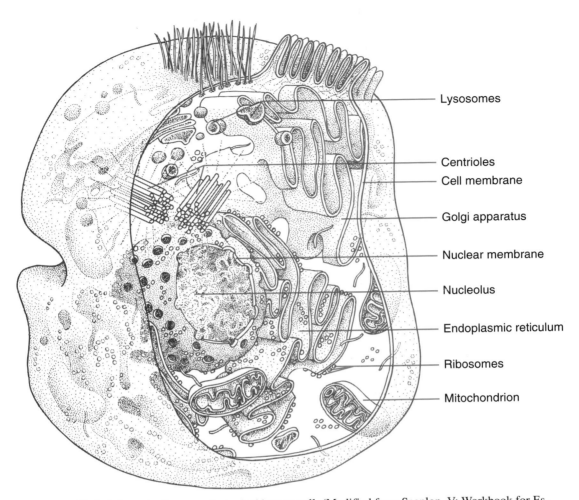

Lysosomes

Centrioles

Cell membrane

Golgi apparatus

Nuclear membrane

Nucleolus

Endoplasmic reticulum

Ribosomes

Mitochondrion

Figure 10–1. Schematic diagram of a typical human cell. (Modified from Scanlon, V: Workbook for Essentials of Anatomy and Physiology, ed 2. FA Davis, Philadelphia, 1995, p 30, with permission.)

This ribosomal RNA is a type of cell organelle called the ribosome and is involved in protein synthesis.

The nucleus is the control center of the cell because it contains the chromosomes. The 46 chromosomes of a human cell are made of DNA and protein. DNA is the genetic code for the characteristics and activities of the cell. Specific regions of DNA are called genes; a gene is the code for one protein. Not all the genes in any cell are active, only the relative few needed for the proteins to carry out their specific functions. These proteins may be structural proteins such as the collagen of connective tissue or functional proteins such as the hemoglobin of red blood cells. Important functional proteins are those that speed the specific chemical reaction that is characteristic of each type of cell.

GENETIC CODE AND PROTEIN SYNTHESIS

The genetic code of DNA is the code for the amino acid sequences needed to synthesize a cell's proteins. This process is shown in Figure 10–2 and may be described simply as

follows. A complementary copy of the DNA's gene is made by a molecule called messenger RNA (mRNA). The mRNA then moves to the cytoplasm of the cell and attaches to the ribosomes. As with any complex process, mistakes are possible. Should there be a mistake in the DNA code, the process of protein synthesis may go on anyway, but the resulting protein will not function normally; this is the basis for genetic diseases. Such DNA mistakes may be acquired during life; these are called mutations. A mutation is any change in the DNA code. Ultraviolet rays or exposure to certain chemicals may cause structural changes in the DNA code. These changes may kill the affected cells or may irreversibly alter their function. Such altered cells may become **malignant,** unable to function normally but very active; this is the basis of some forms of cancer.

MITOSIS

Mitosis is the process by which a cell reproduces itself. One cell, after its 46 chromosomes have duplicated themselves, divides into two cells, each with membrane, cytoplasm, and organelles from the original cell and a complete

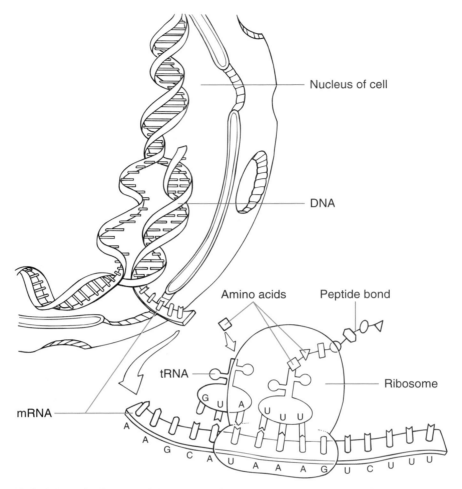

Figure 10–2. Schematic diagram of the process of protein synthesis. (Modified from Scanlon, V: Workbook for Essentials of Anatomy and Physiology, ed 2. FA Davis, Philadelphia, 1995, p 35, with permission.)

set of duplicated or identical chromosomes. Mitosis is necessary for the growth of the body and to replace dead or damaged cells. Some cells are capable of mitosis and others are not. Cells of the epidermis of the skin undergo mitosis continuously to replace the superficial cells that are constantly worn off of the skin surface. The same is true of the cells that line the stomach and intestines. Cells in the red bone marrow also divide frequently; red blood cells have a fixed life span (about 120 days) and must be replaced. Some cells seem to be capable of only a limited number of divisions, and when that limit has been reached, the cells die and are not replaced.

Other cells do not undergo mitosis to any great extent after birth. Nerve cells (neurons) are unable to divide, and muscle cells have very limited mitotic capability. When such cells are lost through injury or disease, the loss of their function in the individual is usually permanent.

CELL CYCLE

The cell life cycle involves a series of changes through which a cell progresses starting from the time it develops until it reproduces itself. The duration of the cell's life, the

time it takes for mitosis to occur, the growth ratio (percentage of cycling cells), the frequency of cell loss, and the doubling time (time for a tumor to double its size) are important concepts related to tumor growth and treatment strategies.

Three functions are noted in the cell cycle, including cells that are actively dividing, those that leave the cycle after a certain point and die, and those that temporarily leave the cycle and remain inactive until reentry into the cycle. Inactive cells continue to synthesize RNA and protein (Fig. 10–3).

CELLS AND TISSUES

A tissue is a group of cells with similar structure and functions. The four groups of human tissues are epithelial, connective, muscle, and nerve.

Epithelial tissues form coverings and linings throughout the body. Often the cells are capable of mitosis, and damage to the tissue may be repaired. The healing of a cut to the skin is a typical example.

Connective tissues are of many kinds with many varied functions. Blood is a connective tissue involved in the transportation of materials throughout the body. Fibrous connective tissue, made mostly of the protein collagen,

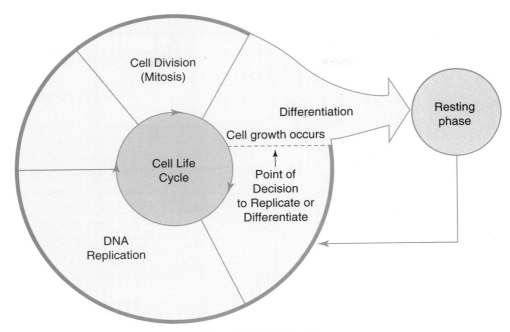

Figure 10–3. Cell cycle.

forms strong membranes such as those around muscles, attaching structures such as ligaments and tendons, and the dermis of the skin. Bone and cartilage are supporting connective tissues. Adipose tissue, another form of connective tissue, stores fat as potential energy. Many kinds of connective tissue cells are capable of mitosis.

There are three kinds of muscle tissue: skeletal muscle, smooth muscle, and cardiac muscle. Skeletal muscle tissue makes up the voluntary muscles attached to the skeleton. Smooth muscle is found in viscera such as the stomach and intestines, the walls of arteries and veins, the walls of the bronchial tubes, and, in women, the uterus. Cardiac muscle forms the walls of the chambers of the heart. As mentioned, the cells of muscle tissue have little ability to reproduce themselves.

Nerve tissue is made of neurons and supporting cells; in the central nervous system these supporting cells are called neuroglia. Although mature nerve cells are not capable of mitosis, many of the neuroglia are capable of mitosis. It is the neuroglia, not neurons, that usually form the tumors that may develop in the central nervous system.

Introduction to Cancer Concepts

Oncology is the branch of medicine dealing with tumors. Oncology nursing is also called cancer nursing, which is an important component of medical-surgical nursing care. A list of cancer resources is provided in Table 10–3. Cancer

is second only to heart disease in mortality rates in the United States. The American Cancer Society reports that an estimated 10 million Americans alive today have a history of cancer.

Early accounts of cancer date back to the seventeenth century BC. Documentation of the benefits of early cancer detection and its impact on treatment exist from the beginning of the nineteenth century. Today, microscopic technology and genetic engineering provide physicians with a better understanding of tumor growth and cell activity and a means for early cancer detection and intervention.

Benign Tumors

Normal cells that reproduce abnormally result in **neoplasms** or **tumors.** *Neoplasm* is a term that combines

Table 10–3. **Cancer Resources**

American Cancer Society
1-800-ACS-2345
http://www.cancer.org

Association of Community Cancer Centers
http://nysernet.org/bcic/accc/index.html

National Cancer Institute
301-496-8531
http://cancernet.nci.nih.gov/
http://www.nci.hih.gov

Oncology Nursing Society
412-921-7373
http://www.ons.org/

---

oncology: onco—mass + logy—word, reason
neoplasm: neo—new + plasm—form

Table 10–4. **Benign and Malignant Tumors**

	Benign	Malignant
Growth Rate	Typically slow expansion	Often rapid with cell numbers doubling normal cell growth; malignant cells infiltrate surrounding tissue
Cell Features	Typical of the tissue of origin	Atypical in varying degrees of the tissue of origin; altered cell membrane; contains tumor-specific antigens
Tissue Damage	Minor	Often causes necrosis and ulceration of tissue
Metastasis	Not seen; remains localized at origin site	Often spreads to form tumors in other parts of the body
Recurrence after Treatment	Seldom recurrence after surgical removal	Recurrence can be seen after surgical removal and following radiation and chemotherapy
Related Terminology	Hyperplasia, polyp, and benign neoplasia	Cancer, malignancy, and malignant neoplasia
Prognosis	Not injurious unless location causes pressure or obstruction to vital organs	Death if uncontrolled

the Greek word *neo,* meaning new, and *plasia,* meaning growth, to suggest new tissue growth. A neoplasm is an enlargement of tissue forming an abnormal mass. A neoplasm develops as cells multiply. Not all neoplasms have cancer cells. However, a neoplastic cell is responsible for producing a tumor and shows a lively growing cell. A new neoplastic growth is very difficult to detect until it contains about 500 cells and is approximately 1 cm in size.

A **benign** tumor is defined as a cluster of cells that is not normal to the body but is noncancerous. Benign tumors grow more slowly and have cells that are the same as the original tissue. An organ containing a benign tumor usually continues to have normal function, whereas an organ affected with a cancerous tumor will eventually cease to function. *Malignant* is a term often used as a synonym for cancer. *Malignant* is defined as a growth that resists treatment. A comparison of benign and malignant tumors is found in Table 10–4.

Cancer

Cancer is a group of cells that grows out of control, taking over the function of the affected organ. Cancer cells are described as poorly constructed, loosely formed, and without organization. A simplistic definition would be "confused cell."

LEARNING TIP

Cancer is not contagious.

PATHOPHYSIOLOGY

Cancer is not one disease, but many diseases with different causes, manifestations, treatments, and prognoses. It is a disease of over 100 different types, caused by mutation of

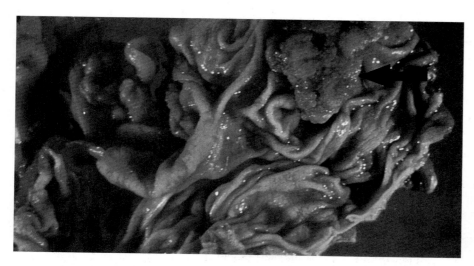

Figure 10–4. Adenocarcinoma of the caecum. Note the cluster of cells at upper right of the caecum. (Photograph courtesy of Dinesh Patel, MD. Medical Oncology, Internal Medicine, Zanesville, Ohio.)

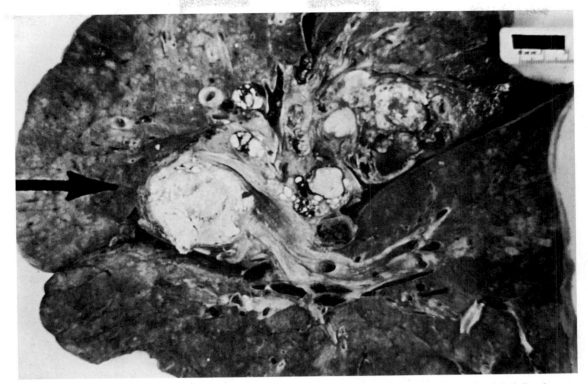

Figure 10–5. Lung cancer. The black arrow marks the tumor site. (Photograph courtesy of Dinesh Patel, MD. Medical Oncology, Internal Medicine, Zanesville, Ohio.)

cellular genes. Cancer takes on the characteristics of the cell it mutates and then takes on characteristics of the mutation. Growth regulating signals in the cell's surrounding environment are ignored as the abnormal cell growth increases. Normal cells are limited to about 50 to 60 divisions before they die. Cancer cells do not have a division limit and are considered immortal.

The progression from a normal cell to a malignant cell follows a pattern of mutation, defective division and abnormal growth cycles, and defective cell communication. Cell mutation occurs when a sudden change affects the chromosomes, causing the new cell to differ from the parent. The malignant cell enzymes destroy the gluelike substance found between normal cells, which disrupts the transfer of information used for normal cell structure.

LEARNING TIP

An individual's cancer risk is viewed as the balance between exposure and susceptibility to **carcinogens.**

CANCER CLASSIFICATION

Cancers are identified by the tissue affected, speed of cell growth, cell appearance, and location. Neoplasms occurring in the epithelial cells are termed *carcinoma.* Carcinoma is the most common type of cancer and includes cells of the skin, gastrointestinal system, and lungs (Figs. 10–4

and 10–5). Cancer cells affecting connective tissue, including fat, the sheath that contains nerves, cartilage, muscle, and bone, are termed *sarcoma. Leukemia* is the term used to describe the abnormal growth of white blood cells. Cancers involving cells of the lymphatic system, lymph nodes, and spleen are termed *lymphoma* (Table 10–5).

SPREAD OF CANCER

Neoplastic cells that remain intact in an area are considered localized or in situ cancers. These tumors may be difficult

Table 10–5. **Tumor Description**

Benign Tumors
• Fibroma—originating from connective tissue • Lipoma—originating from fat tissue

Cancerous Tumors
• Carcinoma—originating from tissue of the skin, glands, and digestive, urinary, and respiratory tract linings • Sarcoma—originating from connective tissue, including bone and muscle • Leukemia—originating from blood, plasma cells, and bone marrow • Lymphoma—originating from lymph tissue • Melanoma—originating from skin cells

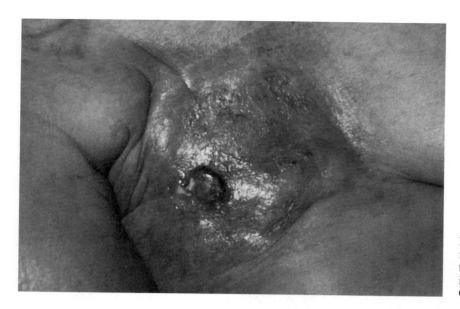

Figure 10–6. Invasive metastasis to skin area following mastectomy for breast cancer. (Photograph courtesy of Dinesh Patel, MD. Medical Oncology, Internal Medicine, Zanesville, Ohio.)

to visualize on clinical examination and are detected through microscopic cell examination. In situ tumors are often removed surgically and require no further treatment. **Metastasis** is the term used to describe the spread of the tumor from the primary site into separate and distinct areas.

Metastasis is the stage when cancer cells acquire invasive behavior characteristics and cause the surrounding tissue to change (Figs. 10–6 and 10–7). Metastasis occurs primarily because cancer cells break away more easily than normal cells and can survive for a time independently from other cells.

There are three steps in the formation of a metastasis. Cancer cells are able to (1) invade blood or lymph vessels, (2) move by mechanical means, and (3) lodge and grow in a new location.

Metastatic tumors carry with them the cell characteristics of the original or primary tumor site. As a result, surgeons are able to determine the original tumor site based on metastatic cell characteristics. For example, lung tissue found in the brain suggests a primary lung tumor with metastasis to brain tissue. Common sites of metastasis are lungs, liver, bones, and the brain.

INCIDENCE OF CANCER

Cancer affects all age groups, although the incidence is higher in individuals 60 to 69 years of age. The second highest age group is 70 to 79 years of age. Men have a higher incidence of cancer than women.[1] Cancer in persons over age 60 is thought to occur from a combination of exposure to carcinogens and weakening of the body's immune system.

Some cancers, such as Wilms' tumor of the kidney and acute lymphocytic leukemia, occur in young people. The cause of tumors in young people is not well understood, but genetic predisposition tends to be a major factor.

The most common type of cancer in adults is skin cancer; it is also considered to be the most preventable. Exposure to ultraviolet radiation (sunlight) increases the risk of skin cancer. Wearing protective clothing and sunscreen can greatly reduce the risk of skin cancer.

Lung cancer is responsible for the highest mortality rate in both men and women and is also considered to be preventable in some cases. Cigarette smoking and air pollution are regarded as possible causes (Fig. 10–8).

Men have a high incidence of prostate cancer between the ages of 60 and 79. The second highest is lung cancer related to chemical agents. Cancer of the colon and rectum has been linked with the consumption of high-fat, low-fiber diets and ranks as the third highest cancer in men (Fig. 10–9).

The highest incidence of cancer in women is found in the lungs, and the second highest involves the breast (Fig. 10–9). Women with a family history of breast cancer have a greater risk than those with no family history of breast cancer. Commercial testing for the oncogene linked with breast cancer is available and marketed for high-risk women, especially those in the Ashkenazi Jewish population. Genetic testing is done through genetic counseling programs, and the cost ranges from $700 to $2400, depending on the geographical region.

MORTALITY RATES

Cancer survival rates have improved over the past 30 years. The American Cancer Society reports a gain in client survival rates from 33% in the 1960s to 40% currently (American Cancer Statistics, 1997). A 5-year time period is used to monitor cancer client progress following diagnosis

metastasis: meta—beyond + stasis—stand

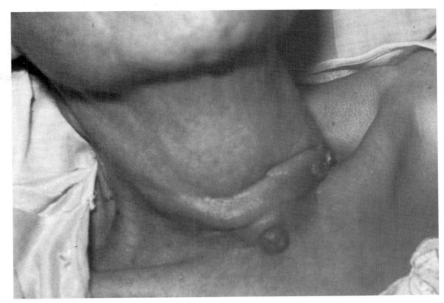

Figure 10–7. Note lesions on neck. These lesions are an example of cancer metastasis. (Photograph courtesy of Dinesh Patel, MD. Medical Oncology, Internal Medicine, Zanesville, Ohio.)

and treatment. Survival statistics are based on persons living 5 years in remission.

ETIOLOGY

Cancer cell growth and reproduction involves a two-step process. The first step in cancer growth is called initiation. Initiation causes an alteration in the genetic structure of the cell (DNA). Cell alteration is associated with exposure to a carcinogen. The cellular change primes the cell to become cancerous.

Promotion is the second type of cancer cell growth and occurs after repeated exposures to carcinogens cause initiated cells to mutate. During the promotion step, a tumor forms from mutated cell reproduction.

A healthy immune system can often destroy cancer cells before they replicate and become cancerous. It is important to remember that any substance that weakens or alters the immune system puts the individual at risk for cell mutation. Medical researchers support the theory that cancer is a symptom of a weakened immune system.

Risk Factors

Increased risk of cancer is linked to several environmental factors. An evaluation of cancer begins with assessment of well-known risk factors such as specific viruses; exposure to radiation, chemicals, and irritants; genetics; diet; and general immunity. Certain racial and ethnic groups also are at higher risks for some types of cancer. (See Cultural Considerations Box 10–1.)

Viruses

Certain viruses, such as the **oncoviruses** (RNA-type viruses) are linked to cancer in humans. Retrovirus is an enzyme produced by RNA tumor viruses and is found in human leukemia cells.

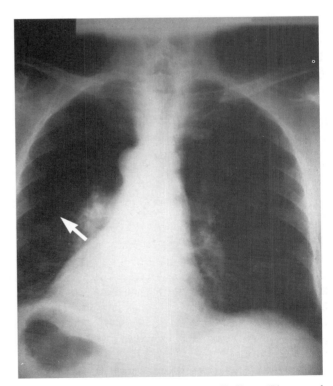

Figure 10–8. Lung x-ray with lung cancer findings. (Photograph courtesy of Dinesh Patel, MD. Medical Oncology, Internal Medicine, Zanesville, Ohio.)

---

oncovirus: onco—bulk + virus

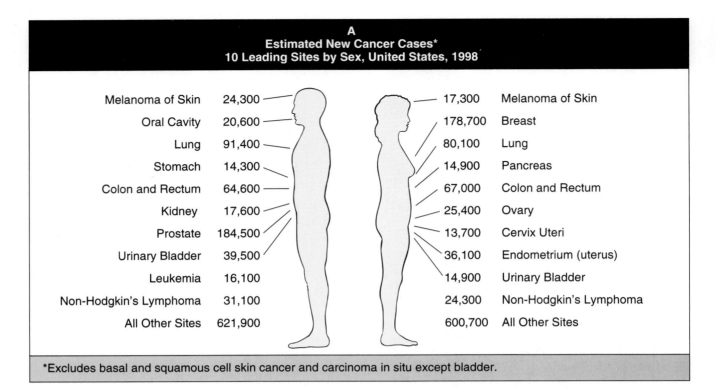

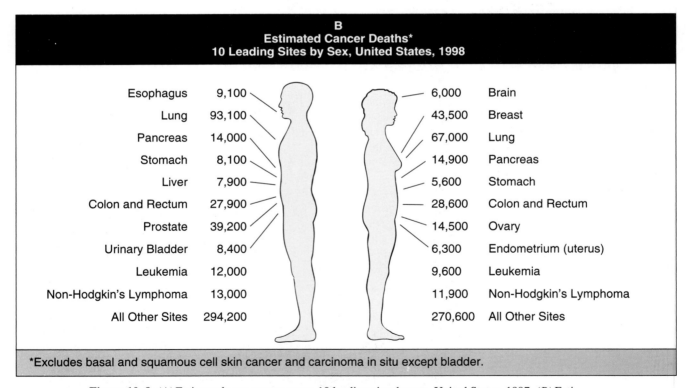

Figure 10–9. *(A)* Estimated new cancer cases, 10 leading sites by sex, United States, 1997. *(B)* Estimated cancer deaths, 10 leading sites by sex, United States, 1997. (Modified from Cancer statistics booklet, American Cancer Society, 1998.)

CULTURAL CONSIDERATIONS BOX 10-1

Many racial and ethnic groups in the United States have high rates of cancer. Whereas risk factors for the development of specific cancers are similar, barriers to prevention and nursing strategies to reduce risk factors vary among ethnicities.

Foreign-born and first-generation white men from Norway, Sweden, and Germany have an increased risk of stomach cancer. This suggests an interrelation among ethnic, geographic, and dietary risk factors as the cause of this high incidence of stomach cancer.[2] Assessing for this data among these populations may assist in the diagnostic process.

Recent Eastern European immigrants may be at risk for thyroid cancer and leukemia because of the current industrial pollution and radiation exposure from the Chernobyl nuclear disaster in 1988. Some contamination occurred in Estonia, Latvia, Lithuania, and Poland. This may constitute a health hazard and may affect both recent immigrants and visitors to these countries. It is essential that health care providers carefully screen individuals for these cancers.

The Appalachian region has the highest rate of cervical cancer in the United States.[3] Thus the nurse needs to encourage Appalachian women to have gynecological examinations on a yearly basis.

Cancer sites among African-Americans include the prostate, breast, lung, colon, rectum, cervix, pancreas, and esophagus. Because African-Americans are overrepresented in the working class, they experience increased exposure to hazardous occupations. For example, African-American men are at a higher risk for developing cancer related to their high representation in the steel and tire industries and in factories manufacturing chemicals and pesticides.[4] They have the highest overall cancer rate, the highest overall mortality rate, and their 5-year survival rate is 30% lower than that of European-Americans. Mortality rates for colorectal cancer declined 12.3% from 1973 to 1989 for European-Americans; however, it increased 7% for African-Americans. In general, African-Americans report later for treatment than European-Americans. Colon tumors are deeper within African-Americans, making detection on digital examination more difficult. Poverty, a diet high in fat and low in fiber, and lower levels of thiamine, riboflavin, vitamins A and C, and iron may increase cancer risk among African-Americans. Additionally, cigarette smoking, inner city living with pollution, obesity, and alcohol consumption increase African-Americans' risk for developing cancer.

Lack of medical care access acts as a barrier to prevention among African-Americans. Survival, not prevention, is the priority. Additional barriers include a lack of cancer risk teaching and detection in some African-American communities, lack of health insurance, and little stigma attached to alcohol consumption and smoking. Strong family ties encourage seeking health care from family members before professionals.[4]

Primary strategies for cancer prevention and increasing survival among African-Americans include using African-American professionals as speakers in community activities, using church-based information dissemination, providing forums in African-American communities, and addressing smoking advertisements in African-American communities. Additional strategies include involving granny healers and ministers, changing food preparation practices and amounts rather than changing cultural food habits, involving extended family members in educational campaigns, and using African-American sports leaders in media campaigns.

Hispanic populations in the United States have an increased incidence for some types of cancer. Cervical cancer is increased among Central and South American women. Pancreatic, liver, and gallbladder cancer is increased among Mexican-Americans. Many Mexican-Americans are less aware of the early warning signs of cancer; many are more fearful of getting cancer than the general public; and many work in mining, factories using chemicals, and farming using pesticides.[5-7]

Barriers to preventive health care among many Hispanics include high poverty rates, low educational rates, a preference for health care providers who understand Spanish, a preference for health care information presented in Spanish, a delay in seeking treatments for symptoms, and using lay healers as a first choice in health care. Additionally, many have a fear of surgical intervention with a body cavity left open to air and have decreased access to health care. For some, an undocumented immigration status creates a fear of reprisal.

Nursing approaches effective among Hispanics include educating lay healers regarding cancer prevention, educating lay healers about early warning signs of cancer, using bilingual health care providers, using Hispanic health care providers whenever available, using respected Hispanic community leaders in educational programs, presenting videos in Spanish using Hispanic actors, educating the entire family because of close family networks, and connecting with Hispanic community churches, restaurants, and stores. Additionally, the nurse can use the 1-800-4-CANCER telephone number for Spanish translation and counseling, become involved with Hispanic community movements, and provide information in community and regional Hispanic newspapers and community publications.

Cervical, liver, lung, stomach, multiple myeloma, esophageal, pancreatic, and nasopharyngeal cancer are higher among Chinese-Americans. Chinese-American women have a 20% higher rate of pancreatic cancer.[8] High rates of stomach and liver cancer in Korea predispose recent immigrants to these conditions. Thus the nurse needs to assess and teach newer immigrants regarding these types of cancer.[9]

High rates of stomach, breast, colon, and rectal cancer common among Japanese people may be related to the high sodium content of the Japanese diet, a genetic predisposition, consumption of salted fish and contaminated grain, hepatitis B, smoking, vitamin A deficiency, low vitamin C intake, chronic esophagitis, and pulmonary sequelae of cigarette smoking.[10] Barriers to prevention include the follow-

continued

ing: prevention models are not native to their culture; there may be a lack of trust in Western medicine; they have decreased access to health care; some are unable to speak the English language; and for some, an undocumented immigration status creates a fear of reprisal.

Nursing approaches to improve cancer risk prevention among Asians and Pacific Islanders include education about prevention versus acute care practice, educating native healers, involvement in community with respected native leaders, videos and literature in native language, and incorporating native healing practices such as traditional Chinese medicine.

Native-American populations have an increased risk for skin, pancreatic, gallbladder, liver, and prostate cancer.[11] Risk factors for the development of cancer include obesity, a diet high in fat, high rates of alcohol consumption, and

high rates of smoking. Barriers to prevention include a lack of Native-American health care providers, health care providers' unfamiliarity with Native-American cultures, lack of financial resources, and a lack of integration of Native-American healing practices into prevention practices. Nursing approaches to decrease cancer risk prevention among Native-American populations include the following: incorporate prevention into Native-American healing practices; educate Native-American lay healers regarding cancer prevention practices; work with tribal community leaders; respect modesty, gender roles, and tribal customs; work with the Indian Health Service and Bureau of Indian Affairs; encourage traditional customs of physical fitness and exercise; and encourage dietary portion control and healthy food preparation practices instead of changing cultural food habits.

The Epstein-Barr virus (EBV), which causes infectious mononucleosis, is also associated with Burkett's lymphoma. Herpes simplex virus II has been associated with cervical and penile cancers. Papillomavirus associated with genital warts is considered one cause of cervical cancer in women. Chronic hepatitis B is linked with liver cancer.

Radiation

There is an increased incidence of cancer in persons exposed to prolonged or high measures of radiation. Ionizing radiation involving x-rays; alpha, beta, and gamma rays; and ultraviolet rays such as sunlight plays a major role in the promotion of leukemia and skin cancers, primarily the melanomas.

Persons exposed to radioactive materials in large doses such as a radiation leak or an atomic bomb are at risk for leukemia, breast, bone, lung, and thyroid cancer. Controlled radiation therapy is used to treat cancer clients by destroying rapidly dividing cancer cells. Radiation can also damage normal cells. The decision to use radiation is made after careful evaluation of the location and tumor vulnerability to other treatments.

Chemicals

Chemicals are present in air, water, soil, food, drugs, and tobacco smoke. Chemical carcinogens are implicated as triggering mechanisms in malignant tumor development. An increased length of exposure time and degree of exposure intensity to chemical carcinogens put individuals at greater risk for cancer development.

Smoking accounts for 87% of lung cancer worldwide.[12] Chemical agents, as in tobacco, are more toxic when used with alcohol. Alcohol and tobacco are the greatest causes of cancers of the mouth and throat. Chemicals used in manufacturing such as vinyl chloride are associated with liver cancer.

Irritants

Chronic irritation or inflammation caused by irritants such as snuff or pipe smoking often cause cancer in local areas. Nevi (moles) that are chronically irritated by clothing, especially clothing contaminated by chemical residue, may turn malignant. Asbestos found in temperature and sound insulation has been proven to cause a particularly virulent type of lung cancer.

Genetics

Genetics plays a large part in cancer formation. Certain breast cancers are linked to a specific gene mutation. Skin and colon cancers have a genetic tendency. People with Down syndrome (a chromosomal abnormality) have a higher risk of developing acute leukemia.

Diet

Diet is a large factor in both cause and prevention of malignancies. People who eat high-fat, low-fiber diets are more prone to develop colon cancers. Diets high in fiber reduce the risk of colon cancer. High-fat diets are linked to breast cancer in women and prostate cancer in men. Consumption of large amounts of pickled, smoked, and charbroiled foods has been linked with esophageal and stomach cancers. A diet low in vitamins A, C, and E is associated with cancers of the lungs, esophagus, mouth, larynx, cervix, and breast. (See Nutrition Notes Box 10–2.)

Hormones

Hormonal agents that cause a disturbance in the balance of the body may also promote cancer. Long-term use of the female hormone estrogen is associated with cancer of the breast, uterus, ovaries, cervix, and vagina. It has been found that young women born of pregnant women who took diethylstilbestrol (DES) have an increased incidence of developing vaginal cancer. DES is a synthetic hormone with estrogen-like properties used in the past to prevent miscarriage.

Tumors of the breast and uterus are tested for estrogen or progesterone influence. If a breast tumor is malignant, the tumor is tested and treatment is varied depending on it being positive for estrogen or progesterone dependence.

Immune Factors

A healthy immune system destroys mutant cells quickly on formation. An individual with altered immunity is more susceptible to cancer formation when exposed to small amounts of carcinogens compared with someone with a healthy immune system. Immune system suppression allows malignant cells to develop in large numbers.

Altered immunity is noted in persons with chronic illness and stress. An increased risk of developing cancer follows a very traumatic stress period in life, such as a loss of a mate or a job. Failure to decrease stress productively contributes to a higher incidence of chronic illnesses. Thus a cycle of stress, illness, and increased cancer risk develops. A decline in the immune system is also noted as the body ages. A weaker immune system contributes to the chronic illnesses and cancer associated with the elderly population.

DETECTION AND PREVENTION

Nurses play an important role in the prevention and detection of cancer. Nurses help provide education concerning risk factors, self-examination, and cancer screening programs. Early diagnosis and initiation of treatment provide time to stop the progression of cancer.

An annual physical examination helps medical personnel assess for cancer's seven warning signals promoted by the American Cancer Society.[13] The warning signals are based on the mnemonic CAUTION:

Change in bowel or bladder habits
A sore that does not heal
Unusual bleeding or discharge
Thickening or lump in breast or other tissue
Indigestion or swallowing difficulties
Obvious change in wart or mole
Nagging cough or hoarseness

Monthly breast self-examination for men and women is recommended after puberty. Mammogram (a specific x-ray of breast tissue used to detect a mass too small for palpation) is recommended once between ages 35 and 39 to provide a baseline and then annually past age 40. Routine pelvic examination and Papanicolaou testing (Pap smear) are recommended annually after 18 years of age to screen for cervical cancer. Cytological examination of cervical cells increases the chances of diagnosing cervical cancer in situ.

Promotion of healthy lifestyle practices, including proper diet and exercise, helps strengthen the immune system and reduce cancer risks. The American Cancer Society promotes "stop smoking" campaigns and supports the effort by stating that smoking is the most preventable cause of death from lung cancer. Secondhand smoke contributes to increased risk of lung cancer in nonsmokers.

The American Cancer Society recommends two courses of action to screen for colorectal cancer, beginning at age 50. The first option includes an annual stool test for blood, with a flexible sigmoidoscopy and digital rectal examination every 5 years. The second option is a total colon examination, either by colonoscopy with digital rectal examination every 10 years or by barium enema and digital rectal examination every 5 to 10 years.[14]

Detection of prostate cancer is significant for men beginning around age 50. Digital rectal examination and prostate-specific antigen (PSA) blood testing is recommended annually for men over 50 who have a life expectancy of at least 10 years and for younger men who are at higher risk.[15] See Gerontological Issues Box 10–3 for early signs of cancer in older adults.

Currently much attention is directed toward genetic testing and identification of persons at risk for cancer. Genetic testing technology poses both legal and ethical questions concerning confidentiality and insurance cost issues. Family member cooperation is important because genetic testing is done after a family member has been diagnosed with cancer. Persons may experience a variety of emotions centered on increased risk for self and guilt concerning the role played in causing an increased risk for their children.

Preventive cancer vaccines are being developed for cancers associated with specific viruses. At present, most cancer vaccines are therapeutic rather than prophylactic and are used to stimulate the client's immune system to destroy cancer cells. Vaccine therapy for malignant melanoma is being tested.

DIAGNOSIS OF CANCER

A diagnosis of cancer can be a very frightening experience. Often people will try to mask symptoms because they are so frightened of the disease. Exploring client attitudes and perceptions about the disease helps the nurse construct an

GERONTOLOGICAL ISSUES BOX 10-3

Early Signs of Cancer in Older Adults

Colorectal Cancer

Rectal bleeding, blood (red or black) in feces, change in usual bowel evacuation patterns, and constipation or diarrhea may be associated with cancerous lesions in the large intestine.

Fatigue, weakness, and anemia can be signs of chronic occult blood loss. These symptoms are often discounted as normal aging.

Breast Cancer

Detection of a small lesion with an annual mammogram and prompt removal increases the probability of cure. A small lump, dimple, or thickened area of the breast or breast discharge may be an early sign of breast cancer.

Prostate Cancer

Rectal examination can detect prostate enlargement. Elevation of prostate-specific antigen can be an early sign of cancer.

Skin Cancer

Examine the skin (especially sun-exposed areas such as the nose, cheeks, top of the ears, head, neck, shoulders, hands, and arms) for dry patches of precancerous actinic keratoses that can be removed.

Be aware of any sores that do not heal and any changes in a wart or a mole. These can be signs of a cancerous lesion.

Other

Unfortunately, there is no effective early detection examination for lung and ovarian cancer. Often, the symptoms are vague, and by the time lung cancer is diagnosed with sputum cytology and ovarian cancer is diagnosed by tissue biopsy, the diseases have significantly advanced.

Incisional biopsy is an invasive procedure that involves the surgical removal of a small amount of tissue for inspection. Tissue can also be removed during endoscopic procedures (insertion of a tube for observing the inside of a hollow organ or cavity), such as a lung biopsy done during a bronchoscopy. Excisional biopsy is used to remove an entire tissue mass. Needle aspiration biopsy involves insertion of a needle into tissue for fluid or tissue aspiration (Fig. 10–10). This procedure is considered less invasive than incisional or excisional biopsy. Transcutaneous aspiration involves the insertion of a fine needle into tissue such as breast, prostate, or salivary glands and is used for diagnosing metastatic cancers.

Frozen-section biopsy provides immediate evaluation of the tissue sample during a surgical procedure. By freezing the tissue sample for microscopic examination, a quick analysis is possible, which helps direct additional surgical intervention. Frozen section biopsy is useful in the diagnosis and surgical intervention of breast cancer.

Stereotactic biopsy is a safe and efficient procedure for evaluating lesions in the brain and breast. The procedure is done by a specially trained radiologist. The biopsy site must be firmly immobilized. The lesion is scanned for location, and a small incision is made for easy insertion of a small fiber-optic instrument (Fig. 10–11). Stereotactic biopsy of the brain involves a local anesthetic for making a small hole in the skull. Breast stereotactic biopsy uses pressure exerted by a mammogram machine to secure the breast; anesthesia may not be necessary.

Laboratory Tests

Blood, serum, and urine values are important in establishing baseline values and general health status. Laboratory values are used with other assessment findings. An elevated white blood cell (WBC) count is expected if the

effective teaching plan. A careful and thorough assessment of the client's present and past medical and surgical history and pertinent family history are obtained. A complete physical examination provides the nurse with both objective and subjective data. The most conclusive information about the health of tissue is by examining cell activity; this is accomplished by biopsy.

Biopsy

Accurate identification can only be done by **biopsy** (the surgical removal of tissue cells). Microscopic examination of a piece of suspected tissue or aspirated body fluid can confirm the presence of mutant cells. A biopsy is often done in the physician's office or outpatient surgery department.

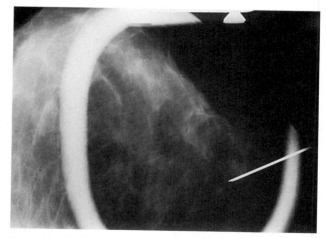

Figure 10–10. Fine-needle breast biopsy. (Photograph courtesy of Dinesh Patel, MD. Medical Oncology, Internal Medicine, Zanesville, Ohio.)

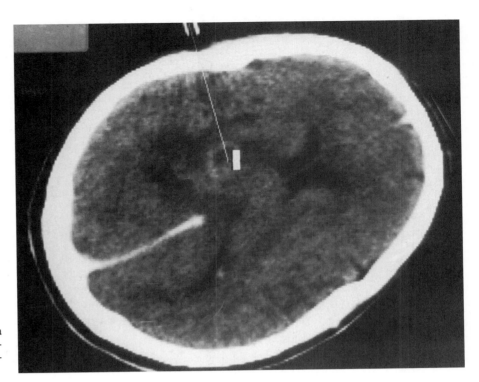

Figure 10–11. Stereotactic biopsy of a brain lesion. (Photograph courtesy of Dinesh Patel, MD. Medical Oncology, Internal Medicine, Zanesville, Ohio.)

client has evidence of infection; however, an increase in WBCs without infection raises suspicion of leukemia. Fifty percent of clients with liver cancer have increased levels of bilirubin, alkaline phosphatase, and glutamic-oxaloacetic transaminase.

Bone marrow aspiration is done to learn the number, size, and shape of red and white blood cells and platelets. Bone marrow aspiration is a major tool for diagnosis of leukemia. (See Chapter 23 for a description of this test and related nursing care.)

Tumor markers, also called biochemical markers, are proteins, antigens, genes, hormones, and enzymes produced and secreted by tumor cells. Tumor markers help confirm a diagnosis of cancer, detect cancer origin, monitor the effect of cancer therapy, and determine cancer remission. Tumor markers include the following:

- Prostatic acid phosphatase (PAP)—high levels noted in prostate cancer
- Prostate-specific antigen (PSA)—elevated levels associated with prostate cancer
- Cancer antigen (CA) 15-3—elevated levels noted in breast cancer; useful in monitoring client response to therapy for metastatic breast cancer
- Cancer antigen (CA) 125—increased levels in ovarian, cervical, liver, and pancreas cancers
- Cancer antigen (CA) 19-9—used to diagnose and evaluate pancreatic and hepatobiliary cancer; levels elevated in cancer
- Carcinoembryonic antigen (CEA)—increased levels suggest tumor activity

Cytological Study

Cytology is the study of the formation, structure, and function of cells. Cytological diagnosis of cancer is obtained primarily through Pap smears of cells shed from a mucous membrane (e.g., a cervical or oral smear). Test results are based on the degree of cell abnormality; normal reflects no cellular changes, slight cellular changes are considered normal with a possible link to abnormal cells seen in infection, and severe cellular changes reflect a higher probability of precancerous or cancerous cellular activity. Infection causes cellular changes and contributes to an increase in abnormal cells detected.

Radiological Procedures

X-ray is a valuable diagnostic tool in detecting cancer of the bones and hollow organs. Routine chest x-ray is one diagnostic test used in detecting lung cancer. Mammography is a reliable and noninvasive low-radiation x-ray procedure for detecting breast masses. Breast tissue is compressed to allow better visualization of the soft tissue. The nurse must alert clients that soft tissue compression causes a degree of discomfort, but the compression is necessary to obtain an accurate picture. The discomfort is over very quickly (Figs. 10–12 and 10–13).

Contrast media x-rays are used to detect abnormalities of bone and the gastrointestinal and urinary systems. Contrast media can be given by various methods. Barium is given orally for visualization of the esophagus and stomach or rectally for visualization of the colon (e.g., a barium

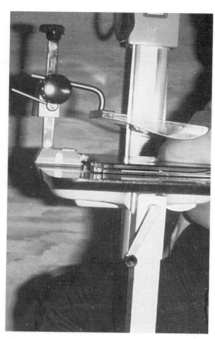

Figure 10–12. Mammogram procedure. (Photograph courtesy of Dinesh Patel, MD. Medical Oncology, Internal Medicine, Zanesville, Ohio.)

enema). Intravenous injection of contrast media is used for lung and brain scans.

Computerized tomography (CT) provides a three-dimensional cross-sectional computerized picture of the body. CT scans are important in the diagnosis and staging of malignancies. CT scans can detect minor variations of tissue thickness. The use of a contrast medium enhances the accuracy of an abdominal CT scan. CT scans are also used to improve the accuracy of inserting a fine needle for biopsy.

Nuclear Imaging Procedures

Nuclear medicine imaging involves camera imaging of organs or tissues containing radioactive media. Radioactive compounds are given intravenously or by ingestion. These studies are highly sensitive and can detect sites of abnormal cell growth months before changes are seen on an x-ray.

Positron emission tomography (PET) provides information about cellular biochemical and metabolic activity. Clients are given biochemical compounds and images are made of the tissue through gamma-camera tomography. PET scans have been useful in brain imaging.

Ultrasound Procedures

Ultrasonography (US) uses high-frequency sound waves to provide images of deep soft-tissue structures in the body. The procedure is noninvasive and does not use x-ray. Echoes from high-frequency sound waves outline tissue density and masses. This technology helps detect tumors of the pelvis and breast. Ultrasound may also be used to distinguish between benign and malignant breast tumors.

Magnetic Resonance Imaging

Magnetic resonance imaging (MRI) creates sectional images of the body. MRI can be done with or without contrast dye and does not use radiation. Clients are placed in a cylinder-shaped magnetic field. The magnetic field aligns the nuclei of body cells in one direction. The magnetized cells are then excited by radio-frequency pulses. Images are made as cell nuclei change their alignment. MRI is valuable in the detection, localization, and staging of malignant tumors in the central nervous system, spine, head, and musculoskeletal system. MRI cannot be used in clients

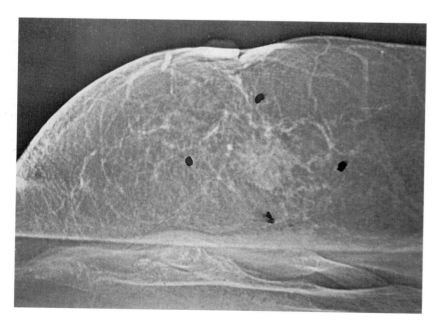

Figure 10–13. Mammogram. (Photograph courtesy of Dinesh Patel, MD. Medical Oncology, Internal Medicine, Zanesville, Ohio.)

with pacemakers, implanted pumps, surgical clips, metal knees or hips, or tattooed eyeliner.

Endoscopic Procedures

An endoscopic examination allows the direct visualization of a body cavity or opening. The procedure involves the insertion of a flexible endoscope containing fiber-optic glass bundles that transmit light and can produce an image. Endoscopy enables the surgeon to biopsy abnormal tissue. Endoscopy is used to detect lesions of the throat, esophagus, stomach, colon, and lungs.

Oral endoscopic procedures require client preparation to reduce the risk of aspirating stomach secretions. The client is given nothing to eat or drink before and immediately after the examination. A local anesthetic is used during the examination to anesthetize the throat. Following the procedure, oral food and fluids are withheld until the gag reflex returns, to prevent aspiration. Assessment of the gag reflex is done by placing a tongue blade on the back of the tongue or by using a cotton-tipped swab at the back of the throat to stimulate the gag reflex after the procedure.

STAGING AND GRADING

Tumor staging is used to determine the stage of solid-tumor masses. It provides valuable information about the potential success of treatment plans. Tumor staging is important in the development of an international system that can compare statistics among cancer centers. The most common system used for staging tumors is called TNM (tumor, node, metastasis).

This staging system classifies solid tumors by size and tissue involvement. TNM stages are T_0 (no tumor), T_{is} (tumor in situ), and T_1 through T_4 (progressive increase in tumor size or involvement). Extent of lymph node involvement ranges from N_0, no nodes, to N_4, a large amount of lymph node involvement. Metastasis is described as M_0, no metastasis, to M_1, metastasis to some area (Table 10–6).

There is also a rating or grading system to define the cell types of tumors. Tumors are classified according to the percentage of cells that are differentiated (mature). If the tissue of a neoplastic tumor closely resembles normal tissue it is called well differentiated. Poorly differentiated refers to a malignant neoplasm that contains some normal cells, but most of the cells are abnormal. The better defined or differentiated the tumor, the easier it is to treat.

TREATMENT FOR CANCER

There are three main types of treatment for cancer: surgery, **radiation therapy,** and **chemotherapy.**

---

chemotherapy: chemo—chemistry + therapy—treatment

Table 10–6. **Tumor, Node, Metastasis (TNM) Classification, Staging, and Tissue Involvement**

Classification	Staging	Tissue Involvement
Primary tumor (T)		
T_{is}	Stage I	Tumor in situ, indicates no invasion of other tissues
T_1, T_2, T_3, T_4	Stage II	Ranges indicate progressive increase in tumor size with local metastasis
Regional lymph node involvement (N)		
N_0		No nodes
N_1, N_2, N_3	Stage III	Metastasis to regional lymph nodes
Metastasis (M)		
M_0		No metastasis
M_1	Stage IV	Distant metastasis

Surgery

Surgery can be used as a cure for cancer when removal of the entire tumor is possible. Skin cancers and well-defined tumors without metastasis can be removed without any additional intervention.

Prophylactic surgery is used to remove moles or lesions that have the potential to become malignant. Colon polyps are often removed to prevent malignancies from developing, especially if the polyps are considered premalignant. An extreme example of prophylactic surgery is a woman who elects to have a mastectomy (surgical removal of the breast) due to high prevalence of breast cancer in her family.

Surgery may also be done for **palliation** (symptom control). Surgical removal of tissue to reduce the size of the tumor mass is helpful, especially if the tumor is compressing nerves or blocking the passage of body fluids. The goal of palliative surgery is that the client will experience less discomfort and an improved quality of life.

Reconstructive surgery can be done for cosmetic enhancement or for return of function of a body part. Facial reconstruction is important for a client's self-image after removal of head or neck tumors. Women can elect to have breast implants after mastectomy surgery.

Surgical intervention for cancer treatment is typically not an emergency intervention, which allows clients and medical personnel time for preplanning. Autologous blood donation (blood donated by the client before surgery) has become very popular and reduces an individual's risks of being exposed to blood-borne infections. The American Red Cross and many hospitals have programs specifically designed for autologous blood donation and will accept donations from 30 days to 72 hours before surgery.

Nurses play a major role in reducing the client's fears about postoperative pain. Patient-controlled analgesia (PCA) provides clients with a measure of control over their pain. Measures such as deep relaxation, imagery, and hypnosis can be used with traditional pain control measures.

It is important to encourage clients to express and discuss their fears. Clients with a limited understanding about cancer may fear that tissues will not heal postoperatively. Information about wound care, including dressing changes and presence of drainage tubes, increases the client's knowledge base and sense of control. Visual aids concerning tumor site and surgical procedures are valuable teaching tools.

Clients who are undernourished are poor surgical candidates and require intervention such as enteral or parenteral nutrition before and after surgery. Clients with cancer are also at increased risk for developing deep vein thrombosis (DVT) postoperatively. Preoperative teaching includes the importance of leg movement, early ambulation, wearing antiembolism stockings, and recognizing symptoms of DVT, such as a cramping sensation in the calf muscle and pain when the foot is dorsiflexed. (See Chapter 18.)

Radiation

Radiation is used commonly in the treatment of cancer. Radiation can be used for cure, control, or palliation. The decision to use radiation is often based on cancer site and size. Radiation treatment may be curative if the disease is localized. Radiation destroys cancer cells by affecting cell structure and the cell environment. It is used in fractionated (divided) doses to prevent destructive side effects; however, side effects can occur in the area being treated because of damage to normal cells.

The size of a large tumor can be decreased with radiation before surgery, making surgical intervention more effective and less dangerous. Palliative radiation is used to reduce the size of a large cancerous lesion and consequently reduce pressure and pain. Radioisotopes inserted into cancerous tissue during surgery help destroy the cancerous cells without removing the organ.

Nursing Care of the Client Receiving Radiation Treatment

Symptoms of tissue reaction to radiation treatment can be expected approximately 10 to 14 days after the start of the treatment program and continue up to 2 weeks after treatment is completed. Typical reactions and appropriate nursing interventions include the following:

- *Fatigue.* Encourage clients to nap frequently and prioritize activities. Reassure them that the feeling will go away when the treatments are completed.
- *Nausea, vomiting, and* **anorexia.** Encourage clients to take prescribed medication for nausea and vomiting. Anorexia can be helped by eating small amounts of high-carbohydrate, high-protein foods and avoiding foods high in fiber.
- **Mucositis** (inflammation of the mucous membranes, especially of the mouth and throat). Encourage the client to avoid irritants such as smoking, alcohol, acidic food or drinks, extremely hot or cold foods and drinks, and commercial mouthwash. Advise the client to do mouth care before meals and every 3 to 4 hours. A neutral mouthwash is appropriate and can be made by using 1 ounce of diphenhydramine hydrochloride (Benadryl) elixir diluted in 1 quart of water or normal saline. Agents that coat the mouth such as Maalox are sometimes used. Lidocaine hydrochloride 2% viscous has an anesthetic effect on the mouth and throat.
- **Xerostomia** (dry mouth). Encourage frequent mouth care. Substitute saliva is available over the counter and is helpful to use especially at night when clients complain of a choking sensation from extreme dryness.
- *Skin reactions.* Skin reactions vary from mild redness to raw moist lesions similar to a second-degree burn. Skin surfaces that are especially warm and moist such as the groin, perineum, and axillae have a poor tolerance to radiation. Prophylactic skin care includes keeping skin dry; free from irritants, such as powder, lotions, deodorants, and restrictive clothing; and protected against exposure to direct sunlight.
- *Bone marrow depression.* Bone marrow depression occurs with both radiation and chemotherapy treatments. Weekly blood counts are done to detect low levels of white blood cells, red blood cells, and platelets. Transfusions of whole blood, platelets, or other blood components may be necessary.

Safety Considerations

Radiation may be administered externally or internally. External radiation treatment is given by a trained medical specialist in a designated area within the hospital or clinic. Internal radiation treatment is administered to clients admitted to a health care facility.

Safety guidelines must be followed when caring for the client with radioactive materials implanted into tissue or body cavities or administered orally or intravenously. Nursing responsibilities include knowledge about (1) the radiation source being used, (2) method of administration, (3) start of treatment, (4) length of treatment, and (5) prescribed nursing precautions. Personnel involved with radiation therapy must recognize the three primary factors in radiation protection: time, distance, and shielding. These three factors depend on the type of radiation used. Time involves the time spent administering care, distance involves the amount of space between the radioisotope and the nurse, and shielding involves the use of a barrier such as a lead apron.

---

anorexia: an—not + orexis—appetite
mucositis muco—mucous (membrane) + itis—inflammation
xerostomia: xero—dry + stoma—mouth

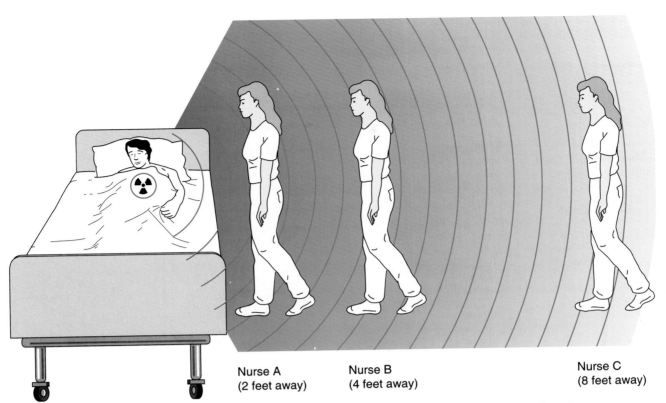

Figure 10–14. Radiation distancing. Nurse B receives less radiation than Nurse A, and Nurse C receives less radiation than Nurse B.

Nurse A
(2 feet away)

Nurse B
(4 feet away)

Nurse C
(8 feet away)

The nurse must work efficiently when providing care for clients who are receiving radioisotopes that are releasing gamma rays. The nurse's exposure to radiation is proportionate to the time spent and the distance from the radiation source. For example, a nurse standing at the foot of the bed of a client with radioisotopes inserted into the head receives less exposure than the nurse standing at the head of the bed (Fig. 10–14). Time and distance are used to protect the nurse, visitors, and other personnel.

It is very important to teach the client and family members the reason nursing care focuses on providing only essential care. Speedy nursing encounters and visitor restrictions are better accepted and less likely to promote feelings of isolation when clients understand the reasons behind them.

Drainage from the site of a radioactive colloid injection is considered radioactive, and the physician must be informed immediately. Dressings contaminated with radioactive seepage must be removed with a long-handled forceps. Radioactive materials must never be touched with unprotected hands; shielding is required to prevent exposure to radiation. Contamination from radioisotope applicators or interstitial implants cannot occur when the cap-sule is intact; contamination occurs when the capsule is broken.

LEARNING TIP

Remember to use the principles of time, distance, and shielding to protect yourself from radiation exposure.

Chemotherapy

Chemotherapy is chemical therapy that uses **cytotoxic** drugs to treat cancer. Cytotoxic drugs can be used for cure, control, or palliation of cancerous tumors. Cytotoxic drugs are described according to how they affect cell activity. For example, alkylating agents bind with DNA to stop the production of RNA; antimetabolites substitute for nutrients or enzymes in the cell life cycle; mitotic inhibitors interfere with cell division; antibiotics inhibit DNA and RNA synthesis; and hormonal agents alter the hormonal structure of the body. Chemotherapy is usually more effective when multiple drugs are given in multiple doses. Specific drugs and side effects are provided in Table 10–7.

The effects of chemotherapy are systemic unless used topically for skin lesions. Chemotherapy is used preoperatively to shrink tumors and postoperatively to treat residual tumors. Factors influencing the effectiveness of chemo-

---

cytotoxic: cyt—cell + toxic—poison

Table 10–7. **Chemotherapy Medications**

Medication	Classification	Method of Administration	Common Side Effects
Bleomycin	Antibiotic	IM or IV	Fever and chills, cough, shortness of breath, in severe cases pulmonary fibrosis
Busulfan	Alkylating	PO	Unusual bleeding or bruising, diarrhea, fatigue, nausea and vomiting
Carmustine (BCNU)	Alkylating	IV	Fever and chills, nausea and vomiting
Chlorambucil (Leukeran)	Alkylating	PO	Unusual bleeding or bruising, nausea and vomiting
Cisplatin	Alkylating	IV	Difficulty in hearing, fever and chills, ringing in ears, nausea and vomiting
Cyclophosphamide (Cytoxan)	Alkylating	IV or PO	Nausea and vomiting, blood in the urine, loss of hair
Cytarabine (Cytosar)	Antimetabolic	IV	Fever and chills, unusual bleeding or bruising, sore throat, tiredness, nausea and vomiting
Dacarbazine (DTIC)	Alkylating	IV	Vesicant, nausea and vomiting, loss of appetite, bleeding or bruising
Dactinomycin (Cosmegen)	Antibiotic	IV	Vesicant, loss of hair, nausea and vomiting, tiredness
Daunorubicin	Antibiotic	IV	Vesicant, red urine, nausea and vomiting, loss of hair
Doxorubicin (Adriamycin)	Antibiotic	IV	Vesicant, red urine, nausea and vomiting, loss of hair, cardiac damage
Estramustine (Emcyt)	Alkylating Estrogenic	PO	Nausea, vomiting, anorexia, edema, breast tenderness or enlargement
Etoposide (VP-16)	Alkylating	IV	Mildly vesicant, nausea and vomiting, loss of hair, numbness and tingling in fingers and toes
Floxuridine (FUDR)	Antimetabolic	IV	Diarrhea, nausea and vomiting, loss of appetite, sores in mouth
Fluorouracil (5-FU)	Antimetabolic	IV	Diarrhea, loss of appetite, loss of hair, nausea and vomiting
Hydroxyurea (Hydrea)	Antimetabolic	PO	Fever and chills, sore throat, drowsiness, diarrhea, nausea and vomiting
Lomustine (CCNU)	Alkylating	PO	Loss of appetite, nausea and vomiting, sore throat
Mechlorethamine (Nitrogen mustard)	Alkylating	IV	Vesicant, nausea and vomiting
Melphalan (Alkeran)	Alkylating	PO	Nausea and vomiting
Methotrexate	Antimetabolite	PO, IV Intrathecal	Blood in urine, sun sensitive, diarrhea, sores in mouth, jaundice, nausea and vomiting
Mitomycin-C (Mutamycin)	Antibiotic	IV	Vesicant, blood in urine, nausea and vomiting, loss of appetite
Mitotane		PO	Dizziness, drowsiness
Mitoxantrone (Novantrone)	Miscellaneous	IV	Blue-green urine, nausea and vomiting, loss of hair
Paclitaxel (Taxol)	Miscellaneous	IV	Nausea, vomiting, muscle aches, cardiac toxicities
Procarbazine	Alkylating	PO	MAO inhibitor, drowsiness, nausea and vomiting
Streptozocin (Zanosar)	Antibiotic	IV	Anxiety, chills, nausea and vomiting
Tamoxifen (Nolvadex)	Hormone	PO	Hot flashes, weight gain, nausea, bone pain
Thiotepa	Alkylating	IV	Nausea, loss of appetite, loss of hair, dizziness
Vinblastine (Velban)	Vinca alkaloid	IV	Muscle pain, nausea and vomiting, loss of hair
Vincristine (Oncovin)	Vinca alkaloid	IV	Constipation, difficulty in walking, tingling in fingers and toes

therapy are tumor type, available chemotherapeutic drugs, and genetics.

Routes of Administration

Drugs may be given via oral, intramuscular, intravenous, or topical routes. The dosage of medication is regulated by the size of the individual and the toxicities of the drug. The administration of intravenous chemotherapeutic drugs requires specialized training and knowledge of antineoplastic drugs.

Vesicant drugs are given only by the intravenous route. These drugs cause blistering of tissue that eventually leads to necrosis if they infiltrate or leak out of the blood vessel into soft tissue (Fig. 10–15). Skin grafts may be necessary if tissue damage is extensive.

CENTRAL LINES. Central lines are intravenous catheters that terminate in the superior vena cava near the right atrium of the heart. This is a large vessel that allows for dilution of vesicant drugs and reduces the risk of infiltration. Central lines may be external, with the distal end of the catheter exiting the skin, or internal, with the distal catheter ending in an implanted port. See Chapter 6 for additional information on central lines.

Side Effects of Chemotherapy

Toxicities in clients receiving chemotherapy vary according to the medications given. However, there are some

---

vesicant: vesicare—to blister

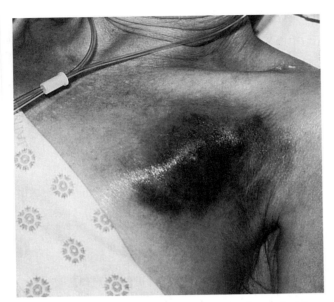

Figure 10–15. Necrosis of skin tissue resulting from administration of a vesicant chemotherapy drug. (Photograph courtesy of Dinesh Patel, MD. Medical Oncology, Internal Medicine, Zanesville, Ohio.)

general side effects that are commonly associated with chemotherapy drugs. Fast-growing epithelial cells such as those of the hair, blood, skin, and gastrointestinal tract are generally affected by both chemotherapy and radiation.

BONE MARROW. Chemotherapy is toxic to the bone marrow where the blood cells are produced. Clients may develop low white blood cell counts (**leukopenia**), increasing their susceptibility to infection and sepsis. A reduction in platelets (**thrombocytopenia**) increases the risk of bruising and bleeding and can require platelet transfusions. Increased risk of **anemia** occurs with the reduction of red blood cells and may require blood transfusions.

GASTROINTESTINAL TRACT. The gastrointestinal tract is susceptible to the toxicity of chemotherapy drugs. Clients often become nauseated and vomit or experience diarrhea. **Stomatitis** is a common complaint and is discussed under side effects of radiation. These side effects can be controlled with medication.

HAIR. Alopecia (hair loss) is common with many drugs. This is a temporary condition, and growth of the new hair will usually start when the chemotherapy medication is stopped. Alopecia involves the entire body and includes eyebrows, eyelashes, and axillary and pubic hair. Hair regrowth may be of different color or texture than the original hair. It is not uncommon for individuals to regrow curly hair when they originally had straight hair.

---

leukopenia: leuko—white cells + penia—lack
thrombocytopenia: thrombo—clot + cyte—cell + penia—lack
anemia: an—not + emia—blood
stomatitis: stoma—mouth + itis—inflammation

REPRODUCTIVE SYSTEM. The effects of chemotherapy or radiation can cause temporary or permanent alterations of the reproductive system. Occasionally, clients are rendered sterile because of the treatment. Issues concerning fertility should be discussed with the client before treatment. Measures such as freezing ova and the use of sperm banks provide options for the client and his or her partner.

NEUROLOGICAL SYSTEM. Drugs may affect the neurological system. An adverse reaction to vincristine is neurotoxicity, which may result in tingling or numbness in the extremities and in severe cases may cause footdrop from muscle weakness.

Less common complications include renal toxicities, such as pain and burning on urination, and hematuria. Adriamycin has been associated with permanent heart damage, and bleomycin can cause pulmonary fibrosis.

Severe toxic side effects can be controlled by carefully limiting the amount of medication given and constantly monitoring the client for complications.

New Treatments Being Researched

Laetrile is a medication made from the pits of peaches or apricots. The main ingredient of this medication is cyanide. The drug is given with very strict dietary guidelines, and conditions are very difficult for the client to manage.

Hyperthermia has been used with radiation and chemotherapy. Hyperthermia has been beneficial in some types of cancer but is seldom used except in investigational studies.

Biological response modifiers (such as interferons) are drugs used to stimulate the individual's immune system. These drugs are used commonly for specific types of cancer and have produced some very beneficial results. They are also being used in many investigational studies.

Nursing Process for the Client with Cancer

ASSESSMENT

Clients are assessed for many different problems associated with cancer and its treatment. (See Nursing Care Plan Box 10–4 for the Client with Cancer.) Assessment of client knowledge concerning the disease, treatment, and expected outcomes helps the nurse provide adequate information about client rights and responsibilities. See Table 10–8 for the Cancer Survivor's Bill of Rights.

Home safety management and coping skills of the client and family are assessed. Client and caregiver strengths and weaknesses related to therapeutic care are determined.

The nurse assesses for side effects of chemotherapy or radiation, as described earlier. Infection and septicemia can occur quickly, especially when the client's white blood cell count is low. The temperature is monitored frequently for

NURSING CARE PLAN BOX 10-4 FOR THE CLIENT WITH CANCER

Risk for ineffective individual coping related to the diagnosis and treatment of cancer as evidenced by behaviors such as denial, isolation, anxiety, and depression

Outcomes
Client will cope effectively as evidenced by identifying stressors related to illness and treatment; communicating needs, concerns, and fears; and use of appropriate resources to support coping.

Evaluation of Outcomes
Is client able to identify stressors and communicate concerns? Does client have and appropriately use support systems?

Interventions	Rationale	Evaluation
Assess effective coping mechanisms used in the past and currently available to the client.	Coping mechanisms that worked in the past may be helpful again, and the nurse can support appropriate choices.	Is the client able to identify and draw on past coping mechanisms?
Use active listening skills to encourage the client to express feelings and fears.	The client must identify fears to be able to cope effectively with them.	Does the client identify fears and concerns?
Assess the meaning of quality of life to the client.	Once identified, the nurse can assist the client to achieve quality-of-life goals.	Is the client able to identify the meaning of quality of life? Are there ways the nurse can assist the client to reach quality-of-life goals?
Assess for suicide risks.	A client who feels hopeless may be at risk for suicide.	Is the client at risk? Are suicide precautions necessary?
Explore outlets that promote feelings of personal achievement.	Personal achievement promotes self-esteem.	Does the client have creative outlets that promote feelings of achievement? Can the nurse assist in implementing these activities?
Promote the use of humor.	Humor can be distracting and therapeutic.	Does the client use humor? Does it provide temporary distraction from concerns?

Pain related to tissue injury from tumor invasion or surgical intervention

Outcome
Client will be pain free as evidenced by client statement of comfort on pain scale.

Evaluation of Outcome
Does client state pain is controlled?

Interventions	Rationale	Evaluation
Ask client to rate pain on a scale from 0 to 10 (0 = absence of pain; 10 = worst pain).	A complete pain assessment should be done before and after any interventions for pain.	Does client use pain assessment scale effectively? Is client in pain?
Educate client on use of patient-controlled analgesic (PCA).	PCA allows the client to be in control of own pain relief.	Does PCA keep client pain free and able to participate in desired activities?
Monitor pain relief from PCA or epidural catheter every 2 to 4 hours.	Alternative medications may be necessary for breakthrough pain.	Is PCA or epidural analgesic effective?
Explain and encourage use of relaxation techniques.	Relaxation techniques can reduce pain intensity by reducing skeletal muscle tension.	Does client use relaxation techniques effectively?

detection of infection. The client is examined daily for signs of inflammation or purulent drainage at potential infection sites such as old aspirate sites, old and new venipuncture sites, mouth and rectal mucosa, perineal area, axilla, under breasts, between toes, incisions, and earlobes if ears are pierced. The client is monitored for signs of respiratory infection such as sore throat, cough, shortness of breath, and purulent sputum. Signs of urinary infection include burning, pain, urgency, frequency, and presence of blood or pus in the urine.

Bleeding can occur when the platelet count is low. Bleeding gums, easy bruising, tarry stools, and blood in the

Table 10-8. *Cancer Survivor's Bill of Rights*

The American Cancer Society promotes the following Survivor's Bill of Rights to promote cancer care.

1. Survivors have the right to assurance of lifelong medical care, as needed. The physicians and other professionals involved in their care should continue their constant efforts to be:
   - sensitive to the cancer survivor's lifestyle choices and need for self-esteem and dignity;
   - careful, no matter how long their patients have survived, to take symptoms seriously, and not dismiss aches and pains, for fear of recurrence is a normal part of survivorship;
   - informative and open, providing survivors with as much or as little candid medical information as they wish, and encouraging their informed participation in their own care;
   - knowledgeable about counseling resources, and willing to refer survivors and their families as appropriate for emotional support and therapy, which will improve the quality of individual lives.
2. Survivors will have the right to the pursuit of happiness. This means they have the right:
   - to talk with their families and friends about their cancer experience if they wish, but to refuse to discuss if that is their choice and not to be expected to be more upbeat or less blue than anyone else;
   - to be free of the stigma of cancer as a "dread disease" in all social relations;
   - to be free of blame for having gotten the disease and of guilt for having survived it.
3. In the workplace, survivors have the right to equal job opportunities. They have the right:
   - to apply for jobs worthy of their skills, and for which they are trained and experienced;
   - to be hired, promoted, and accepted on return to work, according to their individual abilities and qualifications, and not according to "cancer" or "disability" stereotypes;
   - to privacy about their medical histories.
4. Every effort should be made to assure all survivors adequate health insurance, whether public or private. This includes:
   - survivors have the right to be included in group coverage at the place of employment;
   - physicians, counselors, and other professionals must keep themselves and survivors informed and up to date on available group or individual health policy options;
   - social policy makers, both in government and in the private sector, must seek to broaden insurance programs like Medicare to include diagnostic procedures and treatment to help prevent recurrence and lessen survivor anxiety.

Source: From Cancer Survivor's Bill of Rights, American Cancer Society.

urine are all signs that should be reported to the physician immediately.

The client's weight is monitored, and complaints of nausea, vomiting, and diarrhea related to either the disease or treatment are noted. Clients with cancer are at risk for dehydration and wasting syndrome. Pain may also keep the client from eating.

The client's pain may be slight to severe, with both physical and emotional components. Pain assessment includes location, onset, intensity, pattern, duration, mental state, and known relief measures. This may be accomplished with the WHAT'S UP? format presented in Chapter 2. Assessment of intensity is best done by using a pain

scale, such as a 0 to 10 scale with 0 indicating no pain and 10 indicating extreme pain. The client's perceptions about pain management and the impact of pain on performance of activities of daily living are also assessed.

LEARNING TIP

When assessing clients with possible side effects of chemotherapy and radiation, use BITES:

B-Bleeding suggests low platelet count
I- Infection suggests low white blood count and risk for septicemia
T-Tiredness suggests anemia
E-Emesis places the client at risk for altered nutrition, fluid and electrolyte imbalance
S- Skin changes may be evidence of radiation reaction or skin breakdown

NURSING DIAGNOSIS

Individual diagnoses must be determined based on specific client assessment. Possible nursing diagnoses include the following:

- Pain related to disease process and cancer treatment
- Risk for infection related to diminished immunity and bone marrow suppression as a result of chemotherapy or radiation
- Risk for injury related to bleeding tendencies associated with chemotherapy and radiation
- Nutrition, altered: less than body requirements related to anorexia, nausea, or vomiting associated with disease, pain, and treatment
- Self-care deficit related to weakness and fatigue
- Anticipatory grieving related to potential disease outcome
- Risk for caregiver role strain related to client care and anticipated outcome
- Social isolation related to changing relationships
- Altered sexuality pattern related to change in body functions
- Body image disturbance related to surgical procedures such as an ostomy or loss of hair associated with chemotherapy

PLANNING AND IMPLEMENTATION

Short-term and long-term goals must be set. Short-term goals are centered around control of pain and side effects of therapy. Long-term goals are determined by the client.

Pain

Pain intervention involves a multidimensional nursing approach. Cancer pain is associated with (1) surgical interventions, postoperative recovery, and painful procedures;

(2) pressure from a large tumor mass on nerves and blood vessels; (3) psychological depression and anxiety over mortality; and (4) cultural views and perceptions concerning the cancer process.

Pain affects quality of life for the client with cancer. Chronic pain places the client at risk for depression, hopelessness, delirium, loss of control, exhaustion, and suicide. Clients need reassurance that measures will be taken to control their pain and that they will not become addicted to pain medication.

Obstacles to effective pain management include a lack of understanding about pain, inadequate pain assessment, ineffective treatment with analgesics, and fears of addiction, sedation, and respiratory depression. (See Ethical Considerations Box 10–5.)

Cancer pain is treated first with use of analgesics. The goal is effective prevention of pain, rather than treatment of pain once it occurs. Use of medications for pain is discussed in Chapter 9.

ETHICAL CONSIDERATIONS BOX 10–5

Pain Medications for the Client with Cancer

Ms. Parker, LPN, returned to work on the oncology unit after a 2-week vacation. During report, she could hear moans of pain emanating from the room of Mr. Stipe, a 32-year-old male suffering from metastatic bone cancer. She had liked Mr. Stipe when he was admitted for diagnosis and initial treatment several months ago, and now he was back to die. The metastatic growths in his spine were causing intolerable pain, while the metastatic growths in his liver were threatening death.

The goal the oncology team had established for Mr. Stipe was to keep him as pain free as possible, and correspondingly large doses of morphine sulfate had been ordered both by continuous drip and PCA pump boosters. In reviewing Mr. Stipe's chart for the last shift, Ms. Parker noted that he had received 800 mg by drip with 20 mg boosters every hour. She became very concerned that this much morphine would cause respiratory depression and arrest.

The head nurse verified the dose with Ms. Parker and also explained that Mr. Stipe had a very high tolerance to the medication due to his severe pain and long-term use of the medication for pain control. When Mr. Stipe screamed in pain again, the head nurse instructed Ms. Parker to give another 20 mg booster. "Our goal is to keep him comfortable," she said, "and the only way to do that is to give him his medication." Ms. Parker agreed that the pain must be relieved, but she felt very uncomfortable giving more medication on top of the medication he had already gotten. What if he went into respiratory arrest after the next dose of medication? Would she be responsible for his death? But was it right to let him suffer in pain so that she would not feel guilty? What should she do?

Procedures such as anesthetics or nerve blocks are used for intractable pain. Nursing responsibilities associated with these procedures include teaching the client why and how the procedure will be done, potential complications, and expected benefits from the procedure.

Noninvasive therapies may be used in addition to pain medication to increase the client's control over the pain. These may include (1) cutaneous stimulation, which eliminates or decreases pain by using massage and vibration, heat and cold, and menthol application; (2) distraction, such as music therapy or coping statements; (3) relaxation through deep breathing exercises and humor therapy; and (4) imagery.

Risk for Infection

Leukopenia occurs when the white blood cell count is decreased to 2000 (normal range is 5000/mm³ to 10,000/mm³), increasing the client's risk for infection. Clients with leukopenia must be protected against sources of infection such as persons with transmissible illnesses; bird, cat, or dog excreta; stagnant water in flower vases, denture cups, irrigating containers, respiratory equipment, or soap dishes; and fruit peelings.

Signs and symptoms of infection are reported to the physician immediately. Antibiotics and analgesics are administered as ordered. The client is advised to avoid intercourse while the white count is low, in order to prevent secondary infection.

Risk for Injury Related to Bleeding

Thrombocytopenia increases the risk for bleeding or hemorrhage. The normal platelet level is 150,000/mm³ to 300,000/mm³. Potential for bleeding exists when the platelet count is 50,000; risk for spontaneous bleeding occurs when the count is less than 20,000. Bleeding precautions are necessary when the platelet count falls below 50,000.

Bleeding precautions include monitoring platelet counts daily and observing for signs of bleeding such as bruising, petechiae, bleeding gums, tarry stools, and black emesis. Intramuscular and subcutaneous injections are avoided to prevent bleeding into the injection site. Safety measures are instituted to prevent cuts, bruises, and falls. The client is advised to use an electric razor, avoid blowing the nose, and avoid intercourse to prevent bleeding for the duration of the thrombocytopenia.

Altered Nutrition

Clients are instructed about the importance of maintaining proper nutrition. See Nutrition Notes Box 10–6 for criteria for determining whether a client needs nutritional support. The nurse consults with the dietitian and physician for dietary supplements and medications used to control nausea, vomiting, and diarrhea. The environment should be free of odors that might induce nausea, such as strong disinfec-

NUTRITION NOTES BOX 10-6

Adjunct Treatment

Any two of the following findings indicates a need for nutritional support.[16]

Weight loss of 10 percent or more of body weight
Serum albumin less than 3.4 g/dL
Serum transferrin less than 190 mg/dL

NUTRITION NOTES BOX 10-7

Interventions for Problems Related to Nutrition

Early satiety and anorexia: nutrient dense foods; appropriate exercise; attractive food presentations; small, frequent meals; home-cooked food

Bitter or metallic taste: cook in glass utensils in microwave oven; serve cold or at room temperature; eggs, fish, poultry, and dairy products preferred to beef and pork; experiment with sauces and seasonings

Local effects about the mouth:
- Ulcerations—soft, mild foods; cream sauces, gravies, dressings for lubrication; cold foods for numbing; "dunking" encouraged; soda straws for liquids; topical vitamin E oil[17]
- Dry mouth—frequent sips of water; artificial salivas; gravies, butter, margarine, milk, cream, bouillon for lubrication
- Dysphagia—make swallowing conscious act; experiment with head position; foods with smooth, even consistency; thick liquids easier to swallow than thin

Nausea, vomiting: antiemetics on regular prophylactic schedule; dry crackers; liquids between meals to reduce volume in stomach; low-fat meals to facilitate stomach emptying; thorough chewing and slow eating followed by rest period; unconventional meal schedule takes advantage of "feeling better" times; avoidance of favorite foods so will not associate with vomiting

Diarrhea: low-residue diet; lactose-free diet (for temporary intolerance); pectin-containing foods (apples, strawberries, citrus fruits) to absorb water in bowel; active cultures of yogurt to repopulate intestine

Altered immune response: restrict fresh fruits and vegetables (unable to disinfect adequately)

tants, perfumes, deodorizers, and body wastes. Intake and output are monitored every 8 hours, and the client is weighed daily. Room-temperature foods or cold foods and clear liquids may help reduce vomiting. Sour foods such as hard candy, lemon, and pickles might be helpful. Music or relaxation exercises may help distract the client from the nausea. Adding nutmeg to foods may help slow down motility of the gastrointestinal tract. Mouth care is provided before meals to make eating more pleasant. Small, high-calorie meals are better tolerated than large meals. Administration of pain medication before meals will help reduce the impact of pain on the appetite. The client is instructed to avoid fluids with meals to prevent premature feelings of fullness and to avoid exercise before meals to prevent fatigue. See Nutrition Notes Box 10–7 for additional nutrition interventions.

Self-Care Deficit

Psychosocial issues related to cancer are as varied as the persons afflicted with the disease. The nurse can help the client explore perceptions about quality of life. The nurse can help the client rank quality-of-life issues based on an understanding of the disease process, treatment, and specific limitations. Culture and age affect cancer perceptions (e.g., in a culture where life expectancy is short, possible death from cancer in the later years is not a significant threat). See Table 10–9 for findings from a research study about how clients with cancer define quality of life.

It is helpful for the client with cancer to anticipate a time when he or she will no longer be able to care for his or her own needs. The nurse can assist the client to determine resources that can be called on at that time. If the client lives with family members, they can be instructed in how to assist in daily care. Home health nurses and hospice care can also be invaluable.

Anticipatory Grieving

Cancer to many people is synonymous with death. Although some cancers are very aggressive and death occurs quickly after diagnosis, many cancers are controllable and provide clients with years of living after diagnosis and treatment. The nurse should be sure that the client has re-

ceived accurate information about the prognosis; the nurse should never give false hope. The nurse uses therapeutic communication techniques to assist the client to talk about his or her anticipated death. Family members are encouraged to spend time with the client. The nurse can contact the client's minister or clergy if the client agrees.

Risk for Caregiver Role Strain

The emotional issues of the disease can be devastating for clients, family members, and other support persons. Income is lost and lifestyles are changed when the disease affects wage-earning members of the family. When a client's caregiver works outside the home, the stress of dual responsibility takes its toll. Family growth needs are often replaced with meeting basic survival needs such as providing food, clothing, and shelter. This can create many guilt feelings for both the client and family. The nurse can help by providing information about local community resources.

Table 10–9. *Quality of Life*

Greisinger, AJ, Lorimor, RJ, Aday, LA, et al: Terminally ill cancer patients: Their most important concerns. Cancer Pract 5:3, 1997.

In this study, researchers asked clients what concerns most affected their quality of life. Clients expressed the following concerns:
- The need for a sense of hope, meaning, and purpose
- The need to find strength from spiritual beliefs and faith
- The need to feel appreciated by family, to be able to express concerns to family, and to be able to say goodbye to family
- The need for knowledge about symptoms to expect and truthful information about their prognosis

The most frequent emotional concern was feelings of restlessness.

Role changes in the family are sometimes needed and may be a difficult adjustment for the family to make. If the dominant person is the client, the less dominant partner may have to assume new responsibilities that contribute to stress. The nurse's ability to actively listen to family members' concerns is important.

Social Isolation

Isolation can be either self-imposed or imposed by friends and family as terminal illness issues are confronted. It can be very frustrating to see a loved one decline with cancer; often people say they are "afraid of saying or doing the wrong thing" so they "just stay away." Clients may engage in self-blame, and their anger may lead to depression and further isolation. It is important to recognize signs of depression and suicidal tendencies.

Altered Sexuality Patterns

Maintaining healthy sexuality is important to the cancer client. Individual sexual attitudes and practices vary, making it difficult to define what is "normal." Normal can be best described as what the client and partner consider pleasurable.

A decline in sexual desire is not uncommon when clients are undergoing cancer therapy. Anxiety about sexual intercourse includes fears concerning contracting cancer from the client and that sexual intercourse will make the cancer worse.

It is important to stress that cancer is not contagious. It cannot be passed from person to person, even through contact as close as kissing, intercourse, or oral-genital sex. Sexual activity is usually safe during and after cancer treatment. Clients who are advised to abstain from sexual intercourse because of low blood counts are temporarily at risk for secondary infections and bleeding until blood counts return to normal. They do not put their partners at risk.

Closeness and intimacy are often desired even if sexual intercourse is not.

Pain is the most common problem for both male and female clients during intercourse. Pain is associated with pelvic surgery, radiation therapy, or treatment that affects hormone levels. Pain can prevent the male client from achieving an erection. Most obstacles can be overcome if the couple are open and honest about feelings. The nurse must be prepared to address sexuality issues in a timely fashion.

Body Image Disturbance

The loss of any body part can be traumatic to a person's self-image. The nurse can provide information about plastic surgery and prosthetics and help the client through the grieving process related to the loss.

Cancer treatment is costly, and financial aid may be needed. The nurse can provide information about community assistance programs or services. Social service personnel are available in most health care facilities.

EVALUATION

If interventions have been effective, the client will describe known facts about his or her disease and prescribed treatment plan. The client will verbalize relief or a reduction in pain intensity. Pain management should provide the client with periods of rest and an ability to appropriately focus on living. The client or family will demonstrate knowledge of risk factors associated with bleeding and infection. The client remains infection free and maintains intact skin as evidenced by an absence of reddened or ulcerated areas. The client has no signs of bleeding or anemia. The client maintains optimal nutritional status, as reflected by caloric intake adequate to meet body requirements, balanced intake and output, absence of nausea and vomiting, and good skin turgor. The client feels free to share feelings about his or her disease and coping abilities and achieves or maintains control of his or her body.

 CRITICAL THINKING: Mrs. Jones

Mrs. Jones is admitted to your unit following a simple mastectomy for breast cancer. The tumor was staged as a T_2, N_0, M_0. Estrogen and progesterone receptors were negative. A bone scan was negative for metastasis.

Mrs. Jones was told she would need four chemotherapy treatments, 3 weeks apart. The medications prescribed are high doses of Adriamycin and Cytoxan. A central line is inserted for chemotherapy.

1. What does the staging of Mrs. Jones' tumor mean?
2. What major side effects of her medications should you observe for?

3. Why was a central line inserted?
4. What nursing diagnoses are appropriate for Mrs. Jones?

Answers at end of chapter.

Hospice Care of the Client with Cancer

Clients who are considered terminal and have a life expectancy of 6 months or less are eligible for hospice care. Hospice care provides humanistic care for dying people and their families. The dying person is provided care in a home or homelike setting that promotes comfort and quality of life until death. Hospice care is offered as an inpatient or outpatient service.

Inpatient services are used for symptom control and respite care for the family. Family and pets are allowed to stay with clients. Hospice care deals with the family in crisis and extends after the client dies with follow-up counseling, listening, nurturing, and referral.

Outpatient care is given in the home with family members providing the primary care. Support care is given by the hospice staff. Medication and supplies are furnished by the hospice service. The client can enjoy his or her loved ones, pets, plants, music, and other personal possessions for as long as possible.

Oncological Emergencies

SUPERIOR VENA CAVA SYNDROME

Superior vena cava syndrome occurs in clients with lung cancer, when the tumor or enlarged lymph nodes block the circulation in the vena cava. This results in edema of the head and neck and may lead to convulsions. Radiation therapy can be used to shrink the tumor and allow for circulation to resume naturally.

SPINAL CORD COMPRESSION

Spinal cord compression may develop in bone metastasis when the bones collapse and cause compression of the spinal cord. This is a very painful problem and requires pain management while radiation is given to relieve the symptoms. Clients may develop some motor loss when this occurs. Often a myelogram or bone scan is used for diagnosis.

HYPERCALCEMIA

Hypercalcemia occurs when serum calcium reaches a level greater than 11 mg/dL. In clients with cancer, hypercal-

---

HOME HEALTH HINTS

■ The home health or hospice nurse helps manage cancer pain in the home. Intramuscular dosing of pain medication should be avoided because of pain associated with injections and the burden this places on the caregiver. Oral or intravenous analgesics are preferred. For moderate to severe pain, medication dosing should be around-the-clock with prn doses for breakthrough pain. The nurse should anticipate constipation from opioid administration and treat prophylactically.

■ Home health nurses are in key positions for making timely referrals for hospice care. Eligible clients are those who have a life expectancy of 6 months or less, have a desire for supportive care rather than continued treatments, and have a friend or relative who is willing to coordinate the care.

---

cemia is associated with the release of calcium into the blood from bone deterioration. Hypercalcemia is common in clients with bone metastasis, especially breast cancer with metastasis in the bones. It can be treated with intravenous medication to lower the calcium levels.

PERICARDIAL EFFUSION/ CARDIAC TAMPONADE

This is a condition usually caused by direct invasion of the cancer, causing the pericardial sac to fill with fluid. Treatment involves draining the fluid from the heart sac by pericardiocentesis and using sclerosing agents to keep the pericardial sac from refilling with fluid.

DISSEMINATED INTRAVASCULAR COAGULATION

Disseminated intravascular coagulation (DIC) is an abnormal activation of the clot formation and fibrin mechanisms of the blood resulting in the consumption of coagulation factors and platelets. These clients are at a high risk for thrombus formation, infarctions, and bleeding. Treatment includes the administration of fresh frozen plasma and cryoprecipitates with heparin.

Review Questions

1. The hereditary material of cells is
   a. Protein in the ribosomes
   b. DNA in the chromosomes
   c. RNA in the nucleus
   d. Ribosomes in the cytoplasm

2. A mutation in a cell means that
   a. The cell membrane has been punctured
   b. The cell can no longer divide
   c. Proteins can no longer be synthesized
   d. There has been a genetic change

3. Mr. Michaels, age 56, has been recently diagnosed with prostate cancer. He asks the nurse, "How do malignant tumors differ from benign tumors?" Which of the following is the most accurate statement?
   a. Malignant tumors invade surrounding cells.
   b. Malignant tumors are encapsulated.
   c. Malignant tumors remain localized.
   d. Malignant tumors always require surgical intervention.

4. Which of the following is the most accurate definition of cancer?
   a. Cancer is a name for cells that produce toxins that destroy body organs.
   b. Cancer is a name for a large group of diseases characterized by cells that multiply rapidly and invade normal tissue.
   c. Cancer is a name for an inherited disease occurring most often in children.
   d. Cancer is a name given to a disease caused primarily from toxins in the environment and unhealthy lifestyles.

5. A client asks the meaning of alopecia. The most appropriate response is
   a. Itching of skin
   b. Frequent bowel movements
   c. Blood vessel constriction
   d. Hair loss

6. Mrs. Berstein is receiving chemotherapy treatments. She is told that her blood counts are not normal and she will not receive a treatment today. The medical term for low white blood cell count is
   a. Thrombocytopenia
   b. Leukopenia
   c. Anemia
   d. Cytonemia

7. The nurse understands that the cell cycle is important in chemotherapy because
   a. Dividing cells tend to be more vulnerable to chemotherapy
   b. Chemotherapeutic agents act on only the last phase of the cell cycle
   c. Chemotherapeutic agents are unable to destroy all cancer cells
   d. Most normal cells are not affected by chemotherapeutic agents

8. One of the best principles to follow in helping a client through his or her chemotherapy treatment regimen is
   a. Avoid discussing side effects of the drug

   b. Reassure the client that the treatment provides a cure
   c. Be consistent in giving concise, accurate information
   d. Discourage client decision making

9. Mrs. Rosse, a 45-year-old client undergoing chemotherapy, telephones the clinic to complain of a nosebleed. Her last treatment was 2 days ago. Select the most appropriate nursing diagnosis for Mrs. Rosse.
   a. Altered nutrition less than body requirements
   b. High risk for injury related to low platelet count
   c. Self-image disturbance related to effects of chemotherapy
   d. Pain related to pressure from cancerous tumor

10. Mr. West is receiving radiation therapy and notes that the skin over the treated area is slightly reddened. The best care for this area involves
   a. Applying moist normal saline compresses
   b. Lubricating the skin with water-soluble lubricant
   c. Keeping the skin clean and protected from the sun
   d. Applying a heat lamp to the area two times a day

11. Mr. Waist, age 70, admitted for diagnostic tests to confirm cancer of the colon, is restless and uncomfortable. He states that he will need a pain pill soon. Select the most appropriate nursing measure before administering pain medication.
   a. Assess anxiety level.
   b. Assess client understanding concerning the pain medication's side effects.
   c. Determine client's pain tolerance.
   d. Assess success with past pain management measures.

12. Mrs. Hossey, age 40, develops fatigue related to radiation therapy. Which of the following interventions is appropriate to help treat fatigue?
   a. Encourage mild exercise when not taking radiation treatments.
   b. Encourage her to prioritize activities around frequent rest periods.
   c. Encourage larger portions of foods rich with fat and protein.
   d. Discuss her views concerning blood transfusion.

ANSWERS TO CRITICAL THINKING:
Mrs. Jones

1. Mrs. Jones' tumor is beginning to invade surrounding tissue. There is no lymph node involvement and no metastasis.
2. Adriamycin is commonly associated with red urine. Cytoxan can cause blood in the urine. Both medications can cause nausea, vomiting, and alopecia. Both are vesicants.

3. Because the drugs are vesicants, it is important to inject them into a large vein.
4. Many diagnoses are appropriate, including acute pain related to surgical incision, body image disturbance related to loss of a breast and alopecia, altered nutrition related to nausea and vomiting, risk for injury related to side effects of medications, and knowledge deficit about cancer treatment and management of side effects.

REFERENCES

1. American Cancer Statistics. American Cancer Society, Atlanta, 1997.
2. Kneller, RW, McLaughlin, JK, Bjelke, E, et al: A cohort study of stomach cancer in a high-risk American population. Cancer (68):672, 1991.
3. Fisher, S, and Page, A: Women and preventive health care: An exploratory study of the use of Pap smears in a potentially high-risk Appalachian population. Women's Health 11(3/4):83, 1987.
4. Campinha-Bacote, J: African-Americans. In Purnell, L, and Paulanka, B (eds): Transcultural Health Care: A Culturally Competent Approach. FA Davis, Philadelphia, 1998.
5. Grossman, D: Cuban-Americans. In Purnell, L, and Paulanka, B (eds): Transcultural Health Care: A Culturally Competent Approach. FA Davis, Philadelphia, 1998.
6. Jurabe, T: Puerto Ricans. In Purnell, L, and Paulanka, B (eds): Transcultural Health Care: A Culturally Competent Approach. FA Davis, Philadelphia, 1998.
7. Purnell, L: Mexican-Americans. In Purnell, L, and Paulanka, B (eds): Transcultural Health Care: A Culturally Competent Approach. FA Davis, Philadelphia, 1998.
8. Matocha, L: Chinese-Americans. In Purnell, L, and Paulanka, B (eds): Transcultural Health Care: A Culturally Competent Approach. FA Davis, Philadelphia, 1998.
9. Sabet, L: Korean-Americans. In Purnell, L, and Paulanka, B (eds): Transcultural Health Care: A Culturally Competent Approach. FA Davis, Philadelphia, 1998.
10. Sharts-Hopko: Japanese-Americans. In Purnell, L, and Paulanka, B (eds): Transcultural Health Care: A Culturally Competent Approach. FA Davis, Philadelphia, 1998.
11. Still, O, and Hodgins, D: Najavo Indians. In Purnell, L, and Paulanka, B (eds): Transcultural Health Care: A Culturally Competent Approach. FA Davis, Philadelphia, 1998.
12. Genovese, L, and Wholihan, D: The "VANAC team": Establishing a cancer prevention team. Cancer Nurs 18(6):421, 1995.
13. Groenwald, S, Frogge, M, Goodman, M, and Yarbro, C: Cancer Nursing, ed 3. Jones & Barlett, Boston, 1993.
14. American Cancer Society: http://www.cancer.org/media/story/1may14.html. 1997.
15. American Cancer Society: http://www.cancer.org/media/story/1jun12.html. 1997.
16. Daly, HM, and Shinkwin, M: Nutrition and the cancer patient. In Holleb, AI, Fink, DJ, and Murphy GP (eds): American Cancer Society Textbook of Clinical Oncology. American Cancer Society, Atlanta, 1991.
17. Wadleigh, RD, et al: Vitamin E in the treatment of chemotherapy-induced mucositis. Am J Med 92:481, 1992.

BIBLIOGRAPHY

Campbell, M, and Pruitt, J: Radiation therapy: Protecting your patient's skin. RN 59:46, 1996.
Cancer Survivor's Bill of Rights. American Cancer Society, Atlanta, 1990.
Chapman, K: When the prognosis isn't as good. RN 57:55, 1994.
Doenges, M, and Moorhouse, M: Nurse's Pocket Guide: Nursing Diagnoses with Interventions, ed 5. FA Davis, Philadelphia, 1996.
Donegan, W: Tumor-related prognostic factors for breast cancer. CA Cancer J Clin 47:1, 1997.
Gorman, L, Sultan, D, and Raines, M: Davis's Manual of Psychosocial Nursing for General Patient Care. FA Davis, Philadelphia, 1996.
Graydon, J, Bubela, N, Irvine, D, and Vincent, L: Fatigue-reducing strategies used by patients receiving treatment for cancer. Cancer Nurs 18:23, 1995.
Greifzu, S: Chemo quick guide alkylating agents. RN 59:53, 1996.
Greifzu, S: Antimetabolites. RN 59:32, 1996.
Greifzu, S: Antitumor antibiotics. RN 59:35, 1996.
Greisinger, AJ, Lorimor, RJ, Aday, LA, et al: Terminally ill cancer patients: Their most important concerns. Cancer Pract 5:147, 1997.
Janowski, M: Managing cancer pain. RN 58:30, 1995.
Kershner, K: Comedy and cancer. Frontiers Cleveland Clinic, Cleveland, Autumn 1996.
Kornfeld, H: Co-meditation: Guiding patients through the relaxation process. RN 58:57, 1995.
Lynch, H, Fsaro, R, and Lynch, J: Hereditary Cancer in Adults. International Society for Preventive Oncology, 1995.
Miller, K: Cancer and the immune system. Cancer Biotherapeutics Newsletter 1:1, 1997.
Morton, D, and Barth, A: Vaccine therapy for malignant melanoma. CA Cancer J Clin 46:4, 1996.
Parker, S, Tong, T, Bolden, S, and Wingo, P: Cancer statistics, 1997. CA Cancer J Clin 47:1, 1997.
Rustoen, T: Hope and quality of life, two central issues for cancer patients: A theoretical analysis. Cancer Nurs 18:355, 1995.
Schweid, L, Etheredge, C, and McCullough, M: Will you recognize these oncological crises? RN 57:23, 1994.
Schmidt, C: The basics of therapeutic touch. RN 58:50, 1996.
Sommers, M, and Johnson, S: Davis's Manual of Nursing Therapeutics for Diseases and Disorders. FA Davis, Philadelphia, 1997.
Talton, C: Touch—of all kinds—is therapeutic. RN 58:61, 1995.
Thomas, C: Taber's Cyclopedic Medical Dictionary, ed 17. FA Davis, Philadelphia, 1993.
Ward, D: Secrets of the cell. Frontiers Cleveland Clinic, Cleveland, Autumn 1996.

Nursing Care of Clients Having Surgery

Linda S. Williams

Learning Objectives

Upon completion of this chapter, the student will be able to:

1. Identify the three phases of perioperative nursing.
2. Describe the role of the nurse in each perioperative phase.
3. Explain six factors influencing surgical outcomes.
4. Identify the purpose of a preoperative client assessment and data collection.
5. Describe teaching strategies to enhance learning for the elderly preoperative client.
6. Describe surgical asepsis.
7. Identify two priority nursing interventions in the postanesthesia care unit.
8. Describe nursing interventions for common postoperative client needs.
9. Explain signs and symptoms of common postoperative complications.
10. Identify ambulatory discharge criteria.
11. Explain the process for giving discharge instructions.
12. Describe the postoperative role of the home health nurse.

Key Words

adjunct (**ADD**-junkt)
anesthesia (AN-es-**THEE**-zee-uh)
anesthesiologist (an-es-**THEE**-zee-uhl-la-just)
aseptic (ah-**SEP**-tik)
atelectasis (AT-e-**LEK**-tah-sis)
debridement (day-breed-**MAHNT**)
dehiscence (dee-**HISS**-ents)
evisceration (E-**VIS**-sir-a-shun)
hematoma (HEE-muh-**TOH**-mah)
hypothermia (HIGH-poh-**THER**-mee-ah)
induction (in-**DUCK**-shun)
intraoperative (IN-trah-**AHP**-er-uh-tiv)
perioperative (PER-ee-**AHP**-er-uh-tiv)
postoperative (post-**AHP**-er-uh-tiv)

preoperative (pre-**AHP**-er-uh-tiv)
purulent (**PURE**-u-lent)
serosanguineous (SEER-oh-**SANG**-gwin-ee-us)
surgeon (**SURGE**-on)

Table 11–1. **Surgical Procedure Suffixes**

Suffix	Meaning	Word-Building Examples
-ectomy	Removal by cutting	*crani (skull) + ectomy = craniectomy*
		appen (appendix) + ectomy = appendectomy
-orrhaphy	Suture of or repair	*colo (colon) + orrhaphy = colorrhaphy*
		herni (hernia) + orrhaphy = herniorrhaphy
-oscopy	Looking into	*colon (intestine) + oscopy = colonoscopy*
		gastr (stomach) + oscopy = gastroscopy
-ostomy	Formation of a permanent artificial opening	*ureter + ostomy =ureterostomy*
		colo (colon) + ostomy = colostomy
-otomy	Incision or cutting into	*oust (bone) + otomy = osteotomy*
		thoro (thorax) + otomy = thorocotomy
-plasty	Formation or repair	*oto (ear) + plasty = otoplasty*
		mamm (breast) + plasty = mammoplasty

Surgery is the use of instruments during an operation to treat injuries, diseases, and deformities. It is usually invasive and may require an opening being made into the body for accessing the area to be treated. Physicians perform the surgical procedure, including **surgeons,** family practice physicians, or other physicians trained to do certain surgical procedures. Surgery is performed in clinics, physician's offices, ambulatory surgical centers, and hospitals. Laser and scope technology has led to the development of new procedures that offer less risk, less invasion, faster recovery, and reduced hospitalization. Today, surgery is a safe, effective treatment option due to medications such as antibiotics and anesthetics that allow a quicker recovery.

Surgical procedures are named according to the involved body organ, part, or location and a suffix that describes what is done during the procedure (Table 11–1).

Surgery Urgency Levels

Surgery is scheduled based on the urgency required for a successful outcome for the client. Emergency or immediate surgery is needed when life or limb is suddenly threatened and any delay in surgery would jeopardize the client's life or limb. Examples of the need for emergency surgery are ruptured aortic aneurysm, ruptured appendix, traumatic limb amputation, or loss of pulse due to an extremity emboli. Urgent surgery is the need for an operation within 24 to 30 hours. Examples of this are fracture repair or an infected gallbladder. An elective surgery is one that can be planned and scheduled without any immediate time constraints. Examples of this are joint replacement, hernia repair, or skin lesion removal. Optional surgery, such as cosmetic surgery, is done at the request of the client.

Purposes of Surgery

Surgery is done for several reasons. Preventive surgery removes tissue before it causes a problem as in mole or polyp removal to prevent cancer development. Diagnostic or exploratory surgery takes tissue samples for study to make a diagnosis, uses scopes to look into areas of the body, or involves an incision to open an area of the body for examination. Examples of this surgery are a biopsy or exploratory laparotomy performed with a scope or incision. Curative surgery involves the removal of diseased or abnormal tissue as in an inflamed appendix, a tumor, or a benign cyst or the repair of defects such as hernias or cleft palate. Palliative surgery is done when an underlying condition cannot be corrected but symptoms need to be alleviated. Examples of this are removal of part of a tumor that is causing pain or pressure; a rhizotomy, which cuts a nerve root to relieve pain; insertion of a gastrostomy tube (feeding tube inserted into the stomach through the abdominal wall) to provide tube feedings for a client with swallowing problems; and formation of a colostomy (opening of the colon through the abdominal wall for fecal elimination) for an incurable bowel obstruction. Cosmetic or reconstructive surgery is done to improve appearance, as in a face-lift and mammoplasty, or to correct defects, as in repair of scars.

Perioperative Phases

There are three phases in the surgical process: **preoperative, intraoperative,** and **postoperative.** These three phases are referred to collectively by the word **perioperative,** which is defined as the time surrounding and during surgery. Throughout each phase, nurses interact closely with the client, physician, and other members of the health care team to provide perioperative nursing care.

Each of the perioperative surgical phases has distinct time frames and events occurring within them. The preoperative phase begins with the decision to have surgery and ends with the transfer of the client to the operating room. The intraoperative phase begins when the client is transferred to the operating room and ends when the client is admitted to the postanesthesia care unit (PACU). The postoperative phase begins with the admission of the client to the PACU and continues until the client's recovery is completed.

Preoperative Phase

The primary role of the LPN/LVN in the preoperative phase is to assist in data collection for the plan of care development. The LPN/LVN also offers reinforcement of explanations and instructions given to the client and family by the physician and registered nurse. Another important role for the LPN/LVN is providing emotional and psychological support for clients and their families. Studies have shown that clients' families experience anxiety during the surgical procedure even if the client's surgery is elective and of short duration. Helping to reduce the family's anxiety is a major contribution that the LPN/LVN can make. When families are less anxious, they are better able to assist clients in their recovery.

Other health team members assist in preparing the client for surgery. The physician obtains a medical history, performs a physical examination, and orders diagnostic testing. Registered nurses collect a baseline preoperative assessment, provide explanations and instructions, offer clients and families emotional and psychological support to ease anxiety, develop a plan of care, and then verify the client's name, surgical site, allergies, and related information when the client arrives in the surgical waiting area.

FACTORS INFLUENCING SURGICAL OUTCOMES

When preparing a client for surgery, the goal is to identify and implement actions that reduce surgical risk factors. Preoperative care focuses on helping the client achieve the best possible surgical outcome by having the client in the best possible condition for surgery. Several factors can influence the outcome of the surgical experience and should be considered for clients being prepared for surgery.

Emotional Responses

The word *surgery* evokes some common emotional reactions in clients and their families. The nurse needs to be aware of these reactions to assist the client in coping with them. If any of the client's fears are extreme, such as a fear of dying or not awakening after surgery, the physician should be informed.

Surgical clients may experience several common fears. They may be concerned about **anesthesia** issues such as possible brain damage, feeling sensations during surgery, or experiencing a loss of control. Clients may state that they are afraid they will not wake up after anesthesia. These concerns should be discussed by the client with the **anesthesiologist** for reassurance. Listening to music or using guided imagery can help reduce clients' anxiety and calm them.

A concern of being in pain is common among most surgical clients. Clients are told that anesthesia prevents pain during the operation. After surgery, medication is available for pain relief. Other techniques can also help reduce pain, such as guided imagery or focused breathing (see Chapter 4).

Concerns about disfigurement or mutilation may occur in some clients. The thought of bleeding or having a scar causes great anxiety for some individuals. The nurse should understand that alteration of body image may be a great fear for some clients.

Every surgery carries some risk, so a fear of death can occur in any surgical client. Allowing the client to express this concern is an important role of the nurse. The nurse understands the client has been prepared to be in the best possible condition for surgery. Therefore individualized, realistic reassurance is offered to the client based on this.

Age

Surgery can be a positive experience that promotes quality of life for many elderly clients. For healthy older clients, age alone does not mean that they are a greater surgical risk. Complications can occur, however, related to previous health status, immobilization occurring from surgery, normal aging changes reducing the effectiveness of deep breathing and coughing, and the effects of administered medications (Gerontological Issues Box 11–1). Older clients may take longer to recover from anesthetic agents because of changes in drug metabolism and elimination. To reduce complications the elderly client's health problems need to be under control, and the client should be well nourished and hydrated at the time of surgery.

Hydration

Body fluids and electrolytes need to be adequate to decrease complications. Preoperative screening may include assessment of fluid and electrolyte status. Then, if abnormalities are detected, treatment can be ordered. For example, a client on furosemide (Lasix) is at risk for cardiac dysrhythmias if potassium levels are abnormal, so a potassium level is usually drawn preoperatively. If the potassium level is found to be low, a potassium supplement can then be ordered by the physician to correct the abnormality before surgery.

GERONTOLOGICAL ISSUES BOX 11-1

Reducing Postoperative Complications for the Elderly

Pain Control

Provide adequate pain relief so that required postoperative activities such as deep breathing, coughing, position changes, and exercise can be performed more effectively.

Respiratory Function

Reduce respiratory complications by encouraging deep breathing and coughing:

- Time deep breathing exercises and coughing after pain medication has begun to take effect because this will increase the older client's ability to take deeper breaths.
- Use a pillow and instruct the patient to hold it firmly over abdominal or chest incisions to support the incision. Taking a deep breath increases chest expansion along with increasing abdominal pressure, which may pull or stretch an incision.
- Elderly clients perform deep breathing and coughing exercises better if the nurse performs the exercises with them. For example, say the following: "Let's take a deep breath in through the nose, hold it and count to three, then slowly blow it out completely through the mouth. When you blow the air out, shape your lips like they are going to whistle. Great, let's do it again."

Mobility

- Use pillows to support the client's body alignment, assist the patient to ambulate as soon as possible after surgery, and regularly help the client with passive or active range of motion along with flexion and extension exercises for legs and feet.

- Deep vein thrombosis is a risk related to venous pooling in the lower extremities. This risk is increased with postoperative inactivity.
- If clients lie in one position too long, pressure ulcers can develop. When tissues are compressed between bones and the bed surface, blood supply is reduced to the tissue and cells begin to die. This results in painful open wounds.

Bowel Function

- Assess bowel sounds. It is common for clients to feel bloated after surgery. Increasing activity, such as walking (not just sitting in a chair), stimulates peristaltic action of the bowel. This helps expel flatus and reduce discomfort.

Urinary Function

- It is common for individuals to have difficulty emptying their bladder after surgery. Clients who are sleeping but restless should be evaluated for bladder distention. Many people have difficulty voiding on a bedpan or in a urinal in a supine position.
- Older men with an enlarged prostate may have even greater difficulty voiding if they have received medications that have urinary retention side effects.
- Assisting clients to sit or stand to use urinals, use a bedside commode, or ambulate to the bathroom promotes bladder emptying and helps avoid the use of urinary catheters.
- Measure urine output that is voided or from a catheter. Note the color and odor of the urine. The elderly are prone to dehydration, and this provides an indication of their hydration status for intervention.

Nutrition

To adequately heal and recover from surgery, clients need to be well nourished. Higher levels of protein are required to promote tissue repair and healing. Obese or underweight clients may not heal as well and may experience complications. Obese clients have more respiratory problems and wound healing difficulties, such as delayed healing and wound **dehiscence** (opening of the incision). Emaciated individuals may have more infections and delayed wound healing from the lack of nutrients needed for tissue healing. Identifying clients at risk and providing preoperative intervention reduce the risk of surgery for these clients (Nutrition Notes Box 11–2).

Smoking and Alcohol

The use of tobacco and alcohol can increase the surgical client's risks. Smoking thickens and increases the amount of lung secretions and reduces the action of cilia that remove the secretions. Clients should be encouraged to avoid smoking for 24 hours before surgery or as recommended by their physician. This increases the action of the lungs' defense mechanisms. It also reduces elevated carboxyhemoglobin levels so more hemoglobin is available to carry oxygen during surgery.

Long-term alcohol use may cause the client to have nutritional deficiencies and liver damage, which can create bleeding problems, fluid volume imbalances, and drug metabolism alterations. In addition, alcohol can interact with medications. The client should avoid it before surgery.

Diseases and Medications

Chronic disorders may increase the client's surgical risk unless they are well controlled. A preoperative assessment and clearance for surgery by the client's family physician or internist may be needed. Certain diseases require special monitoring or intervention to prevent complications. For example, the stress of surgery can alter the blood glucose levels of diabetics, so they need careful monitoring.

NUTRITION NOTES BOX 11-2

Nourishing the Surgical Client

Healing requires increased vitamin C for collagen formation, vitamin K for blood clotting, and zinc for tissue growth, skin integrity, and cell-mediated immunity. Protein is essential for controlling fluid balance and manufacturing antibodies and white blood cells. Hypoalbuminemia (low serum albumin) impedes the return of interstitial fluid to the venous return system, increasing the risk of shock. Local edema, which accompanies any trauma, even a clean surgical incision, impedes circulation and healing. A serum albumin level, then, becomes a useful, and readily available, measure of protein status.

Before elective surgery, the client may have time to correct some nutritional deficiencies. Many clients are instructed to lose weight to reduce the risk of surgery. If they are anemic, an iron preparation can be administered. At least 2 to 3 weeks are required for objective evidence of the effectiveness of nutritional therapy. In clients identified as high risk, 7 days of preoperative total parenteral nutrition produced a sixfold reduction in major sepsis.[1] Before surgery on the gastrointestinal tract, a low-residue diet may be given for 2 to 3 days to minimize the feces in the bowel.

Clients with chronic lung disorders are at greater risk for pulmonary complications from anesthesia. To prepare for surgery, they should deep breathe and cough and use an incentive spirometer (Fig. 11–1). They should also be encouraged to stop smoking 3 to 4 weeks before surgery.[1]

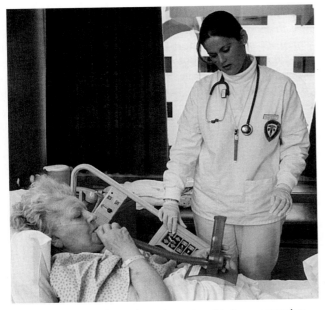

Figure 11–1. An incentive spirometer aids lung expansion.

PREOPERATIVE CLIENT ASSESSMENT

Surgical clients are usually assessed before admission to a surgical facility or hospital. The department that does this screening may be referred to as the preadmission testing (PAT) department. The client is assessed in PAT by nurses and members of the anesthesia department to obtain a health history, identify risk factors, begin client and family teaching, and make necessary referrals to social work, support groups, and educational programs, such as a total joint education program for clients undergoing a total joint replacement. Laboratory tests, electrocardiograms (ECGs), chest x-rays, and other diagnostic testing is done based on the client's individualized needs. A urine or serum pregnancy test for female clients who have begun menstruating but have not yet gone through menopause (ending of menses) and have not had a tubal ligation (tying off of fallopian tubes) or hysterectomy (removal of the uterus) is often done to prevent fetal exposure to anesthetics. Because health information is collected and diagnostic testing is done before surgery, results can be reviewed and interventions ordered for detected abnormalities to place the client in the best possible condition for surgery. The client's health history information is also used to plan preoperative, intraoperative, and postoperative care.

Before having surgery, clients are required by law to be asked if they have signed an advance directive, which indicates their wishes for medical care if they become unable to speak for themselves. If they do not have one, information about advance directives must be offered to them. A health care durable power of attorney and a living will are examples of advance directives. A power of attorney allows clients to place someone of their own choosing, such as a relative or friend, in control of their medical decisions if they are unable to make them. A living will instructs the physician when to provide, withhold, or withdraw treatment that prolongs life and specifies types of treatment the client wishes, such as comfort care only. If clients have an advance directive it is placed in their medical record.

PREOPERATIVE CLIENT ADMISSION

On admission for surgery, the nurse completes a health assessment. Subjective and objective data are collected (Table 11–2). During the interview, the client's emotional reaction to the surgery is assessed. If the client is anxious, the nurse should explore the cause of the anxiety and allow the client to express any concerns. Past experiences of clients or their significant others can influence clients' perception of the surgical experience and their emotional status. The client's usual coping techniques should also be assessed.

Subjective Data

Functional status information, such as marital status, family roles, occupation, diet, elimination patterns, rest pat-

Table 11–2. **Nursing Assessment of the Preoperative Client**

Subjective Data: Health History Questions

Demographic information: Name, age, marital status, occupation, roles?
History of condition for which surgery is scheduled: Why are you having surgery?
Past medical history: Any allergies, acute or chronic conditions, current medications, pain, or prior hospitalizations?
Past surgical history: Any reactions or problems with anesthesia? Previous surgeries?
Tobacco use: How much do you smoke? Pack-year history? (Number of packs per day × number of years.)
Alcohol use: How often do you drink alcohol? How much?
Coping techniques: How do you usually cope with stressful situations? Support systems?
Family history: Hereditary conditions—diabetes, cardiovascular, anesthesia problems?
Female clients: Date of last menses and obstetrical information?

Objective Data: Body System Review

Vital signs, oxygen saturation
Height and weight
Emotional status—calm, anxious, tearful, affect
Nervous system—ability to follow instructions
Skin—color, warmth, bruises, lesions, turgor, dryness, mucous membranes
Respiratory—infection; cough; breath sounds; chronic obstructive pulmonary disease; respiratory rate, pattern, and effort; barrel chest
Cardiovascular—angina, myocardial infarction, heart failure, hypertension, valvular heart disease, mitral valve prolapse, heart rate and rhythm, peripheral pulses, edema, neck vein distention
Abdomen—bowel sounds, distention
Musculoskeletal—deformities, weakness, decreased range of motion, crepitation, pain

---

terns, tobacco use, and alcohol intake, is obtained by the nurse. Dentures, bridges, capped teeth, and loose teeth need to be documented because they can become dislodged during intubation (insertion of endotracheal breathing tube) for general anesthesia. The reason for surgery and the client's perception of this reason is explored. Past medical and surgical information is obtained. Past health data include allergies, acute and chronic conditions, and a detailed list of all medications the client is taking. If clients have rheumatic, congenital, or cardiac valvular heart disease, such as mitral valve prolapse, prophylactic antibiotics may be ordered before surgery to prevent endocarditis. The nurse should ensure that this cardiac history is reported to the physician. For female clients, obstetrical information and the dates of their last menstrual period are recorded.

A family health history is also taken to identify possible conditions that could have an influence on the client. Conditions such as diabetes and heart disease are important to note because they can be hereditary. It is especially important to ask if there have been any family problems with anesthesia. A hereditary muscle disease known as malignant hyperthermia occurs in families and can predispose the client to a serious life-threatening reaction to certain anesthetic agents.

A surgical history is also documented. Information included in this history includes previous surgeries, malignant hyperthermia, or other problems with anesthesia. All surgeries are recorded. Some clients may consider removal of tonsils or an appendix to be minor surgery and fail to mention them. The nurse may need to prompt clients to obtain this information.

Medications

All medications that clients are taking must be reviewed. Alterations in dosages and routes of administration may be required. For example, clients taking an anticoagulant such as Coumadin may be told by their physician to decrease or stop it several days before surgery to avoid bleeding problems during surgery. The nurse should ensure that the client clearly understands these instructions.

Diabetic clients on insulin may be told by their physician to modify their dose on the day of surgery. The client may be told to take either no insulin, their normal dose of insulin, or half of their normal dose. The client should clearly understand these instructions. Blood glucose monitoring is ordered to ensure that blood glucose levels are maintained within a desired range.

Clients on chronic oral steroid therapy cannot stop their medication abruptly if they are told to take nothing by mouth (NPO) before or after surgery. Surgery is a great stressor for the body. Higher steroid levels are needed during this time to deal with the stress. The physician should order oral steroid therapy to be given by a parenteral route if the client is NPO so that it can be continued uninterrupted. Serious complications, including circulatory collapse, can develop if steroids are stopped abruptly. The nurse should ensure that the therapy is ordered and continued for the client via an alternate route.

Clients should be asked about the use of drugs such as cocaine, marijuana, or opioids because these drugs can interact with anesthesia or other medications. To obtain accurate information, clients should be told of this potential interaction. Information and questions should be stated in a nonjudgmental manner by the nurse. For example, the nurse should ask "How much alcohol do you drink daily or weekly?" instead of "Do you drink alcohol?" The first statement assumes that people drink alcohol. This allows the client who does not drink to indicate none and the client who does to state an amount rather than having to say yes and then give an amount on further questioning. This approach generates more accurate responses because it is viewed more positively by the client who consumes alcohol. Another example would be to ask the client "What roles do drugs or alcohol play in your life?"

Objective Data

A physical assessment of body systems is performed. This information can highlight risk factors for surgery, determine the type of anesthesia to be used, and assist in planning interventions to reduce risk factors. Baseline vital signs and height and weight are obtained. Vital signs may be elevated due to anxiety. If an elevated blood pressure or pulse is obtained an additional measurement should be taken at a later time when the client is at ease. A cough, cold, or fever is reported to the physician because surgery may be delayed until the client recovers from an acute infection.

Skin Assessment

The skin is observed for color, bruises, and open areas. It is palpated to check turgor, warmth, and dryness. Mucous membranes are inspected for color and moistness. This assessment is especially important in elderly clients, who are at greater risk for hydration problems.

Sensory Assessment

The client's ability to see and hear are assessed. The use of any assistive devices such as contact lenses, glasses, or hearing aids is documented. It is important for the client to have access to these devices whenever explanations or instructions are given to ensure effective communication.

Nervous System Assessment

Assessing a client's ability to understand and follow directions is important because preoperative instructions such as being NPO after a specified time are given. These instructions must be followed to avoid the delaying of surgery. If cognitive impairments are found, the physician should be informed. A family member may need to be included in teaching sessions to assist the client in following instructions.

Respiratory Assessment

The client's respiratory rate, pattern, and breathing effort should be noted. An oxygen saturation is obtained using an electronic oximeter attached to either the finger, nose, or ear that measures the oxygen saturation of the blood flowing past the sensor. The thorax is inspected for use of accessory muscles. The presence of a barrel chest, which is an increase in the anteroposterior diameter of the chest that makes it look like the shape of a barrel, is noted. Clients who develop barrel chests usually have chronic obstructive lung disease and may be at greater risk for lung problems. Breath sounds are auscultated, and abnormalities are documented and reported to the physician. Pulmonary function tests or arterial blood gases may be done based on the client's history of lung disease and assessment findings such as shortness of breath, inability to tolerate activity without dyspnea (feeling out of breath and laboring to breathe), or abnormal breath sounds such as crackles or wheezes. Crackles are produced by air flowing over secretions or the snapping open of collapsed airways. They sound like the crackling of Velcro being opened and can be fine (soft, short, high pitched) or coarse (loud, long, low pitched). Wheezes are a continuous musical sound caused by airway narrowing.

Cardiovascular Assessment

The apical heart rate and rhythm are auscultated by the nurse. Pulses are palpated. Any edema or neck vein distention is noted and documented.

Musculoskeletal Assessment

The client's gait and mobility are observed. The range of motion of joints and muscular strength are noted. Any deficits or pain is recorded. The joints are inspected and palpated for warmth, redness, swelling, or crepitation (grating with movement). Artificial limbs or prostheses are documented. Positioning in surgery may be affected by any abnormal findings.

Abdominal Assessment

The abdomen is inspected for distention and firmness. Bowel sounds are auscultated. The client's normal elimination pattern obtained during the history is compared with physical assessment findings.

Diagnostic Testing

Client preoperative diagnostic testing is based on the client's age, history, and assessment findings. Institutional protocols for clients of specified age ranges or with certain conditions may guide testing (Table 11–3). Abnormal findings are reported to the physician.

NURSING PROCESS FOR PREOPERATIVE CLIENTS

Nursing Assessment

Data gathered during the nursing assessment are used to make nursing diagnoses to plan care for the surgical client.

Nursing Diagnosis

Common preoperative nursing diagnoses may include but are not limited to the following:

- Anxiety related to potential change in body image, hospitalization, pain, loss of control, and uncertainties surrounding surgery
- Fear related to expectation of pain and surgical risk factors
- Knowledge deficit related to lack of information about surgical routines and procedures

Planning

The client's goals are to have (1) decreased anxiety, (2) reduced fear, and (3) increased knowledge of surgical routines and procedures.

Nursing Interventions

Anxiety

Anxiety is a common reaction to surgery for most clients. Anxiety is a feeling of apprehension or uneasiness from a source that may be unknown. Uncertainties and risks are associated with surgery, so it is natural for anxiety to be felt by clients. Clients should be allowed to express their concerns. Understanding the cause of the anxiety helps the nurse provide interventions to decrease it. Anxiety can be reduced by informing clients about procedures and surgical routines. If the client expresses extreme anxiety, the physician is informed.

Fear

Fear, a feeling of dread from a source known to the client, is an extreme reaction to surgery. Explanations and reassurances about a client's concerns may help reduce fear. However, if fear continues, the physician should be notified because it can result in complication development or even death. When fear is excessive, the physician may reschedule the surgery until the client is better able to cope with it.

Knowledge Deficit

Knowledge deficits occur from a lack of information and experience with surgery. Explanations about procedures and common surgical routines are given. Providing this information to clients decreases their anxiety, promotes informed choice, and increases their self-care abilities. Teaching is caring in action. It is done in preadmission test-

Table 11–3. **Preoperative Diagnostic Tests**

Diagnostic Test	Purpose
Chest x-ray	Detect pulmonary and cardiac abnormalities
Oxygen saturation	Obtain baseline level and detect abnormality
Serum Tests	
Arterial blood gases	Obtain baseline levels and detect pH and oxygenation abnormalities
Bleeding time	Detect prolonged bleeding problem
Blood urea nitrogen	Detect kidney problem
Creatinine	Detect kidney problem
Complete blood count	Detect anemia, infection, clotting problem
Electrolytes	Detect potassium, sodium, chloride imbalances
Fasting blood glucose	Detect abnormalities, monitor diabetes control
Pregnancy	Detect early, unknown pregnancy
Partial thromboplastin time	Detect clotting problem
Prothrombin time, INR	Detect clotting problem, monitor Coumadin therapy
Type and crossmatch	Identify blood type to match blood for possible transfusion
Urine Tests	
Pregnancy	Detect early, unknown pregnancy
Urinalysis	Detect infection, abnormalities

ing, by telephone for outpatient surgery, or on admission for clients admitted the night before surgery.

Teaching sessions should include the client, family members, or others who are assisting the client through the surgical experience. Client anxiety levels should be considered in planning teaching sessions because learning can be affected by high anxiety levels. Knowledge deficits should be identified by both the nurse and client. If clients do not understand that there is a deficit they are not motivated to learn. A variety of teaching methods, such as discussion, written materials and instructions, models, and videos, should be used to allow for different learning styles. Several of these methods should be used in each teaching session to reinforce learning. The depth of the explanations should be individualized so that the client is given enough information without being overwhelmed. All teaching and client understanding is documented.

When teaching elderly clients, it is important to use teaching methods that provide adaptation for aging changes that may affect learning. Gerontological Issues Box 11–3 describes considerations to provide a positive learning experience for the elderly client.

PREOPERATIVE ROUTINES. Preoperative teaching provides information about common surgical preparation procedures and routines:

- Date and time of admission and surgery
- Admission procedures
- Length of stay, items to bring and wear
- Time frames for surgery and recovery
- Family information: where to wait during surgery and who communicates client's status to them
- Discharge criteria

When the client is admitted the same day of surgery arrival time is usually 2 hours before surgery to allow preparation time. If outpatient surgery is being done, a responsible adult must take the client home. When postoperative admission to a specialized area such as a surgical intensive care unit is likely, an explanation about that unit and its routines should be given. Sharing this information preoperatively prevents the family from automatically worrying that there are complications when the client is admitted to an intensive care unit.

PREOPERATIVE INSTRUCTIONS. To reduce the risk of aspiration when anesthesia is started, as well as postoperative nausea and vomiting, the client is told when to stop fluid and food intake (NPO). Clients may brush their teeth if no water is swallowed. The anesthesiologist orders fluid and food restrictions. Typically, the client is made NPO after midnight the night before surgery. If surgery is scheduled for the afternoon, clear liquids in the early morning may be allowed by the anesthesiologist. Cancellation of surgery may result if the client has not been NPO as ordered.

Any medications the client is to take the morning of surgery, with just an ounce or two of water, are explained. A special preparation such as an enema is also described. For

---

GERONTOLOGICAL ISSUES BOX 11–3

Considerations for Elderly Client Teaching Session

Environmental Considerations

Comfortable—anxiety free, quiet, appropriate temperature
Lighting—small, intense, nonglare, soft white light, not fluorescent
Privacy—no distractions, no background noise

Presentation Considerations

Based on assessment data and current knowledge base
Use preferred learning style, using understandable words
Use legible audiovisual materials: large print, black print on white nonglare paper
If use colors—red, orange, yellow best; blue, violet, and green poorest
Ongoing assessment of energy level of client
Answer questions as they occur

Presenter Considerations

Positive attitude and belief in self-care promotion for elderly
Earn trust by being viewed as credible, positive role model
Professional appearance
Use knowledge of aging changes in presentation:
  Speaks slowly in low tone
  Seated near client for best visibility
  Ensures prostheses in place: glasses, hearing aids
  Allows client increased response time, uses memory aids
Uses touch appropriately to convey caring

---

abdominal or intestinal surgery, enemas are ordered to empty the bowel in order to reduce fecal contamination preoperatively and straining or distention postoperatively.

Instructions for postoperative care are given before surgery so the client is alert when being taught and has time to learn. Clients should be told that active participation in postoperative care aids in their recovery. They are instructed to inform the nurse of their pain level using a pain rating scale (such as a 1 [low] to 10 [severe] rating, colors, or pictures of faces showing varying degrees of frowning or smiling that indicate a certain pain level) so that prompt pain relief can be provided. Pain relief methods are described, such as analgesic injections or an epidural catheter. If patient-controlled analgesia (PCA) is ordered for pain control, the client is shown the PCA pump and taught how to use it. Clients are also told that the PCA pump has safety lockouts to prevent overdose and that the nurse monitors the client's vital signs, sedation level, and pain level frequently. Anticipated dressings, tubes, casts, or special equipment such as a continuous passive motion machine for total knee replacement is also described. If needed, crutches are fitted to the client, and their proper use is explained and demonstrated.

Postoperative exercises are taught to decrease complications. They include deep breathing and coughing, use of incentive spirometry, leg exercises, turning, and how to get out of bed. After an exercise is taught the client should perform a return demonstration so the nurse can evaluate understanding and ability to perform the exercise correctly.

Deep breathing helps prevent the development of **atelectasis** (collapse of the lung due to hypoventilation or mucus obstruction that prevents some alveoli from opening and being fully ventilated) by expanding and ventilating the lungs. The client is taught to sit up, exhale fully, take in a deep breath through the nose, hold breath and count to three, and then exhale completely through the mouth. The client is told to repeat this hourly while awake, in sets of five, for 24 to 48 hours postoperatively.

Incentive spirometry may also be ordered postoperatively to prevent atelectasis by increasing lung volume, alveoli expansion, and venous return. Any client can benefit from incentive spirometry, especially those at increased risk for developing lung complications and the elderly. The spirometer sits at the client's bedside for hourly use while awake except around mealtimes. The nurse should offer the spirometer to the client each hour to help ensure that it is used. Teach clients to do the following:

- Sit upright, at 45 degrees minimum, if possible.
- Take two normal breaths. Place mouthpiece of spirometer in mouth.
- Inhale until target, designated by spirometer light or rising ball, is reached and hold breath for 3 to 5 seconds. (See Fig. 11–1.)
- Exhale completely.
- Perform 10 sets of breaths each hour.

Coughing aids clients in moving secretions to prevent pneumonia, so clients are taught how to cough effectively (Table 11–4). Pain medication and reassurance that coughing should not open the incision are given before coughing. Several sets of coughing are performed every 1 to 2 hours while the client is awake.

Leg exercises, if not contraindicated, improve circulation and help prevent complications related to stasis of blood such as emboli formation. Clients are told to lie down, raise the leg, bend it at the knee, flex the foot, extend the leg, and lower it to the bed. Each leg is exercised in sets of five. Foot exercises include flexion and extension of the foot, making circles with the foot, and wiggling the toes. These exercises should be done hourly while awake.

Clients are taught that turning from side to side in bed is aided by bending the leg that is to be on top and placing a pillow between the legs to support the top leg. Clients are told, unless contraindicated, to use the bed rail to pull themselves over to the side. They are encouraged to deep breathe instead of holding their breath while turning to promote comfort.

Table 11–4. *Teaching Clients Coughing Technique*

Procedure	Rationale
Have client sit up and forward.	Promotes lung expansion and ability to generate forceful cough
Show client how to splint incision with hands, pillow, or blanket.	Reduces incision pressure so it does not feel as if incision is opening
Have client inhale and exhale deeply three times through mouth.	Helps expand lungs
Take in deep breath and cough out the breath forcefully with three short coughs using diaphragmatic muscles. Take in quick deep breath through mouth, cough deeply, and deep breathe.	Generates forceful cough and expands lungs to help move secretions

To reduce the strain on the incision and make it easier for clients to get out of bed, clients are instructed to turn to their side, without pillows between their knees. Then they should place their hands flat against the bed and push up while swinging their legs out of bed and into a sitting position. Clients should be told to sit for a few minutes after changing position to avoid dizziness and falling and to deep breathe while sitting up.

Evaluation

- The goal for anxiety is achieved if the client states and demonstrates that anxiety is decreased. If the client is able to learn during teaching sessions, anxiety is not a barrier to learning.
- The goal for fear is accomplished if the client verbalizes fears or states that fear is decreased or gone.
- The goal for knowledge deficit is reached if the client states understanding of the information and accurately performs return demonstrations.

PREOPERATIVE CONSENT

Before performing surgery, it is the physician's responsibility to obtain voluntary, written, informed consent from the client. The consent gives legal permission for the surgery and has two purposes. It protects the client from unauthorized procedures, and it protects the physician, anesthesiologist, hospital, and hospital employees from claims of performing unauthorized procedures.

Informed consent involves three elements: (1) The physician must tell the client in understandable terms about the diagnosis, the proposed treatment and who will perform it, the likely outcome, possible risks and compli-

atelectasis: ateles—imperfect + ektasis—expansion

cations of treatment, alternative treatments, and the prognosis without treatment. If the client has questions before signing the consent, the physician must be contacted to provide further explanation to the client. It is not within the nurse's scope of practice to provide this information. (2) The consent must be signed before analgesics or sedatives are given because clients must demonstrate that they are informed and understand the surgery. (3) Consent must be given voluntarily. No persuasion or threats can be used to influence the client. The client can withdraw consent at any time even after the consent form has been signed.

It is often the nurse's role to obtain and witness the client's or authorized person's signature on the consent form. The nurse should ensure that the person signing the consent form understands its meaning and that it is being signed voluntarily. If the client is unable to read, the entire consent must be read to the client before it is signed. Clients are unable to give consent if they are unconscious, are mentally incompetent, are minors, or have received analgesics or drugs that alter central nervous system function within time frames specified by agency policy. Consent can be obtained in any of these cases from parents, next of kin, or legal guardians.

In a medical emergency, the client may not be able to give consent. In this case, the next of kin or legal guardian may give telephone consent, or a court order can be obtained. If time does not permit this, the physician documents the need for treatment in the chart as necessary to save the client's life or avoid serious harm according to state law and institutional policy.

LEARNING TIP

Witnessing a Consent
1. As the client's advocate the nurse should ensure, before the consent is signed, that the client is informed about the surgery and has no further questions for the physician.
2. If the client does have questions, the consent should not be signed and the physician should be contacted to answer the client's questions.
3. A nurse's signature as a witness on a consent form indicates that the nurse observed the informed client or client's authorized representative voluntarily sign the consent form. It does *not* mean that the nurse informed the client about the surgical procedure, because that is the responsibility of the physician.

PREPARATION FOR SURGERY

Preoperative Checklist

A preoperative checklist is completed and signed by the nurse (per agency policy) before the client is transported from the unit to surgery (Fig. 11–2). The checklist guides the nurse in areas of preoperative preparation for the client:

- An identification band is placed on the client. A hospital gown is given to the client to wear. Underwear may need to be removed, depending on the type of surgery.
- Vital signs are taken and recorded as baseline information and to assess client status.
- Makeup, nail polish, and one artificial nail are removed to allow assessment of natural color and pulse oximetry for oxygenation status during surgery.
- Removal of hair pins, wigs, and jewelry prevents loss or injury. Rings are taped in place if the client does not want to take them off. However, rings on the operative side must be removed in case edema occurs.
- Dentures, contact lenses, and prostheses are removed to prevent injury. Some clients are concerned about body image and do not want family members to see them without dentures or makeup. Interventions to meet this client need should be considered, such as removing dentures after the family goes to the waiting room and inserting them before the family sees the client postoperatively.
- Glasses and hearing aids should go with clients to surgery if they are unable to communicate without them. They should be labeled with the client's name and their disposition documented.
- All orders, diagnostic test results, consents, and history and physical, which is required to be on the chart, are reviewed for completion and documented on the checklist by the nurse.
- Client valuables are recorded and given to a family member or locked up per institutional policy by the nurse.
- Antiembolism devices are applied, if ordered.
- Clients are asked to void before preoperative medications are given, unless a urinary catheter is present, to prevent injury to the bladder during surgery.

Preoperative Medications

The final preparation before surgery is the administration of preoperative medications.

- Meperidine (Demerol), morphine sulfate, and fentanyl (Sublimaze) are narcotics that provide analgesia and enhance postoperative pain relief.
- Diazepam (Valium), midazolam (Versed), and hydroxyzine hydrochloride (Vistaril) are given for sedation and anxiety reduction.
- Secretions are reduced with anticholinergics, either atropine sulfate or glycopyrrolate (Robinul).
- Antiemetics such as droperidol (Inapsine), ondansetron (Zofran), and metoclopramide (Reglan) control nausea and vomiting and may be effective into the postoperative period.
- Cimetidine (Tagamet) and ranitidine (Zantac) are ordered by anesthesiologists to reduce acidic gastric se-

Pre-op Surgical Checklist   **Client Name**

_____   I.D. BAND ON

_____   NPO AS ORDERED   _____

_____   PRE-OP TEACHING COMPLETED

_____   INFORMED CONSENT SIGNED

_____   HISTORY AND PHYSICAL ON CHART

_____   ALLERGIES

_____   LAB RESULTS

_____   CBC: HGB _____ HCT _____ WBC _____ PLATELETS _____

_____   POTASSIUM _____

_____   URINALYSIS _____

_____   PREGNANCY TEST   SERUM _____ URINE _____

_____   PT _____ PTT _____ BLEEDING TIME _____

_____   TYPE AND SCREEN _____ CROSSMATCH _____-___ UNITS

_____   ECG ON CHART

_____   CHEST X-RAY REPORT ON CHART

_____   SHOWERED/BATHED

_____   HOSPITAL GOWN ON

_____   PREPS COMPLETED AS ORDERED

_____   ANTIEMBOLISM STOCKINGS

_____   JEWELRY TAPED/REMOVED: DISPOSITION _____

_____   VALUABLES: DISPOSITION _____

_____   DENTURES, PROSTHESIS REMOVED

_____   HAIR PINS, WIGS, MAKE UP, NAIL POLISH, ONE ACRYLIC NAIL REMOVED

_____   CONTACT LENSES REMOVED

_____   VOIDED

_____   VITAL SIGNS: T _____ P _____ R _____ BP _____

_____   PRE-OP MEDICATIONS GIVEN _____ SIDE RAILS UP _____

_____   IV STARTED _____

_____   EYE GLASSES AND HEARING AID(S) TO OR

_____   OLD CHART TO OR

_____   X-RAYS TO OR

_____   FAMILY LOCATION _____

_____   NEXT OF KIN _____

CLIENT READY FOR SURGERY _____

     TIME _____   (NURSE SIGNATURE)

COMMENTS:

Figure 11–2. Sample preoperative checklist form.

cretions in case aspiration occurs either silently or with vomiting. When acid secretions are aspirated, clients can have an asthmalike attack; develop pneumonitis, pulmonary edema, and severe hypoxia; and require intensive treatment.

Intravenous (IV) antibiotics are given prophylactically to prevent postoperative infection. Research shows that they are most effective if they are given before surgery for surgery lasting less than 3 hours.[3,4] For surgery longer than 3 hours an extended half-life antibiotic or a second dose of the antibiotic should be given. Additional research has shown that preoperative antibiotics are most effective in preventing postoperative wound infections if they are given so that their peak effect occurs when the surgical wound is open.[4] This means that the ideal time to administer the antibiotic is close to the time anesthesia begins. This is more likely to occur if the anesthesia department is responsible for administering the preoperative antibiotics rather than the unit or holding room nurse. If surgery is delayed and preoperative antibiotics have been ordered, an order to reschedule the antibiotics should be obtained.

Preoperative medications may be ordered at a specific time or on call to surgery. This means that when the nurse is notified that surgery is ready for the client the medication is to be given. All medications administered are documented. The bed rails should be raised for safety and the client instructed not to get up after medications are given.

TRANSFER TO SURGERY

When surgery calls for the client, the client is assisted by the transporter into a wheelchair or onto a cart whose side rails are then raised. The client's chart goes to surgery with the client. If clients have asthma, their inhaler medications are usually ordered to be sent to surgery with them. The nurse should ensure that clients, especially the elderly, have their glasses or hearing aids to enable them to communicate in the holding area. The client is then transported to the surgical holding area, accompanied by family members (Fig. 11–3). A family member may be allowed to wait with the client in the holding area until the client goes into the operating room. When the client is transferred to the operating table the next phase of the perioperative period, the intraoperative phase, begins.

The transporter shows the accompanying family where they can wait during surgery. This family waiting area is a communication center that keeps the family informed on the client's status. It allows the physician to easily locate the family when surgery is over to talk with them. Sometimes families are given beepers so that they can walk outside or to other areas of the hospital and still be reached.

After Transfer

The nurse prepares the client's room so it is ready for the client's return after surgery (Table 11–5). Equipment that may be needed for the client after surgery is obtained and set up.

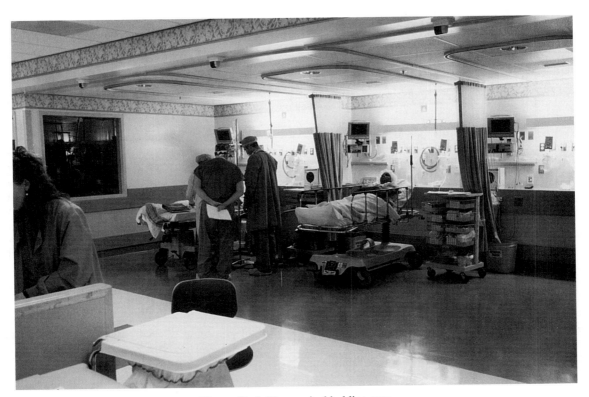

Figure 11–3. The surgical holding area.

Table 11–5. **Postoperative Client Hospital Room Preparation**

After client transfer to surgery, the nurse should prepare the client's room for the client's postoperative care needs to be ready for the client's return from the postanesthesia care unit.

Preparation	Rationale
Bed	
Bed linens should be clean and are changed if used before surgery by client.	Reduces contamination of surgical wound.
Place disposable, absorbent, waterproof pads on bottom sheet if drainage may be expected.	Protects linen from wetness and soiling so a client in pain does not have to be disturbed for linen change.
Apply lift sheet on bed of client needing assistance with repositioning.	Makes lifting and turning easier for client and nurse.
Have extra blankets available.	Client may be cold or have a low temperature.
Fanfold top covers to end of bed or to side of bed away from client transfer side.	Bed ready to receive client on transfer from cart to bed. Allows covers to be easily pulled up over client.
Obtain extra pillows as needed for positioning, elevating extremities, splinting during coughing.	Pillows help maintain position when client is turned, elevate operative extremities for comfort and swelling reduction, or splint an incision during coughing.
Equipment	
Obtain IV pole.	Surgical clients have IV infusions postoperatively.
Have emesis basin at bedside.	Nausea or vomiting may occur, especially after movement during transfer.
Have tissues and washcloths in room.	Promotes comfort: washing face or a cool cloth on forehead.
Have urinal or bedpan available in room.	Clients may be unable to get out of bed for first voiding.
Prepare suction setup for tracheostomy, nasogastric tube, or drains, as ordered.	Suction may be ordered related to surgical procedures:
	Sterile suction: tracheostomy
	Nasogastric tube: thoracic, abdominal, gastrointestinal surgery
	T tube: cholecystectomy
Have oxygen set up, as needed.	After tracheostomy, clients wear humidified oxygen mask.
Obtain special equipment as indicated by the surgical procedure.	Institutional policy and physician orders may require specialized equipment. Examples:
	Jaw surgery: suction, wire cutters, tracheostomy tray
	Tracheostomy: suction, extra tracheostomy set, tracheostomy care supplies
	Transurethral resection of prostate: irrigation supplies.
Have vital sign equipment available.	Promotes ability to promptly obtain vital signs.
Documentation Forms	
Obtain agency postoperative documentation forms and place in room.	Promotes timely and accurate documentation of client data.

Intraoperative Phase

Surgery traditionally takes place in a hospital operating room (OR) (Fig. 11–4). However, advances in technology and new care delivery options have expanded the locations where surgery can be performed. Freestanding ambulatory or outpatient surgical centers for surgery are now common. Additionally, surgery is performed in physician's offices, cardiac catheterization labs, radiology centers, emergency rooms, and specialized units that perform endoscopy procedures.

The OR is designed to enhance **aseptic** technique. Special ventilation systems control dust and prevent air from flowing into the OR from hallways. The temperature and humidity in the room are controlled to discourage bacterial growth. Everyone entering the OR wears surgical scrubs, shoe covers, caps, masks, and goggles to protect the client from infection and themselves from blood-borne pathogens. Traffic in and out of the OR is limited. Strong disinfectants are used to clean the OR after each surgical case, and instruments are sterilized.

Before the client arrives in surgery, the nurse develops a plan of care from preadmission assessment data and prepares the OR based on the plan of care (Nursing Care Plan Box 11–4). Special needs are addressed such as a tall client's need for extra table length or an elderly client's special positioning needs due to osteoporosis. A cart containing sterile instruments required for the client's case is prepared ahead of time. The scrub nurse creates a sterile field and removes the sterile instruments from the cart.

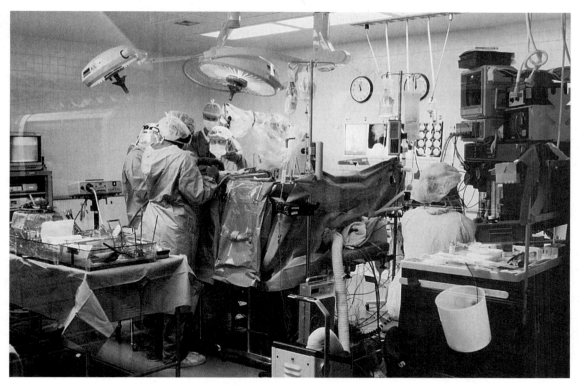

Figure 11–4. The operating room.

Items such as needles and sponges are counted before surgery and again before closure of the incision to account for all of them and ensure that none of them have been left in the client. To ensure safety, electrical equipment is checked for proper functioning.

HEALTH CARE TEAM MEMBER ROLES

The LPN/LVN's major role in this phase is as a scrub nurse who assists the physician during the surgery. Scrub nurses scrub their hands and arms and dress in sterile garb. They maintain the sterile instrument field and hand the sterile surgical instruments to the physician.

Other health care team members involved in this phase may include the physician, surgical assistant, anesthesiolo-gist, certified registered nurse anesthetist (CRNA), registered nurse, and surgical technician. A surgical assistant assists the physician. The assistant can be another physician, a registered nurse, or a physician's assistant. The anesthesiologist is a physician who specializes in anesthesia and supervises certified registered nurse anesthetists in the operating room. The certified registered nurse anesthetist is a registered nurse trained and certified in the administration of anesthesia usually at the master's degree level. Surgical technicians are trained to assist the physician as the scrub nurse does. The registered nurse circulates and is responsible for nonsterile functions such as planning care, client safety, client positioning, monitoring vital signs, providing psychological support and reducing client anxiety, ensuring an antiseptic environment, skin preparation, managing

---

NURSING CARE PLAN BOX 11–4
INTRAOPERATIVE NURSING DIAGNOSES AND OUTCOMES

- Risk for injury related to positioning, chemicals, electrical equipment, restraints, and effect of being anesthetized
  Free from injury
- Risk for impaired skin integrity related to chemicals, positioning, restraints, and immobility
  Skin integrity is maintained
- Risk for fluid volume deficit related to NPO status and blood loss
  Maintains blood pressure, pulse, and urine output within normal limits
- Risk for infection related to incision and invasive procedures
  Is free of symptoms of infection
- Pain related to positioning, restraints, incision, and surgical procedure
  Reports pain is relieved to satisfactory level

equipment such as sponge counts, and communicating with other members of the health care team.

CLIENT ARRIVAL IN SURGERY

When clients are transferred to surgery, they are taken to either a holding room or the operating room. The nurse greets the client; verifies the client's name, age, allergies, surgeon performing the surgery, consent, surgical procedure (especially right or left when applicable), and medical history; answers questions; and alleviates anxiety. The client is introduced to the anesthesiologist and certified registered nurse anesthetist, who also verify client information and explain the type of anesthesia that is to be used. An IV needle and IV fluids are started on all surgical clients either on the nursing unit or in the holding room.

As a client enters the OR, he or she should be told what to expect: "The room may feel cool but you can request extra blankets." "There is a lot of equipment, including a table and large bright overhead lights." "Several health care team members will introduce themselves to you." "The physician will greet you."

Next, the client is assisted onto the operating table and safety straps are applied. Monitoring equipment is applied and readings recorded. Then the anesthesia provider begins anesthesia. When the anesthesia provider gives permission, the client is carefully positioned to prevent pressure points that could cause tissue or nerve damage. Then any necessary tubes that are not already in place such as a nasogastric tube or urinary catheter are inserted by the RN.

After client allergies are checked by the nurse, a prepping solution such as Betadine is used to scrub and cleanse the skin. Some clients may be allergic to a preparation solution, which is why allergies must be checked. An allergic reaction can cause skin redness and blistering wherever the solution was used. After the skin is scrubbed, the nurse applies a sterile drape with the incisional area left exposed.

ANESTHESIA

Anesthesia is used for surgery to prevent pain and allow the procedure to be done safely. The type of anesthesia and the anesthetic agents are selected by the anesthesia provider with input from the client and physician. Considerations for choosing a specific type of anesthesia include the client's medical history and current health, the type of procedure, the client's anxiety level, and the client's preference for being awake or asleep. When the choice is made and client consent is given, the anesthesia provider writes the orders for the anesthesia and preoperative medications (Cultural Considerations Box 11–5).

There are two types of anesthesia: general and local. General anesthesia causes the client to lose sensation, consciousness, and reflexes. It acts directly on the central nervous system. Local anesthesia results in the loss of sensation without the loss of consciousness. It works by blocking the nerve impulses along the nerve where it is injected.

CULTURAL CONSIDERATIONS BOX 11–5

Care of the Client Having Surgery

Chinese people show a greater increase in heart rate in response to atropine than whites. Thus the nurse needs to carefully monitor the pulse after atropine is given as a preoperative medication. Additionally, Chinese people are more sensitive to the sedative effects of diazepam (Valium) and require lower doses.[5] Thus the nurse needs to carefully monitor the Chinese client for untoward effects of diazepam (Valium).

General Anesthesia

General anesthesia is commonly given by an IV or inhalation route. It is the type of anesthesia chosen when clients are very anxious or do not want local anesthesia, when the surgical procedure requires a long time period and there is a need for muscle relaxation, or when the client is unable to cooperate as in head injury, muscle disorders, or impaired cognitive function.

Intravenous Agents

To begin most general anesthesia, the client is induced (to cause anesthesia) with a short-acting IV agent that provides a rapid, smooth **induction** (period when anesthetic is first given until full anesthesia is reached) (Table 11–6). Because these agents last only a few minutes, they are used along with inhalation agents, which maintain anesthesia during surgery. After induction, the client is intubated with an endotracheal (ET) tube (Fig. 11–5). It is essential for the anesthesia provider to check for proper placement of the ET tube after intubation by listening to bilateral breath sounds and monitoring CO_2 levels. The ET tube is used to provide mechanical ventilation and anesthesia. The cuff on the ET tube is inflated to help prevent aspiration and air leakage during mechanical ventilation.

Inhalation Agents

Maintenance of anesthesia is accomplished by using inhalation agents (see Table 11–6). These agents are delivered, controlled, and excreted through mechanical ventilation. Inhalation agents and the ET tube can be irritating to the respiratory tract. Complications that can occur from their use include laryngospasm (sudden violent contraction of the vocal cords), laryngeal edema, irritated throat, or injury to the vocal cords. Suctioning through the ET tube may be needed during surgery. When the tube is removed, the nurse should closely monitor the client and be prepared to provide respiratory support and assist with reintubation if complications arise.

---

induction: inductio—to lead in

Table 11–6. **General Anesthetic and Adjunct Agents**

Intravenous Anesthetic Agents

Propofol (Diprivan)
Methohexital (Brevital Sodium)
Thiopental sodium (Pentothal)
Droperidol/fentanyl (Innovar)
Ketamine (Ketalar)

Inhalation Anesthetic Agents

Desflurane (Suprane)
Enflurane (Ethrane)
Halothane (Fluothane)
Isoflurane (Forane)
Nitrous oxide

Adjunct Agents

Narcotics
Fentanyl (Sublimaze)
Meperidine (Demerol)
Morphine sulfate
Sufentanil (Sufenta)

Muscle Relaxants
Succinylcholine (Anectine)
Vecuronium (Norcuron)
Pancuronium (Pavulon)
Tubocurarine (Tubarine)
Gallamine (Flaxedil)

Sedatives
Midazolam (Versed)
Diazepam (Valium)

Antiemetics
Droperidol (Inapsine)
Metoclopramide (Reglan)
Prochlorperazine (Compazine)

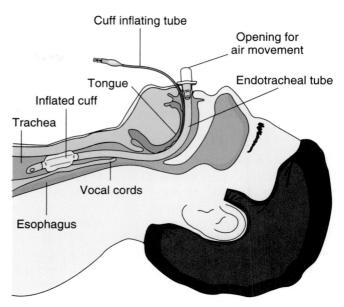

Figure 11–5. Endotracheal tube with cuff inflated.

Adjunct Agents

An **adjunct** agent is a medication that is used along with the primary anesthetic agents. These medications can include narcotics to control pain, muscle relaxers to avoid movement of muscles during surgery, antiemetic to control nausea or vomiting, and sedatives to supplement anesthesia (see Table 11–6).

Malignant Hyperthermia

Malignant hyperthermia is a rare hereditary muscle disease that can be triggered by some general anesthesia agents. It is characterized by hypermetabolism in the muscles, which produces a very high fever and muscle rigidity. Other signs and symptoms include tachycardia, tachypnea, hypertension, dysrhythmias, hyperkalemia, metabolic and respiratory acidosis, and cyanosis. It is life threatening, so immediate treatment is required or death results.

Surgery is stopped and anesthesia discontinued immediately. Oxygen at 100% is administered. The client must be cooled with ice and infusions of iced solutions. Dantrolene sodium (Dantrium), a muscle relaxant that relieves the muscle spasms, is the most effective medication for treating malignant hyperthermia. It is kept readily available in the OR and administered according to the treatment protocol of the Malignant Hyperthermia Association of the United States.

Obtaining a history of anesthesia problems in the client or family members can help detect the potential for development of this condition so that precautions can be taken. Clients with this condition can undergo surgery safely with careful planning and choice of anesthetic agents by the anesthesia provider.

Local Anesthesia

Local anesthesia is selected when the client is not anxious, can tolerate the local agent, and is not required by the surgical procedure to be unconscious or relaxed. It is a good choice for some outpatient procedures or when the client has not been NPO. There is less risk because there is no induction. Recovery time is less, and it is also less expensive. The anesthesia provider, or sometimes the physician, administers local anesthesia.

Local anesthetic agents can include bupivacaine hydrochloride (Marcaine), lidocaine (Xylocaine), dibucaine (Nupercainal) and procaine. These agents can be given topically, with a local injection or by a regional block. Topical administration places the agent directly on the surgical area. Local infiltration is achieved by injecting the medication into the tissue where the incision is to be made. A regional block is done by injecting the local agent along a nerve that carries impulses in the region where anesthesia is desired.

There are several types of regional blocks. A nerve block is the injection of a nerve at a specific point. A Bier block is done by placing a tourniquet on an extremity to remove the blood and then injecting the local agent into the extremity. A field block is a series of injections surrounding the surgical area. A spinal or epidural block is injection of a local agent into an area around the spinal nerves.

Spinal and Epidural Blocks

Injection of a local agent into the subarachnoid space produces spinal block (Fig. 11–6). Epidural block occurs when the local agent is injected into the epidural space. Spinal and epidural blocks are used mainly for lower extremity and lower abdominal surgery. Both motor and sensory function is blocked. Because these blocks are less risky than general anesthesia, they are often chosen for the elderly, who have decreased physiological reserves and may have multiple chronic health problems. The client must be carefully monitored for complications. Hypotension results from sympathetic blockade causing vasodilation, which reduces venous return to the heart and therefore cardiac output. Respiratory depression results if the block travels too far upward. As the block wears off, clients feel as if their legs are very heavy and numb. This is normal and reassurance should be offered to the client that this type of feeling does not last after the block wears off.

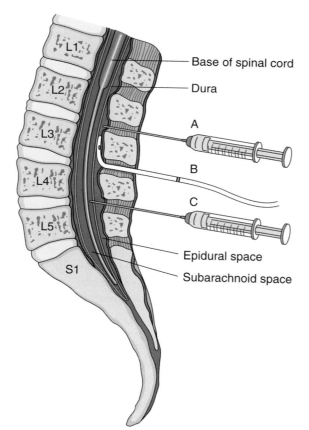

Figure 11–6. Injection of spinal anesthesia. *(A)* Epidural anesthesia. *(B)* Epidural catheter. *(C)* Spinal anesthesia.

COMPLICATIONS. A postdural puncture headache may occur in 10 to 40 percent of clients due to leakage of cerebrospinal fluid (CSF) from the needle hole in the dura that does not close when the needle is withdrawn.[6] The use of a small-gauge spinal needle (<25 gauge) helps prevent headache development. Postanesthesia orders usually include methods to help reduce the pain of a headache, including positioning the client flat and forcing fluids.

If a spinal headache develops, it may be severe and can last for weeks. Lying flat and prone (on abdomen) may help relieve the pain of the headache. Steroids may be helpful. If the headache continues, a blood patch treatment can be used to stop the CSF leakage. This treatment can be done by the anesthesiologist at the bedside or in the PACU. To create a blood patch, about 10 mL of the client's blood is injected into the epidural space at the previous puncture site. The injected blood forms a clot that "patches" the dura hole to prevent further CSF from leaking. Pain relief should happen quickly if the patch is successful. Blood patch treatment can be repeated as needed.

Adjunct Anesthesia Techniques

Several techniques may be used with anesthesia to improve the outcome of surgery. Cryoanesthesia uses cooling or freezing in a localized area to block pain impulses. Deliberately lowering the body temperature to reduce metabolism and oxygen use is referred to as **hypothermia.** Loss of sensation is produced with acupuncture. Controlled hypotension decreases blood loss by lowering the blood pressure.

TRANSFER FROM SURGERY

When surgery is completed and anesthesia stopped, the client is stabilized for transfer. After local anesthesia the client may return directly to a nursing unit. Following general and spinal anesthesia the client goes to the PACU or in some cases the intensive care unit (ICU).

Client safety is an important concern at this time. The client is never left alone. Ensuring a patent airway and preventing falls and injury from uncontrolled movements are a priority. The anesthesia provider and OR nurses transfer the client to the PACU. They monitor the client until the PACU nurse is able to receive the report and assume care of the client. This begins the final client perioperative phase, the postoperative period.

Postoperative Phase

The postoperative phase begins when the client is admitted to the PACU or nursing unit and ends with the client's postoperative evaluation in the physician's office. The PACU is usually located next to surgery to reduce movement of the client and allow anesthesia providers to be nearby to supervise client care and discharge (Fig. 11–7).

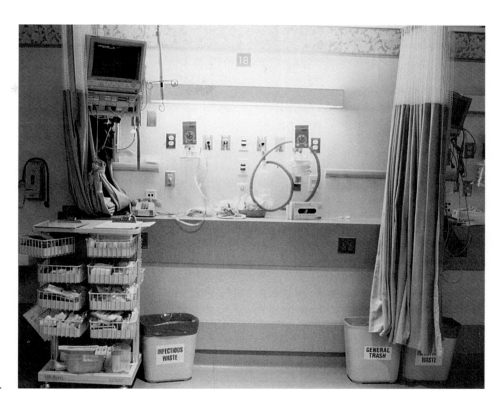

Figure 11–7. Postanesthesia care unit.

Nursing care in the PACU is typically provided by specially trained registered nurses, but LPN/LVNs may also be employed there. The nurse's role in the PACU begins by receiving a client report from the OR nurse and anesthesia provider. The report contains general client information; medical history; intraoperative information, such as type of surgery, vital signs, anesthetics, medications, fluids, drains, catheters, and problems; and the PACU plan of care. The family is updated on the client's status by the physician when the client is admitted to the PACU.

ADMISSION TO THE POSTANESTHESIA CARE UNIT

When the client is admitted to the PACU, an admission assessment is done. The priority areas of assessment are the client's respiratory status, vital signs, level of consciousness, surgical site, and pain level. Oxygen by nasal cannula or mask is started if the client has had general anesthesia, or as ordered. Some clients who are still intubated may require mechanical ventilation. Continuous monitoring is done on all clients for ECG, pulse oximetry, and blood pressure measurements. If the client has a urinary catheter, drains, or a nasogastric tube, they are checked for function and patency. The surgical site incision or dressing is assessed. Drainage or hematoma formation is documented and reported.

The client's body temperature is measured on admission, and then blankets heated in blanket warmers are applied. If the client's temperature is below normal, a warming blanket that can be set to a desired temperature is applied. Body temperature may be decreased as a result of a cool OR environment, anesthesia, cool IV solutions, and incisional openings, which allow heat loss. Client recovery is aided by avoiding a decrease in body temperature during surgery. The nurse should be aware that the elderly are at increased risk of hypothermia. Temperature is measured again before PACU discharge because a normal body temperature is usually one of the discharge criteria.

Shivering may occur from anesthesia or as a result of being cold. It is important to control shivering because it increases oxygen consumption 400 to 500 percent. Demerol is effective in relieving shivering when anesthesia is the cause. Raising the body temperature is helpful to decrease shivering if the client is cold.

PACU nursing responsibilities are listed in Table 11–7. Vital signs and assessment are done at least every 15 minutes, IV fluid infusion is maintained, and IV analgesics are given for pain as needed. Antiemetics are administered for nausea or vomiting. Deep breathing and coughing, if not contraindicated by the surgical procedure, is encouraged. Coughing increases pressure, which could cause harm to some surgical areas. Surgical procedures that prohibit coughing include hernia repair; eye, ear, intracranial, and plastic surgery; and jaw surgery. If the client is no longer NPO, ice chips or sips of water may be offered when the client is fully awake to promote comfort for a dry mouth. If ordered, postoperative therapies such as patient-controlled analgesia (PCA), which allows clients to administer their own pain medication (see Chapter 9), or continuous passive motion machines for joint replacement surgeries are begun in the PACU.

Table 11-7. **Postanesthesia Care Unit Nursing Responsibilities**

Vital signs
Airway maintenance
Respiratory assessment
Neurological assessment
Surgical site status
General assessment
Client safety
Monitoring anesthetic effects
Pain relief
Assessing PACU discharge readiness

NURSING PROCESS FOR POSTOPERATIVE CLIENTS

Several complications may occur after surgery in the PACU or later in the postoperative phase. The cause of these complications may be the surgical procedure, anesthesia, blood and fluid loss, immobility, unrelieved pain, or other diseases the client may have. Nursing care focuses on preventing, detecting, and caring for these complications.

Respiratory Function

Assessment

Normal respiratory function can be altered in the immediate postoperative period by airway obstruction, hypoventilation, secretions, laryngospasm, or decreased swallowing and cough reflexes. Respiratory function assessment includes respiratory rate, depth, ease, and pattern. Breath sounds, chest symmetry, accessory muscle use, and sputum are also observed.

Nursing Diagnosis

Respiratory-related nursing diagnoses for the PACU include the following:

- Ineffective airway clearance related to obstruction, anesthesia medications, and secretions
- Ineffective breathing pattern related to anesthesia medications and pain
- Risk for aspiration related to depressed cough and gag reflexes and reduced level of consciousness

Planning

The client's goals are to (1) have a patent airway at all times; (2) breathe comfortably and maintain normal arterial blood gases, and (3) have clear lung sounds.

Nursing Interventions

The priority nursing responsibility in the PACU is to ensure that clients maintain a patent airway.

- Airway obstruction is usually caused from relaxed muscles allowing the tongue to block the pharynx in the client who has decreased level of consciousness. It may be necessary to manually open a client's airway to prevent obstruction if the client has snoring respirations and has not completely emerged from anesthesia. The jaw-thrust method is used to open the airway.
- Clients are positioned on their side, unless contraindicated, to protect the airway until they are awake. Then, elevating the head in a supine position once they are alert assists respirations.
- Suction equipment is always readily available to clear secretions or emesis. Aspiration is a risk due to the effects of anesthesia, which depress cough and gag reflexes and reduce level of consciousness. As a result, secretions may accumulate and not be effectively controlled.
- Oxygen therapy is started on all general anesthesia clients. Hypoventilation can be an effect of anesthesia medications or analgesics, decreased level of consciousness, or an incision in the thorax causing painful respirations. Medications may be given if hypoventilation is caused by anesthesia.
- Deep breathing is encouraged to expand the lungs. Pain is controlled with carefully administered analgesics to promote deep breathing but avoid respiratory depression. Respiratory depression is reported to the anesthesiologist for prompt treatment.

Evaluation

- The goal for ineffective airway clearance and aspiration is achieved if the client's airway remains patent and lung sounds remain clear.
- The goal for ineffective breathing pattern is met if the client's respiratory rate is within normal limits, no dyspnea is reported, and arterial blood gases are within normal limits.

Cardiovascular Function

Assessment

Alterations in cardiovascular function can include hypotension, dysrhythmias, or hypertension. Hypotension can be the result of blood and fluid volume loss or cardiac abnormalities. Shock can result from significant blood and fluid volume loss (see Chapter 8). Dysrhythmias may occur from hypoxia, altered potassium levels, hypothermia, pain, stress, or cardiac disease. New-onset hypertension can develop from pain, a full bladder, or respiratory distress. Cardiovascular function assessment includes heart rate, blood pressure, ECG, skin temperature, color, and moistness. Vital signs are compared with baseline readings to determine if they are normal. Tachycardia, hypotension, pale skin color, cool, clammy skin, and decreased urine output indicate hypovolemic shock, which requires prompt treatment. Abnormal findings are promptly reported to the physician for intervention.

Tachycardia: An Early Warning Sign. Tachycardia is a compensatory mechanism designed to provide adequate delivery of oxygen in times of altered function. It is usually the earliest warning sign that an abnormality is occurring. It should be a red flag to assess the client and ask what this particular client is likely to be experiencing that is compromising oxygenation so that prompt treatment can be given.

Client Examples	Possible Causes
Postoperative client	Hemorrhage, respiratory depression, pain
Myocardial infarction client	Cardiogenic shock, pain
Respiratory client	Respiratory distress
Trauma client	Hemorrhage, severe pain

Nursing Diagnosis

The PACU cardiovascular-related nursing diagnoses include the following:

- Fluid volume deficit related to blood and fluid loss or NPO status
- Decreased cardiac output related to volume loss, medication effects, or cardiac disease

Planning

The client's goals are to (1) maintain blood pressure, pulse, and urine output within normal limits; and (2) maintain blood pressure, pulse, and rhythm within normal limits.

Nursing Interventions

- Dressings and incisions are checked for color and amount of drainage.
- IV fluids are maintained at the ordered rate to replace lost fluids but avoid fluid overload.
- Intake and output are monitored to detect imbalances.
- Providing pain relief, warming the client, and preventing bladder distention help prevent hypertension.

Evaluation

- The goal for fluid volume deficit is met if vital signs and urine output are within normal limits.
- The goal for decreased cardiac output is achieved if vital signs and rhythm are within normal limits.

Neurological Function

Anesthesia can alter neurological function until its effects wear off. Clients may arrive in the PACU either awake, arousable, or sleeping. If clients are sleeping, they should become more alert during their stay in the PACU. As emergence from anesthesia occurs, clients may become wild or agitated for a short period of time. This is referred to as emergence delirium. Amnesia effects can be caused by anesthesia. Movement, sensations, and perceptions may also be altered by anesthesia. Movement is the first function to return after spinal anesthesia.

For geriatric clients, it is important to review their history to understand if they have any cognitive or neurological deficits. Confused clients may be agitated or frightened when they awaken. It is helpful to know how caregivers normally communicate with the client. The nurse should understand that the client may not be able to report pain or follow commands. If possible, it may be helpful to have a familiar relative or caregiver with the client in the PACU to calm them and help them communicate. The nurse should watch for nonverbal pain cues such as moaning, grimacing, rubbing an area, and restlessness. If clients have limited movements or sensations before surgery, the nurse should know this to obtain an accurate assessment of anesthesia effects.

Assessment

A neurological assessment includes level of consciousness; orientation to person, place, and time; pupil size and reaction to light; and motor and sensory function.

Nursing Diagnosis

The PACU neurological-related nursing diagnoses include the following:

- Risk for injury related to anesthesia effects causing decreased level of consciousness, sensation, and movement.
- Sensory/perceptual alterations related to decreased level of consciousness, amnesiac effects of anesthesia, or spinal anesthesia.

Planning

The client's goals are to maintain safety and be free from injury.

Nursing Interventions

- All client data are verified until clients are awake and can communicate.
- The nurse maintains clients' safety until they are fully awake or movement and sensation return following spinal anesthesia. Side rails are kept up. Extremities are positioned in proper alignment and protected from injury until sensation and movement return.
- Tubes, dressings, and IVs are secured and monitored.
- As clients wake up, orientation explanations are provided and repeated until amnesiac anesthesia effects are no longer present. Examples of explanations include the following: "Mr. Smith, surgery is over, you are in the recovery room." "Your family is waiting for you and knows you are in the recovery room." "The doctor spoke with your family about how you are doing."

Evaluation

The goals for risk for injury and sensory/perceptual alterations are met if the client remains free from injury.

Pain

Assessment

If clients are awake they are asked to rate the presence of pain using a scale, such as 1 to 10, a pain scale using color, or pictures that rate pain. The location and character of the pain are documented. When clients are not fully awake, vital signs and nonverbal indications of pain should be monitored. Nonverbal indications of pain can include abnormal vital signs, restlessness, moaning, grimacing, rubbing, or pulling at specific areas or equipment.

Planning

The client's goal for pain is to report pain is relieved at a satisfactory level.

Nursing Interventions

- Client pain is monitored and promptly relieved. IV narcotic analgesics are used for their rapid onset. If PCA is ordered, it is started in PACU. Pain can result from the surgical procedure, movement, deep breathing, anxiety, or a full bladder. Positioning during surgery and the presence of devices such as nasogastric tubes, catheters, IVs, or ET tubes can also be a source of pain.
- Repositioning the client, providing warmth, and emptying a full bladder may alleviate pain.

Evaluation

After pain medication is given, clients are asked to rate their pain level. The goal for pain is met if they report a decreased level of pain that is satisfactory to them. Clients' responses are documented. For example, the client reports pain of 10 on a scale of 1 to 10. The nurse medicates the client and 30 minutes later the client rates pain as 2 on a scale of 1 to 10.

DISCHARGE FROM THE POSTANESTHESIA CARE UNIT

The length of stay in the PACU is normally 1 hour, if the client remains stable. The anesthesiologist orders the client to be transferred to a nursing unit or discharged home when discharge criteria are met (Table 11–8). The client may be transferred to the ICU if frequent monitoring is needed.

TRANSFER TO NURSING UNIT

The PACU nurse gives a report of the client's condition to the unit nurse when the client is transferred to the nursing

Table 11–8. *Discharge Criteria for Postanesthesia Care Unit or Ambulatory Surgery*

Vital signs stable
Client awake or at baseline level of consciousness
Drainage or bleeding not excessive
Respiratory function not depressed
Oxygen saturation above 90%

Additional Criteria for Ambulatory Surgery

No nausea or vomiting
No IV narcotics within last 30 minutes
Voided if required by surgical procedure or ordered
Ambulatory or baseline mobility
Understands discharge instructions
Provides means of contact for follow-up telephone
    assessment
Released to responsible adult

unit. The client is moved into bed on the nursing unit with assistance to prevent dislodging IVs, tubes, drains, or dressings. After clients are placed in bed, safety interventions are performed. The bed is placed in its lowest position, the side rails are raised, the nurse's call button is placed within easy reach of clients, and clients are instructed that they should be assisted with ambulation when they get up. Clients getting up for the first time may be dizzy and weak. They may also have IVs and equipment that must be moved. One or two nurses should be present, according to institution policy, to ensure client safety with initial ambulation.

NURSING PROCESS FOR POSTOPERATIVE CLIENTS

A complete client assessment is performed after transfer to the nursing unit. Respiratory status, vital signs (including temperature), level of consciousness, surgical site, dressings, and pain assessment are especially noted. IV site and patency are assessed. The IV solution and infusion rate are verified and monitored. Nasogastric tubes are hooked to suction or clamped as ordered. Drains and catheters are positioned to promote proper functioning.

After clients are discharged from the PACU, the nurse's role is to provide interventions to promote recovery. These interventions include monitoring for complications, providing postoperative care, education of clients and their significant others, making necessary referrals, and providing home health care. (See Nursing Care Plan Box 11–6 for the Postoperative Client.) The client is watched for possible problems such as respiratory depression, hemorrhage, and shock, especially during the first 24 hours postoperatively.

NURSING CARE PLAN BOX 11–6 FOR THE POSTOPERATIVE CLIENT

Ineffective airway clearance related to ineffective cough and secretion retention

Client Outcomes
Client maintains a patent airway at all times. Breath sounds remain clear.

Evaluation of Outcomes
Is client able to clear own secretions? Are breath sounds clear?

Interventions	Rationale	Evaluation
Monitor breath sounds.	Abnormal breath sounds such as crackles or wheezes can indicate retained secretions.	Are breath sounds clear?
Encourage deep breathing and coughing and use of incentive spirometer hourly while awake.	Lung expansion helps prevent atelectasis and keeps lungs clear of secretions.	Does client perform breathing and coughing and use incentive spirometer?
Ensure client pain is relieved before activity.	Movement can cause or increase pain.	Does client state pain is controlled before activity?
Encourage movement by turning every 2 hours and ambulating as able.	Movement promotes lung expansion and movement of secretions.	Is client moving?

Pain related to surgery, nausea, and vomiting

Client Outcomes
Client reports pain management relieves pain satisfactorily and describes pain management plan.

Evaluation of Outcomes
Does client report satisfactory pain relief? Is client able to describe pain management plan?

Interventions	Rationale	Evaluation
Assess pain using rating scale such as 1 to 10.	Self-report is the most reliable indicator of pain.	Does client report pain using scale?
Provide analgesics prn.	Analgesics relieve pain.	Is client's pain less after medication?
Provide antiemetics prn.	Antiemetics relieve nausea and vomiting.	Is client's nausea and vomiting less after medication?
Position client comfortably.	Incisions, drains, tubing, equipment, and bed rest can cause discomfort, which positioning can relieve.	Does client report positioning is comfortable?

GERIATRIC

Interventions	Rationale	Evaluation
When assessing pain speak clearly and slowly so elderly client can hear.	If elderly client does not hear or misunderstands, pain may not be reported accurately to ensure appropriate intervention provided.	Does client hear and report pain and relief accurately using pain scale?
Assess elderly clients' pain level regularly, observing nonverbal pain cues (restlessness, grimacing, moaning), especially for those cognitively impaired.	The pain of elderly clients is often underreported and undertreated, especially if cognitively impaired, and noting nonverbal cues can aid in pain treatment.	Are nonverbal cues present in elderly clients, especially those cognitively impaired?

continued

NURSING CARE PLAN BOX 11–6 (continued)

Altered urinary elimination related to surgery, pain, anesthesia, altered positioning

Client Outcomes
Client empties bladder completely and regularly without pain.

Evaluation of Outcomes
Is client able to void completely and regularly?

Interventions	Rationale	Evaluation
Measure and record urine, noting amount.	Hourly urine less than 30 mL or voiding of frequent, small amounts can indicate problems.	Is client voiding sufficient quantity?
Assist client to bathroom, bedside commode, or stand or sit (males) to void.	Natural positioning can promote voiding, but using a bedpan can be difficult for clients and inhibit voiding.	Does client positioning promote voiding?
Use techniques to promote voiding: run water, pour warm water over female client's perineum, offer hot beverage, provide privacy, place client's feet on floor.	Voiding is promoted using techniques that relax the muscles and sphincter.	Is client able to void?
Maintain sterile technique for indwelling catheter.	Catheters can be a source of infection.	Is client free of urinary tract infection?

GERIATRIC

Assist client promptly with voiding needs.	Age-related changes decrease the elderly client's ability to delay voiding.	Does elderly client void without incontinence?

Risk for infection related to inadequate primary defenses from surgical wound

Client Outcomes
Client remains free from infection.

Evaluation of Outcomes
Does client remain free from infection?

Interventions	Rationale	Evaluation
Observe incision for signs and symptoms of infection.	Redness, warmth, fever, and swelling indicate infection.	Are signs and symptoms of infection present?
Monitor drainage and maintain drains.	Drains remove fluid from the surgical site to prevent infection development.	Are drainage amount and color normal for procedure?
Maintain sterile technique for dressing changes.	Sterile technique reduces infection development.	Are drains functioning? Is incision free of signs and symptoms of infection?

Altered nutrition: less than body requirements related to NPO, pain, nausea

Client Outcomes
Client resumes normal dietary intake and maintains weight within normal limits.

Evaluation of Outcomes
Is client able to resume normal diet? Does client maintain normal weight for height?

continued

NURSING CARE PLAN BOX 11–6 (continued)

Intervention	Rationale	Evaluation
Monitor bowel sounds.	After major or abdominal surgery peristalsis stops for 2 to 4 days. Flatus returns in 24 to 72 hours; bowel sounds return in 24 to 96 hours, then bowel movements resume.	Does the client have flatus or bowel sounds?
Provide antiemetics prn.	Antiemetics relieve nausea and vomiting.	Is client's nausea and vomiting less after medication?
Provide frequent oral care.	Good oral hygiene promotes appetite.	Is oral care provided often?
Begin diet with water and clear liquids and advance to soft and solid foods as tolerated.	Foods that are easy to digest are started first to aid tolerance of diet.	Does client tolerate diet without nausea or vomiting?
Maintain tube feedings or total parenteral nutrition as ordered.	Nutrition is maintained when client is NPO with tube feedings or total parenteral nutrition.	Are client's nutritional needs met: weight within normal limits, electrolytes and albumin levels normal?

	GERIATRIC	
Increase activity as tolerated.	Activity stimulates peristalsis and appetite, which are often decreased in the elderly.	Does client have normal bowel sounds and appetite?

Knowledge deficit related to lack of knowledge about surgery and postoperative treatment

Client Outcomes
Client verbalizes knowledge of surgery and ability to comply with postoperative regimen.

Evaluation of Outcomes
Is client able to explain postoperative treatment?

Interventions	Rationale	Evaluation
Explain surgical routine and postoperative care.	Client must have basic knowledge to comply with therapy.	Is client able to verbalize knowledge taught?
Explain medications or therapies ordered.	Compliance and safe use of medications is promoted with an adequate knowledge base.	Can client explain need for ordered medications? Can client explain ordered therapies?

	GERIATRIC	
During teaching sessions, include caregiver or family.	Compliance is increased if support person understands instructions.	Does client or caregiver participate and state understanding of teaching?
Set up teaching environment to promote learning for elderly.	Environmental adjustments for age-related changes increase elderly learning.	Does elderly client report comfortable environment?

Respiratory Function

Assessment

The client's respiratory status is assessed and monitored to ensure that a patent airway is maintained. Chest symmetry is noted. If the client's airway is compromised, immediate action is taken to support the airway and the physician is notified. Breath sounds are auscultated for adequate air exchange and absence of abnormal sounds in all lobes. The client's cough is assessed if it is not contraindicated by the type of surgery, such as hernia repair or eye, ear, intracranial, jaw, or plastic surgery.

Nursing Diagnoses

Postoperative respiratory-related nursing diagnoses include the following:

- Ineffective airway clearance related to ineffective cough and secretion retention
- Ineffective breathing pattern related to analgesic medications and pain

Planning

The client's goals are to have (1) a patent airway and clear breath sounds and (2) normal arterial blood gases. Factors that may inhibit this goal should be identified and discussed with the client.

Nursing Interventions

- Regular monitoring of the client's respiratory rate, depth, and effort; cough strength; and breath sounds should be done. Postoperative clients are at risk for developing atelectasis and pneumonia. They may have a weak cough as a result of being drowsy from anesthesia or analgesics. If fine crackles are heard in the lung bases, the client should be encouraged to deep breathe or cough. Afterwards, the nurse should listen again to see if the crackles have cleared.
- Preoperative teaching of deep breathing and coughing is reinforced and encouraged every hour while the client is awake. Deep breathing and coughing, especially through the first postoperative day, helps prevent atelectasis and keeps lungs clear of secretions. If secretions are retained, mucus plugs can develop and block bronchioles, causing alveoli to collapse. Infection can develop from the stasis of mucus resulting in pneumonia.
- An incentive spirometer also helps prevent atelectasis by encouraging clients to inspire a deep breath, which opens their airways. After the client is taught to use the incentive spirometer, it is placed within the client's reach, and encouragement to use it is given frequently.
- Pain should be controlled so the client does not guard against deep respirations or coughing. An incision near the diaphragm makes deep breathing or coughing painful, so clients avoid it.
- Turning the client at least every 2 hours helps expand the lungs and moves secretions. Bed rest results in decreased movement of secretions, so ambulating the client as soon as possible also aids in keeping the airway clear.

Evaluation

If the client's breath sounds are clear and arterial blood gases remain normal, the goals are met. The client's ability and willingness to deep breathe or cough and use an incentive spirometer every hour while awake is important in achieving the goal.

Circulatory Function

Assessment

The primary concern in monitoring the client's circulatory status is the detection and prevention of hemorrhage,

shock, and thrombophlebitis. Vital signs and skin temperature, color, and moistness are observed and compared with baseline data. The incision or dressing is checked for drainage or hematoma formation. Drainage may leak down the client's side and pool underneath the client. The nurse, while wearing gloves, should feel underneath the client or turn the client to check for bleeding. Any signs of hemorrhage or shock are promptly reported by the LPN/LVN to the RN, who notifies the physician of the client's status.

Institutional policy is followed for client monitoring frequency. A typical protocol for monitoring vital signs is every 15 minutes for the first hour, then every 30 minutes for 2 hours, hourly for four hours, and then every 4 hours, if stable.

The lower extremities of surgical clients are observed. Tenderness or pain in the calf may be the first indication of a deep vein thrombosis. Leg swelling, warmth, and redness, as well as fever, may also be present. Bilateral calf and thigh measurement is done daily if thrombophlebitis is suspected or diagnosed. Peripheral pulses and capillary refill are also checked.

Nursing Diagnosis

Postoperative cardiovascular-related nursing diagnoses include the following:

- Fluid volume deficit related to blood and fluid loss or NPO status
- Altered tissue perfusion: peripheral or pulmonary related to interruption of blood flow

Planning

The client's goals are to (1) maintain blood pressure and pulse within normal limits and (2) maintain normal tissue perfusion.

Nursing Interventions

Vital signs are monitored and abnormal trends noted. Dressings, incisions, drains, and tubes are checked for color and amount of drainage. Bright red drainage or excessive drainage amounts are reported immediately to the physician. Intake and output are monitored to detect imbalances. IV fluids are maintained at the ordered rate.

Slower blood flow during surgery, dehydration, leg straps, and positioning may contribute to venous injury or thrombosis development. Preventive interventions to decrease the development of thrombophlebitis and pulmonary embolism should be used (see Chapter 17). Leg exercises that were taught preoperatively are encouraged hourly while the client is awake. Postoperative early ambulation is a major preventive technique for thrombosis. Clients' pain should be controlled to facilitate their ability to participate in early ambulation. Knee- or thigh-length antiembolism elastic stockings or intermittent pneumatic compression may be ordered. Low-dose heparin, low-molecular-weight heparin (enoxaparin [Lovenox]), warfarin, and plasma expanders such as dextran 40 and dextran

70 reduce clot formation through dilution. It is important to avoid pressure under the knee from pillows, rolled blankets, or prolonged bending of the knee. Leg elevation is helpful in preventing venous stasis.

Evaluation

- The goal for fluid volume deficit is met if vital signs and urine output are within normal limits.
- The goal for altered tissue perfusion is met if tissue blood flow remains normal.

Postoperative Pain

It is common for clients to experience pain after surgery, although each client's pain experience varies. In addition to incisional pain, painful muscle spasms can occur. Nausea and vomiting, ambulation, coughing, deep breathing, and anxiety can cause discomfort and increase postoperative pain. Unrelieved pain has negative physiological effects. It also impairs deep breathing and coughing and hinders early ambulation, which may increase complications, length of hospital stay, and health care costs. Nurses should understand that providing pain relief not only reduces suffering, it also has positive benefits for a quicker recovery. It is important for nurses to stay informed of advances in pain management and ensure that they make pain relief a priority in providing client care (see Chapter 9).

Assessment

Nurses must be proactive and diligent in their provision of pain relief. Studies show that commonly used intramuscular (IM) pain medication orders may not provide adequate pain relief in many clients and can result in the client's waiting for periods of up to 20 minutes for requested pain injections.[7] Anticipating postoperative clients' pain by regularly monitoring their pain level instead of waiting until it is the time for the next pain medication is essential in providing quality nursing care for pain relief.

Elderly clients, including the very oldest, experience postoperative pain. Pain is not a normal part of aging. Careful assessment of elderly clients' unique aging changes, chronic diseases, and pain relief needs is required to appropriately treat their pain.[8] Cognitively impaired adults are at risk for undertreatment of their postoperative pain.[9] Pain relief needs remain even when client communication is impaired.

If clients are not fully awake on transfer, vital signs and nonverbal indications of pain should be monitored. Nonverbal indicators of pain include abnormal vital signs (usually elevated blood pressure, although hypotension can occur in some clients), restlessness, moaning, grimacing, and rubbing or pulling at specific body areas or equipment. Clients who are awake are asked to rate the presence of pain using a scale such as 1 to 10. If clients such as children or the elderly are unable to rate their pain, picture or color pain rating scales can be used.

The client is also asked the location of the pain and to describe the pain quality such as sharp, aching, throbbing, or burning. The rating, quality, and location of the pain are documented.

Nursing Diagnosis

- Pain related to tissue damage from surgery, muscle spasms, nausea, or vomiting

Planning

The client's goal for pain is to report pain relief at a satisfactory level. Clients should be involved in setting the goal for the level of pain relief that is satisfactory to them using the pain rating scale.

Nursing Interventions

- Clients are monitored for pain and provided prompt interventions for relief. If IV analgesics are used initially, such as in the PACU, and then ordered as IM injections on the unit, the nurse should know the length of action of the IV analgesic. IV analgesics usually have a shorter duration than IMs. Clients in pain should not have to wait after an IV analgesic dose for their first dose of an IM analgesic the ordered time interval of IM doses (i.e., 3 hours, if IM order is morphine 10 mg IM q 3 hours prn). Having to wait when the IV analgesic is no longer effective can cause needless pain. The nurse should consult the physician or pharmacist for appropriate timing intervals for IV to IM doses of analgesics.
- PCA may be started in the PACU. The nurse monitors the client's ability to use PCA, response to the medication, and the relief obtained from it. If PCA is not effective or side effects occur, the physician should be notified.
- Comfortable positioning, warming the client, and relieving a client's full bladder can also alleviate pain. Attention to environmental factors such as bright overhead lighting, excessive noise or visitors, and extreme room temperatures also helps promote comfort.
- Antiemetics should be given, as ordered, to relieve the discomfort of nausea and vomiting. If vomiting occurs, clients should be turned onto one side to aid emesis removal and prevent aspiration. A nasogastric tube may be ordered to control vomiting.

Evaluation

Thirty minutes after pain medication is given, clients are asked to rate their pain level. If clients are sleeping at this time, the nurse should allow them to sleep. When they awaken, the nurse can ask them to rate their pain level. The goal for pain is met when clients report a decreased level of pain, as compared with their previous level of pain, that is satisfactory to them. If the client does not report satisfactory pain relief, the physician should be promptly notified of the inadequate pain relief.

CRITICAL THINKING: Mrs. Wood

Mrs. Wood, following a hysterectomy, returns to the unit from the PACU. Mrs. Wood's postoperative vital signs and assessment findings are normal. The LPN/LVN asks Mrs. Wood her pain level, noting that she moans occasionally, moves her legs, and pulls at her covers near her abdominal incision. She is drowsy but says it hurts. In the PACU, she received 10 mg of morphine IV 55 minutes ago. Morphine 5 to 10 mg IM is ordered every 3 hours as needed.

1. What nonverbal pain cues does Mrs. Wood have?
2. How should the LPN/LVN document Mrs. Wood's pain?
3. What action should the LPN/LVN take to relieve Mrs. Wood's pain?
4. When should the LPN/LVN next monitor Mrs. Wood's pain level?
5. If Mrs. Wood indicates that her pain is unrelieved after 30 minutes, what action should the LPN/LVN take?

Answers at end of chapter.

Urinary Function

Assessment

The client's urinary status is monitored to ensure that normal function is maintained because urinary retention can occur after anesthesia. For outpatient surgery, clients may be required to void before being discharged. If the client has a urinary catheter, the amount, color, and consistency of the urine are noted. Otherwise, the nurse monitors the client's first postoperative voiding to prevent bladder distention. Clients should void within 8 hours from their last voiding. For clients having urinary or gynecological procedures, the client may be ordered to void within 4 to 6 hours, to prevent increased pressure on the surgical site. Catheterization may be necessary if the client is unable to void.

If clients report the inability to void, the bladder is palpated for distention. The nurse should be aware that restlessness can be caused by discomfort from a full bladder. A distended bladder requires intervention to empty it. Efforts are made to promote voiding before inserting a urinary catheter because of the risk of infection.

The nurse notes the amount, color, and consistency of the client's urine. The body's stress response to the surgical experience stimulates the sympathetic (fight or flight) nervous system, which saves fluid by reducing urine output. So initially, urine output may be reduced and concentrated. Then it should gradually increase and become less concentrated and lighter in color.

Nursing Diagnosis

Postoperative urinary-related nursing diagnoses include the following:

- Altered urinary elimination related to surgery, pain, anesthesia, altered positioning
- Urinary retention related to surgery, pain, anesthesia, altered positioning

Planning

The client's goals are to (1) completely and regularly empty the bladder and (2) remain free from pain during voiding.

Nursing Interventions

- Output is measured and recorded on most postoperative patients, especially those undergoing major procedures or urological surgery, elderly clients, and those with an IV or urinary catheter.
- If the client's urinary output from the catheter is less than 30 mL for 1 hour, it is reported to the physician.
- Clients who void small, frequent amounts (30 to 50 mL every 20 to 30 minutes) or dribble may have retention overflow and may not be emptying their bladder. This is not normal and may require catheterization to empty the bladder and prevent complications.
- To promote voiding, clients should be assisted to the bathroom or bedside commode, and men should be allowed to stand or sit to void, if possible. If bedpans are used, they should be warmed to prevent reflexive sphincter tightening.
- When clients get up postoperatively, especially for the first time, they may be weak or dizzy. One or two health care workers should assist the client and allow the client to dangle before standing (Fig. 11–8). Call lights should be placed within client reach and answered promptly. These precautions can help prevent falls.
- If the client is unable to void, techniques to promote voiding should be used before catheterization. Running water, pouring warm water over a female client's perineum, or drinking a hot beverage may stimulate voiding. The client is given privacy to void after safety is ensured. Having clients place their feet solidly on the floor relaxes the pelvic muscles to aid voiding.
- If the client is uncomfortable, has a distended bladder, or has not voided within the specified time frame, the physician is notified. An order to catheterize the client after other measures have been unsuccessful, either with a straight or an indwelling catheter, is usually received.

Evaluation

- The goal for altered urinary elimination is met if the client is able to void completely and regularly.

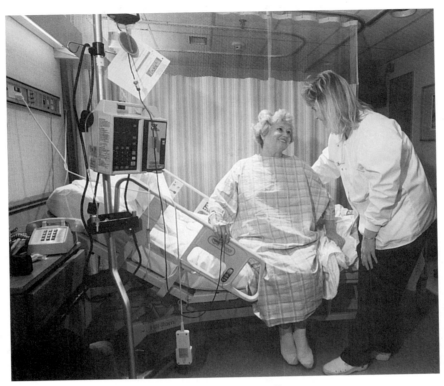

Figure 11–8. Client dangling.

- The goal for urinary retention is met if the client is able to void without pain or complications.

Surgical Wound Care

Assessment

A wound is a break in the skin. An incision is a wound made by a physician with a sharp instrument such as a scalpel. A laceration is an irregular, jagged cut such as glass makes. A puncture wound has a small opening and may be made with a scalpel to insert a tube or drain (Fig. 11–9). Incisions are closed with sutures, staples, or surgical glue, which is painless, is rapidly applied, and produces less scarring (see Fig. 11–9). Wound healing occurs in phases (Table 11–9). As the wound heals, sutures or staples are removed in 7 to 10 days, and Steri-Strips may be applied to continue supporting the wound as it heals.

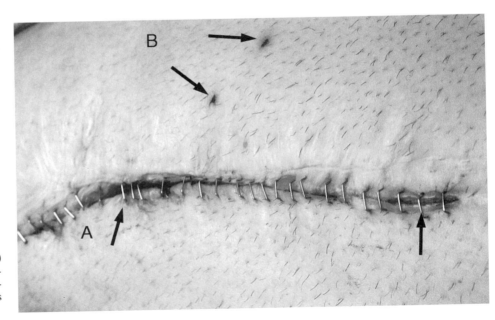

Figure 11–9. A stapled incision. *(A)* Note wound edges not approximated at arrows. *(B)* Arrows indicate puncture sites where drains were inserted. See Plate 17.

Table 11–9. **Wound Healing**

Wound Healing Processes	
First Intention	Wound edges well approximated, little tissue loss
Second Intention	Large tissue loss, granulation tissue fills in area over time
Third Intention	Granulation tissue fills in area with scar formation

Wound Healing Phases			
Phase	**Time Frame**	**Wound Healing**	**Client Effect**
Phase I	Incision to second postoperative day	Inflammatory response	Fever, malaise
Phase II	Third to fourteenth postoperative day	Granulation tissue forms	Feeling better
Phase III	Third to sixth postoperative week	Collagen deposited	Raised scar formed
Phase IV	Months to 1 year	Wound contracts and shrinks	Flat, thin scar

When a wound occurs, it disrupts the integrity of the skin giving bacteria an entry point into the body. Wounds can be clean or dirty. Clean wounds are surgical wounds that are not infected. Contaminated wounds include accidental wounds or surgical incisions exposed to gastrointestinal (GI) contents or unsterile conditions. Infected wounds and dirty wounds contain microorganisms from trauma, ruptured organs, or infection. Necrotic and infected tissue is removed before infected wounds are closed. This is known as **debridement.**

Nursing Diagnosis

Postoperative skin-related nursing diagnoses include the following:

- Impaired skin integrity related to surgical incision
- Risk for infection related to inadequate primary defenses from surgical wound

Planning

The client's goals are to (1) regain skin integrity and (2) remain free from infection. The client should know the signs and symptoms indicating infection that should be reported to the physician.

Nursing Interventions

DRAINS. Drains are inserted into wounds in surgery to prevent accumulation of blood, lymph, or necrotic tissue in wounds that can lead to infection or delayed healing. Drains may work by gravity or suction. Penrose drains are open, soft, flat, rubberlike drains that carry drainage out of the wound. Moderate **serosanguineous** drainage is expected from a Penrose drain that may require frequent dressing changes. Examples of drains that use suction to gently enhance drainage include the Jackson-Pratt, Hemovac, and Mini-Snyder Hemovac (Fig. 11–10). These drains are closed systems that may require periodic emptying and reapplication of the suction by compressing the

drain. Output is recorded when the drainage is emptied. The amount of drainage expected varies with the type of surgery. Specialized drainage systems allow the autotransfusion of bloody drainage back to the client to maintain hemoglobin levels without the risks associated with blood transfusions such as transfusion reactions or transmission of infections.

Surgical wound drainage initially is sanguineous (red) and changes to serosanguineous (pink) and then serous (pale yellow) after a few hours to days. Drainage that is bright red, remains sanguineous after a few hours, or is large in quantity should be promptly reported to the physician because the client may be hemorrhaging.

DRESSINGS. Dressings are applied to surgical wounds for several reasons. They protect the wound, absorb drainage, prevent contamination from body fluids, provide comfort, and apply pressure to reduce swelling or bleeding as in a pressure dressing. The initial dressing is applied in surgery and then usually removed by the physician about 24 hours postoperatively. If drainage appears on the initial dressing, the nurse usually reinforces it with another dressing according to physician orders or institution policy and documents the color, amount, and consistency of the drainage.

After the initial dressing is removed, if the wound is dry and the edges intact (approximated) the physician may not order the dressing to be replaced. This allows easy observation of the wound and avoidance of applying tape to the skin. Draining wounds are dressed with several layers that are changed as needed by the nurse. The Centers for Disease Control and Prevention's Standard Precautions are used when changing dressings. When the old dressing is removed, it should be done carefully to prevent dislodging of tubes or drains. The condition of the wound is documented with each dressing change. It is normal for the inci-

---

serosanguineous: sero—whey + sanguineous—bloody

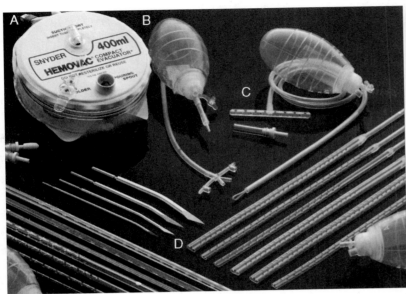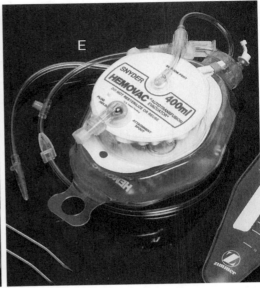

Figure 11–10. Surgical drains. *(A)* Hemovac. *(B)* Mini-Synder Hemovac. *(C)* T drain. *(D)* Flat drains. *(E)* Hemovac autotransfusion system. (From Zimmer Patient Care Products, Dover, Ohio, with permission.)

sion to be puffy and red from the inflammatory response. The surrounding skin should be the client's normal color and temperature. Sterile technique is used to reapply the new dressing. Correct tape application over the dressing is done by gently laying the tape over the dressing and applying even pressure on each side of the wound. Pressure should not be applied on top of the wound by pulling on the tape from one side of the wound to the other side.

Evaluation

- The goal for impaired skin integrity is met if the client's wound heals and skin integrity is regained without complications.
- The goal for risk for infections is achieved if the client remains free from signs and symptoms of infection.

Wound Complications

Wound problems can include **hematoma,** infection, dehiscence, and **evisceration.** A hematoma occurs from bleeding in the wound and into the tissue around the wound. A clot forms from the bleeding. If the clot is large with swelling, the clot may need to be removed by the physician.

Infected wounds may be warm, reddened, and tender and have **purulent** (pus) drainage. The drainage may have a foul odor. A fever and elevated white blood cell (WBC) count may be present. Antibiotics are used to treat the infection. Careful use of sterile technique for incisional care can help prevent infection.

Dehiscence and evisceration are serious wound complications (Fig. 11–11). Wound dehiscence is the sudden bursting open of a wound's edges that may be preceded by

an increase in serosanguineous drainage. Evisceration is the viscera spilling out of the abdomen. They often occur with abdominal incisions in clients who are malnourished, obese, elderly, or who have poor wound healing. Supporting the wound during coughing and activity that pulls on the incision, or applying an abdominal binder on clients who are at risk, helps prevent them from occurring. When evisceration occurs, the client may have pain and vomiting and may report that "something let loose" or "gave way."

If dehiscence or evisceration occurs, the client is placed in a low Fowler's position with flexed knees. The wound is covered with sterile towels moistened with warm sterile normal saline, and the physician is notified immediately of this surgical emergency. The nurse applies gentle pressure over the wound and keeps the client still and calm. Vital signs are monitored to watch for signs of shock (tachycardia, tachypnea, dyspnea, hypotension). IV fluids are infused as ordered, and the client is prepared for immediate surgery to close the wound.

Gastrointestinal Function

Nutritional intake and bowel functioning can be affected by surgery and anesthesia. Being NPO and having bowel preparation often occur preoperatively. Postoperatively, intestinal handling during surgery, the need to rest the GI tract following a procedure, immobility, lack of peristalsis, and complications such as nausea and vomiting, paralytic ileus (from peristalsis stopping), constipation, or obstruction can interfere with normal GI function.

Assessment

Postoperatively, bowel sounds are auscultated every 4 hours. If no bowel sounds are heard initially, the nurse

---

hematoma: heimatos—blood + oma—tumor
evisceration: e—out + viscera—body organs

Dehiscence

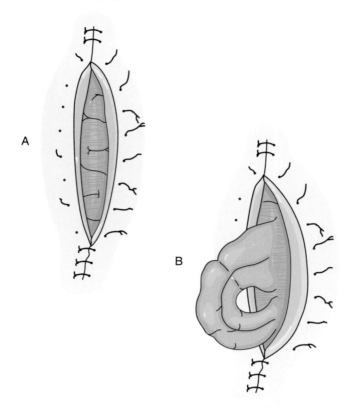

Evisceration

Figure 11–11. *(A)* Wound dehiscence. *(B)* Wound evisceration.

should listen for 5 minutes in each quadrant before documenting that they are absent. Normally, 5 to 30 bowel sounds are heard per minute. Bowel sounds can be absent, hypoactive, normal, or hyperactive. The abdomen is checked to see if it is soft or firm and flat or distended. When the client begins passing flatus or stool, the nurse documents it. Any abnormal findings are reported to the physician by the nurse.

After abdominal surgery, peristalsis and bowel sounds usually stop for 24 to 72 hours. Flatus is usually absent for 24 to 72 hours postoperatively. Clients do not have bowel movements until peristalsis returns. The client is kept NPO until flatus and bowel sounds return or as ordered by the physician. A nasogastric or gastrointestinal tube may be inserted and attached to suction to remove secretions and flatus until peristalsis returns. The client's abdominal girth is measured if distention occurs. Drainage from the decompression tube is observed for amount, color, and consistency. Intake and output are measured. Removal of gastric secretions can cause electrolyte imbalances. Signs and symptoms of electrolyte imbalance can include new-onset confusion or weakness, which should be reported.

Nursing Diagnosis

Postoperative gastrointestinal-related nursing diagnoses include the following:

- Altered nutrition: less than body requirements related to NPO, pain, nausea
- Constipation related to decreased peristalsis, immobility, altered diet, narcotic side effect
- Altered oral mucosal membranes related to NPO status

Planning

The client's goals are to (1) resume normal dietary intake and maintain weight within normal limits; (2) return to normal bowel elimination patterns and report freedom from gas pains and constipation; and (3) maintain intact, moist mucous membranes.

Nursing Interventions

- The primary focus of the nurse is to help restore normal GI functioning. When normal GI function is achieved, dietary intake can be resumed. Until the client can resume a normal dietary intake, as determined by the surgical procedure, IV fluids, total parenteral nutrition, or enteral feedings may be required (Nutrition Notes Box 11–7).

LEARNING TIP

The primary purpose of most IV fluids is to provide hydration. Most IV solutions do not provide enough nutrients or calories to prevent malnutrition. A 1000 mL IV solution containing 5% dextrose provides only about 170 calories. This does not meet an adult's daily caloric needs, especially if healing is occurring. The nurse should ensure that early consideration of other nutritional methods is made to meet the client's dietary needs.

- If nausea and vomiting occur, antiemetics may be given.
- Early ambulation, exercise, and diet promote restoration of GI functioning. The client should be encouraged to be active as much as possible. If gas pains occur, techniques to relieve the pain, as tolerated, include ambulation, having the client lie prone, and pulling the knees up to the chest.
- If the client is NPO, oral care is provided frequently. Good oral hygiene helps promote appetite. A dry mouth is uncomfortable and can cause increased bacterial accumulation and mucous membrane breakdown. Products such as dry mouth toothpaste, moisturing gel, or mouthwash can be used to promote good oral hygiene and decrease dryness. If the client is allowed occasional ice chips, they can be made from

NUTRITION NOTES BOX 11-7

Nourishing the Postoperative Client

After surgery, the usual fluid replacement is 2 L of 5 percent glucose in water in 24 hours. This amount contains 100 g of glucose and delivers 340 calories. Although this does not meet a person's resting energy expenditure, it prevents ketosis from the breakdown of fat for energy. Most adults have nutrient reserves for 3 to 4 days of semistarvation. To prevent excessive muscle protein from being used for energy, adequate nourishment should be provided within 3 days. Clear liquid feedings containing complete nutrition are available commercially.

To avoid abdominal distention, oral feedings are delayed until peristalsis returns. The return of peristalsis is evident by the client passing flatus or the health care worker auscultating bowel sounds. Clients are usually progressed from clear liquids to a regular diet as soon as possible. If "diet as tolerated" is prescribed, the client should be asked what foods sound good. Sometimes a full dinner tray "turns off" the client's appetite if the client does not feel well.

After gastrointestinal surgery, oral food and fluids are deferred longer than with other surgeries, to allow healing. When particular amounts are prescribed, those limits should be strictly implemented to preserve the suture lines. Another precaution is often taken after surgery on the mouth and throat. After tonsillectomy, for example, no red liquids are given, so that vomitus is not mistaken for blood and bleeding is not thought to be the red beverage or food.

normal saline to prevent depletion of electrolytes. Alcohol-containing mouthwashes increase dryness and should be avoided. Lemon glycerin swabs may also increase dryness.

- If a paralytic ileus develops, abdominal distention, absent bowel sounds, and pain may result. If severe peristalsis occurs, nausea and vomiting result. As ordered, a nasogastric tube can be used to decompress the GI tract until peristalsis returns.
- When the client is able to resume oral intake, food is introduced gradually to tolerance. Water and clear liquids are usually started first. Then the diet is advanced to soft and finally solid foods.

Evaluation

- The goal for altered nutrition: less than body requirements is met if clients are able to maintain their baseline weight and resume a normal dietary intake.
- The goal for constipation is met if clients are free from discomfort and establish a regular bowel elimination pattern.

- The goal for altered oral mucous membranes is met if clients maintain intact, moist mucous membranes.

Mobility

Assessment

It is important for the client to move as much as possible to prevent complications and promote healing. Pain, incisions, tubes, drains, dressings, and other equipment may make movement difficult. The nurse determines the client's ability to move in bed, to get out of bed, and to walk. Pain levels that may interfere with movement are assessed. The client's tolerance to activity is observed. Understanding of how to perform exercises is noted.

Nursing Diagnosis

Postoperative mobility-related nursing diagnoses include the following:

- Impaired physical mobility related to surgery, decreased strength, and movement restriction
- Activity intolerance related to immobility and weakness

Planning

The client's goals are to (1) resume normal physical activity and (2) demonstrate increased activity tolerance.

Nursing Interventions

- The nurse assists the client with turning in bed, dangling, and ambulation to ensure that movement occurs.
- Encouraging exercises in bed is important, especially if ambulation is not possible. Exercises should be done hourly while awake to promote normal functioning and prevent complications.
- Deep breathing, range of motion of all joints, and isometric exercises of the abdominal, gluteal, and leg muscles should be performed by the client. Passive joint range of motion is done by the nurse if the client is unable to do active range of motion.
- The client is assisted with positioning in bed. Pillows can be used to support the body in good alignment. Turning should be done at least every 2 hours. Positioning should be alternated from supine to side to side. Clients should move themselves as much as possible for several reasons. Movement increases circulation and promotes lung expansion to prevent complications. Also, clients know where it hurts and are less likely to increase their pain when moving than if the nurse moves them.
- As clients are assisted to sit up, the head of the bed is raised slowly to allow the circulatory system to adjust to the position change. If clients report dizziness or feeling faint, the head of the bed is lowered. Vital

signs and skin color are noted. Clients should rest about 1 hour, as tolerated, before sitting up again. Once clients tolerate a sitting position, they can be dangled on the side of the bed in preparation for ambulation.

- If dangling is tolerated, clients can be ambulated. When getting up, clients should pedal their feet to "wake up" the muscles controlling the arteries, keep their eyes forward, and move slowly until they feel adjusted to being up. Usually, the client ambulates a short distance for the first time and increases distance as tolerated. One or two health care workers should assist the client and use a gait (walking) belt for safety. Walkers with wheels and seats may also be used for support and for resting if the client becomes dizzy or tired. If clients feel faint or dizzy or their vital signs change, they should be assisted back to bed. A wheelchair may be needed to transport them safely back to their room.

Evaluation

- The goal for impaired physical mobility is met if clients are able to increase ambulation and resume normal activities.
- The goal for activity intolerance is met if clients are able to increase activity to desired level and maintain vital signs within normal limits.

POSTOPERATIVE CLIENT DISCHARGE

Discharge planning begins in preadmission testing and continues after admission to ensure that the client is ready for a timely discharge. When the client meets discharge criteria, the physician discharges the client from either the ambulatory setting or the hospital.

Ambulatory Surgery

Discharge Criteria

Generally, the client can be considered as a candidate for discharge 1 hour after surgery if discharge criteria are met (see Table 11–8). Discharge criteria include stable vital signs, no bleeding, no nausea or vomiting, and controlled pain that is not severe. Depending on the type of surgical procedure, such as urological, gynecological, or hernia surgery, the client may be required to void before discharge. The client should be able to sit up without dizziness before discharge. When clients meet discharge criteria and are discharged by the physician, they are released to a responsible adult. They are not permitted to drive themselves home because of the effects of anesthesia and medications they have received.

Discharge Instructions

Clients and their families are given written discharge instructions before discharge. Elderly clients should have a caregiver participate in the discharge instruction session to understand what observations to make and what to do if complications develop. The instruction form is signed by the client or an authorized representative to indicate understanding. Prescriptions and a copy of the instructions, to provide a reference for later, are sent with the client. The client is encouraged to rest for 24 to 48 hours. The client is to avoid operating machinery, driving, drinking alcoholic beverages, and making major decisions for 24 hours because the effects of undergoing surgery can affect energy levels and thinking ability. The physician orders any fluid, dietary, activity, or work restrictions.

Clients are taught wound care, medication information (including side effects), and signs and symptoms of complications to report to the physician. Phone numbers for the physician, surgical facility, and emergency care are provided. Clients are informed of the date for their follow-up visit to the physician and told to call and make an appointment. They are also told that a nurse will call the next day to check on their progress and answer any questions.

Inpatient Surgery

Discharge Criteria

The physician determines the client's readiness for discharge from the hospital. Postoperative length of stays vary based on the surgical procedure and the client's individual needs. Before discharge, a complete assessment of the client is done and documented.

Discharge Instructions

Clients and their families are given prescriptions and a copy of written instructions that are signed by the client to indicate understanding before discharge. All necessary teaching is completed before discharge. If more teaching or reinforcement is needed, a referral to a home health nurse can be requested.

The physician orders any fluid, dietary, activity, or work restrictions. Clients are taught wound care, medication information (including side effects), and signs and symptoms of complications to report to the physician. Clients are informed of the date for their follow-up visit to the physician.

HOME HEALTH CARE

The role of the home health nurse is to assist the client in the recovery process. A referral to the home health nurse is made when the client requires (1) continued assistance with skilled nursing interventions, such as wound care, IV medications, or ostomy care; (2) additional teaching to be able to perform self-care, such as diabetic teaching for a newly diagnosed diabetic client or ostomy care; (3) assessment of the recovery process; or (4) assistance due to weakness, lack of social support, or development of complications. Care provided in the home is adapted to the client's resources and environment to facilitate compliance.

HOME HEALTH HINTS

- When a client comes home from surgery, the home care nurse can help give direction to the family to prepare the room where the client will be staying:
  - It is helpful if the room can be on the same floor with the bathroom, kitchen, and living space.
  - If an extended recovery period or illness is expected, the den or living room might be considered to provide room for equipment and make companionship easier. The client can see activity in the home and be included in family activity. Also caregivers can be more attentive to the client's needs and save countless footsteps.
- Special equipment may be needed that include the following:
  - For the client on bed rest, a hospital bed offers the safety and convenience of full side rails, a variety of position changes, and better height for the caregiver.
  - Draw sheets made of folded twin sheets will be needed, as well as extra pillows for positioning.
  - A bedside stand will be needed for personal and toilet articles.
  - A bedside commode can be placed near the bed if the client cannot walk to the bathroom. A bedpan or urinal may be needed. A functional female urinal is easier to use than a bedpan.
  - A flexible tube with a shower head that connects to the bathtub faucet is convenient and allows the client more independence for bathing.
  - Grab bars, tub stools, and skid-proofing of a shower or tub are important safety measures to help prevent falls.
- If equipment is billed to insurance companies or Medicare, a physician must order it.
- It is helpful for caregivers to keep a notebook in the hospital and continue it at home. Treatments, medicines, observations, procedures, doctor and nurse visits, instructions, and therapies with dates and times can be recorded. This helps prevent confusion, prepares the next caregiver, and affords better organization of time and resources for everyone. It can also be nice to see who visited the client.
- Families of clients recovering from surgery should provide items that will keep the client occupied and comfortable (e.g., talking books, inspirational reading material, pictures, and the client's favorite pajamas, robe and slippers, and coverlet).

Home health care workers can include assistants who help with activities of daily living and household chores, LPNs/LVNs who provide basic nursing care, and registered nurses who perform client assessments, teaching, and complex nursing care. The frequency of visits is determined by the client's needs. The RN can contact the physician from the client's phone for orders for abnormal findings.

Review Questions

1. Which one of the following is a priority LPN/LVN client care role in the preoperative phase?
   a. Assisting in data collection
   b. Explaining the surgical procedure
   c. Obtaining preoperative orders
   d. Providing informed consent

2. When the nurse is caring for a preoperative client who expresses a fear of dying, which of the following is the best action for the nurse to take?
   a. Tell the client everything will be all right
   b. Explain the national death rate from surgery
   c. Allow the client time to express concerns
   d. Ask the family to comfort the client

3. The nurse is reviewing the medication history of a new preoperative client who is NPO. The nurse notes that the client has been on long-term oral steroid therapy. Which of the following actions should be taken by the nurse to reduce potential complications related to steroid use?
   a. Ensure that the physician is informed of steroid history
   b. Hold steroid medication while the client is NPO
   c. Administer the steroid medication topically
   d. Monitor vital signs and document

4. When teaching the elderly preoperative client, which of the following is a teaching strategy that improves learning?
   a. Sit near a window with bright sunlight
   b. Use large black-on-white printed materials
   c. Sit beside client
   d. Use blue and green materials

5. Which one of the following related to the client providing consent for surgery is within the LPN/LVN's scope of practice?
   a. Obtaining informed consent
   b. Providing informed consent
   c. Answering surgical procedure questions
   d. Requesting client questions be referred to physician

6. Which of the following is an intraoperative outcome for the surgical client?
   a. Verbalizes fears
   b. Demonstrates leg exercises

c. Remains free from injury
d. States understanding of discharge instructions

7. Which one of the following is the priority nursing responsibility in the PACU?
   a. Monitoring urine output
   b. Maintaining a patent airway
   c. Assessing readiness for discharge
   d. Administering pain medication

8. Which one of the following may be the earliest indicator of hemorrhage or shock that should be reported?
   a. Tachycardia
   b. Polyuria
   c. Nausea
   d. Fever

9. Which one of the following does early postoperative ambulation help prevent?
   a. Increased peristalsis
   b. Coughing
   c. Thrombophlebitis
   d. Wound healing

10. Which one of the following would indicate that the client's diet could be resumed?
    a. Absence of flatus
    b. Bowel sounds every 8 seconds
    c. Excessive thirst
    d. Absent bowel sounds

11. Which one of the following actions should the nurse take if evisceration occurs?
    a. Have client sit upright in a chair
    b. Discontinue intravenous fluids
    c. Apply sterile saline–moistened dressings
    d. Encourage clear oral fluids

12. Which one of the following should be encouraged by the nurse to help prevent atelectasis?
    a. Incentive spirometry use
    b. Holding breath while moving
    c. Restricting fluids
    d. Leg exercises

13. When the LPN/LVN is assisting the client to use an incentive spirometer, which one of the following client instructions would be most appropriate?
    a. Exhale five times before inhaling
    b. Inhale deeply until target reached
    c. Do not hold breath after inhaling
    d. Exhale deeply until target reached

14. Which one of the following is a criterion for discharge from ambulatory surgery?
    a. Ability to drive an automobile
    b. Ability to ambulate 50 feet
    c. Being pain free
    d. No nausea or vomiting

ANSWERS TO CRITICAL THINKING

CRITICAL THINKING: Mrs. Wood

1. Moaning occasionally, moving legs restlessly, pulling covers near abdominal incision.
2. By actual observations: occasional moaning, restless leg movements, and pulling of covers near abdominal incision. By client's statement: "It hurts."

   Because Mrs. Wood is too drowsy to use the pain scale, other data are used. When Mrs. Wood is more awake, explanation of the pain scale should be reinforced and used.

3. Review pain medication orders to determine if analgesics can be given. Noting that an IV analgesic was given 50 minutes ago and the IM analgesic is ordered every 3 hours, the LPN/LVN should have the physician or pharmacist consulted to determine appropriate time intervals. If the consultation indicates it is time to give the analgesic, the LPN/LVN verifies that vital signs are still stable and then gives the analgesic. The LPN/LVN should also consider other pain relief measures such as client warmth, positioning, or environmental issues such as bright lighting, room temperature, and noise.

4. After administration of the analgesic, Mrs. Wood's pain level should be assessed in at least 30 minutes to determine pain relief. If Mrs. Wood is asleep, she should not be awakened unless the nurse determines it is necessary. Nonverbal cues should be observed and respirations counted and documented. If no indication of pain is noted, Mrs. Wood's pain level should be monitored by the nurse at least hourly or as needed.

5. Document pain level and have the physician notified of inadequate pain relief. The client should not be allowed to wait the 3-hour time interval in pain. Consider other pain relief measures to provide while the physician is being notified.

REFERENCES

1. Mullen, JL: Consequences of malnutrition in the surgical patient. Surg Clin North Am 61:465, 1981.
2. Reilly, JJ, Jr: Preoperative and postoperative care of standard and high risk surgical patients. Hematol Oncol Clin North Am 11(3)449, 1997.
3. Scher, KS: Studies on the duration of antibiotic administration for surgical prophylaxis. Am Surg 63(1):59, 1997.
4. Matuschka, PR, et al: A new standard of care: Administration of preoperative antibiotics in the operating room. Am Surg 63(6):500, 1997.
5. Levy, RA: Ethnic and racial differences in response to medicines: Preserving individualized therapy in managed pharmaceutical programmes. Pharm Med 7:139, 1993.

6. Thomas, C (ed): Taber's Cyclopedic Medical Dictionary, ed 18. FA Davis, Philadelphia, 1997.
7. Acute Pain Management Guideline Panel: Acute Pain Management: Operative or Medical Procedures and Trauma. Clinical Practice Guideline. AHCPR Pub No 92-0032. Agency for Health Care Policy and Research, Public Health Service, US Department of Health and Human Services, Rockville, Md, 1992.
8. Pasero, C, and McCaffery, M: Pain in the elderly. Am J Nurs 96(10):39, 1996.
9. Bell, ML: Postoperative pain management for the cognitively impaired older adult. Semin Perioper Nurs 6(1):37, 1997.

BIBLIOGRAPHY

Acute Pain Management Guideline Panel: Acute Pain Management in Adults: Operative Procedures. Quick Reference Guide for Clinicians. AHCPR Pub No 92-0019. Agency for Health Care Policy and Research, Public Health Service, US Department of Health and Human Services, Rockville, Md, 1992.

Association of Operating Room Nurses: Proposed recommended practices for establishing and maintaining a sterile field. AORN J 63(1):211, 1996.

Association of Operating Room Nurses: Patient outcomes: Standards of perioperative care. AORN J 65(2):408, 1997.

Cunningham, MF, Monson, B, and Bookbinder, M: Introducing a music program in the perioperative area. AORN J 66(4):674, 1997.

Chung, F, Ritchie, E, and Su, J: Postoperative pain in ambulatory surgery. Anesth Analg 85(4):808, 1997.

Heiser, R, et al: The use of music during the immediate postoperative recovery period. AORN J 65(4):777, 1997.

Hopf, HW, et al: Wound tissue oxygen tension predicts the risk of wound infection in surgical patients. Arch Surg 132(9):997, 1997.

Lancaster, K: Patient teaching in ambulatory surgery. Nurs Clin North Am 32(2):417, 1997.

Le, TH, et al: Outpatient bowel preparation for elective colon resection. South Med J 90(5):526, 1997.

Leske, JS: Anxiety of elective surgical patients' family members. AORN J 57:1091, 1993.

Mitchell, M: Patients' perceptions of pre-operative preparation for day surgery. J Adv Nurs 26(2):356, 1997.

Pontieri-Lewis, V: The role of nutrition in wound healing. Medsurg Nurs 6(4):187, 1997.

Ruzicka, S: The impact of normal aging processes and chronic illness on perioperative care of the elderly. Semin Perioper Nurs 6(1):3, 1997.

Stienstra, R, et al: Double-blind comparison of alizapride, droperidol and ondansetron in the treatment of post-operative nausea. Eur J Anaesthesiol 14(3):290, 1997.

Tusek, DL, et al: Guided imagery: A significant advance in the care of patient undergoing elective colorectal surgery. Dis Colon Rectum 40(2):172, 1997.

Tusek, DL, Church JM, and Fazio, VW: Guided imagery as a coping strategy for perioperative patients. AORN J 66(4):644, 1997.

Vernon, S, and Molnar Pfeifer, G: Are you ready for bloodless surgery? Am J Nurs 97(9):40, 1997.

Wattsman, TA, and Davies, RS: The utility of preoperative laboratory testing in general surgery patients for outpatient procedures. Am Surg 63(1):81, 1997.

Webb, MR, and Kennedy, MG: Behavior responses and self-reported pain in postoperative patients. J Post Anesth Nurs 9:91, 1994.

Ziegler, DB, and Prior, MM: Preparation for surgery and adjustment to hospitalization. Nurs Clin North Am 29:655, 1994.

Understanding Aging and Chronic Illness

Influence of Age on Health and Illness

Kathy Culliton

Learning Objectives

Upon completion of this chapter, the student will be able to:

1. Identify aspects of the whole person and ways they affect client care.
2. Define health and illness.
3. Explain the nurse's role in promoting health.
4. Identify eight developmental stages.
5. Explain common health needs in the adolescent and adult developmental stages.

Key Words

developmental stage (DEE-vell-up-**MEN**-tal STAYJ)
health (HELLTH)
illness (**ILL**-ness)

Health and Illness

Nurses often care for individuals who are ill and need assistance to meet their basic needs. Because nurses mainly care for ill clients, it may be difficult to visualize or imagine the client healthy and productive outside of the health care agency. Nurses need to develop a working understanding of **health,** wellness, and **illness** that positively affects their nursing care of clients. A person is made up of physical, psychological, cultural, sociological, and spiritual aspects. All of these aspects need to be considered when studying health, wellness, and illness.

LEARNING TIP

To foster understanding of how an ill client, especially the older client, was once healthy and active, ask family members to bring in photos showing the client at various ages or engaged in favorite activities. Displaying these photos in the client's room or on a hallway bulletin board allows caregivers to see the client in times that are not associated with illness.

Aspects of the Whole Person

PHYSICAL ASPECT OF A WHOLE PERSON

The physical part of the whole person includes all systems and structures of the body. When a person's health or illness is discussed, the person's physical attributes are usually described. Health is often described physically by using such phrases as bright eyes, good posture, "spring in their step," good muscle tone, and glowing skin. An ill person may be described as pale or flushed, swollen or reddened, vomiting or bleeding. Clients describe physical complaints, such as "I have a headache," "My stomach hurts," or "I itch all over," when they are experiencing physical illness.

PSYCHOLOGICAL ASPECT OF THE WHOLE PERSON

The psychological aspect of a person encompasses how individuals think and feel, their self-concept, and their responses to stress. This is often referred to as mental health. Mental health is demonstrated by communication and behavior patterns that are appropriate to the situation, such as eye contact and verbal interaction with the health care worker, use of good judgment in problem solving, and orientation to person, place, time, and environment. Unlike physical health and illness, there usually are no outward physical signs that are clues to a client's mental health. Psychological illness involves problems such as confusion, depression, fear, anger, nervousness, personality disorders, or psychoses. Individuals experiencing psychological illness often report feeling depressed, anxious, or confused. Observing communication and behavior is often the best way to evaluate the psychological aspect of the whole person. Clients who avoid eye contact, refuse to speak or respond to questions, wring their hands, talk to themselves or to people that are not there, or inappropriately use a toothbrush to comb their hair may be experiencing psychological illness. (See Chapter 55.)

CULTURAL ASPECT OF THE WHOLE PERSON

Culture includes race, ethnic background, language, and communication, along with culturally defined habits, customs, and beliefs. Culture also involves values that define acceptable and unacceptable behaviors, taboos, or restrictions. Illness in a cultural context may have nothing to do with the physical or psychological aspects of health. Individuals who are not following culturally defined customs may be shunned or censured by their family or community. Banishment or isolation may be a consequence for breaking cultural codes. People living outside of their cultural community may experience stress due to a lack of resources available to meet cultural customs or traditions. Language barriers may block the ability to communicate cultural needs or beliefs. Cultural health is demonstrated through the ability to express and practice cultural values and beliefs, according to what is defined as acceptable by the family or community. (See Chapter 3.)

SOCIOLOGICAL ASPECT OF THE WHOLE PERSON

Friends, educational background, job skills, social status, and economic resources are all parts of a person's sociological aspect. When individuals have the necessary support and resources to operate effectively within their family and community, they demonstrate sociological health. Sociological illness may be manifested as a lack of resources to meet one's needs, no available family members to provide support, or a lack of money to buy food. Divorce, neighborhood crime, and contaminated water are examples of factors that can contribute to sociological illness. Isolation or ineffective individual coping can result from sociological illness.

SPIRITUAL ASPECT OF THE WHOLE PERSON

Spirituality is how one connects with the world. It involves the soul, a sense of belonging or being a part of the whole, and includes hope, faith, and purpose. The choice and practice of religion are a part of the spiritual aspect of an individual. A strong sense of purpose, direction within life, and a vision for the future are signs of spiritual health. If people are unable to participate in religious services or practices, they may have spiritual distress. One of the best examples of spiritual illness is the expression of hopelessness. Anger or losing a sense of purpose or meaning are also expressions of spiritual illness.

HEALTH AND ILLNESS OF THE WHOLE PERSON

Often health and illness are seen as direct opposites. If people are ill, they cannot be healthy, and if people are healthy, it means they are not ill. Using the concept of the whole person, health is a balance and harmony of the physical, psychological, cultural, sociological, and spiritual aspects of the individual. Words such as *normal* or *perfect* might be used to define this harmony.

Is perfection or perfect harmony the correct definition of health? Are *health* and *illness* really mutually exclusive terms? To answer this consider the following examples. The covers of popular magazines often have pictures of models and celebrities who are the "pictures of health." Outwardly, their physical appearance is one of health, but they may have an eating disorder, marital problems, drug addictions, or bipolar disease. Therefore the picture portraying them as healthy is misleading because there is an imbalance in their life.

Consider the paralysis that Christopher Reeve, an actor, experienced after his fall from a horse. The accident caused him to lose movement of his arms and legs and most sensation. In interviews, he acknowledges the devastating effect of the paralysis on his life. However, since the accident, he directs movies, raises money for spine injury research, and maintains his family role. The physical imbalance is evident here, but there has been an adaptation to the physical disability through the use of medical equipment. A sense of purpose, supportive relationships, productivity, and a hope for a cure contribute to an increase in the balance toward health. Christopher Reeve as an actor was the picture of health. Does Christopher Reeve who is paralyzed also have a level of health?

The concept of illness is one of imbalance or disharmony due to a problem that causes one to be sick. Physical causes of illness are usually easily recognized. Examples include *Escherichia coli*, a bacterium that is eaten in undercooked contaminated meat; exercise that induces an asthma attack in an asthmatic person; or a fall that causes bones to be broken. In applying the concept of the whole person, illness can also be the result of a psychological, sociological, cultural, or spiritual imbalance. After the loss of a spouse, one may experience loneliness and depression and a loss of balance in the social and psychological aspects of life. A hospitalization may increase disharmony if cultural beliefs and practices are not understood or upheld by health care providers. A person faced with a terminal diagnosis may lose hope and direction in life, causing anxiety and despair.

So rather than being exclusive concepts, health and illness are dynamic and ever-changing states of being. The whole person model defines level of wellness on a very personal level. This definition is ever changing depending on the "health balance" that the individual maintains. A health crisis such as a myocardial infarction (MI) overwhelms a client's ability to maintain a normal level of wellness. Two months after the MI, however, this same client could be enjoying a higher level of wellness than before the MI because the client has lost weight, is walking daily, and is eating a nutritious low-fat diet. This client mobilized all of the aspects of his whole person to manage the physical problems with lifestyle changes. Wellness is a very personal expression of the balance between health and illness.

CRITICAL THINKING: Jim

Jim, age 30, was in a motorcycle accident. Luckily, he was wearing a helmet when he lost control of his bike on a patch of sand. Unfortunately, he was only wearing a T-shirt, shorts, and tennis shoes. As a result, he has multiple abrasions and deep cuts that were sutured on his left lateral leg, hip, and buttocks. His right arm was also broken, and surgery was required to stabilize the fracture with pins. His right arm is casted. His hands and left shoulder have deep abraded areas. He is in a lot of pain.

How are these physical changes going to affect the physical, psychological, cultural, sociological, and spiritual aspects of Jim's life?

Answers at end of chapter.

The Nurse's Role in Supporting and Promoting Wellness

When young children are asked "What does a nurse do?" they usually say things like "A nurse gives shots," "A nurse changes bandages," "A nurse helps the doctor," or "A nurse helps people feel better." When a nurse cares for a person, the total picture of that client's wellness is the focus of nursing care. The goal of nursing care can best be defined as helping clients achieve their highest possible level of wellness. To do this, the nurse must consider the client's strengths, assets, and resources, as well as weaknesses, liabilities, and disabilities. The nurse also encourages the client to take a personal inventory and recognize what is required to attain wellness. Working together, the nurse, client, family, and other members of the health care team set wellness goals and develop a plan of action that will help meet those goals. The plan of care focuses on six main areas: (1) mobilizing resources, (2) providing a safe and adaptable environment, (3) assisting the client to learn about his or her health problem and treatment, (4) performing and teaching the client to perform health care procedures, (5) anticipating problems and recognizing potential crises, and (6) evaluating the plan and progress toward the goals with the client and family. (See Home Health Hints at end of chapter.)

Life Span Issues in Health and Illness

Promoting health and high-level wellness does not take place just when someone suffers a major physical trauma or illness. Health promotion occurs throughout life and is aimed at anticipating and preventing potential threats to health. The **developmental stages** of life focus on the balance an individual needs to achieve for high-level wellness within that stage.

Each developmental stage in life is identified by the extremes of total resolution and unresolved conflict. The experiences, changes, and crises of each stage involve a spectrum of dilemmas and developmental tasks that must be addressed and resolved by the well-adjusted individual. Across the life span at various ages and stages of life there are recognized potential threats to the health of the whole person. Risk factors may be related to growth and development, physical attributes, family, behavior, social interactions, environment, lifestyle choices, and ethnic background.

Developmental stages begin at birth and continue through death. Erik Erickson proposed eight stages of development: 0 to 1 year—trust versus mistrust; 2 to 3 years—autonomy versus shame and doubt; 4 to 5 years—initiative versus guilt; 6 to 12 years—industry versus inferiority; 13 to 18 years—identity versus role confusion; young adult—intimacy versus isolation; middle-aged adult—generativity versus self-absorption; old adult—ego integrity versus despair.[1,2] This chapter will examine some of the unique health promotion needs for the developmental stages, beginning with adolescents.

THE ADOLESCENT

Adolescence is the growth and development period that bridges the time between childhood and becoming a young adult. Generally, an adolescent is age 13 to 18. In his theory of psychological development, Erik Erickson identified adolescence as the fifth stage of development, at which time a young person works to develop an identity, or sense of self. The teenage years are also a time of physical growth, increased influence of peers and social forces outside of the family, and sexual maturation.

Common Adolescent Health Concerns

Teenagers are generally concerned about their appearance. Complexion problems such as acne are important to teens. Most teenagers experience increased production of sebum by the sebaceous glands. If the gland is clogged with sebum, it forms a whitehead or blackhead, which are called comedones. The trapped sebum may become infected, leading to redness, pain, and tenderness of the comedones. Teenagers need to be encouraged to gently clean their skin and promote drainage of the sebaceous glands by removing dead skin and debris from the skin. Products that dry the skin and close the openings to the sebaceous glands, such as alcohol, should be avoided. An exfoliating product such as benzoyl peroxide opens up and drains the sebaceous glands and accelerates the shedding of the outer layer of the epidermis. This can cause initial redness and chafing of the skin. Any adolescent who has pustular infected lesions, as with acne vulgaris, should be referred to a dermatologist for treatment, which may include antibiotic therapy. Infected red lesions and lesions that are squeezed or picked can leave permanent areas of scarring.

Nutritional requirements for teens are of concern for health promotion. During periods of growth, the body needs more calories and nutrients to grow effectively. Teenagers are making more independent food choices and need good information about what nutrients their bodies require. Fast food and snack foods are high in fat and calories and contribute to obesity problems for teens. A special dietary need for teens is adequate intake of calcium and vitamin D, which are both necessary for growing bones and teeth. The primary source of calcium and vitamin D is milk that is vitamin D fortified.

Teens should be taught to make nutritionally sound diet choices by choosing fruits and vegetables instead of chocolate bars and potato chips. Distorted body image leads to dangerous restrictive diets and eating behaviors. Rigid dieting can lead to serious malnutrition. Anorexia nervosa and bulimia are life-threatening eating disorders that usually begin during adolescence. Teens who are underweight and are not eating or are eating and then vomiting need to be referred for a medical evaluation.

Sexual identity and sexual expression are another challenge for the adolescent. Boys and girls need to have access to information about sexual development and need to be able to ask questions. Appropriate sexual expression is a struggle for many teens. The way they dress and behave and the people they associate with are part of the exploration to find their identity. Many teens choose to be sexually active, which is a high-risk behavior. Sexually active teens risk contracting sexually transmitted diseases such as chlamydia, gonorrhea, herpes, and human immunodeficiency virus (HIV) and acquired immunodeficiency syndrome (AIDS). Most teens do not plan ahead for sexual intercourse and often do not discuss contraception or safer sex measures with their partner. Sexually active adolescent girls are at high risk for unplanned pregnancies.

The vigorous physical activity that many adolescents engage in increases the risk for traumatic physical injuries. Contact and competitive sports and other physical activities require professional instruction and supervision for adequate warm-ups, appropriate fitness level, and use of proper protective equipment. Teens need positive reinforcement of the good lifestyle practice of exercise and encouragement to make exercise a lifelong habit that is carried on into adulthood.

Trying to determine a sense of identity can create a great deal of stress in teenagers. They are notorious for "going the extra mile" in trying to find an identity separate from their parents and other adults. They test the boundaries of acceptable behavior and often test established rules, social codes, and laws. Involvement in crimes and gangs, using drugs and alcohol, smoking or chewing tobacco, and driving recklessly over the speed limit are high-risk behaviors in this age group. Teens need to be aware of the consequences of high-risk behavior. Programs offered by schools and communities are available to help teens identify and avoid high-risk situations and deal effectively with peer pressure.

The quest for identity for adolescents can be very painful and may lead to depression. One of the most tragic problems for teenagers is the high rate of attempted and actual suicides. Individuals who work or live with teens need to carefully listen and observe for clues that teens have lost hope, purpose, or direction in their young lives. Expressions of the desire to end one's life are always taken seriously. The teen should be immediately evaluated by a mental health professional for diagnosis and treatment.

 CRITICAL THINKING: Marcus

Marcus, age 16, refuses to go to school because he says he "looks like something out of a horror film" due to his acne. His self-image and social interactions are being negatively affected by his complexion problems.

1. What would be helpful to teach Marcus about promoting good skin health?

and developed through fondness, understanding, caring, or love. When this stage is not successfully resolved, the individual often experiences isolation from others. This stage encompasses ages 18 to 45. Physically, growth is usually completed by age 20. Socially, young adults begin to move away from their parents to develop their own families (Fig. 12–1). The young adult begins to work to develop a place in society through school, work, and social activities (Fig. 12–2). This is the stage where intimacy or closeness develops with partners and friends. The decision to marry, have children, or have a pet is demonstration of the individual striving for intimacy. Challenges to intimacy are tasks that must be overcome in this stage. Within a marriage, financial issues, communication, and the needs of children must be successfully met to maintain the marriage.

There are cultural issues facing the young adult. Melding one's traditions and customs with the traditions and customs of a spouse, family, or friends is a major responsibility, as is the passing on of culture to children. Values and beliefs, which arise from an individual's culture or conscience, serve as guidelines for behavior.

Common Health Concerns

As with adolescents, the lifestyle choices of young adults may place their health at risk. Health promotion for this age group is mainly focused on preventing or limiting possible risk factors. Young adults need to understand the importance of diet and exercise in maintaining health. They are also in the position of teaching these lifelong habits to their children. Positive health practices in young adulthood help prevent long-term complications. Maintaining an aerobic exercise program and following a diet that is low in fat helps keep weight down and avoid obesity, along with promoting cardiovascular health. Blood cholesterol should be kept below 200 mg/dL. Avoiding sun exposure and using sunscreen are important to avoid sunburn and permanent sun damage to the skin. Years of sun exposure may

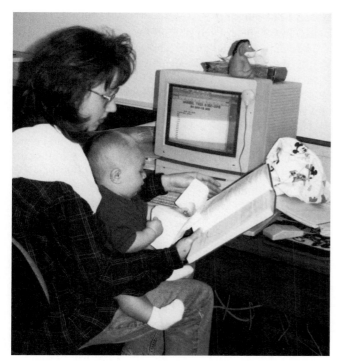

Figure 12–1. Young adults develop their own families. (From Anderson, M: Nursing Leadership, Management and Professional Practice for the LPN/LVN. FA Davis, Philadelphia, 1997, p 191, with permission.)

  2. What are some coping skills Marcus could use to deal with his concerns?

     Answers at end of chapter.

THE YOUNG ADULT

Developing intimacy is the sixth psychological development task. The young adult's task is to develop relationships with a spouse, family, or friends that are warm, affectionate,

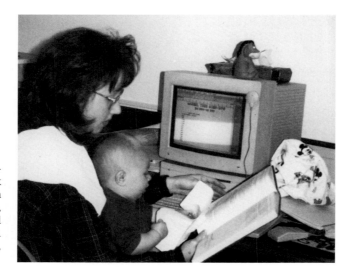

Figure 12–2. A young adult interviewing for a job to fulfill the task of entering the work world. (From Anderson, M: Nursing Leadership, Management and Professional Practice for the LPN/LVN. FA Davis, Philadelphia, 1997, p 65, with permission.)

cause skin cancer. Habits, such as smoking, started in the teen years are carried through young adulthood. More and more information is becoming available that directly links cigarette smoking to chronic bronchitis, emphysema, and lung cancer in later life.

In the early part of young adulthood, the individual is preparing for the work world with a college or vocational education or is in the workforce. Being a novice in the work world and accepting new independence, freedom, and responsibilities can introduce stressors into the young adult's life. Unfortunately, overeating, use of alcohol or drugs, smoking cigarettes, and family violence are all negative lifestyle choices and poor coping mechanisms for stress. Young adults need to be aware of their individual stress and be encouraged to develop positive coping mechanisms for stress. Exercise, support groups, music, and meditation are just a few positive ways to cope with stress.

Although marriage commonly occurs within this age group, it has the highest rate of divorce. Trying to make a marriage work is a hard task. The blending of two people into a couple requires a lot of creative communication and loving care. When the stressors overwhelm the couple's coping mechanisms or coping strategy, the marriage relationship is in trouble. Sometimes because of the high rate of divorce many couples choose to live together without being married. The avoidance of making a commitment often sets these relationships up for failure.

As with the adolescent, if young adults are sexually active with multiple partners, they are at risk for sexually transmitted diseases. Safer sex guidelines and information on birth control should be available for the sexually active young adult.

Pregnancy is a common health occurrence for women in this age group. Because research indicates that a mother's health practices directly affect the health of the developing fetus, nutrition, drug and alcohol use, physical health, and effective stress coping mechanisms are lifestyle issues that need to be discussed with every pregnant woman. Prenatal care should be encouraged and readily available to pregnant women.

CRITICAL THINKING: Rita

Rita, age 25, and her husband are trying to start a family. Rita visits her physician, who confirms that she is pregnant.

What information and health practices should Rita and her husband be instructed in during a prenatal health examination?

Answers at end of chapter.

THE MIDDLE-AGED ADULT

People age 45 to 65 are considered to be in the middle adult years. The psychological developmental task of this age group is developing generativity. Generativity is demonstrated by a concern and support for others along with a vision for future generations. The negative outcome or unresolved conflict would be preoccupation with personal needs or self-absorption. Physically, middle adults start to notice signs of decreased endurance and intolerance for physical exercise if they have not maintained healthy lifestyle choices. Socially, their children are adolescents or young adults who require extra attention and assistance with entering adulthood. Along with this, middle-aged adults may also be faced with the challenging demands of caring for aging parents. Middle adults also look over their lives and assess accomplishments versus unrealized goals. Midlife crisis occurs as this self-inspection leads to a desire to change work, social, or family situations to try to meet unrealized goals. Planning for retirement by developing meaningful pastimes and interests outside of work and preparing for financial security is another important task during this period.

Common Health Concerns

Adverse health choices, such as smoking, use of alcohol, drug use, sedentary lifestyles, diet high in saturated fat, and being overweight, often have serious consequences for middle adulthood. Hypertension and heart disease are major health concerns, as are chronic bronchitis, emphysema, and lung cancer. Cardiovascular disease and cancer cause most of the deaths in this age group. However, middle adulthood is not too late to initiate lifestyle changes that positively affect health. Replacing high-risk habits with lifestyle choices such as regular exercise, healthful eating, weight reduction, and positive stress coping mechanisms are positive challenges. Helping adults recognize the benefits of these lifestyle choices and empowering them to change is the major challenge for health care professionals for this age group.

CRITICAL THINKING: Paul

Fifty-four-year-old Paul calls the doctor's office for the fourth time this month complaining of severe indigestion and requesting a medication that will work to fix it. He has refused to have any x-rays or other diagnostic tests because he "can't fit them into" his "busy schedule." Paul has his own insurance business. His wife quit her job to monitor the activities of their 13-year-old son, who was not going to school every day. The couple's twin daughters are both in college out of state.

1. Why might Paul be experiencing health problems?
2. What is affecting the developmental tasks Paul needs to meet?

Answers at end of chapter.

THE OLDER ADULT

Development and *aging* seem to be terms that are directly opposite because aging is commonly viewed as deterioration or a "downhill slide" to inevitable death. This negative view of aging is supported by cultures that idolize and strive to maintain youthfulness. Being old is equated with outliving one's usefulness. However, individuals are living productive, fulfilling lives even into their eighties, nineties, and one hundreds. Many of these older adults are likely to be found working in their garden, exercising at the gym, participating in church activities, or volunteering at the local community hospital or with other organizations (Fig. 12–3).

The developmental goal for people 65 years of age or older is integrity versus despair. Health state, environment, relationships, and lifestyle choices influence the diversity found in this group of people. Physical health is often a concern for older adults. Chronic health problems that require medication and treatment often also require lifestyle changes or adaptations. Because psychological development for the older adult is characterized by striving for integrity, older adults often spend time reflecting over their lives. Integrity is measured by feeling satisfied with having

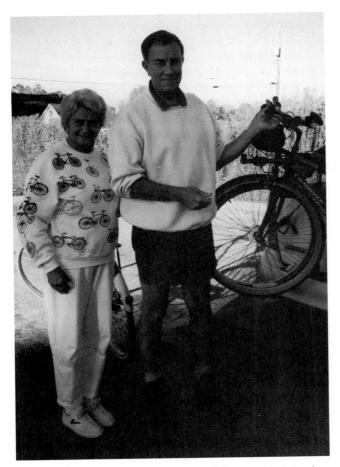

Figure 12–3. Socialization helps older adults maintain integrity.

lived a full and productive life. When this life reflection is characterized by misgivings, missed opportunities, dissatisfaction, and disappointment, the older adult feels hopeless despair.

Coping with loss is a major challenge for older adults. Life events such as retirement, illness, or death of a spouse and changes such as decreased physical ability are losses facing older adults. Coping with aging is also influenced by the individual's cultural beliefs. Cultural viewpoints on the social role and value of aged members affect the health of older adults. Sometimes, the greatest loss for older adults is their lack of connection with the world and a lack being part of a greater purpose.

Common Health Concerns

As a person ages, the incidence of chronic illness and disability increases. Unfortunately, these chronic diseases often limit an older person's ability to be independent in self-care and activities of daily living.

Hypertension is common, as are the incidence of heart disease and strokes in this age group. Managing blood pressure, losing weight, eating a low-fat diet, not smoking, enhancing effective stress coping strategies, and regular exercise decrease the potential for cardiovascular disease. Changes in mobility and chronic pain may limit an older person's activity and impede an active lifestyle. Impaired vision can be caused by decreased peripheral vision, macular degeneration, cataracts, or glaucoma and can severely limit an older adult's function. One of the most dramatic losses for many older adults is not being able to safely drive a car. This is usually associated with a loss of independence and free will. Many older adults continue to drive during the day but not at night because of night vision problems. Decreased hearing is also a common health concern for older adults. Loss of high-pitch discrimination and reduced ability to filter background noises cause older adults to hear background noise and rumbling clearer than they hear a one-to-one conversation in a crowded room. Social stigmas related to memory changes such as forgetfulness, dementia, and senility are a serious worry for many older adults. The elderly often confuse their own depression with senility and attempt to hide their symptoms rather than seek treatment.

As a result of these changes in older people's health, the nurse needs to focus on assisting older adults to meet their physical, psychological, cultural, sociological, and spiritual needs. Nurses can help older adults be more creative in living productive and satisfying lives. Encouraging the use of community services for seniors and promoting self-care are important functions of the nurse. Most older adults continue to live in their own homes or apartments, but impairment in mobility and the ability to carry out instrumental activities of daily living, which include shopping for groceries, preparing meals, and cleaning and maintaining a home, threaten their independence. Having to ask or pay others to perform tasks that they formerly were able to do themselves is seen as a significant loss by many older adults. Adding in the loss of a spouse, the death of friends, or the lack of social contacts may further isolate an older person, leading to depression and hopelessness. The accumulation of losses can overwhelm an older adult's resources and coping mechanisms and is related to a high rate of suicide, especially for older men. Suicide is the ultimate expression of hopelessness.

Older adults need to be encouraged to remain active and to continue to pursue interests. Most communities have transportation services such as buses and vans that operate to meet the needs of older adults. Senior centers offer diverse programs and services to older adults. Some senior groups are focused on community service; others mainly plan trips or sponsor activities such as dances or bowling leagues (Fig. 12–4). Seniors also have opportunities to continue to work in areas of interest as volunteers. Schools, hospitals, nursing facilities, parks, museums, zoos, community theaters, and youth groups all welcome older adult volunteers. Colleges and universities offer discounted tuition for senior citizens, and there are elder hostel programs across the country, which are programs especially designed for older adults. Elder hostels offer a wide variety of programs such as learning photography, Civil War history, nature survival, bird watching, and painting.

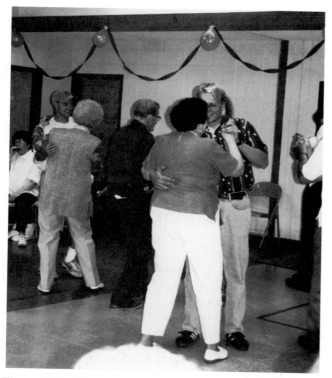

Figure 12–4. Older adults can remain active by participating in activities such as dances. (From Anderson, M: Nursing Leadership, Management and Professional Practice for the LPN/LVN. FA Davis, Philadelphia, 1997, p 200, with permission.)

Falls are a serious concern for older adults. Falls and accidents can be prevented by in-home safety assessments and altering the home environment to ensure the safety of the older adult. Bathrooms should be equipped with grab bars and nonskid mats. Bath chairs or benches make getting into a bath or shower less risky. Removing clutter, throw rugs, small furniture, and electrical cords is necessary to decrease the potential for the older adult to trip and fall.

Fractures of vertebrae, wrists, and hips are common problems from falls for older adults. Osteoporosis can significantly contribute to causing these types of fractures, which are painful and debilitating. Often hip fractures require surgery for hip replacement or pinning of the bone to stabilize the break. Older adults, especially women, need to have a regular dietary intake of calcium and vitamin D. Calcium intake and weight-bearing exercise work together to maintain bone density and help prevent these types of fractures.

Medication safety is also a health promotion issue for older adults. Many older adults have multiple medications with varied time schedules. Having a caregiver set up a weekly medication box helps prevent underdosing or overdosing with medications (Fig. 12–5). Medication boxes can be simple, plastic boxes or elaborate machines that have light and sound alarms to alert the client that it is time to take the dispensed medication. Older adults should be encouraged to use one pharmacy for all of their medications so the pharmacist has a total picture of all of the medications they are taking. This allows pharmacists to be better able to identify potential drug interactions and to serve as a resource for the older adult.

Death is a natural consequence of living. Although individuals can die at any age, as an individual ages, the probability of dying increases with age. A concern for many older adults is death with dignity. Older adults need to be encouraged to express their wishes for their terminal care to family members and their physician. A living will and advance directives are documents designed to allow older adults to make their wishes for their care known. Often an older adult with a terminal illness will request that they not

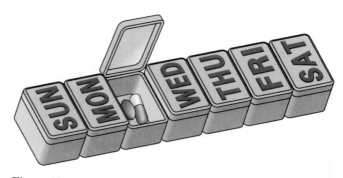

Figure 12–5. Medication boxes can be set up by caregivers to assist with medication compliance.

be resuscitated or placed on life support equipment. Care for these individuals is aimed at providing general high-level comfort care. Caring for older adults who are terminally ill includes supporting a review of their life, promoting pain relief, and assisting them to be as active and involved with their family and their care as they desire and can tolerate.

CRITICAL THINKING: Mrs. Riccardi

Mrs. Riccardi, 87 years old, lives alone in her small apartment. Her daughter and son are both retired and live in the same community. Mrs. Riccardi had a dizzy spell, so her daughter brought her to the hospital emergency department (ED). Upon admission, Mrs. Riccardi's blood pressure was 208/128 and she had blurred vision in the left eye that resolved after 1 hour in the ED. She was diagnosed with hypertension, which had possibly contributed to a small stroke or transient ischemic attack (TIA). Mrs. Riccardi was started on Lasix 20 mg twice a day and Lanoxin 0.125 mg every day. She was discharged to her home. The nurse's discharge plan addressed safety issues.

1. Why might Mrs. Riccardi be at increased risk of falling?
2. What nursing interventions would help promote Mrs. Riccardi's independence and safety?

Answers at end of chapter.

HOME HEALTH HINTS

■ A good way to ease into conversation with clients of various ages who are "quiet" is to give them a manicure. You'll find out a lot about the client's day, his worries, his joys and sorrows. While the home care nurse is "busy with the manicure," rapport is established with the client. Cues will be obtained from the client's conversation regarding needs for care. In addition, a manicure exercises the client's fingers!

■ When the home care nurse teaches a client, it is important to acknowledge the client's knowledge and life experiences. When given a chance, clients tell how they have maintained their health over the years. Use open-ended scenarios for teaching, such as "What would you do if you were alone and fell?" Teaching should occur *with* clients, not *to* them. The nurse is in the client's home, which is a personal place. Client dignity should always remain intact during home care visits and teaching sessions.

Summary

Individuals are composites of the physical, psychological, social, cultural, and spiritual aspects of their lives. The definitions of illness, health, and wellness depend on people's ability to develop and cope with crises and changes in their life. Physical disease, emotional problems, social failures, cultural distance, and spiritual distress are potential life traumas that may challenge clients' health. To effectively care for others, the nurse needs to focus on the whole person. When nurses examine the whole person, they look beyond medical diagnoses and problems to the total being or wellness potential of the individual. Understanding developmental stages and life events that individuals face throughout the life span helps nurses assist the whole client to high-level wellness. The goal, the greatest challenge for clients and nurses, is promoting and achieving the highest level of wellness possible to meet full health potential.

Review Questions

1. Which one of the following may indicate the presence of psychological illness in a client?
   a. Lack of eye contact
   b. Orientation to person, place, time
   c. Ability to problem solve
   d. Verbal interaction with others

2. Which one of the following demonstrates the presence of health?
   a. Physical appearance of health
   b. Balance of the aspects of the whole person
   c. Operate effectively within their family
   d. A strong sense of purpose

3. Which one of the following best defines the goal of nursing care?
   a. To encourage the client to take a personal inventory
   b. To assist in development of a plan of action
   c. To care for physically ill clients
   d. To help clients achieve their highest level of wellness

4. Which one of the following is Erickson's developmental stage for the middle-aged adult?
   a. Generativity versus self-absorption
   b. Identity versus role confusion
   c. Intimacy versus isolation
   d. Integrity versus despair

5. Which one of the following interventions would increase safety for the elderly client?
   a. Restricting driving to the evening
   b. Using the same pharmacy for prescriptions
   c. Setting up one's own weekly medication box
   d. Decreasing intake of calcium and vitamin D

ANSWERS TO CRITICAL THINKING

CRITICAL THINKING: *Jim*

Jim is obviously having physical problems that are affecting his health. As a result of the accident he may fear riding his motorcycle or have nightmares. He may be feeling embarrassed because he had an accident. He may be unable to work or perform any of his usual roles, which may cause financial or family problems. Feelings of being a victim of circumstances may possibly cause some spiritual distress for Jim.

CRITICAL THINKING: *Marcus*

1. Gently clean the skin; remove dead skin and debris from the skin with an exfoliating product such as benzoyl peroxide; avoid alcohol-containing products; see a dermatologist for severe cases; avoid squeezing the skin.

2. Telling a teenager that looks are only skin deep and that every teenager has complexion problems is not helpful. These statements minimize serious concerns about appearance. Concerns should be verbalized by Marcus and discussed with the nurse. Previously used coping skills should be considered for effectiveness. Taking proper care of his skin and remaining active in social activities is important for Marcus to maintain a positive self-image. Planning actions and goals for Marcus's specific concerns should be the focus of the plan of care.

CRITICAL THINKING: *Rita*

Prenatal education information should be offered to Rita and her husband. This education should include an overview of Rita's health needs, what to expect during pregnancy, ways Rita's husband can be supportive, and information on prenatal classes. Rita's physical examination should include a vaginal examination, blood pressure, and blood work. It is important to be aware of any sexually transmitted diseases that may be transferred to the fetus or during birth. A rubella titer (a test for immunity to rubella or measles) is important because of potential birth defects if the mother has rubella while pregnant. Elevated blood glucose may be a sign of diabetes, and low red blood cell counts and low hemoglobin are related to anemia. To prepare a woman for pregnancy, prenatal vitamins or vitamins with iron and folic acid (necessary for effective neural tube development in the first 3 months of pregnancy) are recommended. Because of the increased workload of the heart during pregnancy, blood pressure needs to be closely monitored. A balanced diet, maintaining an exercise program, and continuing to develop effective and positive ways to deal with stress are very important for pregnant women. In preparation for pregnancy, Rita also needs information on the negative effects that cigarette smoking, alcohol use, and drug use can have on the developing fetus.

CRITICAL THINKING: *Paul*

1. Paul's physical health is being affected by poor diet choices, excessive stomach acid secretion, or other gastrointestinal problems and stress.

2. It is easy to recognize the psychological stress related to parenting skills when a child is in trouble. Decreased family income with increased family expenses (two children in college) can cause financial strains and more economic pressure on Paul's business. With family problems or health problems, Paul may be questioning why things are happening to him and his family, causing him spiritual distress.

CRITICAL THINKING: *Mrs. Riccardi*

1. Falls could be caused by environmental problems, such as throw rugs that may move or cause tripping, clutter, electrical cords in walking paths, lack of hand grips in the bathroom, or lack of nonskid mats in the shower or tub. Poor vision and altered depth perception can result in missing a stair step or obstacles. Weakness or orthostatic hypotension can cause an unsteady gait or fall. Lasix can cause urinary urgency and incontinence. If incontinence occurs, falls may result from a wet, slippery floor.

2. It would be important for the nurse to instruct the client and family about home safety. Mrs. Riccardi may even benefit by using a cane or a walker if she is unsteady. Because Mrs. Riccardi lives alone, an emergency alert system, such as a small transmitter that is worn around the neck or wrist with a button that can be activated in emergencies, would be beneficial. When activated, the transmitter alerts an answering service to contact designated individuals to check on the client. Safety with medications is also an important consideration. To avoid forgetting to take medications or taking them too often, a prefilled medication box with daily doses in it is a helpful tool. Clients who take diuretics or other medications that lower blood pressure must be aware of the potential for orthostatic hypotension. Orthostatic hypotension is a drop in blood pressure that happens when a person moves from a lying to sitting or sitting to standing position. It is often accompanied by dizziness or light-headedness. Some people may even faint, causing a fall.

REFERENCES

1. Erickson, EH: Childhood and Society, ed 2. WW Norton, New York, 1963.
2. Erickson, EH: Identity and the Life Cycle. WW Norton, New York, 1980.

BIBLIOGRAPHY

Bakarich, A, McMillan, V, and Prosser, R: The effect of a nursing intervention on the incidence of older patient falls. Aust J Adv Nurs 15(1):26, 1997.

Beers, MH: Explicit criteria for determining potentially inappropriate medication use by the elderly. An update. Arch Intern Med 157(14): 1531, 1997.

Hoeymans, N, et al: Age, time and cohort effect on functional status and self-rated health in elderly men. Am J Public Health 87(10):1620, 1997.

Jones, P, and Meleis, A: Health is empowerment. Adv Nurs Sci 1:1, 1993.

Mueller, C, Schur, C, and O'Connell, J: Prescription drug spending: The impact of age and chronic disease status. Am J Public Health 87(10):1626, 1997.

Mulsant, BH, Ganguli, M, and Seaberg, EC: The relationship between self-rated health and depressive symptoms in an epidemiological sample of community-dwelling older adults. J Am Geriatr Soc 45(8):954, 1997.

Norton, R, et al: Circumstances of falls resulting in hip fractures among older people. J Am Geriatr Soc 45(9):1108, 1997.

Patrick, DL, et al: Validation of preferences for life-sustaining treatment: Implications for advance care planning. Ann Intern Med 27(7):509, 1997.

Pieper, RM, et al: Trends in cholesterol knowledge and screening and hypercholesterolemia awareness and treatment, 1980–1992. The Minnesota Heart Survey. Arch Intern Med 157(20):2326, 1997.

Pender, NJ: Health Promotion in Nursing Practice. Appleton & Lange, Norwalk, Conn, 1996.

Ray, WA, et al: A randomized trial of a consultation service to reduce falls in nursing homes. JAMA 278(7):557, 1997.

Schiffman, SS: Taste and smell losses in normal aging and disease. JAMA 278(16):1357, 1997.

Tremethick, MJ: Thriving, not just surviving. The importance of social support among the elderly. J Psychosoc Nurs Ment Health Serv 35(9):27, 1997.

US Department of Health and Human Services: Healthy People 2000 National Health Promotion and Disease Prevention Objectives. DDHS Pub No (PHS) 91-50212. US Government Printing Office, Washington, DC, 1991.

Nursing Care of Elderly Clients

MaryAnne Pietraniec-Shannon

Learning Objectives

Upon completion of this chapter, the student will be able to:

1. Define aging as a universal yet unique maturational process.
2. Identify basic physiological changes associated with advancing age.
3. Identify basic psychological and cognitive changes associated with advancing age.
4. Discuss how the physiological and psychological changes associated with advancing age affect nursing care for the older client.
5. Identify nursing practices that promote safety for the older client.

Key Words

activities of daily living (ack-**TIV**-i-tees of **DAY**-lee **LIV**-ing)

arrhythmias (uh-**RITH**-mee-yahs)

aspiration (ASS-pi-**RAY**-shun)

cataract (**KAT**-uh-rackt)

constipation (KON-sti-**PAY**-shun)

contractures (kon-**TRACK**-churs)

dementia (dee-**MEN**-cha)

depression (dee-**PRESS**-shun)

edema (uh-**DEE**-muh)

expectorate (eck-**SPECK**-tuh-RAYT)

extrinsic factors (eks-**TRIN**-sik **FAK**-ters)

glaucoma (glaw-**KOH**-mah)

homeostasis (HOH-mee-oh-**STAY**-sis)

intrinsic factors (in-**TRIN**-sik **FAK**-ters)

macular degeneration (**MACK**-you-lar dee-JEN-uh-**RAY**-shun)

nocturia (nock-**TYOO**-ree-ah)

optimum level of functioning (**OP**-teh-mum **LEV**-uhl of **FUNK**-shun-ing)

osteoporosis (AHS-tee-oh-por-**OH**-sis)

perception (per-**SEP**-shun)

pressure ulcer (press-sure **ULL**-sir)

range of motion (RANJE of **MOH**-shun)

reality orientation (ree-**AL**-i-tee OR-ee-en-**TAY**-shun)

sensory deprivation (**SEN**-suh-ree DEP-ri-**VAY**-shun)

sensory overload (**SEN**-suh-ree **OH**-ver-lohd)

urinary incontinence (**YOOR**-i-NAR-ee in-**KON**-ti-nents)

What is Aging?

Over time, it is easy to visually notice changes that occur in the human body. Both the physical structures and the functions that they carry out undergo changes and declines with advancing age. Although there is not one commonly accepted definition or theory to explain these declines over time, there is a common understanding that aging is a universal and normal process that starts at conception and continues until death.

For this chapter, aging is defined as a maturational process that creates the need for individual adaptation because of physical and psychological declines that occur over the period of a lifetime. Even though aging truly begins at conception, the focus in this chapter is on the maturational process that is experienced after the sixth decade of life and will refer to the client at this stage as the older client. This is done with the understanding that the changes dis-

cussed do not suddenly occur in the sixth decade of life, but can and do occur much later in some people and much earlier in others based on a variety of individualized factors.

The individualized factors that determine the occurrence and rate of the declines commonly attributed to aging have been studied from many different perspectives. Although aging is known to be universal, it remains a unique experience when it comes to the individual. Factors that contribute to this process can be grouped into two categories. **Intrinsic factors** focus on such things as the genetic theories of aging, such as biological clock theory or programmed aging theory, and some aspects of physiological theories of aging, such as wear-and-tear theory or stress-adaptation theory. **Extrinsic factors** focus on environmental influences, such as pollutants, free radical theory, and stress-adaptation theory. Regardless of which factors may have the greatest influence on this process of aging, **per-**

ETHICAL CONSIDERATIONS BOX 13-1

Elderly Clients and the Health Care System

Sarah, 93 years old, is admitted through the hospital emergency room (ER) for nonspecific complaints of chest pain and dizziness. This is the fourth time this month that she has come to the hospital with this complaint, and although previous examinations and tests showed no acute disease process, the ER physician believed that because of her age and long history of coronary artery disease, she should be monitored and evaluated more closely. She has no private insurance but is covered under Medicare, parts A and B, with a supplemental from a small insurance company in her state.

Despite her age, Sarah is mentally alert and competent, lives by herself in a small apartment, and manages basic daily care, including shopping and cleaning, with only minimal assistance from friends. She has no living family members except for a few aging cousins in a distant state. She is taking three prescription medications at home.

After a complete physical examination, including several tests and an electrocardiogram, she is scheduled for a cardiac catheterization. A significant block is seen in one of the major coronary arteries, and it is decided to perform angioplasty on the artery. She is admitted to the intensive care unit after the procedure, where she also receives 2 units of blood for an anemia problem. She recovers without incident and is discharged 5 days after her admission. The total cost for her hospitalization, including tests and angioplasty, is more than $18,000.

Sarah is not a typical client for her age group. Many medical experts would categorize the treatment given her as "overtreatment" because of the current emphasis on quality of life, death with dignity, and the futility of treating the hopelessly ill. Yet, as the population of this country continues to age, it is more likely that Sarah will be the norm rather

than the exception. Many ethical and financial issues surround this case.

In an era of cost containment and reform, financial issues are always near the top. The reimbursement system, which is concerned about paying for expensive and complicated procedures, such as angioplasty, which may not necessarily improve the quality of life, and for which there may be less expensive alternatives, causes physicians to select modes of care that the elderly often consider substandard. In general, angioplasty on a 93-year-old would be classified as excessive, yet given this client's mental state and quick return to a normal life, it would appear to be the correct course of action.

The elderly, through the various entitlement programs, consume a relatively large proportion of the national budget. This cost is borne primarily by young and middle-aged workers through their taxes.

The problems posed by an ever-aging population will become worse as the next century approaches. Decisions will have to be made about where it is best to spend the limited resources available for health care. Basic questions, such as whether it is better to spend $0.65 to immunize a 4-year-old or to spend $10,000 to perform an angioplasty on a 103-year-old woman, will challenge health care providers of the future. It would seem that blanket policies, such as are used now, will be inadequate to deal with these complex issues. The development of geriatric consultation teams at all health care facilities to evaluate and make decisions about each client over 65 years of age may be helpful. The decisions would include appropriate care based on the client's input, as well as what could be done to improve the quality of the individual's life. This would allow clients such as Sarah to live their lives to the fullest, and end their days with dignity and respect.

ception and attitude also play key roles in how the changes over time affect the individual. It is through the filter of perception and attitude that the individual identifies, defines, and adapts to the changes that occur in structure and function over time. These factors not only have implications for older clients but also for their families and the health care providers working with them. (See Ethical Considerations Box 13–1.)

Physiological Changes

Over time, cells change and do not function as efficiently as in earlier years (Table 13–1). The physical changes that are seen when looking at the older client are slight as compared with the cellular changes that occur. Cellular decline in structure and function increases in severity and extent over time. Although the body works hard to maintain **homeostasis,** it is often unable to fully adapt to many of the declines that result from aging. Cells that die cannot regenerate themselves. As a result, structures are altered, and the body tries to adapt in making the revised structure meet functional demands.

COMMON PHYSICAL CHANGES IN OLDER CLIENTS AND THEIR IMPLICATIONS FOR NURSING

Key Changes in the Muscular System with Aging

- Decrease in muscle mass so muscles look smaller
- Decrease in muscle tone so muscles look flabbier
- Muscle responses slowed so response time is increased
- Decrease in elasticity of tendons and ligaments restricting movements

Nursing Implications

Changes in the muscular system have implications for movement, strength, and endurance. Restricted movements are most commonly seen in the arms, legs, and neck of the older client, who may demonstrate limited **range of motion** (ROM) in these areas. Because muscle response abilities are slowed, it will take longer for the older client to move. This increased response time has implications on the older individual's confidence level regarding personal abilities to perform routine tasks.

Key Changes in the Skeletal System with Aging

- Eroding cartilage
- Exaggerated bony prominence

- Joint stiffening and decreased flexibility
- **Osteoporosis** due to a thinning and softening of the bone (Fig. 13–1)
- Shortening in height due to water loss in the intervertebral disks of the spinal column, flexion of the spine, and stooped posture

Nursing Implications

Because muscles and bones work together for movement, aging skeletal changes are most obvious when the older client is moving. **Contractures** of the fingers and hands can limit the individual's ability to perform self care tasks called **activities of daily living** (ADL). It is important for the nurse to assist the client with ROM exercises if help is needed to prevent the long-term disabilities that contractures bring (Fig. 13–2). Performing ROM exercises in warm water will help the client who experiences discomfort with these exercises. If the individual has arthritis, anti-inflammatory medications should be given so that their action peaks when the exercises begin. Older clients on anti-inflammatory medicines should be monitored closely for gastrointestinal upset or bleeding and taught the symptoms of bleeding to report.

Decreased bone density is influenced by diet and weight-bearing exercise, so balanced diets rich in calcium and vitamin D and safe and sensible exercise programs should be promoted. Clients should be encouraged to ambulate whenever possible, using sensible shoes that have nonskid soles and sturdy assistive devices if needed, such as handrails, canes, or walkers. When the decreasing density of older bones is considered, it is easy to understand that broken bones do not always result from a fall, but may indeed be the reason for the fall in many older clients.

Key Changes in the Integumentary System with Aging

- Increased dryness of the skin
- Increased pigmentation causing liver or aging spots
- Thinning in the layers of the skin, which makes the skin more fragile
- Decreased elasticity of the skin causing wrinkle development
- Decreased subcutaneous fat layer of skin so older clients have less insulation and less protective cushioning
- Hardness and dryness of nails, making them more brittle
- Decrease in nail growth rate and strength
- Thinning of scalp hair (primarily men)
- Increased growth and coarseness of nose, ear, and facial hair
- Decrease in melanin, which results in gray hair
- Decreased sebaceous and sweat glands, which has implications for dryness and decreased temperature regulation

---

homeostasis: homios—similar + stasis—standing
osteoporosis: osteon—bone + poros—a passage + osis—condition

Table 13–1. **Physiological Aging Changes**

Body System	Aging Change	Effect of Change
Cardiovascular	Increased conduction time	Heart rate slows, unable to increase quickly
	Decreased cardiac output	Less oxygen delivered to tissues
	Decreased blood vessel elasticity	Increased blood pressure increases cardiac workload
	Irregular heartbeats	Poor heart oxygenation, decreased cardiac output, heart failure
	Leg veins dilate, valves less efficient	Varicose veins, fluid accumulation in tissues
Endocrine and Metabolism	Basal metabolic rate slows	Possible weight gain
	Altered adrenal hormone production	Decreased ability to respond to stress
	Decreased insulin release	Hyperglycemia
Gastrointestinal	Reduced taste and smell	Appetite may be reduced
	Decreased saliva	Dry mouth, altered taste
	Decreased gag reflex, relaxation of lower esophageal sphincter	Increased **aspiration** risk
	Delayed gastric emptying	Reduced appetite
	Reduced liver enzymes	Reduced drug metabolism and detoxification
	Decreased peristalsis	Reduced appetite, constipation
Genitourinary	Kidney size decreases	Able to live with 10% renal function
	Decreased bladder size, tone, changes from pear to funnel shaped	Frequency of urination increased
	Muscles weaken	Incontinence
	Decreased concentrating ability	Nocturia
	Less sodium saved	Risk for dehydration
	Reduced renal blood flow	Decreased renal clearance of all medications
Immunological	Decreased function	Infection and cancer risk greater
	Increased autoimmune response	Increased autoimmune diseases
Integumentary	Reduced cell replacement	Healing slower
	Water loss	Dryness of the skin
	Increased pigmentation	Aging spots
	Thinning of skin layers	Skin more fragile
	Decreased subcutaneous fat	Less insulation and protective cushioning
	Decreased sebaceous and sweat glands	Dryness and decreased temperature regulation
	Hard, dry nails	Brittle nails
	Thinning scalp hair	Baldness
	Decreased melanin	Gray hair
	Decreased skin elasticity	Wrinkle development
Musculoskeletal	Decreased muscle mass	Reduced strength
	Decreased muscle tone	Muscles look flabbier
	Decreased elasticity of tendons and ligaments	Movements are restricted
	Muscle responses slowed	Response time increased
	Bone thinning, softening	Decreasing bone density
	Joint stiffening	Decreased flexibility
	Vertebral disk water loss	Decreased height
Neurological		
Central nervous system	Loss of brain cells	Able to maintain function with remaining cells
	Decreased brain blood flow	Short-term memory loss
	Decreased regulation of body temperature	Hypothermia, hyperthermia risk
	Decreased endorphins	Increased depression
Peripheral nervous system	Decreased sensation	Risk for injury, burns
	Increased reaction times	Slow response, injury risk
	Decreased motor coordination	Unsteady, fall risk
Respiratory	Decreased lung capacity	Dyspnea with activity
	Decreased cough and gag reflexes	Aspiration, infection risk
	Reduced lung tissue tone	Shallow, faster respirations
	Reduced lung emptying on exhalation	CO_2 retention
	Decreased fluid and ciliary action	Mucous obstruction, infection risk

continued

Table 13-1. (continued)

Body System	Aging Change	Effect of Change
Sensory		
Eye	Lens less elastic	Decreased near and peripheral vision
	Lens opaque, yellows	Cataracts
	Cornea more translucent	Blurry vision
	Smaller pupil	Decreased dark adaptation
	Decreased violet, blue, green color vision	See red, orange, yellow colors better
	Arcus senilus—blue or milky lipid ring on iris edge	No effect on vision
Ear	Degeneration of auditory nerve	Lose high-frequency tones, deafness
	Excess bone impairs sound conduction	Deafness
Nose	Decreased smell	Decreased ability to smell substances such as smoke, gas causing safety risk; appetite reduced
Sexuality	Availability of partner or privacy decreases	Lack of sexual expression, suppression of desires
	Slower sexual arousal time	Increased time needed for sexual stimulation
Men	Decreased erection, slower ejaculation	Psychologically causes concern
Women	Less vaginal lubrication	Painful intercourse
	Vaginal acidity reduced	Increased vaginal infection risk

aspiration: ad—to + spirate—breathe

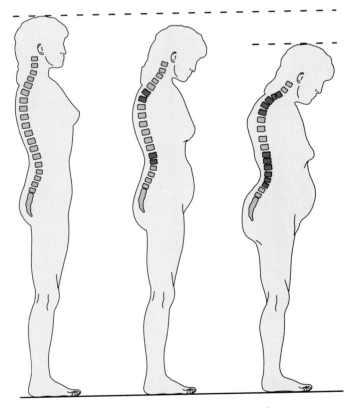

Space decreases between vertebrae

Figure 13–1. Osteoporosis. Note height loss and posture changes from thin, weakened vertebrae and loss of space between vertebrae.

Nursing Implications

The skin, which is the first line of defense against infection and injury, does not work as effectively in older clients (Fig. 13–3). In the elderly, skin injuries take longer to heal, and those longer healing times are usually complicated by the fact that many older clients have multiple chronic diseases such as diabetes and circulatory ailments.

The older client with limited mobility is especially prone to developing pressure ulcers (Fig. 13–4). These ulcers usually develop over a bony prominence of the body (ears, shoulders, elbows, tip of the spine, pelvic bone ridges, knees, heels, or ankles). Pressure ulcers are caused by ischemia that results from continuous pressure on an area of

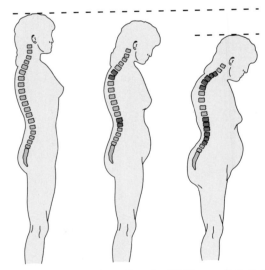

Figure 13–2. Nurse assists client in ROM exercises to prevent contracture development.

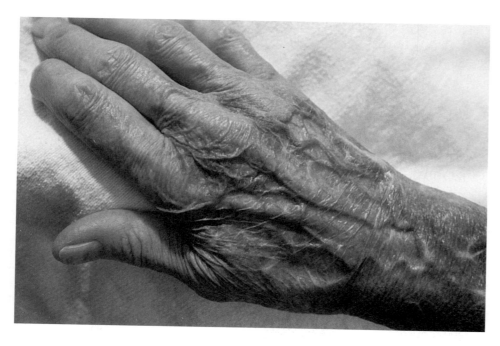

Figure 13–3. Thin, fragile skin of older client. See Plate 17.

the body. Ischemia from unrelieved pressure can develop in 20 to 40 minutes. Early signs of **pressure ulcer** formation are warmth, redness, tenderness, or a burning sensation at the potential ulcer site. These potential ulcer sites are aggravated by lack of activity and the weight of the body. For this reason it is especially important for the nurse to take the time to assess skin integrity daily. Skin care includes gently stimulating nonreddened intact skin sites with massage, moisturizing with creams regularly, avoiding the use of hot water and a complete daily bath, and limiting the use of soap. If able, clients should be taught to shift their weight every 15 minutes when sitting. For im-

mobile clients, consistent repositioning is essential. Repositioning every 30 minutes is the most beneficial to help ensure ulcer prevention. Keeping bed linens clean, dry, and wrinkle free also aids in the prevention of pressure ulcer formation.

As with care of the skin, nail care is important for older individuals. Soaking in warm water helps soften nails to ease in their trimming while encouraging blood flow to the peripheral areas of the body. Filing the nails with an emery board is safer than cutting the nails. To prevent accidental injury to the feet, clients should be instructed not to walk barefooted. Potential pressure points of the feet should be

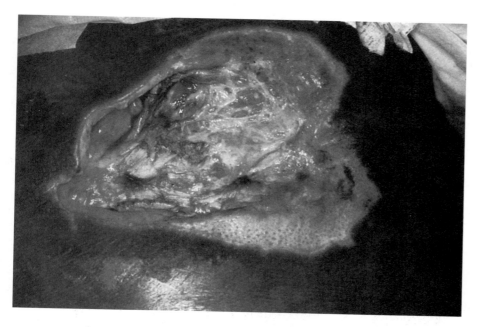

Figure 13–4. Pressure ulcer. (From Goldsmith: Adult and Pediatric Dermatology: A Color Guide to Diagnosis and Treatment. FA Davis, Philadelphia, p 445, with permission.) See Plate 18.

identified, closely monitored, and referred to a podiatrist for treatment should there be any concerns. Diabetics should assess their feet daily because they may have decreased sensation causing lack of awareness of foot irritation or injury.

Key Changes in the Cardiovascular System with Aging

- Heart rate slows.
- Decreased cardiac output caused by less effective functioning of the heart and blood vessels so less oxygen is delivered to body tissues.
- Decreased elasticity of the blood vessels so there is a less efficient circulatory system.
- Resting heart rate remains unchanged with age.
- Heart cannot increase its rate as quickly in response to an emergency situation because of a thickening of the heart valves, left ventricle, and aorta. When the rate finally does increase, the heart takes a longer period of time to return to the resting rate.
- Aged heart exhibits more irregular heartbeats, **arrhythmias,** which leads to poor oxygenation of the heart.
- Classic symptoms of cardiac emergencies are often not present in the older client.
- Increased peripheral vascular resistance in blood vessels increases blood pressure.
- Superficial blood vessels of the legs become more visibly dominant.
- Leg blood vessel valves work less efficiently, creating the risk for an accumulation of excess fluids in the leg tissues.

Nursing Implications

The nurse should be a good observer when it comes to caring for older clients because many early symptoms related to circulatory problems are subtle. Cardiovascular disease, which is separate from the process of aging, accounts for half of all deaths in people over the age of 65 years.[1] Nurses must take the time to educate older individuals in those prevention practices that promote healthy circulation. They need to encourage the older client to take prescribed medications as they are ordered and also encourage them to maintain a balanced intake and output of fluids. Special note should be made of older clients receiving intravenous therapy because the negative effects from fluid overload that affect the circulatory system occur quickly in older individuals.

Special care should be taken to maintain good skin integrity and provide appropriate stimulation. If **edema** is present in the legs they should be elevated to assist the fluid return to the upper body while supportive, nonrestrictive stockings should be appropriately and consistently worn. Concerns of leg circulation should be identified and reported early to the physician before problems develop. It is important to identify whether the circulation problem is arterial or venous before treatment is ordered.

Because quick changes in body position can make the older client feel weak and dizzy, it is important that the nurse stand next to older clients as they dangle their legs over the side of the bed before rising to stand. Changes in body positioning from lying to sitting to standing need to occur gradually to accommodate the less efficient circulatory system that is found in older clients. (See Fig. 11–9.) Older clients may find comfort in the security of an ambulatory belt or walker if they fear unsteadiness when in an upright position. Falls rank as the second leading cause of accidental death in older clients.[2] Every effort should be made by the nurse to decrease the risk of falling for the older client. The fall history of clients should be assessed to identify whether they are at high risk of falling so that preventive measures can be used.

Key Changes in the Respiratory System with Aging

- Decreased lung capacity
- Weaker cough or gag reflex increases risk for upper respiratory infections
- Reduced tone of lung tissue so respirations increase to 16 to 25 per minute and are more shallow in character
- Reduced tone of the diaphragm muscle
- Less complete emptying of the lungs with greater CO_2 retention
- Decreased blood flow to the lungs can contribute to cardiac arrhythmias

Nursing Implications

Because the respiratory system is less efficient with advancing age, the older client has a decreased tolerance for activity in general. Nurses should therefore pace activities for older clients instead of letting them confine themselves to bed. It is important to prevent overexertion, so rest periods should be scheduled. However, the rest periods should not outnumber the activity sessions planned throughout the course of the client's day.

Cough, marked fatigue, and confusion may be early signs of an inadequate oxygen uptake. Respiratory rates greater than 25 per minute may be an early indication of a lower respiratory tract infection. Because overall muscle strength is reduced, the older client performs the O_2-CO_2 exchange in the less efficient upper lobes of the lung instead of the larger lower lobes specifically designed for this purpose. Because lung recoil strength is decreased, mucus may be more difficult for the older client to **expectorate.** This situation is compounded by the fact that older individuals also have less effective cough and gag reflexes, which creates greater po-

---

edema: oidema—swelling
expectorate: ex—out + pectus—breast

tential for lung problems. Because of the normal changes in the respiratory system that occur with aging, it is important for the nurse to include coughing, deep breathing, and position changes in the exercise program designed to stimulate all lobes of the older client's lungs. At the prevention level, the nurse should encourage the older individual to receive a pneumonia vaccine and an annual flu shot. This is important because influenza and pneumonia combine to be the fourth leading cause of death in individuals over the age of 65 years.[3] The nurse should also be aware that lifelong habits, such as smoking and respiratory pollutant exposure in employment settings, secondhand smoke, or paints and glues used in hobbies, are cumulative over time and can contribute to respiratory sensitivity for the older client.

Key Changes in the Gastrointestinal System with Aging

- Changes in taste and smell affect the enjoyment of eating
- Saliva production decreases
- Decreased gag reflex and relaxation of lower esophageal sphincter increase the risk of aspiration
- Delayed gastric emptying
- No functional changes in the small intestine
- Tone in external sphincter decreases
- Marked decline in enzymes of the liver affects drug metabolism and detoxification
- Decreased peristalsis from generalized weakness of muscle activity
- Alteration in bowel habits

Nursing Implications

Many factors can alter appetite, ingestion, digestion, and absorption of nutrients in food, regardless of an individual's age. However, the structural and functional changes that occur with advancing age put the older client at greater risk for not obtaining the nutrients needed to sustain a healthy body. (See Nutrition Notes Box 13–2.)

There is little that the nurse can do to change the physical alterations in the older body that make getting needed nutrients more difficult. However, the nurse can become educated and committed to providing those supports necessary to meet nutritional goals. These supports can take many forms. The nurse should always assist clients in toileting before helping them to eat. An appropriate amount of time for the client to accomplish the task of eating needs to be provided. If the client needs assistance with feeding, the nurse should be sensitive to the client's pace while allowing the client to have as much control as possible.

Additional forms of support can focus on the need to recognize that for some cultures eating has a strong social component. The nurse should encourage the client to eat out of bed and with others as much as possible, while respecting the client's right of refusal to eat in a designated social setting. Some clients may not eat as well when seated next to agitated or confused residents in a common dining hall.

The nurse can offer continuing support by maintaining a calm and comfortable environment that aids digestion. Certain food combinations enhance nutrient absorption, such as vitamin C foods taken with plant foods high in iron which increase the iron's absorption rate. The nurse should

NUTRITION NOTES BOX 13–2

Nutrition in the Older Adult

Energy needs decrease 5 percent for every decade after 40 years of age, so special attention must be given to maximizing nutritional content in fewer calories if a slow weight gain is to be avoided. Many normal physiological changes of aging affect nutritional status in the older adult.

Decreased visual acuity and impaired dexterity may make shopping for food and preparing it difficult or even hazardous. Arthritis affects not only mobility, but also jaw movements, so chewing may be problematic. Skill in the use of dentures may have to be acquired. It is recommended that an individual learn to drink with dentures first, then learn to manipulate soft foods, and last learn to bite and chew with them.

Sensation for sweet and salty tastes is lost before that for sour and bitter. Clients may increase intake of sugar and salt to the detriment of a prescribed diet plan.

Achlorhydria may occur as a result of aging or from chronic ingestion of antacids. In either case, protein digestion and absorption of iron and vitamins B_{12} and C can be impaired by the lack of gastric acid. Although anemia can be caused by poor nutrition, older clients should be evaluated for hidden blood loss, just as younger ones are.

Care should be used in offering high-protein supplements to older individuals because normal aging reduces kidney function significantly, and excretion of nitrogenous products of excessive protein intake could stress the urinary system. In addition, a high protein intake increases calcium excretion. The vitamin necessary for calcium metabolism, vitamin D, may be deficient in older persons who neither drink milk nor spend time outdoors.

Many mature clients are at increased risk for food, nutrient, and drug interactions. Situations associated with these interactions are the use of many drugs, including alcohol; the need for long-term drug therapy in chronic illness; and poor or marginal nutritional status. Identification of any of these factors should prompt a thorough nutritional assessment or referral to a registered dietitian.

offer these selections together whenever possible. Family members can be asked to bring in familiar seasonings clients used at home. If acceptable, familiar seasonings in shakers that clients apply themselves can be used to stimulate a lagging appetite. Nurses need to work closely with the dietitian or nutritionist, who may provide other ideas to promote healthful eating for older clients.

Although many older clients wear dentures or partial plates, it is important not to stereotypically assume that all older individuals wear dentures. Tooth loss is not a normal change of aging. With proper lifelong dental care, teeth should last a lifetime. If the older client does have dentures, the nurse must be aware that any significant change in body weight will affect their fit and comfort and the client's nutritional intake. Because of this, it is important for the nurse to conduct regular assessments of the mouth when assisting the older client during oral care.

Medications may cause taste disturbances or problems with dry mouth that may also affect the older client's ability to meet nutritional needs. Some medications create problems with bowel motility, resulting in **constipation.** Constipation can also result from a change in routine, stress, and anxiety. To gain a greater understanding of the situation, the nurse should talk with the client about previous assistive procedures and establish an expectation baseline for bowel elimination. It is up to the nurse to educate the older client about the important relationship between intake of fiber and water and exercise in the promotion of effective bowel evacuation. Enemas, suppositories, and medications should be considered for use only after dietary management is found to be ineffective.

Key Changes in the Endocrine-Metabolic System with Aging

- Slowing in the basal metabolic rate requiring a 5 percent reduction of calorie consumption to maintain weight
- Alteration in hormone production, including changes in estrogen, progesterone, and adrenal secretions
- Decreased pancreatic insulin release and peripheral sensitivity
- Decreased glucose tolerance with advancing age

Nursing Implications

Increased incidence of metabolic disease such as diabetes occurs with advancing years. Because of this, older clients should be encouraged to participate in screening programs for early detection of metabolic problems.

Because there is a notable decrease in the effectiveness and interaction of all hormones as one ages, it becomes especially difficult for the older body to respond appropriately to any stressful situations. Nurses should spend time addressing the psychological needs of clients by recogniz-

ing and addressing those actual and perceived stressors that affect their care. Preventive care to keep clients free from the stress of illness is also important.

Key Changes in the Genitourinary System with Aging

- Decreased kidney size
- Decreased kidney function, urinary output, and adaptability
- Reduction of blood flow to the kidneys because of decreased cardiac output and increased peripheral resistance
- Diminished kidney filtration rate and tubular function, which causes a decrease in the renal clearance of all medications
- Decreased bladder size and tone
- Increased incidence of urinary tract infection with age, especially in women
- Longer correction times for fluid and electrolyte imbalances

Nursing Implications

Many older individuals have an urge to urinate at night, which is referred to as **nocturia.** Changes in the kidneys, lack of gravity influence when in the recumbent position, fluid retention, and medication use contribute to nocturia. About 30 minutes after lying down many older people need to urinate because fluid that was held in the legs by gravity is circulated through the kidneys and urine is produced, causing the urge to void. It is important for the nurse to plan safe toileting facility access for older clients during the night. Emptying the bladder becomes more difficult to control from weakening of bladder and perineal muscles and also from a change in brain sensation about the need to void. As a result, the older client may have difficulty controlling urination either knowingly or unknowingly, resulting in **urinary incontinence.**

LEARNING TIP

With age, the urge to void is not felt as early as it once was. This aging change combined with other changes in the urinary system, such as the bladder becoming funnel shaped, contribute to the older client's voiding urgency. If the client is not assisted to void promptly on request, incontinence can result.

Incontinence is socially embarrassing and can occur in both male and female clients. It is said to be one of the major reasons that older people are admitted to nursing homes.[3] The incidence in men is most often associated with prostate enlargement; women are more likely candidates because of weakened perineal muscles. Older women are more likely to

nocturia: nocte—night + ouron—urine

experience urinary incontinence because they have short urethras that are not supported by strong perineal muscles and more urinary tract infections than older men.

Management of urinary incontinence needs to be tailored to the particular need of the client. Bladder training programs have been effective when clients are reminded on a regular basis that it is time to urinate. If incontinence results from problems that affect the toileting task itself, such as clothing removal or distance to the bathroom, steps need to be taken to eliminate those obstacles that stand in the way of continence. Clothing with Velcro fasteners can replace buttons or zippers that are difficult for the client to manipulate. Urinary briefs can help instill confidence in older clients who previously restricted activities because of fear of urine leakage. With use of the supportive incontinence brief, the nurse needs to assess for early signs of perineal skin breakdown and proper application of the proper brief to meet individual needs.

Older clients who are aware of their incontinence may try to inappropriately decrease the chance for leakage by severely limiting fluid intake. This approach often results in dehydration, which disturbs the acid-base and electrolyte balance in the body. Over time, dehydrated clients may have problems with vomiting, diarrhea, weakness, and confusion. Because fluid intake needs to be encouraged in older clients, the nurse may wish to focus educational efforts on topics such as liquid intake timing and beverage selection (e.g., teaching that caffeine and alcoholic beverages should be avoided because they normally increase urinary output).

In addition, the nurse should review client medications and personal medication practices, such as taking diuretics late in the day, which then causes nighttime urination. With some older clients, the nurse may find some success with teaching perineal muscle support exercises and techniques. All unexplained urinary incontinence should be referred to a specialist who treats urinary incontinence for further evaluation because it is not a normal condition of aging.

CRITICAL THINKING: Mr. Jones

Mr. Jones, 72 years old, lives at home. His home has wood floors with throw rugs. The bathroom is located in the hall outside his bedroom. Mr. Jones has nocturia and is occasionally incontinent from urgency to void. He takes bumetanide (Bumex) daily.

1. What additional assessment data should the nurse obtain about Mr. Jones regarding his urinary status and home environment?
2. Are safety concerns present in the home environment?
3. What nursing diagnoses would be included in Mr. Jones's nursing care plan?
4. What should be included in a teaching plan for Mr. Jones?

Answers at end of chapter.

Key Changes in the Immunological System with Aging

- Immune response declines.
- Number and function of T cells decreases, leading to impaired ability to produce antibodies to fight disease.

Nursing Implications

Older clients tend to have more chronic diseases that may increasingly depress their immune abilities over time. Although older clients have fewer colds, they are at higher risk for influenza and other complications once they get a cold. It takes a longer time to recover from infections, so clients and their family members need to be told that a prolonged recovery is to be expected. It is also important for the nurse to screen visitors for illness before they visit a recuperating older client.

Efforts at prevention should focus on teaching the older client about the importance of obtaining current immunizations, reducing stress, eating right, exercising, and maintaining a healthful lifestyle. Individuals on medications for conditions that would put them at risk for immunosuppression, such as steroids, should be aware of the need to take additional safety precautions around others who are ill. Nurses can help clients help themselves by encouraging techniques such as proper hand washing that support universal precautions.

Key Changes in the Neurological System with Aging

- Progressive loss of brain cells
- Decreased blood flow and oxygen utilization to the brain
- Decreased protein synthesis
- Decrease in sensitivity and the sensation pathways
- Increased reaction times
- Decreased motor coordination
- Decreased equilibrium
- Decreased ability of the hypothalamus to regulate body temperature
- Change in neurotransmitter secretion levels

Nursing Implications

Changes in the nervous system of the older client can be seen in both the peripheral and central systems. These changes have significant meaning for the older individual, especially in the area of safety. With normal aging there is a slowed response to stimuli and a marked decrease in the speed of the psychomotor response to that stimuli. Because stronger stimuli are required to elicit any neurological response, the older client is unable to perceive early signs of danger. To protect from accidental skin burns, the thermostat on water heaters should be lowered and electrical heating devices such as heating pads, electric blankets, and mattress pads should not be used.

Another safety issue of concern focuses on changes in balance. It is more difficult to maintain balance as one ages, especially when musculoskeletal changes are considered. Special caution should be taken to assist older clients with transferring and ambulation activities so optimal levels of safety can be maintained.

Fine tremors of the hand are a normal finding with advancing age and tend to increase in occurrence when the older client is cold, excited, hungry, or active. Assistive devices provided by an occupational therapist such as handle grips or anchored equipment can help eliminate the unsteadiness created when fine tremors make it more difficult to accomplish activities of daily living (Fig. 13–5). Accompanied by generalized muscle weakness, normal neurological changes that occur with advancing age usually occur on both sides of the body at the same time. One-sided weakness, sensory problems, and performance problems should always be referred for further evaluation.

Coarse tremors of the finger, forearm, head, eyelids, or tongue, which occur when the body part is at rest, may be a sign of a neurological problem such as Parkinson's disease. These generally occur on one side of the body first and should always be referred for further evaluation.

Key Changes in the Sensory System with Aging

- Decreased visual perception
- Decreased elasticity of the eardrum
- Decreased sense of smell
- Decreased taste perception
- Decreased touch sensation

Nursing Implications

Problems that occur with normal changes in the aging sensory system are not inevitable with advancing age. Early identification and prompt referral can minimize sensory loss, which has a strong impact on the older person's psychological health.

Normal aging changes in the eye affect the focus ability of the lens and the maneuverability of the eye muscles to meet the needs of near and far vision. It is especially difficult for older clients to read fine print, although it is usually manageable with reading glasses or a bifocal lens. If the nurse is caring for clients who wear glasses, it is important to remind clients to consistently wear their glasses as needed, helping to keep them clean and in good repair.

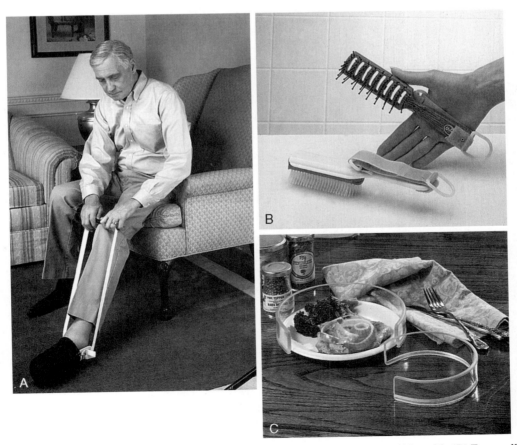

Figure 13–5. Assistive devices for activities of daily living. *(A)* Sock and stocking aid. *(B)* Easy-pull hairbrush. *(C)* Food guard. (Courtesy of Sammons Preston, Inc., Bollingbrook, Ill, with permission.)

When they are removed by the client, they should be accessible and kept in a protective, labeled case.

The older client has a more difficult time adjusting to changes between light and dark settings. Seeing in the dark can be enhanced with the use of a red night-light because red lighting is more easily detected by the cones and rods in the older client's eye. The nurse should also make every effort to reduce glare from bright sunlight because sensitivity to glare is enhanced with the normal changes that occur in the aging eye (Fig. 13–6). The glare from car headlights may impair vision in older clients and reduce their ability to drive at night.

Cataracts are one of the most common pathological problems affecting the aging eye.[4] They cloud the lens and occur at different rates in different people. Cataracts increase the risk for **sensory deprivation** if the cataract grows over the pupil of the eye and causes a distortion in the field of vision. The older client with cataracts may complain of poor vision, eye fatigue, increased sensitivity to light, blurred vision, multiple images, and headache.

Older clients with **glaucoma,** a disease characterized by increased intraocular pressure that can damage the optic nerve, may complain of eyestrain and morning headaches that disappear after rising. Unlike cataracts, the glaucoma client usually does not have symptoms early in the disease process. Loss of peripheral vision is a precursor to blindness if glaucoma is left untreated.

Another common visual condition that occurs later in life is **macular degeneration.** Unlike glaucoma, early stages of this condition result in a loss of central vision while peripheral vision remains intact. Regardless of the means, it must be understood that any visual loss in older clients puts them at risk for developing psychological problems with disorientation, withdrawal, or self-imposed isolation caused by sensory deprivation.

Hearing loss is a common condition found in older individuals. Although the severity of the hearing loss caused by aging is variable, the stigma it carries is the same. For most older clients, the first difficult sounds to discriminate are the high-pitched tones. Therefore it is often more effective to whisper when communicating with the hearing-impaired individual because whispering decreases the pitch of the sounds. Shouting is not helpful because both volume and pitch are increased. It is best to speak to a hearing-impaired person in a moderate volume and a lower tone. It

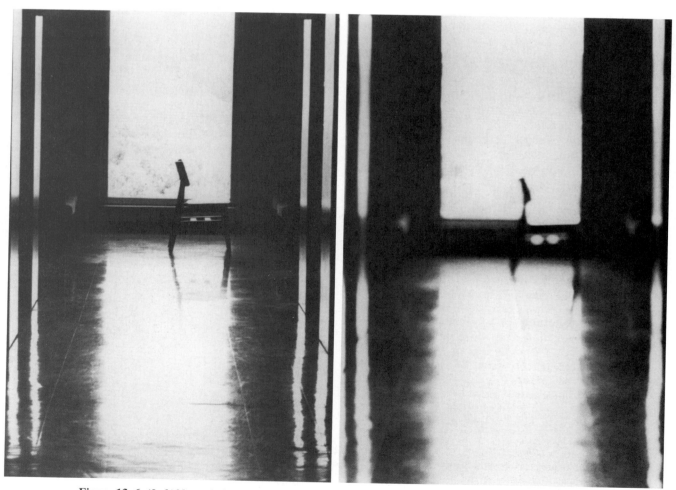

Figure 13–6. *(Left)* Normal view. *(Right)* The effects of glare as seen by an older client. (From Matteson, MA, and McConnell, ES: Gerontological Nursing. WB Saunders, Philadelphia, 1988, p 314, with permission.)

is also helpful to stand in front of hearing-impaired clients so they can see the speaker's face during communication (Table 13–2) (Fig. 13–7).

There are two types of hearing loss that can occur separately or in combination in the hearing-impaired client. Conduction loss is due to blockage or damage to the mechanisms that transmit sound to the middle ear, where it is carried by the acoustic nerve to the brain. Conduction hearing loss can be due to a variety of factors, some as simple as ear wax buildup, and in most cases can be successfully managed. The other type of hearing loss, sensorineural loss, is due to damage to the structures in the inner ear and is much more difficult to manage. This type of loss can result from illness, medication use, or long-term abusive noise pollution that damages the sensitive structures involved with sensation and interpretation of sound. It is important to use hearing protection throughout life because damage to the ear is usually not reversible.

New technology hearing aids can help most people with either type of hearing loss. Clients should be referred to an audiologist for further evaluation if hearing loss is suspected. It is important that the nurse realize that hearing aids are not well accepted by all older persons or their family members because they are a visual sign of a loss. Because of this, the nurse must maintain client privacy if a referral for further evaluation is made. If the older client already has a hearing aid, it should be kept accessible to the client at all times. The hearing aid should be kept clean with soap and water. A cotton swab removes wax buildup in tiny areas of the hearing aid. When not in use, the hearing aid should be stored in a labeled protective container and the battery turned off to conserve it. Extra batteries should be readily available.

As discussed in the gastrointestinal section of this chapter, the senses of taste and smell work closely together. Like other sensory losses, a declining ability to taste is not a problem exclusive to the older individual. Both ill-fitting dentures and poor oral care can contribute to an alteration in the sense of taste, as can certain medications, tobacco substances, and oral disease.

Although they are often treated together as one sensory loss, the incidence in the loss of the sense of smell is more common than the disorder that focuses on the loss of taste.[4] In some cases, the loss of smell may be due to sinus problems, nasal obstruction, or allergies. If olfactory receptors

are the primary cause for losing the sense of smell, there is little that can be done to treat the loss. It is important for the nurse to assess clients' medication charts as well as their oral cavity if they report a recent loss of smell or taste sensation.

Nurses also need to be aware of the care environment they provide for the older client. Overstimulation produced by **sensory overload,** commonly experienced in intensive care hospital settings, can create psychological and physical strains that can make it difficult for the older client to cope. As a client advocate, the nurse must be sensitive to the client's care environment and changes in the client's health care status, identifying and minimizing overload situations early in the recuperation period.

Key Changes in the Sexuality System with Aging

- Functional sexual changes in older men commonly focus on the alteration in abilities to obtain or maintain an erection and ejaculate.
- Functional sexual changes in older women commonly focus on the alteration in abilities for vaginal lubrication.
- Sexual activities for older individuals focus more heavily on nonintercourse intimacy behaviors that include various forms of touch.
- Sexual problems in older individuals more often result from psychological factors rather than physical ones.
- Sexual arousal time in the older client commonly takes longer with advancing age.

Nursing Implications

The older client's sexuality is an important aspect to consider. The nurse must be aware of personal attitudes and values about sex, sexuality, and aging, being careful that

*Table 13–2. **Communicating with Hearing-Impaired Clients***

- Ensure that hearing aids are on with working batteries, if applicable.
- Face client so the speaker's face is visible to client.
- Speak toward client's best side of hearing.
- Speak in a clear, moderate-volume, low-pitched tone.
- Do not shout because this distorts sounds.
- Recognize that high-frequency tones and consonant sounds are lost first—s, z, sh, ch, d, g.
- Eliminate background noise because it can distort sounds.

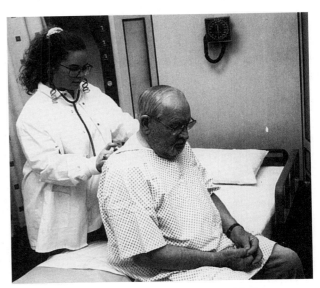

Figure 13–7. Facing a hearing-impaired client during conversation aids communication. (From Anderson, MA: Nursing Leadership, Management, and Professional Practice for the LPN/LVN. FA Davis, Philadelphia, 1997, p 29, with permission.)

personal stereotypes and beliefs do not interrupt the older person's attempt to maintain sexual identity. Because privacy remains a common problem for individuals in health care settings, the nurse should provide the client some scheduled privacy time. It is important to incorporate a sexual history section in the nursing assessment form and recognize that barriers to sexual expression can include such things as cultural or religious beliefs, lack of a suitable partner, fear of failure, fear of consequences, illness, side effects of medications, and certain chronic diseases that may alter libido or sexual functional abilities.

Cognitive and Psychological Changes in the Older Client

COGNITION

In addition to those physiological changes that occur with advancing age, older clients are also experiencing changes that have an effect on cognition. Cognition includes abilities related to intelligence, memory, orientation, judgment, calculation abilities, and learning. The cognitive domain is a complex system that focuses on registration of information, storage, processing, and retrieval of stored information. For the most part, older clients register and store information without much conscious effort. It is when there is difficulty processing and retrieving information that the older person may begin to worry about how the advancing years are affecting routine brain functions. Unless this worry is addressed, the client's concern can create the opportunity for the development of unnecessary psychological problems and fears.

Many factors can affect processing and retrieval of information. A variety of sensory changes brought on with advancing age can cause misinterpretation of the information being collected. For this reason it is important for the nurse caring for the older client to conduct a sensory assessment before conducting a mental status examination. Diseases commonly linked with older persons can also affect cognitive abilities. The pain from chronic diseases, such as arthritis, can limit cognitive functioning as pain takes over body and mind. Sleep deprivation caused by worry or fear can make it more difficult to perform even routine tasks effectively. Medications that cause drowsiness as a side effect to their therapeutic action can also impair brain functioning when it comes to task performance.

Research on the aging brain tells us that long-term memory retrieval is easier to accomplish in old age than short-term memory retrieval is.[3] The nurse can assist the client having short-term memory problems by using written lists, visual cues, and other memory-enhancing systems to assist in strengthening short-term memory skills.

Intelligence does not decline as one ages if it is measured using an appropriate instrument that focuses on accuracy and not on speed of response. Although cognitive abilities do tend to slow down with advancing age, they are not lost. Most of the subtle declines that do occur with information processing and retrieval do not need to interfere with the older client's abilities in performing activities of daily living.

Nurses need to assist in the identification of individual problem situations and work with older clients and their families in developing strategies to better address their needs. It is common knowledge that health, good nutrition, and adequate sleep are important factors for brain functioning. These should be the cornerstones in case management planning with older clients.

COPING ABILITIES

How the individual chooses to adapt to a change in functional ability over time has a significant impact on how that individual will work through the entire maturational process called aging. Nurses must not lose sight of the fact that in addition to the changes caused by some decline in physical functioning, older persons simultaneously work to deal with many societal and culturally perceived losses that are associated with advancing age. Changes in employment status, societal roles, and family roles and shifts from independence to dependence have a strong psychological impact on both older clients and their families when societal norms are considered.

The older individual's personality, attitude, past life experiences, and desire to adapt to change are all intrinsic influencing factors that assist the older client in coping with changes brought on by advancing age. Extrinsic factors include things such as financial status, family support, and support provided by those who directly care for the client. If older clients have the energy, desire, determination, and support of those who care for them, they will be better able to optimize use of their cognitive functions toward health.

DEPRESSION

There are times when the psychological impact of change is too difficult to cope with, and loneliness, grief, or sadness does not easily allow the older person to cognitively focus on health. When this happens, **depression** can result with the potential to disable the older individual's mind and body. Depression is the most common psychiatric problem among older adults.[3] This psychological condition, which causes a disturbance in mood, increases the risk for suicide, physical health complaints, and sleep disturbances.

It is important for the nurse to understand that the frequency and intensity of depression generally increases with advancing age. Depression can result from physical changes in the brain caused by medications or conditions that affect the neurotransmitters in the brain or from psychological changes at an emotional level, such as maladaptive coping from a perceived loss. Regardless of the cause, depression is a condition that has the potential to be reversed with prompt identification and treatment. It is important, therefore, for the nurse to be sensitive to what the older individual is and is not saying during communications. Clients should be referred for treatment if depression is suspected before maladaptive behaviors occur.

DEMENTIA

Unlike depression, **dementia** involves a more permanent progressive deterioration of mental functioning. Dementia is often characterized by confusion, forgetfulness, impaired judgment, and personality changes. There are two main types of dementia: multi-infarct dementia and Alzheimer's disease.

The multi-infarct classification results from repeated strokes that affect the brain tissue. The onset for this condition can be sudden or gradual, but its course is marked by a cyclical worsening and lessening of signs and symptoms that vary with the intensity and location of the brain damage.

The cause of Alzheimer's disease is unknown, but symptoms gradually begin with impaired memory that pro-gresses to language and motor function losses. The course of this disease is marked by stages that can occur up to 14 years before death. It is only on autopsy of the brain that a definitive diagnosis of Alzheimer's disease can be made. Until then, Alzheimer's is suspected after other types of dementia have been ruled out with testing.

With any dementia, it is the nurse's role to help the older client maintain an **optimum level of functioning** in an atmosphere that provides for physical and emotional safety. In efforts to help ground the confused client, the nurse needs to incorporate **reality orientation** or validation into all nursing interventions. Sensory overload should be decreased for confused clients. The nurse should speak calmly and slowly and provide nonthreatening therapeutic touch, if accepted by the client.

In addition, it is important to address the education and support needs of the client's family as they learn to deal with changes in behavior demonstrated by the older client. The nurse should refer any client with confusion for a mental status examination to help in determining whether the person suffers from depression or dementia. It is essential that a sensory status examination be conducted on the older client before a mental status examination is conducted to help ensure the accuracy of the test results.

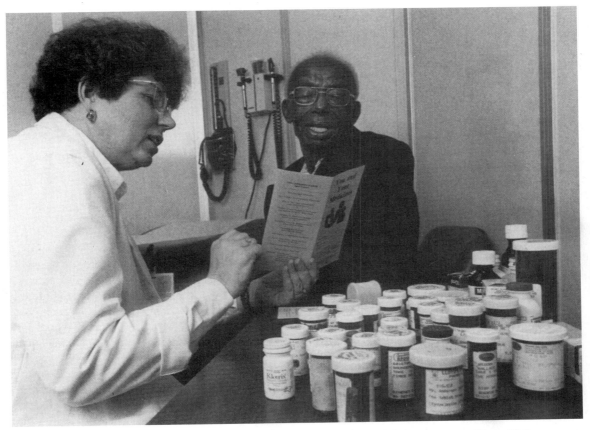

Figure 13–8. Older clients use many medications and must understand their correct use. (From Matteson, MA, and McConnell, ES: Gerontological Nursing. WB Saunders, Philadelphia, 1988, p 588, with permission.)

HOME HEALTH HINTS

- Try to schedule therapy visits and nurse visits on the same day, to decrease fatiguing the older client.

- Because many older clients keep their homes warm, the home health nurse should wear layers of clothing, removing a layer as needed, rather than adjusting the heat in the older client's home.

- Pagers should be placed on a silent mode if possible to avoid startling or confusing the older client.

- Nurses should not assume that the older client remembers them when the client answers the door. Nurses should state their name and why they are there. A large letter name tag should be in clear view.

- To enhance the effectiveness of a visit, the older client should be asked to visit in a quiet room of the home with the primary caregiver invited in at the appropriate time. This may help the older client stay more focused, offer privacy, and assist hearing.

- Making a sign for the door of the home giving visitors instructions may be helpful to the older client, such as ringing the doorbell several times, knocking loudly, or using the other door. Do not provide information that would inform a stranger that an older client lives in the home.

- Limiting visitors or persons with colds can be helpful in preventing illness for the older client.

- Stressors in a client's life, such as annoying visitors, chastisement by caregivers, and bill collectors, are often experienced firsthand by the home health nurse. Document and share them with the home care team so that a coordinated approach can be taken.

- When auscultating lungs, ask the older client to take deep breaths in and out through the mouth. This may stimulate coughing, which is an opportune time to teach deep breathing and coughing exercises.

- If the older client seems fatigued early in the day, ask about sleeping patterns and things that disturb it, such as barking dogs, traffic noise, and visitors. Recommend ear plugs or changing rooms to obtain a good night's rest. A 15- to 30-minute nap in the early afternoon can be helpful.

- One of the first signs of infection in the older client is confusion. Take the client's temperature on every visit.

- One of the first signs of dehydration is tachycardia.

- Assess the older client's environment for safety hazards on each visit and promote safety. Offer to clear pathways and hallways of clients who live alone to prevent falls.

- Take a complete medication history if the older client complains of nausea, bloating, or cramps. The older client may be taking the medication without food or mixing it with another drug that can lead to gastrointestinal disturbances.

- If the older client is taking vitamins, explain that mineral oil makes the vitamins less effective.

- If the older client has dentures, assess whether they are worn for eating. If not, assess why they are not worn (sores, improper fit from weight loss) and discuss solutions.

- Checking the refrigerator for outdated food is helpful. The older client is often on a limited budget and has been taught not to waste food. These factors, along with a decreased sense of smell and taste, can lead to food poisoning in the older client.

- Encourage the use of spices and herbs instead of salt and sugar, such as parsley, oregano, lemon, garlic, and basil. Suggest keeping pared apples and slices of oranges in the refrigerator for snacks.

- If a meals-on-wheels program is available, ask if the older client would like to be placed on the service.

- Use a warming tray when feeding an older client who takes a longer time to eat.

- When swallowing is difficult, freezing liquids helps, so they can be eaten with a spoon or like a popsicle. Examples are milk shakes, high-protein drinks, instant breakfast mix, and eggnog.

- If a female older client wears perineal pads or adult briefs, ask how many are used in a 24-hour period to assess the degree of incontinency or amount of output. Teach Kegel exercises. It is never too late to start Kegel exercises.

- Suggest a bedside commode when a weakened older client is on diuretics or has a history of falling or confusion. Placing it next to the bed at night helps reduce the risk of falls and eases the caregiver burden.

- If older clients have a history of inadequate fluid intake, assess their use of laxatives and teach them to avoid laxatives that require a large amount of fluid to work because such laxatives can increase constipation if clients do not consume enough fluid.

- When drawing blood from the hand of an older client, use the smallest needle possible. Hold light pressure for at least 2 minutes after the needle is removed. Do not use a Band-Aid on the fragile skin of the older client if the bleeding has stopped with pressure.

SLEEP AND REST PATTERNS

The need for sleep in elderly clients does not decrease with advancing age, but the pattern usually varies from earlier times in their lives. As with any age group, the lack of sleep leads to fatigue, irritability, increased sensitivity to pain, and increased likelihood of accidental behaviors. This is why it is important to obtain a baseline sleep and rest history when the older client is admitted to the health care unit. The nurse should consider sleep patterns, bedtime rituals, rest and nap patterns, daily exercise patterns, stress level, dietary intake patterns, and lifestyle issues such as caffeine, alcohol, and nicotine intake when completing the sleep and rest assessment of an older client.

Circulatory problems may disrupt normal sleep patterns for the older person and may be the only clue of an impending health problem. The anxious client who is unable to sleep may be calmed with back rubs, foot rubs, a warm bath, warm milk, or a glass of wine, if not contraindicated, when patterned bedtime rituals prove to be unsuccessful. Sleep medications should be used only as a last resort because they can affect the quality or depth of the sleep the older person receives and may produce unwanted side effects.

MEDICATION MANAGEMENT

One of the most difficult tasks for older clients, their family members, and the health care provider caring for them centers around the topic of medication management. Because older clients are more susceptible to drug-induced illness and adverse side effects for a variety of reasons already addressed in this chapter, nurses need to be especially aware of what the older client is taking, how it is being taken, and what effect it is having.

Older clients use many medicines for various ailments (Fig. 13–8). Most have more than one chronic illness for which they take medications. Sometimes these different medications interact and produce side effects that can be dangerous. Not only do health care providers need to be concerned about prescribed medicines, they also need to look at the types of over-the-counter medicines older clients take, as well as the self-prescribed extracts, elixirs, herbal teas, cultural healing substances, and other home remedies commonly used by individuals of their age cohort.

Health care providers not only need to be concerned about overuse and combinations of medications, but also misuse of them. To have an older client crush a large enteric-coated pill so that it can be taken in food and easily swallowed destroys the enteric protection and can inadvertently cause damage to the stomach and intestinal system. Because the U.S. health care system does not have a universal national health supported medication program for older individuals, some clients intentionally skip prescribed doses in efforts to save money. When prescribed doses are not being taken as expected, problems do not clear up as quickly and new problems may result.

The nurse needs to work closely with older clients and their families on medication education. Clients need to know what each prescribed pill is for, when it is prescribed to be taken, how it should be taken, and side effects to report. As a client advocate, the nurse can work with the pharmacist to remedy administration concerns so that the prescribed dose can be taken as directed. The nurse needs to write down early medication side effects, educating clients or designated care providers to be proactive in their care.

Medication use, abuse, and misuse need to be addressed regularly with older persons. Concerns need to be closely monitored and addressed before they evolve into problem situations. Helping older clients consistently adhere to a prescribed medication routine with visual and verbal supports helps all of those involved in the process of their medication management. This method also encourages self-care and supportive independence, as able, making for easier and safer medication use.

Review Questions

1. Which of the following commonly contributes to individuals becoming shorter with age?
   a. Contractures
   b. Bone degeneration in the legs
   c. Hyperextension of the cervical spine
   d. Water loss from spinal intervertebral disks

2. Pressure ulcers occur at sites of ischemia and can begin to develop in
   a. 5 to 10 minutes
   b. 20 to 40 minutes
   c. 60 minutes
   d. 120 minutes

3. Which of the following contributes to increased blood pressure with age?
   a. Increased peripheral vascular resistance
   b. Decreased peripheral vascular resistance
   c. Increased cardiac output
   d. Decreased cardiac output

4. Which one of the following increases the older client's risk for aspiration?
   a. Increased lung capacity
   b. Decreased lung capacity
   c. Decreased gag reflex
   d. Increased gag reflex

5. Which of the following is an expected taste bud change with advancing age?
   a. No change in salty tastes
   b. Increased sensitivity to sweet tastes
   c. Decreased sensitivity to sweet tastes
   d. Increased sensitivity to salty tastes

6. Which one of the following factors is the most common factor related to sexual problems in older clients?
   a. Social
   b. Financial
   c. Physical
   d. Psychological

7. A client living in an extended care facility has shown progressive memory decline during the past 4 years. The client's memory, judgment, and learning have all been affected in the same way. Which of the following conditions would show these characteristics?
   a. Dementia
   b. Delirium
   c. Depression
   d. Sensory deprivation

ANSWERS TO CRITICAL THINKING

CRITICAL THINKING: Mr. Jones

1. Does he live alone? Fall history? If so, does he wear a device to signal help? What type of night-light is used? How far is it to the bathroom? Does he take his bumetanide (Bumex) early in the day rather than at night? Does he void before going to bed? Does he anticipate needing to void 30 minutes after lying down?

2. Wood floors that are slippery when wet from incontinence. Throw rugs that may slide or cause tripping. Appropriate night-light available.

3. Functional incontinence related to distance to bathroom. Knowledge deficit related to safety, medication administration, and nocturia. Risk for injury related to slippery floors from incontinence, use of throw rugs, lighting.

4. Teaching plan:

• *Safety.* Place urinal at bedside to prevent incontinence on way to bathroom. Use red night-light to improve vision and prevent falls. Use easily cleaned floor covering that is secure and absorbent to avoid falls. Consider need for wearing device that sends signal for help.

• *Medication administration.* Take diuretics early in the day to avoid having to get up frequently at night.

• *Nocturia.* Void before lying down. Anticipate need to void after lying down by reclining in chair for 30 minutes before going to bed and then void on way to bed.

REFERENCES

1. Wallace, RB, and Woolson, RF (eds): The Epidemiologic Study of the Elderly. Oxford University Press, New York, 1992.
2. Eliopoulos, C: Caring for the Elderly in Diverse Care Settings. JB Lippincott, Philadelphia, 1990.
3. Crandall, RC: Gerontology: A Behavioral Science Approach. McGraw-Hill, New York, 1991.
4. Staab, AS, and Hodges, LC: Essentials of Gerontologic Nursing: Adaptation to the Aging Process. JB Lippincott, Philadelphia, 1996.

BIBLIOGRAPHY

Abrams, W, and Berkow, R (eds): The Merck Manual of Geriatrics. Merck Sharp and Dome Research Laboratories, Rahway, NJ, 1995.

Burke, M, and Walsh, M: Gerontologic Nursing: Wholistic Care of the Older Adult. Mosby, St Louis, 1997.

Dellasega, C, et al: Nursing process: Teaching elderly clients. J Gerontol Nurs 20(1):31, 1994.

Loughran, S: Medication use in the elderly: A population at risk. Medsurg Nurs 5(2):121, 1996.

Lutz, C, and Przytulski, K: Nutrition and Diet Therapy. FA Davis, Philadelphia, 1997.

Purnell, L, and Paulank, B (eds): Transcultural Health Care: A Culturally Competent Approach. FA Davis, Philadelphia, 1998.

Redeker, N, and Sadowski, A: Update on cardiovascular drugs and elders. Am J Nurs 95(9):34, 1995.

Reuben, D, Greendale, G, and Harrison, G: Nutrition screening in older persons. J Am Geriatr Soc 43:415, 1995.

Stanley, M, and Beare, P: Gerontological Nursing. FA Davis, Philadelphia, 1995.

Wound, Ostomy and Continence Nurses Society: Standards of Care for Dermal Ulcers. Costa Mesa, Calif, 1996.

Nursing Care of Clients with Chronic or Terminal Illness

14

Linda S. Williams

Learning Objectives

Upon completion of this chapter, the student will be able to:

1. Define chronic illness.
2. Describe the effects of chronic illness.
3. Describe caregiver needs and respite care.
4. Explain health promotion methods.
5. Identify nursing interventions for the chronically ill.
6. Describe care for the terminally ill.

Key Words

chronic illness (**KRAH**-nick **ILL**-nes)
hopelessness (**HOHP**-less-nes)
powerlessness (**POW**-er-less-nes)
respite care (**RES**-pit CARE)
spirituality (SPIHR-it-u-**AL**-it-tee)
terminal illness (**TERM**-in-al **ILL**-nes)

Chronic Illness

Chronic illness is defined as an illness that is long lasting or continues to recur. A chronic illness usually interferes with the client's ability to perform activities of daily living. Medical care and hospitalization, commonly at least once a year, are often required on an ongoing basis. **Terminal illness** could or is expected to cause death. Clients are usually considered terminally ill when they may have less than 6 months to live.

When nurses care for clients with chronic illness, the focus and goal of nursing care is to maintain and improve the client's quality of life. A chronic illness also affects the client's and family's quality of life. Therefore client care planning also includes consideration of the family's needs for adapting to the chronic illness to maintain quality of life.

Fostering hope is an important intervention that should be a primary foundation of care planning for the chronically ill client. A chronic illness may appear to be a hopeless situation if no cure is possible. When recovery from an illness is not possible for the client, the first thought that may occur is that nothing can be done for the client. However, whenever there is life, there is potential for growth. Although this growth may not be growth in the sense that gains toward maturity are made, growth in other areas such as developmental tasks, health promotion, knowledge, or spirit can still occur. Individuals have developmental tasks to perform even as they cope with illness or prepare for death that can make this journey more peaceful.

INCIDENCE OF CHRONIC ILLNESS

The incidence of chronic illness is rising for several reasons. First, people are living longer, in part due to better hygiene, nutrition, vaccinations, antibiotic development, and exercise. This is resulting in a larger elderly population who live long enough to develop many chronic illnesses. Second, medical advances have resulted in reduced mortality from some chronic illnesses so that clients live longer with these illnesses. Third, today's technology and modern lifestyles affect the development of some chronic illnesses. Examples include a sedentary lifestyle, exposure to air and water pollution, chemicals or carcinogens, substance abuse, and stress.

Some of the most common chronic conditions include chronic sinusitis, arthritis, hypertension, orthopedic dysfunction, decreased hearing, heart disease, bronchitis, asthma, and diabetes. This is important to understand so that preventive measures can be taught to clients to reduce the incidence of these conditions.

TYPES OF CHRONIC ILLNESSES

There are a variety of chronic illnesses resulting from several different causes (Table 14–1). These illnesses can have varying degrees of severity and can affect length of life. A chronic illness can lead to the development of others, such as in hypertension that causes chronic renal failure. Chronic illnesses can have onsets at various ages, although the elderly are most commonly affected by chronic illness, often having several chronic illnesses at one time (Table 14–2).

GERONTOLOGICAL INFLUENCE

The elderly are one of the largest age-groups living with chronic illness. As people live longer, elderly spouses or older family members are increasingly being called on to care for a chronically ill family member. Children of elders who themselves are reaching their sixties are being expected to care for their parents. These elderly caregivers

Table 14–1. **Examples of Chronic Illnesses by Causes**

Genetic
Sickle cell anemia
Cystic fibrosis
Muscular dystrophy
Huntington's disease

Congenital
Heart defects
Spina bifida
Malabsorption syndromes

Acquired
Chronic obstructive pulmonary disease
Arthritis
Head or spinal cord injury
Diabetes
Acquired immunodeficiency syndrome (AIDS)
Cancer
Multiple sclerosis
Cataracts
Peripheral vascular disease

Table 14–2. **Examples of Chronic Illnesses in the Elderly**

Arthritis
Diabetes
Hypertension
Heart disease
Peripheral vascular disease
Cerebrovascular accident
Chronic lung disease
Hearing impairments
Cataracts
Visual impairments

may also be experiencing a chronic illness themselves. For elderly spouses, it is usually the less ill spouse that provides care to the other spouse. The elderly family unit is at great risk for ineffective coping or further development of health problems. Nurses should assess all members of the elderly family to ensure that their health needs are being met.

Elderly adults are very concerned about becoming dependent and a burden to others. They may become depressed and give up hope if they feel that they are a burden to others. Establishing short-term goals or self-care activities that allow them to participate or have small successes are important nursing actions that can increase their self-esteem. (See Cultural Considerations Box 14–1.)

Barriers to caring for a chronically ill elderly client include a lack of information about treatments, medications or special diets, and being unfamiliar with supportive services in the community such as meal programs or **respite care.** The nurse should be aware of this and provide this information, as well as a resource number for questions.

EFFECTS OF CHRONIC ILLNESS

For the client to live as normally as possible with a chronic illness, many adjustments are usually necessary. Lifelong routines and habits may need to be changed. Daily living patterns are affected by routines that are established to cope with the illness. Treatment needs such as going

CULTURAL CONSIDERATIONS BOX 14–1

Traditional Appalachians believe that disability is natural with aging and is inevitable.[1] This belief discourages the use of rehabilitation as an option. Thus, in order to promote rehabilitation efforts among Appalachians, the nurse may need to stress self-help and a return to physical function.

to therapy sessions, performing peritoneal dialysis exchanges, or monitoring blood sugars can interrupt daily life.

Spiritual

Clients with chronic illness can experience spiritual distress when faced with the limitations of their illness. Maintaining clients' quality of life includes assisting clients with their spiritual needs. Religious and spiritual needs are important to people whose lives have been disrupted with new challenges from chronic illness. Studies show a positive relationship between clients' coping abilities and their spiritual concerns. Clients must be helped to find meaning in the illness and realistic hope. Interventions that address **spirituality** may need to be performed first to allow success of subsequent nursing care.

The LPN/LVN needs to develop a comfortable approach in assessing and meeting the client's spiritual needs. Several factors may make the nurse uncomfortable in caring for the client's spiritual needs. These factors include a lack of training, a lack of understanding of one's own spiritual needs and beliefs, and not recognizing or believing that this is the nurse's role. Nurses should examine their own spiritual needs to define a personal spiritual view. By doing this, the nurse develops insight into spiritual needs and spiritual resources, as well as a greater understanding of issues surrounding a client's spiritual needs.

Clients use spirituality to cope with chronic illness. It helps give them a sense of wholeness, hope, and peace during a time filled with uncertainty and anxiety. Spirituality plays an important role in empowering clients to handle their condition. It is a source of inner strength that allows the client to experience a sense of unity. In one study, elderly clients reported needing spiritual care.[2] Hospital interventions may include a meditation room for quiet reflection or prayer, chaplain visits, or worship services. The nurse, in helping to meet the client's spiritual needs, should assist the client with transportation to the meditation room or worship services.

Accreditation agencies require the spiritual needs of clients to be addressed and documented by nurses. Nursing diagnoses related to spiritual needs include spiritual distress and potential for enhanced spiritual well-being.

LEARNING TIP

Spiritual needs should not be thought of in only a religious focus. Spirituality is feeling connected with a higher power. The nurse should understand that everyone has spiritual needs that involve hope, peace, and wholeness. Spiritual care goes beyond simply asking the client's religion. It is assessing clients' perceptions of spirituality and then devising ways to assist them to meet their spiritual needs.

Powerlessness

Those with chronic illness often feel powerless because they are uncertain of their ability to control what may happen to themselves (Fig. 14–1). A chronic illness can take an unknown course in relation to its seriousness and controllability. This leaves the client vulnerable to the many phases of a chronic illness (the diagnosis, phase of instability, an acute illness or crisis, remissions, and a terminal phase).

Treatments that the client undergoes can be a new experience that is painful, frightening, and invasive. If clients do not understand what is happening, they can feel overwhelmed and alone. All of this contributes to a feeling of **powerlessness** because the client does not have the authority to control the outcome.[3] Clients with chronic illness are faced with a lack of control throughout their illness. It influences the reactions of the client to the illness. The nursing diagnosis of powerlessness may apply to many chronically ill clients.

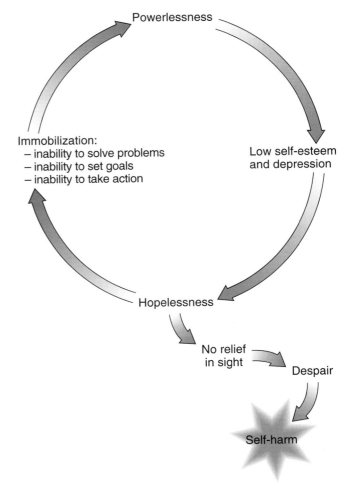

Figure 14–1. Powerlessness-hopelessness cycle. (Modified from Miller, J: Coping with Chronic Illness. Overcoming Powerlessness. FA Davis, Philadelphia, 1992, p 416.)

Coping

Clients can be helped to feel more in control of their illness if nurses remember to include them in their care; listen to their feelings, values, and goals; and explain all procedures before they are done. Complex medical language should be avoided when talking with clients to increase their understanding and feeling of being included instead of isolated. Additionally, coping with a chronic illness can be aided if the client develops a positive attitude toward the illness. This can be accomplished if the client gains knowledge, utilizes a problem-solving approach to difficulties, and becomes motivated to continue adapting to the illness and not succumbing to a defeatist attitude.

A variety of coping techniques can be useful. The nurse should assess the client's perception of the illness and coping techniques that the client has previously used successfully. New coping resources may need to be added as well to effectively deal with the client coping tasks that are associated with chronic illness. Support services in the community should be made available to the client and family. To cope effectively, the client should become comfortable with the newly defined person he or she is to become. The nursing diagnoses of ineffective coping for the client or family may apply to those dealing with chronic illness.

Hope

Before coping resources can be used, hope must be established by the client. False hope is not beneficial and should be replaced with realistic hope. Providing clients with accurate knowledge regarding their fears helps do this. Hope should not be directed toward a cure that may not be possible but rather at living a quality life with the functional capacity that the client has. Over the course of the illness, hope needs to be maintained in both the client and family. The nurse should periodically assess if the client is maintaining hope. Many studies have shown that clients adapt better when hope is high.

Many nursing interventions may increase hope. The use of humor by nurses helps clients be lighthearted and hopeful. Clients should be encouraged to live each moment to the fullest and experience the joy of being alive. Awakening the senses to appreciate the environment can bring a feeling of hope and peace. Simple things, such as the smell of baking bread, the clean scent of the air after a rain, or the scent of pine trees, can make one appreciate the beauty of nature and inspire hope. Family members need to be encouraged to help foster hope for the client. By doing this, the family member may also gain hope as well. During times of acute illness, the client needs to maintain as much control as possible and be told that any loss of control related to treatments is usually temporary. This prevents a continual feeling of loss of power. The use of music or inspirational reading material can reduce stress and help the client find meaning in life. This in turn fosters hope. Hopeful clients are empowered clients who no longer feel powerless. The nursing diagnosis of **hopelessness** may apply to chronically ill clients.

CRITICAL THINKING: Sol

Sol, 88, still lives in his own home with his wife of 60 years. He is in good health except for poor vision, which developed slowly over the last 8 years. He cares for his yard, which is his pride and joy, and grows prize-winning tomatoes each year. He plays golf three times a week and walks every day in the neighborhood to the neighborhood grocery store or bank. The employees know him and assist him due to his vision limitations.

Sol's wife was always the homemaker and he was the provider. His wife is now in the early stages of Alzheimer's disease exhibiting confusion, fatigue, and paranoia. She is unable to perform activities of daily living, so he has assumed the homemaker and caregiver roles. They complement each other's limitations because she can still see and is not always confused.

Over time, Sol's wife declines and must be institutionalized. Sol remains in his home alone. His family is concerned about him being alone and eventually convinces him to move into a studio apartment in senior housing. He is very reluctant to leave his home and does not actively participate in moving and selling his home. Sol rarely leaves his apartment, sleeps 14 hours a day, and eats one daily meal. He tries to visit his wife by taking the bus but finds it difficult, so he rarely goes to see her. Within a year, Sol develops pneumonia and dies.

1. Why did Sol exhibit the described behaviors after he moved?
2. What interventions could have been used to empower Sol?
3. Why might Sol have developed pneumonia and died?

Answers at end of chapter.

Sexuality

Chronic illness can affect a client's sexuality. Sexuality includes femininity or masculinity, as well as sexual activity. Body image changes affect the way clients view themselves and are viewed by others. If clients have a negative body image perception, they may withdraw and become depressed. Nurses can influence the perception clients have of their interactions with each other. As nurses interact with clients, they must be aware of their facial expressions, nonverbal cues such as appearing hurried or keeping a distance, use of or lack of touch, and amount of time spent with the client. When clients believe they have lost their femininity or masculinity, their self-worth decreases. Interventions to enhance sexuality should be used by the nurse, such as obtaining a wig from the wig bank for clients undergoing chemotherapy.

There are many forms of sexual expression. Sexual intimacy can include touching, hugging, or sharing time together. Nurses should provide clients with the opportunity to discuss sexuality concerns or questions. The nurse should assume a professional and confidential approach to this topic, which is usually considered a private matter by clients. Chronically ill clients can be referred to sex counselors for information on ways to cope with sexual issues in relationship to their illness. Support groups can also be helpful.

Clients in extended care facilities should be given private time with their significant other, if appropriate. Elderly clients need to have their sexuality needs met just as younger clients do. Because sexuality is a part of a person's lifelong identity, nurses need to ensure that the elderly client's sexuality is addressed in plans of care. Grooming methods can increase a client's self-esteem and sexual identity. Women may get their hair and nails done; men can be shaved or get a haircut.

Roles

Chronically ill clients are usually faced with altering their accustomed roles in life. Common roles that may be affected for the adult client include that of being a spouse, grandparent, parent, provider, homemaker, or friend. Not only is the client faced with dealing with these role alterations, the family must also adapt to these changes. Family members may have to take on new roles themselves to compensate for roles the client is no longer able to perform. The nursing diagnosis of altered role performance should be included in the plan of care for the client and family.

The client is faced with giving up aspects of old roles at the same time that new roles related to being chronically ill need to be assumed. Grieving accompanies the loss of old roles. If a client is no longer able to participate in social events such as being a golf team member or a committee member, grief work occurs to help the client accept the loss and maintain dignity. With other roles, only certain aspects of the role may change. For example, in the parenting role, clients may still be there as support systems for the child, although they are no longer able to be the disciplinarian. Whatever the role loss, the client needs to be allowed to grieve the loss. The nursing diagnosis of grieving helps in planning care for the client.

The new roles the client may have to assume related to chronic illness include dependency, ongoing health care consumer, self-care agent, and being chronically ill. Clients need to learn how to cope with these new roles. They need to gather knowledge and be given understanding as they become familiar with these roles. For clients used to being independent before the illness, being dependent on others to meet activities of daily living can cause a loss in self-esteem. Navigating the complex health care and financial reimbursement systems can be overwhelming. Transportation needs and waiting times for medical appointments can be difficult for the client who must deal with them on an ongoing basis. Becoming a self-care agent requires assuming responsibility for meeting one's own care needs. Handling chronic illness covers many areas such as living with pain, having altered mobility, or complying with daily treatments. Knowledge deficit is a nursing diagnosis helpful for fostering learning for these new roles.

As clients live with chronic illness over time, they become experts on their own illness. However, today's health care system tends to assume control over clients and does not respect the client's own knowledge. One study reported that clients who are not given this respect take charge of caring for themselves.[4] They seek knowledge and try alternative healing methods to take back control of their care. (See Chapter 4.) Nurses need to be sensitive to the client's knowledge and respect it to improve their relationship with the client. Clients who are treated with respect have increased self-esteem.

Family and Caregivers

Families are affected by the chronic illness of a family member in many ways. Chronic illness care is usually provided in the home so that families become involved in the management of the illness. Family members may have to take on new family roles or assume the role of caregiver. Family life can be altered. Decreased socialization, lost income, and increased medical expenses can increase family stress and tension.

Families must learn to cope with the stress of illness and its often unpredictable course. Most families develop ways to cope with the client's illness the majority of the time and may become closer as a family unit. Children adapt better to a parent's illness when they receive parental support. Families often deal with the illness on a day-by-day basis and take a passive approach for most problems to let them work themselves out. During times of exacerbation or crisis, however, the family may need coping assistance.

Clients are often concerned about being a burden to their families. It is important for the nurse to assess both the family's and the client's feelings about the care required by the client. The family's ability to provide this care adequately must also be considered in care planning. If the family lacks the desire, skills, or resources to adequately care for the client, alternative care options must be explored such as home health care, adult foster care, or extended care facilities.

Client caregivers often have certain ideas about the care that the client should receive. This may come into conflict with the views of health care providers. Caregiver input into the client's plan of care should be sought so that everyone has a clear understanding of goals and expectations for the client's care.

Caregivers often experience depression, role strain, guilt, powerlessness, and grieving due to caregiving.[5] Nurses must be aware of this to detect indications that caregivers are in need of help to deal with these feelings. Chronic care coaches are a resource available to caregivers who can provide insight, encouragement, and support for caring for the chronically ill. A nursing diagnosis useful for caregivers is risk for caregiver role strain.

Respite Care

When caregivers are required to provide 24-hour care for a client, they can experience burnout, fatigue, and stress, which, if extreme, in some cases can lead to client abuse. Caregivers may not be able to leave clients alone even briefly due to wandering behaviors, confusion, or safety issues. They may not ever be able to get a normal night's sleep and suffer from sleep deprivation due to client wandering or around-the-clock treatment needs.

Caregivers must be given periodic relief from their responsibilities of caregiving to reduce the stress of always having to be responsible. Everyone requires private time for reflection or pursuing favorite hobbies. Caregivers may need to get away overnight or for a weekend simply to sleep soundly and be refreshed.

Respite care is designed to provide caregivers with a much-needed break from caregiving by providing someone else to assume the caregiver role. Many communities have respite care services of which the nurse should be familiar to share with caregivers. Unfortunately, there are often not enough respite care services available to meet the needs of caregivers. Most respite care is provided by volunteers who receive training. As the number of chronically ill grow, more respite care programs must be developed to promote the health of the caregiver and in turn the client.

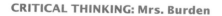

CRITICAL THINKING: Mrs. Burden

Mrs. Burden, 64, is caring for her husband, who has Alzheimer's. He exhibits wandering behaviors. He gets up at night and in freezing winter weather is found walking down the street in only his pajamas. He attempts to cook and burns the pans. He is unable to express his needs. He disrobes frequently and is incontinent around the house. Mrs. Burden quit her job to care for him. She no longer goes to lunch weekly with her friends. Her children live out of town. She places a chair and tin cans in front of the home's doors in case her husband tries to open the doors.

1. What is Mrs. Burden at risk of developing?
2. What nursing diagnoses should be included in a plan of care for Mrs. Burden?

3. What nursing interventions would be beneficial for Mrs. Burden?

Answers at end of chapter.

Finances

Managing a chronic illness can be expensive. Income can be lost if the client is unable to work or caregivers are forced to stay home. Family savings can quickly be wiped out. If the client is covered by insurance, it may not cover all of the client's expenses or it may have caps on lifetime coverage amounts. Expenses may involve medications, medical equipment or supplies, therapy, acute care, or home care. Inadequate funds can place a strain on families. This can lead to the nursing diagnosis of ineffective family coping. Nurses may need to refer clients to a social worker or sources of financial aid to help them meet their financial needs.

HEALTH PROMOTION

Health promotion is possible and necessary at all levels of age or disability. With the increase in elderly population, nurses are challenged to understand the role of health promotion in the elderly who have chronic illness. Promoting health is aimed at increasing the client's optimal wellness level.[6] Clients with chronic illness make daily lifestyle choices that affect their health. For example, the client with chronic lung disease who smokes can make a choice to smoke or quit smoking. Clients with degenerative joint disease can choose whether or not to keep their weight within ideal weight ranges to reduce wear and tear on their joints. Arthritic persons can reduce their fatigue levels by pacing their activities and scheduling daily rest periods.

Those with chronic illness consider health promotion important in maintaining their qualify of life and rehabilitation.[7] The LPN/LVN should encourage health promotion efforts. Clients need to be assisted to strive toward high-level wellness. This can be achieved by looking at the client's strengths and weaknesses holistically to develop a plan of care. The LPN/LVN assesses the client's risk factors to plan methods of promoting health. Providing clients with knowledge to make informed decisions empowers them to take control of their lives and reach for their greatest potential. The nursing diagnosis of health-seeking behaviors can be used to assist clients in promoting their health.

NURSING CARE

Nursing care is primarily devoted to caring for clients with chronic illness. Nurses must develop a sensitivity to understanding that the wishes of the client must be respected even if the nurse does not agree with them. Clients have the right to establish their own goals in partnership with the health care team. Because of the nature of chronic illness, the nurse needs to understand the unique needs of clients and families experiencing chronic illness. These needs differ from acute care as far as depth of knowledge needs and the compounding problems that are usually faced by the client.

Most chronic illness care occurs in the home and community rather than the acute care setting. Therefore family members and caregivers, even more so than in acute care, must be assessed and included in the plan of care. As the numbers of those with chronic illness grow, community support for the chronically ill and their caregivers must be established. Training programs for caregivers must be developed and offered affordably.

A major focus of nursing care for the chronically ill is teaching. These clients and their families have tremendous educational needs if they are to successfully learn to cope with a long-term illness. There are primary tasks that the chronically ill need to perform:

- Being willing and able to carry out the medical regimen
- Understanding and controlling symptoms
- Preventing and managing crises
- Reordering time to meet demands caused by the illness such as treatments, medication schedules, and pacing of activities
- Adjusting to changes in the disease over the course of time, whether positive or negative
- Preventing social isolation from physical limitations or an altered body image
- Compensating for symptoms and limitations in order to be treated as normally as possible by others

Nurses should highlight and explain individualized interventions to deal with these tasks during teaching sessions.

Nurses are in a unique position to interact with chronically ill clients on a long-term basis. Special acute care nursing units can be developed that take a holistic approach to care to foster independence rather than dependence of clients and families on the health care team.[8]

Unique approaches such as this are needed to positively assist chronically ill clients and their families on their long-term journey.

Terminal Illness

Death is a natural occurrence after many illnesses, especially chronic illness. Reactions to death vary by culture and individual's responses. Kubler-Ross described the emotional reactions that people have to dying in five stages: denial and isolation, anger, bargaining, depression, and acceptance.[9] These emotional stages assist the client and family to deal with the news of a terminal illness. Each person experiences these stages uniquely and may move back and forth among them. Denial allows hope to continue after being informed that death may occur. Anger reflects the question, "Why me?" In bargaining, a deal is made with God if the client is allowed to live just a little longer, usually to attend a special event such as a graduation. Depression indicates that the client is sad and feels that nothing more can be done. With acceptance, the client is at peace and simply seeks a comfortable and dignified death.

The main focus of terminal nursing care is providing the client and family with a pain-controlled and dignified death that allows participation by family members. This care is given in many locations: the client's home, a hospice facility, an extended care facility, or a hospital. Nurses should assess the goals of the client and family in dealing with the terminal illness. Families should be taught what to expect and do as death approaches so they do not panic when signs of impending death occur (Table 14–3). If the client becomes comatose and no further medical treatment is desired, comfort care is usually ordered and provided until death occurs. At this time, the nurse's primary focus may become the client's significant others, who need assistance with emotional support and grief work. Nursing diagnoses that may apply at this time include anticipatory grieving or grieving for either the client or family.

Table 14–3. **Signs and Symptoms of Approaching Death**

Signs and Symptoms	Cause	Nursing care
Coolness, mottling	Vasoconstriction	Use blankets
Sleeping	Metabolism changes	Sit quietly, remember hearing is last sense to leave
Disorientation	Metabolism changes	Orient as needed
Incontinence	Muscles relaxing	Keep clean and comfortable
Chest congestion	Weakened cough to remove secretions	Oral care to keep mouth moist
Restlessness	Decreased brain oxygen	Calm and distract client with music, massage, reading
Oliguria	Less fluid intake	Consider if catheter needed (often it is not)
Fluid and food intake decreases	Body is saving energy, may cause natural analgesia	Do not force intake; oral care, sips of ice if desired
Breathing pattern changes	Less circulation to organs	Position in semi-Fowler's or on the side.

HOME HEALTH HINTS

- Home care nurses can strengthen a client's self-care capacity by saying "let me assist you" instead of "let me do this for you," being a partner in caring instead of being a caretaker, and empowering the client instead of doing everything for the client.

- Being attentive to any of the client's efforts or accomplishments, such as number of steps taken, shaving without help, interest in a book or TV show, or decisions on fixing up the house or cleaning, provides opportunities to offer support and praise for accomplishments.

- Using humor can be helpful during a visit, unless the patient is distraught, anxious, or angry. Comics or jokes from magazines can be read. Humor can relieve the client's and caregiver's stress and humanize the care that must be performed. Humor can provide a mechanism for dealing with issues and giving messages that might not be taken as well as if their stressful nature is tempered with humor. However, the nurse should remember that humor might be irritating if it is taken as downplaying the seriousness of a situation.

- Families can be empowered, and the client may feel more secure, if families are taught cardiopulmonary resuscitation (CPR). The nurse can refer families to hospital or community CPR classes.

- The home health social worker should be informed of any client concerns regarding cost of medicines or equipment. There are many programs to assist the chronically ill to obtain resources.

- The home health nurse has an opportunity to increase a client's self-concept by emphasizing the client's existing abilities, joys, and talents. This can be done by observing the home environment for clues: photographs, trophies, hobby paraphernalia, flowers, or homemade items. Each clue observed can be a springboard to discuss triumphs and losses. It can help the nurse understand how the client copes to assist in planning care.

- The home health nurse should always be aware of the client's wishes for resuscitation if it is needed. If the client has a do-not-resuscitate (DNR) status, the DNR should be reviewed with the client and family so everyone has the same understanding.

- The nurse should always carry a pocket mask in the event cardiopulmonary resuscitation is needed for clients desiring resuscitation or another emergency situation.

- To enable emergency medical technicians to get to the client more easily, clients and families should be taught that if an ambulance is called, they should turn on an outside light, open the door, and move furniture, if possible, before the ambulance arrives.

- The nurse can encourage the family of bed-confined clients to purchase an inexpensive portable intercom to give the caregiver freedom to move about the house and hear the client if help is needed.

- When clients have the use of only one hand or arm, provide a sponge for personal grooming instead of a washcloth because a sponge is easier to use and hold.

Review Questions

1. Which one of the following is the primary goal of chronic illness treatment?
   a. Ensuring a cure
   b. Providing comfort care
   c. Maintaining quality of life
   d. Undergoing new experimental treatments

2. Which one of the following is a caregiver barrier to caring for a chronically ill elderly client?
   a. Awareness of support services
   b. Lack of information
   c. Using a meal program
   d. Excess knowledge

3. Which one of the following is most likely to be an effect of a chronic illness?
   a. Powerfulness
   b. Hopefulness

   c. Increased socialization
   d. Spiritual distress

4. Which one of the following is the purpose of respite care?
   a. To provide personal time for the caregiver
   b. To allow the client to rest for several hours
   c. To give the client a vacation
   d. To give the client free time away from a caregiver

5. Which one of the following is a health promotion method used for the chronically ill client?
   a. Making choices for the client
   b. Empowerment with knowledge
   c. Setting goals for the client and family
   d. Asking the family to make decisions for the client

6. Which one of the following is an appropriate nursing intervention for a chronically ill client?
   a. Decreasing educational information
   b. Limiting visiting hours for family members

c. Including family members in teaching sessions

d. Setting goals for the client and family

7. Which one of the following is a sign of impending death?
   a. Warmth of extremities
   b. Increased body temperature
   c. Insomnia during the night
   d. Mottling of lower extremities

ANSWERS TO CRITICAL THINKING

CRITICAL THINKING: Sol

1. He has lost control of his world and feels powerless. His environment, both home and outdoors, is shrinking. He is having to give up his daily routines and interactions with others. His purpose in life is gone now that he is not caring for his wife. He is separated from his loved one. His visual limitations make his new environment unfamiliar and frightening.

2. Options to keep him safely in his home could have been explored with his input. After the move, he should be thoroughly oriented to his environment. He should explain what he would like his life to be like now as he adapts to this new developmental stage. Hobbies and interests should be continued. Visual support services should be contacted for ideas. Transportation should be arranged to allow him to visit his wife. Determine whether phone calls to his wife are possible.

3. He was depressed and slept from a lack of any interests. His lungs were at risk for pneumonia due to his long periods of immobility. He lost hope and gave up on living, which decreased his ability to fight the pneumonia.

CRITICAL THINKING: Mrs. Burden

1. Sleep deprivation, fatigue, stress, and burnout.

2. Sleep pattern disturbance, fatigue, social isolation, risk for caregiver role strain, knowledge deficit.

3. Teaching about Alzheimer's, a chronic care coach, respite care referral, alarm devices for wandering, stress management techniques.

REFERENCES

1. Hansen, M, and Resick, L: Health beliefs, health care, and rural Appalachian subcultures from an ethnographic perspective. Fam Community Health 13(1):1, 1990.
2. Ross, LA: Elderly patients' perceptions of their spiritual needs and care: A pilot study. J Adv Nurs 26(4):710, 1997.
3. Miller, J: Coping with Chronic Illness. Overcoming Powerlessness. FA Davis, Philadelphia, 1999, in press.
4. Lindsey, E: Experiences of the chronically ill. A covert caring for the self. J Holist Nurs 15(3):227, 1997.
5. Ruppert, RA: Psychological aspects of lay caregiving. Rehabil Nurs 21(6):315, 1996.
6. Polan, E, and Taylor, D: Journey across the Life Span. FA Davis, Philadelphia, 1998.
7. Stuifbergen, AK, and Rogers, S: Health promotion: An essential component of rehabilitation for persons with chronic disabling conditions. ANS Adv Nurs Sci 19(4):1, 1997.
8. Byers, JF: Holistic acute care units: Partnerships to meet the needs of the chronically ill and their families. AACN Clin Issues Crit Care Nurs 8(2):271, 1997.
9. Kubler-Ross, E: On Death and Dying. New York, Macmillan, 1969.

BIBLIOGRAPHY

Aguilar, N: Counseling the patient with chronic illness: Strategies for the health care provider. J Am Acad Nurse Pract 9(4):171, 1997.
Bates, M, Rankin-Hill, L, and Sanchez-Ayendez, M: The effects of the cultural context of health care on treatment of and response to chronic pain and illness. Soc Sci Med 45(9):1433, 1997.
Bibou-Nakou, I, Dikaiou, M, and Bairactaris, C: Psychosocial dimensions of family burden among two groups of carers looking after psychiatric patients. Soc Psychiatry Psychiatr Epidemiol 32(2):104, 1997.
Bull, M, and Jervis, LL: Strategies used by chronically ill older women and their caregiving daughters in managing posthospital care. J Adv Nurs 25(3):541, 1997.
Davidhizar, R, and Shearer, R: Helping the client with chronic disability achieve high-level wellness. Rehabil Nurs 22(3):131, 1997.
do Rozario, L: Spirituality in the lives of people with disability and chronic illness: A creative paradigm of wholeness and reconstitution. Disabil Rehabil 19(10):427, 1997.
Eckes Peck, SD: The effectiveness of therapeutic touch for decreasing pain in elders with degenerative arthritis. J Holist Nurs 15(2):176, 1997.
Eliopoulos, C: Chronic care coaches: Helping people to help people. Home Healthc Nurse 15(3):185, 1997.
Fowler, S: Health promotion in chronically ill older adults. J Neurosci Nurs 29(1):39, 1997.
Grunfeld, E, et al: Caring for elderly people at home: The consequences to caregivers. Can Med Assoc J 157(8):1101, 1997.
Hart, BG: Chronic pain management in the workplace. AAOHN J 45(9):451, 1997.
Kane, RA: Being there: Chronic disease management in and by families. J Am Geriatr Soc 44(11):1405, 1996.
Kotchick, BA, et al: The role of parental and extrafamilial social support in the psychosocial adjustment of children with a chronically ill father. Behav Modif 21(4):409, 1997.
Kubusch, S, and Wichowski, H: Restoring power through nursing interventions. Nurs Diagn 8(1):7, 1997.
Lewis, KS: Emotional adjustment to a chronic illness. Lippincotts Primary Care Practice 2(1):38, 1998.
Malone, JA: Family adaptation: Adult sons with long-term physical or mental illnesses. Issues Ment Health Nurs 18(4):351, 1997.
Medaliem, JH: The patient and family adjustment to chronic disease in the home. Disabil Rehabil 19(4):163, 1997.
Newman, DM: Responses to caregiving: A reconceptualization using the Roy adaptation model. Holist Nurs Pract 12(1):80, 1997.
Pierce, LL: The framework of systemic organization applied to older adults as family caregivers of persons with chronic illness and disability. Gastroenterol Nurs 20(5):168, 1997.
Qualey, TL: Assessing the patient's caregiver. Nurs Manage 28(6):43, 1997.
Sharoff, L: Coping with the dis-ease of having a disease: A holistic perspective. J Psychosoc Nurs Ment Health Serv 35(10):43, 1997.
Sidell, NL: Adult adjustment to chronic illness: A review of the literature. Health Soc Work 22(1):5, 1997.
Zerwekh, J: Do dying patients really need IV fluids? Am J Nurs 97(3):26, 1997.

Understanding the Cardiovascular System

Cardiovascular System Function, Assessment, and Therapeutic Measures

15

Linda S. Williams and Valerie C. Scanlon

Learning Objectives

Upon completion of this chapter, the student will be able to:

1. Identify the structures of the cardiovascular system.
2. Describe the functions of the cardiovascular system.
3. List the effects of aging on the cardiovascular system.
4. Describe nursing assessment of the cardiovascular system, including health history and physical assessment.
5. Explain laboratory and diagnostic studies used when evaluating cardiovascular function.
6. Describe therapeutic measures for clients with cardiovascular disease.

Key Words

arteriosclerosis (ar-TIR-ee-oh-skle-**ROH**-sis)

atherosclerosis (ATH-er-oh-skle-**ROH**-sis)

bradycardia (BRAY-dee-**KAR**-dee-yah)

bruit (BROUT)

claudication (KLAW-di-**KAY**-shun)

clubbing (**KLUB**-ing)

dysrhythmias (dis-**RITH**-mee-yahs)

Homans' sign (**HOH**-manz SIGHN)

ischemic (iss-**KEY**-mik)

murmur (**MUR**-mur)

pericardial friction rub (PER-ee-**KAR**-dee-uhl **FRIK**-shun RUB)

poikilothermy (POY-ki-loh-**THER**-mee)

point of maximal impulse (POYNT OF **MAKS**-i-muhl **IM**-puls)

preload (**PREE**-lohd)

pulse deficit (PULS **DEF**-i-sit)

thrill (THRILL)

Review of Normal Anatomy and Physiology

The cardiovascular system consists of the heart and blood vessels, including arteries, capillaries, and veins. Its function is to pump and distribute blood throughout the body.

HEART

Cardiac Location and Pericardial Membranes

The heart is located in the mediastinum, the area between the lungs in the thoracic cavity. It is enclosed by three pericardial membranes that make up the pericardial sac. The outermost of these membranes is the fibrous pericardium, which forms a loose-fitting sac around the heart. The second or middle layer is the parietal pericardium, a serous membrane that lines the fibrous layer. The third and innermost layer, the visceral pericardium or epicardium, is a serous membrane on the surface of the heart muscle. Between the parietal and visceral layers is serous fluid, which prevents friction as the heart beats.

Cardiac Structure and Vessels

The walls of the four chambers of the heart are made of cardiac muscle, myocardium, and are lined with endocardium, which is smooth epithelial tissue that prevents abnormal clotting. The endocardium also covers the valves of the heart and lines the vessels. The coronary vessels include the arteries and capillaries that circulate oxygenated blood throughout the myocardium and veins that return unoxygenated blood to the heart. The two main coronary arteries are the first branches of the ascending aorta, just outside the left ventricle (Fig. 15–1).

The upper chambers of the heart are the thin-walled right atrium and left atrium, which are separated by the interatrial septum. The lower chambers are the thicker-walled right and left ventricles, which are separated by the

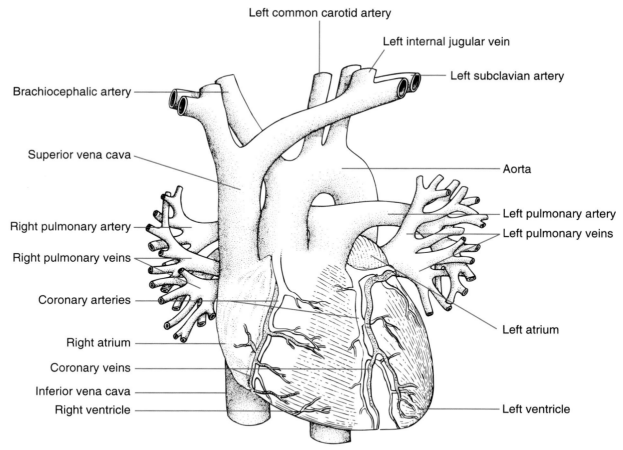

Figure 15–1. Anterior view of the heart and major blood vessels. (Modified from Scanlon, VC, Sanders, T: Workbook for Essentials of Anatomy and Physiology, ed 2. FA Davis, Philadelphia, 1995, p 182, with permission.) See Plate 1.

interventricular septum. Each septum is made up of myocardium that forms a common wall between the two chambers.

The right atrium receives deoxygenated blood from the upper body by way of the superior vena cava and from the lower body by way of the inferior vena cava. (See Fig. 15–1.) This blood flows from the right atrium through the tricuspid valve into the right ventricle. Backflow during ventricular systole is prevented by the tricuspid or right atrioventricular (AV) valve (Fig. 15–2). The right ventricle pumps blood through the pulmonary semilunar valve to the lungs by way of the pulmonary artery. The pulmonary semilunar valve prevents backflow of blood into the right ventricle during ventricular diastole.

The left atrium receives oxygenated blood from the lungs by way of the four pulmonary veins. This blood flows through the mitral or left AV valve into the left ventricle. The mitral valve prevents backflow of blood into the left atrium during ventricular systole. The left ventricle pumps blood through the aortic valve to the body by way of the aorta. The aortic valve prevents backflow of blood into the left ventricle during ventricular diastole.

The tricuspid and mitral valves consist of three and two cusps, respectively. These cusps or flaps are connective tissue covered by endocardium and are anchored to the floor of the ventricle by the chordae tendineae and papillary muscles. The papillary muscles are columns of myocardium that contract along with the rest of the ventricular myocardium. This contraction pulls on the chordae tendineae and prevents inversion of the AV valves during ventricular systole. (See Fig. 15–2.)

Although each ventricle pumps the same amount of blood, the much thicker walls of the left ventricle pump with approximately six times the force of the right ventricle to pump the blood throughout the body. This difference in force is reflected in the great difference between systemic and pulmonary blood pressure.

Cardiac Conduction Pathway and Cardiac Cycle

The cardiac conduction pathway is the pathway of electrical impulses that generates a heartbeat (Fig. 15–3). The sinoatrial (SA) node in the wall of the right atrium is a specialized mass of cardiac muscle that depolarizes rhythmically and most rapidly, 60 to 80 times per minute, and therefore initiates each heartbeat. For this reason it is sometimes called the pacemaker, and a normal heartbeat is

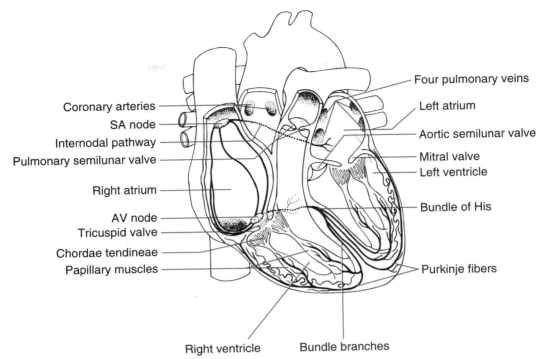

Figure 15–2. Frontal section of the heart showing internal structures and cardiac blood flow. (Modified from Scanlon, VC, Sanders, T: Workbook for Essentials of Anatomy and Physiology, ed 2. FA Davis, Philadelphia, 1995, p 266, with permission.) See Plate 1.

called a normal sinus rhythm. From the SA node, impulses travel to the AV node located in the lower interatrial septum, to the bundle of His in the upper interventricular septum, to the right and left bundle branches in the septum, and to the Purkinje fibers in the rest of the ventricular myocardium. If the SA node becomes nonfunctional, the AV node can initiate each heartbeat, but at a slower rate of 50 to 60 beats per minute. The bundle of His is capable of generating the beat of the ventricles, but at the much slower rate of 15 to 40 beats per minute.

A cardiac cycle is the sequence of mechanical events during one heartbeat. Simply stated, the two atria contract simultaneously, followed a fraction of a second later by the simultaneous contraction of the two ventricles. The contraction, or systole, of each set of chambers is followed by relaxation, or diastole, of the same set of chambers.

The atria in diastole continually receive blood from the veins. As pressure within the atria increases, the AV valves are forced open, causing most of the blood to flow passively into the ventricles. Atrial systole, referred to as atrial kick, pumps the remaining blood into the ventricles, and then the atria relax. Ventricular systole follows. The pressure in the ventricles causes the AV valves to close and forces the semilunar valves to open. Blood is then pumped into the aorta and pulmonary artery. There is no passive blood flow. Any blood leaving the ventricles must be pumped. Toward the very end of ventricular systole, as the pressure drops, the blood tends to flow backward. It is this backflow of blood that closes the semilunar valves. The

ventricles and the atria are then all in diastole; the atria continue to fill until pressure opens the AV valves again, and the cycle is repeated.

The events of the cardiac cycle create the normal heart sounds. The first of the two major sounds (the *lubb* of *lubb-dupp*) is caused by the closure of the AV valves during ventricular systole. The second sound is created by the closure of the aortic and pulmonary semilunar valves.

Cardiac Output

Cardiac output is the amount of blood pumped by the left ventricle in 1 minute (the right ventricle pumps a similar amount); it is determined by multiplying stroke volume by pulse. Stroke volume is the amount of blood pumped by a ventricle in one beat and averages 60 to 80 mL. With an average resting heart rate of 70 beats per minute, an average resting cardiac output is 5 to 6 L (approximately the total blood volume of an individual that is pumped within 1 minute). During exercise, venous return increases and stretches the ventricular myocardium, which in response contracts more forcefully. This is known as Starling's law of the heart, and the result is an increase in stroke volume. More blood is pumped with each beat, and, at the same time, the heart rate increases, causing cardiac output to increase to as much as four times the resting level, and even more for athletes.

The ejection fraction is a measure of ventricular efficiency and is usually about 60 percent. It is the stroke vol-

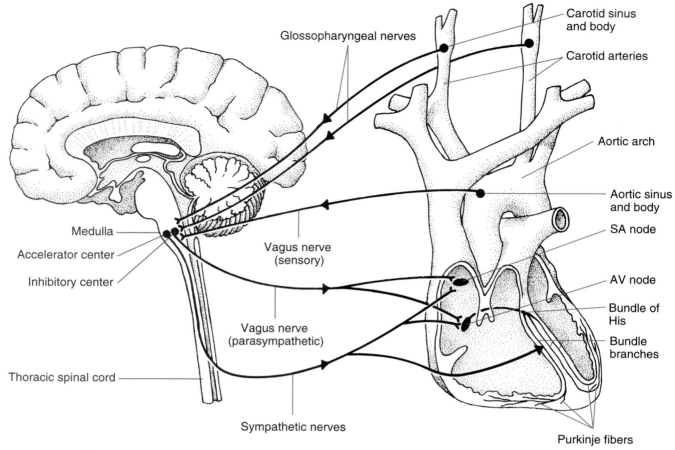

Figure 15–3. Nervous system regulation of the heart. (Modified from Scanlon, VC, Sanders, T: Workbook for Essentials of Anatomy and Physiology, ed 2. FA Davis, Philadelphia, 1995, p 189, with permission.)

ume divided by total blood in the ventricle (also known as the end-diastolic volume, which is approximately 120 to 130 mL). Lower values indicate that the ventricle is not pumping as forcefully and that more blood remains in the ventricle at the end of systole. The normal end-systolic volume is about 50 to 60 mL.

Regulation of Heart Rate

The heart generates its own electrical impulse, which begins at the SA node. The nervous system, however, can change the heart rate in response to environmental circumstances. (See Fig. 13–3.) Within the brain, the medulla contains the cardiac centers: the accelerator center and the inhibitory center. Sympathetic nerve impulses, along sympathetic nerves from the thoracic spinal cord to the SA node, AV node, and ventricular myocardium, increase rate and force of contraction. Parasympathetic impulses, along the vagus nerve to the SA node and AV node, decrease heart rate.

The information for changes necessary in the heart rate comes to the medulla from pressoreceptors and chemore-

ceptors located in the internal carotid arteries and the aortic arch. The pressoreceptors, specialized cells called the carotid and aortic sinuses, detect changes in blood pressure. The chemoreceptors are located in the carotid and aortic bodies and are specialized cells to detect changes in the oxygen content of the blood. In response to either a drop in blood pressure or a decrease in blood oxygen level, the heart will receive sympathetic impulses and will beat faster in an attempt to provide sufficient oxygenation for tissues.

Hormones and the Heart

The hormone epinephrine, secreted by the adrenal medulla in stressful situations, is sympathomimetic in that it increases heart rate and force of contraction (and dilates the coronary vessels). This in turn increases cardiac output and systolic blood pressure.

Aldosterone, a hormone produced by the adrenal cortex, is important for cardiac function because it helps regulate blood levels of sodium and potassium, both of which are needed for the electrical activity of the myocardium. The blood level of potassium is especially critical because even a small deficiency or excess will impair the rhythmic contractions of the heart.

The atria of the heart secrete a hormone of their own called atrial natriuretic peptide (ANP) or atrial natriuretic hormone (ANH). As its name suggests, ANP increases the excretion of sodium by the kidneys, perhaps by inhibiting secretion of aldosterone by the adrenal cortex or renin by the kidneys. Atrial natriuretic peptide is secreted when a higher blood pressure or greater blood volume stretches the walls of the atria. The loss of sodium is accompanied by the loss of more water in urine, which decreases blood volume and perhaps blood pressure as well.

BLOOD VESSELS

Arteries and Veins

Arteries and arterioles carry blood from the heart to capillaries. Their walls are relatively thick and consist of three layers (Fig. 15–4). Arteries carry blood under high pressure, and the outer layer of fibrous connective tissue prevents rupture of the artery. The middle layer of smooth muscle and elastic connective tissue contributes to the maintenance of normal blood pressure (BP), especially diastolic BP, by changing the diameter of the artery. The diameter of arteries is regulated primarily by the sympathetic division of the autonomic nervous system. The lining is simple squamous epithelium, called endothelium, which is very smooth to prevent abnormal clotting.

Veins and venules carry blood from capillaries to the heart. Their walls are relatively thin because there is less smooth muscle (veins do not have as important a role in the maintenance of BP as arteries). Sympathetic impulses can bring about extensive constriction of veins, however, and this becomes important in situations such as severe hemorrhage. The lining of veins is endothelium that prevents abnormal clotting; at intervals it is folded into valves to prevent backflow of blood. Valves are most numerous in the veins of the extremities, especially the legs, where blood must return to the heart against the force of gravity.

Capillaries

Capillaries carry blood from arterioles to venules and form extensive networks in most tissues. The exceptions are cartilage, the epidermis, and the lens and cornea of the eye. Their walls, a continuation of the lining of arteries and veins, are one cell thick to permit the exchanges of gases, nutrients, and waste products between the blood and tissues. (See Fig. 15–4.) Blood flow through a capillary network is regulated by a precapillary sphincter, a smooth muscle cell that contracts or relaxes in response to tissue needs. In an active tissue such as exercising skeletal muscle, for example, the rapid oxygen uptake and carbon dioxide production will cause dilation of the precapillary sphincters to increase blood flow. At the same time, precapillary sphincters in less active tissues will constrict to reduce blood flow. This is important because there is not enough blood in the body to fill all the capillaries at once; the fixed volume must constantly be shunted or redirected to where it is needed most.

The blood pressure in capillaries is 30 to 35 mm Hg at the arterial end of the network, and it drops to about 15 mm Hg at the venous end. This pressure is low enough to prevent rupture of the capillaries but high enough to permit filtration. Tissue fluid is formed from the plasma in capillaries by the process of filtration. Because capillary blood pressure is higher than the pressure of the surrounding tissue fluid, plasma and dissolved materials such as nutrients are forced through the capillary walls to become tissue fluid. Some of this tissue fluid will return to the capillaries, and some will be collected in lymph capillaries. Now called lymph, it too will be returned to the blood, by the system of lymph vessels. Should blood pressure within the capillaries increase, more tissue fluid than usual will be formed, which is too much for the lymph vessels to collect. This is called edema.

BLOOD PRESSURE

Blood pressure is the force of the blood against the walls of the blood vessels and is measured in mm Hg: systolic/diastolic. The normal range of systemic arterial pressure is 90 to 135/60 to 85 mm Hg. Blood pressure decreases in the arterioles and capillaries, and the systolic and diastolic pressures merge into one pressure. As blood enters the veins, BP decreases further and approaches zero in the caval veins. As mentioned previously, the blood pressure in the capillaries is of great importance, and normal BP is high

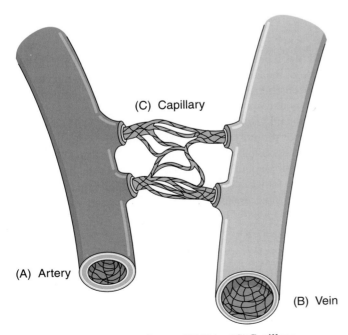

(C) Capillary

(A) Artery

(B) Vein

Figure 15–4. *(A)* Artery, *(B)* Vein, *(C)* Capillary.

enough to permit filtration for nourishment of tissues, but low enough to prevent rupture.

The arteries and veins are usually in a state of slight constriction that helps to maintain normal BP, especially diastolic BP. This is called peripheral resistance and is regulated by the vasomotor center in the medulla, which generates impulses along sympathetic vasoconstrictor nerves to all vessels with smooth muscle to maintain slight constriction. More impulses per second increase vasoconstriction and raise BP; fewer impulses per second bring about vasodilation and lower BP. The information for changes needed in the vessel diameter comes to the medulla from the pressoreceptors and chemoreceptors located in the internal carotid arteries and aortic arch.

Blood pressure is also affected by many other factors. If heart rate and force increase, BP will increase up to a point. If the heart is beating very fast, the ventricles will not be filled before they contract, cardiac output will decrease, and BP will drop. The strength of the heart's contractions depends on adequate venous return, which is the amount of blood that flows into the atria. Decreased venous return will result in weaker contractions.

Venous return depends on several factors: constriction of the veins so that blood does not pool in them, the skeletal muscle pump to squeeze the deep veins of the legs, and the muscles of respiration to compress and expand the veins in the chest cavity. The valves in the veins prevent backflow of blood and thus contribute to the return of blood to the heart.

The elasticity of the large arteries also contributes to normal blood pressure. When the left ventricle contracts, the blood stretches the elastic walls of the large arteries, which absorb some of the force. When the left ventricle relaxes, the walls recoil or snap back and put pressure on the blood. Normal elasticity, therefore, lowers systolic pressure, raises diastolic pressure, and maintains normal pulse pressure. Pulse pressure is the difference between the systolic and diastolic pressures. The usual ratio of systolic to diastolic to pulse pressure is 3:2:1.

Renin-Angiotensin Mechanism

The kidneys are of great importance in the regulation of blood pressure. If blood flow through the kidneys decreases, renal filtration will decrease and urinary output will decrease to preserve blood volume. Decreased BP stimulates the kidneys to secrete renin, which initiates the renin-angiotensin mechanism (Fig. 15–5). Renin splits the plasma protein angiotensinogen (from the liver) to form angiotensin I, which is changed to angiotensin II by a converting enzyme found primarily in lung tissue. Angiotensin II causes vasoconstriction and stimulates secretion of aldosterone, both of which raise BP.

Aldosterone, secreted by the adrenal cortex, increases the reabsorption of sodium ions by the kidneys. Water follows the sodium back to the blood; this increases blood volume

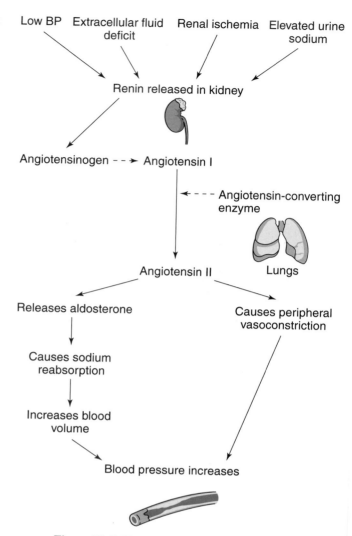

Figure 15–5. The renin-angiotensin mechanism.

and blood pressure. Other hormones that affect BP include those of the adrenal medulla: norepinephrine, which causes vasoconstriction throughout the body, and epinephrine, which increases cardiac output and causes vasoconstriction in skin and viscera. Antidiuretic hormone (ADH), from the posterior pituitary, directly increases water reabsorption by the kidneys, thus increasing blood volume and BP. Atrial natriuretic peptide, secreted by the atria of the heart, is believed to inhibit aldosterone and renin secretion and thereby increase renal excretion of sodium ions and water, which decreases blood volume and subsequently BP.

PATHWAYS OF CIRCULATION

The two pathways of circulation are pulmonary and systemic. (See Fig. 15–2.) Pulmonary circulation begins at the right ventricle, which pumps deoxygenated blood into the pulmonary artery. The pulmonary artery branches into two arteries, one to each lung. The pulmonary capillaries around the alveoli of the lungs are the site of gas exchange. Oxygenated blood returns to the left atrium by way of the pulmonary veins. The blood pressure in the pulmonary circulation is always low because the right ventricle pumps with only about one-sixth the force of the left ventricle. The arterial pressure is about 20 to 25/8 to 10 mm Hg, and the pulmonary capillary pressure is lower still. This is important to prevent filtration in pulmonary capillaries, which prevents tissue fluid from accumulating in the alveoli of the lungs, causing pulmonary edema.

Systemic circulation begins in the left ventricle, which pumps oxygenated blood into the aorta, the many branches of which give rise to capillaries within the tissues. Deoxygenated blood returns to the right atrium by way of the superior and inferior vena cava. The hepatic portal circulation is a special part of the systemic circulation in which blood from the capillaries of the digestive organs and spleen flows through the portal vein and into the capillaries (sinusoids) in the liver before returning to the heart. This pathway permits the liver to regulate the blood levels of nutrients such as glucose, amino acids, and iron and to filter or remove potential toxins such as alcohol or medications from circulation.

AGING AND THE CARDIOVASCULAR SYSTEM

It is believed that the "aging" of blood vessels, especially arteries, begins in childhood, although the effects are not apparent until later in life. **Atherosclerosis** is the deposition of lipids on and in the walls of arteries over a period of years, which narrows their lumens, decreases blood flow, and forms rough surfaces that may stimulate intravascular clot formation. **Arteriosclerosis** is the gradual deterioration of the walls of arteries as a result of the pressure they have withstood over many decades. Average resting blood pressure tends to increase with age and may contribute to stroke or left-sided heart failure. The thinner-walled veins, especially those of the legs, may also weaken and stretch, making their valves incompetent.

With age, the heart muscle becomes less efficient, and there is a decrease in both maximum cardiac output and heart rate, although resting levels may be more than sufficient. The health of the myocardium depends on its blood supply, and with age there is greater likelihood that atherosclerosis will narrow the coronary arteries. Hypertension causes the left ventricle to work harder, and it may hypertrophy and outgrow its blood supply. The heart valves may become thickened by fibrosis, leading to heart **murmur. Dysrhythmias** are more common in the elderly as the cells of the conduction pathway become less efficient.

---

atherosclerosis: athere—porridge + sklerosis—hardness
arteriosclerosis: arteria—artery + sklerosis—hardness
dysrhythmia: dys—difficult or abnormal + rhythmia—rhythm

Nursing Assessment of the Cardiovascular System

Nursing assessment of the cardiovascular system includes a client health history and physical examination. If the client is experiencing an acute problem, the nursing assessment should focus on the most serious signs and symptoms and physical assessment data until the client is stabilized (Table 15–1). An in-depth nursing assessment can be completed when the client is stable. For stable or chronic cardiac conditions, a complete nursing assessment is done on admission. The nurse provides privacy and makes the client as comfortable as possible before beginning the nursing assessment. (See Gerontological Issues Box 15–1.)

SUBJECTIVE DATA

To understand the client's cardiovascular problems the nurse will ask about past and current symptoms; use of pre-

Table 15–1. **Acute Cardiovascular Nursing Assessment**

History	Significance
Allergies	For medication administration, test dyes
Smoking History	Risk factor for cardiovascular disorders
Medications	Toxic levels; influencing symptoms
Pain	Location—chest, calf; radiation—arms, jaw, neck; description—pressure, indigestion, tightness, burning, angina, myocardial infarction, thrombus, embolism
Dyspnea	Left-sided heart failure; pulmonary edema or embolism
Fatigue	Decreased cardiac output
Palpitations	Dysrhythmias
Dizziness	Dysrhythmias
Weight Gain	Right-sided heart failure
Physical Assessment	**Possible Abnormal Findings**
Vital Signs	Bradycardia, tachycardia, hypotension, hypertension, tachypnea, apnea, shock
Heart Rhythm	Dysrhythmias
Edema	Right-sided heart failure
Jugular Vein Distention	Right-sided heart failure
Breath Sounds	Crackles, wheezes with left-sided heart failure
Cough, Sputum	Acute heart failure—dry cough, pink frothy sputum

GERONTOLOGICAL ISSUES BOX 15–1

Older clients often have signs and symptoms atypical for the disorder. For example, the only symptom of myocardial infarction in an older client may be dyspnea. Chest pain may not be present.

scribed and over-the-counter medications; use of recreational drugs; surgeries; treatments; and risk factors such as diet, activity, tobacco use, and recent stressors. Assessment of symptoms includes asking questions for WHAT'S UP: *w*here it is, *h*ow it feels, *a*ggravating and alleviating factors, *t*iming, *s*everity, *u*seful data for associated symptoms, and *p*erception by the client of the problem.

Health History

The entire body can be affected by cardiovascular problems. Some symptoms can have more than one cause. For example, shortness of breath can be the result of either heart failure or chronic obstructive pulmonary disease. The health history can help determine the cause of the symptom. For cardiovascular problems, the assessment focuses on the areas listed in Table 15–2.

Past Medical History

If previous medical records are available, they can provide objective client data that can be supplemented with client responses. If medical records are not available, the client is asked about previous conditions that could affect the cardiovascular system. A history of childhood illnesses that can lead to heart disease, such as rheumatic fever and scarlet fever, is noted. Other conditions include pulmonary disease, hypertension, kidney disease, cerebral vascular accident or brain attack, transient ischemic attack, renal disease, anemia, streptococcal sore throat, congenital heart disease, thrombophlebitis, and alcoholism. Client allergies, previous hospitalizations, and surgeries are documented. Baseline diagnostic tests are helpful for comparison with current tests. Functional limitations that are related to cardiovascular problems, such as performing activities of daily living (ADL), walking, climbing stairs, or completing household tasks, are also assessed.

Medications

Medication use is noted. This includes prescription drugs, over-the-counter medications such as aspirin that can prolong clotting time, and recreational drugs. The medication history includes the client's understanding of the medication and the medication name, dosage, reason for taking, last dose, and length of use.

Family History

A family history of cardiovascular conditions is assessed because many cardiac problems are hereditary. Health histories of close relatives, such as parents, siblings, and grandparents, are the most significant.

Health Promotion

Risk factors such as diet, activity, tobacco use, and recent stressors for the client are assessed in the health history. The client's health promotion activities are noted, especially for risk factors that are modifiable through changes in lifestyle.

OBJECTIVE DATA

Physical Assessment

The client's general appearance is observed. The client's level of consciousness, which is an indicator of oxygenation of the brain, is assessed. Height and weight are recorded. Vital signs are measured.

Blood Pressure

The average adult reading is 120/80 with a normal range of 100/60 to 140/90. For accurate measurement the correct size cuff for the client is used. Readings in both arms are done for comparison. A difference in the readings is reported to the physician. The arm with the higher reading is used for ongoing measurements. The leg may be used if necessary, with a larger blood pressure cuff. The reading in the leg is normally 10 mm Hg higher than in the arm.

Blood pressure measurements are done with the client lying, sitting, and standing to detect abnormal variations with postural changes. When the client sits or stands, a drop in the systolic pressure of up to 15 mm Hg and either a drop or slight increase in the diastolic pressure of 3 to 10 mm Hg is normal. In response to the drop in blood pressure, the pulse increases 15 to 20 beats per minute to maintain cardiac output. Orthostatic hypotension, also referred to as postural hypotension, is a greater than normal change in these pressures and indicates a problem that should be investigated by the physician. The client may experience dizziness when changing positions, so fall-prevention methods should be used during blood pressure measurement.

LEARNING TIP

Orthostatic or Postural Hypotension. Anticipate potential drops in blood pressure with position changes. Orthostatic or postural hypotension is a drop in systolic blood pressure greater than 15 mm Hg, a drop or slight increase in the diastolic blood pressure greater than 10 mm Hg, and an increase in heart rate greater than 20 beats per minute in response to the drop in blood pressure. It can be found in clients of any age but is most

Table 15–2. **Cardiovascular History Assessment**

Question	Rationale
Pain: WHAT'S UP Format	
• **W**here is pain? Does it radiate?	• Cardiac pain may radiate to shoulders, neck, jaw, arms, or back. Vascular disorders cause extremity pain.
• **H**ow does it feel? Discomfort, burning, aching, indigestion, squeezing, pressure, tightness, heaviness, numbness in chest area? Fullness, heaviness, sharpness, throbbing in legs?	• Pain can be associated with angina or MI. The quality of pain varies. Venous pain is a fullness or heaviness. Sharpness or throbbing is arterial pain.
• **A**ggravating/alleviating factors that increase/relieve the pain?	• Activity may cause or increase angina. Rest or medications may relieve angina. Leg activity pain, intermittent claudication, results from decreased perfusion that is aggravated by activity. Rest pain, from severe arterial occlusion, increases when lying. Dangling reduces the pain because blood flow is increased by gravity.
• **T**iming of pain: onset, duration, frequency?	• Pain may be continuous, intermittent, acute, or chronic. Arterial occlusion causes acute pain.
• **S**everity of pain?	• Rate pain on a scale of 1 to 10.
• **U**seful data for associated symptoms?	• Accompanying symptoms and their characteristics guide diagnosis and treatment.
• **P**erception of client about problem?	• Client's insight to problem is helpful in planning care.
Level of Consciousness (LOC)	
• What is your name? What is the month? Year? Where are you now?	• A lack of oxygen caused by cardiac disease can decrease LOC.
Dyspnea	
• Are you short of breath? What increases your shortness of breath? What relieves your shortness of breath?	• Dyspnea can be present with heart failure that reduces cardiac output, on exertion in angina pectoris or from a pulmonary embolus resulting from thrombophlebitis, heart failure, or dysrhythmias.
Palpitations	
• Are you having palpitations or irregular heartbeat? Does your heart ever race, skip beats, or pound?	• Palpitations can occur from dysrhythmias resulting from ischemia, electrolyte imbalance, or stress. Dizziness can be associated with dysrhythmias.
Fatigue	
• Have you noticed a change in your energy level?	• Fatigue occurs from reduced cardiac output resulting from heart failure.
• Are you able to perform activities that you would like to?	• Functional abilities can be limited from fatigue.
Edema	
• Have you had any swelling in your feet, legs, or hands?	• Right-sided heart failure can cause fluid accumulation in the tissues.
• Have you gained weight?	• Fluid retention causes weight gain.
Paresthesia/Paralysis	
• Any numbness, tingling, or other abnormal sensations in extremities?	• Numbness and tingling, pins and needles, and crawling sensations are paresthesia.
• Can you move your extremity?	• Paralysis is inability to move extremity. Reduced nerve conduction from decreased oxygen supply causes paresthesia and paralysis.

commonly found in the older client. The client will often report light-headedness or syncope because the drop in pressure decreases the amount of oxygen-rich blood traveling to the brain. The change from a lying to a sitting or a sitting to a standing position may cause the drop in pressure. This blood pressure drop increases the risk of fainting and falling. Factors that can contribute to orthostatic hypotension include fluid volume deficit, diuretics, analgesics, and pain.

To assess orthostatic hypotension, do the following:

1. Take client's lying blood pressure and heart rate.
2. Assist client to sitting position. Ask if dizzy or light-headed with each position change. If yes, ensure safety from fainting or falling. A gait or walking belt can be used. With any position change, if client experiences additional symptoms with the dizziness and decreased blood pressure and increased heart rate, assist the client into bed, take blood pressure, and notify the physician. Consider the possible cause of the orthostatic hypotension—hemorrhaging, dehydration, diuretics—to plan client care.
3. Wait at least 1 minute, and then take client's sitting blood pressure and heart rate. If client remains dizzy or light-headed, continue sitting position for 5 minutes if tolerated. Do not attempt to stand client. Repeat sitting blood pressure. If blood pressure has increased and client is no longer dizzy, assist client to stand.
4. Assist client to stand. Wait at least 1 minute, and then take client's standing blood pressure and heart rate. If blood pressure drops and client is dizzy or light-headed, continue standing position for 5 minutes, if tolerated. Do not attempt to ambulate client. Repeat standing blood pressure and heart rate.
5. Document all heart rate and blood pressure measurements, including extremity used and client position when reading obtained (e.g., right arm—lying 132/78, sitting 118/68, standing 110/60). Also document client tolerance, symptoms, and nursing interventions, if symptomatic.
6. Report abnormal findings to physician.

Pulses

The apical pulse is auscultated for 1 minute to assess rate and rhythm. Normal heart rate is 60 to 100 beats per minute. In athletic individuals, the heart rate is often slower, around 50 beats per minute, because the well-conditioned heart pumps more efficiently. Apical pulse rhythm is documented as regular or irregular. The apical rate can be compared with the radial rate to assess equality. If there are fewer radial beats than apical beats a **pulse deficit** exists and should be reported to the physician.

Arterial pulses are palpated for volume and pressure quality (Fig. 15–6). They are palpated bilaterally and compared for equality. The normal vessel feels soft and springy. The sclerotic vessel feels stiff. The quality of the pulses is described on a four-point scale as follows: 0 is absent; 1+ is weak, thready; 2+ is normal; and 3+ is bounding. An absent pulse is not palpable. A thready pulse is one that disappears when slight pressure is applied and returns when the pressure is removed. The normal pulse is easily palpable. The bounding pulse is strong and present even when slight pressure is applied. When the normal vessel is palpated, a tapping is felt. In the abnormal vessel that has a bulging or narrowed wall, a vibration is felt, which is called a **thrill.** When auscultating an abnormal vessel, a humming is heard that is caused by the turbulent blood flow through the vessel. This is referred to as a **bruit.**

Respirations

The rate and ease of respirations are observed. Breath sounds are auscultated. Sputum characteristics such as amount, color, and consistency are noted. Pink, frothy sputum is an indicator of acute heart failure. A dry cough can occur from the irritation caused by the lung congestion resulting from heart failure.

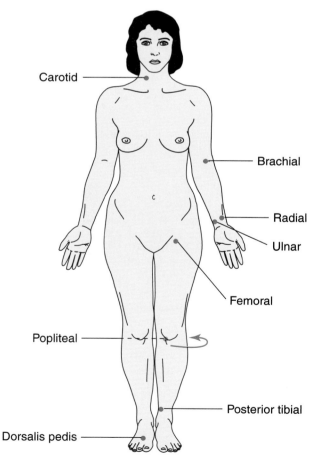

Figure 15–6. Peripheral pulse sites.

Carotid

Brachial

Radial

Ulnar

Femoral

Popliteal

Posterior tibial

Dorsalis pedis

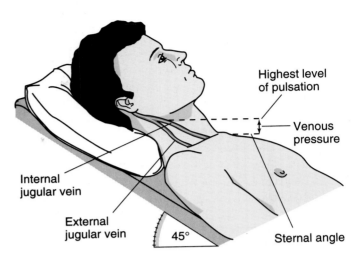

Figure 15–7. Jugular vein distention. Distention of the jugular vein at 45 degrees (arrow).

Inspection

During the health history, inspection begins by noting any shortness of breath when the client speaks or moves. The client's skin is noted for oxygenation status through the color of skin, mucous membranes, lips, earlobes, and nailbeds. Pallor may indicate anemia or lack of arterial blood flow. Cyanosis shows an oxygen distribution deficiency. A reddish-brown discoloration (rubor) found in the lower extremities occurs from decreased arterial blood flow. A brown discoloration and cyanosis when the extremity is dependent may be seen in the presence of venous blood flow problems. Hair distribution on the extremities is observed. Decreased hair distribution; thick, brittle nails; and shiny, taut, dry skin occur from reduced arterial blood flow. Venous blood return is assessed by inspecting extremities for varicose veins, stasis ulcers, or scars around the ankles and signs of thrombophlebitis such as swelling; redness; or a hard, tender vein.

The internal and external jugular neck veins are observed for distention (Fig. 15–7). Normally in the upright position, the veins are not visible. Distention of the veins in an upright position of 45 to 90 degrees indicates an increase in the venous volume. This is most commonly caused by right-sided heart failure. To observe for this, the client is gradually elevated to a 45- to 90-degree position and any distention noted.

Capillary refill time assesses arterial blood flow to the extremities. The client's nailbed is briefly squeezed, causing blanching, and then released. The amount of time that it takes for the color to return to the nailbed after release of the squeezing pressure is the capillary filling time. Normal capillary refill time is 3 seconds or less. Longer times indicate anemia or a decrease in blood flow to the extremity.

ischemic: ischein—hold back + haima—blood
poikilothermy: poikilos—varied + therme—heat

Clubbing of the nailbeds occurs from oxygen deficiency over a period of time. It is often caused by congenital heart defects or the use of tobacco over a period of time. The distal ends of the fingers and toes swell and appear clublike. With clubbing, the normal 160-degree angle where the base of the nail and the skin join is lost, causing the nail to be flat (Fig. 15–8). Later the nail base elevates and the nail feels spongy when squeezed.

Palpation

In addition to palpating the arteries, the thorax can be palpated at the **point of maximal impulse** (PMI). The PMI is palpated by placing the right hand over the apex of the heart. If palpable, a thrust is felt when the ventricle contracts. An enlarged heart may shift the PMI to the left of the midclavicular line.

The temperature of the extremities is palpated bilaterally for comparison. Palpation begins proximally and moves distally along the extremity. In areas of decreased arterial blood flow the **ischemic** area will feel cooler than the rest of the body because it is blood that warms the body. In the absence of sufficient arterial blood flow, the area becomes the temperature of the environment. This is called **poikilothermy**. A warm or hot extremity indicates a venous blood flow problem.

LEARNING TIP

Six Ps characterize peripheral vascular disease: pain, pulselessness, pallor, poikilothermia, paralysis, and paresthesia (decreased sensation).

Edema is palpated in the extremities and dependent areas such as the sacrum for the supine client (Fig. 15–9). Edema can occur from right-sided heart failure, gravity, or altered venous blood return. The nurse assesses the severity of the edema by pressing with a finger for 5 seconds

Clubbing—early

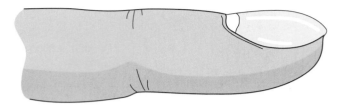

Clubbing—severe

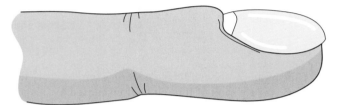

Figure 15–8. Clubbing of the fingers. The nailbed angle is lost (arrow) from clubbing of the distal ends of the fingers.

over a bone, the medial malleolus or tibia, in the area of edema. If the finger imprint or indentation remains, the edema is pitting. Measuring the leg circumference is an accurate method for monitoring the edema.

Homans' sign is an assessment for venous thrombosis; however, in less than 50 percent of clients with thrombosis the test is not positive. A positive Homans' sign is pain in the client's calf or behind the knee when the foot is quickly dorsiflexed with the knee in a slightly flexed position (Fig. 15–10). Homans' sign should not be performed if a positive diagnosis of thrombosis has been made.

Percussion

Percussion is performed by the physician to detect cardiac enlargement. Usually only the left border of the heart can

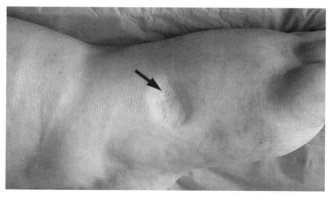

Figure 15–9. Lower extremity pitting edema. Application of pressure over a bony area displaces the excess fluid, leaving an indentation or pit (arrow). Hence the term *pitting edema.*

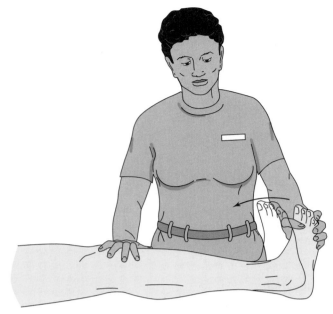

Figure 15–10. Assessment of Homans' sign for venous thrombosis. The foot is quickly dorsiflexed with the knee flexed. Calf or knee pain is noted. This assessment should not be performed if a positive diagnosis of thrombosis has been made.

be percussed. The heart is heard as dullness in contrast to the resonance heard over the lungs.

Auscultation

The normal heart sounds heard with a stethoscope placed on the wall of the chest are produced by the closing of the heart valves. The areas of auscultation are shown in Figure 15–11. These areas indicate where the sounds are best heard because sound in blood-flowing vessels is transmitted in the direction of the blood flow. The first heart sound (S_1) is heard at the beginning of systole as lubb when the tricuspid and mitral (AV) valves close (Fig. 15–12). The second heart sound (S_2) is heard at the start of diastole as dupp when the aortic and pulmonic semilunar valves close. The diaphragm of the stethoscope is used to hear the high-pitched sounds of S_1 and S_2. Extra heart sounds, usually indicating pathology, may be heard with practice. Normally no other sounds are heard between S_1 and S_2. With the bell of the stethoscope placed at the apex, a third heart sound (S_3) or a fourth heart sound (S_4) may be heard. Having clients lean forward or lie on their left side can make the heart sounds easier to hear by bringing the area of the heart where the sound may be heard closer to the chest wall. S_3 is normal for children and younger adults. It sounds like a gallop and is a low-pitched sound heard early in diastole. S_3 may be heard with left-sided heart failure, fluid volume overload, and mitral valve regurgitation. S_4 is also a low-pitched sound, similar to a gallop but heard late in diastole. It occurs with hypertension, coronary artery disease, and pulmonary stenosis.

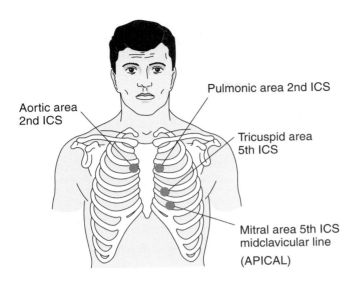

Figure 15–11. Auscultation points of heart.

ICS = intercostal space

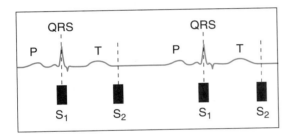

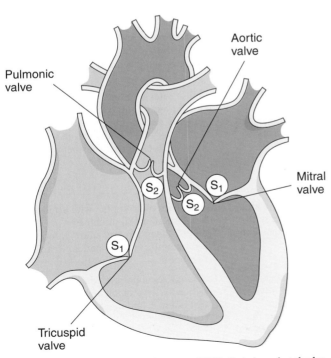

Figure 15–12. Heart sounds shown on ECG. S_1 is heard at the beginning of systole. S_2 is heard at the start of diastole.

Murmurs are caused by turbulent blood flow through the heart and major blood vessels. A murmur is a prolonged sound caused by a narrowed valve opening or a valve that does not close tightly. A swishing sound that ranges in intensity from faint to very loud is produced. The intensity of the murmur is graded by the physician on a scale of 1 to 6. The timing of the murmur in relationship to the cardiac cycle of systole or diastole is also documented by the physician.

A **pericardial friction rub** occurs from inflammation of the pericardium. The intensity of a rub can range from soft and faint to loud enough to be audible without a stethoscope. A rub has a grating sound like sandpaper being rubbed together that occurs when the pericardial surfaces rub together during the cardiac cycle. (See the Learning Tip in Chapter 17.) Having the client sit and lean forward allows a rub to be heard more clearly. The rub is best heard to the left of the sternum using the diaphragm of the stethoscope. A pericardial friction rub may occur after a myocardial infarction or chest trauma.

CRITICAL THINKING: Mrs. Smith

Mrs. Smith, 78, is admitted to the hospital with shortness of breath. Initial assessment findings are BP 152/88, pulse 104, respiration 26, temperature 99.4°F, short of breath at rest, shortness of breath increases with activity, ankles swollen, heart tones sound far away, nailbeds are very light pink, no pain, has not eaten well for 2 weeks, 6-pound weight gain in 1 week, sleeps on three pillows, veins in neck are visible on both sides.

A diagnosis of acute myocardial infarction with heart failure is made by the physician.

1. Why is Mrs. Smith not reporting chest pain with a diagnosis of acute myocardial infarction?
2. How should swollen ankles be assessed to provide complete and measurable data?
3. What should be documented for the assessment of the swollen ankles?
4. How should the assessment findings for the swollen ankles be documented?
5. How should the assessment findings be documented for the additional symptoms Mrs. Smith has?

Answers at end of chapter.

Diagnostic Studies

Diagnostic test results provide valuable assessment information for the nurse (Table 15–3). These data are combined with the health history and physical assessment to plan care for the client.

Table 15–3. **Diagnostic Tests and Procedures**

Procedure	Definition	Nursing Management
	Noninvasive	
Chest X-Ray	Anterior-posterior and left lateral views of chest taken to show heart size and contour and lungs.	Assess x-ray history and whether pregnant. Remove metal items. Teaching—no discomfort.
Magnetic Resonance Imaging (MRI)	Three-dimensional image of heart.	Assess for metallic items and claustrophobia. Give antianxiety medication as ordered before MRI. Teaching—must lie still in long, small cylinder with loud, pounding sounds. Can talk to technician, listen to music.
Electrocardiogram (ECG)	Electrodes on skin carry electrical activity of heart from different views to show rhythm of heart, size of chambers, and heart damage.	Teaching—no discomfort. Explain procedure.
Holter Monitor	Recording of ECG for up to 48 hours to match abnormalities with symptoms recorded in client's diary.	Apply electrodes and leads. Teaching—keep accurate diary; push event button for symptoms. No showers or baths. Return visit.
Transtelephonic Event Recorder	Records ECG events infrequently occurring for transmission over phone to interpreting center for analysis. Pacemaker checks done.	Teaching—explain use of recorder and how to transmit. Ensure good skin contact for best ECG tracing.
Pressure Measurement	Blood pressures taken at several sites along extremity to show area of occlusion or decreased blood flow at rest and with exercise.	Teaching—no discomfort. Explain procedure.
Exercise Treadmill Test (ETT)	Evaluates effects of exercise on heart and vascular circulation; ECG and vital signs are continuously monitored. Test stopped if symptoms develop.	Monitor vital signs and ECG before, during, and after test until stable. Teaching—explain procedure, wear walking shoes and comfortable clothes.
Echocardiogram	Transducer transmits sound waves that bounce off heart to produce heart images and show blood flow. Provides audio and graphic data.	May be done at bedside. Client lies on left side. Teaching—no discomfort, gel applied.
Transesophageal Echocardiogram	Probe with transducer on end inserted into esophagus, depth and angle directed by physician. Shows clearer images of heart because no lung or rib tissue is crossed. Dye injected for blood flow study.	Monitor vital signs and oxygen saturation. Encourage client to relax. Suction continually during procedure. Teaching—NPO 6 hours before test. Sedation and local throat anesthetic given.
	Radioisotopes	
	IV injection of radioactive isotopes, which are taken up by heart and scanned with scintillation camera to show cardiac contractility, injury, and perfusion.	Assist client to lie supine with arms over head for about 30 minutes. Teaching—explain procedure, inform that radioactivity is small and gone within a few hours.
Thallium Imaging	IV injection of thallium 201 to evaluate cardiac blood flow. Cold spots show infarcted areas. With exercise, thallium given 1 minute before end of test to circulate the thallium. Scan done within 10 minutes and repeated in 2–4 hours for comparison.	Teaching—explain procedure, inform that radioactivity is small and gone within a few hours. Light meal only between scans.

continued

Table 15–3. (continued)

Procedure	Definition	Nursing Management
	Radioisotopes	
Dipyridamole Thallium Imaging	Dipyridamole (Persantine) IV is a vasodilator given to increase blood flow to coronary arteries; test is same as thallium imaging.	Teaching—explain procedure, instruct no caffeine or aminophylline 12 hours before. Same as thallium imaging.
Technetium Pyrophosphate Imaging	Technetium 99m pyrophosphate IV given. Shows hot spot in heart injury area. Scanned 2 hours later.	Teaching—explain procedure, inform that radioactivity is small and gone within a few hours.
Blood Pool Imaging	Technetium 99m pertechnetate IV. Studies effects of drugs, recent MI, and congestive heart failure. Serial studies are done over several hours. May be done at bedside.	Teaching—explain procedure.
Positron Emission Tomography (PET)	Nitrogen-13-ammonia IV given and scanned for cardiac perfusion. Then fluoro-18-deoxyglucose IV given and scanned for cardiac metabolic function. In normal heart, scans match; in injured heart, they differ. Exercise may also be used.	Client's blood glucose must be 60 to 140 mg/dL for accuracy. Teaching—explain procedure. Must lie still during scan. If exercise used, NPO and no tobacco use.
Doppler Ultrasound	Sound waves bounce off moving blood, producing recordings. Evaluates PVD.	Teaching—explain procedure.
Plethysmography	After the leg being tested is raised 30 degrees with the client supine, a pressure cuff is inflated on the leg to distend the veins. Blood flow is measured with electrodes. Cuff is then rapidly deflated and venous volume changes recorded. Thrombi detected by less venous volume.	Teaching—explain procedure. No discomfort. Takes 30–45 minutes.
	Serum Enzymes	
Creatine Kinase (CK)	Heart, brain, skeletal muscle contain CK enzymes. Damaged cells release CK. With MI, CK elevates in 6 hours and returns to baseline in 48–72 hours. Normal: male 5–55 U/mL; female 5–25 U/mL.	Avoid IM injections and take baseline CK before inserting IVs to avoid elevating CK from muscle cell damage. Serial sampling done.
CK-MB	Only heart muscle contains MB isoenzyme, which rises with MI in 6 hours and returns to baseline in 72 hours. Normal: 0–7 IU/L.	Same as CK.
Lactic Dehydrogenase (LDH)	Intracellular enzyme found in many tissues, including heart. Elevates with MI after 8 hours and returns to baseline in 7 days. Normal: 80–120 U.	Serial sampling done.
LDH_1 and LDH_2	LDH contains five isoenzymes. Normally $LDH_2 > LDH_1$. In MI, ratio reverses: $LDH_1 > LDH_2$.	Same as LDH.
Serum Aspartate Aminotransferase (AST)	Nonspecific for cardiac damage.	No special care.
Myoglobin	Rises in 8 hours after MI and returns to baseline in 4–8 days; 99% indicative of MI. Rises in 1 hour after MI and peaks in 4–12 hours so must be drawn within 18 hours of chest pain onset. Normal: 250–450 ng/mL.	No special care.

continued

Table 15–3. (continued)

Procedure	Definition	Nursing Management
	Serum Enzymes	
Cardiac Troponin I	Cardiac cell protein. Elevated levels sensitive indicator of MI. Levels elevated up to 7 days.	No special care.
	Serum Lipids	
Cholesterol	Measure CAD risk. Normal: 140–200 mg/dL.	Fasting not required.
Triglycerides	Elevated in cardiovascular disease. Normal: 40–190 mg/dL.	Eat normal diet for 2 weeks before test. Fasting required for 12 hours. Water allowed but no alcohol.
Phospholipids	May elevate in cardiovascular disease. Normal: 125–380 mg/dL.	Same as triglycerides.
Lipoproteins	Electrophoresis done to separate lipoproteins: VLDL, LDL, HDL. HDL protects against CAD; LDL increases CAD risk. Normal lipoproteins: 400 to 800 mg/dL. Desirable: LDL less than HDL (values vary with age).	Same as triglycerides.
	Invasive	
Angiography	Dye injected into vessels to make them visible on x-rays to assess patency, injury, or aneurysms. Coronary—coronary arteries via cardiac catheter. Peripheral—peripheral arteries or veins.	Precare: Informed consent required. NPO 4–18 hours before test. Assess dye allergies. Teaching—sedative and local anesthesia may be used; burning sensation from dye; monitored continuously. Postcare: assess vital signs, circulation mobility sensation, catheter insertion site, or puncture site for hemorrhage, hematoma every 15 minutes for 1 hour, then every 30 minutes to 1 hour. Apply insertion site pressure (dressing, sandbag) as needed. Immobilize extremity for several hours as ordered.
Cardiac Catheterization	Catheter inserted into heart for data on oxygen saturation and chamber pressures. Dye may be injected to visualize structures.	Same as angiography. Sensory teaching—table is hard, cool cleansing solution used, sting felt from local anesthetic, hear monitor beeping, feel pressure of catheter insertion, dye warm, burning feeling, headache, chest pain briefly, hear camera, feel table move.
Hemodynamic Monitoring	Continuous readings of arterial BP, cardiac and pulmonary pressures, CO and SvO_2 obtained with catheter attached to transducer and monitor to diagnose and guide treatment. Normal: BP 120/80; right atrial pressure 2–6 mm Hg; pulmonary artery systolic pressure/pulmonary artery diastolic pressure 20–30/0–10; pulmonary artery wedge pressure 4–12 mm Hg; CO 4–8 L/min; SvO_2 60–80%.	Informed consent signed for insertion. Continuous assessment to ensure proper placement of catheter is maintained and a permanent catheter wedge does not go undetected. Recording of readings and monitoring of insertion site for signs of infection.
Central Venous Pressure (CVP)	Catheter inserted into a vein and threaded into vena cava. Monitors CVP, which reflects fluid volume status. Normal: 2–6 mm Hg.	Informed consent signed for insertion. Recording of readings and monitoring of insertion site for signs of infection.

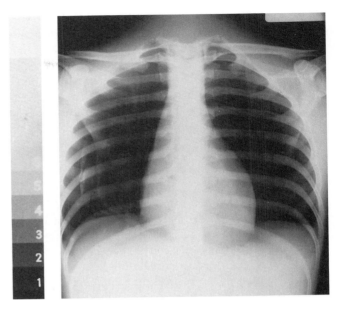

Figure 15–13. Normal chest x-ray. Note white outline of heart borders in center. (From McKinnis, LN: Fundamentals of Orthopedic Radiology. FA Davis, Philadelphia, 1997, p 15, with permission.)

Noninvasive

PULSE OXIMETRY. A transdermal clip or patch placed on a finger, a toe, an ear, or the nose is attached to a monitor and used to assess arterial oxygen saturation. A light in the clip or patch passes through the artery and provides data to measure the oxygen saturation. Normal levels are 95 percent or greater.

CHEST X-RAY. A chest x-ray shows the size, position, contour, and structures of the heart (Fig. 15–13). It will show heart enlargement, calcifications, and fluid around the heart. Heart failure can be confirmed with a chest x-ray. Correct placement of pacemaker leads and pulmonary artery catheters within the heart can be confirmed.

Fluoroscopy uses a luminescent x-ray screen to show cardiac structures and pulsations. It is used as a guide when placing cardiac catheters or pacemaker leads.

MAGNETIC RESONANCE IMAGING. A three-dimensional image of the heart is produced by magnetic resonance imaging (MRI). The client must lie still in a long, small-diameter cylinder with a strong magnetic field. Because of the small cylinder's close proximity to the client, clients can experience claustrophobia. Clients are asked if they are claustrophobic before the test, and antianxiety medication is given 1 hour before the MRI, as ordered. No metallic items are permitted in the machine, so some clients, such as those with pacemakers or metal implants, shavings, or shrapnel, are not candidates for this test.

ELECTROCARDIOGRAM. The electrocardiogram (ECG) assesses the electrical activity of the heart from different views (Fig. 15–14). Abnormalities in cardiac function can be detected and the area of abnormality pinpointed with the

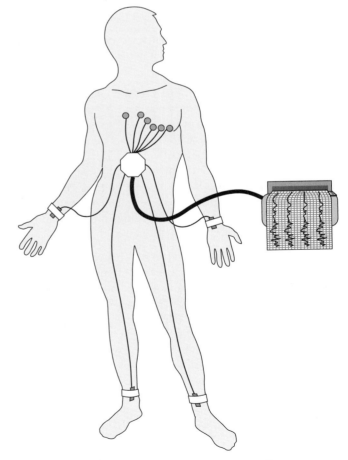

Figure 15–14. Standard 12-lead electrocardiogram.

aid of the different views on the ECG. When an ECG is requested, information that will aid in its interpretation is provided, including the client's sex, age, height, weight, blood pressure, and cardiac medications. The client requires no special preparation but is given an explanation of the procedure and told that the ECG is painless.

Electrodes placed on the skin transmit electrical impulses to the ECG machine for recording. The ECG is seen on an oscilloscope or traced on ECG graph paper. The electrical impulses from the heart appear as waves on the graph paper. A cardiac cycle is represented by the P, Q, R, S, and T waves. A normal ECG tracing is called normal sinus rhythm. (See Chapter 20.)

To obtain an ECG, five electrodes are placed on the skin. One electrode is placed on each limb and on the chest. The right leg is a ground electrode. The chest electrode is moved along the chest to provide different views of the heart. One view of the heart using a combination of electrodes to obtain that view is called a lead. The standard 12-lead ECG provides 12 views of the heart. An 18-lead ECG can be done if necessary by moving the chest electrode across the right side of the chest to visualize the right ventricle and posterior left ventricle, which are not seen on a 12-lead ECG.

The ECG shows abnormalities related to conduction, rate, rhythm, heart chamber enlargement, myocardial ischemia, myocardial infarction, and electrolyte imbalances.

AMBULATORY ELECTROCARDIOGRAM MONITORING. Continuous monitoring of the ambulatory client is possible with the use of tape recorders.

Holter monitoring. A Holter monitor, which weighs two pounds, continuously records one lead for up to 48 hours (Fig. 15–15). The client wears loose-fitting clothing and may only sponge bathe while wearing the monitor. The client records a diary of activities and symptoms and pushes the event button if symptoms occur. Symptoms are documented for later correlation with the ECG recordings. Dysrhythmias or myocardial ischemia that occurs infrequently can be detected. The recordings are scanned by a computer and interpreted by a physician.

Transtelephonic event recorders. This recorder is used for dysrhythmic events that occur so infrequently that they would not likely be captured in 48 hours, or for follow-up evaluation of permanent pacemakers. With this recorder the patient has greater flexibility because the device is worn when needed or when symptoms occur. The disadvantage is that if the event is brief it may be missed before the recorder is on. When an event is recorded the client can transmit it over the telephone for printout and analysis. The telephone mouthpiece is placed over the signal transmitter box for transmission. After transmission the recording can be erased and the recorder reused.

PRESSURE MEASUREMENT. Pressure readings are done to assess areas of occlusion or narrowing in vessels. Blood

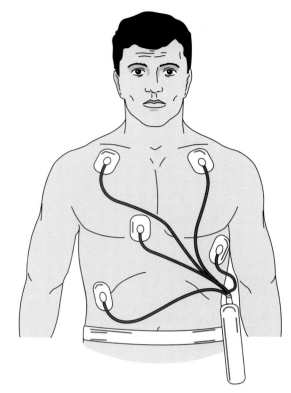

Figure 15–15. Holter monitor.

pressure readings are taken at intervals along the extremity. Reduced readings are found in areas with blood flow problems.

EXERCISE TOLERANCE TESTING. The exercise tolerance test or stress test measures cardiac function or peripheral vascular disease during a defined exercise protocol (Fig. 15–16). Before the test, clients are given an explanation of the test and told not to smoke, eat, or drink for 2 to 4 hours before the test. They are also instructed to wear comfortable walking shoes, a loose top, and for women a supportive bra. After the test, clients should rest and wait to eat. They should also avoid eating or drinking stimulants such as caffeine and temperature extremes such as going out into cold weather for a few hours after the test.

Cardiac stress test. This test simulates sympathetic nervous system (fight or flight) stimulation. It shows the heart's response to increased oxygen needs. Before the test, baseline vital signs are obtained. Then, while the client exercises on a treadmill, on a stationary bicycle, or by climbing stairs, vital signs, oxygen saturation, skin temperature, physical appearance, chest pain, and ECG are monitored to help ensure client safety. The test is completed when the client reaches peak heart rate (client's age subtracted from 220), experiences chest pain, is unable to exercise further, or develops vital sign or ECG changes. Vital signs and ECG continue to be monitored after the test until they return to baseline.

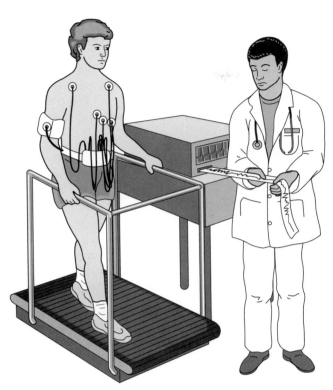

Figure 15–16. Performance of stress test.

The cardiac stress test is used to evaluate coronary artery disease. It aids in diagnosing ischemic heart disease, the cause of chest pain and dysrhythmias. The functional capacity of the heart can also be measured after a cardiac event or to plan a physical fitness or rehabilitation program.

Peripheral vascular stress test. The client walks for 5 minutes at 1.5 miles per hour on the treadmill. At certain intervals, pulse volume measurements are taken, including baseline resting, during the test, and final resting after the test. This test assesses response to activity. If **claudication** occurs the test is stopped.

ECHOCARDIOGRAM. An echocardiogram is an ultrasound test that records the motion of the heart structures, including the valves, as well as the heart size, shape, and position. No preparation is required for a cardiac ultrasound. This test transmits ultrasonic sound waves into the heart so that the returned echoes can be recorded on videotape as audio and visual information. An ECG is recorded at the same time for comparison purposes.

Abnormalities that may be seen on the echocardiogram include heart enlargement, valvular abnormalities, and thickened cardiac walls or septum, the cause of heart murmurs and pericardial effusion.

claudication: claudicare—to limp

TRANSESOPHAGEAL ECHOCARDIOGRAPHY. Transesophageal echocardiography (TEE) provides a clearer picture than echocardiography. It produces images through the chest wall by using a transducer on a probe that is swallowed. The images are clearer because lung and rib tissue does not have to be penetrated by the sound waves. The physician controls the position of the probe as it travels within the esophagus and takes pictures. Clients take nothing by mouth (NPO) for about 6 hours before the test, receive a sedative, and have their throat locally anesthetized. After the procedure, clients remain NPO until their gag reflex returns.

RADIOISOTOPE IMAGING. For this type of imaging, small amounts of radioisotopes are given intravenously. The client is then scanned to determine the radioactivity emitted. Radiation exposure is similar to that of other x-rays. These tests can provide information about myocardial ischemia or infarction, cardiac blood flow, and ventricle size and motion.

Thallium imaging. Thallium 201 is used to detect impaired myocardial perfusion. It is injected intravenously (IV), and after 10 to 15 minutes the heart is scanned to see where the thallium has concentrated. Four hours later the scan is repeated to look for changes. Healthy myocardial cells with good blood flow take up the thallium. Areas in which the thallium is not seen are referred to as cold spots and indicate ischemia or infarction. The patency of a coronary artery graft may also be assessed with this test.

Exercise testing may be combined with thallium injection to detect blood flow changes with activity and after rest. The client exercises and about 2 minutes before stopping is given thallium. Scans are taken immediately and again in 2 to 4 hours. Cold spots on initial images indicate ischemia. If the cold spots are gone in later images it indicates exercise-induced ischemia. If the cold spots are still present in later images, they show scarred areas.

If clients are unable to participate in exercise for the thallium stress test, dipyridamole (Persantine) or adenosine, coronary vasodilators, can be given. These drugs simulate the increased blood flow to healthy myocardial cells that occurs with exercise.

Technetium pyrophosphate scanning. Technetium 99m pyrophosphate is injected for this test. Areas of ischemia or myocardial cell damage take up the radioisotope, and when scanned these areas appear as hot spots. Acute myocardial infarction (MI) size and location can be detected, but old MIs cannot be detected.

Blood pool imaging. Technetium 99m pertechnetate is injected IV and remains in the bloodstream; it is not taken up by myocardial cells. A camera follows the flow of the radioactivity, which shows ventricular function and wall motion and the heart's ejection fraction.

Positron emission tomography. Positron emission tomography (PET) shows myocardial perfusion and viability with three-dimensional images. Nitrogen-13-ammonia is injected IV first and then scanned to show myocardial perfusion. Next, fluoro-18-deoxyglucose IV is given and then scanned to show myocardial metabolic function. If there is ischemia or heart damage, the two scans will be different. For example, in ischemia of viable cells, blood flow will be decreased but metabolism elevated. Treatment to increase blood flow improves cardiac function in this case. Before the test the client's blood glucose should be normal, and caffeine and tobacco should be avoided for 4 hours before the test.

DOPPLER ULTRASOUND. In this test, sound waves are transmitted to an artery or vein to assess blood flow problems. The sound waves bounce off moving blood cells and return a sound frequency in relationship to the amount of blood flow. With decreased blood flow the sounds are reduced. This test requires no client preparation, takes about 20 minutes to complete, and is painless.

PLETHYSMOGRAPHY. With this test, blood volume and changes in blood flow are measured to diagnose deep vein thrombosis and pulmonary emboli and to screen clients for peripheral vascular disease. The leg being tested is raised 30 degrees with the client supine. A pressure cuff is then inflated on the leg to distend the veins. Blood flow is measured with electrodes, and the cuff is then rapidly deflated and venous volume changes are recorded. Thrombi are detected by reduction in venous volume.

Laboratory Blood Tests

CARDIAC ENZYMES. When heart cells are damaged or die, they rupture and release their enzymes into the bloodstream. Levels of these enzymes rise in the serum as a result. Common cardiac enzyme tests are creatine kinase (CK), also referred to as creatine phosphokinase (CPK), and lactic dehydrogenase (LDH). However, these enzymes are also found in body cells other than the heart, so a more organ-specific test, the enzymes' isoenzymes (or different forms), is measured. Serum aspartate aminotransferase (AST) is a nonspecific cardiac test formerly known as serum glutamic-oxaloacetic transaminase (SGOT).

Creatine kinase. Creatine kinase is found in three types of tissue: brain, skeletal muscle, and heart muscle. Isoenzymes of CK contained in these tissues are CK-BB (brain), CK-MM (skeletal muscle), and CK-MB (heart muscle). Levels of CK-MB rise within 4 to 6 hours after cardiac cells are damaged, peak in 12 to 24 hours, and return to normal in 48 to 72 hours. Serial CK levels are drawn at intervals to track trends. It is important to avoid invasive procedures such as IVs and intramuscular (IM) injections before drawing the first CK to prevent elevation in the CK levels from cell trauma caused by the procedure. Medications are often given IV rather than IM to prevent this elevation.

Lactic dehydrogenase. Another intracellular enzyme that is found in a variety of body cells is LDH. There are five types of isoenzymes for LDH: LDH_1 and LDH_2 are found in the heart, kidneys, and red blood cells (RBCs); LDH_3 is specific to the lungs; and LDH_4 and LDH_5 are found in skeletal muscle and the liver. Normally LDH_2 is higher than LDH_1. After an MI, the pattern reverses and LDH_1 rises higher than LDH_2. Levels of LDH rise 8 to 12 hours after an MI, peak at 24 to 48 hours, and return to normal in 5 to 7 days.

Serum aspartate aminotransferase. There are no specific cardiac isoenzymes for AST, so it is not a definitive test for MI. It is found in heart, liver, skeletal muscle, RBCs, and kidneys. In an acute MI, it is usually elevated.

MYOGLOBIN. Myoglobin levels elevate within 1 hour of an acute MI. This test is 99 percent sensitive for an MI. Peak levels are reached 4 to 12 hours after an MI and levels return to normal within 18 hours after the onset of chest pain, so it is a test that must be done early when MI is suspected.

CARDIAC TROPONIN I. Cardiac troponin I is a highly sensitive indicator of myocardial damage. It is a protein found only in cardiac cells. When injured or dead, cardiac cells release this protein, which results in elevated levels. These levels remain elevated for up to 7 days after injury, which is helpful in diagnosing MI.

BLOOD LIPIDS. Lipids are triglycerides, cholesterol, and phospholipids. Lipoproteins are made up of these lipids attached to proteins. Triglycerides are found in very low density lipoproteins (VLDL). Cholesterol is mainly found in low-density lipoproteins (LDL). High-density lipoproteins (HDL) are a mixture of one-half protein and one-half phospholipids and cholesterol.

A lipid profile can screen for increased risk for coronary artery disease (CAD). Clients must fast for 12 hours before the test, and, although water is not withheld, alcohol is restricted for 24 hours before the test. High levels of LDL are linked to an increase in CAD, but high levels of HDL are not. High-density lipoproteins play a protective role against CAD. (See Cultural Considerations Box 15–2.)

CULTURAL CONSIDERATIONS BOX 15–2

Among French-Canadians, familial chylomicronemia (hyperlipoproteinemia type I), an autosomal recessive disorder, occurs with the highest frequency worldwide.[1] Familial hypercholesterolemia can lead to coronary thrombosis. Thus the nurse can improve the health of French-Canadians by encouraging early diagnostic workups for familial chylomicronemia and encouraging healthful lifestyles.

Invasive Studies

ANGIOGRAPHY. Arteriography and venography are the two types of angiography (Fig. 15–17). Arteriography examines arteries. Venography studies veins. Angiography uses dye injected into the vascular system to visualize the vessels on radiographs. This test is used to assess blood clot formation, to assess peripheral vascular disease (PVD), and to test vessels for potential grafting use.

The client must be assessed for allergies, give informed consent, be NPO for about 4 hours before the test, and be informed that the dye produces a hot, burning feeling when injected. After the procedure the client is assessed for several hours. Vital signs, allergic reaction signs, hemorrhage at the injection site, and pulses are assessed after the procedure.

CARDIAC CATHETERIZATION. Cardiac catheterization allows the study of the heart's anatomy and physiology (Fig. 15–18). It is an invasive diagnostic procedure that measures pressures in the heart chambers, great blood vessels, and coronary arteries and provides information on cardiac output and oxygen saturation. Fluoroscopy is used, and dye can be injected once the catheter is in place to visualize the heart chambers and vessels. This procedure is often done before heart surgery.

Right catheterization. A catheter with or without a fiber-optic tip is inserted into the basilic or cephalic vein or the femoral vein and advanced into the vena cava. It is then moved through the right chambers of the heart and into the pulmonary artery. The catheter can be wedged momentarily in the artery by inflating the balloon at the tip of the catheter. This position provides the pulmonary artery wedge pressure (PAWP), which reflects pressures in the left side of the heart. Other pressures obtained with right cardiac catheterization are right atrial pressure, which reflects central venous pressure, pulmonary artery systolic and diastolic pressures, and cardiac output, and mixed venous oxygen saturation (SvO_2) if a fiber-optic catheter is used.

Left catheterization. The left side of the heart can be directly assessed by inserting a catheter into the brachial or the femoral artery. It is advanced against the flow of blood into the aorta, through the aortic valve, and into the left ventricle. Coronary angiography, which visualizes the coronary arteries with dye, can be done with this approach. The catheter is inserted into the opening of the coronary arteries, the dye is injected, and x-rays are taken. Coronary artery disease can be assessed with coronary angiography.

An informed consent must be obtained. The client is assessed for allergies to iodine, seafood, and shellfish and kept NPO before the procedure. Clients should be told that during the test they are awake and a warm, flushing sensation may be felt when the dye is injected; the room has a lot of equipment; a movable table is used; the client's vital signs and ECG are monitored constantly; and the length of the procedure is 2 to 3 hours.

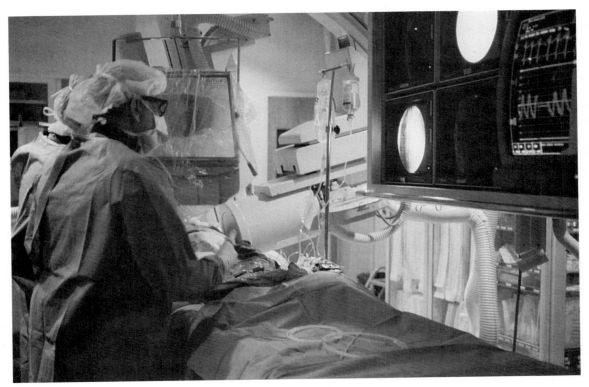

Figure 15–17. Coronary angiography.

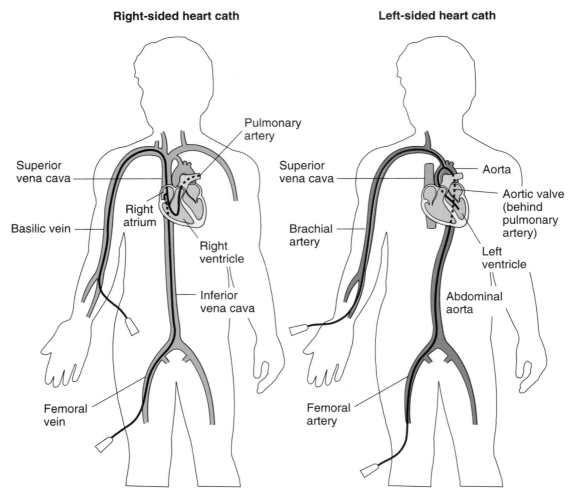

Figure 15–18. *(A)* Right cardiac catheterization. Veins are used to enter the right heart. *(B)* Left cardiac catheterization. Arteries are used to enter the left heart.

Complications of the procedure can be allergic reaction, breaking of the catheter, hemorrhage, thrombus formation, emboli of air or blood, dysrhythmias, MI, cerebrovascular accident (CVA), and puncture of the heart chambers or lungs.

After the catheter is removed, firm pressure must be applied to the insertion site for several minutes to prevent hemorrhage or hematoma formation. A pressure dressing or sandbag may be applied to the site when bleeding is stopped and is removed in several hours. Vital signs are assessed according to the physician's orders and the institution's policies. During vital sign checks, the puncture site is assessed and peripheral pulses are verified. The extremity used for insertion must not be moved or flexed for several hours after the procedure. Clients usually may eat and are instructed to drink fluids to help eliminate the dye from the body. If the client is stable and no significant findings are found, the client may be discharged.

HEMODYNAMIC MONITORING. Bedside monitoring can be done to monitor the pressures in the blood vessels or heart. A catheter attached to a transducer and monitor, called an arterial line, can be inserted into the radial or femoral artery to measure continuous arterial blood pressure.

Ongoing monitoring of cardiac pressures, cardiac output, and central venous pressure (CVP) can be done with either a central catheter or a pulmonary artery catheter. Central venous pressure is measured directly with a central catheter inserted into the vena cava via the brachial, femoral, subclavian, or jugular vein (Fig. 15–19). It is measured indirectly with the pulmonary artery catheter (Fig. 15–20). The right atrial pressure measurement obtained from the pulmonary artery catheter reflects the pressure in the vena cava. Central venous pressure measures **preload** or fluid volume status; CVP readings used in fluid or diuretic therapy have been primarily replaced by pulmonary artery catheter measurements.

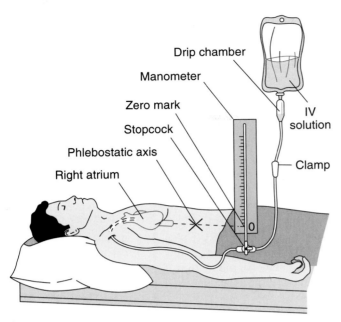

Figure 15–19. CVP measurement.

Therapeutic Measures for the Cardiovascular System

EXERCISE

A prescribed walking program or cardiac rehabilitation program can promote improved cardiovascular functioning. Walking helps promote blood flow by contracting the skeletal muscles.

SMOKING CESSATION

Smoking causes vasoconstriction that can last up to 1 hour after the smoking of one cigarette. For clients with cardiac or vascular disease, blood flow is reduced, which can exacerbate symptoms. Clients should be encouraged to stop smoking and should be provided with support information such as cessation programs and support groups.

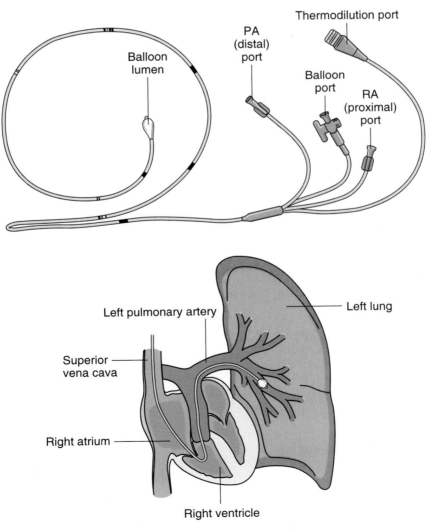

Figure 15–20. Pulmonary artery catheter.

DIET

A diet low in sodium may be prescribed if excess fluid volume is a problem. Weight reduction is encouraged to decrease the heart's workload. If diuretics that promote potassium loss are used, potassium levels must be monitored and adequate amounts of potassium included in the diet. A high-fiber diet for cardiac clients is recommended to reduce straining and subsequently the heart's workload.

OXYGEN

Supplemental oxygen is administered to clients with chest pain to help ensure that the heart receives sufficient oxygen to function. The oxygen can be delivered via a nasal cannula or face mask. The client must be taught safety precautions necessary for home use of oxygen if it is ordered, such as avoiding open flames and smoking while the oxygen is in use.

MEDICATIONS

The primary cardiovascular drugs are cardiac glycosides, vasodilators, antihypertensives, antidysrhythmics, antianginals, anticoagulants, and thrombolytics. They are discussed in further detail where the disorders they are used to treat are explained. (See Chapters 16–22.)

ANTIEMBOLISM DEVICES

Antiembolism devices improve blood flow to prevent the formation of blood clots. They are used for clients with peripheral vascular disease, on bed rest, or after surgery or trauma.

Elastic Stockings

Antiembolism stockings apply pressure over the leg to promote the movement of fluid and prevent stasis of fluid. These stockings may be knee or thigh length. They must be applied correctly so that a tourniquet effect is not produced by the stockings. For ease in application, the stocking is turned inside out to the heel, the foot portion is placed on the client up to the heel, and then the remaining stocking is pulled up over the leg. The tops of the stockings should be 1 to 2 in below the bottom of the kneecap. They should not roll down or they will cause stasis rather than prevent it. The stockings are removed for 20 minutes twice a day and the skin inspected for irritation. Elderly clients may require assistance in applying the stockings if they have impaired manual dexterity.

Intermittent Pneumatic Compression Devices

This system consists of plastic inflatable stockings that are filled intermittently with air by an attached motor. This device promotes fluid movement by simulating the contraction of the leg muscles to prevent thrombosis development.

The compartments in the stockings inflate to 35 to 55 mm Hg of pressure beginning in the ankle compartment and progressing next to the calf compartment and finally the thigh compartment. The nurse should monitor the device for proper pressure inflation.

CARDIOVERSION

When a rapid heart rhythm requires termination, cardioversion can be used. Cardioversion provides a synchronized shock to the heart to restore the heart's own normal pacemaker rate and rhythm. The shock must be synchronized with the R wave, if an R wave is present, to avoid delivering the shock on top of the T wave, which could result in lethal dysrhythmias. (See Chapter 20.) The client is sedated and electrodes are applied to the chest. The machine is synchronized and charged to 25 to 100 J. If the first impulse is not effective, the shock may be repeated with higher joules.

PACEMAKERS

Pacemakers can be temporary or permanent. They are used to provide a normal heart rate and rhythm. The pacemaker generator is the power source that delivers an impulse via an electrode or lead to the heart to cause contraction. The pacemaker may be transcutaneous, in which an electrode is applied to the chest and the impulse delivered to the heart via the electrode through the skin; transvenous, which has a lead inserted via a vein to the heart; or implantable, which is placed into a subcutaneous chest wall pocket surgically with a lead implanted into the heart. Pacemakers are used to treat **bradycardia** with symptoms, tachycardias, heart blocks, and MI.

Review Questions

1. The mitral and tricuspid valves prevent backflow of blood from the
   a. Ventricles to atria when the ventricles contract
   b. Atria to ventricles when the ventricles relax
   c. Ventricles to atria when the atria contract
   d. Atria to ventricles when the atria contract

2. The purpose of the endocardium of the heart is to
   a. Cover the heart muscle and prevent friction
   b. Support the coronary blood vessels
   c. Line the chambers of the heart and prevent abnormal clotting
   d. Prevent backflow of blood from atria to ventricles

3. The function of the coronary blood vessels is to
   a. Prevent abnormal clotting within the heart
   b. Bring oxygenated blood to the myocardium
   c. Carry deoxygenated blood to the lungs
   d. Carry oxygenated blood to the lungs

---

bradycardia: bradys—slow + kardia—heart

4. Which of the following is the location of the cardiac centers in the nervous system?
   a. Cerebrum
   b. Hypothalamus
   c. Spinal cord
   d. Medulla

5. The functions of angiotensin II are to increase which of the following?
   a. Vasodilation and ADH secretion
   b. Vasoconstriction and aldosterone secretion
   c. Heart rate and vasodilation
   d. Heart rate and ADH secretion

6. The increase of resting blood pressure with age may contribute to which of the following?
   a. Dysrhythmias
   b. Thrombus formation
   c. Left-sided heart failure
   d. Peripheral edema

7. Which one of the following is a modifiable cardiovascular risk factor that should be noted during client data collection?
   a. Age
   b. Gender
   c. Ethnic origin
   d. Tobacco use

8. If it takes longer than 3 seconds for the color to return when assessing capillary refill, it may indicate which of the following?
   a. Decreased arterial flow to the extremity
   b. Increased arterial flow to the extremity
   c. Decreased venous flow from the extremity
   d. Increased venous flow from the extremity

9. Which one of the following is an important safety intervention that should be used while assessing a client for orthostatic hypotension?
   a. Reality orientation
   b. Gait or walking belt
   c. Liquids at bedside
   d. Standing client quickly

10. Which one of the following areas is assessed for edema in the supine client?
    a. Arms
    b. Ankles
    c. Sternum
    d. Sacrum

11. Which of the following should be included in client teaching for coronary angiography with femoral catheter insertion site?
    a. Dye injection causes hot, flushing sensation.
    b. General anesthesia is administered.
    c. Claustrophobia may be experienced.
    d. Ambulates immediately after procedure.

12. A high-fiber diet for cardiac clients is recommended to
    a. Increase absorption of nutrients
    b. Reduce cardiac workload
    c. Reduce edema development
    d. Reduce appetite

ANSWERS TO CRITICAL THINKING

CRITICAL THINKING: Mrs. Smith

1. The older client often does not experience typical disorder symptoms. Chest pain is often not present because of reduced nerve sensitivity with aging for an MI. Dyspnea is the classic symptom of MI in the older client.
2. Inspect both legs to determine edematous areas. Determine location and severity of edema by pressing finger for 5 seconds over the medial malleolus and moving up the leg along the tibia until no edema is found. Assess bilaterally. Measure leg circumference.
3. Document location of edema and whether edema is nonpitting or pitting. Document findings for both legs.
4. Bilateral pitting ankle edema with leg circumference measurement number.
5. Dyspnea at rest that increases with exertion, heart tones clear and distant, nailbeds pale, pain free, poor appetite for 2 weeks, 6-pound weight gain in 1 week, three-pillow orthopnea, bilateral neck vein distention.

REFERENCE

1. Ma, Y, et al: A mutation in the human lipoprotein lipase gene as the most common cause of familial chylomicronemia in French Canadians. N Engl J Med 324(25):176, 1991.

BIBLIOGRAPHY

Adams, J, et al: Improved detection of cardiac contusion with cardiac troponin I. Am Heart J 131(2):308, 1996.
Arnold, S: Cardiac stress testing. Nursing 27(1):58, 1997.
Cheney, AM, and Maquindang, ML: Patient teaching for x-ray and other diagnostics. RN 56(4):54, 1993.
Hasemeier, C: Permanent pacemaker. Am J Nurs 96(2):30, 1996.
Jaffe, M, and McVan, B: Davis's Laboratory and Diagnostic Test Handbook. FA Davis, Philadelphia, 1997.
Mee, C, and Possanza, C: Getting a good look: How to record an accurate 12 lead ECG. Nursing 27(3):60, 1997.
Ulak, L, and Millman, F: What to do for patients undergoing transesophageal echocardiography. Am J Nurs 97(1):16K, 1997.
Wei, J: Age and the cardiovascular system. N Engl J Med 327:1735, 1992.
Williams, K, and Morton, P: Diagnosis and treatment of acute myocardial infarction. AACN Clin Issues 6(3):375, 1995.

16

Nursing Care of Clients with Hypertension

Diane Lewis

Learning Objectives

Upon completion of this chapter, the student will be able to:

1. Define hypertension.
2. Explain the pathophysiology, cause, and risk factors associated with hypertension.
3. Identify cause and treatment for primary, secondary, and isolated systolic hypertension.
4. Describe the signs and symptoms of hypertension.
5. Identify laboratory tests used to assist in the diagnosis and treatment of hypertension.
6. Identify four classifications of hypertension in adults and recommendations for follow-up based on blood pressure.
7. Explain the treatment of hypertension, including lifestyle modifications and medications.
8. Identify the common complications of hypertension.
9. Provide teaching and learning strategies to assist the client with hypertension to adjust to a chronic illness.
10. Describe the nursing care of the client with hypertension who is undergoing a procedure.
11. Develop a nursing care plan for a client with hypertension.
12. Define hypertensive crisis.

Key Words

atherosclerosis (ATH-er-oh-skle-**ROH**-sis)

cardiac output (**KAR**-dee-yak **OWT**-put)

diastolic blood pressure (dye-ah-**STAH**-lik BLUHD **PRE**-shure)

essential hypertension (e-**SEN**-shul HIGH-per-**TEN**-shun)

hypertension (HIGH-per-**TEN**-shun)

hypertensive crisis (HIGH-per-**TEN**-siv **CRY**-sis)

hypertrophy (high-**PER**-truh-fee)

isolated systolic hypertension (**EYE**-suh-lay-ted sis-**TAH**-lik HIGH-per-**TEN**-shun)

lifestyle modifications (LYEF-style MAH-di-fi-**KAY**-shuns)

normotensive (nor-mo-**TEN**-siv)

peripheral vascular resistance (puh-**RIFF**-uh-ruhl VAS-kyoo-lar ree-**ZIS**-tense)

plaque (PLAK)

primary hypertension (PRY-mer-ee HIGH-per-**TEN**-shun)

secondary hypertension (**SEK**-un-DAR-ee HIGH-per-**TEN**-shun)

systolic blood pressure (sis-**TAL**-ik BLUHD **PRESS**-ur)

viscosity (vis-**KAH**-si-tee)

Hypertension (HTN), or high blood pressure (BP), is a condition in which the blood pressure, on at least two or more readings on different dates after an initial screening, is found to be higher than normal. If the **systolic blood pressure** (SBP) is above 140 mm Hg or the **diastolic blood pressure** (DBP) is above 90 mm Hg, the adult aged 18 or over should be evaluated for hypertension by a health care provider.[1] In the United States, as many as 60 million people have hypertension.[1]

Pathophysiology of Hypertension

Normally the heart pumps blood through the body to meet the needs of the cells for oxygen and nutrients. The pumping activity of the heart forces the blood through the blood vessels to the vital organs and tissues. The pressure exerted by blood on the walls of the blood vessels is measured as blood pressure. Blood pressure is determined by **cardiac output** (CO); **peripheral vascular resistance** (PVR); the ability of the vessels to stretch; the **viscosity,** or thickness, of the blood; and the amount of circulating blood volume. Decreased stretching ability and increased viscosity and fluid volume increase blood pressure.

Several processes maintain blood pressure by controlling CO and PVR. These processes include the nervous system, the baroreceptors, the renin-angiotensin mechanism, and the balancing of body fluids. One way blood pressure is maintained is through adjustment of the CO, which is the amount of blood that the heart pumps out each minute. Heart rate will increase to pump out more blood in response to either physical or emotional activities to meet the increased oxygen needs of organs and tissue. Another factor that maintains blood pressure, PVR, is the opposition that the blood encounters as it flows through the vessel. Anything causing blood vessels to become narrower will increase the PVR. Any time the PVR is increased, more pressure is needed to push the blood along the vessel, so the blood pressure increases. When PVR is decreased, less pressure is needed, so the blood pressure decreases. Increased arteriolar PVR is the main mechanism that elevates blood pressure in hypertension.

PRIMARY HYPERTENSION

Primary hypertension, or **essential hypertension,** is the chronic elevation of blood pressure that is the result of an unknown cause. These unknown causes influence the factors that control blood pressure, resulting in a hypertensive state.

SECONDARY HYPERTENSION

Secondary hypertension has a known cause. It is high blood pressure that is a sign of another problem such as a kidney abnormality, tumor of the adrenal gland, or congenital defect of the aorta. When the cause of secondary hypertension is treated before permanent structural changes occur, blood pressure usually returns to normal. Treatment of the cause may include surgery or medication.

ISOLATED SYSTOLIC HYPERTENSION

Isolated systolic hypertension (ISH), an SBP of 160 mm Hg or greater and a normal DBP of 90 mm Hg or less, is an abnormal finding. It occurs mainly in the elderly, although it can occur at any age. For people with an SBP > 160 mm Hg and a normal DBP on two separate visits, a referral to a physician for further evaluation is recommended. Treating ISH is recommended to decrease cardiovascular disease, especially the incidence of stroke. **Lifestyle modifications** are usually tried first if the SBP elevation is not too severe. If the SBP is still not controlled, antihypertensive medication is added.

Signs and Symptoms of Hypertension

Often there are no signs or symptoms other than elevated blood pressure readings associated with hypertension. As a result, it is referred to as the "silent killer." It is usually impossible for the client to correlate the absence or presence of symptoms with the degree of elevation of BP. In a small number of cases, the client with hypertension may complain of a headache, bloody nose, or blurred vision. On many occasions, the client newly diagnosed with hypertension is diagnosed while seeking health care for reasons unrelated to hypertension. Most of the signs and symptoms of hypertension are related to the long-term effects of blood pressure elevations on the blood vessels of the heart, kidneys, brain, and eyes, known as target organ disease (TOD).[1] In target organ disease, pathological changes occur in the large and small blood vessels of the heart, kidney, brain, and eyes.

Diagnosis of Hypertension

Diagnosis is based on a health history to assess a client's risk factors for hypertension, any previous diagnosis of hypertension, presence of any signs and symptoms, history of kidney or heart disease, and current use of medications. Although there are no diagnostic studies specifically for hypertension, there are diagnostic tests that can be helpful in

---

hypertension: hyper—excessive + tensio—tension
systolic: systole—contraction
diastolic: diastole—expansion
viscosity: visous—sticky

detecting information, such as damage to organs or blood vessels. The type of diagnostic tests performed depends on the stage of the hypertension or other medical conditions that also may be present at the time of diagnostic evaluation.

The Joint National Committee (JNC) on Prevention, Detection, Evaluation, and Treatment of High Blood Pressure was created by the National Heart, Lung, and Blood Institute of the National Institutes of Health.[1] The sixth report of the JNC defines normal and abnormal blood pressures for adults age 18 years and older and reclassified blood pressure measurement and treatment guidelines for physicians, clinicians, nurses, and community programs to follow (Table 16–1).[1]

DIAGNOSTIC TESTS

Laboratory tests such as urinalysis, blood urea nitrogen (BUN), and creatinine may indicate kidney damage from high blood pressure. Serum levels of sodium, calcium, chloride, potassium, magnesium, and phosphate are essential to evaluate the client's fluid, electrolyte, and acid-base balance. A complete blood count (CBC) detects blood disorders. Blood glucose, uric acid, cholesterol, and triglyceride levels help determine possible causes of cardiovascular and hypertensive disease. An electrocardiogram or chest x-ray may assist in recognizing abnormal heart function. These diagnostic tests are also used to monitor the effects of prescribed treatment.

Risk Factors for Hypertension

A combination of genetic (nonmodifiable) and environmental (modifiable) risk factors are thought to be responsible for the development of hypertension, although the cause remains unknown. Risk factors that are nonmodifiable, or unable to be changed, associated with hypertension include family history of hypertension, age, ethnicity, and diabetes mellitus. Modifiable, or changeable, risk factors include stress, control of glucose levels and blood pressure by weight reduction, improved meal planning, and reduced salt and alcohol intake. Increasing physical activity, not smoking, and managing stress decrease blood pressure.

NONMODIFIABLE RISK FACTORS

Family History of Hypertension

Hypertension is seen more commonly among people with a family history of it. When a family history for hypertension is present, the risk for developing it is almost twice that of persons with no family history. People with a family history of hypertension should be encouraged to have their blood pressure checked regularly. (See Table 16–1.)

Age

Because people age differently due to genetic and environmental risk factors and lifestyle habits, results of the aging process may be reflected in the wide variations of blood pressure among elderly people. As a person ages, **plaque** builds up in the arteries and the blood vessels become stiffer and less elastic, causing the heart to work harder to force blood through the vessels. These vessel changes increase cardiac output to maintain blood flow into the circulation and subsequently raise blood pressure in the elderly.

Race and Ethnicity

The incidence of hypertension among African-Americans is double that of Caucasians, especially for African-American women. This condition is also more severe in African-Americans, especially for African-American men. See Cultural Considerations Box 16–1 for the incidence of hypertension in other ethnic groups.

Table 16–1. **The Four Stages of Hypertension and Recommendations for Follow-up**

Category	Systolic Blood Pressure (mm Hg)	Diastolic Blood Pressure (mm Hg)	Recommended Follow-up
Normal	<130	<85	2 years
High Normal	130–139	85–89	1 year
Hypertension			
Stage 1	140–159	90–99	2 months
Stage 2	160–179	100–109	1 month
Stage 3	≥180	≥110	1 week-immediately

Adapted from The National Heart, Lung, and Blood Institute, The Sixth Report of the Joint National Committee on Prevention, Detection, Evaluation, and Treatment of High Blood Pressure. Arch Intern Med 157(21):2413, 1997.

CULTURAL CONSIDERATIONS BOX 16–1

The incidence of hypertension varies depending on gender, race, and ethnicity. Following is the incidence for selected populations:

Population Group	Women	Men
African-American	19.73%	13.79%
Native-American/ Alaskan Native	13.82%	10.29%
Asian and Pacific Islander	8.35%	9.67%
Hispanic	10.55%	7.86%
European-American	10.96%	10.32%

Data from Chronic Disease in Minority Populations. U.S. Department of Health and Human Services, Washington, DC, 1994, pp 2-17, 5-17.

Hypertension continues to be the most serious health problem for African-Americans in the United States. Over 5 million of the 26 million African-Americans living in the United States are hypertensive.[2] They suffer higher mortality and morbidity rates related to hypertension and at an earlier age.[3] African-Americans from lower socioeconomic backgrounds have higher blood pressure than African-Americans from higher socioeconomic backgrounds. Additionally, African-Americans are 3.2 times more likely to develop kidney failure related to hypertension than European-Americans.

Hypertension among African-Americans is usually caused by an increased renin activity resulting in increases in sodium and fluid retention. Thus African-Americans respond better to diuretics such as furosemide (Lasix) and hydrochlorothiazide (HydroDiuril) than to beta blockers such as propranolol (Inderal). Hypertension among European-Americans is more often caused by chemical imbalances, thus they respond better to beta blockers.[4]

Chinese people are more sensitive than Caucasians to the effects of the beta blocker propranolol (Inderal) on heart rate and blood pressure, requiring only half the blood level of European-Americans to achieve a therapeutic affect.[4] Propranolol is eliminated from the bodies of many Chinese persons at double the rate of European-Americans. They are more likely to suffer fatigue as a side effect. Thus the nurse must carefully monitor the Chinese client for therapeutic and side effects.

Hypertension among Japanese-Americans is primarily related to the high sodium content of the Japanese diet, stress, and a high incidence of cigarette smoking.[5]

High rates of hypertension among Koreans and Filipinos are due to the stress of immigration, preserving foods in salt, and using condiments high in sodium.[6,7]

Diabetes Mellitus

Two-thirds of adults who have diabetes mellitus also have hypertension. The risk of developing hypertension when a family history of diabetes and obesity are present is two to six times greater. Approximately 80 percent of people with non-insulin-dependent diabetes mellitus are overweight. Lifestyle modifications and adherence to therapy are crucial to prevent the heart attacks, strokes, blindness, and kidney failure associated with high glucose and high blood pressure levels.

MODIFIABLE RISK FACTORS

The JNC suggests advising clients with hypertension to use lifestyle modifications. These modifications include weight reduction; meal planning, including moderation of dietary sodium and alcohol intake; increased physical activity; smoking cessation; and stress management (Table 16–2). Lifestyle modifications are most often used in combination with antihypertensive medications to control hypertension and enhance the effect of the medications. (See Nutrition Notes Box 16–2.)

Stress

Groups who are economically deprived often have a high incidence of hypertension. Factors such as poor nutritional habits, low-status jobs, frustration, discontent, and suppression of hostility contribute to stress-related hypertension. Other factors that may affect health include reduced access to quality health care and poor living conditions.

Weight Reduction

There is a strong relationship between excess body weight and increased blood pressure. Weight reduction is one of the most important, if not the most important, lifestyle modifica-

Table 16–2. **Lifestyle Modifications for Hypertension**

- Lose weight.
- Limit alcohol intake.
- Get regular aerobic exercise.
- Decrease amount of salt intake.
- Include daily allowances of potassium, calcium, and magnesium.
- Stop smoking.
- Reduce dietary saturated fat and cholesterol.
- Manage stress.

Adapted from The National Heart, Lung, and Blood Institute, The Sixth Report of the Joint National Committee on Prevention, Detection, Evaluation, and Treatment of High Blood Pressure. Arch Intern Med 157(21):2413, 1997.

NUTRITION NOTES BOX 16-2

Nutrition in Hypertension

WEIGHT REDUCTION. Weight loss of as little as 10 lb has been effective in lowering blood pressure. Exercise, a well-balanced calorie-controlled diet, and behavior modification are necessary parts of a sound and long-lasting weight reduction program.

REDUCED SODIUM INTAKE. A 100 mmol (2.5 g) difference in sodium intake is associated with differences in systolic pressure ranging from 5 mm Hg in those aged 15 to 19 years to 10 mm Hg in those aged 60 to 69 years. Sodium restriction is more effective in hypertensive subjects than in **normotensive** ones.

REDUCED ALCOHOL CONSUMPTION. Blood pressure is positively correlated with an alcohol intake of three or more drinks per day, independent of age, body mass index, and smoking. An estimated 5 to 7 percent of hypertension is attributed to an alcohol intake of three or more drinks per day.[8]

EXERCISE. Activity is inversely related to blood pressure independent of excess weight in both sexes and across all ages. Hypertension is less prevalent in active adults than in age-matched subjects for Caucasians and African-Americans, for both sexes, and for younger and older persons. Increasing physical activity has been shown to decrease both systolic and diastolic pressures by 6 to 7 mm Hg.[8]

OTHER DIETARY COMPONENTS. Low potassium, especially the sodium/potassium ratio, is implicated in hypertension, but potassium supplementation is believed to be less important than controlling weight and sodium intake. Other factors, such as omega-3 fatty acids, calcium, magnesium, protein, and fiber, have been studied as affecting hypertension but with inconclusive or clinically minimal results.[8,9]

tion to lower blood pressure. The health care provider and dietitian should be consulted to assist the client in developing a weight-reduction diet and other methods of weight loss.

Meal Planning

Salt Intake

Research has shown that some people may develop high blood pressure by eating a diet high in salt. Clients whose blood pressure can be lowered by restricting dietary sodium are called salt sensitive. This sensitivity is particularly common among African-Americans, elderly persons, and clients with diabetes and obesity.

The usual dietary recommendations are to restrict sodium intake to 2 g per day. Clients with hypertension should be instructed not to add salt while cooking meals and to avoid

adding table salt to their food. Processed foods or those foods in which salt can be easily tasted (canned soups, ham, bacon, and salted nuts) should also be avoided.

Intake of Potassium, Calcium, and Magnesium

Recent studies are inconclusive as to the role that low dietary potassium, calcium, and magnesium intake play in the development of high blood pressure. A balanced diet that ensures adequate intake of these nutrients is important in maintaining general health. Foods rich in potassium include oranges, bananas, and broccoli. Milk, yogurt, and spinach are calcium-rich foods. Vegetables such as spinach, garbanzo beans, and lima beans are good sources of magnesium. Whenever possible, fresh or frozen foods should be selected rather than canned foods to increase intake of these nutrients.

Alcohol Consumption

The regular consumption of three or more drinks per day can increase the risk of hypertension and cause resistance to antihypertensive therapy. The nurse should counsel hypertensive clients who drink alcohol to avoid it or at least limit their daily intake to 1 oz of alcohol per day (i.e., 2 oz of 100-proof whiskey, 8 oz of wine, or 24 oz of beer).[1] Blood pressure may decrease or return to normal when alcohol consumption is limited or eliminated.

Exercise

People with sedentary lifestyles have an increased risk for the development of hypertension when compared with people who exercise regularly. Exercise has been shown to be beneficial in preventing and controlling hypertension by reducing weight, decreasing peripheral resistance, and decreasing body fat. Moderate activity, such as 30 to 45 minutes of brisk walking three to five times per week, is recommended by the Joint National Committee.[1] Clients with hypertension should be evaluated by a health care provider before starting any exercise program.

Smoking

Smoking is a major risk factor for cardiovascular disease and is associated with a high incidence of stage 3 hypertension. Clients who smoke may show an increase in blood pressure because nicotine constricts the blood vessels. The nurse should instruct clients with hypertension to quit or decrease smoking to reduce the risk of myocardial infarction and stroke. A referral by the nurse to a smoking cessation program can be helpful.

Stress Management

Reducing stress can play a major role in the treatment of clients with hypertension. Stress stimulates the sympathetic (fight or flight) nervous system. This causes the vessels to constrict and activate the renin-angiotensin mechanism. Those who have high stress levels tend to develop hypertension more than those who do not. Additionally, studies have shown that an increase in stress can also raise the body's production of cholesterol, which can lead to cardiovascular disease. It is important for clients to learn how to deal with stress. For many clients, stress management techniques, such as exercise, relaxation therapies, yoga, meditation, and biofeedback, may be useful in controlling their response to stress and lowering their blood pressure.

 CRITICAL THINKING: Mrs. Miller

Mrs. Miller, a 54-year-old African-American, visits a health clinic for headaches she has every morning. The nurse collects data on Mrs. Miller and finds that she is an office manager, smokes a pack of cigarettes a day, eats fast food for lunch at her desk, has two adult children, and is recently divorced. Mrs. Miller has been in good health and takes two aspirin for her headaches daily.

1. What are Mrs. Miller's risk factors for hypertension?
2. What is the most significant client information identified? Why?
3. Why is hypertension referred to as the silent killer?
4. Why should Mrs. Miller be told of the need for lifelong therapy if she is diagnosed with hypertension?

Answers at end of chapter.

Hypertension Treatment

The JNC has guidelines for selecting therapy based on severity of blood pressure risk factors and the presence of target organ disease (TOD) or cardiovascular disease. If the no or low risk hypertensive client's blood pressure remains at or above 140/90 mm Hg during the 6- to 12-month period of lifestyle modifications, the Joint National Committee advises the practitioner to add antihypertensive medications to the client's antihypertensive therapy. The medication is selected by the physician or health care provider in collaboration with the client. For clients with severe hypertension, high risk factors or TOD drug therapy is started immediately along with lifestyle modifications.

The goal of drug therapy is to decrease the DBP to 90 mm Hg or less and the SBP to 160 mm Hg or less. For clients with stage 1 or 2 hypertension, diuretics and beta blockers are recommended by the JNC for initial drug therapy. If the response is inadequate to achieve the blood pressure goal, the drug dose may be increased, another drug

may be substituted, or a drug from a different class may be added. There are eight categories of medications to treat hypertension: diuretics, alpha blockers, beta blockers, calcium channel blockers, angiotensin-converting enzyme (ACE) inhibitors, central agents, peripheral agents, and vasodilators (Table 16–3).

The treatment plan of lifestyle modifications and medications is effective only when clients accept the diagnosis of hypertension and include lifelong treatment in their daily routine. Clients should be instructed that antihypertensive therapy usually must be continued the rest of their lives. Clients should be reminded that although they may be feeling better with the modifications and medications, the hypertension is still present even if it is well controlled. The client should be told that lifelong therapy for hypertension is required and medications should not be discontinued unless a physician or advanced practice nurse instructs the client to do so.

Antihypertensive medications can have unpleasant side effects. Clients should be told what they are and to report them if they do occur so that alterations in the medications can be made, if possible. Impotence can be one of the side effects of these medications. Male clients may be reluctant to discuss this side effect and instead choose to discontinue the medication. The nurse should be proactive and inform male clients about this side effect so they will understand that if impotence does occur and is reported, the physician can make adjustments in their medication.

LEARNING TIP

Hypertension Lifestyle Modifications
L—Limit salt and alcohol.
I—Include daily potassium, calcium, and magnesium.
F—Fight fat and cholesterol.
E—Exercise regularly.
S—Stress management.
T—Try to quit smoking.
Y—Your medications are to be taken daily.
L—Lose weight.
E—End-stage complications will be avoided!

 CRITICAL THINKING: Mrs. Bell

Mrs. Bell, 80 years old and a widow for 15 years, visits her physician. She lives alone in her own home with a bathroom down the hall from the bedroom. She has wood floors with throw rugs in the hall and a tile floor in the bathroom. Her son lives in the same city. She has a 10-year history of hypertension for which she is taking bumetanide (Bumex) and propranolol (Inderal), when she remembers them. She wears glasses and has a cataract. She has an unsteady gait and nocturia. She is 40 lb overweight and is very sedentary.

Table 16–3. **Antihypertensive Agents**

Medications	Action	Side Effects	Nursing Considerations
		Diuretics	
Thiazide and Thiazide-like Diuretics Chlorothiazide (Diuril) Chlorthalidone (Hygroton) Metolazone (Zaroxolyn)	Remove sodium, extracellular fluid, and potassium, reducing cardiac output	Hypokalemia, hyponatremia, dehydration, muscle weakness, dry mouth, hypotension	Monitor electrolytes. Teach need for increased dietary or supplemental potassium. **Geriatric:** Teach about postural hypotension, especially in hot weather and need to get up slowly. Teach to take in morning to avoid getting up in night.
Loop Diuretics Bumetanide (Bumex) Furosemide (Lasix)	Rapid action, block sodium and water reabsorption; diuresis profound	Same as thiazides	Monitor electrolytes. Must replace electrolytes. **Geriatric:** Same as thiazides.
Potassium-Sparing Diuretics Amiloride (Midamor) Spironolactone (Aldactone) Triamterene (Dyrenium)	Remove sodium and extracellular fluid but keep potassium	Hyperkalemia, hyponatremia, nausea, vomiting, diarrhea	Monitor electrolytes. Give after meals to decrease nausea. **Geriatric:** Mental confusion and unsteady gait may occur, so ensure safety.
		Adrenergic Inhibitors	
Beta Blockers Atenolol (Tenormin) Propranolol (Inderal) Pindolol (Visken)	Block beta$_1$ heart receptors to reduce heart rate and blood pressure; some reduce peripheral vascular resistance	Bradycardia, shortness of breath, fatigue, insomnia, numb hands	Assess for signs of heart failure. Teach not to stop agent abruptly. **Geriatric:** Assess for toxicity. Teach about postural hypotension and need to get up slowly.
Alpha Blockers Prazosin (Minipress) Terazosin (Hytrin)	Vasodilate to reduce peripheral vascular resistance	Dizziness, hypotension, headache, nausea, palpitations	Monitor for hypotension. Teach to make position changes slowly. **Geriatric:** May be weak and fatigued, so ensure safety.
Central-Acting Adrenergic Inhibitors Clonidine (Catapres) Methyldopa (Aldomet)	Suppress central nervous system	Drowsiness, sedation, dry mouth, constipation	Caution client not to take alcohol. Suggest gum or hard candy. Encourage a high-fiber diet. **Geriatric:** Assess bowel routine and monitor for constipation.

continued

Table 16–3. (continued)

Medications	Action	Side Effects	Nursing Considerations
		Adrenergic Inhibitors	
Peripheral-Acting Adrenergic Inhibitors Guanadrel (Hylorel) Reserpine (Serpalan) Labetalol (Normodyne)	Decrease production of nor-epinephrine to lower blood pressure	Depression, lethargy, nasal stuffiness, edema	Inform client to report signs of depression: mood swings, insomnia, anorexia. **Geriatric:** Postural hypotension common. Assess for depression.
		Angiotensin-Converting Enzyme Inhibitors	
Captopril (Capoten) Enalapril maleate (Vasotec)	Block conversion of angiotensin I to angiotensin II	Cough, rash	**Geriatric:** Assess for toxicity and recognize need for reduced dose with renal impairment.
		Calcium Channel Blockers	
Nifedipine (Procardia) Diltiazem (Cardizem) Verapamil (Calan, Isoptin)	Block entry of calcium into smooth muscles to reduce afterload	Headache, dizziness	Monitor for hypotension. Treat headache with acetaminophen. **Geriatric:** Decreased dosage may need to be used.
		Vasodilators	
Hydralazine (Apresoline) Minoxidil (Loniten)	Vasodilate arteries, arterioles to reduce afterload	Headache, palpitation	Treat headache with acetaminophen.

1. What are Mrs. Bell's modifiable and nonmodifiable risk factors for hypertension?
2. Why is Mrs. Bell taking bumetanide (Bumex) and propranolol (Inderal) to treat her hypertension?
3. What teaching methods could be used to help ensure that Mrs. Bell will understand and follow her treatment plan?
4. Why should safety needs be addressed in the nursing care plan?
5. What safety interventions should the client and family be taught?

Answers at end of chapter.

Complications of Hypertension

Common complications associated with hypertension are coronary artery disease, **atherosclerosis,** myocardial infarction (MI), strokes, and kidney or eye damage. The severity and duration of the increase in blood pressure determine the extent of the vascular changes causing organ damage. High blood pressure levels may also result in an increase in the size of the left ventricle referred to as **hypertrophy.** Elevated blood pressure damages the small vessels of the heart, brain, kidneys, and retina. The results are a progressive functional impairment of these organs, or target organ disease.

Special Considerations

Blood pressure should be well controlled before any invasive procedure. Hypertensive clients are at greater risk for strokes, MI, kidney failure, and pulmonary edema. These clients should be instructed to continue their blood pressure medications until the time of the procedure, unless otherwise directed by their physician or health care provider. They should resume their antihypertensive medications as soon as possible after the procedure, unless they are given new instructions by the physician.

atherosclerosis: athere—porridge + sklerosis—hardness

Nursing Process

NURSING ASSESSMENT

The assessment of the client with hypertension includes the client's history, medications, and physical assessment. Assessing the knowledge of hypertensive clients and their families about hypertension and associated risk factors is essential for client and family education planning and subsequent lifestyle modification needs.

NURSING DIAGNOSIS

Based on the data and defining characteristics, a nursing diagnosis should be chosen in collaboration with the health care team and the client. Because the risk of hypertension depends on the number and severity of modifiable risk factors, several nursing diagnoses may be applicable. Common diagnoses may include but are not limited to the following:

- Knowledge deficit related to lack of knowledge about hypertension
- Ineffective management of therapeutic regimen related to complexity of therapy, cost of medications, lack of symptoms, side effects of medications, need to alter long-term lifestyle habits, normal blood pressure controlled by therapy

See Nursing Care Plan Box 16–3 for the Client with Hypertension.

PLANNING

After nursing diagnoses have been identified, specific goals for control of blood pressure should be set by the physician, nurse, client, and family. Any barriers to meeting these goals should be discussed with the client and family so that the plan can be carried out more effectively. The client's goals are to (1) understand the disease and its treatment and (2) reduce blood pressure by following therapy.

NURSING INTERVENTIONS

To meet their goals, clients may require more information, guidance, and support from the health care team. Referrals to other resources such as the dietitian, social worker, pharmacist, and home health nurse should be included. The client and family should be allowed to maintain a sense of control, make informed decisions regarding care, and de-

HOME HEALTH HINTS

- For meal planning, most clients eat fast foods occasionally. Assist them in choosing foods that are low in fat, sugar, and salt (e.g., choose chicken salads with low-fat dressing or fajitas without sour cream and guacamole).

- Because medication and electrolyte interaction can occur with salt substitute, which often contains potassium, the physician should be consulted before the client uses it.

- Teach clients how to read labels for fat and salt content. If clients are on a 2 to 3 g sodium diet, instruct them on eating breads or cereals that contain 200 mg or less of sodium per serving, or canned vegetables of 150 mg of sodium per serving. Fresh vegetables are better, but cost and storage must be considered. Providing written suggestions for the caregiver who does the grocery shopping increases compliance with diet therapy.

- Home exercise using weights can be improvised using canned goods and bags of sugar as weights. The amount of weight being used is easily identified for documentation by the labeling on the food item.

- The following suggestions may help a client decrease or stop smoking: use cinnamon mouthwash on arising; put away all ashtrays but one and keep it in a place not normally used for smoking; find ways to keep hands busy at times when usually holding cigarette, such as when drinking coffee or alcohol.

- Encourage clients to put "No Smoking" signs on their door to avoid passive smoking.

- Medication compliance can be a challenge for the elderly hypertensive client. Instruct clients to take medication as prescribed even if they are feeling well or if side effects, which they should report, are present. If the medicines are too expensive for the client, check with the physician and pharmacist for less expensive substitutes.

- During home visits count the amount of pills in a bottle to assess compliance. Remind the client to get refills and keep physician appointments by writing them on the calendar.

- Because many of the antihypertensive medicines can cause bradycardia, teach the client or caregiver to take the client's pulse and to call the nurse if it is below 60 or the parameters defined by the physician or agency.

- Monitor carefully for symptoms of congestive heart failure when the client is on beta blockers. This is a side effect that needs to be caught early and reported to the physician.

- Encourage the client to obtain a home blood pressure monitoring device. Instruct the client or caregiver on proper use and logging the date, time, and reading obtained. The home health nurse should review the log on each visit.

- Clients should be instructed to weigh themselves every morning, wearing the same amount of clothing each time, and keep a log for the nurse to review.

NURSING CARE PLAN BOX 16–3 FOR THE CLIENT WITH HYPERTENSION

Knowledge deficit related to lack of knowledge about hypertension

Client Outcomes
Verbalizes knowledge of hypertension (HTN), risk factors, complications, and treatment.

Evaluation of Outcomes
Is client able to explain HTN, risk factors, complications, and treatment?

Interventions	*Rationale*	*Evaluation*
Use simple terms to define HTN, SBP, DBP, symptoms, and risk factors.	Client must have basic knowledge to comply with therapy.	Is client able to verbalize and understand knowledge of hypertension, SBP, DBP, symptoms, and risk factors?
Teach need to monitor BP regularly.	A sense of control is gained with participation in self-care. Regularly monitoring BP shows trends.	Does client state understanding and willingness to monitor BP?
Explain complications related to target organ disease.	Compliance is increased with understanding and commitment to prevent complications.	Is client able to verbalize complications and importance of preventing them?
Explain medication action, side effects, dosage as ordered.	Compliance and safe use of medications is promoted with an adequate knowledge base.	Can client explain medication usage accurately? Can client state side effects and need to report them?

GERIATRIC

Include caregivers/family in educational sessions.	Compliance increases if support systems understand instructions.	Do caregivers/family participate and offer client support?
Assess ability to take medications daily: financially, obtaining refills, understanding directions.	Elderly clients may be on a fixed income, lack transportation, or lack ability to take several medications several times a day. Simplifying this process, to one medication if possible, can increase compliance.	Is client able to obtain medications? Can client self-administer medications accurately on daily basis?

Ineffective management of therapeutic regimen related to complexity of therapy, cost of medications, lack of symptoms, side effects of medications, need to alter long-term lifestyle habits, normal blood pressure controlled by therapy

Outcomes
Verbalizes ability and willingness to comply with treatment.

Evaluation of Outcomes
Is client able to state how lifestyle will include therapy? Does client identify and problem solve barriers for therapy?

Interventions	*Rationale*	*Evaluation*
Identify client's modifiable risk factors and lifestyle modification needs.	Identifying risk factors is the first step in planning therapy. Client must understand the relationship of these risk factors with hypertension and complication development.	Can client state rationale for modifying risk factors to prevent complication development?
Identify factors that are barriers to client complying with therapy.	Factors such as finances, transportation, aging changes, client motivation, habits, and reading and educational level can be barriers for therapy.	Are barriers present for client?

continued

NURSING CARE PLAN BOX 16–3 *(continued)*

Interventions	Rationale	Evaluation
Develop plan to overcome barriers. Make referrals as needed.	Identified barriers can be overcome with planning and intervention, such as referral to support groups or for financial assistance or prescription delivery service and instructions provided at level of client's learning ability.	Have barriers been eliminated? Is client willing to use referrals?
GERIATRIC		
Assess ability to take medications daily: financially, obtaining refills, understanding directions.	Elderly clients may be on a fixed income, lack transportation, or lack ability to take several medications several times a day. Simplifying this process, to one medication if possible, can increase compliance.	Is client able to obtain medications? Can client self-administer medications accurately on daily basis?
Teach client to take medications as prescribed and not to skip dosages.	Elderly clients may skip dosages to save money, reduce side effects, or reduce need to void.	Does client take dosages as prescribed? Does client express concern over cost, side effects, or frequent voiding?
Teach client to change positions slowly to prevent falls.	Antihypertensive medications can cause hypotension, resulting in dizziness and weakness and possibly leading to falls.	Does client understand how to change positions slowly? Does client experience dizziness or weakness?

velop the skills necessary to make lifestyle modifications. Behavioral changes are the most difficult for the client to initiate and maintain. The nurse plays a major role in therapy and treatment compliance for hypertensive clients.

EVALUATION

One of the best outcome criteria for evaluation is reaching a lowered blood pressure with minimal side effects and no evidence of target organ damage. Other indicators of success in implementing the plan of care are weight loss, maintaining a low-sodium diet, decreasing alcohol intake, decreased or no smoking, and management of stress on a daily basis. If the client is satisfied and comfortable with the quality of life after the modifications, another goal has been met.

Client Education

The use of educational programs in hospitals, clinics, churches, and health fairs helps increase client motivation to adhere to antihypertensive therapy. Instructions provided by the nurse are directed toward helping clients control their blood pressure through self-care measures, as well as the prescribed medical regimen. To effectively control hypertension, clients must be knowledgeable about their condition. They need to be taught about the condition, its treatment, and the need for lifelong commitment to con-

trolling it. (See Nursing Care Plan Box 16–3 for the Client with Hypertension.)

Hypertensive Emergency

Hypertensive crisis is a severe type of hypertension characterized by rapidly progressive elevations in blood pressure with diastolic values above 110 mm Hg. Clients who are untreated, do not comply with antihypertensive therapy, or stop their medication abruptly are at risk for hypertensive crisis. A client with hypertensive crisis may experience morning headaches, blurred vision, dizziness, nosebleeds, and dyspnea. A diminished level of consciousness, weakness, paralysis, palpitations, or complaints of chest pain may also indicate a hypertensive crisis and should be reported immediately. Clients with hypertensive crisis are admitted to the critical care unit. In some cases, the blood pressure may need to be reduced within 1 hour to prevent organ damage.

Review Questions

1. Which one of the following is true of the cause of primary hypertension?
   a. It is caused by a tumor of the adrenal gland.
   b. It is caused by renal artery stenosis.
   c. It is caused by coarctation of the aorta.
   d. There is no known cause.

2. Which one of the following is often the only sign of hypertension?
   a. Sacral edema
   b. Elevated blood pressure
   c. Tachycardia
   d. Neck vein distention

3. Which one of the following is affected by chronic elevations in blood pressure?
   a. Lungs
   b. Liver
   c. Stomach
   d. Eyes

4. The nurse should include which one of the following instructions to a client receiving a thiazide diuretic?
   a. "Eliminate salt in your diet."
   b. "Make position changes slowly."
   c. "Take your medication before bedtime."
   d. "Empty your bladder after taking the first dose."

5. For which one of the following blood pressure readings should a follow-up visit be recommended?
   a. 128/70
   b. 136/76
   c. 140/94
   d. 142/86

6. Which one of the following is the most important lifestyle modification for the hypertensive client who is obese?
   a. Reduce weight
   b. Restrict salt intake
   c. Quit smoking
   d. Decrease alcohol intake

7. For a client with stage 1 hypertension, initial drug therapy would include which one of the following?
   a. Amiloride (Midamor)
   b. Diltiazem (Cardizem)
   c. Labetalol (Normodyne)
   d. Minoxidil (Loniten)

ANSWERS TO CRITICAL THINKING

CRITICAL THINKING: *Mrs. Miller*

1. Gender; age; ethnicity; smoking cigarettes; diet high in fat, salt, and calories; recently divorced; stressful occupation; and morning headaches.
2. Morning headaches. Mrs. Miller may be experiencing an episode of hypertensive crisis and should be evaluated immediately by a health care provider.
3. Silent killer refers to the fact that there are often no signs or symptoms associated with hypertension.
4. Lifelong therapy is required because there is no cure for hypertension and complications need to be prevented.

CRITICAL THINKING: *Mrs. Bell*

1. Nonmodifiable: age, gender, history of hypertension. Modifiable: weight, compliance with antihypertensive therapy.
2. Diuretics remove excess salt and water to decrease the volume of the blood and lower the blood pressure. Beta blockers stop the beta receptors from receiving the message from the brain for the heart to work harder. Therefore the heart rate and blood pressure decrease.
3. Assess client's reading level and primary language. Provide client with written instructions in large letters about medications. Include family members and encourage their support in reinforcing the importance of adhering to the treatment plan.
4. Client is 80 years old, makes frequent trips to the bathroom related to diuretics, and a side effect of propranolol (Inderal) is weakness and fatigue.
5. Make arrangements for a bedside commode to reduce the distance and urgency to get to the bathroom. Encourage the family to place red night-lights in the bedroom, hall, and bathroom. Explain that throw rugs can be a fall risk and that wood or tile floors can be slippery when wet and hard if a fall occurs. Encourage removal of throw rugs and suggest carpeting these areas, if possible. Suggest the use of safety bars in hall and bathroom for support or other walking aids as needed. If incontinence is a concern, suggest wearing an adult brief to prevent a wet, slippery floor. Suggest discussing with the physician an exercise program such as lifting small, lightweight objects (such as canned foods), squeezing a rubber ball, and riding an exercise bike as able to increase strength. These exercises can be done while sitting so they are not a fall risk activity.

REFERENCES

1. The Sixth Report of the Joint National Committee on Prevention, Detection, Evaluation, and Treatment of High Blood Pressure. Arch Intern Med 157(21):2413, 1997.
2. Mallory, D: Compliance and health beliefs in the African American female hypertensive client. J Nat Black Nurses Assoc 1:38, 1988.
3. Gregory, S, and Clark, P: The "big three" cardiovascular risk factors among Americans, Blacks, and Hispanics. J Holistic Nurs 8(1):76, 1992.
4. Levy, RA: Ethnic and racial differences in response to medicines: Preserving individualized therapy in managed pharmaceutical programmes. Pharm Med 7:139, 1993.
5. Sharts Engel, N, Kojima, M, and Martinson, M: A community health center responds to the aging of Japan. J Geriatr Nurs 12(11):12, 1986.

6. Sabet, L, and Sabet, T: Korean Americans. In Purnell, L, and Paulanka, B (eds): Transcultural Health Care: A Culturally Competent Approach. FA Davis, Philadelphia, 1997.
7. Stavig, GR, Igra, A, and Leonard, AR: Hypertension and related health issues among Asians and Pacific Islanders in California. Public Health Rep 103(1):28, 1988.
8. National High Blood Pressure Education Program: Working Group Report on Primary Prevention of Hypertension. National Institutes of Health, No. 93-2669, Bethesda, Md, 1993.
9. Allender, PS, et al: Dietary calcium and blood pressure: A meta-analysis of randomized clinical trials. Ann Intern Med 124:825, 1996.

BIBLIOGRAPHY

Beare, PG, and Myers, JL: Principles and Practice of Adult Health Nursing, ed 2. Mosby, St Louis, 1994, p 721.
Boutain, DM: A research review: Involving the African American family in anti-hypertensive medication management. J Nat Black Nurses Assoc 9(1):22, 1997.
Byers, JF, and Goshorn, J: How to manage diuretic therapy. Am J Nurs 95:2, 1995.
Cuddy, RP: Hypertension: Keeping dangerous blood pressure down. Nursing 25:8, 1995.
Johannsen, JM: Update: Guidelines for treating hypertension. Am J Nurs 93:3, 1993.

Liehr, P, Vogler, R, and Meininger, JC: Guidelines for selecting outcome measures: Lifestyle modification for stage 1 hypertension. Adv Pract Nurs Q 3(2):10, 1997.
Lutz, CA, and Przytulski, KR: Nutrition and Diet therapy, ed 2. FA Davis, Philadelphia, 1997.
McCuiston-Schmidt, LE: Treatment algorithm for hypertension. Medsurg Nurs 3(6):487, 1994.
Nash, CA, and Jensen, PL: When your surgical patient has hypertension. Am J Nurs 94:12, 1994.
Oparil, S, and Calhoun, DA: Managing the patient with hard to control hypertension. Am Fam Physician 57(5):1007, 1998.
Porth, CM: Pathophysiology: Concepts of Altered Health States, ed 4. JB Lippincott, Philadelphia, 1994, p 379.
Redeker, NS, and Sadowski, AV: Update on cardiovascular drugs and elders. Am J Nurs 95:9, 1995.
Shulman, NB, Saunders, E, and Hall, WD: High Blood Pressure. Dell, New York, 1993, pp 1–169.
Trilling, JS, et al: Hypertension in nursing home patients. J Hum Hypertens 12(2):117, 1998.
Whelton, P, et al: Effects of oral potassium on blood pressure: Meta-analysis of randomized controlled clinical trials. JAMA 277(20):1624, 1997.
Whelton, PK, et al: Sodium reduction and weight loss in the treatment of hypertension in older persons: A randomized controlled trial of non-pharmacologic interventions in the elderly (TONE). TONE Collaborative Research Group. JAMA 279(11):839, 1998.

Nursing Care of Clients with Inflammatory and Infectious Cardiovascular Disorders

Linda S. Williams

Learning Objectives

Upon completion of this chapter, the student will be able to:

1. Describe the pathophysiology, etiology, signs and symptoms, diagnostic tests, and medical treatment for rheumatic fever and rheumatic heart disease.
2. Explain nursing care for rheumatic fever and rheumatic heart disease.
3. Describe the pathophysiology, etiology, signs and symptoms, complications, diagnostic tests, and medical treatment for infective endocarditis, myocarditis, and pericarditis.
4. Explain nursing care for infective endocarditis, myocarditis, and pericarditis.
5. Explain the importance of prophylactic antibiotics for infective endocarditis, myocarditis, and rheumatic heart disease.
6. Describe the pathophysiology, etiology, signs and symptoms, complications, diagnostic tests, and medical treatment for dilated, hypertrophic, and restrictive cardiomyopathy.
7. Explain nursing care for dilated, hypertrophic, and restrictive cardiomyopathy.
8. Describe the pathophysiology, etiology, signs and symptoms, complications, diagnostic tests, and medical treatment for thrombophlebitis.
9. Explain nursing care for thrombophlebitis.

Key Words

beta-hemolytic streptococci (**BAY**-tuh-HEE-moh-**LIT**-ick STREP-toh-**KOCK**-sigh)

cardiac tamponade (**KAR**-dee-yak TAM-pon-**AYD**)

cardiomegaly (KAR-dee-oh-**MEG**-ah-lee)

cardiomyopathy (KAR-dee-oh-my-**AH**-pah-thee)

chorea (kaw-**REE**-ah)

Dressler's syndrome (**DRESS**-lers **SIN**-drohm)

emboli (EM-boh-li)

hypercoagulability (HIGH-per-koh-AG-yoo-lah-**BILL**-i-tee)

infective endocarditis (in-**FECK**-tive EN-doh-kar-**DYE**-tis)

international normalized ratio (IN-ter-**NASH**-uh-nul **NOR**-muh-lized **RAY**-she-oh)

myectomy (my-**ECK**-tuh-mee)

myocarditis (MY-oh-kar-**DYE**-tis)

pancarditis (PAN-kar-**DYE**-tis)

pericardial effusion (PER-ee-**KAR**-dee-uhl ee-**FYOO**-zhun)

pericardial friction rub (PER-ee-**KAR**-dee-uhl **FRICK**-shun RUB)

pericardiectomy (PER-ee-kar-dee-**ECK**-tuh-mee)

pericardiocentesis (PER-ee-KAR-dee-oh-sen-**TEE**-sis)

pericarditis (PER-ee-kar-**DYE**-tis)

petechiae (pe-**TEE**-kee-ee)

rheumatic fever (roo-**MAT**-ick **FEE**-ver)

rheumatic heart disease (roo-**MAT**-ick HART di-**ZEEZ**)

thrombophlebitis (THROM-boh-fle-**BYE**-tis)

Cardiac Disorders

The layers of the heart, the endocardium, myocardium, and pericardium, can become infected (Fig. 17–1). Inflammation of the heart structures and layers can result from a cardiac infection or as a complication from a hypersensitivity reaction to antigens of infecting organisms. Systemic infections are the main cause of cardiac infections. The invading organisms are carried to the heart via the blood.

RHEUMATIC FEVER

Pathophysiology and Etiology

Rheumatic fever is a hypersensitivity reaction to antigens of group A **beta-hemolytic streptococci** that mainly occurs in children. Rheumatic fever is a complication of a streptococcal infection, such as a sore throat. The onset of rheumatic fever typically occurs 2 to 3 weeks after the streptococcal infection. Few of those with a streptococcal infection develop rheumatic fever. It can recur, however, if the client develops another streptococcal infection. In rheumatic fever, an inflammatory response results that most often targets the heart and joints. On occasion, the

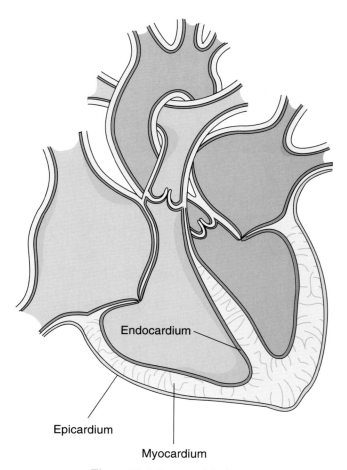

Figure 17–1. Layers of the heart.

Epicardium

Endocardium

Myocardium

skin, central nervous system (CNS), and lungs may also be affected by the inflammatory response.

Signs and Symptoms

Rheumatic fever signs and symptoms include polyarthritis, subcutaneous nodules, **chorea** with rapid, uncontrolled movements, carditis, fever, arthralgia, and pneumonitis. The joints become inflamed one at a time, resulting in polyarthritis. The major joints are most commonly affected, but this inflammation does not cause permanent damage. Subcutaneous nodules that are small, firm, and painless develop over bony prominences. The lungs may also be affected by inflammation, causing pneumonitis. Chorea is a sign of CNS involvement. With chorea involuntary, purposeless contractions of the muscles of the trunk and extremities are seen.

Diagnostic Tests

A throat culture will diagnose a streptococcal infection at the time of the infection, but there is no specific test for rheumatic fever. Because rheumatic fever occurs days to weeks after a streptococcal infection, some test values may have already returned to normal when rheumatic fever begins. A test that will show a recent group A streptococcal infection is an antistreptolysin O titer level greater than 250 IU/mL. Erythrocyte sedimentation rate (ESR) levels may be elevated from inflammation, and the white blood cell (WBC) count may be elevated.

Medical Treatment

Treatment for rheumatic fever is aimed at controlling the symptoms because there is no cure. Anti-inflammatory medications such as aspirin or corticosteroids are used to control the fever and joint inflammation and pain.

Complications

Rheumatic Heart Disease

The most serious complication of rheumatic fever is severe damage to the heart. This complication is referred to as **rheumatic heart disease.** In some clients, all layers of the heart are affected by inflammation, which is referred to as rheumatic **pancarditis.** In other clients, only part of the heart is affected. With rheumatic **pericarditis,** the pericardial layers are covered with an exudate and become thickened. As healing takes place, the pericardial sac can be damaged or destroyed by fibrosis. However, this is usually not serious. In rheumatic **myocarditis,** the inflammatory

---

chorea: choreia—dance
pancarditis: pan—all + kardia—heart + itis—inflammation
pericarditis: peri—around + kardia—heart + itis—inflammation
myocarditis: myo—muscle + kardia—heart + itis—inflammation

process causes nodules to form in the myocardial tissue, and the nodules become scar tissue over time. This can weaken the heart's contractions and may lead to heart failure.

The endocardium is the most serious area of the heart affected in rheumatic fever, and the mitral valve is the structure most often affected. Tiny, pinhead-size vegetations form on the valve leaflets from blood and fibrin. This can lead to thickening, fibrosis, and calcification of the valve leaflets and support structures. If the valve leaflets do not close completely, regurgitation of blood can occur. If the valve leaflets do not open fully, which is referred to as valvular stenosis, blood movement is impaired and severe heart failure may result. Chronic rheumatic carditis can be a complication of rheumatic fever. The valves and their structures can be scarred and damaged. These changes may occur years after an episode of rheumatic fever and can lead to heart failure.

PREVENTION. Preventing rheumatic fever also prevents rheumatic heart disease from developing. Rheumatic fever can be prevented by detecting and treating streptococcal infections promptly with penicillin. The signs and symptoms of a pharynx streptococcal infection include sudden sore throat, fever of 101 to 104°F, chills, throat redness with exudate, sinus or ear infection, and lymph node enlargement. A throat culture is obtained to provide an accurate diagnosis. Prophylactic antibiotics either long term or just before invasive procedures are usually given to clients who have had rheumatic fever because they are at risk for developing a cardiac infection.

SIGNS AND SYMPTOMS. Rheumatic heart disease signs and symptoms depend on the area of the heart involved. A new murmur may be heard; pericarditis symptoms, such as a pericardial friction rub and chest pain, may be present; or the signs and symptoms of heart failure may occur.

DIAGNOSIS. Cardiac involvement can be diagnosed with a chest x-ray showing heart enlargement, an echocardiogram showing valvular damage, and an electrocardiogram (ECG) showing changes in conduction times.

MEDICAL TREATMENT. Activity is limited based on the degree of cardiac involvement. Treatment for cardiac involvement is based on the symptoms, such as those seen in heart failure.

Nursing Process: Rheumatic Fever and Rheumatic Heart Disease

Assessment

A client history is obtained that includes recent illnesses, such as a sore throat, streptococcal infection, or scarlet fever; past episodes of rheumatic fever; heart disease; joint pain; and current medications. A physical assessment is done, noting swelling of joints; nodules under the skin that are painless, firm, and movable; murmurs;

pericardial friction rub; chorea; and heart failure signs, such as JVD, edema, dyspnea, crackles, cough, and fatigue. Vital signs are documented, noting fever and tachycardia.

Nursing Diagnosis

The major nursing diagnosis for rheumatic fever and rheumatic heart disease may include but are not limited to the following:

- Pain related to joint or cardiac inflammation
- Anxiety related to disease process
- Decreased cardiac output related to valvular damage and carditis
- Knowledge deficit related to lack of knowledge about rheumatic fever and rheumatic heart disease and their treatment

Planning

The client's goals are to (1) relieve pain, (2) decrease anxiety, (3) maintain normal cardiac function, and (4) understand the disease and its treatment.

Nursing Interventions

Nursing care focuses on relieving the client's pain and anxiety, maintaining normal cardiac function, and educating the client about the disease. Pain is relieved by giving analgesics, aspirin, or corticosteroids as ordered.

Reducing anxiety is important. It can be accomplished by providing explanations for procedures and educating the client about the disease and its treatment.

Maintenance of normal cardiac function includes monitoring of vital signs and for the presence of symptoms of valvular damage or heart failure. The presence of these symptoms is immediately reported to the physician.

An explanation of the disease and its treatment is provided to promote understanding of procedures and compliance with acute and prophylactic treatment.

Evaluation

The goal for pain is met if the client reports satisfactory pain relief. Satisfactory pain relief is measured by comparing the client's stated level of pain on a rating scale of 1 to 10 with the client's predetermined goal for acceptable level of pain.

The goal for the nursing diagnosis of anxiety is achieved if the client states that anxiety is reduced. Additionally, if the client is able to learn during teaching sessions, anxiety is not a barrier to learning.

The goal for the nursing diagnosis of decreased cardiac output is met if the client's vital signs are within normal range and no symptoms of heart failure are present.

The goal for the nursing diagnosis of knowledge deficit is met if the client explains the disease and states understanding of treatment. A statement of willingness to follow lifestyle changes needed to maintain health also supports goal achievement.

INFECTIVE ENDOCARDITIS

Pathophysiology

Blood flow through the heart can create turbulence. This turbulence promotes the invasion of organisms in damaged areas of the heart. Microorganisms infecting the endocardium of the heart are attracted mainly to the valves of the heart, although any heart endothelial surface can be infected. Damaged valves from conditions such as mitral valve prolapse, rheumatic fever, congenital defects, and valvular surgery are especially prone to invasion by these organisms. The mitral valve is the valve most commonly infected in individuals with a history of heart disease. The tricuspid valve is infected more commonly from intravenous drug abuse.

Damage to the valve's leaflets occurs as the organisms grow. Growths of these organisms are called vegetations. As blood flows through the heart, the vegetations may break off and become **emboli.** These emboli may obstruct blood flow as they travel through the bloodstream and infarct organs such as the brain or kidneys if they are from a left heart infection or the lungs if they are from a right heart infection.

If the infection spreads it can damage the valves and their structures. If it infiltrates the myocardium it can result in cardiac damage. In either case, heart failure may result.

Etiology

Organisms that may infect the endocardium are bacteria (*Staphylococcus aureus,* beta-hemolytic streptococci, *Escherichia coli*), *Streptococcus viridans,* and fungi. These organisms may enter the bloodstream through a variety of ways. Portals of entry include invasive catheters in clients with weakened immune systems, intravenous drug use, and dental or invasive procedures in clients with valvular heart disease. People with weakened immune systems, including the elderly, or valvular heart disease, including those with mitral valve prolapse, valvular replacement surgery, or rheumatic heart disease, as well as immunocompromised clients, are at greater risk for infection.

Prevention

Antibiotic therapy before invasive procedures is recommended for high- and moderate-risk clients.[1] Those at high risk include clients with prosthetic heart valves, prior endocarditis, surgical pulmonary shunts, and complex cyanotic congenital heart disease. Moderate-risk clients include those with mitral valve prolapse with valvular regurgitation, other congenital cardiac malformations, rheumatic heart disease, and hypertrophic cardiomyopathy. Invasive procedures include some dental procedures and some surgical or invasive procedures of the respiratory, genitourinary, or gastrointestinal tracts.

It is important that high- and moderate-risk clients are taught the need for prophylactic treatment. They should in-

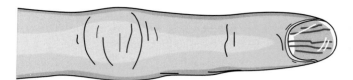

Figure 17–2. Nailbeds with splinter hemorrhages.

form health care team members of their history before a procedure. The nurse should ensure that the history is reported to the physician so that prophylactic therapy can be ordered and given if needed.

Signs and Symptoms

Manifestations of infective endocarditis may develop gradually. Fever is the most common sign in most cases of infective endocarditis. Chills, night sweats, fatigue, malaise, weight loss, weakness, abdominal pain, anorexia, and generalized pain in joints, muscles, or the back may also be present. With left heart endocarditis, a new murmur may be heard as damage to the valves occurs. A vascular sign of infective endocarditis is splinter hemorrhages in the nailbeds (Fig. 17–2). These appear as black or red-brown longitudinal lines or streaks in the nails. **Petechiae** resulting from microembolization of the vegetation may occur on the lips, mouth, conjunctivae, feet, or antecubital area.

Complications

Emboli can be a major complication of endocarditis. If organ embolization occurs, signs and symptoms that reflect the organ that was affected by the emboli may be seen. Brain emboli may produce changes in level of consciousness or stroke. Kidney emboli may produce pain in the flank area, hematuria, or renal failure. Emboli in the spleen may cause left upper quadrant pain. Emboli in the small blood vessels can impair circulation in the extremities. Pulmonary emboli from right-sided endocarditis may lead to pneumonia or abscesses. Heart structures can be damaged or destroyed by endocarditis. Stenosis or regurgitation of a heart valve may also result. As the infection progresses and causes more damage to heart structures, heart failure may occur.

Diagnostic Tests

Table 17–1 summarizes the diagnostic tests and their findings for infective endocarditis. In addition to the client's health history, information about recent invasive procedures or infections should be obtained. Physical examination findings should be noted. Laboratory tests may in-

---

petechiae: petecchia—skin spot

Table 17–1. Diagnostic Tests for Infective Endocarditis

Test	Finding
White blood cell count with differential	Slight elevation
Blood cultures	Identifies causative organism
Erythrocyte sedimentation rate	Elevated
Rheumatoid factor	Positive
Electrocardiogram	Dysrhythmias
Chest x-ray	Heart failure
Echocardiogram	Vegetations on heart valves
Cardiac catheterization	Abnormal heart and valve function

clude a slightly elevated WBC count and an elevated ESR. Some clients may also have a positive rheumatoid factor. In most clients with infective endocarditis, blood cultures are positive and identify the causative organism of infective endocarditis. An echocardiogram can be used to see vegetations attached to the heart valves. Other tests that may be used include cardiac catheterization, ECG, and chest x-ray.

Medical Treatment

Medications to fight the causative organism are the primary focus of treatment (Table 17–2). An antimicrobial drug is selected that is sensitive to the organism identified through the blood culture. For bacterial infections, penicillin is commonly used. In fungal infections, an antifungal agent such as amphotericin B is given. The medication is usually given intravenously over a period of 4 to 6 weeks. Although treatment may begin with a brief period of hospitalization if the client's symptoms are more severe, it is usually started in the client's home. The home care nurse

Table 17–2. Medical Treatment for Infective Endocarditis

Treatment	Purpose
Prophylactic antibiotic therapy	Prevention
Acute Therapy	
IV antimicrobial medications	Cure infection
Antipyretics	Reduce fever
Rest	Decrease cardiac workload
Anticoagulant therapy	Decrease risk of vegetation emboli
Surgical—valve replacement	Restore normal valve function
Complications—Heart Failure	
Digitalis	Strengthen heart contraction
Diuretics	Reduce fluid volume returning to heart (preload)

provides ongoing monitoring of the client's response to the drug. Serum drug levels are monitored and periodic blood cultures are done to determine the response of the organism to the medication. Changes in the medication may be made for side effects, allergies, organism resistance to the drug, and relapses. Rest, fluids, and acetaminophen or aspirin for fever may be used to treat the infection. Prophylactic anticoagulants may be given to prevent emboli resulting from valvular damage. Aspirin should not be used with anticoagulants.

Surgical replacement of valves is usually required for clients with severely damaged heart valves. Prime candidates for this would be clients with fungal endocarditis, prosthetic valve infection, recurrent infection, emboli from damaged valves, or heart failure. Recovery from the disease can be greatly improved with surgery, and antimicrobial therapy is usually continued after surgery.

Nursing Process

Assessment

A client history is obtained that includes risk factors for endocarditis and recent infections or invasive procedures (Table 17–3). Vital signs are measured and recorded, and heart sounds are auscultated to detect murmurs. A thorough physical assessment is done. Petechiae on the chest, conjunctiva, mouth, or legs are noted. Fever, joint pain, and muscle tenderness are assessed. Signs of heart failure and emboli are noted.

Nursing Diagnosis

The major nursing diagnoses for infective endocarditis may include but are not limited to the following:

- Decreased cardiac output related to impaired valvular function or heart failure
- Pain related to fever from cardiac infection
- Activity intolerance related to reduced oxygen delivery from decreased cardiac output
- Diversional activity deficit related to restricted mobility from prolonged intravenous therapy
- Knowledge deficit related to lack of knowledge about infective endocarditis and treatment
- Risk for alteration in tissue perfusion related to emboli

Planning

The client's goals are to (1) maintain normal cardiac function, (2) achieve pain relief, (3) restore quality of life and activity tolerance, (4) participate in satisfying activities, (5) understand the disorder and prevention of complications, and (6) maintain normal tissue perfusion.

Nursing Interventions

Nursing care is aimed at maintaining the client's normal cardiac function, promoting prevention techniques, monitoring symptoms and complications, administering med-

Table 17–3. Nursing Assessment for Clients with Infective Endocarditis

Subjective Data

Health History

Infections (rheumatic fever, previous endocarditis, streptococcal or staphylococcal, syphilis)?
Cardiac disease (valvular surgery, congenital)?
Childbirth?
Invasive procedures (surgery, dental, catheterization, intravenous therapy, cystoscopy, gynecological)?
Malaise?
Anorexia?

Medications

Steroids, immunosuppressants, prolonged antibiotic therapy, IV drug use, alcohol abuse?

Respiratory

Dyspnea on exertion or when lying (orthopnea)?
Cough?

Cardiovascular

Any palpitations, chest pain, fatigue, or activity intolerance?

Musculoskeletal

Weakness, arthralgia, myalgia?

Knowledge of Condition

Objective Data

Fever, Diaphoresis

Respiratory

Crackles, tachypnea

Cardiovascular

Murmurs, tachycardia, dysrhythmias, edema, headache

Integumentary

Nailbed splinter hemorrhages, petechiae on lips, mouth, conjunctivae, feet, or antecubital area

Renal

Hematuria

Diagnostic Test Findings

Anemia, elevated WBC count, elevated ESR, positive blood cultures, ECG showing conduction problems, echocardiogram showing valvular dysfunction and vegetations, chest x-ray showing heart enlargement (cardiomegaly) and lung congestion

---

ications as ordered, and teaching the client about the disease and treatment. See Nursing Care Plan Box 17–1 for the Client with Infective Endocarditis for specific nursing interventions.

Maintenance of normal cardiac function includes the monitoring of vital signs, intake and output, and daily weights. Medications are given as prescribed. Before administering anticoagulants, laboratory values must be assessed to ensure patient safety. For warfarin (Coumadin), prothrombin times and **international normalized ratio** (INR) values are reviewed and compared with the laboratory's normal ranges. Prothrombin times are therapeutic if they are within a range of 1.5 to 2 times the normal values. The INR normal and therapeutic values are provided on the laboratory report.

LEARNING TIP

Interpreting Therapeutic Prothrombin Times. Prothrombin time values are measured in the time interval of seconds. The normal value range gives the seconds required for a fibrin clot to form during the test. If a client is on warfarin (Coumadin), an anticoagulant, the purpose of the warfarin (Coumadin) is to increase the time or seconds required for the blood to clot. It is therefore expected that the prothrombin time will be elevated when warfarin (Coumadin) is taken.

Because therapy, the warfarin (Coumadin), is being given, a prothrombin time range that safely considers the expected effects of the warfarin (Coumadin) is needed. This range is called the therapeutic range.

Remember that a range has a high and a low. The therapeutic range is 1.5 to 2 times the normal prothrombin time range. To monitor the client's therapeutic prothrombin time, compare the client's result with the therapeutic range that you calculate. For example:

Client's value on warfarin (Coumadin): 16 seconds
Normal prothrombin time range: 9–12 seconds

To calculate		
therapeutic	1.5	2
range, multiply	× 9 seconds	× 12
The therapeutic	13.5 seconds	to 24 seconds
range is		

Compare the client's value of 16 seconds with the therapeutic range of 13.5 to 24 seconds to determine that the client is safely within the therapeutic range.

Education to promote understanding of the disorder and prevention of complications is an important nursing intervention. An explanation of the disorder is provided to promote understanding of health maintenance and early recognition of onset of symptoms so that medical care can be sought. It is essential that clients fully understand the need to treat streptococcal infections and to take prophylactic antibiotics before invasive procedures to prevent endocarditis if they have had rheumatic fever or are at risk for endocarditis. Teaching is provided for medications the client is taking. If the client is on anticoagulants, a Medic Alert bracelet should be worn and monthly appointments to monitor prothrombin time and INR values should be maintained.

Interventions that improve the quality of life include activities of daily living that reduce fatigue. Assistance as

NURSING CARE PLAN BOX 17–1
FOR THE CLIENT WITH INFECTIVE ENDOCARDITIS

Decreased cardiac output related to impaired valvular function or heart failure

Client Outcomes
Client has adequate cardiac output as evidenced by vital signs within normal limits (WNL), no dyspnea or fatigue.

Evaluation of Outcomes
Are client's vital signs WNL with no dyspnea or fatigue?

Interventions	Rationale	Evaluation
Assess vital signs, murmurs, dyspnea, and fatigue.	Vital signs, dyspnea, and fatigue are indicators of cardiac output decline.	Are vital signs WNL with no dyspnea or fatigue?
Give oxygen as ordered.	Supplemental oxygen provides more oxygen to the heart.	Are breathing pattern and oxygen saturation WNL?
Provide rest as ordered.	Cardiac workload and oxygen needs are reduced with rest.	Are vital signs WNL and no fatigue reported?
Elevate head of bed 45 degrees.	Venous return to heart is reduced and chest expansion improved.	Are vital signs WNL and respirations easy?

Pain related to fever from cardiac infection

Client Outcomes
Temperature is 97°to 99.5°F; states pain relieved.

Evaluation of Outcomes
Does client state that he or she is free from pain or pain is at tolerable level? Is temperature WNL?

Interventions	Rationale	Evaluation
Monitor temperature every 4 hours and as required (prn).	Documenting temperature shows therapy need and effectiveness.	Is client's temperature remaining WNL?
Assess pain using rating scale such as 1–10.	Self-report is the most reliable indicator of pain.	Does client report pain using scale?
Provide antipyretics prn.	Antipyretics reduce fever and associated pain from chills.	Is client's temperature and pain lower after medication?
Keep client warm with blankets.	Removing blankets to decrease fever results in chills and shivering, which further increases body temperature from muscular activity during shivering.	Does client have chills or is shivering seen?

Activity intolerance related to reduced oxygen delivery from decreased cardiac output

Client Outcomes
Client will state less fatigue in response to activity.

Evaluation of Outcomes
Does client report less fatigue? Is client able to participate in desired activities?

Interventions	Rationale	Evaluation
Assist with activities of daily living (ADL) prn.	Assistance conserves energy.	Are ADLs completed?
Provide rest and space activities.	Cardiac workload and oxygen needs are reduced with rest.	Does client report less fatigue?

continued

NURSING CARE PLAN BOX 17–1 *(continued)*

Diversional activity deficit related to restricted mobility from prolonged intravenous therapy

Client Outcomes
States participation in satisfying diversional activities

Evaluation of Outcomes
Does client participate in diversional activities? Does client state satisfaction with activities?

Interventions	Rationale	Evaluation
Assess client's preferred activities and hobbies.	Activity preference should be known to plan satisfactory diversional activities.	Are client's preferred activities known?
Plan client's schedule around relaxing and fun activities.	Self-esteem is fostered with increased client control.	Does client offer input into scheduled care? Is input followed?
Use pet therapy.	Individuals who can interact with pets live longer and healthier.	Does client state enjoyment of pet therapy?
Provide a mix of physical, mental, and social activities on a rotating schedule.	Rotating stimulating activities and visitors will keep client interested and avoid fatigue.	Does client state satisfaction in activities with no fatigue?

Knowledge deficit related to lack of knowledge about disorder and treatment

Client Outcomes
Verbalizes knowledge of disorder and ability to comply with therapeutic regimen.

Evaluation of Outcomes
Is client able to explain infectious endocarditis and its treatment?

Interventions	Rationale	Evaluation
Explain condition, symptoms, and complications.	Client must have basic knowledge to comply with therapy.	Is client able to verbalize knowledge taught?
Explain need to prevent endocarditis with prophylactic antibiotics.	Antibiotics are necessary before invasive procedures to prevent endocarditis.	Can client state rationale for prophylactic antibiotics?
Explain medications or therapies ordered.	Compliance and safe use of medications are promoted with an adequate knowledge base.	Can client explain medications and therapies?

Risk for alteration in tissue perfusion related to emboli

Client Outcomes
Demonstrates sufficient tissue perfusion with vital signs WNL, no pain reported, and no alteration in level of consciousness (LOC).

Evaluation of Outcomes
Are client's vital signs and LOC WNL with no pain?

Interventions	Rationale	Evaluation
Assess breath sounds, respiratory rate (RR), and respiratory pattern.	Pulmonary emboli decrease breath sounds and increase RR. Brain emboli produce abnormal patterns such as Cheyne-Stokes respirations.	Are client's breath sounds, RR, and respiratory pattern WNL?
Assess confusion, syncope, and altered level of consciousness.	Decreased cerebral perfusion causes these changes.	Is client alert and oriented ×3 without syncope?
Assess abdominal pain.	Splenic emboli cause abdominal pain.	Is client free of abdominal pain?

continued

NURSING CARE PLAN BOX 17–1 *(continued)*

Interventions	Rationale	Evaluation
Assess skin and mucous membranes for petechiae.	Microemboli from vegetative lesions cause petechiae.	Are petechiae present?
Assess for splinter hemorrhages in nailbeds.	Emboli in the hand area produce splinter hemorrhages.	Are splinter hemorrhages present?
Do neurovascular checks (NVCs) on extremities.	Redness, swelling, and calf tenderness show thrombophlebitis.	Are NVCs WNL?
Use elastic stockings and teach client leg exercises.	Venous return is increased and thrombophlebitis is decreased.	Does client use stockings and exercise legs?

needed, frequent rest periods, and energy conservation techniques are planned.

Ongoing monitoring for circulatory complications related to emboli is done by the nurse. The physician should be notified immediately if circulatory impairment, such as cold skin, decreased capillary refill, cyanosis or absent peripheral pulses in an extremity, or symptoms of organ-related emboli are detected.

Evaluation

The goal for the nursing diagnosis of decreased cardiac output is met if the client's vital signs are within normal range and no symptoms of heart failure are present.

The goal for the nursing diagnosis of pain is met if the client reports satisfactory pain relief and the client's temperature is within normal limits. Satisfactory pain relief is measured by comparing the client's stated level of pain on a rating scale of 1 to 10 with the client's predetermined goal for acceptable level of pain.

The goal for the nursing diagnosis of activity intolerance is met if the client reports reduced fatigue. The ability to complete tasks and engage in desired activities also supports goal attainment.

The goal for the nursing diagnosis of diversional activity deficit is met if the client states participation in satisfying diversional activities.

The goal for the nursing diagnosis of knowledge deficit is met if the client explains the disease and states understanding of treatment. A statement of willingness to follow lifestyle changes needed to maintain health also supports goal achievement.

The goal for the nursing diagnosis of risk for alteration in tissue perfusion is met if the client's vital signs are within normal limits, no pain is reported, and no alteration in level of consciousness is observed.

▼ CRITICAL THINKING: Mrs. Jones

Mrs. Jones, 28 years old, is admitted to the hospital with a fever of 102°F, chills, fatigue, anorexia, and pain in her joints. A physical assessment reveals a heart murmur, splinter hemorrhages in her nailbeds, and petechiae on her lips. She is diagnosed with bacterial infective endocarditis.

1. Why is a heart murmur heard with endocarditis?
2. What do splinter hemorrhages look like on inspection?
3. What do petechiae indicate?
4. What type of medication does the nurse expect to be ordered to treat the infection?
5. Why does Mrs. Jones have chills if her temperature is elevated?
6. What signs and symptoms might occur if the complications of heart failure develop?
7. Why does Mrs. Jones need to be taught that she needs prophylactic antibiotics before invasive procedures?
8. Why might prophylactic anticoagulants be ordered for Mrs. Jones?
9. The nurse would evaluate Mrs. Jones as understanding teaching about the anticoagulant warfarin (Coumadin) if Mrs. Jones correctly restated what information about the medication?

Answers at end of chapter.

PERICARDITIS

Pathophysiology

Pericarditis is an inflammation of the pericardium, which is the sac surrounding the heart. Normally, there is about 50 mL of serous fluid in the space between the inner and outer layers of the pericardium. Pericarditis results in an increased amount of pericardial fluid, called a pericardial effusion, and inflammation of nearby tissues. It may be acute or chronic.

Chronic constrictive pericarditis often follows an acute episode, in which there is increased fluid accumulation with fibrin being deposited on the inner pericardial layer. As the fluid decreases, fibrous scarring and calcium deposits occur. The heart is then surrounded by a thickened and stiff sac that can limit the stretching ability of the heart's chambers for filling.

Etiology

Pericarditis can be caused by a variety of factors. Acute pericarditis can be the result of (1) infections, such as viruses, bacteria, fungi, or Lyme disease; (2) acute myocardial infarction or postmyocardial infarction (**Dressler's syndrome**); (3) connective tissue disorders, such as systemic lupus erythematosus, rheumatic fever, or rheumatoid arthritis; (4) uremia; (5) trauma from chest injury or invasive thoracic procedures; (6) drug reactions; (7) dissecting aneurysm or pulmonary disease; and (8) unknown factors. If pericarditis occurs within 48 to 72 hours after a myocardial infarction, it is acute. If it occurs 2 to 4 weeks after a myocardial infarction, it is Dressler's syndrome, or late pericarditis.

Chronic constrictive pericarditis results from (1) neoplastic disease and metastasis; (2) radiation; (3) tuberculosis; and (4) unknown factors.

Signs and Symptoms

Chest pain is the most common symptom of pericarditis. The pain is usually located over the pericordium, which is located over the heart and lower part of the chest, or it may radiate to the clavicle, neck, left scapula, or epigastric area. It is an intense, sharp, stabbing pain that increases with deep inspiration, coughing, moving the trunk, or lying flat. The pain may be relieved by sitting up and leaning forward. The client often assumes this position of comfort to decrease the pain. Other symptoms include dyspnea, fever, and chills. Dyspnea may occur because the client takes shallow, rapid breaths to reduce the chest pain that deep breathing causes and as a result of decreased cardiac output when the heart is unable to fill normally from pericardial compression.

The classic sign of pericarditis is a **pericardial friction rub,** a grating, scratchy, high-pitched sound that is heard when a rub is present. The rub is a result of the friction from the inflamed pericardial and epicardial layers rubbing together as the heart fills and contracts. Depending on the severity of the pericarditis, the rub may be faint when auscultated or loud enough to be audible without auscultation. The rub may be heard intermittently or continuously. It is usually heard during each heartbeat, over the lower left sternal border of the chest.

LEARNING TIP

Pericardial Friction Rub. To simulate the sound of a pericardial friction rub, hold the diaphragm of a stethoscope against the palm of one hand; listen through the stethoscope as you rub the index finger of the opposite hand over the knuckles of the hand holding the diaphragm. The sound you hear is similar to that of a pericardial friction rub.

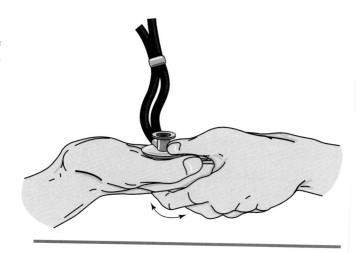

Chronic constrictive pericarditis produces the signs and symptoms of heart failure. Atrial fibrillation may also be seen in some clients with chronic constrictive pericarditis.

Diagnostic Tests

Physical signs and symptoms and ECG waveform changes are used to diagnose pericarditis. Echocardiogram results are also helpful. Serum laboratory tests would focus on possible causes of the pericarditis, such as elevated WBC count indicating a bacterial or viral infection or elevated blood urea nitrogen or creatinine levels indicating uremia. Fluid obtained during **pericardiocentesis** can also be examined to help diagnose the cause.

In chronic constrictive pericarditis, cardiac catheterization, computed tomography, and magnetic resonance imaging results are helpful in diagnosis.

Medical Treatment

Once the cause is determined, appropriate treatment is provided, such as antibiotics for bacterial infections. Bed rest is used to reduce the heart's workload during acute symptoms. Medications may include analgesics for pain control, aspirin for inflammation, pain and fever reduction, and nonsteroidal anti-inflammatory drugs (NSAIDs) such as indomethacin (Indocin) to resolve the inflammation and reduce pain. Corticosteroids are used when NSAIDs are not effective and when systemic lupus erythematosus is the cause.

Chronic effusive pericarditis can be treated with a pericardial window to allow continuous drainage of pericardial fluid. A pericardial window is created surgically by remov-

---

pericardiocentesis: peri—around + kardia—heart + kentesis—puncture

ing a portion of the outer pericardial layer. Fluid can then drain from the pericardial space through the window.

Chronic constrictive pericarditis is treated with a **pericardiectomy,** which is the surgical removal of the entire tough, calcified pericardium. This procedure is done to relieve the constriction of the heart and allow normal filling of the ventricles.

Complications

A buildup of fluid in the pericardial space, referred to as a **pericardial effusion,** is the most common complication of pericarditis. A rapidly developing effusion, such as one occurring from trauma, can produce symptoms at smaller amounts of fluid (250 mL) than slowly developing effusions, such as pericarditis from tuberculosis, with larger amounts of fluid (400 mL). The increasing fluid presses on nearby tissue. Pressure on lung tissue can produce dyspnea, cough, and tachypnea. The heartbeat sounds distant. The body's compensatory mechanisms attempt to maintain blood pressure.

As the fluid accumulation grows, **cardiac tamponade,** a second complication of pericarditis, can occur. Cardiac tamponade is the life-threatening compression of the heart by the fluid accumulating in the pericardial sac surrounding the heart. The increasing pericardial effusion interferes with the heart's filling ability, and as a result cardiac output drops. The blood pressure begins to fall as compensatory mechanisms fail. The client shows symptoms of decreased cardiac output: restlessness, confusion, tachycardia, and tachypnea. Jugular vein distention may be present from increased venous pressure. Cardiac tamponade is a medical emergency requiring immediate treatment with pericardiocentesis to reduce the excess fluid (Fig. 17–3). A pericardiocentesis is the surgical puncture of the pericardium to allow the removal of the excess fluid in the pericardial sac.

When cardiac tamponade occurs, a pericardiocentesis using sterile technique and ECG monitoring is performed. During this procedure fluid is removed from the pericardial space using a 16-gauge needle to reduce heart compression. After the procedure, the client should be monitored for complications, such as dysrhythmias, laceration of a coronary artery, or laceration of the myocardium or pneumothorax.

Nursing Process

Assessment

A client history is obtained that includes any cardiac disease, recent infections, and current medications. A physical assessment is done. Chest pain, pericardial friction rub, heart sounds, and signs of heart failure are noted. Vital signs are documented, noting fever and tachycardia.

---

cardiac tamponade: kardia—heart + tamponade—plug

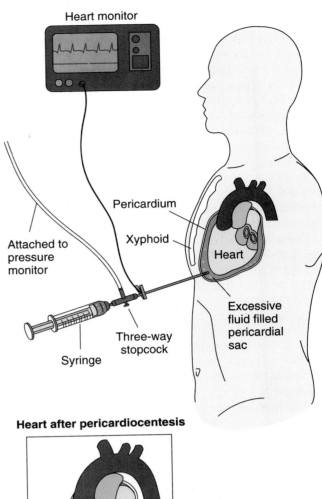

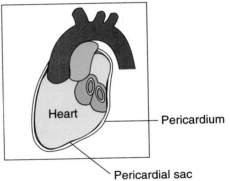

Figure 17–3. Pericardiocentesis.

Nursing Diagnosis

The major nursing diagnoses for pericarditis may include but are not limited to the following:

- Pain related to inflammation of pericardium
- Anxiety related to disease process
- Decreased cardiac output related to cardiac constriction
- Knowledge deficit related to lack of knowledge about pericarditis and its treatment

Planning

The client's goals are to (1) relieve pain, (2) decrease anxiety, (3) maintain normal cardiac function, and (4) understand the disease and its treatment.

Nursing Interventions

Nursing care focuses on relieving the client's pain and anxiety and maintaining normal cardiac function. Symptoms are monitored to detect complications. Teaching the client about the disease and its treatment is important to relieve anxiety and increase the client's understanding of procedures and treatments.

Pain is relieved by giving analgesics, aspirin, NSAIDs, or corticosteroids as ordered. The pain associated with pericarditis may be severe, and relieving it should be a priority nursing intervention. Allowing the client to assume a position of comfort by sitting up and leaning forward also relieves pain. The goal is met if the client reports satisfactory pain relief.

Reducing anxiety is important and can be accomplished by providing explanations for procedures and educating the client about the disease and its treatment. The goal is met if the client states that anxiety is reduced.

Maintenance of normal cardiac function includes monitoring vital signs and the presence of symptoms of cardiac tamponade or heart failure. The presence of these symptoms is immediately reported to the physician. The goal is met if the client's vital signs are within normal range and no symptoms of cardiac tamponade or heart failure are present.

An explanation of the disease and its treatment is provided to promote understanding of procedures and treatment. This may allow clients to feel in control of their lives by being able to make knowledgeable decisions about their health care. The goal is met if the client explains the disease and states understanding of treatment.

Evaluation

The goal for the nursing diagnosis of pain is met if the client reports satisfactory pain relief. Satisfactory pain relief is measured by comparing the client's stated level of pain on a rating scale of 1 to 10 with the client's predetermined goal for acceptable level of pain.

The goal for the nursing diagnosis of anxiety is achieved if the client states that anxiety is reduced.

The goal for decreased cardiac output is met if the client's vital signs are within normal range and no symptoms of heart failure are present.

The goal for the nursing diagnosis of knowledge deficit is met if the client explains the disease to the nurse and states understanding of treatment.

MYOCARDITIS

Pathophysiology

In myocarditis, an inflammation of the myocardium occurs. It may involve a localized or a widespread area of the heart muscle. Healthy heart muscle fibers are essential for effective cardiac function. The amount of muscle destruction and necrosis that occurs as a result of myocarditis de-

termines the extent of damage to the heart. The heart may enlarge in response to the damaged muscle fibers, although most cases of myocarditis are benign, with few signs or symptoms.

Etiology

Myocarditis can be caused by organisms such as viruses, bacteria, parasites, fungi, rickettsiae, and spirochetes. It can also be caused by medications, lead toxicity, autoimmune factors, rheumatic fever, and systemic lupus erythematosus or in association with pericarditis or infective endocarditis. In some cases, no known cause can be found when myocarditis occurs.

Signs and Symptoms

Signs and symptoms of myocarditis can vary from none to severe cardiac manifestations. Fatigue, fever, pharyngitis, malaise, dyspnea, palpitations, muscle aches, gastrointestinal (GI) discomfort, and enlarged lymph nodes may occur early from a viral infection. Cardiac manifestations may occur 7 to 10 days after the viral infection. They can include chest discomfort or pain, tachycardia, or pericardial friction rub if pericarditis is also present.

Diagnostic Tests

An endomyocardial biopsy during the first 6 weeks of inflammation is the best diagnostic test for myocarditis. Small amounts of myocardial tissue are obtained percutaneously from the right ventricle with an instrument called a bioptome to be examined under the microscope for cellular damage and presence of lymphocytes. An ECG shows dysrhythmias if they are present. Serum blood tests can be vague. Leukocytosis may be present. The ESR may be increased. Enzymes such as creatine phosphokinase (CPK) and lactic dehydrogenase (LDH) can be elevated.

Medical Treatment

Treatment is aimed at the cause if it is known. For example, antibiotics are used for bacterial infections. Interventions to reduce the heart's workload, such as bed rest, limited activity, and oxygen, are used. If dysrhythmias are present, cardiac monitoring should be used and emergency equipment should be available for treating life-threatening dysrhythmias. Heart failure is treated with medication to strengthen the heart's contractility and slow the heart's rate, which reduces the heart's workload and oxygen needs. Digoxin is often used to treat heart failure. With myocarditis, the heart is sensitive to digoxin, and toxicity may occur even with small doses. The client should be monitored closely for signs of digoxin toxicity, which may include anorexia, nausea, vomiting, bradycardia, dysrhythmias, or malaise. Immunosuppressant medications such as prednisone or cyclosporine may be used to reduce inflammation and resulting cardiac damage. These drugs should only be used after the acute infection is resolved. Increased tissue necrosis can occur if these drugs are used early in a viral infection.

Complications

Cardiomyopathy, emboli, dysrhythmias, or heart failure may occur depending on the extent of heart damage. In each case, the signs and symptoms would be specific to the disease process exhibited.

Nursing Process

Assessment

A client history is obtained that includes recent illnesses, toxin exposure, cardiac diseases, activity tolerance, and current medications. A physical assessment is done. Signs of heart failure, such as jugular vein distention, peripheral edema, crackles, dyspnea, and chest pain, are noted. Vital signs are documented, noting fever and tachycardia.

Nursing Diagnosis

The major nursing diagnoses for myocarditis may include but are not limited to the following:

- Decreased cardiac output related to heart failure
- Pain related to fever from cardiac infection
- Activity intolerance related to reduced oxygen delivery from decreased cardiac output
- Anxiety related to activity limitations and disease process
- Knowledge deficit related to lack of knowledge about myocarditis and treatment

Planning

The client's goals are to (1) maintain normal cardiac function, (2) relieve pain, (3) restore activity tolerance, (4) decrease anxiety, and (5) understand the disorder and its treatment.

Nursing Interventions

Nursing care is aimed at the client's maintenance of normal cardiac function by monitoring vital signs and symptoms and administering medications as ordered.

Reducing the client's anxiety and knowledge deficit can be achieved by teaching the client about the disease and its treatment.

Determining diversional activities with the client for times when activity is restricted will further reduce anxiety.

Interventions to increase activity tolerance are aimed at reducing fatigue. Providing assistance as needed, scheduling frequent rest periods, and teaching energy conservation techniques are important interventions.

Evaluation

The goal for decreased cardiac output is met if the client's vital signs are within normal range and no symptoms of heart failure are present.

The goal for the nursing diagnosis of pain is met if the client reports satisfactory pain relief and the client's temperature is within normal limits. Satisfactory pain relief is measured by comparing the client's stated level of pain on a rating scale of 1 to 10 with the client's predetermined goal for acceptable level of pain.

The goal for the nursing diagnosis of activity intolerance is met if the client reports reduced fatigue. The ability to complete tasks and engage in desired activities also supports goal attainment.

The goal for the nursing diagnosis of anxiety is achieved if the client states that anxiety is reduced.

The goal for the nursing diagnosis of knowledge deficit is met if the client explains the disease to the nurse and states understanding of treatment.

CARDIOMYOPATHY

Pathophysiology

Cardiomyopathy is a group of diseases that affect the myocardium's structure or function. There are three types of cardiomyopathy: (1) dilated, or congestive; (2) hypertrophic; and (3) restrictive (Fig. 17–4). A consequence of all types of cardiomyopathy can be cardiac enlargement and heart failure.

In dilated or congestive cardiomyopathy the size of the ventricular cavity enlarges and the muscle wall thickness decreases from cell destruction. The atrium enlarges and there is stasis of blood in the left ventricle. Contractile function decreases as the myocardial tissue is destroyed.

Hypertrophic cardiomyopathy is enlargement of the heart muscle, especially along the septum without dilation of the ventricle. The result is a small ventricle that does not easily relax and fill with blood or eject blood. The enlarged septal area may also obstruct outflow of blood into the aorta.

Restrictive cardiomyopathy impairs ventricular stretch, which limits ventricular filling. Cardiac muscle stiffness is present, although systolic emptying of the ventricle remains normal.

Etiology

The cause of cardiomyopathy is unknown. Of the three types, dilated, or congestive, cardiomyopathy occurs most commonly. Dilated, or congestive, cardiomyopathy may follow infectious myocarditis or chronic alcohol or cocaine use.

Hypertrophic cardiomyopathy is a hereditary disorder that is transmitted as a dominant trait. It is often seen in

---

cardiomyopathy: kardia—heart + myo—muscle + pathy—disease

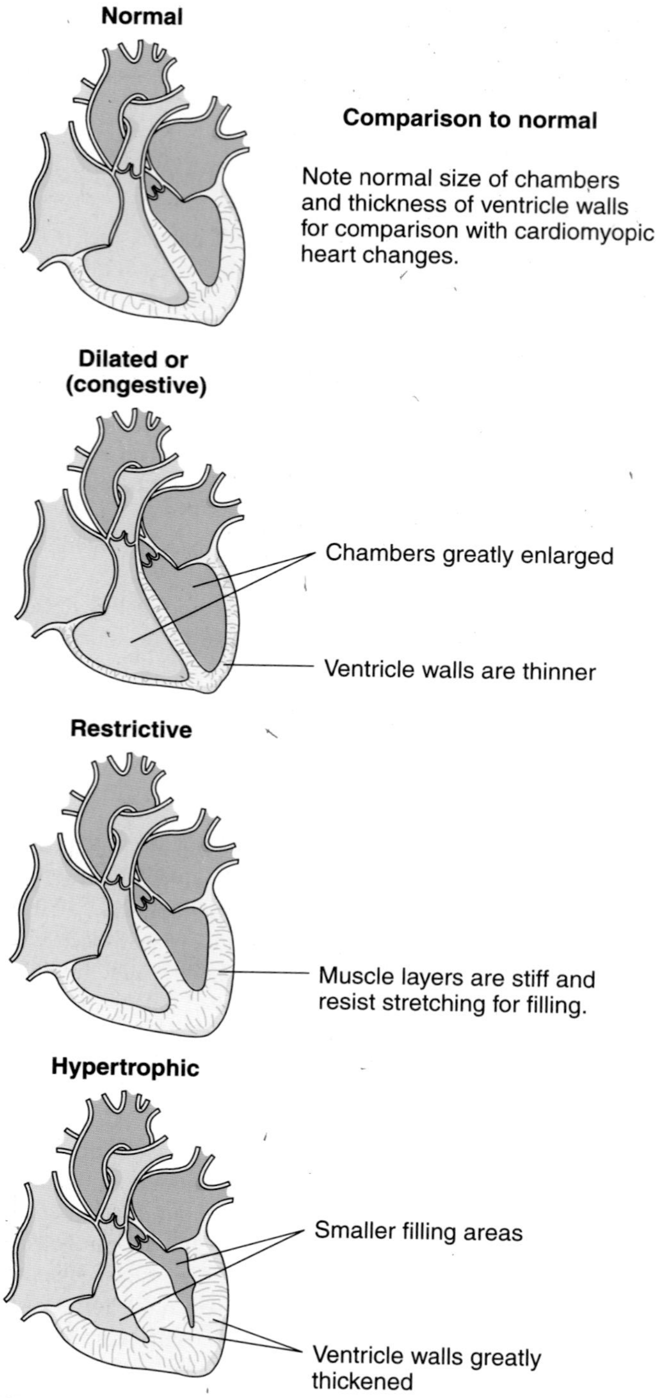

Normal

Comparison to normal

Note normal size of chambers and thickness of ventricle walls for comparison with cardiomyopic heart changes.

Dilated or (congestive)

Chambers greatly enlarged

Ventricle walls are thinner

Restrictive

Muscle layers are stiff and resist stretching for filling.

Hypertrophic

Smaller filling areas

Ventricle walls greatly thickened

Figure 17–4. Comparison of the normal heart structure with each type of the cardiomyopic heart structure.

young, athletic males. Restrictive cardiomyopathy is the rarest form of cardiomyopathy. It may be caused by infiltrative diseases such as amyloidosis that deposit the protein amyloid within the myocardial cells, which makes the muscle stiff.

Signs and Symptoms

Most clients show signs and symptoms of heart failure. Dyspnea on exertion, angina, syncope, and fatigue are other common manifestations of the myopathies that are related to reduced cardiac output.

Diagnostic Tests

Client signs and symptoms and ruling out other causes of heart failure are used to diagnose cardiomyopathy. **Cardiomegaly** can be seen with chest x-ray. Echocardiography is helpful in evaluating muscle thickness and chamber size. Changes related to enlarged chamber size, tachycardia, and dysrhythmias can be seen on the ECG. Cardiac catheterization may also be useful.

Medical Treatment

There is no cure for cardiomyopathy. Treatment is aimed at managing the heart failure. Anticoagulants may be given to prevent emboli formation from the stasis of blood in the ventricle. Antidysrhythmics are given for dysrhythmias. Treatment for any known underlying cause is also provided. For hypertrophic cardiomyopathy, surgical removal of some of the hypertrophied muscle, **myectomy,** can be done. For severe heart failure, a heart transplant may be the only hope for survival. A ventricular assist device may be used until a donor is found. Many clients die while waiting for a donated heart because donated organs are limited.

Complications

All types of cardiomyopathy can lead to cardiomegaly, which is the enlargement of the heart. Severe heart failure and death often result (Fig. 17–5).

Nursing Process

Assessment

A client history is obtained that includes signs and symptoms and assessment of family support systems, due to the chronic nature of the disease. A physical assessment is done, noting any signs or symptoms of heart failure. Vital signs are documented.

Nursing Diagnosis

The major nursing diagnoses for cardiomyopathy may include but are not limited to the following:

- Decreased cardiac output related to impaired myocardial function

---

cardiomegaly: kardia—heart + mega—large
myectomy: myo—muscle + ectomy—cutting out

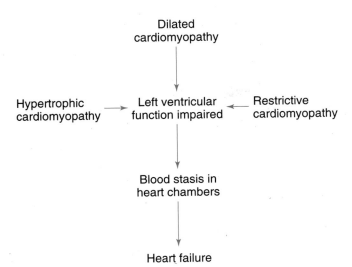

Figure 17–5. Cardiomyopathies leading to heart failure.

- Activity intolerance related to cardiac insufficiency
- Anxiety related to disease process
- Knowledge deficit related to lack of knowledge about cardiomyopathy and its treatment

Planning

The client and family should be included in planning care. The client's goals are to (1) maintain normal cardiac function, (2) maintain desired activities, (3) decrease anxiety, and (4) understand the disease and its treatment.

Nursing Interventions

Nursing care focuses on maintaining normal cardiac function, increasing activity tolerance, relieving anxiety, and educating the client about the disease and its treatment. These clients can be very ill. Symptoms are carefully monitored to detect changes and complications, such as emboli or dysrhythmias. Home health care is often utilized for these clients to maintain their functional ability and reduce hospitalizations.

Maintenance of normal cardiac function includes monitoring of vital signs and the presence of symptoms of heart failure. The presence of these symptoms is immediately reported to the physician.

Increasing activity tolerance includes planning rest periods, scheduling activities in small amounts, avoiding tiring activities, and providing smaller meals that require less energy to digest than large meals.

Reducing anxiety is important and can be accomplished by providing explanations for procedures, as well as educating the client about the disease and its treatment. Meth-

ods to incorporate necessary lifestyle changes such as avoiding fatigue and scheduling rest periods can be helpful. Emotional support is greatly needed by these clients because of the chronic nature of this disease.

An explanation of the disease and its treatment is provided to promote understanding of procedures and treatment. This may allow clients to feel in control of their lives by being able to make knowledgeable decisions about their health care. Lifestyle changes should be made with the least amount of disruption for the client.

Evaluation

The goal for decreased cardiac output is met if the client's vital signs are within normal range and no symptoms of heart failure are present.

The goal for the nursing diagnosis of activity intolerance is met if the client reports reduced fatigue. The ability to complete tasks and engage in desired activities also supports goal attainment.

The goal for the nursing diagnosis of anxiety is achieved if the client states that anxiety is reduced.

The goal for the nursing diagnosis of knowledge deficit is met if the client explains the disease to the nurse and states understanding of treatment.

Client and Significant Other Education

Clients need to be taught the importance of medication compliance to prevent heart failure. The client and family should have emergency telephone numbers readily available. Families should learn cardiopulmonary resuscitation (CPR). In terminal stages of the disease, the client and family should be informed about the availability of hospice care and be emotionally supported during the grieving process.

Venous Disorders

THROMBOPHLEBITIS

Thrombophlebitis is the formation of a clot and inflammation within a vein. Usually the clot forms first and then inflammation occurs. Thrombophlebitis is the most common disorder of veins, with the legs being most often affected. Any superficial or deep vein can be involved. Deep vein thrombosis (DVT) is the most serious because pulmonary emboli can result if the thrombosis detaches.

Pathophysiology

A venous thrombosis is made up of platelets, red blood cells, white blood cells, and fibrin. The platelets attach to a vein wall and then a tail forms as more blood cells and fibrin collect. As the tail grows it drifts in the blood flowing past it. The turbulence of the blood flow can cause parts of

---

thrombophlebitis: thromb—lump (clot) + phleb—vein + itis—inflammation

Table 17–4. **Predisposing Conditions for Thrombophlebitis**

Condition	Type	Examples
Venous Stasis	Reduction of blood flow	Shock, heart failure, myocardial infarction, atrial fibrillation
	Dilated veins	Vasodilators
	Decreased muscle contractions	Immobility, sitting for long periods as in traveling, fractured hip, paralysis, anesthesia, surgery, obesity, advanced age
	Faulty valves	Varicose veins, venous insufficiency
Venous Wall Injury		Venipuncture, venous cannulation at same site for > 48 h, venous catheterization, surgery, trauma, burns, fractures, dislocation, IV medications (potassium, chemotherapy drugs, antibiotics, IV hypertonic solutions), contrast agents, diabetes, cerebrovascular disease
Increased Coagulation of Blood		Anemia, malignancy, antithrombin III deficiency, oral contraceptives, estrogen therapy, smoking, discontinuance of anticoagulant therapy, dehydration, malnutrition, polycythemia, leukocytosis, thrombocytosis, sepsis, pregnancy

the drifting thrombus to break off and become emboli that travel to the lungs.

Etiology

Three factors are believed to be involved in the formation of a thrombosis: stasis of blood flow, damage to the lining of the vein wall, and increased blood coagulation. Clients at risk for any of these factors are at increased risk for developing a thrombus (Table 17–4). Two of these factors must be present for a thrombus to form.

Venous blood in the extremities flows normally when muscles contract and valves are intact to maintain blood flow in one direction. The client is predisposed to venous stasis when blood flow is reduced, veins are dilated, muscle contractions are decreased, or valves are faulty. Examples of conditions leading to venous stasis are listed in Table 17–4.

When the wall of a vein is damaged it provides a site for a thrombus to form. Many conditions can cause injury to the lining of a vein (Table 17–4). Intravenous (IV) therapy and venipuncture cause trauma to the vein, and IV catheters in place longer than 48 hours increase the risk of inflammation and thrombosis.

Increased coagulation of the blood promotes thrombus formation. Clients on oral anticoagulants that are abruptly stopped experience **hypercoagulability,** which is the increased ability of the blood to clot. Smoking, oral contraceptive use, and estrogen therapy also increase blood coagulation.

Hematological disorders can also lead to altered blood coagulation and increased risk of thrombus formation.

Prevention

Identification of risk factors is important to allow the use of preventive interventions for thrombosis. Clients and families should be educated in preventive techniques to reduce risk. Since the elderly are at increased risk for thrombosis formation, a family member should be instructed along with the elderly person in techniques that may be difficult for the elderly person to perform. Dehydration, which is common in the elderly population, should be avoided to reduce thrombus risk.

Immobility

People with sedentary jobs that require long periods of sitting or standing or traveling long distances should change positions, do knee and ankle flexion exercises, or walk at regular intervals to prevent stasis of blood. Clients on bed rest should have legs elevated above the level of the heart if possible to prevent pooling of blood. Active or passive range of motion exercises of the extremities should be done regularly postoperatively and for those on bed rest to increase blood flow. Postoperative early ambulation is a major preventative technique for thrombosis. Clients' pain should be controlled to facilitate their ability to participate in early ambulation. Deep breathing aids in improving blood flow in the large thoracic veins. Smoking should be avoided because nicotine vasoconstricts and contributes to hypercoagulability.

Prophylactic Antiembolism Devices

Clients with peripheral vascular disease, on bed rest, or following surgery or trauma may use antiembolism devices to improve blood flow. Knee- or thigh-length elastic stockings apply pressure to the leg. They must be applied correctly to avoid a tourniquet effect. Older clients with decreased manual dexterity may need assistance. The stockings are removed for 20 minutes twice a day and the skin inspected for irritation. Intermittent pneumatic com-

---

hypercoagulability: hyper—excessive + coagulare—to congeal

pression (IPC) devices use plastic inflatable stockings that are filled intermittently with air via a motor set to move fluid by simulating the contraction of the leg muscles. They may be used in combination with elastic stockings. Research that compares the various preventive measures for DVT and rates of DVT in surgical clients has shown that the lowest incidence of DVT occurs with elastic stockings and IPC devices used together.

Prophylactic Medication

Subcutaneous heparin may be used postoperatively to prevent thrombosis. A common prophylactic dose of heparin is 5000 units subcutaneously every 8 to 12 hours. Clotting values are usually not altered by this prophylactic dose of heparin. Oral anticoagulants such as warfarin (Coumadin) can be used in the high-risk client to decrease thrombosis. The prothrombin time (PT) and international normalized ratio (INR) values are monitored when warfarin (Coumadin) is given.

Intravenous Therapy

Monitoring of venous IV sites should be performed according to institutional policy time frames to detect signs of thrombophlebitis. Venous cannula sites should be changed regularly according to institutional guidelines to prevent thrombus formation.

Signs and Symptoms

Up to 50 percent of clients have no symptoms of thrombophlebitis in the legs. For other clients, the symptoms will vary according to the size and location of the thrombus. If adequate collateral circulation is present near the involved area, symptoms may be reduced. For some clients, a pulmonary embolus is the only evidence of a DVT.

Superficial Veins

Thrombophlebitis in a superficial vein may produce redness, warmth, swelling, and tenderness in the area around the site of the thrombus. The vein will feel like a firm cord, which is referred to as induration. The saphenous vein is the most commonly affected vein in the leg. Varicosity of the vein is usually the cause. In the arm, IV therapy is the most common cause.

Deep Veins

In a deep vein thrombosis of the leg, swelling, edema, pain, warmth, venous distention, and tenderness with palpation of the calf may be present in the affected leg. Obstruction of blood flow from the leg causes edema and varies with the location of the thrombosis. An elevated temperature may also be present. Pain in the calf with sharp dorsiflexion of the foot, a classic sign known as a positive Homans' sign, is present in less than 50 percent of those with thrombophlebitis and is not specific to DVT (Fig. 17–6). Once a

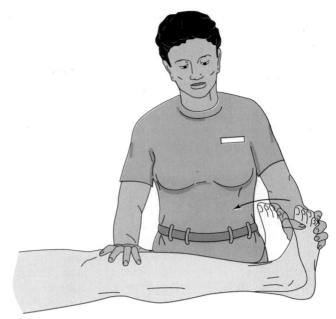

Figure 17–6. Assessment of Homans' sign.

DVT is positively diagnosed, it is important to avoid performing the Homans' sign because it may cause the clot to become dislodged. Cyanosis and edema may occur if the large veins such as the vena cava are involved.

Complications

The most serious complication of deep vein thrombophlebitis is pulmonary embolism, which is a life-threatening emergency. Another complication, chronic venous insufficiency, results from damage to the valves in the vein causing venous stasis. Signs and symptoms from venous insufficiency that may appear years after a thrombosis include edema, pain, brownish discoloration and ulceration of the medial ankle, venous distention, and dependent cyanosis of the leg. This condition can be difficult to treat.

Diagnostic Tests

Coagulation tests, including PT, INR, PTT, platelet count, and bleeding time, will be done to obtain baseline levels for diagnosis and before anticoagulant therapy is started. Noninvasive tests that are used to diagnose thrombophlebitis include venous doppler ultrasonography, duplex venous scanning, impedance plethysmography, and magnetic resonance imaging (MRI). Duplex scanning produces the best information for diagnosis. Invasive techniques using contrast media are venography and [251]I-labeled fibrinogen, a newer test that is limited in detection and costly. To detect pulmonary emboli, a lung scan or pulmonary arteriogram is used.

Medical and Surgical Treatment

The goals of treatment are to prevent thrombus enlargement, pulmonary emboli, and further thrombus development and relieve pain. Superficial thrombophlebitis is treated with bed rest, extremity elevation, warm, moist heat, analgesics, and NSAIDs. Deep vein thrombophlebitis management includes bed rest with extremity elevation above the level of the heart for 5 to 7 days, warm, moist heat, an elastic stocking usually only on the unaffected leg initially, and anticoagulants. A continuous heparin IV infusion is started for up to 10 days to prevent further enlargement of the thrombus and development of new ones; it does not dissolve the clot. An oral anticoagulant is begun 4 to 7 days before the heparin is stopped. This allows the blood level of the oral anticoagulant to move into the therapeutic range before the heparin is discontinued. The oral anticoagulant is continued for several months. In some cases, thrombolytic therapy may be used to dissolve the clot, but the risk of bleeding is much higher than with heparin.

Surgical treatment is used to prevent pulmonary emboli or chronic venous insufficiency when anticoagulant therapy cannot be used or the risk of pulmonary emboli is great. Venous thrombectomy removes the clot through a venous incision. In some cases, a vena cava filter can be placed into the inferior vena cava through the femoral or right internal jugular vein (Fig. 17–7). Once in place, it is opened and attaches to the vein wall. The filter prevents clots from traveling to the lungs without hindering blood flow.

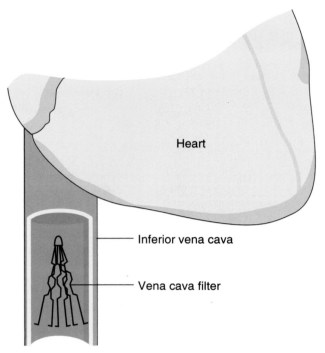

Figure 17–7. Vena cava filter placed in the inferior vena cava to prevent emboli from reaching the lungs.

HOME HEALTH HINTS

- When home health clients complain of dyspnea, the nurse asks them at what point in the activity it occurs. For example, is it when they are sitting, or does it wake them up in the middle of the night? If it is when ambulating, it is important to document the number of feet walked when they become dyspneic. This may be hard for them to do, so the nurse asks if it happens while crossing the room or when walking to the bathroom, kitchen, down the hall, or end of the driveway. The nurse can then estimate the distance and report it to the physician.

- Home health nurses can assist clients to develop energy-conserving techniques by being observant of their lifestyle. For instance, notice the room and chair that they spend most of the day in. Television trays and baskets can be used to hold items they may need or want, such as water pitcher and glass, TV remote, reading material, paper and pen, mail, medicines, telephone and phone book, snacks, washcloth, or tissues. Answering the door should be done by the caregiver. When the client is alone, a note can be placed on the door with instructions; however, the instructions should not convey that the client is alone.

- Other techniques to conserve energy are putting a carrying pouch on the front bar of a walker to carry items such as a portable phone or tissues and if the house has stairs, putting a chair at the top and bottom of the stairs so the client can rest.

- When a client with venous circulation problems is sitting in a recliner with the leg rest up, the nurse notes whether pressure is being applied on the popliteal area or calf muscle. The angle of the recliner and the client's height affect the position of the pressure. A small, flat pillow is placed underneath the knees and lower legs to open the angle and relieve the pressure. A recliner fits everyone differently.

- When the nurse auscultates the chest, the diaphragm is placed firmly on the chest. This can avoid the sound caused by movement of the chest hair or skin, which could sound like a "rub." The nurse asks if the TV or radio can be turned down if it is difficult to hear.

- When performing a venipuncture for a prothrombin time in the home, the nurse puts the labeled tube on ice and transports it to the laboratory within 2 hours.

NURSING CARE PLAN BOX 17–2
FOR THE CLIENT WITH THROMBOPHLEBITIS

Pain related to inflammation of vein

Client Outcome
Reports satisfactory pain relief.

Evaluation of Outcome
Does client report satisfactory pain relief?

Interventions	Rationale	Evaluation
Assess pain using rating scale such as 1–10.	Self-report is the most reliable indicator of pain.	Does client report pain using scale?
Provide analgesics and NSAIDS as ordered.	Pain is reduced when inflammation is decreased.	Is client's rating of pain lower after medication?
Apply warm, moist soaks.	Heat relieves pain and vasodilates, which increases circulation to reduce swelling. Moist heat penetrates more deeply.	Does client report increased comfort with warm, moist soaks? Is swelling reduced?
Maintain bedrest with leg elevation above heart level.	Elevation decreases swelling, which reduces pain.	Is swelling reduced?

Impaired skin integrity related to venous stasis

Client Outcome
Skin remains intact without edema.

Evaluation of Outcome
Does client's skin remain intact? Is edema present?

Interventions	Rationale	Evaluation
Assess skin for edema, skin color changes, and ulcers. Measure extremeties.	Assessment will detect signs of skin integrity impairment and extremity swelling.	Are skin changes seen? Do daily measurements show a change in swelling?
Elevate legs.	Elevation decreases swelling.	Is swelling reduced?
Fit and apply elastic stockings after edema reduced as ordered.	Elastic stockings are fitted after edema is reduced to avoid constriction. They increase venous blood flow to reduce swelling.	Is swelling reduced?
Teach client to avoid crossing legs or wearing constricting clothes.	Crossing legs and constrictive clothes impair venous return.	Does client state understanding if teaching?

Anxiety related to disease process and uncertain prognosis

Client Outcome
States anxiety is reduced.

Evaluation of Outcome
Does client report anxiety reduced?

Interventions	Rationale	Evaluation
Provide explanations for procedures, the disease, and its treatment.	Knowledge allows a feeling of control and reduces anxiety.	Does client state less anxiety?

continued

NURSING CARE PLAN BOX 17–2 *(continued)*

Knowledge deficit related to lack of knowledge about disorder and treatment

Client Outcomes
Verbalizes knowledge of disorder and willingness to comply with therapeutic regimen.

Evaluation of Outcomes
Does client accurately explain therapeutic regimen? Does client express willingness to follow therapeutic regimen?

Interventions	Rationale	Evaluation
Explain condition, symptoms, complications. Explain medications, therapies ordered, monthly lab test monitoring, and need for medic-alert identification. Teach client not to massage extremity.	Client must have basic knowledge to comply with therapy. Compliance and safe use of medications is promoted with an adequate knowledge base. Massage can dislodge an embolus.	Is client able to verbalize knowledge taught? Can client explain medications, therapies, lab tests, and purpose of medic-alert identification? Does client avoid massaging extremity?

Impaired gas exchange related to emboli

Client Outcomes
Vital signs WNL without dyspnea, blood-tinged sputum, chest pain, or changes in level of consciousness.

Evaluation of Outcomes
Are client's vital signs WNL with no dyspnea, level of consciousness normal, no chest pain, or blood-tinged sputum?

Interventions	Rationale	Evaluation
Assess breath sounds and vital signs. Report changes. Assess confusion and altered level of consciousness. Maintain bedrest.	Pulmonary emboli decrease breath sounds and increase vital signs. Decreased oxygenation causes these changes. Bedrest prevents dislodging of clot.	Are client's breath sounds and vital signs WNL? Is client alert and oriented? Does client maintain bedrest?

Nursing Process

Assessment

A client history is obtained that includes recent IV therapy or contrast dyes, surgery, extremity trauma, childbirth, bed rest, recent long trip, cardiac disease, atrial fibrillation, recent infections, and current medications. A physical assessment is done. Pain, tenderness, positive Homans' sign, redness, warmth, swelling, edema, and a firm cordlike vein in the affected extremity are noted. Daily measurements are taken of bilateral thighs and calves and recorded to document swelling. Vital signs are documented and fever is reported. Coagulation tests are monitored.

Nursing Diagnosis

The major nursing diagnoses for thrombophlebitis may include but are not limited to the following:

- Pain related to inflammation of vein
- Impaired skin integrity related to venous stasis
- Anxiety related to disease process and uncertain prognosis
- Knowledge deficit related to lack of knowledge about disorder and treatment
- Risk for impaired gas exchange related to pulmonary emboli

Planning

The client's goals are to (1) relieve pain, (2) maintain skin integrity, (3) decrease anxiety, (4) understand the disease and its treatment, and (5) maintain gas exchange within normal limits.

Nursing Interventions

See Nursing Care Plan Box 17–2 for specific nursing interventions. Pain is relieved by giving analgesics and NSAIDs as ordered. Warm, moist soaks aid in reducing pain.

Skin assessment of the extremities is done to note edema, skin color changes, and ulcers. Legs are elevated to

kings are fitted and applied

reduce edema. Elast̶
when edema is redu̶ortant and can be accomplished
by providing ̶s for procedures and educating
the client ab̶e and its treatment.
Teachi̶bout the disease and treatment is
import̶ice with treatment to prevent com-
plica̶rmal gas exchange includes monitor-
elusive ̶symptoms of pulmonary emboli. The
car̶, tachycardia, tachypnea, blood-tinged
̶, or changes in level of consciousness
eported to the physician.

̶he nursing diagnosis of pain is met if the
̶s satisfactory pain relief. Satisfactory pain re-
̶measured by comparing the client's stated level of
̶n on a rating scale of 1 to 10 with the client's predetermined goal for acceptable level of pain.

The goal for the nursing diagnosis of impaired skin integrity is met if the client's skin remains intact.

The goal for the nursing diagnosis of anxiety is achieved
if the client states that anxiety is reduced.

The goal for the nursing diagnosis of knowledge deficit
is met if the client explains the disease to the nurse and
states understanding of treatment.

The goal for the nursing diagnosis of risk for impaired
gas exchange is met if the client's vital signs are within
normal range and no symptoms of pulmonary emboli are
present.

Review Questions

1. Which one of the following does the nurse understand causes rheumatic fever?
   a. Viral infection
   b. Fungal infection
   c. Bacterial infection
   d. Hypersensitivity response

2. Rheumatic fever can be prevented by treating strepto-coccal infections with which one of the following?
   a. Penicillin
   b. Prednisone
   c. Cortisone
   d. Cyclosporine

3. For clients recovering from infective endocarditis, discharge teaching to prevent recurrence should include which one of the following?
   a. Proper use of isolation techniques
   b. Keeping vaccinations up to date
   c. Need to obtain annual flu injection
   d. Need for antibiotics before invasive procedures

4. Which one of the following signs and symptoms would indicate to the nurse the presence of a deep vein thrombosis in the leg?
   a. Calf swelling
   b. Negative Homans' sign
   c. Crackles
   d. Jugular vein distention

5. Which one of the following is the *most* severe complication of a deep vein thrombosis?
   a. Coronary artery disease
   b. Pulmonary embolism
   c. Pericardial friction rub
   d. Pulmonary edema

6. Which one of the following laboratory tests is monitored for clients taking oral anticoagulants for infective endocarditis or thrombophlebitis?
   a. Partial thromboplastin time (PTT)
   b. Prothrombin time (PT)
   c. Plasma fibrinogen
   d. Thrombin clotting time

7. Which one of the following would be an outcome for the nursing diagnosis of activity intolerance for the client with cardiomyopathy?
   a. Normal cardiac function is maintained.
   b. Client states that pain is relieved.
   c. Client is able to participate in desired activities.
   d. Anxiety is decreased.

ANSWERS TO CRITICAL THINKING

CRITICAL THINKING: Mrs. Jones

1. A heart murmur may be heard with endocarditis because damage to the heart valves occurs.
2. Splinter hemorrhages appear as long black or red-brown lines or streaks in the nails.
3. Petechiae indicate that tiny pieces of a lesion on the endocardium or valves have broken off and become microemboli.
4. Antibiotics IV.
5. Removing blankets to decrease fever results in chills and shivering, which further increases body temperature from the heat generated by muscular activity during shivering. Therefore Mrs. Jones should be kept covered to prevent chills.
6. For left-sided heart failure, crackles, wheezes, cough, or dyspnea might be seen. In right-sided heart failure, peripheral edema or jugular vein distention could be present.
7. Prophylactic antibiotics are needed to prevent another episode of infective endocarditis that can result from bacteria entering the circulation during the invasive procedure, attaching to areas of the endocardium damaged from the current infection, and growing.

8. To prevent emboli, which can be a complication of infective endocarditis.
9. Anticoagulant teaching should include the purpose of the medication; the need for monthly coagulation studies; the need to wear Medic Alert identification; contacting the physician before taking other medications that affect the action of warfarin (Coumadin), especially vitamins and aspirin; avoiding injury that will cause bleeding; reporting signs of bleeding, such as faintness, headaches, bruises, rash, red or black stool, or red or brown urine, to physician; and limiting foods high in vitamin K, such as green leafy vegetables.

REFERENCE

1. Dajani, A, et al: Prevention of bacterial endocarditis: Recommendations by the American Heart Association. JAMA 277(22):1794, 1997.

BIBLIOGRAPHY

Ackley, BJ, and Ladwig, GB: Nursing Di[...] Louis, 1997.

Ahrens, G: Managing heart failure: A bluep[...] 25(12):26, 1995.

Bresler, MJ: Acute pericarditis and myocarditis. E[...]

Bright, LD, and Georgi, S: How to protect your pa[...] Nurs 94(12):28, 1994.

Durack, D: Prevention of infective endocarditis. N Eng[...] 1995.

Jaffe, MS, and McVan, BF: Davis's Laboratory and Diagno[...] book. FA Davis, Philadelphia, 1997.

Kaplan, EL: Acute rheumatic fever. In Schlant, RE, and Ale[...] (eds): Hurst's the Heart, ed 8. McGraw-Hill, New York, 199[...]

Majoros, K, and Moccia, J: Pulmonary embolism: Targeting a[...] enemy. Nursing 26(4):26, 1996.

Spirito, P, et al: Medical progress: The management of hypertrophi[...] diomyopathy. N Engl J Med 336(11):775, 1997.

Nursing Care of Clients with Occlusive Cardiovascular Disorders

Elizabeth Chapman

Learning Objectives

Upon completion of this chapter, the student will be able to:

1. Define arteriosclerosis and atherosclerosis.
2. Identify causes of coronary artery disease.
3. List specific data to include in the nursing data collection for a client with coronary artery disease.
4. Identify signs and symptoms of angina pectoris.
5. List medications used to treat coronary artery disease and angina pectoris.
6. Explain nursing care for clients with coronary artery disease.
7. Identify client education for the client with coronary artery disease.
8. Describe the signs and symptoms of a myocardial infarction.
9. Describe the treatment options for myocardial infarction.
10. Explain nursing care for clients with a myocardial infarction.
11. Identify two peripheral vascular disorders.
12. Explain nursing care for clients with peripheral vascular disorders.

Key Words

aneurysm (**AN**-yur-izm)

angina pectoris (an-**JIGH**-nah **PEK**-tuh-riss)

arteriosclerosis (ar-TIR-ee-oh-skle-**ROH**-sis)

atherosclerosis (ATH-er-oh-skle-**ROH**-sis)

atherosclerosis obliterans (ATH-er-oh-skle-**ROH**-sis uh-**BLI**-ter-anz)

collateral circulation (koh-**LA**-ter-al SIR-kew-**LAY**-shun)

coronary artery disease (KOR-uh-na-ree **AR**-tuh-ree di-**ZEEZ**)

embolism (**EM**-buh-lizm)

high-density lipoprotein (HIGH **DEN**-si-tee LIP-oh-**PROH**-teen)

hyperlipidemia (HIGH-per-LIP-i-**DEE**-mee-ah)

intermittent claudication (IN-ter-**MIT**-ent KLAW-di-**KAY**-shun)

lymphangitis (lim-FAN-je-**EYE**-tis)

myocardial infarction (MY-oh-**KAR**-dee-yuhl in-**FARK**-shun)

peripheral arterial disease (puh-**RIFF**-uh-ruhl ar-**TIR**-ee-uhl di-**ZEEZ**)

Raynaud's disease (ra-**NOHZ** di-**ZEEZ**)

thrombosis (throm-**BOH**-sis)

varicose veins (**VAR**-i-kohn VAINS)

venous stasis ulcers (**VEE**-nus **STAY**-sis **UL**-sers)

Occlusive Cardiovascular Disorders

Cardiovascular disorders are the leading cause of disability and death in the United States. Diseases of the heart and peripheral vessels can affect the ability of the individual to perform tasks of everyday living. The loss of person-hours and cost to businesses are high. Long-term disability can place a burden on families and businesses and can cause high insurance costs. Many factors leading to cardiovascular diseases can be controlled or modified. Education is paramount to preventing and treating these diseases.

Arteriosclerosis and Atherosclerosis

Arteriosclerosis is the most common disease of the arteries. The lining of the walls of the arteries and arterioles becomes thick and hardened, which is commonly referred to as hardening of the arteries. **Atherosclerosis,** a type of arteriosclerosis, is a formation of plaque within the arterial wall. Arteriosclerosis and atherosclerosis are diseases that progress over a long period of time before symptoms are seen. Atherosclerosis usually affects the main arteries in varying degrees. Arteriosclerosis and atherosclerosis have different pathologies but usually occur together.

PATHOPHYSIOLOGY

The exact progression for arteriosclerosis and atherosclerosis development is unknown. It is thought that with atherosclerosis a fatty streak appears on the lining of the artery. This buildup of fatty deposits is known as plaque. Plaque has irregular, jagged edges that allow blood cells and other material to adhere to the wall of the artery. Over time, this buildup becomes calcified and hardened (arteriosclerotic), which damages the vessel. Stenosis, which is a loss of elasticity and compliance, results in a narrowing of the vessel. Stenosis of the vessel leads to partial or total occlusion of the artery. When this occurs, the area distal to the occlusion can become ischemic from a lack of blood flow.

CAUSES

There are many theories as to the causes of these disorders. Genetics is believed to play a role in the development of arteriosclerosis and atherosclerosis. A familial history of these disorders shows a predisposition to **hyperlipidemia,** which is an increase in blood lipids. This leads to formation of fatty plaques within the vessels, even in the presence of normal blood cholesterol levels. Diabetes mellitus is also seen as a common cause of atherosclerosis. Hyper-glycemia is suspected as the cause of arterial damage and the development of peripheral vascular disorders. Other factors contributing to these disorders are hypertension, obesity, a sedentary lifestyle, smoking, and stress. Many of these disorders directly affect blood vessels and cause damage, leading to arteriosclerosis or atherosclerosis.

SIGNS AND SYMPTOMS

Clients with atherosclerosis may not have symptoms of it until later in its development. The nurse checks for signs of decreased blood supply and oxygen to the heart and extremities. This can be evidenced by chest pain or seen as pallor in nailbeds, reddish-purple color to lower extremities, thickened nails, dry skin, or loss of hair on the extremities. Peripheral pulses may be diminished or absent. Skin temperature in the extremities is cooler, and there is prolonged capillary refill, greater than 3 seconds.

DIAGNOSTIC TESTS

Cholesterol and triglycerides are often elevated in clients with atherosclerosis. They can also indicate a risk factor for further development of atherosclerosis. Radiological studies of the arteries can be performed. These procedures require injecting a dye to visualize where the vessels are narrowed or occluded. Examples of these studies are arterial angiography, computed tomography (CT) scan, and magnetic resonance imaging (MRI).

TREATMENT

Cholesterol screening and frequent checkups for clients who are at risk can be helpful in arresting the progress of these disorders. Changes in diet and exercise, as well as a decrease or cessation of smoking, may also aid in the treatment of these disorders, along with a medication regimen prescribed by the physician.

Diet

Saturated fats are the primary cause of increased cholesterol levels, and they promote arteriosclerosis and atherosclerosis. Because the formation of plaque within arteries is primarily caused by fatty deposits, an adherence to a low-fat diet is recommended. There are numerous studies on the types and amounts of fats that should be ingested. The recommendations are to limit fat intake to no more than 30 percent of the total caloric intake. The American Heart Association has complete guidelines and diets for decreasing fat and cholesterol intake. (See Nutrition Notes Box 18–1.)

---

hyperlipidemia: hyper—above + lipos—fat + emia—blood

NUTRITION NOTES BOX 18-1

Nutrition in Occlusive Cardiovascular Diseases

ELEVATED SERUM CHOLESTEROL. Two-thirds of the body's cholesterol is produced by the liver and intestines, but diet also influences serum cholesterol levels. Only foods of animal origin contain cholesterol.

Step 1 diet. The step 1 diet is strict interpretation of the food pyramid. A client is often instructed in the physician's office by the nurse or medical assistant. Daily portion control is critical to the success of this diet: 6 oz of lean meat, fish, shellfish, or poultry; 4 to 6 servings of polyunsaturated or monounsaturated fats; 3 servings of skimmed or 1% milk; 4 to 7 servings of low-fat breads; 3 servings of fruit; and 4 servings of vegetables. A reduction of total and LDL cholesterol of 10 to 20 percent is expected.[1,2]

Step 2 diet. After possibly a 3-month trial, the client's cholesterol is reevaluated. If further instruction or restriction is needed, a dietitian's referral is commonly made.

HYPERLIPOPROTEINEMIAS. Because the six types of hyperlipoproteinemias have different features, the client should receive individualized instruction from a dietitian. So that nurses appreciate some of the variations, the following summary capsules are offered.

Type 1. Food sources of triglycerides are restricted: 20 to 30 g of fat and 3 to 4 oz of lean meat per day.

Type 2A. Less than 200 mg of cholesterol; polyunsaturated and monounsaturated fats outnumber saturated 1.5 or 2 to 1.

Type 2B. Same as type 2A except alcohol and simple sugar are restricted; 40 percent of calories from carbohydrate.

Type 3. From 35 to 40 percent of calories from carbohydrate; reduction of dietary cholesterol if weight loss does not lower serum cholesterol.

Types 4 and 5. From 35 to 40 percent of calories from carbohydrate; sugar and alcohol limited.

Smoking

Smoking contributes to a loss of **high-density lipoprotein** (HDL). These proteins are considered the best cholesterol to have present in the body to decrease the risk of cardiovascular disorders. The rate of progressive damage to blood vessels is increased with smoking. Smoking also causes vasoconstriction, which leads to **angina pectoris** and cardiac dysrhythmias. Education of the dangers of smoking should be presented to clients. The client must be willing and able to make the commitment to stop smoking. The American Cancer Society has many programs to help clients quit smoking.

Exercise

An exercise program has been shown to decrease the risk of developing atherosclerosis by increasing levels of high-density lipoproteins ("good cholesterol"). A planned program of exercise can lead to the development of **collateral circulation.** This collateral circulation allows blood to flow around occluded sites. Before beginning an exercise program, a physician should be consulted by the client.

Medications

Drug therapy is directed at the cause of arteriosclerosis or atherosclerosis. Lowering cholesterol levels is the major treatment for atherosclerosis. When dietary control is not effective, medication is used to help lower cholesterol.

Antilipemic drugs include cholestyramine (Questran), which causes loss of bile acids and prevents cholesterol use, thus lowering cholesterol levels. Gemfibrozil (Lopid), another antilipemic, inhibits synthesis of very low density lipoprotein (VLD) and low-density lipoprotein (LDL), which are responsible for cholesterol development. Nicotinic acid (niacin) is a water-soluble vitamin that prevents conversion of fats into very low density lipoprotein ("bad cholesterol"), and when given in large doses it decreases serum cholesterol levels. Another cholesterol-lowering agent is lovastatin (Mevacor), which reduces cholesterol synthesis. Nursing implications for these drugs are to instruct clients to take them with meals to decrease gastric upset and increase their fluid intake to help flush out their system. With these drugs it can take 4 to 6 weeks before cholesterol levels respond.

Coronary Artery Disease

Coronary artery disease (CAD) is a term applied to obstructed blood flow in the coronary arteries. The primary cause for the development of this disease is atherosclerosis. It is believed to begin early in life and must be recognized, especially in the presence of known risk factors. There is an accumulation of fatty deposits and minerals in the coronary arteries called plaque, which leads to stenosis and eventually occlusion. Over time, the arteries become unable to dilate, which causes a decrease in blood flow to the myocardium. This reduces the amount of oxygen supplied to the myocardium via the coronary arteries so that myocardial oxygen demands are not met. This results in

---

angina pectoris: angina—to choke + pectora—chest

ischemia, which can lead to chest pain. If the ischemia becomes severe and prolonged, irreversible damage from a **myocardial infarction,** a heart attack, can occur.

PATHOPHYSIOLOGY AND ETIOLOGY

As discussed in atherosclerosis and arteriosclerosis, the blockage of arteries causes decreased blood supply distal to the narrowed or blocked area. This helps initiate the formation of collateral circulation, which is the growth of smaller blood vessels surrounding the area of decreased blood supply to supply the area around the occluded vessel with blood. This collateral circulation allows the myocardium to receive the nutrients it needs, and it can be effective for a long period of time before symptoms appear from diminished blood flow. The symptoms usually become apparent when increased activity or workload places an increased demand on the heart. The symptoms of CAD then become apparent. Increased activity causes complaints of chest pain. The pain associated with CAD occurs from a lack of oxygen to the myocardium as a result of the CAD and is referred to as angina pectoris.

RISK FACTORS

Risk factors can be broken down into two components: those that cannot be changed and those that can be changed.

Risk Factors That Cannot be Changed

Risk factors that cannot be changed include heredity, age, gender, and race. Studies have shown that more men are affected by CAD after age 35, with an increased incidence after age 50. Women are not as affected by CAD before menopause but show about equal levels of occurrence after menopause. Heredity increases the chance of acquiring CAD, and African-Americans have higher incidence of hypertension, which contributes to the development of atherosclerosis.

Risk Factors That Can Be Changed

Cigarette Smoking

Cigarette smoking is a major risk factor in the cause of CAD. Smoking is responsible for more deaths from CAD than from lung cancer or pulmonary disease.[3] It is not known exactly how smoking causes CAD. It is believed that smoking increases myocardial oxygen demand. It interferes with oxygen supply to the heart due to vasoconstriction. Smoking has also been linked to decreasing levels of HDL, the good cholesterol.

Hypertension

High blood pressure affects some 60 million people in the United States, including children. The definition of hyper-

tension is a systolic blood pressure greater than 140 mm Hg or a diastolic blood pressure greater than 90 mm Hg on more than two measurements done at different times. Individuals with hypertension show increased risk of cardiovascular disease and death. Lifelong control of hypertension is important in lowering the risk of CAD, strokes, and renal failure.

Elevated Serum Cholesterol

Increased serum cholesterol leads to the development of CAD. It is recommended that cholesterol levels be less than 200 mg/dL. Serum levels greater than 250 mg/dL can double the risk of developing CAD. The body produces two thirds of its cholesterol primarily in the liver and intestine.[4] The body's additional cholesterol is ingested through dietary intake. The American Heart Association recommends decreasing fat content and substituting polyunsaturated fats for saturated fats. Polyunsaturated fats include corn, cottonseed, soy, safflower oils, and margarine. Saturated fats are coconut oil, butterfat, and animal fat. Exercise, low-fat diet, and low-cholesterol diet help diminish the risk of developing CAD.

Diabetes Mellitus

Diabetes is associated with a higher incidence of high blood pressure, obesity, and high blood lipids. As a result, this disease contributes to the development of atherosclerosis, the primary cause of CAD. Controlling diabetes is important in lowering the risk of CAD.

Contributing Factors

Obesity, stress, and a sedentary lifestyle are contributing factors that may also increase the risk of CAD. Obesity increases the workload on the heart. Clients who are obese are more prone to hypertension, diabetes, glucose intolerance, and hyperlipidemia, all of which have been shown to contribute to the development of CAD. A sedentary lifestyle contributes to obesity, hypertension, and increased cholesterol. Stress causes increased blood pressure and an increased workload on the heart. Altering these factors may help protect the client from developing cardiovascular disease.

If coronary artery disease is not prevented or treated early it can progress to more serious cardiac disorders. These include angina, stable or unstable; myocardial infarction; congestive heart failure; cardiac dysrhythmias; and even sudden death.

NURSING PROCESS

Caring for a client with CAD includes monitoring blood pressure, heart rate, reports of chest pain, and any associated symptoms that may point to the presence of complications from CAD. The care of the client is directed at teaching and working with the client to change or modify risk factors that are present.

Hypertension and chest pain are common symptoms that may be present in a client with CAD. A history of hypertension is also a contributing factor to the development of CAD. Thus monitoring and controlling the client's blood pressure is an important part of the care of the client with CAD.

MEDICAL MANAGEMENT

Prevention is the goal for clients with CAD. Educating clients on dietary changes, cessation of smoking, controlling hypertension, and diabetes can decrease their risk of CAD. Dietary changes are made to reduce saturated fats to less than 10 percent of daily food intake. Cholesterol intake on the step 1 diet contains less than 300 mg per day and less than 200 mg per day on the step 2 diet. Medication may be given to reduce cholesterol levels. Anticoagulants are used to prevent the formation of a thrombus.

SURGICAL MANAGEMENT

Percutaneous Transluminal Coronary Angioplasty

Percutaneous transluminal coronary angioplasty (PTCA) is an invasive procedure that helps reduce symptoms of CAD. A catheter is inserted via the femoral or brachial artery and is advanced into the heart. Once the blocked artery is entered, the balloon on the catheter is inflated. This procedure causes plaque to be compressed against the wall of the artery, thus widening the opening of the artery. This helps ease the symptoms of CAD but does not stop the underlying progression of atherosclerosis development. Reocclusion of the artery can, and usually does, occur within 6 months. The number of times a PTCA can be performed on a client is determined by the facility and the physician performing the procedure.

Coronary Artery Bypass Graft

Coronary artery bypass graft (CABG) surgery involves bypassing one or more blocked coronary arteries. Clients who have severe CAD or have had myocardial infarctions may be candidates for a CABG. Established guidelines for clients who are candidates for this surgery are dependent on the facility in which the surgery is to be performed. Clients will usually have had a cardiac catheterization that identifies which coronary arteries are blocked. Once the area of blockage is determined the client is prepared for surgery. The nurse must be knowledgeable in the anatomy of the heart to assist the client in understanding the purpose of the surgery. Refer to Chapter 22 for further discussion of this surgical procedure.

Angina Pectoris

Angina is a symptom of ischemia and is seen with CAD. Atherosclerosis contributes to the development of CAD

and narrowing of the arteries. The decreased blood supply to areas distal to the narrowing produces ischemia and causes the classic symptom of CAD, chest pain.

LEARNING TIP

Angina is not a disease. It is a symptom of ischemia that results from a lack of blood.

PATHOPHYSIOLOGY

Any increased workload placed on the heart as in exercise or activities requires an increased demand for oxygen. Normally, when the heart needs a greater supply of blood, the coronary arteries dilate. However, the narrowed vessels of CAD are unable to dilate and supply the myocardium with extra blood and oxygen. This inadequate blood supply for the increased demand causes myocardial ischemia. When a client is at rest the supply of blood from narrowed vessels may be enough, but the increased workload deprives the myocardium of extra blood and therefore oxygen, and ischemia ensues. Chest pain results from the ischemia but usually lasts only for a few minutes, especially if the activity is stopped. If adequate blood supply to the myocardium is restored with rest, no myocardial damage usually occurs.

SIGNS AND SYMPTOMS

The pain of angina manifests itself in several ways. The pain can be described as a heaviness, tightness, or viselike or crushing pain in the center of the chest. The pain can radiate down one or both arms, with the left arm being more common, into the shoulder, neck, jaw, or back. Clients may describe a heaviness in their arms or a feeling of impending doom. During the episode of pain, the client may be pale, diaphoretic, or dyspneic. The pain is usually brought on by exertion and subsides with rest. It can also be relieved by using a medication that causes vasodilation. Episodes of chest pain can increase in frequency and severity over time. If clients do not heed the warning to stop their activity and rest, they may be risking a myocardial infarction or sudden death.

TYPES

Stable Angina

Stable angina occurs when the atherosclerotic arteries cannot dilate to increase blood flow to the myocardium. When increased physical activity and stress place an added demand on the heart, the client develops midsternal chest pain. The pain of stable angina usually subsides when the activity is stopped or with the use of nitroglycerin sublingually, which is a vasodilator.

Unstable Angina

Unstable angina is seen in clients with worsening CAD. The episodes of chest pain increase in frequency and severity, placing them at risk for myocardial damage or sudden death. Rest does not decrease the chest pain in a client with unstable angina, which can occur even when the client is resting.

Variant Angina (Prinzmetal's Angina)

The pain of variant angina is the same as in stable angina, except it has a longer duration and can occur at rest. This type of angina is often caused by coronary artery spasms and usually does not cause damage to the myocardium.

DIAGNOSTIC TESTS

Electrocardiogram

An electrocardiogram (ECG) may help with the diagnosis of angina. It may remain normal in 20 to 30 percent of clients with angina pectoris. ECGs obtained during an episode of chest pain may identify which coronary artery is involved. ECG changes that may be seen in clients with angina may include a depressed T wave, which indicates ischemia, or an elevated ST segment, which can indicate injury.

Exercise Electrocardiogram (Stress Test)

In an exercise stress test, the client is placed on a treadmill or stationary bicycle. Exercise activity is increased until the client has reached 85 percent of his or her maximal heart rate. If during the test the client experiences chest pain, or if noticeable ECG or vital sign changes occur, it may be an indication of ischemia.

Another type of stress test, the dipyridamole (Persantine) thallium stress test, uses an intravenous medication in place of exercise. This test is used for clients who cannot exercise. Dipyridamole (Persantine) dilates coronary arteries and produces the effect of exercise. The collateral vessels also dilate, taking blood from the coronary arteries, which may cause ischemia if CAD is present. Radiology imaging is then done to determine the area of the heart that has severe ischemia.

Radioisotope Imaging

In radioisotope imaging, the injection of a radioisotope is performed during the stress test. When the maximal heart rate is reached, or other changes take place, the test is stopped and the client is taken to a room with special imaging equipment. Areas that are poorly perfused or ischemic are seen as decreased or absent activity in the areas that are blocked.

Coronary Angiography

This test consists of injecting a dye and viewing the coronary arteries. It identifies the arteries that are partially or totally blocked.

TREATMENTS

Treatment is directed at relieving an acute attack and preventing further attacks that could lead to a myocardial infarction. The risk factors identified for the client determine the course of treatment. Weight reduction; low-fat, low-cholesterol diets; and stress reduction can help decrease the number of attacks.

Most clients with angina are placed on medication that reduces oxygen demand and increases oxygen supply to the myocardium. This is the goal of pharmacological treatment. The three major groups of medication used for angina are vasodilators, calcium channel blockers, and beta blockers. Specific drugs with actions, side effects, and nursing implications are listed in Table 18–1.

Vasodilators

Nitroglycerin is the drug of choice for acute anginal attacks. Nitroglycerin can be administered sublingually, orally, transdermally, intravenously, or as a buccal spray. When administered sublingually it may relieve chest pain within 1 to 2 minutes (Table 18–2).

Long-acting nitrates can be given orally, by ointment, or by transdermal patches. They all act to maintain coronary artery vasodilation. Isosorbide dinitrate (Isordil) and isosorbide mononitrate (ISMO) are examples of long-acting nitrates. A problem with the long-acting nitrates is that a tolerance develops to the drug. It is now recommended that the patch and ointment be removed at bedtime and reapplied in the morning, giving the client 8 to 12 hours that are free of nitrates. This helps reduce the problem of tolerance development.

Calcium Channel Blockers

Calcium is required for electrical excitability of cardiac cells and contraction of the myocardium. Calcium channel blockers relax vascular smooth muscles, which leads to decreased peripheral vascular resistance (afterload) and decreased myocardial oxygen demand. They dilate main coronary arteries, increasing the myocardial oxygen supply. Nifedipine (Procardia) and verapamil (Calan, Isoptin) are potent inhibitors of coronary artery spasms and are used to treat variant (Prinzmetal's) angina. Diltiazem (Cardizem), another calcium channel blocker, has similar actions but has fewer side effects. Calcium channel blockers are also used to decrease systolic and diastolic blood pressures and to slow the heart rate. They are slow acting

Table 18-1. **Pharmacological Treatment for Angina Pectoris**

Class	Drug/Route	Side Effects
Vasodilators	Nitrates/nitroglycerin sublingual/spray Isosorbide dinitrate (Isordil) Isosorbide monotrate (ISMO) orally Nitroglycerin topical (Transderm Nitro, Nitro-Bid)	Headaches, light-headedness, postural hypotension, tachycardia, flushing
Calcium Channel Blockers	Diltiazem (Cardizem) Nifedipine (Procardia) Verapamil (Calan, Isoptin)	Headache, peripheral edema, dysrhythmias, flushing, dizziness, atrioventricular blocks
Beta Blockers	Propranolol (Inderal) Metoprolol (Lopressor) Atenolol (Tenormin)	Dizziness, bradycardia, hypotension, nausea, confusion, fatigue, agranulocytosis, laryngospasm

Nursing Implications

Vasodilators	Monitor blood pressure and heart rate before and after giving. Caution client to rise slowly due to orthostatic hypotension, especially with sublingual nitroglycerin. Take up to three nitroglycerin tablets at 5-minute intervals. If pain is not relieved, call a doctor or emergency medical assistance immediately. Do not remove tablets from bottle. Vasodilators become inactive when exposed to heat, air, light, and moisture. Tell client a burning or tingling sensation may be felt under the tongue with sublingual nitroglycerin.
Calcium Channel Blockers	Monitor blood pressure and heart rate before and after giving. Hold if blood pressure is less than 90 systolic or heart rate is less than 50 and call physician.
Beta Blockers	Assess blood pressure and heart rate before and after giving. Administer with food. Propranolol (Inderal) should not be given to asthmatics. Do not stop abruptly.

and thus are ineffective in relieving acute anginal attacks. These drugs are commonly given in conjunction with other vasodilators and beta blockers.

Beta Blockers

Beta blockers decrease the workload on the heart and the effects of epinephrine and norepinephrine on the heart,

Table 18-2. **Key Points for Use of Nitroglycerin Sublingually**

1. The client must carry it at all times.
2. It must be kept tightly sealed in the original container.
3. It must be replaced every 6 months to be fresh for maximal effect.
4. Client should take nitroglycerin before an activity known to cause chest pain.
5. Take one, then repeat every 5 minutes, if no pain relief, for two more doses.
6. If unrelieved after three doses, call for emergency medical care. Clients should not drive themselves to the hospital.
7. A tingling may be felt under the tongue when used.
8. May cause a headache.
9. May cause light-headedness; teach client to rise slowly.

thus preventing anginal attacks. There is a decreased myocardial oxygen demand secondary to decreased heart rate, decreased myocardial contractility, and decreased blood pressure, which decreases the workload on the heart. Because of these effects, beta blockers should be avoided in clients with any degree of heart failure. Clients with asthma or chronic obstructive pulmonary disease (emphysema, bronchitis, and bronchiectasis) should avoid beta blockers due to the constrictive effect on the bronchial tree. Beta-blocking agents such as propranolol (Inderal), metoprolol (Lopressor), and atenolol (Tenormin) are used to treat chronic angina. Metoprolol and atenolol are more cardioselective and can be used in clients with asthma and chronic obstructive pulmonary disease (COPD). Beta blockers are not effective for coronary artery spasms.

NURSING PROCESS

The nurse must obtain a thorough history on a client admitted with a diagnosis of angina pectoris. Documenting how long the client has had angina and the risk factors present assists in the development of a plan of care. It is important to know what activities trigger the onset of angina and what the client does to relieve the pain. If the client reports chest pain, the nurse needs to assess the type, the location, and if the pain radiates to other areas of the body. Other data to collect include skin color and temperature, blood pressure, pulse, respiratory rate, dyspnea, and nausea. The nurse must promote rest and decrease anxiety for the client with chest pain. Sublingual nitroglycerin should be administered as ordered. Blood pressure and heart rate should be assessed before and after nitroglycerin is given. A client who is experiencing chest pain should never be left alone.

Myocardial Infarction

A myocardial infarction (MI) results in the death of a portion of the heart muscle from a partial or complete blockage of a coronary artery, which decreases the blood supply to the cells of the heart supplied by the blocked coronary artery. This is a broad definition of a potentially devastating condition. The ability of the heart to contract, relax, and propel blood throughout the body requires healthy cardiac muscle. When the client has an MI, part of the heart muscle becomes damaged and can no longer function as it is supposed to. Cardiac conduction and blood flow can be dramatically altered by an MI.

Those with MIs are typically men over 40 with atherosclerosis development. Hypertension is also an increased risk factor. Although MIs can occur at any age in men or women, women who smoke and use oral contraceptives are at greater risk for MI.

PATHOPHYSIOLOGY

Myocardial infarction does not happen immediately. Ischemic injury evolves over several hours before complete necrosis and infarction takes place. The ischemic process affects the subendocardial layer, which is most sensitive to hypoxia. This process leads to depressed myocardial contractility. The body's attempt to compensate for decreased cardiac function triggers the sympathetic nervous system. The sympathetic nervous system increases heart rate, which increases myocardial oxygen demand, which further depresses the myocardium.

Prolonged ischemia can produce severe cellular damage and necrosis of cardiac muscle. Once necrosis takes place, the contractility function of the muscle is permanently lost. The heart has a zone of ischemia and injury around the necrotic area (Fig. 18–1). The zone of injury is next to the necrotic area and is susceptible to becoming necrosed. If treatment is initiated with the first sign of an MI, the area of damage can be minimized. Around the injury zone is the area of ischemia and viable tissue. If the heart responds to treatment, this area can rebuild and maintain collateral circulation. If prolonged ischemia takes place, the size of the infarction can be quite large. The size of the infarction depends on how quickly the blood supply from the blocked artery can be restored.

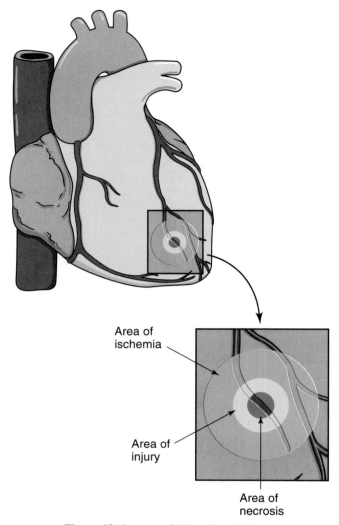

Figure 18–1. Areas of ischemia and injury.

The area that is affected by an MI depends on which coronary artery is involved and the extent of occlusive coronary disease (Fig. 18–2). Being familiar with the anatomy of the heart and the area of the MI helps the nurse anticipate dysrhythmias, conduction disturbances, and heart failure, which are the major complications of MIs (Table 18–3).

The left anterior descending (LAD) branch of the left main coronary artery is the area that feeds the anterior wall of the heart, which also includes most of the left ventricle. An occlusion in this area causes an anterior wall MI. If the left ventricle is affected, there can be severe loss of left ventricular function, which can lead to severe changes in the hemodynamic status of the client.

The right coronary artery (RCA) feeds the inferior wall and parts of the atrioventricular node and the sinoatrial node. An occlusion of the RCA leads to an inferior MI and abnormalities of impulse formation and conduction. Serious dysrhythmias can occur early in an inferior MI and may be life threatening.

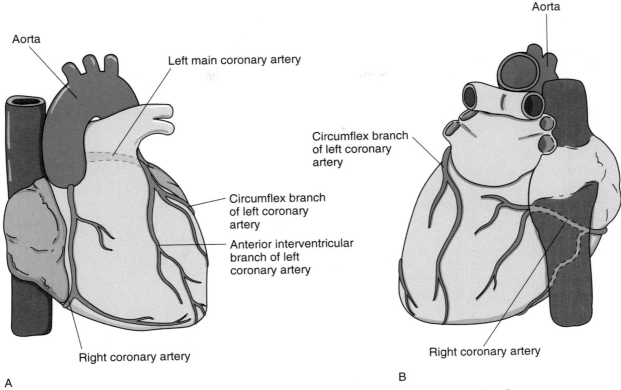

Figure 18–2. *(A)* Coronary arteries, frontal view. *(B)* Coronary arteries, posterior view.

The left circumflex coronary artery feeds the lateral wall of the heart and part of the posterior wall of the heart. A lesion in the circumflex leads to a lateral wall infarction of the left ventricle.

LEARNING TIP

To remember what coronary artery occlusion results in a specific MI location, use coast-to-coast U.S. location initials:

Location	Coronary Artery	Resulting MI Location
Los **A**ngeles =	**L**eft **a**nterior descending artery	Anterior
Cedar **P**oint =	**C**ircumflex artery	Posterior
Rhode **I**sland =	**R**ight coronary artery	Inferior

SIGNS AND SYMPTOMS

Pain is the most common symptom of an MI. The pain begins suddenly and continues without relief with rest or nitroglycerin. The pain is usually described as crushing or viselike. Clients may report that it feels like an elephant standing on their chest. The pain may radiate to one or both arms and shoulders, the neck, or the jaw. The pain can imitate indigestion or a gallbladder attack with abdominal pain and emesis. Clients often deny that they may be having an MI. Other symptoms may include dyspnea, restlessness, a feeling of impending doom, nausea and vomiting, diaphoresis, cold and clammy skin, and an ashen color. When listening to lung sounds, crackles or wheezing may be heard. The pulse may be rapid or irregular, and an extra heart sound (referred to as S_3 or S_4) may be present. The presence of an extra heart sound can mean ventricular failure is imminent.

Gerontological Implications

Some myocardial infarctions occur without the presence of pain. This type of MI is sometimes referred to as a silent MI. When pain is not present, the only symptom that may be present is a sudden onset of shortness of breath, fainting, restlessness, or a fall experienced by the client. This type of MI occurs most often in the elderly client. Atypical presentation of MI symptoms is normal in the elderly client, especially in those over age 85. Because the elderly have had more time to develop collateral circulation than younger people, they often do not have as many complications.

DIAGNOSTIC TESTS

Clients with a strong familial history of MIs should be considered as a risk for an MI until it is ruled out. The four

Table 18–3. **Complications of Myocardial Infarction**

Complication	Types or Symptoms	Interventions
Dysrhythmias	Premature ventricular contractions, ventricular tachycardia, ventricular fibrillation, heart block	Continuous cardiac monitoring Protocols for treatment of dysrhythmias (see Chapter 20)
Cardiogenic shock	Decreased blood pressure; increased heart rate; diaphoresis; cold, clammy, gray skin	Immediate initiation of treatment to decrease infarct size, control pain and dysrhythmias Thrombolytic therapy Dopamine and dobutamine
Heart failure/pulmonary edema	Dizziness, orthopnea, weight gain, edema, enlarged liver, jugular venous distention, crackles	Correct underlying cause, relieve symptoms, increase cardiac contractility, Lasix and digoxin
Ventricular aneurysms, rupture of muscles or valves of the heart, septal rupture	Signs of cardiogenic shock—death	Mortality rate high; immediate treatment of MI to limit extent of damage
Pericarditis (inflammation of the heart muscle)	Chest pain, increased with movement, deep inspiration, or cough; pericardial friction rub (fine grating sound)	Relieved when sits up and leans forward Anti-inflammatory drugs (aspirin, Indocin)

most useful indicators of an MI are client history, ECG, and serum cardiac troponin I and CK-MB levels. (See Chapter 15.) The client's health history is always obtained and used as a primary indicator of an MI along with other diagnostic tests.

An ECG usually shows the area that has infarcted, as well as the ischemic areas of the heart. The damage is seen as ST-segment elevation, the presence of a Q wave, or T wave abnormalities (Fig. 18–3). Serial ECGs are done to watch for changes indicating damage or ischemia.

Cardiac troponin I, a regulatory protein in cardiac muscle cells, is a highly specific indicator of cardiac injury that remains elevated up to 1 week after MI. This is very helpful in diagnosing MIs.

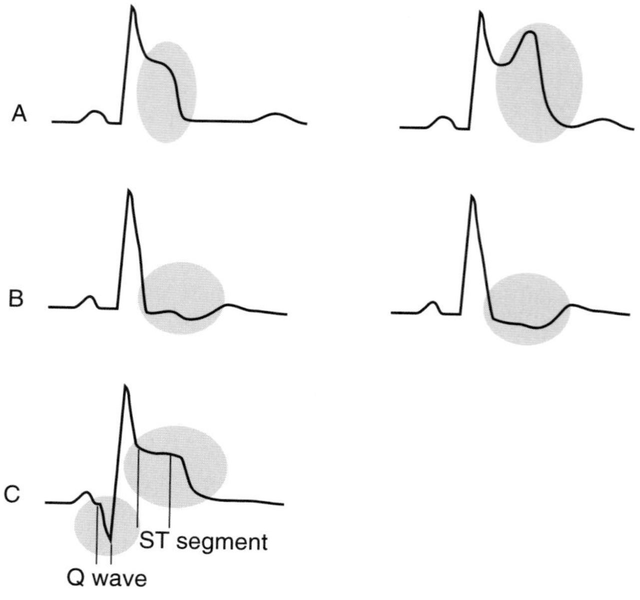

Myoglobin levels elevate within 1 hour of an acute MI and are 99 percent sensitive for an MI. Peak levels are reached 4 to 12 hours after an MI and return to normal within 18 hours after the onset of chest pain.

CK-MB, which is exclusively released into the circulation from heart cells after they die and rupture, indicates cardiac muscle death. CK-MB levels rise within 4 to 6 hours after injury, peak in 12 to 24 hours, and return to normal in 48 to 72 hours. Serial CKs are drawn to track trends in CK levels. Invasive procedures such as intravenous lines and intramuscular injections are avoided before drawing the first CK to prevent elevation in CK levels from cell trauma.

Lactic dehydrogenase (LDH) or aspartate aminotransferase (AST) (formally SGOT) levels are also elevated. LDH rises within 12 to 24 hours and AST after 24 to 48 hours. LDH and AST are not reliable indicators for cardiac damage because they are not cardiac specific and can also be elevated in liver and lung disease.

Figure 18–3. ECG changes during myocardial infarction. *(A)* ST segment elevation—injury. *(B)* ST segment inverted—ischemia. *(C)* Large Q wave—ST segment elevation—necrosis.

TREATMENT

Clients should immediately seek medical treatment for any unrelieved chest pain. The American Heart Association recommends that the client take one 325 mg aspirin at the onset of chest pain. Delays in seeking care can limit treatment options and result in more cardiac damage. Clients need to be educated that "time is muscle." This means that as time passes during an MI, more muscle is lost. Clients should not drive themselves to the hospital if they are having chest pain. They should call for emergency medical care.

Initially, clients are kept on bed rest to decrease myocardial oxygen demand. Clients are medicated promptly for chest pain. The presence of chest pain indicates a lack of oxygen to the myocardium. Medications are used to dilate blood vessels and increase perfusion and oxygen supply to the heart muscle. The use of oxygen also helps increase the supply of oxygen to the heart muscle. Clients reporting chest pain are treated as if they have an MI until it has been ruled out through testing.

Oxygen

Oxygen is placed on the client immediately, usually at 2 liters per minute via nasal cannula. Arterial blood gases (ABGs) are drawn to determine the client's oxygen needs. Oxygen can be administered via mask if higher concentrations are needed. Mechanical ventilation can be provided when indicated by ABGs.

Medication

Table 18–4 summarizes pharmacological treatment of myocardial infarction.

Analgesics

Analgesics are given for relief of chest pain. Morphine sulfate (MS) is the most commonly used narcotic for several reasons. In addition to pain relief, it helps decrease anxiety, opens bronchioles, and reduces preload and afterload, which can help increase blood supply and oxygen to the myocardium. It is given intravenously in small doses that are titrated to meet the client's pain relief needs when needed.

Vasodilators

Nitroglycerin sublingually, topically, or by intravenous (IV) drip can be administered for vasodilation to supply more blood to the myocardium and reduce the heart's workload. In the acute phase, the IV route is usually used.

Individual health care agencies have set protocols for the use of nitroglycerin.

Thrombolytics

Thrombolytic therapy is used to dissolve a blood clot that is occluding a coronary artery. Many communities allow initiation of thrombolytic therapy by paramedics in the field. Studies have revealed a decreased incidence of mortality and morbidity and less extensive MIs when thrombolytic treatment is used. Thrombolytic therapy must be started within a specified time range from the onset of symptoms, usually within 1 to 6 hours, before necrosis results.

Diet

Diet therapy must also be addressed, especially if the client is overweight. During the acute phase, small, easily digested meals are served. Caffeinated beverages are usually restricted because they can increase the heart rate and cause vasoconstriction. Iced or cold beverages should be avoided because they can cause ischemic changes on the ECG. Room temperature liquids are best. Fluids may be restricted if the client is in heart failure as well.

A cardiac diet may be ordered as low cholesterol and low sodium. The number of grams of sodium is prescribed by the physician. If the client is obese, a dietitian may work with the client and family to devise a diet that is suitable and palatable for the client.

Smoking

Smoking should be avoided, and clients are instructed on the hazards of continuing to smoke. The nurse needs to understand that too many major lifestyle changes at one time can increase anxiety and noncompliance. The nurse needs to work with clients to help them understand and accept lifestyle changes.

Table 18–4. **Pharmacological Treatment for Myocardial Infarction**

Drug	Rationale
1. Oxygen (nasal cannula, face mask, face tent)	Decreases myocardial oxygen demand, improves cellular oxygenation
2. Morphine sulfate (IV)	Relieves pain, decreases anxiety, and slows respirations Decreases preload and afterload, allowing increased blood flow to the heart
3. Nitroglycerin (sublingual, spray, topical, and IV infusion)	Dilates coronary arteries, increases blood flow to the heart, and relieves chest pain
4. Xylocaine (Lidocaine) (IV bolus, IV drip)	Used for prevention of ventricular dysrhythmias
5. Beta blockers (Inderal, Lopressor, Tenormin)	Decreases heart rate and force of contraction, decreases oxygen requirements of the heart
6. Thrombolytic therapy (streptokinase, Eminase, tissue plasminogen activator)	Lyses the clot and prevents others from forming
7. Heparin sodium (IV push, subcutaneous, IV infusion)	Prevents more clots from forming No effect on clots already present

NURSING PROCESS

Assessment

A thorough history must be obtained to identify risk factors that may contribute to a myocardial infarction. All clients admitted with chest pain are treated as having a possible MI until it has been ruled out. Monitoring ECGs and laboratory values, such as CK-MB, helps determine the degree of cardiac damage and identify life-threatening dysrhythmias. Controlling chest pain immediately can help diminish anxiety and the negative physiological effects pain has on the body. Until the cause of the chest pain is resolved, there is decreased blood supply and oxygen to the myocardium, making it susceptible to infarction.

Nursing Diagnosis

The nursing diagnoses may include but are not limited to the following:

- Pain related to reduced coronary artery blood flow and increased myocardial oxygen needs
- Decreased cardiac output relating to ischemia or infarction, changes in heart rate and rhythm, and decreased contractility
- Anxiety relating to threat of death, changes in lifestyle, and chest pain
- Activity intolerance relating to imbalance between oxygen supply and demand, weakness, and fatigue
- Knowledge deficit relating to disease process, lifestyle changes, and medication

See Nursing Care Plan Box 18–2 for the Client with Myocardial Infarction.

Planning

The client and family should be included in planning care. They need to understand that the purpose of the treatment is to prevent further myocardial damage. A plan of care should focus on factors that may contribute to increased cardiac workload to reduce them. The client's goals are to (1) report that the pain management regimen relieves pain; (2) maintain palpable pulses, warm and dry skin, and vital signs within normal range; (3) state that anxiety is relieved; (4) maintain desired activities; and (5) understand the disease and its treatment.

Nursing Interventions

Nursing care in addition to relieving pain is aimed at reducing the heart's workload and relieving client and family anxiety. Several interventions to help reduce the heart's workload are important. The client should be positioned for comfort and ease in breathing. Semi-Fowler's position is usually preferred by clients having respiratory distress. Whenever clients are sitting upright, their arms should be supported on pillows to further reduce the heart's workload

from gravity pulling on unsupported arms. The client should be taught to avoid Valsalva's maneuver, which occurs when the client bears down against a closed glottis, mouth, and nose. Valsalva's maneuver increases intrathoracic pressure, slows the heart rate, and decreases blood return to the heart. Valsalva's maneuver can occur when the client moves or turns in bed or strains with defecation. Clients must be taught not to hold their breath whenever moving and also not to strain. Stool softeners are usually ordered by the physician. A record of the client's bowel movements and intake and output is monitored.

Emotional support should be provided. The client should be allowed to verbalize fears. Procedures should be explained. Family support should also be offered. Spouses also experience anxiety and need support such as ongoing information and explanations, being allowed to stay with the client, and being involved in the client's care.[5] Spouses often ignore their own needs to focus on the client. Nurses need to help them meet their needs, so that they are able to support the client, by being supportive and aware of their needs.

Teaching about the therapeutic regimen includes information about the disease, medications, diet, activity, and rehabilitation needs that may require lifestyle changes. Diet, stress reduction, a regular exercise program, cessation of smoking if necessary, and following a medication schedule require extensive client and family teaching. This disease can affect all aspects of a client's lifestyle. Issues about family and job roles and sexual activities need to be addressed. Clients need time to understand presented information and should be encouraged to express their questions, needs, and fears.

Evaluation

The goal for the nursing diagnosis of pain is met if the client reports satisfactory pain relief. Satisfactory pain relief is measured by comparing the client's stated level of pain on a rating scale of 1 to 10 with the client's predetermined goal for acceptable level of pain.

The goal for the nursing diagnosis of alteration in tissue perfusion is met if the client's vital signs are within normal limits, no pain is reported, and no alteration in level of consciousness is observed.

The goal for the nursing diagnosis of anxiety is achieved if the client states that anxiety is reduced.

The goal for the nursing diagnosis of activity intolerance is met if the client reports reduced fatigue and the ability to complete tasks and engage in desired activities.

The goal for the nursing diagnosis of ineffective management of therapeutic regimen is met if the client verbalizes understanding of the disease, medications, and reasons for lifestyle changes and a willingness to follow the regimen.

CARDIAC REHABILITATION

Cardiac rehabilitation is begun when the client's acute symptoms are relieved. The purpose of cardiac rehabilita-

NURSING CARE PLAN BOX 18–2
FOR THE CLIENT WITH MYOCARDIAL INFARCTION

Pain related to decreased coronary blood flow causing myocardial ischemia

Client Outcomes
Client will exhibit signs of decreased pain. Client will exhibit signs of relaxation.

Evaluation of Outcomes
Does client state pain is reduced?

Interventions	Rationale	Evaluation
• Assess for location, duration, intensity, and radiation; use a scale of 1 to 10.	Identifies type and severity of pain.	What is pain level, location, duration, intensity, and radiation?
• Assess blood pressure, pulse, and respiration.	Vital signs may elevate episodes of pain.	Are vital signs within normal limits?
• Obtain ECG as ordered.	Identifies location of infarction or ischemia.	Is ECG normal?
• Administer oxygen as ordered.	Helps prevent hypoxia.	Are ABGs within normal limits? Is oxygen saturation greater than 90 percent?
• Instruct client to report pain at first onset.	Helps control pain quickly to prevent further ischemia.	Does client report pain?
• Instruct client to rest during pain.	Activity increases oxygen demand and can increase chest pain.	Does client remain quiet and relaxed?
• Remain with client during chest pain until it is relieved.	Provides comfort and reassurance to decrease anxiety and fear.	Are anxiety and fear decreased?
• Explain and assist with alternative pain relief measures: • Positioning • Diversional activities • Relaxation techniques	These measures help decrease painful stimuli, allowing the client to focus on other things.	Does client express relief and decreased stress?
• Medicate as ordered.	Helps eliminate pain.	Is pain relieved?

Decreased cardiac output relating to ischemia or infarction, changes in heart rate and rhythm, and decreased contractility

Client Outcomes
Client will maintain adequate cardiac output and tissue perfusion. Client will exhibit signs of improved cardiac output and tissue perfusion.

Evaluation of Outcomes
Does client have heart rate greater than 60 and less than 100, blood pressure greater than 90/60 and less than 140/90, and urine output greater than 30 mL/h?

Interventions	Rationale	Evaluation
• Monitor blood pressure greater than 90/60, heart rate greater than 60 and less than 100, urine output greater than 30 mL/h.	Indirect indicators of cardiac output.	Are indicators within normal limits?
• Listen to lung sounds.	Crackles indicate heart failure.	Are lungs clear?
• Monitor peripheral circulation, pulses, capillary refill, edema, color, and temperature.	Indicators of adequate tissue perfusion.	Does client have strong peripheral pulses, capillary refill less than 3 seconds, no edema, warm skin, pink nailbeds?
• Monitor ECG.	Identifies dysrhythmias.	Is client's ECG within normal limits?
• Administer medications as ordered by physician, such as vasodilators, beta blockers, calcium channel blockers, and cardiac glycosides.	Helps improve contractility, cardiac output, and tissue perfusion.	Does client show signs of improved contractility, increased cardiac output, and tissue perfusion?

continued

NURSING CARE PLAN BOX 18-2 (continued)

Interventions	Rationale	Evaluation
• Promote and provide for adequate rest, quiet environment, bed rest; place in semi-Fowler's position.	Decreases cardiac workload and stress and allows for improved breathing.	Is client relaxed?

Activity intolerance related to insufficient oxygen supply and demand, weakness, and fatigue

Client Outcomes
Client will show improved activity intolerance. Client will exhibit signs of increased energy.

Evaluation of Outcomes
Does client show increase in activities of daily living by participating in care? Does client state less fatigue and increased energy?

Interventions	Rationale	Evaluation
• Monitor for level of fatigue, weakness, changes in vital signs after activity.	Indicates current activity status and allows for progression in activities.	Does client increase activity without difficulty?
• Use oxygen during activity.	Improves oxygen to the heart during increased activities.	Is client free of dyspnea?
• Take vital signs before and after activity.	Indicates response to activity and will help plan necessary changes in activity level if blood pressure increases more than 15 mm Hg during activity or heart rate increases more than 20 beats per minute.	Are vital signs within normal limits?
• Provide for adequate rest between activities.	Allows time for healing, decreases oxygen demand, and promotes rest.	Does client display signs of adequate rest between activities?

Knowledge deficit related to disease process, medication, diet, and lifestyle changes

Client Outcomes
Client will show increased knowledge of disease and treatment. Client will state understanding of care needed to improve cardiac status.

Evaluation of Outcomes
Does client state understanding of purpose of medications? Is client able to state lifestyle changes needed to improve outcome?

Interventions	Rationale	Evaluation
• Check for readiness to learn about disease and lifestyle changes.	Client must be ready and willing to learn about disease and care.	Does client show desire to learn?
• Ask client's usual health practices and beliefs.	Helps promote compliance and facilitate learning.	Does learning fit client's beliefs?
• Perform or provide clear explanations within client's ability to understand. Do not overload with information at one time.	Prevents misunderstanding and allows client time to take in information necessary to comply with treatment.	Does client ask appropriate questions and express understanding of information given?
• Provide a quiet environment for learning.	Prevents distraction that may interfere with learning.	Is client able to learn?
• Use teaching aids such as visual aids, written materials.	Promotes and reinforces learning.	Does client comprehend information given?

tion is to improve cardiac function and assist the client in returning to as normal a life as possible. Cardiac rehabilitation protocols are used in many institutions. The first two periods of rehabilitation occur in the hospital, and activities for each hospital day, such as types and amounts of self-care and activity, are specified in protocols. The third period begins with hospital discharge and focuses on returning to prior levels of activity and function. Outpatient programs are often ordered for clients in this phase. The final period encourages the client to maintain optimal physical fitness and to continue a healthy lifestyle.

CRITICAL THINKING: Sally

Sally, 43, is admitted to the intensive care unit with a diagnosis of atypical chest pain. The patient has a history of midsternal chest pain and chest pressure. The pain radiates from sternum to left and right shoulders down her left arm. Pain increases with activity and decreases with rest. She smokes 1½ packs of cigarettes per day and is 50 pounds overweight. The cardiac monitor shows normal sinus rhythm without dysrhythmias. She has nitroglycerin sublingual ordered prn for chest pain.

One hour after admission, Sally reports midsternal chest pain radiating to left neck and jaw. The cardiac monitor shows sinus tachycardia with occasional premature ventricular contractions. Her blood pressure is 100/70, respirations are 20 and unlabored, and skin is warm and dry.

1. What actions should the nurse take?
2. What is happening?
3. How is angina differentiated from an MI?
4. What are four indicators of an MI?
5. What are medical interventions that can be used for an MI?
6. What patient education is indicated for this client?

Answers at end of chapter.

Peripheral Vascular System

Changes in the peripheral vascular system may occur in anyone but are particularly common in elderly and diabetic clients. These changes result in peripheral vascular disease (PVD), which may be either arterial or venous in origin.

Arterial disease begins, as discussed previously, in clients with arteriosclerosis and atherosclerosis who have impedance of blood flow. There is a reduction in blood flow through the vascular system of the peripheral vessels. As a result, decreased nutrition, cellular waste accumulation, and the development of ischemia occur at the area distal to the obstruction. With the increased debris and sluggish flow, **thrombosis** and **embolism** become a major

problem. If left untreated, the area distal to the obstruction becomes ulcerated, gangrenous, and necrotic. When this occurs, amputation of the limb may become necessary.

Venous disease is the result of venous insufficiency that occurs over time. Damaged or aging valves within the veins prevent blood return to the heart, and pooling of blood occurs.

HISTORY

The nurse obtains data regarding symptoms that pertain to circulation. The nurse should understand if the problem is arterial or venous disease to prevent serious complications. Typically, with arterial disease the client reports leg pain when the legs are elevated or calf pain during activity that then disappears with rest. Venous disease has a slower onset and is not associated with activity. Pain occurs when the legs are positioned dependently causing pooling of blood at the ankles.

The history should include risk factors that contribute to arteriosclerosis and atherosclerosis. A family history of diabetes mellitus, hypertension, coronary artery disease, and known peripheral vascular disease predisposes clients to vascular disease.

Arterial Thrombosis and Embolism

Atherosclerosis, a form of arteriosclerosis, eventually leads to obliteration of the peripheral arterial tree. Regardless of the cause of vessel disease the complication of thrombosis or embolism can occur. The symptoms depend on the artery occluded, the tissue supplied by that artery, and whether collateral circulation has begun.

PATHOPHYSIOLOGY

Thrombus, a blood clot, adheres to the vessel wall. Acute arterial thrombi occur where there is injury to an arterial wall, sluggish flow, or plaque formation secondary to atherosclerotic changes. Other causes of arterial thrombosis are polycythemia, dehydration, and repeated arterial needle sticks. An arterial embolism is the occlusion of a vessel too small to allow the embolism to pass. The difference between arterial thrombosis and embolism is that the embolism usually develops in the heart and passes through healthy arteries. Some of the causes of an arterial embolism are dysrhythmias, prosthetic heart valves, and rheumatic heart disease.

SIGNS AND SYMPTOMS

Usually, there is an abrupt onset of symptoms for acute arterial occlusion. If a client has chronic arterial insufficiency, the symptoms may not occur abruptly because collateral circulation has had time to develop and can supply some blood to the occluded area.

There are six clinical signs of acute arterial occlusion, known as the six P's: pain, pallor, pulselessness, paresthesia (numbness), paralysis, and poikilothermia (temperature). The client experiences pain, numbness, and decreased movement in the extremity, which is pale and without pulses distal to the occlusion. The extremity feels cold because blood normally provides warmth. If treatment is not initiated immediately, ischemia occurs and can progress to tissue necrosis and gangrene development within hours.

TREATMENTS

Early treatment is a necessity to protect and save the affected limb. Anticoagulant therapy is started immediately. Intravenous heparin is the treatment of choice to prevent further clotting. It has no effect on already existing clots. An initial bolus of heparin is given, usually 5000 units. An intravenous infusion is then started at the ordered units per hour. The client will remain on heparin therapy for several days. Daily partial thromboplastin times (PTTs) are monitored for therapeutic levels, and the heparin is adjusted accordingly. After 3 to 7 days warfarin (Coumadin) is added. Coumadin, an oral anticoagulant, takes 3 to 5 days to reach therapeutic levels. The heparin is continued until the therapeutic Coumadin level is reached. To monitor Coumadin, prothrombin times and international normalized ratios (INRs) are done daily, and adjustments in doses are made based on the results.

For clients with severe occlusions, if the risk of limb loss is imminent, surgical procedures, such as emergency embolectomy or thrombectomy, are performed to save the extremity. The artery is cut open, the emboli or thrombus is removed, and the vessel is sutured closed. Thrombolytic agents can also be used to dissolve the thrombus or embolus.

CRITICAL THINKING: Mary

Mary, 68, is admitted with severe rheumatoid arthritis. She has been bedridden for 9 months. She was returning to her room following a whirlpool treatment when she suddenly reported severe pain in her left groin.

1. What is your first action?
2. After assessing the client, what action should be taken next?
3. What are the possible causes of these symptoms?
4. What would the immediate interventions be?
5. What medical interventions would the nurse anticipate?
6. What surgical procedure may need to be done if risk of losing the limb is imminent?

Answers at end of chapter.

Peripheral Arterial Disease

Peripheral arterial disease (PAD) involves progressive narrowing of arterial vessels and eventually obstruction, usually in the lower extremities. Causes may include atherosclerosis, thrombosis, embolism, trauma, vasospasm, and inflammation of the arterial tree. As previously discussed, atherosclerosis is the leading cause of occlusive disease. Chronic arterial occlusion is a slow, progressive disease that is attributed to the atherosclerotic process. The term **atherosclerosis obliterans** is used to describe this disorder.

PATHOPHYSIOLOGY

The purpose of the arterial system is to delivery oxygen-rich blood to the vascular beds. Anything that impedes this flow will cause an imbalance in supply and demand for oxygen. The body has several mechanisms to attempt to compensate for this imbalance. Peripheral vasodilation, development of collateral circulation, and anaerobic metabolism to meet the body demands are the mechanisms used for compensation. However, these mechanisms are not adequate to meet the ongoing blood supply needs of the body. It takes time for collateral circulation to develop, blood vessels eventually reach their limit of dilation, and anaerobic metabolism is only a very short-term compensatory mechanism. Eventually this lack of blood supply produces signs of ischemia, and if not corrected, necrosis of the extremity occurs.

SIGNS AND SYMPTOMS

Symptoms usually occur late in the course of occlusive disease. It is only when diminished blood flow begins to produce changes in the extremities that symptoms occur. **Intermittent claudication** is a common symptom associated with arterial occlusive disease. This is pain in the calves of the lower extremities associated with activity or exercise. If blood supply to the muscles is poor, they are unable to receive adequate oxygen. As ischemia increases, the muscle will develop a cramping-type pain. This pain usually subsides with rest when the activity is stopped. As atherosclerosis and arteriosclerosis worsen, the pain is present at rest, thus indicating severe arterial occlusion.

Skin color changes are associated with decreased blood supply. The extremity is pale if the leg is elevated. If the leg is in a dependent position, it becomes a reddish-purple color or cyanotic. The extremity is cool to touch even in warm environments. As occlusion of the arteries progresses there are diminished or absent arterial pulses. The loss of circulation will lead to death of the tissue and gangrene. See Table 18–5 for stages of peripheral arterial disease.

Table 18–5. *Stages of Peripheral Arterial Disease*

Stage I: Asymptomatic
1. No claudication is present.
2. Bruit (swishing sound over artery or vein) or aneurysm may be present.
3. Physical examination may rarely reveal decreased pulses.

Stage II: Claudication
1. Muscle pain, cramping, or burning is exacerbated by exercise and relieved by rest.
2. Symptoms can be produced by exercise.

Stage III: Rest Pain
1. Pain while resting commonly wakes the client at night.
2. Pain is described as numbness, burning, or toothache-type pain.
3. Pain usually occurs in the distal portion of the extremity and only rarely in the calf or ankle.
4. Pain is relieved by placing the extremity in a dependent position.

Stage IV: Necrosis/Gangrene
1. Ulcers and blackened tissue occur on the toes, forefoot, and heel.
2. A distinctive gangrenous odor is present.

Source: Ignatavicius, DD, and Hausman, KA: Pocket Companion for Medical-Surgical Nursing, ed 2. WB Saunders, Philadelphia, 1995, p 93, with permission.

DIAGNOSTIC TESTS

Several noninvasive studies can be used to diagnose occlusive disorders. The ankle-brachial (arm) blood pressure index is used to determine pressures in the upper and lower extremities. Normally, pressures in the legs and arms should be equal. When an occlusion occurs in the lower extremities, the pressures between the upper and lower extremities become uneven. A Doppler ultrasound is used to measure the velocity of the blood flow. MRI can give definitive images of vessels and degrees of closure.

Arteriography is an invasive procedure that x-rays an artery after dye has been injected. This requires a client's consent. The nurse must also ask whether the client is allergic to iodine. This test is usually done before surgical intervention.

LEARNING TIP
Arterial Insufficiency Risk Assessment:
Ankle-Brachial Index
1. Take brachial blood pressure.
2. Take ankle blood pressure.
3. Divide ankle systolic pressure by brachial systolic pressure (e.g., 98 ÷ 130 = 0.75).
4. 0.8 or less = arterial disease.
5. Do not treat arterial disease like venous disease!

TREATMENT

Conservative medical treatment is initiated with mild to moderate occlusive disease. This includes clients who experience pain on activity that ceases with rest. This type of client usually receives medication for vasodilation and diet management, if necessary. Surgical intervention is used for the client who experiences pain at rest or who has leg ulcers that do not heal. Surgical treatment includes endarterectomy to remove the atherosclerotic lesion or grafting to bypass the occluded area.

Diet

As previously discussed, the diet should be low fat, low cholesterol, and low calorie if the client is overweight. Teaching the client to avoid red meats, fried foods, whole milk, and cheese is important. Avoiding high-cholesterol foods, such as egg yokes, organ meats, animal fats, and shellfish, helps lower lipid levels.

Medications

Drug therapy is geared toward the symptoms and causes of the occlusive disease. The same drugs used to decrease cholesterol and lipid levels in atherosclerosis are used with occlusive disease. Vasodilators can be used, but their effectiveness is not the same for all clients. Pentoxifylline (Trental) is commonly the drug of choice in those clients with occlusive disorders who experience intermittent claudication. This drug makes red blood cells more flexible to improve perfusion. The major side effect is primarily gastrointestinal, so it should be taken with meals.

Invasive Therapies

Percutaneous transluminal angioplasty is a procedure in which a catheter is inserted into a vessel. A balloon is then inflated to dilate a narrowed vessel. One of the complications that can occur with this procedure is a ruptured artery, which is the result of the stretching caused by the balloon. Peripheral atherectomy is used to remove plaque from atherosclerotic arteries. This has fewer complications because it does not overstretch the artery, and the vessel lining becomes smoother to decrease risk of clot formation. Intravascular stents are used as support structures to maintain patency of an artery. Clients are usually placed on dipyridamole (Persantine) or aspirin. These drugs are used to decrease platelet aggregation.

Thrombolytic therapy is used when an occlusion is caused by a thrombus or an embolus. Streptokinase or urokinase is the drug of choice to dissolve clots. These drugs require careful and continuous monitoring.

NURSING PROCESS FOR PERIPHERAL ARTERIAL DISEASES

Assessment

When dealing with clients having arterial occlusive disorders, monitoring the peripheral circulation is paramount. Careful assessment of pulses, temperature, color, and presence of edema helps identify clients at risk for complications.

Nursing Diagnosis

The nursing diagnoses for PAD may include but are not limited to the following:

1. Alteration in tissue perfusion related to decreased arterial perfusion
2. Pain related to decreased blood supply to lower extremities
3. Activity intolerance related to activity pain
4. Knowledge deficit related to complications, medications, or postoperative care

See Nursing Care Plan Box 18–3 for the Client with Peripheral Arterial Occlusive Disorders.

Planning

Arterial occlusive disease is a progressive disorder that can be controlled or at least slowed. Including the client and family in the development of the plan of care will help ensure their understanding of the reasons for the current therapy. The client's goals are to (1) maintain palpable pulses and warm and dry skin, (2) report that pain is relieved, (3) maintain desired activities, and (4) understand the disease and its treatment.

Nursing Interventions

The client should be able to describe symptoms and complications associated with arterial occlusive disorders. Medication cards can be developed to help the client understand the different medications being used and any special considerations they require. (See Nutrition Notes Box 18–4.) The client should be seen by a dietitian before discharge for instructions on a low-fat, low-cholesterol diet. Proper leg positioning should be taught to prevent complications and the potential loss of the extremity. Clients should not elevate their legs, especially if pain is increased. They should keep their legs in a dependent position. Walking programs have been shown to be helpful in maintaining circulation and should be encouraged if ordered by the physician.

Evaluation

The best indicator that outcomes for the client with PAD have been achieved is that the client is experiencing less pain with activity and the absence of complications with activity. If the client states understanding of the disease and the need to comply with treatment, the goal for knowledge deficit is achieved. This disorder requires constant monitoring and evaluation of the progression of this occlusive disease.

Aneurysms

An **aneurysm** is a bulging or dilation at a weakened point of an artery. The artery diameter is often increased by 50 percent. Anything that weakens the artery wall or causes loss of elasticity in the artery can cause an aneurysm. Atherosclerosis is probably the most common cause of an aneurysm. Other causes include hypertension, trauma, and congenital abnormalities.

Aneurysms can occur in any artery in the body. Abdominal aortic aneurysms are common and occur in those with atherosclerosis. Men over the age of 60 have the highest incidence. Hypertension is a risk factor.

TYPES

There are different types of aneurysms (Fig. 18–4). A fusiform aneurysm is the dilation of the entire circumference of the artery. A saccular aneurysm is a bulging on one side only of the artery wall.

A dissecting aneurysm occurs when a cavity is formed from a tear in the artery wall, usually the intimal (inner) layer. The layers of the artery are then separated as blood is pumped into the tear with each heartbeat, expanding the cavity, which is then prone to rupturing.

SIGNS AND SYMPTOMS

Usually there are few if any symptoms. Back pain is the classic symptom; it is caused by the aneurysm pressing against nerves of the vertebrae. Depending on the location and size of the aneurysm, there may be complaints of abdominal pain or nausea caused by pressure on the intestines. There may be a pulsating mass in the abdomen caused by an abdominal aortic aneurysm that is detected during routine physical examination by the physician.

Severe, sudden back or abdominal pain can indicate that the aneurysm may be about to rupture. Intense, constant back pain is a sign of rupture. The client's blood pressure drops and signs of shock are present. The mortality rate is high with a ruptured aneurysm.

DIAGNOSTIC TESTS

Computer tomography and ultrasound are the most common diagnostic tools used to confirm the presence of an aneurysm. Aortography can be performed, and usually is, when surgical intervention is considered. This procedure is

NURSING CARE PLAN BOX 18-3
FOR THE CLIENT WITH PERIPHERAL ARTERIAL OCCLUSIVE DISORDERS

Pain related to impaired circulation to extremities causing intermittent or continuous pain

Client Outcomes
Client will report that pain is controlled.

Evaluation of Outcomes
Does client report relief from pain by nonpharmacological or pharmacological methods?

Interventions	Rationale	Evaluation
• Monitor for intermittent claudication or pain at rest.	Helps determine degree of occlusive disease.	Does client have pain during activity or at rest?
• Note peripheral circulation, pulses, color, temperature, presence of edema, and skin breakdown.	Determines the degree of tissue perfusion and complications.	Does client have pulses, warm skin, capillary refill less than 3 seconds, no evidence of skin breakdown?
• Administer medication as ordered:		Does client show signs of increased circulation and relief of pain following administration of medications?
• Analgesics	Relieves chronic or acute pain.	
• Vasodilators	Increases blood flow to extremities.	
• Calcium channel blockers	Decrease vasospastic episodes.	
• Promote bed rest if pain is present.	Rest decreases muscle contraction and prevents further ischemia in extremities.	Is client able to rest?
• Position lower extremities below heart level.	Increases arterial flow to lower extremities.	Pulses strong, capillary refill less than 3 seconds, extremities pink and warm?
• Protect extremities from cold or trauma.	Extremities with decreased circulation have decreased sensation, which increases risk of injury.	Are extremities injury free?

Altered tissue perfusion related to interruption of arterial flow in arms and legs

Client Outcomes
Client will exhibit signs of increased arterial blood flow and tissue perfusion.

Evaluation of Outcomes
Does client have strong peripheral pulses, capillary refill less than 3 seconds, warm skin, absence of edema?

Interventions	Rationale	Evaluation
• Check peripheral pulses, capillary refill, color, temperature, and presence of edema every 4 hours.	Indication of adequate tissue perfusion.	Are peripheral pulses strong, nailbeds pink, capillary refill less than 3 seconds with no edema noted?
• Check skin for intactness, healed areas, signs of ulceration or infection.	Chronic arterial occlusion leads to decreased blood flow, resulting in tissue damage and poor wound healing.	Is skin intact?
• Place extremities lower than heart, feet on floor in sitting position, head of bed elevated on blocks.	Increases blood flow to the legs and feet.	Does client have adequate tissue perfusion signs?
• Avoid bending knees, pillows under knees, prolonged sitting or crossing legs.	These activities impede blood flow to extremities.	Does client exhibit understanding of improving blood flow?
• Inspect lower extremities frequently. Clean feet with mild soap, dry carefully. Protect from injury.	Cleaning prevents trauma to feet, protecting feet from things that can lead to ulcerations.	Is client free from trauma or breaks in skin of the lower extremities?

continued

NURSING CARE PLAN BOX 18–3 (continued)

Knowledge deficit related to discharge care to increase circulation and to prevent impaired tissue perfusion and skin breakdown

Client Outcomes
Client will be able to state signs of occlusive disease. Client will show compliance with prevention and treatment plan of care.

Evaluation of Outcomes
Does client verbalize symptoms of occlusive disease? Is client free of complications from impaired arterial circulation?

Interventions	Rationale	Evaluation
• Teach client and family the process of diminished arterial circulation. • Teach client risk factors. • Teach daily walking exercises, increasing distance and rest periods as needed. • Teach to avoid constrictive clothing, sitting for long periods, or impeding flow behind knees. • Dietary restrictions of cholesterol and fat. Weight reduction if necessary. • Teach client about medications, including purpose, route, and side effects. • Teach to watch extremities for signs of compromised circulation (increased pain, pallor, cold extremities, cyanosis, edema, or breaks in skin) and report to physician.	Promotes understanding and compliance with treatment. Risk factors contribute to vascular disease and can be modified. Maintains blood flow by increasing collateral circulation. These contribute to decreased blood flow to extremities. Prevents further atherosclerosis that contributes to arterial disease. Promotes compliance with therapy. Allows for early detection of complications.	Are client and family able to verbalize the effects of the disease process? Is client able to express changes in lifestyle to improve circulation? Is client able to walk without pain? Is client able to explain activities that impede blood flow? Is client able to verbalize dietary needs? Is client able to state medications' purpose and side effects? Is client able to state signs of decreased circulation?

NUTRITION NOTES BOX 18–4

ANTICOAGULATION THERAPY. Warfarin (Coumadin) achieves anticoagulation by fooling the liver into using it as vitamin K to manufacture clotting factors. For maximum therapeutic effect, the amount of foods high in vitamin K consumed should be consistent, not excessive one day and scanty the next.
Avoid:
  Kale (except garnish)
  Parsley (except garnish)
  Natto (Japanese)
One serving per day, 1 cup raw or 1/2 cup cooked:
  Broccoli
  Brussels sprouts
  Spinach
  Turnip or other greens
Check with prescriber if large increases or decreases in the following:
  Green vegetables
  Garbanzo beans
  Lentils
  Soybeans or soybean oil
  Liver

done to identify the size and exact location of the aneurysm. Small aneurysms may be watched over time to see if they enlarge.

TREATMENT

Medical treatment consists of medication to maintain lower blood pressures because clients with aneurysms often have hypertension. If the blood pressure is allowed to get too high it can cause the arterial wall to rupture. Surgical treatment, a bypass graft, is performed when the client is experiencing pain or showing signs of circulatory compromise. An aneurysm that is larger than 5 cm requires surgery.

NURSING CARE

The nurse must help clients understand their medications and the importance of taking antihypertensives as prescribed. Stress may be a factor and may need to be addressed. Lifting can increase pressure within the artery and may be restricted even in the individual being treated with more conservative measures. Postoperatively, the client must also avoid lifting heavy objects.

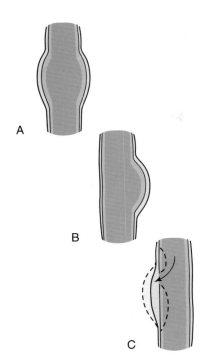

Figure 18–4. Types of aneurysms. *(A)* **Fusiform.** The entire circumference of the artery is dilated. *(B)* **Saccular.** One side of artery is dilated. *(C)* **Dissecting.** A tear in the inner layer causes a cavity to form between the layers of the artery and fill with blood. The cavity expands with each heartbeat.

Raynaud's Disease

A vasoconstrictive response causing ischemia from exposure to cold and stress is known as **Raynaud's disease.** It occurs more often in women who live in cold climates. Raynaud's primarily affects the hands but can also occur in the feet, ears, or nose. To be diagnosed with Raynaud's disease, the client must experience intermittent attacks of ischemia for at least 2 years.

PATHOPHYSIOLOGY

Raynaud's disease is characterized by spasms of small arteries in the digits. These spasms prevent arterial blood from perfusing the fingertips and sometimes the toes. The spasms can occur unilaterally and in one or two digits, but most often it occurs bilaterally and in all digits.

SIGNS AND SYMPTOMS

The hands, when exposed to cold, exhibit vascular spasms and a marked decrease in blood flow to the tissues. The resulting effect to the tissues is ischemic pain. After several minutes of ischemia, hyperemia occurs. This is intense reddening of the hands from dilation of all the vessels of the hands. Pain becomes more intense at this time. Raynaud's disease goes through phases of blanching of the skin, pain,

and reddening of the skin. This disease can progress over time whereby the vessels remain constricted and severe decrease in blood flow can lead to fingers becoming gangrenous and necrotic.

TREATMENT

Conservative treatment is attempted first. The client is instructed to keep the hands warm. Gloves should be worn when going outside, cleaning a refrigerator, or preparing cold foods. Clients are instructed in the importance of protecting the hands from injury. They need to avoid things that can contribute to vasoconstriction, such as smoking, alcohol, and caffeine. Reducing stress levels can also help prevent vasoconstriction. Vasodilators are sometimes prescribed to help the client avoid peripheral vasoconstriction. Low doses of nifedipine (Procardia) or long-acting nitrates can be used.

To treat Raynaud's disease surgically the sympathetic reflex must be blocked. This is accomplished by interrupting the sympathetic nerve impulses from the spinal cord to the hand, which is known as sympathectomy.

NURSING CARE

Education is the primary goal for clients with Raynaud's disease. Teaching the client to protect the hands is very important. Stressing the use of gloves in cold climates, reducing vasoconstrictive activity, and decreasing stress levels will help reduce the number and severity of attacks.

Thromboangitis Obliterans (Buerger's Disease)

Buerger's disease is a recurring inflammation of small and medium arteries and veins of the lower extremities. It is usually the result of occlusion of the vessels by thrombus formation. The cause is unknown, but heavy cigarette smoking is a major contributing factor. Some studies are linking an autoimmune response to tobacco products as a possible cause.

PATHOPHYSIOLOGY

The inflammation and irritation of the vessels contribute to the development of vasospasms. These vasospasms lead to an obstruction in blood flow. The tissues become hypoxic, and the development of ischemic pain can occur. This ischemia, left untreated, can lead to ulceration and gangrene.

SIGNS AND SYMPTOMS

Intermittent claudication and other symptoms of occlusive disease are common in clients with Buerger's disease.

Other symptoms include numbness or decreased sensation and cool extremities. Lower extremities can be red or cyanotic in dependent position, and pulses may be diminished. Depending on the degree of ischemia, ulceration or gangrene may be present.

TREATMENT

Because the primary contributing factor is smoking, there is an urgency in helping the client to cease smoking. The client must be made aware of the effect smoking has on the body and that the disease will progress and further damage other vessels. Therapy for Buerger's disease is the same as those used for other arterial occlusive diseases. Careful inspection of the lower extremities for signs of breakdown is important so early treatment can begin. The use of calcium channel blockers such as diltiazem (Cardizem) promotes vasodilation and may help with intermittent claudication.

NURSING CARE

The care for clients with Buerger's disease is the same as the other arterial occlusive disorders. The care is directed at preserving the integrity of the lower extremities. Promotion of adequate circulation is an ongoing concern.

Varicose Veins

Venous dilation that causes elongated and tortuous veins is called **varicose veins.** The exact cause is unknown. Varicose veins are divided into primary and secondary varicosities.

PATHOPHYSIOLOGY

Primary varicosities are believed to be caused by a structural defect in the vessel wall. Along with the defect, the dilation of the vessel can lead to incompetent venous valves. The valves help prevent blood from refluxing. If reflux occurs, it can cause further dilation of the vessel. The superficial veins are the vessels most often involved in primary varicosities.

Secondary varicosities are caused by an acquired or congenital pathology of the deep venous system. This produces dilation of collateral and superficial veins. As a result, there is an interference of blood return to the heart, which leads to stasis, or pooling, of the blood in the deep venous system. This increases the pressure within the system pushing blood into the collateral vessels, producing varicosities in the superficial veins.

CAUSES

A number of factors can lead to varicose veins. The wall defects have been identified as a familial tendency and may be inherited. Any factor that may contribute to increasing hydrostatic pressure within the leg, such as prolonged standing, pregnancy, and obesity, may promote venous dilation. Incompetent valves within the veins can cause blockage of blood flow and lead to dilated veins.

SIGNS AND SYMPTOMS

The most common manifestation is the disfigurement of the lower extremity with primary varicosities. There may be dull pain, especially after prolonged standing. This usually can be relieved by walking or elevating the extremity. With secondary varicosities, the pain and disfigurement may be more severe. There can be development of edema or ulceration if circulation is severely compromised.

TREATMENT

Treatment is usually not indicated if the problem is merely cosmetic. Conservative treatment is geared to reduction of factors that contribute to varicose veins. Weight reduction, elevation of the extremities, walking, and exercise help increase muscle strength and contraction. One should avoid wearing tight-fitting clothes at tops of legs or waist. The use of support hose assists in blood flow return to the heart. Injection sclerotherapy is used to treat superficial varicosities. Surgical intervention involves stripping the vein to remove incompetent valves. It is performed only if the venous insufficiency cannot be controlled or prevented with conservative treatment.

NURSING CARE

The primary goal is to improve circulation, relieve pain, and avoid complications. Clients are taught the importance of assessing peripheral circulation and avoiding trauma to the lower extremities. Elastic compression stockings should be used as ordered. Risk factors are identified, and the client is helped to reduce factors that contribute to the development of varicose veins.

Venous Stasis Ulcers

Venous stasis ulcers are the end result of chronic venous insufficiency. The valves in the venous system are dysfunctional and prevent or reduce venous return. As the pressure increases, venous stasis occurs. Over time, the congestion and decreased venous circulation lead to changes in the lower extremities. There may be edema, a brownish discoloration of the leg and foot with the surrounding skin hardened and leathery in appearance. The brown color is caused when veins rupture, releasing red blood cells into the tissues; the red blood cells then break down and stain the tissue brown.

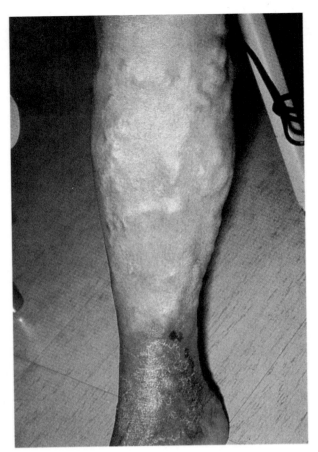

Figure 18–5. Varicose veins and chronic stasis dermatitis of the ankle. (From Reeves J, Maibach H. Clinical Dermatology Illustrated, 2nd ed, 1998. Reproduced with permission: MacLennan & Petty, Sydney.) See Plate 18.

Stasis ulcers develop from the increased pressure and rupture of small veins. Signs of skin breakdown are most commonly seen at the medial malleolus of the ankle (Fig. 18–5). Stasis ulcers are a serious complication of venous insufficiency that are difficult to cure and can affect the client's quality of life.

MEDICAL TREATMENT

The focus of treatment is to decrease the edema and treat the skin ulcerations. Compression wraps such as elastic stockings or Ace wraps to decrease edema are used. It is important to ensure that the wraps are not too tight at the top, which would prevent the return of blood to the heart.

Bed rest and elevation of legs and feet above the heart are important to assist with drainage of lower extremities. Clients are advised not to keep legs dependent and to avoid long periods of standing or sitting. They should elevate the end of their bed about 5 to 6 inches. They should be encouraged to exercise and walk at frequent intervals during nonacute episodes. Clients should be taught not to cross their legs or wear constricting clothing that would decrease venous blood return to the heart.

Skin ulcers are usually cultured and treated with topical antibiotics. Wound care can be chronic and challenging. (See Chapter 51.) An Unna boot, which is a bootlike dressing of gauze with zinc oxide paste, may be used to promote healing in severe ulcers. Zinc promotes wound healing and can be soothing. The Unna boot is changed and reapplied as ordered, usually every 2 to 7 days. Skin grafting may be necessary if ulcerations are severe or do not heal.

NURSING INTERVENTIONS

The client's leg is protected from injury. Heating devices are avoided due to decreased sensitivity. The client is taught treatment measures used to reduce edema and pain. Emotional support is provided to clients with chronic ulcers that affect quality of life and require ongoing wound care.

Lymphatic System

The lymphatic system returns fluid from other tissues in the body to the bloodstream. It is a pumpless system with one-way valves that return the fluid to the heart. Any interruption in the flow of lymph results in edema.

LYMPHANGITIS

Lymphangitis is an inflammation of the lymphatic channels. The infection can occur in the arms or legs and is commonly caused by staphylococcus or streptococcus bacteria.

Signs and Symptoms

Symptoms include pain at the site of the infected area, which may appear reddish in color. There may also be a red streak that follows the lymphatic channel. The client may experience chills and fever. Lymph nodes in the area of infection can be enlarged and painful.

Treatment

Antibiotic therapy is initiated with a broad-spectrum antibiotic as the drug of choice. The use of heat on the extremity, as well as elevating it, can help improve circulation. Physicians may order the use of pneumatic pressure devices to help alleviate congestion.

Nursing Care

Frequent assessment and meticulous wound care, if needed, are performed. The nurse monitors the size of the extremity and notifies the physician of any increase in size or possible spread of infection.

HOME HEALTH HINTS

- If a client reports chest pain, ask what time the pain began. If it is relieved by nitroglycerin within 15 minutes, it indicates angina. If not, it is usually an MI. Ask the client if rest relieves the pain. It will relieve angina but not an MI.

- The elderly client will not usually describe angina as pain, but may say it feels like pressure, or burning, or a butterfly. Ask what the client was doing when the angina began, such as yard work, eating, receiving emotional news, or engaging in sexual activity. Symptoms of accompanying nausea or sweating are common with an MI.

- Post-MI clients will usually come home with a schedule of graduated activities. Review them with the client and caregivers and post it in the home.

- Encourage the caregiver to walk with the client outdoors when the weather is nice, avoiding extreme cold or heat. Caution them to avoid uneven sidewalks and areas with no sidewalks.

- When a client is enrolled in a formal cardiac rehabilitation program, be sure to reinforce the exercises within the formal guidelines, incorporating them into the home health care plan. The nurse should inspect the layout of the house to identify those areas or the daily activities of the client that cause more exertion than the client realizes. Examples are the number of steps or stairs inside and outside and amount of reaching, pushing, or pulling that the client actually does.

- When inquiring about bowel movements, ask if the client has to strain. This should be avoided. Ask the physician to prescribe a laxative or stool softener. Remember that all over-the-counter drugs should be listed on the home health treatment plan.

- A home health social worker may be appropriate for visiting a post-MI or postsurgical cardiac patient and to provide input into the plan of care (anxiety and environmental stress reduction, relaxation techniques).

- When a client reports cardiac symptoms, the nurse should ask about possible precipitating factors such as emotional stress, alcohol or drug abuse, or if a hot bath was taken.

- When a client wears elastic compression stockings and the home health nurse has to check the appearance of the lower extremities, the client should lie down to help remove the compression stockings. They should be put back on while the client is still lying down.

- Remind clients to put the stockings on before getting out of bed in the morning and leave them on all day.

- Compression stockings should be discarded when they become too easy to put on. Because they are expensive, many clients keep them even after they are ineffective.

- Instruct the home health client on these easy exercises to enhance venous return: going up and down on tiptoe when standing, and pedaling (simulating using car brake and gas pedals) when sitting.

- Clients with varicose veins should not jump or lift weights. They should be instructed to avoid wearing high heels or using hot tubs. They should elevate their legs on a regular basis.

- When assessing edema of a bedridden patient, check all dependent areas, especially the sacral area.

- Private mobile x-ray companies will come to a client's home to perform x-rays and ECGs. If the physician orders these tests, inform the client of the service, especially if moving the client will be difficult. Check the yellow pages.

- Niacin is the most inexpensive cholesterol-lowering drug. The side effect of skin flushing from niacin can be very pronounced and distressing for the client. Instruct the client that it will subside with continuous therapy. Aspirin, given 30 minutes before the niacin, will decrease the flushing if ordered by the physician.

Review Questions

1. Which one of the following is a risk factor that can be changed for CAD?
   a. Age
   b. Cholesterol
   c. Heredity
   d. Gender

2. Which of the following is a risk factor that can be controlled to prevent the development of cardiovascular disease?
   a. Family history of cardiovascular disease
   b. Hypertension
   c. Ethnicity
   d. Family history of diabetes mellitus

3. Mr. White was admitted to the hospital a week ago with an acute myocardial infarction. He calls the nurse to his room, reporting chest pain. What action should be performed first?
   a. Administer nitroglycerin sublingually.
   b. Take vital signs.
   c. Raise head of bed 30 to 45 degrees.
   d. Notify physician.

4. The nurse is teaching a client with myocardial infarction how to avoid activity that results in Valsalva's maneuver. Which of the following statements by the client would indicate to the nurse that the teaching has been effective?
   a. "I will breathe normally when moving."
   b. "I will use a straw to drink oral fluids."

c. "I will take fewer but deeper breaths."
d. "I will clench my teeth when moving."

5. Which one of the following is a classic symptom of peripheral arterial occlusive disease?
   a. Stasis ulcers
   b. Edema
   c. Intermittent claudication
   d. Angina

6. Mr. Thomas has arterial insufficiency of the lower extremities. Expected physical findings include which of the following?
   a. Lymphedema
   b. Pedal edema
   c. Absence of pedal pulses
   d. Bluish cast to extremities

7. The nurse is caring for Lou, 64, who has had an MI and has peripheral arterial disease. Lou is being discharged from the hospital. The client is taking furosemide (Lasix) and digoxin (Lanoxin). Which of the following statements by Lou would indicate understanding of discharge instructions for managing the *pain* of peripheral arterial disease?
   a. "I will lie down frequently."
   b. "I will use a reclining chair."
   c. "I will sit with my legs down."
   d. "I will do knee flexion exercises."

ANSWERS TO CRITICAL THINKING

CRITICAL THINKING: Sally

1. Place on bed rest, administer O$_2$ per nasal cannula at 2 liters per minute if not already on, assess blood pressure and pulse, administer nitroglycerin sublingual as ordered, obtain ECG, and notify physician.
2. Having an anginal attack versus acute MI.
3. With angina, nitroglycerin will usually stop chest pain. Rest may also alleviate chest pain. Neither nitroglycerin nor rest will effect an acute MI.
4. Patient history, ECG changes with ST-segment elevation, CPK-MB elevation, and elevated troponin I.
5. Nitroglycerin drip, morphine, and anticoagulant therapy (heparin or thrombolytic agents) to lyse the clot. A cardiac catheterization to determine which coronary artery is blocked. A coronary artery bypass graft may be done to reroute blood.
6. Educate patient about the hazards of smoking and being overweight.

CRITICAL THINKING: Mary

1. Assess leg for pulses, color, and temperature in femoral, popliteal, dorsalis pedis, and posterior tibial.

2. If unable to palpate pulses, use a Doppler that enhances sound to locate pulses.
3. Possible embolism above left femoral artery.
4. Complete bed rest, protect the leg, and notify the physician.
5. Medication for pain. Use of an anticoagulant, such as heparin. If no pulses are present, use of a thrombolytic agent, such as streptokinase or tissue plasminogen activator, which dissolves already formed clots. Surgery.
6. Thrombolectomy or embolectomy.

REFERENCES

1. Sempos, CT, et al: Prevalence of high blood cholesterol among US adults. JAMA 269:3009, 1993.
2. Williams, CL, and Bollella, M: Guidelines for screening, evaluating, and treating children with hypercholesterolemia. J Pediatr Health Care 9:153, 1995.
3. Newton, K, and Froelicher, E: Coronary heart disease risk factors. In Woods, S, et al (eds): Cardiac Nursing, ed 3. JB Lippincott, Philadelphia, 1995.
4. Groff, JL, Gropper, SS, and Hunt, SM: Advanced Nutrition and Human Metabolism, ed 2. West, Minneapolis, 1995.
5. Levin, R: Caring for the cardiac spouse. Am J Nurs 93(11):51, 1993.

BIBLIOGRAPHY

Adams, J, et al: Improved detection of cardiac contusion with cardiac troponin I. Am Heart J 131(2):308, 1996.
Apple, S: New trends in thrombolytic therapy. RN 96(1):30, 1996.
Ashton, K: Perceived learning needs of men and women after myocardial infarction. J Cardiovasc Nurs 12(1):93, 1997.
Conhers, K, and Lamas, G: Postmyocardial infarction patients: Experience from the SAVE trial. Am J Crit Care 4(1):23, 1995.
Corwan, T: Compression hosiery. Prof Nurse 12(12):88, 1997.
Deglin, JH, and Vallerand, AH: Davis's Drug Guide for Nurses. FA Davis, Philadelphia, 1995.
Fowler, JP: How to respond rapidly when chest pain strikes. Nursing 96(4):42, 1996.
Harris, A, Brown-Etris, M, and Troyer-Candle, J: Managing vascular leg ulcers. Part 1: Assessment. Am J Nurs 96(1):38, 1996.
Harris, A, Brown-Etris, M, and Troyer-Candle, J: Managing vascular leg ulcers. Part 2: Treatment. Am J Nurs 96(2):38, 1996.
Harris, T, et al: Carrying the burden of cardiovascular risk in old age: Associations of weight and weight change with prevalent cardiovascular disease, risk factors, and health status in the Cardiovascular Health Study. Am J Clin Nutr 66(4):837, 1997.
Hayes, D: Understanding coronary atherectomy. Am J Nurs 96(12):38, 1996.
Ignatavicius, D, Workman, M, and Mishler, M: Medical Surgical Nursing: A Nursing Process Approach, ed 2. WB Saunders, Philadelphia, 1995.
Ignatavicius, DD, and Hausman, KA: Pocket Companion for Medical-Surgical Nursing, ed 2. WB Saunders, Philadelphia, 1995.
Jaffe, M: Medical-Surgical Nursing Care Plans: Nursing Diagnosis and Intervention, ed 3. Appleton & Lange, Norwalk, Conn, 1996.
Lazure, L, and Baun, M: Increasing patient control of family visiting in the coronary care unit. Am J Crit Care 4(2):157, 1995.
LeMone, P, and Burke, K: Medical-Surgical Nursing: Critical Thinking in Client Care. Addison-Wesley Nursing, Redwood City, California, 1996.

Manune, J, and Giordano, J: Experience with open-heeled Unna boot application technique. J Vasc Nurs 15(2):63, 1997.

Muir, N, et al: The influence of dosage form on aspirin kinetics: Implications for acute cardiovascular use. Curr Med Res Opin 13(10):547, 1997.

Nunnelle, J: Healing venous ulcers. RN 60(11):38, 1997.

Ondrusek, R: Spotting an MI before it's an MI. RN 96(4):26, 1996.

Polaski, A, and Tatro, S: Luckmann's Core Principles and Practice of Medical-Surgical Nursing. WB Saunders, Philadelphia, 1996.

Regensteiner, J, and Hiatt, W: Medical management of peripheral arterial disease. J Vasc Interv Radiol 5(5):669, 1994.

Tyler, D: Activity progression in acute cardiac patients. J Cardiovasc Nurs 12(1):16, 1997.

Williams, K, and Morton, P: Diagnosis and treatment of acute myocardial infarction. AACN Clin Issues 6(3):375, 1995.

Yu, C, Chan, T, Tsoi, W, and Sanderson, J: Heparin therapy in the Chinese—Lower doses are required. Q J Med 90(8):535, 1997.

Nursing Care of Clients with Cardiac Valvular Disorders

Linda S. Williams

Learning Objectives

Upon completion of this chapter, the student will be able to:

1. Describe the pathophysiology, etiology, and signs and symptoms of mitral valve prolapse.
2. Describe the pathophysiology, etiology, and signs and symptoms of mitral valve stenosis.
3. Describe the pathophysiology, etiology, and signs and symptoms of mitral valve regurgitation.
4. Describe the pathophysiology, etiology, and signs and symptoms of aortic valve stenosis.
5. Describe the pathophysiology, etiology, and signs and symptoms of aortic valve regurgitation.
6. Explain the importance of prophylactic antibiotic therapy in preventing endocarditis for clients with valvular disorders.
7. List diagnostic tests for valvular disorders.
8. Describe surgical procedures used to treat valvular disorders.
9. Describe nursing care for clients with valvular disorders.

Key Words

annuloplasty (**AN**-yoo-loh-PLAS-tee)

atrial kick (**AY**-tree-uhl **KIK**)

commissurotomy (KOM-i-shur-**AHT**-oh-mee)

insufficiency (IN-suh-**FISH**-en-see)

murmur (**MUR**-mur)

regurgitation (ree-GUR-ji-**TAY**-shun)

stenosis (ste-**NOH**-sis)

valvuloplasty (**VAL**-vyoo-loh-PLAS-tee)

---

stenosed: stenos—narrow
regurgitation: re—again + gurgitare—to flood
insufficiency: in—not + sufficiens—sufficient

In the normal heart, blood flows in one direction because of the presence of the heart valves. The heart valves open and close to allow one-way flow of blood. There are four valves in the heart: mitral, tricuspid, pulmonic, and aortic. (See Fig. 15–2.) The chordae tendineae and papillary muscles are attachment structures for the mitral and tricuspid valves. They ensure that the valves close tightly. The pulmonic and aortic valves do not have these attachment structures.

Damage to the valves or their surrounding structures can result in abnormal valvular functioning (Fig. 19–1). The valves of the left side of the heart are most commonly affected and are discussed in this chapter. Forward blood flow can be hindered if the valve is narrowed, or **stenosed,** and does not open completely. If the valve does not close completely, blood backs up, which is referred to as **regurgitation** or **insufficiency.** The abnormal blood flow increases the workload of the heart and increases the pressures in the affected heart chamber. With stenosis, afterload is increased due to inadequate emptying of the heart chamber. Preload is increased with regurgitation because extra blood volume reenters the heart chamber.

Valvular damage may occur from congenital defects, rheumatic heart disease, or infections. Congenital defects occur mainly in children, and rheumatic heart disease occurs mainly in adults. Antibiotic therapy helps prevent rheumatic heart disease.

LEARNING TIP

The opening of a stenosed valve and an insufficient valve look very similar, and the results of extra blood building up in a chamber are the same (Fig. 19–1). However, the problem is different. Remember what the defect is in each disorder to understand why the blood is building up in a chamber.

A valve that does not open fully (stenosed) will not allow a chamber to empty normally. Blood will build up in that chamber as a result. For example, mitral stenosis does not allow the left atrium to empty easily, so blood builds up in the left atrium.

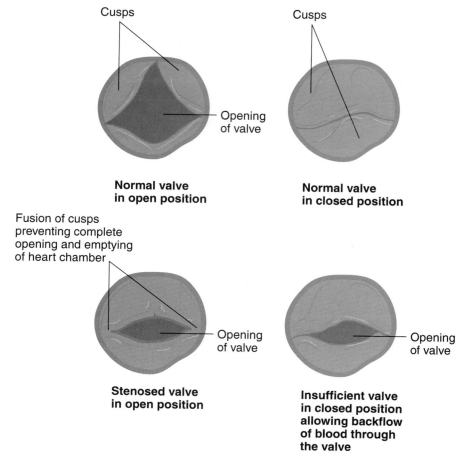

Cusps

Cusps

Opening
of valve

**Normal valve
in open position**

**Normal valve
in closed position**

Fusion of cusps
preventing complete
opening and emptying
of heart chamber

Opening
of valve

Opening
of valve

**Stenosed valve
in open position**

**Insufficient valve
in closed position
allowing backflow
of blood through
the valve**

Figure 19–1. Openings of stenosed and insufficient valves compared with a normal valve.

A valve that does not close fully (insufficient) allows blood to flow back into the chamber that emptied. Blood will build up in that chamber as a result. For example, mitral insufficiency allows blood to backflow from the left ventricle into the left atrium after the left atrium has emptied, so blood builds up in the left atrium.

Valvular Disorders

MITRAL VALVE PROLAPSE

Pathophysiology

During ventricular systole, when pressures in the left ventricle rise, the leaflets of the mitral valve normally remain closed and stay within the atrioventricular junction. In mitral valve prolapse (MVP), however, the leaflets bulge backward into the left atrium during systole. The bulging leaflets may or may not fit together. Often there are no functional problems seen with MVP. However, if the leaflets do not fit together, mitral regurgitation can occur with varying degrees of severity.

Etiology

MVP tends to be hereditary, although the cause is unknown. Infections that damage the mitral valve may be a contributing factor. It is the most common form of valvular heart disease and typically occurs in women 20 to 55 years of age.

Signs and Symptoms

Most clients with MVP do not have symptoms. However, symptoms that may occur include chest pain, dysrhythmias, palpitations, dizziness, or syncope. A **murmur** or click may be heard in some clients. Emotional stress may trigger symptoms.

Diagnostic Tests

Several diagnostic tests can be used for MVP (Table 19–1). An echocardiogram can detect MVP. A normal electrocardiogram (ECG) is usually seen with MVP. A cardiac catheterization shows the bulging leaflets of the mitral valve on angiogram.

Table 19–1. **Diagnostic Tests for Cardiac Valvular Disorders**

History and physical examination
Electrocardiogram
Chest x-ray
Echocardiogram
Cardiac catheterization

Medical Treatment

Unless clients have severe mitral regurgitation, MVP is a benign disorder. No treatment is needed unless symptoms are present (Table 19–2). Stimulants and caffeine should be avoided to prevent symptoms. Stress management may reduce the occurrence of symptoms. Preventive antibiotic therapy before invasive procedures may be needed for some clients.[1]

Client Education

Information on endocarditis prevention is essential for clients with most valvular problems. Damaged cardiac valves are prone to developing infection from organisms such as *Staphylococcus epidermidis* or *Streptococcus viridans*. During invasive procedures these organisms can enter the circulation and attack the damaged valves. Bacteria are attracted to damaged valves, attach to them, and multiply. Clients should be taught the possible need for prophylactic antibiotics before invasive procedures, including dental work or surgery, to prevent the occurrence of endocarditis.[1] If clients are unsure of the need for antibiotics they should ask their physician.

Table 19–2. **Medical Treatment for Cardiac Valvular Disorders**

Prophylactic antibiotic therapy considered
Anticoagulant therapy
Medication therapy
  Digitalis
  Diuretics
  Antidysrhythmics
Low-sodium diet
Percutaneous transluminal balloon valvuloplasty
Surgical
  Valvuloplasty
    Closed commissurotomy
    Open commissurotomy
    Annuloplasty
  Valve replacement

CRITICAL THINKING: Sue

Sue, 32, has a mitral valve prolapse. She reports palpitations when she experiences stress. She drinks three cups of coffee daily. She is admitted for an outpatient cystoscopy.

1. What may the nurse hear when auscultating heart sounds?
2. Why does Sue experience palpitations?
3. What medication might the nurse expect to be ordered preoperatively?
4. Why does Sue need to be taught that she may need prophylactic antibiotics before invasive procedures?
5. What other teaching does Sue need to manage her MVP?

Answers at end of chapter.

MITRAL STENOSIS

Pathophysiology

Mitral stenosis results from thickening of the mitral valve leaflets and shortening of the chordae tendineae, causing narrowing of the valve opening. This narrowed opening obstructs blood flow from the left atrium into the left ventricle. The left atrium enlarges to hold the extra blood volume caused by the obstruction. As a result of this increased blood volume, pressures rise in the left atrium. Pressures then rise in the pulmonary circulation and the right ventricle as blood volume backs up from the left atrium. The right ventricle dilates to handle the increased volume. Eventually, the right ventricle fails from this excessive workload, reducing the blood volume delivered to the left ventricle and subsequently decreasing cardiac output.

Etiology

The major cause of mitral stenosis is rheumatic heart disease. Less common causes include congenital defects of the mitral valve, tumors, rheumatoid arthritis, systemic lupus erythematosus, calcium deposits, and rheumatic endocarditis.

Signs and Symptoms

Mitral stenosis occurs most commonly in 20- to 40-year-old women. Clients may be initially asymptomatic. Then mild symptoms progressing to more severe symptoms develop. Pulmonary symptoms are most commonly seen. Dyspnea, cough, and hemoptysis from pulmonary congestion are the major symptoms. Fatigue and intolerance to activity result from decreased cardiac output. Palpitations from atrial flutter or fibrillation caused by atrial enlargement and chest pain from decreased cardiac output may be experienced. A click or low-pitched murmur may be heard. Complications from emboli formed from the stasis of blood in the left atrium include stroke and seizures. If the right ventricle fails, symptoms related to heart failure are seen. (See Chapter 21.)

Diagnostic Tests

Mitral stenosis is diagnosed with data from the client history and physical examination and findings from diagnostic tests. (See Table 19–1.) The ECG shows enlargement of the left atrium and right ventricle and changes in the P waveform. Atrial flutter or fibrillation may be seen. A chest x-ray confirms enlargement of the affected heart chambers. Echocardiogram shows the narrowed mitral valve opening and decreased motion of the valve. Cardiac catheterization measures the pressures in the heart chambers and pulmonary vessels, as well as cardiac output. Elevated pressures and a reduced cardiac output are found. Angiography during the catheterization reveals the severity of the stenosis.

Medical Treatment

Prophylactic antibiotic therapy may be given to prevent infectious endocarditis, especially before invasive procedures.[1] Anticoagulants are given to clients with atrial fibrillation to prevent development of emboli from stasis of blood in the atrium. If heart failure develops, symptoms are treated with medications such as digitalis and diuretics and other therapies used for heart failure. (See Chapter 21.)

Percutaneous transluminal balloon valvuloplasty (PTBV), which uses a balloon to dilate the stenosed heart valve, is done in a cardiac catheterization laboratory (Fig. 19–2). It is an alternative to surgery for clients who are poor surgical risks, such as older clients. To reach the mitral valve, one or two balloon catheters are inserted via the venous circulation to the right atrium. Then the catheter is threaded through a small hole pierced in the atrial septum into the left atrium through the mitral valve. If two balloon catheters are used they are placed side by side in the valve opening and inflated. Inflation of the balloon opens the stenosed valve leaflets. The septal puncture closes on its own. There are fewer complications with PTBV than with surgery. Complications may include dysrhythmias, emboli, hemorrhage, or cardiac tamponade.

Surgical treatment includes **commissurotomy** or **annuloplasty,** which are forms of valvular repair (**valvuloplasty**) or valve replacement. These procedures usually require major surgery using cardiopulmonary bypass and are palliative, not curative. In commissurotomy, the valve leaflets that have adhered to each other and closed the

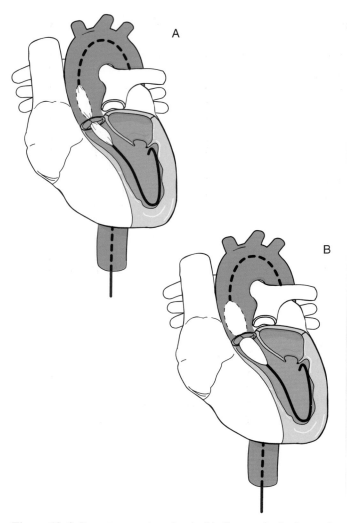

Figure 19–2. Percutaneous transluminal balloon valvuloplasty of aortic valve.

opening between them, known as the commissure, are separated to enlarge the valve opening. A closed commissurotomy is commonly done, which does not require cardiopulmonary bypass. In closed commissurotomy, the valve is not seen directly. Most commonly a dilator or the surgeon's finger is inserted via a midsternal incision and puncture of the apex into the left ventricle. Then the mitral valve is opened with the dilator or finger.

Annuloplasty is the repair or reconstruction of the valve leaflets or annulus. It may involve the use of prosthetic rings. Valve replacement with prosthetic valves has been done since 1952. Valve replacement uses mechanical or biological valves from animal or human tissue (Fig. 19–3). Valvular surgery is discussed in Chapter 22.

---

commissurotomy: commissura—joining together + tome—incision

annuloplasty: annulus—ring + plasty—formed

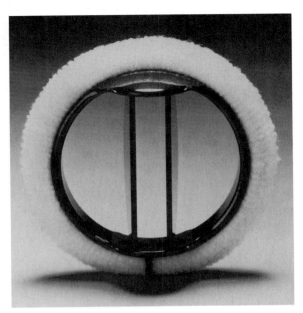

Figure 19–3. Valve prostheses. St. Jude Medical® mechanical heart valve. (Photograph: Courtesy of St. Jude Medical, Inc. All rights reserved. St. Jude Medical® is a registered trademark of St. Jude Medical, Inc.)

MITRAL REGURGITATION

Pathophysiology

Mitral regurgitation, or insufficiency, is the incomplete closure of the mitral valve. It allows some backflow of blood into the left atrium with each contraction of the left ventricle. Factors that prevent the mitral valve leaflets from fitting together tightly may include tearing, shortening or rigidity of a leaflet, or shortening of the chordae tendineae.

When the mitral valve does not close completely, backflow of blood into the left atrium occurs. This blood is then extra volume that is added to the incoming blood from the lungs. With chronic mitral regurgitation, the increase in blood volume dilates and increases pressures in the left atrium. In response to the extra blood volume delivered by the left atrium, the left ventricle compensates by dilating. If the compensatory mechanism of dilation is inadequate, pressures rise in the pulmonary circulation and then in the right ventricle as blood volume backs up from the left atrium. The left ventricle and eventually the right ventricle may fail from this increased strain.

Etiology

The major cause of mitral regurgitation is rheumatic heart disease. Other causes include endocarditis, rupture or dysfunction of the chordae tendineae or papillary muscle, MVP, or congenital defects.

Signs and Symptoms

Initially clients may be asymptomatic. The symptoms of chronic mitral regurgitation are similar to those of mitral stenosis. Dyspnea and cough occur from increased pulmonary congestion. Palpitations and an irregular pulse from atrial fibrillation may result. Weakness and fatigue from decreased cardiac output occur if the left ventricle begins to fail. A high-pitched systolic murmur is heard at the heart's apex, and an extra heart sound, S_3, may be heard.

If acute mitral regurgitation develops, such as in papillary muscle rupture following myocardial infarction, pulmonary edema and shock symptoms will be exhibited.

Diagnostic Tests

The ECG shows enlargement of the left atrium and left ventricle and changes in the P waveform. Atrial flutter or fibrillation may be seen. A chest x-ray confirms hypertrophy of the affected heart chambers. An echocardiogram shows left atrial enlargement and regurgitation of blood. Cardiac catheterization with dye also shows regurgitation.

Medical Treatment

Prophylactic antibiotic therapy may be given to prevent infectious endocarditis, especially before invasive procedures.[1] Vasodilators are given to reduce afterload, making it easier for the left ventricle to eject blood into the aorta, thus decreasing regurgitation. Heart failure symptoms are treated according to heart failure treatment. (See Chapter 21.) Surgical treatment includes mitral valve replacement (Fig. 19–4) or annuloplasty. (See Table 19–2.)

AORTIC STENOSIS

Pathophysiology

Blood flow from the left ventricle to the aorta through the narrowed aortic valve is obstructed. The opening of the aortic valve may be narrowed from thickening, scarring, calcification, or fusing of the valve's leaflets. To compensate for the difficulty in ejecting blood into the aorta, the left ventricle contracts more forcefully. In chronic stenosis, the left ventricle hypertrophies and the left atrium produces a stronger contraction, **atrial kick,** to maintain normal cardiac output. With increased narrowing of the valve opening, the compensatory mechanisms are unable to continue and the left ventricle fails.

Etiology

The major causes of aortic stenosis are congenital defects or rheumatic heart disease. Mitral valve stenosis is often

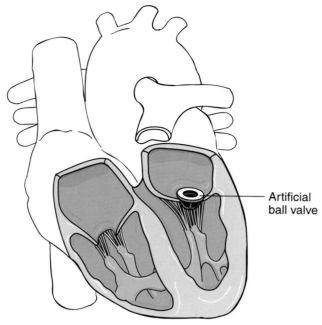

Figure 19–4. Mitral valve replacement with ball valve prosthesis.

also present when the cause is rheumatic heart disease. Calcification of the aortic valve can be related to aging.

Signs and Symptoms

It may take many years or decades before signs or symptoms of aortic stenosis are observed. If the mitral valve is diseased signs and symptoms may appear earlier, allowing the detection of the aortic stenosis.

Angina pectoris is a primary symptom that occurs from the increased oxygen needs of the myocardium. The extra workload of the left ventricle and the hypertrophy of the cardiac muscle require more oxygen. Angina results if these oxygen needs are not met. In the young client, angina indicates severe obstruction.

Other signs and symptoms include a murmur, syncope from dysrhythmias or decreased cardiac output, and heart failure signs and symptoms. Orthopnea, dyspnea on exertion, and fatigue are indicators of left ventricular failure. Progressive heart failure can result in pulmonary edema and right-sided heart failure.

Diagnostic Tests

The ECG shows enlargement of the left ventricle and left atrium. A chest x-ray confirms hypertrophy of the left ventricle. Left atrial enlargement may be seen but occurs primarily when mitral stenosis is also present. An echocardiogram shows thickening of the left ventricular wall and impaired movement of the aortic valve. Cardiac catheteri-

zation will show elevated left ventricular pressure and decreased cardiac output.

Medical Treatment

Prophylactic antibiotics may be given to prevent infectious endocarditis, especially before invasive procedures.[1] Heart failure symptoms are treated with medications such as digitalis and diuretics and other therapies used for heart failure. (See Chapter 21.) Evaluation for surgery is made. The treatment of choice is valve replacement because of the risk of sudden death when even moderate symptoms are present. (See Table 19–2.)

AORTIC REGURGITATION

Pathophysiology

The aortic valve cusps may be scarred, thickened, or shortened in aortic regurgitation. A backflow of blood from the aorta into the left ventricle occurs if the aortic valve cusps do not close completely. The left ventricle's blood volume increases with this backflow of blood, as well as the blood entering from the left atrium. To handle the increased volume, the left ventricle dilates and hypertrophies to deliver a stronger contraction. The stronger contraction ejects more blood volume with each beat. The dilation in aortic regurgitation is greater than dilation in other valvular disorders. In severe regurgitation, the left ventricle may fail, cardiac output drops, and pulmonary edema develops.

Etiology

Rheumatic heart disease is the usual cause of aortic regurgitation. Other causes include congenital defects, syphilis, endocarditis, severe hypertension, and rheumatoid arthritis. More than 70 percent of the clients with aortic regurgitation are men. An acute cause of aortic regurgitation is aortic dissection.

Signs and Symptoms

Exertional dyspnea and fatigue are the first symptoms of chronic aortic regurgitation. They appear after years of progressive valvular dysfunction. The client may report feeling a forceful heart beat. The palpated pulse is forceful and then quickly collapses (Corrigan's pulse). A click and murmur may be heard. The diastolic blood pressure decreases to widen the pulse pressure. This compensates for an increase in systolic blood pressure. Angina pectoris may occur late. The angina is atypical, often happening at night, when a lower pulse rate results in delivery of less oxygen to the myocardium. Eventually heart failure symptoms develop if the left ventricle fails.

In acute dysfunction, profound symptoms of pulmonary distress, chest pain, and shock symptoms occur. The prognosis is poor.

Diagnostic Tests

The ECG shows left ventricle hypertrophy. A chest x-ray confirms hypertrophy of the left ventricle and aorta. With severe regurgitation, left atrial enlargement may be seen. An echocardiogram shows an enlarged left ventricle. Cardiac catheterization reveals elevated left ventricular diastolic pressure and, with dye injection, shows the regurgitation of blood into the left ventricle.

Medical Treatment

Surgical replacement is the treatment of choice even if symptoms are absent. (See Table 19–2.) The surgery should be done before the left ventricle becomes dysfunctional. Prophylactic antibiotic therapy may be given to prevent infectious endocarditis, especially before invasive procedures.[1]

NURSING PROCESS FOR VALVULAR DISORDERS

Nursing Assessment

A history that includes information presented in Table 19–3 is obtained. Vital signs are measured and recorded. Heart sounds are auscultated to detect murmurs. Signs and symptoms of heart failure are noted. (See Chapter 21.)

Nursing Diagnosis

The major nursing diagnoses for all valvular disorders are the same and include those for heart failure as well when heart failure symptoms are present. (See Nursing Care Plan Box 19–1 for the Client with Cardiac Valvular Disorders.) The diagnoses may include but are not limited to the following:

- Pain related to reduced coronary artery blood flow and increased myocardial oxygen needs
- Decreased cardiac output related to valvular stenosis or insufficiency or heart failure
- Activity intolerance related to decreased oxygen delivery from decreased cardiac output

---

Table 19–3. **Nursing Assessment for Clients with Cardiac Valvular Disorders**

Subjective Data
Health History
Infections—rheumatic fever, endocarditis, streptococcal or staphylococcal, syphilis
Congenital defects
Cardiac disease—myocardial infarction, cardiomyopathy
Respiratory
Dyspnea at rest, on exertion, when lying, or that awakens client?
Cough or hemoptysis?
Cardiovascular
Any palpitations, chest pain, dizziness, fatigue, activity intolerance?
Medications
Knowledge of Condition
Coping Skills

Objective Data
Respiratory
Crackles, wheezes, tachypnea
Cardiovascular
Murmurs, extra heart sounds, dysrhythmias, edema, jugular vein distention (JVD), Corrigan's pulse, increased or decreased pulse pressure
Integumentary
Clubbing; cyanosis; diaphoresis; cold, clammy skin; pallor
Diagnostic Test Findings

NURSING CARE PLAN BOX 19–1
FOR THE CLIENT WITH CARDIAC VALVULAR DISORDERS

Pain related to reduced coronary artery blood flow and increased myocardial oxygen needs

Client Outcomes
Client reports that pain management relieves pain satisfactorily and describes total pain management plan.

Evaluation of Outcomes
Does client report satisfactory pain relief? Is client able to describe pain management plan?

Interventions	Rationale	Evaluation
Assess pain using rating scale such as 1 to 10.	Self-report is the most reliable indicator of pain.	Does client report pain using scale?
Provide pain medication such as nitroglycerin prn.	Chest pain is caused by ischemia from reduced cardiac blood flow. Vasodilators improve blood flow.	Is client's rating of pain lower after medication?
Teach pacing of activities with rest periods.	Ischemia is reduced when activities are paced with periodic rest.	Is client able to complete desired activities without pain?

GERIATRIC		
When assessing pain speak clearly and slowly so elderly client can hear.	If elderly client does not hear or misunderstands, pain may not be reported accurately to ensure appropriate intervention provided.	Does client hear and report pain and relief accurately using pain scale?

Decreased cardiac output related to valvular stenosis or insufficiency or heart failure

Client Outcomes
Client has adequate cardiac output as evidenced by vital signs within normal limits (WNL), no dyspnea or fatigue.

Evaluation of Outcomes
Does client have vital signs WNL with no dyspnea or fatigue?

Interventions	Rationale	Evaluation
Assess vital signs, chest pain, and fatigue.	Vital signs, chest pain, and fatigue are indicators of cardiac output decline.	Are vital signs WNL with no chest pain or fatigue?
Give oxygen as ordered.	Supplemental oxygen provides more oxygen to the heart.	Is breathing pattern normal?
Provide bed rest or rest periods as ordered.	Cardiac workload and oxygen needs are reduced with rest.	Are vital signs WNL and no fatigue reported?
Elevate head of bed 45 degrees.	Venous return to heart is reduced and chest expansion improved.	Are vital signs WNL and respirations easy?

GERIATRIC		
Assess for cardiac medication side effects and teach client side effects to report.	Toxic side effects are more common due to altered metabolism and excretion of medications in the elderly.	Are side effects present for medications client is taking? Does client understand side effects to report?

continued

NURSING CARE PLAN BOX 19–1 *(continued)*

Activity intolerance related to decreased oxygen delivery from decreased cardiac output

Client Outcomes
Client will show normal changes in vital signs with less fatigue in response to activity.

Evaluation of Outcomes
Does client have normal changes in vital signs with activity? Does client report decreased fatigue with activity?

Interventions	*Rationale*	*Evaluation*
Assist as needed with activities of daily living (ADL).	Energy is conserved with ADL assistance.	Are all ADL completed?
Provide rest and space activities.	Cardiac workload and oxygen needs are reduced with rest.	Are vital signs WNL with activity?
GERIATRIC		
Slow pace of care and allow client extra time to perform activities.	Elderly clients can often perform activities if allowed time to slowly perform them and rest at intervals.	Is client able to perform activities when allowed extra time?
Ensure safety when mobilizing elderly client.	Orthostatic hypertension is common in the elderly.	Does BP remain WNL when changing position? Does client ambulate without injury?

Fluid volume excess related to heart failure and the secondary reduction in renal blood flow for filtration

Client Outcomes
Client will have clear breath sounds, no edema or weight gain.

Evaluation of Outcomes
Does client have clear breath sounds, no edema, no weight gain?

Interventions	*Rationale*	*Evaluation*
Assess for edema, weight gain, JVD, lung crackles.	Excess fluid is indicated by edema, sudden weight gain, JVD, and crackles in the lungs.	Is edema, weight gain, JVD, or crackles present?
Decrease sodium intake as ordered.	Sodium retains fluid.	Does client restrict sodium intake?
Administer diuretics as ordered.	Diuretics promote fluid excretion.	Does output increase following diuretics?
GERIATRIC		
Recognize that fluid volume excess is particularly serious in elderly.	Normal aging changes of decreased cardiac output and stroke volume increase risk for fluid volume excess.	Are risk factors present for fluid volume excess? Are fluid volume excess signs and symptoms present and reported?

Ineffective management of therapeutic regimen related to lack of knowledge about disorder

Client Outcomes
Client verbalizes knowledge of disorder and willingness to comply with therapeutic regimen.

Evaluation of Outcomes
Does client explain hypertension, treatment, and importance of complying with treatment?

continued

NURSING CARE PLAN BOX 19–1 *(continued)*		
Interventions	**Rationale**	**Evaluation**
Explain condition, symptoms, complications. Explain need to prevent endocarditis with prophylactic antibiotics. Explain medications or therapies ordered.	Client must have basic knowledge to comply with therapy. Antibiotics are necessary before invasive procedures to prevent endocarditis. Compliance and safe use of medications are promoted with an adequate knowledge base.	Is client able to verbalize knowledge taught? Can client state rationale for prophylactic antibiotics? Can client explain medications and therapies?
GERIATRIC		
Include caregivers/family in educational sessions.	Compliance increases if support systems understand instructions and client needs.	Do caregivers/family participate in sessions and offer client support?

- Fluid volume excess related to heart failure and the secondary reduction in renal blood flow for filtration
- Ineffective management of therapeutic regimen related to lack of knowledge about disorder

Planning

The client and family should be included in planning care. The client's goals are to (1) report that the pain management regimen relieves pain, (2) maintain vital signs and oxygen saturation within normal range, (3) maintain desired activities, (4) remain free of edema and maintain clear lung sounds, and (5) understand the disease and its treatment.

Nursing Interventions

Nursing care is aimed at relieving clients' pain, maintaining clients' normal cardiac function, improving clients' ability to participate in activity, maintaining fluid balance, educating clients to understand the therapeutic management of their valvular disorder, promoting prevention techniques, monitoring symptoms, and providing preoperative and postoperative care as needed. See Nursing Care Plan Box 19–1 for the Client with Cardiac Valvular Disorders for specific nursing interventions.

Pain management is achieved by assessing pain on an ongoing basis using a rating scale such as 1 to 10 with 10 being the most severe pain. Providing pain medication such as nitroglycerin as needed can relieve the pain. Teaching the client to pace activities with frequent rest periods can reduce the workload of the heart. This helps prevent ischemia and subsequently angina from occurring.

Maintenance of normal cardiac function includes monitoring of vital signs, intake and output, and daily weights if heart failure is present or diuretics are given. Sodium may be restricted to reduce fluid retention. Smoking cessation information is provided. Medications are given as prescribed.

Interventions that improve the quality of life include activities of daily living that reduce fatigue. Assistance as needed, frequent rest periods, and energy conservation techniques are planned. (See Chapter 21.) Exercise tolerance is assessed and daily exercise is planned according to this tolerance.

Ongoing monitoring for signs or symptoms of excess fluid volume are important to allow early detection and treatment. Daily weights provide the most accurate assessment of weight gain caused by excess fluid. The weights should be obtained at the same time of day, using the same scale and type of clothing for accuracy. Assessment for edema, JVD, lung crackles or wheezes, dyspnea, and orthopnea should be done. Restricting sodium intake and administering diuretics as ordered assist in decreasing fluid volume excess. Monitoring intake and output is also important to detect imbalances. For the elderly client it is important to understand that fluid volume excess develops more easily and can be very serious. Therefore it is important to assess and monitor risk factors for fluid volume excess in the elderly client.

Education to promote understanding of the disorder and prevention of complications is an important nursing intervention. An explanation of the disorder is provided to promote understanding of health maintenance and early recognition of onset of symptoms so medical care can be sought. It is essential that the client fully understands the need to treat streptococcal infections. The client also needs to recognize that prophylactic antibiotics may be needed before invasive procedures to prevent endocarditis. Teaching is provided for any medications the client is taking. If the client is on anticoagulants for atrial fibrillation or valve replacement, a Medic Alert bracelet should be worn, and monthly appointments to check prothrombin time and international normalized ratio (INR) values should be kept. For elderly clients, it is important to include caregivers or family members in teaching sessions to assist with understanding of the information being taught.

Evaluation

The goal for the nursing diagnosis of pain is met if the client reports satisfactory pain relief. Satisfactory pain relief is measured by comparing the client's stated level of pain on a 1 to 10 rating scale with the client's predetermined goal for acceptable level of pain.

The goal for the nursing diagnosis of decreased cardiac output is met if the client's vital signs are within normal range and no symptoms of heart failure are present.

The goal for the nursing diagnosis of activity intolerance is met if the client reports reduced fatigue and the ability to complete tasks and engage in desired activities.

The goal for the nursing diagnosis of fluid volume excess is met if the client remains free of edema, maintains appropriate weight for client, maintains clear lung sounds without dyspnea, has normal vital signs, and has no evidence of neck vein distention.

The goal for the nursing diagnosis of ineffective management of therapeutic regimen is met if the client verbalizes understanding of completed teaching and does not have recurrence of symptoms.

Review Questions

1. Which of the following occurs in mitral stenosis?
   a. Failure of the mitral valve to close tightly
   b. Backflow of blood into the right atrium
   c. Backflow of blood into the left atrium
   d. Impaired emptying of the left atrium

2. Which of the following occurs in aortic regurgitation?
   a. Backflow of blood into the right ventricle
   b. Backflow of blood into the left ventricle
   c. Impaired emptying of the right ventricle
   d. Calcified and narrowed aortic valve

3. Which one of the following can be a complication of any valve disorder?
   a. Rheumatic fever
   b. Heart failure
   c. Rheumatic heart disease
   d. Hypertension

4. Which one of the following causes the dyspnea and cough in clients with chronic mitral regurgitation?
   a. Atrial fibrillation
   b. Heart murmur
   c. Increased pulmonary congestion
   d. Palpitations

5. Which one of the following medications would the client be given to prevent complications associated with atrial fibrillation?
   a. Furosemide (Lasix)
   b. Bumetanide (Bumex)
   c. Penicillin (Bicillin)
   d. Warfarin (Coumadin)

6. Which one of the following diagnostic tests shows the structure and function of cardiac valves?
   a. ECG
   b. Chest x-ray
   c. Echocardiogram
   d. Cardiac catheterization

7. Which one of the following is a client outcome for activity intolerance?
   a. Clear breath sounds, no edema or weight gain
   b. Normal changes in vital signs with less fatigue during self-care
   c. Verbalizes knowledge of disorder
   d. States willingness to comply with therapeutic regimen

ANSWERS TO CRITICAL THINKING

CRITICAL THINKING: Sue

1. A murmur.
2. Stress and caffeine increase the occurrence of palpitations.
3. Prophylactic antibiotics.
4. To prevent infective endocarditis, which can result from bacteria entering the circulation during the procedure, attaching to the damaged valve, and growing.
5. A definition of what MVP is, stress management, caffeine intake reduction with decaffeinated coffee, and symptoms of endocarditis to report to her physician.

REFERENCE

1. Dajani, A, et al: Prevention of bacterial endocarditis: Recommendations by the American Heart Association. JAMA 277(22):1794, 1997.

BIBLIOGRAPHY

Ackley, BJ, and Ladwig, GB: Nursing Diagnosis Handbook. Mosby, St Louis, 1997.
Altman, R: Comparison of high dose with low dose aspirin in patients with mechanical heart valve replacement treated with oral anticoagulant. Circulation 94(9):2113, 1996.
Chamber, J, et al: Pulmonary autograft procedure for aortic valve disease: Long-term results of the pioneer series. Circulation 96(7):2206, 1997.
Cheng, T, et al: Evaluation of mitral valve prolapse by four-dimensional echocardiography. Am Heart J 133(1):120, 1997.

Cowper, T: Pharmacologic management of the patient with disorders of the cardiovascular system. Infective endocarditis. Dent Clin North Am 40(3):611, 1996.

Hahn, C, and Vlahakes, G: Nonreplacement operations for mitral valve regurgitation. Annu Rev Med 48:295, 1997.

Jaffe, M, and McVan, B: Davis's Laboratory and Diagnostic Tests Handbook. FA Davis, Philadelphia, 1997.

Kvidal, P, et al: Long-term follow up study on 64 elderly patients after balloon aortic valvuloplasty. J Heart Valve Dis 6(5):480, 1997.

McGrath, D: Clinical snapshot: Mitral valve prolapse. Am J Nurs 97(5):40, 1997.

Nakano, M, et al: Mitral valve remodeling using valvuloplasty, chordoplasty, and ring annuloplasty. J Cardiol 29(suppl 2):51, 1997.

Okura, H, et al: Planimetry and transthoracic two-dimensional echocardiography in noninvasive assessment of aortic valve area in patients with valvular aortic stenosis. J Am Coll Cardiol 30(3):753, 1997.

Perry, B: Mitral valve prolapse. Am J Nurs 97(8):17, 1997.

Prager, R, et al: The aortic homograft: Evolution of indications, techniques and results in 107 patients. Ann Thorac Surg 64(3):659, 1997.

Waszyrowski, T, et al: Early and long-term outcome of aortic valve replacement with homograft versus mechanical prosthesis—8-year follow-up study. Clin Cardiol 20(10):843, 1997.

20

Nursing Care of Clients with Cardiac Dysrhythmias

Elizabeth Chapman

Learning Objectives

Upon completion of this chapter, the student will be able to:

1. Identify the flow of blood through the heart.
2. Identify sinoatrial node, atrioventricular node, and Purkinje fibers.
3. Identify electrical activity across the heart.
4. Identify the components of a cardiac cycle.
5. Name and describe the major cardiac dysrhythmias.
6. Describe the different treatments of cardiac dysrhythmias.
7. Explain nursing care for clients with dysrhythmias.
8. Discuss the types and uses of cardiac pacemakers.

Key Words

atrial depolarization (**AY**-tree-uhl DE-poh-lahr-i-**ZAY**-shun)

atrial systole (**AY**-tree-uhl **SIS**-tuh-lee)

atrioventricular node (**AY**-tree-oh-ven-**TRICK**-yoo-lar NOHD)

bigeminy (bye-**JEM**-i-nee)

bradycardia (BRAY-dee-**KAR**-dee-yah)

bundle of His (**BUN**-duhl of HISS)

cardioversion (KAR-de-oh-**VER**-zhun)

defibrillate (dee-**FIB**-ri-layt)

dysrhythmia (dis-**RITH**-mee-yah)

electrocardiogram (ee-LECK-troh-**KAR**-dee-oh-GRAM)

fluoroscopy (fluh-**RAHS**-kuh-pee)

hyperkalemia (HIGH-per-kuh-**LEE**-mee-ah)

hypomagnesemia (HIGH-poh-MAG-nuh-**ZEE**-mee-ah)

isoelectric line (EYE-so-e-**LEK**-trick LINE)

multifocal (MUHL-tee-**FOH**-kuhl)

nodal or junctional rhythm (**NOHD**-uhl or **JUNGK**-shun-uhl **RITH**-uhm)

sinoatrial node (SIGH-noh-AY-tree-al NOHD)

trigeminy (try-**JEM**-i-nee)

unifocal (YOO-ni-**FOH**-kuhl)

ventricular diastole (ven-**TRICK**-yoo-lar dye-**AS**-tuh-lee)

ventricular escape rhythm (ven-**TRICK**-yoo-lar es-**KAYP** **RITH**-uhm)

ventricular repolarization (ven-**TRICK**-yoo-lar RE-pol-lahr-i-**ZAY**-shun)

ventricular systole (ven-**TRICK**-yoo-lar **SIS**-tuh-lee)

ventricular tachycardia (ven-**TRICK**-yoo-lar TACK-ee-**KAR**-dee-yah)

Cardiovascular System

The heart beats repeatedly and rhythmically at an average of 60 to 100 times per minute. The heart must contract and relax to propel blood throughout the body. The cardiovascular system picks up oxygen from the lungs and nutrients from the digestive system and delivers them to body tissues. It then picks up and removes metabolic waste from the cells and takes it to the lungs or kidneys for excretion.

The heart is a muscular organ with four chambers. The two upper chambers of the heart are called the atria, and the two lower chambers of the heart are called ventricles. The atria are separated from the ventricles by valves, and the right side of the heart is separated from the left side by the septum.

The heart receives blood returning from the body via the superior vena cava and inferior vena cava and from the coronary veins and empties into the right atrium. When the right atrium contracts it pushes blood through the tricuspid valve into the right ventricle. The right ventricle contracts and propels the unoxygenated blood through the pulmonic valve into the pulmonary artery. Here the blood will circulate into the lungs and become oxygenated. This circulation into the lungs is known as pulmonary circulation. The oxygenated blood leaves the lungs via the pul-monary veins and empties into the left atrium. When the left atrium contracts it pushes the blood through the mitral valve into the left ventricle. The left ventricle is the largest chamber of the heart and has the thickest myocardium. When the left ventricle contracts it propels the blood through the aortic valve into the aorta to carry throughout the body. (See Chapter 15.) The blood is pumped from the left side of the heart through the body. The circulation of blood through the body is known as the systemic circulation.

Any disturbance in the electrical system of the heart impedes the contracting and emptying of the chambers. Diseases of either the valves or the chordae tendineae, which connects edges of the atrioventricular (AV) valves to papillary muscle, will also affect how the chambers empty. An understanding of the movement of the blood through the heart helps understanding of the problems associated with malfunction of the electrical system of the heart.

Cardiac Conduction System

The heart's electrical conduction system (Fig. 20–1) initiates an impulse to stimulate the cardiac muscle to contract. The conduction system can be viewed on a cardiac

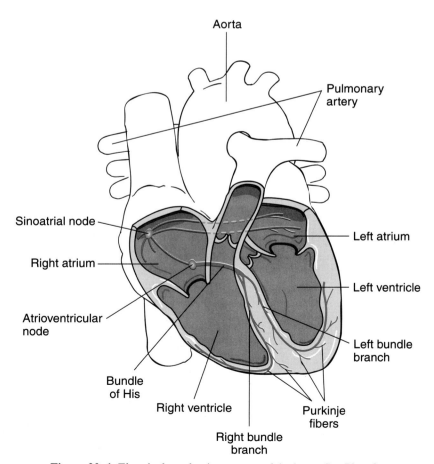

Figure 20–1. Electrical conduction system of the heart. See Plate 2.

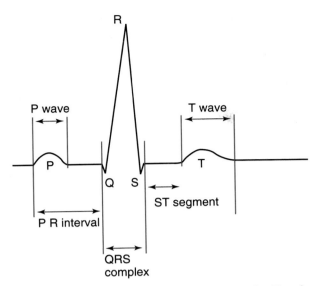

Figure 20–2. Components of the cardiac cycle. See Plate 2.

monitor or recorded on an **electrocardiogram** (ECG) tracing. The origin of the impulses and the time it takes for them to travel through the heart can be seen. The activity seen on the ECG does not mean that the heart has contracted in response to the electrical impulse. To verify that contraction occurs, the client's vital signs and pulses are monitored.

Located in the upper posterior wall of the right atrium is the **sinoatrial (SA) node.** The SA node is also known as the primary pacemaker of the heart because this is the area from which normal initial impulses arise. The SA node fires normally at a rate of 60 to 100 beats per minute. In heart disease, the SA node may not function properly. As a protective mechanism, other areas of the heart can initiate impulses at varying rates to ensure that the heart keeps beating. The **atrioventricular node** rate is 40 to 60 beats per minute, and the ventricular rate is 20 to 40 beats per minute. Treatment is necessary to reestablish a normal heart rate as soon as possible when the SA node is not functioning normally.

After the SA node fires, the impulse travels across both atria, stimulating them to contract. This is known as **atrial systole.** This atrial contraction propels blood out of the atria and into the ventricles. The ventricles are relaxed at this time, which is referred to as **ventricular diastole.** The impulse crosses the atria to the AV node, located in the lower portion of the right atria, where it is delayed briefly. It then travels down the **bundle of His,** which divides into right and left bundle branches. From here the impulse quickly travels through the Purkinje fibers, stimulating both ventricles to contract. This is known as **ventricular systole.**

An ECG monitor or tracing shows the electrical activity of the heart. It is used to verify normal heart functioning and to detect abnormal heart function. Specialized training, usually by physicians, is required to interpret ECG abnormali-

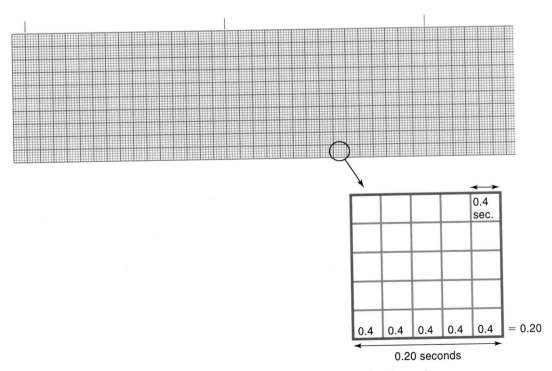

Figure 20–3. Electrocardiogram recording paper, time intervals.

ties. Nurses can learn characteristics of a normal heart rhythm and rules for common **dysrhythmias** to be able to interpret and report them to the nurse in charge or physician.

CARDIAC CYCLE

To interpret rhythms, a cardiac cycle must first be identified. A cardiac cycle is the period of time from the beginning of one heartbeat to the beginning of the next. It is the electrical representation of the impulse that stimulates contraction and relaxation of the atria and ventricles. Within the cardiac cycle, there is a P wave, a QRS complex, and a T wave. To be considered normal, each cycle must consist of each of these components. Figure 20–2 shows the components of a cardiac cycle.

ELECTROCARDIOGRAM GRAPH PAPER

Once a complete cycle is identified, the intervals of each of these components are measured by looking at the ECG graph paper on which the rhythm is recorded. The graph paper is the same for all ECG machines and has many small squares that are measured in seconds of time (Fig. 20–3). Each small box is 0.04 seconds long. There are five small boxes, which equals 0.20 seconds of time, between two heavy vertical black lines. (See Fig. 20–3.)

When the ECG is on but there is no electrical activity detected, a straight line is produced. This straight line, known as the **isoelectric line,** occurs when there is no electrical flow, so there are neither positive nor negative electrical wave deflections. Cardiac cycle waves, depending on how they travel through the heart, are either upright (positive) or downward (negative) from the isoelectric line on the ECG graph paper.

Components of a Cardiac Cycle

P WAVE

The P wave is the first wave of the cardiac cycle and represents **atrial depolarization.** When the SA node fires, it is

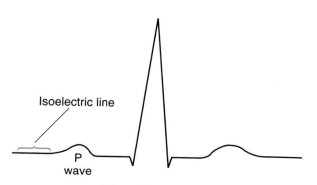

Figure 20–4. P wave.

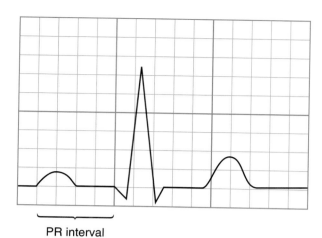

PR interval

Figure 20–5. P-R interval. This P-R interval covers four full boxes. Each box is 0.04 seconds. 0.04 × 4 = 0.16 seconds.

normally shown on the rhythm strip as a rounded, upright deflection from the isoelectric line (Fig. 20–4). There is one P wave in a normal cardiac cycle.

P-R INTERVAL

The P-R interval represents how long it takes the electrical impulse to travel across the atria to the AV node. It starts at the beginning of the P wave and ends at the beginning of the QRS complex. Counting the number of small boxes that the interval covers determines the length of the P-R interval (Fig. 20–5). The normal P-R interval is 0.12 to 0.20 seconds.

LEARNING TIP

To make measuring waves easier, try to find one that starts at the beginning of one small box. (See Fig. 20–5.) If the wave starts in the middle of the box, count it as one-half of a box, which is 0.02 seconds.

QRS COMPLEX

The QRS complex represents ventricular depolarization. The Q wave is the first downward deflection after the P wave but before the R wave. The R wave is the first upward deflection after the P wave. The last part of the QRS complex is the S wave, which is the second negative deflection after the P wave or the first negative deflection after the R wave (Fig. 20–6). Though not every QRS complex has a Q wave, it is still referred to as a QRS complex (Fig. 20–7).

---

dysrhythmia: dys—difficult or abnormal + rhythm—rhythm

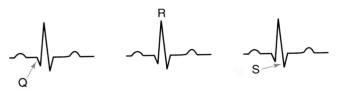

Figure 20–6. QRS complex.

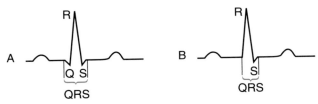

Figure 20–7. *(A)* QRS complex with a Q wave. *(B)* QRS complex without a Q wave.

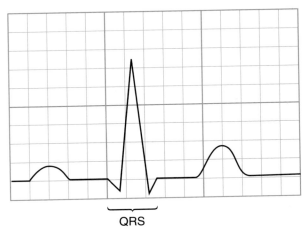

Figure 20–8. QRS interval. This QRS interval covers 2½ boxes. Each full box is 0.04 seconds. One-half box is 0.02 seconds. 2.5 × 0.04 = 0.10 seconds.

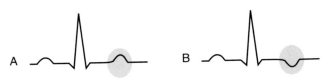

Figure 20–9. *(A)* T wave with positive deflection. *(B)* T wave with inverted, negative deflection.

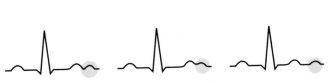

Figure 20–10. Different locations U waves appear.

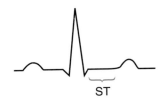

Figure 20–11. ST segment.

QRS INTERVAL

To measure the QR interval, count the number of boxes from the start of the Q wave to the end of the S wave (Fig. 20–8). The normal interval is 0.04 to 0.11 seconds.

T WAVE

The T wave represents **ventricular repolarization,** the resting state of the heart, when the ventricles are filling with blood and preparing to receive the next impulse. The T wave starts at the next upward (positive) deflection, after the QRS complex, and ends with a return to the isoelectric line. The T wave may also be a downward deflection after the QRS complex. This can occur in some leads (different view of the heart), or it can indicate ischemia of the heart (Fig. 20–9).

U WAVE

This waveform is usually not present. It is seen in clients with hypokalemia, which is a low serum potassium level. It occurs shortly after the T wave and can distort the configuration of the T wave (Fig. 20–10).

ST SEGMENT

The ST segment reflects the time from completion of a contraction (depolarization) to recovery (repolarization) of myocardial muscle for the next impulse. The ST segment starts at the end of the QRS and ends at the T wave (Fig. 20–11). The ST segment is examined in clients who are experiencing chest pain. Changes in the ST segment configuration can indicate the presence of ischemia or an injury pattern suggestive of myocardial damage. If a client is experiencing ischemia, the ST segment can be inverted or depressed (Fig. 20–12). If the client is experiencing an injury pattern, the ST segment is elevated (Fig. 20–13).

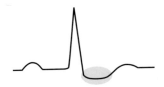

Figure 20–12. ST segment inverted or depressed.

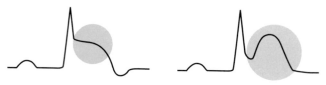

Figure 20–13. ST segment elevated.

Interpretation of Cardiac Rhythms

FIVE-STEP PROCESS

An orderly, systematic method for interpreting ECG rhythms should be used. Following this process, in order, increases understanding of items to examine and ensures that nothing is omitted. Five steps are examined in this process: (1) regularity, (2) heart rate, (3) P waves, (4) PR interval, and (5) the QRS complex (Table 20–1). The findings of these five steps are then used to interpret the ECG rhythm according to the rules for each dysrhythmia.

Regularity of the R Waves

The regularity or rhythm of the heartbeat can be determined by looking at the R-R interval on the ECG. The same spacing between each R-R interval, with a variation of no greater than two small boxes, is seen in a normal rhythm. One way to determine the regularity of a rhythm is to count the number of small boxes between each R wave, which normally should remain the same. A more common way is to use calipers to measure the spacing of the R-R interval. A caliper is a small metal instrument with a sharp

Table 20–1. ***Five-Step Process for Dysrhythmia Interpretation***

1. Regularity or rhythm
   Rhythm regular?
   Rhythm irregular?
   Is there a pattern to the irregularity?
2. Heart rate
   What is heart rate?
3. P waves
   Is there one P wave for every QRS?
   Are P waves regular and constant?
   Do P waves look alike?
   Are P waves upright and in front of every QRS?
4. PR interval
   Is PR interval normal?
   Is PR interval constant or varying?
   Is there a pattern to any variation present?
5. QRS complex
   Is QRS interval normal
   Is QRS interval constant?
   Do QRS complexes all look alike?

point at the end of each side. It is V-shaped when spread apart to measure various distances. To use a caliper, one point is placed at the top of an R wave and the other point is spread apart until it rests on the top of the next R wave. Then, without changing the distance between the points, the calipers are moved from one R wave to the next across the whole tracing (also known as a strip) to see if the distance remains the same for each R-R interval. If the distance is the same, the rhythm is regular. If the distance changes, the rhythm is irregular. An irregular rhythm can be regularly irregular, which means it has a predictable pattern of irregularity, or totally irregular, without any pattern.

LEARNING TIP

If calipers are not available, a piece of paper can be placed on the ECG strip. A mark can be made at the top of one R wave with another mark made at the top of the next R wave. The marks on the paper can then be moved across the R-R intervals on the strip (just as caliper points would be) to determine whether they are regular or irregular.

Heart Rate

After the components of a cardiac cycle are identified and the intervals measured, the heart rate is determined. There are two methods to determine heart rate.

1. At the top of the ECG graph paper there are vertical marks at 3-second intervals (Fig. 20–14). Count the number of R waves within a 6-second strip and multiply the total by 10 (Fig. 20–15). This gives the beats per minute (6 seconds × 10 = 60 seconds or 1 minute). This is used for rapid estimates because it is not very accurate.
2. Count the number of large boxes between two R waves and divide that number into 300. This gives the beats per minute (Fig. 20–16). This method is used only with regular rhythms.

A normal heart rate is 60 to 100 beats per minute, which is generated by the SA node. Other areas of the heart can also initiate an impulse if the SA node is not functioning properly. The AV node and the ventricles have their own inherent (naturally occurring) rates. This is a compensatory mechanism for the heart to keep it pumping. If the SA node fails, the AV node will attempt to initiate an impulse. The inherent rate for the AV node is 40 to 60 beats per minute. The rhythm produced when the AV node initiates the impulse is called a **nodal** or **junctional rhythm.** The body can usually function adequately with this rhythm. If, for some reason, the AV node is unable to initiate an impulse, the ventricles will take over. The rhythm produced when the ventricles initiate the impulse is called a **ventricular escape rhythm**

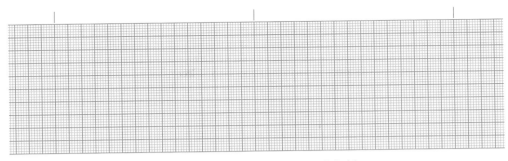

Figure 20–14. Three-second interval dividers.

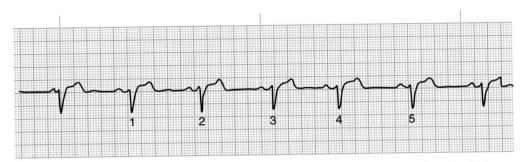

Figure 20–15. Counting R waves in 6-second strip. Five R waves in 6-second strip, 5 × 10 = 50 beats per minute. The first R wave is not counted; the entire complex must fall within the 6-second strip.

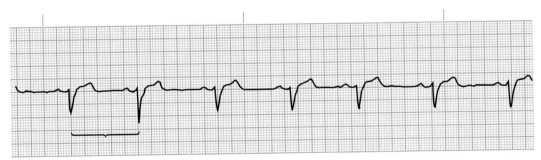

Figure 20–16. Heart rate. Counting large boxes and dividing into 300. Count number of large boxes between two R waves and divide into 300; five large boxes, 300/5 = 60 beats per minute.

or complete heart block. This is a last attempt to compensate for loss of SA and AV node conduction. The ventricular rate is 20 to 40 beats per minute. This is usually not adequate, and the client will begin to show signs of inadequate cardiac output such as dyspnea, abnormal vital signs, and changes in level of consciousness.

P Wave

The P waves on the strip are examined to see if (1) there is one P wave for every QRS complex, (2) they are regular, (3) the P waves all look alike, and (4) they are upright and in front of the QRS. If the P waves all meet these criteria, they are considered normal. If they do not, further exami-

nation of the strip is necessary to determine the type of dysrhythmia.

PR Interval

The PR intervals are measured to determine whether they are all normal and constant. If the PR is found to vary, it is important to note if a pattern to the variation is seen.

QRS Complex

The QRS intervals are measured to determine whether they are all normal and constant. Then the QRS complexes are examined to see if they all look alike.

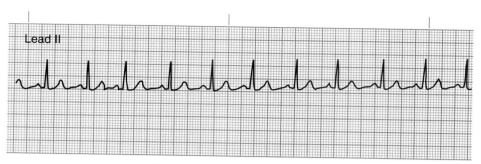

Figure 20–17. Normal sinus rhythm.

Normal Sinus Rhythm

DESCRIPTION

Normal sinus rhythm is the normal cardiac rhythm. It originates in the SA node and represents a series of complete and regular cardiac cycles with a normal heart rate. Each cycle must consist of a P wave, QRS complex, and a T wave. The measurements of the P-R intervals and QRS intervals must fall within normal limits. The heart rate must be 60 to 100 beats per minute and have a regular rhythm. If all these elements exist, it is interpreted as a normal sinus rhythm (NSR) (Fig. 20–17).

ELECTROCARDIOGRAM RULES

1. Rhythm: regular
2. Heart rate: 60 to 100 beats per minute
3. P waves: smoothly rounded and upright in lead II, precedes each QRS complex, alike
4. PR interval: 0.12 to 0.20 seconds
5. QRS interval: 0.06 to 0.11 seconds

Dysrhythmias

Two terms are used for rhythm disturbances: *arrhythmia* and *dysrhythmia*. An arrhythmia is an irregularity or loss of rhythm of the heartbeat, and a dysrhythmia is an abnormal, disordered, or disturbed rhythm.[1] These two terms are used interchangeably, but *dysrhythmia* is the most accurate term for the discussion of abnormal rhythms.

Several mechanisms can cause irregularity or a dysrhythmia. Two examples of these mechanisms can be a disturbance in the formation of an impulse or the conduction of the impulse. When impulse formation is disturbed, the impulse may arise from the atria, the AV node, or the ventricles. This disturbance can be seen as increased or decreased heart rate, early or late beats, or atrial or ventricular fibrillation. With a disturbance in conduction there may be normal formation of the impulse, but it becomes blocked within the electrical conduction system, resulting in abnormal conduction (as in heart block or bundle branch blocks).

DYSRHYTHMIAS ORIGINATING IN THE SINOATRIAL NODE

Rhythms arising from the SA node are referred to as sinus rhythms. The SA node, being the pacemaker of the heart, fires normally at a rate of 60 to 100 beats per minute. Disturbances in conduction from the SA node can cause irregular rhythms or abnormal heart rates. Most dysrhythmias arising from the SA node are rarely dangerous. Clients, especially those with heart, lung, or kidney disease, who cannot tolerate rapid or slow heart rates as determined by symptoms may require treatment.

Sinus Bradycardia

Description

Bradycardia is a slow heart rate. Sinus bradycardia has the same cardiac cycle components as normal sinus rhythm except for a slower heart rate (Fig. 20–18). The impulses originating from the SA node are fewer than normal.

Causes

Medications, myocardial infarction, and electrolyte imbalances can cause bradycardia. Well-conditioned athletes also can have slower heart rates because their hearts work more efficiently.

Electrocardiogram Rules

1. Rhythm: regular
2. Heart rate: less than 60 beats per minute
3. P waves: smoothly rounded and upright in lead II, precedes each QRS complex, alike
4. P-R interval: 0.12 to 0.20 seconds
5. QRS interval: 0.06 to 0.11 seconds

Signs and Symptoms

Sinus bradycardia rarely produces symptoms unless it is so slow that it reduces cardiac output. Symptoms consist of fatigue or fainting episodes. Clients are monitored for their responses to bradycardia.

---

bradycardia: bradys—slow + kardia—heart

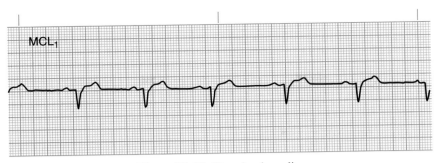

Figure 20–18. Sinus bradycardia.

Treatment

Treatment is not required if the client is asymptomatic. If the client is symptomatic, medications such as atropine sulfate can be given to increase heart rate for a short time. The cause is determined and treated. If necessary, a temporary pacemaker can be inserted to maintain a normal heart rate until the cause is resolved.

Sinus Tachycardia

Description

Tachycardia is defined as a fast heart rate. Sinus tachycardia has the same components as normal sinus rhythm except for a faster heart rate (Fig. 20–19). The impulses originating from the SA node are more than normal.

Causes

Physical activity, hemorrhage, shock, medications, dehydration, fever, myocardial infarction, electrolyte imbalance, or anxiety may cause sinus tachycardia. Tachycardia occurs whenever hypoxia occurs and more cardiac output is needed to deliver oxygen.

Electrocardiogram Rules

1. Rhythm: regular
2. Heart rate: greater than 100 beats per minute
3. P waves: smoothly rounded and upright in lead II, precedes each QRS complex, alike
4. P-R interval: 0.12 to 0.20 seconds
5. QRS interval: 0.06 to 0.11 seconds

Signs and Symptoms

Sinus tachycardia usually produces no symptoms. If the heart rate is very rapid and sustained for long periods of time, the client may experience angina or dyspnea. Elderly clients may become symptomatic more rapidly than younger clients. (See Gerontological Issues Box 20–1.) In clients with myocardial infarction, rapid heart rates can increase the cardiac workload and produce more severe symptoms.

Treatment

Treatment depends on the cause and the client's symptoms. Treating the underlying cause usually corrects the tachycardia. If the client is hemorrhaging, immediate intervention is needed to stop the bleeding and restore normal blood volume. Medications such as digoxin (Lanoxin) or verapamil (Calan) can be given to slow the heart rate.

LEARNING TIP

Tachycardia is often the first sign of hemorrhage. It is a compensatory mechanism to maintain cardiac output. If a client develops sudden tachycardia, consider if hemorrhage could be the cause such as in postoperative clients, clients with gastrointestinal bleeding or cancer, or trauma clients. The bleeding may be external or internal and therefore not visible. Apply pressure to the site if the bleeding is obvious. Report the tachycardia and obvious bleeding promptly.

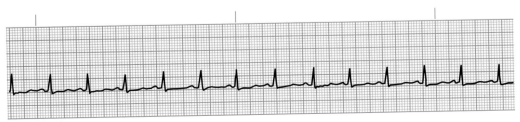

Figure 20–19. Sinus tachycardia.

DYSRHYTHMIAS ORIGINATING IN THE ATRIA

As previously discussed, all the areas of the heart can initiate an impulse. The SA node is the primary pacemaker, but if the atria initiate an impulse faster than the SA node, they become the primary pacemaker. Atrial rhythms are usually faster than 100 beats per minute and can exceed 200 beats per minute. When an impulse originates outside the SA node, the P waves look different (flatter, notched, or peaked), which indicates that the SA node is not controlling the heart rate. The impulse, although not coming from the SA node, still travels to the ventricles to initiate a normal QRS complex after each P wave.

LEARNING TIP

1. If a QRS complex measures less than 0.12 seconds, the dysrhythmia originated above the ventricles. This is known as a supraventricular dysrhythmia.
2. Ventricular dysrhythmias have QRS complexes greater than 0.11 seconds.

Premature Atrial Contractions

Description

The term *premature* refers to an early beat. When the atria fire an impulse before the SA node fires, a premature beat results. If the underlying rhythm is sinus rhythm, the distance between R waves is the same except where the early beat occurs. When looking at the ECG strip, a shortened R-R interval is seen where the premature beat occurs. The R wave preceding the premature atrial contraction (PAC) and the PAC's R wave are close together followed by a pause, with the next beat being regular (Fig. 20–20).

Causes

Hypoxia, myocardial ischemia, enlarged atria, and medications can cause PACs.

Electrocardiogram Rules

1. Rhythm: the premature beat interrupts the underlying rhythm where it occurs.
2. Heart rate: depends on the underlying rhythm. If NSR, 60 to 100 beats per minute.
3. P waves: the early beat will be abnormally shaped and may be inverted or negative.
4. P-R interval: usually appears normal, but the premature beat could have a shortened or prolonged P-R interval.
5. QRS interval: 0.06 to 0.11 seconds indicates normal conduction to the ventricles.

Signs and Symptoms

Premature atrial contractions can occur in healthy individuals, as well as in the client with a diseased heart. No symptoms are usually present. If many PACs occur in succession, the client may report the sensation of palpitations.

Treatment

PACs are usually not dangerous, and no treatment is required. Frequent PACs indicate atrial irritability, which may worsen into other atrial dysrhythmias. Digoxin can be given to a client having frequent PACs to slow the heart rate. Frequent assessment of apical pulse, the client's symptoms, and the ECG assist in determining the need for intervention.

Atrial Flutter

Description

In atrial flutter, the atria contract or flutter at a rate of 250 to 350 beats per minute. The very rapid P waves appear as flutter or F waves on ECG and look like a sawtooth pattern.

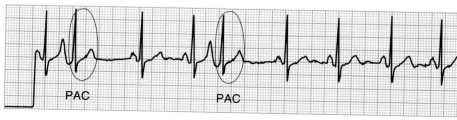

Figure 20–20. Premature atrial contractions.

Some of the impulses get through the AV node and reach the ventricles, resulting in normal QRS complexes. There can be from two to four F waves between QRS complexes. If impulses pass through the AV node at a consistent rate, the rhythm is regular (Fig. 20–21).

The classic characteristics of atrial flutter are more than one P wave before a QRS complex, a sawtooth pattern of P waves, and an atrial rate of 250 to 350 beats per minute.

Causes

Causes of atrial flutter include rheumatic or ischemic heart diseases, congestive heart failure (CHF), hypertension, pericarditis, pulmonary embolism, and postoperative coronary artery bypass surgery. Many medications can also cause this dysrhythmia.

ECG Rules

1. Rhythm: atrial rhythm regular; ventricular rhythm regular or irregular depending on consistency of AV conduction of impulses
2. Heart rate: ventricular rate varies
3. P waves: flutter or F waves with sawtooth pattern
4. P-R interval: none measurable
5. QRS complex: 0.06 to 0.11 seconds

Symptoms

The presence of symptoms in atrial flutter depends on the ventricular rate. If the ventricular rate is normal, usually no symptoms are present. If the rate is rapid, the client can experience palpitations, angina, or dyspnea.

Treatment

Treatment depends on the ventricular rate and cardiac output. Digoxin is used to slow conduction through the AV node and increase cardiac contractility. Other medications, such as quinidine sulfate, procainamide (Pronestyl), or propranolol (Inderal), can also be used to slow the heart rate. A rapid ventricular rate or symptoms of decreased cardiac output usually require cardioversion. If these treatments are unsuccessful, an atrial pacemaker can be inserted to pace faster than the atrial rate and override the dysrhythmia.

Atrial Fibrillation

Description

In atrial fibrillation, the atrial rate is extremely rapid and chaotic. An atrial rate of 350 to 600 beats per minute can occur. However, the AV node blocks most of the impulses, so the ventricular rate is much lower than the atrial rate. There are no definable P waves because the atria are fibrillating, or quivering, rather than beating effectively. No P waves can be seen or measured. A wavy pattern is produced on the ECG. Because the atrial rate is so irregular and only a few of the atrial impulses are allowed to pass through the AV node, the R waves are irregular. The ventricular rate varies.

Atrial fibrillation is easy to identify based on its two classic characteristics. One is the lack of identifiable P waves and the other is the irregularly irregular rhythm or R waves.

The presence of this dysrhythmia indicates heart disease. A complication of this dysrhythmia is the formation of a thrombus in the atria, due to blood stasis from poor emptying of the atria (Fig. 20–22).

Causes

Atrial fibrillation causes include aging, rheumatic or ischemic heart diseases, heart failure (HF), hypertension, pericarditis, pulmonary embolism, and postoperative coronary artery bypass surgery. Medications can also cause this dysrhythmia.

ECG Rules

1. Rhythm: grossly or irregularly irregular.
2. Heart rate: atrial rate not measurable; ventricular rate under 100 is controlled response; greater than 100 is rapid ventricular response
3. P waves: no identifiable P waves
4. P-R interval: none can be measured because no P waves are seen
5. QRS complex: 0.06 to 0.11 seconds

Symptoms

With atrial fibrillation, most clients feel the irregular rhythm. Many describe it as palpitations or a skipping heart-

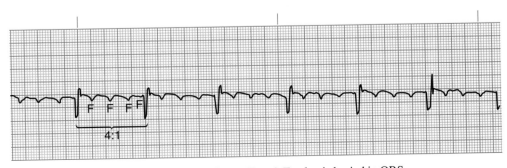

Figure 20–21. Atrial flutter. Fourth F valve is buried in QRS.

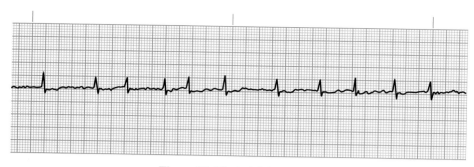

Figure 20–22. Atrial fibrillation.

beat. When checking a client's radial pulse, it may be faint due to a decreased stroke volume (volume of blood ejected with each contraction). If the ventricular rhythm is rapid and sustained, the client can go into left ventricular failure.

Treatment

The underlying cause is treated. Medications such as digoxin (Lanoxin), beta blockers, calcium channel blockers, quinidine, procainamide (Pronestyl), disopyramide (Norpace), and amiodarone (Cordarone) are sometimes used. **Cardioversion,** a synchronized electrical shock, can be delivered to try to return the heart to normal sinus rhythm.

VENTRICULAR DYSRHYTHMIAS

Premature Ventricular Contraction

Description

Premature ventricular contractions (PVCs) originate in the ventricles from an ectopic focus (a site other than the SA node). The ventricles are irritable and fire prematurely or before the SA node. When the ventricles fire first, the im-

pulses are not conducted normally through the electrical pathway. This results in a wide (greater than 0.11 seconds), bizarre QRS complex on an ECG (Fig. 20–23).

PVCs can occur in different shapes and repetitive cycles. The shape of the PVC is referred to as **unifocal** (one focus) if all the PVCs look the same because they come from the same irritable area (Fig. 20–24). **Multifocal** PVCs do not all look the same because they are originating from several irritable areas in the ventricle.

There are several repetitive cycles or patterns of PVCs. **Bigeminy** is a PVC occurring every other beat (a normal beat and then a PVC). **Trigeminy** is a PVC occurring every third beat (two normal beats and then a PVC). Quadrigeminy is one that occurs every fourth beat (three normal beats and then a PVC). When two PVCs occur together, they are referred to as a couplet (pair). If three or more PVCs occur in a row, it is referred to as a run of PVCs or **ventricular tachycardia.** (Fig. 20–25).

Causes

Use of caffeine or alcohol, anxiety, hypokalemia, cardiomyopathy, ischemia, and myocardial infarction are common causes of PVCs.

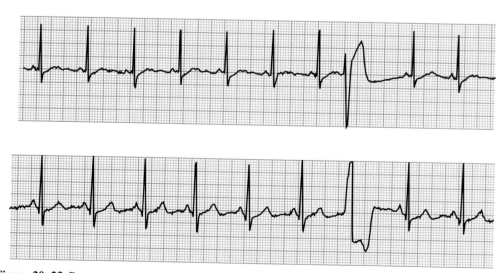

Figure 20–23. Premature ventricular contractions. PVCs may arise from different foci causing them to look differently.

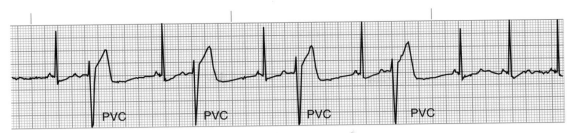

Figure 20–24. Bigeminal premature ventricular contractions.

Electrocardiogram Rules

1. Rhythm: depends on the underlying rhythm; the PVC usually interrupts the rhythm
2. Heart rate: depends on the underlying rhythm
3. P waves: absent before the PVC QRS complex
4. P-R interval: none for the PVC
5. QRS complex: for the PVC greater than 0.11 seconds; the T wave is in the opposite direction of the QRS complex (i.e., QRS upright, T downward; QRS downward, T upright)

Symptoms

PVCs may be felt by the client and are described as a skipped beat or palpitations. With frequent PVCs, cardiac output can be decreased, leading to symptoms of fatigue, dizziness, or more severe dysrhythmias.

Treatment

Treatment depends on the type and number of PVCs and whether symptoms are produced. Xylocaine (Lidocaine) is the drug of choice to suppress ventricular ectopic beats. A loading dose is given IVP and then an infusion is started. If lidocaine (Xylocaine) is not effective, procainamide (Pronestyl), bretylium (Bretylol), or phenytoin (Dilantin) can be used.

 CRITICAL THINKING: Mrs. Mae

Mrs. Mae, 70, is 5 days post–myocardial infarction without complications. She is transferred from the intensive care unit (ICU) to the step-down unit. On admission to step-down, the cardiac monitor shows normal sinus rhythm without ectopy. One hour later, the monitor shows sinus rhythm with bigeminal PVCs, with less than six per minute.

1. What should the nurse do first?
2. What should the nurse do regarding the dysrhythmia?
3. What might some of the causes be for this dysrhythmia?
4. What symptoms, if any, would the nurse expect to be present?
5. What would the nurse do if symptoms were present?

6. What type of orders would the nurse anticipate from the doctor?

Answers at end of chapter.

Ventricular Tachycardia

Description

The occurrence of three or more PVCs in a row is referred to as ventricular tachycardia (VT) (Fig. 20–25). VT results from the continuous firing of an ectopic ventricular focus. During VT, the ventricles become the pacemaker of the heart, rather than the SA node. The pathway of the ventricular impulses is different from normal conduction, producing a wide (greater than 0.11 seconds), bizarre QRS complex.

Causes

Myocardial irritability, myocardial infarction, and cardiomyopathy are common causes of VT. Respiratory acidosis, hypokalemia, digoxin toxicity, cardiac catheters, and pacing wires can also produce VT.

Electrocardiogram Rules

1. Rhythm: usually regular, may have some irregularity
2. Heart rate: 150 to 250 ventricular beats per minute; slow VT is below 150 beats per minute
3. P waves: absent
4. P-R interval: none
5. QRS complex: greater than 0.11 seconds

Symptoms

The seriousness of ventricular tachycardia is determined by the duration of the dysrhythmia. Sustained VT compromises cardiac output. Clients are aware of a sudden onset of rapid heart rate and can experience dyspnea, palpitations, and light-headedness. Angina commonly occurs. The severity of symptoms can increase rapidly if the left ventricle fails and complete cardiac arrest results.

Treatment

If the client is stable, medications can be tried first. The medications used for PVCs are used in VT to decrease ven-

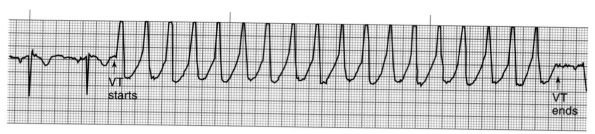

Figure 20–25. Ventricular tachycardia.

tricular irritability. Magnesium can be used to help stabilize ventricular muscle excitability, if the client's magnesium level is low.

If the client is unstable, immediate synchronized cardioversion is indicated. If the client is pulseless or not breathing, cardiopulmonary resuscitation (CPR) and immediate **defibrillation** are required. Current Advanced Cardiac Life Support (ACLS) protocols for VT treatment should be used by individuals certified in ACLS.

CRITICAL THINKING: Mrs. Parker

The LPN/LVN is caring for Mrs. Parker, 66, who had a myocardial infarction and several episodes of ventricular tachycardia while in the ICU. Mrs. Parker is found to be unresponsive with no palpable pulses and in VT on the ECG.

1. Why are there no palpable pulses?
2. What is occurring to the heart when it is in VT?
3. Why is lidocaine (Xylocaine) a drug of choice in treating VT?

Answers at end of chapter.

Ventricular Fibrillation

Description

Ventricular fibrillation occurs when many, many ectopic ventricular foci fire at the same time. Chaotic ventricular activity with no discernible waves is seen (Fig. 20–26). The ventricle quivers and is unable to initiate a contraction. There is a complete loss of cardiac output. If this rhythm is not terminated immediately, death will ensue.

Causes

Hyperkalemia, hypomagnesemia, electrocution, coronary artery disease, and myocardial infarction are all possible causes of ventricular fibrillation. Placement of intracardiac catheters and cardiac pacing wires can also lead to ventricular irritability and then ventricular fibrillation.

Electrocardiogram Rules

1. Rhythm: chaotic and extremely irregular
2. Heart rate: not measurable

3. P waves: none
4. P-R interval: none
5. QRS complex: none

Symptoms

Clients experiencing ventricular fibrillation lose consciousness immediately. There are no heart sounds, peripheral pulses, or blood pressure. These are all indicative of circulatory collapse. Additionally, respiratory arrest, cyanosis, and pupil dilation occur.

Treatment

CPR is started and immediately followed by defibrillation as soon as the defibrillator is available. Immediate defibrillation is the best treatment for terminating ventricular fibrillation and survival. As a result, defibrillators that analyze rhythms and either prompt operators or automatically deliver an electrical shock if necessary are now used by rescue personnel and kept in public places such as malls for immediate access. Medications are given according to ACLS protocols and may include epinephrine, lidocaine (Xylocaine), bretylium (Bretylol), or procainamide (Pronestyl). Intubation supports respiratory function.

Asystole

Description

Asystole is the total absence of electrical activity in the cardiac muscle. It is referred to as cardiac arrest. A straight line is seen on an ECG strip (Fig. 20–27). Ventricular fibrillation usually precedes this rhythm and must be reversed immediately to help prevent asystole.

Causes

Ventricular fibrillation and a loss of a majority of functional cardiac muscle due to a myocardial infarction are common causes of asystole. Hyperkalemia can be another cause of asystole.

---

defibrillation: de—from + fibrillation—quivering fibers
hyperkalemia: hyper—above + kalium—potassium + emia—blood
hypomagnesemia: hypo—below + magnes—magnesium + emia—blood

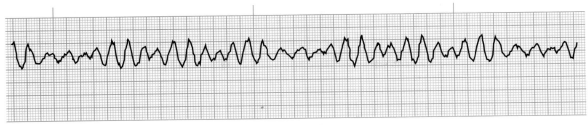

Figure 20–26. Ventricular fibrillation.

Electrocardiogram Rules

1. Rhythm: none
2. Heart rate:none
3. P waves: none
4. P-R interval: none
5. QRS complex: none

Treatment

CPR is started immediately. ACLS protocols for asystole are used. Common medications include epinephrine and atropine. Intubation to support respirations is done.

 CRITICAL THINKING: Mr. Peet

The LPN/LVN is making rounds. Upon entering Mr. Peet's room, the nurse notes that he is having difficulty breathing and is unresponsive.

1. What are the nurse's initial actions?
2. What should the nurse do after assessing and finding no pulse or respirations?
3. What is the LPN/LVN's responsibility during a code?

Answers at end of chapter.

Cardiac Pacemakers

Pacemakers can be temporary or permanent (Fig. 20–28). They are used to override dysrhythmias or to perform the function of the SA or AV node or the ventricles when they can no longer initiate an impulse. Temporary pacemakers are commonly used after an MI to allow the heart time to heal. The diseased myocardium is unable to respond to, or is not receiving, electrical conduction due to damage within the system. The pacemaker becomes the electrical conduction system and stimulates the atria and ventricles to contract to maintain cardiac output.

Temporary pacemakers are used for bradycardias and tachycardias that do not respond to medications or cardioversion. Temporary pacemakers are commonly inserted during valve or open heart surgery. They are also used as emergency treatment until surgery can be scheduled to insert a permanent pacemaker.

Pacemaker insertion is a surgical procedure in which **fluoroscopy,** a screen that shows an image similar to an x-ray, is used. Different types of pacemakers are available that pace either the atria or ventricle, or both. They are set at a prescribed rate, usually 72 beats per minute.

When a client is in a paced rhythm, a small spike is seen on the ECG before the paced beat. This spike is the electrical stimulus. It can precede the P wave, QRS complex, or both depending on what is being paced. Clients may have all paced beats (100% paced), a mixture of their own beats and paced beats, or all of their own beats on an ECG. Clients' own beats occur if their heart initiates an impulse faster than the pacemaker's set rate, which suppresses the pacemaker from firing.

NURSING CARE FOR PACEMAKERS

Clients are usually required to remain on strict bed rest for 12 to 24 hours after insertion of a pacemaker and are placed on a cardiac monitor. The nurse monitors the apical

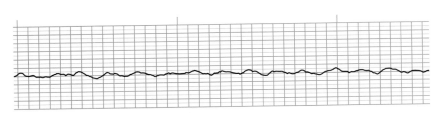

Figure 20–27. Asystole.

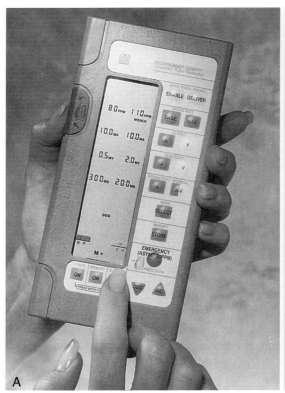
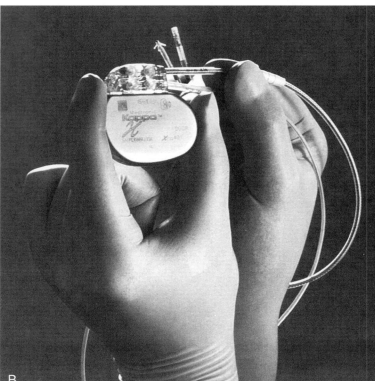

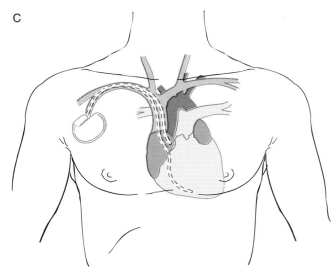

Figure 20–28. *(A)* Temporary pacemaker. *(B)* Permanent pace-maker. *(C)* Insertion of permanent pacemaker. (*A* and *B* courtesy of Medtronics, Inc., Minneapolis, Minn.)

pulse frequently to detect changes in the heart rhythm. Irregular heart rhythms or a rate slower than the pacemaker's set rate can indicate pacemaker malfunction. The nurse observes the dressing at the pacemaker insertion site every 2 to 4 hours for signs of bleeding. Any change in heart rhythm, complaints of chest pain, or changes in vital signs must be reported immediately.

CRITICAL THINKING: Mr. Treacher

Mr. Treacher, 58, is 6 days postoperative pacemaker placement and is being transferred to the medical

floor. After transfer, his vital signs are blood pressure 138/72, heart rate 72 beats per minute, 100% paced rhythm. Thirty minutes later he states that he feels weak and tired. His vital signs are now blood pressure 100/60, heart rate 60 beats per minute and irregular.

1. What is the nurse's first action?
2. What actions should be taken next?
3. What might be happening?
4. What interventions should the nurse anticipate next?

Answers at end of chapter.

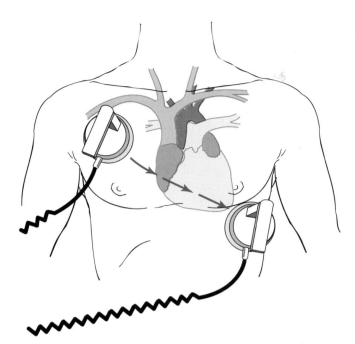

Figure 20–29. Placement of defibrillator paddles on chest.

Defibrillation

The use of defibrillation is reserved for lethal dysrhythmias. It is a lifesaving procedure. Defibrillation can be used to terminate ventricular tachycardia and ventricular fibrillation. ACLS protocols or agency policy specifies the amount and frequency of joules that can be delivered for defibrillation. LPN/LVNs should check their facility's policy on who is allowed to defibrillate a client in a life-threatening situation.

When defibrillation of a pulseless ventricular dysrhythmia is desired, the synchronize switch must be off. This switch is used during cardioversion if an R wave is present to allow the machine to sense the R waves and deliver the shock at the appropriate time to prevent a more life-threatening dysrhythmia from developing. In the defibrillation mode, when the trigger is pressed, the charge is immediately released. In the synchronized mode for cardioversion, there is a delay in the release of the charge while the R wave is sensed for appropriate timing.

Self-adhesive pads, conductive jelly, or saline pads are placed on the client's chest, back, or both to prevent electrical burns from the defibrillator and promote conduction of the electrical charge. After the defibrillator is charged, the paddles are pressed firmly and evenly against the chest wall for defibrillation (Fig. 20–29). If they are not pressed firmly, burns or electrical arcing can result when the shock is delivered. Before discharge, the person defibrillating must announce "all clear." No one, including the person defibrillating, should touch the bed or client during this time to avoid also being shocked.

After defibrillation, if successful, the client is assessed for a pulse and adequate tissue perfusion. Vital signs, peripheral pulses, and level of consciousness should be noted. The client is transferred to the intensive care unit for further treatment.

Emotional support for the client having experienced cardiac arrest and defibrillation is a very important aspect of nursing care. This can be an extremely frightening event for the client. It is important to explain what happened to the client and to listen and allow the client to express any concerns. The client is reassured that continuous monitoring is done in the intensive care unit.

Automatic Implanted Cardioverter Defibrillator

The automatic implanted cardioverter defibrillator (AICD) is surgically implanted in clients who experience life-threatening dysrhythmias and are at risk for sudden cardiac death (Fig. 20–30). The use of AICDs has decreased the number of deaths from these dysrhythmias. Two types of clients are considered to be candidates for the AICDs. One is the client who has had cardiac arrest without having had an acute myocardial infarction, and the other is one who has experienced frequent life-threatening dysrhythmias but has not responded to drug therapy.

An AICD recognizes configurations of complexes, the heart rate, or both. When it recognizes an abnormal complex or detects the heart rate outside of a preset rate, it automatically defibrillates. Most newer units recognize both criteria. If the dysrhythmia does not convert on the initial shock, four or five more shocks are delivered sequentially.

Client and family education is very important in preparing for discharge. Clients are extremely anxious about having another cardiac arrest and receiving shocks from the AICD. Providing emotional support, answering all questions, and correcting any information that has been misunderstood is included in discharge teaching.

CARDIOVERSION

Cardioversion is usually an elective procedure. It is used for dysrhythmias such as atrial fibrillation, atrial flutter, and supraventricular tachycardias that are not responsive to drug therapy.

On the defibrillator, there is a switch labeled "synchronize." This switch should be in the on position during cardioversion to program the defibrillator to recognize the client's R waves. The client is attached to the machine by electrode wires, which enables the ECG to be viewed on a screen. When the defibrillator is in the synchronized position it will mark a highlighted area on the client's R waves. The synchronized defibrillator must recognize R waves in order for it to deliver a shock.

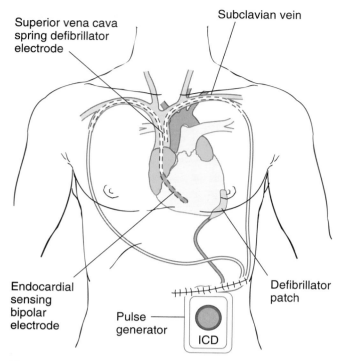

Figure 20–30. Placement of an automatic implanted cardioverter defibrillator.

Before the procedure, the client is usually given a sedative and monitored by anesthesia personnel. The client remains awake during the procedure. The amount of joules delivered with each shock is determined by the physician but usually ranges from 25 to 50 joules. Self-adhesive pads or conduction jelly is placed on the chest. The paddles must be firmly and evenly pressed against the pads or jelly on the chest until the shock is delivered to prevent skin burns and electrical arcing. When the discharge trigger is pressed, the shock is released when the machine senses it is safe to do so. The cardiac monitor screen is observed to see the discharge of the shock and to note the client's ECG response. The client's pulse and vital signs are checked. If cardioversion is successful there should be a return to normal sinus rhythm. If there is not an immediate conversion, more cardioversion attempts can be made as determined by the physician. After the procedure, the client is monitored for skin burns, rhythm disturbances, respiratory problems, hypotension, and changes in the ST segment.

Nursing Process for the Client with Dysrhythmias

ASSESSMENT

Assessment of the cardiac system, respiratory rate, breath sounds, neck veins, and urinary output is important. Monitoring apical and radial pulses at frequent intervals helps detect dysrhythmias. Most dysrhythmias are not life threatening. Careful observation of clients at risk for dysrhythmias aids in detecting them and helping to prevent them from becoming potentially dangerous. A client's complaints of dizziness, chest pain, or palpitations should always be reported.

NURSING DIAGNOSIS

The major nursing diagnoses for dysrhythmias may include but are not limited to the following:

1. Decreased cardiac output related to dysrhythmias or response to medications
2. Alteration in tissue perfusion related to decreased cardiac output
3. Activity intolerance related to decreased cardiac output
4. Anxiety related to fear of dying, knowledge deficit, and diagnostic procedures
5. Knowledge deficit related to dysrhythmias, diagnostic procedures, medications, and treatment

PLANNING

The goal of therapy is to identify clients at risk for dysrhythmias and promote adequate cardiac output. The nurse needs to identify factors that may contribute to increased cardiac workload. Careful assessment of all systems will focus on areas that might be affected by decreased cardiac output.

The client's goals are to (1) maintain vital signs and oxygen saturation within normal range; (2) maintain warm, dry skin, palpable pulses, and normal vital signs; (3) maintain desired activities; (4) decrease anxiety; and (5) understand the disease and its treatment.

IMPLEMENTATION

To implement the plan of care, the client and family should be included. The nurse needs to assist them in understanding the plan and the reasons for the prescribed interventions. The client and family need to be given time to understand the plan of care and to express their needs and fears. See Nursing Care Plan Box 20–2 for the Client with Dysrhythmias for specific nursing interventions.

Family members should be taught CPR or given information on local CPR classes. This training gives the client and family a sense of control and hope. In the event that the client requires CPR, the family can take action instead of simply standing by and feeling helpless. The client will feel more secure in knowing that immediate help is available from family members until medical help arrives.

EVALUATION

Evaluation of the outcome stems from regulation of dysrhythmias. Compliance with medication and therapy is the best indicator of understanding. Involvement of the client and family in asking questions and being involved in the plan of care leads to positive outcomes and control of dysrhythmias.

NURSING CARE PLAN BOX 20–2 FOR THE CLIENT WITH DYSRHYTHMIAS

Decreased cardiac output related to dysrhythmias

Client Outcomes
(1) Client's cardiac status stabilizes. (2) Client tolerates activities of daily living (ADL).

Evaluation of Outcomes
(1) There is an absence of dysrhythmias. (2) Client is able to perform ADL without tachycardia, chest pain, or weakness.

Interventions	Rationale	Evaluation
Assess apical and radial pulses every 2 to 4 hours. Assess blood pressure and urinary output.	Monitors for dysrhythmias, impending cardiac arrest, or shock. Blood pressure, pulse, and urinary output are indicators of cardiac output.	Is the client free of dysrhythmias with vital signs within normal limits?
Monitor mental status every 2 to 4 hours.	Dizziness, confusion, and restlessness may indicate decreased cerebral blood flow.	Does client show signs of decreased cerebral perfusion, such as confusion?
Assess lung sounds every 2 to 4 hours.	Dysrhythmias can cause heart failure.	Are lungs clear with no report of dyspnea?
Administer O$_2$ as ordered.	Increases oxygenation to the heart and brain.	Is client free of chest pain, confusion, and light-headedness?
Ensure that client gets adequate rest and does not exceed activity tolerance.	Reduces dyspnea and decreases O$_2$ demand on the myocardium.	Does client rest and tolerate activity without dyspnea or chest pain?

GERIATRIC

Administer medications as ordered and observe for adverse reactions.	Older clients may have decreased renal and liver function that may lead to rapid development of toxicity.	Does client have signs of toxicity?

Altered tissue perfusion (cardiopulmonary) related to decreased cardiac output

Client Outcomes
Client's vital signs and level of consciousness will be within normal limits.

Evaluation of Outcomes
Client's blood pressure, pulse, respirations, mental status, and urinary output are within normal limits for this client.

Intervention	Rationale	Evaluation
Monitor and document blood pressure, pulse, and urinary output.	These are indicators of cardiac output.	Does client maintain blood pressure > 90/40 or < 140/90; pulse > 60 or < 100; urinary output > 30 mL/h?
Assess peripheral circulation: pulses, color, temperature, and presence of edema.	Changes can mean decreased tissue perfusion.	Peripheral pulses strong, skin warm and dry, absence of edema?
Monitor respiratory rate and breath sounds.	Increased respiratory rate may indicate body trying to compensate for tissue hypoxia.	Respiratory rate > 12 or ≤ 20; lungs clear?
Monitor oxygen therapy.	Oxygen aids in maintaining oxygen saturation.	Oxygen levels normal; absence of cyanosis?

continued

NURSING CARE PLAN BOX 20–2 (continued)

Activity intolerance related to decreased oxygen delivery from decreased cardiac output

Client Outcomes
(1) Client will show normal changes in vital signs with less fatigue in response to activity. (2) Client will tolerate ADL.

Evaluation of Outcomes
(1) Client will have decreased complaints of fatigue and weakness. (2) Client is able to assist with activities of daily living.

Intervention	Rationale	Evaluation
Identify and minimize factors that decrease the client's exercise tolerance.	Helps increase the activity level.	Client identifies factors that increase fatigue.
Encourage client to help plan activity progression.	Participation in planning helps ensure client compliance.	Does client state a desire to increase activity level?
Instruct and help client to alternate periods of rest and activity.	To reduce the body's oxygen demand and prevent fatigue.	Is client able to state understanding of need to gradually increase activity level?
Monitor vital signs with activity—blood pressure, respirations, and heart rate and rhythm.	Detects abnormal changes with activity.	Do blood pressure, pulse, and respirations remain within guidelines during activity?
Teach client exercises to increase strength and endurance.	Helps improve breathing and increase activity levels.	Does client perform exercises?
Support and encourage activity up to client's tolerance.	Helps develop client's independence.	Is client able to express satisfaction with and increase activity?
Upon discharge, teach client and family plan for activity.	Helps reinforce need for increased activity and client's compliance.	Does client understand discharge plan of care?

GERIATRIC

Slow pace of care and allow client extra time to perform activities. Ensure safety when mobilizing elderly client.	Elderly clients can often perform activities if allowed time to slowly perform them and rest at intervals. Orthostatic hypertension is common in the elderly.	Is client able to perform activities when allowed extra time? Does blood pressure remain within normal limits when changing position? Does client ambulate without injury?

Anxiety related to situational crisis

Client Outcomes
(1) Client is able to effectively manage anxiety. (2) Client will report decreased anxiety.

Evaluation of Outcomes
(1) Client uses effective coping mechanisms to manage anxiety. (2) Client expresses decreased anxiety.

Interventions	Rationale	Evaluation
Assess level of anxiety.	Establishes a baseline.	What is client's level of anxiety?
Encourage client and family to verbalize fears.	Helps correct and clarify their concerns.	What are client's feelings or fears?
Explain procedures to client and family.	Lack of knowledge increases anxiety. Also will help with compliance of therapy.	Does client express understanding of therapy with decreased anxiety?
Identify and reduce as many environmental stressors as possible.	Anxiety often results from lack of trust in the environment.	Can client describe two situations that increase tension?

continued

NURSING CARE PLAN BOX 20–2 *(continued)*

Interventions	Rationale	Evaluation
Teach client relaxation techniques to be performed every 4 to 6 hours, such as guided imagery, muscle relaxation, and meditation.	These measures can restore psychological and physical equilibrium and help decrease anxiety.	Is client successful in demonstrating relaxation methods?
Medicate with antianxiety agents as ordered.	Aids the client in decreasing anxiety.	Does client show decreased anxiety?

Knowledge deficit related to dysrhythmias, diagnostic tests, medications, and treatment

Client Outcomes
Verbalizes knowledge of disorder and willingness to comply with therapeutic regimen.

Evaluation of Outcomes
Can client explain dysrhythmias and treatments?

Interventions	Rationale	Evaluation
Explain condition, symptoms, and complications. Explain medications or therapies ordered.	Client must have basic knowledge to comply with therapy. Compliance and safe use of medications are promoted with an adequate knowledge base.	Is client able to verbalize knowledge taught? Can client explain medications and therapies?
Teach family CPR.	CPR increases client survival when promptly provided.	Is family willing to learn CPR?

GERIATRIC		
Include caregivers/family in educational sessions.	Compliance increases if support systems understand instructions and client needs.	Do caregivers/family participate in sessions and offer client support?

HOME HEALTH HINTS

- The nurse should have a pocket mask for CPR available at all times.

- A car phone or portable phone affords a home health nurse safety, convenience, and efficiency, especially if emergency help is needed, because some clients do not have phones.

- Clients prone to dysrhythmias should avoid straining with bowel movements. If the client reports straining, request a laxative or stool softener order from the physician.

- Clients who come home with a pacemaker should be instructed to wear loose tops. Women should not wear tight bras.

- Symptoms to watch for infection after a pacemaker implant are redness, swelling, warmth, and pain at the site.

- Instruct pacemaker clients to take their pulse once a day, in the morning, for a full minute. Assist them in setting up a log to record date, time, and pulse reading. Instruct them to call if the pulse varies outside parameters set by the physician.

- Clients on beta blockers need to know how to take their pulse, because bradycardia is a major side effect. A pulse below 50 warrants a call to the nurse or physician.

- Advise clients who are leaving home for weekend or holidays to refill medicines ahead of time. Also, the physician may write a prescription for clients to keep in their wallet for emergencies.

Review Questions

1. What area in the conduction system initiates the heartbeat?
   a. Atrioventricular (AV) node
   b. Bundle of His
   c. Right atrium
   d. Sinoatrial (SA) node

2. A client has a radial pulse of 58 beats per minute. This rate is called
   a. Tachycardia
   b. Normal
   c. Asystole
   d. Bradycardia

3. A run of three or more PVCs together is known as
   a. Ventricular tachycardia
   b. Bigeminy
   c. Trigeminy
   d. Quadrigeminy

4. If a patient in ventricular tachycardia is hemodynamically stable, the first choice of treatment is
   a. Cardioversion
   b. Pacemaker
   c. Defibrillation
   d. Antidysrhythmic medication

5. After a pacemaker implantation, which is a common complication?
   a. Hemorrhage
   b. Infection at site
   c. Pneumonia
   d. Embolism

6. If cardioversion or medications are not successful in converting atrial flutter, what would be the next treatment?
   a. Synchronized cardioversion
   b. Coronary bypass surgery
   c. Pacemaker insertion
   d. Bed rest

7. What is the total absence of electrical impulse in the cardiac muscle called?
   a. Atrial fibrillation
   b. Ventricular fibrillation
   c. Asystole
   d. Sinus arrest

ANSWERS TO CRITICAL THINKING

CRITICAL THINKING: Mrs. Mae

1. Assess client: vital signs, heart sounds; note symptoms; obtain an ECG per agency protocol.
2. Report the client findings to the registered nurse (RN) or physician.

3. Hypokalemia or ischemia causing irritability of the heart.
4. Light-headedness, feel heart skipping, chest pain, or fatigue.
5. Elevate head of bed for comfort, monitor vital signs, maintain O_2 per nasal cannula at 2 L per minute per agency protocol, remain with client to help alleviate anxiety. Notify the RN.
6. ECG, oxygen, potassium or electrolytes, may consider lidocaine (Xylocaine) starting infusion, if symptomatic.

CRITICAL THINKING: Mrs. Parker

1. A heart in VT has an ectopic focus firing. The heart is unable to maintain adequate cardiac output with such a rapid heart rate. The rapid and irregular heart rhythm does not allow the heart chambers time to adequately fill and empty, therefore reducing the blood volume with each beat. This in turn affects the peripheral circulation, causing the absence of palpable pulses.
2. In VT, one or more sites in the ventricle may be initiating impulses. The rapid rate of VT overrides the normal pacemaker of the heart. The rhythm can be regular or irregular. The inability of the heart to conduct impulses along normal pathways prevents the chambers from emptying and filling properly. This leads to a decreased cardiac output and can lead to cardiac arrest if the rhythm is not converted.
3. Lidocaine (Xylocaine) suppresses ventricular ectopic foci and causes changes in the conduction tissue. This allows the normal pacemaker of the heart to take over and resume normal coverage.

CRITICAL THINKING: Mr. Peet

1. Assess responsiveness, presence of carotid pulse. Check for breathing.
2. Open the airway. Call for assistance or use the client's phone to report a cardiac arrest. Initiate CPR until help arrives.
3. Once help or the code team arrives, the LPN/LVN reports the client's status. The person in charge will delegate responsibilities. Many facilities have protocols for each team member in a code. The LPN/LVN will assist in the code as delegated by the RN in charge.

CRITICAL THINKING: Mr. Treacher

1. Obtain ECG per agency protocol, notify RN and physician.
2. Head of bed elevated, O_2 per nasal cannula at 2 L per minute per protocol. Turn client onto side because this may help float pacemaker wire to chamber wall for better contact. Monitor client's

ECG, vital signs, and symptoms, and remain with client to provide emotional support.
3. Pacemaker malfunction.
4. Transfer to step-down unit or ICU, reprogramming of the pacemaker or a return to surgery for manipulation of the pacemaker wires or replacement.

REFERENCE

1. Thomas, CL (ed): Taber's Cyclopedic Medical Dictionary, ed 18. FA Davis, Philadelphia, 1997.

BIBLIOGRAPHY

Capucci, A, Villani, G, and Aschieri, D: Risk of complications of atrial fibrillation. Pacing Clin Electrophysiol 20(10 pt 2):2684, 1997.

Dunbar, S, and Summerville, J: Cognitive therapy for ventricular dysrhythmia patients. J Cardiovasc Nurs 12(1):33, 1997.

Gilbert, M, Wagna, GS, and Ramo, BV: Ventricular tachycardia. In Waugh, RA, et al (eds): Cardiac Arrhythmias: A Practical Guide for the Clinician, ed 2. FA Davis, Philadelphia, 1994.

Hattori, Y, Atsushi, S, Hiroaki, F, and Toyama, J: Effect of cilazapril on ventricular arrhythmia in patients in congestive heart failure. Clin Ther 19(3):481, 1997.

Hebia, JD: The nurse's role in continuous dysrhythmia monitoring. AACN Clin Issues Crit Care Nurs 5:178, 1994.

Ignatavicius, DD, Workman, ML, and Mishler, MA: Interventions for clients with dysrhythmias. In Ignatavicius, DD, Workman, ML, and Mishler, MA (eds): Medical Surgical Nursing: A Nursing Process Approach, ed 2. WB Saunders, Philadelphia, 1995.

Josephson, ME, and Callins, DJ: Sustained ventricular tachycardia. In Kastor, JA (ed): Arrhythmias. WB Saunders, Philadelphia, 1994.

Kerber, RE: External direct current cardioversion-defibrillation. In Zipes, DP, and Jnlife, J (eds): Cardiac Electrophysiology: From Cell to Bedside, ed 2. WB Saunders, Philadelphia, 1995.

Masoudi, F, and Goldschlager, N: The medical management of atrial fibrillation. Cardiol Clin 15(4):689, 1997.

Meyerburg, RJ, and Kessler, KM: Ventricular fibrillation. In Kastor, JA (ed): Arrhythmias. WB Saunders, Philadelphia, 1994.

Strimike, D, and Wojcik, J: Stopping atrial fibrillation with Ibutilide. Am J Nurs 98(1):32, 1998.

Plate 1 - Atlas of Body Systems Illustrations

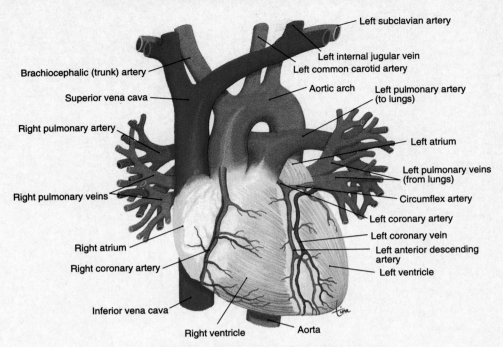

Heart and major blood vessels in anterior view.
(See Fig. 15-1, p.262.)

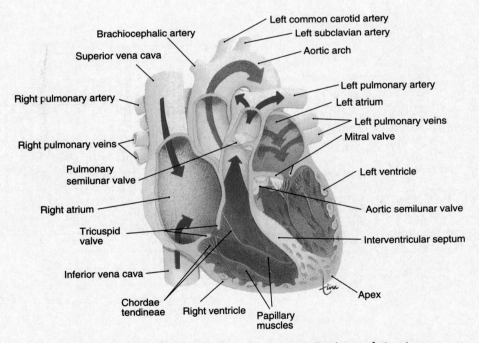

Frontal section of the heart in anterior view showing internal structures.
(See Fig. 15-2, p.263.)

Plate 2 - Atlas of Body Systems Illustrations

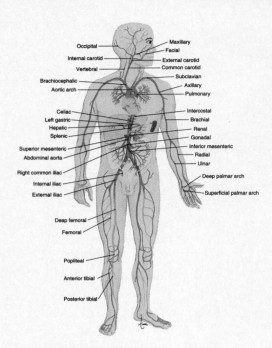

Systemic arteries. The aorta and its major branches are shown in anterior view.
(See Chapter 15.)

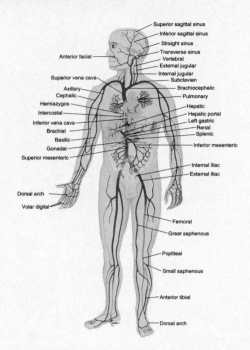

Systemic veins shown in anterior view.
(See Chapter 15.)

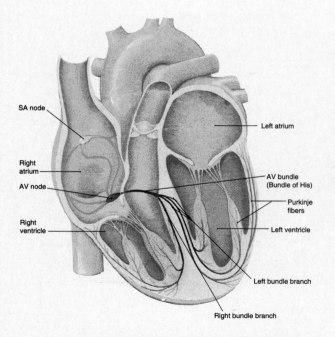

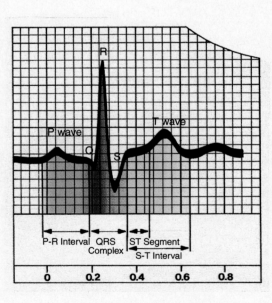

Conduction pathway of the heart. The interior of the heart is shown in anterior view.
The electrocardiogram tracing is of one normal heartbeat.
(See Chapter 20.)

Plate 3 - Atlas of Body Systems Illustrations

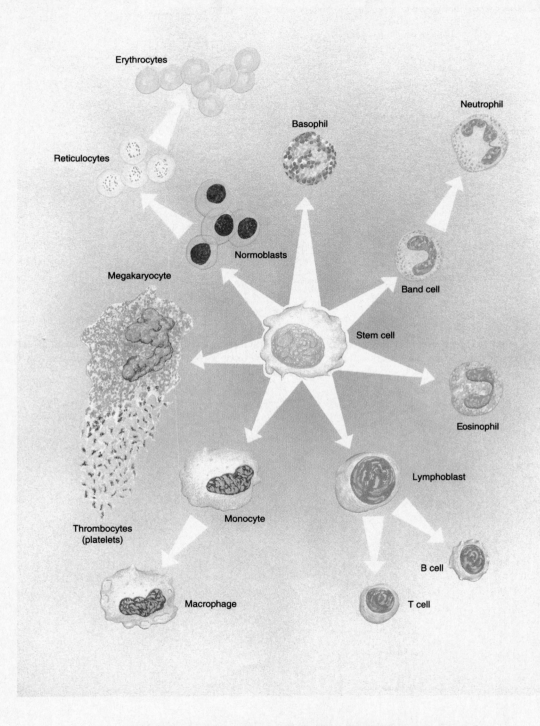

Blood cell production. Stem cells are found in red bone marrow and lymphatic tissue and are the precursor cells for all types of blood cells. (See Chapter 23.)

Plate 4 - Atlas of Body Systems Illustrations

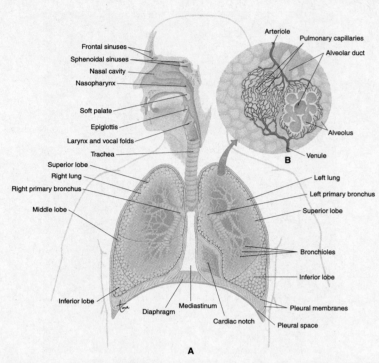

A

Respiratory system. (A) Anterior view of the upper and lower respiratory tracts. (B) Microscopic view of alveoli and pulmonary capillaries. (The colors represent the vessels, not the oxygen content of the blood within the vessels.)
(See Fig. 26-1, p.478.)

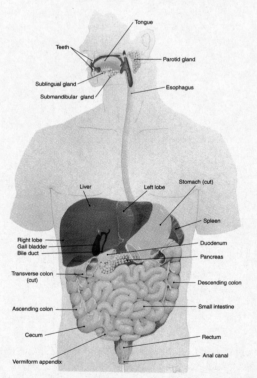

The digestive organs shown in anterior view of the trunk and left lateral view of the head. The spleen is not a digestive organ, but is included to show its location relative to the stomach, pancreas, and colon.
(See Fig. 29-1, p.556.)

Plate 5 - Atlas of Body Systems Illustrations

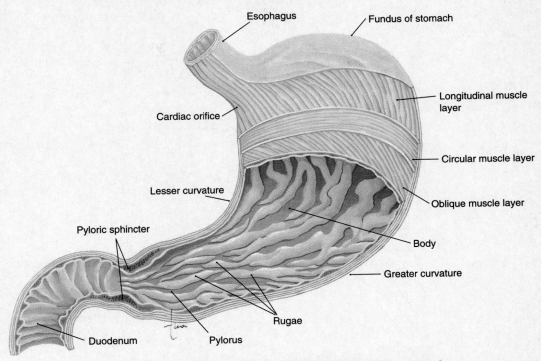

The stomach shown in anterior view. The stomach wall has been sectioned
to show the muscle layers and the rugae of the mucosa.
(See Fig. 29-2, p.557.)

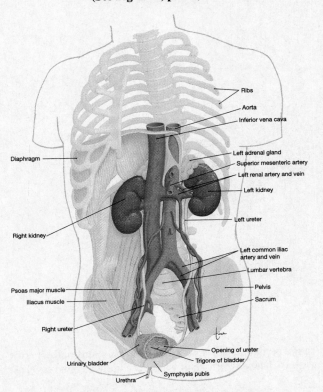

The urinary system shown in anterior view.
(See Chapter 34.)

Plate 6 - Atlas of Body Systems Illustrations

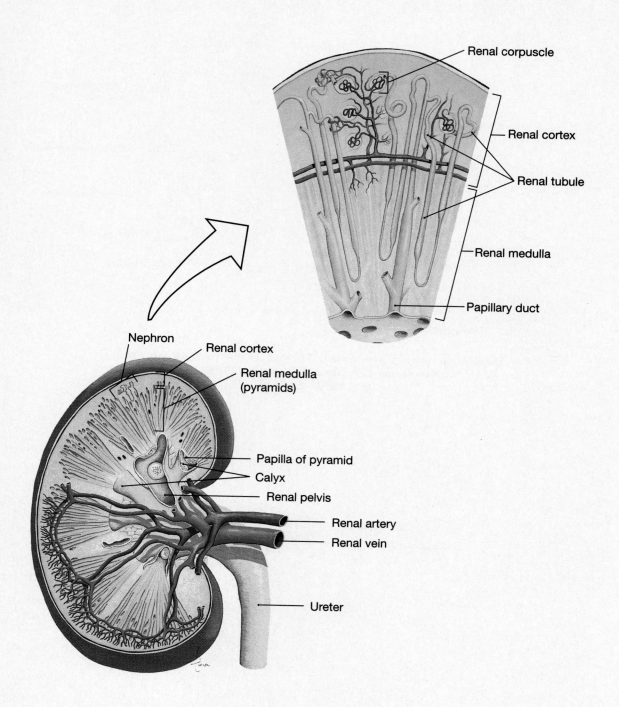

Frontal section of the right kidney showing internal structure and blood vessels. The magnified portion of the kidney shows several nephrons. (See Fig. 34-1, p.672.)

Plate 7 - Atlas of Body Systems Illustrations

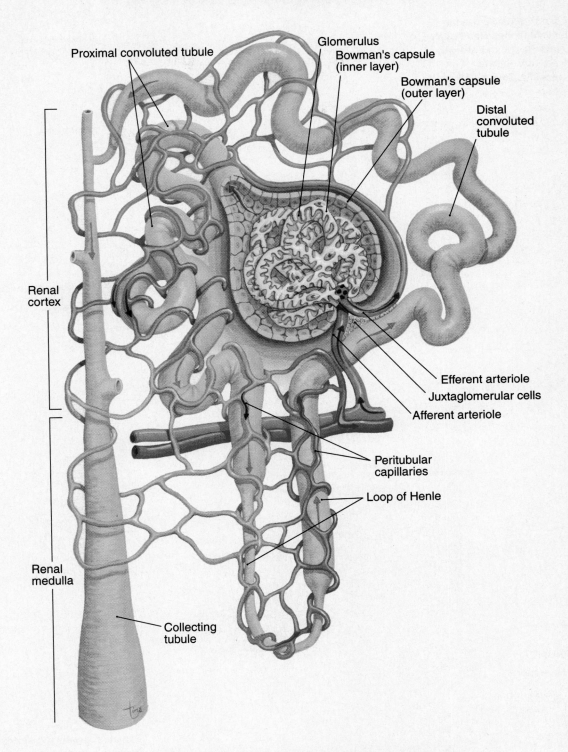

Proximal convoluted tubule

Glomerulus

Bowman's capsule (inner layer)

Bowman's capsule (outer layer)

Distal convoluted tubule

Renal cortex

Efferent arteriole

Juxtaglomerular cells

Afferent arteriole

Peritubular capillaries

Loop of Henle

Renal medulla

Collecting tubule

A nephron and its associated blood vessels. The arrows indicate the
direction of blood flow and the flow of renal filtrafte.
(See Fig. 34-2, p.673 and the text for a description.)

Plate 8 - Atlas of Body Systems Illustrations

Glands of the endocrine system. Both male and female gonads (testes and ovaries) are shown.
(See Fig. 36-1, p.718.)

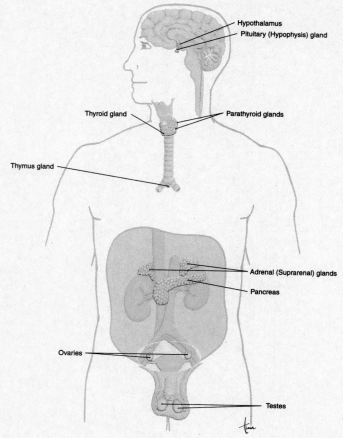

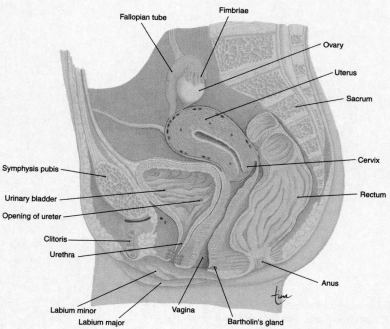

Female reproductive system shown in a midsagittal section through the pelvic cavity.
(See Fig. 39-1, p.774.)

Plate 9 - Atlas of Body Systems Illustrations

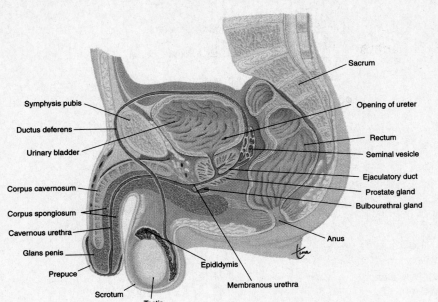

**Male reproductive system
shown in a midsagittal section
through the pelvic cavity.
(See Fig. 39-3, p.777.)**

Symphysis pubis

Ductus deferens

Urinary bladder

Corpus cavernosum

Corpus spongiosum

Cavernous urethra

Glans penis

Prepuce

Scrotum

Testis

Epididymis

Membranous urethra

Sacrum

Opening of ureter

Rectum

Seminal vesicle

Ejaculatory duct

Prostate gland

Bulbourethral gland

Anus

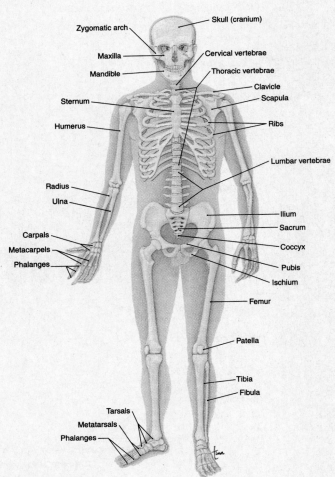

Zygomatic arch

Maxilla

Mandible

Sternum

Humerus

Radius

Ulna

Carpals

Metacarpels

Phalanges

Skull (cranium)

Cervical vertebrae

Thoracic vertebrae

Clavicle

Scapula

Ribs

Lumbar vertebrae

Ilium

Sacrum

Coccyx

Pubis

Ischium

Femur

Patella

Tibia

Fibula

Tarsals

Metatarsals

Phalanges

**Skeleton in anterior view.
(See Fig. 43-1, p.873.)**

Plate 10 · **Atlas of Body Systems Illustrations**

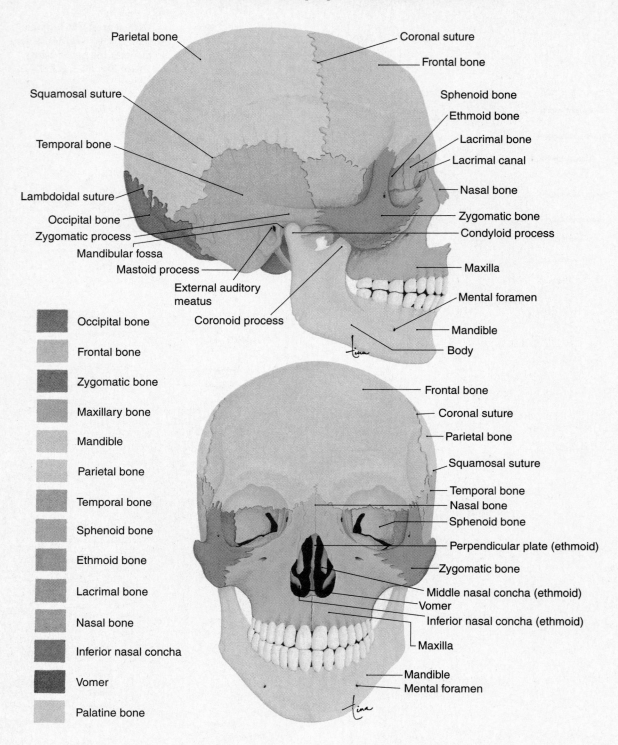

Skull. Lateral view of right side (top) and anterior view (bottom). (See Fig. 43-2, p.874.)

Plate 11 · Atlas of Body Systems Illustrations

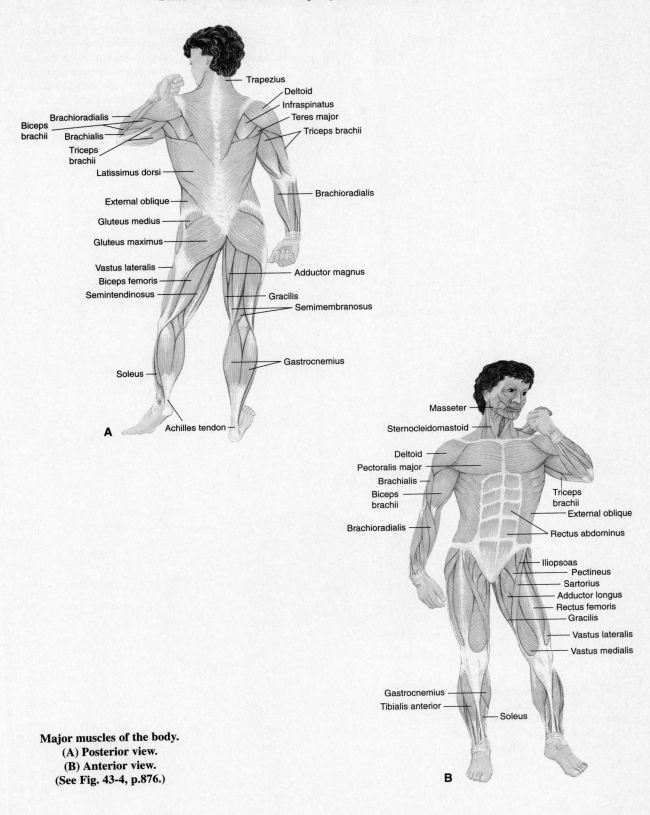

Major muscles of the body.
(A) Posterior view.
(B) Anterior view.
(See Fig. 43-4, p.876.)

Plate 12 · Atlas of Body Systems Illustrations

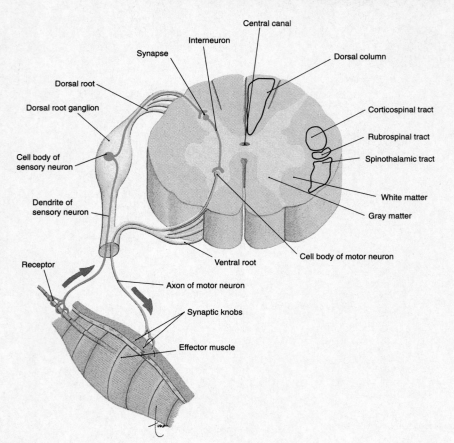

Central canal

Interneuron

Synapse

Dorsal column

Dorsal root

Dorsal root ganglion

Corticospinal tract

Rubrospinal tract

Cell body of
sensory neuron

Spinothalamic tract

White matter

Dendrite of
sensory neuron

Gray matter

Receptor

Ventral root

Cell body of motor neuron

Axon of motor neuron

Synaptic knobs

Effector muscle

**Spinal cord in cross section.
Spinal nerve roots and their
neurons are shown on the left
side. Spinal nerve tracts are
shown in the white matter.
Spinal tracts and nerves
are bilateral.
(See Fig. 45-3, p.929.)**

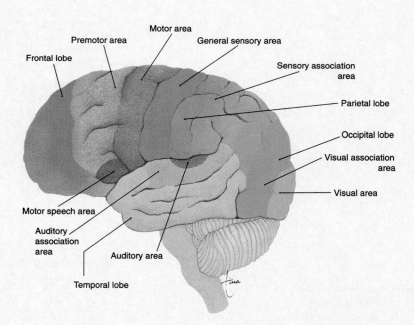

Motor area

Premotor area

General sensory area

Frontal lobe

Sensory association
area

Parietal lobe

Occipital lobe

Visual association
area

Visual area

Motor speech area

Auditory
association
area

Auditory area

Temporal lobe

**Left cerebral hemisphere
showing some of the
functional areas that have
been mapped.
(See Fig. 45-4, p.930.)**

Plate 13 · Atlas of Body Systems Illustrations

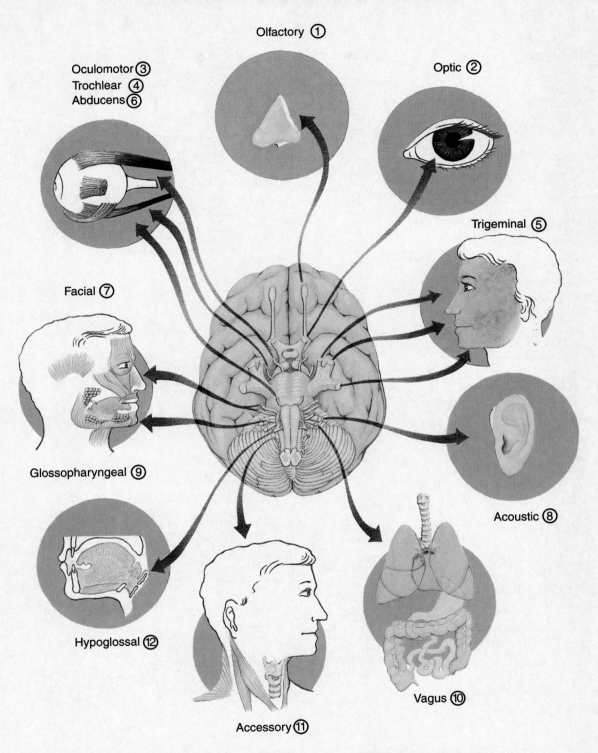

Olfactory ①

Oculomotor ③
Trochlear ④
Abducens ⑥

Optic ②

Trigeminal ⑤

Facial ⑦

Glossopharyngeal ⑨

Acoustic ⑧

Hypoglossal ⑫

Vagus ⑩

Accessory ⑪

Cranial nerves and their distributions. The brain is shown in an inferior view.
(See Table 45-2, p.932.)

Plate 14 - **Atlas of Body Systems Illustrations**

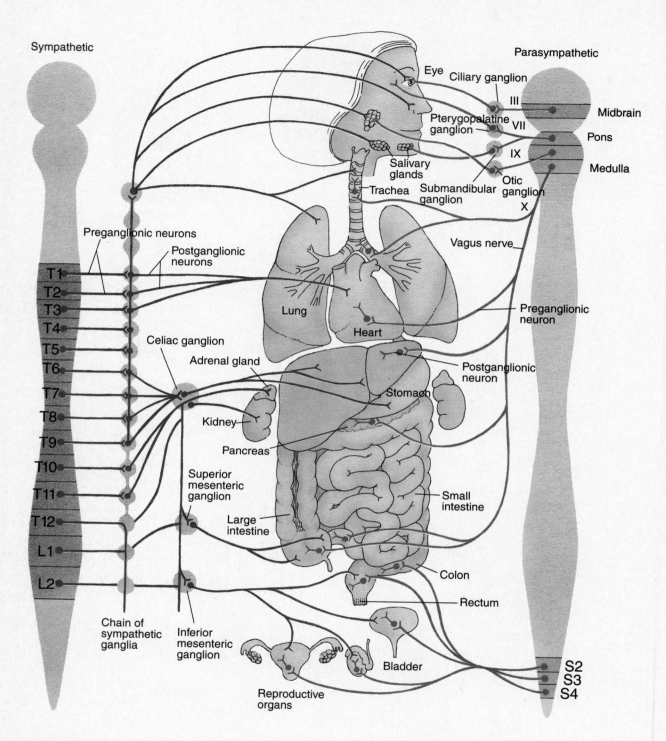

The autonomic nervous systems. Sympathetic division (left) and parasympathetic division (right). Both divisions are bilateral. (See Chapter 45.)

Plate 15 · Atlas of Body Systems Illustrations

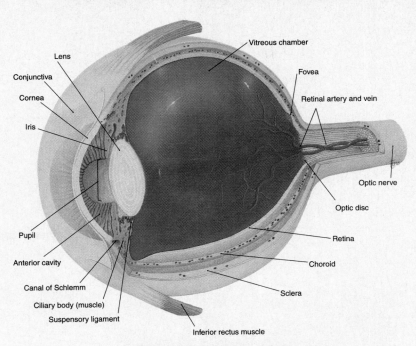

Internal anatomy of the eyeball.
(See Fig. 48-1, p.1022.)

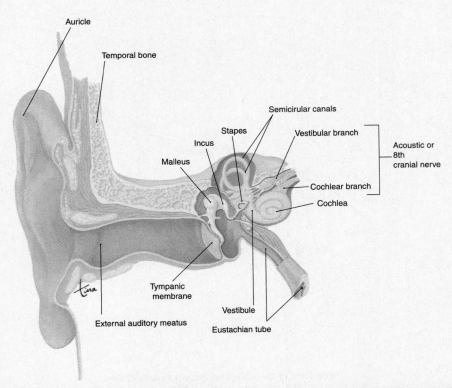

Outer, middle, and inner ear structures as shown in a frontal section through the right temporal bone.
(See Fig. 48-6, p.1031.)

Plate 16 - Atlas of Body Systems Illustrations

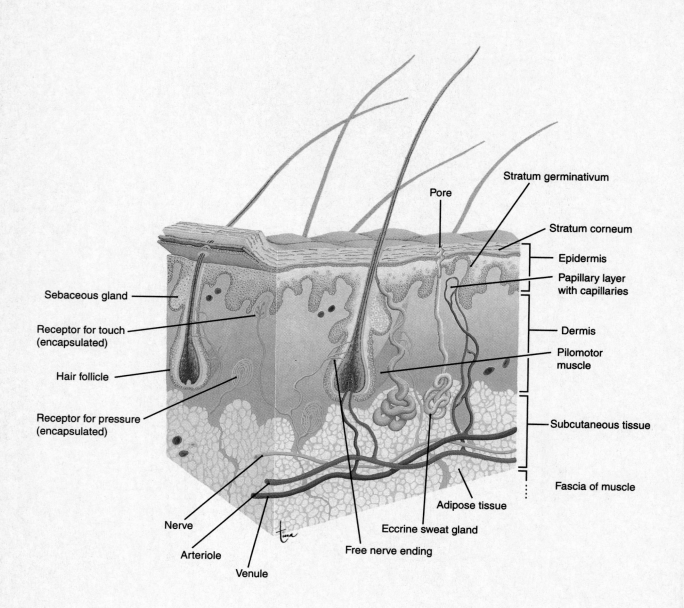

Structure of the skin and subcutaneous tissue.
(See Fig. 50-1, p.1080.)

Nursing Care of Clients with Heart Failure

Linda S. Williams

Learning Objectives

Upon completion of this chapter, the student will be able to:

1. Define heart failure.
2. Identify causes of heart failure.
3. Identify the pathophysiology and signs and symptoms of left- and right-sided heart failure.
4. Describe pathophysiology, signs and symptoms, diagnostic tests, and management of acute heart failure.
5. Describe diagnostic tests and medical management for chronic heart failure.
6. Identify nursing interventions for acute and chronic heart failure.
7. Explain health teaching for clients with heart failure and their families.

Key Words

afterload (**AFF**-ter-lohd)

cor pulmonale (**KOR** PUL-mah-**NAH**-lee)

cyanosis (SIGH-an-**NOH**sis)

hepatomegaly (HEP-uh-toh-**MEG**-ah-lee)

orthopnea (or-THOP-**knee-a**)

paroxysmal nocturnal dyspnea (PEAR-ox-**IS**-mall knock-TURN-al DISP-knee-a)

peripheral vascular resistance (puh-**RIFF**-uh-ruhl **VAS**-kyoo-lar ree-**ZIS**-tense)

preload (**PREE**-lohd)

pulmonary edema (**PULL**muh-NER-ee uh-**DEE**-muh)

splenomegaly (SPLEE-noh-**MEG**-ah-lee)

Heart Failure

Heart failure is a syndrome that occurs from the progressive inability of the heart to pump enough blood to meet the body's oxygen and nutrient needs. It can result in decreased tissue perfusion, fatigue, fluid volume overload in the intravascular and interstitial spaces, and reduced quality and length of life. Causes of heart failure include coronary artery disease, myocardial infarction, cardiomyopathy, heart valve problems, and hypertension. In the elderly, the most common cause of heart failure is cardiac ischemia.

Heart failure is classified according to which side of the heart has weakened and failed: left-sided heart failure, right-sided heart failure, or biventricular heart failure. It may develop rapidly or over time. Cardiogenic shock and **pulmonary edema** are types of acute or rapid-onset heart failure. Chronic heart failure develops over time as a result of another disorder, such as hypertension or pulmonary disease.

The incidence of heart failure is increasing as the elderly population increases. It is the most common reason for hospital admission in the elderly.[1] Quality of life is impaired. The client may experience many functional limitations and symptoms, and there is a high mortality rate. Readmission rates to hospitals for heart failure treatment is high.[2]

PATHOPHYSIOLOGY

The heart is divided into two separate pumping systems. The right side of the heart forms one pump. The left side of the heart forms the other pump. Normally, these pumps work together to ensure that equal amounts of blood enter and leave the heart.

Blood flow through the heart begins in the right atrium. (See Chapter 15.) Unoxygenated blood from the body's venous system enters the right atrium from the inferior and superior venae cavae. Next, the blood enters the right ventricle to be pumped into the pulmonary artery and into the lungs for oxygenation. After receiving oxygen in the lungs, the blood is returned to the left atrium via the four pulmonary veins. The oxygenated blood then enters the left ventricle and is pumped out into the aorta and systemic circulation.

Proper cardiac functioning requires each ventricle to pump out equal amounts of blood over time. If the amount of blood returned to the heart becomes more than either ventricle can handle, the heart can no longer be an effective pump. Conditions that cause heart failure may affect one or both of the heart's pumping systems. Therefore heart failure can be classified as right-sided heart failure, left-sided heart failure, or biventricular heart failure. The ventricle is the area of the heart's pumping system that commonly fails. Of the two ventricles, the left ventricle is typically the one to weaken first because it has the greatest workload. The right and left heart pumping systems work together in a closed system to continuously move blood forward, so failure of one side eventually leads to failure of the other side.

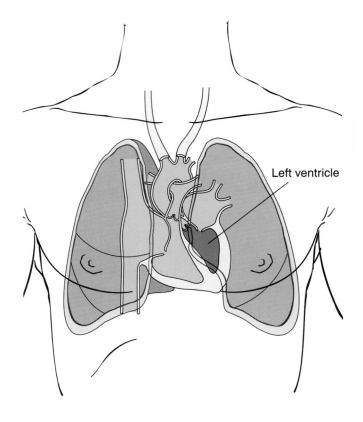

Left ventricle

LEARNING TIP

Heart Failure's Effect on Blood Flow. To visualize and understand the effects of heart failure, trace the flow of blood backward from each ventricle on the diagram. Along the backward path from the failing ventricle, congestion develops and produces the signs and symptoms seen in heart failure. If you understand the backward path of congestion, you can identify the signs and symptoms specifically associated with right- or left-sided heart failure.

LEARNING TIP

Heart Failure Pathophysiology. To understand heart failure, compare it to a river and a dam in the river.

1. In a river without a dam, the water flows freely; in the normal circulatory system, blood flows freely.
2. In a river with a dam, the water is blocked by the dam and builds up behind it; in heart failure, the failing ventricle acts like the dam in the river, causing blood to back up behind it.
3. When the dam on the river malfunctions, too much water builds up behind it and the riverbanks flood; in heart failure, if too much blood builds up behind the failing ventricle, the lungs or peripheral tissues are flooded (edema).

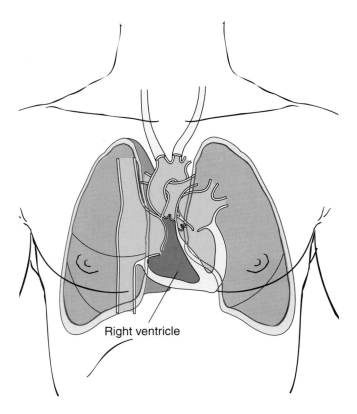

Right ventricle

Heart failure can be the result of systolic (contractile) dysfunction, diastolic (relaxation) dysfunction, or a mixed systolic and diastolic dysfunction. Systolic dysfunction is a contractile problem in which the ventricle is unable to generate enough force to pump blood from the ventricle. Diastolic dysfunction is a problem with the ventricle's ability to relax and fill. Mixed systolic and diastolic dysfunction is a combination of the two defects.

LEFT-SIDED HEART FAILURE

A certain amount of force must be generated by the left ventricle during a contraction to eject blood into the aorta

Table 21-1. **Causes of Left-Sided Heart Failure**

Cause	Primary Effect on Left Ventricular Workload
Hypertension	Resistance increased from elevated pressure
Coarctation of the Aorta	Resistance increased from elevated pressure
Myocardial Infarction	Increased workload from poor contractility
Cardiomyopathy	Increased workload from poor contractility
Aortic Stenosis	Increased volume to pump
Mitral Regurgitation	Increased volume to pump

through the aortic valve. This force is referred to as **afterload.** The pressure within the aorta and arteries influences the force needed to open the aortic valve to pump blood into the aorta. This pressure is called **peripheral vascular resistance (PVR).**

Hypertension is one of the major causes of left-sided heart failure because it increases the pressure within arteries. Increased pressure in the aorta makes the left ventricle work harder to pump blood into the aorta. Over time, the strain caused by the increased workload causes the left ventricle to weaken and fail. Other conditions that can lead to left-sided heart failure are described in Table 21–1 and

Figure 21–1. Among these conditions are disorders that (1) restrict the outflow of blood from the left ventricle, as in aortic valve stenosis or coarctation of the aorta, which is a malformation causing narrowing; (2) impair contractility of the heart, as in myocardial infarction or cardiomyopa-

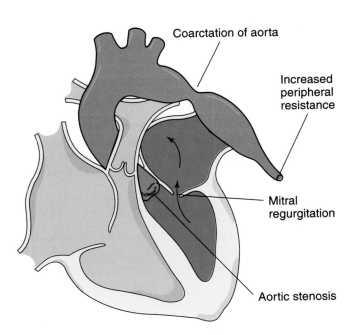

Coarctation of aorta

Increased peripheral resistance

Mitral regurgitation

Aortic stenosis

Major causes of left-sided heart failure.

Figure 21–1. Causes of left-sided heart failure.

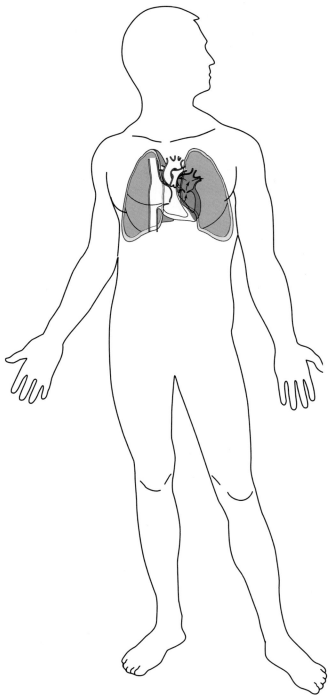

Figure 21–2. Left-sided heart failure. Shaded areas indicate areas of congestion from blood backup from the failing left side of the heart.

thy; and (3) allow blood to flow backward into the left atrium, as in valvular disorders.

With left-sided heart failure, blood backs up from the left ventricle into the left atrium and then into the four pulmonary veins and lungs (Fig. 21–2). This increases pulmonary pressure, causing movement of fluid first into the interstitium and then the alveoli. Alveolar edema is more serious because it reduces gas exchange across the alveolar capillary membrane. Shortness of breath and **cyanosis** may result from the decreased oxygenation of the blood leaving the lungs. If the fluid buildup is severe, pulmonary edema occurs, which requires immediate medical treatment.

RIGHT-SIDED HEART FAILURE

Causes of right-sided heart failure are described in Table 21–2 and Figure 21–3. The major cause of right-sided heart failure is left-sided heart failure. When the left side fails, fluid backs up into the lungs and pulmonary pressure is increased. The right ventricle must continually pump blood against this increased fluid and pressure in the pulmonary artery and lungs. Over time, this additional strain eventually causes it to fail.

Conditions causing right-sided heart failure increase the work of the right ventricle. They increase the amount of contractile force needed or they require pumping of excess blood volume (**preload**). Among these conditions are disorders that (1) increase pulmonary pressures, such as emphysema or congenital heart defects; (2) restrict the outflow of blood from the right ventricle, as in pulmonary valve stenosis; and (3) allow left atrial blood to flow into the right atrium, thereby increasing blood volume in the right ventricle, as in septal defects. When the right ventricle hypertrophies or fails due to increased pulmonary pressures, it is referred to as **cor pulmonale.**

When the right ventricle fails, it does not empty normally and there is a backward buildup of blood in the systemic blood vessels. As the blood backs up from the right ventricle, right atrial and systemic venous blood volume increases. The jugular neck veins, which are not normally visible, become distended and can be seen when the person

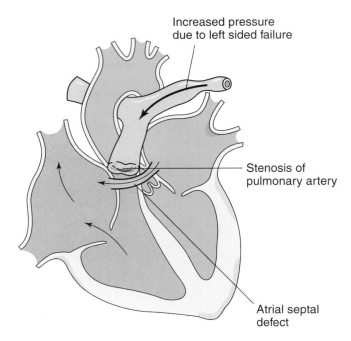

Major causes of right-sided heart failure.

Figure 21–3. Causes of right-sided heart failure.

is in a 45-degree upright position. Edema may occur in the peripheral tissues, and the abdominal organs can become engorged (Fig. 21–4). Congestion in the gastrointestinal tract causes anorexia, nausea, and abdominal pain. As the failure progresses, blood pools in the hepatic veins and the liver becomes congested, known as **hepatomegaly.** Pain in the right upper quadrant and impaired liver function are caused by this liver congestion. Systemic venous congestion also leads to engorgement of the spleen, known as **splenomegaly.**

LEARNING TIP

Heart Failure Signs and Symptoms. To understand the signs and symptoms of left-sided versus right-sided heart failure, remember that left-sided signs and symptoms are found in the lungs. *L*eft begins with *L,* as does *L*ung:

$$Left = Lungs, \quad L = L$$

Any signs and symptoms not related to the lungs (L) are caused by right-sided failure.

Table 21–2. **Causes of Right-Sided Heart Failure**

Cause	Primary Right Ventricular Workload Effect
Pulmonary Hypertension	Resistance increased from elevated pressure
Cor Pulmonale	Resistance increased from elevated pressure
Pulmonary Stenosis	Increased volume to pump
Atrial Septal Defect	Increased volume to pump

cor pulmonale: cor—heart + pulm—lung
hepatomegaly: hep—liver + mega—large
splenomegaly: splen—spleen + mega—large

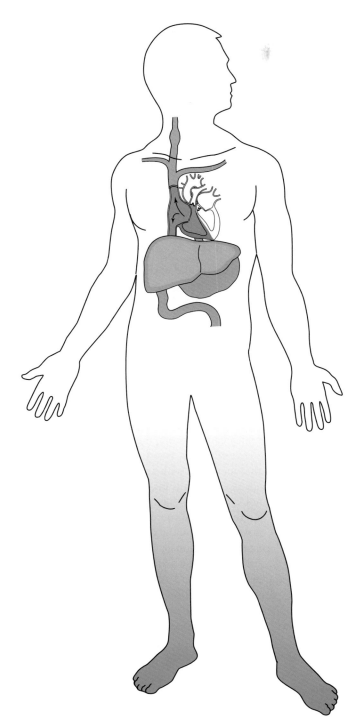

Figure 21–4. Right-sided heart failure. Shaded areas indicate areas of congestion from blood backup from the failing right side of the heart.

orthopnea: orth—straight + pnea—to breathe

Compensatory Mechanisms to Maintain Cardiac Output

Compensatory mechanisms help ensure that an adequate amount of blood is being pumped out of the heart. Although these mechanisms are designed to maintain cardiac output, they can also contribute to heart failure and create a cycle that instead of being helpful leads to further failure.

When the sympathetic nervous system detects low cardiac output, it speeds up the heart rate by releasing epinephrine and norepinephrine. Although this raises cardiac output (Cardiac output = Heart rate × Stroke volume), the increased heart rate also increases the oxygen needs of the heart. In response to low renal blood flow, the kidneys activate the renin-angiotensin-aldosterone system, and antidiuretic hormone is released from the pituitary gland to conserve water, causing decreased urine output. This adds to the fluid retention problem already found in heart failure.

Over time, the heart responds to its increased workload by enlarging its chambers (dilation), and increasing its muscle mass (hypertrophy). In dilation, the heart muscle fibers stretch to increase the force of myocardial contractions, which is known as the Frank-Starling phenomenon. In hypertrophy, the muscle mass of the heart increases, creating more contractile force. Both of these compensatory mechanisms increase the heart's oxygen needs.

Acute Heart Failure (Pulmonary Edema)

Acute heart failure, or pulmonary edema, results in severe congestion in the alveoli of the lungs and is a life-threatening condition. It occurs when the heart suffers an acute event such as a myocardial infarction (MI) or when the heart is severely stressed and unable to compensate, causing the left ventricle to fail. Complications of pulmonary edema include dysrhythmias and cardiac and pulmonary arrest.

PATHOPHYSIOLOGY

In the early phase of pulmonary edema, pressure rises in the lung's venous blood vessels and blood builds up. As pressures continue to rise, fluid moves into the interstitial spaces. With continued pressure increases, fluid containing red blood cells then moves into the alveoli. Finally, the alveoli and airways become filled with fluid.

SIGNS AND SYMPTOMS

Classic signs and symptoms of pulmonary edema include anxiety, restlessness, pale skin or mucous membranes, clammy and cold skin, severe dyspnea, **orthopnea,** use of accessory muscles, rapid respirations, coughing, pink and frothy sputum, crackles, and wheezes. Compensatory mechanisms increase the heart rate and blood pressure; however, as the pulmonary edema worsens, the blood pressure may fall.

DIAGNOSIS

Diagnostic studies may include chest x-ray, arterial blood gases (ABGs), electrocardiogram (ECG), and hemodynamic monitoring. The congested pulmonary system can be seen on x-ray. ABGs will show a decrease in PaO_2 that continues to decrease as the edema worsens and an increase in $PaCO_2$ causing respiratory acidosis (pH < 7.35). The pulmonary artery catheter will show elevated pulmonary pressures and a decreased cardiac output.

MEDICAL MANAGEMENT

Immediate treatment is necessary to prevent clients from drowning in their own secretions (Table 21–3). The goal of therapy is to reduce the workload of the left ventricle in order to improve cardiac output and reduce the client's anxiety. Care for the client is usually provided in an intensive care unit. Treatment for the underlying cause occurs at the same time that the client is being treated for the pulmonary edema.

Treatment includes positioning the client upright to make breathing easier in a semi-Fowler's or high Fowler's position. In a Fowler's position, the lungs can more easily expand. The client should be asked what position is preferred. Oxygen is applied and is usually delivered by mask to provide higher concentrations of oxygen. In severe cases of pulmonary edema, endotracheal intubation and mechanical ventilation may be necessary. Medications administered may include intravenous (IV) morphine to reduce anxiety, relax airways, and increase peripheral blood pooling to decrease preload; diuretics to reduce fluid congestion; vasodilators to reduce preload; and inotropic agents to strengthen heart contractions.

Chronic Heart Failure

SIGNS AND SYMPTOMS

The signs and symptoms of chronic heart failure are influenced by the client's age, the underlying cause and severity of heart disease, and the ventricle that is failing. Heart failure is a progressive disorder, so signs and symptoms may worsen over time. The classic signs and symptoms are dyspnea, dry cough, weight gain, edema, fatigue, weakness, abdominal pain, and nausea and vomiting. Signs and symptoms caused by a specific failing ventricle are listed in Table 21–4.

Fatigue and Weakness

Fatigue and weakness are the earliest symptoms of heart failure. They occur from the decreased amount of oxygen reaching the tissues. During the day the fatigue worsens, especially with activity.

Dyspnea

A failing left ventricle produces prominent respiratory effects. Dyspnea is a common symptom, particularly of left-sided heart failure. It occurs from the pulmonary congestion that impairs gas exchange between the alveoli and capillaries. Dyspnea causes short, rapid respirations. It can be classified in several ways. Exertional dyspnea is shortness of breath that increases with activity, and orthopnea is dyspnea that increases when lying flat. In an upright position, gravity holds fluid in the lower extremities. In a supine position, gravitational forces are removed, allowing fluid to move from the legs to the heart, which overwhelms the already congested pulmonary system. When orthopnea is present, two or more pillows are often used for sleeping, and the documentation should state the number of pillows used. For example, three pillows used would be three-pillow orthopnea. **Paroxysmal nocturnal dyspnea** (PND) is sudden shortness of breath that occurs after lying flat for a

---

Table 21–3. **Medical Management of Acute Heart Failure**

Oxygen by cannula, mask, or mechanical ventilation
Positioning in high Fowler's or semi-Fowler's position
Bed rest
Drug therapy
   Morphine IV
   Diuretics IV
   Inotropic agents IV
   Vasodilators IV
Frequent vital signs, urinary output, pulmonary pressures
Daily weights
Treatment of underlying cause

Table 21–4. **Signs and Symptoms of Heart Failure**

Right-Sided Heart Failure	Left-Sided Heart Failure
Tachycardia	Tachycardia
Jugular vein distention	Dyspnea
Dependent peripheral edema	Dry cough
Ascites	Crackles, wheezing
Weight gain	Orthopnea
Nocturia	Paroxysmal nocturnal dyspnea
Hepatomegaly	Fatigue, weakness
Splenomegaly	Cheyne-Stokes respiration
Gastrointestinal discomfort	Cyanosis
Fatigue, weakness	Nocturia

period of time. It mainly results from excess fluid accumulation in the lungs. The sleeping person awakens with feelings of suffocation and anxiety. Relief is obtained by sitting upright for a short period of time, which reduces the amount of fluid returning to the heart.

Cough

A chronic, dry cough is common in heart failure. The coughing increases when lying down from increased irritation of the lung mucosa. This irritation is due to the increase in pulmonary congestion that occurs when gravity no longer keeps fluid in the legs and more fluid returns to the heart and lungs.

Crackles and Wheezes

Pulmonary congestion causes abnormal breath sounds such as crackles and wheezes. These sounds indicate the presence of increased fluid in the lungs. Crackles are produced from fluid buildup in the alveoli resulting from increased pressure in the pulmonary capillaries. Wheezes occur from bronchiolar constriction caused by the increased fluid.

LEARNING TIP

To simulate the sound of crackles, open a piece of Velcro. This sound is similar to the sound of crackles heard with a stethoscope.

Tachycardia

The sympathetic nervous system compensates for the decreased cardiac output in heart failure by releasing epinephrine and norepinephrine to increase the heart rate. Normally, this is helpful because the increased heart rate increases the amount of blood ejected by the heart to maintain an adequate cardiac output. However, whenever the heart works faster it also requires more oxygen, which a failing heart finds it difficult to supply.

Chest Pain

Chest pain may occur from ischemia in the client with heart failure. Decreased cardiac output results in decreased oxygen delivery to the heart itself, via the coronary arteries. Compensatory mechanisms designed to maintain cardiac output increase the workload and oxygen needs of the heart and are counterproductive in heart failure. Tachycardia increases the oxygen needs of the heart. The kidneys compensate by retaining sodium and fluid, which increases the fluid volume returning to the heart (preload) and therefore the heart's workload and oxygen needs. Pain also increases oxygen requirements, adding further to the cycle of heart failure.

Cheyne-Stokes Respiration

A breathing pattern of shallow respirations building to deep breaths followed by a period of apnea characterizes Cheyne-Stokes breathing. The apneic period occurs because the deep breathing causes carbon dioxide levels to drop to a level that does not stimulate the respiratory center. This apnea may last up to 30 seconds and is then followed by the shallow-to-deeper respiratory pattern of Cheyne-Stokes, as carbon dioxide levels rise again.

Edema

Edema occurs in heart failure as a result of (1) systemic blood vessel congestion and (2) the sympathetic compensatory mechanisms that cause the kidneys to activate the renin-angiotensin system in which antidiuretic hormone is released from the pituitary gland, causing sodium and water to be retained. Several forms of edema can occur in heart failure. The effect of backward buildup of pressure in the systemic blood vessels is seen with distention of the jugular veins (Fig. 21–5), swelling of the legs and feet, sacral edema in the individual on bed rest, and increased fluid within the abdominal cavity and organs. An acute buildup of fluid in the lungs produces pulmonary edema, and weight gain is a sign of fluid retention.

Nocturia

Nocturia is an increase in urine output at night. After lying down, fluid in the lower legs returns to the circulatory system. Renal blood flow and filtration is increased, resulting in greater urine production and the need to urinate frequently during the night. Nocturia may occur up to six times per night, contributing to the client's fatigue.

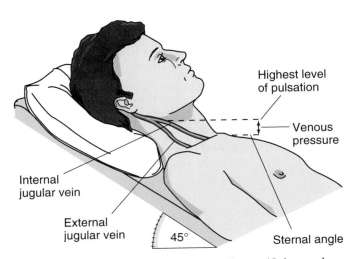

Figure 21–5. Jugular vein distention in a client at 45-degree elevation.

Cyanosis

The skin, nailbeds, or mucous membranes may appear blue, or cyanotic, from decreased oxygenation of the blood. Cyanosis is a late sign of heart failure. It is associated primarily with left-sided heart failure.

Altered Mental Status

A decrease in blood flow from heart failure decreases the amount of oxygen delivered to the brain. As a result, restlessness, insomnia, confusion, and impaired memory may occur. A decrease in the level of consciousness may also be seen.

Malnutrition

Several factors contribute to malnutrition in the person with chronic heart failure. Altered mental status, dyspnea, and fatigue interfere with the ability to eat. Anorexia and gastrointestinal (GI) upset occur from pressure exerted by excess fluid surrounding the GI structures. Absorption of food may also be impaired by this pressure.

CRITICAL THINKING: Mr. Shepard (1)

Mr. Shepard, 66, has a family history of cardiac disease. He has been hypertensive for 10 years and takes nifedipine daily. His baseline vital signs are blood pressure 122/78, pulse 80, respiration 18, height 66 in, and weight 170 lb. During a visit to his physician, he states that he has been short of breath during his daily 2-mile walk and has been using two pillows at night for sleep. As he talks, the physician notes that he has a dry cough. His physical examination shows blood pressure 140/86, pulse 106, respiration 24, weight 178 lb, and bilateral crackles in the lung bases.

1. What signs and symptoms of heart failure does Mr. Shepard have?
2. Do the signs and symptoms reflect right- or left-sided heart failure?
3. Why are each of the signs and symptoms occurring?
4. Why is Mr. Shepard using two pillows for sleeping?

Answers at end of chapter.

COMPLICATIONS OF HEART FAILURE

Complications of heart failure may include hepatomegaly, splenomegaly, pleural effusion, left ventricular thrombus and emboli, and cardiogenic shock. The liver and spleen enlarge from the fluid congestion, which causes impaired function, cellular death, and scarring. Pleural effusion, a leakage of fluid from the capillaries of the lung into the pleural space, can occur. This leakage of fluid is caused by the elevated pressures in the capillaries of the lung. Thrombosis and emboli may occur because of the poor emptying of the ventricles. Whenever blood pools, there is increased risk for thrombus formation and emboli. Aspirin or anticoagulants are often prescribed to prevent thrombus formation for clients with heart failure. Cardiogenic shock occurs when the left ventricle is unable to supply the tissues with enough oxygen and nutrients to meet their needs. The damage to the left ventricle resulting in cardiogenic shock is usually caused by a myocardial infarction.

DIAGNOSTIC TESTS

Diagnostic tests are done to identify the cause of the failure and determine the degree of failure that is present. Table 21–5 lists the common diagnostic methods used for heart failure, in addition to history and physical examination.

A chest x-ray shows the size and shape of the heart and the pulmonary vessels. Early heart disease can be detected with x-ray. Cardiac enlargement or congestion in the pulmonary circulation can also be assessed by x-ray.

Cardiac dysrhythmias that precipitate and contribute to heart failure can be diagnosed with ECG. (See Chapter 20.) Heart failure can also be detected by ECG. Chamber enlargement in the atrium is shown by P wave changes and in the left ventricle by increased voltage and deeper S waves in some V leads. Exercise stress testing and nuclear imaging studies provide information on activity tolerance, which is usually limited in heart failure.

Table 21–5. **Diagnostic Tests for Heart Failure**

History and physical examination
Chest x-ray
Serum laboratory tests: arterial blood gases, electrolytes, liver enzymes, blood urea nitrogen, creatinine
Electrocardiogram
Exercise stress test
Nuclear imaging studies
Echocardiography
Angiography
Cardiac catheterization
Invasive hemodynamic monitoring

Echocardiography measures the size of the heart chambers to detect enlargement and assess valvular function and motion of the ventricles. Cardiac catheterization and angiography are used to detect underlying heart disease that may be the cause of heart failure.

Direct assessment of the heart's pressures is done with invasive hemodynamic monitoring. A catheter is inserted into the heart and pulmonary artery to transmit pressures to a cardiac monitor. These cardiac and pulmonary pressures are then used to diagnose and guide medical therapy (See Chapter 15.)

Serum laboratory tests may show elevated serum sodium from fluid retention, elevated serum blood urea nitrogen (BUN) and elevated serum creatinine from renal failure, and elevated liver enzymes from liver damage.

> ### CRITICAL THINKING: Mr. Shepard (2)
>
> Mr. Shepard's chest x-ray shows an enlarged heart (cardiomegaly).
>
> 1. Why is Mr. Shepard's heart enlarged?
> 2. What is the significance of an enlarged heart?
>
> *Answers at end of chapter.*

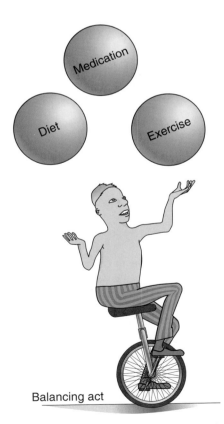

Figure 21–6. Management of heart failure is a balancing act. (Modified from Stanley, M, and Beare, P: Gerontological Nursing. FA Davis, Philadelphia, 1995, p 198, with permission.)

MEDICAL MANAGEMENT

The overall goal of medical treatment for chronic heart failure is to improve the heart's pumping ability and decrease the heart's oxygen demands. Treatment of heart failure focuses on (1) identifying and correcting the underlying cause, (2) increasing the strength of the heart's contraction, (3) maintaining optimal water and sodium balance, and (4) decreasing the heart's workload (Fig. 21–6). Heart failure management requires a team approach that may involve physicians, case managers, nurses, dietitians, physical therapists, occupational therapists, pharmacists, social workers, and clergy. Critical pathways are being used for heart failure to ensure quality-based outcomes while reducing treatment costs.

The severity of heart failure determines the individualized therapy selected. Noninvasive approaches are usually tried first (Table 21–6). If noninvasive treatment is not effective, invasive approaches may be used to achieve the goal of therapy.

Oxygen Therapy

One of the major problems caused by heart failure is a reduction in oxygen delivered to the tissues. The heart failure signs and symptoms related to this are fatigue, dyspnea, altered mental status, and cyanosis. Oxygen therapy assists

Table 21–6. Medical Management of Chronic Heart Failure

Noninvasive
Identification and treatment of underlying cause
Oxygen by cannula or mask
Drug therapy
Diuretics
Inotropic agents
Vasodilators
Nitrates
Angiotensin-converting enzyme inhibitors
Beta blockers
Anticoagulants
Antidysrhythmic agents
Individualized activity plan
Dietary sodium restriction
Fluid restriction
Daily weights

Invasive
Mechanical assistive devices
Intra-aortic balloon pump
Left ventricular assist device
Total artificial heart
Surgery
Cardiomyoplasty
Cardiac transplant

in supplying the oxygen needs of the tissues. In mild heart failure, oxygen may be delivered by nasal cannula. For more severe cases, arterial blood gas values guide oxygen delivery, either with masks that provide high concentrations of oxygen or with mechanical ventilation.

Activity

Activity tolerance depends on the severity of heart failure signs and symptoms. Severe symptoms may require bed rest with restricted activity until treatment reduces the symptoms. For stable heart failure, a regular exercise program can be helpful in improving cardiac function and reducing heart failure effects. Clients should be encouraged to stay as active as possible within the parameters the physician has prescribed. An individualized walking program that increases activity over time is often prescribed. Clients should be taught how to exercise safely without causing symptoms and to understand that overexertion can produce fatigue the next day. Referral to a cardiac rehabilitation program can be helpful for some clients.

Nutrition

Dietary sodium is often restricted to decrease fluid retention. Sodium restrictions are individualized but may begin at 3 g for mild to moderate heart failure. Avoiding table salt, canned foods such as soup, and salty foods such as hot dogs and potato chips will achieve a daily intake limited to 3 g of sodium. For more severe heart failure, dietary sodium may be restricted to 2 g or less per day.

Restricting sodium is challenging. Compliance is often low because low-sodium foods are not very appealing. A referral to a dietitian is important. Diet counseling helps the client and family understand the need for dietary compliance and the need to provide menus that are appealing and easy to use. Salt substitutes often use potassium in place of sodium, so the client and physician should discuss their use. Spices, herbs, and lemon juice may be suggested to flavor unsalted foods. Eating should remain pleasurable for the client to avoid malnutrition.

In severe heart failure with abdominal discomfort present, malnutrition is a concern. The client can be anorexic, but the weight gain that occurs with fluid retention can mask the weight loss occurring from the anorexia. Food intake should be monitored to ensure that fluid retention weight gain does not contribute to malnutrition being undetected.

Drug Therapy

The major classifications of drugs used to treat heart failure include diuretics, which increase fluid output; inotropic agents, which strengthen heart contractions; and vasodila-

tors, which reduce peripheral vascular pressure to decrease the heart's workload.

Diuretics

The purpose of using a diuretic is to reduce fluid volume and decrease pulmonary venous pressure so that the heart does not have to work so hard. Diuretics act on various areas of the kidneys to promote the excretion of edema fluid, which allows the heart to work more efficiently. A combination of diuretics may be used to achieve the desired effect. Electrolytes (especially potassium levels, to prevent hypokalemia) and fluid balance (to prevent dehydration) should be carefully monitored.

Inotropic Agents

Inotropic drugs strengthen ventricular contraction, which allows the heart to function more efficiently. Inotropic agents include the cardiac glycosides (digitalis, digoxin), sympathomimetics (dopamine, dobutamine), and phosphodiesterase inhibitors (amrinone, milrinone). The sympathomimetics and phosphodiesterase inhibitors are usually used short term.

DIGITALIS. In addition to improving contraction strength, digitalis preparations decrease conduction time within the heart, which slows the heart rate to allow more complete emptying of the ventricles. Digitalis may increase myocardial oxygen needs, so it is being used more cautiously. Monitoring of serum drug levels is necessary to detect toxic levels of the drug. If toxic levels are present, the drug is stopped to allow digitalis levels to decrease over time. If digitalis levels are life threatening, a digoxin antibody, digoxin immune FAB (Digibind), can be administered.

Vasodilator Drugs

Vasodilator drugs reduce pressure within blood vessels to reduce cardiac workload in three ways: (1) the amount of fluid returning to the heart is reduced from venous pooling (preload); (2) pulmonary congestion decreases as pulmonary pressures decrease and fluid is reabsorbed; and (3) ventricular workload (afterload) is decreased as peripheral vascular resistance is reduced. Several types of vasodilator drugs are used. Angiotensin-converting enzyme (ACE) inhibitors (captopril, enalapril, lisinopril) are the most commonly used vasodilators.

Mechanical Assistive Devices

Mechanical assistive devices can provide temporary support to clients in cardiogenic shock or awaiting cardiac transplant. These devices increase the cardiac output of the client. Research is ongoing into the development of mechanical pumps that may become heart replacements. These mechanical assistive devices are used primarily in critical care settings.

Intra-Aortic Balloon Pump

The intra-aortic balloon pump (IABP) increases circulation to the coronary arteries. This provides more oxygen to the myocardium and reduces the workload of the heart. The IABP is inserted into the femoral artery and positioned in the descending aortic arch (Fig. 21–7). The IABP is attached to a machine that senses ventricular contraction. During diastole the balloon inflates, forcing increased blood into the coronary arteries. During systole the balloon deflates.

Ventricular Assist Devices

A ventricular assist device (VAD) temporarily supports cardiac output and allows the failing ventricle to rest. VADs are attached to different areas of the heart depending on their type (Fig. 21–8). For example, VADs can pump blood directly from either the right atrium to the pulmonary artery (right ventricular failure) or the left atrium to the aorta (left ventricular failure). Two devices can be used for biventricular failure.

The left ventricular assist device is a pump attached to a heart catheter that is positioned in the left ventricle to assist the failing left ventricle. Blood remaining in the left ventricle after systole is pumped directly into the aorta by the device. This increases cardiac output and rests the left ventricle.

Surgical Management

Cardiomyoplasty

Cardiomyoplasty is a surgical procedure that uses the client's own skeletal muscle (latissimus dorsi) to enhance the function of the heart and improve circulation (Fig. 21–9). The muscle is positioned around the aorta or heart, and a cardiomyostimulator and leads are implanted to stimulate muscle contraction. The muscle is rested for 2 weeks after surgery and then programmed to gradually start stimulation. After 4 months, the muscle can be stimulated either at a 1:1 or 1:2 heartbeat ratio.

For clients with end-stage heart failure, cardiac transplantation is an option. (See Chapter 22.) Mechanical assistive devices may be used to support cardiac function while the client awaits a donor heart.

   CRITICAL THINKING: Mr. Shepard (3)

During Mr. Shepard's visit, the physician tells him to continue the vasodilator, the diuretic, and a 2 g sodium diet.

1. Why is the vasodilator continued?
2. Will the vasodilator affect preload or afterload?
3. Why is the diuretic ordered?
4. Why is a 2 g sodium diet ordered?
5. What is the overall goal of the ordered treatment?

Answers at end of chapter.

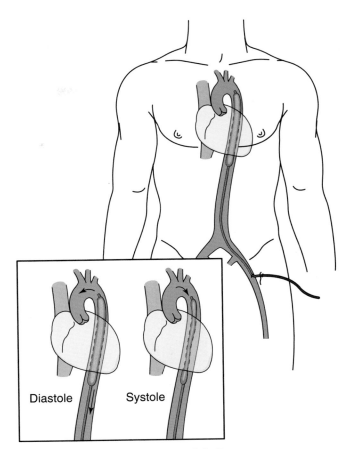

Diastole   **Systole**

Figure 21–7. Intra-aortic balloon pump.

NURSING PROCESS FOR CHRONIC HEART FAILURE

Nursing Assessment

A nursing history and physical examination are done to gather subjective and objective data. While obtaining data, the nurse should focus on areas that might indicate the presence of heart failure (Table 21–7).

Planning

The client and family should be included in planning care. The client's goals are to (1) maintain desired activities, (2) remain free of edema and dyspnea, (3) awaken refreshed with less fatigue, (4) reduce anxiety, and (5) follow a mutually agreed on health maintenance plan.

Nursing Diagnosis

Individualized nursing care plans are developed for the client with heart failure from collected data. See Nursing Care Plan Box 21–1 for the Client with Chronic Heart Failure for common nursing diagnoses. Additional problems may also be identified. These problems should be addressed in the client's individualized nursing care plan.

Left ventricular
assist device

Right ventricular
assist device

Biventricular
assist device

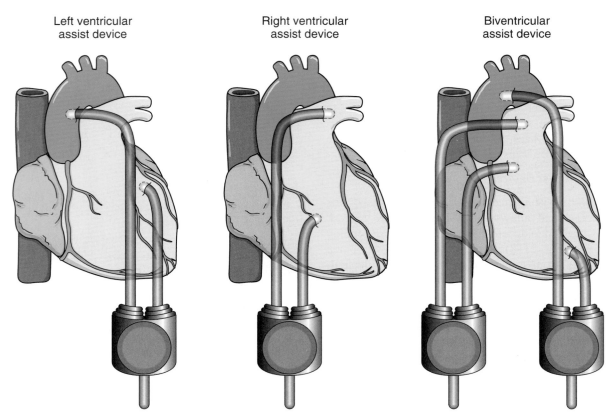

Figure 21–8. Different types of ventricular assist devices. (Modified from Ruppert, S, Kernicki, J, and Dolan, J: Dolan's Critical Care Nursing. FA Davis, Philadelphia, 1996, p 336, with permission.)

Nursing Interventions

The major focus of nursing care for chronic heart failure clients includes (1) improving oxygenation, (2) educating clients about their condition and health maintenance needs, (3) promoting self-care with energy conservation techniques, and (4) facilitating client and family coping.

Oxygenation can be improved with oxygen therapy and a decrease in the body's need for oxygen. Decreased metabolic oxygen needs can be achieved with rest, positioning, medications, fluid balance, and oxygen consumption control.

Oxygen

Oxygen therapy is ordered by the physician and guided by blood gas analysis. Before starting oxygen therapy, the nurse explains the therapy to the client. For chronic heart failure, oxygen is administered at 2 to 6 L/min via nasal cannula. The effects of the oxygen should be monitored carefully. Oxygen should be used cautiously in all clients so that their stimulus to breathe is not diminished.

HOME OXYGEN THERAPY. If a client will be using home oxygen therapy, instructions must be given on the proper use of the oxygen and safety precautions for oxygen use. The family must also understand oxygen safety precautions and be willing to comply with them. Smoking is prohibited when oxygen is in use.

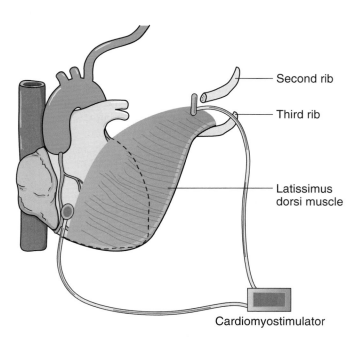

Second rib

Third rib

Latissimus
dorsi muscle

Cardiomyostimulator

Figure 21–9. Cardiomyoplasty. (Modified from Ruppert, S, Kernicki, J, and Dolan, J: Dolan's Critical Care Nursing. FA Davis, Philadelphia, 1996, p 329, with permission.)

Table 21–7. Nursing Assessment for the Client with Chronic Heart Failure

Subjective Data

History
Respiratory
  Lung disease?
  How many flights of stairs can be climbed without dyspnea?
  How many pillows used for sleeping?
  Dyspnea at rest or that awakens from sleeping?
Cardiovascular
  Any cardiac disease history: hypertension, myocardial infarction, valvular problem, anemia, dysrhythmias, palpitations
  Chest pain—precipitating factors, severity, relieving factors
  Can activities of daily living be performed?
  Can activities performed 6 months, 4 months, 2 months, 2 weeks ago still be done?
  Any dizziness (vertigo) or fainting (syncope)?
Fluid retention
  Daily sodium intake?
  Weight gain?
  Are shoes tight? Do ankles swell?
Gastrointestinal
  Is appetite good?
  Any nausea, vomiting, or abdominal pain?
Urinary
  Decrease in daytime urine output?
  How often does client go to the bathroom at night (nocturia)?
Neurological
  Any change in behavior?

Medications

Knowledge of Condition

Coping Skills

Objective Data

Respiratory
  Tachypnea, crackles, wheezing, respiratory effort, dyspnea with exertion
Cardiovascular
  Tachycardia, dysrhythmias, jugular vein distention, peripheral edema—degree of pitting
Gastrointestinal
  Abdominal distention, ascites, hepatomegaly, splenomegaly
Neurological
  Confusion, decreased level of consciousness, restlessness, impaired memory
Integumentary
  Cold, clammy skin; pallor; cyanosis
General
  Weight
Diagnostic test findings

Rest and Activity

Reduction of the body's oxygen demands decreases the workload of the heart. A balance of rest and activity that does not produce signs or symptoms of oxygen deprivation is essential. The activity level of the client is determined by the severity of the heart failure. During times of exertion, the nurse should monitor the client's vital signs and respiratory effort for oxygen deprivation. If activity intolerance develops, the activity should be stopped.

Positioning

Semi-Fowler's or high Fowler's position makes breathing easier. In upright positions, the lungs are able to expand more fully, and gravity decreases the amount of fluid returned to the heart, thereby reducing the heart's workload.

Fluid Retention

Monitoring daily weights for weight gain is important in detecting fluid retention. Edema usually is not observed until there are 5 to 10 lb of extra fluid present. A baseline weight should be obtained when heart failure is diagnosed. Daily weights should be measured on the same scale, at the same time of day, and with the same type of clothing worn to ensure accuracy. A good time to obtain a daily weight is in the morning after the bladder is emptied. Documentation of daily weights should include the date and time of the weight, the scale used, the clothing worn, and the weight measurement.

Oxygen Consumption

Increased oxygen consumption by the heart should be avoided. Tachycardia increases the oxygen needs of the heart and should be reported promptly to the physician for treatment. Elderly clients are especially vulnerable to the effects of tachycardia because of their decreased reserves. Constipation should be prevented because straining during defecation, Valsalva's maneuver, increases the heart's workload by increasing venous return to the heart. Stool softeners should be administered, as ordered, to prevent straining.

Clients should be taught methods of saving energy while performing activities of daily living (ADL). Activities should be alternated with periods of rest. Fatigue should be avoided. A referral to occupational therapy and physical therapy can be helpful in developing techniques that allow the client to conserve energy during self-care. Some suggestions for conserving energy include placing frequently used objects at waist level to avoid reaching overhead, planning bathing activities to include rest periods, and using Velcro fasteners to make dressing easier.

Medications

Because heart failure is a progressive, chronic condition, clients may require lifetime medications. The long-term use of medications has many implications for clients. Financial resources, compliance, and ongoing monitoring are issues that must be considered by the nurse.

Diuretics require monitoring of the client's potassium levels and blood pressure. To prevent hypokalemia, potassium supplements may be prescribed during diuretic therapy, and a diet with high-potassium foods should be encouraged. If too much fluid is removed, the client may become hypotensive. If orthostatic hypotension develops,

NURSING CARE PLAN BOX 21-1
FOR THE CLIENT WITH CHRONIC HEART FAILURE

Activity intolerance related to fatigue caused by oxygen imbalance

Client Outcomes
Client will show increased activity tolerance with vital signs within normal limits (WNL) in response to activity.

Evaluation of Outcomes
Does the client participate in activities and maintain vital signs WNL?

Interventions	Rationale	Evaluation
Provide rest, space activities, and conserve energy.	Myocardial oxygen need is decreased with rest and energy conservation.	Does client participate in activity with no pulse rate or ECG changes?
Assist as needed with activities of daily living (ADL).	Conserve energy by assisting with ADL.	Are client's ADL met?
Teach use of assistive devices and lifestyle changes.	Assistive devices can overcome limitations to increase activity.	Does client incorporate assistive devices into lifestyle changes?
GERIATRIC		
Increase time allowed to complete activities.	Independence and participation are increased if extra time is allowed for tasks.	Does client report greater ability to complete activities with fewer symptoms?

Fluid volume excess related to heart failure and the secondary reduction in renal blood flow for filtration

Client Outcomes
Client remains free from edema and dyspnea, has clear lung sounds, and maintains baseline weight.

Evaluation of Outcomes
Does client have clear lung sounds with baseline weight maintained?

Interventions	Rationale	Evaluation
Monitor for edema, weight gain, jugular vein distention (JVD), lung crackles.	Excess fluid is indicated by edema, sudden weight gain, JVD, and crackles in the lungs.	Is edema, weight gain, JVD, or crackles present?
Decrease sodium intake as ordered.	Sodium retains fluid.	Does client restrict sodium intake?
Administer diuretics or inotropics as ordered.	Diuretics promote fluid excretion. Inotropics increase cardiac contraction strength.	Is output increased and edema or dyspnea reduced?
Monitor intake and output.	Intake and output will show imbalances.	Are intake and output balanced for 24 hours?

Sleep pattern disturbance related to nocturia and inability to lie down and sleep comfortably

Client Outcomes
Client awakens refreshed and is less fatigued during the day.

Evaluation of Outcomes
Does client wake up less frequently during the night and feel more refreshed with less fatigue during the day?

continued

NURSING CARE PLAN BOX 21–1 *(continued)*

Interventions	Rationale	Evaluation
Identify barriers to sleep.	Anxiety, nocturia, diuretics, orthopnea, or paroxysmal nocturnal dyspnea can make sleep difficult.	Does client identify sleep barriers?
Assist client in identifying positions of comfort for sleeping.	Use of pillows or a recliner can decrease orthopnea.	Can client identify a position of comfort?
Teach client cause of dyspnea at night.	Anxiety about falling asleep and waking up short of breath is reduced.	Can client explain cause of dyspnea?
Encourage client to recline for 30 to 60 minutes before bedtime.	Reclining before bedtime redistributes fluid and increases renal perfusion, resulting in increased voiding that can occur before going to sleep instead of after going to sleep.	Is client awakened less shortly after going to bed to void?

GERIATRIC

Interventions	Rationale	Evaluation
Encourage client to take diuretics early in the day.	Nocturia is reduced if diuretics are taken earlier in the day.	Does client take diuretics early and report less nocturia?

Anxiety related to threat of death and dyspnea

Client Outcomes
Client states that anxiety is reduced.

Evaluation of Outcomes
Does client report that anxiety is decreased?

Interventions	Rationale	Evaluation
Ask client to identify reasons for anxiety.	Identifying causes of the anxiety can lead to interventions to reduce it.	Can client list causes of anxiety?
Allow client time to ventilate feelings.	Expression of feelings can reduce anxiety.	Does client share feelings?
Explain procedures before performing them.	Lack of understanding increases anxiety.	Does client understand intent of procedures and how procedures will be done?

GERIATRIC

Interventions	Rationale	Evaluation
Use consistent caregivers.	Elderly clients adapt to changes with more difficulty, especially during illness.	Are caregivers consistent?

Altered health maintenance related to lack of knowledge of heart failure pathophysiology and treatment and cognitive impairment

Client Outcomes
Client follows and meets goals for mutually agreed on health maintenance plan.

Evaluation of Outcomes
Does client follow health maintenance plan without complication development?

continued

NURSING CARE PLAN BOX 21-1 (continued)		
Intervention	**Rationale**	**Evaluation**
Determine client's baseline knowledge.	Following a health plan is difficult without an adequate knowledge base.	Is client able to learn and accept responsibility for health needs?
Include support person in teaching designed for client.	Supportive relationships improve health and increase treatment compliance.	Does client have a support network interested in learning?
Teach heart function, symptoms, drugs, and diet.	To comply and achieve optimal health, client must have basic understanding of condition and treatment plan.	Is information restated correctly? Are return demonstrations accurate?
Refer to support agencies.	Compliance is increased with support systems.	Can client access support groups?
GERIATRIC		
Identify compliance barriers.	Social limitations can interfere with health maintenance.	Does client have means to reach goals?
Recognize resistance to changing life patterns.	Change is a stressor for the elderly, and one lifestyle change affects other areas of lifestyle.	Is client willing to set and follow goals for lifestyle changes?

the client may be dizzy and at risk of falling. Therefore the client should be cautioned to change positions slowly to prevent falls during diuretic therapy.

Inotropic agents such as digitalis strengthen heart contractions and slow the heart rate. Before administration of a digitalis drug, the client's pulse should be counted for 1 minute. If the pulse is below 60 beats per minute the physician should determine if the drug should be given. Some clients are given digitalis even if their heart rates are between 50 to 60 beats per minute as long as their heart's conduction system is normal. When giving digitalis, the nurse should be aware that hypokalemia increases the heart's sensitivity to digitalis. A client can become toxic on a normal dose of digitalis when hypokalemia is present. This is important to note because many people on digitalis also take diuretics, which may lower potassium levels. Monitoring for signs and symptoms of digitalis toxicity should be done routinely during client assessment. Early symptoms of digitalis toxicity are anorexia, nausea, and vomiting. Other signs and symptoms include bradycardia or other dysrhythmias, visual problems, and mental changes. The elderly are especially prone to toxic effects of this drug and may exhibit confusion when levels are toxic.

Vasodilators reduce the heart's workload by decreasing vascular pressure. Therefore blood pressure should be monitored when administering vasodilators.

Clients and their significant others should be taught the purpose, side effects, and precautions for prescribed medications. They should be told to report the occurrence of side effects to the physician. Clients taking a digitalis preparation should be taught to take their pulse rate. They should hold the medication and call their physician if their heart rate is less than 60 beats per minute or the lower limit heart rate set by their physician. Clients on diuretics should

be taught to (1) take them during the day to decrease being awakened at night to void, (2) have a readily available and obstacle-free bathroom or commode to prevent incontinence and falls, (3) eat high-potassium foods if they are taking a potassium-depleting diuretic, and (4) weigh themselves daily and report a 2 to 3 lb weight gain over 1 to 2 days to the physician. Clients should understand the importance of taking their medication as prescribed, even if they do not have symptoms. A schedule should be developed to assist clients to remember to take their medications.

Low-Sodium Diet and Weight Control

A diet assessment should be completed to help establish an appealing diet plan for the client with heart failure. Factors such as the client's food likes and dislikes, cultural influences, economic status, and food preparation resources such as shopping ability, storage, refrigeration, and cooking equipment will influence compliance with any restricted diet and therefore should be assessed. It is helpful to include a dietitian in the planning process, as well as the food preparer or a support person, in order to increase diet compliance.

Excess weight influences heart failure by increasing the heart's workload. For the overweight client, weight reduction may help eliminate the underlying cause of heart failure. Diet counseling and support should be given to the obese client to encourage weight loss.

If anorexia occurs in the later stages of heart failure, the client's intake should be evaluated. Several small meals rather than three large meals will decrease the heart's workload. If the client's nutritional needs are not being met the physician should be informed and a referral to a dietitian considered.

Clients should be taught which foods are high and low in sodium content. With this knowledge, clients can help

Table 21–8. *Client and Family Education*

Heart Failure Signs and Symptoms to Report to the Physician

Shortness of breath
Fatigue
Dry cough
Shortness of breath when lying down (orthopnea)
Episodes of sudden awakening with shortness of breath (PND)
Weight gain of 3 pounds since last visit
Ankle or foot edema
Nocturia
Anorexia

design a daily meal plan using low-sodium foods that are appealing to them. Food preparers should be taught not to salt food during cooking, and table salt should be eliminated. Explaining seasoning alternatives such as spices, herbs, and lemon juice is helpful in making food taste better.

Education

Chronic management of heart failure requires client and family understanding of the disease process, management of home oxygen therapy, diet and weight control, and medications. The client and family must recognize the importance of each of these factors in order to foster a productive

HOME HEALTH HINTS

■ Some clients may not have a scale in their home. It may be necessary to assist them in obtaining one or to leave an agency scale in the home for daily weights.

■ The most objective way to document edema is to use a tape measure on the abdominal girth, thigh, calf, and ankle in centimeters. Measure at the same place each visit, such as measuring the girth of the calf at a specified distance above the medial malleolus.

■ The sacrum, back, and sides of a bedridden client should be checked to note edema. These are dependent areas in the bedridden client, so fluid accumulates in these areas instead of the ankles.

■ Blood drawn for potassium levels needs to be transported to the lab within 1 hour. Ice should not be put directly on the tube because this can cause destruction of the cells and a false elevation in the potassium level.

■ Blood drawn for digoxin levels should be taken to the lab within 2 to 3 hours.

■ Clients on sodium-restricted diets who already have canned vegetables in their home can still use them even though they are not the low-sodium type. They should be instructed to pour off the liquid and rinse the vegetables before heating them for serving. The use of herbs and spices helps make them more flavorful.

■ For the client on a low-sodium diet, an effective diet teaching technique is to have the client name the foods highest in sodium. Asking the client to rename the list on each visit helps knowledge retention and compliance.

■ If clients have a poor appetite, ask their caregiver if they eat well when eating with others. Anorexia could be a sign of loneliness and depression if they eat well with others instead of an effect from the heart failure.

■ Assist clients in taking medications at times that fit their lifestyle. A morning dose of a diuretic may limit what they can do for the next few hours. An afternoon dose might encourage compliance. Lack of compliance is a major factor in the rehospitalization of heart failure clients.

■ The home health nurse should periodically check the contents of medicine bottles. If pills have been cut in half, ask about this. Often it is an attempt by the client to "stretch" the medicine to decrease expenses. There are community or drug company programs that help purchase medicines for clients with financial need. Eligible Medicaid clients can apply for medication cards.

■ Visual disturbances can occur from digitalis toxicity. If the client sees halos around lights or red-green tinting on everything, report this to the physician.

■ Troublesome side effects of an ACE inhibitor such as Capoten or Vasotec are an intractable cough and hypotension. It should be noted how much coughing the client is doing. The physician should set parameters for the blood pressure and reporting of abnormal findings.

■ Oxygen concentrators are widely used in home care. Long tubing allows the client ease in moving about the home. Clients need to be cautioned about keeping the tubing out of their way and not kinking it. If the client also has chronic obstructive pulmonary disease (COPD), the oxygen flow rate is generally limited to 2 L/min, so the client's drive to breathe is not decreased. A note stating this should be placed near the gauge as a reminder to the client.

■ As the home health nurse becomes acquainted with the client, it is easier to pick up on signs of oxygen deprivation and hypoxia, such as confusion, combativeness, or unusual expressions of anger.

■ For clients with orthopnea, a foam wedge can be obtained from a medical equipment company to use under their head when sleeping, instead of pillows.

■ As heart failure clients feel better, they may go back to the old habits that cause an increase in fluid. The home health nurse can help by providing information about the disease and help clients foster their own independence and ways of coping with the condition. Each home health visit is a teaching opportunity that empowers clients with a knowledge base to empower them to take control of their health.

life for the client with chronic heart failure. A discussion using simple terms of the pathology of heart failure should be included in the teaching plan for the client. Signs and symptoms that the client is to report to the physician should also be highlighted (Table 21–8).

Coping

Living with a chronic illness can be frustrating for both clients and their families. An assessment of coping skills used by clients and their families in the past is helpful. The coping skills identified during this assessment can be used and enhanced to successfully cope with this current illness. Available support systems should be identified and explained to clients. A referral to a social worker can be helpful in providing clients with resources that may make living with heart failure easier. An understanding of the chronic nature of heart failure is important for clients, families, and caregivers to positively deal with the emotions and feelings that can result from heart failure.

Evaluation

The goal for the nursing diagnosis of activity intolerance is met if the client reports reduced fatigue and the ability to complete tasks and engage in desired activities.

The goal for the nursing diagnosis of fluid volume excess is met if the client has less edema and no dyspnea and maintains a baseline weight.

The goal for the nursing diagnosis of sleep pattern disturbance is met if the client is able to sleep and wake up refreshed without being fatigued during the day.

The goal for the nursing diagnosis of anxiety is met if the client reports that anxiety levels are reduced.

The goal for the nursing diagnosis of altered health maintenance is met if the client follows the health maintenance plan without complication development.

CRITICAL THINKING: Mr. Shepard (4)

The nurse meets with Mr. Shepard after the physician orders the vasodilator to be continued, a diuretic, and 2 g sodium diet.

1. What information should the nurse teach Mr. Shepard based on the prescribed treatment?
2. What types of foods should be included in Mr. Shepard's diet?
3. Why does the nurse instruct Mr. Shepard to weigh himself daily?
4. Why does the nurse tell Mr. Shepard to weigh himself at the same time of day, on the same scale, and with the same type of clothing?

Answers at end of chapter.

Review Questions

1. The nurse is caring for Tom, 68, who is receiving digoxin 0.125 mg qd. Which of the following assessments of the client would indicate to the nurse that Tom is experiencing a side effect of digoxin that will require follow-up?
   a. Skin flushing
   b. Bradycardia
   c. Hypertension
   d. Constipation

2. The nurse is teaching a client with heart failure how to avoid activity that results in Valsalva's maneuver. Which of the following statements by the client would indicate to the nurse that the teaching has been effective?
   a. "I will breathe normally when moving."
   b. "I will use a straw to drink oral fluids."
   c. "I will take fewer but deeper breaths."
   d. "I will clench my teeth when moving."

3. Joe, 65, is anxious and reports dyspnea. The nurse notes diaphoresis; cold, clammy skin; and pink, frothy sputum. Vital sign data are BP 174/96, P 116, R 32. Which one of the following changes from these vital signs would indicate the client is having a therapeutic response to morphine 4 mg IVP?
   a. Shallow respirations
   b. Increased respirations
   c. Increased blood pressure
   d. Decreased blood pressure

4. Lou, 64, has heart failure and is being discharged from the hospital. He is taking furosemide (Lasix) 20 mg daily. Which of the following statements by Lou would indicate understanding of instructions for his medications?
   a. "I will take the Lasix in the morning."
   b. "I will take the Lasix in the evening."
   c. "I will drink lots of fluids with the Lasix."
   d. "I will drink fewer sweetened beverages."

5. Mr. Smith has heart failure and two-pillow orthopnea. He comes to the emergency department with dyspnea and says he went to bed and awoke with a feeling of suffocation. He says it was frightening. Which of the following responses by the nurse would be *most* appropriate to explain the cause of his dyspnea?
   a. "Using more than one pillow decreases lung expansion."
   b. "Reclining decreases the heart's ability to pump blood."
   c. "Sleeping increases heart rate and the body's oxygen needs."
   d. "Reclining increases fluid returning to the heart and lungs."

ANSWERS TO CRITICAL THINKING

CRITICAL THINKING: Mr. Shepard (1)

1. Shortness of breath, two-pillow orthopnea, dry cough, tachycardia (pulse 106), tachypnea (respiration 24), bilateral crackles.
2. Left-sided heart failure.
3. Shortness of breath: fluid in the lungs impairs gas exchange; orthopnea: lying flat increases fluid accumulation in the lungs, causing dyspnea; dry cough: fluid in the lungs irritates the mucosal lining of the lungs; tachycardia: sympathetic compensation to increase cardiac output; tachypnea: sympathetic compensation to increase blood oxygenation; bilateral crackles: fluid trapped in the lungs.
4. To prevent orthopnea by using a more upright position, which allows gravity to decrease fluid accumulation in the lungs.

CRITICAL THINKING: Mr. Shepard (2)

1. To compensate for the strain caused by increased peripheral vascular resistance from hypertension in order to maintain an adequate cardiac output.
2. An enlarged heart requires more oxygen, which often cannot be supplied in heart failure.

CRITICAL THINKING: Mr. Shepard (3)

1. To vasodilate, which reduces peripheral vascular resistance and decreases the heart's workload.
2. Afterload.
3. To decrease fluid volume, which reduces preload and decreases the heart's workload.
4. To reduce water retention, which decreases preload and decreases the heart's workload.
5. To decrease the heart's workload and increase its efficiency by reducing preload and peripheral vascular resistance.

CRITICAL THINKING: Mr. Shepard (4)

1. After assessment of Mr. Shepard's knowledge base, medication teaching on the vasodilator and diuretic that includes their purpose, side effects, and precautions. A schedule for taking the medications can be planned. An explanation of the purpose of a low-sodium diet and menu planning based on Mr. Shepard's likes and dislikes should be done.
2. Low-sodium foods should be selected to prevent fluid retention, and high-potassium foods should be included to prevent hypokalemia from the diuretic if appropriate. Low-sodium foods include puffed rice, wheat cereals, fruits, chicken, beef, eggs, and potatoes. High-sodium foods include tomato juice, sauerkraut, softened water, buttermilk, cheese, smoked meats, canned tuna, canned soup, pickles, instant rice, and instant potatoes. High-potassium foods include bran products, avocado, bananas, prunes, oranges, baked potato, sweet potato, spinach (cooked), chocolate, nuts, and molasses.
3. To detect a rapid weight gain that would indicate fluid retention (2 to 3 lb over 2 days) and to measure weight loss resulting from the diuretic.
4. To ensure accuracy of the weight so that comparison to the baseline weight will detect a weight gain or loss.

REFERENCES

1. Sackner-Bernstein, J, and Mancini, D: Rationale for treatment of patients with chronic heart failure with adrenergic blockade. JAMA 274:1462, 1995.
2. Venner, G, and Seelbinder, J: Team management of congestive heart failure across the continuum. J Cardiovasc Nurs 10(2):71,1996.

BIBLIOGRAPHY

Ackley, BJ, and Ladwig, GB: Nursing Diagnosis Handbook. Mosby, St Louis, 1997.

Aronow, W: Treatment of congestive heart failure in older persons. J Am Geriatr Soc 45(10):1252, 1997.

Bove, L: Now! Surgery for heart failure. RN 95(5):26, 1997.

Buchanan, A, and Tan, R: Congestive heart failure in elderly patients. The treatment goal is improved quality, not quantity, of life. Postgrad Med 102(4):207, 1997.

Dracup, K, Dunbar, S, and Baker, D: Rethinking heart failure. Am J Nurs 95(7):23, 1995.

Funk, M, and Krumholz, H: Epidemiologic and economic impact of advanced heart failure. J Cardiovasc Nurs 10(2):1, 1996.

Heaney, L, et al: Intermittent inotropic infusions: Critical care in an outpatient setting. Congestive Heart Failure 15 July-Aug, 1995.

Janowski, M: Managing heart failure. RN 96(2):34, 1996.

Konstam, MA, et al: Heart Failure Evaluation and Care of Patients with Left-Ventricular Systolic Dysfunction. AHCPR Pub No 94-0612. US Department of Health and Human Services, Public Health Service, Agency for Health Care Policy and Research, Rockville, Md, 1994.

Krumholz, H, et al: Quality of care for elderly patients hospitalized with heart failure. Arch Intern Med 157(19):2242, 1997.

Lewandowski, D: Congestive heart failure. Am J Nurs 95(5):36, 1995.

Lutz, CA, and Przytulski, K: Nutrition and Diet Therapy. FA Davis, Philadelphia, 1996.

Packer, M, et al: The effect of carvedilol on morbidity and mortality in patients with chronic heart failure. N Engl J Med 334:1351, 1996.

Rich, M: Epidemiology, pathophysiology and etiology of congestive heart failure in older adults. J Am Geriatr Soc 45(8):968, 1997.

Ruppert, S, Kernicki, J, and Dolan, J: Dolan's Critical Care Nursing. FA Davis, Philadelphia, 1996.

Shepard, RJ: Exercise for patients with congestive heart failure. Sports Med 23(2):75, 1997.

Shively, M, Verderver, A, and Fitzsimmons, L: Caring for patients with ventricular assist devices. J Cardiovasc Nurs 8:91, 1994.

Steele, I, et al: Non-invasive measurement of cardiac output and ventricular ejection fractions in chronic cardiac failure: Relationship to impaired exercise tolerance. Cli Sci 93(3):195, 1997.

Zuccala, G, et al: Left ventricular dysfunction: A clue to cognitive impairment in older patient with heart failure. J Neurol Neurosurg Psychiatry 63(4):509, 1997.

Nursing Care of Clients Undergoing Cardiovascular Surgery

Sharon M. Nowak

Learning Objectives

Upon completion of this chapter, the student will be able to:

1. Explain preoperative and postoperative routines and procedures.

2. Explain purpose and flow of cardiopulmonary bypass machine.

3. Describe complications of cardiopulmonary bypass.

4. Describe myocardial revascularization procedure.

5. Explain commissurotomy, annuloplasty, and valve replacement.

6. Identify types of mechanical and biological valves.

7. Explain different types of cardiac traumas and indications for surgery.

8. Define cardiac myxoma and sarcomas and their prognosis.

9. Explain complications of cardiac and valve surgery.

10. Identify complications of cardiac transplantation.

11. Develop preoperative and postoperative care plans for cardiac, valve, and transplant surgery clients.

12. Define embolectomy and endarterectomy.

13. Explain peripheral and great vessel surgery.

14. Develop preoperative and postoperative care plans for the vascular surgery client.

Key Words

anastomose (uh-NAS-tuh-**MOS**)
annuloplasty (**AN**-yoo-loh-PLAS-tee)
atelectasis (AT-e-**LECK**-tah-sis)
cardioplegia (KAR-dee-oh-**PLEE**-jee-ah)
commissurotomy (KOM-i-shur-**AHT**-oh-mee)
encephalopathy (en-SEFF-uh-**LAHP**-ah-thee)
endarterectomy (end-AR-tur-**ECK**-tuh-mee)
gastroepiploic (GAS-troh-EP-i-**PLOH**-ick)
hemolysis (he-**MAHL**-e-sis)
hypothermia (HIGH-poh-**THER**-mee-ah)

hypoxemia (HIGH-pock-**SEE**-mee-ah)
hypoxia (high-**POCK**-see-ah)
leukocytosis (LOO-koh-sigh-**TOH**-sis)
mediastinum (ME-dee-ah-**STYE**-num)
nephrotoxic (NEFF-roh-**TOCK**-sick)
pancreatitis (PAN-kree-uh-**TIGH**-tis)
paresthesia (PAR-es-**THEE**-zee-ah)
pericardiocentesis (PER-ee-KAR-dee-oh-sen-**TEE**-sis)
pericardiotomy (PER-ee-KAR-dee-**AH**-tah-mee)
pericarditis (PER-ee-kar-**DYE**-tis)
sternotomy (stir-**NAH**-tuh-mee)
tachydysrhythmia (TACK-ee-dis-**RITH**-mee-yah)

Cardiac Surgery

As heart disease symptoms increase in severity and frequency or the diagnostic tests show a worsening of the disease process, cardiac surgery may be used as treatment. As cardiac surgery seemingly becomes commonplace, it is still a major surgery with numerous complications, as well as physical, emotional, and social stressors. (See Gerontological Issues Box 22–1.)

PREPARATION FOR SURGERY

For elective heart surgery, clients are usually admitted to the hospital 1 to 3 days before the surgery based on their medical history. A thorough nursing assessment is important for baseline data that can be used for comparison postoperatively and for early discharge planning. In addition to routine admission testing, clients with chronic obstructive pulmonary disease (COPD) may have pulmonary function tests and baseline arterial blood gases (ABGs) done (Table 22–1). Clients with carotid bruits have carotid studies to determine the amount of occlusion in the carotid artery. If the occlusion is significant, a carotid **endarterectomy,** which removes the plaque on the lining of the blocked or diseased carotid artery, is performed, usually several weeks before having cardiac surgery to place the client in the best possible condition for surgery.

Table 22–1. *Routine Admission Testing*

12-lead electrocardiogram (ECG)
Chest x-ray
Complete blood count (CBC)
Coagulation studies
Chemistry profile
Crossmatched for blood

Several types of medication may normally be held before surgery: aspirin, which is often stopped 7 days preoperatively; Coumadin, which may be stopped 4 to 5 days preoperatively; intravenous (IV) heparin, which is stopped 4 hours preoperatively; diuretics, which may be held 1 to 2 days before surgery; and insulin or oral hypoglycemic agents, which are sometimes held the morning of surgery. However, clients should be instructed to check with their physician before they stop taking any medications.

Clients recover more quickly and have less stress postoperatively when they have had thorough preoperative teaching. Brief explanations of IV lines, endotracheal tube (ETT), ventilator, chest tubes, various equipment alarms, urinary catheter, pain management, incisions, and communication methods are provided to the client and family preoperatively. Emphasis should be placed on the fact that clients are not able to talk while the ETT is in place, as well as coughing and deep breathing exercises that must be done after the ETT is removed. Additionally, a preoperative family tour of the client's initial postoperative unit and the waiting area helps prepare them for the surgical experience. A referral to pastoral care, if desired, can be comforting to the client.

The anesthesiologist will see the client the evening before surgery to assess and order the preoperative medications. An antiseptic scrub shower is taken the evening before and morning of surgery. The client receives nothing by mouth (NPO) after midnight. Finally, all preoperative medications are administered as ordered when the operating room calls for the nursing unit to transfer the client to surgery.

CARDIOPULMONARY BYPASS

Almost all cardiac surgeries use cardiopulmonary bypass (CPB). During surgery blood is temporarily diverted away from the heart and lungs to a special pump. This allows for a bloodless and motionless surgical field while the functioning of the heart and lungs is maintained by the pump. After the **sternotomy** is made, the vena cava and ascending aorta are cannulated (a small tube with multiple holes is placed into each of them). The aorta is cross-clamped be-

GERONTOLOGICAL ISSUES BOX 22–1

Elderly clients can benefit from coronary artery bypass and other cardiac surgeries. Clients over 80 years of age have unique needs and bring complex challenges to their care needs. Frail elderly clients require skilled care and understanding of their needs for positive outcomes after surgery.

Before cardiac surgery, the elderly client should have a functional assessment done. This assessment identifies preoperative strengths and deficits. After surgery another functional assessment should be done and compared with the preoperative one to identify functional deficits. Once deficits are identified, care can be provided to meet client needs in these areas of deficits and plan rehabilitation to overcome any deficits, if possible.

Elderly clients have unique respiratory care needs due to aging changes following cardiac surgery. Careful attention to changes in respiratory status is important. The ability of the elderly client to participate in measures to prevent respiratory complications, such as coughing and deep breathing, using an incentive spirometer, and ambulating, needs to be noted. Encouragement and reinforcing how to perform these interventions are important.

endarterectomy: end—inside + arter—artery + ectomy—excision
sternotomy: stern—sternum + otomy—incision into

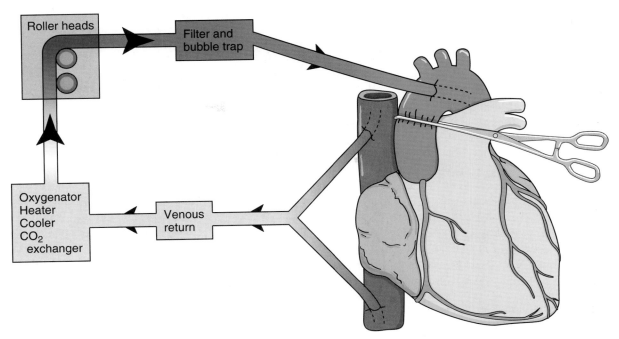

Figure 22–1. Cardiopulmonary bypass machine.

tween the heart and the cannula. Cross-clamping is done by clamping two large hemostats over the aorta in opposite directions. The cannulas are then attached to the pump tubing. Blood flows from the body through the vena cava cannula to the CPB pump. The pump oxygenates the blood and removes carbon dioxide. Then the blood is returned to the body by the force of the pump. The blood flows through the cannula into the ascending aorta, where it then circulates through the body (Fig. 22–1).

Using the CPB can present its own unique set of complications. Before going on the pump, the client is anticoagulated with heparin until the prothrombin time (PT) is five to six times greater than normal. The effects of the heparin are reversed with protamine sulfate, the antidote for heparin, immediately before coming off the pump. However, heparin is absorbed and stored in organs and tissue and can be sporadically released hours after surgery, thus predisposing the client to excessive bleeding. Air embolism is a risk that is minimized by the pump being primed with lactated Ringer's solution and being carefully observed. The priming solution increases circulating volume, which then results in a shifting of fluid into the interstitial tissue and edema formation. These fluid shifts can continue up to 6 hours after surgery and can cause hypotension.

Methods for providing closed-chest cardiopulmonary bypass and **cardioplegia** are being studied.[1] The chest would not have to be opened to provide CPB or cardioplegia. Therefore these techniques might allow less invasive types of cardiac surgery to be performed.

---

cardioplegia: cardio—heart + plegia—paralysis

GENERAL PROCEDURE FOR CARDIAC SURGERY

After the client is placed on CPB, a cardioplegia solution is infused into the aortic root along with iced saline, which is placed around the heart to cause cardiac standstill. Once the surgery is completed, the client's blood is warmed in the CPB circuit and the client is slowly weaned from CPB. The heart starts beating when it is warmed and defibrillated. Temporary pacing wires are sewn onto the myocardium before the pump is discontinued. These wires can be attached to an external temporary pacemaker if bradycardia develops. Once the heart is beating, the CPB is discontinued. Mediastinal chest tubes are placed to drain remaining blood and fluid from the chest, and the sternotomy is closed first with wires through the sternum and then sutures for the layer of skin. While under anesthesia, the client is transferred to an intensive care unit (ICU), usually for 1 to 2 days.

SURGICAL PROCEDURES

Myocardial Revascularization (Coronary Artery Bypass Graft)

Coronary artery bypass graft (CABG) surgery is a procedure used to increase blood flow and oxygen to the myocardium and alleviate anginal symptoms. Significant occlusions in the coronary arteries are bypassed with vein or artery grafts (Fig. 22–2). One or more bypasses can be performed during the procedure (CABG × 4). The saphenous vein from the leg or the right or left internal mammary artery from the chest wall is generally used. The right **gas-**

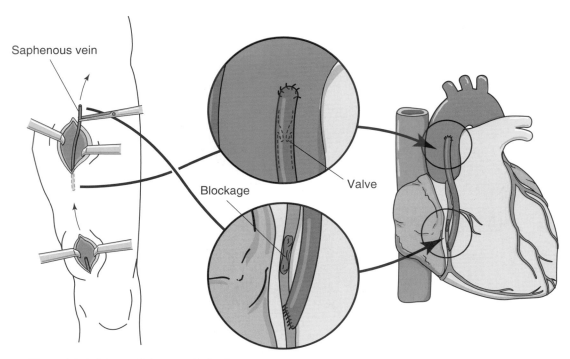

Figure 22–2. Myocardial revascularization: coronary artery bypass graft surgery. (Modified from Rupport, S, Kernicki, J, and Dolan, J: Dolan's Critical Care Nursing. FA Davis, Philadelphia, 1996, p 319, with permission.)

troepiploic artery (RGEA), a branch of the gastroduodenal artery, and the inferior epigastric artery (IEA) have also been used as repeat operations have been increasing.

While the sternotomy is made, the vein graft is harvested (removed from the leg). The graft is flushed with a heparinized solution to check for leaks, then set aside for later use during the surgery. The client is placed on CPB. After cardiac standstill, one end of the graft is **anastomosed,** or joined to the coronary artery distal to the occlusion, while the proximal end of the graft is anastomosed, often to the ascending aorta. The surgery than continues as previously described.

Resecting the mammary arteries for grafting is more difficult and time consuming than the saphenous vein, but the longevity of their patency is greater. The proximal end of the artery is left attached to its origin and the distal end is anastomosed to the coronary artery distal to the occlusion.

Exploration of less invasive types of procedures for CABG is being done. A method using a thoracoscopic procedure to perform the CABG is being studied.[2] As advances are made in cardiopulmonary bypass and cardiac surgery techniques, less invasive surgery will be possible.

Heart Valve Repairs

A mitral **commissurotomy** is one type of valve repair in which the client is placed on CPB and a left atriotomy (incision into the atrium) is made to expose the valve. The valve cusps are either incised with a knife or broken apart with a dilator. The atrium is sewn closed, CPB is discontinued, and surgery continues as previously described.

A second type of valve repair is an **annuloplasty,** which is the repair of the annulus of a valve. The mitral valve is the most common valve that is repaired in this way. Sutures or a ring may be placed in the valve annulus to improve closure of the leaflets. Similar procedures are used on the tricuspid valve, but the aortic valve is not readily repaired in this manner.

Heart Valve Replacement

Valves used for cardiac valve replacement may be either mechanical or biological. There are three types of mechanical valves: caged ball, monoleaflet, and bileaflet (Fig. 22–3). Mechanical valves are very durable but create turbulent blood flow. From the valve's design and its presence as a foreign body, **hemolysis** (destruction of blood cells) can occur. The turbulent flow can lead to clot formation, requiring lifelong anticoagulant therapy.

Biological (tissue) valves come from three sources: porcine (pig), bovine (cow), and allografts (human). Tissue valves have a very low incidence of thrombus formation and do not require lifelong anticoagulant therapy, but they may not last as long as mechanical valves. The

---

gastroepiploic: gastro—stomach + epiploic—pertaining to omentum
commissurotomy: commissur—connecting band of tissue + otomy—incision into
annuloplasty: annulo—annulus + plasty—repair
hemolysis: hemo—blood + lysis—destruction

A. Caged ball valve

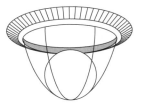

B. Monoleaflet

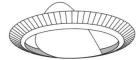

C. Bileaflet

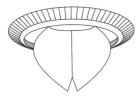

Figure 22–3. Types of mechanical heart valves used in the United States. (Modified from Ruppert, S, Kernicki, J, and Dolan, J: Dolan's Critical Care Nursing. FA Davis, Philadelphia, 1996, p 333, with permission.)

durability and potential for tissue degeneration have not yet been fully determined. (See Cultural Considerations Box 22–2.)

For a mitral valve replacement (MVR), a left atriotomy is made once the client is on CPB. For an aortic valve replacement (AVR), an incision is made above the right coronary artery in the aorta. The diseased valve is excised and the new valve sutured in place. The incision is closed and surgery continues as previously described. Aortic valve replacement is the most common cardiac valve replaced in the elderly.[3]

Ventricular Aneurysm Repair

Indications for ventricular aneurysm surgery are generally persistent angina or symptoms of heart failure, a large aneurysm impeding the heart's function, left ventricular failure, or **tachydysrhythmias.** Once the client is on CPB, an incision is made to expose the heart and then the aneurysm is resected (cut out), leaving a fibrous border (Fig. 22–4). The ventricle is wiped clean and irrigated to ensure that all thrombi are removed. The opening is then sutured closed or patched with a graft. Air is aspirated from the ventricle, and the surgery continues as previously described.

---

tachydysrhythmias: tach—fast + dys—bad + rhythm—regularity + ia—condition

pericardiocentesis: peri—around + cardio—heart + centesis—surgical puncture

Cardiomyoplasty

Cardiomyoplasty uses the client's own skeletal muscle (latissimus dorsi) to improve the contractile function of the heart. (See Fig. 21–9.) The muscle is wrapped around the aorta or heart, and a cardiomyostimulator and leads are implanted to stimulate muscle contraction. The muscle is rested for 2 weeks after surgery and then programmed to gradually start stimulation. After 4 months, the muscle can be stimulated either at a 1:1 or 1:2 heartbeat ratio. Benefits from cardiomyoplasty include the improved contractility of the failing heart and reduced changes in heart failure remodeling from the wrapping or enclosing effects of the muscle.[4] Cardiomyoplasty may reduce the need for heart transplantation by delaying or preventing end-stage heart failure.[5]

Cardiac Trauma

Two types of trauma can occur to the heart: nonpenetrating and penetrating. Nonpenetrating injuries, or contusions, occur from a blunt trauma such as motor vehicle accidents and contact sports where direct compression or a force is applied to the upper torso. Contusions may vary from small bruises to areas of hemorrhage.

There may be few or no external injuries indicating traumatic cardiac injury. The client may be asymptomatic or exhibit the pain and signs and symptoms identical to a myocardial infarction. In severe contusions, laboratory results may show an elevated CK-MB.

If bleeding occurs into the pericardial sac, cardiac tamponade may occur, which is compression of the heart due to this collection of blood. If decompensation occurs, a **pericardiocentesis** may be necessary whereby a puncture of the pericardial cavity is made with a needle and the fluid is aspirated. However, the tamponade may seal the bleeding area with its pressure without restricting cardiac movement and function, so no decompensation occurs. In this case only bed rest and observation are required. There are usually no long-term effects with contusions. With severe contusions, scarring and necrosis of the myocardium may decrease cardiac output and increase the risk for cardiac rupture.

Penetrating traumas may have an obvious external injury to the chest, such as a stab or gunshot wound, or a less

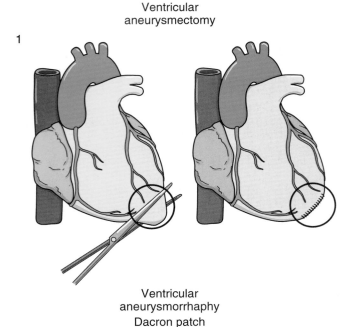

Ventricular
aneurysmectomy

1

Ventricular
aneurysmorrhaphy
Dacron patch

2

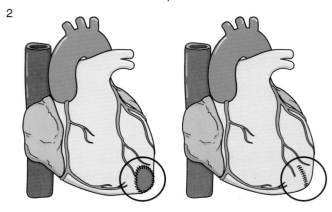

1: Aneurysm is cut and closed.
2: Patch inserted inside incision, then closed.

Figure 22–4. Ventricular aneurysm repair. (Modified from Ruppert, S, Kernicki, J, and Dolan, J: Dolan's Critical Care Nursing. FA Davis, Philadelphia, 1996, p 335, with permission.)

obvious injury as with invasive lines that have penetrated from within the cardiac muscle. Complications vary depending on the size, location, and cause of injury. Tamponade occurs from bleeding into the pericardial sac if the pericardium seals with a clot. A hemothorax develops if blood drains into the pleural space in the chest. Symptoms of hemorrhage and myocardial ischemia may be noted. Treatment is cardiac surgery to repair the damage to regain hemostasis.

Cardiac Tumors

Cardiac tumors may be primary or secondary in origin, with each being either benign or malignant. Primary cardiac tumors are less common than secondary or metastatic cardiac tumors. A large portion of benign primary tumors are myxomas.

A myxoma is a soft, gelatinous, intracavitary mass that is attached to the endocardium by a narrow stalk (peduncle). They can be found in any of the four chambers of the heart but are more common in the left atrium. Symptoms vary depending on the location of the tumor and its impedance on valve function. There is a high risk of emboli formation from this type of tumor because it breaks apart easily. Surgical excision of the tumor offers a good prognosis.

Sarcomas are the majority of malignant primary cardiac tumors. Secondary cardiac tumors are generally carcinomas that have metastasized. The symptoms depend on the location and size of the mass. Treatment consists of palliative measures such as surgery, radiation, and chemotherapy. If **pericarditis** is present, a pericardiocentesis may be performed. Pericarditis may recur, and a pericardial "window" (permanent opening) is cut into the pericardium to allow drainage and prevent fluid buildup and cardiac tamponade. The prognosis is poor with a short life expectancy.

COMPLICATIONS OF CARDIAC SURGERY

Cardiovascular

Postoperative bleeding into the **mediastinum** is common. When drainage is greater than 200 mL per hour, conservative treatment is instituted before taking the client back to surgery for exploration to find the bleeding cause. Bleeding can come from oozing blood vessels within the chest, graft anastomoses, or myocardial incisions. These oozing areas may result from increased blood pressure, which may occur if clients are shivering until they are rewarmed after surgery, or coagulation problems occurring from platelet, fibrin, and other coagulation factors being destroyed in the CPB circuit. Inadequate reversal of the heparin that is given before the client is placed on pump and a delayed release of heparin stored in organs and fatty tissue also can add to postoperative bleeding.

Tamponade can occur if clots form in the chest tubes causing blood to increase in the pericardial sac. If the heart is constricted, which decreases the ability of the heart to contract and fill, it can lead to cardiac arrest without prompt treatment.

Myocardial depression, which results in decreased cardiac output, is usually a transient finding caused by **hypoxemia,** acidosis, interstitial fluid accumulation, or electrolyte imbalance. Hemodilution and diuretics can cause hypomagnesemia and hypocalcemia, which also depress myocardial function.

A perioperative myocardial infarction can occur from graft thrombosis, an embolus, inadequate myocardial preser-

---

mediastinum: medi—middle + stinum—sternum
hypoxia: hypo—below normal + ox—oxygen + ia—condition

vation during aortic cross-clamping, or inadequate revascularization.

Dysrhythmias are fairly common. They can be due to **hypoxia,** hypoxemia, acidosis, electrolyte imbalance (especially hypokalemia), and pain or anxiety. Other causes include inflammation from the **pericardiotomy** and CPB cannulas and gastric distention. Varying degrees of heart block are associated with valve replacement due to the close proximity of the AV node to all of the valves.

Pericarditis, an inflammation of the pericardial sac, is due to the manipulation of the pericardium. This inflammation may occur immediately postoperatively or months later. Should it recur numerous times, it is termed *postpericardiotomy syndrome.*

Pulmonary

The most common postoperative problem is **atelectasis,** which is the collapse of airways due to hypoventilation. This can occur from pain, exhaustion, prolonged anesthesia leading to shallow breathing, poor cough effort, and decreased ambulation and movement. These atelectatic areas contribute to hypoxemia and become sites for infections.

Pleural effusions occur when fluid accumulates within the pleural lining. Heart failure, inflammation, and hypoalbuminemia (low serum albumin) cause changes in cell wall permeability and pressures that lead to an imbalance in the production and reabsorption of pleural fluid. Treatment involves the insertion of a chest tube to drain the fluid and allow lung reexpansion.

The phrenic nerve conducts the motor impulses to the diaphragm. Phrenic nerve paralysis can occur from direct injury during the resection of the internal mammary artery (IMA) or from the cold saline used while on CPB. Symptoms include dyspnea and paradoxical (contradictory) abdominal breathing. On chest x-ray, the diaphragm is elevated on inspiration. The paralysis may be unilateral or bilateral. Clients with preexisting pulmonary disease require continued ventilator support. Phrenic nerve paralysis resolves itself, but the length of time varies.

Renal

Low arterial pressure on CPB activates the renin-angiotensin-aldosterone system, creating vasoconstriction, which decreases renal perfusion and function. Other factors that decrease renal function are **nephrotoxic** antibiotics, **hypothermia,** and hemolysis from CPB. If the kidneys do not recover, the client may be started on hemodialysis until the kidney's functioning improves.

Gastrointestinal

Postoperative complications in the gastrointestinal (GI) tract can range from the minor annoyance of medication-induced diarrhea (quinidine or various antibiotics) to a life-threatening bowel infarction. Gastric distention can occur if the nasogastric tube is not properly functioning while the client is on the ventilator. This distention can be uncomfortable and may impede the lungs' ability to expand, causing decreased ventilation. As with any surgery, a paralytic ileus can develop, necessitating a longer gastric decompression time with a nasogastric tube and NPO status.

Bowel infarction secondary to ischemia of the mesenteric vasculature is rare, yet life threatening. It can be caused from low blood flow while the client is on CPB, myocardial depression, or emboli. These clients are extremely ill and may have sepsis, respiratory distress, severe abdominal pain, metabolic acidosis, or diarrhea. Surgery to resect the necrotic bowel may be indicated. This low blood flow state while the client is on CPB or postoperatively can also cause a necrotic injury to the pancreas, producing **pancreatitis.**

Immune and Humoral Systems

As blood passes along the foreign surfaces of the CPB circuit, the complement system (an immune response involving plasma proteins and immunoglobulins) is activated. This leads to fever, **leukocytosis,** vasodilation, and increased vascular permeability resulting in interstitial fluid accumulation.

Neurological

Peripheral nerve injury is associated with improper and prolonged positioning on the operating room (OR) table. Symptoms of brachial plexus injury are weakness, numbness, and burning in the hand. Symptoms of ulnar nerve injury are numbness and tingling in the fourth and fifth fingers. **Paresthesia** and burning can occur in the extremity from which the saphenous vein was harvested.

Central nervous system deficits include **encephalopathy,** or brain embolism from dysrhythmias or aortic cross-clamping. Encephalopathy involves the entire brain, unlike an embolism, which produces a localized problem. There can be an altered level of consciousness and confusion with these conditions. Causes include medication such as morphine, hypoxic and hypoperfusion episodes, and volume overload resulting in brain tissue edema.

Pain is individualized and subjective. Chest pain is usually due to the sternotomy during which there is retracting

---

pericardiocentesis: peri—around + cardio—heart + centesis—surgical puncture

atelectasis: atel—imperfect + ectasis—stretching

nephrotoxic: nephro—kidney + tox—poison + ic—pertaining to

hypothermia: hypo—below normal + therm—temperature + ia—pertain to

pancreatitis: pancreat—pancreas + itis—inflammation

paresthesia: para—abnormal + esthes—sensation + ia—pertaining to

encephalopathy: en—inside + cephalo—head + pathy—disease

of the ribs and stretching of the muscles and ligaments. Anterior or posterior chest pain can be considerable with IMA grafts due to manipulation and resection of the mammary artery.

Psychological

Clients may experience varying degrees of memory loss, depression, immobilizing fear, frustration in role adjustments, hallucinations, cognitive dysfunction, or sexual dysfunction. Sleep disturbances such as insomnia, nightmares, and waking frequently are common and tend to prolong the symptoms.

Valve Replacement Complications

Tissue valves, over time, can undergo degenerative changes and calcification, leading to failure. Mechanical valves can fail due to structure, but more commonly failure is due to thrombus formation. Thromboembolism occurs when thrombi form on the mechanical valve and then become dislodged. This rarely occurs with tissue valves. It is prevented when mechanical valves are used with anticoagulant therapy.

It is vitally important for a PT and international normalized ratio (INR) to be drawn regularly when the client is on Coumadin therapy. Ideally the client's PT should be 1½ to 2 times higher than the normal level. If the PT is less, the client is at risk for thrombus formation. If the PT is higher, the client is at risk for hemorrhage. Client education is crucial, along with follow-up evaluation and instruction about anticoagulation therapy.

Other complications can include anemia and endocarditis. Anemia is due to hemolysis of red blood cells (RBCs) as they come in contact with mechanical valve structures. Endocarditis is an infection of the inner lining of the heart. Microorganisms tend to grow on the valve leaflets or the sewing ring of mechanical valves. These growths can make valves incompetent and break off and become emboli.

▼ CRITICAL THINKING: Mr. Jones

Mr. Jones, 68, is transferred to the nursing unit 12 hours after a CABG × 4. Preoperative vital signs are blood pressure 164/88, apical pulse 62 regular, respiratory rate 18, temperature 98.4°F.

Assessment findings are blood pressure 100/56, apical pulse 105 and irregular, respiratory rate 28 and shallow, temperature 99.8°F, chest and leg dressings dry and intact, no Foley, and is being monitored for first voiding postoperatively (due to void), lung sounds diminished with crackles in bilateral bases, and pedal pulses weak bilaterally.

1. Which finding(s) may indicate pulmonary problems?

2. List four nursing interventions for the altered pulmonary status.
3. What are three reasons why the apical pulse could be elevated?
4. What are two reasons why the blood pressure could be low?

Answers at end of chapter.

Cardiac Transplantation

Cardiac transplantation is reserved for clients with end-stage cardiac disease. Strict criteria for the selection of recipients and donors is applied in order to optimize survival (Table 22–2). Preoperative teaching is done once the recipient is accepted into the transplant program.

SURGICAL PROCEDURE

Once a donor heart is found, the recipient is notified, admitted to the hospital, and immediately prepared for surgery. The general procedures for this surgery are similar to those described in the cardiac surgery section. Two types of cardiac transplant procedures can be performed: orthotopic and heterotopic. In the orthotopic procedure, once the client is on CPB, the recipient's diseased heart is removed, leaving the posterior wall of the atria, superior vena cava and inferior vena cava, and pulmonary vein (Fig. 22–5). The aorta and pulmonary artery are cut. The donor's atria, aorta, and pulmonary artery are then anastomosed to the recipient's atria, aorta, and pulmonary artery. Surgery continues as previously described. The heterotopic procedure joins the donor heart and vessels to the recipient's heart and vessels without removing the recipient's heart. The donor heart rests in the right side of the chest.

Immunosuppressive therapy begins preoperatively with high loading doses of cyclosporine, azathioprine, steroids,

Table 22–2. **Cardiac Transplant Criteria**

Donor Criteria	Recipient Criteria
Less than 40 years of age	Less than 55 years of age
No significant cardiac or malignant disease	Class IV cardiac disease (not treatable with other medical or surgical treatment, less than 6–12 months survival)
No active infections	No irreversible pulmonary hypertension
No severe hypertension or diabetes mellitus	No unresolved pulmonary infarcts
Only ± 20 lb difference in weight between donor and recipient	No systemic disease limiting survival
	No drug addiction or peptic ulcer disease

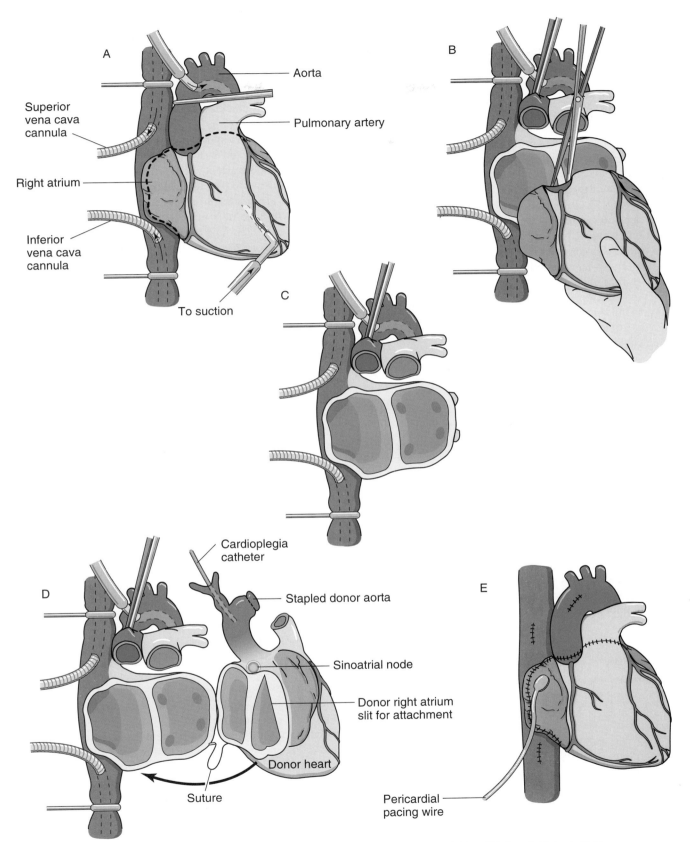

Figure 22–5. Heart transplantation. (Modified from Ruppert, S, Kernicki, J, and Dolan, J: Dolan's Critical Care Nursing. FA Davis, Philadelphia, 1996, p 339, with permission.)

and other medications. The risk for rejection is highest immediately after surgery and decreases with time, so doses of immunosuppressive medication are also highest initially after surgery and decrease with time. (See Nutrition Notes Box 22–3.)

COMPLICATIONS

Complications following heart transplantation include all of those stated for cardiac surgery in addition to rejection, which is the major cause of death in the first year, and infection and malignancies due to postoperative immunosuppressive therapy. Cyclosporine is nephrotoxic and hepatotoxic. Hypertension commonly occurs, related to the renal dysfunction resulting from the use of nephrotoxic medications. The use of steroids can cause osteoporosis, hyperglycemia, sodium and water retention, gastritis, hypertension, and cataract formation. Azathioprine is also hepatotoxic. The client may develop bone marrow depression or a skin sensitivity to the sun. Orthoclone OKT3, an immunosuppressant used to treat rejection, can cause fever, malaise, and headaches.

CRITICAL THINKING: Mrs. Eden

Mrs. Eden, 45, a single mother of two, is transferred to a surgical unit 5 days after a cardiac transplant. She is withdrawn and having a poor appetite. Her vital signs are stable. However, on ambulating to the bathroom, she is very weak, requiring two nurses to help her. Her respiratory rate increases from 20 to 32, is slightly labored, and her apical pulse increases from 88 to 103.

1. Is Mrs. Eden tolerating this activity? Why or why not?
2. List four reasons why Mrs. Eden could have a poor appetite.
3. Give four nursing interventions for Mrs. Eden's poor appetite.
4. Give three reasons why Mrs. Eden may be withdrawn.

Answers at end of chapter.

NUTRITION NOTES BOX 22–3

The potency of antirejection medications may be reduced if clients drink grapefruit juice with them. Grapefruit increases body metabolism.

Individuals who drink wine may not get the desired therapeutic effects of certain immunosuppressive medications.

MEDICAL MANAGEMENT

The client receives a diuretic when coming off CPB to aid in excretion of the excessive circulating fluid obtained while on CPB. Intake and output are monitored hourly, and the client is observed for fluid overload. Lung sounds are monitored for crackles. Daily weights and electrolytes are ordered.

Postcardiotomy syndrome (PCS) may occur on day 2 to 5 after surgery and last a few weeks. Clients may arouse normally and be oriented but will exhibit anywhere from a mild confusion to psychosis. Pupillary reaction and motor response are assessed. The safety of the client is maintained with side rails up, bed in low position, and equipment out of reach. The client is given as much rest and decreased sensory stimulation as possible. The family is kept informed and involved in the client's recovery.

Due to the continuous and high level of activity in the ICU and pain, it is difficult to promote sleep. Allowing for 90-minute intervals of sleep by dimming lights and decreasing all sensory stimulation near the client helps in promoting sleep. Listening to a favorite soothing tape with earphones and the use of ordered narcotics may help sedate and relax the client.

Temperature is ordered to be taken every 4 hours. Complete blood count (CBC) and white blood cell (WBC) results are monitored for indications of infection. If oral thrush (white patches) develops, an antifungal agent is ordered. A urine culture is ordered if urinary changes such as cloudy urine or urinary tract burning occurs.

Nursing Process

The client who is undergoing cardiac or vascular surgery has preoperative and postoperative needs in addition to those discussed here that are presented in Chapter 11 for the client having surgery.

PREOPERATIVE CARDIAC SURGERY OR CARDIAC TRANSPLANT

Assessment

A thorough routine baseline assessment is important for postoperative comparison and to begin discharge planning (Table 22–3). Specific data about pain control needs and circulatory status are essential items covered in the assessment. The nurse checks to see that results of x-rays or other studies are available for surgery. Results of any tests such as a CBC, electrolytes, PT, partial thromboplastin time (PTT), or a bleeding time are reviewed, reported if abnormal, and placed on the chart by the registered nurse. The nurse also ensures that any physician's orders to type or crossmatch up to 4 units of blood placed are available on hold. Additional assessment items, tests, and preoperative considerations are discussed in the preparation for surgery section.

Table 22–3. **Preoperative Nursing Assessment**

Past and present medical conditions and surgeries
Present medications
Allergies: medications, foods, other
Description of anginal pain and symptoms
Vital signs with blood pressure taken in both arms
Client's usual functioning level
Client's and family members' current knowledge of procedure
Family roles and support
Financial, transportation, or home life concerns

Nursing Diagnosis

The nursing diagnoses for preoperative cardiac surgery or transplant may include but are not limited to the following:

- Anxiety related to threat of death, pain, powerlessness, or lifestyle changes
- Knowledge deficit related to lack of knowledge of preoperative and postoperative procedures

These nursing diagnoses and their planning, intervention, and evaluation are presented in Nursing Care Plan Box 22–4 for the Preoperative Client Undergoing Cardiac or Transplant Surgery.

POSTOPERATIVE CARDIAC SURGERY OR CARDIAC TRANSPLANT

Assessment

The client is accompanied to the ICU by the anesthesiologist, who gives the nurse a report of the procedure, complications, and hemodynamic and ventilatory management of the client. The client is attached to the cardiac monitor and the mechanical ventilator, which may be used for 12 to 48 hours. A thorough head-to-toe assessment of the client, dressings, tubes and IVs is done after transfer. Pupils are checked, and signs of awakening, shivering, or pain are assessed. Lung and heart sounds are auscultated, and the entire chest and neck are palpated for crepitus (a crackling sound from air being in subcutaneous tissue). A temporary pacemaker is attached to the epicardial pacing wires as a precaution if bradycardia develops. Blood is drawn for a CBC, electrolytes, coagulation studies, and arterial blood gases. Vital signs and cardiac pressures are monitored and recorded every 15 minutes initially. Body temperature is monitored continuously. The nasogastric tube is placed to suction, and the urinary catheter drains by gravity. Intake and output is usually done at the same time intervals as the vital signs. The client is placed under a warming device, such as a warming light or warming blanket. A 12-lead ECG is done to rule out perioperative myocardial infarction. A chest x-ray is done to check any central line and endotracheal tube placement and to rule out a pneumothorax or hemothorax, diaphragm elevation, or mediastinal widening from bleeding. At this point, the family may see

the client and have care explained. Cardiac transplant clients may be in isolation for their own protection, depending on the agency's policy.

Nursing Diagnosis

The nursing diagnoses for the client who has had cardiac surgery may include but are not limited to the following:

- Pain related to surgical incision or reperfusion of tissue
- Ineffective airway clearance related to intubation, anesthesia, pain, or sedation
- Impaired gas exchange related to volume overload, atelectasis, phrenic nerve injury, or preexisting pulmonary dysfunction
- Decreased cardiac output related to myocardial depression, hypothermia, or dysrhythmias
- Risk for infection related to surgical incisions or immunosuppression
- Knowledge deficit related to lack of knowledge about therapeutic regimen

Nursing diagnoses for postoperative cardiac surgery or transplant are discussed in Nursing Care Plan Box 22–5 for the Postoperative Client Undergoing Cardiac or Transplant Surgery.

Planning

The client's goals are to (1) report pain management regimen relieves pain, (2) maintain a patent airway and clear lung sounds, (3) maintain oxygen saturation within normal limits, (4) maintain vital signs within normal limits, (5) remain free from infection, and (6) understand the surgery and the therapeutic regimen.

Nursing Interventions

Pain

After cardiac surgery, pain is assessed in relation to the client's preoperative anginal or infarction-associated pain. Experiencing chest pain after surgery can be very frightening for clients. They need to be told that chest pain occurs from the surgical incision. Otherwise they may not associate it with surgical incision pain, but rather their previous angina or infarction pain and become concerned. Any pain is promptly relieved to a tolerable level.

Decreased Cardiac Output

Trends in cardiac output are monitored. Body temperature is continuously monitored until warming measures are discontinued when the core body temperature nears 37°C. While clients are being rewarmed, they are assessed for shivering, which may be felt as a fine vibration at the mandibular angle of the jaw. Paralyzing agents given with narcotics eliminate shivering.

NURSING CARE PLAN BOX 22–4 FOR THE PREOPERATIVE CLIENT UNDERGOING CARDIAC OR TRANSPLANT SURGERY

Anxiety related to threat of death, potential changes in lifestyle, pain, and powerlessness

Outcomes
Client will verbalize a decrease in anxiety. Client will identify stressors.

Evaluation of Outcomes
Does client report a decrease in anxiety? Does client identify stressors?

Interventions	Rationale	Evaluation
• Assess anxiety level.	Anxiety is an individualized response to life events.	Does client rate anxiety?
• Assist client in identifying stressors.	Helps evaluate the threat and plan ways to deal with it.	Can client identify stressors?
• Spend unhurried time with client and family.	Relaxed atmosphere fosters trust and verbalization.	Does trust develop between client and family and nurse?
• Use open-ended questions.	Requires client to provide details.	Does client provide detailed information?
• Identify previous successful coping mechanisms.	Previously used skills will aid client under stress.	Does client identify coping skills?
• Be accepting of defenses, rationalizations, and fears.	Client needs to feel accepted to continue to verbalize.	Does client continue to verbalize feelings and ideas?
• Keep explanations short and simple.	Easily understood explanations are less anxiety producing.	Does client understand explanations?

GERIATRIC

• Provide elderly client with a quiet, safe, and consistent environment.	Unfamiliar, noisy environments increase anxiety.	Does elderly client report less anxiety and satisfaction with environment?

Knowledge deficit related to inadequate knowledge of preoperative and postoperative procedures and expectations

Outcomes
Client and family will verbalize understanding of preoperative and postoperative procedures.

Evaluation of Outcomes
Do client and family report understanding of explained procedures?

Interventions	Rationale	Evaluation
• Assess current level of knowledge.	Able to build on knowledge already known.	Does client provide prior knowledge information?
• Assess literacy of client and family.	Verification of reading ability is necessary for appropriate teaching method selection.	Client verbalizes understanding of written material.
• Use lay terms, not medical terms.	Most clients do not understand medical terms.	Does client understand terms used?
• Periodically assess understanding through return verbalization.	Periodic confirmation of teaching is needed to ensure knowledge building.	Can client verbalize understanding of information?
• Reinforce prior explanations about procedures.	Repeating information aids in retention.	Can client remember explanations?
• Review team members that will visit client.	Explains visits to expect from multiple services.	Can client state team member?
• Review tests (blood work, ECG, and x-rays).	Relates normalcy of routine tests to increase client comfort.	Does client verbalize understanding of tests?

continued

NURSING CARE PLAN BOX 22-4 *(continued)*		
Interventions	*Rationale*	*Evaluation*
• Review what client will experience during preoperative scrub, NPO, IVs, ETT, chest tubes, ventilator, equipment alarms, Foley catheter, pain management, communication, coughing, and deep breathing exercises.	Clients are often more concerned with what sensations will be experienced than why something is done.	Does client report comfort with sensations that may be experienced during procedures?

Ineffective Airway Clearance

Coughing and deep breathing and using incentive spirometry every hour while awake are important. Elevating the head of the bed, splinting the chest incision with a pillow or blanket roll, and relieving pain increase the client's ability to cough and deep breathe. Elderly clients have a weakened cough force. They should be encouraged and assisted to cough as effectively as possible. Sitting upright while deep breathing allows greater lung expansion for the elderly client.

Impaired Gas Exchange

Daily chest x-rays are monitored for diaphragm elevation, atelectasis, pulmonary effusions, and pneumothorax or hemothorax. The client is given oxygen and suctioned as needed. Respiratory treatments with bronchodilators may be given while the client is on the ventilator and after extubation. Diuretics and steroids may also be given to reduce excess fluids to improve air exchange.

Risk for Infection

Hand washing is very important to prevent infection. The temperature is monitored every 4 hours. Dressings are kept dry and intact, and incisions are assessed with every dressing change. Sterile technique is used to change dressings. The client should cough and deep breathe and use the incentive spirometer every 1 to 2 hours while awake. Sputum color is noted, and a sputum culture is requested by the registered nurse if changes occur. Urine consistency is noted, and a request for a urine culture is made if changes occur.

For the immunosuppressed client, the risk of infection development is greater. Fever is usually low grade in an immunosuppressed client because the suppressed immune system cannot produce a normal response to an infection. The client's oral mucosa is checked every shift for sores or thrush resulting from immunosuppression. All IV solutions and tubing are changed according to the agency's protocol for immunosuppressed clients. Discontinuing IVs and invasive lines should be done as early as possible. The cardiac transplant client may be in varying degrees of reverse (protective) isolation. Observation is a key to the early detection of infection because fever may be low grade in an immunosuppressed client.

Knowledge Deficit

Awakening with many questions, strange auditory and tactile sensations, and being unable to speak are very frightening and frustrating to the client. Keeping eye contact with the client and using touch appropriately can be very soothing. If lip reading is unsuccessful, using simple closed-ended questions, nonverbal gestures, communication boards, and magic slates may be effective. When the client is awake, keep explanations regarding procedures and how the client can help simple and in lay terms.

The family is allowed to assist with the client's care in such a way that self-care of the client is fostered. Cardiac transplant clients commonly have memory deficits, cognitive dysfunction, and short attention spans due to long-term decreased cerebral perfusion. Information must be given in small increments. Family involvement in teaching sessions is important to promote understanding and retention.

Studies have shown that discharge teaching should include treatment and complications, activity permitted, medications, and how to enhance quality of life. Sexual questions and concerns should be discussed with the client and his or her significant other. In addition to written materials, audiotapes can be used to provide discharge information.

Additional Nursing Care for Cardiac Transplant Clients

Cardiac transplant clients may have feelings of sadness and grief for the donor and her or his family. These feelings may be offset with great elation, relief, and hope after a long waiting period for the transplant. Clients should be told that these feelings are normal. They should be encouraged to ventilate their feelings. Emotional support may be needed if clients display or express these types of feelings.

Transplant rejection is a possible complication of this surgery and is monitored. Clients need to understand the importance of following instructions regarding medications and testing that are related to preventing or detecting rejection.

Cardiac transplant clients are followed in an exercise rehabilitation program that closely monitors their activity progression in relation to myocardial oxygen consumption

NURSING CARE PLAN BOX 22–5 FOR THE POSTOPERATIVE CLIENT UNDERGOING CARDIAC OR TRANSPLANT SURGERY

Pain related to sternotomy, leg incisions, internal mammary artery resection, or pericarditis

Outcomes
Client will state pain is relieved or tolerable. Client is able to rest and perform respiratory treatments.

Evaluation of Outcomes
Does client state pain is within acceptable levels? Is client able to rest and perform respiratory therapies?

Interventions	Rationale	Evaluation
• Assess characteristics of pain with each episode.	A thorough description is needed to determine cause and plan actions.	Does client describe pain on scale of 1 to 10?
• Splint chest incision with all movement and coughing and deep breathing.	Stabilizes sternum and incision to increase comfort.	Can client splint chest incision independently?
• Encourage client to report pain even when pain is mild.	It is easier to keep pain under control when mild.	Does client report pain when mild?
• Turn, reposition every 2 hours.	Changes muscle position, relieving stiffness.	Is client comfortable without stiffness?
• Offer back rubs frequently.	Relaxes tense muscles retracted during operation.	Is client able to rest in comfort?
• Instruct client to take a deep breath before movement and exhale slowly during movement.	Keeps muscles relaxed, minimizing tension with guarding and pain.	Can client perform coughing and deep breathing techniques as instructed?

Ineffective airway clearance related to intubation, sternotomy, pain, fatigue, sedation, anesthesia, and neurological deficits

Outcomes
Client will maintain a patent airway without signs of dyspnea or cyanosis.

Evaluation of Outcomes
Does client maintain a patent airway?

Interventions	Rationale	Evaluation
• Assess lung sounds every 2 to 4 hours.	Recognize changes early.	Are lungs clear on auscultation?
• Assess sputum color and character.	Changes may indicate need for cultures, antibiotics, or treatment to liquefy secretions.	Are sputum changes recognized and reported immediately?
• Monitor ABGs as ordered.	Acidosis may lead to decreased CO and hypoxemia to myocardial ischemia.	Do ABGs remain within normal limits (WNL)?
• Suction ETT as needed.	Assists in removing secretions from airways.	Does ETT or airway remain clear and free of secretions?
• Cough and deep breathe, use incentive spirometer hourly while awake.	Opens alveoli and mobilizes secretions.	Are lungs clear on auscultation and chest x-ray?
• Assess for pain, medicate, and evaluate effectiveness.	Comfort enhances client's ability to cough and deep breathe.	Is client's pain level acceptable to client?
• Turn every 2 hours, head of bed up 30 to 45 degrees.	Mobilizes secretions and drains lung fields.	Are lungs clear on auscultation and on chest x-ray?
• Give bronchodilators, O_2 prn or as ordered.	Opens airways and increases inspired oxygen to increase O_2 exchange in lungs.	Is client free of wheezes and hypoxemia?

continued

Impaired gas exchange related to anesthesia, sedation, volume overload, atelectasis, phrenic nerve injury, pneumothorax, gastric distention, or preexisting pulmonary dysfunction

Outcomes
Client will have clear lungs. Respirations and ABGs will be WNL.

Evaluation of Outcomes
Does client have clear lungs? Are respirations and ABGs WNL?

Interventions	Rationale	Evaluation
• Assess lung sounds and oximeter every 2 to 4 hours.	Identify changes early to prevent major complications.	Are lungs clear and is O_2 saturation WNL?
• Monitor chest x-ray daily as ordered.	Monitoring trends on x-ray aids in anticipating needs.	Are problems prevented due to early recognition?
• Turn, cough, and deep breathe every 1 to 2 hours.	Mobilizes secretions and opens alveoli.	Are lungs clear on auscultation and chest x-ray?
• Suction ETT as needed.	Assists in removal of secretions.	Is airway clear of secretions?
• Give supplemental O_2 and bronchodilators as ordered.	Facilitates O_2 exchange in lungs, opens airways.	Does client have clear lung sounds?
• Check nasogastric tube (NGT) patency and placement every 4 hours.	Significant gastric distention can impede ventilation.	Is client free of gastric distention?
• Splint chest incision with movement, coughing, and deep breathing.	Stabilizes sternum and chest incision, increasing comfort.	Does client splint chest incision independently?
• Assess chest tubes every 2 to 4 hours.	Chest crepitus indicates air leak; tubing kinks prevent drainage and reexpansion of lungs.	Are lungs reexpanding without signs of hemothorax or pneumothorax?
• Daily weights.	Assesses fluid retention.	Is weight within 5 lb of preoperative weight by discharge?
• Monitor hemoglobin, hematocrit, and RBCs as ordered.	Anemia from hemolysis or hemorrhage decreases O_2 carrying capacity of blood.	Are hemoglobin, hematocrit, and RBCs WNL?

Decreased cardiac output related to myocardial depression, hypothermia, bleeding, unstable dysrhythmias, or hypoxemia

Outcomes
Client will remain free of major side effects of pharmacological support. Client will maintain vital signs WNL, palpable peripheral pulses, urine output greater than 30 mL/h, and normal sinus rhythm.

Evaluation of Outcomes
Is client free of major side effects? Are vital signs WNL?

Interventions	Rationale	Evaluation
• Monitor vital signs.	Trends reflect problems.	Are vital signs WNL?
• Assess peripheral circulation.	Mottling or weak pulses may indicate poor cardiac output (CO).	Do peripheral pulses remain strong with normal skin color, temperature, capillary refill?
• Monitor intake and output.	Fluid deficit or excess can alter CO.	Does total intake equal output?
• Assess lung sounds and character of sputum.	Wet lung sounds may indicate heart failure or pulmonary edema.	Are lungs clear?
• Monitor temperature closely while rewarming the client.	Febrile state increases HR and myocardial oxygen consumption.	Does temperature remain less than or equal to 38°C?
• Assess for shivering.	Shivering increases the blood pressure, decreasing CO and increasing risk for bleeding.	Is client's shivering controlled?

continued

NURSING CARE PLAN BOX 22–5 *(continued)*

Interventions	Rationale	Evaluation
• Monitor chest tube drainage for increase or sudden decrease.	Drainage >200 mL/h may lead to hypovolemia and a decrease in CO.	Is client free from tamponade and hypovolemia?
• Monitor ECG.	Premature ventricular contractions and atrial fibrillation decrease CO.	Does client remain in normal sinus rhythm or controlled dysrhythmia?
• Monitor electrolytes.	Low Ca and Mg and high K decreases contractility and CO.	Are electrolytes WNL?
• Monitor ABGs.	Acidosis decreases heart function, and a low CO may lead to further acidosis.	Are ABGs WNL?

Risk for infection related to inadequate primary defenses from surgical wound or immunosuppression (transplants)

Client Outcomes
Client will remain free from infection.

Evaluation of Outcomes
Does client remain free from infection?

Interventions	Rationale	Evaluation
• Observe incision for signs and symptoms of infection.	Redness, warmth, fever, and swelling indicate infection.	Are signs and symptoms of infection present?
• Monitor drainage and maintain drains.	Drains remove fluid from the surgical site to prevent infection development.	Are drainage amount and color normal for procedure?
	Sterile technique reduces infection development.	Are drains functioning?
• Maintain sterile technique for dressing changes.		Is incision free of signs and symptoms of infection?
• Monitor and report abnormal findings for temperature, lung sounds, sputum, and urine consistency.	Low-grade (immunosuppressed) or high-grade fever, crackles, yellow-green sputum color, or cloudy urine can indicate infection.	Is the client's temperature WNL and lung sounds, sputum, and urine clear?
	Lung infections can be prevented with lung expansion and secretion removal.	
• Encourage coughing and deep breathing and incentive spirometer use.		Does client perform coughing and deep breathing and use incentive spirometer?

Knowledge deficit related to complex postoperative routines and rehabilitation expectations (strict posttransplant routines and monitoring)

Outcomes
Client and family will demonstrate understanding of therapeutic regimen: dietary restrictions, activity goals and restrictions, medications, incision care, resources, importance of frequent vital sign monitoring, physician visits, heart biopsies, and catheterizations for transplant clients.

Evaluation of Outcomes
Is client able to manage the therapeutic regimen?

Interventions	Rationale	Evaluation
• Frequently inform clients that surgery is over. Inform them of their status, and reorient to time, person, and place.	Short attention spans and short-term memory difficulties occur while sedated, requiring frequent orientation.	Does client awaken calmly?
• Keep explanations short and simple.	Simple explanations are less confusing for client.	Does client understand explanations?
• Instruct client before procedure what is to be done, sensations, and how to help.	Understanding and preparation facilitate cooperation.	Does client cooperate with care and acknowledge understanding of procedures?

continued

NURSING CARE PLAN BOX 22–5 *(continued)*

Interventions	Rationale	Evaluation
• Once awake and extubated begin instructing on medications, activity, and diet.	Start teaching early to allow for maximum repetition, time.	Does client have a beginning knowledge of medications, diet, and activity by transfer?
• Instruct mechanical valve replacement clients on specifics of Coumadin therapy: action, dose, side effects, diet, complications, over-the-counter drug interactions, exercise precautions, and importance of scheduled PT/INR draws.	Importance of information is stressed with repetition.	Does client have a beginning knowledge of Coumadin therapy on transfer and verbalize adequate knowledge regarding Coumadin on discharge from hospital?
• Instruct transplant client and family together.	Families must be involved for support and assistance at home.	Are client and family willing to learn?
• Explain immunosuppressive medications, physician visits, vital sign monitoring, heart biopsies, and catheterizations for cardiac transplant clients.	Immunosuppressive medications have major side effects that must be monitored; early rejection is seen with heart biopsies and chronic rejection through catheterizations.	Does client demonstrate adequate knowledge of discharge teaching through verbalization, demonstration, and appropriate questions before discharge?

and signs of activity intolerance. Their progression may be slow depending on their condition and strength before surgery, but most reach an activity level allowing them to participate in most recreational sports.

Evaluation

Evaluation of these nursing diagnoses for postoperative cardiac surgery or transplant is presented in Nursing Care Plan Box 22–5 for the Postoperative Client Undergoing Cardiac or Transplant Surgery.

Vascular Surgeries

Vascular impairments requiring surgery may be acute or chronic and involve arteries, veins, or lymphatic vessels.

SURGICAL PROCEDURE

Embolectomy and Thrombectomy

When an artery becomes completely occluded by an embolus or thrombus, it is considered a surgical emergency. Surgical removal to restore blood flow and oxygenation to the tissue distal to the occlusion is imperative to decrease ischemia and necrosis. Fogerty catheters (long narrow catheters with an inflatable balloon tip) are used to remove the thrombus or embolus. The catheter is inserted into the blood vessel lumen through a small incision located near the blood vessel occlusion. The tip is inserted past the occlusion, the balloon is inflated, and the catheter (with the occlusive material) is drawn back through the incision. The blood vessel and wound are sutured as circulation is assessed.

Vascular Bypasses and Grafts

Vascular bypass surgery involves the use of either autografts, such as the client's own saphenous vein, or a synthetic graft material that resembles the diseased vessel. The graft is anastomosed to the artery proximal to the occlusion and tunneled past the occlusion, where the distal end of the graft is anastomosed to the artery (Fig. 22–6). The graft is assessed for hemostasis and function, and then the wound is sutured closed.

A diseased area of a blood vessel, as in an aortic abdominal aneurysm, can be resected and replaced with a graft (aortic aneurysmectomy). This is usually an elective procedure. However, if the aneurysm is dissecting or ruptures, it is a surgical emergency.

New advances in bypass surgery are being tried. One technique being explored uses video-assisted aortofemoral bypass without laparotomy (opening the abdomen).[6] This method may reduce length of hospital stay and the need for postoperative analgesia. Client recovery times with less invasive surgical approaches may be reduced.

Arteriovenous (AV) shunts or fistulas are made for frequent, easy circulatory access, such as is needed with hemodialysis. A shunt is formed when one end of a synthetic graft is anastomosed to a selected artery and the other end to a selected vein (Fig. 22–7). An AV fistula is formed when a selected artery and vein are directly anastomosed to each other. The radial artery and cephalic vein in the forearm are most commonly used for these procedures. Local anesthesia is usually used during these procedures.

Endarterectomy

Arteriosclerotic plaques are dissected from the lining of the arterial wall and removed in a procedure called an en-

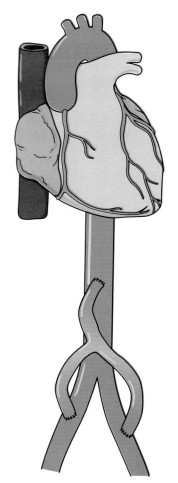

Figure 22–6. Aortic-femoral bypass.

darterectomy. This is most commonly performed on the carotid artery. The artery is clamped on both sides of the occlusion, and an incision is made into the artery. The plaque is removed with forceps. The artery is irrigated to remove any further debris and then sutured. The clamps are removed and the skin is closed. A drain may be placed.

COMPLICATIONS OF VASCULAR SURGERIES

Bleeding and reocclusion are complications with all vascular surgeries. Thrombi or emboli can develop and create a

surgical emergency to restore blood flow through the vessel. Drainage is usually small when peripheral vessels are involved. When the great vessels are involved, however, drainage is usually heavier, and drains are more often placed to remove this drainage.

A complication with carotid surgery is hematoma formation, which can compress and compromise the airway. Neurological dysfunction may occur if a piece of plaque embolizes to the brain during surgery. Extensive surgeries may also result in significant blood loss leading to volume deficit or shock.

MEDICAL MANAGEMENT

Daily weights and abdominal girths (for aortic aneurysm) are ordered. An increase in abdominal girth needs to be reported to the physician because it may indicate hemorrhage. Neurological checks following carotid surgery are ordered hourly initially. Neurovascular checks of extremities are ordered, usually every 1 to 4 hours. Changes are reported immediately to the physician. A loss of a pulse can indicate that circulation has been impaired in the vessel and may need to be restored with an emergency embolectomy. The nurse should anticipate the client's possible need to return to surgery if signs of impaired circulation are found. The incisional area is monitored for hematoma formation. CBC, PT, PTT, and electrolytes may be ordered daily. Intake and output may be ordered hourly initially. Imbalances in fluid status should be reported. Blood, volume expanders, and IV crystalloid solutions may be ordered for fluid deficits.

Nursing Process

PREOPERATIVE VASCULAR SURGERY

Assessment

As with cardiac surgery, a thorough routine baseline assessment is important for postoperative comparison and to begin discharge planning. Specific data about pain control needs and circulatory status are addressed in the assessment. The results of angiograms, arteriograms, or other special studies need to be available in surgery. Laboratory tests, such as CBC, electrolytes, PT, PTT, and bleeding

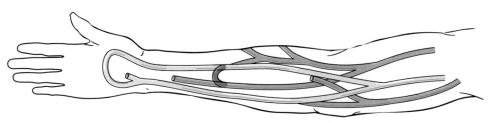

Figure 22–7. Arteriovenous shunt.

time results, are reviewed. The client may also be cross-matched with up to 4 units of blood placed on hold, which the nurse can ensure is available before surgery.

Nursing Diagnosis

The nursing diagnoses for preoperative vascular surgery may include but are not limited to the following:

- Pain related to ischemia of tissue distal to occlusion or aneurysm
- Anxiety related to unknown outcome, pain, powerlessness, or threat of death
- Knowledge deficit related to preoperative and postoperative procedures

These nursing diagnoses and their planning, intervention, and evaluation are presented in Nursing Care Plan Box 22–6 for the Preoperative Client Undergoing Vascular Surgery.

POSTOPERATIVE VASCULAR SURGERY

Assessment

On transfer to either the ICU or a surgical unit, the client is positioned comfortably and assessed. Findings are documented. If the client is hemodynamically stable, the head of the bed is placed in semi-Fowler's position. Once a patent airway is ensured, vital signs are monitored according to institutional policy, or a minimum of every 15 minutes or more frequently if they are unstable, low, or high. The client's pain level is rated on a scale of 1 to 10 and recorded.

Frequent airway and neurological checks are done for carotid surgeries. Airway checks involve assessment of respirations and tracheal position. Any respiratory distress is reported for prompt intervention. If the trachea is not midline, the shift to either side is noted and reported immediately. Impaired respiratory function may occur rapidly with tracheal shifting from bleeding or hematoma development in the neck. These checks usually include level of consciousness, orientation, pupil size and reaction, temporal pulses (located at the hairline by the outer end of the eyebrow), cranial nerve function such as eye and tongue movements, movement, strength and sensation of extremities, and speech. These are done hourly as ordered or according to institutional policy. Deficits are reported immediately to the registered nurse, who informs the physician.

Neurovascular checks are done for aortic or extremity vascular surgery. These checks include extremity movement and sensation, presence of numbness or tingling, temperature, color, capillary refill (less than 3 seconds normally), and pulses. Initially they are checked as frequently as hourly. Peripheral pulses are palpated, checked with a Doppler if not palpable, marked, and compared with the unaffected extremity as frequently as hourly. If a pulse is absent or weak and the extremity cool or dusky, the registered nurse should be informed so the physician can be notified immediately. A possible return to surgery for an embolectomy or other procedure should be anticipated by the nurse. Comparison with the opposite extremity may be helpful in detecting deficits.

Arteriovenous shunts and fistulas are assessed for patency by palpating for a thrill (a tremor) and auscultating for a bruit (swishing sound) at the site of the shunt or fistula. If a thrill or bruit is not present, the registered nurse should be informed so the physician can be notified immediately. Dressings or incisions are checked, and any drainage or hematoma development is noted and marked. Any drains or IVs are checked for proper functioning.

A client with extensive surgery may have a nasogastric tube to be monitored. Measurement of intake and output is usually done hourly. Laboratory tests such as CBCs and electrolytes may also be monitored.

LEARNING TIP

Extremity Neurovascular Checks. Neurovascular checks refer to the assessment of an extremity. Neurological checks refer to assessment of the central nervous system and involve different areas to assess. The following are areas to check on an extremity when doing neurovascular checks. They are identified under the category for which they are providing information.

Neurological	Vascular
Movement	Pulses
Sensation	Capillary refill
Numbness	Color (nailbed or skin)
Tingling	Temperature

Nursing Diagnosis

The nursing diagnoses for postoperative vascular surgery may include but are not limited to the following:

- Pain related to surgical incision or reperfusion of tissue
- Ineffective airway clearance related to intubation, anesthesia, pain, or sedation
- Risk for infection related to surgical incisions
- Risk for altered tissue perfusion related to hypotension, hypothermia, emboli, or vascular reocclusion
- Knowledge deficit related to lack of knowledge about surgical recovery needs

These nursing diagnoses and their planning, intervention, and evaluation are presented in Nursing Care Plan Box 22–7 for the Postoperative Client Undergoing Vascular Surgery.

Planning

The client and family should be included in planning postoperative care goals. The client's goals are to (1) report pain

NURSING CARE PLAN BOX 22–6 FOR THE PREOPERATIVE CLIENT UNDERGOING VASCULAR SURGERY

Pain related to preoperative ischemia of tissue distal to occlusion or aneurysm pressure on adjacent tissue

Outcomes
Client will verbalize pain is relieved or maintained at a tolerable level.

Evaluation of Outcomes
Is client's pain level as desired?

Interventions	Rationale	Evaluation
• Thoroughly assess characteristics of pain and compare with previous episodes.	Different qualities can mean different things; be specific when informing surgeon.	Are changes in pain noted with appropriate actions to prevent major complications?
• Administer pain medications when pain mild or on a schedule.	Easier to keep pain under control when mild.	Does client state pain is controlled?
• Position client for comfort; position extremity appropriately: peripheral arterial disease—dependent, peripheral vascular disease—elevated.	Gravity promotes arterial blood flow; elevation increases venous return.	Does client state increased comfort with positioning?
• Check circulation of extremity every hour if acute, every 2 to 4 hours if chronic.	Early recognition of emergency, necrosis from total occlusion can be rapid.	Are changes in circulatory status noted with appropriate actions to prevent problems?

Anxiety related to unknown, powerlessness, potential pain, and survival (extensive surgery)

Outcomes
Client will verbalize a decrease in anxiety. Client will exhibit coping behaviors to diminish anxiety.

Evaluation of Outcomes
Does client state decreased anxiety? Does client exhibit coping behaviors?

Interventions	Rationale	Evaluation
• Sit when interviewing client and use touch when allowed.	Conveys a genuine concern for client and their needs.	Is client relaxed and verbalizing freely?
• Allow sufficient time to thoroughly investigate causes of anxiety.	Information is missed when hurried.	Are causes of anxiety identified and plan for resolution made?
• Identify causes of anxiety.	Anxiety increases catecholamine release and vasoconstriction, decreasing blood flow through vascular occlusions.	Is pain decreased during or following interview?
• Obtain a social work referral when appropriate.	Social workers can assist clients with many anxiety-provoking social situations.	Is client willing to talk with social worker?
• Use pastoral care services when appropriate.	Pastoral services assist with spiritual needs.	Are client's spiritual needs met and used to reduce anxiety?

Knowledge deficit related to surgery and preoperative and postoperative procedures

Outcomes
Client and family will verbalize understanding of diagnosis, surgery, complications, and preoperative and postoperative tests and procedures.

Evaluation of Outcomes
Do client and family verbalize understanding of surgery and procedures?

continued

NURSING CARE PLAN BOX 22-6 *(continued)*

Interventions	Rationale	Evaluation
• Instruct client on the frequency and importance of neurological checks (carotid endarterectomy) and circulatory checks (peripheral surgery).	Relate normalcy of these postoperative procedures to minimize anxiety so client will not wonder what is wrong when repeatedly asked similar questions.	Does client state understanding, cooperate, and not become anxious when repeatedly asked similar questions after surgery?

management regimen relieves pain, (2) maintain vital signs and oxygen saturation within normal range, (3) remain free from infection, (4) maintain peripheral pulses and tissue perfusion, (5) remain free of edema and maintain clear lung sounds, and (6) understand the disease and its treatment.

Nursing Interventions

Pain

Pain is usually mild and easily controlled after peripheral surgery. If the pain is severe, it may indicate ischemia due to spasm or reocclusion. Severe pain is experienced with great vessel surgery, requiring more than one pain management method for relief. All characteristics of the pain are assessed to compare with previous pain episodes. The surgeon is informed of changes by the registered nurse.

Ineffective Airway Clearance

Clients with carotid endarterectomy must have the head of the bed elevated 30 to 45 degrees. This minimizes venous oozing and helps prevent hematoma formation in the neck, which can shift the trachea and compromise respiratory function. Clients are encouraged to deep breathe to help clear airways. Coughing should be avoided to prevent increased pressure on the surgical site.

Risk for Infection

Dressings are kept dry and intact and incisions assessed with every dressing change. The temperature is monitored every 4 hours. Oral mucosa is checked every shift for sores or thrush (white patches). Sterile technique is used to change dressings. Hand washing is very important to prevent infection. The client should cough and deep breathe and use the incentive spirometer every 1 to 2 hours while awake. Sputum color is noted, and a sputum culture is requested by the registered nurse if changes occur. Urine consistency is noted, and a request for a urine culture is made if changes occur.

Risk for Altered Tissue Perfusion

If possible, when care is turned over to another nurse, circulatory parameters should be double-checked between the two nurses in order for the oncoming nurse to have a baseline for comparison. The presence of a pulse, whether pal-

pated or heard with a Doppler, should be noted, as well as its quality. The quality of a pulse is its strength and its occlusion pressure, which is the amount of pressure required that causes the pulse not to be felt or heard. The registered nurse and then surgeon are notified immediately of any changes.

Knowledge Deficit

The client's and family's understanding regarding the postoperative recovery period is assessed. Physician's orders and routines regarding ambulation, exercise or restrictions, pain management, incision care, coughing and deep breathing, medications (Heparin or Coumadin), prevention and early signs and symptoms of thrombus or embolus formation are explained. Written as well as verbal information should be given for future reference by the client in the home setting. Audiotapes are also a helpful method of providing discharge information. The client can listen to the tapes in the hospital and have questions answered by the nurse, then they can take the tape home to review as needed or share with other family members that may not have been able to participate in hospital teaching sessions.

Evaluation

Evaluation of these nursing diagnoses for postoperative vascular surgery is presented in Nursing Care Plan Box 22–7 for the Postoperative Client Undergoing Vascular Surgery.

 CRITICAL THINKING: Mr. Smith

Mr. Smith has just returned to the surgical unit from the postanesthesia recovery room after undergoing a right carotid endarterectomy. He is sleepy but arousable; he is oriented to person, place, and time; his pupils are equal and reactive to light; and he is moving all extremities spontaneously and in response to command equally and strongly. His right neck dressing is dry and intact. His blood pressure is 146/82, apical pulse is 74, and respiratory rate is 16.

1. How should Mr. Smith be positioned?

   One hour later Mr. Smith is very sleepy but arouses to verbal and tactile stimulation. His pupils are equal, but the right one reacts slower than the left.

text continues on page 429

NURSING CARE PLAN BOX 22–7
FOR THE POSTOPERATIVE CLIENT UNDERGOING VASCULAR SURGERY

Pain related to surgical incision and reperfusion of tissue

Outcomes
Client will state that the pain is relieved or is tolerable. Client will rest comfortably, perform respiratory treatments as necessary, and perform activities of daily living (ADL).

Evaluation of Outcomes
Does client state pain is relieved or acceptable? Is client able to rest and participate in respiratory treatments and ADL?

Interventions	Rationale	Evaluation
• Assess severity of pain, as well as all other qualities.	Peripheral vascular surgery pain is usually mild, and severe pain may indicate reocclusion. Major vascular surgery pain is severe.	Does client state pain is at a tolerable level with a patent vessel?
• Ask client to rate pain after analgesic is given.	Pain relief is individualized.	Does client state pain is controlled at a tolerable level?
• Notify physician if pain is unrelieved.	Different analgesic may be needed to give relief.	Are client's pain relief needs met?

GERIATRIC

• Ensure that elderly client's pain is relieved.	Pain is not a normal part of aging, and elderly clients need and are entitled to adequate pain relief.	Does client rate pain as none or at a tolerable level using a scale of 1 to 10?
• Use opioid pain medications cautiously. Consider reducing frail elderly client's first opioid dose by 25%–50%, and increase as safe, needed and as ordered.	Elderly clients are more susceptible to peak effects and duration of analgesia of opioids.	Are client's vital signs and sedation levels WNL?

Ineffective airway clearance related to intubation, anesthesia, incisional and ischemia pain, sedation, and neurological deficits

Outcomes
Client will maintain a patent airway without signs of dyspnea or cyanosis.

Evaluation of Outcomes
Is client's airway patent?

Interventions	Rationale	Evaluation
• Assess vital signs, dressing, and neck for swelling as ordered (carotid surgery).	Increased BP may cause bleeding into neck tissue, compressing the trachea.	Are client's vital signs WNL, with no neck swelling or excessive bleeding from incision?
• Head of bed elevated 30 to 45 degrees at all times initially for carotid surgery.	Elevation will minimize venous stasis and oozing at neck incision, minimizing risk for hematoma formation and tracheal compression.	Is client's trachea midline with no pulmonary compromise due to hematoma at surgical wound?

continued

NURSING CARE PLAN BOX 22–7 *(continued)*

Risk for infection related to inadequate primary defenses from surgical wound

Client Outcomes
Client will remain free from infection.

Evaluation of Outcomes
Does client remain free from infection?

Interventions	Rationale	Evaluation
• Observe incision for signs and symptoms of infection.	Redness, warmth, fever, and swelling indicate infection.	Are signs and symptoms of infection present?
• Monitor drainage and maintain drains.	Drains remove fluid from the surgical site to prevent infection development.	Are drainage amount and color normal for procedure? Are drains functioning?
• Maintain sterile technique for dressing changes.	Sterile technique reduces infection development.	Is incision free of signs and symptoms of infection?
• Monitor and report abnormal findings for temperature, lung sounds, sputum, and urine consistency.	Elevated temperature, crackles, yellow-green sputum color, or cloudy urine can indicate infection.	Is the client's temperature WNL and lung sounds, sputum, and urine clear?

Risk for altered tissue perfusion related to hypotension, hypothermia, emboli, vascular spasm, or reocclusion

Outcomes
Client will have palpable peripheral pulses; adequate capillary refill; and normal color, temperature, motor, and sensory function of extremities. Client will have reactive pupils and baseline cognitive function.

Evaluation of Outcomes
Is client's circulatory status WNL? Does client have reactive pupils and baseline cognitive function intact?

Interventions	Rationale	Evaluation
• Assess circulation, movement, and sensation to extremities every 1 to 4 hours.	Early detection of spasm or reocclusion minimizes risk of ischemia and necrosis.	Does graft or vessel remain patent?
• Mark location of pulses on affected extremity.	Allows for quick location of pulses.	Are pulses located easily?
• Neurological checks every 2 to 4 hours (carotid).	Allows early detection of complications.	Are major neurological or circulatory problems detected?
• Circulation or neurological check between nurses when changing caregiver.	Subtle changes can be detected and new caregiver has baseline for comparison.	Is baseline assessment done?
• Abdominal girths every shift (abdominal aortic surgery).	Increasing girths may indicate bleeding into abdomen.	Does abdominal girth remain unchanged?
• Take temperature every 4 hours.	May indicate infection or hypothermia with need for further warming.	Does client remain normothermic?
• Monitor CBC as ordered.	RBC count, hemoglobin, and hematocrit decrease with insidious bleeding into abdomen or significant hematoma formations.	Is CBC WNL?
• Avoid constricting measures on affected extremity: knee gatch of bed, adhesive tape, tight dressings.	Prevent further decrease in blood flow to compromised extremity.	Is blood flow to affected extremity maintained?
• Auscultate AV shunts and grafts for bruits and palpate for thrills.	Any decrease or cessation of bruit or thrill indicates occlusion.	Does AV shunt or fistula remain patent?

continued

NURSING CARE PLAN BOX 22–7 *(continued)*

Knowledge deficit related to lack of knowledge about vascular surgery and therapeutic regimen

Outcomes
Client verbalizes knowledge of disorder and willingness to comply with therapeutic regimen.

Evaluation of Outcomes
Does client verbalize knowledge of disorder and comply with regimen?

Interventions	*Rationale*	*Evaluation*
• Explain condition, symptoms, and complications.	Client must have basic knowledge to comply with therapy.	Is client able to verbalize knowledge taught?
• Explain medications, therapies ordered, monthly lab test monitoring, and need for Medic Alert identification for anticoagulation therapy.	Compliance and safe use of medications is promoted with an adequate knowledge base.	Can client explain medications, therapies, lab tests, and purpose of Medic Alert identification?
• Teach client not to massage extremity.	Massage can dislodge an embolus.	Does client avoid massaging extremity?
GERIATRIC		
• Include caregivers/family in educational sessions.	Compliance increases if support systems understand instructions and client needs.	Do caregivers/family participate in sessions and offer client support?

HOME HEALTH HINTS

■ A copy of the discharge instructions should be reviewed with the client and family to ensure consistent understanding between the nurse and the family of the plan of care.

■ A home health social worker visit to a postsurgical cardiac client may be useful to help the client and family plan for lifestyle changes to reduce anxiety and environmental stress.

■ The ability of the client's caregiver to provide necessary care should be assessed. The support and resources available to the caregiver should be explored to prevent caregiver role strain.

■ The need for caregiver respite care should be assessed, especially over time. If respite care is needed, assist the caregiver in identifying respite care resources in the family or community.

■ Assist the caregiver to identify a plan to distribute the care workload among family members, if possible.

■ Teach the caregiver stress management techniques to use.

■ The importance of taking medications as prescribed needs to be reinforced, especially for immunosuppressive medications for cardiac transplant clients.

■ Advise clients who are leaving home for the weekend or holidays to refill medicines ahead of time to ensure that they do not run out. The physician can write a prescription for the client to have for emergency refills.

■ Clients with cardiac transplants should not be exposed to people with illnesses such as colds or the flu. This should be explained to family members and visitors.

■ Monitor the client following cardiovascular surgery for complication development such as incisional infection, pneumonia, thrombophlebitis, or pulmonary emboli. Report any abnormal findings.

■ Chest pain from esophageal reflux can mimic cardiovascular symptoms. The home health nurse should ask if the pain is related to consuming large meals, lying down, or bending over or if it is relieved with antacids or food. Inform the physician of these findings.

He is moving all extremities only to repeated commands, and the left ones are weaker than the right. There is a 2 cm shadow of drainage on the right neck dressing. His blood pressure is 176/88, apical pulse is 64, and respiratory rate is 26.

2. What are seven areas of concern found during this assessment of Mr. Smith?
3. What should the nurse's first action be?
4. List four priority items the nurse should continue assessing while awaiting physician orders.

Answers at end of chapter.

Review Questions

1. Mr. Jones asks what the cardiopulmonary bypass pump does. Which one of the following is the best explanation by the nurse about its purpose?
   a. "It removes the end products of metabolism."
   b. "It removes carbon dioxide and oxygenates blood."
   c. "It filters the blood to remove any medications."
   d. "It adds extra fluid volume to the circulatory system."

2. Thrombus formation is primarily a complication of which one of the following types of valves?
   a. Mechanical valves
   b. Porcine valves
   c. Allograft valves
   d. Bovine valves

3. Which one of the following conditions results from brain tissue edema and causes altered level of consciousness and confusion?
   a. Encephalopathy
   b. Cardiomyopathy
   c. Neuropathy
   d. Retinopathy

4. Which one of the following is the time frame after a cardiac transplant for the highest risk of rejection?
   a. Immediately after surgery
   b. Ten months after surgery
   c. One year after surgery
   d. Two years after surgery

5. Which one of the following is the purpose of coronary artery bypass graft (CABG) surgery?
   a. Cure coronary artery disease
   b. Increase blood flow to the myocardium
   c. Prevent spasms of the coronary arteries
   d. Decrease blood flow to the coronary arteries

6. Which one of the following conditions can occur immediately postoperatively or months later from manipulation of the heart's pericardium during surgery?
   a. Angina
   b. Pericarditis
   c. Dysrhythmias
   d. Endocarditis

7. Which one of the following can cause postoperative bleeding?
   a. Coronary artery spasm
   b. Hypotension
   c. Hypertension
   d. Reversal of heparin

8. Following a CABG, Mr. Jones' cardiac assessment was within normal limits. Over the last hour the nurse has observed an increase in dysrhythmias on the monitor, slightly blue nailbeds, and a blue color around his lips. He is restless and working against the ventilator. Which one of the following could be causing Mr. Jones' assessment changes?
   a. Hypoxemia
   b. Hypertension
   c. Hypocalcemia
   d. Vasodilation

9. Which one of the following signs or symptoms results from a sudden occlusion of an artery?
   a. Brisk capillary refill
   b. Redness
   c. Edema
   d. Pain

10. When assessing the patency of an AV fistula or shunt, which one of the following should be done?
    a. Check the pulse proximal to the fistula or shunt.
    b. Palpate the skin temperature proximal to the fistula or shunt.
    c. Check skin color and capillary refill proximal to the fistula or shunt.
    d. Palpate the thrill and auscultate the bruit over the fistula or shunt.

Answers to Critical Thinking

CRITICAL THINKING: Mr. Jones

1. Apical pulse 105, respirations shallow, lung sounds diminished with crackles, respiratory rate 28, temperature 99.8°F, irregular apical pulse.
2. Turn, cough and deep breathe, incentive spirometry, head of bed elevated, sputum culture, pain medication, splinting incision, possible diuretics, assess lungs every 2 to 4 hours.
3. Hypovolemia, hypoxemia, febrile.
4. Hypovolemia, irregular rhythm.

CRITICAL THINKING: Mrs. Eden

1. No. Increased respiratory rate and apical rate.
2. Steroids, immunosuppressive therapy, depression, fatigue.
3. Changes in lifestyle, extreme fatigue and how to raise children, grieving for donor, fear of rejection.

4. Small frequent meals, favorite foods from home, rest before meals, oral hygiene before meals, administer antiemetics before meals, give high-calorie meal at peak appetite.

CRITICAL THINKING: Mr. Smith

1. Elevate head of bed 30 to 45 degrees.
2. Increased blood pressure, increased respiratory rate, decreased apical pulse, drainage on dressing, more difficult to arouse, unequal movement, unequal pupillary reaction.
3. Have the registered nurse notify the physician and stay with the client.
4. Respiratory status (rate, depth, stridor), bleeding (increased drainage, swelling around neck, tracheal shift to left), neurological (decreased level of consciousness, movement of extremities), vital signs (increased blood pressure, decreased apical pulse).

REFERENCES

1. Peters, W, et al: Closed-chest cardiopulmonary bypass and cardioplegia: Basis for less invasive cardiac surgery. Ann Thorac Surg 63(6):1748, 1997.
2. Soulez, G, et al: Catheter-assisted totally thoracoscopic coronary artery bypass grafting: A feasibility study. Ann Thorac Surg 64(4):1036, 1997.
3. Rossi, M: The octogenarian cardiac surgery patient. J Cardiovasc Nurs 9(4):75, 1995.
4. Patel, H, et al: Dynamic cardiomyoplasty: Its chronic and acute effects on the failing heart. J Thorac Cardiovasc Surg 114(2):169, 1997.
5. Chachques, J, et al: Study of muscular and ventricular function in dynamic cardiomyoplasty: A ten-year follow-up. J Heart Lung Transplant 16(8):854, 1997.
6. Fabiani, J, et al: Video-assisted aortofemoral bypass: Results in seven cases. Ann Vasc Surg 11(3):273, 1997.

BIBLIOGRAPHY

Ackley, BJ, and Ladwig, GB: Nursing Diagnosis Handbook: A Guide to Planning Care. Mosby, St Louis, 1997.
Alexander, J: Phrenic nerve dysfunction following coronary artery bypass grafting: An aggravation or a real problem? Chest 113(1):2, 1998.
Barnason, S, and Zimmerman, L: A comparison of patient teaching outcomes among postoperative coronary artery bypass graft (CABG) patients. Prog Cardiovasc Nurs 10(4):11, 1995.
Bernat, J: Smoothing the CABG patient's road to recovery. Am J Nurs 97(2):23, 1997.
Bezanson, J: Respiratory care of older adults after cardiac surgery. J Cardiovasc Nurs 12(1):71, 1997.
Blum, A, and Aravot, D: Heart transplantation—an update. Clin Cardiol 19(12):930, 1996.
Bove, L: Now! Surgery for heart failure. RN 95(5):26, 1997.
Camp, P: Having faith: experiencing coronary artery bypass grafting. J Cardiovasc Nurs 10(3):55, 1996.
Daly, KA: Post anesthesia care of the vascular surgical patient. In Drain, CB (ed): The Post Anesthesia Care Unit: A Critical Care Approach to Post Anesthesia Nursing, ed 3. WB Saunders, Philadelphia, 1994.

Darovic, GO: Hemodynamic Monitoring: Invasive and Noninvasive Clinical Approach, ed 2. WB Saunders, Philadelphia, 1995.
Davids, D, and Verderber, A: Functional outcomes of cardiac surgery for the elderly. J Cardiovasc Nurs 9(4):96, 1995.
Doran, K, et al: Clinical pathway across tertiary and community care after an interventional cardiology procedure. J Cardiovasc Nurs 11(2):1, 1997.
Duits, A, et al: Prediction of quality of life after coronary artery bypass graft surgery: A review and evaluation of multiple, recent studies. Psychosom Med 59(3):257, 1997.
Earp, JK: The gastroepiploic arteries as alternative coronary artery bypass conduits. Crit Care Nurse 14(1):24, 1994.
Fleury, J, Thomas, T, and Ratledge, K: Promoting wellness in individuals with coronary heart disease. J Cardiovasc Nurs 11(3):26, 1997.
Gaw-Ens, B: Informational support for families immediately after CABG surgery. Crit Care Nurse 14(1):41, 1994.
Goldman, M: Pocket Guide to the Operating Room. FA Davis, Philadelphia, 1996.
Goral, S, et al: Long-term renal function in heart transplant recipients receiving cyclosporine therapy. J Heart Lung Transplant 16(11):1106, 1997.
Hall, RJ, et al: Neoplastic heart disease. In Schlant, RC, and Alexander, RW (eds): The Heart: Arteries and Veins, ed 8. McGraw-Hill, New York, 1994.
Hunt, SA, Schroeder, JS, and Billingham, ME: Cardiac transplantation. In Schlant, RC, and Alexander, RW (eds): The Heart: Arteries and Veins, ed 8. McGraw-Hill, New York, 1994.
Jesurum, J: Tissue oxygenation and routine nursing procedures in critically ill patients. J Cardiovasc Nurs 11(4):12, 1997.
Jickling, J, and Graydon, J: The information needs at time of hospital discharge of male and female patients who have undergone coronary artery bypass grafting: A pilot study. Heart Lung 26(5):350, 1997.
Kretzer, K, and Kinney, M: Managing heart and lung transplant patients. Am J Nurs 96(suppl 5):20, 1996.
La Forge, R: Mind-body fitness: Encouraging prospects for primary and secondary prevention. J Cardiovasc Nurs 11(3):53, 1997.
LeDoux, D, and Shinn, J: Cardiac surgery. In Woods, SL, et al (eds): Cardiac Nursing, ed 3. JB Lippincott, Philadelphia, 1995.
Lindsay, P, et al: Educational and support needs of patients and their families awaiting cardiac surgery. Heart Lung 26(6):458, 1997.
Matula, P: Aortic rupture. RN 96(11):38, 1996.
Medich, C, Stuart, E, and Chase, S: Healing through integration: Promoting wellness in cardiac rehabilitation. J Cardiovasc Nurs 11(3):66, 1997.
Moore, S: Effects of interventions to promote recovery in coronary artery bypass surgical patients. J Cardiovasc Nurs 12(1):59, 1997.
Moore, S: The effects of a discharge information intervention on recovery outcomes following coronary artery bypass surgery. Int J Nurs Stud 33(2):181, 1996.
Roach, G, et al: Adverse cerebral outcomes after coronary bypass surgery. N Engl J Med 335:1857, 1996.
Ruppert, S, Kernicki, J, and Dolan, J: Dolan's Critical Care Nursing. FA Davis, Philadelphia, 1996.
Soehren, P: Stressors perceived by cardiac surgical patients in the intensive care unit. Am J Crit Care 4:1, 1995.
Symbas, PN: Traumatic heart disease. In Schlant, RC, and Alexander, RW (eds): The Heart: Arteries and Veins, ed 8. McGraw-Hill, New York, 1994.
Winkel, E, and Piccione W: Coronary artery bypass surgery in patients with left ventricular dysfunction: Candidate selection and perioperative care. J Heart Lung Transplant 16(6):S19, 1997.
Zimmerman, L, Nieveen, J, Barnason, S, and Schmaderer, M: The effects of music interventions on postoperative pain and sleep in coronary artery bypass graft (CABG) patients. Scholar Inq Nurs Pract 10(2):153, 1996.

Understanding the Hematopoietic and Lymphatic Systems

23

Hematopoietic and Lymphatic System Function, Assessment, and Therapeutic Measures

Valerie C. Scanlon and Cheryl L. Ivey

Learning Objectives

Upon completion of this chapter, the student will be able to:

1. Identify the components of the blood.
2. Describe how changes in the blood or blood-producing processes are manifested as disease processes.
3. Describe the sequence of events in the process of blood clotting.
4. Describe nursing assessment of the client with a disorder of the hematological or lymphatic system.
5. Explain the laboratory and diagnostic studies used when evaluating the hematological and lymphatic systems.
6. Describe common therapeutic measures for clients with hematological and lymphatic disorders.
7. Describe the role of the LPN in administering blood products.

Key Words

ecchymoses (ECK-uh-**MOH**-sis)
lymphedema (LIMPF-uh-**DEE**-mah)
petechiae (puh-**TEE**-kee-eye)
purpura (**PUR**-pur-uh)
thrombocytopenia (THROM-boh-SIGH-toh-**PEE**-nee-ah)

Review of Normal Anatomy and Physiology

BLOOD

Hematology is the study of blood, its parts, its uses, and its abnormalities. Review of the lymphatic system includes studying the specialized network of nodes and nodules that serve to remove foreign invaders from the body directly. The lymphatic system is involved in the creation of most of the white cells that fight infection and the process that returns the cleansed lymph fluid back to the blood via an intricate vessel system.

The general functions of blood are transportation of nutrients for cellular growth and development, transportation of cellular waste products for disposal, overall body temperature regulation, and the production of cells that offer the body protection. Specific aspects of these functions will be discussed with the particular part of the blood that is responsible for each.

A person has from 4 to 6 L of blood; 52 to 62 percent is plasma, and 38 to 48 percent is cells. The blood cells are the red blood cells (RBCs or erythrocytes), white blood cells (WBCs or leukocytes), and platelets (thrombocytes). All of these blood cells are produced by the red bone marrow (RBM), a hematopoietic (blood-producing) tissue found in flat and irregular bones. The red bone marrow contains the undifferentiated stem cells that are the precursor cells for all blood cells. The other hematopoietic tissue is the lymphatic tissue of the lymph nodes, lymph nodules, spleen, and thymus, which produces only lymphocytes and monocytes. (See Table 23–1 for normal cell counts and other values.)

PLASMA

Plasma is the liquid portion of the blood and is approximately 91 percent water. The plasma serves as the trans-

Table 23–1. **Blood Cells—Normal Values**

Test	Normal Value	Sample disorders
	Red Blood Cells	
Number of circulating RBCs	4.1–6.0 million/mm³	Increased in chronic hypoxia; decreased in anemia or blood loss
Hematocrit (cellular portion of blood)	38–48%	Increased in dehydration or chronic hypoxia; decreased in anemia or blood loss
Hemoglobin (reflects oxygen carrying capacity of blood)	12–18 g/100 mL	Increased in chronic hypoxia; decreased in blood loss or anemia
Reticulocytes (number of circulating immature RBCs)	0–1.5%	Increased in hypoxia or anemia; decreased in RBC maturation defect
	White Blood Cells	
Number of circulating WBCs	5000–10,000/mm³	Increased in infection
Neutrophils	55–70%	Increased in infection
Eosinophils	1–3%	Increased in allergic response, some leukemias
Basophils	0.5–1%	Increased in hyperthyroidism, some bone marrow disorders, ulcerative colitis
Lymphocytes	20–35%	Increased in viral infections, chronic bacterial infection, some leukemias
Monocytes	3–8%	Increased in chronic inflammatory disorders, some leukemias
	Platelets	
Number of circulating thrombocytes	150,000–300,000/mm³	Increased from trauma; decreased with blood disorders; low platelet count causes risk for bleeding

porting medium for nutrients, wastes, hormones, antibodies, and carbon dioxide. The plasma proteins include the clotting factors, albumin, and the globulins. Clotting factors such as prothrombin and fibrinogen are synthesized by the liver and circulate until activated in the clotting mechanism. Albumin is also synthesized by the liver, and it helps maintain blood volume and blood pressure by pulling tissue fluid into the venous ends of the capillary networks. Alpha and beta globulins are synthesized by the liver to be carrier molecules for substances such as fats, and gamma globulins are the antibodies produced by lymphocytes.

The plasma is also important in temperature maintenance in that blood carries heat. The water of plasma is warmed by passage through active organs, such as the liver or skeletal muscles, and distributes this heat as blood circulates throughout the body. The overall goal is to keep the body temperature more or less even. One example of temperature regulation includes the blood seeking the surface of the skin when in need of cooling off as may be seen with the flushed face of the person with a fever or the person who has exercised vigorously. Conversely, the client whose body temperature has dipped to the lowest readings will often have a very pale color to the face and extremities, because the blood has begun being stored in the warmest parts of the body—the organs.

The normal pH range of blood is 7.35 to 7.45, which is slightly alkaline. The chemical buffer system in the blood prevents sudden fluctuations in pH and contributes to acid-base balance of the body as a whole.

RED BLOOD CELLS

Mature RBCs are biconcave disks without nuclei; they carry oxygen bonded to the iron in hemoglobin (Hgb). Oxyhemoglobin is formed in the pulmonary capillaries where the hemoglobin combines with the oxygen from the lungs. Once hemoglobin gives up its oxygen to the cells of the body it becomes reduced hemoglobin. The amount of hemoglobin in RBCs and the amount of iron in that hemoglobin are (in addition to the number of RBCs) the determining factors for the amount of oxygen the blood can carry. Any lack of iron, hemoglobin, oxygen, or red blood cells will result in the client experiencing the side effects of anemia, including shortness of breath and weakness.

The rate of production of RBCs by the red bone marrow is most influenced by blood oxygen level. Hypoxia stimulates the kidneys to secrete erythropoietin, which increases the rate of RBC production and thereby the oxygen-carrying capacity of the blood. At such times, immature RBC stages may be found in greater abundance in peripheral blood. A normoblast is the last RBC stage with a nucleus; a reticulocyte has visible fragments of its endoplasmic reticulum. These cells usually remain in the red bone marrow until mature; their presence in large numbers in peripheral blood indicates an insufficient amount of mature RBCs to meet the oxygen demands of the body.

Other requirements for the normal production of RBCs include sufficient dietary intake of protein and iron to synthesize hemoglobin. The vitamins folic acid and vitamin B_{12} are necessary for DNA synthesis in the stem cells of the red bone marrow. The continuous mitosis of these cells depends on their ability to produce new sets of chromosomes. Vitamin B_{12} is also called the extrinsic factor because its source is food. The parietal cells of the stomach lining produce the intrinsic factor, a chemical that combines with vitamin B_{12} to prevent its digestion and promote absorption in the small intestine.

Red blood cells live for approximately 120 days and then become fragile and phagocytized by fixed macrophages in the liver, spleen, and red bone marrow. The iron is returned to the red bone marrow for synthesis of new hemoglobin or is stored in the liver. The heme portion of the hemoglobin is converted to bilirubin, a bile pigment that the liver excretes into bile to be eliminated in the feces. Diseases such as malaria and specific liver disorders such as cirrhosis or cancer cause a more rapid than usual destruction of red blood cells. This hemoglobin release may cause the blood level of bilirubin to rise. When the bilirubin level is elevated, it stains the body fluids bright yellow to dark orange, depending on the bilirubin levels. This staining is known as jaundice and is a reliable indicator that there is an underlying medical problem.

Each client has a hereditary blood type, which refers to the antigens present on the RBCs. The two most important types are the ABO group and the Rh factor. The ABO type (A, B, O, or AB) indicates the antigens present (or not present, as in the case of type O) on the RBCs. In the plasma are antibodies for those antigens *not* present; these can interact with antigens in transfused blood if the donor's blood does not match the recipient's blood (Table 23–2). To be Rh positive means the D antigen is present on the RBCs; Rh negative means the antigen is not present. Rh negative people do not have natural antibodies to the D antigen but will produce them if given Rh positive blood.

WHITE BLOOD CELLS

White blood cells are larger than RBCs and all have nuclei when mature. The granular WBCs (neutrophils, eosino-phils, and basophils) are produced only in the red bone marrow. The agranular WBCs (lymphocytes and monocytes) are produced in the lymphatic tissue as well as the red bone marrow. (See Table 23–1 for normal value and percent of each kind in a different count.) WBCs carry out their functions in tissue fluid as well as the blood, and all are involved in immunity or inflammation (response to injury).

Monocytes become macrophages, which phagocytize pathogens and dead tissue; neutrophils are more numerous but phagocytize only pathogens. Eosinophils detoxify foreign proteins during allergic reactions and parasitic infections. Basophils release histamine as part of inflammatory reactions. There are two groups of lymphocytes: T cells and B cells. T cells may be helper, suppressor, killer, or memory T cells. B cells become plasma cells, which produce antibodies to foreign antigens, and also become memory cells.

PLATELETS

Platelets are formed in the red bone marrow; they are pieces of large cells called megakaryocytes. Platelets are involved in all mechanisms of hemostasis: vascular spasm, platelet plugs, and chemical clotting.

When a blood vessel is damaged platelets release serotonin, which promotes contraction of smooth muscle and thereby vasoconstriction of an artery or a vein. Such constriction makes the break smaller, perhaps small enough to be covered by a clot. The clot is more likely to stay in place and stop any continued bleeding because it covers a smaller area. Because capillaries have no smooth muscle to be constricted by the action of serotonin, another process for clotting is necessary. This process in ruptured capillaries is simple; platelets become sticky, adhering to the rough edges of the broken capillary and one another, and eventually form a platelet plug that stops the bleeding.

Platelets also produce platelet factors, chemicals whose release is stimulated by contact of blood with a rough surface (either a break or damaged vessel lining) and which are necessary for the first of the three stages of chemical clotting. In stage 1, platelet factors, clotting factors from the liver, tissue thromboplastin, and calcium ions react to form prothrombin activator. In stage 2, prothrombin activator converts prothrombin (synthesized by the liver) into thrombin. In stage 3, thrombin converts soluble fibrinogen (also from the liver) to insoluble fibrin, strands of which form the clot. Calcium ions are also required for stages 2 and 3.

Excessive clotting within the vascular system is prevented in several ways. The very smooth endothelial lining of blood vessels repels platelets so that they do not stick to intact vessel walls. Heparin produced by mast cells inhibits the clotting mechanism. Antithrombin (synthesized by the liver) inactivates excess thrombin to prevent the clotting mechanism from becoming a vicious cycle.

*Table 23–2. **ABO Blood Types***

Type	Antigens Present on RBCs	Antibodies Present in Plasma
A	A	Anti-B
B	B	Anti-A
AB	Both A and B	Neither anti-A nor anti-B
O	Neither A nor B	Both anti-A and anti-B

The Lymphatic System

The lymphatic system consists of lymph (the specialized fluid), the system of lymph vessels, the lymph nodes and nodules, the spleen, and the thymus. Functions of the lymph system are to return tissue fluid to maintain blood volume and to protect the body against pathogens and other foreign material (the latter is called immunity and will be covered in a separate chapter).

LYMPHATIC VESSELS

Lymph is tissue fluid that has entered lymph capillaries (tissue fluid is formed from plasma by filtration in blood

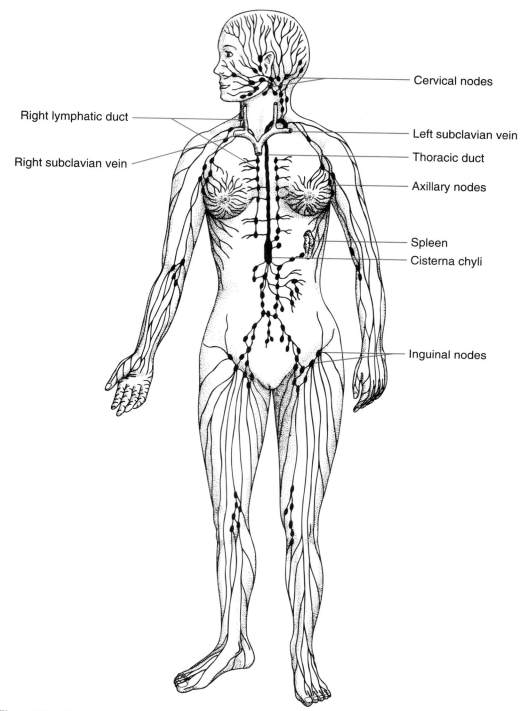

Figure 23–1. System of lymph vessels and major groups of lymph nodes. (Modified from Scanlon, VC, Sanders, T: Workbook for Essentials of Anatomy and Physiology, ed 2, FA Davis, Philadelphia, 1995, p 219, with permission.)

capillaries); it must be returned to the blood to maintain blood volume and blood pressure. Lymph capillaries are found in most tissue spaces; they anastomose, forming larger and larger lymph vessels, which have valves to prevent backflow of lymph. Lymph from the lower body and the upper left quadrant enters the thoracic duct (in front of the vertebral column) and is returned to the blood in the left subclavian vein (Fig. 23–1). Lymph from the upper right quadrant enters the right lymphatic duct and is returned to the blood in the right subclavian vein.

LYMPH NODES AND NODULES

Lymph nodes are masses of lymphatic tissue (producing lymphocytes and monocytes) along the pathways of the lymph vessels. As lymph flows through the nodes, the WBCs produced enter the lymph, foreign materials are phagocytized by fixed macrophages, and fixed plasma cells produce antibodies to foreign antigens. The major paired groups of lymph nodes are the cervical, axillary, and inguinal nodes. These areas are located at the junction of the head (cervical) and extremities (axillary and inguinal) with the main portion of the abdomen to remove pathogens in the lymph from the extremities before the lymph is returned to the blood.

Lymph nodules are small masses of lymphatic tissue found just beneath the epithelium of all mucous membranes. The body tracts lined with mucous membranes are those that have openings to the environment: the respiratory, digestive, urinary, and reproductive systems. Any natural body opening is a potential portal of entry for pathogens; any pathogens that penetrate the epithelium will usually be destroyed by the macrophages in the lymph nodules. The tonsils, which protect the oral and nasal portions of the pharynx, are familiar examples of lymph nodules, although most lymph nodules do not have names.

SPLEEN

The spleen is located in the upper left quadrant of the abdominal cavity, just below the diaphragm, behind the stomach. The lower rib cage protects the spleen from mechanical injury. In the fetus, the spleen produces red blood cells, a function assumed by the red bone marrow after birth. The functions of the spleen after birth are as follows:

- The spleen produces lymphocytes and monocytes, which enter the blood.
- The spleen contains fixed plasma cells that produce antibodies to foreign antigens.
- The spleen contains fixed macrophages that phagocytize pathogens or other foreign material in the blood. These macrophages also phagocytize old red blood cells and form bilirubin. By way of portal circulation, the bilirubin is sent to the liver for excretion in the bile.
- The spleen acts as a blood reservoir.

The spleen is not considered a vital organ because other organs compensate for its functions if the spleen must be removed (a person without a spleen is somewhat more susceptible to certain bacterial infections such as pneumonia and meningitis). The liver and red bone marrow will remove old red blood cells from circulation, and the many lymph nodes and nodules will produce lymphocytes and monocytes and phagocytize pathogens (as will the liver).

THYMUS

The thymus is located below the thyroid gland on the front of the trachea; in the fetus or infant it extends under the sternum. With increasing age the thymus shrinks, and relatively little thymus tissue is found in adults. The thymus produces lymphocytes, called T lymphocytes or T cells, and hormones that contribute to the maturation of the immune system, that is, the ability to destroy foreign material. This ability is usually established by the age of 2 years. Immunity will be covered in a later chapter.

Nursing Assessment

HISTORY

A thorough nursing assessment starts with an in-depth client history. After establishing a rapport with the client, the nurse should be sure to ask about diet, medication, and occupational history, as well as recent travel, living arrangements, and perhaps even use of herbs or alternative therapies. These factors can play important roles in hematological disorders.

The nurse asks the client why he or she needs medical help or what brings the client to seek medical attention as part of the thorough history. Document the response in the client's own words. Because signs and symptoms from hematological problems can occur in any body system, complaints will often be nonspecific, such as lack of energy, light-headedness, or nosebleeds. These symptoms are not diagnostic by themselves but become an important part of the overall complete nursing history. If the client complains of more than one problem, ask which is the most bothersome and explore that complaint first. Specific problems usually seen in clients with hematological disorders include abnormal bleeding, **petechiae** (small purplish hemorrhagic spots under the skin), and **ecchymoses** (larger areas of discoloration from hemorrhage under the skin) spread over the body's skin surfaces, as well as fatigue, weakness, shortness of breath, and fever.

The next area to explore is the present illness. Begin by obtaining biographical data, marital status, occupation, religion, client age, sex, and ethnic background. These areas can give the nurse valuable clues as to risk factors. For example, even though hemophilia almost always occurs in males, females may carry the gene. Sickle cell anemia occurs mostly in African-Americans but also affects people of Mediterranean or Asian ancestry. Pernicious anemia occurs most often in people of northern European ancestry. By carefully documenting this information, the nurse may be documenting important clues that will help pinpoint the client's problem. Finally, focus on the assessment of symptoms by using the WHAT'S UP format presented in Chapter 2.

A complete review of past illnesses and family history is always indicated and can net some valuable information. The social history is also useful. If the nurse has developed a good rapport with the client, the nurse may be able to explore the client's dietary and alcohol intake habits, any drug use or possible drug abuse, and sexual habits, all of which may cause changes in the hematological system.

An occupational review could reveal exposure to some hazardous substances that may cause bone marrow dysfunction. Certain occupations, such as working in a paint factory, tool and dye processing, and even dry cleaning are sometimes implicated in the formation of some hematological cancers. Military information may also reveal sources of exposure that would help during the diagnostic phase for hematological and lymphatic disorders.

PHYSICAL EXAMINATION

The physical examination is an important aspect of the nursing assessment. Hematological disorders can involve almost every body system, so the nurse will not want to skip a system during the assessment. First, assess the vital signs, which can give the nurse important clues. Frequent fevers are indicative of a poorly functioning immune system. Subnormal temperatures may indicate an overwhelming gram-negative infection which combined with other abnormal assessment data. Heart and respiratory rate abnormalities may indicate decreased blood volume or decreased oxygen supply. Finally, checking the level of consciousness may yield changes brought on by hypoxia, fever, and intracranial bleeding.

An inspection of physical structures most relevant to the blood and lymph systems includes the skin, mucous membranes, fingernails, eyes, lymph nodes, liver, and spleen. Specifically, perform these functions for each of the areas listed.

Observe for the client's skin color, noting pallor (indicating anemia), cyanosis (indicating poor oxygenation of red cells), or jaundice (indicating liver disease or hemolysis). Observe the face, neck, and hands for areas of local inflammation, enlargements, or obvious sites of infection. Check the entire skin surface for **purpuric** lesions (hemorrhages into the skin, mucous membranes, and other tissues), and examine the oral mucosa for color changes and petechiae or ecchymoses. These findings may indicate a bleeding disorder. Other important findings can be found after careful examination of the skin, looking for dryness and coarseness, which might indicate an anemia. Inquire about itchiness, which may also indicate blood or lymph disorders.

Fingernails can give the nurse important clues to the health of the client. For instance, long striations, or lines, on the nails may indicate anemia. Spoon-shaped nails may also indicate anemia. Clubbed fingertips and raised nail beds may indicate long-term hypoxia, the cause of which could be anemia or heart disease.

Abdominal assessment should include the use of auscultation, or listening with the stethoscope. Listen intently and try to identify high-pitched, tinkling sounds, which might indicate intestinal obstruction, versus the regular, gurgling, and lower-pitched noises heard in the intestines. In some cases, it would be a good idea to measure the abdominal girth and record the measurement in the nurses notes. This baseline measurement might be useful if the client begins to exhibit abdominal enlargement secondary to the buildup of ascites or bleeding.

Next progress to palpation, making sure that the client is comfortable and that the client's privacy is protected. Also, the nurse makes sure to warm his or her hands. Start with an examination of the lymph nodes. The nodes of the neck can be gently palpated while the client is sitting by simply running the hands over the neck and axillary surfaces. When examining the axillary nodes, the client may lie down. Any nodes that are palpable with or without **lymphedema** indicate some type of lymphatic disorder. Make sure to note the location, size, tenderness, texture, and fixation of the node groups. Enlarged or tender nodes indicate current or previous inflammation. Sternal tenderness may or may not be present. If present, this finding indicates that the bone marrow is being "packed" with an abnormal number and type of cells that are causing recognizable symptoms of anemia, leukemia, or an immunoproliferative disease.

Diagnostic Tests

A number of diagnostic tests can help rule out or confirm a suspected diagnosis based on the analysis of the formed elements of the blood and the bone marrow. Specific studies include tests for RBCs and platelet studies, coagulation, agglutination studies, bone marrow aspiration, and needle biopsy.

BLOOD TESTS

Examples of laboratory studies routinely done for clients with hematological disorders include the complete blood count (CBC), total hemoglobin concentration (Hgb), hematocrit levels (Hct), and platelet levels. (See normal values in Table 23–1.)

---

lymphedema: lymph—fluid found in lymphatic vessels + edema—swelling

LEARNING TIP

When a client has a bacterial infection, the neutrophils, which are one type of WBC, rise to help fight it. There are two forms of neutrophils: segmented (mature) and bands (immature). Initially, the segmented neutrophils go up. Then, as the infection becomes more severe, the bands begin to rise.

An easy way to remember this is that the WBCs are part of the body's defenses, just like the military is part of a country's defenses. When needed, Sargents who are fully trained or mature are called to battle first. If they are unable to fight off the invading enemy, new recruits being trained in boot camp are called in to help.

So segmented neutrophils (**S**egs) are like the **S**argents, fully mature and ready to fight. The **B**ands are like **B**oot camp recruits, immature and not fully trained. However, in an acute infection bands are necessary to prevent the body from being overwhelmed by the infection and losing the battle.

As you look at the differential WBC count, if the segs are elevated but the bands are normal, it is probably a new infection. If the bands are also elevated, the infection is worsening. The more elevated they are the more severe the infection.

Lymphocytes fight viral infections and are elevated during a virus.

A common pattern in the WBCs is produced for either a bacterial or viral infection. If the infection is acute bacterial:

Segs ↑ Bands ↑ Lymphocytes ↓

If the infection is viral:

Segs ↓ Bands ↓ Lymphocytes ↑

This can be remembered as the bone marrow producing the cells that are needed most during this time and reducing production of the cells least needed at this time. When the infection is resolved all the cells should return to their normal production levels.

COAGULATION TESTS

Tests in this category include bleeding times, capillary fragility test, prothrombin time (PT), partial thromboplastin time (PTT), and thrombin clotting time (TCT) (Table 23–3). Agglutination tests include ABO blood typing, Rh typing, crossmatching blood samples, and direct antiglobulin tests (also known as a Coomb's test).

CRITICAL THINKING: Mrs. Brown

Mrs. Brown is on warfarin (Coumadin) therapy following a blood clot in her leg. She has a PT drawn at the lab, and the result is 12 seconds. Will the physician most likely increase her daily dose of Coumadin, decrease it, or leave it the same?

Answers at end of chapter.

BONE MARROW BIOPSY

Biopsy information may be obtained through bone marrow aspiration, which in most states is obtained by a physician. Aspiration of the bone marrow is done to obtain a specimen that can be viewed under the microscope. Purposes of this test include the diagnosis of hematological disorders; monitoring the course of treatment; discovery of other dis-

Table 23–3. *Coagulation Studies*

Test	Normal Value	Comments
Prothrombin time (pro time, PT; affected by activity of clotting factors V, VII, X, prothrombin, and fibrinogen)	Men 9.6–11.8 seconds Women 9.5–11.3 seconds	Desired results 1.5 to 2 times longer for client on warfarin (Coumadin) therapy
International normalized ratio (INR)	2.0–3.0 seconds for client using anticoagulants (3.0–4.5 for recurrent problems)	Monitored with PT for warfarin therapy Standardized test adopted by World Health Organization
Partial thromboplastin time (PTT; affected by activity of clotting factors, prothrombin, and fibrinogen)	30–45 seconds	Desired results 1.5 to 2 times longer for client on heparin therapy
Thrombin clotting time (TCT; measures time for fibrin clot to form after addition of thrombin)	10–15 seconds	Desired results 1.5 to 2 times longer for client on heparin therapy
Bleeding time (measures time for small puncture wound to stop bleeding)	2.5–9.5 minutes	Indicates platelet function
Capillary fragility test	Fewer than 10 petechiae appearing in a 2-inch circle after application of a blood pressure cuff at 100 mg Hg for 5 minutes	Tests ability of capillaries to resist rupture under pressure Excessive fragility may be associated with thrombocytopenia

orders such as primary and metastatic tumors, infectious diseases, and certain granulomas; and isolation of bacteria and other pathogens by culture.

An accurate bone marrow specimen in an adult can be obtained from the sternum, the spinous processes of the vertebrae, or the anterior or posterior iliac crests. If a biopsy is also required, the latter are the preferred sites. Bone marrow biopsy, as well as aspiration, must be considered a minor surgical procedure and carried out under aseptic conditions. The client is placed comfortably on the side (for iliac crest aspiration) with the back slightly flexed and drawn slightly toward the chest. The posterior iliac crest is cleansed and covered with antiseptic solution. The skin, the subcutaneous tissue, and the periosteum are anesthetized using 1 or 2 percent lidocaine (Xylocaine). A 2 to 3 mm incision is made to facilitate penetrations with a 14 gauge, 2 to 4 cm bone marrow needle. More important, the incision is made to avoid introducing a skin plug into the marrow cavity, which could cause infection.

The nurse's role in bone marrow biopsy is multifaceted. First, it is often the nurse who will help coordinate between the laboratory and the physician for a time to do the procedure and for procuring the supplies, such as the disposable bone marrow aspiration tray or other specialized needles from the central supply area. The nurse administers an analgesic before the procedure according to the physician's order; helps position the client in a position that is helpful to the physician while ensuring comfort for the client as much as possible; holds the client in a particular position or coaches the client to stay in the necessary position; observes the aspiration site for excess bleeding and infection; and medicates the client for the expected discomfort that accompanies the procedure. The nurse often is called on to give emotional support before, during, and after the procedure.

LYMPHANGIOGRAPHY

Disorders of the lymph system can be evaluated using lymphangiography. This procedure involves injection of a dye into the lymphatic vessels of the hand or foot. Various x-ray views are then taken to determine lymph flow or blockages. X-rays are repeated in 24 hours to assess lymph node involvement.

Following the procedure, the physician may order a pressure dressing and immobilization of the injected extremity to prevent leakage at the site. The nurse monitors the extremity for swelling, circulatory status, and changes in sensation. The client is warned that the skin, urine, or feces may be blue tinged from the dye for about 2 days.

LYMPH NODE BIOPSY

If a lymph node is enlarged it may be biopsied to determine whether the cause is infection or malignancy. A biopsy may be done with a needle aspiration or surgical incision. A small dressing or Band-Aid is applied. Following the procedure the nurse instructs the client in signs of bleeding or infection at the site to report to the physician.

Therapeutic Measures

Therapeutic nursing measures are based on information the nurse obtained during the nursing assessment. Nursing diagnoses commonly used in clients with hematological disorders include fatigue related to anemia secondary to decreased hemoglobin and hematocrit levels. The nurse would want a client with this nursing diagnosis to conserve energy through careful planning of rest and activity cycles, reduction of stress, structuring the client's environment, enhancing client dietary intake of iron and minerals; and avoiding highly emotional situations that can aggravate the client's fatigue level.

A second nursing diagnosis is self-protection deficit: risk for bleeding, which may be associated with the medical diagnosis of hemophilia, **thrombocytopenia,** or disseminated intravascular coagulation. Interventions would include monitoring vital signs every 4 hours and assessing sites of bleeding for change or increase. Assess for changes in mental status, hypotension, and tachycardia, which may indicate bleeding and impending shock. Take measures to prevent bleeding, if not already present. This can best be accomplished by avoiding invasive measures such as injections, rectal suppositories or enemas, or even urinary catheterization. Avoid aspirin-containing products because they can increase bleeding, shave client with electric razors only, and give oral care with soft toothbrushes. The nurse may need to ask the physician to order a stool softener daily to maintain regularity and avoid straining at stool.

BLOOD ADMINISTRATION

Administration of blood is done by the registered nurse. The LPN/LVN may be called on to assist with proper identification procedures and monitoring of vital signs during the transfusion. See Table 23–4 for blood components that may be ordered. The main goal is to give them safely and avoid mistakes. Make sure to use proper identifying information to ensure that the right client is receiving the right blood products. The fail-safe system most often used in health care institutions is outlined next.

Safety Steps

Identification

Before administering any blood product, the nurse will need to make safety the first priority. This safety check includes the need to check and double-check the client's

---

thrombocytopenia: thrombocyte—platelet + penia—lack

Table 23–4. **Blood Products**

Product	Use
Packed red blood cells	Severe anemia or blood loss
Frozen red blood cells	Autotransfusion (blood taken from client and saved for future surgery), prevention of febrile reactions
Platelets	Bleeding due to thrombocytopenia
Albumin	Hypovolemia due to hypoalbuminemia
Fresh frozen plasma	Provides clotting factors for bleeding disorders, occasionally used for volume replacement
Cryoprecipitates	Bleeding from specific missing clotting factors

identity. Do not take this identification step for granted, because if the nurse makes a mistake and accidentally transfuses blood that does not match the client's blood type, the results may be fatal. Great care has been taken in the blood bank to match the donor's blood type with the recipient's blood type. After obtaining the unit of blood but before hanging the unit, two nurses (one of them a registered nurse) will need to check the following information at the client's bedside with the continued focus on safety (Fig. 23–2). The client is asked to say his or her name if alert and able to speak. Next use the client's identification band to confirm the client's identity and compare with the information on the paperwork obtained from the blood bank. After confirming the client's identity, examine the blood bag and verify that the client information and other information such as the ABO type, the Rh type, and the unit number all match. Finally, make sure to check the expiration date on the blood bag. Do not give the unit of blood if all information does not match. Notify the blood bank immediately of any discrepancies, and delay the transfusion until the differences are cleared up. Remember, there is no room for error when transfusing blood products.

Filtering

Most often, the filter that comes with the transfusion tubing is sufficient for each unit of packed red blood cells. Filters are commonly used with those clients who have specific problems, such as pulmonary impairments. It is thought that these finer filters remove many more of the microclots that could cause the client to have more problems breathing. In addition, many of these additional filters remove white blood cells and platelets and can decrease the occurrence or severity of some febrile reactions. However, these smaller filters also make the transfusion flow much slower. Because of their superior filtering ability, make sure that these microfilters are used on only whole blood or packed red cell transfusions, never on platelet transfusions, because they will become occluded with the platelets.

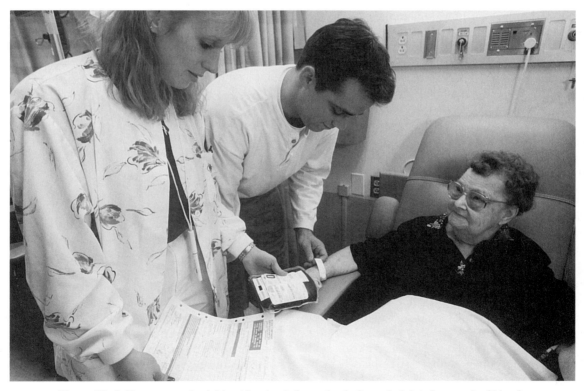

Figure 23–2. Two nurses check identification information before administering a unit of blood.

Washed or Leukocyte Depleted

There are instances when packed red blood cells (PRBCs) are ordered as "washed," often coming up from the blood bank in a round bag. The washing process removes almost all of the plasma and can decrease the occurrence or severity of a febrile reaction. In addition, leukocyte filters may also be used to completely remove all white blood cells. This removal process is used in cases where many transfusions are anticipated and decreases the chances of antigen sensitization as well as transmission of certain viruses, such as cytomegalovirus (CMV).

Warmed

If the client has had a severe bleeding episode and the nurses are helping to give replacement therapy through rapid, multiple transfusions, the physician may consider ordering the use of a blood warmer. The blood warmer works just as the name implies, warming the cold blood from the blood bank to the standard body temperature of 98.6° F. This warming helps prevent hypothermia, which can cause heart dysrhythmias, and shivering, which destroys blood cells and platelets.

Administration

Guidelines

The correct intravenous needle size is necessary to infuse blood because of its viscosity. The best sizes are 18- and 20-gauge needles. In a pinch, a 22-gauge cannula can be used, but be aware that an infusion pump may be needed to assist the thick blood through the smaller lumen of the 22-gauge cannula. Additionally, make sure to use only normal saline solutions to help dilute the blood and to flush the intravenous lines before and after the transfusions. Any other type of fluid or medication may cause the blood product to clump, clot, or not infuse at all. Two hours is usually a good time frame to transfuse each unit of packed cells. If the nurse must transfuse slower, make sure that the unit does not hang longer than 4 hours. After that time period, the blood is too warm and will begin to deteriorate.

Monitoring

Careful monitoring of the client's response to the transfusion is done to prevent complications or to detect and treat them quickly if they occur. Vital signs are taken and documented before initiating the transfusion, after the blood has begun to infuse, and following its completion. Some institutions require monitoring vital signs every 15 to 30 minutes during the infusion. The client is assessed for signs and symptoms of transfusion reactions. The nurse should carefully follow the policy at the institution where the blood is being administered.

Complications

The nurse must stay alert to the possibility of complications. Many health care workers think of transfusing blood components as a routine procedure. After reviewing these complications, the nurse will never think of a transfusion as being a routine procedure again. Complications may include febrile reactions, hypersensitivities, hemolytic reactions, anaphylaxis, and circulatory overload.

Febrile Reaction

By far the most common reaction is the febrile (fever) reaction, occurring up to 2 percent of the time. The risk of a febrile reaction goes up with each unit of PRBCs given to the client. Many times, febrile reactions occur after the transfusion is completed, but they can occur at any time. For this reason, the nurse will want to obtain pretransfusion vital signs, including the temperature. Usually, the most common signs are fever and shaking chills, which can be severe. Other symptoms may include chest pain, headache, hypotension, and nausea or vomiting. If these symptoms occur, stop the transfusion and notify the physician. The nurse can usually expect to treat the reaction symptomatically with acetaminophen for the fever. Often, the physician will want to continue the transfusion once the client is more comfortable. Make sure that the 4-hour hang rule is not violated.

Urticarial Reaction

Urticarial (hive) reactions are also seen about 2 percent of the time and are usually associated with antigens in the plasma accompanying the transfusion. There may be a fever, but the cardinal sign is the appearance of hives or a hivelike rash. On discovery of this reaction, notify the physician. Most likely, the client will be given a dose of Benadryl (diphenhydramine) and then the transfusion will be restarted.

Hemolytic Reaction

The most deadly and, fortunately, most rare of the possible reactions is the acute hemolytic reaction. The most common cause of this reaction is transfusion of incompatible blood. The result is hemolysis (destruction) of red blood cells. Usually this reaction will be noticed within minutes of starting the transfusion. Early symptoms may include back pain, chest pain, chills, fever, shortness of breath, and nausea or vomiting. As the reaction progresses, the client begins to show signs of shock, hypotension, and oliguria. Finally, signs and symptoms of disseminated intravascular coagulation occur, and the client begins to bleed uncontrollably from many different sites at the same time, usually ending in death. At the first sign of this type of reaction, stop the transfusion and notify the physician and the blood bank. Keep the vein open with normal saline using another administration set to administer the drugs that are ordered. Expect to deliver high volumes of fluids (to decrease shock and hypotension) and high doses of diuretics to promote urine flow, because the kidney is the most likely organ system to be damaged. Dialysis may be instituted to help save the client.

Anaphylactic Reaction

Anaphylactic reactions are not a common occurrence but may be seen more often in clients who have received many transfusions or have had many pregnancies. Usually the source of the anaphylaxis is from sensitization to immune globulins passed from the donor's unit of blood product. Usually, the very first milliliters of blood to pass into the client's system will be enough to cause the client to develop respiratory or cardiovascular collapse. Other symptoms include severe gastrointestinal cramping, instant vomiting, and uncontrollable diarrhea. If the client exhibits these signs and symptoms, stop the transfusion at once and have someone else notify the registered nurse and the physician. Emergency resuscitation measures must be instituted until the code team arrives. Expect the client to be intubated and continue with oxygen, steroids, and other drugs as needed to support life. After the emergency has passed, this client will likely need to receive transfusions from frozen, deglycerolized blood cells. There is no way to know in advance or to test for this type of RBC incompatibility, so it is best to monitor the client closely according to hospital policy and procedure.

Circulatory Overload

Circulatory overload is caused by rapid transfusion in a short period of time, particularly in elderly and debilitated clients. Usual signs and symptoms include chest pain, cough, frothy sputum, distended neck veins, crackles and wheezes in the lung fields, and increased heart rate. If symptoms occur, stop the transfusion and notify the physician. Anticipate administration of diuretics, which will help get rid of the excess fluid. Later, the transfusion may be restarted, but at a much slower rate. (See Gerontological Issues Box 23–1.)

Review Questions

1. Clotting factors such as prothrombin are produced by the
   a. Red bone marrow
   b. Liver
   c. Spleen
   d. Lymph nodes

2. The function of erythropoietin is to
   a. Increase production of platelets to promote clotting
   b. Decrease production of platelets to prevent abnormal clotting
   c. Increase RBC production to correct hypoxia
   d. Decrease RBC production to prevent hypoxia

3. The waste product of RBC destruction is
   a. Thrombin
   b. Iron
   c. Bilirubin
   d. Intrinsic factor

4. The lymph nodes that remove pathogens in the lymph coming from the legs are called
   a. Thoracic nodes
   b. Axillary nodes
   c. Cervical nodes
   d. Inguinal nodes

5. The return of tissue fluid to the blood is important to maintain normal
   a. Blood clotting
   b. Blood volume
   c. White blood cell formation
   d. Red blood cell formation

6. The portion of the blood in which cellular elements are suspended is referred to as the
   a. Cytoplasm of cells
   b. Platelets
   c. Plasma
   d. Hemoglobin

7. Which of the following anatomical sites is used to obtain a bone marrow specimen?
   a. Posterior iliac crest
   b. Long bones in the legs
   c. Ribs
   d. Humerus

8. What is the normal value for a platelet count?
   a. 50,000–75,000/mm^3
   b. 100,000–150,000/mm^3
   c. 150,000–300,000/mm^3
   d. 200,000–400,000/mm^3

GERONTOLOGICAL ISSUES BOX 23–1

Elderly clients have less cardiac and renal ability to adapt to changes in blood volume, so they have a much higher risk of fluid overload when receiving blood transfusions. The nurse should carefully monitor lung sounds and vital signs both before and during a transfusion. New onset of dyspnea, crackles, hypertension, or bounding pulse should be reported to the registered nurse or physician immediately.

ANSWERS TO CRITICAL THINKING

CRITICAL THINKING: Mrs. Brown

The physician will most likely increase Mrs. Brown's Coumadin dose. Note in Table 23–3 that the PT for a client on Coumadin therapy should be 1.5 to 2 times longer than normal. That is the reason the Coumadin is ordered—to prolong the time it takes for blood to clot. If a normal PT is 9.5 to 11.3 seconds, a therapeutic PT for Mrs. Brown would be 14.25 (or 9.5 × 1.5) to 22.6 (or 11.3 × 2). Her result of 12 seconds is not therapeutic.

BIBLIOGRAPHY

Baldy, CM: Hematologic disorders. In Price, SA, and Wilson, LM (eds): Pathophysiology: Clinical Concepts of Disease Processes, ed 4. Mosby, St Louis, 1992.

Bodnar, RM: Hematologic care. In Illustrated Manual of Nursing Practice, ed 2. Springhouse, Springhouse, Pa, 1993.

Harmening, DM: Clinical Hematology and Fundamentals of Hemostasis, ed 3. FA Davis, Philadelphia, 1997.

Kier, S: Caring for people with blood disorders. In Luckmann, J (ed): Saunders Manual of Nursing Care, ed 1. WB Saunders, Philadelphia, 1997.

Nettina, SM: Hematologic disorders. The Lippincott Manual of Nursing Practice, ed 6. JB Lippincott, Philadelphia, 1996.

Watson, J, and Jaffe, MS: Nurse's Manual of Laboratory and Diagnostic Tests, ed 2. FA Davis, Philadelphia, 1995.

24

Nursing Care of Clients with Hematopoietic Disorders

Cheryl L. Ivey

Learning Objectives

Upon completion of this chapter, the student will be able to:

1. List three ways anemias develop.
2. Describe causes of commonly occurring anemias.
3. Identify common signs and symptoms of anemia.
4. Use the nursing process to plan care for the client with anemia.
5. Explain nursing management of the client with sickle cell anemia.
6. List signs and symptoms of clotting disorders.
7. Describe precautions to prevent bleeding in clients with clotting disorders.
8. Use the nursing process to plan care for the client with hemophilia.
9. List the most common physical findings in the client with leukemia.
10. Use the nursing process to plan care for the client with leukemia.
11. State two places where the client can find information about leukemia.
12. Describe the pathophysiology, signs, and symptoms of multiple myeloma.
13. Use the nursing process to plan care for the client with multiple myeloma.

Key Words

anemia (uh-**NEE**-mee-yah)

disseminated intravascular coagulation (dis-**SEM**-i-NAY-ted IN-trah-**VAS**-kyoo-lar koh-AG-yoo-**LAY**-shun)

ecchymosis (eck-uh-**MOH**-sis)

glossitis (glah-**SIGH**-tis)

hemarthrosis (HEEM-ar-**THROH**-sis)

hemolysis (he-**MAHL**-e-sis)

hemophilia (HEE-moh-**FILL**-ee-ah)

idiopathic thrombocytopenic purpura (ID-ee-oh-**PATH**-ik THROMB-boh-SIGH-toh-**PEE**-nik **PUR**-pew-rah)

leukemia (loo-**KEE**-mee-ah)

pancytopenia (PAN-sigh-toh-**PEE**-nee-ah)

panmyelosis (PAN-my-e-**LOH**-sis)

pathological fracture (PATH-uh-**LAH**-jik-uhl **FRAHK**-chur)

petechiae (pe-**TEE**-kee-ee)

phlebotomy (fle-**BAH**-tuh-mee)

polycythemia (PAH-lee-sigh-**THEE**-me-ah)

thrombocytopenia (THROM-boh-SIGH-toh-**PEE**-nee-ah)

Clients with hematopoietic disorders have problems related to their blood. Some problems are caused by too many cells, others by too few or defective cells. When red blood cells are affected, oxygen transport is also affected, causing symptoms of poor oxygenation. When white blood cells are affected, the client is unable to effectively fight infections. If platelets or clotting factors are affected, bleeding disorders occur.

Disorders of Red Blood Cells

ANEMIAS

The term **anemia** describes a condition in which there is a deficiency of red blood cells, hemoglobin, or both in the circulating blood. Because hemoglobin carries oxygen, this results in a reduced capacity to deliver oxygen to the tissues. The result is symptoms such as weakness and shortness of breath, which lead the client to seek medical help.

Pathophysiology

Clients with anemia have an abnormally low number of circulating red blood cells (RBCs), or a reduced amount of hemoglobin in the RBCs. The decrease in the numbers of RBCs can be traced to three different conditions: (1) impaired production of RBCs, such as is seen in aplastic anemia and nutrition deficiencies; (2) increased destruction of RBCs, as in hemolytic or sickle cell anemia; or (3) massive or chronic blood loss. Some anemias are related to genetic problems in certain cultures (see Cultural Considerations Box 24–1). It is important to remember that the general term *anemia* refers to a symptom or a condition secondary to another problem and is not a diagnosis in itself. Different types of anemia are discussed below.

Etiology

Dietary Deficiencies

Iron, folic acid, and vitamin B_{12} are all essential to production of healthy red blood cells. A deficiency of any of these nutrients can cause anemia. Pernicious anemia is associated with a lack of intrinsic factor in stomach secretions, which is necessary for absorption of vitamin B_{12}. See Nutrition Notes Box 24–2 for more information.

Hemolysis

Hemolysis is the destruction, or lysis, of red blood cells. Destruction of red cells leads to anemia and is termed *hemolytic anemia*. This may be a congenital disorder, or it may be caused by exposure to certain toxins.

CULTURAL CONSIDERATIONS BOX 24–1

In the past, Iranian cross-cousin marriages have resulted in an increased incidence of several forms of anemia and hemophilia. These marriages are now being addressed through premarital screening for carriers and genetic counseling. People are also tested for vitamin B_{12} or folic acid deficiencies linked to an enzyme deficiency.[1]

A sex-linked genetic disease common in the Chinese is glucose-6-phosphate dehydrogenase (G6PD) deficiency, an enzyme deficiency affecting the person's red blood cells and resulting in anemia. Mediterranean G6PD is common, causing a hemolytic crisis when fava beans are eaten, when aspirin or certain other drugs are taken, or in acidotic or hypoxemic states. Mediterranean-type G6PD deficiency is an inherited disorder most fully expressed in males with a carrier state in females.[2]

Among Asian Indians, sickle cell disease is highly prevalent; the gene is detected in 16.5 percent of selected populations. Sickle cell anemia is the most common genetic disorder among African-American populations. Sickle cell anemia also is found in individuals where malaria is endemic, such as the Caribbean, the Middle East, the Mediterranean region, and Asia.

Other

Thalassemia anemia is a hereditary anemia found in persons from Southeast Asia, Africa, Italy, and the Mediterranean Islands. Individuals with thalassemia do not synthesize hemoglobin normally. Individuals with chronic disease also develop anemia (see Gerontological Issues Box 24–3). Additional causes of anemia are discussed under the separate headings of aplastic and sickle cell anemias.

Signs and Symptoms

Symptoms of anemia include pallor, tachycardia, tachypnea, irritability, and lethargy (Table 24–1). In addition to these symptoms, the client with pernicious (vitamin B_{12}) anemia may experience a sore tongue, numbness of the hands or feet, and weakness, because vitamin B_{12} is necessary for normal neurological function.

Diagnostic Tests

A complete blood count is done to determine the number of red blood cells and white blood cells (WBCs) per cubic millimeter. The size, color, and shape of the blood cells are

---

anemia: a—not + emia—blood

hemolysis: heme—blood + lysis—dissolution

NUTRITION NOTES BOX 24-2

Nutritional Causes of Anemia

Although not its only cause, nutritional deficiencies can produce anemia. Nutrients vital to the construction of red blood cells include iron, folic acid, and vitamin B_{12}. Even if the cause of the anemia is dietary, other therapies may be employed in addition to nutritional interventions.

Iron deficiency anemia, the most common nutritional deficiency in the world, is characterized by microcytic, hypochromic red blood cells. Insufficient intake of iron, excessive blood loss, or lack of stomach acid can lead to iron deficiency anemia. Individuals at greatest risk are women of childbearing age and young children. Even before frank anemia is seen, cognitive abilities can be impaired.

In early iron deficiency anemia, serum transferrin, a blood protein that carries iron, rises in an attempt to increase iron-carrying capacity. Later the hemoglobin and hematocrit levels drop.

Foods high in iron include liver and other organ meats, blackstrap molasses, oysters, and red meat. In addition, vitamin C enhances absorption of iron. Iron supplements are prescribed to treat iron deficiency. Iron therapy should be continued for several months after hemoglobin and hematocrit levels return to normal to enable the body to rebuild iron stores.

Macrocytic anemia can be produced by folic acid or vitamin B_{12} deficiencies. Although their functions are interwoven, both are necessary for normal RBC production.

Folic acid aids in the formation of DNA and heme, the iron-containing portion of hemoglobin. Conditions that increase the metabolic rate increase the need for folic acid. Many drugs, including alcohol, anticonvulsants, oral contraceptives, and aspirin, interfere with its absorption, metabolism, or excretion and can contribute to development of anemia.

Good food sources of folic acid include liver, leafy green vegetables, and legumes. Clients with anorexia or alcoholism often have a less than balanced diet. Other clients may not make food choices that include adequate folic acid. Occasionally, the nurse may find that the client is overcooking the foods in such a way that the folic acid is destroyed. Clients with inflammatory bowel diseases may eat the right foods but not absorb the nutrient. Because of the importance of folic acid in the diet, it has recently joined the list of nutrients added to enriched foods in the United States.

Vitamin B_{12} is required in a series of reactions preceding the use of folic acid in DNA replication. It is essential for the manufacture of red blood cells and for synthesis and maintenance of myelin.

Vitamin B_{12} requires a highly specific protein binding factor called intrinsic factor, secreted by glands in the stomach, to be absorbed. Intrinsic factor and vitamin B_{12} (also called extrinsic factor) combine in the stomach to form a complex that transports vitamin B_{12} to the ileum, where it is absorbed.

Lack of intrinsic factor may occur after extensive gastric surgery, resulting in pernicious anemia. Because the deficiency is not dietary, neither is the treatment. Vitamin B_{12} is given by injection so it can be absorbed without intrinsic factor.

Symptoms of vitamin B_{12} deficiency are, in usual order of appearance, numbness or tingling in the hands and feet, followed by red blood cell changes. Moodiness, confusion, depression, delusions, and overt psychosis appear next. Last, irreparable nerve damage occurs, and eventually death. Vitamin B_{12} deficiency should be considered in any person being evaluated for dementia.

If a person with pernicious anemia consumes ample folic acid, the body will manufacture red blood cells in the correct size and number. In this way folic acid is said to mask vitamin B_{12} deficiency. Unfortunately, the neurological deterioration continues unabated.

Vitamin B_{12} is found in animal sources, such as meat, fish, shellfish, poultry, and milk. Anyone eating these foods regularly is not at risk of deficiency, but strict vegetarians are at risk. A dietary supplement is the treatment.

determined by microscopic examination. Hemoglobin and hematocrit are below normal in anemia. Serum iron, ferritin, and total iron binding capacity measurements are done to diagnose iron deficiency anemia. Serum folate is measured if folic acid deficiency is suspected. A bone marrow analysis may also be done.

Clients with pernicious anemia have low gastric acid levels, and many have antibodies to intrinsic factor. Both abnormalities are associated with poor absorption of vitamin B_{12}. If blood loss is suspected, additional tests may be done to determine the source of bleeding.

Medical Treatment

Treatment begins with elimination of the contributing causes. Intake of the deficient nutrient can sometimes be increased in the diet or by administration of a supplement. Changing cooking habits, taking dietary supplements, decreasing alcohol intake, or controlling chronic diarrhea can help correct folic acid deficiency. If symptoms of anemia are acute, a blood transfusion may be necessary.

Nursing Process for the Client with Anemia

Assessment

The nurse monitors hemoglobin and hematocrit levels and other laboratory studies as ordered and reports any downward trend. Responses to therapy are monitored. The client's fatigue level and ability to ambulate safely and perform activities of daily living (ADL) are assessed. Degree

GERONTOLOGIC ISSUES BOX 24-3

Anemia of chronic disease is often diagnosed in an older client who has a chronic inflammation or a cancerous tumor. Unfortunately, this disease is often mistaken for iron deficiency anemia. The older client may be pale, weak, and confused with both diseases. The complete blood count for both diseases will show a low hemoglobin, low reticulocyte count, and low serum iron. The diseases can be differentiated only by the results of total iron binding capacity (TIBC). The TIBC is lowered in iron deficiency anemia but is normal in the anemia of chronic disease. This is important, because taking supplemental iron will not improve the symptoms of anemia of chronic disease. Treatment of the associated chronic disease is the only way to treat this anemia.

of dyspnea is monitored. Pallor may be noted in the skin and conjunctivae.

Nursing Diagnosis

Nursing diagnoses are based on assessment data and may include the following:

- Activity intolerance related to tissue hypoxia and dyspnea
- Altered nutrition: less than body requirements related to disease, treatment, and lack of knowledge of adequate nutrition
- Risk for injury: falls related to weakness and dizziness
- Altered oral mucous membranes related to vitamin B_{12} deficiency

Planning and Intervention

ACTIVITY INTOLERANCE. Care is planned to conserve energy after periods of activity. The client is assisted with self-care activities as needed. Articles are placed within easy reach of the client to reduce physiological demands on the body. The client is encouraged to limit visitors, telephone calls, and unnecessary interruptions. Rest should be allowed between activities.

Vital signs are monitored to evaluate tolerance to activity. If the pulse or respiratory rate increases over 20 percent from baseline during activity, the activity is too strenuous. Oxygen is administered as ordered to increase oxygenation. Blood transfusions may be ordered if hemoglobin levels are very low or symptoms are severe.

ALTERED NUTRITION. If the anemia is caused by a dietary deficiency, the dietitian should be consulted to provide diet modifications and instruction. The client with folic acid deficiency is taught that daily requirements can be met by including foods from each food group at every meal. If the client has a severe deficiency, dietary folic acid will not be enough and supplementation is the only way to correct the imbalance. The nurse instructs the client to continue taking the supplements until instructed to stop by the physician.

Vitamin B_{12} is administered by intramuscular injection. The client with pernicious anemia will need B_{12} injections for life.

The client with iron deficiency is instructed in the use of iron supplements and side effects, which include nausea, diarrhea or constipation, and dark stools. If liquid supplements are used, they should be given with a straw to avoid staining the teeth. Iron is sometimes given as an intramuscular injection (Imferon). It should be given by the Z-track method to avoid staining at the site. Foods high in iron

Table 24–1. *Clinical Manifestations of Anemia*

Body System	Mild (Hgb = 10–14 g/dL)	Moderate (Hgb = 6–10 g/dL)	Severe (Hgb < 6 g/dL)
Skin	None	None	Pallor, jaundice, pruritis
Eyes	None	None	Jaundiced conjunctiva and sclera, retinal hemorrhages, blurred vision
Mouth	None	None	Glossitis, smooth tongue
Cardiovascular	Palpitations	Increased palpitations	Tachycardia, increased pulse pressure, systolic murmurs, angina, congestive heart failure, myocardial infarctions
Lungs	Exertional dyspnea	Frank dyspnea	Tachypnea, orthopnea, dyspnea at rest
Neurological	None	None	Headache, vertigo, irritability, depression, impaired thought processes
Gastrointestinal	None	None	Anorexia, hepatomegaly, splenomegaly
Musculoskeletal	None	None	Bone pain
General	None	Fatigue	Sensitivity to cold, weight loss, lethargy

should be included in the diet; Vitamin C enhances absorption of iron (see Nutrition Notes Box 24–2).

RISK FOR INJURY. The client is assisted to change positions slowly to decrease dizziness and risk of falls. The nurse assists with ambulation as needed. The client with pernicious anemia must be protected from injuries because of decreased sensation. Care must be taken with heating pads, turning and positioning, and other potential sources of injury because the client may not feel pain.

ALTERED ORAL MUCOUS MEMBRANES. If the client has **glossitis,** the nurse provides good oral hygiene and soft, bland foods until healing occurs. The client is instructed to use a very soft toothbrush and perform oral care after each meal and at bedtime.

EVALUATION. When successfully treated, the client will tolerate a normal level of activity. The client should be able to explain the correct treatment plan and therapeutic measures for long-term prevention.

Aplastic Anemia

Pathophysiology

This type of anemia differs from other types of anemia in that the bone marrow becomes fatty and incapable of production of the necessary numbers of red blood cells. Also known as hypoplastic anemia, the cells that are produced are normal in size and shape, but there are not enough of them to sustain life. The resulting **pancytopenia** (reduced numbers of all of the formed elements from the bone marrow—red blood cells, platelets, and white blood cells) is the indicator that something is wrong with the bone marrow. Left untreated, aplastic anemia is almost always fatal.

Causes

Aplastic anemia may be congenital—that is, the person is born with bone marrow incapable of producing the correct number of cells. It may be due to exposure to toxic substances such as industrial chemicals (e.g., benzenes and insecticides), chemotherapy medications, or use of cardiopulmonary bypass during surgery. Other causative agents include some bacterial and viral infections, including tuberculosis and hepatitis.

Signs and Symptoms

The clinical features of aplastic anemia vary with the severity of the bone marrow failure. As with other anemias, early symptoms include progressive weakness, fatigue, pallor, shortness of breath, and headaches. As the disease progresses and the anemia and pancytopenia worsen, other

symptoms such as tachycardia and heart failure may appear. **Ecchymoses** and **petechiae** appear on the skin surface because of the reduced platelet count (Fig. 24–1; see also Fig. 24–5). The nurse may observe oozing of blood from mucous membranes. Puncture sites may progress from oozing to frank bleeding. Often there is overt bleeding into vital organs. When aplastic anemia is left untreated, most clients die from infection or bleeding, secondary to the lack of production of white blood cells and platelets.

Diagnostic Tests

The diagnosis of aplastic anemia begins with a complete blood count (CBC). Usually all values are reported as very low, with the occasional exception of the red blood count, in part because of the longer life span of the red cells. Eventually the red blood cells are also depleted. If the patient is having gross bleeding internally or externally, the RBC level will drop rapidly and dramatically. The most definitive test is the bone marrow biopsy. Because the bone marrow is essentially dead, the result is often described as a "dry tap," in which pale, fatty, yellow, fibrous bone marrow is extracted instead of the red, gelatinous bone marrow normally seen. Not surprising, the more fatty and pale the marrow is at the bone marrow biopsy, the more dysfunctional the bone marrow is. Other diagnostic tests include the total iron binding capacity (TIBC) and the serum iron level. It is common to find both of these levels elevated because the red blood cells are not being produced to use up the stores of iron in the production of hemoglobin.

Treatment

Early identification of the cause of the anemia and correction of the underlying problem are important to survival.

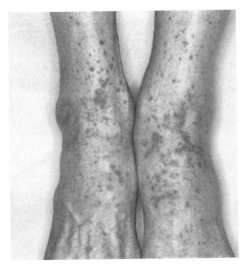

Figure 24–1. Petechiae on the skin from thrombocytopenia. (From Goldsmith, LA, et al: Adult and Pediatric Dermatology. FA Davis, Philadelphia, 1997, p 61, with permission.)

---

glossitis: gloss—tongue + itis—inflammation

pancytopenia: pan—all + cyto—cell + penia—poverty

Unfortunately, it is often difficult to determine the cause, and there is no way to reverse the damage already done. Aggressive supportive measures may be the only treatment. Most of these measures are aimed at prevention of infection and bleeding.

Today the most effective treatment for aplastic anemia is bone marrow transplantation. Another common therapy is the administration of steroids to stimulate production of cells in the weakened bone marrow. Occasionally the administration of hormones may work to increase the viability of the marrow. Steroid and other hormone treatments may be tried before attempting a bone marrow transplant.

A new line of therapy is also available. In many treatment institutions, limited success is being obtained with the use of colony-stimulating factors, natural elements now being produced synthetically. For example, erythropoietin (Epogen) stimulates the production of red blood cells and filgrastim (granulocyte colony stimulator, Neupogen) stimulates the production of white blood cells. The major drawback to this type of therapy is the high cost. Many of the pharmaceutical manufacturers have client-access programs that help with the costs of these medications.

Nursing Interventions

Nursing care of clients with symptoms of reduced hemoglobin levels is presented under Nursing Process for the Client with Anemia, above. If the client's platelet count is low (usually less than 20,000) the client is placed on bleeding precautions (Table 24–2). If the white count is low, the client must be protected from infection (Table 24–3).

Table 24–2. *Interventions to Prevent Bleeding in the Client with Thrombocytopenia*

1. Use an electric razor instead of a safety razor for shaving.
2. Use a soft toothbrush or gauze to clean the teeth.
3. Avoid invasive procedures as much as possible, including enemas, douches, suppositories, and rectal temperatures.
4. Avoid intramuscular injections.
5. To avoid injury when checking blood pressure, pump cuff up only until pulse is obliterated.
6. Avoid blood draws whenever possible. Use established access sites or group draws into once daily.
7. Maintain pressure on IV, blood draw, and other puncture sites for 5 minutes.
8. Encourage use of shoes or slippers when out of bed.
9. Keep area clutter free to prevent bumps and bruises.
10. Avoid use of drugs that interfere with platelet function, such as aspirin products and nonsteroidal anti-inflammatory drugs.
11. Administer stool softeners as ordered to prevent straining to have a bowel movement.
12. Move and turn client gently to avoid bruising.
13. Instruct client to avoid blowing the nose.

Table 24–3. *Interventions for the Client at Risk for Infection*

1. The client should be in a private room.
2. All personnel and visitors should wash hands before entering the room.
3. The client should be taught to wash hands before and after using the toilet and before and after eating.
4. The client and family should be instructed to wash hands before touching.
5. Staff or visitors with known infections should not enter the client's room.
6. The client should not handle flowers or plants brought into the room.
7. Raw fruits, vegetables, and milk products should be avoided.
8. Foley catheters and other invasive devices should be avoided.
9. If invasive procedures are necessary, strict aseptic technique should be used.
10. Use acetaminophen if an antipyretic is necessary; aspirin may induce bleeding.

Sickle Cell Anemia

Pathophysiology

Sickle cell anemia is an inherited anemia in which the red blood cells have a specific mutation that makes the hemoglobin in the red cells very sensitive to oxygen changes. Any time a decrease in the oxygen tension is sensed, the cells begin an observable physical change process from their usual spherical shape to a sickle or crescent shape (Fig. 24–2). Sickled cells are very rigid and easily cracked and broken. The abnormal shape also causes the cells to become tangled in the vessels, veins, and organs. The result is congestion, clumping, and clotting.

As red cells are broken the cellular contents spill out into the general circulation. The resulting increase in the bilirubin level causes jaundice. Gallstones (cholelithiasis) may develop because of the increased amounts of bile pig-

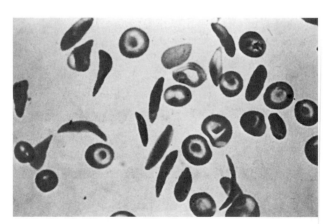

Figure 24–2. Sickled cells in sickle cell disease.

ments. The spleen and liver may enlarge because of the increase in retained cells and cellular materials.

Because of the differences in shape and texture, there is a significant decrease in life span of the red blood cells in clients with sickle cell anemia. Normal red cells live about 120 days. Sickled cells survive only about 15 to 20 days, an 80 to 90 percent decrease in cell survival.

Etiology

Sickle cell disease is an autosomal recessive hereditary disorder. This means that if both parents pass on the abnormal hemoglobin, the child will have the disease. If only one parent passes on the abnormal hemoglobin, the child will have the sickle cell trait and will be able to pass the trait on to his or her child (or the disease, if the other parent is also affected).

In the United States, sickle cell anemia is most frequently found in those of African heritage and people of Eastern Mediterranean origin. Worldwide, many persons residing in Asia, the Caribbean, the Middle East, and Central America are affected. In African Americans, nearly 10 percent have the sickle cell trait; 1 out of every 400 infants born has inherited the two sets of abnormal genes necessary to have the disease. Symptoms do not appear in infants until after the age of 6 months, because up to that age the infant is using hemoglobin manufactured during fetal life, which is not affected by the sickling process.

Signs and Symptoms

The sickling changes described above are a daily occurrence. The rapid return of the oxygen level to normal returns the cells to their normal shape for the most part.

Occasionally, the sickling process cannot be reversed and the problem continues unabated. This sudden and severe sickling is termed *sickle cell crisis.* As more and more sickling occurs, the blood becomes very sluggish and does not flow easily. It tends to collect in the capillaries and the veins of the organs of the chest and abdomen, as well as joints and bones, and cause infarcts (tissue necrosis due to lack of blood supply). Tissue necrosis results in pain, fever, and swelling.

Factors that contribute to the development of a sickle cell crisis include those related to decreased oxygenation. Some examples include pneumonia with hypoxia, exposure to cold, diabetic acidosis, or severe infection. Sickle cell anemia presents problems for the client who needs surgery. Anesthesia and blood loss during surgery and postoperative dehydration can trigger a crisis.

Common symptoms produced during sickle cell crises include severe pain and swelling in the joints, especially of the elbows and knees as the sickled cells impede circulation. Abdominal pain is common with the swelling of the spleen and engorgement of the vital organs. Hypoxia occurs as fever and pain increase, causing the client to breathe rapidly. The male client may have a continuous, painful erection (priapism) from impaired blood flow through the penis. Symptoms of renal failure are common as the kidneys become clogged with cellular debris and the circulation is slowed.

Repeated crises and infarcts lead to chronic manifestations such as hand-foot syndrome, an unequal growth of fingers and toes from infarction of the small bones in the hands and feet (Fig. 24–3). Additional manifestations of sickle cell disease are shown in Figure 24–4.

The client with sickle cell anemia has impaired quality of life. Often strenuous exercise or more exotic activities such as scuba diving are ruled impossible. Dehydration exacerbates the symptoms of sickle cell disease. Crises may occur without any apparent cause. In general, crises last from 4 to 6 days. They may occur in cycles close together for a period of time and then may become dormant for months to years. The cause of death is usually infection, stroke, or organ involvement.

Diagnostic Tests

The most telling feature is a blood smear that shows sickle-shaped red blood cells in circulation. The Sickledex test is a screening test that shows sickling of red blood cells when

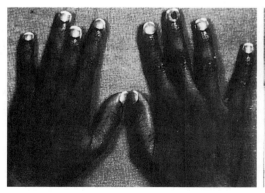
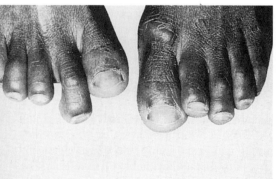

Figure 24–3. Hand-foot syndrome. Note different lengths of fingers and toes. (Courtesy of the Sandoz Pharmaceutical Corporation, East Hanover, NJ.)

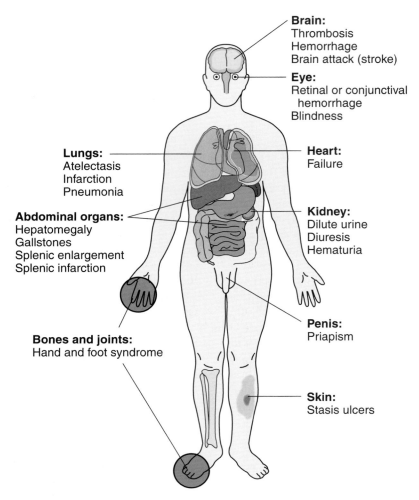

Brain:
Thrombosis
Hemorrhage
Brain attack (stroke)

Eye:
Retinal or conjunctival
hemorrhage
Blindness

Lungs:
Atelectasis
Infarction
Pneumonia

Heart:
Failure

Abdominal organs:
Hepatomegaly
Gallstones
Splenic enlargement
Splenic infarction

Kidney:
Dilute urine
Diuresis
Hematuria

Penis:
Priapism

Bones and joints:
Hand and foot syndrome

Skin:
Stasis ulcers

Figure 24–4. Clinical manifestations of sickle cell anemia.

oxygen tension is low. Hemoglobin electrophoresis is a test used to determine the presence of Hgb S, the abnormal form of hemoglobin. Also, there will be a decreased amount of hemoglobin, a lowered red blood cell count, an elevated white blood cell count, and a decreased erythrocyte sedimentation rate.

Treatment

No cure is available for sickle cell anemia. Treatment is aimed at continual client education to prevent crises and supportive care when crises occur. Some clients may be placed on low-dose oral penicillin to help prevent infections to decrease the risk of crises.

During acute crises, the client is admitted to the hospital for 5 to 7 days. The nurse can anticipate that the client will probably require sedation and analgesia for severe pain and blood transfusions to replace the sickled red cells lost by being caught, crushed, and destroyed. Oxygen therapy decreases the dyspnea caused by the anemia, and large amounts of oral and intravenous fluids are given to flush

the kidneys of the by-products of the many broken cells' debris. Antibiotics are used to treat infection that may have triggered the crisis.

New treatments are being developed to treat sickle cell disease. Frequent blood transfusions, often monthly, are one of the newest treatment recommendations. A drug, hydroxyurea, has been shown to decrease crises, but it can cause life-threatening side effects. Bone marrow transplantation is also being investigated as a potential cure.

Nursing Care

The nurse assesses circulation in the extremities every 2 hours, including pulse oximetry, capillary refill, peripheral pulses, and temperature. Frequent pain assessment is also necessary.

The LPN/LVN assists the RN to monitor IV fluids and encourages oral fluids. Opioid analgesics such as morphine are administered as ordered for acute pain. They are often given intravenously by the nurse or through use of patient-controlled analgesia (PCA). Warm compresses to the painful areas, covering the client with a blanket, and keeping the room temperature above 72°F reduce the vasoconstricting effects of cold. Cold compresses are contraindicated because they decrease circulation and increase the number of sickled cells caught in the painful area. Restrictive clothing and raising the knee gatch of the bed are avoided, because these can also restrict circulation. Tylenol is administered to control fever; aspirin is avoided because it may increase acidosis, which can worsen the crisis. Bed rest is encouraged during the acute phase.

Client Teaching

During remission, the nurse teaches the client how to prevent acute episodes. The client is advised to avoid tight-fitting clothing that restricts circulation. The client should avoid strenuous exercise, which increases oxygen demand, and cold temperatures and smoking, which cause vasoconstriction. Alcoholic beverages can also trigger a crisis and should be avoided. Clients should never fly in unpressurized aircraft or undertake mountain climbing or other sports that can cause hypoxia. Clients are encouraged to get yearly flu and pneumococcal vaccines. Fluids are encouraged to maintain hydration and reduce blood viscosity. Genetic counseling is important to prevent passing the trait or disease on to children.

Polycythemia

Pathophysiology and Etiology

Polycythemia (which literally means "too many cells") is really two separate disorders that are easily recognizable by similar characteristic changes in the red blood cell count. In both forms of polycythemia, the blood becomes so thick with an overabundance of red blood cells that it more closely resembles sludge. This thickness does not allow the blood to move easily. Laboratory tests show a hemoglobin over 18 mg/dl, the red blood cell mass over 6 million, and the hematocrit over 55 percent.

Polycythemia vera (PV) is known as primary polycythemia. Its cause is unknown. Because the red blood cells, platelets, and white blood cells are overproduced, the bone marrow becomes packed with too many cells. As this overabundance of cells spills out into the general circulation, the organs become congested with cells and the tissues become packed with blood. The skin takes on a ruddy appearance from the buildup of red cells. PV is usually found in clients over the age of 50.

In contrast, secondary polycythemia is the result of long-term hypoxia. Common coexisting conditions that

---

polycythemia: poly—many + cyt—cells + emia—in the blood

panmyelosis: pan—all + myel—marrow + osis—condition

phlebotomy: phleb—vein + otomy—incision (for the purpose of removing blood)

---

may predispose a client to develop secondary polycythemia include pulmonary diseases such as chronic obstructive pulmonary disease (COPD), cardiovascular problems such as chronic heart failure, living in high altitudes, and smoking. The body makes more red cells in response to the low oxygenation associated with these conditions. Secondary polycythemia is a compensatory mechanism rather than an actual disorder.

Signs and Symptoms

The client with PV commonly presents with hypertension, visual changes, headache, vertigo, tinnitus, and dizziness. Laboratory results show an increased level of all of the bone marrow components (RBCs, WBCs, platelets), which is called **panmyelosis.** The client may exhibit nosebleeds and bleeding gums, retinal hemorrhages, exertional dyspnea, and chest pains because of the increased pressure exerted by the excess cells. The client with PV usually has a ruddy (or reddish) complexion and abdominal pain with an early feeling of fullness because of the enlarged liver and spleen. Nearly all of the symptoms in PV are due to the major problems of hypervolemia, hyperviscosity, and engorgement of capillary beds. Without treatment, clients with PV die of thrombosis or hemorrhage.

Treatment

Treatment of PV takes place in two stages. The first stage is to decrease the hyperviscosity problem. The most common first-line treatment is therapeutic **phlebotomy.** Phlebotomy involves withdrawal of blood, which is then discarded. From 350 to 500 mL of blood are removed each time on an every-other-day basis, with the goal being a Hct of 40 to 45 percent. This reduces the RBC levels, and the client usually feels more comfortable quickly. Repeated phlebotomies will eventually cause iron deficiency anemia, which in turn stabilizes RBC production; phlebotomies can then be reduced to every 2 to 3 months.

The problem that remains is the increased white cell and platelet counts because phlebotomy does very little to correct these overloads. Chemotherapeutic agents or radiation therapy may be used to suppress production of these cells in some clients. Leukemia is a side effect of this therapy, so it is used only if the benefits outweigh the risks.

Nursing Care

The nurse explains the phlebotomy procedure and reassures the client that the treatment will relieve the most distressing symptoms. The procedure is the same as that used for donating blood. The client is taught to watch for and report any signs of iron deficiency anemia such as pallor, weight loss, and dyspnea. The client should be kept active and ambulatory to help prevent thrombus formation. When bed rest is necessary, passive and active range of motion exercises should be implemented. The client is monitored for complications such as hypovolemia and bleeding. Advise the client to report any signs or symptoms of bleeding immediately.

If the client has more advanced manifestations such as an enlarged liver or spleen, the nurse can offer several small meals each day so that the client will be more comfortable while ensuring adequate nutrition. In addition, the client is encouraged to increase his or her daily intake of fluids in order to reduce the viscosity of the blood.

If the client is on drug therapy the nurse monitors CBC and platelet counts. The nurse should emphasize the need for continued follow-up with the physician once the client begins to feel better, and instructs the client on specific symptoms to report, such as chest pain, increased joint pain, decreased activity tolerance, and fever. A dietitian can be consulted to discuss ways to maintain good nutrition.

Client Education

The client is instructed to drink at least 3 L of water daily to reduce blood viscosity. Tight or restrictive clothing should be avoided, and feet are elevated when resting, to prevent impairment of circulation. Use of support hose when up and around also promotes circulation. Anticoagulants are taken as ordered, and the client is instructed to follow instructions for routine laboratory tests and side effects to watch for. Routine bleeding precautions are implemented (see Table 24–2). The client is warned to stop activities at the first sign of chest pains.

Hemorrhagic Disorders

DISSEMINATED INTRAVASCULAR COAGULATION

Disseminated intravascular coagulation (DIC) involves a series of events that result in hemorrhage.

Pathophysiology

As its name implies, this syndrome is a catastrophic, overwhelming state of accelerated clotting throughout the peripheral blood vessels. In a short period of time all of the clotting factors and platelet supplies are exhausted, and clots can no longer be formed. This results in bleeding from nearly every route possible. DIC is not a disease but is more of a syndrome that develops secondary to some other severe physical problem. Once this deadly syndrome develops the progression of symptoms is rapid.

Massive clotting in blood vessels leads to organ and limb necrosis. Organs most often affected include the kidneys and the brain, but other blood-engorged organs, such as the lungs, the pituitary and adrenal glands, and the gastrointestinal mucosa, are commonly involved.

DIC is usually acute in its onset, although in some patients it becomes a chronic condition. The prognosis depends on early diagnosis and intervention and the severity of the hemorrhaging. Not surprisingly, DIC has a very high mortality rate.

Etiology

DIC can develop after any condition in which the body has sustained major trauma. The sources of trauma are varied and may include an overwhelming infection and sepsis with either gram-positive or gram-negative organisms or an overt viral infection. Obstetric complications such as abruptio placentae, amniotic fluid embolism, or a retained dead fetus can trigger the onset of DIC. Cancer-based causes of DIC include acute leukemia and widely metastatic cancers of the lung. Massive tissue necrosis found in severe crush or burn injuries may increase the risk for development of DIC. Tissue necrosis secondary to extensive abdominal surgery with leakage of the intestinal contents can be related to DIC onset. Rarer causes of this condition have included heatstroke, shock, and poisonous snakebites, as well as fat embolism secondary to broken long bones.

Signs and Symptoms

Abnormal bleeding without a history of a serious hemorrhagic disorder is a cardinal sign of DIC. Early signs of bleeding include petechiae, ecchymoses (Fig. 24–5), and bleeding from venipuncture sites. Bleeding may progress to IV sites, skin tears, surgical sites, incisions, and the gastrointestinal tract and oral mucosa. Pain and enlargement of joints develop if bleeding occurs into the joints. All of these signs and symptoms may occur at the same time. Massive bleeding may also be accompanied by nausea, vomiting, dyspnea, oliguria, convulsions, coma, shock,

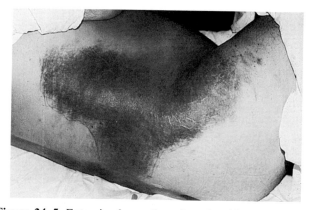

Figure 24–5. Extensive hemorrhage into the skin in DIC. Note how the area is outlined in pen so the nurse can assess if the area is spreading. (From Harmening, DM: Clinical Hematology and Fundamentals of Hemostasis, ed 3. FA Davis, Philadelphia, 1997, p 520, with permission.)

major organ system failure, and severe muscle, back, and abdominal pain.

Diagnostic Tests

Initial laboratory findings in DIC include a prolonged prothrombin time (PT) and partial thromboplastin time (PTT), decreased platelet count, and increased evidence of fibrin degradation products. A decrease in hemoglobin is the result of spilled hemoglobin from the increased numbers of broken red cells. Blood urea nitrogen and serum creatinine levels increase if the kidneys become involved. See Table 24–4 for additional findings.

Medical Treatment

Effective treatment of DIC is dependent on early recognition of the condition. Treatment is first aimed at correcting the underlying cause. Additional treatment consists of supportive interventions, including administration of blood, fresh frozen plasma, and platelets and the infusion of cryoprecipitates to support hemostasis. Some health care organizations include the use of intravenous heparin to help prevent the initial microembolization, but this practice is controversial. Additional therapies are being investigated.

Nursing Care

Care of the client with DIC is a nursing challenge. Early intervention requires early recognition and reporting of signs of bleeding. Besides delivering supportive care, the nurse must focus on the prevention of further bleeding episodes. Care should be taken to avoid any trauma that might cause bleeding. The nurse also should not dislodge clots from any site because another clot may not form, and the client will hemorrhage. See Table 24–2 for bleeding precautions.

Client Teaching

Because a client with DIC will often be placed in the intensive care unit, there will be many chances for client and family teaching. Explain all diagnostic tests to the client if he or she is alert. If not, keep the family informed. A large part of family education will be preparing the family for what the client may look like in terms of bleeding and bruising, as well as specific equipment that may be in place such as IV lines, nasogastric (NG) tube, and a Foley catheter. It may be helpful to enlist the aid of social workers,

idiopathic thrombocytopenic purpura: idio—unknown + pathic—disease + thrombo—clot + cyto—cell + penic—lack + purpura—hemorrhage in the skin
thrombocytopenia: thrombo—clot + cyto—cell + penia—lack

Table 24–4. *Laboratory Abnormalities in Disseminated Intravascular Coagulation*

Screening Test	Finding
Prothrombin time (PT)	Prolonged
Partial thromboplastin time (PTT)	Prolonged
Activated partial thromboplastin time (APTT)	Prolonged
Thrombin time (TT)	Prolonged
Fibrinogen	Reduced
Platelets	Reduced
Fibrin split products (FSP) (also known as fibrin degradation products, FDP)	Elevated
Protamine sulfate	Strongly positive
Dimers (cross-linked fibrin fragments)	Elevated
Antithrombin III	Reduced
Factor assays (for factors V, VII, VIII, X, and XIII)	Reduced

chaplains, and other members of the health care team to help support the family and the nurse.

CRITICAL THINKING: Mrs. Johns

Mrs. Johns is admitted to your unit with DIC following the difficult delivery of her new baby.
1. What will you assess as you care for Mrs. Johns?
2. What treatment do you anticipate?
3. What concerns is Mrs. Johns likely to have?
Answers at end of chapter.

IDIOPATHIC THROMBOCYTOPENIC PURPURA

Pathophysiology and Etiology

This disease results from increased platelet destruction by the immune system. Acute **idiopathic thrombocytopenic purpura** (ITP) usually affects children between the ages of 2 and 6, whereas chronic ITP mainly affects adults under the age of 50. The major population affected is women between the ages of 20 and 40.

Acute ITP usually occurs after an acute viral illness such as rubella or chickenpox. It may also be drug induced or associated with pregnancy. ITP is generally thought to be related to an immune system dysfunction. Antibodies responsible for platelet destruction have been found in nearly all diagnosed clients.

Signs and Symptoms

ITP produces clinical changes that are common to all forms of **thrombocytopenia**: petechiae, ecchymoses, and bleeding from the mouth, nose, or gastrointestinal (GI) tract. Bleeding may occur in vital organs, such as the brain, which may prove fatal. In the acute type, onset may be sudden and without warning, causing easy bruising, nosebleeds, and bleeding gums. Onset of chronic ITP is usually insidious.

Diagnostic Tests

A platelet count of less than 20,000/mm^3 and a prolonged bleeding time suggest ITP. The greatly decreased platelet level places the client at serious risk for hemorrhage. Examination of the platelets under the microscope shows them to be small and immature. Anemia may be present if there has been a bleeding episode. If a bone marrow aspiration is performed, the results show an adequate amount of the precursor cells for platelets, the megakaryocytes. However, instead of the 7 to 10 day life span that platelets usually have, these immature platelets have a life span of just a few hours.

Treatment

Most cases of acute ITP resolve spontaneously without treatment. Initial treatment, if necessary, is often the administration of steroids. The purpose of the steroids is to prolong the life of the platelets and strengthen the capillaries, making them less likely to break and cause bleeding. Some institutions use chemotherapy drugs. The spleen may be removed, because it is the primary site involved in platelet destruction. Often, the client undergoing splenectomy has tried all other courses of treatment unsuccessfully and may be experiencing bleeding episodes. Acute bleeding episodes are treated with transfusions of blood, platelets, and vitamin K.

Nursing Interventions

Care for the client with ITP is the same as any client with a bleeding disorder. See Table 24–2 for bleeding precautions. The client is taught to observe for and report signs and symptoms of bruising and bleeding (Table 24–5). The

Table 24–5. **Client Teaching: Signs and Symptoms of Bleeding**

Notify your health care provider if the following occur:
- Easy bruising of skin
- Petechiae (small red spots on skin)
- Blood in urine
- Black tarry stools
- Bleeding from nose or gums
- New onset of painful joints

client should avoid trauma and restrict activity during severe episodes.

HEMOPHILIA

Hemophilia is a group of hereditary bleeding disorders that result from a severe lack of specific clotting factors. The two most common are hemophilia A (classic hemophilia) and hemophilia B (Christmas disease). Von Willebrand's disease is another related bleeding disorder, but it represents a minority of cases and will not be discussed in this chapter.

Pathophysiology

Hemophilia A accounts for 80 percent of all types of hemophilia and results from a deficiency of factor VIII. Hemophilia B is a factor IX deficiency and affects about 15 percent of hemophiliacs. The severity and prognosis of hemophilia depend on the degree of deficiency of the specific clotting factors. It follows that mild hemophilia has the best prognosis because it does not cause spontaneous bleeding and joint deformities as does severe hemophilia.

After an injury, the person with hemophilia forms a platelet plug (which differs from a clot) at the site of an injury as would normally be expected, but the clotting factor deficiency keeps the client from forming a stable fibrin clot. Continued bleeding washes away the platelet plug that initially formed. Contrary to popular myths, people with hemophilia do not bleed "faster" and are not at risk from small scratches.

Etiology

Hemophilia A and B are inherited as X-linked recessive traits. This means that the female carrier (daughter of an affected father) will have a 50 percent chance of transmitting the gene to each son or daughter. Daughters who receive the gene are carriers, and sons who receive the gene are born with hemophilia. It is technically possible for daughters to be affected with hemophilia, although it is very rare.

Signs and Symptoms

Bleeding occurs as a result of injury, or in severe cases, spontaneously (unprovoked by injury). Bleeding into the muscles and joints (**hemarthrosis**) is common. Severe and repeated episodes of joint hemorrhage cause joint deformities, especially in the elbows, knees, and ankles, which decreases the client's range of motion and ability to walk.

---

hemophilia: hemo—blood + philia—to love
hemarthrosis: hem—bleeding + arthr—joint + osis—condition

In mild hemophilia, excessive bleeding is usually associated only with surgery or significant trauma. However, once a person with mild hemophilia begins to bleed, the bleeding can be just as serious as that of the client with a more severe form.

The client with moderate hemophilia has an occasional bout of spontaneous bleeding. In severe hemophilia, spontaneous bleeding occurs more frequently. It would be possible for the client to develop hemarthrosis or bleeding into the brain without any precipitating trauma. Severe episodes may produce large subcutaneous and deep intramuscular hematomas. Major trauma can cause bleeding so severe that it becomes life threatening.

Another unfortunate problem related to hemophilia treatment is related to the frequent transfusion of replacement clotting factors and other blood products. Before 1986, blood banks and other centers did not routinely test for human immunodeficiency virus (HIV) antibodies. Depending on the client's age and frequency of treatment, she or he may have been exposed to HIV or hepatitis. Blood banks and pharmacies have checked their blood supplies for the presence of HIV since 1986. Today the plasma proteins are artificially created or thoroughly cleansed to prevent transmission of disease.

Diagnostic Tests

Laboratory data reveal a prolonged PTT. The various factor levels are then measured to determine which is missing. Once the missing factor is identified, the type of hemophilia is named and necessary treatments can be implemented.

Medical Treatment

Hemophilia is not curable. However, treatment advances have improved outcomes and many clients can now live a normal life span. Treatment is aimed at the prevention of crippling deformities and at increasing life expectancy. Treatment involves stopping bleeding episodes by increasing the blood levels of the missing clotting factors. Hemophilia A is treated with factor VIII; hemophilia B is treated with factor IV. Each is available in a freeze-dried powder that is reconstituted with water and administered intravenously. The newest treatment is factors made using recombinant DNA technology, without the use of any human blood products. Blood transfusions are uncommon but may be necessary after severe trauma or surgery.

Complications related to therapy are usually because therapy is started too late. Generally speaking, minor trauma needs to be treated with at least 72 hours of added clotting factors; major traumas and surgeries may require up to 14 days of added factors to prevent sudden bleeding. Health care workers should pay careful attention to the client who says that bleeding is starting, even when no outward signs are evident. The client generally knows from experience if bleeding is starting. If treatment is delayed at this time, the results can be disastrous. Some clients with severe disease are treated prophylactically to prevent bleeding.

Nursing Process

Assessment

Because one goal is prevention of bleeding episodes, the client and family are assessed for knowledge of the disease and its treatment and understanding of preventive measures. Most clients care for themselves at home, starting their own IVs and administering treatment independently. Hospitalization is necessary only for surgery or major trauma. During an acute episode of bleeding, the hemoglobin and hematocrit are carefully monitored. Factor VIII or IX levels are monitored to determine if factor replacement has reached adequate levels. Vital signs are monitored for falling blood pressure and rising pulse rate, which are signs of hypovolemic shock. All body systems are assessed for signs of bleeding (see Table 24–5). A pain assessment is done using the WHAT'S UP? format.

Nursing Diagnosis

Priority nursing diagnoses include the following:

- Pain related to bleeding into tissues
- Risk for injury related to effects of bleeding
- Risk for ineffective management of therapeutic regimen related to knowledge deficit

Planning and Implementation

Goals of treatment are to prevent bleeding and to access quick treatment and prevent complications if bleeding occurs.

PAIN. Pain during acute bleeding episodes is managed with opioids as prescribed. Use of patient-controlled analgesia is helpful, especially because this uses the intravenous route. Intramuscular injections are contraindicated because of the risk of causing bleeding into the muscle.

RISK FOR INJURY. Routine precautions to prevent bleeding are summarized in Table 24–2. In the event of an acute episode of bleeding, the client is transfused with factor concentrates (or in rare circumstances, fresh frozen plasma, cryoprecipitate, blood, or a combination of these). See Chapter 23 for transfusion of blood products. Ice or pressure on bleeding sites may help slow bleeding. Special preventive care is exercised if the client requires surgery or dental procedures; these can be life-threatening events for the client with hemophilia.

RISK FOR INEFFECTIVE MANAGEMENT OF THERAPEUTIC REGIMEN. The LPN/LVN assists the RN to instruct the client and family in care of the disorder. They must learn to prevent bleeding episodes, recognize signs and symptoms of bleeding, and obtain emergency care in the event that bleeding does occur. Many clients are taught to administer treatment at home. A nationwide system of comprehensive hemophilia treatment centers coordinates care for these clients. Periodic multidisciplinary clinics are held, at which social service, dental, rehabilitation, nursing, financial, and medical needs can be addressed.

Evaluation

If nursing care is effective, the client will be comfortable, and bleeding will be prevented or complications minimized. The client and family will be able to state appropriate measures to prevent and treat bleeding episodes.

Disorders of White Blood Cells

LEUKEMIA

The term **leukemia** literally means "white blood." It was first identified in 1845 when the blood of victims was examined and found to have an excess of "colorless" cells.

Pathophysiology

Leukemia is a malignant disease of the white blood cells that affects all age-groups. The immature white blood cells (blast cells) generate themselves in an explosive fashion in the bone marrow, the lymph tissue, and the spleen. These cells are abnormal and unable to effectively fight infection. There are so many abnormal cells developed and dumped into the peripheral circulation that they tend to collect in the body organs and tissues, especially where circulation is sluggish. Areas especially prone to infiltration with these immature white blood cells are the oral mucosa, the anus, the sinuses, and the lungs. At the time of diagnosis, these areas are often inflamed, painful, and infected. It is common for some clients to be diagnosed only after suffering with an infection that does not clear up easily.

As the disease progresses, the bone marrow continues to produce large numbers of the useless cells, the peripheral circulation is filled with the abnormal cells, and the bone marrow is packed with the blast cells; production of most other normal cells is impossible. The client becomes anemic because of the lack of RBC production, and bleeding becomes a problem as fewer and fewer platelets are manufactured. But most important, even though the white blood cell count is very high, there are very few normal, mature, and active white cells with which to fight infection. Thus the client often begins to have raging infections that do not respond to antibiotics. Without treatment, the leukemia leaves the client unable to fight infec-

tion, unable to control bleeding, and in a downward spiral of fatigue and anorexia. Leukemia, untreated, is almost always fatal.

Classifications

Leukemias are classified as either acute or chronic and either lymphoid or myeloid. Symptoms of the acute leukemias begin very suddenly, and the client is very sick; chronic leukemias develop very slowly. Lymphoid leukemias affect the lymphocytes. Myeloid leukemias originate in the stem cells of the bone marrow that develop into monocytes, granulocytes, erythrocytes, and platelets. The most common leukemias are discussed below.

Acute Leukemias

Acute lymphocytic leukemia (ALL) commonly affects children under the age of 15 and involves abnormal growth of the lymphocyte precursors (lymphoblasts). Acute myelogenous (myeloblastic) leukemia (AML) usually affects persons over the age of 20 and has a poor prognosis. The client with acute leukemia may present with sudden onset of high fevers, abnormal bleeding from the mucous membranes, petechiae, ecchymoses, and easy bruising after minor trauma. Death is usually from infection.

Chronic Leukemia

Chronic lymphocytic leukemia (CLL) predominantly affects the B and T lymphocytes and usually affects adults over 40. Chronic myelogenous leukemia (CML) is characterized by the Philadelphia chromosome and occurs most often between the ages of 40 and 45.

Chronic leukemia usually develops in a three-stage process. First is the insidious phase characterized by anemia and mild bleeding abnormalities. During this stage, the client often feels well and is not even aware that he or she is sick. After several years, the disease progresses to the accelerated and acute phases in which the scenarios are similar to the events seen in acute leukemias. Chronic leukemia is almost always fatal; the average survival time is 3 to 4 years after onset of the chronic phase and 3 to 6 months after onset of the acute phase. It is not uncommon to encounter patients who have been diagnosed nearly 10 years.

Etiology

The cause of leukemia is unknown. Risk factors are thought to include certain viruses, because remnants of viruses have been found in leukemic cells. Often there are genetic and immunological factors involved. For example, persons with Down syndrome are more likely to develop

---

leukemia: leuk—white + emia—blood

leukemia. Other authorities point to exposure to radiation, in part because radiologists have been found to have a higher-than-average development of leukemias. Some clients have developed leukemia after being treated for another unrelated malignancy using radiation or chemotherapy. Researchers note the higher occurrence rate in persons who lived through the Hiroshima and Nagasaki bombings during World War II. Other authorities cite water pollution with benzenes and other chemicals. There is not one clear-cut cause for the development of leukemia.

Signs and Symptoms

Symptoms are similar for all types of leukemia and include low-grade fever caused by infection, and pallor, weakness, lassitude, and malaise caused by anemia. These symptoms may be present weeks or months before the appearance of other symptoms. The client may also have dyspnea, fatigue, tachycardia, palpitations, and abdominal pain. Sternal pain and rib tenderness may result from crowding of bone marrow. If the leukemia has invaded the central nervous system, the client may experience confusion, headaches, and personality changes. During the acute phase the client may exhibit high fevers from worsening infection and abnormal bleeding because of thrombocytopenia.

Diagnostic Tests

Although a simple CBC will often point toward the diagnosis, only bone marrow aspiration can show the degree of proliferation of the malignant WBCs and confirm the diagnosis of leukemia. The complete blood count may also show a decrease in the numbers of platelets, red blood cells, and mature white blood cells. A lumbar puncture helps determine if the central nervous system is involved. Genetic analysis of the peripheral blood and bone marrow components often shows the presence of the Philadelphia chromosome in CML.

Medical Treatment

Systemic chemotherapy aims to eradicate the leukemic cells and induce a remission. Remission means that the bone marrow is free to produce normally occurring cells in normal proportions without production of the immature WBCs. Chemotherapy types vary with the types of leukemia and the level of involvement. Radiation therapy is also sometimes used for initial treatment of leukemia.

The overall goal of the first treatments is to get the client to a state of remission. Occasionally, partial remission is achieved when everything looks good except for an occasional leukemic cell seen in the bone marrow. Remission is not the same as cure.

There are four phases to the treatment of leukemia: induction, intensification, consolidation, and maintenance. Induction is the period of time in which an attempt to get the client into remission is made. This first phase is very difficult because chemotherapy is given in high doses and on a very aggressive timetable. Often the client becomes quite ill with the complications from the treatment. The client may become very depressed because the treatment seems worse than the disease at this stage. The nurse must help the client deal with the side effects of anemia, thrombocytopenia, and leukopenia (see Tables 24–2, 24–3, and Chapter 10).

If the first remission is accomplished, the other phases of treatment are begun. Intensification is similar to the initial induction phase, using the same drugs at even higher doses. The next phase, consolidation, is used to ensure that all leukemic cells have been eradicated from the body. Finally, the client graduates to maintenance therapy in which the client is kept free of leukemic cells (and in remission) for a period of years (and hopefully, a lifetime). This requires years of continued chemotherapy treatments, often on a monthly basis. Radiation therapy may be used all along this course of treatment in order to decrease the size of the liver or spleen or to decrease the numbers of leukemic cells in the central nervous system.

Bone marrow transplantation (BMT) is also sometimes done for leukemia. Often, the precursor to BMT is total body irradiation so that all of the client's malignant bone marrow can be destroyed and then, at the last possible moment, replaced by a donor's bone marrow (allogenic transplant) or from bone marrow harvested and stored earlier from the client's own body (autologous transplant). This stage of bone marrow replacement is sometimes called bone marrow rescue. Transplanted bone marrow is given to the client like a blood transfusion. Once infused into the bloodstream, the new marrow travels to the bones where it belongs.

Bone marrow transplants are being performed at more and more centers across the United States. Common reasons for BMT include leukemias, lymphomas, breast cancer, aplastic anemia, and congenital immunodeficiency disorders.

Nursing Care

The client with leukemia is at risk for many problems, including fatigue, anxiety, bleeding, infection, and other complications of the disease and its treatment. The client must understand his or her disease process and treatment regimen in order to participate in self-care. See Nursing Care Plan Box 24–4 for the Client with Leukemia for interventions to deal with these problems. Table 24–6 provides a list of resources for clients and families with leukemia. See also Chapter 10 for general care of the client with cancer.

NURSING CARE PLAN BOX 24–4 FOR THE CLIENT WITH LEUKEMIA

Risk for injury from infection or bleeding related to pancytopenia

Client Outcomes

The client is free from infection and bleeding. Signs and symptoms of infection or bleeding are reported promptly.

Evaluation of Outcomes

Is the client free from infection and bleeding, or are problems reported so that quick intervention can prevent further complications?

Interventions	Rationale	Evaluation
Monitor vital signs every 4 hours and prn.	Elevated temperature is a sign of infection. Falling blood pressure and elevated pulse rate may indicate sepsis or blood loss.	Are vital signs stable?
Monitor for swelling, redness, purulent drainage.	These are signs of infection and should be reported promptly.	Are signs of infection present?
Protect client from sources of infection (see Table 24–3).	Client is at risk for infection because of ineffective WBCs.	Are precautions being observed to prevent infection?
Observe for tarry stools, petechiae, ecchymosis (see Table 24–5).	These are signs of bleeding and should be reported promptly.	Are signs of bleeding present?
Protect client from injury that could cause bleeding (see Table 24–2).	Client is at risk for bleeding because of reduced platelet count.	Are precautions being observed to prevent injury and bleeding?

Knowledge deficit related to new diagnosis of leukemia, disease process, and treatment plan

Client Outcomes

The client and significant other state satisfaction with understanding the diagnosis and treatment plan.

Evaluation of Outcomes

Do the client and significant other state satisfaction with understanding of the diagnosis and treatment plan? Are they able to relate correct information as instructed?

Interventions	Rationale	Evaluation
Assess the client's readiness to learn.	The shock of a new diagnosis may make learning difficult.	Is client able to learn at this time?
Assess the client's and significant other's understanding of the disease process and treatment.	New information should build on previous knowledge.	Does the client have baseline information? Where should further instruction begin?
Reinforce instructions from physician related to disease process and treatment regimen.	The client may not understand or remember instructions given during a stressful time.	Does client state understanding of instructions?
Assess and use client's preferred style of learning—discussion, reading materials, videos.	People learn in different ways; some clients may not have good reading skills, making alternative methods necessary.	What is client's preferred learning style? Are appropriate materials provided? (Table 24–6 lists resources that may be contacted for materials.)
Explain common terminology.	Medical terminology can be confusing to clients.	Does client state understanding of common terms?
Explain the roles of the different health team members (nurse, physician, dietitian, social worker, etc.) and how to access each member.	The client must understand the roles of the many different providers he or she will come in contact with in order to utilize them effectively.	Does client state understanding of who team members are, their roles, and how to contact them?
Provide a calendar of planned treatments and follow-up tests.	Knowing plans ahead of time increases the client's feeling of control over the situation.	Does client state understanding of scheduled care?

continued

NURSING CARE PLAN BOX 24–4 (continued)

Fatigue related to decreased red cell count and oxygenation and effects of treatments

Client Outcomes
Client is able to participate in activities that are important to him or her.

Evaluation of Outcomes
Is client able to identify and participate in activities that are important to him or her?

Interventions	Rationale	Evaluation
Assess fatigue using the WHAT'S UP? format.	A good assessment establishes a baseline and aids in planning.	Is fatigue present? To what degree?
Assist client to identify activities that are important to him or her. (ADL? Attending a child's wedding? Taking a trip?) Assist in setting goals to work toward the desired activity.	If the client cannot do everything he or she wishes, it may help to focus on the most important things.	Can client identify important activities? What are they? How can the nurse assist the client to reach activity goals?
Encourage a balanced diet. Contact dietitian as needed.	Poor nutrition contributes to fatigue.	Is client eating a balanced diet? Is weight stable?
Allow periods of rest between activities.	Any activity (ADL, x-rays, even talking) can increase fatigue.	Is client able to rest?
Ensure adequate sleep. Obtain order for sleeping aid if indicated.	Lack of sleep worsens fatigue.	Does client state feeling rested on awakening? Is medication needed?
Provide for ADL when client is unable to do so independently.	Extreme fatigue may prevent the client from participating in self-care.	Does client need total assistance?

Altered oral mucous membranes related to chemotherapy and pancytopenia

Client Outcomes
The client's oral mucous membranes will remain intact.

Evaluation of Outcomes
Are oral mucous membranes intact, without lesions?

Interventions	Rationale	Evaluation
Assess mouth daily for redness, edema, and lesions.	Routine assessment helps identify problems early so treatment can be implemented.	Are mucous membranes intact?
Encourage adequate nutrition and fluids.	Poor nutrition and dehydration increase the risk of oral lesions.	Is client eating and drinking?
Encourage client to brush teeth after meals with a soft toothbrush. If irritation is severe or if the client is at risk for bleeding, use swabs or sponge Toothettes instead of a toothbrush.	Brushing the teeth controls tooth and gum disease; a toothbrush may be too harsh if the client is at risk for bleeding.	Is mouth care being provided after meals? Is mouth care irritating? Are alternative methods needed?
Avoid use of lemon-glycerin swabs for mouth care.	Lemon-glycerin swabs are drying to oral mucosa.	Are products used appropriate?
Obtain an order for a mouthwash such as 1 oz of diphenhydramine (Benadryl) elixir diluted in 1 qt of water or normal saline.	Benadryl reduces inflammation; anesthetics reduce pain.	Does mouthwash soothe pain?
Obtain an order for a topical anesthetic if mouth is very inflamed and painful.		
Encourage the client to avoid smoking, alcohol, acidic food or drinks, extremely hot or cold foods and drinks, and commercial mouthwash.	These things can be irritating to the mucosa.	Does client state understanding of things to avoid?

continued

NURSING CARE PLAN BOX 24-4 (continued)

GERIATRIC

Advise client to remove dentures for cleaning and at bedtime.	Dentures left in for long periods can impair circulation and increase risk of lesions.	Are dentures removed for cleaning and at night?

Anxiety related to diagnosis, treatment, and fear of dying

Client Outcomes
Client's anxiety is controlled as evidenced by the following: client states anxiety is controlled, identifies measures to cope with anxiety.

Evaluation of Outcomes
Does client state anxiety is controlled? Is client able to identify measures to cope with anxiety?

Interventions	*Rationale*	*Evaluation*
Assess anxiety using the WHAT'S UP? format.	Assessment helps guide specific interventions.	Is client experiencing anxiety?
Use empathy to reassure client that some anxiety is normal.	Anxiety is a normal response to a serious diagnosis.	Does client state that some anxiety is expected?
Explain all tests and procedures.	Not knowing what is happening contributes to anxiety.	Does client state understanding of tests and procedures?
Avoid or limit use of caffeine and stimulant drugs.	These substances can increase symptoms of anxiety.	Are stimulants avoided?
Teach the client deep breathing and relaxation exercises.	These activities can interrupt the anxiety response.	Do deep breathing and relaxation help?
Help client identify potential concerns and how he or she can deal with them if they arise.	Knowing ahead of time what to do in the event a problem arises helps reduce anxiety.	Can client identify concerns and strategies for dealing with them?
Consult with social worker or pastoral care.	These individuals are trained to assist with anxiety responses.	Are referrals indicated? Are they helpful?

CRITICAL THINKING: Mr. Washington

Mr. Washington is on your unit undergoing initial treatment for leukemia. You enter his room today and find a room full of visitors.

1. What concerns do you have?
2. What do you do?

Answers at end of chapter.

Multiple Myeloma

Multiple myeloma is a deadly cancer of the plasma cells in the bone marrow. When the disease is caught in its early stages, treatment can prolong life by 3 to 5 years. More important, early detection can decrease the amount of pain and disability due to bony destruction and pathological fractures. Unfortunately, almost half of the clients die within the first 3 months after diagnosis because of the silent and deadly nature of the disease. Another 40 percent

of clients die within 2 years after diagnosis. Because early diagnosis is not often made, only 10 percent of clients can expect to live to the 5-year mark. Multiple myeloma usually affects men 50 to 70 years of age.

PATHOPHYSIOLOGY AND ETIOLOGY

In this disorder, cancerous plasma cells in the bone marrow begin reproducing uncontrollably. These cells infiltrate bone tissue all over the body and produce hundreds of tumors that begin to devour the bone tissue. On x-ray examination the nurse may notice many holes in the bones, forming a Swiss cheese type of pattern (Fig. 24–6). As more and more of these holes are formed, the bone integrity becomes compromised and weak. Multiple myeloma usually affects the bones of the skull, pelvis, ribs, and vertebrae.

As the disease continues, the plasma cells infiltrate the major organs, including the liver, spleen, lymph nodes, lungs, adrenal glands, kidneys, skin, and GI tract. Because the diagnosis usually occurs only after widespread inva-

Table 24-6. **Resources for Clients with Hematological Malignancies**

National and Local Organizations	What the Client Can Receive
American Cancer Society 1599 Clifton Road NE Atlanta, GA 1-800-ACS-2345	All types of client education materials; information on support groups, I Can Cope Education Sessions, limited financial help
Leukemia Society of America 600 Third Avenue New York, NY 10016 1-800-955-4572	Client education materials, support group locations, client aid and financial assistance for clients with leukemia, Hodgkin's and non-Hodgkin's lymphomas, and multiple myeloma
National Coalition for Cancer Survivorship 1010 Wayne Avenue, 5th floor Silver Spring, MD 20910 1-301-650-8868	Networking related to survivorship issues such as insurance and employment; sponsors the National Cancer Survivor's Day Event and published the *National Cancer Survivor's Almanac to Resources*
National Leukemia Association, Inc. 585 Stewart Avenue, Suite 536 Garden City, NY 11530 1-516-222-1944	Information and financial aid for clients
National Marrow Donor Program 3433 Broadway Street NE Minneapolis, MN 55413	Information for clients and information on accessing volunteer donors for bone marrow transplantation
Office of Cancer Communications National Cancer Institute Bldg. 31, Room 10A24 Bethesda, MD 20892 1-800-4-CANCER	National telephone hotline for client and professional education materials, research reports, psychosocial support groups, and wellness groups
BMT Newsletter 1985 Spruce Avenue Highland Park, IL 60035 1-708-831-1913	Information about bone marrow transplants

sion of the bones is well underway, the overall prognosis of clients with this disease is very poor. Although the overall result of the disease is the devastating destruction of the bone and widespread osteoporosis, death is often from sepsis.

ETIOLOGY

The cause of multiple myeloma is unknown, although it is being researched. Some authorities believe this disease to be related to chronic allergies and hypersensitivity reactions. This line of thought stems from the fact that plasma cells are the first line of defense and are the producers of the immunoglobulins that help fight foreign bodies. For some reason these defenders go out of control and begin to attack the host as well as foreign invaders.

SIGNS AND SYMPTOMS

Skeletal pain is the most common complaint. The client may describe the pain as constant, severe back pain that in-

creases with exercise or movement. The client may complain about pain in the ribs. Other signs and symptoms include achiness of the long bones, joint swelling and tenderness, low-grade fever, and general malaise. Sometimes there is evidence of early peripheral neuropathy secondary to vertebral collapse and mild spinal cord compression. The client may be unable to feel the true temperature of bath water (and end up with a burn) or may be unable to feel wounds and infections on the feet. In more severe cases of cord compression, the patient may lose control of bladder and bowels. This is a true oncologic emergency. Prompt emergency treatment is necessary to keep the patient from becoming paralyzed.

Occasionally the client will have **pathological fractures** of the long bones. These are fractures that occur with no trauma, such as the person who breaks a leg just turning over in bed, or breaks a rib while sneezing. In advanced disease there is anemia, weight loss, thoracic spinal deformities from multiple rib destruction, and a loss of height because of pathological fractures and compacting of the vertebrae.

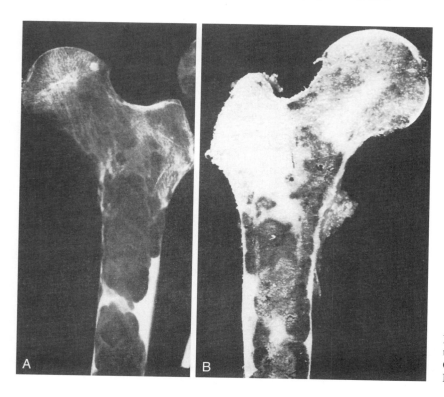

Figure 24–6. X-ray of bone destruction in multiple myeloma. (From Huether, SE, and McCance, KL: Understanding Pathophysiology. Mosby, St Louis, 1996, p 548, with permission.)

Kidney stones are a common occurrence in clients with the diagnosis of multiple myeloma because the calcium released from bone is excreted by the kidneys. Clients often progress to kidney failure as the filtering capacity of the kidney is blocked with calcium.

DIAGNOSTIC TESTS

A CBC shows moderate to severe anemia. Examination of the white blood cell count may show an increase in the number of white cells, secondary to infection, particularly of the respiratory tract. Pneumonia is a common finding in the patient with multiple myeloma. X-ray examinations may show changes in the lungs and diffuse osteoporosis in the bones not already riddled with holes. Urine studies are positive for the M-type globulins (Bence Jones proteins) in 40 percent of clients.

Blood chemistries will often show an increased amount of calcium in the blood. Hypercalciuria results as the calcium released out of the bones is flushed out in the urine. An intravenous pyelogram may be done to see how much calcium is blocking the kidneys.

MEDICAL TREATMENT

Long-term treatment of multiple myeloma consists of a two-prong approach: (1) managing the disease and (2) managing the symptoms. To manage the disease, high-dose steroids (prednisone) and oral or intravenous chemotherapy agents (specific medications usually include cyclophosphamide or melphalan) are given. The goal of drug therapy is to suppress the plasma cell proliferation, which then helps decrease the amount and speed of bone destruction.

The second approach is control of symptoms. The nurse monitors the client for signs and symptoms of hypercalcemia, hyperuricemia, dehydration, respiratory infection, renal problems, and pain. External beam irradiation may be given to especially painful areas of bone involvement. Fortunately, this treatment is quite effective, usually decreasing pain intensity in just a few days. The client can expect to have a daily (or perhaps a twice-daily) therapy treatment over a course of 10 to 14 days. Vigorous attention to pain medications during the early course of treatment will greatly reduce the client's pain levels.

The client may need a laminectomy if vertebral collapse occurs. Because of demineralization of the bone with resulting large amounts of calcium in the blood and urine, surgery for kidney stones and eventual dialysis for acute or chronic kidney failure may be necessary.

NURSING CARE

The nurse assesses for fever or malaise that can signal the onset of infections. Other conditions to be alert for include anemia, hypercalcemia, fractures, and renal complications. Intake and output are monitored, and urine is strained for stones.

Keeping the client mobile is very important. The physical therapist and occupational therapist can help the client continue to be active. Bones in use are strongest, so the client should remain up and moving as much as possible to

HOME HEALTH HINTS

- Clients with sickle cell anemia usually have lower blood pressures. It is important to report even mild hypertension for these clients.

- To prevent bruising, have the client cut the feet off of white sport socks and wear them on the arms. This can be hidden under long-sleeve shirts and blouses, and provides a cushion when doing housework.

- Clients who are at risk for infection can place a sign on the front door of their homes to limit visitors or ask persons with colds to come back when they are well. The client may appreciate the home nurse giving permission to be assertive in such circumstances.

help stimulate calcium resorption and decrease demineralization. An additional important effect of keeping the patient up and active is that it helps decrease the likelihood of respiratory complications. Urination also is enhanced in the patient who does not need to rely on the use of a bedpan.

If the client is bedridden, he or she should be repositioned every 2 hours to prevent complications related to immobility; a lift sheet should be used to move the client gently and decrease the risk of pathological fractures. The nurse provides passive range of motion and encourages deep breathing exercises.

One of the most important things that the nurse can monitor and can teach the client is the importance of good hydration at all times. To minimize complications of hypercalcemia, fluids are administered so that daily output is never less than 1500 mL. Depending on time of year and the type and level of client activities, the client may need to have an intake of over 4 L daily.

One effect that is difficult to manage is hypercalcemia. The signs and symptoms include mental changes, especially confusion, and weakness and fatigue. There may be explosive diarrhea as the body tries to rid itself of the extra calcium, polyuria as the kidneys try to flush the extra calcium out of the body, and renal changes as the extra calcium begins to clog the kidneys.

If hypercalcemia occurs, the physician will order an IV of normal saline to infuse at a high rate followed by regular administration of diuretics. The goal is to get the serum calcium level below 10 mg/dl. Oral compounds are also available to help keep the calcium level down once the client is able to go home.

The nurse stresses the importance for the client to drink 3 to 4 L of fluid per day. The client is advised of the importance of walking to help decrease bone demineralization. The client is never allowed to walk alone because of the risk of pathological fractures of the long bones. If the

client is unsteady, a walker or a support belt should be used. Care of the client having a laminectomy is discussed in Chapter 46.

Review Questions

1. Which assessment finding would the nurse expect to find in the client who has anemia?
   a. Pain
   b. Dyspnea
   c. Vision changes
   d. Skin rash

2. Which question by the nurse helps evaluate the client's response to treatment for anemia?
   a. "Is your appetite improving?"
   b. "Are you sleeping all night?"
   c. "Are you keeping up with your work schedule?"
   d. "Are you requiring many analgesics?"

3. Which of the following activities would be contraindicated for the client with sickle cell anemia?
   a. Riding in an elevator
   b. Taking a long car trip
   c. Running in a marathon
   d. Listening to a concert

4. Which explanation for bleeding should the nurse give to the wife of a client with DIC?
   a. "He is bleeding because he does not have enough red blood cells."
   b. "He is bleeding because his white cells are depleted."
   c. "He is bleeding because his blood pressure is so high that it forces blood from mucous membranes."
   d. "He is bleeding because his body's clotting factors have all been used up."

5. Which instruction will help the mother of the child with hemophilia prevent bleeding episodes?
   a. "Your son should avoid contact sports."
   b. "Your son will have to avoid all potentially irritating foods."
   c. "Your son must never shave."
   d. "Your son should always live near a major hospital system."

6. Which family member should not be permitted to visit the client with newly diagnosed leukemia?
   a. The daughter, who has a new baby at home
   b. The son, who has a history of asthma
   c. The mother, who has received recent radiation for cancer
   d. The sister, who has a runny nose

7. Which of the following assessment findings is encountered in clients with multiple myeloma?
   a. Pathological fractures
   b. Mental status changes

c. Raging infections

d. Bleeding tendencies

8. Which of the following interventions is appropriate when caring for a patient with hypercalcemia secondary to multiple myeloma?

a. Provide bed rest

b. Force fluids

c. Administer antibiotics

d. Withhold meat products

ANSWERS TO CRITICAL THINKING

CRITICAL THINKING: Mrs. Johns

1. Monitor Mrs. Johns' vital signs and report falling blood pressure and rising pulse immediately. Inspect her skin for petechiae and ecchymoses. Monitor urine for signs of blood. Test stools for occult blood. Monitor vaginal discharge for increasing bleeding.

2. Anticipate assisting the RN with administration of blood or blood products. Instruct Mrs. Johns in the importance of preventing injury that could cause further bleeding. Other care will be supportive.

3. Mrs. Johns will be concerned for her new baby, who is most likely on another unit or already discharged home. Allow Mrs. Johns to talk about her concerns. Arrange visits with her family and baby if permitted by her condition and her physician.

CRITICAL THINKING: Mr. Washington

1. Because of his leukemia, Mr. Washington is at risk for infection. If he develops an infection, he will have great difficulty getting over it. With so many visitors in the room, it is likely that one or more has a cold or virus. They may not be aware of the risk this poses to Mr. Washington. Mr. Washington is probably also fatigued due to his disease and treatment, and visiting requires energy.

2. You should kindly explain that he is very susceptible to catching colds or other illnesses and that it would be best to limit visitors to one or two at a time who are fairly certain that they do not have any infections. Visits should also be brief, to prevent overtiring the client.

REFERENCES

1. Lipson, J, and Hafizi, H: Iranians. In Purnell, L, and Paulanka, B (eds): Transcultural Health Care: A Culturally Competent Approach. FA Davis, Philadelphia, 1998.
2. McCance, K, and Huether, S: Pathophysiology: The Biological Basis for Diseases in Adults and Children. Mosby, St Louis, 1994.

BIBLIOGRAPHY

Ackley, BJ, and Ladwig, GB: Nursing Diagnosis Handbook: A Guide to Planning Care, ed 3. Mosby, St Louis, 1997.

Groff, JL, Gropper, SS, and Hunt, SM: Advanced Nutrition and Human Metabolism, ed 2. West, Minneapolis, 1995.

Harmening, DM: Clinical Hematology and Fundamentals of Hemostasis, ed 3. FA Davis, Philadelphia, 1997.

Kier, S: Caring for people with blood disorders. In Luckmann, J (ed): Saunders Manual of Nursing Care, ed 1. WB Saunders, Philadelphia, 1997.

Lutz, CA, and Przytulski, KR: Nutrition and Diet Therapy, ed 2. FA Davis, Philadelphia, 1997.

Neff, C, and Spray, M: Introduction to Maternal and Child Health Nursing, ed 1. JB Lippincott, Philadelphia, 1996.

Watson, J, and Jaffe, MS: Nurse's Manual of Laboratory and Diagnostic Tests, ed 2. FA Davis, Philadelphia, 1995.

25

Nursing Care of Clients with Lymphatic Disorders

Cheryl L. Ivey

Learning Objectives

Upon completion of this chapter, the student will be able to:

1. Identify the one most distinguishing feature of Hodgkin's disease.
2. Contrast non-Hodgkin's lymphoma with Hodgkin's disease in terms of age of onset, symptoms, and curability.
3. Use the nursing process to plan care for the client with a lymphatic disorder.
4. Identify teaching needs for the client with a lymphatic disorder.
5. Describe nursing care of the client undergoing a splenectomy.
6. List the most important client teaching need for the client undergoing therapeutic splenectomy.

Key Words

lymphoma (lim-**FOH**-mah)
pathological fractures (PATH-uh-**LAH**-jik-uhl **FRAK**-churs)
splenectomy (sple-**NEK**-tuh-mee)
splenomegaly (SPLEE-noh-**MEG**-ah-lee)

Lymphatic disorders include Hodgkin's disease and the non-Hodgkin's lymphomas. Because the spleen is part of the lymph system, this chapter will also discuss splenectomy.

Hodgkin's Disease

Despite the name, Hodgkin's disease (HD) is a **lymphoma,** which is a cancer of the lymph system. Its distinguishing feature is Reed-Sternberg cells, which make it different than all the other forms of lymphomas. HD is more prevalent in men than in women and occurs most often in young adults, ages 15 to 35. After a decrease in incidence in persons aged 35 to 50, the incidence peaks again in adults over the age of 50. Of all the lymphomas, HD is the most curable type, even when the disease is widely spread at the time of diagnosis.

PATHOPHYSIOLOGY

Lymph nodes are made of tightly bound fibers and cells that serve as filtering devices for the body's immune system. Most often, HD begins as a single changed lymph node, usually in the cervical lymph nodes of the neck. As the disease progresses, the cancer invades the lymph node chains, node by node. The path of cancer infiltration is usually the same as the path for lymph fluid flow. Left untreated, other lymphoid tissues such as the spleen become infiltrated with HD. The major organs eventually become involved with Hodgkin's disease. Common complaints of clients with organ involvement may include shortness of breath, feelings of fullness, weakness, and malaise. These organ-related symptoms usually motivate the client to seek medical help.

A tentative diagnosis of HD is based on one or more painlessly enlarged nodes in the cervical, axillary, or inguinal areas. A biopsy of several of the enlarged nodes is performed with the intent of searching for the presence of Reed-Sternberg cells, which confirms the diagnosis.

---

lymphoma: lymph + oma—tumor

ETIOLOGY

The exact cause of HD is unknown. A possible viral origin has been proposed. Sometimes it occurs in families, suggesting a genetic link.

SIGNS AND SYMPTOMS

Painless swelling in one or more of the common lymph node chains is a usual presentation (Fig. 25–1). This swelling can range from barely perceptible to a size similar to that of a softball, occasionally even larger. The client may complain of generalized pruritis. One other curious event, alcohol-induced pain, may be present. With just a few sips of any type of alcohol-containing beverage (beer, wine, or liquor), the client may complain of an intense pain at the site of disease. Because the lymph nodes in the upper chest and neck are often involved, the client may have symptoms of obstruction such as cough, dysphagia, and even stridor.

Other common symptoms may include persistent low-grade fever, night sweats, fatigue, weight loss, and malaise. The presence of these additional symptoms predicts a worse prognosis. In older adults, there may be no enlarged lymph nodes visible and these secondary symptoms may be the only presenting symptoms. Other symptoms associated with late-stage disease include edema of the neck and face, possible jaundice, nerve pain, enlargement of the retroperitoneal nodes, and infiltration of the spleen; liver and bones may be involved.

DIAGNOSTIC TESTS/STAGING

Diagnosis usually begins with a lymph node biopsy of the easiest lymph node to access. Lymph node biopsies are done to check for abnormal histiocyte proliferation, nodular fibrosis, and necrosis. Other tests include bone marrow biopsy and aspiration, liver and spleen biopsies, routine chest x-ray, abdominal computed tomography (CT) scan to check for presence of disease in the liver and spleen, lung scan, and bone scan. In some larger cancer centers, lymphangiography may be performed to view the flow of lymph in the lymph network. This test is accomplished by a skilled physician injecting dye into the lymph tracts located between the toes. The dye is then observed as it migrates up the lymph chains signaling blockages where present.

Hematological tests (complete blood count [CBC]) may show wide variability with red cells indicating mild to severe anemia. The white blood cell count is often abnormal and extreme (either extremely high or very low) because of bone marrow infiltration by disease. This places the client at increased risk for infection.

These same tests are used for staging. HD is staged based on the Ann Arbor Clinical Staging Classification and is as follows:

- Stage I disease is limited to a single lymph node or site.
- In Stage II disease, two or more nodes are involved on the same side of the diaphragm. Limited organ involvement may or may not be present.
- Stage III disease is characterized by nodes on both sides of the diaphragm with or without organ involvement.
- Stage IV, the most serious form of the disease, and the least curable, includes widely disseminated disease in several organs or tissues with or without associated lymph node involvement.

MEDICAL TREATMENT

Appropriate therapy includes the use of radiation and chemotherapy, depending on the stage of the disease. Radiation therapy, administered on an outpatient basis over a 4- to 6-week period, can cure most clients with stage I or stage II disease. Combinations of chemotherapy and radiation therapy are used for clients with stage III and stage IV disease, with results based on the location and the stage of disease.

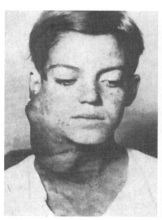
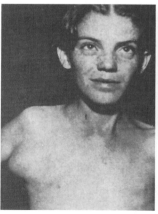
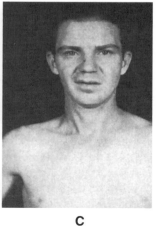

A **B** **C**

Figure 25–1. Cervical Hodgkin's disease. (*A*) Young boy with extensive cervical Hodgkin's disease. (*B*) Appearance several years later, when axillary manifestation developed. (*C*) Appearance 23 years after initial treatment with radiation. (From del Regato, JA, Spjut, HJ, and Cox, JD: Cancer: Diagnosis, Treatment, and Prognosis, ed 6. Mosby, St Louis, 1985, with permission.)

NURSING CARE

Most nursing interventions are aimed at symptom management. If the patient is experiencing pruritis or night sweats, nursing interventions are aimed at alleviation of discomfort. These may include changing the gown and bed linens several times a night and helping the patient remain clean and dry. Keeping the patient and family involved in the plan of care may relieve anxiety.

After the diagnosis is established, the LPN/LVN will collaborate with the RN to teach the patient and the family about the treatments that will be required. Specific information regarding chemotherapy and radiation therapy will be necessary. Most oncology units have pamphlets or other printed material that can be helpful. Type and length of therapy will be based on the stage of the cancer at the time of diagnosis.

Later, nursing interventions are tailored to alleviate problems that arise secondary to chemotherapy and radiation therapy. See Chapter 10 for nursing interventions for these problems. Also see Nursing Care Plan Box 25–1 for the Client with Lymphoma.

CLIENT TEACHING

In addition to the teaching needs outlined above, make sure that the client and the family know about local chapters of the American Cancer Society and the Leukemia Society of America. Both of these organizations have information, financial assistance, and counseling referral sources, which most clients will find valuable. Another source for chemotherapy and radiation therapy information is the National Cancer Institute (NCI). The NCI can send as much information regarding all aspects of treatment as the client requests at no charge. See Table 25–1 for more information.

> ### CRITICAL THINKING: Jeanine
>
> Jeanine is a 60-year-old nurse diagnosed with stage II Hodgkin's disease. She wishes to continue working at her job on a respiratory unit at the local hospital while she undergoes treatment. What concerns do you have with this desire?
>
> *Answers at end of chapter.*

Non-Hodgkin's Lymphomas

All of the other types of lymphomas are clumped into a diverse classification known as the non-Hodgkin's lymphomas (NHL). It is possible to sort these other types of lymphomas into different categories based on the degree of malignancy. Non-Hodgkin's lymphomas arise in the lymphoid tissues of the body, just as Hodgkin's disease does, but they differ in several ways. See Table 25–2 for a comparison of Hodgkin's and non-Hodgkin's lymphomas.

PATHOPHYSIOLOGY

The most distinguishing difference is the absence of the Reed-Sternberg cells in non-Hodgkin's lymphomas. Instead, many of these lymphomas arise from the B cells and the T cells. The B cells are involved in recognizing and destroying specific antigens. Cells specifically involved include the memory B cells and the plasma cells. The T cells also are involved in registering antigens, but there are many more kinds of T cells. These include the amplifier T cells, helper T cells, suppressor T cells, memory T cells, cytotoxic T cells, and delayed hypersensitivity T cells. An abnormality in any of these cells can result in a type of NHL. Most cases of NHL are of B cell origin.

ETIOLOGY

The cause of non-Hodgkin's lymphomas is unclear, but viruses, such as the Epstein-Barr virus and the herpesvirus, are thought to play a role in the development in some types of these cancers.

SIGNS AND SYMPTOMS

Clinical features of malignant lymphomas include swollen lymph glands, enlarged tonsils and adenoids, painless rubbery nodes in the cervical and supraclavicular areas, and occasional symptoms of dyspnea and cough. As the disease progresses, the client may report fatigue, malaise, weight loss, and night sweats, similar to Hodgkin's disease.

DIAGNOSTIC TESTS

Diagnosis is confirmed by histological evaluation of biopsied lymph nodes, tonsils, bone marrow, liver, bowel, skin, or any other affected tissues. Other relevant tests include bone scans, chest x-ray, lymphangiography, liver and spleen scan, CT of the abdomen, and an intravenous pyelogram, to determine the extent of the disease. Laboratory tests include a CBC, which often indicates anemia, serum uric acid level, and liver function studies. Serum calcium level may be elevated if bone lesions are present.

MEDICAL TREATMENT

Treatment usually involves multimodal therapy, including the use of chemotherapy and radiation therapy given in combination. Chemotherapy treatments are given on a set schedule of approximately once every month for about 6 months. These treatments may be performed on an inpatient or an outpatient basis. Radiation therapy is given to affected areas in advanced stages of NHL.

NURSING CARE

The nurse provides emotional support by keeping the client and family informed during the testing phase. Symptoms

NURSING CARE PLAN BOX 25–1 FOR THE CLIENT WITH LYMPHOMA

Activity intolerance related to fatigue and anemia

Client Outcomes
Client will have activities of daily living (ADL) needs met by self or caretaker.

Evaluation of Outcomes
Is client able to carry out ADL, or are ADL needs met by a caretaker?

Interventions	Rationale	Evaluation
Assess amount of activity that causes fatigue.	Assessment helps guide plan of care.	How much can client do before becoming fatigued?
Assist client with activities as necessary.	The client may need assistance with ADL if fatigue is extreme.	Does the client need assistance? Can family members assist?
Provide oxygen therapy as ordered.	Oxygen therapy can increase oxygen levels and activity tolerance.	Does client tolerate activity better with oxygen therapy?
Instruct client to space rest with activities.	Rest periods decrease oxygen need and allow client to conserve energy for next activity.	Is client able to tolerate activity better after a rest period?

Risk for infection related to bone marrow involvement and side effects of treatment

Client Outcomes
Client will have no signs or symptoms of infection.

Evaluation of Outcomes
Are signs and symptoms of infection absent? Is temperature within normal limits?

Interventions	Rationale	Evaluation
Assess client for risk factors for infection.	The white blood cell count may be very high or very low, placing the client at risk for infection.	Is the client at risk? Are additional interventions indicated?
Monitor client for signs and symptoms of infection, such as cough, fever, malaise, erythema, pain, or drainage and report immediately.	Early detection and treatment of infection provides the best results.	Are signs and symptoms of infection present?
Teach client and significant other signs and symptoms of infection to watch for and report.	The client must be involved in monitoring for infection when at home.	Does client verbalize understanding of signs and symptoms of infection and importance of reporting?
Teach the client to avoid exposure to others with influenza or other infections.	Exposure increases risk for infection, especially with compromised immune function.	Does client verbalize understanding of sources of infection to avoid?
Teach client proper hand washing and good oral and personal hygiene.	These activities reduce risk of infection.	Does client demonstrate proper hand washing and hygiene?

Risk for ineffective individual coping related to new diagnosis and potential lifestyle changes to accommodate treatments

Client Outcomes
The client states ability to manage lifestyle changes and medical management of condition.

Evaluation of Outcomes
Does client carry out self-care necessary to manage treatment?

continued

NURSING CARE PLAN BOX 25–1 *(continued)*		
Interventions	*Rationale*	*Evaluation*
Assess client's level of distress related to uncertainty of the future, bothersome symptoms, changes in self-concept, and past coping mechanisms.	Obtaining information regarding past experiences helps the nurse identify and correct misconceptions. The nurse can support effective coping mechanisms that worked in the past.	Is client able to identify sources of anxiety? Are past coping mechanisms effective?
Assess for signs of maladaptive behaviors that interfere with responsible health practices, such as missed appointments or failure to attend to symptoms.	Long-term survival depends on keeping therapy schedule. The ability to manage and report symptoms early keeps the client out of the hospital and in control of his or her own life.	Does the client keep appointments? Does the client participate in self-care activities and report symptoms promptly?
Assist the client to identify support systems and resources. Refer to social worker or other community resources prn.	Resources can assist with participation in treatment plan, home care, or financial assistance.	Are resources identified and helpful?
Refer client and family to a cancer survivors' support group.	There is no better support for the cancer client than others who have been through treatment themselves.	Does the client state that the support group is helpful?

Table 25–1. **National Sources for Information on Lymphatic Disorders**

Source	Booklets
American Cancer Society National Office 1599 Clifton Road NE Atlanta, GA 30329 404-320-3333	*Nutrition and Cancer: Cause and Prevention* *Sexuality and Cancer* *Helping Children Cope When a Parent Has Cancer* *Unproven Methods of Cancer Management* *Cancer: Your Job, Insurance and the Law* *Questions and Answers about Pain Control: A Guide for People with Cancer and Their Families* *Caring for the Client with Cancer at Home: A Guide for Clients and Families*
National Cancer Institute Public Inquiry Section Office of Cancer Communications Building 31, Room 10 A 24 Bethesda, MD 20892 1-800-4-CANCER (Cancer Information Service)	*What You Need to Know about Non-Hodgkin's Lymphoma* *What You Need to Know about Hodgkin's Lymphoma* *Good News, Better News, and Best News: Cancer Prevention* *Diet, Nutrition and Cancer Prevention: A Guide to Food Choices* *Taking Time: Support for the People with Cancer and the People Who Care about Them* *What Are Clinical Trials All About?* *Radiation Therapy and You: A Guide to Self-Help during Therapy* *Chemotherapy and You: A Guide to Self-Help during Treatment* *Eating Hints: Tips and Recipes for Better Nutrition during Cancer Treatment* *Facing Forward: A Guide for the Cancer Survivor* *When Cancer Recurs: Meeting the Challenge Again* *Advanced Cancer: Living Each Day*
Leukemia Society of America National Headquarters 733 Third Avenue New York, NY 10017 1-800-955-4LSA	*Hodgkin's Disease and the Non-Hodgkin's Lymphomas*
Peer Support Groups National Coalition for Cancer Survivorship 1010 Wayne Avenue Silver Springs, MD 20910	

Table 25–2. **Hodgkin's Disease vs. Non-Hodgkin's Lymphoma**

	Hodgkin's Disease	**Non-Hodgkin's Lymphomas**
Age	Younger	Older
Degree of Debilitation (Overall)	Less	More
Presence of Fever, Night Sweats (Indicating More Advanced Disease)	More likely	Less likely
Spread to Other Areas at Time of Diagnosis	Local to regional area of spread	Advanced cancer—spread to many different areas
Types	Just one	Many different types

such as night sweats can be managed with frequent linen and gown changes. If the client has severe anemia and is symptomatic, arrange his or her daily schedule to conserve energy. Transfuse packed red blood cells as ordered.

Give antibiotics as ordered if the patient has an infection or if the white blood cell count is especially low. Observe Standard Precautions and teach the client and family about the need for hand washing and avoiding large crowds of people. Teach the client to avoid others with colds and flu in order to decrease the chance of infection.

Help the client maintain nutrition with attractively prepared meals. Involve other professionals in the care of the client. Include the chaplain, if available and the client is exhibiting spiritual distress. The nurse spends time listening to the client's concerns. Refer the client and family to resources available for more information, including the American Cancer Society, the Leukemia Society of America, and the National Cancer Institute.

Splenic Disorders

The spleen is involved in a number of disorders, including cancers of the blood, lymph, and bone marrow; hereditary conditions such as sickle cell disease; and acquired problems such as idiopathic thrombocytopenia. Under normal circumstances, the spleen is not paid much attention; it generally performs its functions without much fanfare.

If the spleen enlarges markedly it is referred to as **splenomegaly.** Other times, the spleen may or may not be enlarged, but the function is out of control so that too many red cells and platelets are removed from the peripheral circulation. Sometimes the spleen is not able to perform its job because of bleeding into the pulp of the organ, rendering it useless. Regardless of the nature of the malfunction, an occasional alternative is splenectomy.

SPLENECTOMY

Splenectomy is the surgical removal of the spleen. This treatment is sometimes used to treat select hematological

disorders while being used, under different circumstances, to stage (or determine spread) in lymphomas. It is a surgery that is performed fairly often in the United States, but it is not a surgery that is without risk.

Client Teaching

Explain to clients that this surgery will remove the spleen, usually under general anesthesia. Inform clients that they will be able to live a normal life after the surgery but that they may be more prone to infection and that they should get the influenza vaccine each year.

Preoperative Care

Before the surgery, the nurse should ensure that the CBC and coagulation profile are completed and reported to the physician. If ordered, the nurse will assist in the transfusion of blood to correct the underlying anemia and to prepare for the loss of a great deal of blood stored in the spleen. Vitamin K is often ordered to correct clotting factor deficiencies.

Take the client's vital signs and perform a baseline respiratory assessment. Note especially any signs of respiratory infections such as fever, chills, crackles, wheezes, or cough. If any of these are noted, make sure that the physician is aware of them because surgery may need to be delayed. Teach the client routine coughing and deep breathing techniques to help prevent postoperative respiratory complications.

Postoperative Care

During the early postoperative period, watch carefully for bleeding, either external or internal. The nurse should be prepared to administer narcotics for pain, usually on an

---

splenomegaly: splen—spleen + megaly—enlargement
splenectomy: splen—spleen + ectomy—excision

around-the-clock schedule so the client will be comfortable enough to deep breathe, cough, and ambulate. Afterwards be sure to observe for side effects, which may include incomplete pain relief or hypoventilation. Monitor for fever every 4 hours and expect a mild, low-grade, transient fever postoperatively. A persistent fever may indicate abscess or hematoma formation.

If the surgery was performed to decrease the numbers of cells being removed from the peripheral circulation, monitor the platelet count. Often, the count will begin to rise in just a few days, but it may take up to 2 weeks for the platelets to normalize.

Complications

A splenectomy can cause complications such as bleeding, pneumonia, and atelectasis. Respiratory problems occur because of the spleen's position close to the diaphragm. This placement requires the need for a high surgical incision that is very painful. Often the client tries to restrict lung expansion after surgery to keep from hurting, but this splinting behavior may leave the client at risk for pneumonia and respiratory problems. In addition, splenectomy clients are usually more vulnerable to infection, especially influenza infections, because the spleen's role in the immune response is no longer present.

Other possible complications from splenectomy include the development of pancreatitis and fistula formation. This is due to the fact that the tail of the pancreas is very close to the spleen, and irritation may have occurred.

Another serious complication that can occur is that of overwhelming postsplenectomy infection (OPSI). The causative agents in OPSI include streptococci, *Neisseria,* and influenza bacteria. Patients at greatest risk of OPSI may include clients who had a splenectomy secondary to a cancer condition or during childhood.

Early symptoms of OPSI include fever and malaise that seems unremarkable. But the infection may progress within a few hours to sepsis and death. Unfortunately, OPSI has a mortality rate as high as 70%. Being alert to the possibility of the onset of OPSI, the nurse should include the signs and symptoms of OPSI in presplenectomy client education. Also the nurse should stress the need for prompt action in getting the client to medical attention with the first signs and symptoms of OPSI. The client should be directed to continue to receive lifetime use of vaccinations against these bacteria.

Review Questions

1. Hodgkin's disease, a lymphoproliferative disease, will usually be diagnosed by
   a. A blood test
   b. A tissue biopsy
   c. Both a and b

2. Stage III Hodgkin's disease is defined as which of the following?
   a. Lymphatic involvement on both sides of the diaphragm
   b. Localized involvement of more than two adjacent or nonadjacent regions on one side of the diaphragm
   c. Diffuse involvement of one or more extralymphatic organs or tissues such as the bone marrow or liver
   d. Localized involvement of a single lymph node site, usually located in the cervical or supraclavicular area

3. Which of the following interventions is appropriate for the client at home who is at risk for infection?
   a. Advise the client to stay indoors
   b. Encourage the client to avoid crowds
   c. Maintain strict isolation
   d. Instruct the client to avoid blood draws

4. Which of the following circumstances most places the client at risk for respiratory complications following a splenectomy?
   a. Disturbance of clotting factors
   b. NPO status
   c. Need for frequent dressing changes
   d. Location of surgical incision

5. Which of the following postsplenectomy symptoms should the client report *immediately?*
   a. Fever and malaise
   b. Pain at the incision site
   c. Presence of cough
   d. Fatigue

 ANSWER TO CRITICAL THINKING: Jeanine

Jeanine will probably be fatigued from her disease, and fatigue may increase further from side effects of treatment. Staff nursing jobs can be tiring even for healthy nurses. In addition, she will be around patients with respiratory diseases, many of which are contagious. This is not a good idea for someone at risk for infection. Jeanine might want to take a leave of absence during treatment or ask to be reassigned to a different area that is less demanding and away from patients.

BIBLIOGRAPHY

Baldy, CM: Hematologic disorders. In Price, SA, and Wilson, LM (eds): Pathophysiology: Clinical Concepts of Disease Processes, ed 4. Mosby, St Louis, 1992.

Conrad, KJ: Cancer care. In Illustrated Manual of Nursing Practice, ed 2. Springhouse, Springhouse, Pa, 1993.

Kier, S: Caring for people with blood disorders. In Luckmann, J (ed): Saunders Manual of Nursing Care, WB Saunders, Philadelphia, 1997.

Nettina, SM: Hematologic disorders. In The Lippincott Manual of Nursing Practice, ed 6. JB Lippincott, Philadelphia, 1996.

Understanding the Respiratory System

Respiratory System Function and Assessment

Paula D. Hopper

26

Learning Objectives

Upon completion of this chapter, the student will be able to:

1. Identify the structures of the respiratory system.
2. Describe the functions of the respiratory system.
3. List the effects of aging on the respiratory system.
4. Describe nursing assessment of the respiratory system, including health history and physical assessment.
5. Explain laboratory and diagnostic studies used when evaluating respiratory function.
6. Describe common therapeutic measures for clients with respiratory disorders.

Key Words

adventitious (ad-ven-**TI**-shus)
apnea (ap-**NEE**-ah)
crepitus (**KREP**-i-tuss)
cyanosis (SIGH-uh-**NOH**-sis)
dyspnea (**DISP**-nee-ah)
respiratory excursion (**RES**-pi-rah-TOR-ee eks-**KUR**-zhun)
thoracentesis (THOR-uh-sen-**TEE**-sis)
tidaling (**TIGH**-dah-ling)
tracheostomy (TRAY-key-**AHS**-tuh-me)
tracheotomy (TRAY-key-**AH**-tuh-me)

Normal Anatomy and Physiology

The respiratory system consists of the nose, nasal cavities, pharynx, larynx, trachea and bronchial tree, and the lungs and respiratory muscles. The parts outside the chest cavity are collectively called the upper respiratory tract, and those within the chest cavity make up the lower respiratory tract (Fig. 26–1). The lungs are the site of gas exchange between the air and the blood; the rest of the system moves air into and out of the lungs.

NOSE AND NASAL CAVITIES

The nose is made of bone and cartilage covered with skin; hairs inside the nostrils block the entry of dust. The two nasal cavities are within the skull and are separated by the nasal septum, which is made of the ethmoid and vomer bones. The nasal mucosa is ciliated epithelium that is highly vascular; it warms and moistens inhaled air. Dust and microorganisms are trapped on mucus produced by goblet cells and swept backward and down to the pharynx by the cilia.

The paranasal sinuses are air cavities in the maxillae, frontal, sphenoid, and ethmoid bones that open into the nasal cavities. They are lined with ciliated epithelium, and the mucus produced usually drains into the nasal cavities. Their functions are to make the skull lighter in weight and to provide resonance for the voice.

PHARYNX

The pharynx is posterior to the nasal and oral cavities and has three parts. The nasopharynx is an air passage only and is above the level of the soft palate, which is elevated to block it during swallowing. The eustachian tubes from the middle ear cavities open into the nasopharynx; the adenoid is a lymph nodule on its posterior wall. The oropharynx is behind the oral cavity and is both an air and a food passage. The palatine tonsils are on the lateral walls, and together with the lingual tonsils on the base of the tongue and the

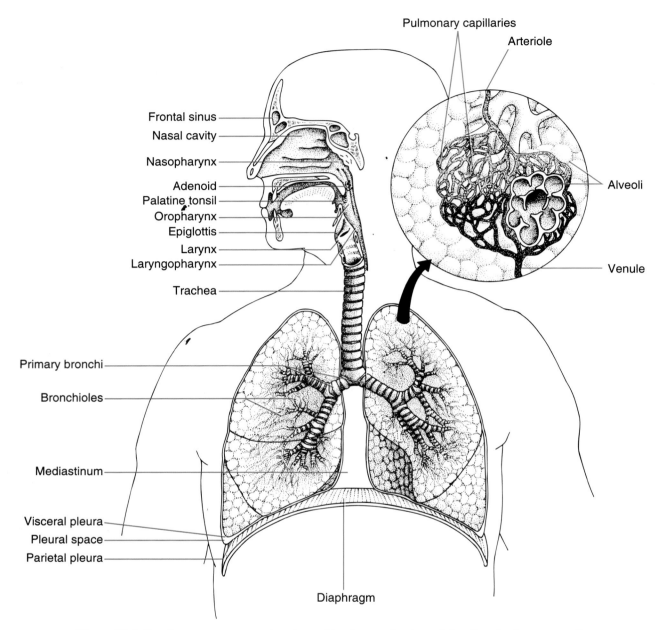

Figure 26–1. Respiratory system, anterior view, with microscopic view of alveoli and pulmonary capillaries. (Modified from Scanlon, VC, Sanders, T: Workbook for Essentials of Anatomy and Physiology, ed 2. FA Davis, Philadelphia, 1995, p 236, with permission.) See Plate 4.

adenoid, they form a ring of lymphatic tissue around the pharynx and destroy pathogens that penetrate the mucosa. The laryngopharynx is both an air and a food passage; it opens anteriorly into the larynx and posteriorly into the esophagus.

LARYNX

The larynx is the voice box and the airway between the pharynx and trachea. It is made of nine pieces of cartilage, a firm yet flexible tissue that keeps the airway open, and is lined with ciliated epithelium. The thyroid cartilage, commonly called the Adam's apple, is the largest and is palpable on the front of the neck. The epiglottis is the uppermost

cartilage and covers the larynx like a flap when the larynx is elevated during swallowing. On either side of the glottis (the airway) are the vocal cords. When pulled together across the glottis and vibrated by exhaled air, the vocal cords produce sounds that may be turned into speech. The vagus and accessory cranial nerves are the motor nerves to the larynx.

TRACHEA AND BRONCHIAL TREE

The trachea is a tube 4 to 5 inches long that extends from the larynx to the primary bronchi. C-shaped pieces of cartilage in the wall keep the trachea open. The mucosa is ciliated epithelium; mucus with trapped dust and microorganisms is swept upward toward the pharynx and is usually swallowed.

The bronchial tree is the series of air passages within the lungs, a succession of progressively smaller tubes that terminate in the alveoli. The right and left primary bronchi are branches of the trachea. Each gives rise to secondary bronchi; their structure is like that of the trachea. The bronchioles, however, have no cartilage in the walls to maintain patency, and they may be closed completely by contraction of their smooth muscle.

LUNGS AND PLEURAL MEMBRANES

The lungs fill the chest cavity on either side of the heart, extending from the clavicles to the diaphragm. On the medial surface of each lung is an indentation called the hilus, where the primary bronchus and the pulmonary artery and veins enter the lung.

The pleural membranes are the serous membranes of the thoracic cavity. The visceral pleura is the membrane that covers the lungs; the parietal pleura lines the chest cavity. A small amount of serous fluid between these membranes prevents friction and keeps the membranes together during breathing.

The functional units of the lung are the millions of alveoli, the air sacs that are the site of gas exchange. Both the alveoli and the surrounding pulmonary capillaries (Fig. 26–1) are made of simple squamous epithelium, that is, their walls are only one cell in thickness, to permit diffusion of gases.

Each alveolus is lined with a thin layer of tissue fluid that is essential for the diffusion of gases, but the surface tension of the fluid tends to make the walls of an alveolus stick together internally. Certain alveolar cells secrete pulmonary surfactant, a lipoprotein that mixes with the tissue fluid and decreases surface tension to permit inflation. Also in the alveoli are the alveolar macrophages, which phagocytize pathogens or bits of particulate matter (such as air pollution) that have not been trapped and swept out by the cilia.

Between clusters of alveoli is elastic connective tissue; it is capable of recoil when stretched (during inhalation) and contributes significantly to normal exhalation. The recoil of this tissue ensures that normal exhalation is a passive process that does not require the expenditure of energy.

MECHANISM OF BREATHING

Ventilation is the term for the movement of air into and out of the alveoli. Air moves from high-pressure to low-pressure areas (pressure gradients), some of which are created by the respiratory muscles, which in turn are controlled by the nervous system. The respiratory centers are in the medulla and pons. The main respiratory muscles are the diaphragm below the lungs and the external and internal intercostal muscles between the ribs. Accessory muscles of respiration are used during exercise and times of respira-

tory distress; these include the sternocleidomastoid and scalene muscles.

Pressures important to breathing include atmospheric pressure, intrapleural pressure, and intrapulmonic pressure. Atmospheric pressure is the pressure of the air around us, which at sea level is 760 mm Hg, and decreases as altitude increases. Intrapleural pressure is in the potential pleural space between the pleural membranes. Serous fluid causes the two membranes to adhere to each other, and because the elastic lungs are always tending to collapse and pull the visceral pleura away from the parietal pleura, the pressure in this potential space is always below atmospheric pressure (about 756 mm Hg). This is called a negative pressure. Intrapulmonic pressure is the pressure within the alveoli and bronchial tree. This pressure fluctuates below and above atmospheric pressure during each cycle of breathing.

Inhalation

Inhalation, also called inspiration, occurs when motor impulses from the medulla cause contraction of the respiratory muscles. Impulses along the phrenic nerves cause the diaphragm to contract and move downward (its dome shaped flattens). Impulses along the intercostal nerves cause the external intercostal muscles to pull the ribcage upward and outward. The chest cavity is thereby expanded in all directions, which expands the pleural membranes. Intrapleural pressure becomes even more negative, but the serous fluid keeps the membranes together and the lungs are expanded as well. As the lungs expand, intrapulmonic pressure falls below atmospheric pressure and air enters the nose and respiratory passages. Entry of air continues until intrapulmonic pressure equals atmospheric pressure; this is a normal inhalation. A deeper inhalation requires a more forceful contraction of the respiratory muscles to expand the chest cavity and lungs even further and permit the entry of more air.

Exhalation

Normal exhalation is a passive process that begins when motor impulses from the medulla decrease and the diaphragm and external intercostal muscles relax. The lungs are compressed as the chest cavity becomes smaller, and the recoil of the elastic lung tissue further compresses the alveoli. Intrapulmonic pressure rises above atmospheric pressure, and air is forced out of the lungs until the two pressures are again equal. Under normal circumstances, energy is not required for exhalation (as it is for inhalation) because the elasticity of the lungs causes recoil and forces air out. A forced exhalation beyond the normal amount is an active process that requires contraction of the internal intercostal muscles to pull the ribcage downward and inward, and contraction of the abdominal muscles to force the dome of the diaphragm upward to compress the lungs still further.

TRANSPORT OF GASES IN THE BLOOD

Oxygen is carried in the blood by the iron in the hemoglobin (Hgb) of the red blood cells (RBCs). The iron-oxygen bond is formed in the lungs, where the PO_2 is high. In tissues where the PO_2 is low, hemoglobin releases much of its oxygen.

Most carbon dioxide is carried in the blood in the form of bicarbonate ions in the plasma. These ions are formed when carbon dioxide enters RBCs and is converted to carbonic acid (H_2CO_3), which ionizes to bicarbonate ions (HCO_3^-) and hydrogen ions (H^+). The bicarbonate ions leave the RBCs for the plasma, and the remaining hydrogen ions are buffered by the hemoglobin in the RBCs. When the blood reaches the lungs, an area of lower PCO_2, these reactions are reversed—carbon dioxide is reformed and diffuses into the alveoli to be exhaled.

REGULATION OF RESPIRATION

Respiration is regulated by both nervous and chemical mechanisms. The medulla contains an inspiration center and an expiration center. The inspiration center generates impulses that bring about contraction of the respiratory muscles; the result is inhalation. Sensory impulses from baroreceptors in the inflating lungs to the medulla depress the inspiration center; this is called the Hering-Breuer inflation reflex and helps prevent overinflation of the lungs. In the pons, the apneustic center prolongs inhalation, and the pneumotaxic center helps bring about exhalation. These four centers provide a normal breathing rhythm, 12 to 20 breaths per minute with exhalation slightly longer than inhalation. When there is a need for more forceful exhalations, the inspiration center activates the expiration center, which brings about contraction of the internal intercostal muscles.

Normal breathing is essentially a reflex, but because the respiratory muscles are skeletal (or voluntary) muscles, it is possible to make changes. The cerebral cortex may bypass the medulla to permit faster or slower breathing, holding one's breath, singing, and so on. Eventually, however, the medulla will resume control and breathing will again become a reflex.

Chemical regulation of respiration involves the blood levels of oxygen and carbon dioxide. Decreased blood oxygen is detected by chemoreceptors in the carotid body and aortic body; the response by the medulla is increased respiration to take more air into the lungs. Increased blood carbon dioxide is detected by central chemoreceptors in the medulla itself (actually responding to the lowered pH); the response is increased respiration to exhale more carbon dioxide to raise the pH back toward normal.

Carbon dioxide is usually the major regulator of respiration because even small changes in its level in the blood will change the pH. Fluctuations in oxygen level have no effect on pH, and an adequate oxygen level in the blood can be maintained even if breathing ceases for a few minutes. The residual air in the lungs is a contributing factor, as is the fact that air contains much more oxygen than we usually use (exhaled air is 16% oxygen) but that is available if necessary. Oxygen becomes the major regulator only when its blood level is very low, as may occur with severe, chronic pulmonary disease.

RESPIRATION AND ACID-BASE BALANCE

Because of its role in regulating the amount of CO_2 in body fluids, the respiratory system is important in the maintenance of normal pH, also called acid-base balance, of these fluids, especially the blood. Any decrease in the rate or efficiency of respiration permits excess carbon dioxide to accumulate, resulting in the formation of excess hydrogen ions, which lower pH. This is called respiratory acidosis and is a consequence of pulmonary disease or any impairment of gas exchange in the lungs. Respiratory alkalosis occurs when the rate of respiration increases and carbon dioxide is very rapidly exhaled. Less carbon dioxide in the blood means that fewer hydrogen ions will be formed, and the pH will rise. Although not a common condition, respiratory alkalosis may occur during states of anxiety accompanied by hyperventilation, or when accommodating to a high altitude before RBC production increases to provide sufficient oxygenation of tissues.

The respiratory system may also help compensate for pH changes that are said to be metabolic, that is, of any cause other than a respiratory one. Metabolic acidosis may be caused by kidney disease, untreated diabetes mellitus, or severe diarrhea, all of which raise the hydrogen ion concentration of body fluids. Respiratory compensation involves an increase in the rate and depth of respiration to exhale more carbon dioxide to decrease hydrogen ion formation and raise the pH toward normal. Metabolic alkalosis may be caused by overingestion of antacid medications or by vomiting of stomach contents only. Respiratory compensation involves a decrease in the breathing rate to retain carbon dioxide in the body to increase the formation of hydrogen ions, which will lower the pH toward normal.

Respiratory compensation for an ongoing metabolic pH imbalance (such as kidney failure) cannot be complete, because there are limits to the amounts of carbon dioxide that may be exhaled or retained. At most, respiratory compensation is only about 75 percent effective.

EFFECTS OF AGING ON THE RESPIRATORY SYSTEM

The respiratory muscles, like all skeletal muscles, weaken with age. Lung tissue loses its elasticity, and even alveoli are lost as their walls deteriorate. All of these result in decreased ventilation and lung capacity and a decreased blood oxygen level. Chronic alveolar hypoxia from diseases such as emphysema or chronic bronchitis may lead to pulmonary hypertension, which in turn overworks the right ventricle of the heart. The cilia of the respiratory mucosa deteriorate with age, and the alveolar macrophages are not as efficient, which makes elderly people more prone to respiratory infections.

Table 26–1. **Questions Asked during Nursing Assessment of the Respiratory System**

Question	Rationale
Do you often have headaches or sinus tenderness?	These may indicate sinusitis.
Do you often experience nosebleeds?	A history of nosebleeds may indicate an abnormality that can predispose to future nosebleeds.
Has your voice changed?	A voice change may indicate a variety of disorders of the nose or throat. Further investigation is necessary.
Do you ever feel short of breath, like you can't get enough air?	Many respiratory and cardiac problems result in shortness of breath.
Do you have a cough? Is it productive? What does the sputum look like?	A cough indicates respiratory irritation or excessive secretions. Yellow or green sputum may accompany an infection. Blood in the sputum may occur with tuberculosis, pulmonary embolism, or cancer.
Have you recently experienced night sweats, chills, fever?	These are symptoms of tuberculosis.
Do you ever feel confused, light-headed, or restless?	These symptoms might indicate a low Po_2, reducing oxygen to the brain.
Have you had any chest surgeries?	This may reveal problem areas the client has not yet mentioned.
Do you have any allergies that cause respiratory symptoms? How do you treat them?	The client may take over-the-counter medications for allergies that affect respiratory function or interact with prescribed medications.
Do you smoke? How many packs per day? For how many years? Are you exposed to secondhand smoke?	Many respiratory disorders are caused or aggravated by exposure to tobacco smoke.
Are you or have you been exposed to airborne pollutants at work?	Pollutants such as asbestos, coal dust, or chemicals can cause lung disease.
Do you take any medications or use inhalers (prescribed or over-the-counter) for your respiratory problems?	Information about medications gives further information about disorders, severity, and treatment. The nurse should also consider drug interactions and side effects.
Do you use home oxygen or other home respiratory treatments?	This helps the nurse determine the severity of disease and the treatment.
Do any of your blood relatives have emphysema, asthma, or tuberculosis?	Some respiratory disorders have a hereditary tendency. Tuberculosis is contagious.

Nursing Assessment

HEALTH HISTORY

Many factors in a client's personal and family history affect respiratory function. Questions the nurse should ask while assessing the client with a history of respiratory dysfunction are presented in Table 26–1. If at any time during the history the client relates a specific symptom, the nurse should redirect the line of questioning to further assess that symptom. One such line of questioning, as presented in Chapter 2, is WHAT'S UP? For example, if the client admits to shortness of breath (SOB), the nurse would respond with the following questions (**W**here is it? doesn't apply to shortness of breath, so it may be skipped):

How does it feel? Does breathing feel tight, gasping, suffocating?

Aggravating and alleviating factors. How much activity causes the SOB? Does anything else aggravate it? What relieves it?

Timing. How long have you had this problem? Does it happen more at any particular time of day or year?

Severity. How bad is it on a scale of 1 to 10, with 0 being normal breathing and 10 being severe dyspnea?

Useful other data. Do you have any other symptoms that occur along with the shortness of breath?

Patient's perception. What do you think is causing your shortness of breath?

The nurse must also be aware of cultural influences on the client's health. See Cultural Considerations Box 26–1.

PHYSICAL ASSESSMENT

Inspection

Inspection begins during the nursing history and continues during the physical assessment. Inspection starts with the nose, which is observed for symmetry, swelling, or other abnormality.

The nurse notes whether the client is short of breath during speaking or movement. If the client is very **dyspneic,** he or she may speak in short sentences.

The client is observed for use of accessory muscles of breathing. Use of the sternocleidomastoid muscles causes the shoulders to raise during labored inspiration. During forced expiration, the abdominal and intercostal muscles contract. The use of accessory muscles for breathing indicates respiratory distress. Retraction of the chest wall between the ribs can indicate serious distress.

---

dyspneic: dys—bad + pnea—breathing

CULTURAL CONSIDERATIONS BOX 26-1

Pulmonary diseases associated with Japanese people include asthma related to dust mites in the straw mats that cover floors in Japanese homes, air pollution from living in urban aras, and cardiac and pulmonary sequelae of cigarette smoking, which is high among Japanese.[1] The nurse should encourage clients who have straw mats and who wish to keep them to have them sterilized.

Clients coming from Poland, Ireland, or other countries where mining is a primary occupation may have an increased incidence of respiratory disease. Mining and heavy industry are health risk factors related to the development of pulmonary diseases. It is essential that health care providers carefully screen Polish and Irish immigrants for respiratory conditions.

Health care practitioners should be aware of the variations among ethnic peoples of color when assessing for cyanosis. Cyanosis and decreased blood hemoglobin levels in darker-skinned individuals gives the skin an ashen color instead of a bluish color. Thus the nurse must examine the sclera, conjunctiva, buccal mucosa, tongue, lips, nailbeds, and palms and soles of the feet to assess for lowered oxygen levels.

Smoking is deeply ingrained in the Arab-American culture. Offering cigarettes is a rite of Arab hospitality. Arabs may have difficulty stopping smoking because of these cultural rituals.[2]

Populations living in inner cities are at increased risk for respiratory diseases related to pollution.[3] Strategies to increase the effectiveness in getting African-Americans to stop smoking include working with community and church groups in African-American communities.

Appalachians, with a preponderance of jobs in pottery making, mining, furniture making, textiles, and fabricated materials, are at increased risk for respiratory diseases.[4] Nurses can improve the health status of their Appalachian clients by encouraging the use of face masks when working in these industries.

Color of skin, lips, mucous membranes, and nailbeds is noted. A bluish color is called **cyanosis** and is a late sign of oxygen deprivation. The trachea and chest are observed for symmetry. Respirations per minute are counted, noting depth and rhythm. Irregular respirations, or periods of **apnea,** can indicate pathology and are described in Figure 26–2. The shape of the chest is observed. Normally, the chest is about twice as wide (side to side) as it is deep (front to back). If it is more rounded, it is called a barrel chest, which is associated with air trapping.

Palpation

The frontal and maxillary sinuses are palpated if sinus inflammation is suspected. See Figure 26–3 for location of the sinuses. The nurse uses the thumbs to palpate gently below the eyebrows and below each cheekbone. Tenderness indicates sinus inflammation or infection.

The nurse can palpate **respiratory excursion.** This is a rough measurement of chest expansion on inspiration. It is not necessary to palpate expansion on every client, but it may be helpful if hypoventilation or asymmetry is suspected. See Figure 26–4 for how to palpate respiratory excursion.

The nurse can also palpate for **crepitus** (also called subcutaneous emphysema). Crepitus feels like Rice Krispies under the skin when felt with the fingers. It occurs when air leaks into subcutaneous tissues because of pneumothorax or around a chest tube site. Palpation for crepitus is not done routinely, but rather when the possibility of an air leak exists.

Percussion

Percussion is done by the experienced nurse. The nurse taps on the anterior and posterior chest, in each interspace, comparing sounds from side to side. A normal chest sounds resonant and is the same on both the right and left sides, except over the heart. If other percussion notes are heard, they may indicate pathology and should be reported. See Chapter 2 for additional information on percussion.

Auscultation

Auscultation provides valuable information about respiratory status. The nurse uses the diaphragm of the stethoscope to listen to the anterior and posterior chest during an entire inspiration and expiration at each interspace (Fig. 26–5). Auscultation of the posterior chest is easiest if the client is sitting, but if necessary it may be done with the client in a side-lying position. Asking the client to breathe deeply through the mouth can help enhance the sounds. The nurse should allow the client to rest at intervals to prevent hyperventilation. Regular and frequent practice helps the nurse distinguish normal from abnormal breath sounds. Abnormal (another term is **adventitious**) sounds indicate pathology and are described in Table 26–2.

Diagnostic Tests

LABORATORY TESTS

Blood Tests

Measurement of red blood cells and hemoglobin can give information about the oxygen-carrying capacity of the blood. Dyspnea can be caused by a reduction in RBCs or Hgb. See Table 26–3 for normal values.

---

cyanosis: cyan—dark blue + osis—condition
apnea: a—not + pnea—breath

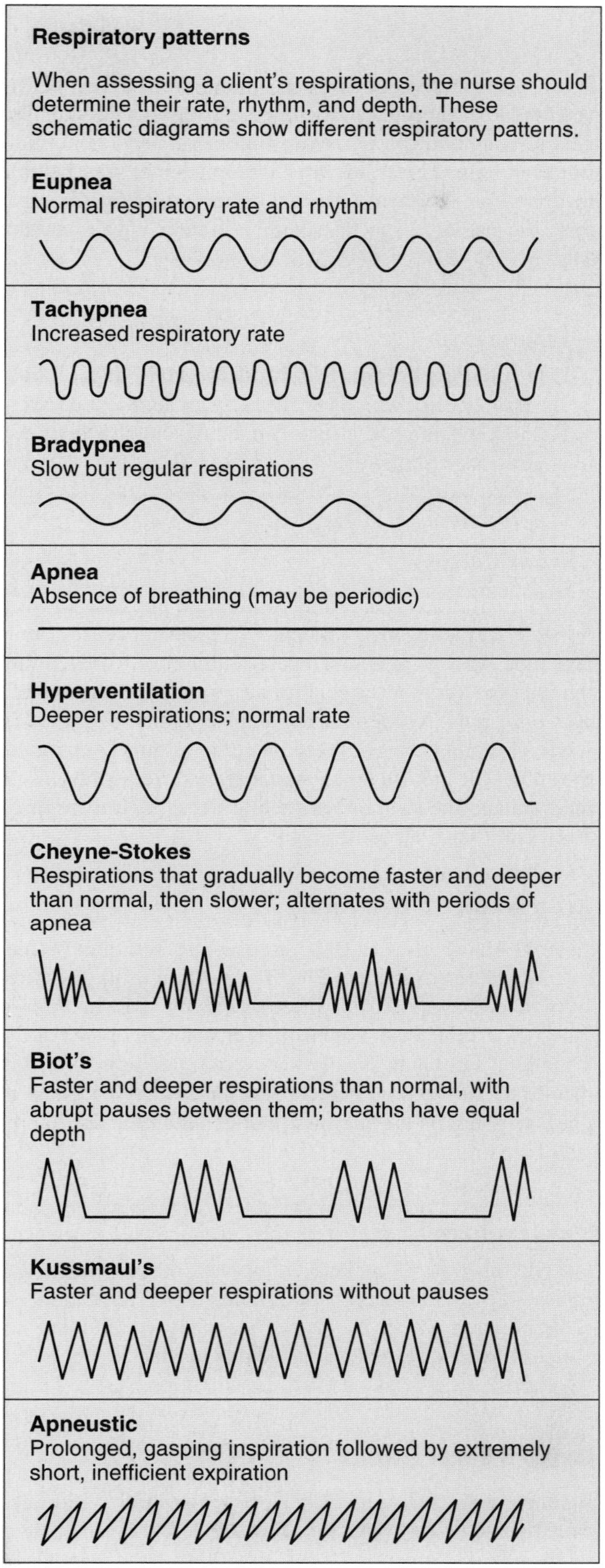

Respiratory patterns

When assessing a client's respirations, the nurse should determine their rate, rhythm, and depth. These schematic diagrams show different respiratory patterns.

Eupnea
Normal respiratory rate and rhythm

Tachypnea
Increased respiratory rate

Bradypnea
Slow but regular respirations

Apnea
Absence of breathing (may be periodic)

Hyperventilation
Deeper respirations; normal rate

Cheyne-Stokes
Respirations that gradually become faster and deeper than normal, then slower; alternates with periods of apnea

Biot's
Faster and deeper respirations than normal, with abrupt pauses between them; breaths have equal depth

Kussmaul's
Faster and deeper respirations without pauses

Apneustic
Prolonged, gasping inspiration followed by extremely short, inefficient expiration

Figure 26–2. Abnormal respiratory patterns. (Modified from Morton, PG: Health Assessment in Nursing, ed 2. FA Davis, Philadelphia, 1993, p 98, with permission.)

Sinus locations

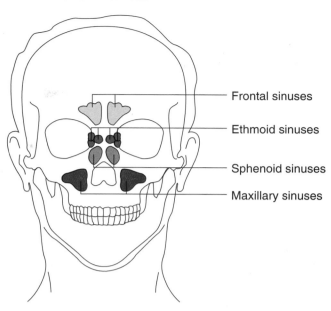

- Frontal sinuses
- Ethmoid sinuses
- Sphenoid sinuses
- Maxillary sinuses

Figure 26–3. Paranasal sinuses. (Modified from Morton, PG: Health Assessment in Nursing, ed 2. FA Davis, Philadelphia, 1993, p 194, with permission.)

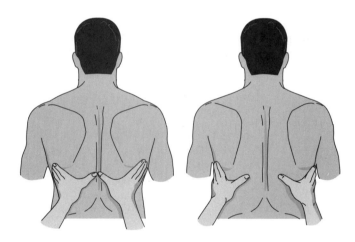

Posterior respiratory excursion
Stand behind the client and place your thumbs in the infrascapular area on either side of the spine at the level of the tenth rib. Grasp the lateral rib cage and rest your palms gently over the lateroposterior surface. Avoid applying excessive pressure to prevent restricting the client's breathing.

As the client inhales, the posterior chest should move upward and outward and your thumbs should move apart. When the client exhales, your thumbs should return to midline and again touch.

Figure 26–4. Palpation of respiratory excursion. (Modified from Morton, PG: Health Assessment in Nursing, ed 2. FA Davis, Philadelphia, 1993, p 267, with permission.)

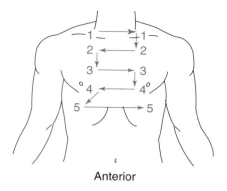

Anterior

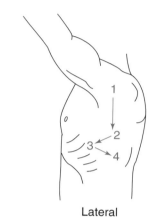

Lateral

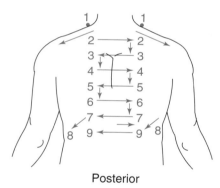

Posterior

Figure 26–5. Auscultation of the chest. Use a systematic approach to auscultate the chest, comparing sounds from side to side. (Modified from Morton, PG: Health Assessment in Nursing, ed 2. FA Davis, Philadelphia, 1993, p 268, with permission.)

Sputum Culture and Sensitivity

A sputum culture identifies pathogens present in the sputum. The sensitivity test determines which antibiotics will be effective. To obtain a sputum specimen, the nurse obtains a sterile container. Some institutions have special containers for sputum that help prevent transmission of infection to the health care worker (Fig. 26–6). The client is instructed to take several deep breaths and cough sputum into the sputum container. It is important that the client does not simply spit saliva or sinus drainage into the cup. The specimen must come from the lungs. It may be easiest to obtain a specimen first thing in the morning (after mouth

care) because secretions build up during the night. The specimen is sent to the lab immediately. If the client is unable to cough up sputum, extra fluids or a bedside humidifier may help. The respiratory therapist (RT) may be able to obtain a specimen with a nebulized mist treatment or with the use of a special suction catheter with a sputum trap.

Throat Culture

A throat culture is done to determine the presence of viral or bacterial pathogens in the pharynx. The nurse uses a culture tube with an attached swab (Culturette) to reach into the pharynx (without touching the mouth) and rub the red area or lesions. A tongue blade helps hold the tongue down while obtaining the culture. Once the culture is obtained, the end of the culture tube is squeezed to release the culture medium and the swab is returned to the tube. It is immediately sent to the lab for analysis.

Arterial Blood Gas Analysis

Arterial blood gases (ABGs) are done to determine effectiveness of gas exchange. The "Pa" portion of the ABG results refer to the partial pressure of the gas in arterial blood. See Table 26–4 for basic interpretation of the ABGs. The blood sample is usually taken from the radial artery in the wrist. This can be painful. The nurse may be asked to place pressure on the site for 5 minutes after the test to prevent bleeding.

Oxygen Saturation

A simple noninvasive test is the oxygen saturation test (also called pulse oximetry, O_2 sat, and SaO_2). A sensor is placed on the client's finger or ear that measures the percentage of hemoglobin that is saturated with oxygen. Oxygen saturation can be measured at rest, or while the client is walking to determine the client's exercise tolerance. It is also often done with and without supplemental oxygen to determine

Table 26–2. **Abnormal Lung Sounds**

Abnormal (Adventitious) Sound	Cause of Sound	Description	Associated Disorders
Coarse crackles (sometimes called rales)	Fluid in airways	Moist bubbling sound, heard on inspiration or expiration	Pulmonary edema, bronchitis, pneumonia
Fine crackles (rales)	Alveoli popping open on inspiration	Velcro being torn apart, heard at end of inspiration	Heart failure, atelectasis
Wheezes	Narrowed airways	Fine high-pitched violins mostly on expiration	Asthma
Stridor	Airway obstruction	Loud crowing noise heard without stethoscope	Obstruction from tumor or foreign body
Pleural friction rub	Pleura rubbing together	Sound of leather rubbing together	Pleurisy, lung cancer, pneumonia, pleural irritation
Diminished	Decreased air movement	Lung sounds faint	Emphysema, hypoventilation, obesity, muscular chest wall
Absent	No air movement	No sounds heard	Pneumothorax, pneumectomy

the client's need for oxygen supplementation at home. See Table 26–4 for normal values. A value of $SaO_2 < 95$ percent should be reported to the physician. If the SaO_2 is less than 75 percent, the nurse should prepare for emergency intervention.

DIAGNOSTIC TESTS

Chest X-Ray

A chest x-ray is ordered to help diagnose a variety of pulmonary disorders. Usually posterior-anterior (PA) and side views (PA and lateral) are taken. If a hospitalized client is too ill to go to the radiology department, a portable chest x-ray can obtain a PA view.

Ventilation-Perfusion Scan

During a ventilation-perfusion scan (also called a lung scan or VQ scan), a radioactive substance is injected intravenously, and a scan is done to view the blood flow to the lungs (perfusion). Another radioactive substance is in-

haled, and scanning shows how well oxygen is distributed in the lungs (ventilation). If an area of the lungs is well ventilated but with no blood supply, a pulmonary embolism is suspected. Chronic lung disease may cause poor ventilation and perfusion.

Pulmonary Function Study

This series of tests is done to determine lung volume, capacity, and flow rates. It is commonly used to help diagnose and monitor restrictive or obstructive lung disease. For this test the client is asked to use a special mouthpiece to blow into a cylinder that is connected to a computer. A computer printout is generated with results. See Table 26–5 for normal values.

Table 26–3. **Common Laboratory Tests**

Test	Normal Values	Associated Conditions
Red blood cell (RBC) count	Male: 4.5–6.2 million; female: 4.2–5.4 million cells/mm³ venous blood	↑ in chronic lung disease, dehydration ↓ in anemia, hemorrhage, overhydration with IV fluids
Hemoglobin (Hgb)	Male: 13.5–18 g/dL Female: 12–16 g/dL	Same as RBC count
White blood cell (WBC) count	5000–10,000 cells/mm³ venous blood	↑ in infection

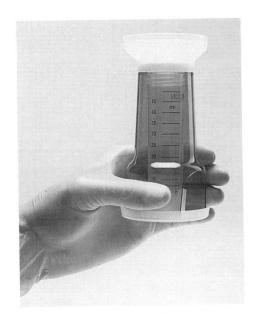

Figure 26–6. A special container that helps prevent transmission of infection is often used to collect sputum for culture. (Photo courtesy of Becton Dickinson Microbiology Systems.)

Table 26–4. **Arterial Blood Gas Analysis**

	Normal Value	Interpretation
PaO_2	75–100 mm Hg	↑ in hyperventilation ↓ in impaired respiratory function
$PaCO_2$	35–45 mm Hg	↑ in impaired gas exchange ↓ in hyperventilation
pH	7.35–7.45	↑ in respiratory alkalosis with low $PaCO_2$ ↓ in respiratory acidosis with high $PaCO_2$
HCO_3^-	22–26	↑ to buffer $PaCO_2$ in acidosis ↓ to buffer $PaCO_2$ in alkalosis
Oxygen Saturation	95–100%	↑ in hyperventilation ↓ in impaired respiratory function

Pulmonary Angiography

Pulmonary angiography involves x-ray of the pulmonary vessels after intravenous (IV) administration of a radiopaque dye. A catheter is inserted into the femoral, brachial, or jugular vein and threaded through the heart to the pulmonary artery, where the dye is injected. Pulmonary angiography is used to help diagnose pulmonary embolism or other pulmonary vessel disorders. Clients receive nothing by mouth (NPO) for 4 to 8 hours before the procedure. The nurse should question the client about allergies to x-ray dyes. As with any procedure involving dye, the client is informed that the dye may cause a warm feeling on injection.

After angiography, the client is placed on flat bed rest for 3 to 8 hours. The nurse monitors vital signs and observes the injection site for bleeding. A sandbag may be used to place pressure on the site. Fluids are encouraged to promote excretion of dye.

Bronchoscopy

A bronchoscopy involves the use of a flexible endoscope to examine the larynx, trachea, and bronchial tree. A bronchoscopy can be used diagnostically for visualization or to obtain a biopsy for examination. It can be used therapeutically to remove an obstruction, foreign body, or thick secretions. The client is told that he or she will be able to breathe through the nose and that oxygen can be administered through the tube if necessary. A signed consent is necessary for this procedure.

The client is NPO for 6 to 8 hours before the procedure. The client is given a sedative before the procedure, and often an injection of atropine to dry excess secretions. An anesthetic spray may be used to numb the throat. After the test, vital signs are monitored, and the client is monitored for laryngeal edema. Sputum may be blood tinged. The client is NPO until return of the gag reflex. The nurse checks for the gag reflex by touching the pharynx with a cotton swab. The client is asked to swallow a sip of water before additional foods or fluids are offered. A sore throat may be relieved by lozenges.

Therapeutic Measures

DEEP BREATHING AND COUGHING

Effective coughing can keep the airways clear of secretions. An ineffective cough is exhausting and fails to bring up secretions. The nurse instructs the client to take two or three deep breaths, using the diaphragm. This helps get the air behind the secretions. After the third deep inhalation, the client holds the breath and coughs forcefully. This is repeated as necessary.

BREATHING EXERCISES

Breathing exercises are essential for clients with chronic lung disease. Diaphragmatic and pursed-lip breathing in-

Table 26–5. **Pulmonary Function Values**

Test	Definition	Normal Values*
Tidal volume (TV)	Air inspired and expired in one breath	400–600 mL at rest
Residual volume (RV)	Air remaining in lungs after maximum exhalation	1000–1500 mL
Functional residual capacity (FRC)	Air remaining in lungs after normal expiration	2300 mL
Vital capacity (VC)	Maximum amount of air expired after maximum inspiration	4600 mL
Inspiratory reserve	Amount of air beyond tidal volume that can be taken in with the deepest possible inhalation	2000 to 3000 mL
Expiratory reserve	Amount of air beyond tidal volume in the most forceful exhalation	1000 to 1500 mL
Forced vital capacity (FVC)	Maximum amount of air expired forcefully after maximum inspiration	3000–5000 mL
Peak expiratory flow rate (PEFR)	Maximum flow of air expired during FVC (this is a rate rather than a volume)	450 L/min

*Normal values are approximate—computer determines normal based on client's height and weight.

crease the effectiveness of breathing and help reduce panic when dyspnea occurs.

Diaphragmatic Breathing

The diaphragm is the major muscle of breathing, but clients often use less efficient accessory muscles when they are short of breath. Conscious use of the diaphragm during breathing can be relaxing and conserve energy. With practice, the client should be able to use diaphragmatic breathing all the time without thinking about it. The client is taught to do the following:

1. Place one hand on the abdomen and the other on the chest.
2. Concentrate on pushing out the abdomen during inspiration and relaxing the abdomen on expiration. The chest should move very little.

Pursed-Lip Breathing

This technique can be used any time the client feels short of breath. It helps keep airways open during exhalation, which promotes carbon dioxide excretion. It should be done with diaphragmatic breathing. Counting during breathing also distracts the client, reducing panic. The client is taught to do the following:

1. Inhale slowly through the nose to the count of two.
2. Exhale slowly through pursed lips to the count of four.

LEARNING TIP

An excellent resource for clients is the *Better Breathers Club Panic Control Workbook II,* by Kim Golemb, RRT. It is presented in an easy-to-read cartoon format. It is available from California College Press, 222 West 24th Street, National City, CA 91950. Phone: (619) 477-4800.

POSITIONING

The client who is short of breath should be positioned to conserve energy while allowing for maximum lung expansion. The client in bed should use a Fowler's or semi-Fowler's position. Most clients do not tolerate lying flat. Some clients prefer to sit in a chair while leaning forward and placing their elbows on their knees. Others may sit at a desk or use an overbed table with a pillow on it to lean on. Recent research shows that in clients with unilateral (one-sided) lung disease, oxygen saturation is increased in the "good lung down" lateral position. This is a side-lying position with the good lung in the dependent position. It is theorized that gravity causes greater blood flow to the dependent, "good" lung, thereby increasing oxygenation. Any of these positions can be used with the breathing exer-

cises described previously for the client who is acutely dyspneic.

OXYGEN THERAPY

Oxygen therapy is ordered by the physician when the client is unable to maintain oxygenation. Many clients are placed on supplemental oxygen when their oxygen saturation is less than 90 percent on room air. The order should include the method of administration and the flow rate. A variety of delivery methods are described in the following subsections. The role of the nurse in oxygen therapy includes monitoring the flow rate, ensuring that the cannula and tubing or other device remains properly placed, and monitoring the client's response to treatment. If the client becomes short of breath while on oxygen therapy, the RT or physician should be notified. The nurse instructs the client to avoid smoking, avoid using electrical equipment, and avoid other activities that can cause fire in the presence of oxygen. The RT is knowledgeable about oxygen therapy and is an excellent resource when questions arise.

LEARNING TIP

If a client suddenly becomes confused, check the oxygen delivery system. The client may have taken off the cannula, or the tubing may be kinked or disconnected, resulting in hypoxia and confusion.

Low-Flow Devices

Nasal Cannula

The nasal cannula is the most common method of oxygen administration. Oxygen is delivered through a flexible catheter that has two short nasal prongs (Fig. 26–7). For the nasal cannula to be most effective, the client must breathe through his or her nose. The cannula allows the client to eat and talk, and it is generally more comfortable than other methods of administration. If the nasal mucous membranes become dry, the RT can place a water source on the system to humidify the oxygen. Oxygen is delivered at 1 to 6 L/min via a nasal cannula.

Masks

Masks are used when a higher flow rate is needed (Fig. 26–8). A disadvantage to masks is that they make some clients feel claustrophobic. Also, a mask must be replaced by a cannula for eating.

SIMPLE FACE MASK. A rate of 5 to 10 L/min can deliver oxygen concentrations from 40 to 60 percent with a simple face mask.

PARTIAL REBREATHER MASK. A partial rebreather mask uses a reservoir to capture some exhaled gas for rebreathing. Vents on the sides of the mask allow room air to mix

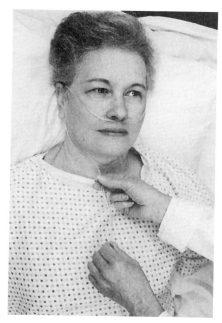

Figure 26–7. Nasal cannula for oxygen delivery.

with oxygen. It can deliver oxygen concentrations of 50 percent or greater.

NONREBREATHER MASK. A nonrebreather mask has one or both side vents closed to limit the mixing of room air with oxygen. The vents open to allow expiration, but remains closed on inspiration. The reservoir bag has a valve to store oxygen for inspiration but does not allow entry of exhaled air. It is used to deliver oxygen concentrations of 70 to 100 percent.

When a client is using a partial rebreather or nonrebreather mask, the nurse ensures that the reservoir is never allowed to collapse to less than half full.

High-Flow Devices

Venturi Mask

A Venturi mask is used for the client who requires precise percentages of oxygen, such as the client with chronic lung disease with CO_2 retention. A combination of valves and specified flow rates determines oxygen concentration.

Transtracheal Catheter

A transtracheal catheter is a small tube that is surgically placed through the base of the neck directly into the trachea to deliver oxygen (Fig. 26–9). This is an attractive alternative for many clients who are on long-term oxygen at home, because it does not obstruct the nose or mouth and can be easily covered with a scarf or collar. The client is taught to remove and clean the catheter two or three times a day to prevent mucus obstruction. The nurse should check institution policy and procedure and the respiratory care department for specific care instructions.

Risks of Oxygen Therapy

Clients with chronic airflow limitation (CAL) have chronically high CO_2 levels. Therefore they depend on low O_2 levels to stimulate breathing. High supplemental oxygen flow rates can depress respirations. Clients with CAL should be maintained on no more than 1 to 2 L of O_2 per minute.

In addition, any client can suffer lung damage from high oxygen concentrations delivered for over 24 hours. If a client exhibits symptoms of dry cough, chest pain, numbness in the extremities, lethargy, or nausea, the physician should be contacted. A PaO_2 greater than 100 mm Hg should also be reported.

NEBULIZED MIST TREATMENTS

Nebulized mist treatments (NMTs) use a nebulizer to deliver medication directly into the lungs (Fig. 26–10). Topical use of medication reduces systemic side effects. Bronchodilators such as albuterol or metaproterenol, mixed with normal saline and sometimes with supplemental oxygen, are most commonly administered. Other medications, including corticosteroids, mucolytics, and antibiotics, may also be given. The RT or a specially trained nurse administers the NMT. The client uses a handheld reservoir with tubing and a mouthpiece to breathe in the medication. The NMTs are commonly ordered every 4 to 6 hours and as needed. The nurse may call for a prn NMT when a client with chronic pulmonary disease becomes acutely dyspneic. Some clients are taught to administer their own NMTs at home.

METERED DOSE INHALERS

Metered dose inhalers (MDIs) are another way to administer topical medication directly into the lungs, reducing systemic side effects. Medications delivered in this way include corticosteroids, bronchodilators, and mast cell inhibitors (cromolyn sodium). See Figure 26–11 for correct use of an MDI. It is important that the RT or nurse carefully instruct the client, because improper use can reduce effectiveness of the medication. It is also important to teach the client to never overuse inhalers. Clients with chronic disease tend to use extra puffs when they feel short of breath. Adrenergic bronchodilators, when used too often, can cause severe bronchoconstriction and even death.

INCENTIVE SPIROMETRY

Incentive spirometers (IS) are devices used to encourage deep breathing in clients at risk for collapse of lung tissue (atelectasis) (Fig. 26–12). They are often ordered for postoperative clients. Clients are instructed to use the spirometer 10 times each hour they are awake. Because a variety of spirometers are available, the nurse should consult with the RT and read package inserts for specific directions for use.

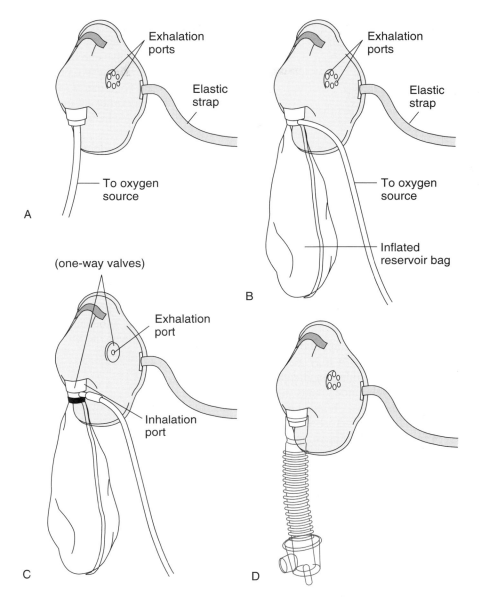

Figure 26–8. Oxygen masks. *(A)* Simple mask. *(B)* Partial rebreather mask. *(C)* Nonrebreathing mask. *(D)* Venturi mask.

CHEST PHYSIOTHERAPY

Chest physiotherapy (CPT) includes postural drainage, percussion, and vibration (Fig. 26–13). Chest physiotherapy helps move secretions from deep within the lungs. It is indicated for the client who has a weak or ineffective cough and who is therefore at risk for retaining secretions. Clients with chronic obstructive pulmonary disease, cystic fibrosis, or bronchiectasis and clients on ventilators benefit from CPT.

The CPT is performed by an RT or specially trained nurse. For postural drainage, the client is placed in various positions (head down, to help drain secretions), and turned periodically during the treatment so all lung fields are drained. The therapist uses cupped hands to strike the chest repeatedly (percussion), producing sound waves that are transmitted through the chest, loosening secretions. The therapist may also use vibration on the client's chest, using the hands or a vibrator, to loosen secretions. A nebulizer treatment should be given before CPT to humidify secretions. The client is instructed to cough and deep breathe at intervals during and after the treatment.

THORACENTESIS

Thoracentesis involves the insertion of a needle into the pleural space. It is often done to aspirate fluid in clients with pleural effusion. The procedure may be diagnostic to

---

thoracentesis: thoraco—chest + centesis—puncture

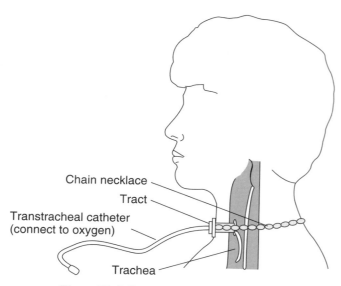

Figure 26–9. Transtracheal oxygen catheter.

Labels in figure:
- Chain necklace
- Tract
- Transtracheal catheter (connect to oxygen)
- Trachea

determine the source of fluid, or therapeutic to remove fluid and reduce respiratory distress. It may also be performed to aspirate blood or air or to inject medication.

The nurse verifies that the client understands the procedure and that written consent has been obtained if required by institution policy. The client voids before the procedure. The client should be aware that a sensation of pressure may be felt, but that severe pain is rare. An analgesic may be administered if ordered before the procedure. A special procedure tray is obtained that has the equipment needed by the physician. The client is placed in a sitting position, bending over the bedside table, or side lying if unable to sit. It is helpful if the nurse is positioned in front of the client and encourages relaxation during the procedure. The

physician uses a local anesthetic before inserting a needle into the client's back through the desired interspace. Specimens are drawn through the needle, labeled, and sent to the lab. If the thoracentesis is being done for therapeutic reasons, a sterile container will be used to collect the remaining fluid. Sometimes as much as 2 L or more can be removed, and the client will state immediate reduction of dyspnea.

After the procedure, the nurse assesses vital signs, breath sounds, and puncture site according to institution policy (for example every 15 minutes times two, every 30 minutes times two, then every 4 hours for 24 hours). The client is usually maintained on bed rest for 1 hour after the procedure.

CHEST DRAINAGE

Continuous chest drainage involves insertion of one or two chest tubes by the physician into the pleural space to drain fluid or air. The tubes are connected to a chest drainage system that collects the fluid or allows escape of the air.

Indications

Chest tubes and a chest drainage system are used when fluid or air has collected in the pleural space. This can occur with a pneumothorax, pleural effusion, or penetrating chest injury or during chest surgery. These conditions are covered in Chapter 28.

Chest Tube Insertion

The physician inserts drainage tubes through the chest wall into the pleural space, either in surgery or at the bedside. If

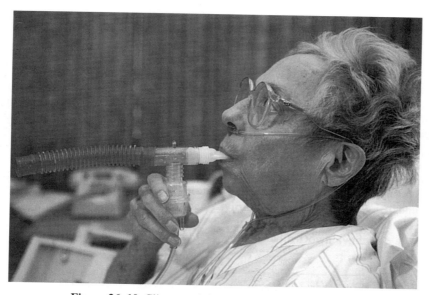

Figure 26–10. Client receiving nebulized mist treatment.

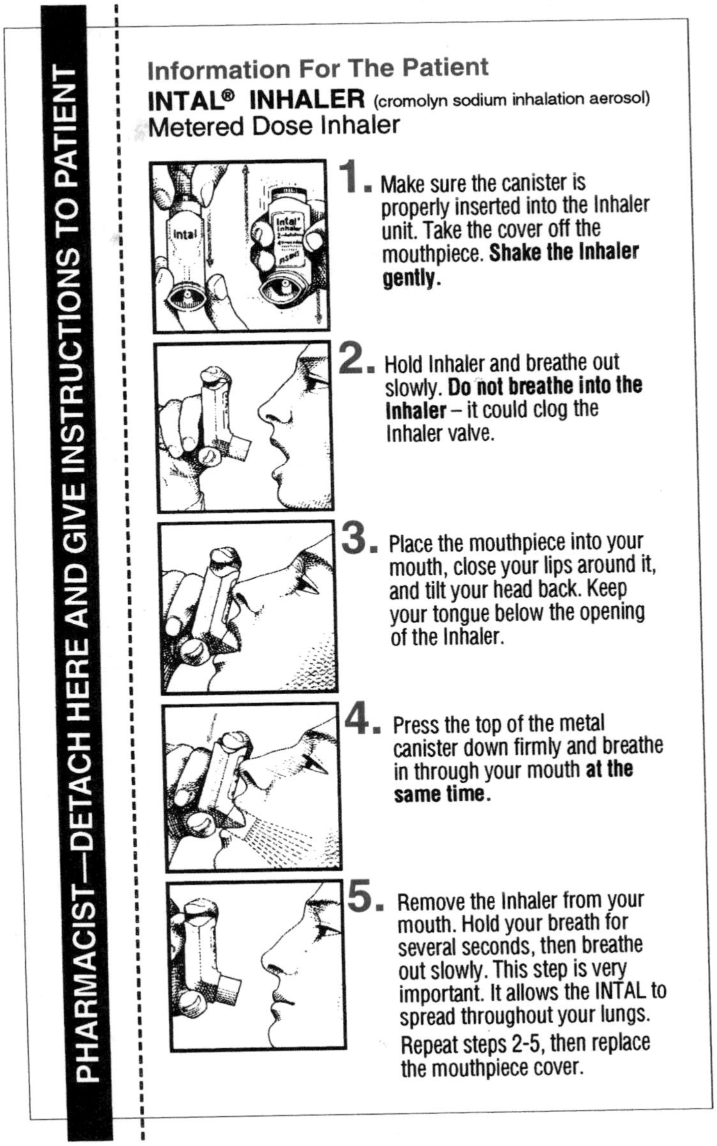

Information For The Patient
INTAL® INHALER (cromolyn sodium inhalation aerosol)
Metered Dose Inhaler

1. Make sure the canister is properly inserted into the Inhaler unit. Take the cover off the mouthpiece. **Shake the Inhaler gently.**

2. Hold Inhaler and breathe out slowly. **Do not breathe into the Inhaler** – it could clog the Inhaler valve.

3. Place the mouthpiece into your mouth, close your lips around it, and tilt your head back. Keep your tongue below the opening of the Inhaler.

4. Press the top of the metal canister down firmly and breathe in through your mouth **at the same time.**

5. Remove the Inhaler from your mouth. Hold your breath for several seconds, then breathe out slowly. This step is very important. It allows the INTAL to spread throughout your lungs. Repeat steps 2-5, then replace the mouthpiece cover.

Figure 26–11. Sample instructions for use of a metered dose inhaler. Patient instructions for Intal® inhaler. (Reprinted with permission from Rhône-Poulenc Rorer Pharmaceuticals, Inc. © 1996, Fisons Corporation, a Rhône-Poulenc Rorer company. All rights reserved. See package insert for specific product instructions.)

removal of air is the goal, the tube is inserted into the upper anterior chest, in the second to fourth intercostal space. If removal of fluid is the goal, the tube is inserted in the lower lateral chest, in the eighth or ninth intercostal space. If a client has both air and fluid to drain, two tubes are inserted and may be joined with a Y connector before connecting to the tubing that leads to a drainage system. The nurse assists the physician by obtaining a chest tube insertion tray and chest drainage system, and preparing it according to the manufacturer's directions. The nurse also ensures that the client understands the procedure and that written consent has been obtained according to institutional policy. An analgesic is administered if ordered. Chest tube insertion is sometimes an emergency intervention, which necessitates that the nurse prepare the client quickly.

Once the tube has been inserted and the system is in place, the nurse ensures that each connection is securely taped with adhesive tape, to prevent a break in the system. Vaseline gauze and a sterile occlusive dressing are applied over the insertion site to prevent air leakage.

The nurse obtains two padded clamps to keep at the bedside. These are used to clamp the chest tube if the chest drainage system becomes accidentally disconnected from the tubing, for changing the drainage system, or for a trial period before chest tube removal. The tubes are never clamped for more than a few seconds, however, because this prevents air escape and causes buildup of air in the pleural space. This creates a tension pneumothorax, which is a life-threatening emergency. (See Chapter 28.)

Chest Drainage System

The drainage system has evolved from a set of glass bottles to a one-piece molded plastic system with chambers that

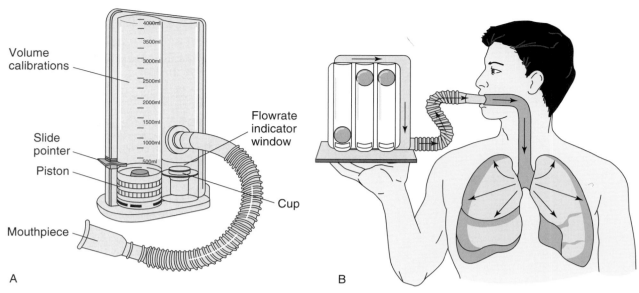

A   B

Figure 26–12. Incentive spirometers. *(A)* Voldyne volumetric deep breathing exerciser. *(B)* Triflo II incentive breathing exerciser. (Modified from Barnes, TA: Respiratory Care Principles. FA Davis, Philadelphia, 1991, p 434, with permission.)

correspond to the bottles. Some physicians, however, continue to use the bottle system. Studying the bottle system helps the nurse understand the one-piece system (Fig. 26–14).

Water Seal Bottle

Each time the client exhales, air trapped in the pleural space travels through the chest tube to the water seal bottle or chamber, under the water, and bubbles up and out of the

bottle. The water acts as a seal, allowing air to escape from the pleural space, but preventing air from getting back in during the negative pressure of inspiration. Water in the tube fluctuates up with each inspiration and down with each expiration, as much as 5 to 10 cm. This is called **tidaling.** When the lung is reinflated, tidaling stops. If tidaling stops before the lung is reinflated, the tubing should be checked for kinks or occlusion. If constant bubbling occurs in the water seal chamber, the system should be checked immediately for leaks.

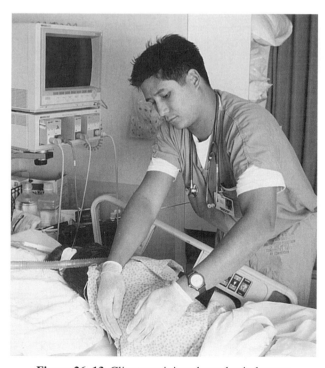

Figure 26–13. Client receiving chest physiotherapy.

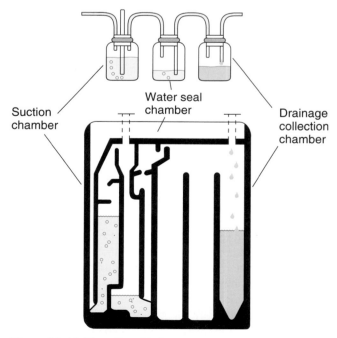

Suction chamber   Water seal chamber   Drainage collection chamber

Figure 26–14. Pleur-Evac™ chest drainage system. (Courtesy of Deknatel Snowden Pencer, Inc., Tucker, Ga.)

Suction Bottle

Sometimes a suction source is used to speed lung reinflation. A separate bottle with tubing attached to suction is used. The amount of suction is dependent on the level of water in the bottle, not the amount of suction set on the machine. The suction level is ordered by the physician and is almost always −20 cm of water. The suction should be turned on far enough to cause gentle bubbling in the suction bottle or chamber. Vigorous bubbling will cause water evaporation and alter the amount of suction. If water evaporates, more must be added to maintain the correct amount of suction.

Drainage Bottle

Sometimes a third bottle is needed to drain fluid from the pleural space. Drainage may be from pleural effusion, chest trauma, or surgery. Sometimes a small amount of drainage occurs because of the insertion of the chest tube. The drainage chamber is *not* emptied to measure drainage. Rather, the drainage level in the bottle or chamber is marked and timed each shift to monitor the amount. It is documented as output on the intake and output record. If drainage suddenly increases, or becomes very bloody, the physician should be notified.

Nursing Care

Nursing care of a client with a chest tube involves regular assessment of the client and the drainage system. See Table 26–6 for specific assessment and care. If permitted by the physician, clients can be free to move around with the chest tube and drainage system. The drainage system must *always* be kept upright and below the level of the chest. If the client must be transported, the drainage system is transported with the client. The nurse must ask the physician if the client can be safely transported without suction. The suction control chamber is then left open to allow air to escape. Tubing is not clamped for transport.

If a chest tube is accidentally pulled out before the pneumothorax is resolved, air can reenter the pleural space. Some physicians want an occlusive dressing placed over the site to prevent air from reentering. However, an occlusive dressing increases the risk of trapped air building up and placing pressure on the heart. The nurse should be aware of the preferences of the client's physician.

Stripping and Milking

In the past it was routine to strip and milk the tubing from the client to the drainage system, to dislodge clots and maintain patency. Stripping is done by holding the proximal end of the tubing and using the other hand to squeeze the tubing between two fingers while sliding the fingers toward the drainage system. This is repeated on small sections of tubing until all have been stripped. It is now known, however, that this process can create negative pressure at the openings in the tubing that are within the pleural

Table 26–6. *Care of the Client with a Chest Drainage System*

Assess the client according to institution policy. Start with the client and move toward the drainage system.
1. Observe respiratory rate, effort, and symmetry.
2. Assess shortness of breath, pain, or other discomforts.
3. Auscultate lung sounds (lung sounds may initially be muffled or absent on the side of a collapsed lung but should gradually return to normal as the lung reinflates).
4. Confirm that dressing is intact; observe for drainage. If necessary, reinforce the dressing and notify the physician. Do *not* change the dressing.
5. Palpate insertion sites for crepitus.
6. Check all tubing for kinks, breaks, or broken connections. Verify that all connections are securely taped.
7. Ensure that there are no dependent loops of tubing. Excess tubing should be coiled on the bed.
8. Verify that drainage system is below level of client's chest at all times.
9. Check drainage system or bottles for cracks or leaks.
10. Check water seal chamber for correct water level and for tidaling (unless lung reinflated). Add water if evaporation has decreased level. If continuous bubbling is present, check entire system for leaks and notify physician.
11. Check suction control chamber for gentle bubbling (or open to air). Confirm correct amount of water if indicated. Add water if needed.
12. Check and mark amount of drainage in collection chamber every 8 hours and prn or as ordered. Report any marked increase in bloody drainage.
13. Document findings.

Notify physician if
• *The client suddenly complains of increasing dyspnea.*
• *The drainage chamber is full and needs to be changed.*

space, which can suck lung tissue in and cause damage. Stripping should be done only if it is ordered by the physician.

Milking is done by gently squeezing portions of tubing from the client to the system, without any sliding motion. This is somewhat safer for the client, but is still not done routinely. If tubing appears to be occluded, the nurse should consult with the physician for specific orders.

Removal of Chest Tube

When the reason for the chest tube is resolved, the physician will remove it and place a Vaseline gauze and a sterile occlusive dressing over the site(s). The nurse continues to watch for development of crepitus and to monitor respiratory status and the dressing site.

   CRITICAL THINKING: Miss Israel

Miss Israel has a chest tube in place for a spontaneous pneumothorax. The nurse notes that the water seal chamber is bubbling vigorously. What should the nurse do?

Answer at end of chapter.

TRACHEOSTOMY

A **tracheotomy** is a surgical opening through the base of the neck into the trachea. It is called a **tracheostomy** when it is more permanent and has a tube inserted into the opening to maintain patency (Fig. 26–15). The client breathes through this opening, bypassing the upper airways. A tracheostomy is performed for a variety of reasons, including clients who have had a laryngectomy for cancer, clients with airway obstruction caused by trauma or tumor, clients who have difficulty clearing secretions from the airway, or clients who need prolonged mechanical ventilation.

The tracheostomy tube consists of three parts: an outer cannula, an inner cannula, and an obturator (Fig. 26–16). The obturator is a guide that is used only during insertion of the tube. After insertion, the obturator is immediately removed and kept at the bedside (often taped to the wall above the bed) for emergency use if the tracheostomy tube is accidentally removed. The outer cannula remains in place at all times and is secured by ties to prevent dislodging. The inner cannula is removed at intervals, usually every 8 hours and as needed for cleaning. Some newer tracheostomy tubes eliminate the need for an inner cannula. The tube may be metal or plastic. Plastic tubes generally have disposable inner cannulas, which can be replaced rather than cleaned. Plastic tubes may also have balloon-like cuffs that are inflated to prevent air escape during mechanical ventilation and to prevent aspiration of food or secretions. Institution policy may dictate that cuffs be de-flated routinely to prevent tissue damage. See Table 26–7 for routine tracheostomy cleaning.

Communication is problematic for the client with a tracheostomy tube, because air is diverted out the tube rather than past the vocal cords and out the mouth. Fenestrated tubes are tubes with openings (fenestra) in the cannula to allow air to flow up into the larynx for speaking. The client is taught to plug the opening of the tube while speaking to divert air through the fenestra. A newer option is the Passy-Muir tracheostomy speaking valve. This is a special valve that allows air into the tracheostomy during inspiration but closes and redirects air up and out of the nose and mouth on expiration, allowing the client to speak. For the valve to work, the tracheostomy tube must be small enough for air to flow around it, or it must be fenestrated.

A client is weaned from the tracheostomy tube when the condition has improved enough to allow breathing without it. The physician may replace the tube with a smaller tube to prepare the client for its removal. In addition, a plug may be inserted into the tracheostomy tube at intervals, to force the client to breathe through the nose and mouth. When the tracheostomy tube has been removed, the opening may be taped shut and covered with gauze until it is healed. The gauze usually becomes saturated with secretions and is changed as needed.

Nursing Process for the Client with a Tracheostomy

See Nursing Care Plan Box 26–2 for the Client with a Tracheostomy.

CRITICAL THINKING: Mr. Smith

Mr. Smith had a plastic cuffed tracheostomy tube that was small enough to allow flow of air around it for talking. The cuff was inflated for lunch to prevent him from aspirating. A friend stopped by for a chat and assisted Mr. Smith to plug his tracheostomy so he could talk. Mr. Smith's face turned dark red, and his expression showed extreme anxiety.

1. What happened?
2. How could the nurse help prevent this in the future?

Answers at end of chapter.

SUCTIONING

Suctioning involves the use of a flexible catheter to remove secretions from the respiratory tract of a client who is un-

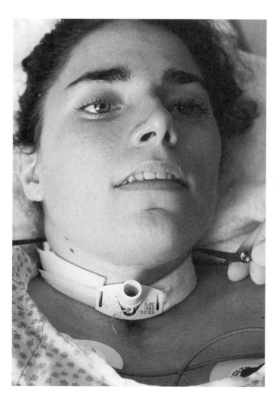

Figure 26–15. Client with tracheostomy.

tracheostomy: trache—trachea + ostomy—opening or mouth

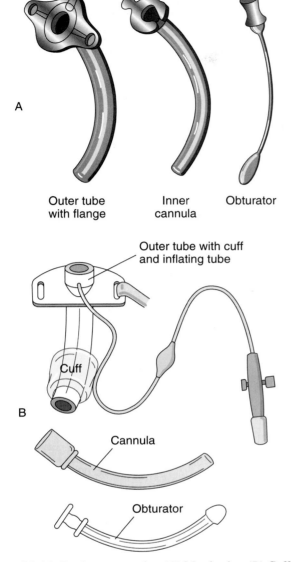

Figure 26–16. Tracheostomy tube. *(A)* Metal tube. *(B)* Cuffed plastic tube.

able to cough effectively. This may be the client with a tracheostomy or endotracheal tube, or one with overwhelming secretions.

The procedures for suctioning are presented in Tables 26–8 and 26–9. A procedure manual should be consulted for more detailed instruction. The nurse should remember that suctioning is both frightening and uncomfortable for a client. Clients sometimes feel as though oxygen is being "vacuumed" from their lungs. Suctioning can cause hypoxia, vagal stimulation with resulting bradycardia, and even cardiac arrest. It is done only when necessary, rather than on a routine basis. Coughing is the most effective way to clear secretions, and should be encouraged if the client is capable. Each step should be explained to the client, even if he or she is unresponsive.

Table 26–7. *Tracheostomy Cleaning Procedure*

1. Assemble equipment: tracheostomy care kit, sterile water or saline, suction equipment, hydrogen peroxide.
2. Explain the procedure to the client.
3. Suction inner cannula if necessary. See Table 26–9.
4. Open and prepare the kit, keeping all equipment sterile. Fill one side of basin with half peroxide and half saline and the other with saline.
5. Don clean gloves.
6. Remove old tracheostomy dressing.
7. Remove inner cannula from tracheostomy tube and place it in peroxide solution.
8. While inner cannula is removed, the client may be suctioned if necessary.
9. Don sterile gloves.
10. Use brush and pipe cleaners to clean inner cannula. Place in water or saline to rinse. Dry inside of cannula with pipe cleaner. Reinsert into tracheostomy tube.
11. Use cotton swab and sterile gauze with sterile peroxide and saline to clean around tracheostomy site. Rinse with saline to prevent skin irritation.
12. Replace ties. Remove old ties after new ties are securely in place.
13. Apply sterile tracheostomy dressing (drain sponge or "trach pants"). Use precut or folded dressing. Cutting gauze creates fibers that can enter the tracheostomy.

Note: A procedure manual should be consulted for more detailed instruction.

LEARNING TIP

Hold your own breath while suctioning your client. It will keep you mindful of how the client feels because suctioning not only removes secretions, but also oxygen, from the respiratory tract.

INTUBATION

Some clients are unable to breathe effectively because of airway obstruction or respiratory failure. These clients are intubated with a special endotracheal (ET) tube through the nose or mouth and into the trachea (Fig. 26–17). Clients in cardiopulmonary arrest are intubated during advanced cardiac life support. Most intubated clients are also mechanically ventilated. Some clients have advance directives that indicate that they do not wish to be intubated. The nurse should be familiar with the client's wishes and draw them to the attention of the physician if necessary.

Because intubation can damage the vocal cords and surrounding tissues, it is usually a short-term intervention. Clients who need long-term support will have a tracheostomy tube placed.

Nursing care of the intubated client includes regular assessment of the client's respiratory status and tube placement. Lung sounds are auscultated bilaterally to ensure that the tube has not been displaced into one bronchus. The tube is carefully secured with tape or a Velcro holder to

NURSING CARE PLAN BOX 26–2 FOR THE CLIENT WITH A TRACHEOSTOMY

Risk for ineffective airway clearance related to increase in secretions

Client Outcome
Airway is free of secretions.

Evaluation of Outcome
Is airway free of secretions?

Interventions	Rationale	Evaluation
• Assess lung sounds every 4 hours and prn.	Coarse crackles or wheezes may indicate secretions in airways.	Are coarse crackles or wheezes present?
• Encourage client to deep breathe and cough as able.	Clients may be able to clear own secretions without suctioning.	Is client able to cough up secretions effectively?
• Encourage fluids if not contraindicated.	Fluids help hydrate secretions, making them easier to cough up.	Is client taking adequate fluids? Are secretions thin?
• Encourage ambulation as able, or turn every 2 hours.	Movement helps mobilize secretions.	Is client mobilized as much as possible?
• Suction client using sterile technique prn. Suction only when necessary.	Suctioning clears secretions from airways. Unnecessary suctioning irritates airways.	Is suction necessary? Is airway free of secretions after suctioning?
• Monitor and document amount, color, and character of secretions. Report increase in secretions accompanied by fever.	Purulent sputum accompanied by fever may indicate pneumonia.	Is sputum clear or white, and scant in amount? Does purulent sputum need to be reported?

Risk for infection related to bypass of normal respiratory defense mechanisms

Client Outcome
Client is free from symptoms of infection.

Evaluation of Outcome
Is client free from symptoms of infection?

Interventions	Rationale	Evaluation
• Use good hand-washing practice.	Hand washing is important in preventing infection.	Do all caregivers use good hand-washing technique?
• Monitor and report signs and symptoms of infection: fever, increased respiratory rate, purulent sputum, elevated white blood cell (WBC) count.	Early recognition and treatment of infection enhances outcome.	Are signs of infection present?
• Protect tracheostomy opening from foreign material: food, sprays, powders.	Foreign materials in the tracheostomy may cause pneumonia.	Is tracheostomy adequately protected?
• Use meticulous sterile technique for all tracheostomy care and suctioning.	Use of nonsterile technique may introduce microorganisms into the respiratory tract.	Is sterile technique used by all caregivers?
• Encourage a well-balanced diet. Consult dietitian prn.	A well-balanced diet enhances immune function.	Is client eating a balanced diet or receiving adequate supplementation?
• Take measures to prevent aspiration of food or secretions.	Aspiration can cause pneumonia.	Is there evidence that the client is aspirating?

Impaired verbal communication related to presence of tracheostomy tube

Client Outcomes
Client uses alternate methods of communication effectively. Client expresses satisfaction with ability to communicate needs.

continued

NURSING CARE PLAN BOX 26–2 *(continued)*

Evaluation of Outcome
Is client able to use alternative methods to express needs? Does client express satisfaction with ability to do so?

Interventions	Rationale	Evaluation
• Take time to allow client to communicate needs.	Communication takes time; client may become frustrated if hurried.	Does client feel he or she is given adequate time for communication of needs?
• Watch for client's nonverbal cues.	Gestures and facial expression can provide valuable cues.	Is the client attempting to communicate with nonverbal cues?
• Offer pen and paper or magic slate (if client is literate).	The client may be able to write out his or her needs/concerns.	Is client able to write out needs?
• Use picture board.	The client can point to a picture (water, toileting) that indicates his or her need.	Is client able to point appropriately to needs?
• Teach client with fenestrated or small tracheostomy tube how to cover opening with a clean finger in order to talk.	Covering opening diverts air into larynx and allows speech.	Is client able to communicate in this manner?
• Consult with speech therapist.	Speech therapist may have additional methods for communicating with client.	Did speech therapist provide alternative communication techniques?

Body image disturbance related to presence of tracheostomy

Client Outcomes
Client verbalizes acceptance of tracheostomy. Client is willing to participate in tracheostomy care.

Evaluation of Outcomes
Does client verbalize acceptance of tracheostomy? Does client participate in learning to care for tracheostomy?

Interventions	Rationale	Evaluation
• Assess client's feelings about tracheostomy.	Assessment provides basis for care.	Are the client's feelings within an expected range for such a change in body image?
• Approach client with an accepting attitude.	The client will be aware of the nurse's nonverbal body language.	Does the client indicate a feeling of acceptance from the nurse?
• Allow client opportunity to verbalize concerns about tracheostomy.	Verbalizing concerns helps the client to sort out feelings and problem solve.	Does the client verbalize feelings as needed? (Note: Some clients do not wish to share feelings and should not be forced to do so.)
• Refer client to support group if available.	The client may benefit from talking with others with tracheostomies.	Is client receptive to a support group referral?
• Assist client in finding attractive ways to conceal tracheostomy if desired.	Loose scarves or collars can help conceal and protect the tracheostomy.	Is client satisfied with appearance of tracheostomy?

Knowledge deficit related to care of new tracheostomy

Client Outcomes
Client and significant other will verbalize understanding of self-care, demonstrate tracheostomy self-care procedures, and state resources for help after discharge.

continued

NURSING CARE PLAN BOX 26-2 *(continued)*

Evaluation of Outcomes

Are client and significant other able to verbalize self-care actions and rationale? Are client and significant other able to correctly demonstrate care procedures? Is client able to state how to obtain help after discharge?

Interventions	*Rationale*	*Evaluation*
• Assess client's and significant other's baseline knowledge of self-care. • Instruct client and significant other in the following (see text for specific instruction): • Tracheostomy cleaning • Deep breathing and coughing • Suctioning • Prevention of infection and symptoms to report to health care provider • Protection of tracheostomy from pollutants, water (no swimming, careful showering)	Teaching should only be initiated if a knowledge deficit exists. The client will need to care for self after discharge.	Does client exhibit knowledge of self-care? Is client able to verbalize understanding of self-care and demonstrate all procedures correctly?
• Provide follow-up with home health nurse after discharge.	A home health nurse can provide reinforcement of instruction at home.	Is client receptive to having a home health nurse assist?

---

avoid dislodging. Oral tubes are repositioned to the opposite side of the mouth and resecured every 24 hours or according to institution policy to prevent tissue damage. An adhesive skin barrier should be applied under the tape. If the client is alert, he or she is instructed to be careful not to pull on the tube. The nurse may obtain an order for soft

Table 26-8. *Oropharyngeal or Nasopharyngeal Suctioning Procedure*

1. Gather equipment: sterile suction catheter, sterile gloves, sterile container (these items may be found in a single "cath and glove" kit); sterile water or saline, suction machine with tubing.
2. Explain procedure to client.
3. Connect catheter to suction tubing, keeping catheter inside sterile sleeve. Turn on suction to level specified by institution policy (usually 80–120 mm Hg for wall suction).
4. Pour saline into sterile container.
5. Put on sterile gloves. Keep dominant hand sterile at all times.
6. Suction small amount of saline into catheter to rinse catheter and test suction.
7. Have client take several deep breaths.
8. With thumb control uncovered to stop suction, insert suction catheter through mouth or nose into the trachea until resistance is met or client coughs.
9. Slowly withdraw catheter, suctioning intermittently while rotating it. The entire procedure should take no more than 10 to 15 seconds.
10. After allowing client to rest, repeat steps 6 through 9 two more times if needed.

Note: A procedure manual should be consulted for more detailed instruction.

Table 26-9. *Suctioning Procedure for the Client with a Tracheostomy*

1. Gather equipment: sterile suction catheter, sterile gloves, sterile container (these items may be found in a single "cath and glove" kit); sterile water or saline, suction machine with tubing, manual resuscitation bag.
2. Explain procedure to client.
3. Connect catheter to suction tubing, keeping catheter inside sterile sleeve. Turn on suction to level specified by institution policy (usually 80–120 mm Hg for wall suction). Connect oxygen source to manual resuscitation bag.
4. Pour saline into sterile container.
5. Put on sterile gloves. Keep dominant hand sterile at all times.
6. Suction small amount of saline into catheter.
7. Oxygenate client with three ventilations using a manual resuscitation bag connected to an oxygen source, using the nonsterile hand. If the client is mechanically ventilated, use manual sigh.
8. With thumb control uncovered to stop suction, insert suction catheter through tracheostomy tube until client coughs or resistance is met.
9. Slowly withdraw catheter, suctioning intermittently while rotating it. The entire procedure should take no more than 15 seconds.
10. Allow client to rest.
11. Repeat steps 6 through 10 two more times if needed.

Some older sources recommend instilling sterile saline into the tracheostomy to loosen secretions. *This should be avoided.* It is now known that this procedure is not effective and may actually cause a drop in the client's SaO_2.

Note: A procedure manual should be consulted for more detailed instruction.

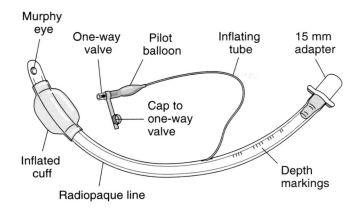

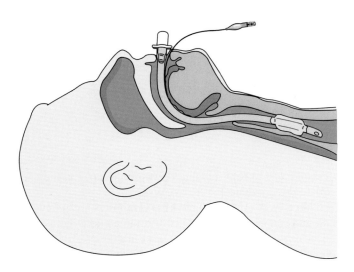

Placement of tube in airway

Figure 26–17. Endotracheal tube. (Modified from Barnes, TA: Respiratory Care Principles. FA Davis, Philadelphia, 1991, p 425, with permission.)

wrist restraints if absolutely necessary for the confused client. Restraints can be avoided if a family member is available to sit with the client. Some nursing interventions for the client with a tracheostomy are also appropriate for the intubated client. (See Nursing Care Plan Box 26–2 for the Client with a Tracheostomy.)

Endotracheal tubes have a cuff (a balloonlike area around the tube) to help maintain proper placement and to prevent leakage of air around the tube. The RT usually inflates the cuff and maintains a specific cuff pressure, and should be consulted for assistance with this activity.

Clients with ET tubes may need suctioning if they are unable to cough. The nurse is aware that the client needs to be suctioned if he or she is unable to cough effectively. Visible secretions in the tube, crackles or wheezes heard with or without the stethoscope, or a drop in SaO$_2$ without another obvious cause are signs that suctioning is necessary. The ET tube suctioning procedure is sterile and is the same as suctioning a tracheostomy tube. Some institutions

have in-line suctioning devices, which are connected to the ET tube within a sterile sleeve (Fig. 26–18). This maintains sterility, protects the nurse, and simplifies the suctioning procedure. Oral suction keeps the mouth free of secretions. Meticulous mouth care is done every 4 hours and as needed.

The intubated client is often extremely anxious, especially if he or she is alert. The nurse explains the purpose of all care activities. Suctioning is particularly anxiety producing and should be explained carefully. Because the ET tube passes between the vocal cords, the client is unable to speak. The nurse provides paper and pencil or a picture board for communication. Yes/no questions can be answered by a nod or shake of the head.

The nurse monitors arterial blood gas and oxygen saturation values and notifies the physician of changes. If O$_2$ values drop or the client becomes confused or agitated, the client should be immediately inspected for a disconnected oxygen source or excessive secretions.

If the physician determines that the client can breathe effectively without the tube, the tube will be removed. Before removal, the client's mouth and tube are suctioned and the cuff is deflated. After removal, the client is observed closely for laryngeal edema or respiratory distress. The client is maintained in high Fowler's position to maximize chest expansion.

MECHANICAL VENTILATION

Ventilators are devices that provide ventilation (respirations) for clients who are unable to breathe effectively on their own (Fig. 26–19). Ventilators use positive pressure to push oxygenated air via a cuffed ET or tracheostomy tube into the lungs at preset intervals. Clients may need mechanical ventilation after some surgeries, after cardiac or respiratory arrest, for declining arterial blood gases related to worsening respiratory disease, or for neuromuscular disease or injury that affects the muscles of respiration.

Nursing Responsibilities

Before initiating mechanical ventilation, it is important that the health care team be aware of advance directives and consult with the client and family, because many clients do not wish to be mechanically ventilated. Some clients will accept mechanical ventilation if it is a temporary measure, but not if it might be a permanent intervention.

Until recently, ventilators were used only in intensive care units. Now, ventilators are seen on medical-surgical units, nursing homes, and even in clients' homes. It is important that a team approach be used when caring for a mechanically ventilated client. The social worker; respiratory therapist; physical, occupational, and speech therapists; dietitian; nurse; and physician all work together to provide the comprehensive care needed by this client. Respiratory

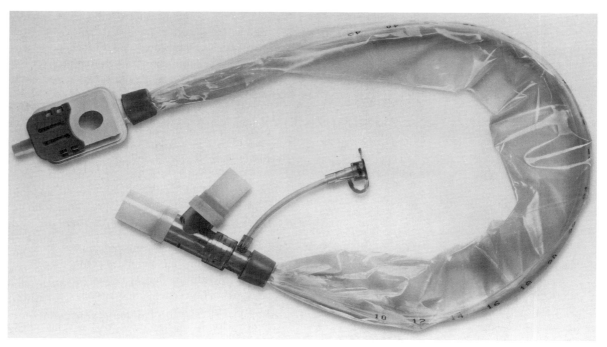

Figure 26–18. In-line suction catheter. (Courtesy of Hudson RCI, Temecula, Calif.)

therapists usually take responsibility for routine monitoring and equipment maintenance. The nurse is responsible for monitoring the client, ensuring that ventilator settings are maintained as prescribed, providing initial response to alarms, keeping tubing free from water accumulation, and keeping the client's airway free from secretions. In addition, the nurse keeps a manual resuscitation bag at the bedside for emergencies.

Clients who are mechanically ventilated are unable to talk and can become very uncomfortable and anxious with no easy way to communicate. See Table 26–10 for one nurse's tips for making ventilated clients feel more secure.

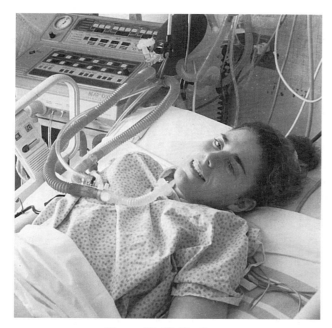

Figure 26–19. Ventilator.

Table 26–10. **Tips for Caring for Mechanically Ventilated Clients**

- Introduce yourself to the client each time you enter the room. Make sure he or she can see you.
- Explain everything you are about to do.
- Check ventilator settings regularly.
- Give sedatives or antianxiety drugs as ordered. Request an order if necessary. Find out cause of unexplained anxiety (client may be hypoxemic).
- Reassure the client that anxiety is normal and that relaxing will help the ventilator to work with him or her.
- Assess for comfort and reposition at regular intervals. Be careful not to pull on the ventilator tubing. (Pulling hurts.)
- Suction quickly and smoothly, without jabbing. Avoid the use of saline with suctioning.
- Provide good oral care, moistening the lips with a cool washcloth and water-based lubricant. (Clients get thirsty.)
- Use restraints only as a last resort.
- Take the time to communicate with the client. Talk to him or her, and provide a magic slate or pen and paper for the client to talk to you. Make sure the call light is within reach at all times.
- Answer client's call light and ventilator alarms promptly.

Adapted from Jablonski, RAS: If ventilator patients could talk. RN, Feb 1995, p 32.

These tips were developed after the author interviewed 12 clients who had been intubated. They shared their fears, anxieties, and physical discomforts.

Ventilator Modes

Ventilators can control ventilation or assist the client's own respirations. See Table 26–11 for terms that help aid understanding of ventilator function. The nurse is wise to consult with the respiratory care department for an explanation of a client's ventilator and how to troubleshoot alarms that may sound.

Ventilator Alarms

Several types of alarms are found on ventilators. Low-pressure alarms sound if the ventilator senses reduced pressure in the system. This can be caused by disconnected tubing, leaks in tubing or around the ET tube, or an under-inflated cuff. A low-pressure alarm may also sound if the client has attempted to remove the tube.

High-pressure alarms sound for higher than normal resistance to air flow. This might occur if the client needs to be suctioned; if the client is biting on the tube, coughing, or trying to talk; if tubing is kinked or otherwise obstructed; or if worsening respiratory disease causes decreased lung compliance. In addition, the high-pressure alarm may be triggered if the client is anxious and is unable to time his or her breaths with those of the ventilator. Water in the tubing might also cause a high-pressure alarm. The nurse can consult with the respiratory care department for guidance in disconnecting and draining the tubing.

A loss of power alarm may signal a power failure or a disconnected plug. The nurse should be aware of emergency power sources and be prepared to manually ventilate if necessary.

Volume and frequency alarms sound when tidal volume or number of breaths per minute fall outside preset parameters.

When an alarm sounds, the nurse always checks the client first. If the client is stable, the machine may then be checked. The nurse must determine why the alarm is sounding and correct the problem quickly. If no cause can be found, the client is disconnected from the ventilator and a manual resuscitation bag is used until the RT arrives.

NONINVASIVE POSITIVE-PRESSURE VENTILATION

Noninvasive positive-pressure ventilation (NIPPV) is an alternative to intubation and mechanical ventilation for clients who are able to breathe on their own, but are unable to maintain normal blood gases. Instead of the invasive endotracheal or tracheostomy tube, NIPPV uses an external masklike device that fits over the nose or mouth (Fig. 26–20). It can be successful in clients who are alert, able to cooperate, do not have excessive secretions, and are able to breathe on their own for periods of time.

Two basic types of NIPPV are available: continuous positive airway pressure (CPAP) and bilevel positive airway pressure (BiPAP®, registered mark of Respironics, Inc.). In CPAP, the same amount of positive pressure is maintained throughout inspiration and expiration, to prevent airway collapse. In BiPAP, a different amount of positive pressure is used on inspiration and expiration.

Problems the nurse must be alert for in clients receiving NIPPV include skin irritation from the mask and gastric distention from swallowing air. An adhesive skin barrier can be applied to the areas that come in contact with the mask to prevent irritation. To prevent gastric distention, the client is placed in semi-Fowler's position, and the nurse consults with the RT to adjust air delivery pressure if necessary. Another problem is client acceptance of NIPPV. Many clients do not like the tight mask covering their nose or mouth. The nurse must be patient in explaining the reason for this treatment and check the client frequently to help control anxiety. The nurse also assesses the client's goals for therapy. Some clients may choose not to use NIPPV, but they must be fully aware of possible consequences.

Clients can use NIPPV nearly continuously, removing it to eat or use the bathroom. Other clients use it only when

Table 26–11. **Ventilator Terminology**

FIO$_2$	Fraction of inspired oxygen.
Tidal volume	Amount of air delivered with each breath.
Rate	Frequency of breaths delivered.
Assist control mode (AC, also called continuous mechanical ventilation, or CMV)	Ventilator delivers a breath each time the client begins to inspire. If the client does not breathe, the machine continues to deliver a preset number of breaths per minute.
Synchronized intermittent mandatory ventilation (SIMV)	Allows client to breathe on own, but delivers a minimum number of ventilations per minute as necessary. Synchronized to client's own respiratory pattern.
Pressure support (PS)	Provides positive pressure on inspiration to decrease the work of breathing.
Continuous positive airway pressure (CPAP)	Provides positive pressure on inspiration and expiration in order to decrease work of breathing in a spontaneously breathing client.
Positive end-expiratory pressure (PEEP)	Provides positive pressure on expiration, to help keep small airways open.

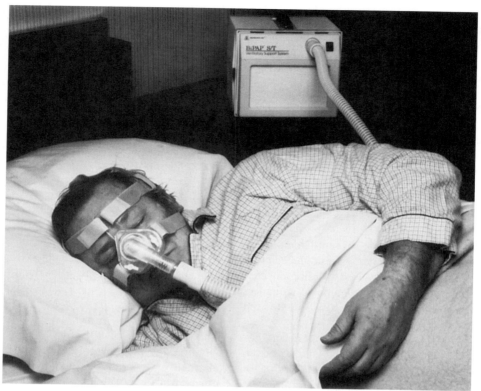

Figure 26–20. Noninvasive positive-pressure ventilation. (Courtesy of Respironics, Inc.)

they are sleeping, and are able to breathe effectively on their own during the day. Some use it for a few days until an acute exacerbation of disease is resolved, and others continue its use indefinitely at home.

Review Questions

1. During inhalation, which of the following muscle contractions takes place to enlarge the chest cavity from top to bottom?
   a. Diaphragm moves down.
   b. External intercostal muscles move down.
   c. Diaphragm moves up.
   d. Internal intercostal muscles move up.

2. The air remaining in lungs after normal expiration is called
   a. Vital capacity
   b. End-expiratory volume
   c. Tidal volume
   d. Functional residual capacity

3. Deteriorating cilia in the respiratory tract predispose the elderly to
   a. Chronic hypoxia
   b. Pulmonary hypertension
   c. Respiratory infection
   d. Decreased ventilation

4. Which of the following terms is used for violinlike sounds heard on chest auscultation?
   a. Crackles
   b. Wheezes
   c. Friction rub
   d. Stridor

5. Which of the following is a normal value for oxygen saturation?
   a. <60%
   b. 61 to 85%
   c. 86 to 95%
   d. >95%

6. The purpose of pursed-lip breathing is to promote
   a. Carbon dioxide excretion
   b. Carbon dioxide retention
   c. Oxygen excretion
   d. Oxygen retention

7. Which of the following actions by the nurse is appropriate when vigorous bubbling is noted in the suction control chamber of a chest drainage system?
   a. Check the tubing for leaks.
   b. Notify the physician.
   c. Reduce the level of wall suction.
   d. Clamp the chest tube.

8. Which of the following actions by the nurse is appropriate when suctioning a client with a tracheostomy tube?
   a. Instill a small amount of saline to liquefy secretions.

b. Have the client hold his or her breath while inserting the suction catheter.

c. Limit suction time to 15 seconds.

d. Move the catheter up and down several times while it is in the trachea.

Answers to Critical Thinking

CRITICAL THINKING: Miss Israel

Bubbling in the water seal chamber indicates a leak in the system. Vigorous bubbling may indicate a large leak, and the physician should be contacted immediately. The nurse should check the entire system for cracks or leaks and correct any problems discovered.

CRITICAL THINKING: Mr. Smith

1. Mr. Smith plugged his tracheostomy while the cuff was still inflated, so no air could get to his lungs. If the plug is not removed immediately he will be totally unable to breathe. Whenever the plug is in place, air must be able to travel around the tracheostomy tube or through the opening of a fenestrated tube in order for the client to breathe.

2. To prevent this from happening in the future, Mr. Smith should be taught how his tracheostomy tube works and how to care for it.

REFERENCES

1. Sharts-Hopko, N: Japanese-Americans. In Purnell, L, and Paulanka, B (eds): Transcultural Health Care: A Culturally Competent Approach. FA Davis, Philadelphia, 1998.

2. AbuGharbieh, P: Arab-Americans. In Purnell, L, and Paulanka, B (eds): Transcultural Health Care: A Culturally Competent Approach. FA Davis, Philadelphia, 1998.

3. Campinha-Bacote, J: African-Americans. In Purnell, L, and Paulanka, B (eds): Transcultural Health Care: A Culturally Competent Approach. FA Davis, Philadelphia, 1998.

4. Purnell, L, and Counts, M: In Purnell, L, and Paulanka, B (eds): Transcultural Health Care: A Culturally Competent Approach. FA Davis, Philadelphia, 1998.

BIBLIOGRAPHY

Ackley, BJ, and Ladwig, GB: Nursing Diagnosis Handbook: A Guide to Planning Care. Mosby, St Louis, 1995.

Barnes, TA: Respiratory Care Principles. FA Davis, Philadelphia, 1991.

Bell, SD: Use of Passy-Muir tracheostomy speaking valve in mechanically ventilated neurological patients. Crit Care Nurse 16:1, 1996.

Calianno, C, et al: Oxygen therapy: Giving your patient breathing room. Nursing 25:33, 1995.

Campolo, S: Spontaneous pneumothorax. Am J Nurs 2, 1997.

Carroll, P: A med/surg nurse's guide to mechanical ventilation. RN 58:26, 1995.

Carroll, P: Chest tubes made easy. RN 58:46, 1995.

Chang, VM: Protocol for prevention of complications of endotracheal intubation. Crit Care Nurse 15:19, 1995.

Fowler, S, et al: The ABCs of tracheostomy care. J Pract Nurs 44, March 1995.

Golemb, K: Better Breathers Club Panic Control Workbook II. California College Press, National City, Calif, 1993.

Jablonski, RAS: If ventilator patients could talk. RN 58:32, 1995.

Lasater-Erhard, M: The effect of patient position on arterial oxygen saturation. Crit Care Nurse 15:31, 1995.

Misasi, RS, and Keyes, JL: Matching and mismatching ventilation and perfusion in the lung. Crit Care Nurse 16:23, 1996.

Morton, PG: Health Assessment in Nursing, ed 2. FA Davis, Philadelphia, 1993.

Somerson, SJ, et al: Mastering emergency airway management. Am J Nurs 96:24, 1996.

Watson, J, and Jaffe, MS: Nurse's Manual of Laboratory and Diagnostic Tests, ed 2. FA Davis, Philadelphia, 1995.

Nursing Care of Clients with Upper Respiratory Tract Disorders

27

Paula D. Hopper

Learning Objectives

Upon completion of this chapter, the student will be able to:

1. Describe pathophysiology, etiology, signs and symptoms, and treatment of disorders of the nose and sinuses.
2. Discuss nursing care of clients with disorders of the nose and sinuses.
3. Apply the nursing process to the care of the client with an infection of the upper respiratory tract.
4. Describe pathophysiology, etiology, signs and symptoms, prevention, and treatment of cancer of the larynx.
5. Discuss physiological and psychosocial needs of the client with a laryngectomy.
6. Apply the nursing process to the care of the client with a laryngectomy.

Key Words

dysphagia (dis-**FAYJ**-ee-ah)

epistaxis (EP-iss-**TAX**-iss)

exudate (**EKS**-yoo-dayt)

laryngectomee (lare-in-**JEK**-tah-mee)

myalgia (my-**AL**-jee-ah)

rhinitis (rye-**NIGH**-tis)

rhinoplasty (**RYE**-noh-plass-tee)

Disorders of the upper respiratory tract generally include problems occurring in the nose, sinuses, pharynx, larynx, and trachea. Many of these problems are minor illnesses that can be cared for at home. Others can become serious if they are not recognized and treated in a timely manner.

Disorders of the Nose and Sinuses

EPISTAXIS

Pathophysiology

Epistaxis is more commonly known as a nosebleed. The nose can bleed either from the anterior or posterior region. Anterior bleeds are much more common and originate from a group of vessels called the Kiesselbach plexus. Anterior bleeds are easier to locate and treat than posterior bleeds, because the posterior nose has larger vessels, and bleeding can be severe and difficult to control.

Etiology

The most common cause of epistaxis is dry, cracked mucous membranes. Trauma, forceful nose blowing, nose picking, and increased pressure on fragile capillaries from hypertension are also factors. Anything that reduces the blood's ability to clot, such as hemophilia or leukemia, regular aspirin use, anticoagulant therapy, or chemotherapy, can also predispose a client to nosebleeds.

Treatment

The nurse instructs the client with a nosebleed to sit in a chair and lean forward slightly, to avoid aspirating or swallowing blood. If the client swallows blood, it will be difficult to assess the extent of bleeding. Pressure is placed on the nares for 5 to 10 minutes to stop bleeding. Pressure is avoided if it is possible that the nose is broken, to avoid further trauma. Ice packs to the nose and eye area may be used to constrict the vessels causing the bleeding. Once bleeding is stopped, the client is instructed to avoid blowing the nose for several hours to prevent further bleeding.

If first aid measures are ineffective, the physician may attempt more invasive treatment. Local application of epinephrine causes constriction of the bleeding vessels. If the bleeding vessel can be located, the physician may cauterize it by use of an electrical cauterizing device, or by application of silver nitrate.

Gauze may be used to pack the anterior or posterior nasal cavity. The anterior cavity is packed firmly but gently, usually with half-inch petroleum gauze. To pack the posterior cavity, the physician must use a catheter and string via the nose to draw the packing through the mouth and into the posterior nasal cavity (Fig. 27–1). The strings are then brought out the mouth and taped to the client's face so they can be used 2 to 4 days later to remove the packing. Placement of packing can be very uncomfortable for the client. If there is time, administration of an analgesic before the procedure is helpful. Petroleum jelly on the packing helps prevent gauze from adhering to the nasal mucosa. If the packing is to remain in place for a prolonged period, it is coated with an antibiotic ointment to reduce the risk of infection.

Another method to stop bleeding is a nasal balloon catheter. This device employs a catheter with a balloon on the end that is inflated after placing it near the bleeding vessels in the nasal cavity. The balloon places pressure on the bleeding vessels, which stops bleeding.

If the client has lost a significant amount of blood, a transfusion may be necessary. Nosebleeds rarely cause death, because blood loss lowers blood pressure, which slows bleeding. Ultimately, the cause of the epistaxis is determined and corrected if possible.

Nursing Care

The nurse monitors the client for further bleeding, noting amount and color of drainage. Vital signs and hemoglobin level are monitored for signs of excessive blood loss. If the client swallows repeatedly, the nurse inspects the back of the throat for bleeding. If bleeding continues or worsens, the physician is notified immediately.

If posterior packing has been used, the client is monitored for airway obstruction from slipped packing. The nurse should be aware of how to remove the packing in case of emergency. The nurse also institutes comfort measures and maintains the placement of the strings that will be used to remove the packing. Once bleeding is controlled, the client is cautioned not to blow the nose for several hours and to avoid nose picking.

CRITICAL THINKING: Mr. Jondahl

Mr. Jondahl is brought to the emergency room with a nosebleed. His vital signs are 140/90, 92, 20. He states that he has never had a nosebleed before. He denies any history of coagulation disorders. His medications at home include captopril (Capoten), furosemide (Lasix), and ibuprofen (Motrin). What are two areas the nurse should assess further in trying to determine a cause? (Hint: If you are not familiar with Mr. Jondahl's medications, look them up.)
Answers at end of chapter.

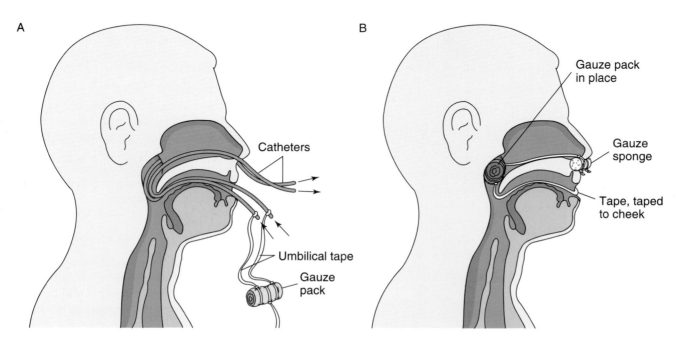

Figure 27–1. Nasal packing. *(A)* Catheters are used to pull packing into place. *(B)* Nasal packing in place.

NASAL POLYPS

Pathophysiology and Etiology

Polyps are grapelike clusters of mucosa in the nasal passages. They are usually benign, but they can obstruct the nasal passages. Though the exact cause is unknown, people with allergies are prone to developing polyps. Some clients with nasal polyps also have asthma and are allergic to aspirin. This is called triad disease because the three components often occur together.

Treatment

Control of allergy symptoms may help control polyp development. If polyps obstruct breathing, they can be removed. This is done as an outpatient procedure under local anesthesia, using laser or endoscopic surgery. Clients are taught to avoid aspirin products following surgery because they increase the risk of postoperative bleeding.

DEVIATED SEPTUM

Pathophysiology and Etiology

The septum dividing the nasal passages is slightly deviated in most adults. This may result from nasal trauma but often has no cause. Some may be so deviated as to block sinus drainage or interfere with breathing.

Signs and Symptoms

The client may complain of a chronically stuffy nose, or discomfort from blocked sinus drainage. Some clients have headaches and nosebleeds.

Medical Treatment

If the deviated septum is causing chronic discomfort, a submucous resection (SMR) or nasoseptoplasty is done. This surgery involves making an incision through the mucous membrane covering the septum and removing the deviated portion. Nasal packing is then placed to reduce bleeding. It is generally done as an outpatient procedure, under local anesthetic.

Nursing Care

Vital signs and bleeding are monitored until the client is stable following surgery. Excessive swallowing alerts the nurse to check for blood running down the back of the throat. The client will have nasal packing and a "mustache dressing" of folded gauze under the nose to catch drainage.

Most clients are discharged home once they are stable, so teaching is very important. The client should maintain a semi-Fowler's position as much as possible and avoid anything that might cause bleeding, such as sneezing, coughing, or straining to move the bowels. Stool softeners and cough suppressants may be ordered by the physician if necessary. Aspirin and related medications are avoided because they increase the risk of bleeding. The physician should be contacted for specific orders if the client is on anticoagulant therapy at home. Ice can be used to reduce swelling and bruising. The client should be instructed to contact the physician if fever, excessive pain, swelling, or bleeding occur and to return in 24 to 48 hours for removal of nasal packing. See Table 27–1 for client teaching after nasal surgery.

RHINOPLASTY

Rhinoplasty is the surgical reconstruction of the nose, usually for cosmetic purposes. It may also be done to correct deformity caused by trauma. Nursing care is similar to that for the client after SMR, described previously and in Table 27–1.

SINUSITIS

Pathophysiology and Etiology

Sinusitis is inflammation of the mucosa of one or more sinuses. It can be either acute or chronic. Chronic sinusitis is diagnosed if symptoms are present for more than 2 months and are unresponsive to treatment. The maxillary and ethmoid sinuses are the most commonly affected. The inflammation is often the result of a bacterial infection and may follow a viral upper respiratory illness. Because the mucous lining of the nose and sinuses is continuous, nasal organisms easily travel to the sinuses. When the infected mucous lining of the sinuses swells, drainage is blocked. Bacteria that normally reside in the sinuses multiply in the retained secretions. The most common infecting organisms are *Streptococcus pneumoniae* and *Haemophilus influenzae*. Other causes of sinusitis include swelling due to aller-

---

Table 27–1. **Client Teaching after Nasal Surgery**

1. Your nose will feel stuffy and may drain. Change the moustache dressing as often as needed. *Do not* blow your nose. If you must sneeze, do so with your mouth open.
2. Drink plenty of fluids unless your physician advises otherwise.
3. Use a cool mist vaporizer to humidify air and prevent nasal drying.
4. Keep your head elevated on two pillows or sleep in a recliner chair.
5. An ice pack on your face may help reduce swelling.
6. Take pain medication as prescribed.
7. Call your physician if you have a fever over 101°F.
8. Return to see your physician in _____ days.

---

rhinoplasty: rhin—nose + plasty—to mold

gies, fungal infection, or intubation with a nasotracheal or nasogastric tube.

Signs and Symptoms

The client usually has pain over the region of the affected sinuses and purulent nasal discharge. If a maxillary sinus is affected, the client will experience pain over the cheek and upper teeth. In ethmoid sinusitis, pain will occur between and behind the eyes. Pain in the forehead indicates frontal sinusitis. Fever may be present in acute infection, with or without generalized fatigue and foul breath.

Complications

The client who has not complied with treatment, or who has received inadequate treatment, is at risk for complications. Uncontrolled sinusitis may spread to surrounding areas, causing osteomyelitis, cellulitis of the orbit (infection of the soft tissues around the eye), abscess, or meningitis.

Diagnostic Tests

Uncomplicated sinusitis may be diagnosed based on symptoms alone. If repeated episodes occur, x-rays, a computed tomography (CT) scan, or magnetic resonance imaging (MRI) may be done to confirm the diagnosis and determine the cause. Nasal discharge may be cultured in order to determine appropriate antibiotic therapy.

Medical Treatment

Treatment is aimed at relieving pain and promoting sinus drainage. Adrenergic nasal sprays such as oxymetazoline (Afrin, Allerest) constrict blood vessels and therefore reduce swelling, but they should be used cautiously in individuals with heart disease or hypertension. Sprays may be used for up to 3 days; longer use may cause rebound congestion. Hot moist packs over the affected sinus for 1 to 2 hours twice a day may help decrease inflammation. Acetaminophen is given for pain and fever. Codeine or meperidine may be used if pain is severe. Expectorants such as guaifenesin (Robitussin), fluids, and room humidification help liquefy secretions. Antihistamines dry and thicken secretions and are generally avoided. Antibiotics are used only if bacterial infection is suspected, as in the client with purulent drainage and fever. If conservative treatment does not relieve symptoms, the physician may surgically drain the affected sinus and irrigate it with normal saline or an antibiotic solution.

One drainage procedure is the Caldwell-Luc procedure. The surgeon enters the maxillary sinus above the upper teeth, under the upper lip. The infected mucosa and bone are removed, and a new, larger opening is made to drain the sinus. Newer procedures use endoscopy to open and drain a chronically infected sinus.

Nursing Care

Clients with uncomplicated sinusitis are cared for at home. The nurse instructs the client to increase water intake to 8 to 10 glasses per day unless contraindicated. Pressure may be relieved if the client maintains a semi-Fowler's position, as in a reclining chair. Use of hot moist packs, acetaminophen, and prescribed medications is explained. The client is instructed to finish the antibiotic prescription even if he or she is feeling better before it is completed, and to call the physician if pain becomes severe or if signs of complications such as a change in level of consciousness occur.

Infectious Disorders

RHINITIS/COMMON COLD

Pathophysiology and Etiology

Rhinitis (also called coryza) is inflammation of the nasal mucous membranes. The release of histamine and other substances causes vasodilation and edema, which result in symptoms. It may occur as a reaction to allergens (sometimes called hay fever) such as pollen, dust, or some foods, or it may be caused by viral or bacterial infection. Viral rhinitis is another name for the common cold.

Signs and Symptoms

Common symptoms include nasal congestion, localized itching, sneezing, and nasal discharge. Viral or bacterial rhinitis may also be accompanied by fever and generalized malaise.

Diagnostic Tests

If allergic rhinitis is suspected, skin testing may be done to determine the offending allergens.

Treatment

Treatment of viral rhinitis is symptomatic. Because the majority of colds are caused by viruses, antibiotics are not effective. In one study however, researchers found that 60 percent of clients who visited their physician for cold symptoms received a prescription for an antibiotic.[1] This practice is not only expensive, it also increases the risk of developing strains of bacteria that are resistant to antibiotics. The nurse can help explain to the client that requesting antibiotics for a viral infection is not only ineffective, but potentially dangerous. The nurse teaches the client that rest and fluids are the most effective treatment.

---

rhinitis: rhin—nose + itis—inflammation

Antihistamines may be used to help control symptoms by inhibiting the histamine response. Decongestants cause vasoconstriction, which reduces swelling and congestion. *Any drugs that cause vasoconstriction should be used cautiously in clients with heart disease or hypertension.* Severe allergies may be treated with desensitization ("allergy shots"). See Nursing Care Plan Box 27–1 for the Client with an Upper Respiratory Infection.

PHARYNGITIS

Pathophysiology and Etiology

Inflammation of the pharynx is usually related to bacterial or viral infection. It may also occur as a result of trauma to the tissues. The most common bacterial infection is caused by β-hemolytic streptococci, commonly referred to as strep throat. If strep throat is not treated with antibiotics, it can lead to rheumatic fever, glomerulonephritis, or other complications.

Signs and Symptoms

The most common symptom of pharyngitis is a sore throat. Some clients may also experience **dysphagia** (difficulty swallowing). The throat appears red and swollen, and **exudate** (drainage or pus) may be present. Exudate usually signifies bacterial infection and may be accompanied by fever, chills, headache, and generalized malaise.

Diagnostic Tests

The physician may order a throat culture and sensitivity (explained in Chapter 26) to identify the causative organism and determine which antibiotic will be effective.

Treatment

If the pharyngitis is bacterial, antibiotics are ordered. Acetaminophen or throat lozenges may be used to relieve discomfort. Saltwater gargles help reduce swelling, and increased fluids (if not contraindicated) and rest are encouraged. See Nursing Care Plan Box 27–1 for the Client with an Upper Respiratory Infection.

LARYNGITIS

Pathophysiology and Etiology

Laryngitis is an inflammation of the mucous membrane lining the larynx (voice box). It can be caused by irritation from smoking, alcohol, or chemical exposure; or a viral,

fungal, or bacterial infection. If often follows an upper respiratory infection.

Signs and Symptoms

The most common symptom is hoarseness of the voice. Cough, dysphagia, or fever may also be present.

Diagnostic Tests

The physician may use a laryngeal mirror to view the larynx. If hoarseness persists for more than 2 weeks, a laryngoscopy is done to rule out cancer of the larynx.

Treatment

Treatment includes rest, fluids, humidified air, and aspirin or acetaminophen. Antibiotics are used if bacterial infection is present. The nurse encourages the client to avoid speaking in order to rest the voice. A magic slate or paper and pen may be used to communicate. Throat lozenges may help increase comfort. The nurse instructs the client to identify and avoid causative factors. See Nursing Care Plan Box 27–1 for the Client with an Upper Respiratory Infection.

TONSILLITIS/ADENOIDITIS

Pathophysiology and Etiology

The tonsils are masses of lymphoid tissue that lie on each side of the oropharynx. They filter microorganisms, thus protecting the lungs from infection. Tonsillitis occurs when the filtering function becomes overwhelmed with a virus or bacteria, and infection results. The adenoids, a mass of lymphoid tissue located at the back of the nasopharynx, can also become involved. Tonsillitis is more common in children, but it is more serious when it occurs in adults. The most common organisms causing tonsillitis are *Streptococcus, Staphylococcus aureus, Haemophilus influenzae,* and *Pneumococcus.*

Signs and Symptoms

Tonsillitis usually begins suddenly with sore throat, fever, chills, and pain on swallowing. Generalized symptoms include headache, malaise, and **myalgia.** On examination, the tonsils appear red and swollen and may have yellow or white exudate on them. The voice may sound like the client has a "hot potato" in his or her mouth. If the adenoids are involved, the client may have complaints of snoring, nasal obstruction, and a nasal tone to the voice.

Diagnostic Tests

A throat culture is done to discover the causative organism and determine effective treatment. A white blood cell count

---

dysphagia: dys—bad + phagia—to swallow
exudate: to sweat out
myalgia: myo—muscle + algia—pain

NURSING CARE PLAN BOX 27–1
FOR THE CLIENT WITH AN UPPER RESPIRATORY INFECTION

Altered comfort related to infectious process

Client Outcomes
Client will be comfortable as evidenced by (1) statement of increased comfort and (2) ability to sleep at night.

Evaluation of Outcomes
(1) Does client express comfort? (2) Is client able to sleep?

Interventions	Rationale	Evaluation
• Assess for cause of discomfort: malaise, muscle aches, fever.	Knowing cause of discomfort helps guide intervention.	Can interventions be directed toward specific symptoms?
• Offer acetaminophen or other analgesic/antipyretics as ordered.	Analgesics relieve pain. Antipyretics relieve fever, which may contribute to discomfort.	Do analgesics/antipyretics relieve discomfort?
• Offer throat lozenges and saltwater gargles as ordered for irritated throat.	Lozenges soothe irritated mucous membranes. Saltwater gargles may reduce swelling.	Do measures relieve throat irritation?
• Encourage rest.	Physical stress increases need for sleep. Rest boosts immune function	Is client resting comfortably?

Hyperthermia related to infectious process

Client Outcomes
(1) Temperature below 103°F. (2) No signs/symptoms of dehydration.

Evaluation of Outcomes
(1) Is fever controlled at safe level? (2) Is client well hydrated?

Interventions	Rationale	Evaluation
• Monitor temperature daily; every 4 hours if fever present.	Screening helps detect temperature changes early.	Is client febrile?
• If client begins chilling, recheck temperature when chilling subsides.	Chilling indicates rising temperature.	Is chilling present? Should temperature be checked more often?
• Monitor for signs of dehydration: dry skin and mucous membranes, thirst, weakness, hypotension.	Fever causes loss of body fluids.	Are signs of dehydration present?
• Encourage oral fluids if not contraindicated.	Fluids prevent or treat dehydration.	Is client taking fluids well?
• Administer antipyretic such as acetaminophen if fever over 102.5°F or for discomfort.	Antipyretics reduce fever. Fever enhances immune function, so should only be treated if very high, if client has a history of febrile seizures, or if client is uncomfortable.	Is fever over 102.5°F? Are antipyretics indicated? Are they effective?

Risk for infection: transmission to others related to presence of infectious disease

Client Outcomes
Risk for infection of others is reduced, as evidenced by the following: (1) Client states measures to prevent transmission. (2) Client takes precautions against spread.

Evaluation of Outcomes
Is transmission to others prevented?

continued

NURSING CARE PLAN BOX 27-1 *(continued)*		
Interventions	*Rationale*	*Evaluation*
• Assess client's understanding of infection transmission. • Based on client's previous knowledge, teach client and all caregivers the importance of good hand washing after contact with client or client's belongings, covering nose and mouth when coughing or sneezing, and not sharing eating or drinking utensils.	Understanding of mode of transmission is essential to prevention. The nurse should build on client's previous understanding and not repeat information. Hand washing prevents spread of infection. Covering nose and mouth prevents spread of infectious droplets. Many infections are transmitted via contaminated objects.	Does client understand how infection is transmitted? Does client take precautions to prevent spread of infection?

helps determine whether the infection is viral or bacterial. A chest x-ray may be done if respiratory symptoms are present.

Treatment

Antibiotics are prescribed for bacterial infection. Acetaminophen, lozenges, and saline gargles help promote comfort. For care of the client who is not having a tonsillectomy, see Nursing Care Plan Box 27–1 for the Client with an Upper Respiratory Infection.

If tonsillitis becomes chronic, or if an abscess occurs, a tonsillectomy may be performed. An adenoidectomy may be performed at the same time. After the tonsillectomy, the client is maintained in a semi-Fowler's position to reduce swelling and promote drainage. The nurse monitors the client for bleeding and airway patency and provides comfort measures. Fluids are encouraged for hydration; cold fluids may help reduce pain and bleeding. Red-colored drinks are avoided because they interfere with observation for bleeding. Suction equipment should be available for emergencies.

 CRITICAL THINKING: Mrs. Hiler

You are assessing Mrs. Hiler after a tonsillectomy. She is sleeping, but you notice that she swallows every few seconds. How do you respond?
Answer at end of chapter.

INFLUENZA

Pathophysiology and Etiology

Influenza, commonly referred to as the flu, is a viral infection that affects the respiratory tract. Many different viruses have been identified, and new strains appear each year, making immunization difficult. It is the cause of millions of lost work days each year. The elderly are particularly at risk for complications and even death from influenza, because of compromised immune function.

Influenza is easily transmitted via droplets from coughs and sneezes of infected individuals, or it may be transmitted by physical contact with a person or object that harbors the virus. The incubation period from time of exposure to onset of symptoms is 1 to 3 days.

Prevention

Yearly immunization is recommended for prevention of influenza, especially for the elderly and others at risk for complications. Immunization of healthy adults has also been shown to reduce the incidence of influenza and to decrease absenteeism from work.[2] Immunization of health care workers helps prevent spread to at-risk clients. Other preventive measures include hand washing and avoidance of individuals with influenza.

Signs and Symptoms

Symptoms include abrupt onset of fever, chills, myalgia, sore throat, cough, general malaise, and headache. It can last for 2 to 5 days, with malaise lasting up to several weeks.

Complications

The most common complication of influenza is pneumonia, which may be caused by the same virus as the flu, or by a secondary bacterial infection. This should be considered if the client experiences persistent fever and shortness of breath or if the lungs develop crackles or wheezes.

Diagnostic Tests

Sputum or throat cultures may be done to determine the cause of symptoms.

Medical Treatment

Treatment is symptomatic. Acetaminophen is given for fever, headache, and myalgia. Aspirin is avoided in children because it increases the risk for Reye's syndrome. Rest and fluids are essential. Antibiotics are used only if a secondary bacterial infection is present. Antiviral drugs such as amantadine may be helpful for high-risk clients if given within 48 hours of exposure.

Nursing Care

The elderly or other high-risk client may be hospitalized for influenza. These clients should be closely monitored for signs of complications. The nurse assesses lung sounds and vital signs every 4 hours and reports changes to the physician. Rest and fluids (if not contraindicated) are encouraged, and comfort measures are provided. Parents are educated about avoiding aspirin to treat influenza symptoms, to prevent Reye's syndrome. See Nursing Care Plan Box 27–1 for the Client with an Upper Respiratory Infection.

Malignant Disorders

CANCER OF THE LARYNX

Pathophysiology

Cancer of the larynx usually develops in the mucosal epithelium. It is evaluated based on the TNM staging system. (See Chapter 10.) It is usually a primary cancer and may spread to the lungs, liver, or lymph nodes. The prognosis for a client with laryngeal cancer is often poor because metastasis (spread) may have occurred before the client sought help.

Etiology

Risk factors for cancer of the larynx include a history of alcohol and tobacco use. Exposure to industrial chemicals, hardwood dust, and chronic overuse of the voice are also factors. Men are five times as likely to be affected as women.

Prevention

Prevention begins with education; the nurse can help educate clients about the relationship between cancer of the larynx and abuse of alcohol and tobacco. It is also important to teach clients to seek help when symptoms first occur, because a delayed diagnosis may mean metastasis of the cancer and a poor prognosis. Any hoarseness of the voice for longer than 2 weeks should be investigated.

Signs and Symptoms

The most common symptom is hoarseness of the voice, because the vocal cords are located within the larynx. The client may also have pain, shortness of breath, a chronic cough, and difficulty swallowing. Stridor may indicate a tumor obstructing the airway. Late symptoms include weight loss and halitosis (foul breath).

Diagnostic Tests

The larynx can be examined with a laryngeal mirror. Laryngoscopic examination with biopsy is used to diagnose and determine the stage of laryngeal cancer. A CT scan or MRI may be done to determine the presence or extent of metastasis.

Medical Treatment

If laryngeal cancer is diagnosed early in the disease, it may be treatable with radiation therapy; this treatment can preserve the client's voice. In more advanced cases, surgical intervention is necessary. The larynx will be either partially or completely removed (Fig. 27–2). If cancer has spread beyond the larynx, a radical neck dissection, which removes adjacent muscle, lymph nodes, and tissue, may be done. Surgery can be done using laser technology, endoscopy, or traditional methods. After a partial laryngectomy the client may have a permanently hoarse voice. If a total laryngectomy is done, the client will have a permanent tracheostomy and no voice. Alternative methods of communication must be learned.

Nursing Process: The Client Undergoing Laryngectomy

Assessment

The nurse provides ongoing assessment of the client's physical and psychosocial status. Assessment of comfort, nutritional status, and ability to swallow is important both before and after surgery. After surgery, assessment of respiratory function and airway patency is vital. The nurse monitors lung sounds, pulse oximetry, and arterial blood gases. In addition, the nurse assesses the client's understanding of the disease process and self-care needs after surgery. It is important to evaluate the client's support systems and ability to cope with the partial or total loss of voice after surgery.

Nursing Diagnosis

Possible diagnoses include altered comfort related to surgical procedure, ineffective airway clearance related to excessive secretions and new tracheostomy, altered health maintenance related to knowledge deficit regarding self-care, impaired communication related to loss of vocal cords, altered nutrition related to absence of oral feeding, impaired swallowing related to edema or laryngectomy tube, grieving related to loss of voice, and body image disturbance related to change in body structure and function. Many more nursing diagnoses may also be identified based on individual assessment, because of the many implications of this disease and surgery.

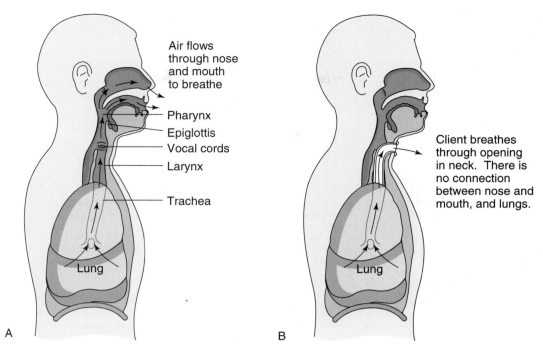

Figure 27–2. Laryngectomy. *(A)* Before laryngectomy. *(B)* After laryngectomy.

Planning, Implementation, and Client Education

ALTERED COMFORT RELATED TO SURGICAL PROCEDURE. Analgesics are given as ordered, on an around-the-clock basis or via a client-controlled pump rather than prn, for the first few days after surgery. If the liver has been damaged from alcohol abuse, dosages are adjusted by the physician. Narcotics are given carefully because they may reduce the cough reflex, which is vital to clearing the airway. Distraction and relaxation are also helpful.

INEFFECTIVE AIRWAY CLEARANCE RELATED TO EXCESSIVE SECRETIONS AND NEW TRACHEOSTOMY. The client will have a laryngectomy tube in place after surgery. A laryngectomy tube is shorter and has a larger diameter than a tracheostomy tube, but care is the same. Routine tracheostomy care and suctioning are done according to hospital policy to keep the airway clear. (See Chapter 26.) Strict sterile technique is essential. The client is encouraged to deep breathe and cough every hour. A special tracheostomy collar may be used to provide oxygen and humidification. The nurse monitors and records amount, color, and consistency of secretions; vital signs; lung sounds; and signs of respiratory distress. Signs of infection or respiratory distress are reported to the physician immediately.

ALTERED HEALTH MAINTENANCE RELATED TO KNOWLEDGE DEFICIT REGARDING SELF-CARE. The client must be taught self-care measures for his or her tracheostomy. See Chapter 26 for this procedure. The nurse should involve the significant other or family whenever possible. Referral to home nursing after discharge will provide assessment of the home environment as well as follow-up instruction. A social service referral may be made for financial concerns if needed. The nurse should consult with the physician or check the local phone directory for **laryngectomee** support groups, and refer the client to them if appropriate.

IMPAIRED COMMUNICATION RELATED TO LOSS OF VOCAL CORDS. A variety of techniques and devices are available to assist the client with communication needs. The speech therapist can provide a picture board, magic slate, or paper and pencil before surgery. The client is instructed to point to the picture that corresponds with his or her need or to write out his or her concern. This can help prevent panic after surgery when the client has a need and cannot speak.

After surgery, the nurse, speech therapist, and physician work together to provide the client with a method of communication that best fits his or her needs (Fig. 27–3). Esophageal speech involves swallowing air and forming words as it is regurgitated back up the esophagus. Also available are electronic devices that the client places next to the neck or mouth. These devices use sound waves to help the client form words. Another alternative is a special surgically implanted voice prosthesis that creates a valve between the trachea and esophagus. If the client holds a finger over the tracheostomy, air is diverted into the esophagus, and the client forms words as the air exits via the

---

laryngectomee: larng—larynx + ectome—excision (person who has undergone laryngectomy)

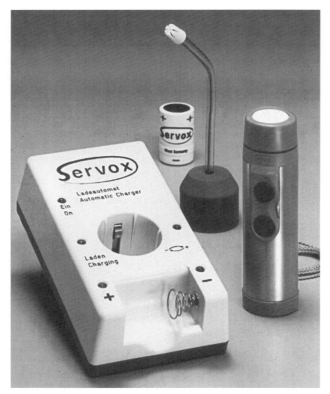

Figure 27–3. Devices to aid speech in laryngectomy client. (Courtesy of Siemens Hearing Instruments, New York.)

mouth. All of these devices take time to adjust to, and the client will need support after discharge to continue to develop skill in communication.

ALTERED NUTRITION RELATED TO ABSENCE OF ORAL FEEDING. Most clients receive parenteral nutrition or tube feedings after surgery until the neck has begun to heal and swallowing can be evaluated. If the client has a history of alcohol abuse, he or she may have been undernourished before surgery. The nurse must advocate for the client and ensure that he or she is receiving adequate calories for healing. It is also important to keep the client's head elevated a minimum of 30 degrees during and at least 30 minutes after tube feedings to prevent aspiration. Some institutions add blue dye to tube feedings to help identify whether tracheostomy secretions are due to aspiration. The nurse should be aware that this may cause a blue-green tinge to urine and stool as well.

IMPAIRED SWALLOWING RELATED TO EDEMA OR LARYN-GECTOMY TUBE. The client should be carefully assessed for ability to swallow safely before initiating oral feeding. The physician may order special swallowing studies to determine how well the client can swallow. The speech therapist can also be helpful in evaluating swallowing. The nurse should be sure to obtain and follow specific instructions provided by the professional who has evaluated the client's swallowing, and be sure that the client and family have received the same instructions before discharge. Of-

ten such instructions are posted above the client's bed so they are available to everyone.

The nurse should have the client sit upright for feeding and remain upright for 30 to 45 minutes after eating. It is often helpful to have the client swallow each bite twice. Thin liquids are avoided because they are more easily aspirated. Special thickening agents are available to add to thin liquids. Suction equipment should be kept nearby in case of aspiration. The new laryngectomee should *not* be left alone while eating.

GRIEVING RELATED TO LOSS OF VOICE. Inability to speak is a loss that cannot be overemphasized. Clients will grieve as they do any other loss. In addition to voice loss, the client may also be facing a career change, if job-related exposure contributed to the disease, or if loss of voice prevents returning to the previously held job. Assessing and involving support systems is important. The family is encouraged to communicate with the client even though it is often difficult, and to be patient as the client learns to communicate with them. Local support groups may have names of individuals who have had similar experiences who are willing to visit with the client. Of course whenever referring to this type of visitor, it is important that the visitor has a positive attitude and has dealt effectively with a similar loss.

BODY IMAGE DISTURBANCE RELATED TO CHANGE IN BODY STRUCTURE AND FUNCTION. In addition to changes in voice, the laryngectomee also now breaths through a hole in his or her neck. In time, the client may not need a tracheostomy tube, but the hole remains intact. This causes a change in body image. Again, a visitor who has been through this experience, and much support from staff and family, can be helpful. The nurse portrays an accepting attitude and allows the client to share his or her feelings if the client indicates a need to do so.

The client must also be instructed to perform gentle range of motion exercises of the neck. Some clients may avoid extending the neck because of the location of the incision, causing muscle contracture and eventual inability to do so.

Evaluation

When evaluating the client's progress toward goals, the nurse asks the following questions: Does the client verbalize an acceptable level of comfort? Is the airway clear, without signs of infection? Do the client and significant other demonstrate understanding of self-care at home or have referrals to continue learning self-care at home? Does the client indicate that he or she is satisfied with the level and quality of communication? Are nutritional needs met as evidenced by albumin levels greater than 3.0 and stable weight? Is the client able to swallow without aspirating if taking oral nutrition? Is the client able to grieve appropriately, and does the client have someone to talk to if he or she wishes? Finally, does the client show acceptance of the laryngectomy by learning to look at it and care for it? It should be noted that many of these evaluative criteria are long term and may not be seen while the client is hospitalized.

Review Questions

1. Which of the following positions is recommended for a client experiencing a nosebleed?
   a. Lying down with feet elevated
   b. Sitting up with neck fully extended
   c. Lying down with a small pillow under the head
   d. Sitting up leaning slightly forward

2. Which of the following is the best explanation by the nurse for why the physician did not prescribe antibiotics for influenza?
   a. Most cases of influenza are caused by antibiotic-resistant bacteria.
   b. Most cases of influenza are caused by viruses.
   c. Antibiotics have too many serious side effects.
   d. Antibiotics can interact with other medications used for influenza.

3. After a laryngectomy, which of the following assessments takes *priority?*
   a. Airway patency
   b. Nutritional status
   c. Lung sounds
   d. Client acceptance of surgery

4. The nurse can assist the laryngectomy client to communicate by all of the following *except:*
   a. Having the client place a finger over the stoma
   b. Providing a special valve that diverts air into the esophagus
   c. Obtaining a picture board
   d. Teaching the client esophageal speech

5. Which of the following statements best explains why the nurse is careful when administering narcotics to a laryngectomee?
   a. Most laryngectomees have been drug addicts in the past.
   b. Even low doses of narcotics may cause respiratory arrest in the laryngectomee.
   c. Narcotics can depress the cough reflex.
   d. Laryngectomy clients have no pain after surgery.

ANSWERS TO CRITICAL THINKING

CRITICAL THINKING: Mr. Jondahl

The nurse should consider the possibility of hypertension as a contributing factor. Mr. Jondahl's blood pressure is currently 140/90, which may be lower than normal for him because he has been bleeding. He is also on an antihypertensive drug and a diuretic. The nurse should also explore the amount of Motrin being taken daily, because nonsteroidal anti-inflammatory agents, such as aspirin, can prolong clotting.

CRITICAL THINKING: Mrs. Hiler

Mrs. Hiler may be swallowing blood. Examine the back of her throat with a flashlight. Check vital signs for signs of impending shock. Notify the physician if bleeding is confirmed.

REFERENCES

1. Mainous, AG, et al: Antibiotics and upper respiratory infection. J Fam Pract 42:4, 1996.
2. Nichol, KL, et al: The effectiveness of vaccination against influenza in healthy, working adults. N Engl J Med 333:14, 1995.

BIBLIOGRAPHY

Ackley, BJ, and Ladwig, GB: Nursing Diagnosis Handbook: A Guide to Planning Care. Mosby, St Louis, 1995.
Ferguson, BJ: Acute and chronic sinusitis. Postgrad Med 97:5, 1995.
Fried, MP, and Girdhar-Gopal, HV: Advanced cancer of the larynx. In Bailey, BJ (ed): Head and Neck Surgery—Otolaryngology. JB Lippincott, Philadelphia, 1993, p 1347.
Harding, M: Preparing patients for the effects of laryngectomy. Nurs Times 90(32):36, 1994.
Isselbacher, KJ, et al: Harrison's Principles of Internal Medicine. McGraw-Hill, New York, 1994.
McCance, CL, and Huether, SE: Pathophysiology: The Biologic Basis for Disease in Adults and Children, ed 2. Mosby, St Louis, 1994.
Schuller, DE, and Schleuning, AJ: DeWeese and Saunders' Otolaryngology—Head and Neck Surgery. Mosby, St Louis, 1994.
Viducich, RA, et al: Posterior epistaxis: Clinical features and acute complications. Ann Emerg Med 25:5, 1995.
Watson, J, and Jaffe, MS: Nurse's Manual of Laboratory and Diagnostic Tests, ed 2. FA Davis, Philadelphia, 1995.

28

Nursing Care of Clients with Lower Respiratory Tract Disorders

Paula D. Hopper

Learning Objectives

Upon completion of this chapter, the student will be able to:

1. Describe the pathophysiology, etiology, signs and symptoms, diagnosis, and treatment of disorders of the lower respiratory tract.

2. Use the nursing process to develop a plan of care for a client with an infectious disorder of the lower respiratory tract.

3. Describe the disorders that cause chronic airflow limitation.

4. Use the nursing process to develop a plan of care for a client with chronic airflow limitation.

5. Relate tobacco use as a cause of many respiratory diseases.

6. Describe care of the client who has experienced chest trauma.

7. Describe warning signs of respiratory failure.

8. Identify risk factors for lung cancer.

9. Describe preoperative and postoperative nursing care for clients undergoing thoracic surgery.

10. Identify interventions with rationale for clients experiencing impaired gas exchange, ineffective airway clearance, and ineffective breathing pattern.

Key Words

adjuvant (ad-**JOO**-vant)

anergy (**A**-ner-jee)

antitussive (AN-tee-**TUSS**-iv)

atelectasis (AT-e-**LEK**-tah-sis)

atypical (ay-**TIP**-i-kuhl)

bleb (BLEB)

bronchiectasis (BRONG-key-**EK**-tah-sis)

bronchitis (brong-**KIGH**-tis)

bronchodilator (BRONG-koh-**DYE**-lay-ter)

bronchospasm (**BRONG**-koh-spazm)

bulla (**BUHL**-ah)

compliance (kom-**PLIGH**-ens)

ectopic (ek-**TOP**-ik)

embolism (**EM**-boh-lizm)

emphysema (EM-fi-**SEE**-mah)

empyema (EM-pigh-**EE**-mah)

expectorant (ek-**SPEK**-tuh-rant)

exudate (**EKS**-yoo-dayt)

hemoptysis (hee-**MOP**-ti-sis)

hemothorax (HEE-moh-**THAW**-raks)

hypostatic (HIGH-poh-**STA**-tik)

immunocompromised (IM-yoo-noh-**KAHM**-prah-mized)

induration (IN-dyoo-**RAY**-shun)

lobectomy (loh-**BEK**-tuh-mee)

mucolytic (MYOO-koh-**LIT**-ik)

paradoxical respirations (PAR-uh-**DOK**-si-kuhl RES-pi-**RAY**-shuns)

pleurodesis (PLOO-roh-**DEE**-sis)

pneumonectomy (NEW-moh-**NEK**-tuh-mee)

pneumothorax (NEW-moh-**THAW**-raks)

polycythemia (PAH-lee-sigh-**THEE**-mee-ah)

status asthmaticus (**STAT**-us az-**MAT**-i-kus)

tachypnea (TAK-ip-**NEE**-uh)

thoracotomy (THAW-rah-**KAH**-tah-mee)

Disorders of the lower respiratory tract include problems of the lower portion of the trachea, bronchi, bronchioles, and alveoli. These disorders may be related to infection, noninfectious alterations in function, neoplasm, or trauma. Any pathology of the lower respiratory tract can seriously impair carbon dioxide and oxygen exchange.

Infectious Disorders

ACUTE BRONCHITIS

Pathophysiology

Bronchitis is an inflammation of the bronchial tree, which includes the right and left bronchi, secondary bronchi, and the bronchioles. When the mucous membranes lining the bronchial tree become irritated and inflamed, excessive mucus is produced. The result is congested airways.

Etiology

Bronchitis may be caused by irritation or infection. Irritation can result from smoking, inhalation of fumes or particulate matter, or air pollution, among other causes. Viral infections are the most common cause, which may then lead to a secondary bacterial infection. Bacterial infection causes mucus to become purulent.

Signs and Symptoms

A harsh cough is the most characteristic symptom of bronchitis. The cough often produces thick sputum, with the largest amounts being produced in the morning. If bronchitis is infectious, a fever and general malaise will likely be present. Wheezes and crackles may be heard on auscultation, because the airways are narrowed from inflammation and the accumulation of mucus. The client may also experience chest pain or dyspnea and a hoarse voice.

Diagnostic Tests

Sputum cultures, chest x-ray, and symptoms reported by the client are used to diagnose bronchitis. The white blood cell count may be elevated, and arterial blood gases may show evidence of impaired gas exchange.

Medical Treatment

Antibiotics are used if bronchitis is caused by bacterial infection. The client who has underlying chronic respiratory disease may be hospitalized for intravenous antibiotic therapy. **Expectorants** such as guaifenesin (Robitussin, Humibid) can help the client bring up sputum. An **antitussive** may be helpful in suppressing a dry and aggravating cough. A productive cough should not be suppressed, because expectorating secretions is desirable. Theophylline or adrenergic **bronchodilators** help open airways and relieve dyspnea. Tylenol may be used for comfort and fever.

BRONCHIECTASIS

Pathophysiology

Bronchiectasis is a dilation of the bronchial airways (Fig. 28–1). These dilated areas form sacs that can remain localized or spread throughout the lungs. Secretions pool in these sacs and frequently become infected.

Etiology

Bronchiectasis usually occurs secondary to another chronic respiratory disorder, such as cystic fibrosis, asthma, tuberculosis, bronchitis, or exposure to a toxin. Infection and inflammation of the airways weakens the bronchial walls and reduces ciliary function. Airway obstruction from excessive secretions then predisposes the client to development of bronchiectasis.

Signs and Symptoms

The client with bronchiectasis has recurrent lower respiratory infections. Sputum is copious and purulent and pools in the dilated airways. The accompanying cough can produce as much as 200 mL of thick, foul-smelling sputum at any one time. Extreme airway inflammation may cause sputum to be bloody. If bronchiectasis is widespread, the client may experience dyspnea even with minimal exertion. Wheezes and crackles may be auscultated. Fever is present during active infection. Cor pulmonale and clubbing of the fingers may develop with chronic disease.

Diagnostic Tests

A chest x-ray may be done, but it may not show early disease. A computed tomography (CT) scan provides a better view of the dilated airways. Sputum cultures determine infecting organisms and guide antibiotic therapy. Additional testing is done to determine the cause of bronchiectasis.

---

bronchitis: bronch—airway + itis—inflammation
expectorant: ex—out + pect—breast
antitussive: anti—against + tussive—cough
bronchodilator: broncho—airway + dilator—to expand
bronchiectasis: bronch—airway + ectasis—dilation or expansion

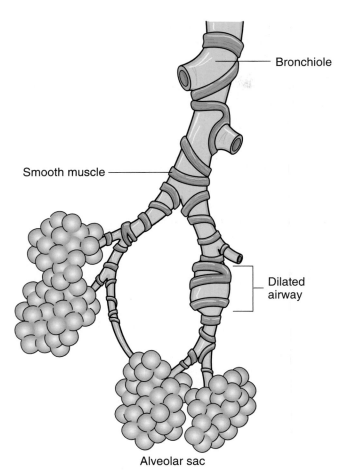

Figure 28–1. Bronchiectasis. Note dilated airway.

Medical Treatment

Treatment of bronchiectasis is aimed at keeping the airway clear of secretions, controlling infection, and correcting the underlying problem. Antibiotics may be used intermittently or for prolonged periods. Bronchodilators improve airway obstruction. **Mucolytic** agents may help thin secretions, and chest physiotherapy helps mobilize secretions so they can be more effectively expectorated. Oxygen is used if hypoxemia is present. If the affected area of the lung is localized and symptoms are severe, surgery may be considered to remove the diseased area.

PNEUMONIA

Pneumonia is the cause of more than 10 percent of hospital admissions each year and is the most common cause of death from infection.

---

mucolytic: muco—mucus + lytic—to break up
immunocompromised: immune—referring to immune system + compromised—lacks resistance
exudate: to sweat out

Pathophysiology

Pneumonia is an acute infection of the lungs, occurring when an infectious agent enters and multiplies in the lungs of a susceptible person. Infectious particles can come from the cough of an infected individual, from contaminated respiratory therapy equipment, from infections in other parts of the body, or from aspiration of stomach or oropharyngeal bacteria. Organisms from the oropharynx may be related to poor oral hygiene or may be present because of a cold or influenza virus. In a healthy person, normal respiratory defense mechanisms and the immune system prevent the development of infection. In a person who is **immunocompromised,** however, even microorganisms that are normally present in the oropharynx can develop into an infection. Persons at risk for pneumonia are the very young, the elderly, and those who are immunocompromised, such as people with acquired immunodeficiency syndrome (AIDS) or other chronic illness.

When the microorganisms multiply, they release toxins that cause inflammation in the lung tissue, causing damage to mucous and alveolar membranes. This causes the development of edema and **exudate,** which fill the alveoli and reduce the surface area available for exchange of carbon dioxide and oxygen. Some bacteria also cause necrosis of lung tissue.

Pneumonia may be confined to one lobe, or it may be scattered throughout the lungs. If it affects only one lobe, it is called lobar pneumonia. Generalized pneumonia is much more serious and is called bronchopneumonia. Bronchopneumonia occurs more often as a nosocomial (hospital-acquired) infection in hospitalized clients, the very young, or very old.

Etiology

Pneumonia has a variety of causes, listed below.

Bacterial Pneumonia

The most common cause of bacterial pneumonia acquired in the community is *Streptococcus pneumoniae.* This is often termed *pneumococcal* pneumonia. This organism accounts for approximately 90 percent of all bacterial pneumonias. Other community-acquired infections are caused by *Staphylococcus aureus* and *Mycoplasma pneumoniae.* Hospital-acquired pneumonias are often more serious, and may be caused by *Escherichia coli, Haemophilus influenzae,* and *Pseudomonas aeruginosa,* among others.

Viral Pneumonia

Influenza viruses are the most common cause of viral pneumonia. The presence of viral pneumonia increases the client's susceptibility to a secondary bacterial pneumonia. Generally, clients are less ill with viral pneumonia than with bacterial pneumonia, but they may be ill longer because antibiotics are ineffective against viruses.

Fungal Pneumonia

Candida and aspergillus are two types of fungi that can cause pneumonia. *Pneumocystis carinii* is also a fungal infection that typically causes pneumonia in clients with AIDS.

Aspiration Pneumonia

Some pneumonias are caused by aspiration of foreign substances. This most often occurs in clients with decreased levels of consciousness or an impaired cough or gag reflex. These conditions might occur due to alcohol ingestion, stroke, general anesthesia, seizures, or other serious illness. Aspiration pneumonia increases the risk for subsequent bacterial pneumonia.

Hypostatic Pneumonia

Clients who hypoventilate over a period of time due to bed rest, immobility, or shallow respirations are at risk for **hypostatic** pneumonia. Secretions pool in dependent areas of the lungs and can lead to inflammation and infection.

Chemical Pneumonia

Inhalation of toxic chemicals can cause inflammation and tissue damage, which can lead to chemical pneumonia.

CRITICAL THINKING: Mr. Smith

Mr. Smith is an 86-year-old gentleman who was watching television when he couldn't sleep one night. After seeing a commercial for toilet cleaner, he decided his own toilet could use some attention. He used bleach and ammonia, "to get it really clean." The combination created toxic fumes, which caused a severe chemical pneumonia. He was brought to the emergency room in acute respiratory distress.

1. As his nurse, what questions might you ask as you further assess the cause of his pneumonia?
2. What will you teach Mr. Smith related to prevention of similar episodes in the future?

Answers at end of chapter.

Prevention

A vaccine is available to help prevent pneumonias caused by *Streptococcus pneumoniae* and *Haemophilus influenzae* type B. It is effective about 80 to 90 percent of the time and requires only a one-time injection.

Nursing care plays an important role in the prevention of nosocomial pneumonia. Regular coughing and deep breathing for clients on bed rest or after surgery, prevention of aspiration for clients at risk, and good hand-washing practices by health care personnel can help prevent many cases. (See Gerontological Issues Box 28–1.)

GERONTOLOGICAL ISSUES BOX 28–1

Advanced age is a significant risk factor for serious complications from respiratory infections such as influenza and pneumococcal pneumonia. Therefore it is recommended that people over the age of 65 and individuals with chronic disease have yearly influenza vaccines and a once-in-a-lifetime pneumococcal vaccine.

Signs and Symptoms

Clients with pneumonia present with fever, shaking chills, chest pain, dyspnea, and a productive cough. Sputum is purulent or may be rust colored or blood tinged. Crackles and wheezes may be heard on lung auscultation.

Some bacterial and many viral pneumonias cause **atypical** symptoms. The client may experience fatigue, sore throat, dry cough, or nausea and vomiting.

Elderly clients may not exhibit expected symptoms of pneumonia. Confusion or lethargy in an elderly client can indicate reduced oxygenation and should alert the nurse to look for other symptoms or request further testing. New onset of fever or dyspnea should also cause suspicion of possible pneumonia in the elderly.

Complications

Complications from pneumonia most commonly occur in clients with other underlying chronic diseases. Pleurisy and pleural effusion (discussed later in this chapter) are two of the most common complications and generally resolve within 1 to 2 weeks. Atelectasis can occur due to trapped secretions and may be resolved with efforts to keep the airways clear. Other complications result from spread of infection to other parts of the body, causing meningitis, septic arthritis, pericarditis, and endocarditis. Treatment for each of these is antibiotics. Although antibiotics have greatly reduced the incidence of death related to pneumonia, it is still a common cause of death in the elderly.

Diagnostic Tests

A chest x-ray is done to identify the presence of pulmonary infiltrate (fluid leakage into the alveoli from inflammation). In addition, a sputum culture is obtained to identify the organism causing the pneumonia and determine an appropriate treatment. Whenever possible, the sputum sam-

hypostatic: hypo—below + static—standing
atypical: a—not + typical—usual

ple should be obtained before antibiotics are started, to avoid altering culture results. If the client is unable to produce a specimen, a nebulized mist treatment may be ordered to promote sputum expectoration. If this is unsuccessful, a bronchoscopy may be done in the very ill client to obtain a specimen. Blood cultures may also be done to help determine the source of infection.

Medical Treatment

Broad-spectrum antibiotics are initiated before sputum culture results are completed (though the nurse should be sure to obtain the specimen before starting the antibiotics). Once the culture and sensitivity report is available, specific antibiotics are ordered if the cause is bacterial. Many clients can be treated with oral antibiotics as outpatients, but hospitalization and intravenous therapy may be necessary in the elderly, chronically ill, or acutely ill individual.

Expectorants, bronchodilators, and analgesics may be given for comfort and symptom relief. Nebulized mist treatments or metered dose inhalers may be used to deliver bronchodilators. Supplemental oxygen via nasal cannula or mask is used as necessary.

TUBERCULOSIS

Pathophysiology

Tuberculosis (TB) is an infectious disease caused by *Mycobacterium tuberculosis*. TB primarily affects the lungs, although other areas, such as the kidneys, liver, brain, and bone, may be affected as well. *M. tuberculosis* is an acid-fast bacillus (AFB), which means that when it is stained in the laboratory and then washed with an acid, the stain remains, or stays fast. *M. tuberculosis* can live in dark places in dried sputum for months, but a few hours in direct sunlight will kill it. It is spread by inhalation of the tuberculosis bacilli from respiratory droplets (droplet nuclei) of an infected person. Once the bacilli enter the lungs, they multiply and begin to disseminate to the lymph nodes and then to other parts of the body. The client is then infected, but may or may not go on to develop clinical (active) disease. During this time the body develops immunity, which keeps the infection under control. The immune system surrounds the infected lung area with neutrophils and alveolar macrophages. This process creates a lesion called a tubercle, which seals off the bacteria and prevents spread. The bacteria within the tubercle die or become dormant, and the client is no longer infectious. If the client's immune system becomes compromised, however, some of the dormant bacteria can become active again, causing reinfection and active disease. Only 5 to 10 percent of infected individuals in the United States actually develop the disease, and even then it may not occur for many years. (See Gerontological Issues Box 28–2.)

LEARNING TIP

If the physician orders "sputum culture for AFB," tuberculosis is suspected. Ask whether precautions should be taken while waiting for culture results.

Etiology

Crowded or poorly ventilated living conditions place people at risk for becoming infected with tuberculosis. Although tuberculosis can infect any age group, the elderly are especially at risk. Elders may have contracted the disease many years before, but it reactivates as the aging process diminishes immune function. Clients with AIDS have a very high risk due to their compromised immune function. In the United States, tuberculosis is also prevalent among the urban poor and minority groups.

Before 1985, the incidence of TB was steadily decreasing. Now it is again on the rise, due in part to the prevalence of AIDS and the development of antibiotic-resistant strains of the TB bacillus.

Prevention

Clean, well-ventilated living areas are essential to the health of all people. If a hospitalized client is known or suspected to have tuberculosis, he or she is placed in respiratory isolation to prevent spread to staff or other clients. Special isolation rooms are ventilated to the outside. Staff should wear special high efficiency filtration masks when in the client's room. The nurse should verify with the institution's infection control department that the masks provided are effective for use with TB clients. If the client must travel through the hallway for tests or other activities, the client must wear a mask. Additional protective barriers are used when contact with sputum is likely.

A vaccine against tuberculosis is available and is used in areas where TB is prevalent. It is safe, but its effectiveness has been questioned.

Ultimately, prevention will come from adequate treatment of clients with TB. A current concern is the development of antibiotic-resistant strains of the tuberculosis bacillus, which develop when clients are noncompliant with drug therapy. When antibiotics are taken intermittently or discontinued early, the more virulent bacteria survive and multiply and are resistant to the drugs being used. This drug-resistant bacteria can then be passed on to someone else. It is therefore vital to teach all clients the importance of strict compliance with drug therapy. Clients who are noncompliant with drug therapy must have a visiting nurse or other health professional observe each dose of antibiotic taken. This is called directly observed therapy (DOT).

Signs and Symptoms

Active tuberculosis is characterized by a chronic productive cough, blood-tinged sputum, and drenching night sweats. A low-grade fever may be present. If effective treatment is not initiated, a downhill course occurs, with pulmonary fibrosis, hemoptysis, and progressive weight loss.

Complications

Spread of the tuberculosis bacilli throughout the body can result in pleurisy, pericarditis, peritonitis, meningitis, bone and joint infection, genitourinary or gastrointestinal infection, or infection of many other organs.

Diagnostic Tests

Routine screening for tuberculosis infection is usually done with the purified protein derivative (PPD) skin test. The PPD is injected intradermally; the test is considered positive if a raised area of **induration** occurs within 48 to 72 hours. A red area without induration is not considered a positive result. A positive result indicates that a person has been exposed; it does not mean that active TB is present. A chest x-ray is used as a screening tool in someone with a known positive test. Diagnosis is made based on sputum culture results.

LEARNING TIP

Some institutions use candida or mumps skin tests along with a PPD skin test. This does not mean the client is being tested for candida or mumps, because everyone generally reacts to these. Rather, the client is being tested for **anergy,** or the inability of the immune system to react to an antigen. If the candida or mumps tests produce positive results, the TB results are considered to be reliable.

Medical Treatment

Treatment consists of specific antibiotic therapy. First-line drugs (Table 28–1) have the fewest side effects. However,

Table 28–1. **Antibiotics Used in Treatment of Tuberculosis**

First-line Drugs	Second-line Drugs
Isoniazid	Ethionamide
Rifampin	Kanamycin
Streptomycin	Para-aminosalicylic acid
Ethambutol	Cycloserine
Pyrazinamide	

these drugs can be toxic to the liver and nervous system, as well as having other side effects. Second-line drugs are more toxic and are reserved for cases that do not respond to first-line drug therapy. Generally two or three antibiotics are given simultaneously to allow lower doses of each individual drug and to reduce the incidence of serious side effects. Drugs must be taken for 6 months or longer. Because of the long-term therapy needed and the incidence of side effects, compliance is often a problem and must be anticipated by the nurse.

Nursing Care

The nurse performs a thorough respiratory and psychosocial assessment of the client with TB. The severity of the disease determines the impact on the client's lifestyle. It is also imperative to determine the client's knowledge of the disease and treatment and his or her compliance with drug treatment.

Possible nursing diagnoses include impaired gas exchange, ineffective airway clearance, ineffective breathing pattern, anxiety, altered nutrition, risk for infection of client's contacts, and possible noncompliance with drug therapy or ineffective management of therapeutic regimen. Diagnoses should be chosen based on individual client data.

Nursing interventions for impaired gas exchange, airway clearance, and breathing pattern are found in Nursing Care Plan Box 28–3 for the Client with a Lower Respiratory Tract Disorder. Anxiety may be reduced by educating the client in self-care measures and by reassurance that the disease can be controlled by careful compliance with treatment. The client who is emaciated due to the disease will benefit from a dietitian consultation to provide specific recommendations or supplements. To prevent infection of others, the client is taught to use a tissue to cover the mouth and nose when coughing or sneezing. Tissues should be flushed down the toilet or disposed of carefully in the trash, and all family members are instructed on the importance of careful hand washing. The client and family must

---

induration: in—in + durus—hard

NURSING CARE PLAN BOX 28–3
FOR THE CLIENT WITH A LOWER RESPIRATORY TRACT DISORDER

Note: The three most commonly used nursing diagnoses related to respiratory disorders are presented in the following care plan. This is not a care plan for any one respiratory disorder. Rather, the student should use it as a reference for use when one of the nursing diagnoses applies to the client, based on a thorough respiratory assessment.

Impaired gas exchange related to decreased ventilation or perfusion

Client Outcomes

The client will experience improved gas exchange, as evidenced by (1) improving arterial blood gases or pulse oximetry and (2) statement of acceptable level of dyspnea.

Evaluation of Outcomes

(1) Are blood gases or SaO_2 improving? (2) Does client state that dyspnea is gone or controlled at an acceptable level?

Interventions	Rationale	Evaluation
• Assess lung sounds, respiratory rate and effort, use of accessory muscles.	Respiratory rate < 12 or > 24 or use of accessory muscles indicates distress. Diminished lung sounds indicate possible poor air movement and impaired gas exchange.	Are lung sounds clear and audible? Is respiratory rate 12 to 20 per minute and unlabored?
• Observe skin and mucous membranes for cyanosis.	Cyanosis indicates poor oxygenation. Oral mucous membrane cyanosis indicates serious hypoxia.	Are skin and mucous membranes pink?
• Assess degree of dyspnea on a scale of 1 to 10, 0 = no dyspnea, 10 = worst dyspnea.	The client's subjective report is the best measure of dyspnea.	Is client's degree of dyspnea within parameters that are acceptable to client?
• Monitor for confusion or changes in mental status.	Changes in mental status can signal impaired gas exchange.	Is client alert and oriented? If not, could poor gas exchange be the reason?
• Monitor arterial blood gas values and pulse oximetry as ordered.	PaO_2 < 80 mm Hg, $PaCO_2$ > 45 mm Hg, or SaO_2 < 90 indicate impaired gas exchange.	Are values within client's baseline values?
• Elevate head of bed or help client to lean on overbed table.	Upright positioning promotes lung expansion.	Did change of position relieve some distress?
• Position with good lung dependent ("good lung down").	This position allows the healthier lung to be better perfused and increases gas exchange.	Is SaO_2 improved in this position?
• Administer supplemental oxygen as ordered.	Supplemental oxygen decreases hypoxia.	Is oxygen placed properly on client? Does it provide relief from dyspnea?
• Teach client relaxation exercises.	Relaxation exercises decrease perceived dyspnea.	Does client use relaxation effectively?
• Teach client diaphragmatic and pursed-lip breathing.	Breathing exercises promote relaxation and increase CO_2 excretion.	Does client use breathing exercises correctly? Do they help?
• Encourage client to stop smoking if client is a current smoker.	Smoking is damaging to lungs and respiratory function.	Is client receptive to smoking cessation? Are resources available?
• For severe dyspnea, ask physician about an order for intravenous morphine sulfate.	Low doses of IV morphine cause vasodilation, which helps relieve pulmonary edema and anxiety.	Does morphine provide relief from dyspnea?

Ineffective airway clearance related to excessive secretions

Client Outcomes

The client will have improved airway clearance as evidenced by (1) clear breath sounds and (2) ability to cough up secretions.

continued

NURSING CARE PLAN BOX 28–3 *(continued)*

Evaluation of Outcomes
(1) Are breath sounds clear? (2) Is client able to effectively cough up and expectorate secretions?

Interventions	Rationale	Evaluation
• Assess lung sounds q4h and prn.	Crackles and wheezes may indicate excess secretions in airways.	Do lung sounds indicate retained secretions?
• Monitor amount, color, and consistency of sputum.	Thick, purulent sputum indicates infection and should be reported to the physician.	Does sputum indicate infection?
• Encourage oral fluids; use cool steam room humidifier.	Hydration decreases viscosity of secretions and aids expectoration.	Is client able to take oral fluids? Are secretions thin and easily expectorated?
• Turn client q2h or encourage to ambulate if able.	Movement mobilizes secretions.	Is client mobile?
• Encourage client to cough and deep breathe every hour and prn.	Controlled coughing following deep breaths is more effective.	Does client cough and deep breathe effectively?
• Administer expectorants as ordered.	Expectorants help liquefy secretions and trigger the cough reflex.	Are expectorants effective?
• If client is unable to cough up secretions, suction per institution policy.	Suctioning is necessary to remove secretions when the client is unable to cough effectively.	Is suctioning necessary? Does it help remove secretions?
• Obtain order for chest physiotherapy if indicated.	Percussion and postural drainage help mobilize secretions.	Is chest physiotherapy effective and well tolerated by the client?

Ineffective breathing pattern related to anxiety or pain

Client Outcomes
The client will maintain an effective breathing pattern as evidenced by (1) respiratory rate between 12 and 20 per minute, even, and unlabored; and (2) arterial blood gas and oxygen saturation results within client's normal range.

Evaluation of Outcomes
(1) Is client's respiratory rate within normal limits and unlabored? (2) Does breathing pattern support normal blood gas and SaO_2 values?

Interventions	Rationale	Evaluation
• Assess respiratory rate, depth, and effort q4h and prn.	Respirations < 12 or > 20 may indicate an ineffective pattern.	Is respiratory pattern ineffective?
• Monitor blood gas and oxygen saturation values.	An ineffective breathing pattern will not maintain oxygenation.	Is breathing pattern adversely affecting oxygenation?
• Determine and treat the cause of ineffective breathing pattern.	Pain or anxiety can cause a client to change the breathing pattern, and should be treated.	Is a contributing factor identifiable and correctable?
• Place client in Fowler's or semi-Fowler's position.	This allows for maximal chest expansion.	Is the client in a comfortable position that enables the client to breathe effectively?
• Teach client to use diaphragmatic breathing, with a regular 2 second in, 4 second out pattern.	Breathing exercises promote relaxation and increase CO_2 excretion.	Is the client able to demonstrate an effective breathing pattern?

be instructed on how to manage drug therapy and when to report side effects. They are forewarned that rifampin turns the urine red.

A visiting nurse is essential to evaluate the home environment and assess the client's ability to comply with therapy. If the client is unable to comply with therapy, measures must be instituted to ensure that medications are taken, to protect both the client and the public. Directly observed therapy at a local health clinic or by a home health nurse may be necessary.

The client will be followed periodically by the physician for sputum cultures and drug monitoring. Once sputum cultures are negative, the client is no longer contagious.

Nursing Process: The Client with a Lower Respiratory Infection

ASSESSMENT

The nurse questions the client about a history of respiratory disorders, smoking history, and symptoms of the current illness using the WHAT'S UP? format presented in Chapter 2. The client is questioned about dyspnea, cough, and sputum presence, including amount, consistency, and color. Whenever possible, the nurse should observe the sputum. Degree of dyspnea can be rated by the client on a scale of 0 to 10. Physical assessment includes vital signs, lung sounds, color of skin and mucous membranes (including presence of cyanosis), use of accessory muscles, and observation of adaptive measures such as positioning to ease respiratory distress. (See Chapter 26.)

NURSING DIAGNOSIS

Possible nursing diagnoses include ineffective airway clearance related to increased mucus production, impaired gas exchange related to reduced ventilation, fever, and activity intolerance related to dyspnea.

PLANNING

Nursing care is aimed at relieving symptoms and promoting comfort. The airway should be free of secretions, dyspnea and fever should be controlled, and the client should receive assistance with activities of daily living (ADL) until activity tolerance improves.

IMPLEMENTATION

Oral or intravenous fluids, a room humidifier, expectorants, and reminders to cough and deep breathe every 1 to 2 hours help the client to raise sputum. Chest physiotherapy may be ordered to help loosen secretions if necessary. Pain control will assist the client in taking deep breaths and coughing. Suction is used if the client is unable to cough effectively.

A Fowler's or semi-Fowler's position promotes lung expansion and reduces dyspnea. Oxygen and antibiotics are administered as ordered. Acetaminophen may be used for fever and malaise. The nurse offers assistance with ADL and allows frequent rest periods until the client is able to tolerate an increase in activity.

CLIENT EDUCATION

The client is instructed in use of medications at home and the importance of finishing the antibiotic prescription. The nurse explains the benefit of pacing activities to prevent fatigue and dyspnea and teaches measures to prevent recurrence of infection. The client should also be aware of signs and symptoms to report to the physician.

EVALUATION

If the plan has been effective, dyspnea will be controlled at a level that is acceptable to the client. The client will be able to effectively cough up secretions, which will progressively become less purulent. The client will verbalize correct understanding of medication use at home, and activity tolerance will improve. (Also see Nursing Care Plan Box 28–3 for the Client with a Lower Respiratory Tract Disorder.)

CRITICAL THINKING: Jim

Jim is a 36-year-old accountant with bronchiectasis secondary to cystic fibrosis. He has frequent bouts of uncontrollable coughing, producing up to 300 mL of sputum at a time. Even after coughing, his lungs sound congested from retained secretions.

1. What questions can you ask Jim to assess his cough?
2. What nursing diagnosis is most appropriate for Jim?
3. What nursing care can you provide to enhance secretion removal?

Answers at end of chapter.

Restrictive Disorders

Restrictive disorders are those problems that limit the ability of the client to expand his or her lungs. These are caused by a decrease in the **compliance** (or elasticity) of the lungs or chest wall.

PLEURISY (PLEURITIS)

Pathophysiology

Recall that the visceral and parietal pleura are the membranes that surround the lungs. Between these membranes is a serous fluid that prevents friction as the pleurae slide over each other during respiration. If the membranes become inflamed for any reason, they do not slide as easily. Instead of sliding, one membrane may "catch" on the other, causing it to stretch as the client attempts to inspire. This causes the characteristic sharp pain on inspiration. The irritation causes an increase in the formation of pleural fluid, which in turn reduces friction and decreases pain.

Etiology

Pleurisy is usually related to another underlying respiratory disorder, such as pneumonia, tuberculosis, tumor, or trauma.

Signs and Symptoms

Pleurisy causes a sharp pain in the chest on inspiration. Pain also occurs during coughing or sneezing. Breathing may be shallow and rapid, because deep breathing increases pain. The client may also exhibit fever, chills, and an elevated white cell count if the cause is infectious. A pleural friction rub is heard on auscultation.

Complications

As pleural membranes become more inflamed, serous fluid production increases, which may result in pleural effusion. If pleuritic pain is not controlled, clients will have difficulty breathing deeply and coughing, which may lead to atelectasis. If infection goes untreated, empyema can result.

Diagnostic Tests

Diagnosis is based on signs and symptoms, including auscultation of a pleural friction rub. A chest x-ray and complete blood count (CBC) may also be done.

Medical Treatment

Treatment is aimed at correcting the underlying cause. Narcotics are given to control pain and facilitate deep breathing and coughing. The physician may perform a nerve block, injecting anesthetic near the intercostal nerves to block pain transmission.

PLEURAL EFFUSION

Pathophysiology

When excess fluid collects in the pleural space, it is called a pleural effusion. Fluid enters the pleural space from surrounding capillaries and is reabsorbed by the lymphatic system. When pathology causes an increase in fluid production or inadequate reabsorption of fluid, excess fluid collects. Several liters of fluid may collect at one time. The effusion may be either transudative, forming a watery fluid from the capillaries, or exudative, with fluid containing white blood cells and protein from an inflammatory process.

Etiology

Like pleurisy, pleural effusion is generally caused by another lung disorder. It is a symptom rather than a disease. Transudative effusions may result from heart failure, liver disorders, or kidney disorders. Exudative effusions more commonly occur with lung cancer, infection, or inflammation.

Signs and Symptoms

Symptoms depend on the amount of fluid in the pleural space. Pleuritic pain may or may not be present. Increasing shortness of breath occurs because of the decreasing space for lung expansion. A dull sound is heard when the affected area is percussed. Lung sounds are decreased or absent over the effusion, and a friction rub may be auscultated.

Diagnostic Tests

A chest x-ray is done to determine whether pleural effusion is present. If a thoracentesis is done, fluid samples are sent to the laboratory for culture and sensitivity and cytologic examination. Further tests may be done to determine the cause of the effusion.

Medical Treatment

Bed rest is recommended to enhance spontaneous resolution of the effusion. If symptoms are severe, a therapeutic thoracentesis is done to remove the excess fluid from the pleural space and relieve the client of dyspnea. If the fluid accumulation is large or recurring, a chest tube might be placed to continuously drain the pleural space. Treatment of the underlying cause of the effusion is necessary to prevent recurrence.

EMPYEMA

Empyema is the collection of pus in the pleural space. It is a pleural effusion that is infected. Empyema is usually a complication of pneumonia, tuberculosis, or a lung abscess.

Symptoms, diagnosis, medical treatment, and nursing care are the same as the care of the client with a pleural effusion, with emphasis on resolving the infection. A chest tube or surgery may be necessary to drain the area.

ATELECTASIS

Atelectasis is the collapse of alveoli. It most commonly occurs in postsurgical clients who do not cough and deep

---

atelectasis: atel—imperfect + ectasis—expansion

breathe effectively, though it can be caused by anything that causes hypoventilation. Areas of the lungs that are not well aerated become plugged with mucus, which prevents inflation of alveoli. As a result, alveoli collapse. Compression of lung tissue from effusion or a tumor can also cause atelectasis. The focus of nursing care is on prevention. Clients should be taught the importance of coughing and deep breathing whenever there is the risk for hypoventilation. Frequent position changes and ambulation are also important.

Nursing Process: The Client with a Restrictive Disorder

ASSESSMENT

A routine respiratory assessment is done. Lung sounds are monitored for friction rub or decreasing breath sounds in any of the lobes. Pain level is monitored. The nurse promptly reports any increase in dyspnea, changes in vital signs or pulse oximetry, increased white blood cell count, or increase in temperature.

NURSING DIAGNOSIS

Most clients experience fear or anxiety related to dyspnea. Impaired gas exchange occurs if atelectasis or hypoventilation are present. Risk for infection occurs when there is stasis of pleural fluid. Ineffective breathing pattern is identified when the client is unable to take a deep breath due to pain on inspiration or buildup of fluid.

PLANNING AND IMPLEMENTATION

The nurse stays with the client during acute dyspneic episodes and encourages an effective breathing pattern. (See Chapter 26.) Analgesics reduce pain so that the client will be better able to take deep breaths, though opioids are used cautiously because of their ability to depress respirations. Coughing and deep breathing help prevent infection and atelectasis. Oxygen is administered as ordered. Bed rest is maintained during acute episodes of dyspnea. Fluids are encouraged unless contraindicated. The client should be instructed to report early signs and symptoms of recurrence to the physician.

If a thoracentesis is performed, the nurse explains the procedure to the client and positions the client in a sitting position, leaning over the bedside table. If the client is unable to sit, a side-lying position is used. Preprocedure pain medication is helpful. After the procedure, specimens are labeled and sent to the lab. The site is observed for drainage or subcutaneous emphysema. Lung sounds are monitored, and a postprocedure chest x-ray may be ordered to ensure that the procedure did not cause a pneumothorax.

EVALUATION

If interventions have been effective, the client should report a decrease in dyspnea and anxiety. Pain will be controlled so that the client is able to take deep breaths and cough effectively, and the client will be free of signs and symptoms of infection.

Chronic Airflow Limitation

Chronic airflow limitation (CAL) refers to a group of pulmonary disorders that are characterized by difficulty exhaling because of narrowed or blocked airways. More effort is required to push air out through obstructed airways (Fig. 28–2). Emphysema, chronic bronchitis, asthma, and cystic fibrosis are disorders that limit airflow. These disorders are sometimes referred to as chronic airway obstruction disorders, chronic obstructive pulmonary disease (COPD), or chronic obstructive lung disease (COLD).

A client with CAL often has more than one disorder at the same time. Emphysema and chronic bronchitis may be present simultaneously. Asthma may also be present to some degree. Generally one disorder predominates. Treatment is aimed at the specific disorders represented. Each disorder is discussed separately below, for ease of understanding.

CHRONIC BRONCHITIS

Pathophysiology

Chronic bronchitis is similar to acute bronchitis, with symptoms occurring for at least 3 months out of the year for two consecutive years. The bronchial tree becomes inflamed from inhaled irritants, and impaired ciliary function reduces the ability to remove the irritants. The mucus-producing glands in the airways become hypertrophied, producing excessive thick, tenacious mucus, which obstructs airways and traps air (Fig. 28–3). These changes lead to chronic low-grade infection.

Etiology

Smoking is the single most important risk factor for chronic bronchitis. Other factors include air pollution, passive (secondhand) smoking, and exposure to industrial chemicals. Some familial predisposition to chronic bronchitis has been demonstrated. Children of smoking parents are also at higher risk due to secondhand smoke exposure.

Prevention

Prevention is important because no cure for chronic bronchitis is currently available. Avoidance of smoking and

AIR TRAPPING IN CHRONIC AIRFLOW LIMITATION

A. Air trapping from
   excess mucous

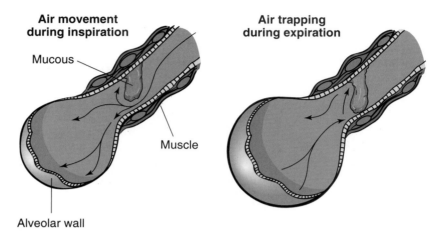

B. Air trapping from
   decreased elastic recoil

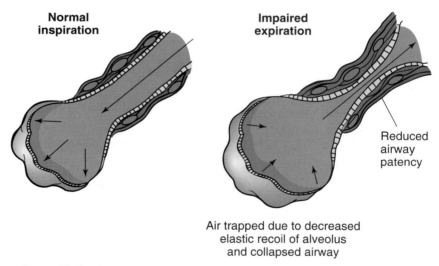

Air trapped due to decreased
elastic recoil of alveolus
and collapsed airway

Figure 28–2. Air trapping in chronic airflow limitation.

other inhaled irritants is vital, especially in those individuals with parents or siblings with CAL.

Signs and Symptoms

The client with chronic bronchitis exhibits a chronic productive cough, shortness of breath, and activity intolerance. Symptoms may initially be worse in the winter months. Crackles and wheezing are often noted on auscultation and may improve after coughing. Expiration is prolonged due to obstructed air passages. Arterial blood gases (ABGs) show an increase in $PaCO_2$ and often a low PaO_2. The client develops **polycythemia** in response to reduced

oxygenation, which results in a ruddy color. Cyanosis may also be present. Right-sided heart failure may develop. (See the section on cor pulmonale in Chapter 21.) Due to the ruddy, cyanotic coloring, and edema related to cor pulmonale, the client with chronic bronchitis may be referred to as a "blue bloater" (Fig. 28–4).

Though the client with chronic bronchitis tends to be overweight, progressive dyspnea may result in an inability to eat an adequate number of calories. As a result, malnutrition and weight loss may occur.

---

polycythemia: poly—many + cyt—cells + emia—in the blood

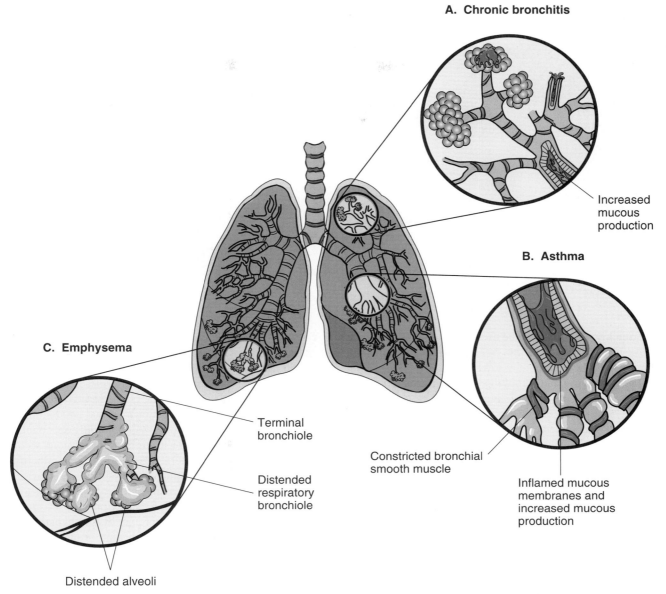

Figure 28–3. *(A)* Chronic bronchitis. Note inflamed airways and excessive mucous. *(B)* Asthma. Note narrowed bronchial tubes and swollen mucous membranes. *(C)* Emphysema. Note distended respiratory bronchioles and alveoli.

Diagnostic Tests

Information from a chest x-ray, blood gas analysis, CBC, and pulmonary function studies is correlated with the history and physical examination to diagnose chronic bronchitis.

Medical Treatment

The most important treatment measure is the cessation of smoking. Even late in the disease process, symptom progression can be slowed by stopping smoking. Exposure to other respiratory contaminants should also be minimized. Hair spray, body powder, and other household aerosols should be avoided.

A pneumococcal vaccine and yearly influenza vaccine are recommended to reduce the risk of respiratory infection. Avoidance of crowds and exposure to people with respiratory infections is advised.

Medications commonly used include adrenergic, anticholinergic, or theophylline bronchodilators; expectorants; and, intermittently, antibiotics. Because the risk for infection is high, the client is taught to report the onset of purulent sputum as soon as it begins so treatment can be initi-

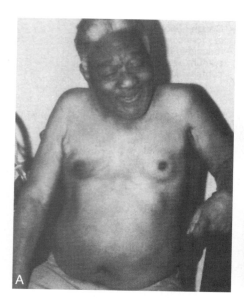
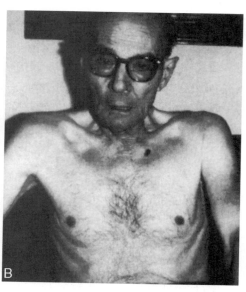

Figure 28–4. *(A)* The client with chronic bronchitis is often called a "blue bloater." *(B)* The client with emphysema is called a "pink puffer." (From Black and Matassarin-Jacobs: Medical-Surgical Nursing, ed 4. WB Saunders, Philadelphia, pp 1027, 1030, with permission.)

ated quickly. Steroids may be used late in the disease to decrease airway inflammation. See Table 28–2 for medications used in the treatment of CAL.

Good hydration and a cool mist humidifier help keep secretions loose. Chest physiotherapy may be used to help the client remove excessive secretions. Nebulized mist treatments and metered dose inhalers are commonly used to administer bronchodilators. Clients with hypoxemia receive supplemental oxygen at home, especially at night. A dietitian consultation is helpful for the client who is unable to maintain a desirable weight. Pulmonary rehabilitation programs can help the client increase exercise tolerance and maintain a sense of well-being.

ASTHMA

The incidence of asthma is on the rise. Nearly 12 million individuals in the United States have asthma. It is more prevalent in African-Americans than in whites. Nearly 5000 individuals die from asthma each year. Asthma deaths are more prevalent in lower socioeconomic groups, presumably because of lack of compliance with treatment regimens. With careful monitoring and treatment, however, clients with asthma can control their symptoms and lead normal lives.

Pathophysiology and Etiology

Asthma is characterized by inflammation of the mucosal lining of the bronchial tree and spasm of the bronchial smooth muscles (**bronchospasm**). This causes narrowed airways and air trapping (Fig. 28–3). Symptoms are intermittent and reversible, with periods of normal airway function. About 50 percent of asthmatics develop the disorder in childhood, but contrary to popular belief, most children do not outgrow asthma. Instead, symptoms just diminish, and often return later in life.

The tendency to develop asthma is inherited. Some sources classify asthma as either allergic or idiosyncratic (unexpected). Allergic asthma is triggered by allergens such as pollen, foods, medications, animal dander, air pollution, molds, or dust mites. It is commonly seasonal. Individuals who developed asthma as children tend to have allergic asthma. Idiosyncratic asthma is generally diagnosed in adults and is related to environmental or other nonallergic factors, such as environmental irritants, smoking, and respiratory infection. Emotional upset and exercise can also trigger symptoms in some asthmatics. Asthma frequently complicates chronic bronchitis or emphysema.

Prevention

Although asthma cannot be prevented, individual episodes can be. It is important that the client identify triggers of asthma symptoms and avoid them whenever possible. Compliance with prophylactic and maintenance therapy is also important.

Signs and Symptoms

Asthma symptoms are intermittent and are often referred to as "attacks," which may last from minutes to days. The client complains of chest tightness, dyspnea, and difficulty moving air in and out of the lungs. Once initial symptoms

---

bronchospasm: broncho—airway + spasm—convulsion, narrowing

Table 28-2. **Medications Used for Chronic Airflow Limitation**

Drug Class and Examples	Route	Action	Side Effects and Nursing Implications
		Glucocorticoids	
Methylprednisolone (Medrol, Solumedrol)	PO IV	Potent anti-inflammatory agents, reduce inflammation in airways	Cushingoid side effects with prolonged use: moon face, sodium and water retention, buffalo hump, osteoporosis, hyperglycemia. May be given IV, PO, or inhaled. Inhaled route causes fewer side effects. Never discontinue abruptly.
Prednisone triamcinolone acetonide (Azmacort)	PO Inhaled		
Beclomethasone (Vanceril, Beclovent)	Inhaled		
		Bronchodilators	
Adrenergic		Stimulate beta receptors to dilate bronchioles	Adrenergic agents cause increased heart rate, tremor, anxiety. Use with care in clients with cardiac disease. Overuse can cause rebound bronchospasm. Serevent is long acting, used bid only.
Albuterol (Ventolin, Proventil)	PO, Inhaled		
Metaproterenol (Alupent, Metaprel)	PO, Inhaled		
Pirbuterol (Maxair)	Inhaled		
Salmeterol (Serevent)	Inhaled		
Anticholinergic		Blocks parasympathetic response, causing bronchodilation	
Ipratropium (Atrovent)	Inhaled		
Methylxanthines		Relax bronchial smooth muscle to dilate airways	Most frequent side effects are tremor, anxiety, tachycardia, nausea, vomiting. Therapeutic theophylline level 5–15 μg/ml.
Theophylline (Slo-Bid, Theolair, Theo-Dur)	PO		
Aminophylline	PO, IV		
		Mast Cell Stabilizers	
Cromolyn sodium (Intal)	Inhaled	Stabilize mast cells to reduce histamine release	Few side effects. Effective for allergic asthma. May be used prophylactically before exercise or allergen exposure.
Nedocromyl (Tilade)			
		Expectorants	
Guaifenesin (Robitussin, Humabid)	PO	Liquefy secretions and stimulate cough	Few side effects. Encourage fluids.
		Antileukotrienes	
Zafirlukast (Accolate)	PO	Inhibit leukotriene synthesis or activity, a mediator of inflammation in asthma	No serious side effects. Possible elevation of liver enzymes.
		Antitussives	
Codeine	PO	Suppress cough reflex	Related to opioids; may be sedating at high doses. Avoid giving to client who has secretions that need to be expectorated.
Dextromethorphan (DM suffix in cough preparations)			

Note: This table is an overview. A drug guide should be consulted for complete administration guidelines.

are controlled, airways may remain hypersensitive and prone to asthma symptoms for many weeks.

On examination, the nurse notes an increased respiratory rate as the client attempts to compensate for narrowed airways. Inspiratory and expiratory wheezing is heard be-cause of turbulent airflow through swollen airways with thick secretions, and may sometimes be heard even without a stethoscope. Air is trapped in the lungs, and expiration is prolonged. A cough is common and may produce thick, clear sputum. Use of accessory muscles to breathe is a sign that the attack is severe and warrants immediate attention.

The nurse should be aware that an absence of audible wheezing may not signal improvement, but rather may be an ominous sign that the client is moving very little air. If wheezing is not heard, use of accessory muscles and peak expiratory flow rate values must be carefully evaluated. Once treatment begins to be effective and the client is moving more air, wheezing may become audible.

Complications

Status asthmaticus occurs if bronchospasm is not controlled and symptoms are prolonged. As the client increases the respiratory rate to compensate for narrowed airways, respiratory alkalosis occurs. If the attack is not resolved and the client begins to tire, the client will no longer be able to compensate and $PaCO_2$ will rise and result in respiratory acidosis. This can lead to respiratory failure and death if untreated.

Diagnostic Tests

Diagnosis is based on the client's report of symptoms, physical examination, and pulmonary function studies. Peak expiratory flow rate is reduced. Arterial blood gases may initially show decreased $PaCO_2$. Late in the course of an attack, PaO_2 decreases and $PaCO_2$ increases. Allergic skin testing and increased serum IgE and eosinophil levels indicate allergic involvement and may help determine treatment.

Medical Treatment

Monitoring

Some clients monitor their peak expiratory flow rate (PEFR) at home (Fig. 28–5). This is a measure of the amount of air the client can blow into a peak flowmeter from fully inflated lungs and is measured in liters per minute. The client determines his or her normal PEFR during symptom-free times. If the PEFR begins to fall below the client's personal norm, treatment that has been predetermined with the health care provider should be initiated. Often PEFR results indicate the onset of asthma before the client experiences any symptoms. (See Home Health Hints Box 28–4.)

Avoidance of Triggers

The client is instructed to identify and avoid asthma triggers. If triggers cannot be avoided, the client can use bronchodilator or mast cell inhibitor metered dose inhalers (MDIs) as prescribed before exposure. MDIs can be especially useful before exercise. Animal dander and foods that cause symptoms are best avoided when possible. Dust mite

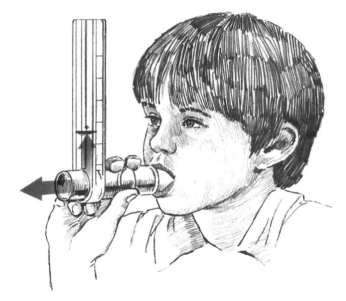

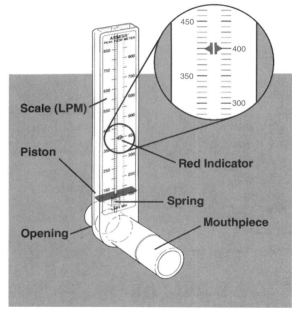

Figure 28–5. Client with asthma using a peak flowmeter to monitor peak expiratory flow rate. (Courtesy of Respironics Health-Scan Asthma & Allergy Products, Cedar Grove, NJ 07009.)

exposure can be reduced by eliminating carpets and curtains in bedrooms, using vinyl mattress covers, and installing a portable or central air filter. Maintenance of indoor humidity between 40 and 50 percent can reduce mold growth. If cold air triggers symptoms, the client should keep the nose and mouth covered when outside in cold weather. Smoking and exposure to secondary smoke are strongly discouraged.

Aspirin and nonsteroidal anti-inflammatory drugs can cause asthma symptoms in some individuals. Beta-blocking medications (propranolol, metoprolol), used com-

HOME HEALTH HINTS BOX 28-4

- When a client is using oxygen by nasal cannula, the area around the ears can become irritated or excoriated. A small sponge-type hair roller can be placed around the tubing to protect the ears.

- When a home health client has an MDI, the nurse should not assume he or she is using it correctly. The client should be observed using it. (Review procedure in Chapter 26.)

- When a client requires more than one MDI, the canisters can be numbered in the order they are to be taken.

- The way to tell if an inhaler is empty is to put the canister in a bowl of water. A full canister will sink and an empty canister will float.

- The home health client who uses inhaled steroids should be instructed to rinse his or her mouth after each use to prevent thrush.

- To help the CAL/COPD client conserve energy, he or she can be encouraged to sit on a stool when cooking at the stove or doing dishes. Personal care activities should be spaced throughout the day (shampoo, bath, etc.).

- If the CAL/COPD client is tempted to adjust his or her own oxygen flow rate, equipment suppliers can put on a locking flowmeter. Increasing flow rate can reduce hypoxic drive and cause hypoventilation.

- Nebulizer parts should be cleaned three times a week or every other day, using warm soapy water in a common home disinfectant solution for 30 minutes.

monly for hypertension, block beta receptors in the lungs, preventing the sympathetic nervous system from promoting bronchodilation. These drugs should be avoided if they make symptoms worse.

Medications

Medications for asthma treatment may be continuous or intermittent, depending on the chronicity of symptoms. See Table 28–2 for a summary of medications used in the treatment of CAL. For clients with only occasional symptoms, adrenergic bronchodilators such as albuterol (Proventil, Ventolin) may be administered via MDI when symptoms occur, or before exercise or other events that trigger asthma.

If the client needs to use an adrenergic MDI more than three times a week, a mast cell inhibitor such as cromolyn sodium (Intal) or nedocromil sodium (Tilade) MDI, or an

emphysema: to inflate

inhaled steroid (Azmacort, Beclovent) may be added. Steroids delivered via metered dose inhalers have become popular and effective therapy in recent years. Because they are used topically, side effects are minimal. The nurse must instruct the client that mast cell inhibitors and steroids must be used regularly to prevent symptoms and will not provide immediate symptom relief.

If inhaled medications do not control symptoms, or if the client has nocturnal symptoms, oral theophylline bronchodilators such as Theodur or Slobid may be added. Immunotherapy (allergy shots) may be used for some clients with allergic asthma.

An acute asthma attack may be treated with an inhaled (nebulized) or subcutaneous adrenergic bronchodilator or intravenous aminophylline. Intravenous or oral corticosteroids (methylprednisolone, prednisone) are potent anti-inflammatory agents that are useful in an acute episode but are avoided for long-term therapy if possible, because of their chronic cushingoid side effects (see the section on Cushing's syndrome in Chapter 37). Corticosteroids must be tapered before discontinuing, to prevent withdrawal symptoms (see the section on Addisonian crisis in Chapter 37).

Oxygen is not often necessary, because many clients hyperventilate. If the attack is prolonged and the client becomes cyanotic or PaO_2 levels begin to fall, oxygen therapy will be used.

LEARNING TIP

Instruct the client to contact the health care provider if the client is using more than two adrenergic MDI canisters per month. This has been associated with an increased risk of death.

EMPHYSEMA

Pathophysiology

Emphysema affects the alveolar membranes, causing destruction of the alveolar walls and loss of elastic recoil. This also causes damage to adjacent pulmonary capillaries. Because of the loss of elastic recoil, passive expiration is impaired, and air is trapped in the alveoli (Fig. 28–3). Reduction in pulmonary capillaries reduces gas exchange. Emphysema can occur primarily in the respiratory bronchioles (centrilobular emphysema) with delayed alveolar damage, or in the respiratory bronchioles and alveoli (panlobular emphysema) (Fig. 28–6).

Etiology

Smoking is the most important cause of emphysema. Air pollution and occupational exposures also contribute to

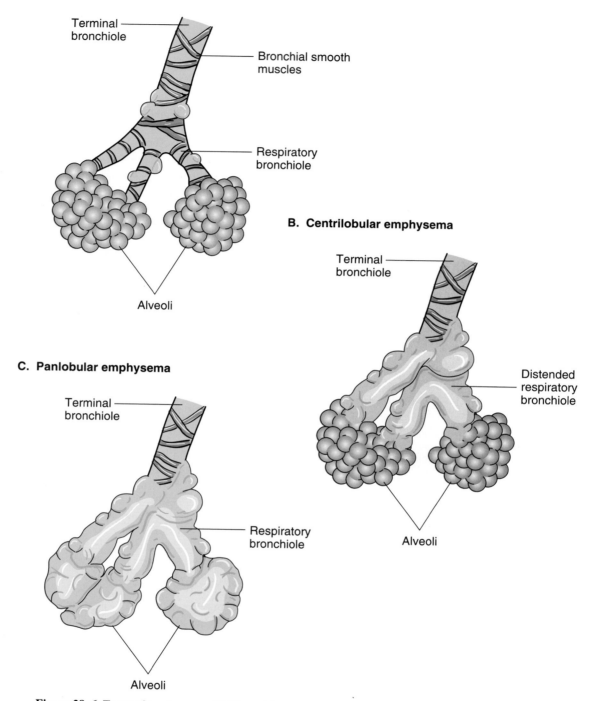

Figure 28–6. Types of emphysema. *(A)* Normal lungs. *(B)* Centrilobular emphysema. *(C)* Panlobular emphysema.

the development of emphysema. A small number of individuals have an inherited deficiency of the enzyme α-antitrypsin, which causes a predisposition to the development of emphysema. Clients with the inherited tendency who also smoke have a very high risk of developing the disease.

Prevention

Avoidance of smoking is the most important preventive factor, especially in those individuals who have relatives with emphysema. The nurse is in a position to teach clients about the importance of preventing this disabling disease.

Signs and Symptoms

The most characteristic symptom of emphysema is progressive shortness of breath, accompanied by activity intolerance. Use of accessory muscles is evident. A barrel chest occurs because of the trapping of air, and expiration is prolonged. Auscultation reveals diminished breath sounds. Because of nearly normal PaO_2 levels early in the disease combined with dyspnea, this client is sometimes referred to as a "pink puffer" (Fig. 28–4). Later in the course of the disease, a productive cough may occur.

LEARNING TIP

The client with emphysema is referred to as a pink puffer, and the client with chronic bronchitis as a blue bloater. This is easy to remember because **b**lue **b**loater and **b**ronchitis all start with **b**.

Complications

Some clients develop large air spaces within the lung tissue (**bullae**) or adjacent to the pleurae (**blebs**) that can rupture and cause the lung to collapse. Cor pulmonale is rare in the client with emphysema but may occur late in the course of the disease. Death may result from respiratory infection.

Diagnostic Tests

A chest x-ray or CT scan will show evidence of air trapping. Pulmonary function studies show a decreased forced expiratory volume and an increase in functional residual capacity and forced vital capacity (FVC). Blood gas analysis is done to monitor gas exchange, and a CBC is done to monitor infection and effectiveness of treatment.

Medical Treatment

Oxygen is administered as ordered at a flow rate of 1 to 2 L. Higher flow rates are avoided to prevent suppression of the hypoxic drive. Pulmonary rehabilitation can help the client increase exercise tolerance. Breathing exercises help improve oxygenation and reduce anxiety. Bronchodilators and expectorants may be helpful. Table 28–2 lists other medications that may be used in the treatment of CAL.

An important measure in the client with emphysema is prevention of infection. Infection can cause an acute exacerbation of symptoms and may require hospitalization. Clients are taught to avoid crowds and other individuals with known infections and to employ good hand-washing practices.

A newer treatment is the surgical removal of some of the emphysematous lung tissue (sometimes called lung re-

duction), which increases the space available for good lung tissue to expand, reducing dyspnea and increasing exercise tolerance. This is a high-risk procedure, but it has allowed some clients to return to a more normal activity level.

CYSTIC FIBROSIS

In the past cystic fibrosis (CF) was thought to be just a childhood disease, because most affected children did not survive past puberty. However, with new treatments, clients with CF are living longer and more productive lives. Some CF clients now marry, have careers, and live well into their thirties.

Pathophysiology

CF is a disorder of the exocrine glands that affects primarily the lungs, gastrointestinal (GI) tract, and sweat glands. The disease varies in severity; some clients have no GI involvement. Abnormal sodium and chloride transport across cell membranes, causing thick, tenacious secretions, is responsible for many of the characteristic symptoms.

The presence of thick, sticky respiratory secretions that are difficult to remove causes airway obstruction, resulting in frequent respiratory infections. Causative organisms are typically *Staphylococcus aureus* and *Pseudomonas aeruginosa.*

Similar abnormalities in the pancreas cause blocked ducts and retained digestive enzymes. These retained enzymes digest and destroy the exocrine pancreas. The absence of digestive enzymes in the intestines causes malabsorption of essential nutrients, frequent foul-smelling, fatty stools, and excess flatus.

Clients with CF secrete sweat that is high in sodium and chloride, because these electrolytes are not reabsorbed as they pass through the sweat ducts.

Etiology

CF is a genetic disorder. Both parents must be carriers of the defective gene for CF to be present in a child. Clients who marry are counseled on the risk of the disease to potential offspring.

Signs and Symptoms

Symptoms usually first appear in infancy or childhood, though a few individuals are not diagnosed until adulthood. Respiratory symptoms are often the first visible manifestation of the disease and range from chronic sinusitis to production of thick, tenacious sputum. Clients with CF are at risk for frequent respiratory infections, manifested by an increase in cough and purulent sputum. Finger clubbing is common. Late in the disease, **hemoptysis** may

---

hemoptysis: hem—blood + ptysis—to spit

occur related to damaged blood vessels within the lungs. Over time, exacerbations of CF due to infection become more frequent, with eventual loss of lung function and respiratory failure.

Frequent foul-smelling stools result from the lack of enzymes in the small intestine. Inability to absorb fat-soluble vitamins and poor appetite due to respiratory disease result in malnutrition. Bowel obstruction, cirrhosis, cholecystitis, and cholelithiasis are associated findings.

Chronic disease causes delayed sexual maturation in both males and females, and infertility is common.

Complications

Clients with CF are at risk for a variety of complications, including bronchiectasis, pneumothorax, cor pulmonale, and respiratory failure. Bowel obstructions can occur due to thick mucus binding with poorly digested fecal matter. Diabetes from pancreatic islet cell involvement may be present late in the disease. Death is usually the result of pulmonary complications.

Diagnostic Tests

Because so many different gene mutations can occur in CF, genetic testing is not helpful at this time. The standard diagnostic test is the sweat chloride test. If respiratory symptoms are accompanied by excessive amounts of sodium chloride in sweat, CF is diagnosed. The reader may recall public health campaigns that advise parents to kiss their babies and report any salty taste to their physicians.

Medical Treatment

Because there is no cure for CF, treatment is aimed at relieving symptoms. Removal of thick sputum is promoted with hydration, postural drainage, and percussion up to four times a day. A hot shower may be an easy occasional alternative to loosen secretions. Nebulized mist treatments using saline or mucolytic medications may be used before chest physiotherapy. Medications to decrease the viscosity of secretions have not yet been entirely successful, but new drugs are constantly being tested. Breathing exercises, incentive spirometry, and effective coughing techniques are also helpful. Lung transplant is a potentially promising treatment.

Prevention of infection is vital to slowing progression of lung damage. Antibiotics must be administered as soon as signs of infection occur. Prophylactic antibiotic therapy may be used. Some clients use home intravenous antibiotic therapy. Antibiotic-resistant infections are a deadly threat to the CF client.

Pancreatic enzyme replacement (Pancrease, Viokase) helps reduce symptoms related to malabsorption and im-

prove nutritional status. An increase in calorie requirements necessitates a high-calorie, nutrient-dense diet.

Nursing Care

The nurse must remember the special needs of the adolescent client with this chronic, debilitating disease. Not only are normal physical growth and development delayed, but psychosocial development is also affected by repeated hospitalizations and the necessity of routine daily medication and treatments.

Nursing Process: The Client with Chronic Airflow Limitation

ASSESSMENT

The nurse does a complete respiratory assessment as presented in Chapter 26. Frequency of assessment is dictated by the severity of the client's condition. Level of consciousness is noted, because poor gas exchange causes confusion and lethargy. Skin and mucous membranes are observed for cyanosis. Lung sounds are auscultated for adventitious sounds. Cough and color and amount of sputum are monitored. Exercise tolerance is noted, and degree of dyspnea can be measured on a scale of 1 to 10. Arterial blood gases are monitored. Careful documentation of findings allows the nurse to monitor and report trends in the client's progress.

NURSING DIAGNOSIS

A number of nursing diagnoses are appropriate for the client with chronic airflow limitation. As always, the nurse must choose diagnoses based on defining characteristics and the client's individual assessment findings. Impaired gas exchange due to poor ventilation or damaged alveoli is common, and can be easily identified when dyspnea is accompanied by abnormal ABGs. Ineffective airway clearance related to copious thick secretions is also a common occurrence, especially in clients with chronic bronchitis and cystic fibrosis. Ineffective breathing pattern may occur related to anxiety. Activity intolerance related to hypoxia is often present. Related diagnoses may include altered nutrition: less than requirements related to dyspnea and poor appetite, and anxiety related to dyspnea. (See Nursing Care Plan Box 28–3 for the Client with a Lower Respiratory Disorder.)

PLANNING

To increase client acceptance of the plan of care, he or she must be involved in identifying goals. The airway should remain clear of secretions. Anxiety should be manageable.

Dyspnea should be controlled to allow the client to maintain his or her desired activity level, within appropriate limitations. Nutrition status should be stable.

IMPLEMENTATION

Impaired Gas Exchange

During acute episodes of dyspnea due to impaired gas exchange, clients can become very anxious and may fear that they are going to die. Oxygen is administered as ordered, and the client is placed in a semi-Fowler's or Fowler's position to aid in thoracic expansion. A Venturi mask may be used to deliver an accurate oxygen flow rate. Rates greater than 2 L are generally avoided to prevent impairing the hypoxic drive. Pursed-lip breathing and relaxation exercises may help reduce dyspnea and the associated anxiety. Small doses of intravenous morphine (usually 2 to 4 mg) can also be very helpful in reducing acute dyspnea and anxiety. The nurse should stay with the client until his or her breathing and anxiety have stabilized.

Ineffective Airway Clearance

Increased fluid intake is encouraged if it is not contraindicated. A cool steam humidifier will also help loosen secretions for expectoration. Expectorants are given as ordered. The client is encouraged to cough and deep breathe regularly. (Occasionally, if a client is in acute respiratory distress, coughing can cause further bronchospasm and is not encouraged.) If able, the client is encouraged to ambulate, or at least turn side to side every 2 hours to prevent secretions from pooling. The nurse may request an order for chest physiotherapy if other measures do not produce the desired results. If a client is unable to cough up secretions due to altered level of consciousness or extreme weakness, suctioning may be necessary.

Ineffective Breathing Pattern

Anxiety, fatigue, and pain are common causes of an ineffective breathing pattern. If a client's breathing pattern is too fast or shallow, the nurse first determines the cause and identifies measures to eliminate it. In addition, relaxation and deep breathing exercises can help improve the breathing pattern.

Activity Intolerance

The client is encouraged to rest between activities. Even talking or eating can cause dyspnea in a client with end-stage disease. A bedside commode prevents unnecessary trips to the bathroom. If the client is able to ambulate, a portable oxygen source should be used. The client should be allowed to sleep without interruptions at night as much as possible. Activity level is slowly increased if the client is able. Referral to a pulmonary rehabilitation program can help increase exercise tolerance.

Altered Nutrition

The cause of altered nutrition must first be identified. If the client is too dyspneic to eat, scheduling rest periods and nebulized mist treatments or MDI administration before meals may be helpful. A poor appetite can be improved by creating a pleasant eating environment, providing smaller, more frequent meals of the client's favorite foods, or encouraging family members to bring food from home for the hospitalized client. Liquid supplements may be necessary to maintain weight. A specialized supplement such as Pulmocare provides less carbon dioxide when metabolized and is recommended for clients with respiratory disease. (See Nutrition Notes Box 28–5.)

Anxiety

The nurse should remain with the client who is acutely anxious. A calming voice reminding the client to breathe slowly in through the nose and out through pursed lips can be very helpful. Relaxation exercises, learned during times when anxiety is minimal, may be used at this time. Antianxiety medications are given as ordered. Intravenous morphine helps acute dyspnea and anxiety, but it is usually reserved for clients with end-stage disease.

CLIENT EDUCATION

The client must be aware of the contributing factors to the disease and eliminate them if at all possible. The client who is a smoker should not simply be told to quit smoking; he or she should be referred to a smoking cessation program and be provided with nicotine patches or other resources and support as necessary to quit. Techniques for effective breathing and anxiety control should also be taught. An excellent resource available to clients is the *Better Breathers Workbook* available from California Press, phone: (619) 477-4800.

EVALUATION

If interventions have been effective, the airway will be clear of secretions. The client will be able to manage anxiety symptoms and complete ADL or other desired activity without dyspnea. The client's intake should be adequate to maintain a stable weight. If any of the client's goals have not been met, the plan of care should be revised.

REHABILITATION OF THE CLIENT WITH CHRONIC AIRFLOW LIMITATION

Many institutions now have pulmonary rehabilitation departments. These programs help clients learn effective

Nutrition in Persons with Diseases of the Lower Respiratory Tract

Factors affecting nutrition include the following:

- Clients with respiratory disease commonly have an inadequate food intake because of anorexia, shortness of breath, or gastrointestinal distress.
- Calorie requirements are often increased in clients with pulmonary disease. The caloric cost of breathing ranges from 36 to 72 kcal/day in normal individuals; the caloric cost of breathing increases to 430 to 720 kcal/day in clients with chronic obstructive pulmonary disease. Both decreased food intake and increased energy requirements may contribute to the weight loss commonly seen in these clients.
- When calorie intake is decreased, the body begins to break down muscle stores, including the respiratory muscles. The gastrointestinal distress common in these clients may be related to malnutrition of the gastrointestinal tract.
- Malnutrition, and the resulting decrease in antibody production, lowers the client's resistance to infection. Also, the malnourished client's lungs produce less pulmonary phospholipid, a fatlike substance that assists in lubricating lung tissue and helps protect the lungs from inhaled pathogens.

- Improved nutritional status has been associated with an increased ability to wean clients from respirators or ventilators. To some extent, all the respiratory muscles atrophy due to inactivity when a machine does the work for the client. Nutrition support improves the likelihood of successful weaning in clients on artificial respiration.
- Many clients with chronic obstructive pulmonary disease suffer from carbon dioxide retention and oxygen depletion. The medical goal for these clients is to decrease the level of carbon dioxide in their blood. Because fat calories produce less carbon dioxide than carbohydrate calories, a diet high in fat is often prescribed. As much as 50 percent of the calories may be given as fat. Several companies produce complete nutritional supplements with higher fat content formulated for clients with respiratory disease. Medical opinion is not unanimous on this issue, because some evidence has related a high fat intake to immunosuppression in some clients.

FEEDING TECHNIQUES. Many of these clients are breathless and lack the energy to eat. Small, frequent feeding of foods with much nutrition in a small volume should be encouraged. Foods that require little or no chewing may help with difficulties chewing and swallowing. To lessen abdominal pressure on the diaphragm, these clients are encouraged to avoid gaseous foods.

---

breathing techniques and how to slowly increase their exercise tolerance. The nurse can request this referral when appropriate.

Pulmonary Vascular Disorders

PULMONARY EMBOLISM

Pathophysiology

An **embolism** is a foreign object that travels through the bloodstream. It may be a blood clot, air, or fat. A pulmonary embolism (PE), sometimes called pulmonary thromboembolism (PTE), is usually a blood clot that has traveled into a pulmonary artery. Resulting obstruction of blood flow causes a ventilation-perfusion mismatch, which in this case means that an area of the lung is well ventilated, but has no blood flow or perfusion. Because reduced or no blood supply is available to pick up the oxygen in the affected portion of the lung, it becomes pulmonary "dead space."

Occasionally, damage occurs to a portion of the lung due to lack of oxygen. This is called lung infarction, and it is not common because oxygen is delivered to lung tissue not only from the pulmonary arteries, but also the bronchial arteries and the airways.

Etiology

Most pulmonary emboli originate in the deep veins of the lower extremities (deep vein thrombosis, or DVT). Some risk factors of DVT, and therefore PE, include surgical procedures done under general anesthesia, heart failure, fractures of the lower extremities, bed rest, obesity, and a previous history of DVT or PE. Less common causes of PE include fat emboli from compound fractures, amniotic fluid embolism during labor and delivery, and air embolism from entry of air into the bloodstream.

Prevention

Prevention of thrombi in the deep veins of the legs is the most important factor in the prevention of a pulmonary embolism. Regular ambulation is advised if the client is able. If a client is at risk for DVT or PE, low-dose heparin, warfarin (Coumadin), or intermittent compression stockings are used to prevent thrombus formation. If a DVT is diagnosed, prompt treatment is essential in order to prevent a PE.

Signs and Symptoms

The most common symptom of PE is a sudden onset of dyspnea for no apparent reason. The client may be gasping for breath and may appear anxious. The nurse should be alert to the presence of risk factors and obtain immediate assistance if the cause of dyspnea might be PE. If lung infarction has occurred, hemoptysis and pleuritic chest pain may also be present. Many clients have no symptoms at all.

Complications

High blood pressure within the pulmonary circulation (pulmonary hypertension) may result from arterial occlusion and lead to right ventricular failure. This occurs because the right ventricle is unable to push blood into the occluded artery. As a result, the contraction becomes weak, cardiac output falls, and the client becomes hypotensive.

Diagnostic Tests

A lung scan (ventilation and perfusion scan) assesses the degree of ventilation of lung tissue and the areas of blood perfusion. If an area is well ventilated but poorly perfused (i.e., a mismatch), PE is suspected.

A pulmonary angiogram can outline the pulmonary vessels with a radiopaque dye injected via a cardiac catheter. This can show where blood flow is diminished or absent, suggesting an embolism.

Chest x-ray, electrocardiogram (ECG), arterial blood gas analysis, CT scan, or MRI may also be done. However, many of these show changes only in the presence of a very large embolism or infarction.

Medical Treatment

The body naturally dissolves clots in 7 to 10 days. Treatment is aimed at preventing extension of the clot and the formation of additional clots. Heparin, a potent anticoagulant medication, is administered via continuous intravenous infusion for 7 to 10 days. Sometimes an intermittent IV or subcutaneous route is used. Heparin is never given intramuscularly because of the risk of hematoma development. Clotting studies (PTT, TCT) are monitored and maintained at 1.5 to 2 times the control value. Oxygen is administered as ordered.

Sometimes heparin therapy is initiated even before a diagnosis of PE is made. It is believed that it is safer to begin therapy and then stop if PE is not confirmed than to wait until all test results are available.

Warfarin sodium (Coumadin), an oral anticoagulant, is used for approximately 12 weeks following the embolism to prevent recurrence. It can also be used for long-term prevention of repeated clots in clients who have risk factors that cannot be resolved. Coumadin therapy can be initiated 2 to 3 days after the initiation of heparin therapy. Because it has a slow onset of action, it may require several days for the full anticoagulant effect to occur. The client will be on both anticoagulants for a period of time. Coumadin therapy is monitored with regular prothrombin times (PT). See Table 28–3 for education for clients on anticoagulant therapy.

Agents that dissolve clots (thrombolytic agents), such as streptokinase, urokinase, and tissue plasminogen activator (TPA), are very effective and are becoming more widely used. However, they must be used within 4 to 6 hours of the clot's occurrence and are associated with a risk for hemorrhage.

Sometimes a filter is placed via the jugular or femoral vein into the inferior vena cava. One filter that is commonly used is the Greenfield filter, which filters out clots traveling from the lower extremities in clients at risk for repeated emboli or in clients who cannot take anticoagulants.

In clients with life-threatening symptoms, a surgical embolectomy can be performed. This is a rare procedure that is reserved for emergency situations.

Nursing Care

Assessment

The client is assessed for respiratory distress, including respiratory rate and effort, cyanosis, confusion, and subjective feelings of dyspnea and anxiety. Lung sounds are auscultated. Sputum color and amount are noted. Arterial blood gases are monitored. Heart sounds and peripheral

Table 28–3. **Education for Clients Receiving Anticoagulant Therapy**

Anticoagulants prolong the time it takes blood to clot, so it is important to prevent injury and to recognize and report signs of bleeding to the physician.

To Prevent Injury
- Wear shoes or slippers; avoid going barefoot.
- Use an electric razor to shave.
- Use a soft toothbrush.

Signs of Bleeding to Report to Physician
- Easy bruising
- Nosebleeds
- Bleeding that does not stop
- Blood in urine
- Blood in sputum
- Blood in stools, or black stools

Additional Instructions
- Avoid use of aspirin because it further prolongs clotting time.
- Have your lab work done as prescribed by your physician to monitor your clotting time and medication dosage.

edema are monitored for signs of heart failure. Contributing factors, such as calf pain, are assessed.

Nursing Diagnosis

The priority nursing diagnosis for a client with a pulmonary embolism is impaired gas exchange. Because of the impaired perfusion of the affected area of the lung, oxygen and carbon dioxide exchange are limited. Anxiety occurs related to dyspnea. Risk for injury related to anticoagulant therapy is a concern once treatment is initiated.

Planning and Implementation

IMPAIRED GAS EXCHANGE. Oxygen is administered as ordered. Bed rest is maintained to decrease oxygen demand. Assisting the client with turning, coughing, and deep breathing will further facilitate gas exchange.

ANXIETY. The nurse stays with the client during acute episodes of dyspnea. The client's questions are answered, and information about pulmonary embolism and its treatment is provided at a level appropriate to the client's need and tolerance, because knowledge may help decrease anxiety.

RISK FOR INJURY. Coagulation studies are monitored and reported to the physician. The client is protected from injury, so that excessive bleeding will not occur. Shoes or slippers are encouraged when ambulating. A soft toothbrush and an electric razor are used. The client is instructed to report any signs of bleeding, such as hematuria or easy bruising. (See also Table 28–3.)

Evaluation

The client should state that dyspnea and anxiety are controlled, and verbalize understanding of anticoagulant therapy and precautions.

PULMONARY HYPERTENSION

Pulmonary hypertension is defined as pressures in the pulmonary arteries above 30 mm Hg systolic, or a mean arterial pressure above 15 mm Hg.

Pathophysiology and Etiology

Primary pulmonary hypertension occurs when the arteries that carry deoxygenated blood from the heart to the lungs become narrowed as a result of changes in the vascular smooth muscle. The result is elevated pressure in the pulmonary arteries, causing the right ventricle to work harder to push blood into them. Eventually the right ventricle fails. The reason for these vascular changes is not known. Primary pulmonary hypertension is more common in females between the ages of 20 and 40 and has a hereditary tendency.

Secondary pulmonary hypertension results from other disorders, such as coronary artery disease or mitral valve disease, both of which increase pressures in the left side of the heart. The pulmonary arterial pressure then rises to push blood into the left heart. Capillary destruction related to alveolar damage in chronic airflow limitation can also lead to secondary pulmonary hypertension. Right ventricular failure (cor pulmonale) eventually occurs as the heart works to push blood against high pulmonary arterial pressures.

Signs and Symptoms

The most common symptoms include dyspnea and fatigue, which worsen over time. Crackles and decreased breath sounds are heard on auscultation. Cyanosis and tachypnea (rapid respiratory rate) are noted. If cor pulmonale is present, peripheral edema and distended jugular veins are seen. Angina may result from right ventricular ischemia. Death usually occurs within 2 to 3 years of diagnosis, unless a transplant is done.

Diagnostic Tests

Arterial blood gases commonly show hypoxemia and hypocapnia. Cardiac catheterization can be done to determine high pulmonary arterial pressures. An ECG may show right ventricular hypertrophy. A chest x-ray, pulmonary function tests, lung scan, and a pulmonary angiogram may be done to determine underlying causes in secondary pulmonary hypertension.

Treatment

No cure is available for pulmonary hypertension, except for lung or heart and lung transplant. In secondary pulmonary hypertension, the underlying disorder is treated. Supportive care includes a low-sodium diet and diuretics to reduce blood volume (and therefore pressure), oxygen, and cardiac monitoring. Vasodilators such as calcium channel blockers may be beneficial in some clients to reduce pulmonary artery pressure. Warfarin (Coumadin) may be used to prevent clotting. Nursing care is collaborative and focuses primarily on client assessment. Fowler's or high Fowler's position may help reduce dyspnea, and bed rest and comfort measures are helpful in treating fatigue and anxiety.

Trauma

PNEUMOTHORAX

The term **pneumothorax** literally means "air in the chest" and is used to describe conditions in which air has entered the pleural space, outside of the lungs. If the pneumothorax

---

pneumothorax: pneumo—air + thorax—chest

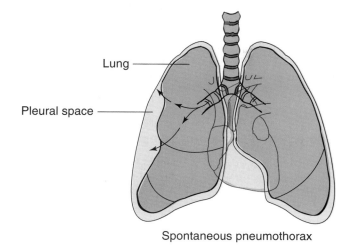

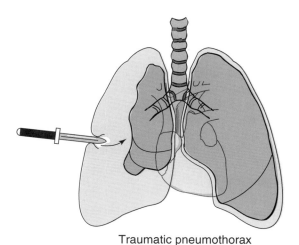

Figure 28–7. Pneumothorax.

Spontaneous Pneumothorax

If no injury is present, the pneumothorax is considered spontaneous. This occurs mostly in tall, thin individuals and in smokers. Clients who have had one spontaneous pneumothorax are at greater risk for a recurrence. Clients with underlying lung disease (especially emphysema) may have blisterlike defects in lung tissue, called bullae or blebs, that can rupture, allowing air into the pleural space. Weakened lung tissue from lung cancer can also lead to pneumothorax.

Traumatic Pneumothorax

Penetrating trauma to the chest wall and parietal pleura allows air to enter the pleural space. This can occur due to a knife or gunshot wound, or from protruding broken ribs.

Open Pneumothorax

If air can enter and escape through the opening in the pleural space, it is considered open.

Closed Pneumothorax

If air collects in the space and is unable to escape, a closed pneumothorax results.

Tension Pneumothorax

If a pneumothorax is closed, air, and therefore tension, builds up in the pleural space. As tension increases, pressure is placed on the heart and great vessels, pushing them away from the affected side of the chest. This is called a mediastinal shift (Fig. 28–8). When the heart and vessels are compressed, venous return to the heart is impaired, resulting in reduced cardiac output and symptoms of shock. Tension pneumothorax is often related to the high pressures present with mechanical ventilation. It is a medical emergency.

occurs without an associated injury, it is called a spontaneous pneumothorax. A secondary spontaneous pneumothorax may occur due to underlying lung disease. Traumatic pneumothorax may result from a traumatic chest injury.

Pathophysiology and Etiology

Recall that the pleural cavity has visceral and parietal pleurae. These membranes normally are separated only by a thin layer of pleural fluid. Each time a breath is taken in, the diaphragm descends, creating negative pressure in the thorax. This negative pressure pulls air into the lungs via the nose and mouth. If either the visceral pleura or the chest wall and parietal pleura is perforated, air enters the pleural space, negative pressure is lost, and the lung on the affected side collapses (Fig. 28–7). Each time the client takes a breath, the temporary increase in negative pressure draws air into the pleural space via the perforation. During expiration air may or may not be able to escape through the perforation.

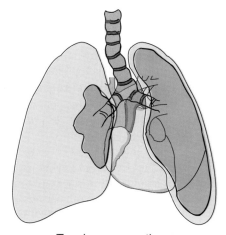

Tension pneumothorax

Figure 28–8. Tension pneumothorax with mediastinal shift.

Hemothorax

The term **hemothorax** refers to the presence of blood in the pleural space. This can occur with or without accompanying pneumothorax (hemopneumothorax) and is often the result of traumatic injury. Other causes include lung cancer, pulmonary embolism, and anticoagulant use.

Signs and Symptoms

Sudden dyspnea, chest pain, **tachypnea,** restlessness, and anxiety occur with pneumothorax. On examination, asymmetrical chest expansion on inspiration may be noted. Breath sounds may be absent or diminished on the affected side. In a "sucking" chest wound, air can be heard as it enters and leaves the wound.

If tension pneumothorax develops, the client becomes hypoxemic and hypotensive as well. The trachea may deviate to the unaffected side. Bradycardia and shock will occur if emergency intervention is not provided.

Diagnostic Tests

History, physical examination, and chest x-ray are used to diagnose pneumothorax. Chest x-rays are repeated to monitor the resolution of the pneumothorax with treatment. Arterial blood gases are monitored throughout the course of treatment.

Medical Treatment

A small pneumothorax may absorb with no treatment other than rest, or the trapped air may be removed with a small-bore needle inserted into the pleural space. Chest tubes connected to a water seal drainage system are used to remove larger amounts of air or blood from the pleural space. See Chapter 26 for complete information about chest drainage. Some injuries require surgical repair before the pneumothorax can be resolved.

If the pneumothorax is recurrent, other treatments can be used to prevent additional episodes. Sterile talc or certain antibiotics (such as tetracycline) can be injected into the pleural space via thoracentesis, irritating the pleural membranes and making them "stick together." This is called **pleurodesis,** or sclerosis, and prevents recurrent pneumothorax. Pleurodesis is painful; the nurse should prepare the client with an analgesic before the procedure.

Nursing Care

Nursing care of the client with a pneumothorax involves close monitoring of the condition. A frequent and thorough assessment should be done, including level of consciousness, skin and mucous membrane color, vital signs, respiratory rate and depth, and presence of dyspnea, chest pain, restlessness, or anxiety. Regular auscultation of lung sounds provides information about reinflation of the affected lung. Any signs of increasing or tension pneumothorax are reported to the physician immediately. Additional attention is given to monitoring the water seal drainage system if present.

RIB FRACTURES

Etiology and Signs and Symptoms

Chest trauma is often accompanied by fractured ribs. Ribs can also be fractured by uncontrolled coughing, especially in the presence of osteoporosis or cancer. The fourth through ninth ribs are the most commonly affected. Broken ribs can be very painful, and often prevent the client from breathing deeply or coughing effectively, which can result in atelectasis or pneumonia. Displaced ribs can also damage lung tissue, causing pneumothorax.

Treatment

In the past, elastic rib belts were used to stabilize the ribs while healing took place. This is no longer done, because it further restricts deep breathing. Pain control is the most important treatment. Keeping the client comfortable allows coughing and deep breathing, which in turn prevents complications such as pneumonia and atelectasis. If traditional pain control measures are ineffective, intercostal nerve blocks may be used. Ribs generally heal in about 6 weeks.

FLAIL CHEST

Pathophysiology and Etiology

When multiple ribs are fractured, the structural support of the chest is impaired. As a result, the affected part of the chest collapses with inspiration and bulges with expiration. This is called **paradoxical respiration,** which is ineffective in ventilating the lungs and results in hypoxia.

Signs and Symptoms

The client with a flail chest exhibits chest movement that is opposite to that usually seen with respiration. The client will be dyspneic, anxious, tachypneic, and tachycardic.

Treatment

The client is given supplemental oxygen. Intubation and mechanical ventilation may be necessary. If lung damage has occurred, chest tubes may be necessary for reinflation.

---

hemothorax: hem—blood + thorax—chest
tachypnea: tachy—rapid + pnea—breathing
pleurodesis: pleur—pleural membrane + desis—binding

Nursing Process: The Client with Chest Trauma

The following nursing process is based on the stabilized client. For emergency care of the client with chest trauma, see Chapter 54.

ASSESSMENT

When caring for the client following chest trauma, it is important to monitor respiratory status. Any sign of worsening status, such as a change in vital signs or lung sounds, change in respiratory rate, increase in dyspnea, chest pain, pallor, or cyanosis, development of tracheal deviation, or onset of anxiety, should be reported to the physician immediately. If a chest wound is present, it is cared for and closely monitored. Additional assessment may be necessary depending on the type of injury sustained.

NURSING DIAGNOSIS

Nursing diagnoses for the client with chest trauma may include impaired gas exchange, pain, ineffective breathing pattern, and anxiety. Additional diagnoses may be appropriate depending on the individual client's assessment.

PLANNING AND IMPLEMENTATION

Gas exchange is maintained with supplemental oxygen. Mechanical ventilation may be necessary. The client is positioned for comfort and maximum chest expansion and is encouraged to take deep breaths. Pain is controlled so the client is able to breathe deeply. The nurse must remember that narcotics depress respirations, so respiratory rate is carefully monitored. Splinting the chest for coughing may also be helpful to reduce pain. Additional care will be necessary if the client has chest tubes.

EVALUATION

Are pain, anxiety, and dyspnea controlled? Is the respiratory rate within normal limits? Are vital signs stable? Frequent evaluation is essential so that failure to progress can be reported to the physician.

Respiratory Failure

ACUTE RESPIRATORY FAILURE

Pathophysiology

Acute respiratory failure is diagnosed when the client is unable to maintain adequate blood gas values. Hypoxemia may result from inadequate ventilation (air movement in and out of lungs) or poor oxygenation (adequate ventila-tion, but inability to get the oxygen into the blood and therefore the cells). Some clients with chronic respiratory disease have adapted to impaired gas exchange. In these clients, a drop in PaO_2 of 10 to 15 mm Hg is considered acute failure.

Etiology

An acute respiratory infection in a client with chronic airway obstruction is often the precipitating factor in acute respiratory failure. Other causes include central nervous system disorders that affect breathing, such as a stroke or myasthenia gravis, inhalation of toxic substances, and aspiration.

Prevention

Avoidance of respiratory infections in clients with chronic respiratory disease is important. If sputum does become purulent, clients should be instructed to notify their physician immediately so treatment can be initiated.

Sedatives and narcotics should be used carefully or avoided in clients with chronic respiratory disease, because these are respiratory depressants and can precipitate failure.

Signs and Symptoms

The client with impending respiratory failure may become restless, confused, agitated, or sleepy. Arterial blood gases show decreasing PaO_2 and pH and increasing $PaCO_2$. The nurse must carefully assess the client and report significant findings to the physician immediately. It is easy to mistakenly treat symptoms of agitation or confusion with sedatives, which will speed the onset of respiratory failure.

Diagnostic Tests

Arterial blood gas analysis is important in determining the presence of respiratory failure. A drop in PaO_2 of 10 to 15 mm Hg or a pH of less than 7.30 with associated elevated $PaCO_2$ indicates respiratory failure. Sputum cultures or chest x-rays may be used to determine the cause and guide treatment.

Medical Treatment

Oxygen therapy via nasal cannula or mask is provided at a flow rate of 1 to 2 L, to prevent interference with the hypoxic drive. Antibiotics or other treatments are ordered to correct the underlying cause of the failure. Aminophylline and beta-adrenergic bronchodilators are used to dilate the bronchioles, promoting ventilation and secretion removal. The client is instructed to cough and deep breathe if able. Suctioning is indicated if the client is unable to cough effectively. Mechanical ventilation may be required.

ACUTE RESPIRATORY DISTRESS SYNDROME

Acute respiratory distress syndrome (ARDS), also called adult respiratory distress syndrome, is a group of disorders that has diverse causes but very similar pathophysiology, symptoms, and treatment. It is called ARDS to differentiate it from neonatal respiratory distress syndrome.

Pathophysiology and Etiology

The most common cause of ARDS is sepsis. Other causes include pneumonia, trauma, shock, narcotic overdose, inhalation of irritants, burns, pancreatitis, and aspiration, among others. Each of these causes begins a chain of events leading to alveolocapillary damage and noncardiac pulmonary edema (pulmonary edema that is not caused by heart failure). ARDS usually affects clients without a previous history of lung disease.

The alveolocapillary membranes become inflamed and damaged either by direct contact with an inhaled irritant or by chemical mediators that are released when systemic injury occurs. The membranes become leaky, so that proteins, blood cells, and fluid move from the capillaries into the interstitial space, and then into the alveoli. Surfactant, a substance that reduces surface tension in the alveoli, is reduced. Alveoli collapse (atelectasis) and fibrotic changes take place. These changes cause the lungs to become stiff, or less compliant, making the client work very hard to inspire. Blood supply to the alveoli may be adequate, but collapsed, wet alveoli are unable to oxygenate it. In other areas of the lungs, vasoconstriction reduces the ability of the vessels to pick up oxygen from functioning alveoli. Tired respiratory muscles, in combination with edema and atelectasis, reduce gas exchange and result in hypoxia. As the condition progresses, atelectasis and edema worsen, and the lungs may hemorrhage. A chest x-ray appears to be white due to the excessive fluid in the lungs. These changes explain some of the older names for what is now known as ARDS: wet lung, white lung, shock lung, and stiff lung.

Prevention

Early recognition and treatment of underlying disorders is important in prevention of ARDS. Good nursing care can help reduce aspiration and some types of pneumonia.

Signs and Symptoms

Initially the client may experience dyspnea and an increase in respiratory rate. Respiratory alkalosis results from hyperventilation. Fine inspiratory crackles may be auscultated. As the condition worsens, breathing becomes more rapid and labored, and the client becomes cyanotic. The client is no longer able to oxygenate the blood and get rid of carbon dioxide, and respiratory acidosis occurs. Oxygen therapy does not reverse the hypoxemia. If ARDS is not reversed, eventually hypoxemia leads to decreased cardiac output and death.

Complications

Complications that can result from ARDS include heart failure, pneumothorax related to mechanical ventilation, infection, and disseminated intravascular coagulation (DIC). The death rate for ARDS in the past was 100 percent. With newer treatments, it is now between 50 and 60 percent. Most clients who survive ARDS recover completely.

Diagnostic Tests

Diagnosis is made based on history of a causative injury, physical examination, chest x-ray, and blood gas analysis. An ECG is done to rule out a cardiac-related cause.

Medical Treatment

The client with ARDS is cared for in an intensive care unit. Treatment begins with oxygen therapy that is adjusted based on repeated ABG results. Intubation and mechanical ventilation is necessary in most cases, with the use of positive end-expiratory pressure (PEEP) to keep the airways open. Diuretics may be used to reduce pulmonary edema, but care must be taken to prevent fluid depletion. A pulmonary artery catheter may be used to monitor hemodynamic status. If infection is the underlying cause, antibiotics are administered. Parenteral nutrition may be given to maintain nutritional status while the client is acutely ill. Positioning the client with the less involved lung in the dependent position ("good lung down") allows the better lung to be well perfused with blood and may increase PaO_2.

Nursing Process: The Client Experiencing Respiratory Failure

ASSESSMENT

The nurse assesses the client's degree of dyspnea on a scale of 1 to 10, if the client is able to participate. Respiratory rate, effort, and use of accessory muscles is noted. Arterial blood gases and oxygen saturation values are monitored as ordered. The presence of cyanosis is noted.

Mental status, including restlessness, confusion, and level of consciousness, is also assessed, because reduced oxygenation can produce central nervous system (CNS) symptoms. Symptoms of the underlying cause of respiratory failure are monitored. If the cause is infectious, sputum amount and color, temperature, and white blood cell counts are monitored.

All assessment findings should be compared with earlier data. Even subtle changes in the assessment findings can be significant and should be reported.

NURSING DIAGNOSIS

Possible diagnoses include impaired gas exchange, ineffective airway clearance, and altered breathing pattern. Related diagnoses include activity intolerance, anxiety, altered thought processes, and self-care deficit.

PLANNING AND IMPLEMENTATION

The client is maintained either in a semi-Fowler's position to aid ventilation or in a side-lying position with the good lung in the dependent position. Relaxation exercises may help reduce anxiety and relieve dyspnea. Breathing exercises may be helpful if the client is able to cooperate. Bed rest is important to reduce the demand for oxygen. Because any movement can trigger an increase in dyspnea, the nurse helps position the client in bed and anticipates needs to prevent unnecessary exertion by the client. Meals and treatments should be spaced to allow the client time to rest. It is often helpful to provide NMTs or MDI therapy before meals so that the client is able to eat without excessive dyspnea. Oxygen therapy is maintained as ordered. Fluids (if not contraindicated) and coughing and deep breathing help remove secretions. Suctioning may be ordered if necessary.

LEARNING TIP

The "good lung down" position can help increase oxygenation in clients with lung disease. Gravity results in more blood in the dependent lung, where it can receive oxygen from the healthier lung tissue. If both lungs are diseased, the right lung down position may be beneficial, because the right lung has a larger surface area.[1]

EVALUATION

If interventions have been effective, the client will state that dyspnea is controlled. Mental status will be normal for the client. Airways will be kept clear at all times, and the client's respiratory rate will be regular and within normal limits.

Lung Cancer

Lung cancer is the leading cause of cancer death in the United States. An estimated 178,000 new cases were pre-

dicted for the United States in 1997. About 29 percent of cancer deaths are from lung cancer. The 5-year survival rate for all lung cancers is 14 percent. This rate increases to 48 percent if lung cancer is diagnosed and treated early.[2] The incidence of lung cancer among men is decreasing, whereas it is on the rise in women; this is thought to be related to an increase in the number of women who smoke.

PATHOPHYSIOLOGY

Lung cancers originate in the respiratory tract epithelium; most originate in the lining of the bronchi. The four major types of lung cancer are identified by the type of cells that are affected. These include small cell lung cancer (SCLC), large cell carcinoma, adenocarcinoma, and squamous cell carcinoma. The latter three types are classified as non–small cell lung cancer (NSCLC).

About 20 percent of lung cancers are SCLC, sometimes called oat cell carcinoma. SCLC grows rapidly and often has metastasized by the time of diagnosis. It is usually caused by smoking and is most often found centrally, near the bronchi. The client with small cell carcinoma has a poor prognosis, with survival time averaging only 9 to 10 months.

Large cell carcinoma is a rapidly growing cancer that can occur anywhere in the lungs. It metastasizes early in the disease, so these clients also have a poor prognosis. It accounts for about 10 percent of lung cancers.

Adenocarcinoma occurs more often in women, and most often in the peripheral lung fields. It accounts for about 40 percent of lung cancers. It is slow growing, but often is not diagnosed until metastasis has occurred. It is less closely linked with smoking. Prognosis may be better than other lung cancer types.

About 30 percent of lung cancers are squamous cell carcinomas. These usually originate near the bronchi and metastasize late in the disease. They are associated with a history of smoking. The prognosis for individuals with squamous cell carcinoma may also be better than for some other lung cancers.

ETIOLOGY

The most common cause of lung cancer is tobacco smoke. Cigarettes contain chemicals that cause DNA to mutate, creating changes in cells and development of tumors. Smokers have an approximately 13 times greater risk for developing lung cancer than nonsmokers. If a client stops smoking, risk for lung cancer decreases significantly. Unfortunately, even with all of this information, 26 percent of Americans continue to smoke.[3]

Environmental tobacco smoke (ETS) has also been shown to cause lung cancer. A recent study by the American Cancer Society showed that women who were married to smokers, but who had never smoked themselves, were 20 percent more likely to die of lung cancer.[4]

Other factors that contribute to increased lung cancer risk are asbestos exposure; coal, uranium, and iron mining; air pollution; diesel exhaust; and radiation. Genetic predisposition and a diet poor in vitamins A, C, and E may also be factors.

PREVENTION

The single most important way to prevent lung cancer is to reduce smoking. Many programs educate schoolchildren about the dangers of smoking. Smoking cessation programs are available for people who desire to quit. The nurse is encouraged to contact a local American Cancer Society chapter for smoking cessation programs that can be recommended to clients.

SIGNS AND SYMPTOMS

Manifestations of lung cancer depend on the location of the tumor. Commonly, clients exhibit a cough with sputum production. These symptoms may be ignored by the client, because they are also associated with smoking. Repeated respiratory infections may occur, producing thick, purulent sputum. Sputum may become bloody (hemoptysis). The client may experience dyspnea. If the airway becomes obstructed by the tumor, wheezing or stridor may be heard. Late signs include chest pain, weight loss, anemia, and anorexia.

COMPLICATIONS

Pleural Effusion

Fifty percent of clients with lung cancer develop pleural effusion. Pleural fluid collects in the pleural space as a result of pleural irritation or obstruction of lymphatic or venous drainage by the tumor.

Superior Vena Cava Syndrome

If the tumor obstructs the superior vena cava, blood flow is interrupted, causing distention of the jugular veins and swelling of the chest, face, and neck. Diuretics may help relieve the fluid buildup. Radiation may be used to shrink the obstruction.

Ectopic Hormone Production

Some lung cancers produce **ectopic** hormones that mimic the body's own hormones. Ectopic production of antidiuretic hormone (ADH) can produce a syndrome of inappropriate ADH production (SAIDH), which is associated with fluid retention. Ectopic production of adrenocorti-

Table 28–4. **Stages of Lung Cancer**

Stages of Non–Small Cell Lung Cancer
Stage I
• No metastasis to lymph nodes.
• Atelectasis or pneumonia may be present.
Stage II
• Cancer has spread to local lymph nodes.
Stage III
• Cancer has invaded chest wall and usually has spread to lymph nodes.
Stage IV
• Tumor has metastasized to distant organs and lymph nodes.
Stages of Small Cell Lung Cancer
Limited Stage
• Cancer is limited to one side of the chest.
Extensive
• Cancer cells are found outside one side of the chest or in pleural fluid.

cotropic hormone (ACTH) can cause Cushing's syndrome. These disorders are discussed in Chapter 37.

Atelectasis and Pneumonia

Atelectasis occurs when tumor growth prevents ventilation of areas of the lung. Clients with lung cancer also have a greater risk for pneumonia.

Metastasis

Common sites of lung cancer metastasis include the brain, bones, opposite lung, liver, adrenal gland, and lymph nodes.

DIAGNOSTIC TESTS

A complete medical history and physical examination are done to look for symptoms and risk factors for lung cancer. A chest x-ray is done to identify a mass. However, all tumors may not show up on chest x-ray. A CT scan and a lung scan may be done to provide more specific information about the size and location of a tumor. Sputum is analyzed for abnormal cells. Brain and bone scans are done to find metastatic lesions.

Diagnosis is confirmed with a biopsy of the lesion. A biopsy may be obtained via bronchoscopy, percutaneous bi-

ectopic: displaced

opsy (a needle through the skin guided by x-ray), or mediastinoscopy (use of a scope into the mediastinum to look for changes in mediastinal lymph nodes).

MEDICAL AND SURGICAL TREATMENT

Tumors are staged based on the TNM staging system. (See Chapter 10.) Staging helps determine appropriate treatment. See Table 28–4 for stages of lung cancer. If the NSCLC is localized and in an early stage, it may be cured with surgical removal of the tumor. This can be accomplished with a segmental or wedge resection, which removes only the affected lung segment. A lobectomy (removal of a lobe), or removal of an entire lung may be done in more advanced cases (Fig. 28–9). Surgery is contraindicated if the cancer has spread to the other lung or has metastasized to distant areas.

Chemotherapy is the treatment of choice in SCLC, because it has generally metastasized and is widespread by the time of diagnosis. Radiation may be used in combination with chemotherapy. Surgery is not indicated. The goal of treatment is not cure, but rather palliation of symptoms.

Radiation may be used to shrink the tumor to reduce symptoms in clients who are unable to undergo surgery. Both radiation and chemotherapy may be used before or after surgery as **adjuvant** treatments.

Nursing Process: The Client with Lung Cancer

ASSESSMENT

The nurse does a complete biopsychosocial assessment of the client with lung cancer. The nurse assesses and docu-

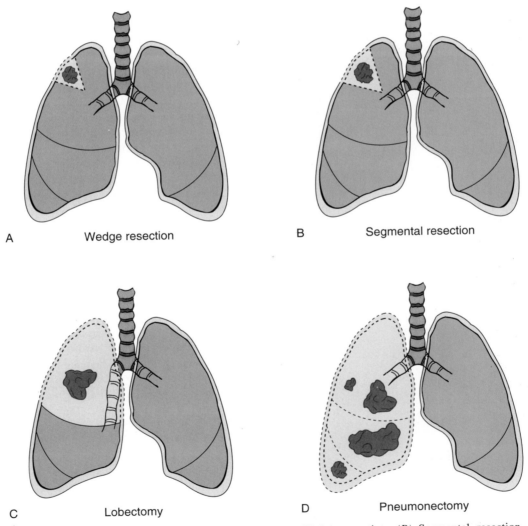

Figure 28–9. Types of surgeries for lung cancer. *(A)* Wedge resection. *(B)* Segmental resection. *(C)* Lobectomy. *(D)* Pneumonectomy.

ments respiratory rate and depth, skin and mucous membrane color, lung sounds, cough, and sputum amount and character. The client is asked to rate the degree of pain and dyspnea on appropriate scales. The client is questioned about appetite and weight loss, as well as symptoms of other complications. Activity tolerance and fatigue are noted.

In addition, the client may be grieving about his or her illness and impending death. Assessment of the client's coping strategies and support systems will help the nurse plan care for psychosocial needs. When the nurse recalls the prognosis for clients with lung cancer, the need to consider planning for terminal care becomes obvious. The presence of a living will or durable power of attorney should be noted. (See Ethical Considerations Box 28–6.)

ETHICAL CONSIDERATIONS BOX 28-6

The Client with Lung Cancer

Mr. David H., 88 years old, is admitted to a room on the surgical unit. Mr. H. has been diagnosed with a metastatic tumor of the lung, but does not yet know the diagnosis. The physician, Dr. Lester I., and the family have discussed the diagnosis. Dr. I. decided not to tell Mr. H. the diagnosis because he believes that Mr. H. would become very upset or depressed by the knowledge. Dr. I. has written an order that the patient is not to be told his diagnosis.

Mr. H. was taken to surgery for a thoracotomy. For the past 2 days after surgery, the patient has been asking all the nurses, staff, and family what the physician found in surgery, and what the results of the pathology reports were. The physician has visited Mr. H. several times, but has avoided talking about the diagnosis by saying that all the lab tests were not back yet. The family has been avoiding visiting the patient so that he will not ask them about the diagnosis. The family frequently asks the nurse when Mr. H. will be told his diagnosis. They believe the physician should tell him.

The nurse believes that the patient should be told, but is fearful of violating the physician's written order. She too has been carefully avoiding answering Mr. H.'s questions by telling "white lies" but feels very uncomfortable doing it. How should the nurse handle this situation?

The basic dilemma in this particular situation is the patient's right to know and the nurse's obligation for veracity or truth telling versus the physician's right to write an order that contradicts that. Possible actions the nurse may take include (1) continue to lie to the patient; (2) encourage the physician to tell the truth to the patient; or (3) go ahead and tell the truth to the patient, and then live with the consequences of contradicting a physician's written order. Remember, telling a patient the medical diagnosis is not really a nursing function except for the obligation to tell the truth. What should the nurse do? Why?

NURSING DIAGNOSIS

Possible diagnoses that may be experienced by the client with lung cancer include impaired gas exchange, ineffective airway clearance, altered nutrition: less than body requirements, pain, constipation related to opioid use, grieving, and activity intolerance, among others.

PLANNING

A plan is formulated that will help the client control episodes of dyspnea, maintain a clear airway, reduce anorexia and maintain body weight, promote comfort, and maintain regular bowel habits. Clients who are terminal are assisted in coping with their impending death.

IMPLEMENTATION

The experience of dyspnea related to impaired gas exchange is very frightening to clients and their families. Home oxygen therapy may be necessary. Positioning, relaxation, and breathing exercises can help reduce dyspnea and feelings of panic. Antianxiety drugs or morphine may also be helpful. Resting between activities will reduce the demand for oxygen. The client is encouraged to avoid smoking and exposure to secondary smoke.

A clear airway can be promoted with a room humidifier and oral fluids to reduce viscosity of secretions, and regular coughing and deep breathing exercises. A nagging, nonproductive cough can be treated with an antitussive as ordered by the physician. The client is instructed to notify the physician if hemoptysis is persistent. Exposure to powders, tobacco smoke, and aerosols increases airway irritation and should be eliminated. Suctioning may be necessary if the client becomes too weak to cough effectively.

Anorexia is common in the client with cancer. Nutrition may be maintained by eating frequent small meals. Nutritional supplements that are high in calories but easy to eat or drink may be helpful. A dietitian consultation is helpful. Antiemetics before meals may help control nausea. Use of spices to enhance flavor of foods may be used as the client prefers. Mints may help reduce the metallic taste left in the mouth by some chemotherapeutic medications. Good mouth care is essential. Total parenteral nutrition may be necessary late in the disease. (See Nutrition Notes Box 28–4.)

Pain is controlled by opioids and supportive noninvasive therapies. See Chapter 9 for more information on pain control. The nurse is also directed to the AHCPR guidelines for treatment of cancer pain (Chapter 9).

Use of opioids for pain control necessitates attention to bowel function. Constipation should be prevented with the use of high-fiber foods and extra fluids if tolerated. If these conservative measures are ineffective, bulk-forming agents, stool softeners, and laxatives can be used.

Fatigue is battled with frequent rest periods and assistance with activities of daily living. The client is encouraged to identify and engage in those activities that are most important to him or her and to avoid unnecessary or undesirable activities.

The client who is grieving should be allowed the opportunity to talk about his or her life and impending death and to express anger or sadness. The nurse should be physically present but should not force verbalization unless the client wishes to talk. The family is encouraged to stay with the client as much as the client wishes. A minister or spiritual counselor is helpful if the client desires a referral.

Hospice care is available for the client who is terminal. This allows the family to have the support needed to care for the client in his or her home or a homelike environment.

EVALUATION

The nurse looks carefully at the client's individual goals when evaluating care. Is the client comfortable and free from unnecessary dyspnea? Is the airway clear, and is nutrition maintained? Are medication side effects manageable? Have terminal clients come to terms with their impending death, and have they been able to do those things most important to them before their death?

Thoracic Surgery

A surgical incision made into the chest wall is called a **thoracotomy.** A thoracotomy may be performed for a number of reasons.

REASONS FOR THORACIC SURGERY

Thoracic surgery may be performed for biopsy; for removal of tumors, lesions, or foreign objects; to repair trauma following penetrating or crushing injuries; or to repair or revise structural problems. Open heart surgery also requires a thoracotomy and is discussed in Chapter 22.

TYPES OF THORACIC SURGERY

Pneumonectomy

A **pneumonectomy** is the surgical removal of a lung. This is usually done to treat lung cancer. It may also be done to treat severe cases of tuberculosis, bronchiectasis, or lung abscesses. Chest drainage is not usually used following a pneumonectomy, because once the lung is removed, the air in the thoracic cavity is absorbed and the cavity fills with serosanguineous fluid. At about 6 months after sur-

gery, the fluid is coagulated and the thoracic cavity is stabilized.

Lobectomy

Lobectomy refers to the surgical removal of one lobe. This also may be done for lung cancer, tuberculosis, or another localized problem.

Resection

Resection refers to removal of a smaller amount of lung tissue, that is, less than one lobe. A segmental resection is the removal of one segment of a lobe; a wedge resection is removal of a small wedge of lung tissue.

Lung Transplantation

Lung transplant can benefit clients with a variety of serious pulmonary disorders, including pulmonary hypertension, emphysema, cystic fibrosis, and bronchiectasis. Either a single lung, both lungs, or heart and lungs have been successfully transplanted. Better criteria for selecting clients and donors, as well as advancements in surgical techniques, have improved outcomes for these clients.

Nursing Process: The Client Undergoing Thoracic Surgery

PREOPERATIVE NURSING CARE

A nursing assessment is done preoperatively, with a focus on the respiratory system. This gives a baseline against which to judge changes postoperatively. Routine preoperative teaching is done by the nurse and physician. The client should understand that he or she will wake up in an intensive care environment. If at all possible, it is helpful to have the client and family tour the intensive care unit before the surgery, to decrease anxiety postoperatively. The client should be prepared for the possibilities of waking up after surgery with an endotracheal tube connected to a ventilator, oxygen, chest tubes, intravenous fluids, a cardiac monitor, a Foley catheter, and possibly an epidural catheter for pain control. The surgeon should be consulted for specific plans.

The client is advised that position changes and early ambulation will help prevent complications following surgery. The client is also instructed in the use of an incentive spirometer and coughing and deep breathing techniques.

POSTOPERATIVE NURSING CARE

Assessment

Following thoracic surgery, clients will initially be in an intensive care unit. Larger hospitals have special intensive

---

pneumonectomy: pneum—lung + ectomy—excision
lobectomy: lobe—lobe (of lung) + ectomy—excision

care units specifically for surgical or thoracic clients. Here clients can be closely monitored for signs of complications. Frequent assessment of vital signs; respiratory rate, depth, and effort; and lung sounds is performed. Remember that lung sounds will be absent on the side of a pneumonectomy. An increase in pulse rate or a falling blood pressure may indicate internal bleeding and should be reported immediately. Oxygen saturation is monitored continuously. Often clients report an immediate improvement in breathing, because the pulmonary blood supply is no longer being routed to diseased lung tissue.

Assessment for tracheal deviation alerts the nurse to the possible complication of mediastinal shift. The trachea is normally positioned straight above the sternal notch. If the trachea deviates from the midline position, the surgeon should be notified immediately. Secretions are monitored and reported to the physician if they become thick, yellow or green, or foul smelling. Arterial blood gases are monitored closely. Chest tubes are usually present (except following pneumonectomy) and are monitored as in Chapter 26. Pain is assessed using a pain rating scale, and incision sites are monitored for redness, edema, or drainage. If the client is mechanically ventilated, additional assessment of the endotracheal tube and ventilator settings will be necessary.

Nursing Diagnosis

After thoracic surgery, many respiratory diagnoses may be appropriate. The client may experience an ineffective airway clearance due to increased secretions and a weak or painful cough. Ineffective breathing pattern may result from pain on inspiration and fatigue. Impaired gas exchange may occur due to increased secretions or hesitance to breathe deeply. Impaired physical mobility results from the client's hesitance to move the arm and shoulder on the affected side. Pain and risk for infection are always concerns following surgery.

Planning and Implementation

Ineffective Airway Clearance

Regular suctioning is necessary while the client is intubated to keep the airways free of secretions. Once extubated, the client is reminded to cough and deep breathe regularly. Postoperative pain must be controlled for the client to be able to cough effectively. Intravenous or oral fluids, humidified oxygen, and a room humidifier will help keep secretions thin.

Acute Pain

Pain control is important in order for the client to be able to deep breathe and cough effectively and ambulate. Some institutions are successfully using epidural analgesia following thoracotomy. Because narcotics depress respirations, it is important to monitor respiratory rate before their admin-

istration. The client is also taught to splint the incision while coughing.

Impaired Gas Exchange

Maintaining a Fowler's position and use of an incentive spirometer will encourage the client to deep breathe and maximize oxygenation. Oxygen and bronchodilators are administered as ordered. Some authorities believe clients should be positioned with the operative side up, others with the operative side down. The surgeon should be consulted for specific positioning orders.

Impaired Physical Mobility

Range of motion exercises are performed to prevent contracture of the arm and shoulder on the affected side. This may be done passively at first, then actively when the client is able. The client is out of bed on the first or second postoperative day and ambulates as tolerated.

Risk for Infection

Sterile technique for suctioning and standard infection control precautions are used. The client is extubated as soon as possible to reduce the risk of postoperative infection.

Evaluation

The client's airway should remain clear, and secretions should be easily coughed up. The client should report an acceptable comfort level and be able to cough, deep breathe, and ambulate without excessive discomfort. The client's breathing should be unlabored, with a respiratory rate of 12 to 20 per minute. The client's affected arm and shoulder should maintain full range of motion. Signs of infection should be absent.

Review Questions

1. Which of the following assessment findings in the client with pneumonia most indicates a need to remind the client to cough and deep breathe?
   a. The client complains of chest pain.
   b. The client has removed her oxygen.
   c. The nurse auscultates wheezes and crackles.
   d. The nurse notes a fever of 101°F.

2. Which of the following clients should be placed in respiratory isolation?
   a. The client with chronic bronchitis
   b. The client with tuberculosis
   c. The client who is coughing
   d. The client with severe dyspnea

3. Which of the following assessment findings does the nurse expect in the client with emphysema?
   a. Purulent sputum
   b. Diminished breath sounds

c. Generalized edema
d. Dull chest pain

4. Which of the following best describes the pathophysiology of asthma?
   a. Damaged alveoli with impaired gas exchange
   b. Pulmonary edema with decreased compliance of the alveoli
   c. Dilated bronchial sacs containing large amounts of sputum
   d. Inflammation and constriction of bronchioles

5. Which of the following assessment findings in the client with pneumothorax does the nurse report immediately?
   a. Diminished breath sounds over the affected area
   b. Frequent dry cough
   c. Moderate pain at the chest tube site
   d. Positioning of the trachea toward the unaffected side

6. As the nurse enters Mr. Jones' room, he notes that the client has become confused and combative over the past hour. Which of the following actions is appropriate first?
   a. Assess Mr. Jones; check to see if his oxygen is flowing correctly.
   b. Page the physician stat.
   c. Put up Mr. Jones' side rails and apply soft restraints.
   d. Administer an oral sedative.

7. Which of the following interventions is most appropriate for the client with an ineffective breathing pattern?
   a. Encourage the client to cough and deep breathe.
   b. Encourage oral fluids.
   c. Teach the client controlled diaphragmatic breathing.
   d. Allow the client to rest between activities.

8. The nurse develops a plan for ineffective airway clearance for Mrs. Brown. Which of the following findings best helps the nurse to know when the goal has been reached?
   a. Mrs. Brown is alert and oriented.
   b. Mrs. Brown is able to clear her airway with coughing.
   c. Mrs. Brown correctly demonstrates coughing and deep breathing techniques.
   d. Mrs. Brown's respiratory rate is 16 per minute and unlabored.

9. Mrs. Jackson had an abdominal hysterectomy yesterday. The nurse enters her room and finds her acutely short of breath, with a look of panic in her eyes. Which of the following additional symptoms is most important as the nurse decides what to do?
   a. Mrs. Jackson complained of pain in her left leg earlier this morning.
   b. Mrs. Jackson states that she also has a headache.
   c. Mrs. Jackson has a recent history of an upper respiratory infection.
   d. Mrs. Jackson has not eaten in 24 hours.

Answers to Critical Thinking

CRITICAL THINKING: Mr. Smith

1. A complete respiratory history is taken as described in Chapter 26. An open-ended question such as "What happened to bring you to the hospital?" will elicit information about the incident. In addition, questions to determine mental status and ability to make decisions and function safely on his own would be appropriate. If any concerns arise, a social service consult might be helpful for discharge planning.

2. Mr. Smith should be instructed to always read label warnings before using any cleaning products in the future, and to *never* mix bleach and ammonia!

CRITICAL THINKING: Jim

1. Ask questions based on the WHAT'S UP? format:
   Where (not applicable)
   How does it feel? Does the coughing cause chest pain? Are you short of breath?
   Aggravating and alleviating factors. What makes the cough worse? What seems to help? Do you use any techniques at home that are helpful?
   Timing. How often do you cough during a day? Is it interfering with sleep and rest?
   Severity. How bad is it on a scale of 1 to 10? How much sputum are you coughing up? What color is it?
   Useful other data. Are you experiencing any other symptoms with your cough (such as shortness of breath, nausea, loss of appetite)?
   Patient's perception. Is it better or worse than usual today? How can I help? (The client with long-standing disease often knows what will help but is hesitant to ask.)

2. The most appropriate nursing diagnosis is ineffective airway clearance related to excessive secretions and ineffective cough.

3. Provide hydration with oral liquids and a room humidifier to liquefy secretions. Administer expectorants as ordered. Instruct the client in coughing and deep breathing exercises to increase the effectiveness of his cough. Provide good oral care following expectoration of sputum to freshen the client's mouth. Obtain an order for chest physiotherapy to help loosen and drain secretions.

REFERENCES

1. Yeaw, E: How position affects oxygenation: Good lung down? Am J Nurs 92:26, 1992.

2. American Cancer Society: Cancer Facts and Figures. American Cancer Society, Atlanta, 1997.
3. American Cancer Society: Cancer Risk Report. American Cancer Society, Atlanta, 1997.
4. Cardenas, VM, Thun, MJ, Austin H, et al: Environmental tobacco smoke and lung cancer mortality in the American Cancer Society's Cancer Prevention Study II. Cancer Causes and Control 8:57, 1997.

BIBLIOGRAPHY

Ackley, BJ, and Ladwig, GB: Nursing Diagnosis Handbook: A Guide to Planning Care. Mosby, St Louis, 1995.
Brenner, ZR, and Addona, C: Caring for the pneumonectomy patient: Challenges and changes. Crit Care Nurse 15:65, 1995.
Borkgren, MW, and Gronkiewicz, CA: Update your asthma care from hospital to home. Am J Nurs 96:26, 1995.
Colice, GL: Pulmonary tuberculosis. Postgrad Med 97:4, 1995.
Dibble, SL, and Savedra, MC: Cystic fibrosis in adolescence: A new challenge. Pediatr Nurs 14:4, 1988.

Handler, JA, and Feied, CF: Acute pulmonary embolism. Postgrad Med 97:1, 1995.
Held, JL: Caring for a patient with lung cancer. Nursing Oct 1995.
Huether, SE, and McCance, KL: Understanding Pathophysiology. Mosby, St Louis, 1996.
Isselbacher, KJ, et al: Harrison's Principles of Internal Medicine. McGraw-Hill, New York, 1994.
Martinez, FJ, et al: Lung-volume reduction improves dyspnea, dynamic hyperinflation, and respiratory muscle function. Am J Respir Crit Care Med 6:155, 1997.
McKinney, B: Under new management: Asthma and the elderly. J Gerontol Nurs 21:39, 1995.
O'Byrne, PM, et al: Antileukotrienes in the treatment of asthma. Ann Intern Med 127:6, 1997.
Repasky, TM: Tension pneumothorax. Am J Nurs 94:47, 1994.
Swanlund, SL: Body positioning and the elderly with adult respiratory distress syndrome: Implications for nursing care. J Gerontol Nurs 22:46,1996.
Wason, J, and Jaffe, MS: Nurse's Manual of Laboratory and Diagnostic Tests, ed 2. FA Davis, Philadelphia, 1995.

Understanding the Gastrointestinal System

Gastrointestinal System Function, Assessment, and Therapeutic Measures

Sharon Ivy Gordon and Valerie C. Scanlon

Learning Objectives

Upon completion of this chapter, the student will be able to:

1. Identify the structures of the gastrointestinal system.
2. Describe the functions of the gastrointestinal system.
3. List the effects of aging on the gastrointestinal system.
4. Perform a gastrointestinal assessment on a client with actual or potential problems of the mouth, esophagus, stomach, and intestines.
5. Describe the client preparation, teaching, and follow-up care for clients having diagnostic tests of the gastrointestinal tract.
6. Describe general therapeutic measures for clients with gastrointestinal disease.

Key Words

basal cell secretion test (**BAY**-zuhl SELL see-**KREE**-shun TEST)

bowel sounds (BOW'L SOWNDS)

carcinoembryonic antigens (**KAR**-sin-oh-EM-bree-ah-nik **AN**-ti-jens)

colonoscopy (KOH-lun-**AHS**-kuh-pee)

endoscope (**EN**-doh-skohp)

esophagoscopy (ee-soff-ah-**GAHS**-kuh-pee)

fluoroscope (**FLAW**-or-oh-skohp)

gastric acid stimulation test (**GAS**-trik **ASS**-id STIM-yoo-**LAY**-shun TEST)

gastric analysis (**GAS**-trik ah-**NAL**-i-sis)

gastroscopy (gas-**TRAHS**-kuh-pee)

gastrostomy (gas-**TRAHS**-toh-mee)

gavage (gah-**VAZH**)

guaiac (**GWY**-ak)

impaction (im-**PAK**-shun)

lavage (lah-**VAZH**)

lower gastrointestinal series (**LOH**-er GAS-troh-in-**TES**-ti-nuhl **SEER**-ees)

occult blood test (ah-**KULT** BLUHD TEST)

peripheral parenteral nutrition (puh-**RIFF**-uh-ruhl par-**EN**-te-ruhl new-**TRISH**-un)

proctosigmoidoscopy (PROK-toh-SIG-moy-**DAHS**-kuh-pee)

steatorrhea (STEE-ah-toh-**REE**-ah)

upper gastrointestinal series (**UH**-per GAS-troh-in-**TES**-ti-nuhl **SEER**-ees)

The authors acknowledge the contribution to this chapter by Gary Sanders Lott.

Review of Normal Gastrointestinal Anatomy and Physiology

The alimentary tube is part of the digestive system (Fig. 29–1). It extends from the mouth to the anus and consists of the oral cavity, pharynx, esophagus, stomach, small intestine, and large intestine (or colon). Digestion takes place within the oral cavity, stomach, and small intestine; most absorption of nutrients takes place in the small intestine. Undigestable material, mainly cellulose, is eliminated by the large intestine.

ORAL CAVITY AND PHARYNX

The boundaries of the oral cavity are the hard and soft palates superiorly, the cheeks laterally, and the floor of the mouth inferiorly. Within the oral cavity are the teeth and tongue and the openings of the ducts of the salivary glands.

The teeth begin mechanical digestion, the physical breakup of food into smaller pieces to create more surface area for the chemical digestion brought about by enzymes. The roots of the teeth are in sockets in the jawbones (the mandible and maxillae). The gums, or gingiva, cover the jawbones and surround the bases of the crowns (top) of the teeth. The tooth sockets are lined with a periodontal membrane that produces a bonelike cement to anchor the teeth.

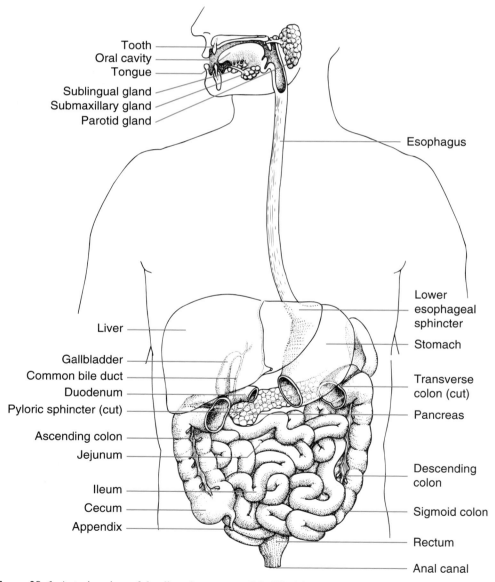

Figure 29–1. Anterior view of the digestive system. (Modified from Scanlon, VC, Sanders, T: Workbook for Essentials of Anatomy and Physiology, ed 2. FA Davis, Philadelphia, 1995, p 252, with permission.) See Plate 4.

The tongue is made of skeletal muscle innervated by the hypoglossal nerve (twelfth cranial). The papillae on the upper surface of the tongue contain taste buds, innervated by the facial and glossopharyngeal nerves (seventh and ninth cranial). The tongue is important for chewing because it keeps food between the teeth. Elevation of the tongue is the first step in swallowing.

The three pairs of salivary glands are the parotid, submandibular, and sublingual glands. Their ducts carry saliva to the oral cavity. The presence of anything in the mouth increases the rate of secretion; this is a parasympathetic response mediated by the facial and glossopharyngeal nerves. Saliva is mostly water, which is important to dissolve food for tasting and moisten food for swallowing. The only digestive enzyme in saliva is amylase, which digests starch to maltose. Usually, however, food does not remain long enough in the mouth for amylase to have any significant effect.

The pharynx is a muscular tube that is a passageway for food from the oral cavity to the esophagus. When a mass of food is pushed backward by the tongue, the constrictor muscles of the pharynx contract as part of the swallowing reflex. This reflex is regulated by the medulla.

ESOPHAGUS

The esophagus is about 10 inches long and carries food from the pharynx to the stomach. No digestion takes place.

Peristalsis of the muscle layer in the wall of the esophagus is one-way; food reaches the stomach even if the body is upside down. At the junction with the stomach, the lumen of the esophagus is surrounded by the lower esophageal sphincter (LES) (gastroesophageal sphincter, or cardiac sphincter), a circular smooth muscle. The LES relaxes to permit food to enter the stomach and then contracts to prevent the backup of stomach contents. Incomplete closure of the LES may allow gastric juice to splash up into the esophagus.

STOMACH

The stomach is in the upper left abdominal quadrant, to the left of the liver and in front of the spleen. It is a saclike organ that extends from the esophagus to the duodenum of the small intestine. Some digestion takes place in the stomach, and it also serves as a reservoir for food so that digestion may take place gradually.

The parts of the stomach are shown in Figure 29–2. The cardiac orifice is the opening of the esophagus; the fundus is the part above the level of this opening. The body of the stomach is the large, central portion, bounded laterally by the greater curvature and medially by the lesser curvature. The pylorus is adjacent to the duodenum, and the pyloric sphincter surrounds the junction of the two organs.

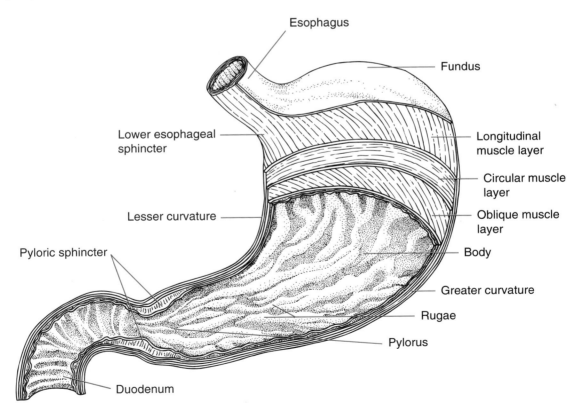

Figure 29–2. Stomach, anterior view and partial section. (Modified from Scanlon, VC, Sanders, T: Workbook for Essentials of Anatomy and Physiology, ed 2. FA Davis, Philadelphia, 1995, p 256, with permission.) See Plate 5.

When the stomach is empty, the mucosa has folds called rugae. The rugae flatten out as the stomach fills and permit expansion of the lining. The mucosa contains gastric pits, the glands of the stomach that produce gastric juice. Gastric juice is mostly water, and contains mucus, pepsinogen, and hydrochloric acid. Pepsinogen is an inactive enzyme that is changed to active pepsin by hydrochloric acid; pepsin begins the digestion of proteins to polypeptides. Hydrochloric acid creates the pH of 1 to 2 that is necessary for pepsin to function and also kills most microorganisms that enter the stomach.

Gastric juice is secreted at the sight or smell of food; this is a parasympathetic response. The presence of food in the stomach stimulates the secretion of the hormone gastrin by the gastric mucosa. Gastrin increases the secretion of gastric juice.

The stomach wall has three layers of smooth muscle: circular, longitudinal, and oblique layers. These provide for very efficient mechanical digestion to change food to a thick liquid called chyme. The pyloric sphincter is usually contracted when the stomach is churning food. It relaxes at intervals to allow small amounts of chyme to pass into the duodenum, then contracts again to prevent the backup of intestinal contents into the stomach.

SMALL INTESTINE

The small intestine is about 1 inch in diameter and approximately 20 feet long. Within the abdominal cavity, the coils of the small intestine are encircled by the colon. The small intestine extends from the stomach to the cecum of the colon. The duodenum is the first 10 inches and contains the hepatopancreatic ampulla (ampulla of Vater), the entrance of the common bile duct. The jejunum is about 8 feet long, and the ileum is about 11 feet in length.

Digestion is completed in the small intestine, and the end products of digestion are absorbed into the blood and lymph. Bile from the liver and enzymes from the pancreas function in the small intestine (Table 29–1). When chyme enters the duodenum the intestinal mucosa produces the enzymes sucrase, maltase, and lactase, which complete the digestion of disaccharides to monosaccharides, and the peptidases, which complete the digestion of proteins to amino acids.

The absorption of nutrients requires a large surface area, and the small intestine has extensive folds for this purpose. The circular folds (plica circulares) are macroscopic folds of the mucosa and submucosa. Villi are folds of the mucosa, and microvilli are microscopic folds of the cell membranes on the free surface of the intestinal epithelial cells. Within each villus is a capillary network and a lymph capillary called a lacteal. Water-soluble nutrients (monosaccharides, amino acids, minerals, water-soluble vitamins) are absorbed into the blood in the capillary networks. Fat-soluble vitamins and fatty acids and glycerol are absorbed into the lymph in the lacteals.

LARGE INTESTINE

The large intestine extends from the ileum of the small intestine to the anus. It is about 5 feet long and 2.5 inches in diameter. The cecum is the first part, and at its junction with the ileum is the ileocecal valve, which prevents backup of colon contents into the small intestine. Attached to the cecum is the small, dead-end appendix, apparently a vestigial (an incompletely developed structure that was more developed in a previous stage of the species) organ for people, but one that may become a site of infection.

The other parts of the colon are the ascending, transverse, and descending colon, which encircle the small intestine; the sigmoid colon, which turns medially and downward; the rectum, which is about 6 inches long; and the anal canal, the last inch that surrounds the anus (clinically, the terminal end of the colon is usually referred to as the rectum).

Although no digestion takes place in the colon, its functions are important. The colon temporarily stores and then eliminates undigestible material. The mucosa absorbs sig-

Table 29–1. **Digestive Secretions**

Organ	Enzyme or Other Secretion	Function	Site of Action
Salivary Glands	Amylase	Converts starch to maltose	Oral cavity
Stomach	Pepsin	Converts proteins to polypeptides	Stomach
	Hydrochloric acid	Changes pepsinogen to pepsin; maintains pH 1–2; destroys pathogens	Stomach
Liver	Bile salts	Emulsifies fats	Small intestine
Pancreas	Amylase	Converts starch to maltose	Small intestine
	Lipase	Converts emulsified fats to fatty acids and glycerol	Small intestine
	Trypsin	Converts polypeptides to peptides	Small intestine
Small Intestine	Peptidases	Converts peptides to amino acids	Small intestine
	Sucrase, maltase, lactase	Converts disaccharides to monosaccharides	Small intestine

nificant amounts of water and minerals, as well as the vitamins produced by the normal bacterial flora.

Elimination of feces is accomplished by the defecation reflex, a spinal cord reflex over which voluntary control may be exerted. When peristalsis propels feces into the rectum, receptors in the smooth muscle layer detect the stretching and generate impulses to the spinal cord. The returning motor impulses cause contraction of the smooth muscle of the rectum, and relaxation of the internal anal sphincter, which surrounds the anus. Surrounding the internal sphincter is the external anal sphincter, which is made of skeletal muscle and may be voluntarily contracted to prevent defecation.

AGING AND THE GASTROINTESTINAL SYSTEM

Many changes occur in the aging gastrointestinal (GI) system. The sense of taste becomes less acute, and there is greater likelihood of periodontal disease or oral cancer. Secretions throughout the GI tract are reduced, and the effectiveness of peristalsis diminishes. Indigestion may become more common, especially if the LES loses its tone, and there is greater chance of peptic ulcer. In the colon, diverticula may form and may be asymptomatic or become infected. Constipation may be a problem, as may hemorrhoids. The risk of colon cancer also increases with age.

Nursing Assessment

Nursing assessment of the GI system includes a client history and physical examination. The nurse notes the client's general GI system health status and characteristics of the present illness.

SUBJECTIVE DATA

Health History

Assessment of current signs and symptoms includes asking questions for the acronym WHAT'S UP: where it is, how it feels, aggravating and alleviating factors, timing, severity, useful data for associated symptoms, and perception by the client of the problem. Also documented are the client's normal bowel pattern; changes in bowel patterns or habits; a history of any gastrointestinal diseases, such as ulcers, cancer, Crohn's disease, or colitis; or an unexplained weight loss or gain. Information about previous gastrointestinal surgeries is obtained. Serious signs or symptoms of disease, such as bloody or tarry stools, rectal bleeding, stomach pain, or abdominal pain, are also noted.

Medications

The client is asked about medication use such as nonsteroidal anti-inflammatory drugs (NSAIDs), aspirin, vitamins, laxatives, enemas, or antacids. Heavy use of medications that can cause irritation and bleeding in the GI tract such as NSAIDs (e.g., ibuprofen [Motrin]) or aspirin should be carefully noted. Elderly clients with arthritis often use these types of medications for pain control. The client's knowledge of the side effects of these medications should be assessed to identify teaching needs. Elderly clients may use laxatives regularly and develop a dependence on them. Teaching may be needed on normal bowel patterns and laxative use.

CRITICAL THINKING: Mrs. Todd

Mrs. Todd, 74, has arthritis and takes eight aspirin daily for pain control. She is admitted for GI bleeding due to bright red stools.

1. What is a likely cause of the GI bleeding?
2. What could the nurse do to help prevent future bleeding episodes for Mrs. Todd?

Answers at end of chapter.

Nutritional Assessment

A diet history should include usual foods and fluids, allergies, appetite patterns, swallowing difficulty, and use of nutritional supplements. (See Cultural Considerations Box 29–1.) A client food diary can be used to provide more detailed information. Gerontological clients may be on fixed incomes, which limits their food budget and may result in meal skipping or purchasing of inadequate food such as outdated food or pet food for them to eat. The elderly client's daily food intake should be explored, especially if malnutrition or financial limitations are seen.

CULTURAL CONSIDERATIONS BOX 29-1

Questions to ask when performing a cultural nutritional assessment:

1. What types of your cultural foods are available in your community?
2. What are your preferred foods over foods available and eaten?
3. What is the nutrient value of the foods you eat?
4. Which foods do you most commonly consume?
5. How and where are your foods chosen and purchased?
6. Who prepares the food in your household?
7. Who purchases the food in your household?
8. How is your food stored for future use?
9. How is your food prepared before eaten?
10. How is any uneaten food discarded?

Also explored during a nutritional assessment are patterns of gastric acid reflux, indigestion, heartburn, nausea, vomiting, diarrhea, constipation, flatulence, and bowel incontinence, which may interfere with proper nutrition. (See Gerontological Issues Box 29–2.) Acid reflux can be assessed by asking clients if they experience reflux with a bile taste or awaken with an unpleasant taste in their mouth.

Family History

Any family history of conditions that may influence the client's gastrointestinal status is assessed. Some gastrointestinal problems such as colon cancer are thought to be hereditary. Health histories of close relatives, such as parents, siblings, and grandparents, are most important.

Cultural Influences

Many cultures have special dietary practices and restrictions. (See Cultural Considerations Box 29–3.) The nurse needs to understand these cultural influences and respect them. As a client advocate the nurse should assist the client to maintain desired cultural practices, as able. Nutrition can be better maintained when client's likes and dislikes regarding food customs are followed.

OBJECTIVE DATA

Height and Weight

When the GI system is assessed, the client's height and weight are obtained. The nurse notes if the client is overweight, underweight, or has a body weight within the normal range for planning care. The client's ideal body weight according to height can be obtained using current

---

GERONTOLOGICAL ISSUES BOX 29-2

A complete bowel history should be obtained for older clients before beginning a bowel program. A bowel history includes the following:

Normal bowel evacuation pattern
Characteristics of stool
Presence of any bleeding or mucus with the stool
Use of products and medications to stimulate or slow bowel function
Report of usual diet
Amount of fluids—number and size of beverages glasses per day (beverages containing caffeine, such as coffee, tea, and sodas, do not count as fluids because of the diuretic effect of caffeine)
Exercise and physical activity
Rituals and practices related to bowel function

---

reference charts. The client's body build is also noted for abnormalities.

Oral Cavity

Gastrointestinal assessment begins with the oral cavity. The lips are examined for lesions, abnormal color, and symmetry. With a penlight and tongue blade, the oral cavity is inspected for inflammation, tenderness, ulcers, swelling, bleeding, and discolorations. Any odor of the client's breath is noted. A foul odor may indicate infection or poor oral care. The client's gums should be pink without swelling, redness, or irregularities. The teeth or dentures are examined for loose, broken, or absent teeth and the fit of the dentures or dental work. Ill-fitting dentures can affect the client's nutritional intake and obstruct the airway. Loose teeth can become dislodged and aspirated into the airway. Broken teeth can be a source of pain and contribute to poor nutritional intake. The client's knowledge of dental and oral care is assessed. The ability of the client to perform oral care is noted and included in the plan of care if there are deficits.

Abdomen

Inspection

To inspect the abdomen, clients are placed in a supine position with their arms at their sides. The abdomen is visually inspected to note the condition of the skin and the contour. The contour may be rounded, flat, concave, or distended, depending on the client's body type. Irregularities in contour may be due to distention, tumors, a hernia, or previous surgeries.

Auscultation

When auscultating the client's abdomen, the client's upper right quadrant is auscultated first (Fig. 29–3). Then a clockwise direction is followed to listen to the other quadrants. The stethoscope is pressed lightly on the abdomen to listen for **bowel sounds,** which are soft clicks and gurgles that may be heard every 5 to 15 seconds. These sounds at this rate are considered to be normal. Bowel sounds are made when peristalsis moves air and fluid through the GI tract. They are categorized as normal, hyperactive, hypoactive, or absent. Hyperactive bowel sounds are usually rapid, high pitched, and loud and may occur with hunger or gastroenteritis. Hypoactive bowel sounds are bowel sounds that are infrequent and can occur in clients with a paralytic ileus or following abdominal surgery. Bowel sounds are considered absent after the nurse has listened to all four quadrants for a minimum of 5 minutes in each quadrant and no sounds are auscultated. With a bowel obstruction, bowel sounds may be a high-pitched tinkling sound proximal to the obstruction and absent distal to the obstruction. Abnormal or absent bowel sounds are important findings. These findings must be confirmed, documented in the chart, and reported to the physician.

CULTURAL CONSIDERATIONS BOX 29–3

Most societies of the world use various foods and herbs for maintaining health. With increased attention to herbal therapies in the United States, the U.S. National Institutes of Health is studying 40 foods that are thought to fight disease. Among them are garlic, carrots, soy, cranberry juice, licorice, and green tea. Green tea has been used in Japan and China for centuries as a means of maintaining health and preventing disease.

Many Arabs eat food only with their right hand because it is regarded as clean. The left hand, commonly used for toileting, is considered unclean. Thus the nurse should feed the Arab client with the right hand regardless of the nurse's dominant handedness. Additionally, some may not drink beverages with their meals because some individuals consider it unhealthy to eat and drink at the same meal. Likewise, mixing hot and cold foods may be seen as unhealthy.

Muslim Arabs may refuse to eat meat that is not Halal (slaughtered and prepared in a ritual manner). Because Muslim Arabs are prohibited from ingesting alcohol or eating pork, they may refuse medication that includes alcohol, such as mouthwashes, toothpaste, and alcohol-based syrups and elixirs, and products derived from pigs, such as insulin, gelatin-coated capsules, and skin grafts. However, if no substitute is available, Muslims are permitted to use these preparations.[1]

Good health to Mexican-Americans, which is largely a part of "God's will," can be maintained by dietary practices that keep the body in balance.[2] In order to provide culturally competent care, the nurse must be aware of the hot-and-cold theory of disease when offering health teaching. Many diseases are thought to be caused by a disruption in the hot-and-cold balance theory of the body. Thus, by eating foods of the opposite variety, one may either cure or prevent specific hot-and-cold illnesses and conditions.

Examples of hot disease conditions include infection, diarrhea, sore throats, stomach ulcers, liver conditions, kidney problems, gastrointestinal upsets, and febrile conditions. Foods that are considered "cold" are therefore viewed as remedies for hot illness conditions. Cold foods include fresh fruits and vegetables, dairy products, barley water, fish, chicken, goat meat, and dried fruits. However, there are significant differences in what are considered hot and cold foods and illnesses among Mexican-American families depending on their native region in Mexico.

Examples of cold illness conditions include cancer, malaria, earaches, arthritis and related conditions, pneumonia and other pulmonary conditions, headaches, menstrual cramping, and musculoskeletal conditions. Hot foods used to treat these conditions typically include cheeses, liquor, beef, pork, spicy foods, eggs, grains other than barley, vitamins, tobacco, and onions.

Among Jews, the laws regarding food are commonly referred to as the laws of Kashrut or the laws of what foods are permissible in accordance with the religious law. The term *kosher* means fit for eating; it is not a brand or form of cooking.[3]

Foods are divided into those that are permitted (clean) and forbidden (unclean). The kosher slaughter of animals prevents undue cruelty to the animal and ensures the animal's health for its consumer. Care must be taken that all blood is drained from the animal before eating it.

Among the more conservative and Orthodox Jews, milk and meat may not be mixed together, whether in cooking, serving, or eating. This involves separating the utensils used to prepare foods and the plates used to serve them. To avoid mixing foods, religious Jews have two sets of dishes, pots, and utensils: one set for milk products and one for meat.

Cheeseburgers, meat lasagna, and grated cheese on meatballs and spaghetti are not acceptable. Milk cannot be used in coffee if served with a meat meal. Nondairy creamers can be used as long as they do not contain sodium caseinate, which is derived from milk.

Fish, eggs, vegetables, and fruits are considered neutral and may be used with either dairy or meat dishes. A U with a circle around it or a K is used on food products to indicate kosher.

When working in a Jewish person's home, the nurse should not bring food into the house without knowing whether the client is kosher. If the client is kosher, do not use any cooking items, dishes, or silverware without knowing which are used for meat and which are used for dairy. It is important for the nurse to understand the dietary laws so as not to offend the client. The nurse should advocate for kosher meals if they are requested and plan medication times accordingly. Frozen kosher meals are available by contacting the local Jewish synagogue for a supplier.

Although liberal Jews decide for themselves which dietary laws, if any, they follow, many still avoid pork and pork products out of a sense of tradition and symbolism. It would be insensitive to serve pork products to Jewish clients unless they specifically request it.

Kosher meals are available in hospitals and long-term care facilities. Even though the organization may not have a kosher kitchen, frozen kosher meals can be obtained from several organizations, most of which are located in large cities with large Jewish populations. The kosher kitchen closest to your organization can be obtained by calling the Jewish synagogue nearest the organization to obtain the address and telephone number. Kosher meals arrive on paper plates and with plastic utensils sealed in plastic. The nurse should not unwrap the utensils if the client is able to do so or change the foodstuffs to another serving dish. Determining a client's dietary preferences and practices regarding dietary laws should be done during the admission assessment.

Among Asian Indians, nutritional deficiencies are patterned from their region of emigration. For example, beriberi (thiamine deficiency) is found in people emigrating from rice-growing areas. Pellagra (niacin deficiency) causing skin and mental disorders and diarrhea is found in people emigrating from maize-millet areas. Thiamine defi-
continued

CULTURAL CONSIDERATIONS BOX 29–3 (continued)

ciency is common among people mostly dependent on rice. Thorough milling of rice, washing rice before cooking, and allowing the cooked rice to remain overnight before consumption the following day result in the loss of thiamine.[4]

Commitment to the sacred cow concept has an impact on Hindus by encouraging dairy and milk use. However, lactose intolerance affects more than 10% of adults. The adequacy or inadequacy to digest lactose may be due to genetic differences among Asian Indians.

Goiter is prevalent among some Asian Indian immigrants resulting from an iodine deficiency in food and water from their homeland. Fluorosis occurs in other parts of India resulting from drinking water high in fluoride. Osteomalacia is prevalent where diets are deficient in calcium and vitamin D. Endemic dropsy is prevalent among Asian Indians emigrating from West Bengal, resulting from using mustard oil for cooking. The nurse needs to be aware of these conditions and their causes when working with Hindus and Asian Indians and teach clients prevention.

There is an increase in gastrointestinal distress among Brazilians when they first come to the United States, partially because many have a lactose intolerance and partially because of different methods of milk pasteurization.[5] The nurse can assist the client in identifying alternative food sources for Brazilian clients to obtain needed calcium in their diet.

The condition of the alimentary tract has priority over all other body parts in the Arab's perception of health. Gastrointestinal complaints are the most common reason Arab-Americans seek care.[6]

Obesity is seen as positive among many African-Americans. They often view individuals who are thin as "not having enough meat on their bones." One needs to have adequate meat on his or her bones so that when an illness occurs, one can afford to lose weight. Many African-American diets are high in animal fat and fried foods and low in fiber, fruits, and vegetables.[7]

The diet of some Appalachians is deficient in vitamin A, iron, and calcium.[8] The nurse working with this population needs to do a dietary assessment and teach clients food selections that include adequate vitamin A, iron, and calcium.

LEARNING TIP

In a total bowel obstruction, air and fluid are propelled forward by peristalsis proximal to the obstruction. This produces proximal high-pitched bowel sounds when the air and fluid create turbulence as they hit the obstruction and are unable to pass. Absent bowel sounds are heard distal to the obstruction.

Palpation

Using the same quadrant approach as mentioned previously, the LPN/LVN may lightly depress the abdomen to check for distention. The nurse notes any pain, tenderness, or rigidity. Abdominal girth is measured by placing a tape measure around the client's abdomen at the iliac crest. A mark can be made at the measurement site so that measurements obtained by others are made at the same location for comparison. Abdominal girth is increased in clients with distention or conditions such as ascites (accumulation of fluid in the peritoneal cavity). Daily measurements should be obtained and recorded to monitor changes when abdominal girth is abnormal.

Usually, the advanced nurse practitioner or physician performs all other types of palpation. The liver is not normally palpable but if enlarged, it may be felt below the right lower rib cage. Rebound tenderness is determined by pressing down on the abdomen a few inches and quickly releasing the pressure. If the client feels a sharp pain during this procedure, it can indicate appendicitis (especially in the right lower quadrant).

Percussion

Percussion is the technique of translating physical force into sound. It is performed by the physician or advanced nurse practitioner. Striking the abdominal wall using percussion produces a sound that identifies the density of the organs below. Percussion is used to detect fluid, air, and masses in the abdomen. It is also used to identify size and location of abdominal organs. Tympanic high-pitched sounds indicate the location of air, and dull thudlike

Quadrants of the abdomen

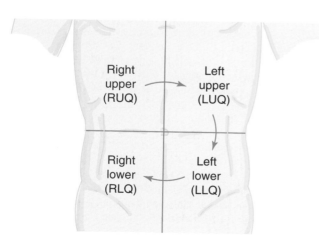

Right upper (RUQ)

Left upper (LUQ)

Right lower (RLQ)

Left lower (LLQ)

Figure 29–3. Abdomial quadrants are auscultated from the right quadrant in a clockwise manner.

sounds indicate fluid or solid organs. Percussion is most helpful in determining the size and position of the liver and spleen.

Diagnostic Tests

Commonly used tests associated with diseases of the GI tract include the following:

- Laboratory tests (Table 29–2)
- Radiographic tests
- Endoscopy
- Gastric analysis
- Cytologic studies
- Magnetic resonance imaging

Whenever the nurse obtains specimens of body fluids, substances, or blood, universal precautions must be used to protect the nurse and clients. Hand washing before and after the procedure, wearing gloves, and using goggles if splashing may occur are important aspects of universal precautions.

LABORATORY TESTS

Carcinoembryonic Antigen

Carcinoembryonic antigen (CEA) is a serum protein normally found in first or second trimester fetuses whose production stops before birth. The presence of CEA levels in children or adults may indicate colorectal or other cancer. Increased CEA levels are also found in clients with cirrhosis, hepatic disease, and alcoholic pancreatitis and in heavy smokers. Elevated CEA levels are used to determine cancer treatment effectiveness. An elevated CEA level after treatment can indicate residual or recurrent cancer.

Stool for Occult Blood

Stool samples can be tested for **occult blood,** which is blood that cannot be seen with the naked eye. It is detectable by two methods: microscopic examination or chemical reaction using **guaiac** (a tree resin). For microscopic examination, the stool specimen is sent to the laboratory, and results are usually returned within 24 hours.

Table 29–2. **Common Laboratory Tests Used to Assess Gastrointestinal Function**

Test	Normal	Significance
Complete Blood Count		
Red Blood Cell Count	4.2–5.2 million/mm³ (women) 4.5–6.2 million/mm³ (men)	Decreased values indicate possible anemia or hemorrhage
Hemoglobin	12–16 g/dL (women) 14–18 g/dL (men)	Increased values indicate possible hemoconcentration, caused by dehydration
Hematocrit	38–46% (women) 42–54% (men)	
Electrolytes		
Potassium	3.5–5.0 mg/dL	Decreased values indicate possible GI suction, diarrhea, vomiting, intestinal fistulas
Calcium	8.0–10.5 mg/dL	Decreased values indicate possible malabsorption
Sodium	135–145 mg/L	Decreased values indicate possible malabsorption and diarrhea
Carcinoembryonic Antigen		
	Less than 5 ng/mL (nonsmokers)	Increased values indicate possible colorectal cancer and inflammatory bowel disease
Fecal Analysis		
Stool for Occult Blood	Negative	Presence indicates possible peptic ulcer, cancer of the colon, ulcerative colitis
Stool for Ova and Parasites	Negative	Presence indicates infection
Stool Cultures	No unusual growth	Presence of pathogens may indicate shigella, salmonella, *Staphylococcus aureus,* or *Bacillus cereus*
Stool for Lipids	2–5 g/24 h (normal diet)	Increased values indicate possible malabsorption syndrome or Crohn's disease

There are several brands of guaiac tests, and it is important to read the directions that come with a kit before beginning the test so that it is done and timed properly. One brand of the guaiac test is the Hemoccult test. This test is inexpensive, noninvasive, and easy to perform. A series of three tests in a row are usually done to increase the chances of detecting blood, if any is present. To guaiac a stool specimen, a wooden applicator is used to smear a small amount of stool on one side of the guaiac paper. A developing solution is then applied and the color is immediately noted. A blue coloration denotes a positive reaction (occult blood is present). No coloration denotes a negative reaction (no blood is present). The results are documented and reported to the physician.

Factors that can give a false-positive occult blood result include the following:

- Bleeding gums following a dental procedure
- Ingestion of red meat within 3 days before testing
- Ingestion of fish, turnips, or horseradish
- Drugs, including anticoagulants, aspirin, colchicine, iron preparations in large doses, nonsteroidal antiarthritics, and steroids

Stool for Ova and Parasites

Stool for ova (eggs) and parasites is collected to detect intestinal infections caused by parasites and their ova. The test usually requires a series of three stool specimens collected every second or third day. The stool specimen is collected using a tongue blade in a container with a preservative and sent immediately to the laboratory. The stool must be examined within 30 minutes of collection. False-negative results can occur from urine in the specimen or a lack of a fresh specimen.

Stool Cultures

Stool cultures are done to determine the presence of pathogenic organisms in the GI tract. It is noted if the client has been taking antibiotics. The stool should be collected using sterile technique. A sterile tongue blade is used to put the stool into the sterile specimen container, and then it is sent to the laboratory.

Stool for Lipids

Stool can also be examined for lipids (fat). Usually dietary lipids are absorbed in the small intestine. Excessive secretion of fecal fats (**steatorrhea**) may occur in various digestive and absorptive disorders. The client is instructed to eat a high-fat diet and to avoid alcohol for 3 days before and during the 3-day stool collection period. The client should avoid drugs that could interfere with the results, such as mineral oil, neomycin, and potassium chloride. The stools are collected for 72 hours and stored on ice if necessary before being sent to the laboratory.

RADIOGRAPHIC TESTS

Flat Plate of the Abdomen

A flat plate of the abdomen is an x-ray giving an anterior-to-posterior view. It is used to visualize abdominal organs and can detect such abnormalities as tumors, obstructions, and strictures. For this procedure, the client should be dressed in a hospital gown without any metal such as zippers, belts, or jewelry. As with any x-ray, pregnant clients or those thought to be pregnant should avoid x-rays. The nurse should inform the physician if the client is or might be pregnant.

Upper Gastrointestinal Series (Barium Swallow)

An **upper gastrointestinal series** (UGI series) is an x-ray of esophagus, stomach, duodenum, and jejunum using an oral liquid radiopaque contrast medium (barium) and a **fluoroscope** to outline the contours of the organs. A UGI series is used to detect such things as strictures, ulcers, tumors, polyps, hiatal hernias, and motility problems.

The client receives nothing by mouth (NPO) for 6 to 8 hours before the procedure. Usually, the client eats a clear liquid supper the night before the procedure and is then NPO until the procedure is done. Because smoking can stimulate gastric motility, the client is discouraged from smoking the morning of the procedure. Client teaching includes information about the client's diet before and after the procedure, the barium ingestion, and the appearance of stools afterward.

During the procedure, the client drinks the thick, chalky barium while standing in front of a fluoroscopy tube. X-ray films are taken at specific intervals to visualize the outline of the organs and to note the passage of the barium through the GI tract.

A laxative is usually ordered after the procedure to expel the barium and prevent constipation or a barium **impaction.** The client is instructed to drink twelve 8-ounce glasses of water per day for several days to prevent dehydration, which can lead to constipation. The abdomen is assessed for distention and bowel sounds. The stool is monitored to determine whether the barium has been completely eliminated. Initially, the client's stool will be white in color (the barium), but it should return to its normal color within 3 days. Constipation with distention indicates a barium impaction.

Lower Gastrointestinal Series (Barium Enema)

The **lower gastrointestinal series** is performed to visualize the position, movements, and filling of the colon. This test is used to detect tumors, diverticula, stenosis, obstructions, inflammation, ulcerative colitis, and polyps. The client is placed on a low-residue or clear liquid diet for 2 days before

---

fluoroscope: flu—flow + skopein—to examine

the test to empty the bowel. Cathartics, laxatives (such as GoLYTELY), and enemas may be administered the evening before the test. This is necessary for adequate visualization during the procedure. An inadequate bowel prep may result in poor test results or test cancellation. (See Fig. 32–2.) The client either receives a clear liquid diet the morning of the test or is NPO past midnight the night before. The area around the rectum should be clean before the client is sent for the procedure. If the client has active inflammatory disease of the colon or suspected perforation or obstruction, a barium enema is contraindicated. Active gastrointestinal bleeding may also prohibit the use of laxatives and enemas.

During the procedure, barium is instilled rectally, and x-rays are taken with or without fluoroscopy. The procedure takes about 15 minutes, and the client is allowed to use the bathroom immediately after the procedure.

The client's stools are monitored after the procedure to note if all the barium is passed as with the UGI. Constipation development is monitored. The client is encouraged to drink at least one 8-ounce glass of liquid per hour for the next 24 waking hours to help remove the barium. The client is told to report any abdominal pain, bloating, or absence of stool, all of which could indicate constipation or bowel obstruction, as well as any rectal bleeding.

Computed Tomography

Computed tomography (CT) uses a beam of radiation to allow three-dimensional visualization of abdominal structures. Dilute oral barium or other contrast media may be used to distinguish normal bowel from abnormal masses. The client may have a clear liquid diet the morning of the test. If a contrast medium is to be used, any allergies to iodine or shellfish are assessed, a consent may be signed, and the client is NPO for 2 to 4 hours before the procedure.

ENDOSCOPY

Upper Gastrointestinal Endoscopy

Endoscope is a general term used to describe a device consisting of a tube and a fiber-optic system for observing the inside of a hollow organ or cavity. Upper GI tract endoscopy includes the visualization of the esophagus (**esophagoscopy**), the stomach (**gastroscopy**), or the esophagus, stomach, and the duodenum (esophagogastroduodenoscopy [EGD]). Fiberoscopy of the upper GI tract allows for direct visualization of the gastric mucosa through an endoscope. It is used to visualize abnormalities such as inflammation, cancer, bleeding, injury, and infection.

The client is NPO for 8 hours before the procedure to prevent aspiration of stomach contents into the lungs dur-

ing the procedure if vomiting occurs. Sedatives, such as diazepam (Valium), meperidine (Demerol), or midazolam (Versed), may be given before the procedure to help relax the client. A local anesthetic in spray or gargle form is administered just before the scope is inserted to inhibit the gag reflex.

After being medicated, the client is placed on the left side to allow the scope to curve around the fundus of the stomach by gravity (Fig. 29–4). The flexible, fiber-optic endoscope tube is passed orally into the esophagus, stomach, and duodenum. Some endoscopes are equipped with a camera or a video processor, which allows permanent pictures or videotapes of the procedure to be made. Biopsy forceps to obtain tissue specimens or cytology brushes to obtain cells for microscopic study can be passed through the endoscope.

After the procedure, vital signs are checked frequently as ordered. Clients are placed on one side to prevent aspiration while sedation and the local anesthetic wear off. Clients are NPO until the gag reflex returns (usually within 4 hours). Clients are assessed for signs of perforation, which include bleeding, fever, and dysphagia. Midesophageal perforation can cause referred substernal or epigastric pain. Blood loss secondary to perforation can lead to hematoma formation, which in turn can result in cyanosis and referred back pain. Distal esophageal perforation may result in shoulder pain, dyspnea, or symptoms similar to those of a perforated ulcer.

Lower Gastrointestinal Endoscopy

Proctosigmoidoscopy

Proctosigmoidoscopy is the examination of the distal sigmoid colon, the rectum, and the anal canal using a rigid or flexible endoscope, in this case a sigmoidoscope. This procedure can detect ulcerations, punctures, lacerations, tumors, hemorrhoids, polyps, fissures, fistulas, abscesses,

---

endoscope: endo—within + skopein—to examine
esophagoscopy: oisophagos—esophagus + skopein—to examine
gastroscopy: gaster—stomach + skopein—to examine

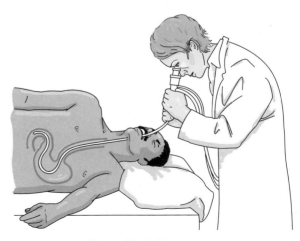

Figure 29–4. Gastroscopy.

and other abnormalities. This procedure can detect malignancy at an early stage and is therefore recommended as an annual examination for clients 40 years old and older.

This procedure requires the lower bowel to be cleaned out. The client usually receives a clear liquid diet 24 hours before the test and a warm tap-water enema or sodium biphosphate (Fleet) enema until returns are clear. In clients with bleeding or severe diarrhea, the bowel preparation may not be ordered by the physician.

The client is positioned in a knee-chest position, which allows the sigmoid colon to straighten by gravity. A left lateral Sim's position can be used for clients unable to tolerate the knee-chest position, such as elderly or debilitated clients. A rigid proctoscope is usually used first to visualize the rectum. A flexible scope is then used to permit visualization above the rectosigmoid junction. Clients are told they may feel pressure as though they are going to have a bowel movement. During the procedure, one or more small pieces of intestinal tissue may be removed for histological study. This is called a biopsy and is performed with small cutting forceps introduced through the flexible scope. Rectal or sigmoid polyps may be removed with a snare. An electrocoagulating current can be used to cauterize sites to prevent or stop bleeding. Specimens are labeled and sent to the pathology laboratory immediately for examination.

After the procedure, the client is allowed to rest for a few minutes in the supine position to avoid orthostatic hypotension when standing. The client is observed for signs of perforation such as bleeding, pain, and fever. A sitz bath may be ordered for comfort after the procedure.

Colonoscopy

Colonoscopy provides visualization of the lining of the large intestine through a flexible endoscope, which is inserted rectally. The colonoscope is used to visualize the same abnormalities as the proctosigmoidoscope.

For this procedure, the client is usually sedated and positioned on the left side with the knees bent. The colonoscope is lubricated with a water-based jelly and inserted into the anus. A small amount of air is instilled to help the physician visualize the bowel. The air causes pressure and may be uncomfortable for the client. The client is encouraged to relax and take slow deep breaths through the nose and out the mouth. The physician may request that the client be moved to the supine position once the colonoscope reaches the sigmoid junction. This makes it easier to move the colonoscope past the curve in the bowel. Vital signs throughout the procedure are monitored to watch for a vasovagal response, which can lead to hypotension and bradycardia.

GASTRIC ANALYSIS

Gastric analysis measures the secretions in the stomach. This procedure is used to aid in the diagnosis of duodenal ulcer, gastric carcinoma, pyloric or duodenal obstruction, and pernicious anemia. A diagnosis of pernicious anemia is ruled out by the finding of acid. A diagnosis of gastric carcinoma may be made by the presence of cancer cells in the gastric secretions. There are two tests performed in gastric analysis: the **basal cell secretion test** and the **gastric acid stimulation test.**

Before the basal cell secretion test the client should avoid taking any drugs that could interfere with gastric acid secretion such as cholinergics and antacids. The client is NPO past midnight the night before the test. For the procedure, a nasogastric (NG) tube is inserted and the contents of the stomach are suctioned out through the tube using a syringe. The NG tube is connected to wall suction, and stomach contents are collected every 15 minutes for 1 hour. The specimens are labeled according to the time they were collected and the order in which they were obtained. The gastric acid is tested for pH using indicator paper or a pH meter. The amount of gastric acid is also measured. Too much hydrochloric acid may indicate a peptic ulcer; too little could be a sign of cancer or pernicious anemia.

The gastric acid stimulation test measures the amount of gastric acid for 1 hour after subcutaneous injection of a histamine drug. If abnormal results occur, radiographic tests or endoscopy can be done to determine the cause.

MAGNETIC RESONANCE IMAGING

Magnetic resonance imaging (MRI) is a noninvasive test that uses magnetic fields to produce cross-sectional images of soft tissue and blood vessels. The test is used to study blood flow and identify tumors and infections. It is usually contraindicated in clients who are claustrophobic, obese, or who have pacemakers, internal metal such as shrapnel or shavings, or orthopedic hardware.

The client remains NPO for 6 hours before the procedure. All jewelry and metal is removed from the client, including bobby pins, dental appliances, and clothing snaps. The client must be able to remain alert but lie still for the procedure, which may take up to 90 minutes. The client is informed that there is a loud clanging noise during the procedure. There is no follow-up care.

Therapeutic Measures

GASTROINTESTINAL INTUBATION

Gastrointestinal intubation refers to the placement of a tube within the gastrointestinal tract for therapeutic or diagnostic purposes (Fig. 29–5). When the gastrointestinal tube is inserted from the nares into the stomach, it is referred to as a nasogastric tube. A nasoenteric tube is a tube inserted from the nares into the intestines. Nasogastric and

---

colonoscopy: kolon—colon + skopein—to examine

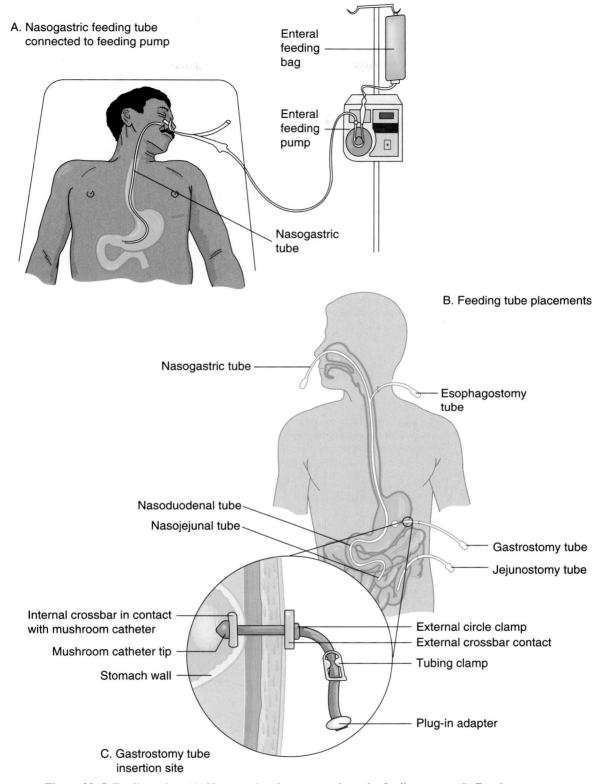

A. Nasogastric feeding tube connected to feeding pump

Enteral feeding bag

Enteral feeding pump

Nasogastric tube

B. Feeding tube placements

Nasogastric tube

Esophagostomy tube

Nasoduodenal tube

Nasojejunal tube

Gastrostomy tube

Jejunostomy tube

Internal crossbar in contact with mushroom catheter

Mushroom catheter tip

Stomach wall

External circle clamp

External crossbar contact

Tubing clamp

Plug-in adapter

C. Gastrostomy tube insertion site

Figure 29–5. Feeding tubes. *(A)* Nasogastric tube connected to tube feeding pump. *(B)* Esophagostomy, gastrostomy, and jejunostomy. *(C)* Gastrostomy tube insertion site.

Table 29–3. **Gastrointestinal Tubes**

Tube	Uses and Description	Nursing Considerations
	Gastric	
Levine Tube	Single lumen, may be used for gastric decompression, irrigations, lavages, and feedings	Tube is not vented, so use with low intermittent suction to prevent injury to stomach lining.
Sump Tube (Salem Sump)	Double lumen, "pigtail" acts as an air vent and prevents excess suction, which could damage stomach lining; used for decompression, irrigations, and lavages	May be used with low continuous suction because of air vent.
Weighted, Flexible Feeding Tubes with Stylets (Nutriflex, Keofeed)	Small-bore tubes for tube feedings only; less injury, remains in place for extended periods of time	Suction collapses tube. If injecting air into tube, use a 10 mL syringe or greater, because smaller syringe creates too much pressure and possible rupture of tube.
Balloon Tamponade Tube (Sengstaken-Blakemore Tube)	Triple-lumen tube (one lumen for gastric aspiration, one lumen to inflate esophageal balloon, one lumen to inflate gastric balloon); used to treat hemorrhages from esophagus and upper stomach by compressing and holding pressure against bleeding sites	Inserted by physician. Maintain pressures in balloon at prescribed levels (excess pressure causes damage). Monitor for respiratory distress because this may indicate that gastric balloon has deflated or ruptured and that tube has moved up and esophageal balloon is obstructing the airway. Scissors are kept at bedside to cut tube in case this occurs.
	Intestinal	
Miller-Abbott Tube	Double-lumen tube used to drain and decompress the small intestine in cases of partial or complete obstruction; one lumen for aspiration, the other to inflate the balloon with mercury so that the tube is weighted and moves by gravity and peristalsis into the small intestine	This tube is inserted by the physician or a specially trained nurse. Tube is not secured with tape, but passed through gauze taped to client's forehead to allow tube to advance into intestines. Usually the tube is advanced 1 to 2 inches every 2 hours; turning and ambulating the client, if possible, facilitates tube's advancement.

nasoenteric tubes are inserted for a variety of reasons, but the main purposes for their use include the following:

- To remove gas and fluids from the stomach or intestines (decompression)
- To diagnose gastrointestinal motility and to obtain gastric secretions for analysis
- To relieve and treat obstructions or bleeding within the gastrointestinal tract
- To provide a means for nutrition (**gavage** feeding), hydration, and medication when the oral route is not possible or is contraindicated
- To promote healing after esophageal, gastric, or intestinal surgery by preventing distention of the gastrointestinal tract and strain on the suture lines
- To remove toxic substances (**lavage**) that have been ingested either accidentally or intentionally and to provide for irrigation

A variety of tubes are used to accomplish these purposes, each designed for specific purposes.

Feeding tubes also include esophagostomy, **gastrostomy,** or jejunostomy tubes. (See Fig. 29–5.) Nasogastric

tubes are usually temporary. Esophagostomy, gastrostomy, or jejunostomy tubes are generally used for longer-term nutrition delivery.

Clients who require a gastric or intestinal tube for the diagnosis or treatment of their condition are usually very ill to begin with, and the added stress of having a tube inserted through their nose or mouth into their stomach or intestines may be overwhelming. The nurse must provide much emotional support and explanation to the client and significant others to facilitate the process of tube insertion and maintenance. Knowledge of the specific tube being inserted and the reason for the tube's use is required by the nurse in order to provide effective nursing care and observations (Table 29–3). General nursing care measures for insertion and maintenance of gastrointestinal tubes are given in Table 29–4. Agency policies regarding nursing roles for insertion and care of GI tubes should be consulted.

gastrostomy: gaster—stomach + ostium—little opening

Table 29–4. *Nursing Care for Insertion and Maintenance of Gastrointestinal Tubes*

1. Explain the procedure and the reason for the tube to the client. Inform the client how he or she can help by swallowing when instructed to do so, either by taking deep breaths or drinking water, if indicated.
2. The client is placed in a high Fowler's position (right side-lying position as alternative). The tube is measured for the correct length to be inserted, by holding the tube from nose to earlobe to xyphoid process, and marked with a piece of tape. The client's head is tilted back if not contraindicated. The nare that is the straightest and from which the client breathes the easiest is selected because the tube can be inserted more easily in a nare that is straight.
3. Lubricate the tube with a water-soluble lubricant and insert it into the selected nare. As the tube is inserted, aim it along the floor of the nare for client comfort. If the client is alert, when the tube stimulates the gag reflex, encourage swallowing to advance the tube down the throat. Water in a glass with a straw or ice chips may be given to facilitate the swallowing process, if the client is allowed and able. Advance the tube whenever the client swallows. Stop when the client breathes to avoid inserting the tube into the trachea while the epiglottis is open. If the client is unconscious, position his or her chin as close to the chest as possible to help prevent the tube from passing into the trachea. Always observe for coiling of the tube in the client's mouth. If at any time the client begins to cough uncontrollably, becomes cyanotic, or begins to experience any respiratory distress, remove the tube, allow rest time, and then reattempt insertion.
4. When the tube has been inserted to the tape marking the premeasured length, confirm gastric placement by injecting air in the tube while auscultating at the epigastric region for a swishing or bubbling sound and by aspirating gastric contents. Measuring the pH of the secretions obtained is even more conclusive for gastric placement confirmation because gastric and intestinal pH range is acidic, usually 3 to 5.6, whereas respiratory secretions are alkaline, with a pH range of 7 or greater. If any doubts about gastric placement exist, the physician should be notified and an order for x-ray obtained to confirm tube placement.
5. Secure the tube in place with tape so that pressure is not put on the nare, and pin coiled excess tubing to the client's gown.
6. Provide frequent care to the nares and mouth, keeping the oral mucous membranes moist. Avoid intake of excessive amounts of ice chips because water may result in electrolyte imbalances. Normal saline instead of water can be made into ice chips to help prevent imbalances. Hard candy may be used to stimulate salivation to keep the mouth moist, unless contraindicated.
7. Keep an accurate intake and output record, including drainage, vomitus, and any irrigation solution instilled. If suction is used, low intermittent suction is preferred as ordered. Gastric placement is periodically confirmed, especially before instilling anything into the tube. The tube should be flushed at intervals (often every 2 to 4 hours) to maintain patency.

TUBE FEEDINGS

The purpose of a tube feeding is to supply the client with nutrition when oral intake is not possible. Some feedings are given to the client as a supplement, and others are provided to meet the client's total nutritional needs. Tube feedings are delivered into the duodenum or proximal jejunum when the esophagus and stomach need to be bypassed. The reasons for administering tube feedings include inability to swallow, severe burns or trauma to the face or jaw, debilitation, mental retardation, and oropharyngeal or esophageal paralysis. Complications associated with tube feedings are presented in Table 29–5.

Tube Feeding Formulas

Most clients receive commercially prepared formulas, which are composed of protein, carbohydrates, and fats. Products such as Ensure Plus, Sustacal, and Isocal are samples. Pulmocare is high in fat and low in carbohydrates. It is ideal for clients who require fluid restriction, and is often used for clients with chronic obstructive pulmonary disease. Jevity and Enrich are formulas that are high in fiber and can help reduce the occurrence of diarrhea. Tube feeding formulas are chosen by the physician depending on the client's nutritional needs, consistency of the formula, the size and location of the tube, the method of delivery, and the convenience for the client at home.

When clients receive tube feedings, their daily water needs in addition to any water supplied by the feeding should be considered. Dietitians can be helpful in calculating the client's water needs. The water used to flush the tube or administer medications can be calculated toward the client's daily total water needs. Dehydration can occur if the client's water needs are not met.

CRITICAL THINKING: Jackie

Jackie, 32, is receiving a tube feeding due to dysphagia, the cause of which is being investigated. Jackie is not receiving any medications. The nurse notes that Jackie's tongue is bright red with deep furrows. Her skin remains tented when skin turgor is checked.

1. What do Jackie's assessment findings indicate?
2. Why might Jackie be exhibiting this condition?
3. What actions could the nurse take for this condition?

Answers at end of chapter.

Method of Delivery

Feedings are administered either by gravity or by a controlled pump that delivers continuous volume through the feeding tube. Gravity feedings are placed above the level of the stomach and dripped in by gravity slowly or given as a bolus feeding over a few minutes. Bolus feedings are often not well tolerated. Intermittent feedings are defined as either being delivered by a pump that runs continuously throughout the day and is discontinued each night, or as a 4- to 6-hour volume of feeding given over 20 to 30 minutes.[9] Intermittent feedings via a pump allow the stomach

Table 29–5. ***Common Mechanical Gastrointestinal, and Metabolic Complications of Tube-Fed Clients and Prevention Strategies***

Complication	Prevention Strategies
Mechanical	
Tube irritation	Consider using a smaller or softer tube
	Lubricate the tube before insertion
Tube obstruction	Flush tube after use
	Do not mix medications with the formula
	Use liquid medications if available
	Crush other medications thoroughly
	Use an infusion pump to maintain a constant flow (Fig. 29–5)
	Feeding should not be started until tube placement is radiographically confirmed
Aspiration and regurgitation	Elevate head of client's bed greater than or equal to 30 degrees at all times
	Discontinue feedings at least 30 to 60 minutes before treatments where head must be lowered (e.g., chest percussion)
	If the client has an endotracheal tube in place, keep the cuff inflated during feedings
	Test pH of aspirate with pH paper or meter
	a. pH of tracheobronchial secretions is alkaline, >7.4
	b. pH of gastric secretions is acidic <5.0
	c. As the tube moves from the acid stomach to the alkaline duodenum, pH will change from acid to alkaline
	Place a black mark at the point where the tube, once properly placed, exits the nostril
Tube displacement	Replace tube and obtain physician's order to confirm with x-ray imaging
Gastrointestinal	
Cramping, distention, bloating, gas pains, nausea, vomiting, diarrhea*	Initiate and increase amount of formula gradually
	Bring formula to room temperature before feeding
	Change to a lactose-free formula
	Decrease fat content of formula
	Administer drug therapy as ordered (e.g., Lactinex, kaolin-pectin, Lomotil)
	Change to formula with a lower osmolality
	Change to formula with a different fiber content
	Practice good personal hygiene when handling any feeding product
	Evaluate diarrhea-causing medications the client may be receiving (e.g., antibiotics, digitalis)
Metabolic	
Dehydration	Assess client's fluid requirements before treatment
	Monitor hydration status
Overhydration	Assess client's fluid requirements before treatment
	Monitor hydration status
Hyperglycemia	Initiate feedings at a low rate
	Monitor blood glucose
	Use hyperglycemic medication if necessary
	Select low-carbohydrate formula
Hypernatremia	Assess client's fluid and electrolyte status before treatment
	Provide adequate fluids
Hyponatremia	Assess client's fluid and electrolyte status before treatment
	Restrict fluids
	Supplement feeding with rehydration solution and saline
	Diuretic therapy may be beneficial
Hypophosphatemia	Monitor serum levels
	Replenish phosphorus levels before refeeding
Hypercapnia	Select low-carbohydrate, high-fat formula
Hypokalemia	Monitor potassium levels
	Supplement feeding with potassium if necessary
Hyperkalemia	Reduce potassium intake
	Monitor potassium levels

* The most commonly cited complication of tube feeding is diarrhea.

From Lutz, CA, and Przytulski, KR: Nutritional and Diet Therapy, ed 2. FA Davis, Philadelphia, 1997, p 280. Reprinted with permission.

to rest at night and more closely simulate normal eating and nutrient absorption patterns. A continuous feeding administered 24 hours a day through a pump allows for small amounts to be given over a long period of time. Pumps are set at the specified rate to control the speed of the feeding being delivered to the client.

When feedings are administered, clients must be positioned in a sitting or high-Fowler's position to reduce the risk of aspiration. The nurse must carefully monitor the rate to avoid administering feedings too rapidly and watch for signs that the feeding is not being absorbed. Abdominal distention, client report of a feeling of fullness, and nausea or vomiting are indicators that the feeding is not being absorbed and should be stopped to prevent aspiration. A residual check to see how much feeding has not been absorbed is done hourly when the feeding is initiated, then every 4 hours or before giving any medications or adding more feeding for infusion. If there is more than 100 mL or the specified amount by the agency or physician, the feeding should be stopped to prevent vomiting or aspiration and the physician notified. Continuous or intermittent feedings reduce the risk of aspiration, distention, nausea, vomiting, and diarrhea.

If medications are administered during tube feedings, the nurse needs to understand possible drug-nutrient interactions. Some medications cannot be given with certain substances. Other medications, such as enteric-coated or sustained-release medications, should not be crushed. Liquid medications should be used when possible to reduce clogging of the tube. Pharmacists and dietitians should be consulted for special considerations.

GASTROINTESTINAL DECOMPRESSION

Gastrointestinal decompression is necessary when the stomach or small intestines become filled with air or fluid. Swallowed air and gastrointestinal secretions enter the stomach and intestines and collect there if they are not propelled through the GI tract by peristalsis. The accumulating air or fluid causes distention, a feeling of fullness, and possibly pain in the abdomen. Gastric distention may occur after major abdominal surgery. Ambulating or turning the client frequently can help prevent this. However, when gastrointestinal decompression is necessary, a nasogastric tube is inserted and applied usually to low intermittent suction. Low intermittent suction helps prevent trauma to the stomach wall. The nasogastric tube remains in place until full peristaltic activity (active bowel sounds and passage of flatus) has returned. The diet is then progressed as ordered and tolerated by the client.

TOTAL PARENTERAL NUTRITION (INTRAVENOUS HYPERALIMENTATION)

Total parenteral nutrition (TPN) is a method of supplying nutrients to the client by an intravenous (IV) route. TPN solutions usually contain dextrose (sugar), amino acids (protein), vitamins, minerals, and fat (intralipid) emulsions. TPN solutions are designed to improve the client's nutritional status, achieve weight gain, and enhance the healing process. The client with conditions such as burns, trauma, cancer, acquired immunodeficiency syndrome (AIDS), malnutrition, anorexia nervosa, fever, or major surgery may need TPN.

Usually, registered nurses are responsible for administering TPN. A filter must be used with TPN solutions but not with the lipid solution, which is given separately several times a week over 6 to 8 hours. The TPN is started slowly to give the pancreas time to adjust to increasing insulin production for the high amounts of glucose in the TPN. The TPN rate is increased until the ordered rate, as tolerated by the client, is reached. When TPN is discontinued it must be gradually weaned off to allow the pancreas to adjust to decreasing glucose levels. The client, if ordered, is fed before stopping the TPN to help prevent hypoglycemia. Signs of hypoglycemia include weakness, shakiness, sweating, and confusion.

During TPN administration, the following laboratory values, as ordered, are usually monitored:

- Complete blood count (CBC)
- Albumin
- Platelet count
- Prothrombin time (PT)
- Electrolytes
- Magnesium
- Glucose

LEARNING TIP

Some clients respond to TPN with an elevated serum glucose level even though they are not diabetics. This is due to the high concentration of glucose used in TPN, which for example may be 50%. These elevated serum glucose levels do not necessarily mean that the client has become a diabetic. Usually once the TPN is discontinued the serum glucose levels return to baseline or normal levels.

Regular insulin can be administered, as ordered, to control the elevated serum glucose. The insulin is ordered either on a sliding scale (regular insulin units ordered based on blood glucose levels measured at ordered intervals over 24 hours) or to be added to the TPN solution by the pharmacist.

It is important to monitor glucose levels as ordered and to look for signs of hyperglycemia in the client receiving TPN. Refer to agency policy for obtaining glucose levels when a hyperglycemic reaction is suspected in the client receiving TPN.

TPN can be irritating to the peripheral veins because it is five or six times more concentrated than blood. Therefore

HOME HEALTH HINTS

- When palpating a client's abdomen, the nurse should ask if any particular area hurts and check that area last.

- The nurse should become familiar with community nutritional support services: how to refer and referral criteria. Examples of these support services include women, infants, children (WIC), elderly feeding sites, meals-on-wheels, school feeding programs, and government surplus food programs.

- The home health nurse should assess the client's food preparation facilities to ensure that the client's nutritional needs can be met. Elderly clients may have outdated or spoiled food in their refrigerators or cupboards because they are unable to see dates or mold growing on foods.

- If elderly clients use appliances to heat food, ensure that they are able to use them safely. Elderly clients may not see gas flames and can ignite their clothing. If clients are confused, they may heat delivered meals still in their boxes on the stove. If the elderly client is able to obtain and learn to use a microwave, it may be a safer cooking appliance alternative.

- To stiffen a nasogastric tube for easier insertion, it can be put in cold water. To relax the tube, it can be placed in warm water.

- A feeding tube can be prevented from kinking by placing a split straw lengthwise around the area that tends to kink and lightly taping over the split in the straw.

- The end of the feeding tube can be kept clean by putting folded gauze at the end and wrapping a rubber band around it.

- Wire coat hangers make good hooks for enteral feeding solutions bags. They can be bent and hung over doorways or closet bars.

- If the nurse or client does not have a 60 mL feeding syringe for a bolus tube feeding or tube flushing, a measuring cup and funnel can be used.

- When the home health nurse is in need of an enema bucket but does not have one, a 16 Foley catheter (used as the enema tubing) can be connected to a 60 mL irrigating syringe. The syringe can be filled with enema solution, and then raised and lowered when connected to the catheter to control the flow of water into the rectum.

TPN dextrose over 12% is administered through a central venous catheter into a large vein such as the subclavian or internal jugular vein. (See Fig. 6–6.) The TPN solution is diluted by the volume in the large vein so it is less irritating.

PERIPHERAL PARENTERAL NUTRITION

Peripheral parenteral nutrition (PPN) is a method of supplying nutrients to the client by an IV route that is not a central vein. PPN is used for less than 10 days when the client does not need more than 2000 calories daily. PPN solutions can contain a mixture of dextrose (of less than 12%), amino acids, and lipids, in addition to electrolytes or water, which can be found in routine IV solutions. The all-in-one PPN system mixes dextrose, amino acids, and lipids all in one container, which is tolerated better by the veins.

LEARNING TIP

Clients with the following may need to be considered for TPN or PPN:

1. Any significant weight loss (10% or more of weight when healthy)
2. A decrease of oral food intake for longer than 1 week
3. Any significant sign of protein loss: serum albumin levels below 3.2 g/dL
4. Muscle wasting
5. Decreased tissue healing
6. Persistent vomiting and diarrhea

Review Questions

1. Which of the following prevents backup of chyme from the small intestine to the stomach?
   a. Pyloric sphincter
   b. Fundus
   c. Duodenal sphincter
   d. Duodenal ampulla

2. Which of the following increases peristalsis in the alimentary tube?
   a. Sympathetic impulses
   b. The ninth cranial nerve
   c. The hormone epinephrine
   d. Parasympathetic impulses

3. Which of the following is the stimulus for the defecation reflex?
   a. Contraction of the rectum
   b. Contraction of the internal anal sphincter
   c. Relaxation of the external anal sphincter
   d. Stretching of the rectum

4. Bowel sounds heard at an irregular rate every 5 to 15 seconds are considered
   a. Abnormal
   b. Hyperactive
   c. Hypoactive
   d. Normal

5. After an EGD procedure the client is NPO until which of the following occurs?
   a. Four hours have passed
   b. The gag reflex returns
   c. Vital signs return to normal
   d. Client can take liquids without vomiting

6. To ease the client's anxiety about insertion of an NG tube, the nurse can
   a. Explain what to expect during insertion and how the NG tube will benefit the client
   b. Assess the client's gag reflex to ease insertion
   c. Restrain the client so he or she does not get too agitated during insertion
   d. Administer a narcotic to calm the client

7. Which of the following clients would most likely require TPN?
   a. Mrs. Norris, who is malnourished due to cancer
   b. Mr. Gibson, who has just returned from surgery for an appendectomy
   c. Miss Russell, who has been admitted with chest pain
   d. Mr. Dawson, who has respiratory distress related to his COPD

ANSWERS TO CRITICAL THINKING

CRITICAL THINKING: Mrs. Todd

1. Daily aspirin use.
2. Medication teaching including side effects. Assessment of pain relief needs and consultation with the physician.

CRITICAL THINKING: Jackie

1. Dehydration.
2. Her daily water needs are not being met. She is not receiving medications that would incidentally provide water during their administration.
3. Consult dietitian or review Jackie's daily water needs. Divide the water needs over 24 hours and ensure that the water is administered. Ensure tubing is flushed per agency policy, and calculate water used toward daily water needs. Monitor intake and output. Continue assessing Jackie's signs and symptoms, and report abnormal findings.

REFERENCES

1. AbuGharbieh, P: Arab Americans. In Purnell, L, and Paulanka, B (eds): Transcultural Health Care: A Culturally Competent Approach. FA Davis, Philadelphia, 1998.
2. Monrroy, LS: Nursing care of Raza/Latino patients. In Block, MS, and Monrroy, LSA (eds): Ethnic Nursing Care: A Multicultural Approach. Mosby, St Louis, 1983.
3. Selekman, J: Jewish Americans. In Purnell, L, and Paulanka, B (eds): Transcultural Health Care: A Culturally Competent Approach. FA Davis, Philadelphia, 1998.
4. Jambanathan, J: Hindus. In Purnell, L, and Paulanka, B (eds): Transcultural Health Care: A Culturally Competent Approach. FA Davis, Philadelphia, 1998.
5. Coler, M: Brazilian Americans. In Purnell, L, and Paulanka, B (eds): Transcultural Health Care: A Culturally Competent Approach. FA Davis, Philadelphia, 1998.
6. Lipson, J, Reizian, A, and Meleis, A: Arab-American patients: A medical record review. Soc Sci Med 24(2):101, 1987.
7. Campinha-Bacote, J: African Americans. In Purnell, L, and Paulanka, B (eds): Transcultural Health Care: A Culturally Competent Approach. FA Davis, Philadelphia, 1998.
8. Purnell, L, and Counts, M: In Purnell, L, and Paulanka, B (eds): Transcultural Health Care: A Culturally Competent Approach. FA Davis, Philadelphia, 1998.
9. Lutz, C, and Przytulski, K: Nutrition and Diet Therapy. FA Davis, Philadelphia, 1997.

BIBLIOGRAPHY

Barnie, DC, and Currier, J: What's that GI tube being used for? RN 95(8):45, 1995.
Belknap, D, Seifert, C, and Petermann, M: Administration of medications through enteral feeding catheters. Am J Crit Care 6(5):382, 1997.
Emery, E, et al: Banana flakes control diarrhea in enterally fed patients. Nutr Clin Pract 12(2):72, 1997.
Grem, J: The prognostic importance of tumor markers in adenocarcinomas of the gastrointestinal tract. Curr Opin Oncol 9(4):380, 1997.
Harrison, A, et al: Nonradiographic assessment of enteral feeding tube position. Crit Care Med 25(12):2055, 1997.
Jaffe, M, and McVan, B: Davis's Laboratory and Diagnostic Test Handbook. FA Davis, Philadelphia, 1997.
Lord, LM: Enteral access devices. Nurs Clin North Am 32(4):685, 1997.
Mateo, MA: Nursing management of enteral tube feedings. Heart Lung 25(4):318, 1996.
Metheny, N, and Clouse, R: Bedside methods for detecting aspiration in tube-fed patients. Chest 111(3):724, 1997.
Nowak, TJ, and Handford, AG: Essentials of Pathophysiology: Concepts and Applications for Health Care Professionals. WC Brown, Dubuque, Iowa, 1994.
Pectasides, D, et al: CEA, CA 19-9 and CA-50 in monitoring gastric carcinoma. Am J Clin Oncol 20(4):348, 1997.
Polaski, AL, and Tatro, SE: Luckmann's Core Principles and Practice of Medical-Surgical Nursing. WB Saunders, Philadelphia, 1996.
Schmieding, N, and Walding, R: Gastric decompression in adult patients. Survey of nursing practice. Clin Nurs Res 6(2):142, 1997.
Schmieding, N, and Walding, R: Nasogastric tube feeding and medication administration: A survey of nursing practices. Gastroenterol Nurs 20(4):118, 1997.
Thomas, CL (ed): Taber's Cyclopedic Medical Dictionary, ed 17. FA Davis, Philadelphia, 1997.
Varella, L, Jones, E, and Meguid, MM: Drug-nutrient interactions in enteral feeding: A primary care focus. Nurse Pract 22(6):98, 1997.

Nursing Care of Clients with Upper Gastrointestinal Disorders

Sharon Ivy Gordon

Learning Objectives

Upon completion of this chapter, the student will be able to:

1. Define anorexia, anorexia nervosa, bulimia nervosa, and obesity, and describe their medical management and nursing care.

2. Describe the nursing management of clients with stomatitis.

3. Define acute and chronic gastritis and their nursing management.

4. Explain the pathophysiology, signs and symptoms, and diagnostic testing for hiatal hernia, peptic ulcer disease, gastric bleeding, and gastric cancer.

5. Describe the pharmacologic treatment of peptic ulcer disease.

6. Define the surgical procedures for hiatal hernia and gastric cancer, and describe the complications and nursing care for them.

7. Describe the nursing care for hiatal hernia, peptic ulcer disease, gastric bleeding, and gastric cancer.

Key Words

anorexia (AN-oh-**REK**-see-ah)

anorexia nervosa (AN-oh-**REK**-see-ah ner-**VOH**-sah)

aphthous stomatitis (**AF**-thus STOH-mah-**TIGH**-tis)

bulimia nervosa (buh-**LEE**-mee-ah ner-**VOH**-sah)

gastrectomy (gas-**TREK**-tuh-mee)

gastritis (gas-**TRY**-tis)

gastroduodenostomy (GAS-troh-DOO-oh-den-**AHS**-toh-mee)

gastrojejunostomy (GAS-troh-JAY-joo-**NAHS**-toh-mee)

gastroplasty (**GAS**-troh-PLAS-tee)

Helicobacter pylori (**HE**-lick-co-back-tur **PIE**-lori)

hiatal hernia (high-**AY**-tuhl **HER**-nee-ah)

obesity (oh-**BEE**-si-tee)

peptic ulcer disease (**PEP**-tick **UL**-sir di-**ZEEZ**)

steatorrhea (STEE-ah-toh-**REE**-ah)

stomatitis (STOH-mah-**TIGH**-tis)

Eating Disorders

ANOREXIA

Simple **anorexia,** which is a lack of appetite, is a common symptom of many diseases and can be caused by noxious food odors, certain drugs (as an intended or side effect), emotional stress, fear, psychological problems, and infections. Prolonged anorexia with an inadequate nutritional intake can lead to serious electrolyte imbalances, which in turn can lead to cardiac dysrhythmias. Although eating is the preferred method of weight gain, other measures such as tube feedings and intravenous infusion can be used. The nurse should ask clients what causes them to lose their appetite and what makes it improve to plan care for them. Nursing actions for the client with anorexia include documenting accurate intake and output; monitoring vital signs, electrolytes, and electrocardiograms; and monitoring the rate of the intravenous infusion and tube feeding.

ANOREXIA NERVOSA

Anorexia nervosa is an eating disorder that is recognized by the American Psychiatric Association (Table 30–1). This disease most commonly occurs in females between the ages of 12 and 18 who are from the middle and upper classes of Western culture. Males account for 5 to 10 percent of the population with anorexia nervosa. Young women with low self-esteem seem to be at highest risk. Anorexia nervosa is thought to be psychological in origin. Clients may have a phobia of weight gain, are afraid of a loss of control, and are mistrusting.

Signs and Symptoms

Early signs and symptoms of anorexia nervosa include severe weight loss, low self-esteem, compulsive dieting, and an altered body image (imagining oneself as fat when within normal weight range). As the disease progresses, additional symptoms include amenorrhea in females, elec-

Table 30–1. *Diagnostic Criteria for Anorexia Nervosa*

1. Refusal to maintain body weight over a minimum normal weight for age and height
2. Intense fear of gaining weight or becoming fat, even though underweight
3. Disturbance in the way in which one's body weight, shape, or size is experienced
4. In females, the absence of at least three consecutive menstrual cycles when otherwise expected to occur

trolyte imbalance, cardiac dysrhythmias, constipation, dry skin, lanugo (downy hair covering body), bradycardia, hypothermia, hypotension, muscle wasting, and facial puffiness. Often these clients deny the existence of any problem. They may develop bizarre food rituals and sometimes weigh themselves several times a day. Anorexia nervosa sometimes overlaps with **bulimia nervosa** (compulsive eating with self-induced vomiting).

Medical Management

Because up to 18 percent of anorexia clients die as a result of the disease, the most important intervention for anorexia nervosa is the restoration of nutritional health. During the crisis period, when severe weight loss, life-threatening electrolyte imbalances and dysrhythmias, or other symptoms occur, this can be accomplished by intravenous infusions containing electrolytes. Additional supplements can include tube feedings, oral feedings, and oxygen given to assist with respiration.

The client's damaged self-image and self-esteem are underlying problems and must be addressed in conjunction with the nutritional aspect (Nutrition Notes Box 30–1). Both self-image and nutrition issues require treatment over a long period of time. Psychotherapy and behavior modification that includes participation by the client's significant other(s) are often used to treat anorexia nervosa.

Nursing Care

Gaining the client's genuine cooperation by using therapeutic communication and setting realistic, mutual goals is important in establishing trust and preventing relapse. Nurses working with clients diagnosed with anorexia nervosa need to develop a therapeutic relationship with them for effective interactions. The nurse should use empathy, acceptance of the client, trust, and warmth and be nonjudgmental when interacting with clients.[1] Caring for clients with anorexia nervosa is challenging. Nursing actions for these clients include regular vital signs, daily weights, and strict accurate documentation of intake and output of food and fluids.

BULIMIA NERVOSA

Bulimia nervosa is compulsive eating with self-induced vomiting, which is commonly known as "binge-purge." The bulimic client typically eats massive amounts of food at one sitting and then purges the food by intentionally in-

---

NUTRITION NOTES BOX 30–1

Nutrition in Upper Gastrointestinal Conditions

ANOREXIA NERVOSA AND BULIMIA. Anorexia nervosa and bulimia are eating disorders requiring multidisciplinary treatment. Although correcting the nutritional consequences of these conditions is of major importance, to achieve a cure, it is essential to treat the underlying psychological causes.

OBESITY. Candidates for gastric stapling or gastric bypass surgery should be carefully selected. The procedure should be seen as one tool to assist with weight control, along with behavioral changes. It is not done to permit overeating because in time the constructed pouch can be stretched, thus negating the surgery. Guidelines include eating three to six small balanced meals per day, chewing thoroughly and eating slowly, consuming fluids between meals, exercising regularly, and taking a multivitamin-multimineral supplement. Among potential complications of these surgeries are nausea, vomiting, bloating, heartburn, staple disruption, obstruction, dumping syndrome, and osteoporosis.

HIATAL HERNIA. The client with hiatal hernia may find symptoms alleviated by protein foods, which tighten the cardiac sphincter. Substances that should be avoided because they relax the sphincter include fat, caffeine, peppermint, spearmint, chocolate, alcohol, and nicotine.

DUMPING SYNDROME. The recommended meal pattern for the dumping syndrome includes six small feedings per day, high in protein and low in simple sugars; fluids between rather than with meals; and reclining for 30 minutes after meals. Supplementation with the vitamins B_{12}, D, and folic acid and the minerals calcium and iron may be necessary to prevent deficiencies.

GASTRIC CANCER. If the client has a poor prognosis following a total gastrectomy for cancer, dietary interventions should focus on symptoms the client wishes to control. An overly restricted diet causing the client discomfort or distress is inappropriate.

ducing vomiting so weight is not gained. Laxatives can also be used by the bulimic client to purge the body of food to avoid weight gain. As in anorexia nervosa, bulimic clients are extremely thin, to the point of starvation. A high percentage of them are young women.

Signs and Symptoms

Clients with bulimia nervosa usually exhibit the same signs and symptoms as clients with anorexia nervosa, but with a few exceptions. Bulimic clients often have enamel erosion of the front teeth due to the acid content of the emesis. They also spend a great deal of time locked in the bathroom vomiting, especially after meals. As the electrolyte imbalance worsens, they develop metabolic alkalosis as a result of the loss of gastric acid in the stomach contents.

Medical Management

The treatment for bulimia nervosa is essentially the same as for that of the client with anorexia nervosa (see above).

OBESITY

Obesity is defined as a weight that is 20 percent or greater than the desirable weight for an adult of a given gender and height. Simply put, obesity is caused by a caloric intake that exceeds the energy expenditure. Only a small percent of obesity is associated with a metabolic or endocrine abnormality within the body. As adults age, their metabolism slows and activity often lessens, which results in a weight gain. Obesity that interferes with activities of daily living, such as breathing or walking, is known as morbid obesity. Morbid obesity applies to people who are more than 100 pounds over their ideal body weight. Diseases that are associated with obesity include atherosclerosis (arterial hardening), diabetes mellitus, hypertension, osteoarthritis, and certain types of cancer.

Medical Management

Initial treatment for obesity centers on weight loss through exercise and dieting. It is important to have the client's cooperation and sustained motivation. This can be maintained through support groups such as Take Off Pounds Sensibly (TOPS) and Weight Watchers.

Clients who do not respond to dietary methods of weight loss or who are morbidly obese may have a surgical procedure to reduce their weight. There are several types of surgical procedures, each having certain advantages and disadvantages (see Nutrition Notes Box 30–1). One example is a **gastroplasty** (gastric stapling) in which a portion of

the stomach is stapled, allowing food to enter the smaller stomach slowly. This makes it necessary for the client to eat only small amounts (30 mL) of food at each meal. Nutritional reeducation is necessary, in addition to the surgery to maintain weight loss.

Inflammatory Disorders

STOMATITIS

Stomatitis is the general term for inflammation of the oral cavity. There are many causes of stomatitis. It can be caused by an infection, or it can be the symptom of a systemic disease. The most common types are **aphthous stomatitis** (canker sores) and herpes simplex virus type I (also known as cold sores or fever blisters).

Aphthous Stomatitis (Canker Sores)

Aphthous stomatitis appears as small, white, painful ulcers on the inner cheeks, lips, tongue, gums, palate, or pharynx and typically lasts for several days to 2 weeks. Self-trauma such as biting the lips and cheeks can cause these ulcers to develop, as well as stress and exposure to certain irritating foods. Application of topical tetracycline several times a day usually shortens the healing time. A topical anesthetic such as benzocaine or lidocaine provides pain relief and makes it possible to eat with minimal pain.

Herpes Simplex Virus Type I

Herpes simplex virus type I (HSV-I) may appear as painful cold sores or fever blisters on the face, lips, perioral area, cheeks, nose, or conjunctiva (Fig. 30–1). These lesions recur over time but last only for a few days each time. The

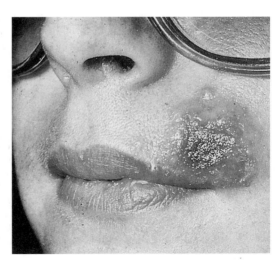

Figure 30–1. Herpes simplex. (From Reeves J, Maibach H. Clinical Dermatology Illustrated 2nd ed, 1998. Reproduced with permission: MacLennan & Petty, Sidney.) See Plate 18.

---

gastroplasty: gastro—stomach + plasty—repair
stomatitis: stoma—mouth + itis—inflammation

onset can be provoked by such things as fever or stress. Acyclovir ointment can be used to ease the pain, but it does not cure the lesions. Oral acyclovir may reduce recurrences. These lesions are infectious, and Standard Precautions should be used when ointment is applied or oral care is given.

Oral Cancer

Oral cancer can occur anywhere in the mouth or throat. If detected early enough, it is curable. Oral cancer is found most commonly in clients who use alcohol or any form of tobacco. The highest incidence of oral cancer is found in the pharynx (throat), with the lowest incidence on the lips. Any oral sore that does not heal in 2 weeks should be assessed by the client's physician. Cancerous ulcers are often painless but may become tender as the cancer progresses. In the later stages, the client may complain of difficulty in chewing, swallowing, or speaking or swollen cervical lymph glands.

Biopsies are taken to determine the presence of cancer. Treatment varies depending on the individualized diagnosis. Radiation, chemotherapy, and surgery are used alone or in combination to treat oral cancer. Radical or modified neck dissection is done if the cancer has metastasized to cervical lymph nodes (Fig. 30–2). The tumor is removed along with lymph nodes, muscles, blood vessels, glands, and part of the thyroid, depending on the extent of the cancer. Drains are inserted into the incision to prevent fluid accumulation. A tracheostomy is usually performed to protect the airway and prevent obstruction. The airway must be monitored and secretions controlled to prevent aspiration. Tube feedings are usually given to meet the client's nutritional needs because swallowing is difficult.

Esophageal Cancer

As with oral cancer, esophageal cancer is associated with the use of tobacco or alcohol. Esophageal cancer is usually

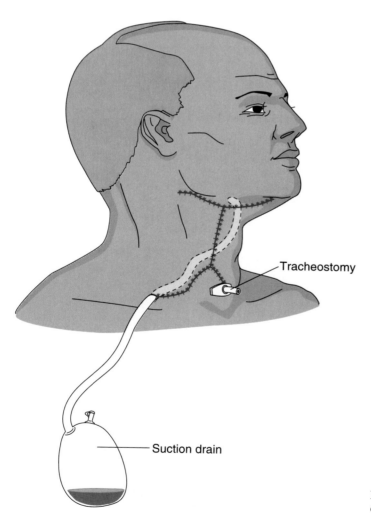

Tracheostomy

Suction drain

Figure 30–2. Radical neck dissection with tracheostomy and drains inserted.

detected late because of its location near many lymph nodes that allow it to metastasize. As the cancer progresses, obstruction of the esophagus can occur, with possible perforation or fistula development that may cause aspiration. The appearance of signs and symptoms usually means that the cancer is in the late stages. Signs and symptoms may include difficulty swallowing, a feeling of fullness, pain in the chest area after eating, foul breath, or regurgitation of foods if there is obstruction.

Diagnosis of esophageal cancer is usually made by esophagogastroduodenoscopy (EGD) and biopsy. Mediastinoscopy (endoscopic examination of mediastinum) is used to determine if the cancer has spread to the lymph nodes and surrounding structures. Treatment for esophageal cancer includes radiation, chemotherapy, and surgery alone or in combination. Surgical procedures include esophageal resection (esophagogastrostomy), Dacron esophageal replacement, or use of a section of colon to replace the esophagus (esophagoenterostomy). If the tumor is inoperable, esophageal dilation or stent placement can be done to relieve dysphagia and allow food to pass through the esophagus.

Hiatal Hernia

The esophagus passes through an opening in the diaphragm called the hiatus. A **hiatal hernia** is a condition in which the lower part of the esophagus and stomach slides up through the hiatus of the diaphragm into the thorax (Fig. 30–3). It occurs most commonly in women, those over age 60, obesity, and pregnancy. A small hernia may not produce any discomfort or require any treatment. However, a large hernia can cause pain, heartburn, a feeling of fullness, and reflux, which can injure the esophagus with possible ulceration and bleeding. Hiatal hernias are diagnosed by x-ray studies and fluoroscopy.

MEDICAL MANAGEMENT

Treatment includes antacids; having the client eat small meals that can pass easily through the esophagus; advising the client not to recline for 1 hour after eating; avoiding bedtime snacks, spicy foods, alcohol, caffeine, and smoking; and elevating the head of the bed 6 to 12 inches to pre-

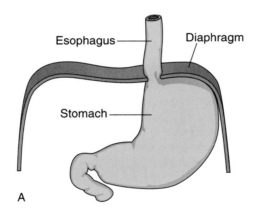

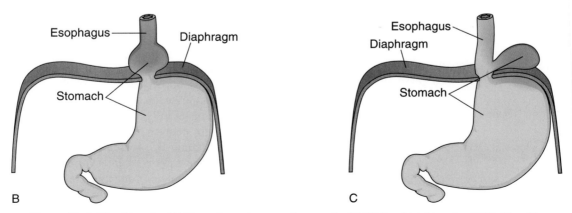

Figure 30–3. Hiatal hernia. *(A)* Normal esophagus and stomach. *(B)* Sliding hiatal hernia. *(C)* Rolling hiatal hernia.

vent reflux (see Nutrition Notes Box 30–1). Surgical procedures can be done to affix the herniated portion of the stomach in place to prevent it from moving upward through the hiatus. Fundoplication is the basic surgical procedure that is done, which is the wrapping of the stomach fundus around the lower part of the esophagus (Fig. 30–4). Following this repair, clients should be assessed for dysphagia during their first postoperative meal. If dysphagia occurs, the physician should be notified because the repair may be too tight and obstructing the passage of food.

Gastroesophageal Reflux Disease

Gastroesophageal reflux disease (GERD) is a condition in which gastric secretions reflux into the esophagus. The esophagus can be damaged by the acidic secretions and exposure to digestive enzymes. It is caused primarily by conditions that affect the ability of the lower esophageal sphincter to close tightly, such as hiatal hernia. It often occurs in the elderly. Signs and symptoms include heartburn, regurgitation, dysphagia, and bleeding. Aspiration is a concern. Scar tissue can develop from the inflammation. Diagnostic tests include a barium swallow, esophagoscopy, or pH monitoring of the normally alkaline esophagus.

MEDICAL MANAGEMENT

Interventions to decrease the reflux of gastric secretions into the esophagus are used. Medications may include antacids, H_2 receptor antagonists, cytoprotective agents (sucralfate), and cholinergic drugs that improve gastric emptying and function of the lower esophageal sphincter. Obese clients should be encouraged to lose weight. A low-fat, high-protein diet is recommended because fat promotes decreased functioning of the lower esophageal sphincter. Caffeine, milk products, and spicy foods should

be avoided. If surgery is necessary to alleviate symptoms, a fundoplication can be done.

NURSING MANAGEMENT

Clients need to be educated about managing their condition. They are told to sleep with the head of the bed elevated 4 to 6 inches and avoid lying down for 2 hours after eating. Small meals should be eaten. Smoking and alcohol intake should be avoided because they decrease functioning of the lower esophageal sphincter. Foods that cause discomfort should be identified by the client and avoided. Teaching about medication is included in the client's plan of care.

Gastritis

ACUTE GASTRITIS

Acute **gastritis** is the inflammation of the stomach mucosa and is sometimes called heartburn or indigestion. It is most often caused by overeating or direct irritation of the stomach lining by food that is too spicy or contaminated with pathogens. Other causes may include ingestion of alcohol, aspirin, acids, and alkalis. If severe, the gastric mucosa can become gangrenous and perforate, which can lead to peritonitis (infection of the peritoneum). Scarring may also occur, resulting in pyloric obstruction.

SYMPTOMS AND MEDICAL MANAGEMENT

The major symptom of gastritis is abdominal pain, which is often accompanied by nausea and anorexia. Treatment is to remove the irritating substance and provide a bland diet of liquids and soft foods along with antacids. With a bland diet, the client usually recovers in about a day.

CHRONIC GASTRITIS TYPE A

Chronic gastritis occurs over a period of time and is classified as type A or type B. Type A is often referred to as autoimmune gastritis. It results from changes in the cells of the stomach mucosa and most often occurs in the fundus or body of the stomach. Chronic gastritis type A is diagnosed by endoscopy, upper gastrointestinal x-ray examination, and gastric aspirate analysis (see Chapter 29). Clients with type A gastritis usually do not secrete enough intrinsic factor from their stomach cells and as a result have difficulty absorbing vitamin B_{12}, which leads to pernicious anemia. This type of gastritis is often asymptomatic except for the symptoms of pernicious anemia. These symptoms include anemia, weakness, sore tongue, numbness and tingling,

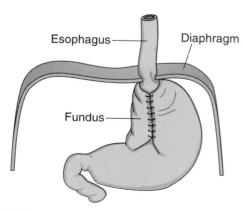

Figure 30–4. Hiatal hernia repair. Nissen fundoplication wraps the stomach fundus around the esophagus and then sutures it onto itself to hold it in place.

---

gastritis: gastr—stomach + itis—inflammation

and gastrointestinal upset. Pernicious anemia is treated with vitamin B$_{12}$ injections.

CHRONIC GASTRITIS TYPE B

Type B gastritis affects the antrum and pylorus (lower end of the stomach near the duodenum) and is associated with the **Helicobacter pylori** (*H. pylori*) bacterium. Infection with *H. pylori* causes type B gastritis (also known as *H. pylori* gastritis). Signs and symptoms include poor appetite, heartburn after eating, belching, sour taste in the mouth, and nausea and vomiting. Type B gastritis can also be diagnosed by endoscopy, upper gastrointestinal x-ray examination, and gastric aspirate analysis. It can be treated with antibiotics such as tetracycline or amoxicillin.

Peptic Ulcer Disease

ETIOLOGY

Until 1982 the cause of peptic ulcer was poorly understood and thought to be related to stress, diet, and alcohol or caffeine ingestion. However, research identified that peptic ulcer disease is primarily caused by infection with the gram-negative bacterium *H. pylori*. This bacterium is responsible for 80 percent of gastric ulcers and over 90 percent of duodenal ulcers.[2] With two thirds of all people infected with *H. pylori,* it occurs more commonly in the elderly, Hispanics, African-Americans, and lower socioeconomic groups in the United States.[2] This discovery has led to changes in treating and curing peptic ulcers. It is not known how *H. pylori* is transmitted, although the oral-oral or fecal-oral route is likely. Contaminated water may also play a role. Vaccines to prevent peptic ulcers are being developed.

Peptic ulcer development is also influenced by smoking, which has many effects, including increasing the harmful effects of *H. pylori,* affecting protective mechanisms, and decreasing gastric blood flow.

LEARNING TIP

Most peptic ulcers are caused by an infection that can be cured with antibiotics.

PATHOPHYSIOLOGY

Peptic ulcer disease (PUD) is a condition in which the lining of the stomach, pylorus, duodenum, or the esophagus is eroded, usually from infection with *H. pylori*. The erosion may extend into the muscle layers or the peritoneum. Ulcers are named by their location: esophageal, gastric, or duodenal ulcer.

Peptic ulcers occur in the portions of the gastrointestinal tract that are exposed to hydrochloric acid and pepsin. The erosion is due to an increase in the concentration or activity of hydrochloric acid and pepsin. The damaged mucosa is unable to secrete enough mucus to act as a barrier against the hydrochloric acid. Some individuals have more rapid gastric emptying, which, combined with hypersecretion of acid, creates a large amount of acid moving into the duodenum. This is why peptic ulcers occur more frequently in the duodenum.

SIGNS AND SYMPTOMS

Clients with peptic ulcers most commonly experience aching, burning, and gnawing pain in the epigastric region. There is more pain and discomfort on an empty stomach and in the middle of the night. This intermittent pain may be relieved by the ingestion of food or antacids. Anorexia and nausea and vomiting may also occur. Bleeding occurs when the ulcer erodes through a blood vessel with massive hemorrhaging or slow oozing. These clients often have low hematocrit and hemoglobin levels, and stool for occult blood or gastroccult of stomach secretions may be positive, depending on where the ulcers are located.

DIAGNOSIS

H. pylori can be diagnosed with several tests. The urea breath test is performed by having the client drink carbon-labeled urea. The urea is metabolized rapidly if *H. pylori* is present, allowing the carbon to be absorbed and measured in exhaled CO_2. An IgG antibody detection test for *H. pylori* identifies if the client is infected with *H. pylori*. These are both noninvasive detection tests. Biopsy specimens can be obtained during esophagogastroduodenoscopy (EGD) to perform the *Campylobacter*-like organism (CLO) biopsy urease test and histological examination. Biopsy is the most conclusive test for *H. pylori*. Cultures can be done but take time.

Peptic ulcers are diagnosed on the basis of symptoms, upper gastrointestinal (GI) series (barium swallow), and EGD.

MEDICAL MANAGEMENT

The first antibiotic treatment for ulcer disease caused by *H. pylori* was approved by the Food and Drug Administration (FDA) in 1996. There are several treatment options approved that can cure the infection without recurrence. For effectiveness, studies show these options should include triple therapy with two antibiotics and a proton pump inhibitor or an H$_2$ antagonist. Two antibiotics are used to decrease possible resistance of the bacteria. Recommended antibiotics include tetracycline, clarithromycin, metronidazole, and amoxicillin. Proton pump inhibitors are powerful agents that stop the final step of gastric acid secretion to reduce mucosa erosion and aid in healing the ulcer. Examples of proton pump inhibitors include omeprazole and lansoprazole. H$_2$ antagonists, such as ranitidine, block H$_2$

Table 30-2. **Medications Used to Promote Healing of Peptic Ulcers**

Medication	Action	Side Effects	Nursing Interventions
Hyposecretory Agents—Histamine (H$_2$) Receptor Blocking Agents			
Cimetidine (Tagamet)	Inhibits gastric acid secretion by blocking H$_2$ receptors on gastric parietal cells	Fever, rash, headaches, dizziness, somnolence, confusion (especially in elderly), hypotension, diarrhea, neutropenia, gynecomastia, and impotence	Monitor mental status of elderly; do not take antacids within 1 hour of Tagamet; take with meals and at bedtime; interacts with theophylline, phenytoin, warfarin, and beta blockers; continue treatment for at least 8 weeks to ensure healing
Ranitidine (Zantac)	Inhibits gastric acid secretion by blocking H$_2$ receptors on gastric parietal cells	All side effects rare, including nausea, constipation, bradycardia, increased liver enzymes, and headache	Give antacids at least 1 hour before or 2 hours after Zantac; can be given in single bedtime dose; use cautiously in clients with liver or renal disease; absorption not affected by food; interacts minimally with other drugs
Famotidine (Pepcid)	Inhibits gastric acid secretion by blocking H$_2$ receptors on gastric parietal cells	Headache, diarrhea, constipation, nausea, flatulence, increased blood urea nitrogen and creatinine, and rash	Should not be taken longer than 8 weeks without physician's order; may be given with antacids; can be given in single bedtime dose; has no significant drug interactions
Nizatidine (Axid)	Inhibits gastric acid secretion by blocking H$_2$ receptors on gastric parietal cells	Diarrhea, rash, bronchospasms, somnolence, joint pain, and sweating	Give as single bedtime dose or, if given twice a day, one dose at bedtime; assess for excessive drowsiness; monitor and record stools; do not give antacids within 1 hour of Axid; must be taken 4 to 8 weeks for ulcer healing; notify physician if somnolence or rash develops
Proton Pump Inhibitor—Gastric Acid Pump Inhibitor			
Omeprazole (Prilosec)	Binds to enzyme on gastric parietal cells to prevent final transport of hydrogen to block gastric acid secretion	Abdominal pain, diarrhea, rash, chest pain, and weakness	Give before meal in morning; swallow capsule whole; assess for abdominal pain and bleeding; monitor CBC and liver enzymes; may give with antacids; must be taken 4 to 8 weeks for ulcer healing; notify physician if bleeding, diarrhea, headache, or abdominal pain develops
Antacids			
Aluminum-Magnesium Combinations (Riopan, Maalox, Mylanta, Gelusil)	Increases gastric pH to reduce pepsin activity; strengthens gastric mucosal barrier and esophageal sphincter tone	Mild constipation or diarrhea	Do not give to clients with renal disease; monitor bowel movements and signs of hypermagnesemia; Riopan low in sodium; do not give within 1 to 2 hours of H$_2$ receptor antagonists, tetracycline, or enteric-coated tablets
Calcium Carbonate (Tums, Titralac)	Increases gastric pH to reduce pepsin activity; strengthens gastric mucosal barrier and esophageal sphincter tone	Constipation, gastric distention, rebound hyperacidity, hypercalcemia, and hypophosphatemia	Do not give to clients with renal disease; do not give with milk; monitor for symptoms of hypercalcemia and constipation; do not give within 1 to 2 hours of H$_2$ receptor antagonists, tetracycline, or enteric-coated tablets
Mucosal Barrier Fortifiers			
Sucralfate (Carafate)	In presence of mild acid condition, forms viscid and sticky gel and adheres to ulcer surface, forming a protective barrier	Dizziness, constipation, sleepiness, nausea, and gastric discomfort	Take on an empty stomach, 1 hour before meals and at bedtime; monitor for constipation; urge client to take entire prescription

receptors to decrease acid secretion, although not as powerfully as gastric acid pump inhibitors. Bismuth subsalicylate (Pepto-Bismol) is also used in treatment.

Additional treatment for acute peptic ulcers focuses on assisting the ulcerated area to heal, which may take several weeks. There are many other medications designed to provide ulcer management, although antibiotics are now the first-line drug (Table 30–2). They help protect the mucosa, neutralize hydrochloric acid, inhibit acid secretion, and decrease the activity of pepsin and hydrochloric acid. A bland diet may also be recommended, and foods known to cause discomfort to the client, such as spicy foods, carbonated drinks, and caffeine, should be avoided until the ulcer heals.

LEARNING TIP

The basic types of medications for the stomach:

1. Proton pump inhibitors such as omeprazole (Prilosec) inhibit gastric acid from forming.
2. H_2 antagonists such as cimetidine (Tagamet), famotidine (Pepcid), and ranitidine (Zantac) reduce gastric acid secretion.
3. Antacids such as Maalox and Mylanta neutralize gastric acid that has already formed.
4. Sucralfate (Carafate) is the "Band-Aid" for ulcers. Carafate forms a sticky gel that adheres to the ulcer, providing a protective barrier.

NURSING PROCESS

Assessment

The primary focus of nursing care for peptic ulcer disease is to educate clients that ulcers are caused by an infection and can be cured with antibiotics. Clients may still believe that ulcers are caused by stress, lifestyle, or diet. The nurse needs to assess the client's knowledge base and provide accurate information to assist the client in recovering.

Nursing Diagnosis and Planning

Nursing Care Plan Box 30–2 discusses nursing diagnoses for peptic ulcer disease.

Interventions

Clients should be taught about their medications. They need to understand the importance of taking all of their medication as directed, even if they feel better. Client noncompliance with treatment is a major cause of ulcer recurrence. Other interventions are presented in Nursing Care Plan Box 30–2.

Evaluation

The client's goals are met if treatment is understood and followed and there is no recurrence of the ulcer.

Stress Ulcers

Clients who are critically ill may develop ulcers from the severe stress caused by the illness. This is referred to as a stress ulcer. The stress causes reduced blood flow to the stomach resulting in ischemia and damage to the mucosa. This allows the acid secretions to cause ulcers. It occurs commonly in clients with burns, infections, cerebral trauma, or major surgery. To prevent stress ulcers in the critically ill, prophylactic medications are usually ordered to keep the gastric pH above 5 so it is less acidic. The nurse monitors the gastric pH around the clock and administers antacids as indicated, or an H_2 antagonist may be given.

Gastric Bleeding

Gastric bleeding may be caused by ulcer perforation, tumors, gastric surgery, or other sources. Bleeding peptic ulcers are the most common cause of blood loss into the stomach or intestine. Blood loss can be minimal, manifested by occult blood in the stool (melena), or massive, in which the client vomits bright red blood. The usual symptoms of GI tract bleeding are vomiting blood (hematemesis) and the passing of tarry stools (melena). When blood mixes with hydrochloric acid and enzymes in the stomach, a dark, granular material resembling coffee grounds is produced. This can be vomited or passed through the GI system and mixed with stools.

SIGNS AND SYMPTOMS

In mild bleeding, the client may experience only slight weakness and diaphoresis. Severe blood loss (more than 1 L in 24 hours) may result in hypovolemic shock, with signs and symptoms such as hypotension, a weak thready pulse, chills, palpitations, and diaphoresis.

MEDICAL MANAGEMENT

The treatment for a massive GI bleed aims at preventing and treating hypovolemic shock and preventing dehydration, electrolyte imbalance, and further bleeding. The client is kept on nothing-by-mouth (NPO) status. An intravenous (IV) line is started to replace lost fluids and administer blood, if necessary. A complete blood count is obtained to determine the amount of blood lost. A urinary catheter is inserted to monitor output. A nasogastric (NG) tube is inserted to assess the rate of bleeding, to decompress the stomach, to monitor the pH of gastric secretions, and to administer saline lavage, if ordered. Oxygen therapy may be required if the client has lost a large amount of blood. To prevent aspiration from vomiting, the nurse should elevate the head of the bed. The physician may perform endoscopy to help control the bleeding. Drugs may also be instilled into the GI tract by use of the endoscope. For severe cases, surgery may be needed to remove the bleeding area or lig-

NURSING CARE PLAN BOX 30–2
FOR THE CLIENT WITH PEPTIC ULCER DISEASE

Pain related to gastric mucosal erosion

Client Outcomes
Client's pain is relieved as evidenced by no report of pain and absence of nonverbal pain cues.

Evaluation of Outcomes
Is pain relieved to client's satisfaction?

Interventions	Rationale	Evaluation
Ask client to assess pain level on scale of 1 to 10 every 3 hours and prn. Assess location, onset, intensity, characteristics of pain, and nonverbal pain cues.	Prompt assessment can lead to timely intervention and relief of pain.	Does client rate pain using scale and describe pain?
Assess for factors precipitating and relieving pain.	Peptic ulcer pain may be relieved by food, antacids, or other interventions.	Is client able to state precipitating and relieving pain factors?
Ask client to help identify techniques for pain relief	Gaining the client's cooperation increases compliance.	Is client willing to participate in planning how to relieve pain?
Administer medications as ordered.	H_2 receptor antagonists reduce amount of gastric acid produced, and antacids neutralize gastric acid to help relieve pain.	Do medications reduce client's symptoms?
Provide small, frequent meals four to six times a day.	Small, frequent meals dilute and neutralize gastric acid.	Does client report relief of gastric pain between meals?
Encourage nonacidic fluids between meals.	Nonacidic fluids decrease irritation to gastric mucosa.	Does client identify and drink nonacidic fluids?

Risk for injury related to complications of peptic ulcer activity such as hemorrhage and perforation

Client Outcomes
Client's vital signs will be maintained within normal limits and bleeding or hemorrhage will be promptly detected.

Evaluation of Outcomes
Are client's vital signs within normal limits?

Interventions	Rationale	Evaluation
Assess for signs and symptoms of hemorrhage such as hematemesis (vomiting blood) and melena (blood in the stool).	Rapid assessment can lead to prompt intervention.	Does client have any bleeding?
Monitor vital signs: blood pressure, pulse, respirations, and temperature.	Severe blood loss of more than 1 L per 24 hours may cause manifestations of shock such as hypotension; weak, thready pulse; chills; palpitations; and diaphoresis.	Are vital signs normal?
Maintain IV infusion as ordered.	Normal fluid balance prevents hypovolemia and shock due to hemorrhage.	Are intake and output balanced?
Monitor hematocrit and hemoglobin levels as ordered.	Decreased hematocrit and hemoglobin levels indicate a decrease in circulating blood volume and reduced oxygen-carrying capacity to the tissues.	Are hematocrit and hemoglobin levels normal?

continued

NURSING CARE PLAN BOX 30–2 *(continued)*

Knowledge deficit related to lack of information concerning diagnosis of peptic ulcer disease and management of ulcers

Client Outcomes
Client states understanding of information about peptic ulcer disease.

Evaluation of Outcomes
Does client follow health maintenance plan without complication development?

Interventions	Rationale	Evaluation
Assess client's education level.	This allows the nurse to use appropriate terminology using language the client can understand.	Is teaching material presented within the client's education level?
Assess client's motivation and willingness to learn.	Increased motivation in the client produces maximum learning.	Is client willing to learn?
Determine client's knowledge base about peptic ulcer disease.	The nurse can build on existing knowledge.	Does the client discuss knowledge about peptic ulcer disease?
Identify misconceptions client may have about peptic ulcer disease.	Clearing up misconceptions allows the client and nurse to work with accurate information.	Does client have any misconceptions?
Determine any client cultural influences for health teaching.	This allows the nurse and the client to adapt to the client's cultural influences concerning diet, health care, gender roles, the sick role, etc.	Does client work with nurse to adapt cultural influences to the teaching session?
Provide physical comfort for the learner.	If client is comfortable, it reduces the stress of handling new information and allows client to concentrate on what is being taught.	Is client comfortable?
Provide a quiet atmosphere without interruption.	This allows client to concentrate on the material being taught.	Is client able to concentrate on learning?
Establish goals for learning at the beginning of the session such as medications for peptic ulcer disease and diagnostic procedure.	Goals allow clients to know what will be discussed and expected during the learning session to reduce fear and anxiety.	Does client understand goals?
Assist the learner in integrating new information into daily life.	Compliance is increased if client is helped to make adjustments in daily life that will result in desired changes in behavior.	Does client have a plan for complying with treatment?
Encourage questions from the client.	Participation engages the client in the teaching session.	Does client ask questions?
Teaching sessions should include signs and symptoms of gastric bleeding, medication actions, dosage and side effects, and gastric lining irritants such as smoking, caffeine, and spicy foods.	Providing essential information allows client to control illness.	Does client understand essential disease knowledge?
Encourage smoking clients to stop smoking and provide information on methods for stopping.	Smoking cessation will increase the client's comfort.	Is client interested in quitting smoking?
Allow the client to practice new knowledge.	Demonstration allows client to use new information immediately to enhance retention and obtain feedback from nurse.	Does client practice new knowledge accurately?
Document progress of teaching and learning.	Documentation allows additional teaching to be based on what the client has completed, enhancing the client's self-confidence.	Does client demonstrate learning progression before discharge?

ate bleeding vessels. Drugs such as ranitidine are given to decrease the secretion of gastric acid.

Gastric Cancer

Gastric cancer refers to malignant lesions found in the stomach and is the second most common cancer in the world.[2] It is more common in men than in women. *H. pylori* infection plays a role in gastric cancer development.[3,4] Studies are being done to see if preventing *H. pylori* infection reduces the development of gastric cancer.[3] Other factors that may be associated with gastric cancer development include pernicious anemia, exposure to occupational substances such as lead dust, grain dust, glycol ethers, or leaded gasoline, or a diet high in smoked fish or meats. There is usually a poor prognosis associated with gastric cancer, with most clients having metastasis at the time of diagnosis (see Nutrition Notes Box 30–1).

SIGNS AND SYMPTOMS

Gastric cancer is rarely diagnosed in its early stages because the symptoms occur late in the disease. In the early stages there may not be any symptoms at all, and metastasis to another organ such as the liver may have already occurred. The symptoms of gastric cancer are often mistaken for peptic ulcer disease: indigestion, anorexia, pain relieved by antacids, weight loss, and nausea and vomiting. Anemia from blood loss commonly occurs, and occult blood in the stool may be present.

DIAGNOSIS

Diagnosis of gastric cancer is made by upper gastrointestinal x-ray, gastroscopy, gastric fluid analysis, and serum gastrin levels.

MEDICAL MANAGEMENT

Surgical removal of the cancer is the most effective treatment for gastric cancer. Most often the cancer has already metastasized, and surgery is done only to relieve the symptoms. Chemotherapy and radiation are sometimes used in conjunction with surgery, although they are not very effective against the cancer. Biological therapies, new cytotoxic agents, and new delivery methods are being studied for use with gastric cancer.[5]

Gastric Surgeries

SUBTOTAL GASTRECTOMY

Two types of surgical interventions are used to treat upper gastrointestinal diseases. The first is the subtotal **gastrectomy,** which is used to treat cancer in the lower two thirds of the stomach. The term *subtotal gastrectomy* is a general term used to describe any surgery that involves partial removal of the stomach. There are two types of subtotal gastrectomies: the Billroth I procedure and the Billroth II procedure.

Billroth I Procedure (Gastroduodenostomy)

In the Billroth I procedure, also known as a **gastroduodenostomy,** the surgeon removes the distal portion (75%) of the stomach. The remainder of the stomach is anastomosed (surgically attached) to the duodenum (Fig. 30–5). This procedure is used to treat gastric problems.

Billroth II Procedure (Gastrojejunostomy)

The Billroth II procedure, **gastrojejunostomy,** involves removal of the distal 50 percent of the stomach and reanastomosis of the proximal remnant of the stomach to the proximal jejunum (see Fig. 30–5). Because it bypasses the duodenum, this procedure is used to treat duodenal ulcers. Pancreatic secretions and bile are necessary for digestion and continue to be secreted into the duodenum from the common bile duct even after the partial gastrectomy.

TOTAL GASTRECTOMY

Total gastrectomy, the total removal of the stomach, is the treatment for extensive gastric cancer. This surgery involves removal of the stomach, with anastomosis of the esophagus to the jejunum (Fig. 30–6).

VAGOTOMY

A vagotomy, in which a section of the vagus nerve is cut, may be performed with gastric surgery. Vagotomy eliminates the vagal stimulation for hydrochloric acid and gastrin hormone secretion and slows gastric motility.

NURSING MANAGEMENT AFTER GASTRIC SURGERY

The nurse monitors the client's vital signs postoperatively as ordered. Respiratory status is monitored because the high location of the surgical incision may cause pain, which interferes with deep breathing and coughing. Atelectasis or pneumonia can develop as a result. The client's pain is assessed

---

gastrectomy: gastr—stomach + ectomy—to remove
gastroduodenostomy: gastro—stomach + duoden—duodenum + ostomy—mouth or opening
gastrojejunostomy: gastro—stomach + jejun—jejunum + ostomy—mouth or opening

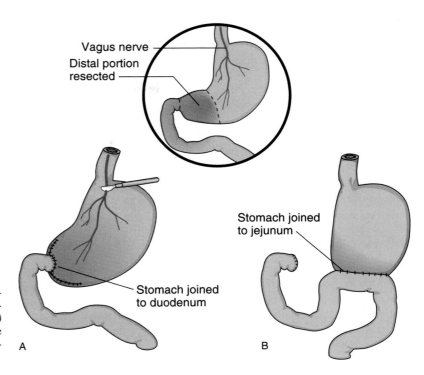

Figure 30–5. Subtotal gastrectomy involves removing the distal portion of the stomach. The remaining portion of the stomach is then sutured (A) to the duodenum (Billroth I procedure) or (B) to the proximal jejunum (Billroth II procedure). Vagotomy may also be performed.

and relieved. This also helps the client's ability to deep breathe or cough without pain. The client's IV site and infusion are monitored, and intake and output are recorded. The incisional site and dressings are observed for drainage and bleeding.

Bowel sounds are assessed. Clients may have an NG tube inserted in surgery. The nurse applies suction as ordered, which is usually low intermittent suction to prevent trauma to the gastric mucosa. The drainage from the NG tube is monitored for color and amount. If bleeding or excessive amounts of drainage are noted, they are reported to the physician. The nurse should not irrigate or reposition the NG tube following gastric surgery to prevent damaging the suture line. The client should be assessed for abdominal distention. If this occurs abdominal girth should be measured and the physician notified.

As clients recover, it is important to teach them how to assist in their recovery. This includes incisional care, any activity or dietary restrictions, and information about prescribed medications. Clients are encouraged to ambulate early because it promotes a quicker recovery by improving respiratory and gastrointestinal function. They must also be taught the lifelong need for vitamin B_{12} injections if any of the stomach was removed.

COMPLICATIONS OF GASTRIC SURGERY

Complications that can occur after gastric surgery include hemorrhage, acute gastric distention, nutritional problems,

steatorrhea (fat in stools), pyloric obstruction, and dumping syndrome.

Hemorrhage

The incidence of hemorrhage after gastric surgery is very low and is most often caused by a dislodged clot at the surgical site or slippage of a suture. The client experienc-

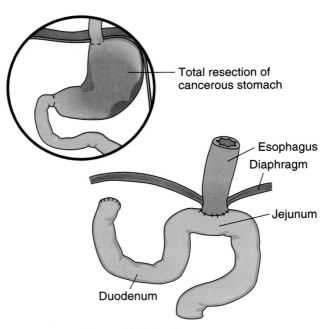

Figure 30–6. Total gastrectomy.

---

steatorrhea: steatos—fat + rhoia—flow

ing hemorrhage exhibits restlessness, cold skin, increased pulse and respirations, and decreased temperature and blood pressure. In addition, the client may vomit bright red blood.

Following gastric surgery, clients usually have an NG tube that was inserted in the operating room. The drainage from the tube should be assessed for color and amount. A small amount of pink or light red drainage may be expected for the first 12 hours, but moderate or excessive bleeding should be immediately reported to the physician. The abdominal dressing should also be assessed for any drainage or bleeding.

Gastric Distention

In the immediate postoperative period, distention of the stomach can occur if an inserted NG tube is clogged or an NG tube has not been inserted. Symptoms of gastric distention include an enlarged abdomen, epigastric pain, tachycardia, and hypotension. The client may complain of feeling full and may hiccup or gag repeatedly. These symptoms must be reported to the physician.

The physician usually inserts the NG tube in surgery so that the suture line is not damaged. The nurse should have an order for suction to be used, and avoid irrigating or repositioning the NG tube so the suture line is not harmed. Any problems with distention or an improperly functioning NG tube should be reported to the physician. The physician may need to reposition the NG tube. The client's vital signs should be monitored until the client's distention is relieved and the client is stable.

CRITICAL THINKING: Mr. Wong

The nurse is working the evening shift on a surgical unit. Mr. Wong has had gastric surgery earlier that morning. He has an intravenous infusion of dextrose 5%/.45 normal saline running at 83 mL per hour and a nasogastric tube to low intermittent wall suction. Mr. Wong is restless and complaining of pain. His bowel sounds are absent and his abdomen is distended. The suction canister contains no gastric output.

1. What nursing interventions would be needed to help Mr. Wong? Prioritize your interventions.
2. What equipment do you need? Make a list.

Answers at end of chapter.

Nutritional Problems

Nutritional problems that commonly occur after removal of part or all of the stomach include B_{12} and folic acid defi-

ciency and reduced absorption of calcium and vitamin D. Also, rapid entry of food into the bowel often results in inadequate absorption of food.

Vitamin B_{12} deficiency can occur after some or all of the stomach is removed because intrinsic factor secretion is reduced or gone. Normally, vitamin B_{12} combines with intrinsic factor to prevent its digestion in the stomach and promote its absorption in the intestines. Lifelong administration of vitamin B_{12} injections is required to prevent the development of pernicious anemia. Injections must be used because oral vitamin B_{12} cannot be absorbed. The vitamin B_{12} is given daily initially, then monthly for life. Clients must be taught the importance of complying with this treatment for the rest of their lives.

Following gastric surgery, clients are usually NPO until bowel sounds return (usually 24 to 48 hours) or the physician orders them to have a diet. They have an IV line infusing for hydration. However, if they are to be NPO for a period of time, they may need additional nutritional intake provided by total parenteral nutrition (TPN) through a central line. TPN is an intravenous solution given to meet caloric needs and provide fluids lost in drainage or emesis. Many clients with gastric cancer are malnourished and may require several days of TPN therapy.

After the return of bowel sounds and the removal of the nasogastric tube, clear fluids may be ordered with progression to full liquids, then soft foods as the client tolerates. It is important to remember that foods and fluids must be introduced into the diet gradually following gastric surgery. If the client eats too much or too fast, regurgitation may result.

Steatorrhea

Steatorrhea is the presence of excessive fat in the stools and is the result of rapid gastric emptying, which prevents adequate mixing of fat with pancreatic and biliary secretions. In most cases, steatorrhea can be controlled by reducing the intake of fat in the diet.

Pyloric Obstruction

Pyloric obstruction can occur after gastric surgery as a result of scarring, edema, inflammation, or a combination of these. The signs and symptoms are vomiting, feeling of fullness, gastric distention, nausea after eating, loss of appetite, and weight loss. As the obstruction increases, it gradually becomes more difficult for the stomach to empty, and symptoms worsen. Conservative methods are used first, such as replacing fluids and electrolytes through intravenous fluids and decompressing the distended stomach using a nasogastric tube. Surgery may be necessary if conservative measures do not relieve the signs and symptoms. Pyloroplasty widens the exit of the pylorus to improve emptying of the stomach.

HOME HEALTH HINTS

- Encourage a healthy diet such as cooking with skinless chicken, using herbs and spices instead of pepper, or drinking other kinds of flavored drinks instead of carbonated beverages.

- Areas to explore with regard to adequate nutrition of the elderly who live alone or with other elderly should include the choosing and preparing of food, such as reading labels, actually obtaining the groceries, opening cans or packages, following the instructions, working a stove or microwave safely, and proper storage (especially the storage and reheating of leftovers).

- Check to see if elderly patients have anything ordered for constipation if on antacids, pain medicine, antihistamines, or iron.

- Warming prune juice may stimulate the bowel a bit faster.

- When visiting clients with anorexia nervosa, checking their weight can be distressing to them. Read the scale quickly and then put it away, noting the weight in the record after leaving the home. Do not dwell on the weight issue during the visit.

- An inexpensive treatment of aphthous ulcers (canker sores) that relieves pain temporarily is to place a Tums on the ulcer or swish Maalox in the mouth.

- If home health clients have pernicious anemia, assess their feet each visit for paresthesia (from myelin degeneration).

- At times, a social worker referral is appropriate for clients with gastric problems. Stress decreases mucus production. Encourage clients to talk about concerns and frustrations. Teaching them about the disease and how to manage it may minimize anxiety. Caring goes a long way in reducing stress.

- Teach client that frequent eating, and foods or liquids such as chocolate, alcohol, and caffeine stimulate gastric juice production.

- For clients with a hiatal hernia or esophageal reflux, use a foam wedge to elevate the client's head. Also, placing 6- to 8-inch blocks under the head of the bed can alleviate heartburn by using gravity.

Dumping Syndrome

Dumping syndrome occurs with the rapid entry of food into the jejunum without proper mixing of the food with digestive juices. On entering the jejunum, the food draws extracellular fluid into the bowel from the circulating blood volume to dilute the high concentration of electrolytes and sugars. This rapid shift of fluids decreases the circulating blood volume and causes symptoms to occur. The symptoms occur 5 to 30 minutes after eating and include dizziness, tachycardia, fainting, sweating, nausea, diarrhea, a feeling of fullness, and abdominal cramping. Additionally, the blood sugar rises, and excessive insulin is excreted in response. This release of insulin causes the client to have symptoms of hypoglycemia about 2 hours later. Symptoms include weakness, sweating, anxiety, shakiness, confusion, and tachycardia. The client should immediately eat some candy or drink juice containing sugar to relieve the symptoms.

The treatment for dumping syndrome includes teaching the client to eat small, frequent meals that are high in protein and low in carbohydrates, especially refined sugars (see Nutrition Notes Box 30–1). The client is also taught to avoid fluids 1 hour before, with, or 2 hours after meals to prevent rapid gastric emptying. It is best for the client to lie down after meals to delay gastric emptying. The client is told that these symptoms may last for up to 6 months after gastric surgery but usually slowly subside over time.

 CRITICAL THINKING: Mrs. Lindsay

Mrs. Lindsay has had gastric surgery. You have taught her about dumping syndrome and she is concerned about what she will eat. Make a 1-day meal plan for Mrs. Lindsay.
Answers at end of chapter.

Review Questions

1. Which one of the following is the most important intervention for anorexia nervosa?
   a. Weighing the client daily
   b. Restoring nutritional health
   c. Providing psychotherapy
   d. Documenting intake and output

2. In the bulimic client, chronic vomiting can lead to which one of the following complications?
   a. Metabolic acidosis
   b. Metabolic alkalosis
   c. Fluid overload
   d. Weight gain

3. Which one of the following is the priority nursing diagnosis for a client with peptic ulcer disease?
   a. Activity intolerance related to epigastric pain

    b. Knowledge deficit related to lack of information on ulcers
    c. Pain related to epigastric erosion and acid buildup
    d. Ineffective individual coping related to diagnosis of peptic ulcers

4. Which one of the following can be used to diagnose peptic ulcers?
    a. Colonoscopy
    b. Barium enema
    c. Gastric aspirate analysis
    d. Esophagogastroduodenoscopy

5. Which one of the following is the purpose of H_2 antagonists?
    a. Neutralize gastric acid
    b. Form a protective paste
    c. Determine gastric pH levels
    d. Inhibit secretion of gastric acid

6. Which one of the following is usually the cause of peptic ulcers?
    a. Eating spicy foods
    b. A stressful life
    c. A bacterial infection
    d. Excessive caffeine intake

7. Which one of the following actions should the nurse take first for a client who has just returned from surgery after a total gastrectomy and begins to vomit bright red blood?
    a. Increase the IV rate
    b. Administer oxygen
    c. Place client on side
    d. Irrigate nasogastric tube

8. Which of the following statements would indicate that a client understands teaching about preventing dumping syndrome?
    a. "I need to eat small, frequent meals."
    b. "I will drink lots of fluids with my meals."
    c. "I need to sit up for two hours after each meal."
    d. "I will eat a high-carbohydrate diet."

ANSWERS TO CRITICAL THINKING

CRITICAL THINKING: Mr. Wong

1. Prioritize your interventions:
    a. Take Mr. Wong's vital signs to determine if he is stable. Pain can sometimes increase the blood pressure and pulse rate. It is usual for clients to have an increased temperature for a day or so following surgery. However, gastric distention can cause pain, and once the distention is relieved, the pain caused by distention subsides.

    b. Listen to Mr. Wong's bowel sounds. Manipulation of internal organs during abdominal surgery can produce a loss of normal peristalsis for 24 to 48 hours. Expect to hear absent or hypoactive bowel sounds for the first 1 or 2 days.

    c. Next, check placement of Mr. Wong's nasogastric tube by inserting 10 mL of air with a 60 mL catheter-tip syringe into the nasogastric tube while auscultating inferiorly to the xiphoid process on his abdomen. The nurse should hear a pop or gurgling sound as air passes into the stomach. This tells the nurse that the nasogastric tube is in the stomach. It is important to check for abdominal placement of Mr. Wong's nasogastric tube to make sure it is not misplaced in the lungs. After abdominal placement is determined, if there is a physician's order, the nasogastric tube can be connected to suction equipment, usually set on low, intermittent suction.

    d. Next, check the suction equipment for ordered settings and to ensure that it is turned on. The suction setting normally is ordered to be on low. A whistling sound is heard when the tube is disconnected from the suction setup. The seals should be tight on the suction canister. When the tubing is hooked to suction, gastric contents should be moving into the suction canister. It is important to make sure equipment is functioning properly to ensure client safety. The nurse discovers while checking Mr. Wong's equipment that the suction machine is not turned on.

    e. Check the nasogastric tube for clogs only if the physician orders aspiration or irrigation to be done. The tube is gently aspirated with a 60 mL catheter-tip syringe. If the tube remains clogged, it is gently flushed as ordered with 10 to 20 mL of sterile normal saline.

    f. After the gastric distention has been relieved, Mr. Wong's pain level is reassessed to determine if he needs pain medication. Considering that he is less than 1 day postoperative, he probably needs it.

2. Necessary equipment includes: stethoscope, 60 mL catheter tip syringe, gloves, goggles, and normal saline for irrigation.

CRITICAL THINKING: Mrs. Lindsay

Although there are many variations, the following is an example of a 1-day meal plan for Mrs. Lindsay:

Breakfast—one egg, any style, ½ orange, one glass milk

Snack—one slice toast with apple butter, jelly, or jam
Lunch—two ounces of ham, ½ cup cottage cheese, four asparagus spears
Snack—½ serving chicken salad on bed of lettuce
Dinner—2 ounces broiled fish, ½ serving corn, ½ serving broccoli
Snack—½ cup yogurt or sherbet

REFERENCES

1. George, L: The psychological characteristics of patients suffering from anorexia nervosa and the nurse's role in creating a therapeutic relationship. J Adv Nurs 26(5):899, 1997.
2. Http://www.cdc.gov/ncidod/dbmd/media.htm. *Helicobacter pylori*. Facts for Health Care Providers. Sept 1997.
3. Miehlke, S, et al: Identifying persons at risk for gastric cancer? Helicobacter 2(suppl 1):S61, 1997.
4. Cheong, H, et al: The association of *Helicobacter pylori* with intestinal type gastric adenocarcinoma in a Hawaii population. Hawaii Med J 56(12):348, 1997.
5. Waters, J, et al: New approaches to the treatment of gastrointestinal cancer. Digestion 58(6):508, 1997.

BIBLIOGRAPHY

Andersen, L, et al: An analysis of seven different methods to diagnose *Helicobacter pylori* infections. Scand J Gastroenterol 33(1):24, 1998.

Aronson, B: Update on peptic ulcer drugs. Am J Nurs 98(1):41, 1998.

Bonavina, L, et al: Mechanical effect of the Angelchik prosthesis on the competency of the gastric cardia: pathophysiologic implications and surgical perspectives. Dis Esophagus 10(2):115, 1997.

Chow, W, et al: An inverse relation between cagA+ strains of *Helicobacter pylori* infection and risk of esophageal and gastric cardia adenocarcinoma. Cancer Res 58(4):588, 1998.

Cooper, J: Current role of esophageal function studies. Semin Thorac Cardiovasc Surg 9(2):157, 1997.

Dhar, R, et al: Evaluation and comparison of two immunodiagnostic assays for *Helicobacter pylori* antibodies with culture results. Diagn Microbiol Infect Dis 30(1):1, 1998.

Deglin, JH, and Vallerand, AH: Davis's Drug Guide, ed 4. FA Davis, Philadelphia, 1995.

Eastwood, G: Is smoking still important in the pathogenesis of peptic ulcer disease? J Clin Gastroenterol 25(suppl 1):S1, 1997.

Figura, N: *Helicobacter pylori* factors involved in the development of gastroduodenal mucosal damage and ulceration. J Clin Gastroenterol 25(suppl 1):S149, 1997.

Fraser, A, et al: Can the urea breath test for *H. pylori* replace endoscopy for the assessment of dyspepsia in primary care? N Z Med J 111(1058):11, 1998.

Gregoire, A, and Fitzpatrick, E: Esophageal cancer: multisystem nursing management. Dimens Crit Care Nurs 17(1):28, 1998.

Kahrilas, P: Anatomy and physiology of the gastroesophageal junction. Gastroenterol Clin North Am 26(3):467, 1997.

Keltner, NL, Schwecke, LH, and Bostrom, CE: Psychiatric Nursing. Mosby, St Louis, 1995.

Lee, H, and O'Morain, C: Who should be treated for *Helicobacter pylori* infection? A review of consensus conferences and guidelines. Gastroenterology 113(suppl 6):S99, 1997.

Luketich, J, et al: Future directions in esophageal cancer. Chest 113(suppl 1):120S, 1998.

Matsukura, N, et al: Role of *Helicobacter pylori* infection in performation of peptic ulcer: an age- and gender-matched case-control study. J Clin Gastroenterol 25(suppl 1):S235, 1997.

Middlemiss, C: Gastroesophageal reflux disease: A common condition in the elderly. Nurse Pract 22(11):51, 1997.

Parent, M, Siemiatycki, J, and Fritschi, L: Occupational exposures and gastric cancer. Epidemiology 9(1):48, 1998.

Riemann, J, et al: Cure with omeprazole plus amoxicillin versus long-term ranitidine therapy in *Helicobacter pylori*–associated peptic ulcer bleeding. Gastrointest Endosc 46(4):299, 1997.

Sjostedt, S, et al: Prolonged and profound acid inhibition is crucial in *Helicobacter pylori* treatment with a proton pump inhibitor combined with amoxicillin. Scand J Gastroenterol 33(1):39, 1998.

Tan, R, and Young, A: The role of chemoradiotherapy in maintaining quality of life for advanced esophageal cancer. Am J Hosp Palliat Care 15(1):29, 1998.

Thomas, CL (ed): Taber's Cyclopedic Medical Dictionary, ed 18. FA Davis, Philadelphia, 1997.

Triadafilopoulos, G, and Sharma, R: Features of symptomatic gastroesophageal reflux disease in elderly patients. Am J Gastroenterol 92(11):2007, 1997.

Tsuju, S, et al: *Helicobacter pylori* and gastric carcinogenesis. J Clin Gastroenterol 25(suppl 1):S186, 1997.

Trotter, K: Nutrition and eating disorders. Nurs Times 93(suppl 46):1, 1997.

Wiseman, C, Harris, W, and Halmi, K: Eating disorders. Med Clin North Am 82(1):145, 1998.

Wisniewski, R, and Peura, D: *Helicobacter pylori:* Beyond peptic ulcer disease. Gastroenterologist 5(4):295, 1997.

Nursing Care of Clients with Lower Gastrointestinal Disorders

Deborah J. Mauffray

Learning Objectives

Upon completion of this chapter, the student will be able to:

1. Identify signs, symptoms, and causes of constipation and diarrhea.
2. Describe nursing interventions for clients with constipation or diarrhea.
3. Describe inflammatory and infectious disorders.
4. Discuss medical treatment and nursing care of clients with inflammatory and infectious bowel disorders.
5. Identify signs and symptoms related to abdominal hernias that should be reported to the physician.
6. Describe nursing care of clients with absorption disorders.
7. Recognize signs and symptoms of intestinal obstruction.
8. Describe causes, treatments, and nursing interventions for intestinal obstruction.
9. Identify signs and symptoms, causes, and medical and nursing interventions for lower gastrointestinal bleeding.
10. Describe nursing care of the client with an ostomy.

Key Words

appendicitis (uh-PEN-di-**SIGH**-tis)
colectomy (koh-**LEK**-tuh-me)
colitis (koh-**LYE**-tis)
colostomy (koh-**LAH**-stuh-me)
constipation (KON-sti-**PAY**-shun)
diarrhea (DYE-uh-**REE**-ah)
diverticulitis (DYE-ver-tik-yoo-**LYE**-tis)
diverticulosis (DYE-ver-tik-yoo-**LOH**-sis)
enteritis (en-ter-**EYE**-tis)
fissure (**FISH**-er)
fistula (**FIST**-yoo-lah)
hematochezia (HEM-uh-toh-**KEE**-zee-uh)
hemorrhoids (**HEM**-uh-royds)
hernia (**HER**-nee-uh)

ileostomy (ILL-ee-**AH**-stuh-me)
impaction (im-**PAK**-shun)
intussusception (IN-tuh-suh-**SEP**-shun)
megacolon (**MEG**-ah-KOH-lun)
melena (muh-**LEE**-nah)
obstipation (OB-sti-**PAY**-shun)
peristomal (PER-i-**STOH**-muhl)
peritonitis (per-i-toh-**NIGH**-tis)
steatorrhea (STEE-ah-toh-**REE**-uh)
stoma (**STOH**-mah)
volvulus (**VOL**-view-lus)

Lower Gastrointestinal Disorders

The lower gastrointestinal (GI) system includes the small and large intestines, rectum, and anus. Disorders associated with this system are discussed in this chapter.

PROBLEMS OF ELIMINATION

Constipation

Pathophysiology

Constipation is a condition that occurs when the fecal mass is held in the rectal cavity for a period of time that is not usual for the client. When the feces are held for a prolonged time in the rectum the amount of water being absorbed increases, making the feces drier, harder, more difficult to pass, and sometimes painful to pass.

Sometimes a client ignores the urge to have a bowel movement, and the musculature and rectal mucous membrane become insensitive to the presence of feces. Eventually a stronger stimulus is required to produce the peristaltic rush needed for defecation. A prolonged period of constipation is called **obstipation.**

Etiology

The possible causes of constipation are many. A client with rectal or anal conditions such as **hemorrhoids** or **fissures** may delay defecation because of the associated pain. Metabolic or neurological conditions such as diabetes mellitus, multiple sclerosis, lupus erythematosus, or scleroderma may interfere with normal bowel innervation and function. Cancer in the colon may cause an obstruction that prevents normal bowel function and leads to constipation. The use of medications such as narcotics, tranquilizers, and antacids with aluminum decreases motility of the large intestine and may contribute to constipation. Low intake of dietary fiber and fluids decreases the bulk of the feces and causes constipation. Decreased mobility, weakness, and fatigue, especially in the elderly, reduce the strength of the muscles used for defecation, increasing the probability of constipation. Also, chronic laxative use can contribute to constipation because the laxative overrides the bowel's ability to recognize the urge to defecate.

Prevention

A diet high in fiber and fluids and regular exercise are the best preventive measures for constipation. Laxatives should be avoided except for occasional use.

Signs and Symptoms

Abdominal pain and distention, indigestion, rectal pressure, a sensation of incomplete emptying, and intestinal rumbling are indications of constipation. The client may also complain of headache, fatigue, decreased appetite, straining at stool, and the elimination of hard, dry stool.

Complications

A variety of problems can occur as a result of constipation. Fecal **impaction** may result when the fecal mass is so dry it cannot be eliminated. Pressure on the colon mucosa from a mass of stool may cause ulcers to develop. Many times the client has small amounts of liquid stool that get around the fecal mass and seep from the rectum. This can result in incontinence of liquid stools and lead to being treated with an antidiarrheal medication, which will worsen the constipation. Straining to have a bowel movement (Valsalva's maneuver) can result in cardiac, neurological, and respiratory complications. If the client has a history of heart failure, hypertension, or recent myocardial infarction, straining can lead to cardiac rupture and death.

Another complication of constipation is the grossly dilated loops of the colon known as **megacolon** that occurs proximal to the dry fecal mass and obstructs the colon. The abdomen becomes very distended, and in extreme cases an outline of the loops of bowel can be seen and palpated on the exterior abdominal wall.

Chronic laxative abuse can lead to colonic mucosal atrophy, muscle thickening, and fibrosis. Both of these conditions can result in perforation of the colon and necessitate an emergency **colectomy.**

Diagnostic Tests

Constipation is usually self-diagnosed or diagnosed by history and physical examination. If complications are suspected a radiographic examination, sigmoidoscopy, and stool testing for occult blood may be necessary.

Medical Treatment

Treatment of constipation depends on the cause. Fiber should be added to the diet, and exercises to strengthen abdominal muscles should be done. Behavior changes can help establish a more normal bowel pattern. These changes include setting a daily defecation time, appropriately responding to the urge to defecate, and drinking 8 ounces of warm water every morning and 2 to 3 liters of water every day if not contraindicated for other reasons. Abusive laxative use should be discontinued. Bulk-forming agents such as psyllium (Metamucil) or stool softeners such as docusate sodium (Colace) should be used instead of laxatives if necessary. Enemas and rectal suppositories are used only in extreme cases and are discontinued when the acute episode is resolved.

Nursing Process

ASSESSMENT. When being interviewed about bowel habits and history, the client may feel self-conscious or embarrassed. The nurse should be considerate of the client's feelings and postpone the discussion until there has been ample time for the client and nurse to build a rapport with

---

megacolon: mega—large + colon—colon
colectomy: col—pertaining to colon + ectomy—surgical excision

each other. The nurse needs to identify the onset and duration of the client's constipation, as well as past elimination pattern, current elimination pattern, occupation, lifestyle (stress, exercise, nutrition), history of laxative or enema use, past medical-surgical history, and current medications being taken. The nurse should ask the client to describe the color, consistency, and odor of the stool along with any intestinal symptoms that may be occurring.

After the interview, auscultation of the client's abdomen should be done to listen for bowel sounds. Notice should be made of infrequent, absent, high-pitched, or gurgling sounds. The abdomen is inspected and palpated for distention and symmetry. Inspection of the perianal area may reveal evidence of external hemorrhoids, fissures, or irritation.

NURSING DIAGNOSES. Once the assessment data are obtained, the major nursing diagnoses may include constipation and anxiety related to concern about irregular elimination pattern. Perceived constipation may be diagnosed in clients who abuse laxatives. Knowledge deficit about health maintenance practices to prevent constipation may also be a problem.

PLANNING. Once the nursing diagnoses are identified, the nurse and client can participate in establishing goals and deciding on interventions that will assist in meeting those goals. The family or caregiver should be included in this process, especially if the client is dependent in any way on anyone else. If the client is a resident of a skilled nursing facility or nursing home or at home, a representative from the facility or home care agency assisting in the client's care should be included in this phase of the nursing process.

IMPLEMENTATION AND CLIENT EDUCATION. Client and family or caregiver education is one of the most important aspects of treatment of constipation. Prevention of constipation may be as simple as correcting the contributing factors. The client should be instructed in the causative factors leading to constipation and the interventions necessary to prevent it. An explanation of the physiology of defecation and the purpose of obeying the urge to defecate, when it occurs, is an important point in which to instruct the client and family. Setting a specific time for defecation, such as after a meal, may facilitate the urge reflex. To ensure the appropriate posture during defecation a footstool can be used to promote flexion of the hips.

What the client may consider a normal diet may not be appropriate for the correction or prevention of constipation. If the constipation is caused by decreased motility or muscle tone, the client should eat a high-fiber, high-residue diet, including fresh fruits and vegetables and whole grains. In the older client, adding 2 g of bran to cereal daily can significantly increase the number of bowel movements and therefore decrease the number of laxatives, enemas, or

stool softeners used. (See Nutrition Notes Box 31–1.) For the client who believes that a daily bowel movement is absolutely necessary, reassurance needs to be given. Inform the client that some foods may increase the transit time of the feces whereas other foods normally stay in the intestinal tract as long as 48 hours after ingestion. The client should be assured that having a bowel movement every day is sometimes not necessary.

Instructions also should include the importance of increasing the client's activity through abdominal exercises designed to improve the muscle tone and a daily walking program. These will improve peristalsis, promoting more spontaneous defecation.

The dangers of regular laxative use should be stressed. By increasing the fiber in the diet, exercise, and the amount of fluids taken in, the client should be able to discontinue use of the laxative. (See Ethical Considerations Box 31–2.)

EVALUATION. If the plan has been effective, a regular bowel function pattern has been established (Table 31–1). With increased physical activity, the client should also experience less abdominal discomfort. The client should verbalize understanding of self-care measures and express satisfaction with the outcomes.

CRITICAL THINKING: Jessie

Jessie is a 93-year-old nursing home resident. You note on her chart that she has not had a bowel movement in a week. How do you respond?
Answer at end of chapter.

Diarrhea

Diarrhea occurs when fecal matter passes through the intestine rapidly, resulting in decreased absorption of water, electrolytes, and nutrients and causing frequent, watery stools. Classification and severity of diarrhea are based on the number of unformed stools in 24 hours. Large-volume diarrhea occurs when the volume of feces is increased. Small-volume diarrhea is caused by an increase in peristalsis, without an increase in fecal volume.

NUTRITIONAL NOTES BOX 31–1

Constipation may be successfully treated with 1 to 2 ounces of the following mixture taken with the evening meal: 1 cup applesauce, 1 cup All-Bran, and ½ cup 100 percent prune juice. May be stored in the refrigerator for 5 days and then should be discarded. In all cases of constipation, especially when increased fiber is given, adequate fluid intake is essential.

---

diarrhea: dia—through + rhea—to flow

ETHICAL CONSIDERATIONS BOX 31-2

The Client Who Abuses Laxatives

Mr. Thomas is an 86-year-old retired professor who lives by himself in a small apartment. He is admitted to the medical-surgical unit of the community hospital with a diagnosis of weakness, dehydration, electrolyte imbalance, and malnutrition. He has no close family, but a neighbor who accompanied Mr. Thomas to the hospital informed the nurse that she felt he had a preoccupation with his bowel movements and took large amounts of over-the-counter laxatives.

During the admission interview, Mr. Thomas was mildly disoriented to place and time, but denied taking any over-the-counter medications. He was started on IV electrolyte and fluid replacement and placed on a high-calorie diet and bed rest. He was very compliant with the treatments except that he frequently visited the bathroom for bowel movements.

On entering the room, one of the LPNs on the evening shift noticed that Mr. Thomas was hurriedly returning what appeared to be a small bottle of laxative pills to his shaving kit. The nurse asked him about it, but was told: "It's none of your business—just stay out of my stuff!" The LPN later informed Mr. Thomas's physician of the episode. The physician ordered the nurse to obtain the shaving kit and see if there were any laxatives in it. He reasoned that if the patient was taking large doses of laxatives and having diarrhea, all the treatments being given him would do no good.

Initially the nurse agreed with the physician, but after thinking about the situation further and remembering some basic principles of ethics she had been taught in school, she questioned her right to search a patient's belongings without his permission. What should she do? What ethical principles might she be violating by searching this patient's belongings without his permission?

Pathophysiology and Etiology

The most common cause of acute diarrhea is bacterial or viral infection. Bacteria are normally found in the intestines. If these bacteria grow out of control, or if bacteria or viruses are ingested in contaminated food or water, infection will result. Some bacteria release toxins that irritate the intestinal mucosa, causing an inflammatory response and an increase in mucus production. Hyperperistalsis occurs, which lasts until the irritants have been excreted. The most common infectious agents are *Escherichia coli, Campylobacter jejuni, Shigella, Clostridium difficile, Giardia,* and *Salmonella.*

Poor tolerance or allergies to certain foods may cause diarrhea. Foods that most commonly cause diarrhea are additives (such as nutmeg or sorbitol), caffeine, milk products, meats, wheat, and potatoes. Acute diarrhea usually resolves in 7 to 14 days.

Chronic diarrhea may result from inflammatory disease, osmotic agents, excessive secretion of electrolytes, or increased intestinal motility. Inflammatory diseases such as Crohn's disease or ulcerative **colitis** (described later in this chapter) may impair absorption, resulting in frequent, watery stools. Osmotic diarrhea results from ingestion of lax-

atives or other agents that prevent absorption of water or nutrients in the intestine. Additional causes of malabsorption include surgical resection or disease of certain areas of the intestinal tract, such as the terminal ileum or pylorus. Radiation therapy for cancer also may induce a malabsorption syndrome. Enteral tube feedings commonly cause diarrhea, especially when malnutrition has caused edema in the gut wall, which decreases absorption.

Increased secretion of water and electrolytes by the intestinal mucosa associated with some hormonal disorders results in high-volume output. Motility problems may be related to an irritable bowel or a neurological disorder. As mentioned earlier, diarrhea may sometimes indicate fecal impaction.

Prevention

Ensuring that handling of all fresh foods is done appropriately and with proper storage and refrigeration will minimize contact with infectious agents. Milk and milk products must be kept refrigerated and protected against exposure. It is extremely important to rigorously clean the kitchen and anything used in preparing or serving food.

With clients who are being fed enterally, it is best to start slowly with full-strength formula and then gradually increase the rate rather than dilute the formula. This will limit contamination of the formula through the manipulation that occurs with adding to the mixture.

Signs and Symptoms

The initial stools are foul smelling and may have undigested food particles and mucus. The stools also may contain blood or pus. If the diarrhea is due to food poisoning,

Table 31-1. Criteria for Regular Bowel Function

1. A regular time for defecation is routine.
2. A regular exercise program is followed.
3. Laxative use is avoided.
4. Water consumption is 2 to 3 L per day.
5. High-fiber and high-residue foods are added to the diet.
6. Consistency of stools reported are soft and formed.
7. Frequency of stools is every 1 to 3 days.

---

colitis: col—pertaining to colon + itis—inflammation

onset usually is explosive and may be accompanied by nausea and vomiting. Usual client complaints include abdominal cramping, distention, anorexia, intestinal rumbling, and thirst. Fever indicates infection. Weakness and dehydration from fluid loss may occur. (See also Gerontological Issues Box 31–3.)

Diagnostic Tests

Diagnostic evaluation of diarrhea hinges on the onset and progression of the disease, absence or presence of fever, laboratory examinations, and visual inspection of the stool. Evidence of bacteria, pus, and blood will be checked. Diarrhea mixed with red blood cells and mucus is associated with cholera, typhoid, typhus, large bowel cancer, or amebiasis. Diarrhea mixed with white blood cells and mucus is associated with shigellosis, intestinal tuberculosis, salmonellosis, regional enteritis, or ulcerative colitis. Bulky, frothy stool is seen in sprue and celiac disease. Pasty stools usually have a high fat content, which may be associated with common bile duct obstruction, sprue, and celiac disease. "Butter stool" appearance is seen in clients with cystic fibrosis.

Medical Treatment

Replacing fluids and electrolytes is the first course of action. This is done by increasing oral fluid intake, using solutions with glucose and electrolytes if ordered by the physician. Intravenous fluid replacement may be necessary in the very young or very old for rapid hydration. The elimination diet can be tried to identify foods that may contribute to diarrhea. This is done by eliminating foods that are known to cause diarrhea and seeing if the client has a change in bowel function. Then each food item is added one at a time into the diet to see which one(s) cause diarrhea. The client should be encouraged to increase fiber and bulk in the diet.

If the client has three or more watery stools per day, motility of the intestines can be decreased with the use of drugs, such as diphenoxylate (Lomotil) and loperamide (Imodium). If diarrhea is thought to be caused by antibiotics changing the normal flora of the bowel, Lactinex (Lactobacillus granules dietary supplement) may be used to restore the normal flora. In the presence of documented infectious disorders, antimicrobial agents are prescribed.

Nursing Process

ASSESSMENT. The nurse will assist in the diagnosis of what causes diarrhea by observing the client's behavior, symptoms, and complaints. Have the client describe any symptoms, when they started, and how long they have been present. Is there any abdominal pain, urgency, or cramping? What time of the day does it happen? Stool consistency, color, odor, and frequency need to be documented.

The abdomen is inspected for distention. Auscultation for hyperactive bowel sounds or rumbling is performed. Assess the client's usual dietary habits and any changes or recent exposure to contaminated food or water. Find out if the client is on any medication that may contribute to diarrhea. If the client has traveled recently, discover location and any exposure to other persons who may have been infected or are having similar symptoms.

Assess for symptoms of dehydration, such as tachycardia, hypotension, decreased skin turgor, weakness, thready pulse, dry mucous membranes, and oliguria. Abnormal laboratory studies may include increased serum osmolality, increased specific gravity of urine, and increased hematocrit, all of which indicate dehydration. Decreased serum potassium may result from intestinal loss.

NURSING DIAGNOSIS. Possible nursing diagnoses include the following:

- Diarrhea related to infection or possible ingestion of irritating foods
- Risk for fluid volume deficit related to frequent passage of stools and insufficient fluid intake
- Risk for transmission of infection related to fecal contamination
- Risk for impairment of skin integrity related to passage of frequent liquid stools
- Anxiety related to uncontrolled elimination
- Pain related to increased peristalsis

PLANNING. Planning of care for the client includes settings goals. The chief goals will include control of diarrhea, prevention of fluid volume deficit, avoidance of spread of infection, keeping skin intact, decreasing anxiety, and controlling pain.

IMPLEMENTATION. The nurse must implement measures to decrease the diarrhea episodes. Caffeine stimulates intesti-

---

GERONTOLOGICAL ISSUES BOX 31–3

Diarrhea can cause older people to quickly become dehydrated and hypokalemic, because both fluid and potassium are lost in stools. The signs and symptoms of hypokalemia include muscle weakness, hypotension, anorexia, paresthesia, and drowsiness. It can also cause cardiac dysrhythmias, such as atrial and ventricular tachycardia, premature ventricular contraction, and ventricular fibrillation, which can cause death.

If the older person has decreased mobility, quick access to the bathroom will be important. Because of poor muscle control, the older client may be incontinent. This might embarrass the client or cause him to hurry, which increases chances of the client falling and causing other problems, such as fracture, dislocation, or hematoma. Also, because the older client's skin is more sensitive due to poor turgor and a reduction in subcutaneous fat layers, skin irritation from the enzymes in the diarrheal stool may be a problem.

nal motility, therefore intake is limited. During acute diarrhea, the client may receive nothing by mouth (NPO) for bowel rest. Clear liquids, such as water, juices, bouillon, and gelatin, are added, followed by a progression to a low-residue diet. (See Nutrition Notes Box 31–4.) Rest is also important because of the weakness associated with the loss of fluids and electrolytes. A record of intake and output (including diarrhea stools) is kept to determine if an appropriate balance is maintained. If there is more output than intake, intravenous fluid replacement may be ordered. Antidiarrheal medications are administered as directed. Control of diarrhea will help control pain.

Identification of potential infected persons or foods is done to try to prevent the spread of the infection. Thorough hand washing by client, family, and nurse is essential. A private room may be necessary. The perianal skin is protected from contact with the liquid stools and the enzymes contained within by keeping the skin clean, dry, and then protected with a moisture barrier, such as petrolatum or medicated ointment, after each bowel movement.

By allowing the client to express fears or anxiety regarding possible incontinence of liquid stools and the embarrassment associated with that, the nurse will intensify the client's coping mechanisms. Adult briefs may be used during acute episodes. Being understanding and tolerant will also help.

CLIENT EDUCATION. The client must be educated in the importance of identification of the source of the diarrhea, such as possible infected persons (family, neighbors) or foods. Also, instruct the client and others in proper hand washing before and after toileting and handling foods for preparation and serving to prevent the spread of the disease. Instruct the client in signs and symptoms of dehydration to be aware of and report to the nurse or doctor.

NUTRITION NOTES BOX 31–4

Diarrhea in healthy adults at minimal risk of electrolyte imbalance may be treated as follows:
FOR THE FIRST 12 HOURS: NPO. Anything additional in the GI tract will stimulate peristalsis.
FOR THE SECOND 12 HOURS: Clear liquids. If more than 5 percent of body weight is lost, seek medical attention.
FOR THE THIRD 12 HOURS: Full liquids. Experiment with milk in case temporary lactose intolerance has developed due to intestinal inflammation.
FOR THE FOURTH 12 HOURS: Soft diet. Include applesauce or banana for pectin and also rice, pasta, and bread without fat, which are digested by enzymes usually unaffected in gastroenteritis.
BY THE FORTY-EIGHTH HOUR: Regular diet. If diarrhea has not resolved and regular diet is not tolerated, seek medical treatment.

EVALUATION. Goals have been met if fluid and electrolyte balance is achieved, frequency of diarrhea stools is decreased, skin integrity is maintained, and anxiety is controlled. The client should report an increase in comfort and verbalize understanding of measures to prevent infection.

INFLAMMATORY AND INFECTIOUS DISORDERS

Many diseases of the lower GI tract are a result of inflammation in the bowel. Sometimes these inflamed areas also become infected, causing a worsening of symptoms and necessitating antimicrobial therapy.

Appendicitis

Pathophysiology

Appendicitis is the inflammation of the appendix, the small, fingerlike appendage attached to the cecum of the large intestine. Due to the size of the appendix, an obstruction may occur, making it susceptible to infection. Typically the appendix is filled with feces. The resulting inflammatory process causes an increase in the intraluminal pressure, which leads to the symptoms described next.

Signs and Symptoms

Signs and symptoms of appendicitis include fever, increased white blood cells, and generalized pain in the upper abdomen. The pain usually becomes localized to the right lower quadrant at McBurney's point (Fig. 31–1) (midway between the umbilicus and the right iliac crest) within hours of onset. This is one of the classic symptoms of appendicitis. Nausea, vomiting, and anorexia are usually present.

Physical examination reveals slight abdominal muscular rigidity, normal bowel sounds, and local rebound tenderness (intensification of pain when pressure is released after palpation) in the right lower quadrant of the abdomen. Sometimes there is pain in the right lower quadrant when the left lower quadrant is palpated. This is called Rovsing's sign. The client may keep the right leg flexed and have increased pain if it is straightened.

Complications

Perforation, abscess of the appendix, and **peritonitis** are the major complications that may occur. With perforation, the pain is severe and the temperature is elevated to at least 37.7°C (100°F). An abscess is a localized collection of pus separated from the peritoneal cavity by the omentum or small bowel. This is usually treated with parenteral antibi-

---

appendicitis: appendic—pertaining to appendix + itis—inflammation
peritonitis: periton—pertaining to peritoneum + itis—inflammation

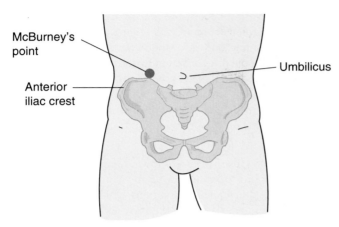

Figure 31–1. Pain at McBurney's point is a syptom of appendicitis.

otics and surgical drainage of the abscess. An appendectomy is done in about 6 weeks. Management of peritonitis is discussed later in this chapter.

Diagnostic Tests

A complete blood count (CBC) reveals an elevated leukocyte count and neutrophil count. Ultrasound or computed tomography (CT) scan will reveal an enlargement in the area of the cecum.

Medical Treatment

The client is NPO, and surgery will be done immediately unless there is evidence of perforation or peritonitis. If the appendix has ruptured, intravenous fluids and antibiotic therapy are started and surgery is delayed for 8 hours or more. Fever is controlled by aspirin or Tylenol. Laxatives and enemas are avoided because they may trigger or complicate rupture. The use of a heating pad on the abdomen is avoided because the warmth may increase inflammation and risk of rupture. Once the inflamed appendix is excised, the patient is discharged from the hospital the day of surgery if he or she is afebrile and pain is controlled. However, if there is evidence of rupture, the patient is hospitalized for 5 to 7 days to observe for signs of peritonitis or ileus.

Nursing Care

The client with suspected appendicitis is given nothing by mouth until diagnosis is confirmed, in case surgery is necessary. Ice to the painful site and a semi-Fowler's position may help reduce pain while the diagnosis is being made. The client is often readied for an appendectomy by emergency department staff, and time for preoperative teaching is limited.

Following surgery, the client may have a nasogastric tube and will remain NPO until bowel sounds return, to prevent abdominal distention and vomiting. Diet will initially consist of clear liquids and is advanced as tolerated by the client. The nurse monitors vital signs and abdominal assessment findings for signs and symptoms of peritonitis.

Early ambulation and turning, coughing, and deep breathing are encouraged to prevent respiratory complications. The client is instructed to splint the incision while coughing and deep breathing to reduce pain and stress on the incision. Routine dressing changes are performed.

Peritonitis

Pathophysiology and Etiology

Trauma, ischemia, or tumor perforation in any abdominal organ will cause leakage of the organ contents into the peritoneal cavity. The most common cause of peritonitis is a ruptured appendix, but it may also occur after perforation of a peptic ulcer, gangrenous gallbladder, intestinal diverticula, incarcerated hernia, or gangrenous small bowel. It may also be a complication of peritoneal dialysis. Peritonitis results from inflammation or infection caused by the leakage. The tissues become edematous and begin leaking fluid. This fluid is filled with increasing amounts of blood, protein, cellular debris, and white cells. Initially, the intestinal tract responds with hypermotility but soon is followed by paralysis (paralytic ileus).

Signs and Symptoms

Generalized abdominal pain evolves into localized pain based on the site of the perforation or leakage. The area of the abdomen that is affected will be extremely tender and aggravated by movement. Rebound tenderness and abdominal rigidity are present. Decreased peristalsis results in nausea and vomiting. Infection causes fever, increased white blood cells, and an elevated pulse.

Complications

One complication of peritonitis is intestinal obstruction (discussed later in this chapter). Hypovolemia may occur because of the shift of fluid into the abdomen. Septicemia may result from bacteria entering the blood stream. Either of these may lead to shock and ultimately to death. Another complication is the development of wound dehiscence or evisceration if the client has had abdominal surgery.

Medical Treatment

The client is NPO because of the impaired peristalsis. Fluid and electrolyte replacement is crucial to correct hypovolemia. Abdominal distention is relieved through insertion of an intestinal tube and suction. Large doses of antibiotics are used to treat or prevent sepsis. Depending on the cause of the peritonitis, surgery may be performed to excise, drain, or repair the cause. Sometimes an ostomy is formed to divert the feces and allow clearing of the infection. Following surgery the client usually has a wound drain, nasogastric (NG) tube, and a Foley catheter. Pain medication is essential to overall recovery. If the client is severely compromised, total parenteral nutrition (TPN) may be administered to meet nutritional needs for immune function and healing.

Nursing Process for the Client with Peritonitis

ASSESSMENT. The nurse assesses the pain according to the WHAT'S UP? format (Table 31–2). Abdominal distention and bowel sounds are monitored and recorded. Vital signs are monitored for fever or signs of septic shock. Intake and output are monitored and recorded accurately so that appropriate fluid replacement therapy is ordered.

NURSING DIAGNOSIS. Nursing diagnoses for the client with peritonitis include acute pain related to inflammatory process, risk for fluid volume deficit related to shifting of fluid from circulation to the peritoneal cavity, risk for injury related to complications of peritonitis, and altered nutrition: less than body requirements related to nausea and NPO status.

PLANNING. Goals for the client include pain control, stable fluid balance, early recognition and reporting of possible complications, and maintenance of nutrition.

IMPLEMENTATION. Narcotics in conjunction with noninvasive measures such as relaxation exercises are provided for pain. A semi-Fowler's position may reduce tension on the abdomen. Frequent mouth care is done if a nasogastric (NG) tube is in place.

Reduced urinary output, dropping blood pressure, and rising pulse rate may indicate fluid volume deficit. If a fever is also present, the client may be developing sepsis. All symptoms are reported to the physician promptly.

Respiratory complications can be prevented with coughing, deep breathing, and regular turning. Splinting the abdomen during coughing and moving may help reduce discomfort. Oxygen may be administered if the O_2 saturation is less than 95 percent. If the client has had surgery, observation of any drains that were placed is done. Documentation of the color, volume, odor, and consistency of all drainage is important. Care should be taken in moving the patient so that the drains are not dislodged.

If nausea occurs, the NG tube should be checked for patency. Antiemetics are administered as ordered. If the client is NPO for a prolonged period of time, total parenteral nutrition (TPN) should be considered to maintain nutritional status.

EVALUATION. Observations of lower temperature and pulse rate are indicators that the peritonitis is improving. The abdomen is less distended and softens with return of normal bowel sounds and passing of flatus. If nursing care is effective, the client should report that pain is controlled, vital signs are stable, complications are prevented, and nutrition is maintained.

Diverticulosis and Diverticulitis

Pathophysiology

A diverticulum is a herniation or outpouching of the bowel mucous membrane due to a defect in the muscle layer. **Diverticulosis** is a condition in which multiple diverticula are present without evidence of inflammation (Fig. 31–2). Many people have diverticulosis without knowing it because it develops gradually. When food and bacteria are trapped in a diverticulum, inflammation and infection develop. This is called **diverticulitis.**

Etiology

Chronic constipation usually precedes the development of diverticulosis by many years. When the client is chronically constipated, pressure within the bowel is increased, leading to development of diverticula. A major cause of the disease is a decreased intake of dietary fiber. Diverticulosis is most common in the sigmoid colon. Approximately 20% of all clients with diverticulosis develop diverticulitis at some point. The most common age group to experience diverticulitis is people over 60.

Prevention

Prevention of the development of diverticulitis is done by increasing dietary fiber, preventing constipation and the onset of diverticulosis.

Signs and Symptoms

The client with diverticulosis is generally asymptomatic. When diverticulitis is present, the client will exhibit bowel changes, possibly alternating between constipation and diarrhea. Crampy pain in the left lower quadrant of the abdomen is the most common symptom of acute diverticulitis.

Table 31–2. **Symptoms Associated with Diverticulitis**

W—Where is the pain?	Usually in the left lower quadrant
H—How does it feel? (Describe quality)	Tender, crampy
A—Aggravating and alleviating factors	Constipation and low-fiber diet may aggravate; treatment of constipation may alleviate
T—Timing (onset, duration, frequency)	Gradual onset, intermittent, gradual increase in frequency of pain events
S—Severity (1–10)	Usually 5–7
U—Useful other data/associated symptoms	Intermittent rectal bleeding, straining at stool, constipation alternating with diarrhea, elevated white blood cells and sedimentation rate, elevated temperature and pulse rate, and pus, mucus, and blood in stool
P—Patient's perception	Fear of diagnosis of cancer

---

diverticulosis: diveticul—blind pouch + osis—condition
diverticulitis: diveticul—blind pouch + itis—inflammation

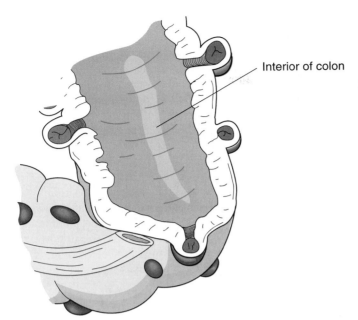

Interior of colon

Figure 31–2. A diverticulum is a herniation or outpouching of the bowel mucous membrane. Multiple diverticuli are called diverticulosis. If they become inflamed or infected, the condition is called diverticulitis. (Modified from Lewis, Collier, and Heitkemper: Medical-Surgical Nursing: Assessment and Management of Clinical Problems, ed 4. Mosby, St Louis, 1996, p 1249, with permission.)

As the condition worsens, bleeding may occur, along with weakness, fever, fatigue, and anemia. Guarding and rebound tenderness may be present. If an abscess develops, the diverticulum may rupture, leading to peritonitis. (See Gerontological Issues Box 31–5.)

Diagnostic Tests

Diagnosis is confirmed with a combination of sigmoidoscopy or colonoscopy and barium enema. If an abscess is suspected, a CT scan is done. Barium enema shows irregular narrowing of the colon and thickened muscle walls. Colonoscopy or sigmoidoscopy can visualize the specific areas of inflammation. A stool specimen may show occult blood if the blood is not visible to the naked eye.

Medical Treatment

Diverticulosis is managed by preventing constipation. In diverticulitis, oral antibiotics may be prescribed, as well as mild tranquilizers or antispasmodics. If pain is severe the client may be hospitalized for intravenous antibiotics and pain control. A nasogastric tube, intravenous fluids, and NPO status may be ordered if nausea or vomiting is present. In the presence or absence of perforation, surgical resection with anastomosis or a diverting temporary **colostomy** is done to allow the diseased portion of colon to rest

---

colostomy: colo—pertaining to colon + stoma—mouth or opening

---

and inflammation to subside. More information regarding colostomies is included later in this chapter.

Nursing Process

ASSESSMENT. The client is assessed for signs and symptoms of diverticulitis. (See Table 31–2.) Physical examination is done to assess for abdominal distention and tenderness. A firm mass may be palpated in the sigmoid area.

NURSING DIAGNOSIS. Constipation related to low-fiber dietary habits may be a nursing diagnosis. Other nursing diagnoses may include pain related to inflammation or infection and alteration in gastrointestinal tissue perfusion related to infection secondary to perforation, peritonitis, or abscess.

PLANNING. Normal bowel elimination, especially without straining, is a goal for the client. Pain should be controlled and risks related to infection and inflammation prevented.

IMPLEMENTATION. Implement interventions that will alleviate and prevent constipation. Fluid intake should be increased to at least 2 to 3 L per day, if not otherwise contraindicated. Dietary considerations for a client with diverticulosis (without evidence of inflammation) include foods that are soft but high in fiber, such as prunes, raisins, and peas. Unprocessed bran can be added to soups, cereals, and salads to give added bulk to the diet. Fiber should be increased in the diet slowly to prevent excess gas and cramping. Some authorities recommend avoiding foods with small seeds that can get caught in diverticuli, such as tomatoes and raspberries, but this has not been proven to help. Interventions for prevention of constipation are implemented as discussed at the beginning of this chapter.

If the client is experiencing pain, administer analgesics or antispasmodic drugs as prescribed. During periods when the client is having acute pain, a diet low in fiber is recommended. Monitor the client closely for any worsening of the pain, especially when associated with abdominal rigidity, and report to the physician immediately. This may indicate that the bowel has ruptured and peritonitis is inevitable.

CLIENT EDUCATION. The nurse instructs the client in dietary changes that will alleviate constipation and prevent further episodes to decrease the likelihood of developing diverticulitis. Clients should also be warned that laxatives or enemas may increase motility and pressure in the bowel and cause further complications. The client needs to be instructed in the signs and symptoms of diverticulitis to be aware of and report to the nurse or physician.

EVALUATION. Having a normal pattern of elimination is a positive desired outcome. When the client reports that there is no pain when having a bowel movement, there is less abdominal pain and cramping, and infection has been prevented, the outcomes have been accomplished.

INFLAMMATORY BOWEL DISEASE

Crohn's Disease/Regional Enteritis

Pathophysiology

Crohn's disease, also known as regional **enteritis** or granulomatous enteritis, is an inflammatory bowel disease (IBD) that involves any part of the intestine, but most commonly the terminal portion of ileum. The inflammation extends through the intestinal mucosa, which leads to the formation of abscesses, **fistulas,** and fissures. As the disease progresses, obstruction occurs because the intestinal lumen narrows with inflamed mucosa and scar tissue.

Etiology

Although the exact cause is unknown, many theories exist, including heredity, infection, or immune disease. Environmental agents such as pesticides, tobacco, radiation, and food additives may also precipitate the onset of the disease. It is characterized by periods of remissions and exacerbations. Exacerbations may be triggered by physical or psychological stress. Crohn's disease is most often diagnosed between the ages of 15 and 30 and occurs more often in women. (See Cultural Considerations Box 31–6.)

Signs and Symptoms

Crampy abdominal pains (unrelieved by defecation), weight loss, and diarrhea are prevalent with the onset of symptoms being insidious. Because the crampy pains occur after eating, the client often does not eat in order to avoid the pain. This, in addition to poor absorption of nutrients, results in malnutrition and weight loss. Chronic diarrhea contributes to fluid and electrolyte imbalance, and the inflamed intestine may perforate, leading to the formation of intra-abdominal or anal fissures, abscesses, or fistulas. Some nongastrointestinal symptoms may also occur, including arthritis, skin lesions, inflammatory disorders of the eyes, and abnormalities of liver function.

Complications

Aside from the malnutrition, the development of the fissures, abscesses, or fistulas is the most common complication. Fistulas may include enterovaginal (small bowel to vagina), enterovesicle (small bowel to bladder), enterocutaneous (small bowel to skin), enteroentero (small bowel to small bowel), or enterocolonic (small bowel to colon) (Fig. 31–3). The fistulas leading to organs that drain externally can lead to tremendous skin irritation, as well as to increased risk of developing infections, such as cystitis. Fistulas are corrected surgically.

Diagnostic Tests

A barium study is the most conclusive diagnostic test for Crohn's disease. This study identifies the classic "cobblestoning" effect on x-ray, and as the disease progresses it reveals the "string sign" indicating constriction in an area of the intestine. Sigmoidoscopy is done to identify if any inflammation is present in the rectosigmoid area. If not, ulcerative colitis is ruled out. An elevated sedimentation rate and leukocytosis are present, and serum albumin may be low due to poor absorption of protein. Bowel sounds are hyperactive over the right lower quadrant, and a stool examination reveals fat and occult blood.

Medical Treatment

Management of Crohn's disease is aimed at relieving symptoms, such as inflammation and diarrhea, and the effects of those symptoms, such as dehydration and malnutrition. Antidiarrheal medications and sedation reduce peristalsis. Sulfasalazine (Azulfidine) or sulfisoxazole (Gantrisin) are used to decrease inflammation, and antibiotics are used if there are abscesses or evidence of peritonitis. Corticosteroids are used during an acute inflammatory phase. Sometimes the symptoms return after the steroids are stopped or reduced.

Surgery may be indicated if obstruction, stricture, fistula, or abscess is present. Surgical procedures include resection of the affected area with anastomosis, colectomy with **ileostomy,** or colectomy with ileorectal anastomosis, depending on the area of bowel involved. See details regarding intestinal ostomies later in this chapter.

CULTURAL CONSIDERATIONS BOX 31–6

Ulcerative colitis and Crohn's disease are more common in whites, Jews, and upper-middle-class urban populations. The incidence of Crohn's disease is increasing rapidly in Western Europe and North America. These findings support possible hereditary or environmental risk factors for IBD.

---

enteritis: entero—intestine + itis—inflammation
ileostomy: ileo—pertaining to ileum + stoma—mouth or opening

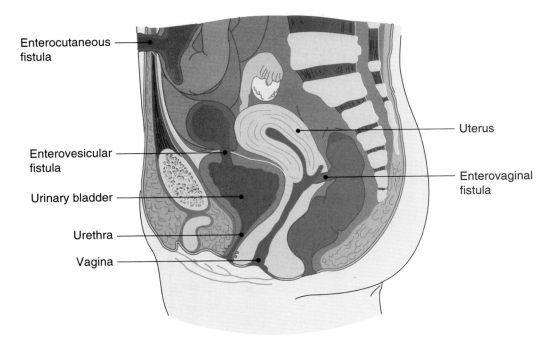

Enterocutaneous fistula

Enterovesicular fistula

Urinary bladder

Urethra

Vagina

Uterus

Enterovaginal fistula

Figure 31–3. Fistulas are a common complication of Crohn's disease.

Due to the similarities between Crohn's disease and ulcerative colitis, the nursing process for both will be discussed together.

Ulcerative Colitis

Pathophysiology

This inflammatory bowel disease is similar to Crohn's disease, but whereas Crohn's disease can occur anywhere in the gastrointestinal system, ulcerative colitis only occurs in the colon or rectum. The epithelial lining of the colon is shed, leading to multiple ulcerations and diffuse inflammations in the superficial mucosa of the colon. The lesions spread throughout the large intestine and usually involve the rectum. The client with ulcerative colitis has increased risk of developing colorectal cancer.

Etiology

Ulcerative colitis is thought to be caused by the same things as Crohn's disease. The tendency to develop ulcerative colitis may be inherited; an autoimmune response may also be a factor. For several years, it was suggested that there was a psychological component in the etiology of ulcerative colitis. However, anyone who experiences chronic intestinal cramps and frequent, sometimes painful bowel movements is going to be discouraged, anxious, and depressed. These traits or behaviors may be a result and not the cause of the disease. Psychological stress may, however, trigger or worsen an attack of symptoms. Ulcerative colitis usually begins between the ages of 15 and 40.

Signs and Symptoms

Abdominal pain, diarrhea, rectal bleeding, and straining at stool are frequent complaints. The client may experience anorexia, weight loss, cramping, vomiting, fever, and dehydration associated with passing 10 to 20 liquid stools a day. Along with potential electrolyte imbalance, there is a loss of calcium, and anemia commonly develops because of the bleeding. Serum albumin may be low because of malabsorption and liver dysfunction. Symptoms are usually intermittent, with periods of remission lasting from months to years.

Complications

Malnutrition and its associated problems is one complication of ulcerative colitis. Another complication is the potential for hemorrhaging during an acute phase of the colitis. Bowel obstruction, perforation, and peritonitis may occur. The client with ulcerative colitis also has an increased risk for colon cancer. Additional symptoms outside of the GI tract may also occur, such as arthritis, skin lesions, and inflammatory disorders of the eyes.

Diagnostic Tests

Examination of stool specimens is done to rule out any bacterial or amebic organisms. The stool is positive for blood. Anemia is often present because of blood loss. Leukocytes and erythrocyte sedimentation rate are elevated because of the chronic inflammation. Electrolytes are depleted from the chronic diarrhea. There is a protein loss because of liver dysfunction and malabsorption. Sigmoidoscopy and barium enema x-ray help differentiate ulcerative colitis from other diseases of the colon with similar symptoms. Biopsies taken during the sigmoidoscopy typically show abnormal cells.

Medical Treatment

Foods that cause gas or diarrhea are avoided. Because the offending foods may be different for each client, foods are tried in small amounts if they are thought to cause symptoms. In general, high-fiber foods, caffeine, spicy foods, and milk products are avoided. Total parenteral nutrition may be needed during acute exacerbations.

As with Crohn's disease, sulfasalazine and anti-inflammatory agents may be given. Corticosteroids are used if necessary.

If medical treatment is ineffective, surgery is considered. Because ulcerative colitis usually involves the entire large intestine, the surgery of choice is total proctocolectomy with formation of an ileostomy. Ileostomies are discussed later in this chapter.

Nursing Process for the Client with Inflammatory Bowel Disease

ASSESSMENT. The nurse obtains a history from the client that includes identification of symptoms, including the onset, duration, frequency, and severity. Ask the client if there has been any correlation between exacerbations of symptoms related to dietary changes or stress. Ascertain any food allergies, such as milk, because some may increase diarrhea. Also, the daily and weekly use of caffeine, nicotine, and alcohol and the quantity of each are noted because all of these stimulate the bowel and can cause cramping and diarrhea.

An assessment of nutritional status is necessary. The amount of weight loss in 2 months can be 10 to 20 pounds. Perianal skin should be assessed for irritation and excoriation.

Assessment of emotional status and coping skills is essential. Because of the frequent bowel movements, the client tends to withdraw from family and friends. The client may be depressed or in denial. Sleep disturbances, depression, and anxiety can be a problem. The nurse needs to assess the client's verbal and nonverbal behaviors. If surgery that results in an ileostomy is planned, the client is at risk for problems with body image.

NURSING DIAGNOSIS. Nursing diagnoses for the client with IBD include the following:

- Diarrhea related to inflammatory process
- Alteration in nutrition, less than body requirements, related to anorexia and malabsorption
- Fluid volume deficit related to anorexia, nausea, and diarrhea
- Pain related to increased peristalsis and cramping
- Impaired skin integrity related to frequent loose stools
- Risk for ineffective individual coping related to repeated episodes of diarrhea

PLANNING. Goals for the client include achieving normal bowel elimination, maintenance of nutrition, prevention of fluid volume deficit, relief of abdominal pain and cramping, and effective coping with the disease.

IMPLEMENTATION. Record characteristics of stools, including color, consistency, amount, frequency, and odor. Make sure the client has quick access to the bathroom, or provide a bedside commode nearby. Keep the environment clean and odor free to help alleviate anxiety. Administer antidiarrheal medication as prescribed. Encourage bed rest to decrease peristalsis.

The client is instructed to avoid high-fiber foods such as whole grains and raw fruits and vegetables to reduce diarrhea. Caffeine, alcohol, and nicotine should also be avoided because they stimulate the GI tract. If symptoms are severe, the client may be given a special liquid (elemental) formula that is absorbed in the upper bowel, allowing the colon to rest. If the client is unable to tolerate oral intake, total parenteral nutrition may be necessary.

Signs of fluid volume deficit are assessed, and daily weights are obtained. An accurate record of intake and output is needed so the physician can order adequate IV fluid replacement. The output record should reflect volume of stools, fistula drainage, vomitus, and urine. Signs of dehydration are documented and reported to the physician.

Document the onset, duration, and severity of pain, and medicate as prescribed. Describe the character of the pain (dull, cramping, burning) and if the pain is associated with meals or activity.

Perianal skin should be kept clean and dry to prevent excoriation from frequent stools. Sitz baths may be helpful. A skin barrier ointment such as A and D emollient ointment or other product especially made for this purpose should be applied after each stool to help protect the area.

Anxiety aggravates the symptoms of inflammatory bowel disease and therefore needs to be reduced. Answer questions; talk in a calm, confident manner; and actively listen to the client. If surgery that may involve an ostomy is being discussed, obtain a consultation for an enterostomal therapy nurse, if available. If not, explain the surgical procedure in basic terms, show the client a picture of a stoma, and allow time to handle an ostomy appliance to become familiar with it. If available, give the client a pamphlet or show a video regarding ostomy management. Allow the client to decide if these information activities are important to see. Include the client's family or significant other. More details about ostomy care are provided later in this chapter.

See also Nursing Care Plan Box 31–7 for the Client with an Intestinal Ostomy.

CLIENT EDUCATION. Information about IBD must be given to the client to promote positive reinforcement and reassurance. Nutrition and dietary considerations need to be discussed. If the client is on medications, instructions regarding when and how to take the drug, why it was ordered, what dose, and potential effects and side effects should be given. Clients who have been on steroids will probably be

---

NURSING CARE PLAN BOX 31–7
FOR THE CLIENT WITH AN INTESTINAL OSTOMY

Body image disturbance related to new ostomy

Outcomes
Client will verbalize acceptance of intestinal ostomy before discharge.

Evaluation of Outcomes
Is the client able to verbalize acceptance of the ostomy?

Interventions	Rationale	Evaluation
• Assess knowledge of self-care of ostomies.	Many people have misconceptions regarding ostomies. Identification of misconceptions and "hearsay" knowledge is important to clarify or correct.	Does the client verbalize appropriate knowledge of ostomy care?
• Encourage client to verbalize feelings about the stoma.	Allowing the client to express his or her feelings provides opportunity to identify and verbalize concerns which then can be addressed by health care providers.	Does the client discuss his or her feelings regarding the stoma to the nurse or significant other?
• Explain the normal characteristics of the stoma before the client's first look.	Helping the client understand what to expect will help relieve anxiety. Being available to answer questions immediately also relieves anxiety.	Does the client look at the stoma without hesitation?
• Demonstrate ostomy appliance change and daily care and encourage client participation.	When the client observes and participates in self-care, his or her self-concept improves.	Is the client participating in self-care? Has the client performed return demonstration of appliance change and emptying of pouch?

---

weaned off of these after surgery. The client needs to know not to stop taking steroids suddenly, to prevent adrenocortical insufficiency. If the client has an ileostomy or colostomy, instructions in daily care are given.

EVALUATION. With the interventions in place, one outcome will be a decrease in the frequency and amount of diarrheal stools. Nutritional status should improve as evidenced by maintenance of ideal weight. The client should maintain a positive fluid and electrolyte balance. The client is experiencing less pain, the client's skin is intact, and the client is able to cope with the disease and treatment.

IRRITABLE BOWEL SYNDROME

Pathophysiology and Etiology

Irritable bowel syndrome (IBS) is a disorder characterized by altered intestinal motility and an increased sensitivity to visceral sensations. Symptoms may be triggered by psychological stress or food intolerances. It is more common in women and in young to middle age.

Signs and Symptoms

IBS is characterized by complaints of gas, bloating, and constipation or diarrhea. Sometimes constipation may alternate with diarrhea. The feelings of bloating are due to the increased sensitivity to visceral sensations; actual ab-

dominal distention is not usually seen. Diarrhea is usually worst first thing in the morning or after breakfast. Weakness, faintness, and palpitations may also be present.

Diagnostic Tests

Diagnosis is made based on history and physical examination. Stool cultures and sigmoidoscopy may be done to rule out other disorders. A trial of avoiding milk products may be advised to rule out lactose intolerance.

Treatment

IBS is a chronic condition, but symptoms can generally be controlled. Relaxation exercises may help control stressors that worsen symptoms. Bran or bulk-forming laxatives such as psyllium (Metamucil) may be used to normalize stools. Foods that cause gas formation are avoided. Mild tranquilizers may help alleviate anxiety. Anticholinergic drugs may reduce intestinal motility and diarrhea.

ABDOMINAL HERNIAS

Pathophysiology and Etiology

A **hernia** is an abnormal protrusion of an organ or structure through the wall of the cavity normally containing it, in this case referring to the abdominal wall.

Hernias are caused by a weakness in the abdominal wall along with sustained increased intra-abdominal pressure, such as the pressure from coughing, straining, and heavy lifting. Obesity and pregnancy are also risk factors. The hernial sac is formed by the peritoneum protruding through the weakened muscle wall. The contents of the hernia can be small or large intestine or the omentum. Indirect hernias are sacs formed from the peritoneum with a portion of the intestine or omentum. Direct hernias arise from a weakness in the abdominal wall, usually at old incisional sites.

There are many types of hernias (Fig. 31–4). Inguinal hernias are located in the groin where the spermatic cord in males or round ligament in females emerges from the abdominal wall. This is the most common type of hernia and is seen most often in males.

Umbilical hernias are seen most often in obese women and in children. They are caused by a failure of the umbilical orifice to close. Ventral (incisional) hernias usually result from a weakness in the abdominal wall following abdominal surgery, especially if a drainage system was used or the client experienced poor wound healing, inadequate nutrition, or is obese.

Prevention

The best way to prevent hernias is to improve the musculature in the abdomen. If a client is going to have abdominal surgery, proper deep breathing and coughing techniques are taught. The client who works at a job that requires heavy lifting, tugging, or pushing should wear a support binder.

Signs and Symptoms

Unless complications occur, there are very few symptoms associated with hernias. An abnormal bulging is seen in the affected area of the abdomen, especially when straining or coughing. It may disappear when the client lies down. If the intestinal mass easily returns to the abdominal cavity or can be manually placed back in the abdominal cavity, it is called a reducible hernia. When adhesions or edema occurs between the sac and its contents, the hernia becomes irreducible or incarcerated; the herniated bowel is trapped and cannot be returned to the abdomen.

Complications

An incarcerated hernia may become strangulated if the blood and intestinal flow are completely cut off. This leads to an intestinal obstruction and possibly gangrene and perforation of the bowel. Symptoms are pain at the site of the strangulation, nausea and vomiting, and colicky abdominal pain. Treatment is emergency surgery.

Diagnosis

Hernias are diagnosed by physical examination.

Medical Treatment

Surgery is indicated if there is strangulation or the threat of obstruction. Surgical treatments of hernias include herniorrhaphy and hernioplasty. Herniorrhaphy involves making an incision in the abdominal wall, replacing the contents of the hernial sac, and then closing the opening. This is the surgery of choice. Hernioplasty involves the surgeon replacing the hernia into the abdomen and also reinforcing the weakened muscle wall with wire, fascia, or mesh. Bowel resection or a temporary colostomy may be necessary if the hernia is strangulated. If the client is not a good surgical candidate, the physician may order the use of a truss or binder once the hernia is manually reduced. A truss is an external restraining device held in place with a belt used to push the hernia into the abdomen.

Nursing Care

If surgery is not planned, the nurse instructs the client to avoid activities that increase intra-abdominal pressure, such as lifting heavy objects. The client is taught to recognize signs of incarceration or strangulation and the importance of notifying the physician immediately. If a truss has

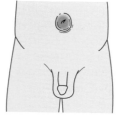
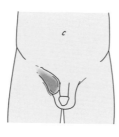
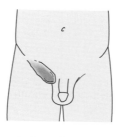
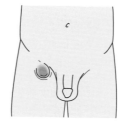

| Umbilical hernia | Direct inguinal hernia | Indirect inguinal hernia | Femoral hernia |

Figure 31–4. Types of hernias. (Modified from Lewis, Collier, and Heitkemper: Medical-Surgical Nursing: Assessment and Management of Clinical Problems, ed 4. Mosby, St Louis, 1996, p 1251, with permission.)

been ordered, the nurse teaches the client to apply it before arising from bed each morning, while the hernia is not protruding. Special attention should be paid to maintenance of skin integrity beneath the truss.

Preoperative Care

A simple herniorrhaphy is generally done as an outpatient surgery. The client is instructed in routine preoperative deep breathing and coughing techniques. Holding the abdomen with a splint, such as a pillow, helps support the weakened abdominal muscles during coughing and moving.

Postoperative Care

Care following surgery is similar to any postoperative care. Following inguinal hernia repair, the male client may experience swelling of the scrotum. Ice packs and elevation of the scrotum may be ordered to reduce swelling. The nurse monitors intake and output and observes for difficulty voiding, which is not uncommon following hernia surgery. As with any abdominal surgery, peristalsis may stop temporarily following surgery. Bowel sounds are monitored, and the client is instructed to report discomfort or distention. Because most clients are discharged the same day as surgery, they are taught to change the dressing and report any signs and symptoms of infection, such as redness, incisional drainage, or fever. The client is also instructed to avoid lifting for 2 to 6 weeks. Specific activity limitations are provided by the surgeon. Most clients can return to work within 2 weeks.

ABSORPTION DISORDERS

The process of digestion reduces nutrients to a form that can be absorbed through intestinal mucosa into the portal bloodstream. Most of the over 8000 mL of liquids with nutrients and electrolytes are absorbed proximal to the ileocecal valve.

Pathophysiology and Etiology

Malabsorption occurs when the gastrointestinal system is unable to absorb one or more of the major nutrients (carbohydrates, fats, or proteins). Some causes of malabsorption are ileal dysfunction, jejunal diverticula, parasitic diseases, celiac diseases, enzyme deficiencies, and inflammatory bowel diseases such as Crohn's disease and ulcerative colitis. The primary malabsorption disorders are tropical sprue, adult celiac disease, and lactose intolerance.

The cause of tropical sprue has not been specifically identified but is thought to be related to bacterial infection of the intestine. In adult celiac disease (sometimes called nontropical sprue), an allergic reaction to gluten is thought to cause malabsorption of protein. Gluten is a protein

---

> ### NUTRITION NOTES BOX 31–8
>
> Gluten enteropathy, or celiac disease, requires permanent elimination of wheat, rye, oats, and barley from the diet. Careful selection of prepared foods is mandatory. If gluten is ingested, damage to the intestine continues even in the absence of symptoms. Instruction from and follow-up by a dietitian is indicated.

found in wheat, barley, oats, and rye. (See Nutrition Notes Box 31–8.)

A deficiency in lactase, an enzyme that breaks down lactose (milk sugar), causes lactose intolerance. Because the lactose is not digested, a high concentration of lactose in the intestines occurs, causing an osmotic retention of water resulting in watery stools. (See Cultural Considerations Box 31–9 and Nutrition Notes Box 31–10.)

Signs and Symptoms

Weight loss, weakness, and general malaise with resulting malnutrition are associated with malabsorption disorders. Signs and symptoms of sprue include frequent loose, bulky, foul stools that are gray in color and have an increased fat content (increased fat in stool is called **steatorrhea**). Lactose intolerance causes abdominal cramping, excessive gas, and loose stools after eating milk products.

Complications

Vitamin K deficiency and resulting hypoprothrombinemia can cause risk for bleeding. Calcium deficiency can be severe enough to cause neuromuscular hyperirritability, including tetany.

Diagnostic Tests

See Table 31–3 for the diagnostic studies used to identify malabsorption diseases.

> ### CULTURAL CONSIDERATIONS BOX 31–9
>
> African-Americans, Asians, Pacific Islanders, Indochinese, and Hispanics have an increased incidence of lactose intolerance resulting in diarrhea, indigestion, and bloating when milk and milk products are consumed. Reduced-lactose milk is available in supermarkets. Calcium can be supplied in other foods such as tofu, soybean curd, and leafy green vegetables.

---

steatorrhea: steat—fat + orrhea—to flow

NUTRITION NOTES BOX 31-10

Lactose-intolerant clients manage their conditions through education and experience. A dietitian's services may be advised. Moderate amounts of many foods can be tolerated when taken with a mixed meal. Ingredients to avoid include milk, milk solids, lactose, and whey. Low-lactose foods (0 to 2 g per serving) include sherbet, aged cheese, processed cheese, and milk treated with lactase enzyme. Some brands of yogurt, a high-lactose food, may be tolerated because of the bacterial lactase present.

Medical Treatment

Folic acid and broad-spectrum antibiotics are given to clients with tropical sprue. For adult celiac disease, eliminating gluten from the diet will eliminate the symptoms. However, gluten is used as a filler or binder in many products, even those labeled "wheat free"; therefore the client must be diligent in identifying potentially offending foods.

Removing foods that contain lactose is the treatment for lactose intolerance. This includes milk and many milk products. Some fermented milk products, such as cheese and yogurt, may be lower in lactose and better tolerated.

Table 31–3. Diagnostic Tests for Disorders of Malabsorption

Diagnostic Test	Test Result and Associated Malabsorption Syndrome
Mean corpuscular volume	Decreased values are found with malabsorption of vitamin B_{12}.
Upper GI series	Thickening of the intestinal mucosa, narrowed mucosa of the terminal ileum, or a change in fecal transit time are indicative of malabsorption syndrome.
Serum carotene level	Decreased values are associated with fat and steatorrhea malabsorption syndrome.
Hemoglobin and hematocrit	Decreased if anemia is present.
D-Xylose absorption test	Decreased excretion of xylose after 5 hours is indicative of malabsorption.
Sudan stain for fecal fat	Malabsorption can be distinguished from maldigestion if this test shows abnormally large numbers of fat droplets.
72-hour stool collection for fat	Stool fat greater than 5 g/24 h after ingestion of 80 g of fat in 2 days implies a fat digestion disorder.

Lactaid is an over-the-counter lactase substitute that clients may take when milk products cannot be avoided. It can be added to milk in liquid form or taken as a tablet before eating a food containing lactose. Lactaid digests about 70 percent of the lactose in the foods, making them more tolerable.

Nursing Care

Nursing care involves monitoring fluid and electrolyte balance, nutrition status, and skin integrity. Daily weights and intake and output help determine if fluid loss is occurring. Intake of electrolyte-rich fluids is encouraged to replace losses. Antidiarrheal agents are given if ordered. Electrolyte levels, especially potassium, are monitored as ordered. The client is instructed in dietary limitations. Nutritional supplements may be ordered if necessary. Perianal skin is kept clean and dry, and barrier ointments are used as needed to protect the skin from excoriation.

INTESTINAL OBSTRUCTIONS

Intestinal obstructions occur when the flow of intestinal contents is blocked. There are two types of intestinal obstruction—mechanical and paralytic. Either can be partial or complete.

Mechanical obstruction occurs when there is a blockage within the intestine from pressure on the intestinal walls from conditions such as adhesions, twisting of the bowel, or a strangulated hernia. Paralytic obstruction occurs when the peristalsis is impaired and the intestinal contents cannot be propelled through. This is seen following abdominal surgeries, trauma, mesenteric ischemia, or infection. The severity of the obstruction depends on the area of bowel affected, the amount of occlusion within the lumen, and the amount of disturbance in the blood flow to the bowel.

Small Bowel Obstruction

Pathophysiology

When obstruction occurs in the small bowel, a collection of intestinal contents, gas, and fluid occurs proximal to the obstruction. The distention that results stimulates gastric secretion but decreases the absorption of fluids. As distention worsens, the intraluminal pressure causes the venous and arterial capillary pressure to decrease. As a result, edema, necrosis, and eventually perforation of the intestinal wall may occur.

Etiology

Following abdominal surgeries, loops of intestine may adhere to areas in the abdomen that may not be healed. This may cause a kink in the bowel that occludes the intestinal flow. These are called adhesions and are the most common cause of small bowel obstruction. Hernias and neoplasms

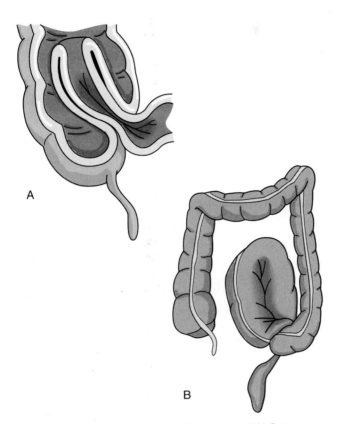

Table 31–4. Causes of Nonmechanical Obstruction

- Abdominal surgery and trauma
- Pneumonia
- Spinal injuries
- Hypokalemia
- Myocardial infarction
- Peritonitis
- Vascular insufficiency

of bowel sounds. In mechanical obstructions, the bowel sounds are usually high pitched proximal to the obstruction and absent below the obstruction.

Due to the loss of fluid and electrolytes, dehydration occurs with the associated symptoms of extreme thirst, drowsiness, aching, and general malaise. The lower in the gastrointestinal tract the obstruction occurs, the more abdominal distention will be evident. If the obstruction is not corrected, shock and possibly death will ensue.

Diagnostic Tests

Dilated loops of bowel will be evident in radiographic studies. If strangulation or perforation occurs, leukocytosis is noted. The hematocrit will be elevated if the client is dehydrated, and the serum electrolytes will be decreased.

Medical Treatment

In the majority of cases, the client is made NPO and the bowel is decompressed using a nasogastric or intestinal tube. This significantly relieves the symptoms. An IV solution with electrolytes is initiated to correct the fluid and electrolyte imbalance. Sometimes IV antibiotics are begun. If complete obstruction is evident, surgical intervention is done to correct the cause of obstruction, such as repair of a hernia, the release of adhesions, or a bowel resection with anastomosis.

Large Bowel Obstruction

Pathophysiology

Obstruction in the large bowel is not usually as dramatic as small bowel obstructions because of the colon's ability to absorb its fluid content and distend well beyond its normal full capacity; therefore dehydration occurs more slowly. If the blood supply to the colon is cut off, the client's life will be in jeopardy due to strangulation and necrosis.

Etiology

Most large bowel obstructions occur in the sigmoid colon and are caused by carcinoma, inflammatory bowel disease, diverticulitis, or benign tumors. Impaction of stool may also cause obstruction.

Signs and Symptoms

Unlike small bowel obstruction, symptoms of large bowel obstruction develop and progress slowly and depend on the

Figure 31-5. Mechanical bowel obstructions. *(A)* Intussusception. *(B)* Volvulus. (Modified from Lewis, Collier, and Heitkemper: Medical-Surgical Nursing: Assessment and Management of Clinical Problems, ed 4. Mosby, St Louis, 1996, p 1236, with permission.)

are the next most common causes. Inflammatory bowel disease, foreign bodies, strictures, **volvulus,** and **intussusception** are other causes. A volvulus obstruction occurs when the bowel twists and the lumen of the intestine is occluded. Intussusception occurs when the intestine telescopes into itself, usually with peristalsis (Fig. 31–5). These conditions are mechanical obstructions. A nonmechanical obstruction occurs when the intestinal peristalsis decreases or stops because of vascular or neuromuscular pathology (Table 31–4). This is also known as paralytic or adynamic ileus.

Signs and Symptoms

The client initially complains of wavelike pain and vomiting. Blood and mucus may be passed, but no feces or flatus. As the obstruction worsens or becomes complete, the symptoms progress. As the peristaltic waves become more extreme, they reverse, propelling the intestinal contents toward the mouth, eventually leading to fecal vomiting. If the pain is sharp and sustained, it may indicate perforation. If the obstruction is nonmechanical, there is an absence

---

intussusception: intus—within + suscept—to receive

location of the obstruction. If the obstruction is in the rectum or sigmoid, the only symptom may be constipation. As the loops of bowel distend, the client may complain of crampy lower abdominal pain, and outlines of the bowel may be visible through the abdominal wall. Eventually, fecal vomiting will develop.

Large bowel obstructions, if not diagnosed and treated, can lead to perforation and ultimately peritonitis (discussed earlier in this chapter).

Diagnostic Tests

Radiologic examination reveals a distended colon.

Medical Treatment

If impact is present, enemas and manual disimpaction may be effective. Other mechanical blockages may require surgical intervention.

Surgical resection of the obstructed colon may be necessary. A temporary colostomy may be indicated to allow the bowel to rest and heal. Sometimes an ileoanal anastomosis is done. In clients who are poor surgical risks, a cecostomy (an opening from the cecum to the abdominal wall) may be done to allow diversion of stool.

Nursing Process

ASSESSMENT. The nurse auscultates the abdomen for 5 minutes in each quadrant before documenting the absence of bowel sounds. The abdomen is palpated for distention. Amount and character of stool, if any, are documented. Pain is assessed on the institution's pain scale and described according to location and character, such as cramping or wavelike. Daily weights and intake and output are monitored, and skin turgor is assessed for fluid deficit. If a nasogastric tube is in place, amount, color, and character of effluent are documented. Vital signs are monitored for signs of infection or shock.

NURSING DIAGNOSIS. Possible diagnoses include acute pain related to abdominal distention and altered tissue perfusion and fluid volume deficit related to collection of fluid in the intestine and vomiting.

PLANNING. Goals for the client include pain control and prevention of dehydration and electrolyte imbalance.

IMPLEMENTATION. The nasogastric tube is maintained on low intermittent suction to relieve discomfort from distention. NPO status is maintained in order to rest the bowel, and frequent mouth care is provided. Medication for pain is administered as ordered. Opioids are given cautiously because they may mask symptoms of perforation and decrease intestinal motility. The client is placed in semi-Fowler's position to reduce tension on the abdomen.

The LPN/LVN assists the registered nurse to monitor IV fluid replacement, which may be ordered based on NG output. Ice chips may be given if ordered by the physician, but they are used sparingly because the melted ice mixes with electrolytes and hydrochloric acid and is removed from the stomach by the suction, resulting in electrolyte imbalance and alkalosis.

If surgery is anticipated, routine care for abdominal surgery is implemented.

EVALUATION. Goals have been met if the client states that pain is controlled, weight and skin turgor show evidence of fluid balance, and electrolytes are within normal limits.

CRITICAL THINKING: Mrs. Loos

Mrs. Loos is admitted for abdominal pain. You note that she has a history of diabetes mellitus. As you do your morning assessment, you find her abdomen large, firm, and tender to touch. She states that she feels nauseated. What do you do? What do you think is happening?

Answers at end of chapter.

ANORECTAL PROBLEMS

Hemorrhoids

Pathophysiology

Hemorrhoids are varicose veins in the anal canal. They are caused by an increase in pressure in the veins, often from increased intra-adominal pressure. Internal hemorrhoids occur above the internal sphincter, and external hemorrhoids occur below the external sphincter.

Etiology

Most hemorrhoids are caused by straining during bowel movements. They are very prevalent during pregnancy. Prolonged sitting or standing may also cause hemorrhoids. Portal hypertension related to liver disease may also be a factor.

Signs and Symptoms

Internal hemorrhoids are usually not painful unless they prolapse. They may bleed during bowel movements. External hemorrhoids cause itching, bleeding during bowel movements, and pain when inflamed and filled with blood (thrombosed). Inflammation and edema occur when the blood within the hemorrhoids clots and becomes infected. This causes severe pain.

Medical Treatment

Prevention of constipation, avoiding straining during defecation, and good personal hygiene relieve hemorrhoid symptoms and discomfort. Astringents such as witch hazel can be used for symptom relief. Sitz baths increase circulation to the area and aid in comfort and healing. Stool softeners can be used to reduce the need for straining. Other anti-inflammatory medications are sometimes tried, such as steroid creams or suppositories. Rotation of ice and heat helps relieve edema and pain with thrombosed hemorrhoids.

If hemorrhoids are prolapsed and are no longer reduced by palliative measures, surgery can be done. Surgical interventions include cryosurgery, which uses cold to freeze the hemorrhoid tissue. Sclerotherapy involves injection of a sclerosing agent into the tissues around the hemorrhoids to cause them to shrink. Rubber band ligation utilizes rubber bands placed on the hemorrhoids until the tissue dies and breaks off. Surgical hemorrhoidectomy involves surgical removal of hemorrhoids and is used in severe cases.

Nursing Care

The client should be instructed to consume a high-fiber diet and at least 2 L of fluids a day to promote regular bowel movements. The effects and side effects, proper dosage, and frequency of local or topical treatments should be explained. If the client has had surgery, the nurse should medicate the client as needed, because the many nerve endings in the anal canal can cause severe pain. A side-lying position and fresh ice packs also promote comfort. After the first postoperative day, sitz baths may be ordered. A side effect of opioid analgesics is constipation, which needs to be avoided, especially in the immediate postoperative period. Because the first bowel movement can be painful and anxiety producing, stool softeners are given and analgesics administered before the bowel movement.

Anal Fissures

Anal fissures are cracks or ulcers in the lining of the anal canal. They are most commonly associated with constipation and stretching of the anus with passage of hard stool, although Crohn's disease or other factors may also play a role. The client may experience bright red bleeding. Pain may be so severe that the client delays defecation, leading to further constipation and worsening symptoms. Treatment of anal fissures involves measures to ensure soft stools, to allow fissures time to heal. Sitz baths may be used to promote circulation to the area to aid in healing. Anesthetic suppositories and nonopioid analgesics may be ordered for comfort. If conservative measures are not helpful, surgical excision may be necessary.

Anorectal Abscess

An anorectal abscess is a collection of pus in the perianal area. Common causative organisms include *E. coli,* staphylococci, or streptococci bacteria. Symptoms include pain, redness, and swelling of the area, drainage, and fever.

Abscesses are treated by antibiotics and surgical incision and drainage of pus. The area may be left open to drain and packing placed to assist with drainage and healing. Nursing care includes daily dressing or packing changes. Sitz baths are used to keep the area clean and promote healing, especially following bowel movements. The client is instructed in the importance of keeping the area clean and dry. Other postoperative care is similar to care following hemorrhoidectomy.

LOWER GASTROINTESTINAL BLEEDING

Etiology

Major causes of lower gastrointestinal bleeding are diverticulitis, polyps (growths in the colon), anal fissures, hemorrhoids, inflammatory bowel disease, and cancer. Bleeding may also occur in the upper GI tract. This is discussed in Chapter 30.

Signs and Symptoms

Bleeding from the GI tract is evident in the stools. **Melena** is the term for black tarry stools from blood that has been in the GI tract for more than 8 hours and come in contact with hydrochloric acid. The presence of melena usually indicates bleeding above or in the small bowel. Bleeding from the colon or rectum is usually bright red (**hematochezia**).

Significant blood loss causes hypotension, light-headedness, nausea, and diaphoresis. The client is pale and has cool skin. The onset of tachycardia and worsening hypotension indicate hypovolemic shock and should be reported immediately to the physician.

Diagnostic Tests

A thorough history is necessary to determine underlying disorders that may be causing the bleeding. Loss of blood is evident in a drop in hemoglobin and hematocrit. The blood urea nitrogen (BUN) may be elevated due to breakdown of proteins in the blood by the GI tract. Stool can be tested for occult blood if bleeding is not immediately visible. Digital examination or sigmoidoscopy may be performed by the physician.

Medical Treatment

Treatment depends on the cause of the bleeding. Mild bleeding may resolve with conservative measures. If bleeding continues, surgery to correct diverticulosis, inflammatory bowel disease, or cancer may be considered.

Nursing Care

The nurse monitors stools for amount and presence of blood. Vital signs are monitored for signs of shock. Declining blood pressure and rising heart rate are reported to the physician immediately. The nurse prepares the client for

---

hematochezia: hemat—blood + chezia—in stool

diagnostic tests. Nursing care for the underlying disorder is provided.

CANCER

Colorectal cancer is one of the most common types of internal cancer in the United States. People with a family history of colon cancer or ulcerative colitis are at higher risk of developing it themselves. The American Cancer Society estimates 131,600 new cases and 56,500 deaths from colorectal cancer in 1998.[1]

Pathophysiology and Etiology

Colorectal cancer originates in the epithelial lining of the intestine. It can occur anywhere in the large intestine.

People with personal or family history of ulcerative colitis or family history of colon cancer are at higher risk of developing cancer. Colon cancer in the elderly has been closely associated with dietary carcinogens. A major causative agent is lack of fiber in the diet, which prolongs fecal transit time and in turn prolongs exposure to possible carcinogens. Also, bacterial flora is believed to be altered by excess fat, which converts steroids into compounds that have carcinogenic properties.

Signs and Symptoms

Change in bowel habits is the most common symptom. Bloody stools is the second most common symptom. Other signs and symptoms include mucus in the stool, abdominal or rectal pain, weight loss, anemia, obstruction, and perforation.

Complications

Complete obstruction of the colon could result in abscess, perforation, or peritonitis. Colorectal cancer can metastasize to the lymphatic system and liver.

Diagnostic Tests

Many colorectal cancers are identified by sigmoidoscopy. Other tests, besides abdominal and rectal examination, include fecal occult blood testing, barium enema, proctosigmoidoscopy, and colonoscopy. Carcinoembryonic antigen (CEA) levels were thought to be good indicators in diagnosing colon cancer. Now, however, they are used more for predicting prognosis.

Medical Treatment

Surgery is performed to either resect the tumor and anastomose the remaining bowel or divert the fecal stream by forming a colostomy. In rectal cancer, an abdominal perineal resection is done with the formation of a permanent end colostomy (Fig. 31–6). An abdominal perineal resection is a procedure in which the anus, rectum, and part of the sigmoid colon are removed. A perineal wound is left where the anus had been. Medical management includes radiation therapy and chemotherapy. When both are used, along with surgery, longer survival rates have been demonstrated.

Nursing Process

ASSESSMENT. Identification of the client's risk factors associated with the diagnosis of colon or rectal cancer is done by asking questions related to the client's personal and family history. Is there a history of inflammatory bowel disease? What were the client's dietary habits, such as the types of foods usually eaten and the amount of liquids usually consumed? Before the client's diagnosis, did the client experience constipation or diarrhea, and has there been a change? Has mucus or blood been noted in the stools? What social habits does the client have, such as smoking, alcohol intake, and exercise? If there has been a recent weight loss, how much and in what time frame? Does the client admit to unusual fatigue or insomnia? Stool should be checked for mucus or blood.

NURSING DIAGNOSIS. Nursing diagnoses identified based on the assessment data may include pain related to tissue compression from the tumor; anxiety related to diagnosis of cancer; alteration in nutrition, less than body requirements, related to nausea and anorexia; and knowledge deficit related to surgery and postoperative self-care.

PLANNING. The goals of the client will include relief from or reduction in pain, alleviation of anxiety, and achievement of optimal nutrition status. The client should also understand self-care following surgery.

IMPLEMENTATION. Administer analgesics as prescribed. Limit visitors and telephone calls if client prefers; provide a quiet, relaxing atmosphere to help alleviate anxiety. If the client wants to talk about the diagnosis and planned surgery, set aside time to allow the client who desires to ventilate, cry, or ask questions.

Provide the client with a high-protein, high-calorie diet that is low in residue to decrease excessive peristalsis and minimize cramping. Total parenteral nutrition may be necessary to provide depleted vitamins, minerals, and nutrients if the client has been anorexic for any length of time or has had a significant weight loss. If the client is anemic, blood transfusions may be necessary.

See later in this chapter for education needs of the client with a new ostomy.

EVALUATION. Expected outcomes are that the client verbalizes less anxiety, verbalizes control of pain, attains an optimal level of nutrition, and verbalizes understanding of the disease and any procedure that was done. If the client

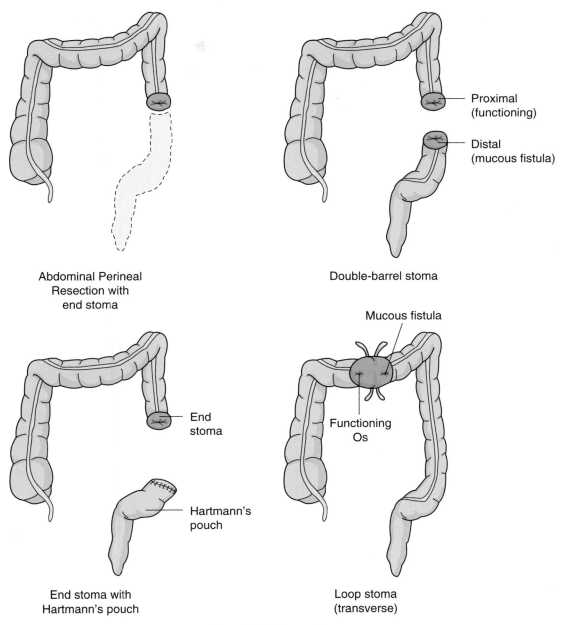

Proximal (functioning)

Distal (mucous fistula)

Abdominal Perineal Resection with end stoma

Double-barrel stoma

Mucous fistula

End stoma

Functioning Os

Hartmann's pouch

End stoma with Hartmann's pouch

Loop stoma (transverse)

Figure 31–6. Types of stomas.

has a colostomy, the stoma is observed by the client and a return demonstration of the appliance change is done before discharge.

OSTOMY MANAGEMENT

An ostomy is a surgically created opening that diverts stool (or sometimes urine) to the outside of the body through a **stoma** on the abdomen. A stoma is the portion of bowel that is sutured onto the abdomen to allow stool to exit. The types of abdominal ostomies that can be performed are colostomy, ileostomy, and urostomy (urinary ostomies are discussed in Chapter 35). The stomas can be end, loop, or double-barrel. See Figure 31–6 for types of ostomies.

Ileostomy

An ileostomy is an end stoma formed by bringing the terminal ileum out to the abdominal wall following a total colectomy. Two types of ileostomies can be formed: the conventional ileostomy (also known as a Brooke ileostomy) or a continent ileostomy (also known as a Kock pouch). The conventional ileostomy is a small stoma in the right lower quadrant that requires a pouch at all times due to the continuous flow of effluent.

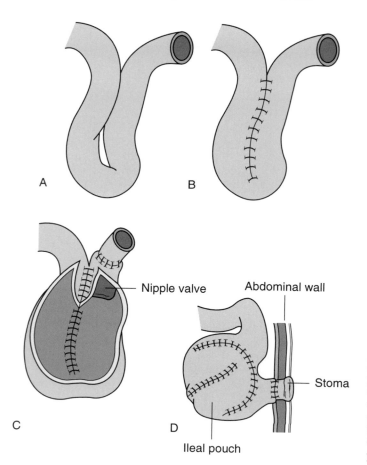

Figure 31–7. Surgical formation of continent ileostomy (Kock pouch). *(A)* Loop of terminal ileum. *(B)* Both limbs of ileum are brought together and sutured into a U shape. *(C)* Pouch created with nipple valve. *(D)* Pouch sutured to abdominal wall. (Modified from Lewis, Collier, and Heitkemper: Medical-Surgical Nursing:Assessment and Management of Clinical Problems, ed 4. Mosby, St Louis, 1996, p 1226, with permission.)

A continent ileostomy is done by taking a portion of the terminal ileum to construct an internal reservoir with a nipple valve (Fig. 31–7). The stoma is flush to the skin and usually located near the suprapubic area. The client is instructed to insert a catheter into the stoma three or four times a day to empty the reservoir. A continent ileostomy is not done as often as a conventional ileostomy for several reasons. One is because there are not as many surgeons who know how to do the procedure. Others are that the procedure is much more involved, has more risks, and the candidates have to be chosen carefully due to the length of surgery time and the difference in the education needed for the client to do self-care.

If the client is totally opposed to having an ileostomy, an ileoanal anastomosis can be done, to connect the ileum to the anus and avoid having a stoma. This procedure is usually done in two steps. The first surgery involves removal of the diseased bowel and formation of a reservoir from part of the ileum, which is connected to the anus. At this time a temporary ileostomy is also formed, to divert stool while the reservoir heals. After 2 to 3 months, the ileostomy is reversed, and the client can have bowel movements from the anus. However, the client may have more problems with perianal skin irritation due to the frequent liquid stools. An ileorectal anastomosis can also be performed, but this will not be a curative procedure for a client

with ulcerative colitis, because the rectum may still be diseased.

Colostomy

End Colostomy

An end stoma is where the proximal end of the bowel is brought to the outside abdominal wall. If an abdominal perineal resection is done (usually for low rectal cancer), the rectum is removed and the proximal sigmoid or descending colon is brought out as a stoma. Another procedure may be done in which a segment of diseased or injured bowel is removed and the proximal limb is brought to form the stoma. The remaining limb of bowel is sutured closed and left in the peritoneal cavity so that the rectum is intact. This is called the Hartmann's pouch and may be permanent or temporary depending on the diagnosis. Because the rectum is intact, the client may feel the urge to defecate. This is normal because the colon continues to produce mucus. As the rectal stump fills with this mucus, the sphincter is triggered and alerts the patient as if it were stool.

A colostomy is named according to where in the bowel it is formed: it may be an ascending, transverse, descending, or sigmoid colostomy. The type of effluent (drainage) to be

Table 31–5. **Location of Stoma and Type of Effluent**

Location of Stoma	Type of Effluent
Ileostomy	Liquid to mushy
Cecostomy, ascending colostomy	Liquid to mushy, foul odor
Right transverse colostomy	Mushy to semiformed
Left transverse colostomy	Semiformed, soft
Descending or sigmoid colostomy	Soft to hard formed

expected is dependent on the location of the bowel used (Table 31–5).

LEARNING TIP

As stool travels through the colon, water is absorbed. Therefore the ileostomy produces the most liquid effluent, followed by an ascending colostomy. A descending or sigmoid colostomy produces more formed stool.

Loop Stoma

To create a loop stoma, the surgeon pulls up a loop of bowel, usually the transverse colon, slips a bridge under the loop to hold it to the outside abdominal wall, and then makes an incision in the top portion of the exposed colon to allow stool to exit. The entire loop of bowel is not cut through. With a double-barrel colostomy, the bowel is completely dissected and both ends of the colon are brought to the outside abdominal wall to form two separate stomas. The proximal stoma will be the functioning stoma where feces will pass. The distal stoma is called a mucous fistula because mucus will pass from it. Both of these procedures are usually done as temporary colostomies, often for the client who has had a bowel resection for diverticulitis, to rest the repaired part of ther bowel during healing. However, sometimes they wind up being permanent.

Preoperative Care

The nurse should consult an enterostomal therapist (ET) before surgery. The ET can help prepare the client both emotionally and physically for the surgery. In addition, the ET has expertise in marking the stoma site for the surgeon. This involves observing the abdomen as the client assumes different positions, and noting how clothing is worn, such as where the belt rides. The site for the stoma can then be chosen to avoid skin or fat folds, or where clothing will interfere with an appliance. Good stoma placement can prevent much agony over leaking or poorly fitting appliances postoperatively.

Routine preoperative instruction, including the importance of coughing and deep breathing, splinting, and early ambulation, is provided. The nurse carries out orders for cleansing of the bowel, to reduce the risk for infection following surgery. Unless the client has chronic diarrhea related to IBD, an oral agent to cleanse the bowel (Go-Lytely) will be given. Antibiotics will be ordered both orally and intravenously.

Nursing Process

ASSESSMENT. The client with a new ostomy has many nursing care needs. In addition to routine postoperative assessment, the stoma should be inspected at least every 8 hours. The stoma should be pink and moist (similar to the inside of the mouth), and should be well attached to the surrounding skin. A bluish stoma indicates inadequate blood supply; a black stoma indicates necrosis. Either complication should be reported to the physician immediately. Initially, the stoma will be swollen. The size will gradually decrease over the first few weeks following surgery. See Figure 31–8 for types of stomas.

Skin is assessed for irritation around the pouch and under the pouch each time it is changed. Ostomy discharge (effluent) is monitored and documented. Unexpected changes, such as liquid stool from a descending ostomy, are reported.

NURSING DIAGNOSIS. A variety of diagnoses may be applicable for the client with a new ostomy. See the section on implementation, later in this chapter. A sample care plan is shown for a nursing diagnosis of disturbance in body image related to new ostomy care. (See Nursing Care Plan Box 31–7 for the Client with an Intestinal Ostomy.)

PLANNING. Goals for the client include the ability to perform self-care measures necessary for safe discharge home. The physical, emotional, psychosocial, economic, and rehabilitative aspects must be considered and the related education must be provided so that the client will learn to live with his or her ostomy. Discharge planning should be done with assistance of the social worker, dietitian, pharmacist, home health nurse, and ET nurse. Some communities also have an ostomy club that sends trained visitors with ostomies to help the new ostomate adjust.

Implementation

Knowledge Deficit Related to New Ostomy

It is important for the nurse to be aware of the client's readiness and ability to learn. When a client is experiencing a lot of pain, nausea, or vomiting, he or she may not be very receptive to looking at the ostomy or learning about ostomy care. If the client has severe arthritis or other physical conditions that may limit his or her ability to perform self-care, the need for a specific type of ostomy appliance

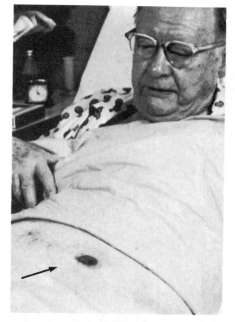

Man at right has a descending or "dry" colostomy.

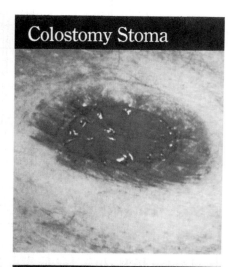

Colostomy Stoma

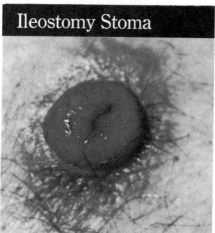

Ileostomy Stoma

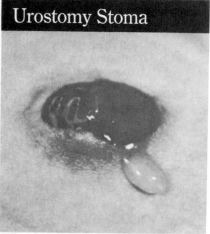

Urostomy Stoma

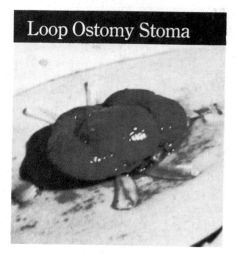

Loop Ostomy Stoma

Figure 31–8. Types of stomas. Note moist, pink to red appearance of healthy stoma. (Reproduced with permission of Hollister Incorporated.)

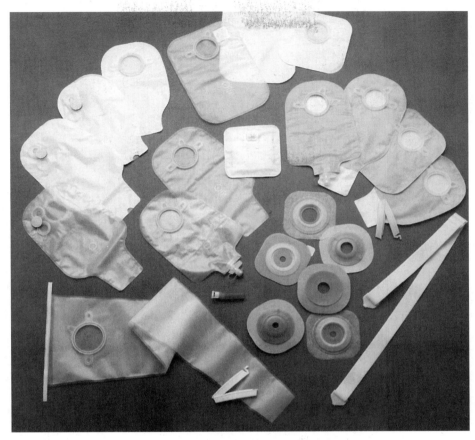

Figure 31–9. Appliances used for ostomies. The long sleeve at the lower left of the photo is used to drain the bowel following irrigation. (Reproduced with permission of Hollister Incorporated.)

may be necessary. The client may be blind or deaf or have a language barrier, which will necessitate special instructional methods.

Unfortunately in the current health care environment, the client will not be in the hospital long enough to wait long to begin learning self-care. If the client is not ready or able to learn, it will be even more important that a family member or caregiver be included in the teaching. A home care nurse can be consulted for continued instruction at home. An enterostomal therapist or equipment supplier can suggest appliances suited to individual clients' needs. See Figure 31–9 for types of appliances.

APPLIANCE CHANGE. Depending on the type of appliance used, the appliance will need to be changed as frequently as every 3 days or as long as every 10 to 14 days. If leakage occurs, the appliance should be changed as soon as possible to avoid **peristomal** skin irritation. The skin barrier that is placed over the stoma onto the skin should fit within one-sixteenth to one-eighth inch of the base of the stoma to prevent skin contact with stool. Because most stomas are not round, a pattern should be made to teach the client

proper size and shape. An open-end or drainable pouch should be used for all colostomies or ileostomies, especially during the first 8 weeks after surgery. See Figure 31–10 for the pouch application procedure.

If the client has a left-sided (descending or sigmoid) colostomy, the bowel can be regulated either by diet or by regular irrigation of the stoma. Once bowel regulation has been achieved, the client may use a closed-end pouch or a stoma cap.

DAILY CARE AND HYGIENE. The client is instructed to empty the pouch when it gets to be one-third to one-half full. The amount of effluent and frequency of emptying will depend on the location of the stoma in the bowel. If the pouch is allowed to get over half full of stool, the weight of the effluent will pull on the pouch and weaken the seal of the skin barrier. Once the pouch is emptied, the inside of the tail of the pouch must be cleaned and dried before the clamp is replaced. Otherwise, there will be odor. If a two-piece system is used, the pouch can be taken off, washed out, and replaced. The client can bathe or shower with the appliance in place, but needs to check the seal and retape if it is loosening. Spray deodorants or chlorophyll tablets can be placed in the pouch for odor control. The chlorophyll is more effective if taken by mouth.

---

peristomal: peri—surrounding + stoma—mouth or opening

Preparation of the Stomahesive Wafer with Sur-Fit Flange

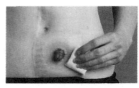

1. Cleanse the peristomal area with water and pat thoroughly dry. Measure your stoma size with the measuring guide provided and trace the proper opening on the white paper backing of the Stomahesive® disc.

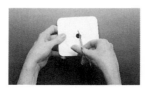

2. Leaving the white paper backing of the wafer in place, cut a hole in the wafer to the same shape and size as the base of the stoma. The best result is usually obtained by cutting from the reverse side of the wafer, using curved, short-bladed scissors.

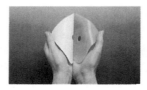

3. Peel the white paper backing from the wafer just prior to application.

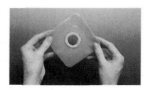

4. Gaps between the wafer and the base of the stoma may be further protected by applying Stomahesive® Paste to the wafer.

Application of the Stomahesive Wafer with Sur-Fit Flange

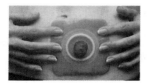

5. Center the enlarged hole over the stoma, place on abdomen, and apply light pressure

Figure 31–10. Preparation to apply an ostomy appliance. (Courtesy of ConvaTec, a Bristol-Myers Squibb Company, Princeton, NJ, with permission.)

DIETARY CONSIDERATIONS. The client needs to be aware of foods that contribute to odor and gas. If foods that are known to cause odor or gas are eaten, the client will know to empty the pouch more often of flatus and to be aware of the possibility of more odor. The foods that contribute to and control diarrhea are important to know, as well as what to do for constipation. A list of foods that may contribute to ileostomy blockage needs to be given to the

Table 31–6. Foods That Can Cause Ileostomy Blockage

Green leafy vegetables	Mushrooms
Spinach	Nuts
Collards	Dried fruits
Mustards	Raisins
Cole slaw	Figs
Celery	Apricots
Corn, popcorn	Chinese vegetables
Foods with nondigestible peels	Meats with casings
Apples	Sausage
Grapes	Wieners
Potatoes	Bologna
Coconut	

ileostomy client (Table 31–6). (See also Nutrition Notes Box 31–11.)

COLOSTOMY IRRIGATION. Colostomy irrigation is rarely done for the purpose of regulation anymore. However, it is done sometimes as a bowel prep for procedures. An irrigation is done similar to an enema, except that special equipment is used to instill fluid into bowel via the stoma. Because the stoma does not have a sphincter, when an irrigation is done, specially designed tubing with a cone at the end is used to help block the fluid being infused from backing back out of the stoma.

Body Image Disturbance

Loss of body image, fear of the unknown, and concerns regarding acceptance by significant others can take control of the client with an ostomy. Overcoming those fears will be crucial to how well the client will adjust. The idea of feces being expelled from the abdomen in full view of the client can make him or her feel dirty and abnormal. The spouse or significant other should be encouraged to view the stoma with the client and allowed to ask questions and participate in care. Attitude and behaviors of the nursing staff caring for the client with an ostomy can significantly affect his or her ability to adapt, either positively or nega-

NUTRITION NOTES BOX 31-11

Ostomy clients receive a soft diet progressing to a general diet as the surgeon prescribes. Stringy, high-fiber foods are avoided initially until tolerance is demonstrated. These include celery, coconut, corn, cabbage, coleslaw, membranes on citrus fruits, peas, popcorn, spinach, dried fruit, nuts, sauerkraut, pineapple, seeds, and skins of fruits and vegetables. Some clients avoid fish, eggs, beer, and carbonated beverages because they produce excessive odor.

tively. In addition, a trained visitor with an ostomy can help the client see that there is hope for a normal life. (Check a local phone directory for The United Ostomy Association or ostomy club.)

One of the most common fears expressed by clients with ostomies is the fear of gas and odor. Because the stoma does not have a sphincter, flatus will be expelled unexpectedly. When the client is wearing clothes, the noise is usually muffled, as opposed to wearing a loose hospital gown after surgery. The client can be reassured by informing him or her of this. The quality of the appliances available now allow for control of odor. If the client notices an odor, something is wrong, and there are several things he or she needs to check: (1) Was the pouch just emptied of feces or "burped" of air? (2) Is there feces on the drainage spout of the pouch? (3) Are there signs of leakage under the skin barrier? (4) If a two-piece system is used, is the pouch snapped onto the skin barrier appropriately?

Leakage of an appliance can occur at any time, and the client needs to be prepared for an emergency pouch change. Encourage the client to always carry an extra appliance. If leakage does occur in a public place, such as the grocery store, church, or a friend's house, the client may not want to go out again. Try to determine the cause of the leak and instruct the client in ways to decrease the likelihood of leakage problems. If leakage is a continuous problem, the enterostomal therapy nurse should be consulted.

Risk for Sexual Dysfunction

Feared change in body image can also lead to sexual dysfunction. If the male client had an abdominal perineal resection for cancer of the rectum, there is a chance that he will be impotent. This impotence may be transient, depending on the severity of nerve damage or edema associated with the surgery. If the client is impotent, a urologist may be consulted for interventions that may help. Encouraging the client and spouse or sexual partner to discuss these concerns will help them work through fear and possible embarrassment. Alternative sexual positions can be suggested. There are pouch covers the client can purchase that can be worn over the pouch to help disguise the pouch and its contents.

Risk for Ineffective Management of Therapeutic Regimen

The client may have difficulty carrying out self-care measures for a variety of reasons. The cost and availability of ostomy supplies is problematic for many clients. Most insurances, including Medicare, will pay for ostomy supplies, although some limit the amount allowed per month. Medicaid even specifies the type of appliance covered. Each state-funded Medicaid system is different; some may not cover expenses at all. Many times the type of appliance needed to eliminate leakage is not covered, and the client

either pays the difference or wears what the insurance will provide. If the client has no insurance, the cost can be astronomical. Sometimes ostomy appliances will be purchased instead of prescriptions. Fortunately, the pouches in most two-piece systems can be washed out and reused to save money. See the Home Health Hints at the end of this chapter.

In some areas, the availability of supplies is very limited. Fortunately, there are many mail-order companies available now. Also, local retail pharmacists can order smaller quantities of supplies through their wholesalers so that they do not have to keep a large number of supplies in their inventory.

Risk for Injury

Complications related to ostomies include skin problems and stomal problems. If there are any complications associated with the care of the ostomy, the ET nurse should be consulted, if available. This nurse has specialized training in caring for the stoma and peristomal skin and has a wealth of information to offer to the client, as well as the staff.

PERISTOMAL SKIN IRRITATION. The skin around the stoma may become irritated if the opening in the skin barrier around the stoma is cut too large, thereby leaving skin exposed to gastrointestinal effluent. Prolonged contact with gastrointestinal effluent on the skin can lead to a reaction similar to chemical burns. The removal of tape and adhesives, especially frequently, can lead to skin shearing. Occasionally, there may be an allergic dermatitis related to sensitivities to the adhesive itself. To prevent irritation, a skin barrier such as Stomahesive should be used, and it should be carefully cut to fit around the stoma with a minimum of skin exposed. Pouches are left on for several days or until leakage begins, to prevent skin shearing from frequent removal.

PERISTOMAL HERNIA. Hernias may develop around the stoma due to weakened abdominal muscles. This can pose a problem with appliance leakage due to the change in body contours associated with the hernia. A more flexible ostomy appliance may be helpful.

STOMAL PROLAPSE. Sometimes the weakened muscles in the abdomen will contribute to the falling down (or out) of the intestinal mucosa. This is called a prolapse and most commonly occurs in the elderly. Pouching a prolapsed stoma can be difficult. A prolapsed stoma should be reported to the physician.

STOMAL NECROSIS. Stomal necrosis occurs when there is circulatory compromise. This may arise due to vascular collapse or blockage in the mesentery of the intestines or edema in the intestine from obstruction proximal to the stoma. If new onset of necrosis is noted, it should be reported to the physician immediately. Most of the time the necrosis is only at the very end of the stoma, and the necrotic tissue will eventually slough off, revealing viable mucosa. Odor may be a problem due to the necrotic tissue.

ILEOSTOMY BLOCKAGE. The client with an ileostomy may have a blockage if he or she complains of having no bowel movement or has the passage of a large quantity of hot liquid through the stoma, which is associated with abdominal cramping. The stoma will become edematous, and the color may be pale to dusky. Once the signs and symptoms are recognized, the client needs to consider what was eaten in the past 24 hours. Certain foods are considered to be high risk for stomal blockage. (See Table 31–6.)

The nurse instructs the client in the signs and symptoms of blockage. Once the client recognizes the problem, instruct him or her to get in a tub full of warm water (not too hot or cold), get in a knee-chest position, and sip on warm liquid, such as coffee, hot tea, bouillon or broth, or chocolate. If the blockage is partial, relief will occur fairly shortly after these measures are taken. If the blockage is complete, an ileostomy lavage will need to be done by a physician or ET nurse.

Evaluation

The plan of care has been effective if the client or significant other is able to competently care for the ostomy, is able to accept the change in body image, and can describe self-care measures to prevent or treat complications.

Rehabilitative Needs

One of the goals of care for the ostomy client is to assist the client to return to activities of daily living. In addition to the ET, a home care nurse may be able to assist the client in

Table 31–7. **Support Groups**

United Ostomy Association, Inc. (UOA)
19772 MacArthur Blvd., Suite 200
Irvine, CA 92612-2405
(714) 660-8624 (voice)
(714) 660-9262 (fax)
(800) 826-0826 (toll free)

Celiac Sprue Association
PO Box 31700
Omaha, NE 68131
(402) 558-0600

Crohn and Colitis Foundation of America, Inc.
386 Park Ave. South
17th Floor
New York, NY 10016-8804
(212) 685-3440 (voice)
(212) 779-4098 (fax)
(800) 932-2423 (toll free)
Info@ccfa.org (e-mail)

American Cancer Society (ACS)
(800) ACS-2345

HOME HEALTH HINTS

- Ostomy bag deodorizers can increase the cost of care. Alternatives include the following: (1) Place tissue or cotton balls saturated in almond or vanilla extract inside the appliance and replace as needed. (2) Put mouthwash in the water that is used to rinse the appliance. (3) Spray a light coat of cooking spray inside the clean bag to make later cleanup easier.

---

becoming comfortable with self-care. Being able to perform the ostomy appliance change and daily care is important, but ensuring that the client returns to work or civic activities as before is also important.

The client can generally do any activity he or she was able to do before he had the ostomy. Resources available, if needed, are the United Ostomy Association, the Crohn's and Colitis Foundation of America, and the American Cancer Society (Table 31–7).

Review Questions

1. Jennie has chronic diarrhea. Which of the following nursing diagnoses should be treated as a priority?
   a. Impaired skin integrity
   b. Altered coping
   c. Fluid volume deficit
   d. Pain

2. Mr. Samuelson has ulcerative colitis. Which foods should he avoid in his diet?
   a. Fresh fruits and vegetables
   b. White bread and cereals
   c. Sweets
   d. Meats and proteins

3. The nurse notes an inguinal hernia as he assesses Mr. Jenks. Which of the following findings should be reported immediately to the physician?
   a. The hernia slides into the abdomen when Mr. Jenks lies down and pops out when he stands up.
   b. Mr. Jenks has an odd-looking belt that he uses to hold the hernia in.
   c. Mr. Jenks has not had a bowel movement in 2 days.
   d. The hernia appears to be stuck outside Mr. Jenks' abdomen, and he complains of nausea.

4. Mr. Smith has a history of diverticulitis. Which of the following symptoms would indicate rupture and the need for immediate medical care?
   a. Explosive diarrhea
   b. Constipation leading to obstipation
   c. Abdominal rigidity and rebound tenderness
   d. Pain at McBurney's point

5. You are listening to Mrs. Patel's abdomen and do not hear bowel sounds. How long must you listen before determining that bowel sounds are absent?
   a. 2 minutes in each quadrant
   b. 5 minutes in each quadrant
   c. 7 minutes in each quadrant
   d. 10 minutes in each quadrant

6. Which of the following is the term to describe black tarry stools?
   a. Melena
   b. Hematochezia
   c. Hematemesis
   d. Steatorrhea

7. Which class of medications may decrease peristalsis and should be used cautiously in clients with gastrointestinal problems?
   a. Cholinergics
   b. Opioid analgesics
   c. Histamine blockers
   d. Diuretics

8. Which of the following dietary habits may increase the risk for development of colon cancer?
   a. High fat, low fiber intake
   b. High intake of milk and milk products
   c. Low meat and protein intake
   d. Low fat, high carbohydrate intake

9. Which of the following ostomies will most likely have formed stool and may be able to be cared for without a pouch?
   a. Ileostomy
   b. Ascending colostomy
   c. Transverse loop ostomy
   d. Descending colostomy

10. A client with a colostomy should routinely avoid which foods?
    a. Fresh fruits and vegetables
    b. Red meats
    c. High-fat foods
    d. No foods should be routinely avoided

ANSWERS TO CRITICAL THINKING

CRITICAL THINKING: Jessie

You need to assess the situation before intervening. First, ask Jessie or other caregivers if she had a bowel movement that was inadvertently not charted. Next, ask Jessie if she feels constipated or if she has abdominal discomfort. Assess Jessie's abdomen for distention and presence or absence of bowel sounds. A digital examination may be necessary to determine if a fecal impaction is present. If simple constipation appears to be the problem, the medical record should be checked for prn laxative or enema orders. Once Jessie has had a bowel movement, laxatives should be discontinued and preventive measures such as regular fluids, fiber, and exercise should be instituted.

CRITICAL THINKING: Mrs. Loos

You need to further assess Mrs. Loos before deciding what to do. Begin by asking the WHAT'S UP? questions, including exactly where the pain is occurring, how it feels, if there is anything that aggravates or alleviates the pain, when it started, how bad it is on a scale of 1 to 10, whether there are associated symptoms, and if Mrs. Loos has some insight as to the cause of her problem. Listen for bowel sounds for 5 minutes in each quadrant. Find out when her last bowel movement was. Because of her history of diabetes, you suspect that neuropathy may be causing a nonmechanical bowel obstruction. If assessment findings confirm the possibility, the physician should be contacted. Because of the nausea and the potential need for surgery, withhold food and fluids until the physician can be contacted.

REFERENCE

1. 1998 Facts and Figures. American Cancer Society. http://www.cancer.org/org/cf98/selectedcancers.html (5 Feb 1998).

BIBLIOGRAPHY

Ackley, E, and Ladwig, G: Nursing Diagnosis Handbook. Mosby, St Louis, 1997.

Belknap, D, Davidson, LJ, and Smith, CR: Diarrhea with enteral feedings: The effects of psyllium hydrophilic mucilloid on diarrhea in enterally fed patients. Heart Lung 26:3, 1997.

Broadwell, DC, and Jackson, BS: Principles of Ostomy Care. Mosby, St Louis, 1982.

Burns, GW: The Science of Genetics: An Introduction to Heredity, ed 5. Macmillan, New York, 1983.

Burns, PE, and Jairath, N: Diarrhea and the patient receiving enteral feedings. A multifactorial problem. J Wound Ostomy Continence Nurs 21, 1994.

Campinha-Bacote, J: African Americans. In Purnell, L, and Paulanka, B, (eds): Transcultural Health Care: A Culturally Competent Approach. FA Davis, Philadelphia, 1997.

Cox, J: Inflammatory bowel disease: Implications for the med-surg nurse. Medsurg Nurs 4:6, 1995.

Gallagher-Allred, CR: Nutritional Care of the Terminally Ill. Aspen, Gaithersburg, Md, 1989.

Lutz, C, and Przytulski, K: Nutrition and Diet Therapy. FA Davis, Philadelphia, 1997.

Martin, FL. Ulcerative colitis. Am J Nurs 97:38, 1997.

Mobarhan, S, and DeMeo, M: Diarrhea induced by enteral feedings. Nutr Rev 53:67, 1995.

Nazarko, L: Preventing constipation in older people. Prof Nurse 11:12, 1996.

Reese, JL, et al: Diarrhea associated with nasogastric feedings. Oncol Nurs Forum 23:59, 1996.

Spiro, CM, Grant, EG, and Gilley, MT: Diverticular disease: Surgical options, patient management. AORN J 59:3, 1994.

Understanding the Liver, Gallbladder, and Pancreas

32

Liver, Gallbladder, and Pancreas Functions and Assessment

Elaine Bishop Kennedy

Learning Objectives

Upon completion of this chapter, the student will be able to:

1. Identify the location of the liver, gallbladder, and pancreas.
2. Describe the functions of the liver, gallbladder, and pancreas.
3. List the effects of aging on the liver, gallbladder, and pancreas.
4. Identify the elements in a nursing history for a client with liver, gallbladder, or pancreas disease.
5. Describe the techniques used in a physical examination of the abdomen conducted for a client with possible liver, gallbladder, or pancreas disease.
6. Describe normal findings from a physical examination of the abdomen conducted for a client with possible liver, gallbladder, or pancreas disease.
7. Describe nursing care for clients undergoing common diagnostic tests for liver, gallbladder, or pancreatic disease.

Key Words

caput medusae (**KAP**-ut mi-**DOO**-see)
cholecystokinin (KOH-lee-sis-toh-**KYE**-nin)
esophagogastroduodenoscopy (e-SOFF-uh-go-GAS-troh-DOO-od-e-**NOS**-kuh-pee)
icterus (**ICK**-ter-us)
jaundice (**JAWN**-diss)
retrograde cholangiopancreatography (**RET**-roh-grayd koh-LAN-jee-oh-PAN-kree-ah-**TOG**-rah-fee)
spider angioma (**SPY**-der AN-jee-**OH**-mah)
striae (**STRIGH**-ee)

Review of Normal Anatomy and Physiology

The liver, gallbladder, and pancreas are called accessory organs of digestion because they produce or store digestive secretions but are not sites of the digestive process, which takes place in parts of the alimentary tube.

LIVER

The liver fills the right and center of the upper abdominal cavity just below the diaphragm. The two main lobes of the liver are called the right and left lobes.

The blood supply of the liver differs from that of other organs. The liver receives oxygenated blood by way of the hepatic artery. By way of the portal vein, blood from the abdominal digestive organs and the spleen is brought to the liver before being returned to the heart. This special pathway is called hepatic portal circulation and permits the liver to regulate blood levels of nutrients or to remove potentially toxic substances such as alcohol from the blood before the blood circulates to the rest of the body.

The only digestive function of the liver is the production of bile by the hepatocytes (liver cells). Bile flows through small bile ducts, then through larger ones, and leaves the liver by way of the hepatic duct (Fig. 32–1), which joins the cystic duct of the gallbladder to form the common bile duct, which carries bile to the duodenum.

Bile is mostly water and has an excretory function in that it carries bilirubin and excess cholesterol to the intestines for elimination in feces. The digestive function of bile is accomplished by bile salts, which emulsify fats in the small intestine. Emulsification is a type of mechanical digestion in which large fat globules are broken into smaller globules but are not chemically changed. Production of bile is stimulated by the hormone secretin, which is produced by the duodenum when food enters the small intestine.

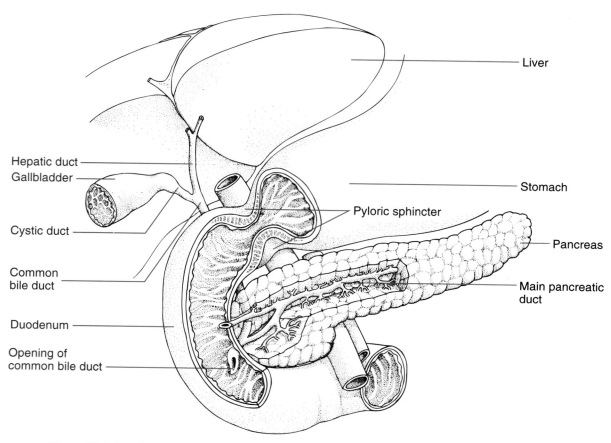

Figure 32–1. The liver, gallbladder, pancreas, and duodenum. (Modified from Scanlon, VC, Sanders, T: Workbook for Essentials of Anatomy and Physiology, ed 2. FA Davis, Philadelphia, 1995, p 257, with permission.)

Functions of the Liver

The liver is involved in a great variety of metabolic functions, most of which involve the synthesis of specific enzymes. For the sake of simplicity these functions may be grouped into categories.

Carbohydrate Metabolism

The liver regulates the blood glucose level by storing excess glucose as glycogen and changing glycogen back to glucose when the blood glucose level is low. The liver also changes other monosaccharides such as fructose and galactose to glucose, which is more readily used by cells for energy production.

Amino Acid Metabolism

The liver regulates the blood levels of amino acids based on tissue needs for protein synthesis. Of the 20 amino acids needed for the production of human proteins, the liver is able to synthesize 12, called the nonessential amino acids, by the process of transamination. The other eight amino acids, which the liver cannot synthesize, are called the essential amino acids. Essential amino acids are required in the diet.

Excess amino acids (those not needed for protein synthesis) undergo the process of deamination in the liver; the

amino group is removed and the remaining carbon chain is converted to a simple carbohydrate that is used for energy production or converted to fat for energy storage. The amino groups are converted to urea, a nitrogenous waste product that is removed from the blood by the kidneys and excreted in urine.

Lipid Metabolism

The liver forms lipoproteins for the transport of fats in the blood to other tissues. The liver also synthesizes cholesterol and excretes excess cholesterol into bile to be eliminated in feces.

The liver is also the main site of the process called beta oxidation, in which fatty acid molecules are split into two-carbon acetyl groups. These acetyl groups may be used by the liver to produce energy, or they may be combined to form ketones to be transported to other cells for energy production.

Synthesis of Plasma Proteins

The liver synthesizes albumin, clotting factors, and globulins. Albumin, the most abundant plasma protein, helps maintain blood volume by pulling tissue fluid into capillaries. Clotting factors produced by the liver include prothrombin and fibrinogen, which circulate in the blood until needed for chemical clotting. The globulins synthesized by the liver become part of lipoproteins or act as carriers for other molecules in the blood.

Formation of Bilirubin

The fixed macrophages of the liver phagocytize old red blood cells (RBCs) and form bilirubin from the heme portion of their hemoglobin. The liver also removes from the blood the bilirubin formed in the spleen and red bone marrow, and excretes it into bile to be eliminated in feces.

Phagocytosis by Kupffer Cells

The fixed macrophages of the liver are called Kupffer cells; they phagocytize pathogens that circulate through the liver. Many of the bacteria that get to the liver come from the colon, after being absorbed as the colon absorbs water. These bacteria are normal flora of the colon but would be very harmful elsewhere in the body. Portal circulation brings this blood to the liver first, however, and the bacteria are phagocytized by Kupffer cells.

Storage

The liver stores the minerals iron and copper, the fat-soluble vitamins A, D, E, and K, and the water-soluble vitamin B_{12}.

Detoxification

The liver synthesizes enzymes that will change harmful substances to less harmful ones. Alcohol and medications are examples of potentially toxic chemicals. The liver also converts ammonia from the colon bacteria to urea, a less toxic substance.

GALLBLADDER

The gallbladder is a muscular sac about 3 to 4 inches long located on the undersurface of the right lobe of the liver. Bile in the hepatic duct from the liver flows through the cystic duct (Fig. 32–1) into the gallbladder, which stores bile until it is needed in the small intestine. The gallbladder also concentrates bile by absorbing water.

When fatty foods enter the duodenum, the duodenal mucosa secretes the hormone cholecystokinin. One function of cholecystokinin is to stimulate contraction of the smooth muscle of the wall of the gallbladder. Contraction of the gallbladder forces bile into the cystic duct, then into the common bile duct, which empties into the duodenum.

PANCREAS

The pancreas is about 6 inches long, between the curve of the duodenum and the spleen in the upper right abdominal quadrant (Fig. 32–1). The digestive secretions of the pancreas are produced by exocrine glands called acini. The small ducts of these glands unite to form larger ducts, and finally the main pancreatic duct (there may be an accessory duct also), which emerges from the medial side, or head, of the pancreas and joins the common bile duct.

The pancreatic digestive enzymes are involved in the digestion of all three food types. The enzyme amylase digests starch to maltose; lipase converts emulsified fats to fatty acids and glycerol. Trypsinogen is an inactive enzyme that is changed to active trypsin in the duodenum. Trypsin digests polypeptides to shorter chains of amino acids.

The pancreas also produces a bicarbonate juice, which is alkaline because of its high sodium bicarbonate content. The function of bicarbonate juice is to neutralize the hydrochloric acid in gastric juice as it enters the duodenum from the stomach. The pH of duodenal chyme is raised to about 7.5, which prevents corrosive damage to the mucosa.

Secretion of pancreatic juice is stimulated by the hormones of the duodenal mucosa. Secretin stimulates the production of bicarbonate pancreatic juice, and cholecystokinin stimulates secretion of the pancreatic enzyme juice.

AGING AND THE LIVER, GALLBLADDER, AND PANCREAS

The liver usually continues to function well into old age, unless damaged by pathogens such as the hepatitis viruses or by toxins such as alcohol. There is a greater tendency for gallstones to form, sometimes necessitating removal of the gallbladder. In the absence of specific pathologies, the pancreas usually functions well, although acute pancreatitis of unknown cause is somewhat more likely in the elderly.

Nursing Assessment

The nurse assessing the client with disease of the liver, pancreas, or gallbladder uses the same systematic approach as when assessing other organ systems. The client is made as comfortable as possible before beginning the assessment process.

NURSING HISTORY

A client history is obtained. Elements of the client history include a complete description of any abdominal pain or tenderness. The client is asked what events cause or provoke pain; what actions, if any, relieve or palliate the pain; the quality of the pain, such as sharp, dull, boring, or burning; the location or in what region the pain occurs; the severity of the pain; and the timing or when the pain occurs. Using the WHAT'S UP? model (presented in Chapter 2) will help the nurse remember all the elements that need to be included in a complete symptom assessment.

The client is questioned about any nausea, vomiting, or abdominal distention. Information about the timing or other frequent triggers of episodes of nausea or vomiting may help the physician identify their cause. Such information may also help determine appropriate treatment for any future nausea or vomiting. Abdominal distention in the presence of nausea and vomiting may indicate intestinal obstruction. Clients with liver, gallbladder, or pancreatic disease may also complain of feeling bloated, of having gas or belching frequently, or of right upper quadrant (RUQ) tenderness.

The client is questioned about any observed changes in bowel elimination. Diarrhea may be caused by irritation of the bowel. Constipation may indicate decreased water intake or excessive water loss. The client's stool is observed for evidence of bacteria (a foul smell), fat (stool floats on the water surface and appears greasy), pus, blood, or mucus. Clients with liver or gallbladder disease may have pale or clay-colored stools.

Clients with disease of the liver, pancreas, or gallbladder commonly have changes in appetite such as anorexia or changes in eating preferences. The client is questioned about any abnormal weight loss or unexpected weight gain and changes in food tolerance, including the type or amount of offending foods. For example, clients with gallbladder disease may report that they feel nauseated or bloated after eating fried or greasy foods.

The client's history should note whether there is a family history of liver, pancreas, or gallbladder diseases such as diabetes mellitus, alcoholism, cancer, heart disease, or bleeding tendencies. These diseases have a high incidence within families.

A social history is obtained. The nurse needs to determine whether the client ingests alcohol or uses other recreational drugs. If the client does acknowledge using alcohol or other drugs, the type, frequency, and amount used are recorded. The nurse also needs to ask the client what medications are being taken with or without a physician's prescription. Many people do not consider over-the-counter preparations, herbal, or natural products that they purchase without a prescription important enough to report, and must be asked specifically to do so. Clients are particularly questioned about the use of antacids, laxatives, vitamins, or pain relievers such as aspirin or nonsteroidal anti-inflammatory drugs (NSAIDs).

The nurse asks about the client's usual work activities and work setting. Exposure to chemicals such as paint fumes, industrial dyes, acids, farm pesticides, or other liver-toxic substances is documented.

The client's activities other than work are investigated. Reports of fatigue are documented along with information about when the fatigue occurs. The client is questioned about stressors such as financial concerns, problems dealing with the health care environment, and any family or personal problems. The nurse attempts to determine what coping mechanisms the client usually employs to deal with stressors.

PHYSICAL ASSESSMENT

The nurse assists with a thorough physical assessment of the client. Instead of following the usual inspect-palpate-percuss-auscultate (IPPA) format, the abdomen is assessed starting with inspection, then auscultation, percussion, and palpation. This is to prevent palpation from changing other assessment findings.

Inspection

Assessment begins with inspection of the client's skin for scars, **striae** (light silvery-colored or thin red lines on the abdomen), bruising, **caput medusae** (bluish-purple swollen vein pattern extending out from the navel), and **spider angiomas** (thin reddish-purple vein lines close to the skin surface). The client's abdomen is observed for any visible masses, visible movement or peristalsis, **jaundice,** or **icterus** (yellowing of the skin and the sclera of the eye).

Jaundice

Jaundice (also called icterus) is a cardinal symptom of liver or gallbladder disease and red blood cell disorders. Old red blood cells are cleared from the circulatory system by phagocytes in the spleen, liver, lymph nodes, and bone marrow. In the process, the compound heme (part of hemoglobin) is split into iron and another substance that is metabolized to bilirubin. The liver is then responsible for converting bilirubin to a water-soluble compound that can be excreted in bile. If the liver is unable to convert or conjugate bilirubin to a water-soluble compound, or if bile drainage is obstructed, serum bilirubin will elevate and pigments will be deposited in body tissues.

When serum bilirubin levels elevate, the client's skin color changes to yellow. The yellow color varies from pale yellow to a striking golden orange. The color intensity is directly related to the amount of elevation of the serum bilirubin. Jaundice can be seen in nearly every body tissue and fluid where there is any amount of albumin. Pigment may occasionally be seen in cerebrospinal fluid or joint fluid. Pigment is not seen in saliva or tears. Urine becomes dark, and if bile flow to the bowel is obstructed, stools will be a light clay color. (See Cultural Considerations Box 32–1.) The nurse should describe any abnormal finding completely in the client's record and report the information promptly.

Auscultation

Inspection should be followed with auscultation of bowel sounds with a stethoscope. All four quadrants should be

---

**CULTURAL CONSIDERATIONS
BOX 32–1**

The nurse should be aware of the variations of assessing for jaundice among people of color. To assess for jaundice in a dark-skinned client, the nurse needs to look at the sclera, conjunctiva, palms of hands, soles of feet, and in the buccal mucosa for patches of bilirubin pigment.

auscultated, at least 1 minute in each quadrant. Normal bowel sounds are heard every 5 to 15 seconds. Bowel sounds are considered normal if they occur within a range of 5 to 30 per minute and are soft gurgles or clicking sounds. If the client has recently had surgery, bowel sounds may be absent or occur less frequently than five per minute. High-pitched, frequent sounds may indicate hypermotility of the bowel or early bowel obstruction. It may be possible to hear circulatory sounds if the stethoscope is placed over the abdominal aorta. Clients with chronic liver failure may have a humming sound over their liver. This finding usually indicates overloaded venous circulation in the liver.

Percussion

The experienced practitioner may percuss the abdomen to determine the presence of masses, fluid, or air in the abdominal cavity. The normal sounds heard during percussion of the abdomen are tympany (musical drumlike sound over hollow air-filled space) or dull (a soft thudding sound over solid organs such as the liver). If an abnormal amount of fluid has collected in the peritoneal cavity, a sloshing sound may be heard when the client turns side to side or shifts position.

Palpation

Light palpation of the abdomen concludes the physical assessment. The nurse depresses the abdomen not more than ½ to 1 inch during the palpation. Any muscle tension, rigidity, masses, or expressions of pain are noted. Deep palpation of the abdomen is done only by physicians and highly skilled nurses such as nurse practitioners.

Diagnostic Studies

Various blood, urine, and stool specimen tests in addition to other radiologic, endoscopic, and ultrasonographic procedures are able to reveal abnormalities of the liver, gallbladder, and pancreas.

LABORATORY TESTS

Laboratory tests and normal values listed in Table 32–1 are the common tests performed to detect problems with the liver, gallbladder, and pancreas. Bilirubin is an excellent measure of liver and gallbladder functioning. In addition, certain enzymes such as alanine aminotransferase (ALT), aspartate aminotransferase (AST), and lactic dehydroge-

Table 32–1. **Laboratory Tests for Liver, Gallbladder, and Pancreas Disorders**

Test	Normal Range	Significance
	Blood	
Alanine aminotransferase (ALT)	5–35 IU/dL	↑ in chronic liver failure and hepatitis
Albumin	3.1–4.3 g/dL	↓ in liver disease
Amylase	53–123 U/L	↑ in pancreatitis, gallstones
Ammonia	12–55 mol/L	↑ in chronic liver failure, hepatitis
Aspartate aminotransferase (AST)	8–20 units/L	↑ in chronic liver failure, viral hepatitis, acute pancreatitis
Bilirubin		
Total serum	0.1–1.0 mg/dL	↑ in liver and gallbladder disease with red blood cell destruction
Conjugated (direct)	0.0–0.4 mg/dL	↑ in gallbladder obstruction
Unconjugated (indirect)	0.1–1.0 mg/dL	↑ with red blood cell destruction or liver disease
Calcium	9–10.5 mg/dL	↓ with acute pancreatitis or malabsorption
Cholesterol	150–200 mg/dL	↑ in pancreatitis, gallbladder disease; ↓ may indicate severe liver disease
Lactic dehydrogenase (LDH)	110–250 IU/L	↑ in liver disease
Potassium	3.5–5.0 mEq/L	↓ with diarrhea, intestinal fistulas, vomiting, suctioning
Prothrombin time	11–12.5 s	↑ in liver disease, vitamin K deficiency
	Urine	
Urine amylase	Depends on test	↑ in acute pancreatitis
Urine bilirubin	Negative	↑ in chronic liver failure, hepatitis, biliary obstruction
Urobilinogen	0.3–1.0 Ehrlich units in 2 h	↑ with destruction of red blood cells, hepatitis, chronic liver failure, obstructive jaundice
	Feces	
Fecal fat malabsorption	Negative	↑ in pancreatic disease
Occult blood	Negative	Positive in cancer, bleeding tendencies from ↓ vitamin K

nase (LDH) are released by damaged liver cells. Elevations in these blood values in the absence of known trauma are excellent indicators of liver damage.

CRITICAL THINKING: Mr. Lee

Mr. Lee is admitted with acute pancreatitis. You note that his amylase level is quite elevated. Why do you think amylase is elevated in the client with pancreatitis?

Answer at end of chapter.

RADIOLOGY

A flat-plate x-ray of the abdomen is usually the first diagnostic radiologic procedure the physician will order. The flat-plate x-ray may show abdominal structures, abnormal masses, or blockage of normal bowel action. There is no client preparation required.

Upper Gastrointestinal Series

This test is usually ordered for clients complaining of nausea, vomiting, weight loss, or abdominal pain. These complaints are common for clients with liver, gallbladder, or pancreas disorders. The client is allowed nothing by mouth after midnight before the test. The nurse answers any client concerns and explains that the client will be asked to swallow a large measure of barium (a substance that is opaque on x-rays) during the procedure. The client will be placed on an x-ray table, and x-rays will be taken in various positions and times during the procedure. The client should understand that the procedure may take several hours depending on the rate at which the barium moves through the client's gastrointestinal tract. A laxative such as milk of magnesia may be given after the procedure to aid in the evacuation of the barium.

Lower Gastrointestinal Series

The physician may order a barium enema (BE, or LGI series) if the client has reported any changes in bowel functioning, such as diarrhea or constipation, or blood or mucus in the stool (Fig. 32–2). The client is asked to eat a low-residue diet for 2 days before the scheduled procedure, then a clear liquid meal the night before the exam. The client is allowed nothing by mouth after midnight before the test. Further, the client is asked to use a powerful laxative such as bisacodyl (Dulcolax) or magnesium citrate (Citrate of Magnesia) to cleanse the bowel for clearer and more accurate x-ray views. Enemas may also be ordered. During the procedure barium is given by enema and the client is asked to retain the barium while x-rays are taken. The client may experience some abdominal cramping and an urge to have a bowel movement during the procedure. The client is told to take slow, deep breaths and to tighten the anal sphincter. The rate of flow of the barium is slowed until the cramping diminishes.

After the procedure, the client is instructed to drink plenty of fluids and that a mild laxative may be necessary to eliminate the barium, because barium left in the bowel tends to harden and become difficult to evacuate. The stool should be observed for complete evacuation of the barium to prevent an impaction. Stools will change from clay colored or white to a brown color when the barium is gone.

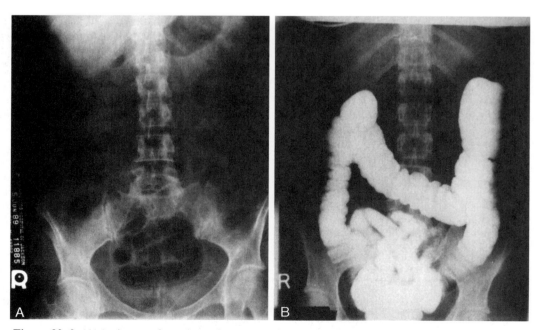

Figure 32–2. *(A)* An image of a patient who was poorly prepared for a barium enema. *(B)* An image of a patient who was adequately prepared for a barium enema. (Courtesy of Dr. Russell Tobe.)

Oral Cholecystogram

An oral **cholecystogram** (gallbladder series) may be ordered if the physician suspects gallstones. The client is asked to ingest a radiopaque dye that collects in bile in the gallbladder. The dye then shows up when the client has x-rays, showing the gallbladder, ducts, and any gallstones. In preparation, the client is asked to eat a high-fat diet for 2 days before the test. The client is asked to eat a low-fat diet the day before the exam. Depending on agency protocol, the client takes radiopaque tablets, usually six, the evening before the exam. Some agencies ask the client to take the pills for two nights before the exam. The client takes them with water about 5 minutes apart. The client then has nothing by mouth after midnight of the day of the exam. The radiopaque tablets contain iodine, so clients are asked about any allergies to iodine or shellfish (which contain iodine). The client is also told that the tablets may cause diarrhea. The procedure will take about ½ hour in the x-ray department.

Computed Tomography

A computed tomography (CT) scan may be ordered for any suspected abnormalities of liver, gallbladder, or pancreas functioning. The computer-enhanced x-rays may be taken with or without contrast medium. There is no client preparation necessary. The client is told that he or she will be on a narrow, hard x-ray table that is closely surrounded by a noisy metal shell. Clients with fear of closed spaces may have to make arrangements for a CT scan at an "open" scanner. There are no follow-up care requirements.

CRITICAL THINKING: Mrs. Pearl

Mrs. Pearl is a 95-year-old woman undergoing an LGI series for complaints of abdominal pain. As her nurse, what additional concerns might you have for Mrs. Pearl as she undergoes this test?

Answer at end of chapter.

ANGIOGRAPHY

Intravenous cholangiography may be ordered for clients with symptoms of biliary obstruction or after a cholecystectomy. This exam permits the radiologist to see the gallbladder and biliary ducts by injecting a contrast medium intravenously, which then collects in those structures. The injection of contrast medium is done about 1 hour before the exam. X-rays are taken about every 20 minutes for 1

hour or until the structures are readily viewed. The radiopaque material is iodine based, so the client is asked about any allergies to iodine. There are no follow-up care requirements after the procedure.

LIVER SCAN

This test involves injecting a slightly radioactive medium that is taken up by the liver. An instrument is passed over the liver that records the amount of material taken up by the liver and forms a composite "picture" of the liver. The physician may be able to determine tumors, masses, and abnormal size and patterns of blood vessel. The procedure takes a short time.

ENDOSCOPY

The physician may order an endoscopic examination of the gastrointestinal tract for client complaints such as bleeding or if cancer or obstruction is suspected. Endoscopic examination permits the physician to directly view the structures of portions of the gastrointestinal tract with an instrument that contains flexible optic fibers. In addition to viewing the structures, the physician can also remove polyps, take biopsies, and coagulate bleeding sites that are identified.

Esophagogastroduodenoscopy

An **esophagogastroduodenoscopy** (EGD) will let the physician view the esophagus, stomach, and duodenum. The client is asked not to take anything by mouth after about 8 P.M. the night before the examination. Clients may be asked to sign an operative consent form, and a preoperative checklist may be necessary, depending on institution policy. Just before the procedure, the client is asked to remove dentures. At the start of the procedure, the client is given medication such as midazolam hydrochloride (Versed) or diazepam (Valium) for relaxation. Doses of the medications may be given at intervals during the procedure. The client may be given atropine sulfate to dry secretions in the mouth. The physician will usually spray the back of the throat with a topical anesthetic to ease passage of the endoscope.

Follow-up care includes placing side rails up until the client is fully alert. The client is not given anything by mouth for up to 2 hours or until the gag reflex returns. The nurse checks the gag reflex and observes the client for any bleeding, complaints of pain, or signs of perforation such as abdominal pain, tenderness, or guarding.

Endoscopic Retrograde Cholangiopancreatography

Endoscopic **retrograde cholangiopancreatography** (ERCP) will permit the physician to visualize the liver, gallbladder, and pancreas (Fig. 32–3). The procedure allows both direct viewing and use of contrast medium. An

---

cholecystogram: chole—bile + cysto—bladder + gram—writing
esophagogastroduodenoscopy: esophago—esophagus + gastro—stomach + duoden—duodenum + oscopy—to examine
retrograde cholangiopancreatography: retro—backward + grade—step + chol—bile + angio—via the vessels + pancreat—pancreas + ography—writing

endoscope is passed through the esophagus to the duodenum, where dye is injected that outlines the pancreatic and bile ducts.

The client is prepared for an ERCP the same as for an EGD, with nothing by mouth after 8 P.M. the night before the exam. In addition, the client is asked about any allergies to iodine. The nurse ensures that any ordered laboratory studies such as a prothrombin time have been done before the procedure and that the client has removed any dentures. Follow-up care is similar to an EGD. In addition, the nurse is alert to client complaints such as increased right upper quadrant pain, fever, or chills, which may indicate infection. Hypotension, tachycardia or rapid heart rate, increasing RUQ pain, nausea, or vomiting may indicate perforation or the onset of pancreatitis.

ULTRASONOGRAPHY

The use of high-frequency sound waves through the abdomen allows the physician to view soft-tissue structures. The sound waves reflect varying images based on the density of the soft tissues in the abdomen. The client is asked not to take anything by mouth after midnight on the day of the exam. A clear gel is applied to the abdomen and to the transducer on the sonograph. The gel improves the conduction of sound waves and thus improves the images obtained. The transducer is placed on the skin and moved over the abdomen while the technician views the sonograph screen and takes periodic pictures. The procedure takes about ½ hour and requires no follow-up care.

PERCUTANEOUS LIVER BIOPSY

If less invasive tests do not aid in diagnosis of liver disease, a liver biopsy may be done. This may be done to identify cancer, cirrhosis, hepatitis, or other causes of liver disease. The physician generally uses a needle through the skin and into the liver to withdraw a small sample for examination. This procedure places the client at risk for

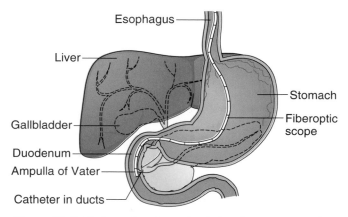

Figure 32–3. Endoscopic retrograde cholangiopancreatography. (Modified from Watson and Jaffe: Nurses Manual of Laboratory and Diagnostic Tests. FA Davis, Philadelphia, 1995, p 525, with permission.)

bleeding, because the liver is highly vascular and because many clients with liver disease have faulty clotting ability.

Before the biopsy, the nurse ensures that the client understands the procedure and that a consent has been signed if required by institution policy. The nurse also ensures that lab work such as a complete blood count and coagulation studies has been completed and reviewed as ordered. The client may be NPO (nothing by mouth) for 6 to 8 hours before the procedure. Baseline vital signs are taken, and a sedative is given if ordered.

During the procedure the nurse assists the physician to position the client on his or her back or left side and assists the client to hold very still while the needle is being introduced. The physician may also ask the client to exhale and hold his or her breath during the needle insertion.

After the biopsy, the client should remain on bed rest for 24 hours. The client lies on the right side for the first 2 hours with a small pillow or rolled towel under the biopsy site to provide pressure and prevent bleeding. Vital signs and the site are monitored for signs of bleeding. The client is advised to avoid coughing or straining. Analgesics are offered for comfort if ordered.

Review Questions

1. Which of the following is NOT stored in the liver?
   a. Fat
   b. Iron
   c. Glycogen
   d. Vitamins D and E

2. Bile is stored and concentrated by which of the following?
   a. Liver
   b. Gallbladder
   c. Hepatic duct
   d. Cystic duct

3. The enzymes of the pancreas are involved in the digestion of which foods?
   a. Starch and fat only
   b. Starch, fat, and protein
   c. Fat and protein only
   d. Starch and protein only

4. Which of the following complications should the nurse monitor for after a liver biopsy?
   a. Headache
   b. Muscle cramps
   c. Bleeding
   d. Respiratory distress

5. Which of the following nursing measures is most important after an upper or lower GI series?
   a. Offer a laxative as ordered.
   b. Place pressure on the puncture site.
   c. Check for return of a gag reflex.
   d. Monitor vital signs.

ANSWERS TO CRITICAL THINKING

CRITICAL THINKING: Mr. Lee

Pancreatitis is an inflammation of the pancreas. The pancreas normally secretes the digestive enzyme amylase. The inflammation causes an increase in the secretion of this enzyme into the pancreas and thus into the bloodstream. This test is often used to monitor the progress of pancreatitis.

CRITICAL THINKING: Mrs. Pearl

Mrs. Pearl is at risk for dehydration and electrolyte loss due to the laxative and enema prep and NPO status. This risk is increased because of her age. The nurse will need to monitor fluid and electrolyte status closely.

Mrs. Pearl will likely have a concern about "making it" to the bathroom during the prep, and should have a bedside commode placed within easy reach. The nurse should answer the call light promptly. If enemas are ordered "until clear," Mrs. Pearl will be at greater risk for fluid and electrolyte loss. If more than two or three enemas are required, the physician should be notified.

Elderly clients can become very fatigued during testing and test preps. Mrs. Pearl should be allowed plenty of rest before and after the test. She may also have a concern about being able to hold the barium in her bowel during the test without having an "accident." She should be assured that the barium is held in with a balloon on the end of the enema catheter and that bathrooms are nearby.

BIBLIOGRAPHY

Beare, PG, and Myers, JL: Principles and Practice of Adult Health Nursing, ed 2. Mosby, St Louis, 1994.

Ignatavicius, DD, Workman, ML, and Mishler, MA: Medical-Surgical Nursing: A Nursing Process Approach, ed 2. WB Saunders, Philadelphia, 1995.

Markell, EK, Voge, M, and John, DT: Medical Gastrology. WB Saunders, Philadelphia, 1992.

Monroe, D: Patient teaching for x-ray and other diagnostics. RN 52, April 1990.

Watson, J, and Jaffe, MS: Nurse's Manual of Laboratory and Diagnostic Tests, ed 2. FA Davis, Philadelphia, 1995.

Nursing Care of Clients with Liver, Gallbladder, and Pancreatic Disorders

33

Elaine Bishop Kennedy

Learning Objectives

Upon completion of this chapter, the student will be able to:

1. Explain the causes, risk factors, and pathophysiology of acute and chronic liver failure.
2. Describe the diagnostic tests and values used to identify acute and chronic liver failure and their complications.
3. Discuss causes, prevention, and treatment of complications in acute and chronic liver failure.
4. Discuss the treatment of clients with acute and chronic liver failure, including diet, medications, surgery, and practices to control bleeding.
5. Describe five common complications of chronic liver failure.
6. Describe the diagnostic tests and values used to identify cancer of the liver and its complications.
7. Discuss treatment of clients with cancer of the liver.
8. Explain the causes, risk factors, and pathophysiology of various types of viral hepatitis.
9. Describe the causes, prevention, and medical and nursing treatment of viral hepatitis.
10. Use the nursing process to plan care for the client with a disorder of the liver.
11. Describe the diagnostic tests and values used to identify acute and chronic pancreatitis and its complications.
12. Discuss the medical and nursing care of the client with acute or chronic pancreatitis.
13. Describe the diagnostic tests and values used to identify cancer of the pancreas and its complications.
14. Describe causes, prevention, medical and nursing treatment, and treatment of complications of cancer of the pancreas.
15. Use the nursing process to plan care for the client with a disorder of the pancreas.
16. Describe the diagnostic tests and values used to identify cholecystitis and cholelithiasis and their complications.

17. Describe causes, prevention, medical and nursing treatment, and treatment of complications of cholecystitis and cholelithiasis.
18. Describe the diagnostic tests and values used to identify cancer of the gallbladder and its complications.
19. Describe causes, prevention, complications, and medical treatment of cancer of the gallbladder.
20. Use the nursing process to plan care for the client with a disorder of the gallbladder.

Key Words

ascites (a-**SIGH**-teez)
asterixis (AS-ter-**ICK**-sis)
cholecystitis (KOH-lee-sis-**TIGH**-tis)
choledochoscopy (koh-LED-oh-**KOS**-koh-pee)
choledocholithiasis (koh-LED-oh-koh-li-**THIGH**-ah-sis)
cholelithiasis (KOH-lee-li-**THIGH**-ah-sis)
cirrhosis (si-**ROH**-sis)
colic (**KAH**-lick)
encephalopathy (en-SEFF-uh-**LAHP**-ah-thee)
extracorporeal shock-wave lithotripsy (ECKS-trah-koar-**POR**-ee-uhl SHAHK-wayv LITH-oh-**TRIP**-see)
fetor hepaticus (**FEE**-tor he-**PAT**-i-kus)
hepatitis (HEP-uh-**TIGH**-tis)
hepatorenal syndrome (hep-**PAT**-oh-REE-nuhl **SIN**-drohm)
laparoscopy (LAP-uh-roh-**SKOP**-ee)
pancreatectomy (partial, total) (PAN-kree-uh-**TECK**-tuh-mee)
portal hypertension (**POR**-tuhl HIGH-per-**TEN**-shun)
steatorrhea (STEE-ah-toh-**REE**-ah)
T-tube (**TEE**-toob)
transjugular intrahepatic portosystemic shunts (**TRANZ**-jug-u-lar in-tra-hep-**PAT**-ick por-to-sis-**TEM**-ick SHUNT)
varices (**VAR**-i-seez)

Disorders of the Liver

HEPATITIS

Hepatitis is an inflammation of the cells of the liver, usually caused by a virus. Less commonly, hepatitis may be caused by drugs. Symptoms of hepatitis may range from nearly no symptoms to life-threatening symptoms from liver necrosis or death of liver tissue.

Pathophysiology

Hepatitis is usually caused by one of five viruses:

Hepatitis A virus (HAV), sometimes called infectious hepatitis

Hepatitis B virus (HBV), sometimes called serum hepatitis

Hepatitis C virus (HCV), sometimes called non-A, non-B (NANB) hepatitis

Hepatitis D virus (HDV)

Hepatitis E virus (HEV)

The viral agents vary by mode of infection, incubation period, symptoms, diagnostic tests, and preventive vaccines (Table 33–1). The response to viral infection is similar to the inflammatory response to other viruses, infecting organisms, or foreign matter. The body attempts to rid itself of the invader virus by redness, organ swelling, and the resulting loss of function.

There are approximately 60,000 new cases of hepatitis in the United States yearly. The incidence of HAV increased nearly 27 percent in the mid-1980s and is the most common cause of hepatitis. Hepatitis A virus has a low mortality rate. However, HBV is more common among some groups, including health care workers and intravenous drug users; it has a mortality rate of about 5 percent.

Prevention

The hepatitis viruses are very resistant to a wide range of anti-infective measures such as drying, heat, ultraviolet light exposure, freezing, and bleach and other disinfectants. The hepatitis viruses require at least 30 minutes in boiling water to guarantee their destruction. The best methods for preventing the transmission of the hepatitis viruses are careful attention to cleanliness and the use of vaccines such as immune serum globulin (ISG) or vaccines to HBV and HAV. Health care workers must use universal precautions at all times. Infection control precautions should reflect the usual mode of transmission of the particular hepatitis virus.

Immune serum globulin is a temporary, passive, nonspecific immunity to hepatitis. Permanent, active immunity is acquired from the body's own antibodies in response to actual viral infection. The active immunity is to the specific virus to which the body has developed antibodies. Vaccines

to HBV are available and provide permanent, active immunity to HBV. Health care workers are strongly encouraged to be vaccinated for HBV. A vaccine for HAV has also been developed.

Public health measures such as health education programs, licensing and supervision of public facilities, screening of blood donors, and careful screening of food handlers are general measures to prevent the transmission of hepatitis viruses.

Signs and Symptoms

Hepatitis usually shows a typical pattern of loss of liver function. There are generally three stages in hepatitis:

1. The prodromal, or preicteric (prejaundice), stage lasts about 1 week. The client complains of flulike symptoms of malaise, headache, anorexia, low-grade fever, and possibly dull right upper quadrant (RUQ) pain.
2. The icteric stage lasts 4 to 6 weeks. The client complains of more severe fatigue, anorexia, nausea, vomiting, and malaise. The client is also likely to have jaundice or noticeable yellowing of the skin, sclera of the eyes, and other mucous membranes. The liver is usually enlarged and tender on examination.
3. The posticteric, or convalescent, stage lasts from 2 to 4 weeks to months. The client usually feels well during this time, but full recovery as measured by the return to normal of all liver function tests may take as long as 1 year.

Hepatitis is considered a reversible process if the client complies with a medical regimen of adequate rest, good nutrition, and abstinence from alcohol or other liver toxic agents. See Chapter 32 for a more complete discussion of signs and symptoms of jaundice.

Complications

Hepatitis may lead to fulminant or acute liver failure. About 5 percent of hepatitis clients progress to chronic liver failure. Some clients become asymptomatic carriers of the virus; HBV-infected carrier clients have a greater risk of developing cancer of the liver.

Diagnostic Tests

Serum liver enzymes are elevated. Serum bilirubin and urobilinogen may be elevated. The erythrocyte sedimentation rate will usually be elevated from the inflammatory process. There may be possible elevation of the prothrombin time with severe hepatitis (Table 33–2). Serologic tests may be ordered to determine the specific virus caus-

---

hepatitis: hepat—liver + itis—inflammation
necrosis: necr—death + osis—condition

Table 33–I. Comparison of Types of Viral Hepatitis

	Hepatitis A Virus (HAV)	Hepatitis B Virus (HBV)	Hepatitis C Virus (HCV)	Hepatitis D Virus (HDV)	Hepatitis E Virus (HEV)
Mode of transmission	Oral-fecal contamination of water, shellfish, eating utensils, or equipment	Blood or body fluids such as saliva, semen, and breast milk; equipment contaminated by blood	Blood transfusions, intravenous drug use, unprotected sex	Blood or body fluids as with HBV; strongly linked as a coinfection with HBV	Usually contaminated water
Incubation period	3 to 7 weeks	2 to 5 months	1 week to months	Same as HBV	2 to 9 weeks
Symptoms	Early (prodromal): fatigue, anorexia, malaise, nausea, or vomiting Icteric: jaundice, pale stools, amber or dark urine, RUQ pain	May have no early symptoms Early (prodromal): 1–2 months of fatigue, malaise, anorexia, low-grade fever, nausea, headache, abdominal pain, muscle aches Icteric: jaundice, rashes	Same as HBV, usually less severe	Similar to HAV and to HBV but more severe	Similar to HAV
Diagnostic tests	Elevated serum liver enzymes (ALT, AST), elevated serum bilirubin, hepatitis A antigen	Elevated serum liver enzymes (ALT, AST), elevated serum bilirubin, hepatitis B antigen	Elevated serum liver enzymes (ALT, AST), elevated serum bilirubin	Elevated serum liver enzymes (ALT, AST), elevated serum bilirubin, hepatitis D antigen	Elevated serum liver enzymes (ALT, AST), elevated serum bilirubin
Preventive vaccine	Immune globulin (IG)	Immune globulin (IG) or HBIG	None	HBIG	None

Table 33–2. **Laboratory Tests for Hepatitis**

Test	Normal Range	Significance
Alanine aminotransferase (ALT)	5–35 IU/mL	Found in high concentrations in liver cells; released with death of liver cells
Aspartate aminotransferase (AST)	8–20 U/L	Found in high concentrations in liver cells; released with death of liver cells

Erythrocyte sedimentation rate	Adult:
	    Women, 1–20 mm/h
	    Men, 1–13 mm/h
		Increased with inflammation and tissue damage

Prothrombin time	Control: 8.8–11.6 s Therapeutic: 1.2–1.5 times control	Liver can no longer make prothrombin
Serological tests		
Anti-HAV	Negative titer	Indicates exposure and probable infection with virus
Anti-HBV	Negative titer	Indicates exposure and probable infection with virus
Anti-HCV	Negative titer	Indicates exposure and probable infection with virus

ing the hepatitis. Each virus has specific antigen markers that serological study can reveal. The antigen markers can be further used to determine the degree of healing from the hepatitis. Abdominal x-ray may show an enlarged liver.

Medical Treatment

Medical treatment is aimed at providing rest and adequate nutrition for healing. There are no specific drugs or other medical therapies for hepatitis. With proper rest and nutrition, the liver should recover.

Clients are restricted from any alcohol or drugs that are known to be toxic to the liver (Table 33–3). In addition, clients are generally placed on limited activity with bathroom privileges. Because the client usually experiences malaise, fatigue, and anorexia, rest is advised. As the client improves, activity may be increased if the client does not become fatigued.

Table 33–3. **Common Hepatotoxic Substances**

Ethyl alcohol
Acetaminophen (Tylenol)
Acetylsalicylic acid (aspirin)
Anesthetic agents
    Halothane
Diazepam (Valium)
Erythromycin estolate (Ilosone)
Isoniazid (INH)
Methyldopa (Aldomet)
Oral contraceptives
Phenobarbital (Luminal)
Phenytoin (Dilantin)
Tranquilizers
    Chlorpromazine (Thorazine)
Industrial chemicals
    Carbon tetrachloride
    Trichloroethylene
    Toluene

Nursing Process

Assessment

The nurse assesses the client for subjective complaints such as malaise, fatigue, pruritus (itching), nausea, anorexia, and RUQ pain. Objective data, such as vomiting, pale stools, amber or dark-colored (tea-colored) urine, and jaundice, are recorded. The client's vital signs are taken, and a low-grade fever or any abnormal bruising or bleeding is reported immediately.

Nursing Diagnosis

Common nursing diagnoses for the client with viral hepatitis are as follows:

- Alteration in nutrition, less than body requirements related to anorexia, nausea, or vomiting
- Alteration in comfort, itching related to bilirubin pigment deposits in skin
- Pain related to inflammation and enlargement of the liver
- Risk for ineffective management of therapeutic regimen related to lack of knowledge of hepatitis and the treatment regimen

Planning

Major goals for the client with viral hepatitis include that the client will have adequate nutrition, describe pain and other discomforts as tolerable, and be able to self-manage the treatment regimen for viral hepatitis.

Implementation

ALTERATION IN NUTRITION. The usual ordered diet is a high-calorie, high-protein, high-carbohydrate, low-fat diet. There are no restrictions on what the client may eat, but the focus is to provide a well-rounded, nutritious diet. The nurse gives any antiemetic drug as ordered. Larger meals are given earlier in the day because nausea tends to increase during the day. The client is placed in an upright or sitting position for meals to decrease abdominal discomfort. Meals are served with attention to a quiet, pleasing environment without unpleasant noise or odors that may decrease appetite.

ALTERATION IN COMFORT. The physician may order an antihistamine to decrease the itching related to bilirubin pigment deposits in skin. The nurse encourages the client not to scratch, but to press firmly on the itching area. The client is encouraged to keep fingernails trimmed short so that vigorous scratching does not tear the skin. Room temperature is kept at a comfortable level to decrease perspiration, which may increase itching.

PAIN. The physician may order analgesics to decrease the pain related to inflammation and enlargement of the liver. The analgesics are administered as ordered. The client is evaluated frequently for abdominal pain and the extent of any RUQ tenderness.

RISK FOR INEFFECTIVE MANAGEMENT OF THERAPEUTIC REGIMEN. Clients are taught the necessity of proper home cleanliness, including hand washing after toileting and soap and hot water cleaning of eating utensils, cookware, and food preparation surfaces. Clients need to be taught how hepatitis affects their body and the importance of adequate rest and proper nutrition. Clients are also taught to avoid alcohol and other liver-toxic drugs.

Evaluation

Successful management of the client with hepatitis can be claimed if the client

Maintains body weight to within 2 pounds of preillness weight.

Remains free of breaks, cuts, or tears on skin.

Reports that abdominal pain or other discomfort is not greater than 2 on a 5-point scale.

Can state the effects of hepatitis and the necessity of adequate rest, proper nutrition, and necessary sanitation measures.

CRITICAL THINKING: Mrs. Rogers

Mrs. Rogers, a 28-year-old woman, is admitted to a medical-surgical nursing unit. During the admission process, Mrs. Rogers, who works as a nurse on the same unit, talks about her trip to a South American country with her husband about 4 weeks ago. Mrs. Rogers asks her nurse about several of the cancer patients she cared for, including administering intravenous chemotherapeutic drugs and blood transfusions, before leaving on her trip. Mrs. Rogers states that since her trip she has lost nearly 8 pounds, is frequently nauseated, has frequent headaches, and tires easily. Mrs. Rogers also tells the nurse that she is very irritable, which is different from her usual easygoing manner.

1. What information might lead Mrs. Rogers' nurse to suspect hepatitis A? Hepatitis B?
2. What precautions should be instituted for Mrs. Rogers?
3. What nursing actions might the nurse implement to help Mrs. Rogers improve her nutrition?
4. What medication orders for Mrs. Rogers would the nurse question?
5. What information should be included in a discharge teaching plan for Mrs. Rogers?

Answers at end of chapter.

FULMINANT (ACUTE) LIVER FAILURE

Fulminant, or acute, liver failure is a rapidly fatal liver disorder. Signs and symptoms of the disorder include hepatic **encephalopathy** or central nervous system dysfunction that develops within 8 weeks of the first symptoms of liver failure. Acute liver failure is an uncommon but gravely serious complication of liver disease and has a mortality rate as high as 50 percent.

Pathophysiology

Acute liver failure results from the sudden massive loss of liver tissue or necrosis. The cause of liver damage is usually drug toxicity or HBV in the presence of HDV. The outcome of the disease may be decided within 48 to 72 hours of diagnosis. Possible outcomes are reversal, need for transplantation, or death.

Etiology

Clients are usually admitted to the hospital with a diagnosis of viral hepatitis. Some clients are admitted through the emergency department with a diagnosis of drug toxicity.

Prevention

Acute liver failure may be evaded by avoiding exposure to hepatitis B or hepatotoxic, liver-damaging substances. Hepatitis B can be transmitted through body fluids such as blood or semen from unprotected sex, intravenous drug use, and dialysis. See Table 33–3 for a list of hepatotoxic substances.

Signs and Symptoms

Signs and symptoms of acute liver failure include a sudden lapse into extremely serious illness in a period of a few hours. The profound illness is characterized by confusion progressing to coma. In a matter of hours, the liver shows a rapid reduction in size. The change in liver size is a typical sign of onset of acute liver failure. In addition, there is a sudden elevation of liver enzymes, bilirubin, and pro-

---

encephalopathy: encephalo—brain + pathy—disease

thrombin time. Marked elevation in the prothrombin time is an ominous sign.

Diagnostic Tests

Early diagnosis of acute liver failure is essential so that the process of organ procurement may begin. An otherwise healthy client may be a priority organ recipient, depending on age and whether or not the client is alcohol dependent.

Laboratory tests include serum liver enzymes, alanine aminotransferase (ALT) and aspartate aminotransferase (AST). Levels of ALT and AST may rise to more than 1000 mU/mL to as high as 4000 mU/mL. The serum bilirubin level is above 2.5 mg/dL. Urobilinogen levels may be elevated. Serum potassium levels will drop below 3.5 mEq/L. Blood sugar will drop below 70 mg/dL. The prothrombin time will elevate above 25 seconds.

Abdominal x-rays may document the change in size of the liver.

Medical Treatment

Medical treatment is directed toward stopping and reversing the damage to the liver. An attempt is made to put the liver completely at rest. The client is put on complete bed rest. All drugs are eliminated. Dialysis may be ordered if the liver damage is a result of an overdose of a hepatotoxic substance. The client is ordered a high-calorie, low-sodium, low-protein diet. Lactulose, neomycin, magnesium citrate, or sorbitol may be given to decrease ammonia levels, but they may not be helpful. (For information on how these drugs work, see the section on medical treatment for chronic liver failure.) The client will need intensive amounts of supportive care. It may be possible to support the client long enough to stabilize him or her for transplantation.

Complications

The client with acute liver failure will experience metabolic alkalosis, hypokalemia, hypoglycemia, disruption of blood clotting, and possible sepsis. Metabolic alkalosis is related to disruption of the urea production cycle and the resulting accumulation of bicarbonate. Acute liver failure clients will also experience electrolyte imbalances. The client's kidneys will excrete potassium rather than hydrogen ions in an attempt to correct the alkalosis. The client will usually have hypoglycemia from loss of glycogen stores in the damaged liver, impaired gluconeogenesis (the manufacture of glucose from other nutrients), and an elevated insulin level caused by the stress response. Further, blood clotting disorders that can lead to disseminated intravascular coagulation (DIC) develop when the prothrombin time elevates.

Finally, the client is at risk for sepsis because of poor white blood cell migration and other responses to infection. Sepsis, abscess formation, endocarditis, and meningi-

tis account for nearly a quarter of the deaths from acute liver failure. Renal failure accounts for about 30 percent of the deaths. Respiratory problems and hypotension also contribute to the deaths from acute liver failure. The client will progress through encephalopathy to a comatose state and death.

Nursing Process

Nursing care of the client with acute liver failure is essentially the same as for the client with terminal chronic liver failure.

Assessment

A complete history and physical assessment are done. The nurse is alert to subjective symptoms of acute liver malfunction, such as malaise, anorexia, indigestion, nausea, and aching RUQ pain. The client is assessed for objective evidence of liver problems, such as weight loss; diarrhea or constipation; and an enlarged, firm, and tender liver.

The nurse observes the client for bruising of the skin; bleeding gums; anemia; and any evidence of alterations in thinking ability, such as confusion, disorientation, or inability to make decisions. The client's vital signs are monitored every 4 hours, especially the temperature.

Nursing Diagnosis

Common nursing diagnoses for acute liver failure include the following:

- Alteration in nutrition: less than body requirements related to the inability of the liver to manufacture nutrients
- Risk for altered thought processes related to elevated ammonia levels
- Risk for ineffective breathing pattern related to metabolic alkalosis
- Risk for fluid volume deficit related to clotting disorders
- Risk for infection related to impaired immune responses

Planning

The nurse, together with the client and other health team members, must plan care to maintain adequate nutrition, maintain or improve the client's thought processes, maintain an effective breathing pattern, maintain a normal fluid volume, and prevent infection.

Implementation

NUTRITION. The client with acute liver failure usually experiences anorexia. The nurse assesses the client's bowel sounds or evidence of any bleeding at least once every 8 hours. Weight loss of greater than 0.5 pounds from previous measurement is reported. The nurse monitors the client's diet to ensure that any ordered protein restriction is carried out. The client is offered frequent small high-calorie feedings. The nurse ensures that odors or other unpleasant situations are eliminated. Frequent mouth care is offered. The nurse administers as scheduled vitamins or other medications that may be ordered for the client.

ALTERED THOUGHT PROCESSES. The nurse assesses the client's level of consciousness, speech, and behavior frequently. Lactulose, neomycin, magnesium citrate, or sorbitol, all of which decrease serum ammonia levels, is given as scheduled. The nurse questions giving medications such as sedatives, narcotics, and tranquilizers that may increase the serum ammonia levels. The client is given simple, clear explanations of care and is given time to understand the explanation. The nurse makes every effort to maintain a safe environment for the confused and possibly unsteady client.

INEFFECTIVE BREATHING PATTERN. The nurse assesses the client's respiratory rate, rhythm, chest movement, and skin color frequently. The nurse makes sure that oxygen and respiratory treatments are carried out as ordered. Further, the nurse makes sure that the client is responding to the treatments as desired. Client care is carried out in an unhurried, quiet manner. Care is timed to allow the client to rest and to avoid fatigue.

SAFETY. The client with acute liver failure is at risk for hemorrhage from the lack of blood clotting factors. The nurse needs to assess gastric secretions, stool, and urine for blood at least every 8 hours. The nurse monitors the blood clotting laboratory studies, such as the prothrombin time, and reports any abnormal values. The client is cautioned to use a soft-bristle toothbrush and an electric rather than straight razor. The nurse uses a small-gauge needle for injections and applies direct pressure to all puncture sites to avoid bleeding. The client should not eat hot, spicy, or irritating foods. If bleeding occurs, the nurse must be ready to monitor the client receiving blood, blood products, and fluids. The nurse administers vasopressin and vitamin K as ordered.

The client is also carefully observed for evidence of infection. Any rise in temperature or sudden increase in pulse and respiratory rate is reported. Laboratory studies such as the white blood cell count need to be carefully evaluated. The white blood cell count may not elevate or may elevate slowly because the white cell activity is impaired. The earliest warning signs of infection may be subtle changes in the client's behavior, such as sudden restlessness, an increase in confusion, or irritability.

Client Education

Clients and their families are taught how acute liver failure is affecting the client's body. They need to observe for and report any confusion, tremors, or personality changes. Clients are taught the importance of total bed rest. They are instructed about diet restrictions and are advised to avoid narcotics, sedatives, and tranquilizers. Clients and their families should know to promptly report any bleeding; any sign of low potassium, such as muscle cramps, nausea, or vomiting caused by diuretics; changes in mental status, such as confusion or personality changes; or any increase in the current symptoms. All should know that the client is gravely ill.

Evaluation

Successful management of the client with acute liver failure can be claimed if the client

- Maintains body weight.
- Remains alert and oriented.
- Has a respiratory rate between 16 and 20 respirations per minute with no cyanosis or changes in level of consciousness.
- Has no bleeding, injuries, or infection.
- States knowledge of acute liver failure accurately and describes proper disease management requirements.

CHRONIC LIVER FAILURE

Chronic liver failure is also called Laënnec's **cirrhosis** or portal, nutritional, or alcoholic liver disease. Chronic liver failure is the fourth leading cause of death in the United States among people aged 35 to 55 years. Chronic liver failure is the ninth leading cause of death among the total population and is more common among men than women. (See Cultural Considerations Box 33–1.)

CULTURAL CONSIDERATIONS BOX 33–1

The incidence of liver disease is more common among Mexican-Americans. Risk factors include working in occupations such as mining, factories using chemicals, and farming using pesticides. Additionally, the use of alcohol is increased with the machismo of society, and cigarette smoking is high.[1]

Egyptian-Americans may suffer from schistosomiasis, known as bilharziasis in Egypt. Schistosomiasis can lead to cirrhosis, liver failure, portal hypertension, esophageal varices, bladder cancer, and renal failure. Thus the nurse may need to screen newer Egyptian-American immigrants for this disease.[2]

Alcohol use and abuse is common among African-American communities. For many it is a socially accepted behavior and carries no stigma.[3] The mortality rate from cirrhosis of the liver among African-Americans is nearly twice that of European-Americans.[4] The nurse needs to provide counseling, teaching the detrimental effects of alcohol, and work with African-American churches and community leaders to help prevent the detrimental effects of alcohol abuse.

---

cirrhosis: cirrh—orange yellow + osis—condition

Etiology

Chronic liver failure may be caused by chronic excessive alcohol ingestion, especially when excess alcohol is combined with a lack of dietary protein. Additional types of liver failure include postnecrotic, biliary, and cardiac.

- Postnecrotic liver failure may result from massive exposure to hepatotoxins or viral hepatitis.
- Biliary liver failure is caused by chronic inflammation and obstruction of the gallbladder and bile ducts.
- Cardiac liver failure is caused by chronic severe congestion of the liver from heart failure. The liver congestion causes death of liver cells from lack of nutrients and oxygen.

Pathophysiology

Chronic liver failure is a progressive disease. Healthy liver cells respond to toxins such as alcohol by becoming inflamed. The liver cells are infiltrated with fat and white blood cells and are then replaced by fibrotic tissue. As the disease progresses, more and more liver cells are replaced by fatty and scar tissue. The lobes of the liver are disrupted and the liver becomes hardened and lumpy. Early in the disease, the liver is enlarged, firm, and hard from the inflammatory process. Later, the liver shrinks and is covered with gray connective tissue.

Prevention

Chronic liver failure may be prevented by abstinence from alcohol, eating a balanced diet with adequate amounts of protein, and avoiding exposure to infections or hepatotoxic chemicals. Clients are advised that total abstinence from alcohol should be a lifelong goal.

Signs and Symptoms

Signs and symptoms of impaired liver function include malaise, anorexia, indigestion, nausea, weight loss, diarrhea or constipation, and dull, aching RUQ pain. The liver may be enlarged, firm, and tender. Bruising of the skin, bleeding gums, anemia, and jaundice, also known as icterus, may be present. Jaundice is a more common finding with hepatitis. The client's skin may be dry or contain abnormal pigmentation. The client may complain of severe pruritus (itching). Laboratory values reflect progressive loss of liver function. As chronic liver failure progresses, signs and symptoms of increasing loss of liver function and complications related to the increasing loss of function will develop.

Complications

Complications of chronic liver failure include **hepatorenal syndrome,** blood clotting defects, **ascites, portal hypertension,** and hepatic encephalopathy. Hepatorenal syndrome occurs in about one-third of liver failure clients.

Symptoms of hepatorenal syndrome include oliguria without detectable kidney damage, reduced glomerular filtration rate (GFR) with essentially no urine output or less than 200 mL/24 h, and nearly total sodium retention. Hepatorenal syndrome is considered an ominous sign.

LEARNING TIP

Complications of Chronic Liver Failure. Remember CHEAP:

    C—clotting disorders
    H—hepatorenal syndrome
    E—encephalopathy
    A—ascites
    P—portal hypertension

Blood clotting defects may develop because of impaired prothrombin and fibrinogen production in the liver. Further, the absence of bile salts prevents the absorption of fat-soluble vitamin K, which is essential for some blood clotting factors. The client has a tendency to bruise easily and may progress to DIC or hemorrhage.

Ascites is an accumulation of serous fluid in the abdominal cavity. The fluid accumulates primarily because of low production of albumin by the failing liver. An insufficient amount of protein in the capillaries causes plasma to seep into the abdominal cavity. The accumulated fluid causes a markedly enlarged abdomen. The fluid may cause severe respiratory distress caused by elevation of the diaphragm.

Portal hypertension is a persistent blood pressure elevation in the portal circulation of the abdomen. Liver damage causes a blockage of blood flow in the portal vein. Increased resistance from delayed drainage causes enlargement of the visible abdominal veins around the umbilicus (caput medusae), rectal hemorrhoids, enlarged spleen, and esophageal **varices** (Fig. 33–1).

The most serious result of portal hypertension is bleeding esophageal varices (dilated veins). The walls of the esophageal veins are thin and tear easily. Varices usually develop from the fundus of the stomach upward and may extend into the upper esophagus. The blood-filled, thin-walled varices may tear easily from sudden excessive pressure such as the intra-abdominal pressure that results from coughing, lifting, or straining, causing severe bleeding.

Hepatic encephalopathy is caused by the accumulation of noxious substances in the circulation. The failing liver is unable to make the toxic substances water soluble for excretion in the urine. Ammonia, which is a by-product of protein metabolism, is the most common substance to cause symptoms. Signs and symptoms of hepatic encephalopathy include progressive confusion; **asterixis,** or

---

hepatorenal syndrome: hepato—liver + renal—kidney + syndrome—group of symptoms

asterixis: a—not + sterixis—fixed position

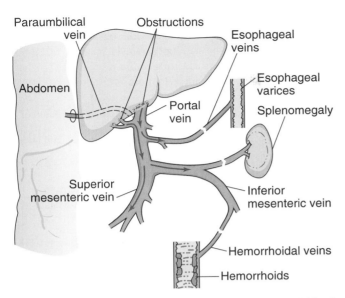

Figure 33–1. Portal hypertension. Obstruction of normal blood flow through the liver causes blood to back up into the venous system, causing esophageal varices, splenomegaly, hemorrhoids, and caput medusae.

flapping tremors in hands caused by toxins at peripheral nerves; and **fetor hepaticas,** or foul breath caused by metabolic end products related to sulfur. Stages of hepatic encephalopathy are early, stuporous and confused, and comatose. Signs and symptoms of the stages are as follows:

- Early—the client exhibits subtle changes in personality, fatigue, drowsiness, and changes in handwriting (the best assessment for the early stage).
- Stuporous and confused state—the client is often belligerent and irritable and develops asterixis, muscle twitching, and marked confusion.
- Comatose—the client gradually loses consciousness and becomes comatose.

If toxic levels can be decreased and managed, the client will gradually regain consciousness. Hepatic encephalopathy represents end-stage liver failure and has a high mortality rate, as much as 90 percent, once coma begins.

Diagnostic Tests

Liver serum enzymes, serum bilirubin, urobilinogen, serum ammonia, and prothrombin times are elevated (Table 33–4).

Clients with chronic liver failure may be expected to have abdominal x-rays that show the enlargement of the liver and ascites. Upper gastrointestinal (UGI) series may

---

fetor hepaticas: fetor—offensive odor + hepat—liver + icas—related to

transjugular intrahepatic portosystemic shunt: trans—across + jugular—jugular vein + intra—within + hepatic—liver + porto—portal—portal (liver) circulation + systemic—systemic circulation + shunt—to divert

reveal esophageal varices or evidence of gastric inflammation or ulcers. If the client is bleeding, other arterial radiologic examinations may be done to locate the specific source of bleeding.

Liver scans may be done to show abnormal liver masses or thickening. The physician may order an esophagogastroduodenoscopy (EGD) to detect any bleeding and to directly observe the esophagus, stomach, and duodenum. Small surface vessels that are bleeding can be treated by injection sclerotherapy. The procedure uses sclerosing agents, which are chemical substances that cause the veins to inflame and scar shut.

The physician may do a liver biopsy to determine the extent and nature of the liver damage. Clients with chronic liver failure undergoing a liver biopsy will need careful observation for bleeding after the procedure. (See Chapter 32.)

Medical Treatment

Medical treatment for chronic hepatic failure seeks to remove or to treat the underlying causes of the disease. In addition, medical treatment seeks to support liver regeneration and to treat the complications of liver failure.

Ascites is treated with diuretics, albumin infusions, and sodium restriction. Paracentesis is sometimes considered as an emergency measure to remove accumulated abdominal fluid. Paracentesis is not commonly done because it removes serous fluid, which contains a large amount of albumin that the liver cannot easily replace. Ascites may be treated by the nonsurgical placement of a shunt between the portal and systemic venous systems, called a **transjugular intrahepatic portosystemic shunt** (TIPS).

The purpose of the shunt is to sidetrack venous blood around the liver to the vena cava. Shunts are used for clients with severe respiratory compromise and are not as successful as originally hoped. Surgical shunts, sometimes called portacaval shunts, may be used to relieve portal hypertension (Fig. 33–2). When shunts are used, less venous blood circulates through the liver and fewer protein end products are metabolized. For this reason, clients are put on a low-protein diet.

The medical goals for managing bleeding from esophageal varices are to

- Stop the bleeding.
- Treat the fluid volume deficit caused by the bleeding.
- Prevent further fluid loss.
- Maintain fluid and electrolyte balance.

Bleeding varices are treated with vasoconstrictors such as vasopressin, with tamponade (direct pressure on the bleeding veins), or with emergency sclerotherapy to close the veins.

Tamponade is usually a temporary measure and is done with a multilumen esophagogastric tube such as the Sengstaken-Blakemore tube (Fig. 33–3). Other multilumen tubes such as the Minnesota tube may be used. The Sengstaken-Blakemore tube is inserted through the nose or

Table 33–4. **Laboratory Tests for Chronic Liver Failure**

Test	Normal Range	Significance
	Blood	
Alanine aminotransferase (ALT)	5–35 IU/mL	Found in high concentrations in liver cells; released with death of liver cells
Albumin	3.5–5.5 g/dL	Decreased because of impaired protein synthesis; edema and ascites may result
Ammonia	15–19 μg/dL	Increased because liver cannot metabolize protein end product; contributes to hepatic encephalopathy
Bilirubin	0.3–3.0 mg/dL	Increased from increased breakdown of red blood cells
Aspartate aminotransferase (AST)	8–20 U/L	Found in high concentrations in liver cells; released with death of liver cells
Prothrombin time	Adult: Women, 1–20 mm/h Men, 1–13 mm/h	Liver can no longer make prothrombin; client bleeds easily
	Urine	
Urobilinogen	<4.0 mg/24 h	Increased urine amounts from filtration of excessive bilinogen in blood

mouth to the stomach. First, the gastric balloon is inflated with 200 mL of air, to secure the tube in its proper location. The esophageal tube is then inflated with 50 mL of air to produce tamponade. One to two pounds of traction may be applied to the tube. Occasionally, the client may wear a football helmet so that the tube can be secured to the face guard rather than putting pressure on the client's nose. The Sengstaken-Blakemore tube is then connected to nasogastric suction.

Complications that may occur from the use of esophagogastric tamponade include (1) aspiration, (2) erosion of esophageal gastric mucosa, and (3) suffocation. With the balloons inflated, the client cannot swallow saliva. Oral suction with a Yankauer catheter should be available. Sometimes a Salem sump tube is placed in the upper esophagus before the esophageal balloon is inflated in order to drain secretions.

Inflation pressure of the esophageal balloon should be maintained between 20 and 25 mm Hg. Agency procedures

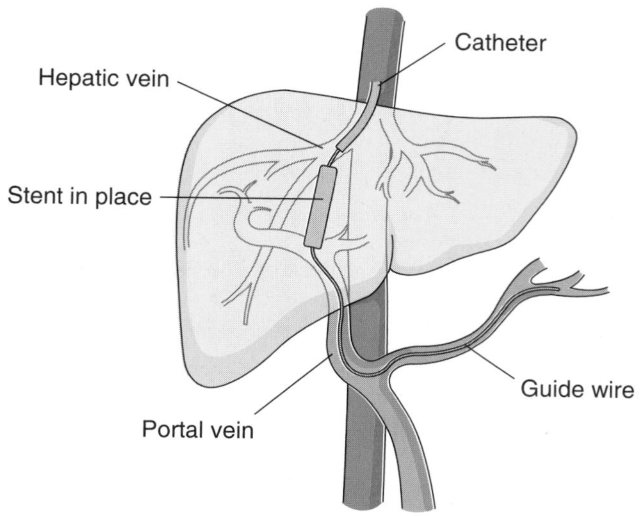

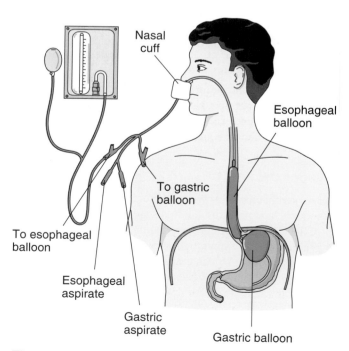

Figure 33–2. Transjugular intrahepatic portosystemic shunt (TIPS). A stent is placed to shunt blood from the portal vein to the systemic circulation to divert blood flow around the diseased liver.

Figure 33–3. Balloon tamponade for bleeding esophageal varices. Esophageal balloon compresses bleeding vessels.

should clearly state how long the tube may remain in place and how often (and for how long) the esophageal balloon should be deflated. The gastric balloon remains inflated at all times until the procedure is stopped.

If the gastric tube dislodges into the esophagus, the client can be suffocated. The nurse must keep a pair of scissors at the bedside when esophagogastric tamponade is in progress. The nurse must cut the inflation ports of the gastric and esophageal balloons if the gastric balloon dislodges.

Unfortunately, recurrence of bleeding occurs in about 20 to 60 percent of clients after successful tamponade. With each new bleeding episode, the mortality rate increases. Sclerotherapy may be undertaken to prevent recurrence of bleeding. Sclerotherapy can be done without general anesthesia, which is an advantage for the client with a severely damaged liver. The procedure is usually done as part of an EGD while the client is sedated with diazepam (Valium) or midazolam hydrochloride (Versed). A topical anesthetic is used, such as benzocaine (Cetacaine). The varices are injected with a sclerosing agent that causes thickening and closing of the dilated vessels. The procedure usually takes 1 hour. After the procedure the client may complain of chest pain for up to 72 hours. The nurse gives the prescribed analgesics and monitors the client for pain relief. Severe pain unrelieved by the prescribed analgesic is reported immediately because the client may be experiencing an esophageal perforation or ulceration, which are complications of sclerotherapy.

Hepatic encephalopathy is treated by trying to remove the toxic waste material. Saline or magnesium sulfate ($MgSO_4$) enemas may remove some of the toxic waste. The enemas may be given to cleanse the bowel of the noxious substances. Neomycin, an intestinal antibiotic, may be given by mouth, nasogastric tube, or enema. The antibiotic inhibits ammonia formation by reducing colonic bacteria that change ammonium to ammonia. Lactulose may be given by mouth to reduce the pH of the intestine and to "trap" ammonia, allowing it to be excreted in the stool. Hepatic encephalopathy is also treated by restricting or eliminating dietary protein. In severe cases, dialysis may be considered to remove ammonia. See Nutrition Notes Box 33–2.

Nursing Process

Assessment

A complete history and physical assessment are done. The nurse is alert to subjective symptoms of liver slowdown such as malaise; anorexia; indigestion; nausea; severe itching; and dull, aching RUQ pain. The client is assessed for objective evidence of liver problems, such as weight loss; diarrhea or constipation; and an enlarged, firm, and tender liver. The nurse also observes the client for dryness and bruising of the skin; bleeding gums; anemia; jaundice; and any evidence of alterations in thinking

---

NUTRITION NOTES BOX 33–2

A registered dietitian may modify the diet of the client with liver disease daily. For early or mild disease, protein is encouraged to support healing. For esophageal varices, foods are soft, in addition to other restrictions. For liver failure, protein is restricted according to the client's ability to metabolize it; complete-protein foods are selected to provide all the essential amino acids; adequate carbohydrate is given to prevent deaminization of protein for energy; and fluid and sodium are usually restricted if ascites is present.

For hepatic encephalopathy, foods producing high ammonia levels are avoided (chicken, salami, ground beef, ham, bacon, gelatin, peanut butter, potatoes, onions, lima beans, egg yolk, buttermilk, blue and cheddar cheeses), as are branched-chain amino acids (leucine, isoleucine, and valine) in vegetable proteins. Hepatic-Aid II and Travasorb-Hepatic are favored over aromatic amino acids (phenylalanine, tryptophan, and tyrosine), which interfere with formation of dopamine and norepinephrine.

---

ability, such as confusion, disorientation, or inability to make decisions.

Nursing Diagnosis

Common nursing diagnoses for chronic liver failure include the following:

Fluid volume excess related to portal hypertension (ascites)

Alteration in nutrition: less than body requirements related to disinterest in food

Pain related to abdominal pressure

Risk for altered thought processes related to elevated ammonia levels

Risk for ineffective breathing pattern related to abnormal amounts of fluid in the abdomen

Risk for fluid volume deficit related to bleeding (esophageal varices, clotting disorders)

Planning

Major goals for the client with chronic liver failure include that the client will experience no fluid excess or deficit, have adequate nutrition, be able to think clearly, and breathe effectively.

Implementation

FLUID BALANCE. The nurse weighs the client on admission to obtain a baseline weight. The client is weighed, and abdominal girth or circumference is measured daily and recorded. Any weight gain or increase in girth is reported promptly. The nurse monitors the client's low-sodium diet and maintains any ordered fluid restrictions. If intravenous fluids or albumin have been ordered, the LPN/LVN assists in careful monitoring of the rate of infusion. The client's vital signs are taken every 4 hours, and any evidence of difficulty breathing or changes in mental status are reported promptly. The nurse administers any ordered diuretics as scheduled. The nurse assists with a paracentesis as required.

NUTRITION. The client with chronic liver failure usually experiences anorexia in addition to impaired metabolism of needed nutrients. The client's bowel sounds, abdominal distention, and evidence of any bleeding should be assessed at least once every 8 hours. Weight loss of greater than one-half pound from previous measurement is reported. The nurse monitors the client's diet to ensure that any ordered protein restriction is carried out. The client is offered frequent small high-calorie feedings. If the client has been ordered to have total parenteral nutrition (TPN) or tube feedings, the nurse administers the treatment and monitors the client's response closely. The nurse makes sure that odors and other unpleasant stimuli are eliminated. Frequent mouth care is offered. The nurse administers vitamins or other medications as ordered.

ALTERED THOUGHT PROCESSES. The nurse assesses the client's level of consciousness, speech, behavior, and neuromuscular function frequently. Neuromuscular function can be assessed by asking the client to hold his or her arms out straight in front and steady. If asterixis or liver flap is present, the client's hands will unwillingly dip and return to the horizontal position in a flapping motion. The nurse also looks for changes in the client's handwriting. Lactulose, neomycin, magnesium citrate, or sorbitol, all of which are given to decrease serum ammonia levels, is given as scheduled. The nurse is aware that lactulose causes loose stools and does not hold the medication when the client develops diarrhea. The nurse questions giving medications such as sedatives, narcotics, and tranquilizers that may increase the serum ammonia levels. The nurse reorients the client to time and place frequently. The client is given simple, clear explanations of care and given time to understand the explanation. The nurse provides a safe environment for the confused and possibly unsteady client.

INEFFECTIVE BREATHING PATTERN. The nurse assesses the client's respiratory rate, rhythm, chest movement, and skin color frequently. The client is assisted in using an incentive spirometer and in coughing gently every 2 to 4 hours. The head of the client's bed is elevated so that the client's lungs have maximum room for expansion. The client is repositioned at least every 2 hours. The nurse avoids suctioning the client if possible because bleeding may occur. The nurse makes sure that oxygen and respiratory treatments are carried out as ordered. The nurse ensures that the client is responding to the treatments as desired. The nurse assists with a thoracentesis if required. Client care is carried out in an unhurried, quiet manner.

Care is timed to allow the client to rest and to avoid fatigue.

SAFETY. The client with chronic liver failure is at risk for hemorrhage from bleeding esophageal varices, gastrointestinal bleeding, and lack of blood clotting factors. The nurse assesses gastric secretions, stool, and urine for blood at least every 8 hours. The nurse also monitors the blood clotting laboratory studies such as the prothrombin time and reports any abnormal values. The client is cautioned to use a soft-bristle toothbrush and an electric rather than straight razor to avoid injury. The nurse uses a small-gauge needle for injections and applies direct pressure to all puncture sites to avoid bleeding. The client should not eat hot, spicy, or irritating foods. The client also should not cough, forcefully blow the nose, strain, vomit, or gag if at all possible. If bleeding occurs, the nurse monitors the client receiving blood, blood products, and fluids. The nurse may need to assist with esophagogastric tubes if needed. The nurse administers vasopressin and vitamin K as ordered.

Client Education

Clients are taught how chronic liver failure is affecting their body. In particular, clients need to know about portal system hypertension and hepatic encephalopathy. Clients and their families need to observe for and report any confusion, tremors, or personality changes. Clients are taught to get adequate rest and to avoid strenuous activity. Clients are instructed about a diet high in calories, low in sodium, and high in protein if hepatic encephalopathy has not developed. Clients should know to avoid narcotics, sedatives, and tranquilizers. Clients and their families should know to promptly report any bleeding; any sign of low potassium, such as muscle cramps, nausea, or vomiting caused by diuretics; changes in mental status, such as confusion or personality changes; changes in weight; and any increase in current symptoms. The client and the family should know that the client must avoid alcohol. The client should also know the importance of frequent follow-up care and laboratory studies.

Evaluation

Successful management of the client with chronic liver failure can be claimed if the client

- Has no weight gain or increase in abdominal girth.
- Maintains body weight.
- Remains alert and oriented.
- Has a respiratory rate between 16 and 20 respirations per minute with no cyanosis or changes in level of consciousness.
- Has no bleeding or injuries.
- States knowledge of chronic liver failure accurately and describes proper disease management requirements.

See also Nursing Care Plan Box 33–3 for the Client with Chronic Liver Failure.

text continues on page 650

NURSING CARE PLAN BOX 33–3
FOR THE CLIENT WITH CHRONIC LIVER FAILURE

Fluid volume excess related to electrolyte imbalances and portal hypertension

Outcome
Client experiences no increase in fluid volume as evidenced by stable or decreasing weight and abdominal girth.

Evaluation of Outcome
Are weight and abdominal girth stable or decreasing?

Interventions	Rationale	Evaluation
Assess the client for evidence of fluid volume excess: Weight gain Intake greater than output Increase in abdominal girth	Weight gain of 1 lb is equal to approximately 500 mL of fluid. Fluid in the peritoneum will cause the abdomen to expand.	Does the client have a weight gain of greater than 0.5 lb? Has the client's abdominal girth increased from baseline measurement?
Maintain sodium-restricted diet.	Decreasing sodium lessens water retention by kidneys.	Does client adhere to sodium restriction?
Maintain fluid restrictions as ordered	Limited intake decreases the amount of water to be retained.	Does client maintain fluid restriction?
Administer diuretics as ordered.	Increases water and sodium excretion by the kidneys.	Are diuretics effective? Is output greater than intake?
Encourage the client to rest in the recumbent position if tolerated.	The recumbent position can help reshift abdominal fluid into the portal circulation.	Does client tolerate this position?

Alterations in nutrition: less than body requirements related to disinterest in food

Outcome
Client has improved nutritional status as evidenced by stable hemoglobin, hematocrit, and albumin levels.

Evaluation of Outcome
Are laboratory values stable or improving?

Interventions	Rationale	Evaluation
Assess the client for evidence of poor nutrition: Weight greater than 20% below ideal body weight (IBW) Low serum albumin, hemoglobin, hematocrit Complaints of weakness and fatigue	These are evidence of impaired protein metabolism.	Does the client maintain or increase body weight without evidence of fluid excess?
Encourage a rest period before meals.	Minimizes fatigue.	Is the client able to carry out activities of daily living without complaints of weakness or fatigue?
Consult dietitian to determine the foods that the client prefers that are also the most nutritious—those low in salt, high in protein, and high in carbohydrates.	The client will tend to eat more preferred foods. The liver needs high protein and high carbohydrate content to regenerate. If client has encephalopathy, protein is limited because of ammonia by-products.	Is the client able to eat a variety of nutritious foods?
Serve small portions in a clean, relaxed, pleasant atmosphere.	Food is more appealing in such an atmosphere.	Does client state that atmosphere is pleasant for eating?
Place client in high semi-Fowler's or high Fowler's position.	Relieves pressure from ascites on the diaphragm and decreases subjective feelings of fullness.	Does client state that position relieves sense of fullness?

continued

NURSING CARE PLAN BOX 33–3 (continued)

Interventions	Rationale	Evaluation
Administer diet supplements such as vitamin B–complex vitamins, fat-soluble vitamins, and trace minerals such as zinc as ordered.	The client may need additional supplements, especially if unable to consume enough of a nutritious diet.	Are vitamins administered as ordered?
Teach the client to eat a diet that is high in carbohydrates, moderate to high in protein, and low in sodium and to take dietary supplements ordered by the physician.	The client should understand that the liver needs nutrients to heal and that meals should not be skipped.	Does the client verbalize understanding of diet recommendations for home?

Pain related to abdominal pressure

Outcome
Client states pain from abdominal pressure is less than 2 on a scale of 0 to 5.

Evaluation of Outcome
Does client state that interventions maintain pain at less than 2?

Interventions	Rationale	Evaluation
Assess the client frequently for evidence of pain: Ask the client to quantify the pain on a scale of 0 to 5. Observe the client for facial grimacing, reluctance to move, and refusal to enter into care activities.	These are evidence of pain.	Does the client state that pain is 2 or less on a pain scale of 0 to 5? Does the client appear to be relaxed and moving freely in bed? Does the client enter into activities without hesitation?
Maintain fluid and sodium restrictions.	Prevents or slows the buildup of abdominal fluid.	Are restrictions followed?
Assist the client to a position of comfort, and support the client with pillows.	A position of comfort will provide relief, and pillows will prevent excessive fatigue.	Does client state that positioning relieves discomfort?
Provide a restful, peaceful environment with diversional activities.	Diversional activities and a quiet environment will help the client relax and divert attention from discomfort.	Are diversional activities effective?
Give pain medication as ordered. Monitor carefully.	The damaged liver is less able to detoxify narcotics. Acetaminophen (Tylenol) may be ordered rather than acetylsalicylic acid (aspirin) even though acetaminophen is more toxic to the liver. Aspirin may increase gastric irritation and the chance of bleeding.	Is pain medication effective?
Teach the client alternative methods for pain control such as relaxation techniques.	Relaxation techniques may lower the need for narcotics or other analgesics, thus lowering the potential for increased liver damage.	Does client use alternative methods effectively?

Risk for altered thought processes related to elevated ammonia levels

Outcome
Client experiences improved thought processes as evidenced by alertness and orientation to person, place, and time.

Evaluation of Outcome
Is client alert and oriented to person, place, and time?

continued

NURSING CARE PLAN BOX 33–3 *(continued)*

Interventions	Rationale	Evaluation
Assess the client's level of consciousness, speech, and behavior.	These indicate adequate functioning of the central nervous system.	Is the client alert and oriented? Is the client able to carry on a sensible conversation? Is the client calm and relaxed?
Assess for asterixis.	Asterixis is evidence of elevated serum ammonia levels.	Does the client exhibit asterixis? Are medications administered?
Give lactulose, neomycin, magnesium citrate, or sorbitol as ordered.	These drugs decrease ammonia levels.	Are ammonia levels decreasing? Are orders appropriate?
Question orders for medications such as sedatives, narcotics, and tranquilizers.	The liver may be unable to detoxify these drugs.	
Give simple, clear directions to the client. Reorient the client frequently.	The client may be unable to retain information. The nurse may have to repeat information frequently.	Does the client follow instructions?

Risk for ineffective breathing pattern related to abnormal amounts of fluid in the abdomen

Outcome
Client will maintain an effective breathing pattern as evidenced by a regular respiratory rate between 16 and 20 respirations per minute.

Evaluation of Outcome
Is respiratory rate even, unlabored, and between 16 and 20 respirations per minute?

Interventions	Rationale	Evaluation
Assess the client for respiratory rate and rhythm, depth of respirations, chest movement, and skin color.	These are evidence of effective breathing patterns if client maintains a regular, easy, nonshallow breathing pattern and has no pallor or cyanosis.	Does the client have a respiratory rate between 16 and 20 respirations per minute? Are respirations unlabored and deep? Does the client have pallor or cyanosis?
Have client positioned in high Fowler's position.	This prevents ascites from compressing the diaphragm.	Does positioning relieve respiratory distress?
Maintain fluid and sodium restrictions.	Prevents excessive fluid buildup.	Are restrictions maintained?
Have the client deep breathe and cough gently every 2 hours. If incentive spirometry is ordered, use with deep breathing and coughing.	Encourages lung expansion and prevents secretions from pooling in the lungs.	Does client deep breathe and cough effectively?
Avoid tracheal suctioning if possible.	May rupture esophageal varices and cause severe bleeding.	Is suctioning avoided?
Assist with paracentesis if necessary.	A paracentesis will remove fluid and pressure for the short term.	Does paracentesis relieve symptoms?
Teach the client the importance of deep breathing, gentle coughing, and changing positions.	The client should understand that these measures will prevent secretions from pooling in the lungs and causing further difficulties with breathing.	Does the client verbalize understanding of the importance of these measures?

Risk for fluid volume deficit related to bleeding (esophageal varices, clotting disorders)

Outcome
Client experiences no bleeding; if bleeding occurs, it is recognized and reported quickly.

Evaluation of Outcome
Does bleeding occur: Is it recognized and reported immediately?

continued

NURSING CARE PLAN BOX 33–3 (continued)

Interventions	Rationale	Evaluation
Assess client's gastric secretions, stool, and urine for blood at least every 8 hours, as well as the client's pulse rate and blood pressure.	These show evidence of bleeding.	Are the client's stool, urine, and gastric secretions free from blood? Are the client's blood pressure and pulse within 10% of baseline?
Assess client's prothrombin time when available.	An elevated prothrombin time indicates an increased chance of bleeding. An abnormal value should be reported.	Is the client's prothrombin time within the agency's accepted normal limits?
Avoid using intramuscular or subcutaneous injections whenever possible. Use a small-gauge needle if injections cannot be avoided.	May cause bleeding at the intramuscular or subcutaneous site.	Are alternatives to injections tried first? Is bleeding at sites avoided?
Give vasopressin or vitamin K as ordered.	May prevent acute hemorrhage by causing vasoconstriction or improving clotting.	Are medications effective in preventing bleeding?
Teach the client to Use a soft-bristle toothbrush and brush gently. Avoid spicy, hot, or irritating foods. Avoid forcefully blowing the nose or coughing violently. Avoid straining, gagging, or vomiting. Use an electric razor rather than a straight razor.	A firm-bristle brush may start gingival bleeding. Vigorous coughing, nose blowing, gagging, straining, or vomiting may increase pressure on esophageal varices. Spicy, hot, irritating foods may start gastric bleeding. Anything that can cause injury should be avoided.	Does the client bleed easily from the gums after oral hygiene? Does client verbalize understanding of measures to prevent injury and bleeding?

CRITICAL THINKING: Jonathan

Jonathan, a 56-year-old physically disabled construction worker, has lived alone for the past 15 years since the death of his wife. He has had a long history of depression and poor nutritional habits. He drinks one to one and one-half pints of alcohol a day. During a recent visit to his physician, he was diagnosed with early chronic liver failure.

1. What risk factors does Jonathan have for chronic liver failure?
2. What symptoms would the nurse expect Jonathan to exhibit with early chronic liver failure?
3. What values does the nurse expect to see for serum albumin? Prothrombin time?
4. What are the two greatest concerns with portal hypertension?
5. What is the usual treatment for ascites?
6. What complication of esophageal tamponade requires that a pair of scissors be at the bedside at all times while tamponade is in progress?

Answers at end of chapter.

TRANSPLANTATION

Clients with liver disease who do not respond well to medical or surgical treatment may be candidates for a liver transplant. Clients who have chronic liver failure from hepatitis or biliary disease, metabolic disorders, or hepatic

vein obstruction may be evaluated for a liver transplant. In general, clients who have cancer are not considered for liver transplantation; the drugs used to suppress tissue rejection by the immune system may cause the cancer cells to grow at an increased rate. (See Cultural Considerations Box 33–4.)

The client with end-stage liver failure who does not have hypertension, bleeding esophageal varices, infection, or severe cardiac disease is placed on a national list as a po-

CULTURAL CONSIDERATIONS BOX 33–4

Jewish law views organ transplantation from the recipient, the living donor, the cadaver donor, and the dying donor.[5] If the recipient's life can be prolonged without considerable risk, transplant is ordained. For a living donor to be approved, the risk to the life of the donor must be considered. One is not obligated to donate a part of himself or herself unless the risk is small. This includes kidney and bone marrow donations. The use of a cadaver for transplant is usually approved if it is saving a life. The use of skin for burns is acceptable, although there is no agreement on the use of cadaver corneas. The nurse may need to help the Jewish client obtain a rabbi when making a decision regarding organ donation or transplantation.

tential liver recipient. The client must be as physically and emotionally stable as possible.

The client must be closely observed for evidence of donor organ rejection after the surgical implant of a donor liver. The client will be placed on drugs such as cyclosporine (Cyclosporin A), azathioprine (Imuran), and prednisone (Deltasone) to suppress the immune system responses to foreign protein or tissue rejection. The nurse watches for the following signs of impending rejection:

- Pulse greater than 100 beats per minute
- Temperature greater than 101°F (38°C)
- Complaints of RUQ pain
- Increased jaundice
- A decrease in bile from the T-tube or a change in bile color

In addition, laboratory studies may show increased serum transaminases (ALT and AST), serum bilirubin, alkaline phosphatase, and prothrombin time. Symptoms of acute tissue rejection usually develop between the 4th and 10th postoperative days.

The client who has received an organ transplant will need extended medical follow-up. The client is taught to promptly report to the physician any symptoms of infection, bleeding episodes, or RUQ pain. (See Ethical Considerations Box 33–5.)

CANCER OF THE LIVER

Cancer of the liver is usually the result of metastasis of a primary cancer at a distant location. The liver is a likely area to be involved if cancer originated in the esophagus, lungs, breast, stomach, or colon. Clients with malignant melanoma may also have liver involvement. For some clients, liver cancer is the primary tumor site. Clients with a history of chronic hepatitis B, nutritional deficiencies, or exposure to hepatotoxins may develop cancer of the liver.

ETHICAL CONSIDERATIONS BOX 33–5

Organ Transplantation

Despite widespread public and medical acceptance of organ transplantation as a highly beneficial procedure, ethical questions remain. Whenever a human organ is transplanted, a large number of people are involved, including the donor, the donor's family, and medical and nursing personnel, as well as the recipient and the recipient's family. Society in general could also be added to this mix because of the high cost of organ transplantation that is usually borne directly by tax monies or indirectly in the form of increased insurance premiums. Each one of these persons or groups has rights that may conflict with others' rights.

Most institutions that perform transplants, or organizations that are involved in obtaining organs, have developed elaborate, detailed, and involved procedures to help deal with the ethical and legal issues involved in transplantation. Despite these efforts, there are still some ethical issues that should be considered whenever the issue of organ transplantation is raised.

Despite the best efforts of the medical and legal community to establish criteria for death, there are still some ethical questions about when a person is really dead. Does brain death, the most widely accepted criterion for death, really indicate that a person no longer exists as a human being? Or are there other criteria that should be examined? Such organs as hearts, lungs, and liver must come from a donor with a beating heart. Might there not be the tendency to declare brain death before it actually occurs?

One of the most difficult ethical issues involved in organ transplantation is the selection of recipients. There are many fewer organs available than there are people who need them. Many potential ethical dilemmas arise from this fact. Should someone receive an organ because he or she is rich or famous or knows the right people? The national organ recipient list attempts to list and rank all persons who need organs in a nondiscriminatory manner. Some of the important criteria include need, length of time on the list, potential for survival, prior organ transplantation, value to the community, and tissue compatibility.

Nurses can be and often are involved in some aspect of the organ donation process. Many states have passed laws that require health care workers to ask family members of potential organ donors if they have ever thought about organ donation for their dead or dying loved one. Many nurses, particularly nurses in critical care units, provide care for clients who are potential organ donors. Nurses in operating rooms may help in the surgical procedures that remove organs from a cadaver and that transplant them into a recipient's body. Many floor nurses provide postoperative care for clients who have received a transplanted organ. Home health care nurses provide follow-up care for these clients at home.

Nurses working with organ transplantation need to be sensitive to the potential for manipulation. Most people who are seeking organ transplantations are desperately ill or near death. They, and their families, can be very easily manipulated or can be very manipulating. On the other side, the families of potential organ donors are usually emotionally distraught because of the sudden and traumatic loss of a loved one. They too are very vulnerable to manipulation. As a general rule, neither the donor nor the donor's family should play any part in the selection of a recipient. Nurses must avoid making statements or giving nonverbal indications of approval or disapproval of potential recipients.

Symptoms of cancer of the liver include encephalopathy, abnormal bleeding, jaundice, and ascites. Laboratory tests show an elevated serum alkaline phosphatase. Radiologic examinations may include abdominal x-rays or radioisotope scans, which will show tumor growth. Liver cancer is definitely diagnosed with a positive needle biopsy combined with an ultrasonogram of the liver.

The client with liver cancer may be a candidate for surgical removal of the affected portion of the liver. Care of the postsurgical client is similar to other abdominal surgery clients. If surgery is not an option, the client may receive chemotherapeutic (anticancer) drugs by injection directly into the affected lobe of the liver or into the hepatic artery. Intra-arterial injection of chemotherapeutic drugs has the advantage of being less toxic to the rest of the body. (See Chapter 10 for care of the client receiving chemotherapy.)

Disorders of the Pancreas

PANCREATITIS

Pancreatitis is an inflammation of the pancreas that may be mild or severe. Pancreatitis appears in one of two forms, either acute or chronic. The two forms of pancreatitis have different courses and are considered two different disorders.

ACUTE PANCREATITIS

Pathophysiology

Inflammation of the pancreas appears to be caused by a process called autodigestion. For reasons not fully understood, pancreatic enzymes are activated while they are still within the pancreas and begin to digest the pancreas itself. In addition, large amounts of the enzymes are released by inflamed cells. Alcohol appears to act directly on the acinar cells of the pancreas and the pancreatic ducts to irritate and inflame the structures. Gallstones may plug the pancreatic duct and cause inflammation from excessive fluid pressure on sensitive ducts. The irritant effect of bile itself may cause inflammation. Trauma to the abdomen or infection may trigger the process by causing ischemia, inflammation, and activation of the pancreatic enzymes.

As the pancreas digests itself, chemical cascades occur. Trypsin destroys pancreatic tissue and causes vasodilation. As capillary permeability increases, fluid is lost to the retroperitoneal space, causing shock. In addition, trypsin appears to set off another chain of events that causes the conversion of prothrombin to thrombin so that clots form. The client may develop DIC.

Etiology

Pancreatitis is most commonly associated with excessive alcohol consumption. Biliary disease such as cholelithiasis (gallstones) or cholangitis (inflammation of the bile ducts) may trigger pancreatitis. Blunt trauma to the abdomen, infection, drugs such as thiazide diuretics (HydroDiuril), estrogen, and excessive serum calcium from hyperparathyroidism are less common causes of pancreatitis. Elderly clients and clients with a first diagnosis of pancreatitis have a higher mortality rate. In addition, clients who have pancreatitis associated with biliary disease have a higher mortality rate than clients with excessive alcohol ingestion.

Prevention

Clients are cautioned to stop drinking alcohol. Clients with biliary disease need to seek medical treatment for these conditions so that pancreatitis does not develop as a complication. Clients, especially the elderly, need to be carefully monitored for any abdominal complaints when they are placed on thiazide diuretic or estrogen therapy. (See Cultural Considerations Box 33–6.)

Signs and Symptoms

Clients with acute pancreatitis are very ill with dull abdominal pain, guarding, rigid abdomen, hypotension or shock, and respiratory distress from accumulation of fluid in the retroperitoneal space. The abdominal pain is generally located in the midline just below the sternum with radiation to spine, shoulders, or low back. The location and degree of pain indicate the area of the pancreas involved and to some extent the amount of involvement. For example, if the client complains primarily of RUQ pain, the head of the pancreas is most likely involved. Respirations are likely to be shallow as the client attempts to splint painful areas.

The client may have a low-grade fever, dry mucous membranes, and tachycardia. If the primary cause is biliary, the client may complain of nausea and vomiting, and jaundice may be evident. The islets of Langerhans in the terminal one-third of the pancreas are usually not impaired.

Complications

It may be useful to think of pancreatitis as a chemical burn to the organ. As with other severe burns, death is likely to

CULTURAL CONSIDERATIONS BOX 33–6

The incidence of pancreatic disease is more common among Mexican-Americans and Chinese-Americans. Risk factors include working in occupations such as mining, factories using chemicals, and farming using pesticides. The high use of alcohol and cigarette smoking add to the risk of pancreatic disease.[1]

occur from secondary causes. From the onset of symptoms, cardiovascular, pulmonary (including acute respiratory distress syndrome), and renal failure are the most likely causes of death. Hemorrhage, peripheral vascular collapse, and infection are also major concerns for clients with pancreatitis. A purplish discoloration of the flanks (Turner's sign) or a purplish discoloration around the umbilicus (Cullen's sign) may occur with extensive hemorrhagic destruction of the pancreas.

Diagnostic Tests

Serum amylase (normal 56–190 IU/L) and serum lipase (normal 0–110 U/L) may be elevated from 5 to 40 times normal. The levels will usually drop within 72 hours. Urine amylase will elevate and stay elevated longer. Glucose, bilirubin, alkaline phosphatase, lactic dehydrogenase, ALT, AST, cholesterol, and potassium are all elevated. Decreases are measured in serum albumin, calcium, sodium, and magnesium.

X-rays may show pleural effusion from local inflammatory reaction to pancreatic enzymes, pulmonary infiltrates, or changes in the size of the pancreas. Computed tomography and ultrasonography can provide more complete information about the pancreas and surrounding tissues.

Medical Treatment

Medical treatment depends on the intensity of the symptoms. Treatment will be concerned with the maintenance of life support until the inflammation resolves. The physician will order intravenous fluids, either crystalloid, electrolyte, or colloid (such as albumin) solutions if the client experiences hypovolemic shock. Blood or blood products may also be ordered if the client has massive blood loss from hemorrhage.

The client may be given antianxiety agents to decrease oxygen demand. The client may require supplemental oxygen if abdominal pressure, pleural effusion, or acidosis causes a severe decrease in circulating oxygen.

The physician will usually order meperidine hydrochloride (Demerol) for pain. Pain and anxiety increase pancreatic secretion by stimulating the autonomic nervous system. Morphine sulfate, long contraindicated as an analgesic because it was thought to cause smooth muscle spasm in the biliary and pancreatic ducts, may also be ordered.

The physician will try to put the gastrointestinal tract at rest. The client is usually ordered to have nothing by mouth (NPO). Further, the client may need to have a nasogastric tube inserted into the stomach and attached to low suction to empty gastric contents and gas. The physician will generally order histamine (H_2) antagonists such as ranitidine hydrochloride (Zantac) to prevent stress ulcers and to decrease acid stimulation of pancreatic secretion. If the NPO therapy is prolonged or if the client is malnourished, the client will receive TPN. (See Nutrition Notes Box 33–7.)

NUTRITION NOTES BOX 33-7

Pancreas

Acute pancreatitis: TPN or IV feedings; NPO with nasogastric suction. (Ice chips made with electrolyte solutions are less likely to stimulate gastric secretions.)

Chronic pancreatitis: six small meals; clear liquids progressing to high-carbohydrate, low-fat diet; vitamin supplements, including parenteral B_{12}. Medium chain triglyceride oil may be better tolerated than other fats. Increasing serum amylase levels may necessitate return to more restricted diet.

Additional typical drug orders include sodium bicarbonate to reverse the acidosis caused by shock, electrolytes such as calcium and magnesium to replace losses, regular insulin to combat hyperglycemia, and antibiotics to treat sepsis.

Nursing Process

Assessment

The nurse frequently measures and records vital signs (especially blood pressure and pulse), skin color and temperature, and urinary output. Episodes of nausea and vomiting are recorded. The client is observed for evidence of respiratory distress, such as restlessness, irritability, use of accessory muscles, or dyspnea. The nurse evaluates the client for pain frequently.

Nursing Diagnosis

The most common nursing diagnoses for the client with acute pancreatitis are as follows:

- Pain related to edema and inflammation
- Altered nutrition: less than body requirements related to vomiting, pain, nothing by mouth, gastric suction
- Risk for ineffective breathing pattern related to abdominal pressure
- Risk for injury related to disturbed blood clotting mechanisms and fluid and electrolyte imbalances

Planning

The nurse, the client, and other members of the health team need to consider acceptable methods for achieving pain control, adequate nutrition, and prevention of cardiorespiratory complications.

Implementation

PAIN. The nurse administers analgesics as ordered. The client is evaluated for pain at least every 2 hours initially. The client may be advised to sit in an upright or slightly forward-leaning position to decrease abdominal discomfort.

Nursing care activities are spaced to allow the client to rest. The nurse keeps the client's immediate surroundings quiet, restful, and free from anxiety-producing stimuli.

ALTERED NUTRITION: LESS THAN BODY REQUIREMENTS. The nurse weighs the client regularly and evaluates laboratory tests such as serum albumin (normal is 3.5–5.5 g/dL) and other pancreatic function tests. If the serum albumin level drops below 3.2 g/dL, the physician may order intravenous albumin as replacement. The client is assessed at least every 8 hours for bowel sounds, nausea, and vomiting.

The nurse monitors TPN therapy, including daily blood sugar results. Clients may be ordered to have finger-stick blood glucose tests done every 6 hours. The nurse administers regular insulin as ordered for an elevated blood sugar.

Histamine (H$_2$) antagonists and antacids are given as ordered. If the client has a nasogastric tube, the amount and character of the drainage is noted and recorded every 8 hours.

The client is usually slowly progressed to solid foods starting with carbohydrate supplements through the nasogastric tube. The client is slowly progressed to tube feedings with protein and fats as they are tolerated. Finally, bland, soft foods will be ordered. Any nausea, vomiting, or increase in complaints of abdominal discomfort is reported immediately. Clients who are progressed too quickly may have a relapse of the pancreatitis.

HIGH RISK FOR INEFFECTIVE BREATHING PATTERN. The client is carefully observed for any signs of respiratory distress such as tachypnea, tachycardia, dyspnea, use of accessory muscles, or presence of abnormal breath sounds or crackles. Evidence of poor oxygenation, including any changes in mental status (e.g., irritability, confusion, or increasing sleepiness), is reported promptly. Supplemental oxygen is administered as ordered. The client is in an upright or slightly forward-leaning position. Good pain control enables the client to breathe more effectively.

HIGH RISK FOR INJURY. The client is assessed for evidence of disturbed electrolyte balance. Laboratory values for sodium, potassium, calcium, and magnesium are monitored daily. Evidence of hypokalemia includes muscle weakness, diminished bowel sounds, apathy, and hypotension. Evidence of hypocalcemia includes nausea, vomiting, irritability, abdominal pain, and neuromuscular irritability. Neuromuscular irritability can be determined by Chvostek's sign, which is an involuntary facial twitch after the facial nerve is gently tapped on the cheek just in front of the ear. The client is also assessed for evidence of abnormal bleeding. The abdomen is observed for Turner's and Cullen's signs. The nurse evaluates the client's vital signs for tachycardia, tachypnea, and hypotension, which may indicate bleeding. Initially, urinary output is measured hourly using a urometer. Urine output should be greater than 30 mL/h. Any evidence of bleeding, such as a urinary output of less than 30 mL/h or frank bleeding, is reported promptly. The nurse monitors the administration of volume replacement solutions or blood infusions as ordered.

Client Education

The client is taught about pancreatitis. The client needs to know the treatment regimen and the reason for slow dietary progression from NPO to a normal diet. The client needs to know that rest is a vital part of the treatment plan and that gradual progression to full activities is normal. The client may never have another episode of pancreatitis but must exercise moderation in food, exercise, and alcohol ingestion.

If the pancreatitis is the result of chronic excessive alcohol ingestion, the client is counseled about abstinence. The client and family are referred to support organizations such as Alcoholics Anonymous.

Evaluation

The plan of care for the client with acute pancreatitis is successful if the client has

- Pain at or less than 2 on a scale of 0 to 5.
- Weight loss of less than 5 percent of total body weight.
- Respirations 16 to 20, unlabored, regular.
- No elevated temperature.
- No abnormal bruising.
- No restlessness.
- Urinary output greater than 30 mL/h.
- Blood pressure within 5 percent of baseline.

See also Nursing Care Plan Box 33–8 for the Client with Acute Pancreatitis.

 CRITICAL THINKING: Mr. Vickers

Mr. Vickers, a 45-year-old construction worker, is admitted to the nursing unit from the emergency department with severe midepigastric pain that radiates to his back. On admission, he is noted to have guarding of the abdomen, and the abdomen is full and tense. His medical record documents that he was seen in the emergency department 3 days ago after an accident at work in which he was struck in the abdomen by a swinging beam. He denies any history of excessive alcohol intake.

1. What is the most common cause of acute pancreatitis? Does Mr. Vickers fit the description?
2. Why do patients like Mr. Vickers have difficulty breathing?
3. Why is Mr. Vickers at risk for hemorrhage?
4. What laboratory test is most likely to be abnormal in early acute pancreatitis?
5. Why are narcotics commonly ordered for acute pancreatitis?
6. Why will the physician usually order a histamine (H$_2$) antagonist?

Answers at end of chapter.

NURSING CARE PLAN BOX 33–8 FOR THE CLIENT WITH ACUTE PANCREATITIS

Pain related to edema and inflammation

Outcome
Client experiences an increase in comfort as evidenced by statement of pain level less than 2 on a scale of 0 to 5.

Evaluation of Outcome
Does client state pain level is less than 2 on a pain scale of 0 to 5?

Interventions	Rationale	Evaluation

Assess the client every two hours for pain by
  Asking the client to rate pain on a scale of 0 to 5.
  Observing the client for acute pain behaviors such as grimacing, irritability, reluctance to move, or inability to lie quietly.
	Intense pain is likely to occur with acute pancreatitis.
	A pain scale allows for a consistent and individual evaluation of pain.
	Observation of acute pain behaviors such as reluctance to move, shallow respirations, grimacing, or irritability may be a reliable indicator of pain. Some clients with pain may deny their discomfort. However, the client in pain may have no observable pain behaviors.
		Does the client state that pain is less than 2 on a pain scale of 0 to 5, where 0 = no pain and 5 = worst possible pain?
		Does the client exhibit pain behaviors that differ from his or her report of pain?

Administer any analgesics as ordered.	Analgesics are most effective if given before pain becomes too great.	Are analgesics effective?
Assist the client to a position of comfort, usually high Fowler's or leaning forward slightly.	Upright position keeps abdominal organs from pressing against the inflamed pancreas.	Does positioning promote comfort?
Keep the environment free from excessive stimuli.	A quiet, restful, anxiety-free atmosphere permits the client to relax and may decrease pain perception.	Does client state atmosphere is relaxing?
Teach the client alternative pain control strategies such as guided imagery and relaxation techniques.	Successful use of pain control strategies may decrease the amount of analgesics needed and give the client a greater sense of control.	Are alternative strategies effective?

Altered nutrition: less than body requirements related to pain, medical restrictions (NPO), and treatment (suction).

Outcome
Client will experience improved nutrition as evidenced by stable weight, albumin greater than 3.5 g/L.

Evaluation of Outcome
Is weight stable? Is albumin level greater than 3.5 g/L?

Interventions	Rationale	Evaluation

Assess the client's nutritional status by
  Weighing the client every other day.
  Checking serum albumin levels on laboratory studies.
  Auscultation for bowel sounds.
  Observing for nausea or vomiting.
  Monitoring blood sugar at least every 6 hours if the client is on total parenteral nutrition (TPN).
  Observing for diarrhea, bloating, or steatorrhea (fatty stools).
	A loss of 1 lb of body weight occurs when the body uses 3500 calories more than is taken in.
	Serum albumin of 3.5–5.5 g/L indicates normal protein metabolism in the absence of liver or renal disease.
	Nausea, vomiting, and pain are risk factors for inadequate intake.
	Clients on TPN are more likely to have high blood glucose.
	Diarrhea, bloating, or fatty stools may indicate malabsorption syndrome.
		Has the client lost less than 5% of total baseline body weight? Is the client's sodium albumin below 3.5 g/dL?
		Does the client have sufficient energy and strength to carry out activities of daily living?

continued

NURSING CARE PLAN BOX 33–8 (continued)

Interventions	Rationale	Evaluation
Administer nutritional supplements, including pancreatic enzymes, as ordered.	Provides adequate nutrition.	Does client take any supplements?
Teach the client to avoid alcohol.	Alcohol may trigger another episode of pancreatitis.	Does client verbalize understanding of importance of avoiding alcohol?
Teach the client and family the signs and symptoms of diabetes mellitus.	Clients with pancreatitis are at great risk for developing diabetes mellitus, which also causes high blood glucose levels.	Does client verbalize signs and symptoms of diabetes to report?
Teach the client and family to self-monitor for symptoms of malabsorption syndrome, such as fatty stools, weight loss, dry skin, or bleeding.	The absence of pancreatic enzymes causes problems with the digestion of fats, carbohydrates, and proteins.	Does client verbalize understanding of symptoms of malabsorption to report?

Risk for ineffective breathing pattern related to abdominal pressure and pain

Outcome

Client has an effective breathing pattern as evidenced by respirations unlabored, 16–20 per minute.

Evaluation of Outcome

Are respirations unlabored, 16–20 per minute?

Interventions	Rationale	Evaluation
Assess the client's breathing patterns: Observe respirations for depth, regularity, and rate. Observe respiratory effort.	Abdominal pressure from inflammation and tissue damage under the diaphragm may cause the client to take shallow, rapid respirations, which can tire the client.	Are the client's respirations between 16 and 20 per minute, unlabored, and regular? Is the client alert and oriented? Has there been a change in the level of the client's arousal?
Observe for evidence of respiratory distress, such as use of accessory muscles, use of intercostal muscles, and rapid or difficult breathing.	Abdominal pressure can force the use of additional muscles to aid in breathing.	Does the client exhibit signs of distress?
Administer oxygen as ordered.	Oxygen can decrease the amount of effort the client must expend to breathe.	Does oxygen help client breathe easier?
Place client in an upright or slightly forward-leaning position.	Relieves pressure on the diaphragm.	Is positioning effective?
Prepare client's food by opening cartons and lids. Cut food into bite-size portions.	Decreases the demand for oxygen.	Does client accept assistance with food preparation?
Teach the client to move slowly and to take frequent rests.	Helps decrease the demand for oxygen.	Does client tolerate activity?

Risk for injury related to disturbed blood clotting mechanisms, fluid, and electrolyte imbalances

Outcome

Client experiences no injury.

Evaluation of Outcome

Is there evidence of injury? Are signs and symptoms of impending injury recognized and reported early?

continued

NURSING CARE PLAN BOX 33–8 (continued)		
Intervention	*Rationale*	*Evaluation*

Assess the client's fluid, electrolyte, and blood clotting mechanisms by
  Monitoring laboratory values of sodium, potassium, calcium, and magnesium daily.
  Evaluating neuromuscular status by checking Chvostek's sign.
	Sodium, potassium, calcium, and magnesium need to be replaced.	Has the client any abnormal bruising, bleeding gums, or pink urine? Is urinary output greater than 30 mL/h? Is the client's blood pressure within 5% of baseline? Do laboratory studies show that client's electrolyte, hemoglobin, hematocrit, and blood clotting values are within acceptable ranges?

Monitoring client's hematocrit, hemoglobin, and blood clotting times frequently.	Clients are likely to bleed.	

Observing abdomen and flanks for Cullen's and Turner's signs.
  Weighing the client daily.
  Measuring and recording intake and output every shift.
  Observing for nausea and vomiting.
	Clients may lose fluids because of nausea, vomiting, diarrhea, and hemorrhage.	

Report any drop in blood pressure greater than 5% of client's baseline.	May indicate severe fluid loss.	Are vital signs stable?
Monitor total parenteral nutrition (TPN) and report any difficulties.	TPN must not be stopped abruptly. Client's blood glucose may drop sharply.	Are blood glucose levels stable?
Teach the client to report any weakness or muscle twitching.	May indicate electrolyte imbalance.	Does client verbalize understanding of signs and symptoms of electrolyte imbalance to report?

CHRONIC PANCREATITIS

Chronic pancreatitis is continuing pancreatic cellular damage and decreased pancreatic enzyme functioning usually following repeated occasions of acute pancreatitis.

Pathophysiology

Chronic pancreatitis is a continuous, progressive disease that replaces functioning pancreatic tissue with fibrotic tissue as a result of inflammation. Toxins from alcohol irritate the pancreatic ducts. The ducts become obstructed, dilated, and finally atrophied. The acinar or enzyme-producing cells of the pancreas ulcerate in response to inflammation. The ulceration causes further tissue damage and tissue death, and it may cause cystic sacs filled with pancreatic enzymes to form on the surface of the pancreas. The pancreas becomes smaller and hardened, and progressively smaller amounts of the enzymes are produced.

Etiology and Incidence

The major cause of chronic pancreatitis in men is excessive alcohol ingestion that causes repeated attacks of acute pancreatitis. The major cause of pancreatitis in women is chronic obstructive biliary disease that causes persistent inflammation of the pancreatic ducts. Other conditions known to cause chronic pancreatitis are prolonged malnutrition, cancer of the pancreas or duodenum, and prolonged use of enteral feedings, which can cause atrophy of the pancreas. The usual age for chronic pancreatitis to develop is between 45 and 60 years. The client's mean life span is 25 years after the diagnosis of chronic pancreatitis is made. Death is often not related to pancreatic failure.

Prevention

Clients with an episode of acute pancreatitis from excessive alcohol ingestion are advised that abstinence could prevent recurrence of the pancreatitis and prevent the possibility of chronic pancreatitis. All clients with obstructive biliary disease are advised to seek medical treatment for their condition to prevent the progression from acute to chronic pancreatitis. Clients who are unable to feed themselves need to be carefully monitored for nutritionally adequate diets. The nurse monitors routine laboratory values of pancreatic functioning. Any trend toward poorer functioning of the pancreas is reported.

Signs and Symptoms

The signs and symptoms of chronic pancreatitis are less severe than acute pancreatitis, but more long term. The client's history will show a pattern of remissions and exacerbations over a period of years. The client will complain of epigastric or RUQ pain, weight loss, and anorexia. Malabsorption and fat intolerance occur late in the disease. Usually, the islets of Langerhans function until late stages of the disease, so diabetes is a late-occurring symptom.

Complications

Complications of chronic pancreatitis include the development of abscesses or fistulas, malabsorption syndrome, and diabetes mellitus. Abscesses and fistulas may develop when cysts filled with pancreatic enzymes burst into the abdominal cavity, causing severe inflammation and tissue necrosis. Pleural effusion may develop from inflammation just under the diaphragm. Malabsorption syndrome with fatty stools and diarrhea may develop in response to the limited amount of pancreatic enzymes produced. In addition, biliary obstruction may further complicate fat absorption. The enzymes are essential for normal absorption of nutrients from the intestines. As the terminal third of the pancreas becomes involved and the islets of Langerhans are destroyed, the client will exhibit the classic pattern of insulin-dependent diabetes mellitus.

Diagnostic Tests

Serum amylase (normal is 59–190 U/L) and serum lipase (normal is 0–110 U/L) will be less than normal. Fecal fat analysis will show higher than normal amounts of fat.

Both computed tomography and ultrasonography will show characteristic pancreatic structural changes such as masses, calcification of ducts, cysts, and change in pancreatic size.

Endoscopic retrograde cholangiopancreatography (ERCP) can locate specific obstructions and detect ductal leaks.

Medical Treatment

Medical treatment is aimed at promoting comfort and maintaining adequate nutrition. Pain is managed with analgesics. Nutrition is improved with the careful replacement of pancreatic enzymes and specially prepared nutritional supplements.

Surgery may be necessary to repair fistulas, drain cysts, or repair other damage. In some cases, ducts or sphincters may be surgically repaired. In other instances, part or all of the pancreas may be removed.

Nursing Process

Assessment

The nurse needs to thoroughly assess the client frequently for pain. The client is weighed frequently. Laboratory values are monitored to determine the adequacy of nutrition, including the serum albumin (normal is 3.5–5.5 g/dL) and blood glucose levels.

Nursing Diagnosis

Common nursing diagnoses for the client with chronic pancreatitis include the following:

- Pain related to edema and inflammation
- Altered nutrition: less than body requirements related to inability to absorb nutrients

Planning

The client and family, in collaboration with other health care providers, need to develop methods to manage chronic pain and to improve the client's nutritional status.

Implementation

PAIN. The nurse determines with the client what events and patterns cause or help the pain. The nurse attempts to determine how pain is affecting the client's eating habits and lifestyle. The nurse administers analgesics as ordered. The client may have chronic pain with periodic episodes of severe acute pain. The possibility exists that the client may develop dependence on the analgesic agent. The nurse can best help by careful assessment of the client so that medication regimens can be tailored to the client's need.

ALTERATION IN NUTRITION: LESS THAN BODY REQUIREMENTS. The client is weighed daily. All nutritional supplements, including pancreatic enzymes, are administered as ordered. The client receives histamine (H_2) antagonists or antacids as ordered. The nurse monitors the client's blood sugar and observes the client carefully for evidence of diabetes mellitus. The client with less than adequate amounts of insulin would show excessive thirst, frequent urination, hunger, and weight loss. (See Chapter 38 for management of the client with diabetes mellitus.) Further, the client is observed for diarrhea, bloating, or **steatorrhea** (fatty stools). Any evidence of continuing difficulty with digestion is reported immediately.

Client Education

The client is counseled to avoid alcohol. The client and family are given the warning signs and symptoms of diabetes mellitus. The client needs to be taught to monitor himself or herself for malabsorption syndrome. The client should check for fatty stools; report any weight loss; and report any evidence of vitamin A, D, E, or K deficiencies. Vitamin A deficiency may be evidenced by dry, scaly skin or changes in skin pigment. Vitamin D deficiency may be detected by client complaints of bone pain. Vitamin E deficiency may be associated with anemia. Vitamin K deficiency can be detected from abnormal bruising and a prolonged clotting time. The client should know that sudden increases in abdominal pain, increased difficulty breathing, or radiating back pain may indicate development of pan-

---

steatorrhea: steat—fat + orrhea—flow

creatic cysts, abscesses, or fistulae and should be reported promptly.

Evaluation

The plan of care for the client with chronic pancreatitis is successful if the client

- Has pain no more than 2 on a pain scale of 0 to 5.
- Has no weight loss or gain of more than one-half pound per week.
- Has no diarrhea or steatorrhea.
- Can state signs and symptoms of diabetes mellitus to report.
- Can state signs and symptoms of pancreatic cysts, abscesses, or fistulae.

CANCER OF THE PANCREAS

Cancer of the pancreas is the fifth leading cause of cancer death in the United States, killing more than 20,000 people each year. More than 25,000 new cases of cancer of the pancreas are diagnosed yearly; it most often affects people between the ages of 65 and 79 years of age. About 70 percent of cancers of the pancreas occur in the head of the pancreas. About 30 percent of cancers are located in the body and tail of the pancreas.

Pathophysiology

Most primary tumors of the pancreas are ductal adenocarcinomas and occur in the exocrine parts of the pancreas. The tumors in the head and body of the pancreas tend to be large. Cancer of the pancreas spreads rapidly by direct extension to the stomach, gallbladder, and duodenum. Cancer located in the body of the pancreas usually spreads more, and more rapidly, than do masses in the head. Cancer of the pancreas may spread by the lymphatic system and through the vascular system to distant organs and lymph nodes. The pancreas may also be the site of cancer spread from the lung, breast, kidney, thyroid gland, or malignant melanomas of the skin.

Etiology

The cause of cancer of the pancreas is not known. Cancer of the pancreas has been associated with chemical carcinogens such as high-fat diets and cigarette smoking, diabetes mellitus, excessive alcohol intake, and chronic pancreatitis.

Signs and Symptoms

The client with cancer of the pancreas usually complains of vague symptoms early in the disease process. Weight loss, pain, anorexia, nausea, vomiting, and weakness are among the vague early symptoms of cancer of the pancreas. Detection is often difficult because of the nonspecific complaints offered by the client. The client may complain of abdominal pain that is often worse at night. The pain is described as gnawing or boring, and it radiates to the back. The pain may be lessened by a side-lying position with the knees drawn up to the chest or by bending over when walking. The pain becomes increasingly severe and unrelenting as the cancer grows.

The client may complain of a bloated feeling or fullness after eating. If the cancer obstructs the bile duct, the client may have jaundice, dark urine, pruritus, and light-colored stools. The client frequently complains of fatigue and depression. The client's health history may include a recent diagnosis of diabetes mellitus.

Complications

Complications may occur before or after surgical treatment. Preoperative complications include malnutrition, spread of the cancer, and gastric or duodenal obstruction. Postoperative complications include infection, breakdown of the surgical site, fistula formation, diabetes mellitus, and malabsorption syndrome. If the client has chemotherapy or radiation therapy, complications specific to those therapies may also occur.

Thrombophlebitis is a common complication of cancer of the pancreas. As the tumor increases, by-products of the tumor growth appear to increase the levels of thromboplastic or blood clotting factors in the blood, making clotting easier. The potential for thrombophlebitis increases if the client is confined to bed or has surgery.

Diagnostic Tests

Serum amylase, lipase, alkaline phosphatase, and bilirubin levels are elevated. Blood coagulation tests, such as clotting time, may be ordered. Carcinoembryonic antigen (CEA) may be ordered to confirm the presence of cancer (normal is <5 ng/mL).

Abdominal x-rays may be ordered to determine the size of the pancreas and the presence of masses. Computed tomography and ultrasonography may be ordered to more precisely locate any masses in the pancreas.

Endoscopic retrograde cholangiopancreatography may be done to visualize the common ducts and to take tissue samples for microscopic analysis.

A tissue sample may be done by needle aspiration during ultrasonography. The procedure may cause seeding of the tumor along the needle pathway.

Medical Treatment

Medical treatment depends on the staging of the cancer. If diagnosed early, treatment may be aimed at cure. If the client's cancer has progressed to distant involvement of other organ structures and lymph nodes, treatment will be directed at easing symptoms, thus making the client more comfortable.

Surgery may include a total or partial **pancreatectomy** or removal of all or part of the pancreas. A Whipple procedure is done to remove the head of the pancreas, parts of the stomach nearby, the lower portion of the common bile duct, and the duodenum (Fig. 33–4). Sometimes the gallbladder is also removed. Potential postoperative problems after a Whipple procedure include failure of the suture lines to hold with leakage of pancreatic enzymes and bile into the abdomen, pneumonia or atelectasis from shallow breathing because the incision line is directly under the diaphragm, paralytic ileus, gastric retention or ulceration, wound infection, fistula formation, unstable diabetes mellitus, and renal failure.

Other surgical procedures may remove the entire pancreas, stomach, gallbladder, duodenum, and regional lymph nodes, or merely the distal portion of the pancreas and the spleen for smaller, more localized tumors. Postoperative complications similar to those that occur after the Whipple procedure may develop.

Relief of biliary obstruction can sometimes be accomplished by implanting a stent or plastic tube in the common bile duct during an endoscopic procedure. Pain can be helped by surgical removal of a portion of the greater splanchnic nerve.

Surgery may be followed by chemotherapy or radiation therapy or a combination of chemotherapy and radiation. In some instances, either radiation therapy or chemotherapy may be used for relief of symptoms if the cancer has become too widespread for surgery. (See Chapter 10 for care of the client with radiation or chemotherapy.)

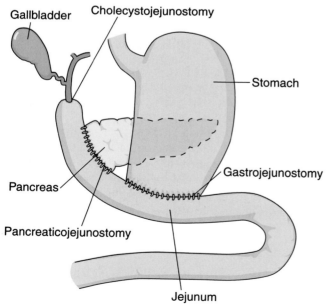

Figure 33–4. Pancreatoduodenectomy (Whipple's procedure) for cancer of the head of the pancreas.

Nursing Process

Assessment

The client with cancer of the pancreas must be observed for evidence of malnutrition and fluid imbalance, including weight loss, inelastic skin turgor, vomiting, fatty stools, and complaints of anorexia or nausea. Laboratory tests, especially blood glucose, liver function studies, and clotting time, are commonly reviewed. The client is evaluated every 2 to 4 hours for pain, including what triggers and what helps relieve the pain. The skin is observed for bruising, scaling, and yellowing, and the client is questioned about itching. The client's mental status is evaluated for evidence of depression.

Nursing Diagnosis

The common nursing diagnoses for the client with cancer of the pancreas include the following:

- Altered nutrition: less than body requirements related to inability to digest food, anorexia, nausea, and vomiting
- Pain related to pancreatic tumor or surgical incision
- Risk for fluid volume deficit related to nasogastric tube drainage, hemorrhage
- Risk for impaired skin integrity related to malabsorption, leakage of pancreatic or bile drainage postoperatively

Planning

The client and health team plan to ensure that the client has adequate nutrition, remains free of excessive pain, and does not develop complications from treatment.

Implementation

ALTERED NUTRITION: LESS THAN BODY REQUIREMENTS. The client is frequently assessed for nausea or vomiting. Bowel sounds are auscultated every 4 to 8 hours. Total parenteral nutrition, if ordered, is monitored carefully. The nurse assesses blood glucose levels by finger stick every 6 hours when TPN is administered. Regular insulin is administered according to the ordered sliding scale.

The nurse administers nasogastric tube feeding or other enteral feedings, such as through a gastrostomy or jejunostomy tube, as scheduled. The client is observed for evidence of intolerance to feedings, such as diarrhea, nausea, or vomiting. Pancreatic enzyme replacements are given as ordered. Steatorrhea (fatty stools) may indicate that the enzyme replacement doses are not meeting the client's needs. Steatorrhea is reported immediately.

PAIN. The pain associated with pancreatic cancer is intense. The client is evaluated for pain every 2 to 4 hours and

---

pancreatectomy: pancreat—pancreas + ectomy—excision

given analgesics as ordered. Opioids such as meperidine hydrochloride (Demerol) or morphine sulfate are usually ordered. For adequate pain relief, dosages of analgesics may need to be very high. The analgesics are given without concern for dependence because the outcome of the disease is so poor. Other medications, such as antidepressants, are administered as ordered.

The client is placed in the position of most comfort. The usual position is a semi-Fowler's position so that the diaphragm has the most expansion room. However, if the client is most comfortable in a side-lying position with legs drawn up, he or she is supported in that position. Additional methods of pain relief, such as guided imagery, distraction, or massage, may assist the client to greater comfort.

RISK FOR FLUID VOLUME DEFICIT. The nurse monitors the client's intake and output carefully. Tachycardia, tachypnea, and low blood pressure may indicate excessive fluid loss. Laboratory values are monitored, especially serum sodium, potassium, calcium, and chloride levels. If electrolyte values are low, the physician may order intravenous replacement solutions. Serum albumin should be between 6 and 8 g/dL. If the albumin level is lower, the nurse reports the value and monitors intravenous albumin therapy if ordered.

Coagulation studies may reveal a lowered clotting time from vitamin K deficiency. The nurse carefully observes the client for any abnormal bruising, bleeding gums, or pink-tinged urine. The client's abdomen and flanks are inspected for Cullen's sign (bluish discolorations around the umbilicus) and Turner's sign (bluish discolorations on the flanks), which are indications of bleeding into the retroperitoneum. If the client has tubes or drains, the nurse carefully inspects around the incision sites and the drainage tubing for any bleeding. The client is taught to use a soft-bristle toothbrush. If the client is male, he is encouraged to use an electric razor rather than a straight razor. The physician may order vitamin K.

HIGH RISK FOR IMPAIRED TISSUE INTEGRITY. The client is assessed for any complaints of itching. The nurse helps the client keep fingernails short, provides frequent skin care with products free of soap or alcohol, and protects skin around drains with skin-protective barrier products and ostomy bags. Products such as calamine lotion may be ordered to decrease itching.

The nurse needs to exercise special care of any drains to prevent unnecessary tension that may cause the sutures to give way. All drains are kept patent, and drainage tubing and bags are kept free from kinks. If the nasogastric tube must be irrigated, 10 to 20 mL of normal saline or air may be gently instilled, unless agency policy calls for a differ-

ent procedure. The client is placed in a semi-Fowler's position to help with gravity drainage.

Client Education

The client and family are educated on self-care measures for decreased pancreatic functioning such as blood glucose monitoring, insulin administration, signs and symptoms of hyperglycemia and hypoglycemia (see Chapter 38), and the regimen for pancreatic enzyme replacement. If the client is discharged with tubes or drains, instructions are given on how to manage dressing changes. The client and family should know the signs and symptoms of hemorrhage, gastric ulceration, infection, and fistula formation. The client should be referred to the appropriate community health care agency for assistance with pain management. The client is also given the opportunity for referral for hospice care.

Evaluation

The plan of care for the client with pancreatic cancer is successful if the client

- Maintains body weight within 5 percent of normal body weight and experiences no nausea or vomiting.
- States that pain remains at 2 or less on a pain scale of 0 to 5.
- Has urinary output greater than 40 mL/h, skin turgor is elastic, mucous membranes are moist, and pulse and blood pressure remain within 10 percent of client's baseline.
- Has no complaints of sudden, excessive abdominal pain or rigidity; incisions healed at the expected rate.
- Can demonstrate the appropriate self-care procedures for tubes, drains, dressings, medication administration, and states the signs and symptoms of complications that are to be reported immediately.

See also Ethical Considerations Box 33–9.

Disorders of the Gallbladder

CHOLECYSTITIS, CHOLELITHIASIS, AND CHOLEDOCHOLITHIASIS

Gallstones and inflammations of the gallbladder and common bile duct are the most common disorders of the biliary system. These disorders are also common health problems for people in the United States: Nearly 25 million people have gallstones, and about 1 million new cases are diagnosed each year.

Pathophysiology

Cholecystitis is an inflammation of the gallbladder. The inflammation is most often a response to obstruction of the common duct resulting in edema and inflammation. Often

---

cholecystitis: chole—bile + cyst—bladder + itis—inflammation

ETHICAL CONSIDERATIONS BOX 33-9

How Much Information Is Enough?

Mr. Golden, a 55-year-old college professor, was admitted to the hospital for nausea, weight loss, and diarrhea. After several tests were performed, a pancreatic mass was suspected, and the physician recommended that an exploratory laparotomy be performed to remove the mass. Mr. Golden, after receiving his preoperative instructions, signed the general surgical permit for an exploratory laparotomy that listed a subtotal pancreatectomy as a possible surgical procedure.

After performing the initial incision, the physician realized that the cancer was metastasized to many of the abdominal organs and, in addition to removing the pancreas, he had to remove part of the stomach, part of the small intestine, and part of the colon. When Mr. Golden returned from the recovery room, he was admitted to the surgical intensive care unit; was intubated; was put on ventilator support; and had multiple drains, a nasogastric tube, and a Foley catheter. When Mr. Golden began to regain consciousness, Ms. Brand, a licensed practical nurse (LPN) who worked in the unit, tried to explain what the machinery and tubings were for and how they would help maintain Mr. Golden's body functions. Mr. Golden seemed very confused and alarmed and soon started expressing his anger and frustration with his condition by way of a pad and pencil. He had not been warned before surgery that he would be in this condition after surgery.

The physician came in briefly during the shift; looked over the machines, tubes, and dressings; and told Mr. Golden that he was doing fine for the surgery he had had. Then he left without answering any of Mr. Golden's questions. In the hall, the physician told Ms. Brand that he didn't think Mr. Golden would make it and that she should keep him comfortable and quiet. Later in the shift, Mr. Golden wrote to Ms. Brand that if he had known that he would be in this condition after surgery, he would have never signed the permit. He also wanted to know just what exactly the physician had found during the surgery.

Ms. Brand believes that she has an ethical obligation to let the client know what was found and what his prognosis is, but she questions whether this is her responsibility. And what about the issue of the permit? Did Mr. Golden really give informed consent? Should she report this to the medical board? What are her obligations and duties in this situation?

---

bacteria invade the bile and add to the inflammation and irritation of the gallbladder. Chronic cholecystitis may be the result of repeated attacks of acute cholecystitis or chronic irritation from gallstones. The gallbladder becomes fibrotic and thickened and does not empty easily or completely.

Cholelithiasis, or stones in the gallbladder, are most often composed primarily of cholesterol. **Choledocholithiasis** refers to gallstones in the common bile duct. Although the exact cause of gallstones is unknown, one theory suggests that cholesterol may supersaturate the bile in the gallbladder. After a period of time, the supersaturated bile crystallizes and begins to form stones. Another type of gallstone is a pigment stone. Pigment stones appear to be composed of calcium bilirubinate, which occurs when free bilirubin combines with calcium.

Etiology and Incidence

Pooling, or stasis, of bile within the gallbladder, appears to contribute to the formation of stones. Stasis may be caused by a decreased gallbladder emptying rate or a partial obstruction in the common duct. Excessive cholesterol intake combined with a sedentary lifestyle is linked with an increased incidence of cholelithiasis.

Some low-fat diets have been linked to cholelithiasis because the diet appears to free cholesterol from body tissues; the cholesterol then crystallizes in the gallbladder before it is excreted. Further, a family history of cholelithiasis,

obesity, diabetes mellitus, pregnancy, some hemolytic blood disorders, and bowel disorders such as Crohn's disease have also been linked to a higher incidence of cholelithiasis.

Cholelithiasis is responsible for about 90 percent of the cases of cholecystitis, or inflammation of the gallbladder. Women between the ages of 20 and 50 years are about three times more likely to have gallstones than men. After the age of 50 years, the rate of gallstones is about the same for men and women. (See Cultural Considerations Box 33–10.)

Signs and Symptoms

Signs and symptoms of cholecystitis and cholelithiasis are similar. Objective symptoms include evidence of inflammation, such as an elevated temperature, pulse, and respiration; vomiting; and jaundice. Subjective symptoms include client complaints of epigastric pain, RUQ tenderness, nausea, and indigestion. The client may have a positive Murphy's sign, which is the inability to take a deep breath when an examiner's fingers are pressed below the liver margin.

The epigastric pain caused by cholelithiasis may also be called biliary **colic.** The pain is a steady, aching, severe

---

cholelithiasis: chole—bile + lith—stone + iasis—condition
choledocholithiasis: chole—bile + docho—duct + lith—stone + iasis—condition
colic: colic—spasm

pain in the epigastrium and RUQ that may radiate back to behind the right scapula or to the right shoulder. The pain usually begins suddenly after a fatty meal and lasts for 1 to 3 hours. If the pain is caused by a stone in the common bile duct (choledocholithiasis), the pain may last until the stone has passed into the duodenum. Jaundice is more commonly present with acute choledocholithiasis because the common bile duct is blocked or inflamed.

The biliary colic caused by cholecystitis typically lasts 4 to 6 hours. The pain is made worse with movement such as breathing. The client will usually have nausea, vomiting, and a low-grade fever with the pain.

Client complaints of heartburn, indigestion, and flatulence are more common with chronic cholecystitis. The client will usually report a medical history that suggests repeated attacks of acute cholecystitis (Table 33–5).

Family history of either cholecystitis or cholelithiasis; dietary habits such as high fat intake or a recent low-fat diet; and complaints of flatulence (gas), eructation (belching), nausea, vomiting, or abdominal discomfort after a high-fat meal are common evidence of a gallbladder disorder.

Complications

Complications of cholecystitis include inflammation of the bile ducts (cholangitis), necrosis or perforation of the gallbladder, empyema (a collection of purulent drainage in the gallbladder), fistulas, and adenocarcinoma of the gallbladder. A major complication of choledocholithiasis is acute pancreatitis if the pancreatic duct is obstructed.

Diagnostic Tests

The client may have an elevated white blood cell count (normal is 5000–10,000 cells/mm^3). The serum amylase may be elevated (normal is 59–190 IU/L) if the pancreas is involved or if there is a stone in the common duct.

An abdominal x-ray is done to determine whether the gallstone is primarily calcium. Calcium-based stones are less responsive to medical treatments. Cholesterol stones are highly responsive to medical therapy. Further radiologic examinations may include an oral cholecystography. The client is given a contrast medium either by mouth or intravenously. X-rays then show the presence of gallstones. Any cholesterol stones usually float to the top of the bile. Clients are then given a high-fat meal, and the radiologist can see the gallbladder contract and empty. Oral cholecystography is not used with clients who are jaundiced because the liver cannot transport the contrast medium to the obstructed gallbladder.

Sonograms can detect stones and may be able to determine whether the walls of the gallbladder have thickened.

Table 33–5. **Symptoms of Gallbladder Disorders**

	Acute Cholecystitis	*Chronic Cholecystitis*	*Cholelithiasis and Choledocholithiasis*
Biliary colic	Last 4–6 hours Worse with movement	Only during acute attack	Sudden onset Lasts 1–3 hours Radiates to right scapula or shoulder
Jaundice	√ (if common bile duct is inflamed or blocked)	√	
Low-grade fever	√	√	√
Nausea, vomiting	√	Only during acute attack	√
Repeated attacks		√	
Heartburn, indigestion, and flatulence		√	
Complications	Cholangitis Necrosis or perforation Fistulas	Empyema Fistulas Adenocarcinoma	Acute pancreatitis

√ = usually present or commonly found on assessment

An ERCP can be done to directly visualize the pancreatic ducts and bile ducts to determine the presence of stones in the common duct, and occasionally to remove stones from the common duct.

Medical Treatment

Medical management for an acute episode of cholecystitis centers on pain control, prevention of infection, and maintenance of fluid and electrolyte balance. Pain control is achieved by using opioid analgesics. The analgesic agent most often ordered is meperidine hydrochloride (Demerol) because morphine sulfate may cause spasms of the gallbladder, biliary ducts, and the sphincter of Oddi. Antispasmotics or anticholinergic drugs such as propantheline bromide (Pro-Banthine) and dicyclomine hydrochloride (Bentyl) may be ordered to decrease the biliary colic. If the client has nausea and vomiting, an antiemetic such as prochlorperazine (Compazine) may be ordered. Clients are placed on high-protein, low-fat diets after the nausea and vomiting subside. (See Nutritional Notes Box 33–11.)

Treatment for cholelithiasis usually involves surgical removal of the gallbladder. The surgical procedure may be a **laparoscopic** cholecystectomy or a traditional cholecystectomy. A laparoscopic cholecystectomy may be done through four small puncture wounds in the abdomen. The client is usually discharged within 24 hours. A traditional cholecystectomy is done through a long, transverse, right subcostal incision. The client has a **T-tube** inserted into the common duct for a period of several days postoperatively to ensure that bile drainage is not obstructed (Fig. 33–5). The client with a traditional cholecystectomy has incisional pain that creates difficulty with coughing and deep breathing postoperatively because with a deep breath, the diaphragm presses on the operative site. Clients are hospitalized for 2 to 3 days with a traditional cholecystectomy and 24 hours or less with a laparoscopic cholecystectomy.

Some clients are poor surgical risks and have stones in the gallbladder or biliary duct that cannot be removed easily by other methods. Such clients may have a cholecys-

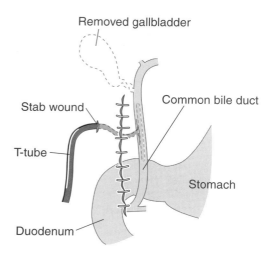

Figure 33–5. T-tube. A T-tube is used to drain bile after a cholecystectomy until swelling of the duct subsides.

tostomy, which is an incision directly into the gallbladder to remove a stone. If the stone is in the biliary ducts, a choledocholithotomy may be done. The client will usually have a T-tube in place to help remove bile from swollen structures for several days.

Other methods of treatment include **choledochoscopy, extracorporeal shock-wave lithotripsy** (ESWL), dissolving stones with oral drugs, and direct contact dissolving drugs. The procedure for a choledochoscopy involves the use of an endoscope to explore the common bile duct and in some instances to snare and remove any stones found.

Extracorporeal shock-wave lithotripsy uses shock waves as a noninvasive method to destroy stones in the gallbladder or biliary ducts. Clients who are considered poor surgical risks and who have few cholesterol stones that are not calcified are the most likely candidates for ESWL. The client lies face down on a water bag over a lithotriptor (Fig. 33–6). A conductive gel is placed between the client and the water bag. Ultrasound is used to locate the stone or stones and to monitor the destruction of the stones. The client requires sedation and strong analgesics during the procedure to reduce the pain and discomfort of the shock waves. After ESWL, the client is usually put on a course of oral dissolution drugs to ensure complete removal of all stones and stone fragments.

Dissolution of stones with drugs may be attempted with chenodeoxycholic acid (chenodiol) or ursodeoxycholic acid (ursodiol). Clients who are poor surgical risks because of advanced age or severe health problems and who have cholesterol stones may use oral dissolution drugs. The major disadvantages to the use of these drugs are that abnormal liver function studies and diarrhea are common side

---

NUTRITION NOTES BOX 33–11

Gallbladder

Acute attacks: full liquids with minimal fat.

Chronic disease: correct obesity; eat breakfast or at least drink two glasses of water on arising to empty gallbladder; avoid troublesome and gas-forming foods; decrease daily dietary fat by

Selecting skim milk dairy products

Limiting fats or oils to 3 teaspoons

Consuming no more than 6 ounces of very lean meat

---

laparoscopic: laparo—pertaining to flank + scopic—to examine
choledochoscopy: chole—bile + docho—duct + scopy—to examine
extracorporeal shock-wave lithotripsy: extra—outside + corporeal—body + litho—stone + tripsy—rub or crush

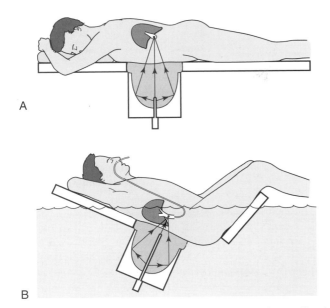

Figure 33–6. Extracorporeal shock-wave lithotripsy. Shock waves are transmitted through water to break up gallstones. *(A)* Position for stones in gallbladder. Client is lying on a fluid-filled bag. *(B)* Position for stones in common bile duct. Client is in a water bath.

effects. Clients may also have an increase in serum cholesterol while taking the drugs. Treatment with the dissolution drugs may take from 4 months to 2 years. Clients may need to take cholesterol-lowering drugs such as cholestyramine (Questran) in addition to the dissolution drugs to lower serum cholesterol and to decrease the probability of stones reforming.

Direct contact dissolution drugs are administered directly into the gallbladder through a percutaneous transhepatic catheter. The physician inserts a catheter through the wall of the abdomen into the gallbladder and then injects and aspirates the dissolution agent repeatedly during the treatment. Candidates for this procedure are clients who are poor surgical risks and whose gallbladder can be seen during oral cholecystography. Disadvantages of the procedure include abnormal liver function studies, pain at the catheter site, nausea, and elevations in the white blood cell count.

Nursing Process

Assessment

The nurse assesses the client frequently for pain, including location, intensity, and relieving and intensifying events. The client's vital signs, particularly the temperature and pulse, are taken frequently to monitor for signs of infection. The client is weighed, and mucous membranes, skin turgor, and urinary output are observed for signs of dehydration. Intake and output are measured, including any emesis or drainage from nasogastric tubes or T-tubes. Stools and urine are observed for color and consistency.

Obstruction of bile flow may result in stools that are clay colored or have a foul, greasy appearance or urine that is dark amber or tea colored. Either finding is reported immediately. Laboratory studies are evaluated for any elevation in the white blood cell count or abnormalities in electrolytes or serum bilirubin levels.

Nursing Diagnosis

Common nursing diagnoses for the client with cholecystitis include the following:

- Pain related to biliary colic
- Risk for fluid volume deficit related to anorexia, nausea, vomiting, or excessive tube drainage

Additional nursing diagnoses for the client with cholelithiasis who has a surgical procedure include the following:

- Risk for impaired skin integrity related to surgical incision and T-tube drainage
- Risk for ineffective breathing pattern related to abdominal incision

Planning

Goals for the client with cholecystitis or cholelithiasis include pain management so that biliary colic is tolerable, management of the nausea and vomiting to prevent excessive fluid loss, management of the surgical incision to prevent infection or tissue damage from drainage, and close monitoring to detect and treat any infection.

Implementation

PAIN. The client is assessed frequently for pain. The pain should be controlled at not more than 2 on a pain scale of 0 to 5. The client is given meperidine hydrochloride as ordered. Antispasmotics or anticholinergics are given as ordered. The client is placed in a position of comfort and supported.

RISK FOR FLUID VOLUME DEFICIT. Intravenous fluids and electrolytes are administered as ordered while the client is on restricted oral intake. Antiemetics are given as ordered if the client experiences nausea and vomiting. After surgery, a nasogastric tube may be inserted to prevent an ileus from developing. The nurse frequently assesses for the return of bowel sounds and flatus. After the nasogastric tube is removed, the client is slowly reintroduced to a solid diet, usually a high-protein, low-fat diet. T-tube drainage is monitored. About 250 to 500 mL of yellowish-green bile is common within the first 24 hours after surgery. The amount of bile diminishes over the next several days. The T-tube drainage unit is carefully observed to prevent kinking of the tubing. Pressure in the biliary drainage system from poor drainage may greatly increase the client's pain and the risk of infection.

RISK FOR IMPAIRED SKIN INTEGRITY. The client's position is changed frequently. The client is encouraged to stay in a low semi-Fowler's position as much as possible. The cholecystectomy incision is inspected frequently for excessive drainage or evidence of infection such as redness, edema, or warmth. The skin around the incision site is protected by changing dressings frequently. Montgomery straps will prevent skin irritation from repeated or prolonged exposure to adhesive bandages. If bile is leaking around the T-tube site, the skin is protected with a skin barrier product or bag such as those used with colostomies. An enterostomal therapist can be consulted for the best choice of dressing if the facility has such a specialist. The client's skin and sclera of the eyes are inspected frequently for jaundice. Client complaints of excessive itching are noted and reported.

RISK FOR INEFFECTIVE BREATHING PATTERN. Deep breathing and coughing after any surgical procedure will help prevent respiratory tract infections and atelectasis. Clients with high abdominal incisions are particularly reluctant to cough and deep breathe. Clients are instructed in the proper techniques before surgery and given the opportunity to practice. After surgery, the nurse encourages the client to cough and deep breathe at every encounter. If the client is reluctant to cough because of pain, the pain medication regimen may need to be evaluated. The client is assisted with splinting and is encouraged to walk when permitted.

Client Education

Client education focuses on diet. Clients are put on high-protein, low-fat diets. Obese clients ar encouraged to lose weight. After a cholecystectomy, there is a slow reintroduction of fat in the diet. Once the duodenum becomes accustomed to constant infusion of bile, the client's individual tolerance for fat becomes the only restriction for diet.

Evaluation

The plan of care for a client with cholecystitis or cholelithiasis is successful if the client

- Reports that pain is not greater than 2 on a pain scale of 0 to 5 or that the pain is tolerable.
- Has no weight loss, urinary output greater than 50 mL/h, mucous membranes moist, skin turgor elastic, and no complaints of excessive thirst.
- Has intact skin with no warmth, redness, swelling, or purulent drainage at the wound site, no jaundice, complaints of itching.
- Has clear breath sounds and a normal white blood cell count.

▼ **CRITICAL THINKING: Donna**

Donna, a 43-year-old mother of six, is diagnosed with possible acute cholecystitis. She is 5 ft 6 in tall and weighs 200 lb. Her physician wishes to delay surgery until her inflammation has subsided.

HOME HEALTH HINTS

- For clients with hepatitis, home health nurses are concerned with proper treatment to prevent transmission in the community and to prevent permanent liver damage to the client.
- If possible, the client should have a separate bedroom and bathroom. The person cleaning the bathroom should wear rubber gloves and then clean the gloves with a 10 percent bleach solution. The family is advised to use liquid soap instead of bar soap.
- Contaminated linens should be washed separately from household laundry, in hot water. One cup of bleach should be added with the detergent to each load. Rubber gloves should be worn to wash the client's laundry.
- Clients with abdominal ascites need a hospital bed at home so the client can be positioned to aid in breathing. A physician's order must be obtained.
- The measurement of abdominal girth should be taken at each visit and recorded in the nurse's notes. The client should weigh on the same scale, first thing in the morning, and record the weight so the nurse can document the findings.

1. What risk factors does Donna have for cholecystitis?
2. What diagnostic tests might be ordered to confirm Donna's diagnosis of cholecystitis?
3. What medications can the nurse anticipate that the physician will order for Donna?
4. What type of diet will Donna need to eat after discharge?
5. When the diagnosis of cholecystitis is confirmed, what type of surgical treatment might Donna's surgeon select?

Answers at end of chapter.

Review Questions

1. The client with ascites related to liver failure most likely has which of the following laboratory findings?
   a. Low bilirubin
   b. High amylase
   c. High hematocrit
   d. Low albumin

2. Jack has an episode of bleeding from esophageal varices. Which of the following conditions placed Jack at risk for varices?
   a. Portal hypertension
   b. Altered nutrition

c. Elevated liver enzymes
d. High-fiber diet

3. Janet has cholelithiasis. Most gallstones are composed of
   a. Calcium
   b. Cholesterol
   c. Sodium
   d. Phosphorus

4. Thelma develops jaundice and clay-colored stools. The cause is most likely
   a. Encephalopathy
   b. Pancreatitis
   c. Bile duct obstruction
   d. Cholecystitis

5. Mr. Jones is scheduled for an incisional cholecystectomy. Postoperatively you place *highest* priority on encouraging which patient activity?
   a. Coughing and deep breathing
   b. Performing leg exercises
   c. Learning to change the dressing
   d. Choosing low-fat foods from the menu

6. Jeff is a 26-year-old health care worker who is diagnosed with hepatitis B virus; HBV is transmitted by which of the following routes?
   a. Fecal-oral route
   b. Blood and body fluids
   c. Casual contact
   d. Respiratory droplets

7. Judy, age 43, is admitted to your unit with acute pancreatitis. You recognize that an elevation in which diagnostic test indicates acute pancreatitis?
   a. Serum bilirubin
   b. Serum calcium
   c. Serum triglycerides
   d. Serum amylase

8. In planning care for the newly admitted client with acute pancreatitis, you assign the highest priority to which patient outcome?
   a. Client expresses satisfaction with pain control.
   b. Client verbalizes understanding of medications for home.
   c. Client increases activity tolerance.
   d. Client maintains normal bowel function.

ANSWERS TO CRITICAL THINKING

CRITICAL THINKING: Mrs. Rogers

1. Information that suggests hepatitis A virus is foreign travel within the past 2 months, fatigue, nausea, and irritability. Information that suggests hepatitis B virus is recent exposure to blood and possibly body fluids, fatigue, headache, and nausea.

2. Careful hand washing and universal precautions when handling any body fluids or feces should be instituted.

3. The nurse should plan to give an antiemetic if Mrs. Rogers is nauseated. Larger meals should be given early in the day, with Mrs. Rogers in an upright or sitting position. The nurse should also ensure that the environment is free of noxious stimulants such as unpleasant odors. The diet should be a high-calorie, high-protein, high-carbohydrate, low-fat diet.

4. Any medication that is known to be hepatotoxic, such as acetaminophen, aspirin, and diazepam (Valium), should be avoided.

5. Mrs. Rogers should be reminded that cleanliness, especially with food preparation, is essential. She should also be reminded that frequent hand washing is crucial. Mrs. Rogers needs to know that alcohol and other liver-toxic substances should be avoided.

CRITICAL THINKING: Jonathan

1. Jonathan has a history of prolonged excessive alcohol consumption and poor diet. His age and sex also put him at risk.

2. Jonathan may report malaise; poor appetite; nausea; weight loss; change in bowel habits; and dull, aching RUQ pain.

3. Serum albumin is usually less than 3.2 g/dL. The prothrombin time is greater than 25 seconds.

4. Esophageal varices and ascites are the two greatest concerns with portal hypertension.

5. The physician will usually order diuretics, intravenous albumin infusions, and a sodium-restricted diet.

6. Suffocation from having the gastric tube dislodge into the esophagus.

CRITICAL THINKING: Mr. Vickers

1. The most common cause of acute pancreatitis is excessive alcohol intake. Mr. Vickers does not fit the description because he denies excessive drinking.

2. Respiratory distress may result from excess fluid accumulation in the retroperitoneal space and from shallow respirations that seek to decrease pressure from the diaphragm on the inflamed pancreas and surrounding tissues.

3. Pancreatitis is similar to a chemical burn and may cause erosion of major blood vessels in surrounding tissue.

4. Serum amylase may be elevated as much as 40 times normal early in acute pancreatitis.

5. Narcotics are ordered because pain is intense, and pain with anxiety stimulates the autonomic ner-

vous system, which may stimulate greater production of pancreatic enzymes.

6. Stomach acid stimulates the production of pancreatic enzymes. The histamine antagonists decrease stomach acidity.

CRITICAL THINKING: Donna

1. Donna has the following risk factors: female, obesity, and multiple pregnancies.
2. White blood cell count, sonogram, endoscopic retrograde cholangiopancreatography, abdominal x-ray, and cholecystogram may be ordered.
3. Meperidine hydrochloride for pain, antispasmodics such as propantheline bromide, prochlorperazine for nausea, and possibly antibiotics may be ordered.
4. Donna will be encouraged to eat a high-protein, low-fat diet.
5. Either a laparoscopic cholecystectomy or traditional cholecystectomy may be selected because Donna does not appear to have any contraindications to surgery.

REFERENCES

1. American Cancer Society: Cancer Facts and Figures for Minority Americans. Publication 91-75M-No. 5623. American Cancer Society, Atlanta, 1991.
2. Meleis, A, and Meleis, M: Egyptian-Americans. In Purnell, L, and Paulanka, B (eds): Transcultural Health Care: A Culturally Competent Approach. FA Davis, Philadelphia, 1998.
3. Goddard, L: An Afrocentric Model of Prevention for African-American High Risk Youth. Institute for the Advanced Study of Black Family Life and Culture, 1990.
4. Jaynes, D, and Williams, R: A Common Destiny: Blacks and American Society. National Academy Press, Washington, DC, 1989.
5. Selekman, J: Jewish-Americans. In Purnell, L, and Paulanka, B (eds): Transcultural Health Care: A Culturally Competent Approach. FA Davis, Philadelphia, 1998.
6. Still, O, and Hodgins, D: Navajo Indians. In Purnell, L, and Paulanka, B (eds): Transcultural Health Care: A Culturally Competent Approach. FA Davis, Philadelphia, 1998.

BIBLIOGRAPHY

Beare, PG, and Myers, JL: Principles and Practice of Adult Health Nursing, ed 2. Mosby, St Louis, 1994.

Brozenec, SA, and Russell, SS (eds): Core Curriculum for Medical-Surgical Nursing. Academy of Medical Surgical Nurses, Pitman, NJ, 1995.

Greifzu, S, and Dest, V: When the diagnosis is pancreatic cancer. RN 54(9):38, 1991.

Grindel, CG, and Costello, MC: Nutritional screening: An essential assessment parameter. Medsurg Nurs 5(3):145, 1996.

Grindel, CG: Fatigue and nutrition. Medsurg Nurs 3(6):475, 1994.

Herreid, J: Hepatitis C: Past, present, and future. Medsurg Nurs 4(3):179, 1995.

Ignatavicius, DD, Workman, ML, and Mishler, MA: Medical-Surgical Nursing: A Nursing Process Approach, ed 2. WB Saunders, Philadelphia, 1995.

Lutz, CA, and Przytulski, KR: Nutrition and Diet Therapy, ed 2. FA Davis, Philadelphia, 1997.

Markell, EK, Voge, M, and John, DT: Medical Gastrology. WB Saunders, Philadelphia, 1992.

Monroe, D: Patient teaching for x-ray and other diagnostics. RN 53(4):52, 1990.

Office of Minority Health Resource Center: Liver cancer is high among American Chinese. Author, Washington, DC, 1994.

Olsen, S, and Frank-Stromberg, M: Cancer prevention and early detection in ethnically diverse populations. Semin Ocol Nurs 9(3):189, 1993.

Ondrusek, RS: Cholecystectomy: An update. RN 56(1):28, 1993.

Rudman, D, et al: Ammonia content of food. Am J Clin Nutr 26:487, 1973.

Sichiere, R, Everhart, JE, and Rothe, H: A prospective study of hospitalization with gallstone disease among women: Role of dietary factors, fasting period, and dieting. Am J Public Health 81:880, 1991.

Smith, A: When the pancreas self-destructs. Am J Nurs 38, Sept 1991.

Willis, DA, Harbit, MD, and Julius, LM: Gallstones: Alternatives to surgery. RN 53(4):44, 1990.

UNIT 9

Understanding the Renal System

Urinary System Function, Assessment, and Therapeutic Measures

34

Betty J. Ackley

Learning Objectives

Upon completion of this chapter, the student will be able to:

1. Identify the structures of the urinary system.
2. Describe the functions of the urinary system.
3. List the effects of aging on the urinary system.
4. State normal and oliguric 24-hour urinary output.
5. Recognize basic assessment information that should be obtained regarding renal function.
6. Identify how to collect a midstream, clean-catch urine specimen and 24-hour creatinine clearance specimen.
7. Explain the meaning of an elevated serum creatinine, blood urea nitrogen, and uric acid.
8. Describe preparation and aftercare for various diagnostic tests of the urinary system.
9. Identify nursing actions that can be taken to decrease the incidence of infection in catheterized clients.
10. Describe nursing care of clients who are incontinent.

Key Words

cystoscopy (sis-**TAHS**-koh-pee)

dysuria (dis-**YOO**-ree-ah)

hematuria (HEM-uh-**TYOOR**-ee-ah)

percutaneous (PER-kyoo-**TAY**-nee-us)

pyelogram (**PIE**-loh-GRAM)

uremia (yoo-**REE**-mee-ah)

Review of Anatomy and Physiology

The urinary system consists of the two kidneys, two ureters, the urinary bladder, and the urethra. The kidneys form urine, and the rest of the system eliminates urine. Although the obvious purpose of urine formation is the removal of potentially toxic waste products from the blood, the work of the kidneys has other equally important functions:

1. Regulation of the volume of blood by the excretion or conservation of water
2. Regulation of the electrolyte balance of the blood by the excretion or conservation of minerals
3. Regulation of acid-base balance of the blood by the excretion or conservation of ions such as hydrogen ions or bicarbonate ions
4. Regulation of all of the above in tissue fluid

The process of urine formation thus helps maintain the normal composition, volume, and pH of both blood and tissue fluid.

KIDNEYS

The two kidneys are located in the upper abdominal cavity behind the peritoneum on each side of the vertebral column. The upper portions of both kidneys rest on the lower surface of the diaphragm and are enclosed and protected by the lower rib cage. The kidneys are cushioned by surrounding adipose tissue, which is in turn covered by a fibrous connective membrane called the renal fascia; both help hold the kidneys in place. On the medial side of a kidney is an indentation called the hilus where the renal artery enters and the renal vein and ureter emerge (Fig. 34–1). The renal artery is a branch of the abdominal aorta, and the renal vein returns blood to the inferior vena cava. The ureter carries urine from the kidney to the urinary bladder.

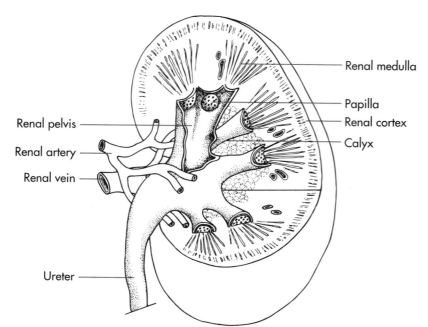

Renal pelvis
Renal artery
Renal vein
Ureter

Renal medulla
Papilla
Renal cortex
Calyx

Figure 34–1. Frontal section of the left kidney. (Modified from Scanlon, VC, Sanders, T: Workbook for Essentials of Anatomy and Physiology, ed 2. FA Davis, Philadelphia, 1995, p 285, with permission.) See Plate 6.

Internal Structure of the Kidney

A frontal section of the kidney shows three distinct areas (Fig. 34–1). The outermost area is the renal cortex and contains the parts of the nephrons called renal corpuscles and convoluted tubules. The middle area is the renal medulla, which contains loops of Henle and collecting tubules. The renal medulla consists of wedge-shaped pieces called renal pyramids; the apex, or papilla, of each pyramid points medially. The third area is a cavity called the renal pelvis; it is formed by the expansion of the ureter within the kidney at the hilus. Funnel-shaped extensions of the renal pelvis, called calyces, enclose the papillae of the renal pyramids. Urine flows from the pyramids into the calyces, then to the renal pelvis, and finally into the ureter.

Nephron

The nephron is the structural and functional unit of the kidney. It is in the approximately 1 million nephrons in each kidney that urine is formed. The two major parts of a nephron are the renal corpuscle and the renal tubule; these and their subdivisions and blood vessels are shown in Fig. 34–2.

A renal corpuscle consists of a glomerulus surrounded by a Bowman's capsule. The glomerulus is a capillary network that arises from an afferent arteriole and empties into an efferent arteriole. The diameter of the efferent arteriole is smaller than that of the afferent arteriole, which helps maintain a fairly high blood pressure in the glomerulus. Bowman's capsule is the expanded end of a renal tubule; it

encloses the glomerulus. The inner layer of Bowman's capsule has pores and is highly permeable; the outer layer has no pores and is not permeable. The space between the inner and outer layers contains renal filtrate, the fluid that is formed from the blood in the glomerulus and that will eventually become urine.

The renal tubule continues from Bowman's capsule and consists of the proximal convoluted tubule, the loop of Henle, and the distal convoluted tubule. The distal convoluted tubules from several nephrons empty into a collecting tubule. Several collecting tubules then unite to form a papillary duct that empties urine into a calyx of the renal pelvis. All of the parts of the renal tubule are surrounded by the peritubular capillaries, which arise from the efferent arteriole and receive the materials reabsorbed by the renal tubules.

Blood Vessels of the Kidney

The pathway of blood flow through the kidney is an essential part of the process of urine formation. Blood from the abdominal aorta enters the renal artery, which branches extensively within the kidney into smaller arteries. The smallest arteries give rise to afferent arterioles in the renal cortex. From the afferent arterioles, blood flows into the glomeruli (capillaries), to efferent arterioles, to peritubular capillaries, to veins within the kidney, to the renal vein, and finally to the inferior vena cava. In this pathway are two sets of capillaries, that is, two sites of exchanges between the blood and the surrounding tissues (in this case, the parts of the nephrons). The exchanges that take place in

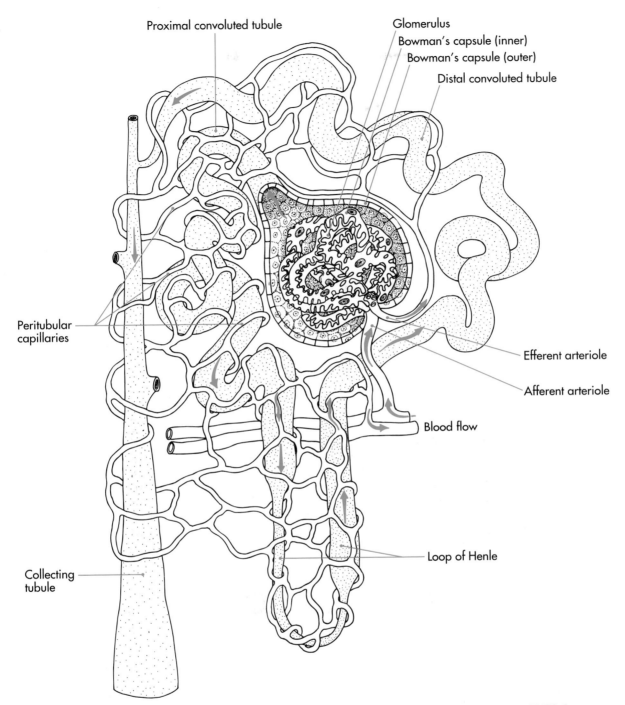

Proximal convoluted tubule

Glomerulus

Bowman's capsule (inner)

Bowman's capsule (outer)

Distal convoluted tubule

Peritubular capillaries

Efferent arteriole

Afferent arteriole

Blood flow

Loop of Henle

Collecting tubule

Figure 34-2. A nephron and its associated blood vessels. (Modified from Scanlon, VC, Sanders, T: Workbook for Essentials of Anatomy and Physiology, ed 2. FA Davis, Philadelphia, 1995, p 287, with permission.) See Plate 7.

the capillaries of the kidneys will form urine from blood plasma.

FORMATION OF URINE

The formation of urine involves three major processes: glomerular filtration in the renal corpuscles, tubular reabsorption, and tubular secretion.

Glomerular Filtration

Filtration is the process in which blood pressure forces plasma and dissolved materials out of capillaries. In glomerular filtration, blood pressure forces plasma, dissolved substances, and small proteins out of the glomeruli and into Bowman's capsules. This fluid is now called renal filtrate.

The blood pressure in the glomeruli is relatively high, about 60 mm Hg. The pressure in Bowman's capsule is very low, and its inner layer is very permeable, so that approximately 20 to 25 percent of the blood that enters glomeruli becomes renal filtrate in Bowman's capsules. The larger proteins and blood cells are too large to be forced out of the glomeruli; they remain in the blood. Waste products such as urea and ammonia are dissolved in plasma, so they pass to the renal filtrate, as do dissolved nutrients and minerals. Renal filtrate is very similar to blood plasma except that there is far less protein and no blood cells are present.

The glomerular filtration rate (GFR) is the amount of renal filtrate formed by the kidneys in 1 minute and averages 100 to 125 mL per minute. The GFR may change if the rate of blood flow through the kidney changes. If blood flow increases, the GFR increases, and more filtrate is formed. If blood flow decreases, the GFR decreases, less filtrate is formed, and urinary output decreases.

Tubular Reabsorption

Tubular reabsorption is the recovery of useful materials from the renal filtrate and their return to the blood in the peritubular capillaries. Approximately 99 percent of the renal filtrate formed is reabsorbed, and normal urinary output per 24 hours is 1 to 2 L. Most reabsorption takes place in the proximal convoluted tubules, whose cells have microvilli that greatly increase their surface area. The distal convoluted tubules and collecting tubules are also important sites for the reabsorption of water. The mechanisms of reabsorption are active transport, passive transport, osmosis, and pinocytosis.

Active transport requires energy in the form of adenosine triphosphate (ATP); the cells of the renal tubule use energy to transport useful materials such as glucose, amino acids, vitamins, and positive ions back to the blood. For many of these substances there is a threshold level of reabsorption, that is, a limit to how much the renal tubules can remove from the filtrate. The level of a substance in the renal filtrate is directly related to its blood level. If the blood level of a substance such as glucose is normal, the filtrate level will be normal, the threshold level will not be exceeded, and no glucose will appear in the urine.

Passive transport is the mechanism by which negative ions are reabsorbed. They are returned to the blood after the reabsorption of positive ions, because unlike charges attract.

The reabsorption of water is by osmosis following the reabsorption of minerals, especially sodium. The conservation of water is very important to maintain normal blood volume and blood pressure. The hormones that influence the reabsorption of water or minerals are summarized in Table 34–1.

Small proteins in the filtrate are reabsorbed by pinocytosis; the proteins become adsorbed to the membranes of the

Table 34–1. **Effects of Hormones on the Kidneys**

Hormone (Gland)	Function
Aldosterone (Adrenal Cortex)	Promotes reabsorption of sodium ions from the filtrate to the blood and excretion of potassium ions into the filtrate. Water is reabsorbed following the reabsorption of sodium.
Antidiuretic Hormone (Posterior Pituitary)	Promotes reabsorption of water from the filtrate to the blood.
Atrial Natriuretic Hormone (Atria of Heart)	Decreases reabsorption of sodium ions, which remain in the filtrate. More sodium and water are eliminated in the urine.
Parathyroid Hormone (Parathyroid Glands)	Promotes reabsorption of calcium ions from the filtrate to the blood and excretion of phosphate ions into the filtrate.

tubule cells and are engulfed and digested. Normally all proteins in the filtrate are reabsorbed; none are found in urine.

Tubular Secretion

In tubular secretion, substances are actively secreted from the blood in the peritubular capillaries into the filtrate in the renal tubules. Waste products, such as ammonia and creatinine, and the metabolic products of medications may be secreted into the filtrate to be eliminated in urine. Hydrogen ions may be secreted by the tubule cells to help maintain the normal pH of the blood.

In summary, tubular reabsorption conserves useful materials, tubular secretion may add unwanted substances to the filtrate, and most waste products simply remain in the filtrate and are excreted in urine.

THE KIDNEYS AND ACID-BASE BALANCE

The kidneys are the organs most responsible for maintaining the normal pH range of blood and tissue fluid. They have the greatest ability to compensate for or correct the pH changes that are part of normal body metabolism or the result of disease.

At its simplest, this function of the kidneys may be described as follows. If body fluids are becoming too acidic, the kidneys will secrete more hydrogen ions into the renal filtrate and return more bicarbonate ions back to the blood. This will help raise the pH of the blood back to normal. In the opposite situation, the body fluids becoming too alkaline, the kidneys will return hydrogen ions to the blood and excrete bicarbonate ions in urine. This will help lower the pH of the blood back to normal.

OTHER FUNCTIONS OF THE KIDNEYS

Some functions of the kidneys are not related to the formation of urine. These include the activation of vitamin D and production of erythropoietin. The production of renin influences urine formation and will be considered first.

When blood pressure decreases, the juxtaglomerular cells in the walls of the afferent arterioles secrete the enzyme renin. Renin then initiates the renin-angiotensin mechanism, which results in the formation of angiotensin II. (See Chapter 15.) Angiotensin II stimulates vasoconstriction and increases the secretion of aldosterone, both of which help raise blood pressure.

Vitamin D exists in several structural forms, which are converted to calciferol, the most active form, by the kidneys. Vitamin D is important for the efficient absorption of calcium and phosphate from food in the small intestine.

Erythropoietin is a hormone secreted by the kidneys during states of hypoxia; it stimulates the red bone marrow to increase the rate of red blood cell (RBC) production. With more RBCs in circulation, the oxygen-carrying capacity of the blood is greater, and the hypoxic state may be corrected.

ELIMINATION OF URINE

The ureters, urinary bladder, and urethra do not change the composition or volume of urine, but are responsible for its periodic elimination.

Ureters

The ureters are behind the peritoneum of the dorsal abdominal cavity. Each ureter extends from the hilus of a kidney to the lower, posterior side of the urinary bladder. The smooth muscle in the wall of the ureter contracts in peristaltic waves to propel urine toward the urinary bladder. As the bladder fills, it expands and compresses the lower ends of the ureters to prevent backflow of urine.

Urinary Bladder

The urinary bladder is a muscular sac below the peritoneum and behind the pubic bones. In women, the bladder is inferior to the uterus; in men, the bladder is superior to the prostate gland. The functions of the bladder are the temporary storage of urine and its elimination.

When the bladder is empty the mucosa appears wrinkled; these folds are called rugae, which permit expansion of the bladder without tearing the lining. The trigone, a triangular area on the bladder floor, has no rugae and does not expand (Fig. 34–3). The points of the trigone are the openings of the two ureters and the urethra.

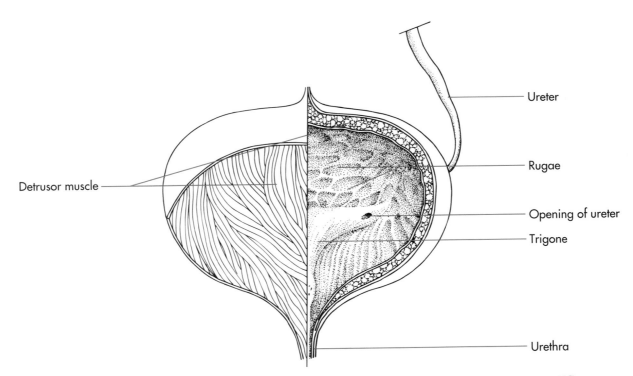

Figure 34–3. Anterior view of urinary bladder; frontal section of left side. (Modified from Scanlon, VC, Sanders, T: Workbook for Essentials of Anatomy and Physiology, ed 2. FA Davis, Philadelphia, 1995, p 293, with permission.)

The smooth muscle layer of the wall of the bladder is called the detrusor muscle, a muscle in the shape of a sphere. When it contracts it becomes a smaller sphere, and its volume diminishes. Around the opening of the urethra the muscle fibers of the detrusor form the internal urethral sphincter, which is involuntary.

Urethra

The urethra carries urine from the bladder to the exterior. Within its wall is the external urethral sphincter, which is made of skeletal muscle and is under voluntary control.

In women, the urethra is 1 to 1.5 inches long and is anterior to the vagina. In men, the urethra is 7 to 8 inches long and extends through the prostate gland and penis. The male urethra carries semen as well as urine.

The Urination Reflex

Urination (micturition) is a spinal cord reflex over which voluntary control may be exerted. The stimulus is the stretching of the detrusor muscle as urine accumulates in the bladder. Sensory impulses travel to the sacral spinal cord, and motor impulses return along parasympathetic nerves to the detrusor muscle, causing contraction. At the same time, the internal urethral sphincter relaxes. If the external urethral sphincter is voluntarily relaxed, urine flows into the urethra and the bladder is emptied.

CHARACTERISTICS OF URINE

Amount

Normal urinary output per 24 hours is 1 to 2 L. Any changes in fluid intake or other fluid output (such as sweating) will change this volume.

Color

The color of urine is often referred to as straw or amber. Dilute urine is a lighter color (straw) than is concentrated urine. Freshly voided urine is also clear rather than cloudy.

Specific Gravity

The normal range of specific gravity of urine is 1.010 to 1.025; this is a measure of the dissolved materials in urine. (The specific gravity of distilled water is 1.000.) The higher the specific gravity, the more dissolved material is present. Specific gravity of urine is a measure of the concentrating ability of the kidneys; the kidneys must excrete the waste products that are constantly formed in as little water as possible.

GERONTOLOGICAL ISSUES BOX 34-1

Renal Function, Assessment, and Medications

With most drugs excreted through the kidneys, renal function becomes a serious consideration when older adults are taking medications. Decreased renal function could slow the excretion of some medications, keeping them in the body longer. This can increase the incidence of adverse drug reactions, such as toxicity and overdose.

pH

The pH range of urine is 4.6 to 8.0, with an average of 6.0. Diet has the greatest influence on urinary pH. A vegetarian diet will result in a more alkaline urine; a high-protein diet results in a more acidic urine.

Constituents

Urine is approximately 95 percent water, which is the solvent for waste products and salts. Nitrogenous wastes include urea, creatinine, and uric acid. Urea is formed by liver cells when excess amino acids are deaminated to be used for energy production. Creatinine comes from the metabolism of creatine phosphate, an energy source in muscles. Uric acid comes from the metabolism of nucleic acids, that is, the breakdown of DNA and RNA.

AGING AND THE URINARY SYSTEM

With age, the number of nephrons in the kidneys decreases, often to half the original number by the age of 70 to 80. The glomerular filtration rate also decreases; this is in part a consequence of arteriosclerosis and diminished renal blood flow. The urinary bladder decreases in size, and the tone of the detrusor muscle decreases. This may result in the need to urinate more frequently or in residual urine in the bladder after voiding. The elderly are also more subject to infections of the urinary tract.

See also Gerontological Issues Box 34–1.

Nursing Assessment

HEALTH HISTORY

When doing the client health history, the following minimum information should be obtained:

1. Past history of renal or urinary problems.
2. Family history of urinary disorders, diabetes, or hypertension. (Diabetes and hypertension are major contributors to renal failure.)

3. Presence of pain either with voiding or over the kidney. Pain over the kidneys is called flank pain.
4. Voiding pattern.
5. New onset of symptoms of edema, shortness of breath, or other symptoms of renal failure. (Refer to Chapter 35, Figure 35–6.)
6. Current medications.
7. Functional ability to take care of own toileting needs.

Any symptoms should be further assessed using the WHAT'S UP? format found in Chapter 2.

LEARNING TIP

To find the kidneys, put your hands on your hips with your thumbs pointing back and upward. Your thumbs are pointing to the bottom of the kidneys. This is called the flank area. Pain in this area is called flank pain.

If the client has impaired kidney function or is in kidney failure, a complete head-to-toe assessment is needed because kidney failure (renal failure) affects every system of the body (Chapter 35, Figure 35–6).

PHYSICAL ASSESSMENT

The nurse first inspects the skin for color and texture. The client with chronic renal failure may have a yellow or gray cast to the skin. The presence of crystals on the skin is called uremic frost and is a sign of waste products building up in the blood (**uremia**). When the wastes are not filtered by the kidneys, they can come out through the skin, and look like a coating of frost.

Palpation and percussion of the kidneys is done by physicians and advance practice nurses. Gentle palpation and percussion of the bladder may be done by the LPN/ LVN if urine retention is suspected. If the client has a feeling of fullness but is unable to urinate, the nurse gently palpates the suprapubic area for a full bladder. Normally, the bladder is not palpable. The bladder may also be percussed. The percussion note sounds dull over a fluid-filled bladder.

Most assessment of the urinary system is done using indirect measures. Assessment of vital signs, lung sounds, edema, daily weights, and intake and output can provide valuable data related to urinary function.

Vital Signs

If renal disease is suspected, blood pressure should be assessed and documented while the client is lying, sitting,

and standing. Usually 1 minute is allowed between each reading. A drop in blood pressure accompanied by a rise in pulse rate as the client rises to sitting or standing positions is called orthostatic or postural hypotension and may indicate fluid deficit. (See Chapter 15 for a more complete discussion of orthostatic hypotension.) A rapid respiratory rate may indicate fluid retention in the lungs.

Lung Sounds

If the client retains more fluid than the heart can effectively pump, fluid may be retained in the lungs. This is manifested as crackles, which are popping sounds heard on inspiration and sometimes expiration when the chest is auscultated. Wheezes may also be present. New-onset crackles and wheezes should be reported to the physician. (See Chapter 26 for assessment of the respiratory system.)

Edema

Fluid retention may be manifested as edema (excess fluid in tissues). The nurse assesses and documents the degree and location of edema. Edema may be generalized in renal failure. The nurse also looks for edema in the area around the eyes (periorbital edema). Assessment of edema is discussed in detail in Chapter 15.

Daily Weights

Weight is the single best indicator of fluid balance in the body. Clients with renal disease often have fluid imbalances. The client should be weighed at the same time each day, in the same or similar clothing. The nurse is careful not just to document the weight, but also to look at trends in weight gain or loss. If the client's weight is steadily increasing, fluid retention is suspected and should be reported. A client being diuresed is expected to have decreasing weights.

Intake and Output

All clients with renal disease should have careful measurement of intake and output. Totals are generally analyzed and documented every 8 hours, or more often for an unstable client. The nurse measures and records all liquids taken in, including oral, intravenous, irrigation, or other fluids. Output includes urine, emesis, nasogastric effluent, wound drainage if it is copious, and any other drainage. As part of measuring output, the nurse should examine the urine for any abnormalities. Often problems show up readily in the urine, with changes such as **hematuria**, cloudiness and foul odor seen with infection, or concentrated dark-amber urine seen with dehydration.

As with daily weights, the nurse notes trends in retention or loss of fluid and reports significant changes to the physi-

---

uremia: ur—urine + emia—blood
hematuria: hemat—blood + uria—urine

cian. Accurate documentation is also vital, because the physician may base medication and intravenous fluid orders on intake and output results.

CRITICAL THINKING: Mr. Nurmii

It is the end of the shift. As you attempt to empty Mr. Nurmii's indwelling catheter bag, you find that it has only 50 mL of concentrated urine in it. What do you do?

Answers at end of chapter.

Diagnostic Tests of the Renal System

LABORATORY TESTS

Urine Tests

Urinalysis

A urinalysis (urine analysis) is a commonly performed diagnostic test for the renal system. The results of the urinalysis give a lot of information regarding kidney function, but can also give information about function of the entire body.

To collect a specimen for urinalysis, the nurse has the client wash the perineum using soap and water, or special towelettes from a clean-catch midstream urine collection kit. Women should be directed to wash from the front to the back of the perineum. The client is instructed to begin to void into the toilet, then void into the collection container, then finish voiding into the toilet. This is called a clean-catch midstream specimen and is used to obtain the cleanest possible specimen. Female clients should be told to separate the labia with one hand and keep it separated while washing and collecting the specimen to decrease the risk of contamination of the specimen. If the female client is menstruating, this should be specified on the laboratory form. A tampon may be used to prevent contamination of the specimen. The uncircumcised male client should be directed to retract the foreskin with one hand and keep it retracted while cleansing and voiding. At least 10 mL of urine should be collected. Table 34–2 lists normal and abnormal findings on a urinalysis.

Urine Culture

A urine culture is done to determine the number of bacteria present in the urine and identify the organism causing infection in the urine. The urine should be collected before antibiotic treatment is begun, to avoid affecting results.

The midstream clean-catch system is used to obtain voided specimens. The physician may order a catheterized specimen to be collected if there is a risk for contamination from the vagina, if the female client is menstruating, or if the client is incontinent. As a general rule, a bacterial count of 100,000 or more per milliliter indicates a urinary tract infection. Less than that may be due to contamination during specimen collection. The urine is cultured to grow and identify the kind of bacteria present. Often a sensitivity test will also be ordered to determine what kind of antibiotic will be most effective in eradicating the offending bacteria.

Renal Function Tests

A number of blood tests reflect kidney function. If the kidneys are not functioning adequately, these test results will be elevated.

Serum Creatinine

Creatinine is a waste product from muscle metabolism and is released into the bloodstream at a steady rate. Creatinine levels are a very good indicator of kidney function (normal results = 0.6–1.5 mg/dL). An elevated creatinine level above 1.5 mg/dL means there is some kidney dysfunction. The higher the creatinine level, the more impaired the kidney function.

Blood Urea Nitrogen

Urea is a waste product of protein metabolism. The blood urea nitrogen (BUN; normal results = 8–25 mg/dL) is not as sensitive an indicator of kidney function as the creatinine level. This is because it is readily affected by increased protein intake, dehydration, and other factors in the body. An elevated BUN can be caused by the following factors:

- Kidney dysfunction or failure.
- Decreased kidney blood supply, such as when the client is in a state of shock or in severe heart failure.
- Dehydration. The loss of water makes the blood more concentrated.
- High-protein diet, which increases urea formation.
- Gastrointestinal bleeding. The blood is absorbed as a protein and converted into urea.
- Steroid use, because steroids increase the rate of protein breakdown in the body.

A decreased BUN is seen with overhydration.

Uric Acid

Uric acid is an end product of purine metabolism and the breakdown of body proteins. The uric acid is not as diagnostic as creatinine because many factors can cause an elevated uric acid level (normal results = 2–7 mg/dL). An ele-

Table 34–2. **Urinalysis Results**

Test	Normal Results	Abnormal Results and Significance
Color of Urine	Pale yellow to amber	Dark-amber urine suggests dehydration. Yellow-brown to green urine indicates excessive bilirubin. Cloudiness of freshly voided urine indicates infection. Nearly colorless urine is seen with a large fluid intake or diabetes insipidus.
Odor of Urine	Aromatic	With infection, urine becomes foul smelling. In diabetic ketoacidosis, the urine has a fruity odor. Urine that has been standing for a while develops a strong ammonia smell.
pH	4.6–8.0	The pH is greatly affected by the food eaten. pH below 4.6 is seen with metabolic and respiratory acidosis. pH above 8.0 is seen when urine has been standing or with infection because bacteria decompose urea to form ammonia.
Specific Gravity	1.010–1.025	Low specific gravity indicates excessive fluid intake or diabetes insipidus. High specific gravity is seen with dehydration. A specific gravity fixed at 1.010 indicates kidney dysfunction.
Protein	0–18 mg/dL	Persistent proteinuria is seen with renal disease from damage to the glomerulus. Intermittent protein in the urine can result from strenuous exercise, dehydration, or fever. As a general rule, protein in the urine is a significant sign of renal problems.
Glucose	None	Glucose in the urine indicates diabetes mellitus, excessive glucose intake, or low renal threshold for glucose reabsorption.
Ketones	None	Ketones in the urine indicates diabetes mellitus with ketonuria or starvation from breakdown of body fats into ketones.
Bilirubin	None	Bilirubin in the urine indicates liver disorders causing jaundice. Bilirubin may appear in the urine before jaundice is visible.
Nitrite	Negative	Nitrites in the urine indicate infection in the urine. Bacteria in the urine convert nitrate to nitrite, which gives a positive reading.
Leukocyte Esterase	Negative	A positive leukocyte esterase in the urine indicates infection in the urine. It determines the presence of an enzyme released by WBCs in the urine.
Red Blood Cells	0–4/hpf*	Blood in the urine may be caused by kidney stones, infection, cancer, renal disease, or trauma.
White Blood Cells	0–5/hpf	WBCs in the urine indicate infection or inflammation in the urinary tract.
Casts	None to occasional hyaline cast	Casts are formed when abnormal urine contents settle out into molds of the renal tubules and may be made of protein, WBCs, RBCs, or bacteria. A few hyaline casts may be found in normal urine. The presence of casts generally indicates renal damage or infection

*hpf: high-power field.

vated uric acid level can be caused by the following factors:

- Kidney disease
- Gout (clients with gout metabolize uric acid abnormally)
- Malnutrition
- Leukemia
- Use of thiazide diuretics (by impairing uric acid clearance by the kidney)

Creatinine Clearance Test

The creatinine clearance test measures the amount of creatinine cleared from the blood in a specified period of time, by comparing the amount of creatinine in the blood with the amount of creatinine in the urine. It is an excellent indicator of renal function.

To carry out the test, urine is collected for a 24-hour period; a serum creatinine is collected sometime during the 24 hours. The following procedure should be followed:

1. When the test is begun, the client is directed to void and discard that urine.
2. Urine is collected for 24 hours, keeping the urine in a large container provided by the laboratory. The container is kept on ice.
3. Twenty-four hours after the test was begun, the client is instructed to void again. This urine is added to the collection container.
4. The laboratory collects a serum creatinine during this 24-hour period.

The creatinine clearance is computed in the laboratory and is expressed in volume of blood that is cleared of creatinine in 1 minute. Normal is 85 to 125 mL per minute. A minimum creatinine clearance of 10 mL/min is needed to live without dialysis.

LEARNING TIP

A handy approximation to determine kidney function is to equate the creatinine clearance result to percent of renal function. For example, a creatinine clearance of 100 mL/min = 100 percent renal function; 30 mL/min = 30 percent renal function; and 5 mL/min = 5 percent renal function.

RADIOLOGIC STUDIES

Kidneys-Ureter-Bladder

A kidneys-ureter-bladder (KUB) is an x-ray of the kidney, ureters, and bladder. This test is also known as a flat plate of the abdomen. It shows the outline of the renal structure and can show cancer, swollen kidneys, and calcium kidney stones. No special care is necessary for this test.

Intravenous Pyelogram

The intravenous pyelogram (IVP) (also called antegrade pyelography) is a commonly done test that can be very diagnostic. During the test a radiopaque dye is injected into a large vein. The dye is cleared from the blood by the kidneys. Because the x-rays cannot penetrate the dye, the dye outlines the renal structures. X-rays are taken at frequent intervals to see the dye filling the kidney pelvis and going down the ureters into the bladder. Figure 34–4 shows an IVP x-ray.

The preparation for an IVP is to have the client take laxatives to cleanse the bowel the day before the test, following agency policy. The client is NPO (nothing by mouth) at midnight the evening before the test. Before the test, the client should be questioned for allergies to iodine and shellfish. The dye can cause allergic and anaphylactic reactions in people who are allergic to these substances. This is a less common phenomenon since the introduction of a newer radiopaque dye. The client should also be warned that he or she will feel a warm flushing sensation up the arm and sometimes all over the body when the dye is injected. A strange taste in the mouth may also occur.

Aftercare for an IVP includes having the client drink a lot of fluids. This is necessary to clear the dye from the kidneys. On rare occasions people can develop acute renal failure because the dye is very concentrated and can obstruct the kidney tubules.

Renal Angiography

A renal angiogram is a test to visualize the renal arteries. The femoral artery is pierced with a needle, and a catheter is

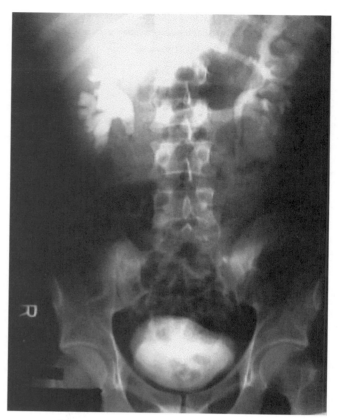

Figure 34–4. Intravenous pyelogram image.

threaded up through the femoral and iliac arteries into the aorta and then the renal artery. A contrast agent is injected to make the renal arterial supply visible on x-ray. Angiography is done in the x-ray department with the client awake during the procedure. The test helps the physician see blood flow to the kidneys to determine the cause and treatment of kidney disease.

Before the procedure the client will be NPO for 4 to 8 hours. Client care following angiography includes bed rest for up to 12 hours to prevent bleeding at the injection site. The extremity is immobilized with a sandbag, and a pressure dressing is applied. The client is instructed not to bend the leg, and the head of the bed is not raised more than 45 degrees. The nurse monitors vital signs, dressing, and pulses in the affected extremity frequently. Institution policy is consulted for specific care guidelines.

ENDOSCOPIC PROCEDURES

Cystoscopy and Pyelogram

A **cystoscopy** and **pyelogram** (C&P) is a minor surgical procedure that involves a rigid or fiber-optic instrument

---

cystoscopy: cysto—bladder + scopy—to examine
pyelogram: pyelo—pelvis of the kidney + gram—x-ray

(cystoscope) inserted into the bladder through the urethra. A light at the end of the instrument allows the physician to visualize the interior of the bladder. Commonly a pyelogram is done also. This involves insertion of a ureteral catheter into the pelvis of the kidney. Radiopaque dye is injected through the catheter and x-rays are taken. A C&P is done for both diagnostic and therapeutic reasons. As part of diagnosing the physician can do the following:

- Inspect the inside of the bladder
- Collect a urine specimen from either kidney
- Visualize the renal structure with x-rays
- Biopsy any suspicious growths in the bladder

Therapeutic interventions that can be done during a C&P include the following:

- Removal of small bladder tumors
- Removal of stones from the bladder
- Removal of stones from the ureters
- Dilation of the ureters

The preparation for a C&P is the same as for any surgery. Care following a C&P includes measuring urine, to ensure that the client has not developed urinary retention from swelling of the urinary meatus, and encouraging fluid intake. The client should expect some **dysuria** for 24 hours following a C&P, and the first one or two voidings may be blood tinged.

ULTRASOUND EXAMINATION OF THE KIDNEYS

Renal Ultrasound

A renal ultrasound, also known as ultrasonography, is a noninvasive study using sound waves to examine the anatomy of the urinary tract. A transducer is passed over the skin, which has been covered with a conductive gel. Structures of the urinary system can be visualized on a screen. A renal ultrasound is used to look for enlargement of the kidneys, kidney stones, and changes of renal structures with chronic infection and to help diagnose tumors of the kidney. There is no special preparation or aftercare, and there are no known complications.

RENAL BIOPSY

A renal biopsy may be done to diagnose or gain more information about kidney disease. Most renal biopsies are **percutaneous** (done with a needle through the skin), though some are open (done through a surgical incision). A percutaneous biopsy may be done in the operating room, the radiology department, or the client's room. A computed tomography (CT) scan or ultrasound is done first to locate the kidney for biopsy. The client is in a prone position, usually with a sandbag under the abdomen, and the biopsy is taken through the flank area. The physician obtains a sample of tissue, which is examined in the laboratory.

Before the biopsy, the client is NPO for 6 to 8 hours, and a mild sedative is given. A complete blood count and coagulation studies are checked. For a percutaneous biopsy, a local anesthetic is used.

Following the biopsy, the client is observed closely for bleeding, because the kidney is very vascular. A pressure dressing is applied to prevent bleeding, and the client is maintained on bed rest for 24 hours. A sandbag may be used under the flank to place additional pressure on the biopsy site. Urine is inspected for blood with each voiding. Vital signs are monitored frequently according to agency policy for 24 hours. Grossly bloody urine, falling blood pressure, and rising pulse are signs of bleeding and are reported immediately. Fluids are encouraged if not contraindicated.

Therapeutic Measures

MANAGEMENT OF URINARY INCONTINENCE

Urinary incontinence is defined as the involuntary passing of urine and is very common. It is estimated that 10 million Americans (mostly women) suffer from incontinence; most clients do not seek treatment. At times incontinence can be prevented by client teaching or physician intervention. Incontinence that cannot be prevented is managed by the use of padding and absorptive products worn by the client. With all kinds of incontinence it is helpful for the nurse or client to keep a urinary diary for at least several days to determine when incontinence occurs and to look for any predisposing events. The client should be referred to a urologist specializing in the area of incontinence for a careful examination to determine the cause and identify potential medical or surgical treatment. Some areas of the country have continence clinics, which can be very helpful for clients with this problem. There are several types of incontinence, discussed below.

Stress Incontinence

Stress incontinence is the involuntary loss of urine associated with increasing abdominal pressure during coughing, sneezing, laughing, or other physical activities. Stress incontinence is commonly seen in women following childbirth and after menopause.

Urge Incontinence

Urge incontinence is the involuntary loss of urine associated with an abrupt and strong desire to void. The client of-

---

dysuria: dys—difficult or painful + uria—urination
percutaneous: per—through + cutaneous—skin

ten complains that he or she is "unable to make it to the bathroom in time." With both stress incontinence and urge incontinence, the client can be taught Kegel exercises to increase perineal muscle tone. Table 34–3 explains how to teach clients to perform Kegel exercises.

Functional Incontinence

Functional incontinence is caused by chronic impairment of physical function or ability to think, leaving the client unable to get to the toilet in time to maintain continence. This is a common cause of incontinence in the elderly.

Total Incontinence

Total incontinence is a continuous and unpredictable loss of urine. Bladder training has been tried and proven ineffective. Often the client with total incontinence is neurologically impaired. In these situations, the nurse's priority is keeping the client clean and dry using absorptive products. For the male client, an external condom catheter can be effective in some situations.

Nursing Process

The medical diagnoses of stress incontinence and urge incontinence are also nursing diagnoses. Many nursing interventions can be helpful to decrease these kinds of incontinence. See Nursing Care Plan Box 34–2 for the Client with Stress Incontinence or Urge Incontinence. See Nursing Care Plan Box 34–3 for the Client with Functional Incontinence.

URINARY CATHETERS

Indwelling Catheters

Indwelling urinary catheters (Foley catheters) are routinely inserted into hospitalized clients. As a general rule, catheters should be avoided if at all possible. Urinary incontinence is *not* justification for insertion of a catheter. Urinary catheters result in infection of the urinary tract in up to 44 percent of clients within 72 hours of catheterization, and up to 90 percent have significant bacterial infection with indwelling catheters in a total of 17 days.[1]

Bacteria enter the bladder mainly in one of two ways with an indwelling catheter: (1) through the outlet at the end of the drainage bag contaminating the urine, which is then inadvertently drained back into the bladder; or (2) around the catheter up the urethra and into the bladder. It has been demonstrated that the incidence of infection is decreased when intermittent straight catheterization is used instead of indwelling Foley catheters. Table 34–4 outlines guidelines that should be followed to decrease infection in the catheterized client.

For any client with an indwelling catheter, the nursing diagnosis of risk for infection is appropriate. The nursing interventions listed in Table 34–4 are methods to decrease the incidence of infection in the catheterized client.

Intermittent Catheterization

For the client who is unable to void without a catheter, the best intervention is intermittent catheterization. The

---

Table 34–3. **Client Education for Kegel Exercises**

The purpose of Kegel exercises is to decrease the incidence of incontinence by strengthening the pubococcygeal muscle, which supports the pelvic organs. By increasing the tone of this muscle, the client has an increased ability to tighten the muscle that encircles the urinary meatus and stop the flow of urine. This exercise can also help prevent uterine prolapse, enhance sensation during sexual intercourse, and hasten postpartum healing. It may be used by the elderly male client to control dribbling.

1. Establish awareness of pelvic muscle function by instructing the client to "pull in" the muscles in the perineum as if to control urination or defecation. The muscles of the buttocks, inner thigh, and abdomen are not used to do Kegel exercises.
2. To help identify the correct muscles to tighten, ask the client to tighten the muscles that control urination. It can be helpful to use an analogy of an elevator: start squeezing at the bottom floor and then squeeze upward to the top floor.
3. Instruct the client to tighten the pelvic muscles for 10 seconds, followed by at least 10 seconds of relaxation.
4. Advise the client to perform these exercises 30 to 80 times per day. Help the client determine cues to remind the client to perform the exercises, such as stopping the stream of urine 10 times each time the client urinates.

Adapted from Urinary Incontinence in Adults: Clinical Practice Guideline. Agency for Health Care Policy and Research, Public Health Service, US Department of Health and Human Services (AHCPR Pub No 92-0038), Rockville, Md, 1992.

Table 34–4. **Guidelines for Care of the Client with an Indwelling Catheter**

1. Maintain a closed system. Do not separate the catheter from the tubing of the bag. Instead, collect specimens and irrigate through the sample port in the tubing.
2. Keep the catheter securely taped or fastened to the leg. This decreases traction on the catheter with back-and-forth movement of the catheter that can help bacteria enter the bladder.
3. Encourage fluids to internally irrigate the catheter, if fluids are not contraindicated because of heart or kidney disease.
4. Use good aseptic technique when emptying the drainage bag by hand washing, wearing clean gloves, and using a container designated for that client only to collect the urine.
5. Wash the perineum with soap and water at least one time per day, and again if there is any bowel incontinence.
6. Keep the tubing coiled on the bed and positioned to allow free flow of urine. *Keep the catheter bag below the level of the bladder at all times.*
7. Do not clamp catheters. Clamping a catheter results in obstruction, which increases infection. Periodic clamping has not been found to be effective in bladder retraining.
8. Remove indwelling catheters as soon as possible.

NURSING CARE PLAN BOX 34–2 FOR THE CLIENT WITH STRESS INCONTINENCE OR URGE INCONTINENCE

Stress incontinence or urge incontinence related to decreased tone of perineal muscles

Outcomes
Client will be continent of urine. Client will state three actions that can be taken to decrease incidence of stress or urge incontinence.

Evaluation of Outcomes
Is the client continent? Is the client able to state three actions that can be taken to decrease the incidence of stress or urge incontinence?

Interventions	Rationale	Evaluation
STRESS INCONTINENCE AND URGE INCONTINENCE		
• Assess history of incontinence; have client keep a voiding journal.	A journal helps identify the severity and timing of incontinence.	Does client complete the voiding journal?
• Instruct client on how to perform Kegel exercises (Table 34–3).	Kegel exercises increase perineal muscle tone and help prevent incontinence.	Does client explain how to perform Kegel exercises?
• Work with the client to incorporate Kegel exercises into normal activities of daily living (e.g., do 10 pelvic muscle contractions with each voiding).	An excellent time to perform Kegel exercises is when voiding because the correct muscles are used.	Does client perform Kegel exercises when voiding, or at other cued times during the day?
• Encourage client to drink at least 2000 mL of fluid per day, preferably 3000 mL per day unless medical reason for fluid restriction.	Concentrated urine is irritating to the urinary tract and can increase the incidence of urge incontinence and dribbling.	Is urine dilute?
• Encourage client to avoid alcohol and caffeine.	Alcohol serves as a diuretic, and caffeine is irritating to the urinary tract.	Does client explain the need to avoid alcohol and fluids containing caffeine?
• Discuss use of and provide small adhesive peripads to wear in underclothing.	Peripads provide protection in case of incontinence.	Does client have and use peripads if desired?
• Refer client to a continence clinic or to a physician specializing in incontinence.	Specialists in the area of incontinence can use medical or surgical interventions to decrease the incidence of incontinence.	Does the client know resources available to further assist with treatment of incontinence?
• Refer client to supportive and educational groups such as Help for Incontinent People (HIP) (see Verdell in Bibliography).	Support groups can help clients deal with the embarrassment of incontinence and learn methods and resources to prevent incontinence.	Does the client know the names and addresses of support groups to help with incontinence?
URGE INCONTINENCE		
• Teach client to void at frequent intervals (every 2 hours), then gradually increase length of time between voidings.	By emptying the bladder at frequent intervals, the incidence of urge incontinence can be decreased.	Does the client follow a frequent voiding schedule?
• Teach urge inhibition techniques (distraction), such as counting back from 100 by 7s and relaxation breathing.	These distraction techniques can help the client reach the bathroom in time to prevent incontinence.	Do distraction techniques help client prevent incontinence?

client who has a neurological disorder, the client with urinary retention, or the postoperative client may benefit from intermittent catheterization. Use of intermittent catheterization greatly reduces the risk of infection, as long as the bladder is prevented from overfilling. A full bladder stretches the muscle fibers, which in turn reduces circulation to the bladder and increases risk for infection.

NURSING CARE PLAN BOX 34–3
FOR THE CLIENT WITH FUNCTIONAL INCONTINENCE

Functional incontinence related to interference with rapid voiding

Outcomes
Client will be continent of urine. Client will state three measures to increase continence.

Evaluation of Outcomes
Is the client continent of urine? Is the client able to state three measures to increase continence?

Interventions	Rationale	Evaluation
• Assess history of incontinence. Keep a voiding log of when client is incontinent.	A voiding log helps demonstrate when incontinence is most likely to occur and can help determine the cause of incontinence.	Does the client cooperate so that a voiding log can be kept?
• Determine any acute causes of incontinence, including new onset of urinary tract infection, constipation or impaction, medication effect, or poor fluid intake.	These may be readily treatable causes of incontinence.	Does the client have any easily treatable causes of incontinence?
• Determine if clothing is inhibiting timely voiding. If necessary, Velcro fasteners can be appropriate, or sweat shirts and sweat pants.	Clothing can be difficult to remove for the elderly, resulting in voiding before the clothing can be removed. Clothing can be modified so that it comes off quickly.	Does the client have easy-to-remove clothing?
• Determine if there are any obstacles to reaching appropriate urine receptacle, such as poor lighting, busy bathroom, lack of assistive devices.	Obstacles can make it impossible for the client to reach the voiding receptacle in time to prevent incontinence.	Does the client have ready access to a voiding receptacle?
• Provide appropriate urinary receptacles, such as a three-in-one commode, female or male urinal, or no-spill urinal.	Assistive devices can be helpful for the client to increase continence.	Does the client need and have access to an appropriate assistive device?
• Initiate a voiding schedule of every 2 hours, or base schedule on voiding log. Always assist client to the toilet when client first awakens and before sleep. Use prompted voiding techniques: check client regularly, provide positive reinforcement if dry, prompt client to toilet, praise client after toileting, return client to toilet in a specified time.	Frequent scheduled voiding using prompting techniques can increase continence.	Does the client receive help to do bladder training with prompted voiding?
• Teach client to set up schedule of voiding using environmental cues such as meals, bedtime, and television shows.	Environmental cues help the client remember when it is time to void.	Can the client indicate cues throughout the day that prompt voiding?

Intermittent catheterization involves the use of a straight, usually firm plastic catheter that is inserted into the urethra every 3 hours or more to empty the bladder. Once the bladder is empty, the catheter is removed. Clients may be taught to do intermittent self-catheterization (ISC) at home. Clients doing ISC may be taught to wash and reuse the same catheter repeatedly. In the hospital, sterile technique is used.

Suprapubic Catheter

After some surgeries of the urinary tract, and in some long-term situations, a suprapubic catheter may be used. This is an indwelling catheter that is inserted through an incision in the lower abdomen directly into the bladder. Once the surgical site is healed, the catheter may be removed.

HOME HEALTH HINTS

■ The home health nurse should always have a sterile specimen container in a client's home. This provides a quick way to get a specimen to the physician's office without the nurse having to obtain the container, saving time and money.

■ For the client who is incontinent or confused and unable to give a clean midstream urine specimen, a solution is to perform a single in-and-out catheterization of the bladder.

■ When catheters plug and irrigation fails, families can be taught to take the catheter out. A syringe for removing water from the balloon should be left in the home for this purpose. The family is instructed to avoid cutting the valve stem. The family should contact the nurse to reinsert the catheter, but in the meantime, the client's bed or chair can be padded with towels or diapers. Garbage or cleaners' bags can be used to line the mattress. If the catheter is being used to treat urine retention, the family must be instructed to notify the nurse immediately if the catheter is plugged or has been removed.

■ Not all homes have adequate lighting, which is a must for inserting a catheter. If lighting is inadequate, a caretaker can be asked to hold a flashlight while the nurse inserts the catheter. The nurse should always have a flashlight with him or her. Having two catheters and catheter trays is also wise in case of a defect or contamination.

■ Urinary drainage bags and leg bags should be changed a minimum of every 2 weeks in the home setting to prevent infection. The family is instructed not to clean and reuse the bags.

■ To encourage fluid intake, the client should keep a large container of water (1 to 2 quarts) next to the place the client sits most of the day. The goal is to drink 2 quarts of water by the end of the day, unless contraindicated by other medical problems. This also simplifies measuring intake.

Nursing care of a suprapubic catheter involves keeping the area clean and dry, changing the dressing when the site is new, and keeping the catheter taped to prevent tension. A skin barrier such as Stomahesive may help protect the skin from urine leakage. All other care is the same as for any indwelling catheter.

Review Questions

1. Mr. Cole is scheduled for an intravenous pyelogram. The nurse should expect the preparation for an IVP to include restricting the client's
   a. Salt intake
   b. Fluid intake
   c. Use of tobacco
   d. Physical activities

2. Mr. Cole is scheduled for a cystoscopy and pyelogram (C&P). Postoperative nursing care following this kind of surgery includes
   a. Observation for signs of renal failure
   b. Limiting fluid intake
   c. Measuring urine output
   d. Daily weights

3. The physician has ordered a midstream urine specimen for culture and sensitivity. Client teaching should emphasize which of the following?
   a. A second voided specimen is preferred.
   b. Women should keep labia separated while voiding.
   c. As soon as the urine starts to flow, it should be collected in a sterile container.
   d. A 24-hour urine specimen is needed.

4. A renal biopsy is performed. Nursing care for a client in the period immediately following this procedure should include
   a. Encouraging coughing and deep breathing
   b. Frequent vital signs
   c. Maintaining bed rest for 48 hours
   d. Positioning the client on the right side

5. Mrs. Jones is experiencing stress incontinence with frequent involuntary loss of urine. Which of the following directions would be most appropriate when teaching Mrs. Jones how to perform Kegel exercises?
   a. "Tighten the rectum at frequent intervals throughout the day."
   b. "Keep the abdominal muscles tightened; do this every time you stand up."
   c. "When urinating, stop and start the stream of urine by tightening the perineal muscles."
   d. "You should do at least 20 sit-ups per day."

6. Which of the following is the most important nursing action that the nurse should take to prevent urinary tract infection in the catheterized client?
   a. Force fluids to 4000 mL/24 hours.
   b. Empty the Foley bag every 4 hours around the clock.
   c. Maintain a closed system with the catheter kept connected to the tubing.
   d. Wash the perineum every 8 hours.

7. Which of the following is the most accurate way to assess fluid balance in the client with renal failure?
   a. Voiding pattern
   b. Daily weight
   c. Laboratory studies
   d. Skin turgor

8. Mrs. Tish has urge incontinence. Which of the following should be taught to help her deal with the incontinence?
   a. Practice voiding at increasingly longer intervals to train the bladder to hold urine.
   b. Decrease fluid intake to decrease loss of urine.
   c. Drink cranberry juice to keep the urine acidic.
   d. Void every 2 hours.

ANSWERS TO CRITICAL THINKING

CRITICAL THINKING: *Mr. Nurmii*

You should realize that 50 mL of concentrated urine after 8 to 12 hours is not normal. Further investigation is necessary to determine the cause and seriousness of the problem. Some items to assess follow.

1. Consider Mr. Nurmii's diagnosis. Is he in renal failure? Is he severely dehydrated and retaining water?
2. Ask if anyone emptied Mr. Nurmii's bag earlier in the shift.
3. Look at the trends in Mr. Nurmii's intake and output record. Has his output been decreasing? Is this a change?
4. Has Mr. Nurmii been taking in enough fluids?
5. Look at trends in daily weights. Is Mr. Nurmii's weight increasing? Is this an expected finding?
6. Listen to Mr. Nurmii's lung sounds. Check for edema. Do findings indicate fluid retention?
7. Percuss and palpate Mr. Nurmii's bladder. Is it distended? Maybe the catheter is blocked.
8. If a problem is identified, the physician should be contacted.

REFERENCE

1. Crow, R, et al: Study of Clients with an Indwelling Urinary Catheter and Related Nursing Practice. Nursing Practice Research Unit, University of Surrey, Guildford, 1986.

BIBLIOGRAPHY

Ackley, B, and Ladwig, G: Nursing Diagnosis Handbook: A Guide to Planning Care. Mosby, St Louis, 1995.

Bierwirth, W: Which pad is for you? Urol Nurs 12:75, 1992.

Burns, P, et al: Treatment of stress incontinence with pelvic floor exercises and biofeedback. J Am Geriatr Soc 38:341, 1990.

Getliffe, K: Informed choices for long-term benefits: The management of catheters in continence care. Prof Nurse 19:122, 1993.

Karlowicz, KA (ed): Urologic Nursing: Principles and Practice. WB Saunders, Philadelphia, 1995.

McCormick, KA, et al: Urinary incontinence in adults. Am J Nurs 92:75, 1992.

McCormick, KA, and Palmer, M: Urinary incontinence in older adults. Annu Rev Nurs Res 10:25, 1992.

McDowell, B, et al: An interdisciplinary approach to the assessment and behavior treatment of urinary incontinence in geriatric outclients. J Am Geriatr Soc 40:370, 1992.

McKinney, BC: Cut your clients' risk of nosocomial UTI. RN 58(11):20, 1995.

Moore, K, et al: Bacteriuria in intermittent catheterization users: The effect of sterile versus clean reused catheters. Rehabil Nurs 18:306, 1993.

Resnick, B: Retraining the bladder after catheterization. Am J Nurs 93:46, 1993.

Retzky, SS, and Rogers, RB: Urinary incontinence in women. Clin Sym 47(3):1, 1995.

Urinary Incontinence Guideline Panel: Urinary Incontinence in Adults: Clinical Practice Guideline. Agency for Health Care Policy and Research, Public Health Service, US Department of Health and Human Services (AHCPR Pub No 92-0038), Rockville, Md, 1992.

Verdell, L (ed): Help for Incontinent People (HIP): Resource Guide of Continence Products and Services, ed 6. HIP, Union, SC, 1994.

Warren, JW; Catheter-associated bacteriuria. Clin Geriatr Med 8:805, 1992.

Watson, J, and Jaffe, MS: Nurse's Manual of Laboratory and Diagnostic Tests, ed 2. FA Davis, Philadelphia, 1995.

35

Nursing Care of Clients with Disorders of the Urinary Tract

Betty J. Ackley and Jeanette Acker

Learning Objectives

Upon completion of this chapter, the student will be able to:

1. Identify predisposing causes, symptoms, and treatment of urinary tract infections (UTIs).
2. Identify laboratory abnormalities associated with UTIs.
3. List predisposing causes, symptoms, and treatment of kidney stones.
4. Explain education for clients with kidney stones.
5. Identify symptoms of cancer of the bladder and cancer of the kidneys.
6. Explain nursing care of a client with an ileal conduit or continent reservoir.
7. Explain the pathophysiology associated with diabetic nephropathy, nephrosclerosis, nephrosis, and glomerulonephritis.
8. Describe nursing care for clients with diabetic nephropathy, nephrosclerosis, nephrosis, and glomerulonephritis.
9. Identify common nephrotoxic substances and when kidney damage is most likely to occur from nephrotoxins.
10. Differentiate acute renal failure from chronic renal failure.
11. Identify common symptoms experienced by the client in renal failure.
12. Describe nursing care of the client in renal failure.
13. Explain in simple terms how hemodialysis and peritoneal dialysis work to replace the function of the kidney.
14. Describe nursing care of hemodialysis blood access sites.

Key Words

anuria (an-**YOO**-ree-ah)

asterixis (AS-ter-**ICK**-sis)

azotemia (AY-zoh-**TEE**-me-ah)

calculi (**KAL**-kyoo-lye)

cystitis (sis-**TIGH**-tis)

dysuria (dis-**YOO**-ree-ah)

glomerulonephritis (gloh-MER-yoo-loh-ne-**FRY**-tis)

hemodialysis (HEE-moh-dye-**AL**-i-sis)

hydronephrosis (HIGH-droh-ne-**FROH**-sis)

nephrectomy (ne-**FREK**-tuh-mee)

nephrolithotomy (NEFF-roh-li-**THOT**-uh-mee)

nephropathy (ne-**FROP**-uh-thee)

nephrosclerosis (NEFF-roh-skle-**ROH**-sis)

nephrostomy (ne-**FRAHS**-toh-mee)

nephrotoxin (NEFF-roh-**TOK**-sin)

oliguria (AH-li-**GYOO**-ree-ah)

peritoneal dialysis (PER-i-toh-**NEE**-uhl dye-**AL**-i-sis)

polyuria (PAH-lee-**YOOR**-ee-ah)

pyelonephritis (PYE-e-loh-ne-**FRY**-tis)

stent (STENT)

uremia (yoo-**REE**-mee-ah)

urethritis (YOO-ree-**THRIGH**-tis)

urethroplasty (yoo-**REE**-throh-PLAS-tee)

urosepsis (yoo-roh-**SEP**-sis)

Disorders of the urinary tract include a variety of problems involving the kidneys, ureters, bladder, and urethra. These problems may arise from infection, obstructions, cancer, hereditary disorders, or chronic diseases. Some may lead to renal failure if not treated or controlled.

Urinary Tract Infections

Urinary tract infection is a general term that refers to invasion of the urinary tract by bacteria. The abbreviation UTI is commonly used to refer to this condition.

PREDISPOSING FACTORS FOR URINARY TRACT INFECTIONS

Urinary tract infections are almost always caused by an ascending infection, starting at the external urinary meatus and progressing toward the bladder and kidneys. Predisposing factors for UTIs include the following:

1. Stasis of urine in the bladder. This can be caused from obstruction such as a clamped catheter or simply from not voiding frequently enough. Urine overdistends the bladder, decreasing the blood supply to the wall of the bladder, which keeps white blood cells (WBCs) from fighting any contamination that may have entered the bladder. The standing urine serves as a culture medium for bacterial growth.
2. Contamination in the area. This can be from fecal soiling, from intercourse in which bacteria are massaged into the urinary meatus as part of the act, or from infection in the area such as vaginitis, epididymitis, or prostatitis.
3. Instrumentation, or having instruments or tubes inserted into the urinary meatus. The most common cause is urinary catheterization. Bacteria ascend around or within the catheter, causing infection. Many clients develop a UTI after 2 weeks of having an indwelling catheter.
4. Reflux of urine from the urethra to the bladder or the bladder to the ureter because of faulty valves to maintain one-way flow. Reflux can be congenital, or it may be acquired as a result of previous infections.

Female clients are more likely to develop UTIs because of the shorter length of the urethra and the proximity of the anal orifice. The majority of UTIs are caused by the bacteria *Escherichia coli,* which is commonly found in the stool. Elderly men are predisposed to infection because of enlarged prostates causing obstruction of urine flow.

SYMPTOMS

UTIs are characterized by common symptoms of **dysuria,** urgency, frequency, and cloudy, foul-smelling urine. Infec-

tion may be found in three different anatomical parts of the urinary tract: the urethra, resulting in **urethritis;** the bladder, with a diagnosis of **cystitis;** or in the kidneys, with a diagnosis of **pyelonephritis.**

Urethritis

Pathophysiology and Etiology

Urethritis is inflammation of the urethra. It may be due to bacterial infection or a chemical irritant, or it may be sexually transmitted. Bubble bath and bath salts are common irritants and should not be used by anyone with a history of UTIs. Urethritis can also be caused by spermicidal agents. Gonorrhea and chlamydia are sexually transmitted diseases that can cause urethritis in men. If it is caused by chlamydia it is called nongonococcal urethritis (NGU) or nonspecific urethritis (NSU). It is also common to have some degree of urethritis in association with bladder or prostatic infections.

Signs and Symptoms

Symptoms of urethritis include urinary frequency, urgency, and dysuria. The male client may have discharge from the penis.

Diagnostic Tests

A urinalysis or urine culture is done to diagnose urethritis.

Treatment

The treatment of urethritis is removal of the cause, if it is caused by a chemical irritant. If urethritis is caused by a bacteria, an antibiotic will be prescribed based on the results of a culture. Phenazopyridine (Pyridium), a urinary analgesic, is often used to treat dysuria. The client should be forewarned that his urine will turn orange while on phenazopyridine. If urethritis is sexually transmitted, it is important that the sexual partner also be treated.

Cystitis

Pathophysiology/Signs and Symptoms

Cystitis is inflammation and infection of the bladder wall. Symptoms include dysuria, frequency, urgency, and cloudy urine.

---

dysuria: dys—painful + uria—urination

urethritis: urethra—a canal for the discharge of urine from the bladder to the outside + itis—inflammation

cystitis: cyst—a closed sac that contains fluid + itis—inflammation

pyelonephritis: pyelo—pelvis + nephr—kidney + itis—inflammation

Diagnostic Tests

Cystitis infection acquired outside of the hospital is diagnosed with a routine urinalysis collected as a clean catch midstream specimen. Changes seen in the urinalysis include cloudy urine and the presence of WBCs, bacteria, and sometimes red blood cells (RBCs) in the specimen. Nitrites are usually positive. Some laboratories also examine for leukocyte esterace, which is positive if infection is present in the urine.

For the complicated UTI, such as one acquired in the hospital or a repeat infection, a urine culture and sensitivity should be done. Hospital-acquired UTIs are often caused by bacteria that are resistant to the usual antibiotics used for UTIs. A sensitivity test can identify which antibiotics will be effective against the offending organism.

Treatment

The treatment of uncomplicated cystitis is most often a combination sulfa medication, sulfamethoxazole and trimethoprim (Bactrim, Septra). Complicated cystitis is often treated with ciprofloxacin (Cipro). Other antibiotics may be prescribed depending on the results of the urine culture and sensitivity. The client should be told to take all medications until gone, force fluids unless contraindicated, and return in a week for a follow-up urinalysis or culture to ensure that the urine is sterile.

Pyelonephritis

Pathophysiology

Pyelonephritis is infection of the kidneys. Pathophysiology includes formation of small abscesses throughout the kidney and gross enlargement of the kidney. The cause is usually an ascending bacterial infection. On occasion, kidney infection is caused by bacteria spreading from a distant site through the bloodstream and entering the kidney through the glomerulus.

Signs and Symptoms

Symptoms include urgency, frequency, dysuria, flank pain, fever, and chills. The urine is cloudy with increased WBCs, bacteria, casts, RBCs, and positive nitrites. In contrast to cystitis, the client with pyelonephritis is much sicker and shows signs of systemic disease.

Diagnostic Tests

To differentiate pyelonephritis from cystitis several tests are helpful. With kidney infection, the urinalysis will show casts. Casts are microscopic particles formed in the kidney from abnormal constituents in the urine such as WBCs, RBCs, or pus. The presence of casts always indicates a problem in the kidneys. The complete blood count (CBC) will show an elevated white blood count. The client will also have costovertebral tenderness and tenderness over the flank area. To test for costovertebral tenderness, the experienced examiner places one hand palm down over the kidney area, and the back of the hand is struck with the opposite hand. If this elicits severe pain, pyelonephritis is usually diagnosed.

Treatment

Treatment of pyelonephritis includes antibiotics prescribed based on the results of the culture and sensitivity. With severe gram-negative infections, the client may be hospitalized for intravenous (IV) antibiotics. The client with acute pyelonephritis generally heals completely after treatment and has no lasting kidney damage.

Complications

Repeated kidney infections can result in scarring and loss of kidney function, leading to renal failure. It is also possible for the bacteria to invade the bloodstream, causing septicemia. This is called **urosepsis,** and in the elderly it can be the cause of a new onset of confusion. The elderly or immunocompromised client may develop septic shock from infection in the urinary tract that has invaded the bloodstream. This can result in death.

NURSING PROCESS: THE CLIENT WITH A URINARY TRACT INFECTION

Assessment

The nurse questions the client about pain on urination, flank pain, or general symptoms of infection such as fever, chills, and malaise. The urine is examined for cloudiness, blood, or foul odor. The presence of a catheter, recent instrumentation, or other predisposing factor is determined. Urinalysis and culture results are examined.

It is important that the nurse listen to the client's concerns about the diagnosis. Often there is acute embarrassment and feelings of shame associated with the diagnosis of a UTI.

Nursing Diagnosis

Possible nursing diagnoses include pain: dysuria and flank pain; hyperthermia; altered pattern of urinary elimination: dysuria, frequency, urgency, or incontinence; and risk for repeat infection.

Planning

The plan for the client focuses on promotion of comfort, treatment of symptoms of infection, and educating the client to prevent future infections.

---

urosepsis: uro—urine + sepsis—infection in the blood

Implementation

Discomfort may be treated with urinary or other analgesics. Fever is treated with acetaminophen. A heating pad as ordered by the physician may be helpful.

Fluids are encouraged to help flush bacteria from the bladder. The nurse answers the hospitalized client's call light promptly for assistance to the bathroom, to avoid incontinence related to urgency. A bedside commode may be helpful. If the client is incontinent, an adult brief and frequent perineal care are provided. Use of an indwelling catheter is avoided, because this increases the risk of further infection.

CLIENT EDUCATION

It is very important that clients be advised to take all of the prescribed antibiotic until it is gone. Commonly clients take medication for several days until they no longer have symptoms and then stop. This allows infection to continue, and the infection can become chronic and resistant to antibiotics.

Clients who have one UTI commonly develop repeat infections. It is important that they receive health teaching to prevent repeated infections of the urinary tract. Refer to Table 35–1 for measures that can help prevent urinary tract infections. See also Nutrition Notes Box 35–1.

Evaluation

Goals have been met if the client states that pain, urgency, and frequency are relieved and fever is controlled. It is also important to have the client verbalize back to the nurse what was taught to ensure that correct learning has taken place.

Table 35–1. **Client Teaching to Prevent Urinary Tract Infection**

1. Void frequently; at least every 3 hours while awake.
2. Drink up to 3000 mL of fluid a day if there are no fluid restrictions from the physician. Preferably drink water.
3. Drink one glass of cranberry juice (10 ounces) per day.
4. Take showers; avoid tub baths.
5. Wipe perineum from the front to the back after toileting.
6. Urinate after intercourse.
7. Avoid bubble bath and bath salts, perfumed feminine hygiene products, synthetic underwear, and constricting clothing such as tight jeans.
8. Take prescribed medication for UTIs until it is all gone.
9. If UTI is associated with another source of infection such as vaginitis or prostatitis, ensure that both infections are treated.

NUTRITION NOTES BOX 35-1

Urinary Tract Infections

Instructions to increase fluid intake should specify amounts to consume or amount of urine resulting. Clients have developed electrolyte imbalances by over-enthusiastically forcing fluids.

An effective intervention for urinary tract infections is increasing fluid intake (with the precaution cited above) both for its flushing effect and to excrete urinary drugs. Daily intake of cranberry juice to prevent UTI has reduced bacteriuria, but agreement is lacking on the mechanism for this effect.[1,2] Nevertheless, 10 ounces of cranberry juice cocktail daily is a readily accepted intervention without apparent ill effects.

  CRITICAL THINKING: Mrs. Milan

Mrs. Milan is a 25-year-old woman who recently spent a 3-day romantic weekend with her husband. On Monday she notices that she has symptoms of dysuria, frequency, and urgency. She visits her family practitioner and is diagnosed with a UTI.

1. What could have predisposed her to developing a UTI?
2. What should Mrs. Milan be taught to prevent further occurrences of a UTI?
3. What abnormal constituents would you expect to see in Mrs. Milan's urine?

Answers at end of chapter.

Urological Obstructions

Obstruction of urine flow in the urinary tract is always significant because if urine does not drain from the kidney, the resulting backup of urine will eventually destroy the kidney by compressing the kidney structures with stagnant urine. The causes of urological obstructions include strictures and stones. Tumors of the urinary tract, covered in the following section, can also obstruct urine flow.

URETHRAL STRICTURES

Pathophysiology and Etiology

A urethral stricture is a narrowing of the lumen of the urethra due to scar tissue. Common causes of strictures are urethral injury caused by insertion of catheters or surgical instruments. Strictures can also be caused by trauma from straddle injuries, a result of direct application of force to the perineal area. Additional causes include untreated gonorrhea and congenital abnormalities.

Signs and Symptoms

The client with a urethral stricture has a diminished urinary stream and is prone to develop UTIs because of obstruction of urine flow. Urethral strictures are often seen in elderly men. The problem becomes more apparent when the nurse attempts to insert a Foley catheter and is unable to do so because of the narrowed lumen.

Treatment

Initially the treatment of a urethral stricture is mechanical dilation by a urologist, by inserting instruments termed *sounds* or *bougies* into the urethra. The urologist begins with thin sounds and then progresses to using larger instruments inserted into the bladder until the obstructed area is gradually dilated and an indwelling catheter can be inserted.

If the stricture continues to be a problem after dilation, the area can be surgically repaired with a surgical procedure called a **urethroplasty.**

Nursing Care

The dilation process is often done at the bedside when the client is awake. This is a painful experience for the client, and it is helpful for the nurse to encourage the urologist to order pain medication that can be given before the procedure. The nursing diagnosis of pain is very relevant. Because an indwelling catheter is generally inserted after the dilation, the nursing diagnosis of risk for infection is also present. Clients need health teaching on how to prevent UTIs. This information is found in Table 35–1.

RENAL CALCULI

Renal **calculi** (kidney stones; singular form is calculus) are hard, generally small stones that form somewhere in the renal structures. When stones are found in the kidneys, the condition is called nephrolithiasis. Stones in the ureters are called ureterolithiasis and usually originate in the kidney.

Pathophysiology

Normally the dissolved substances in urine, including urinary salts, are diluted and readily excreted from the body.

urethroplasty: urethro—urethra + plasty—surgical repair

Calculi are formed when urinary salts are concentrated enough to settle out; there is often a nucleus around which the salts collect and deposit. Substances that can serve as a nucleus include pus, blood, dead tissue, a catheter, or crystals. Following are common urinary salts arranged in order of their frequency of composing renal calculi:

1. Calcium oxalate
2. Calcium phosphate
3. Magnesium ammonia
4. Uric acid
5. Cystine

The majority of renal calculi are calcium, either in the form of calcium oxalate or calcium phosphate, but it is also possible to have combination stones. Figure 35–1 shows a diagram of renal calculi in the kidney.

Etiology

Causes of calculi formation include a family history of stones, chronic dehydration (causing more concentrated urinary salts), and infection, because it provides a nucleus for stone formation. Additional causes of calcium stones include dietary factors. (See Nutrition Notes Box 35–2.) Immobility predisposes to stone formation because of the resulting urinary stasis and because calcium leaves the bones and more is filtered through the kidneys. Excessive amounts of calcium in the water in some areas may also be a factor.

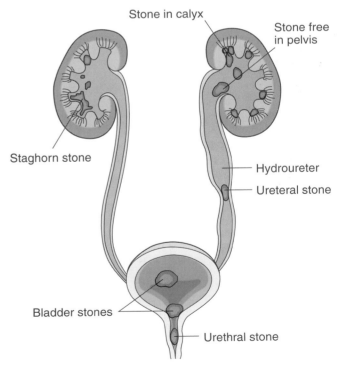

Figure 35–1. Location of calculi in the urinary tract.

NUTRITION NOTES BOX 35-2

Renal Calculi

Sufficient fluid to produce 2000 mL of urine per day should be ingested to prevent concentrated urine, which enhances precipitation of crystals.

About 80 percent of kidney stones are composed of calcium oxalate, which led to early prescriptions of low-calcium diets. A large prospective study correlated higher calcium intake with fewer kidney stone occurrences, possibly because a high calcium intake inhibits gastrointestinal absorption of oxalate and consequently decreases the amount to be excreted in urine.[3] Tables of nutritive composition of foods often are incomplete regarding oxalates; thus implementing a low-oxalate diet is problematic, but recommended. Additionally, in the Curhan[3] study, known high-oxalate foods (chocolate, nuts, tea, and spinach) were not associated with risk of kidney stones; however, intake of animal protein was directly associated and potassium and fluid intakes inversely associated with the risk of kidney stones.

Uric acid kidney stones can be a complication of gout, which is a disorder of purine metabolism. Purines are end products of digestion of certain proteins and are present in some medications. High-purine foods include organ meats, anchovies, herring, sardines in oil, meat extracts, consomme, and gravies. Low-purine foods include fruits, milk, cheese, eggs, refined grains, sugars, coffee, tea, carbonated beverages, tapioca, yeast, and vegetables (except asparagus, beans, cauliflower, mushrooms, peas, and spinach).

Signs and Symptoms

Symptoms of renal calculi include excruciating flank pain and renal colic; when the stone is lodged in the ureter it is common to have pain radiate down to the genitalia. The pain results when the stone prevents urine from draining. Additional symptoms include hematuria from irritation by the stone, dysuria, frequency, urgency, and enuresis. Some clients develop nausea, vomiting, and diarrhea due to the proximity of the gastrointestinal structures.

Diagnostic Tests

The diagnosis of renal calculi may be made initially by doing a kidney, ureter, and bladder (KUB) (flat plate of the abdomen) or an intravenous pyelogram. The client may also have costovertebral tenderness (as explained with the diagnosis of pyelonephritis).

Treatment

Renal calculi are treated medically if possible. The majority of stones are urinated out of the body. Clients can urinate stones if they are 5 mm in size or smaller; larger stones will not pass. If the client experiences severe renal colic, he or she will be admitted to the hospital. Intravenous fluids are administered to hydrate the client and help flush the stone out of the body. All urine is strained to detect passage of stones, and pain medication such as meperidine (Demerol) is given. If the client is unable to pass the stone, surgery is necessary.

The type of surgery done depends on the location of the stone. If the stone is in the bladder, a litholapaxy may be done. For this procedure an instrument is inserted through the urethra to the bladder to crush the stone; it is then washed out with an irrigating solution. If the stone is lodged in a ureter, the urologist may insert an instrument into the ureter through a cystoscope and attempt to catch the stone in a small wire basket. Postoperative care following these procedures is similar to care following any cystoscopy (Chapter 34). In addition to routine care, the nurse should find out if the stone was removed. If the stone is still present, the nurse should continue to strain all urine.

If the urologist is unable to snare the stone, the client may be scheduled for an extracorporeal shock wave lithotripsy (ESWL). For this procedure the client is immersed in a tub of water and ultrasonic shock waves are used to break up the stone into sand (Fig. 34–2), which is then urinated out. The client is anesthetized for the procedure. After the procedure the client is generally discharged home after being told to increase fluid intake and notify the urologist if there are any problems.

If the stone is large and lodged in the pelvis of the kidney, it may be necessary to do a **nephrolithotomy,** which is a surgical incision into the kidney to remove the stone. A major complication with this surgery is bleeding, because the kidney is very vascular.

The client may be advised to avoid foods that increase the risk of recurrent calculus development. Nutrition Notes Box 35–2 discusses foods that may contribute to calculi. (See also Cultural Considerations Box 35–3.) The nurse should consult with the physician and dietitian to determine which foods should be avoided, depending on the type of stone found.

Complications of Renal Calculi

The presence of renal calculi increases the risk for UTIs because of obstruction of free flow of urine. Untreated obstruction of a stone in a ureter or the urethra can also result

---

nephrolithothomy: nephro—kidney + lith—stone + otomy—incision

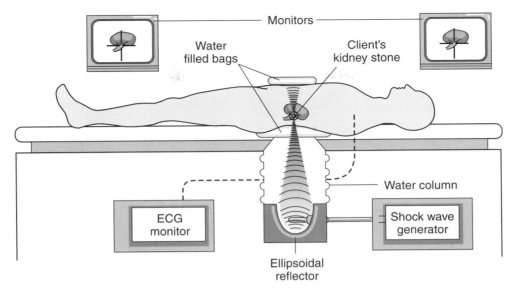

Figure 35–2. Extracorpeal shock wave lithotripsy.

in retention of urine and damage to the kidney. This process is called **hydronephrosis** (discussed next).

Nursing Process

Assessment

Nursing care of a client with a renal calculus always involves careful measurement of intake and output and observation of the urine for abnormalities such as hematuria, pyuria, or passage of a stone. Temperature is monitored for onset of fever, which would indicate infection. The nurse uses a special strainer to strain all urine for stones. If a stone is found it is saved for analysis in the laboratory. Clients with stones are often in extreme pain and should be assessed routinely for pain. The nurse also questions the client about a recent history of infection, dietary or activity changes, or other risk factors for renal calculi. If the cause can be identified, teaching can be done to help prevent recurrent calculi.

Nursing Diagnosis

Pain is a priority nursing diagnosis for any client with renal calculi. Risk for injury or infection from urine retention and risk for recurrent calculi are also concerns.

Planning

Planning should focus on pain relief, prevention of injury and infection, and teaching to prevent recurrent calculi.

Implementation

Analgesics such as meperidine (Demerol) are given to relieve pain. Fluids are encouraged to facilitate passage of

the stone and to prevent dehydration if nausea and vomiting are present. Antipyretics and antibiotics may be used if infection is present. The physician is notified immediately if gross hematuria, oliguria, or anuria develops. The client is instructed about the importance of fluids, activity increase, and diet changes if ordered.

Evaluation

Does the client state that pain is controlled? Are fever and other complications recognized and reported promptly? Does the client verbalize understanding of self-care measures to prevent recurrent stones?

HYDRONEPHROSIS

Hydronephrosis is a condition that results from untreated obstruction in the urinary tract. It is usually treatable once the condition is detected.

CULTURAL CONSIDERATIONS
BOX 35-3

Recurrent Calculus Development

Filipino immigrants are at high risk for developing renal stones, hyperuricemia, and gout.[4] A shift from a traditional Filipino diet to an American diet increases the occurrence of hyperuricemia with some older Filipinos developing gout.[5] The nurse may need to assist Filipino clients to identify food choices that will help prevent these conditions.

---

hydronephrosis: hydro—pertaining to water + nephrosis—degenerative change in the kidney

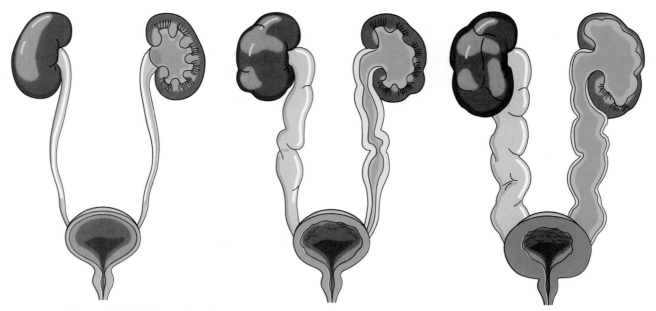

Figure 35–3. Hydronephrosis. Progressive thickening of bladder wall and dilatation of ureters and kidneys results from obstruction of urine flow.

Pathophysiology and Etiology

The obstruction of urine flow can be from stenosis or a stricture in a ureter or the urethra, from kidney stones, from a tumor, or from an enlarged prostate. Because of the unrelieved obstruction, urine backs up and distends the ureters, and then progresses to the kidney (Fig. 35–3). This enlargement of the kidney can be either unilateral or bilateral. The unrelieved pressure on the kidneys from the urine causes the kidneys to become bags filled with urine instead of functioning kidneys.

Symptoms

If the onset of obstruction is gradual, the client may initially be asymptomatic. Clients often develop UTIs because of the obstruction of urine flow and may have symptoms of frequency, urgency, and dysuria. As the disease progresses, flank and back pain may occur. Eventually the client will develop symptoms of renal failure.

Treatment

The treatment of hydronephrosis always involves relieving the obstruction. Initial removal of the obstruction may be done by insertion of an indwelling (Foley) catheter. Long-term correction of the obstruction depends on the cause and includes treatments and surgeries to relieve obstruction from strictures, stones, tumor, or an enlarged prostate. At times the obstruction cannot be relieved because a stone is too large or removal of tumor growth would result in death of the client. In these situations, **stents,** which are tiny

tubes, may be placed inside the ureters during a cystoscopy and pyelogram (C&P) to hold them open, or a **nephrostomy** tube may be inserted directly into the kidney pelvis to drain urine. A nephrostomy tube exits through an incision in the flank area and allows urine to drain into a collecting bag so that function of the kidney can be maintained. Figure 35–4 shows a stent in place in a ureter and a nephrostomy tube.

Complications

Complications associated with hydronephrosis include increased incidence of UTIs because of obstruction of urine flow and kidney failure from unrelieved pressure on the kidneys.

Nursing Care

The nurse carefully measures intake and output. Urine retention can worsen the condition and must be recognized and reported promptly. If the client has a nephrostomy tube, the nurse ensures that it is draining adequately and prevents kinking or clamping of the tube. Kinking of the tube will result in continuation of the hydronephrosis; the resulting pressure will destroy kidney function. If both a nephrostomy tube and Foley catheter are present, output from each should be measured and documented separately.

---

nephrostomy: nephro—pertaining the kidney +ostomy—a surgically formed artificial opening to the outside

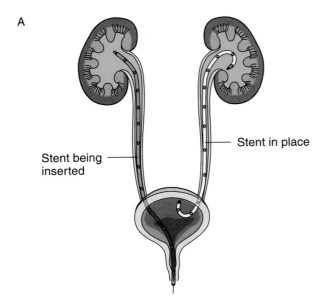

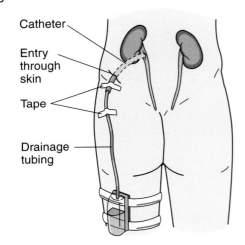

Posterior view

Figure 35–4. *(A)* Ureteral stents. *(B)* Nephrostomy tube inserted into renal pelvis; catheter exits through an incision on flank.

Tumors of the Renal System

CANCER OF THE KIDNEY

Pathophysiology and Etiology

Cancer of the kidney is a rare but serious kind of cancer. Risk factors include smoking, exposure to industrial pollution, obesity, and dialysis. Often the cancer has metastasized before it is diagnosed because the kidney has such a large volume of blood going through it, which increases the risk for spread of the tumor. In addition, there are few early symptoms of the disease.

---

nephrectomy: nephr—kidney + ectomy—excision

Signs and Symptoms

The usual first sign of cancer of the kidney is painless hematuria. Unfortunately the tumor may have metastasized by then. The three classic symptoms of kidney cancer are hematuria, dull pain in the flank area, and a mass in the area. Symptoms of metastasis may be the first manifestation of kidney cancer and include weight loss and increasing weakness.

Diagnostic Tests

A number of diagnostic tests will be done, including an intravenous pyelogram (IVP), C&P, ultrasound examination of the kidneys, and computed tomography (CT) scans. A definitive diagnosis is made with a renal biopsy.

Treatment

A radical **nephrectomy** is the preferred treatment for cancer of the kidney. The kidney is removed along with the adrenal gland and other surrounding structures, including fascia, fat, and lymph nodes, in the area. Radiation therapy, hormonal therapy, immunotherapy, or chemotherapy may be used following surgery.

Nursing Care

Nursing care of the nephrectomy client is similar to postoperative care following any major surgery (Chapter 11). Because the kidney is a very vascular organ, it is essential that the nurse observe for onset of bleeding and any signs of hypovolemic shock. Urine output is monitored; changes in amount or color, bleeding, and signs of infection are reported.

Cancer of the Bladder

Cancer of the bladder is the most common kind of cancer of the urinary tract. It is more commonly seen in elderly men ages 50 to 70.

Etiology

There is a strong correlation between smoking and bladder cancer. Exposure to industrial pollution such as aniline dyes, benzidine and naphthylamine, leather finishings, metal machinery, and petroleum processing products also increases the incidence.

Pathophysiology

Cancer of the bladder often starts as a benign growth on the bladder wall that undergoes cancerous changes. Common sites for metastasis include the liver, bones, and lungs.

Diagnostic Tests

Diagnosis of cancer of the bladder is made with a cystoscopy and biopsy, as well as from laboratory tests such as a urinalysis. The client is also examined for metastasis to other parts of the body utilizing bone scans and x-rays.

Signs and Symptoms

Cancer of the bladder usually causes painless hematuria. Blood in the urine is one of the seven warning signs of cancer from the American Cancer Society. Initially the bleeding is intermittent, which often results in people delaying seeking treatment. As the disease progresses, the client experiences frank hematuria, bladder irritability, urinary retention from clots obstructing the urethra, and fistula formation (an opening between the bladder and an adjoining structure such as the vagina or bowel).

Treatment

Treatment depends on the kind of bladder cancer and the severity. For small confined tumors, chemotherapy is instilled into the bladder through a Foley catheter, allowed to dwell, and then removed along with the catheter. Treatments are given at intervals. Systemic chemotherapy is also used and can be helpful to prolong life when other treatments are no longer indicated.

Surgical treatment of cancer of the bladder includes a number of procedures. A cystoscopy and pyelogram with fulguration (destruction of tissue with electrical current) may be done, to burn off cancerous tissue. For larger tumors, a portion of the bladder may be removed, along with the cancerous tumor (bladder resection).

If it has been determined that the client has potentially curable disease with much bladder involvement, complete removal of the bladder and creation of a urinary diversion may be done. This means that urine is diverted to leave the body in a different manner.

A common surgery for urinary diversion is called an ileal conduit, an involved surgery in which a section of the ileum or colon is removed and used as a conduit for urine. The remaining portions of the bowel are stitched back together. The surgeon is careful to keep the blood and neurological supply intact to the section of bowel that has been removed. The isolated section of bowel is closed off on one end, the ureters are stitched into it, and the other end is brought out as a stoma on the abdomen that almost continuously drains urine (Fig. 35–5). The urine will contain mucus because it comes through the ileum, which secretes mucus. The client will wear an ostomy appliance at all times over the stoma to collect urine. Table 35–2 explains how to apply an appliance to an ileal conduit stoma.

Several newer surgeries are being done for client convenience. The Kock pouch, or continent internal ileal reservoir, is created from a segment of ileum that has been made

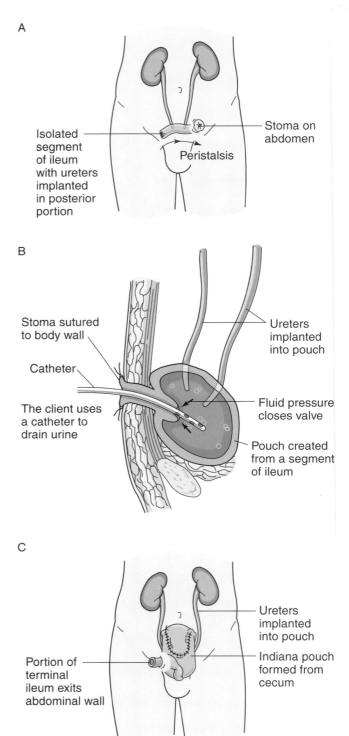

Figure 35–5. Urinary diversion surgery. *(A)* Ileal conduit. *(B)* Kock pouch. *(C)* Indiana pouch.

into a reservoir for urine (Fig. 35–5). The ureters are implanted into the side of the reservoir. A special nipple valve is constructed and is the passageway through which the client inserts a catheter at frequent intervals to drain urine. Another newer surgery is called the Indiana pouch. A reservoir is created using a portion of the ascending colon and

Table 35–2. *Application of a Disposable Pouch to an Ileal Conduit*

1. Gather all supplies: a washcloth and towels and water, a pouch to apply with a stomahesive flange and wicks such as Kerlix gauze to absorb urine. The nurse should wear clean gloves.
2. Empty the old pouch.
3. Gently remove soiled pouch by pushing down on skin while lifting up on the flange. Discard soiled pouch and flange.
4. Place a towel around the stoma to catch urine.
5. Cut an opening in the flange that is only 1/16 to 1/8 inch larger than the stoma. Once stomal shrinkage is complete, a pre-sized pouch can be used that fits the stoma.
6. Remove paper backing from the stomahesive and set the flange to one side.
7. Clean the skin around the stoma with water. Pat dry. Immediately wrap the stoma in wicks to absorb urine. Otherwise urine will leak onto the skin, and the flange will not adhere.
8. Center the flange over the stoma, remove the wick, and immediately apply the flange. Then snap the pouch onto the flange. NOTE: The flange and pouch may be snapped together before application to the stoma.
9. Use the heat of your hand to compress the flange to ensure a good seal.
10. Ensure that the bottom of the pouch is closed off, or connect to a Foley catheter bag for nighttime or for the client in bed most of the time.

Data from Hampton, BG, and Bryant, RA: Ostomies and Continent Diversions: Nursing Management. Mosby, St Louis, 1992.

terminal ileum, making a larger pouch than the Kock pouch.

Nursing Care

Nursing care of the postoperative client is similar to care following any major surgical procedure (Chapter 11). It is important that the nurse ensure that there is adequate urinary output and detect and report any obstruction of urine drainage early to prevent complications. The client will need instruction on how to care for the urinary diversion after surgery, either by frequent draining with a catheter or by wearing an appliance. The nurse should be sensitive to the client's anxiety about caring for the urinary diversion. Body image disturbance may occur because of the change in body function. A consultation with an enterostomal therapist or ostomy support group may be helpful both before and after surgery.

Polycystic Kidney Disease

PATHOPHYSIOLOGY AND ETIOLOGY

Polycystic kidney disease is a hereditary disorder that can result in renal failure. The disease is characterized by for-

nephropathy: nephro—pertaining to the kidney + pathy—disease

mation of multiple cysts in the kidney that can eventually replace normal kidney structures. The cysts are grapelike and contain serous fluid, blood, or urine.

SIGNS AND SYMPTOMS

The client generally first shows signs of the disease in adulthood. The initial symptoms include a dull heaviness in the flank or lumbar region and hematuria. As the disease progresses, the client develops symptoms of renal failure (see Renal Failure, later in this chapter).

TREATMENT

There is no treatment to stop the progression of polycystic kidney disease. Complications such as urinary tract infections are treated as needed. As the disease progresses, treatment for hypertension and eventual renal failure may be necessary.

Because polycystic disease is hereditary, clients should be counseled about the risks of children inheriting it.

Chronic Renal Diseases

DIABETIC NEPHROPATHY

Diabetic **nephropathy** is the most common cause of renal failure. It is a long-term complication of diabetes mellitus in which the effects of diabetes result in damage to the small blood vessels in the kidneys. Renal damage shows up approximately 15 to 20 years after onset of type 1 (insulin-dependent) diabetes, but it may also be a complication of type 2 (non-insulin-dependent) diabetes. Careful control of blood glucose levels will decrease the development of nephropathy in diabetic clients.

Pathophysiology

Multiple factors contribute to diabetic nephropathy. Widespread atherosclerotic changes occur in the blood vessels of clients with diabetes. These atherosclerotic changes decrease the blood supply to the kidney. Abnormal thickening of glomerular capillaries damages the glomerulus, allowing protein to leak into the urine. Diabetic clients also commonly develop pyelonephritis and renal scarring. Another complication of diabetes, neurogenic bladder, causes incomplete bladder emptying. This results in retention of urine, which can cause infection or obstruction of urine, further damaging the kidneys.

Initially clients lose only small amounts of protein in their urine (microalbuminuria); this disease can be detected only with careful watching by the physician, utilizing frequent examinations of the urine. As the disease progresses, high-output renal failure (nonoliguric) can develop, in which a large amount of dilute urine is excreted without the usual amounts of waste product dissolved in the urine. The client can lose large amounts of protein in the urine and may develop nephrotic syndrome, which causes massive edema because of low levels of albumin in the blood. As renal function decreases, the client will need smaller doses of insulin because the kidney normally degrades insulin. Because the kidney is no longer able to break insulin down and excrete it, small doses of insulin circulate in the body for long periods of time.

Symptoms

As diabetic nephropathy progresses, urine output decreases, toxic wastes accumulate, and the client develops chronic renal failure. Symptoms of chronic renal failure are found in Figure 35–6.

Diagnostic Tests

Diabetic nephropathy is diagnosed by careful watching of the diabetic client for onset of protein spillage in the urine, which is an early sign of the disease. Serum creati-

nine levels and 24-hour creatinine clearance tests are then done to confirm the presence and extent of diabetic nephropathy.

Treatment

In the early stages of diabetic nephropathy, strict control of blood glucose levels and blood pressure and a restricted-protein diet can help slow the progress of the disease and reduce symptoms. As the disease progresses into renal failure, the client will need dialysis to maintain life. Unfortunately, other complications related to diabetes cause clients to tolerate dialysis less well than clients with renal failure from other causes. Kidney or kidney-pancreas transplant when available is the treatment of choice for the client with diabetic nephropathy and often improves the client's chance for a healthier life.

Complications

Clients with diabetic nephropathy often have a guarded prognosis because they are vulnerable to all the complica-

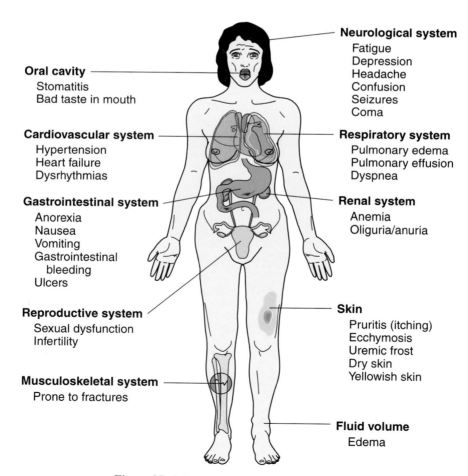

Figure 35–6. Symptoms of chronic renal failure.

tions of long-term diabetes in addition to kidney disease (see Chapter 38).

NEPHROSCLEROSIS

Pathophysiology

Hypertension damages the kidneys by causing sclerotic changes, such as arteriosclerosis with thickening and hardening of the renal blood vessels (**nephrosclerosis**). The arteriosclerotic changes in the kidney blood vessels result in a decreased blood supply to the kidney (ischemia of the kidney) and can eventually destroy the kidney.

Signs and Symptoms

Symptoms of nephrosclerosis include proteinuria, hyaline casts in the urine, and as it progresses symptoms of renal failure.

Treatment

The treatment of nephrosclerosis is treatment of hypertension. The client is placed on antihypertensive medications, or if already on these, changed to stronger antihypertensive medications. The client is placed on a low-sodium diet. If the client develops renal failure, dialysis will be used to maintain life.

Complications

The prognosis is often poor because by the time the client has developed nephrosclerosis, there is widespread arteriosclerosis throughout the body. Arteriosclerosis makes the client prone to myocardial infarctions or cerebrovascular accidents.

Nursing Care

The major nursing diagnosis that is relevant when the client develops nephrosclerosis is altered health maintenance, and the priority is to help the client learn as much about the control of hypertension as possible. The client should also be taught the symptoms of renal failure. Once the client has lost renal function, the nursing care plan for renal failure is appropriate.

---

nephrosclerosis: nephro—pertaining to the kidney + slcerosis—hardening

glomerulonephritis: glomerulo—glomerulus + neph—kidney + itis—inflammation

oliguria: olig—small + uria—urine

> ### CRITICAL THINKING: Mr. White
>
> Mr. White is a 35-year-old African-American gentleman admitted to the intensive care unit with uncontrolled hypertension. His blood pressure is controlled by intravenous medication. His lab tests show protein and hyaline casts in the urine. He is diagnosed with nephrosclerosis.
>
> 1. What should the nurse assess as part of the morning evaluation of the client's condition?
> 2. What other renal function tests are appropriate for the nurse to check?
> 3. What teaching does Mr. White need when his condition is more stable?
>
> *Answers at end of chapter.*

Glomerulonephritis

PATHOPHYSIOLOGY

Glomerulonephritis is an inflammatory disease of the glomerulus. Inflammation occurs as a result of the deposition of antigen-antibody complexes in the basement membrane of the glomerulus or from antibodies that specifically attack the basement membrane. The resulting immune reaction in the glomerulus causes inflammation, which in turn causes the glomerulus to be more porous, allowing proteins, white blood cells, and red blood cells to leak into the urine.

ETIOLOGY

Glomerulonephritis can be caused by a variety of factors but is most commonly associated with a group A hemolytic streptococcus infection following a streptococcal infection of the throat or skin. This is the most common cause in children. Antibodies form complexes with the streptococcal antigen and are deposited in the basement membrane of the glomerulus. Glomerulonephritis generally develops about 6 to 10 days after the preceding infection. Viruses can also be the offending infectious agent.

Occasionally glomerulonephritis is caused by an autoimmune response, in which the person for some unknown reason forms antibodies against his or her own glomerular basement membrane. Glomerulonephritis caused by an autoimmune response usually progresses rapidly and often leads to renal failure.

SYMPTOMS

The symptoms of glomerulonephritis include fluid overload with **oliguria,** hypertension, electrolyte imbalances, and edema. Edema may begin around the eyes (periorbital edema) and face and progress to the abdomen (ascites), lungs (pleural effusion), and extremities. Flank pain may be present. Blood urea nitrogen (BUN) and creatinine may be elevated. Urinalysis shows red blood cells, white blood cells, albumin, and casts. The urine is dark, smoky, or cola colored from old red blood cells and may be foamy because of proteinuria.

TREATMENT

Most cases of acute glomerulonephritis resolve spontaneously in about a week, but some progress to renal failure. Treatment is primarily symptomatic. Sodium and fluid restrictions may be ordered along with diuretics to treat fluid retention. Medications may be given to control hypertension. If associated with a streptococcus infection, antibiotics are given to treat any remaining infection. If fluid overload is severe, dialysis may be done.

COMPLICATIONS

The prognosis is good with acute glomerulonephritis acquired in childhood, and the majority of children recover completely. Adults who develop glomerulonephritis may recover renal function or progress to chronic glomerulonephritis. Some clients develop rapidly progressive glomerulonephritis, which can progress quickly to renal failure. Chronic glomerulonephritis is a slow process characterized by hypertension, slow loss of renal function, and eventual renal failure, discussed next.

Renal Failure

Renal failure, also called kidney failure, is diagnosed when the kidneys are no longer functioning adequately to maintain normal body processes. This results in dysfunction in almost all other parts of the body. Renal failure can be an acute episode, which has a sudden onset of symptoms, or chronic and occur gradually over a period of time.

ACUTE RENAL FAILURE

Acute renal failure (ARF) occurs when loss of kidney function is sudden, with a rapid onset of hours to days.

Pathophysiology and Etiology

In acute renal failure, rapid damage to the kidney causes waste products to accumulate in the bloodstream, resulting in the symptoms of renal failure. The client becomes oliguric with urine output decreasing to less than 20 mL per hour. The exact incidence is unknown, but it is estimated that ARF affects at least 10,000 people a year. Many of these clients recover completely with treatment directed toward correcting the cause, supporting the client with dialysis, and prevention of complications that may lead to permanent damage. Approximately 50 percent die related to complications of infection, pneumonia, or septicemia.

Three categories of causes can lead to acute renal failure. Each category is associated with the location of the cause in the kidney.

Prerenal failure (before the kidney) is associated with a decrease or interruption of blood supply to the kidneys. The causes may include a decrease in blood pressure due to dehydration, blood loss, shock, or a blockage in the arteries that carry blood to the kidneys. When the nephrons receive an inadequate blood supply, they are unable to make urine and the waste products are not adequately removed.

Prerenal failure can be diagnosed by evaluating possible causes. An arteriogram of the renal arteries is helpful to determine if the blood supply to the kidneys is decreased or blocked; angioplasty may be used to open the blockage.

Intrarenal failure (inside the kidney) occurs when there is damage to the nephrons inside the kidney. The most common causes are from infectious processes causing glomerulonephritis, exposure to **nephrotoxins** (Table 35–3), allergic reactions to x-ray dyes, and severe muscle injury, which releases substances that are harmful to the kidneys.

A number of substances can be nephrotoxic to the kidneys when they enter the body. Kidney damage is most likely to occur when these substances enter the body in high concentrations or when there is preexisting kidney damage for some other reason. Environmental nephrotoxins such as insecticides and lead paint may be ingested by children, or by adults as a suicide attempt. Many commonly administered medications can be nephrotoxic. Aminoglycosides are nephrotoxic antibiotics; when they are administered blood levels of the drugs are carefully monitored to avoid toxic levels.

Contrast media used during tests such as intravenous pyelograms and CT scans can cause kidney damage when the client is dehydrated or has preexisting renal damage. The medium can precipitate out in the tubules, damaging the kidney. It is important for the client to be adequately hydrated after any diagnostic test using a contrast medium, to decrease the incidence of toxicity.

Postrenal failure (after the kidney) is associated with an obstruction that blocks the flow of urine out of the body. In this case, the blood supply to the kidneys and nephron function may initially be normal, but urine is unable to drain out of the kidney, resulting in backup of urine and impaired nephron function. Common causes are kidney

---

nephrotoxin: nephro—kidney + toxin—poison

Table 35–3. *Common Nephrotoxins*

Antibiotics
Aminoglycosides
Tetracyclines
Cephalosporins
Sulfonamides

Analgesics
Nonsteroidal anti-inflammatory drugs
Acetaminophen
Phenacetin
Salicylates

Other Drugs
Dextran
Mannitol
Interleukin-2
Cisplatin
Amphetamines
Heroin

Heavy Metals
Lead
Mercury
Arsenic
Copper
Gold
Lithium

Contrast Dyes
Dyes used for diagnostic testing such as intravenous pyelograms, cardiac catheterizations

Organic Solvents
Gasoline
Glycols
Kerosene
Turpentine
Tetrachloroethylene

stones, tumors of the ureters or bladder, or an enlarged prostate that blocks the flow of urine.

Diagnosis of causes of postrenal failure can be done with x-rays of kidneys, ureters, and bladder. Cystoscopy will show presence of tumors, stones, or prostate enlargement. Surgical intervention may be needed to correct the problem.

Treatment

Acute renal failure is treated by relieving the cause. Temporary dialysis may be necessary to treat renal failure and to prevent permanent damage. The care of the acute renal failure client is similar to care of the chronic renal failure client, as explained in the next section.

---

uremia: ur—urea + emia—in the blood

CHRONIC RENAL FAILURE

Chronic renal failure (CRF) affects approximately 75,000 people in the United States. Chronic renal failure occurs with a gradual decrease in the function of the kidneys over a period of time. This loss of function is not reversible.

Etiology

The causes of chronic renal failure are numerous; common ones include diabetes mellitus resulting in diabetic nephropathy, chronic high blood pressure causing nephrosclerosis, glomerulonephritis, and autoimmune diseases.

Pathophysiology

When a large proportion of the nephrons are damaged or destroyed due to acute or chronic kidney disease, renal failure occurs. As the nephrons die off, the undamaged ones increase their work capacity and take over the work previously done by the dead ones, so the client may experience significant kidney damage without showing symptoms of renal failure.

Chronic renal failure is a progressive disease process. In the early, or silent, stage, the client is usually without symptoms, even though up to 50 percent of nephron function may have been lost. This stage is often not diagnosed.

The renal insufficiency stage occurs when the client has lost 75 percent of nephron function and some signs of mild renal failure are present. Anemia and the inability to concentrate urine may be present. The BUN and creatinine levels are slightly elevated. These clients are at risk for further damage caused by infection, dehydration, drugs, heart failure, and diagnostic x-ray dyes.

End-stage renal disease (ESRD) occurs when 90 percent of the nephrons are lost. Clients at this stage experience chronic and persistent abnormal kidney function. The BUN and creatinine levels are always elevated. This client may make urine but not filter out the waste products, or urine production may cease. Dialysis or a kidney transplant is required to survive.

Uremia, urea in the blood, is present in chronic renal failure. Clients eventually develop problems in all body systems. Table 35–4 shows the effect of renal failure on body systems.

SYMPTOMS OF RENAL FAILURE AND NURSING INTERVENTIONS

Clients in either acute or chronic renal failure have multiple symptoms. Some of the more common symptoms associated with renal failure are explained next. (See Figure 35–6 for symptoms of chronic renal failure.)

Table 35–4. **Effects of Renal Failure on Body Systems**

Body System	Disease Process
Cardiovascular System	Edema due to fluid overload and a decrease in osmotic pressure Dysrhythmias due to electrolyte imbalance, coronary artery disease Angina due to coronary artery disease, anemia Hypertension due to fluid overload and accelerated arteriosclerosis Congestive heart failure/pulmonary edema due to fluid overload, increased pulmonary permeability, left ventricular failure
Pulmonary	Pleurisy/pleural effusion due to the waste products in the pleural space causing inflammation with pleurisy pain and also a collection of fluid resulting in an effusion
Hematopoietic	Anemia due to impaired synthesis of erythropoietin, a substance needed by the bone marrow to stimulate formation of RBCs; also due to decreased life span of RBCs due to uremia and interference in folic acid action Bleeding tendency due to abnormal platelet function from effects of uremia Prone to infection due to a decrease in immune system function from uremia; renal patients can rapidly become septic and die from septic shock
Integumentary System	Dry, itchy, inflamed skin due to urochrome, a pigment of uremia causing skin to be pale gray, yellow bronze; skin will have odor of urine because skin is an organ of excretion and the body attempts to remove toxins; there is also a decrease in function of oil and sweat glands Stomatitis due to fluid restriction, presence of waste products in the mouth, and secondary infections
Gastrointestinal System	Anorexia, nausea, vomiting due to uremia Gastritis/gastrointestinal bleeding due to urea decomposition in gastrointestinal tract releasing ammonia that irritates and ulcerates the stomach or bowel; client is also under stress, increasing ulcer formation, and may have platelet dysfunction Constipation due to electrolyte imbalances, decrease in fluid intake, decrease in activity, phosphate binders Diarrhea, hypermotility due to electrolyte imbalance
Neurological System	Confusion due to uremic encephalopathy from an increase in urea and metabolic acids Peripheral neuropathy due to effects of waste products on neurological system
Skeletal System	Bone disease due to renal osteodystrophy from hyperphosphatemia and hypocalcemia
Reproductive System	Loss of libido, impotence, amenorrhea, infertility due to a decrease in hormone production

Disturbance in Water Balance

Clients with renal failure experience disturbances in the removal and regulation of water balance in the body and show signs of fluid accumulation. An early symptom is edema (swelling) of the extremities, sacral area, and abdomen. Clients may complain of being short of breath. Crackles and wheezes may be present on auscultation of the lungs, which are signs of fluid accumulation in the lungs. The blood vessels in the neck may be distended and the client may be hypertensive. These clients may produce a large amount of dilute urine (**polyuria**), small amounts of urine (oliguria), or no urine (**anuria**).

Nursing care for disturbances in water balance involves monitoring the client's weight at the same time each day. The client who is retaining fluid will have an increase in weight. Intake and output are measured, and a fluid restriction will be ordered by the physician, generally 1000 mL per 24 hours. Lung sounds are monitored for crackles and wheezes. Symptoms of fluid retention are reported.

Disturbance in Electrolyte Balance

As kidney function decreases, the kidneys lose their ability to absorb and excrete electrolytes. Important electrolytes are sodium, potassium, and magnesium. When the kidneys are unable to maintain normal amounts of electrolytes in the blood, these substances accumulate at high levels and may be life threatening.

When the kidneys are unable to regulate sodium levels adequately, the client may show signs of hypernatremia, an excessive sodium level in the blood, which causes water retention, edema, and hypertension. Hyponatremia, too little sodium, may occur when too much sodium is lost. This can occur when the client has experienced prolonged episodes of vomiting or diarrhea or is urinating large amounts of dilute urine. Clients with hyponatremia may show signs of confusion.

---

polyuria: poly—much + uria—urine
anuria: an—without + uria—urine

Hyperkalemia (high level of potassium) presents a life-threatening situation. The client may exhibit signs of cardiac rhythm irregularities and cardiac arrest if the potassium level is too high. Clients complain of muscle weakness, abdominal cramping, and diarrhea. The nurse may identify that the client is confused or demonstrates disinterest in care. Hyperkalemia exists when the potassium level exceeds 5 mEq/L. These clients should be placed on a cardiac monitor and observed for cardiac dysrhythmias. A potassium level above 7 mEq/L may be life threatening. A high potassium level in the renal failure client may be caused by the client eating a diet high in potassium-rich foods, injuries, or blood transfusions. Nursing care should include monitoring daily laboratory levels, restricting potassium intake, and reporting abnormalities. Insulin or sodium bicarbonate may be used as a temporary measure to drive excess potassium into the cells. Sodium polystyrene sulfonate (Kayexalate) may be given either orally or as a retention enema; it causes the potassium to be eliminated through the bowels. The definitive treatment for hyperkalemia is hemodialysis to remove potassium from the body. Dietary education is extremely important. The client is instructed to avoid foods that are high in potassium (Table 35–5).

Calcium levels decrease because the kidneys are unable to produce the hormone that activates vitamin D, the vitamin that is necessary for the absorption of calcium. Hypocalcemia exists when the calcium level falls below 8.5 mg/dL. Also associated with a low calcium level is hyperphosphatemia, an elevated phosphorous level above 5 mg/dL. These imbalances cause the bones to release calcium, causing clients to be prone to fractures. These clients should ambulate regularly to prevent further calcium loss from the bone.

Phosphates are supplied by some foods. The increase in phosphorous levels may result in severe itching, and clients may have open sores as a result of scratching, placing them at risk for infections. Clients complain of muscle cramps and aches. Medications to bind phosphate are given to clients with high phosphate levels. Tums (calcium carbonate) and aluminum-based antacids are examples of commonly ordered phosphate binders. These must be given to the client immediately after meals with a full glass of water so that the medication can bind with the phosphates in the bowel and be eliminated. If the client is on nothing by mouth (NPO) status or is unable to eat a meal, the phosphate binder is not necessary for that meal.

Table 35–5. **Foods High in Potassium**

Potatoes, sweet and white
Citrus fruits and juices
Bananas
Excessive dairy products
Excessive meats
Chocolate
Salt substitutes

Disturbance of Removal of Waste Products

When the kidneys are unable to remove the waste products of metabolism, **azotemia** occurs. This is an increase in the serum urea level (measured by the BUN), and often elevated creatinine levels also. These substances are the result of protein metabolism. The client may show signs of weakness and fatigue, confusion, seizures, twitching movements of extremities (**asterixis**), nausea, vomiting, and lack of appetite and may complain of a bad taste in the mouth. The nurse may smell urine on the client's breath. The client may have yellowish-pale skin and complain of itching.

Nursing care for clients with azotemia includes monitoring laboratory results and treating and reporting symptoms. Adequate nutrition is important; the dietitian should be consulted to recommend the appropriate low-protein diet to decrease formation of these waste products.

Special care is given to provide adequate oral care and skin care. The nurse offers mouth care frequently and inspects the mouth for sores. Lotion is used for itching, and the skin is observed for open areas and signs of infection. The client is protected from injury if confusion or seizures occur. Dialysis to remove the excessive waste products in the blood is the only treatment of the underlying causes of these symptoms.

Disturbance in Maintaining Acid-Base Balance

Renal failure affects hydrogen ion excretion, causing a disturbance in acid-base balance that results in metabolic acidosis. Clients may complain of a headache, fatigue, weakness, nausea, vomiting, and lack of appetite. As the acidosis progresses the client shows signs of lethargy, stupor, and coma. Respirations become fast and deep as the lungs attempt to blow off carbon dioxide to correct the acidosis. See Chapter 5 for a more detailed discussion of acid-base balance.

Disturbance in Hematological Function

Failing kidneys do not produce adequate erythropoietin, the hormone that stimulates red blood cell production. Nu-

---

azotemia: azo—nitrogenous waste products + temia—blood
asterixis: abnormal muscle tremors consisting of involuntary jerking movements, especially of the hands

tritional deficiencies and blood loss during dialysis also contribute to anemia. Regular injections of epoetin alpha (Epogen), a synthetic form of erythropoietin, helps restore red cell production and prevent anemia.

Impaired white blood cell and immune function contribute to an increased risk for infection. The client should be protected from potential sources of infection.

Impaired platelet function creates a risk for bleeding. The client should be protected from injury, and signs of bleeding, such as blood in stool or emesis, should be reported.

TREATMENT OF RENAL FAILURE

Renal insufficiency and early renal failure are treated symptomatically with restricted diet and fluids, medications, and careful monitoring for onset of serious problems that warrant initiation of dialysis. In later stages, dialysis is necessary to replace lost kidney function. A kidney transplant, when available, may return the client to a nearly normal state of health.

Diet

Dietary recommendations are individualized by the dietitian and physician, based on the client's needs. Calories are high to maintain weight and energy needs. Protein is usually restricted to limit nitrogen intake but may be increased for the client on dialysis, because protein is lost during the dialysis process. Sodium is restricted to minimize sodium and fluid retention. Potassium is restricted, especially later in the disease when the kidneys are unable to eliminate it. Calcium is increased or supplemented because of poor absorption related to faulty vitamin D activation. Phosphorus is restricted because of high blood levels related to hypocalcemia. Saturated fat and cholesterol are restricted for clients with hyperlipidemia. Fluids are restricted to prevent overload. Most clients are given iron, vitamins, and minerals to supplement the restricted diet. (See also Nutrition Notes Box 35–4.)

Because restrictions are many and complex, the diet is a source of frustration for many clients. The nurse should assist the client to identify foods that are palatable, yet within the diet plan. The dietitian should be consulted for instruction and assistance.

Medications

Early in the disease, diuretics are given to increase output, and angiotensin-converting enzyme (ACE) inhibitors, calcium channel blockers, or beta blocking agents may be used to control hypertension. Phosphate binders are given with meals to reduce phosphate levels. Calcium and vitamin D supplements are used to raise calcium levels. Agents

NUTRITION NOTES BOX 35-4

Kidney Disease

Clients with impaired renal function require careful coordination of diet with current physiological status, which may change frequently. Nutritional care of renal patients is a specialty practice for dietitians.

- Caloric intake is maintained to avoid catabolism of tissue for energy. Simple carbohydrates and monounsaturated and polyunsaturated fats are given freely because their end products of carbon dioxide and water are less likely than protein to burden the kidney. Clients with diabetes and uremia may receive higher amounts of sugar than usual because treatment of the uremia may take precedence over the diabetes. Clients with type IV hypertriglyceridemia may have to limit carbohydrate intake.
- Protein may be decreased or increased. Those of high biological value (eggs, meat, and dairy products) are preferred sources because they are more easily converted to body protein than those of low biological value. Protein may be less restricted when the client is treated with dialysis to compensate for losses in the dialysate.
- Sodium may be restricted depending on blood pressure, edema, and laboratory findings.
- Potassium may be restricted for oliguric clients. Salt substitutes are often potassium compounds, so they are avoided. Potassium content in foods varies with processing and preparation methods. Clients should choose from prescribed foods only.
- Fluid restriction may be altered daily according to output. Renal insufficiency patients may receive 500 mL plus the amount of the previous day's output.

to lower potassium levels are used if necessary. All drug therapy is closely monitored because diseased kidneys are unable to effectively remove medications from the body.

Dialysis

Dialysis is started when the client develops symptoms of severe fluid overload, high potassium levels, acidosis, or symptoms of uremia that are life threatening.

Hemodialysis

Hemodialysis involves the use of an artificial kidney to remove waste products and excess water from the client's blood. The blood flows from the client's body through

hemodialysis: hemo—blood + dialysis—the passage of a solute through a membrane

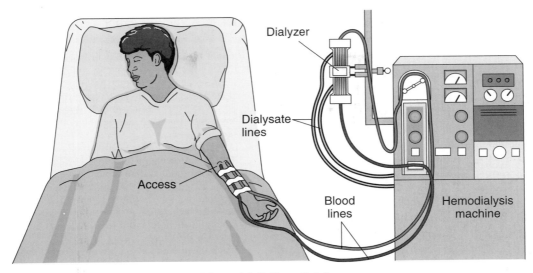

Figure 35–7. Hemodialyis.

tubes into an artificial kidney called a dialyzer. The artificial kidney has specialized chambers that allow the client's blood to flow through while the waste products and excess fluids pass into a dialysate solution that circulates around the chambers. The dialysate solution carries the waste products away, and the cleansed blood is returned back into the client's body through another tube (Fig. 35–7). A hemodialysis treatment takes 3 to 4 hours and is done three or four times a week. Hemodialysis can be done at a hemodialysis center (Fig. 35–8) or at home. At a center the treatment is done by nurses or trained technicians. At home the treatment is done by the client with the help of a specially trained family member or by a technician who comes into the home.

Hemodialysis provides a rapid and efficient way to remove waste products from the blood. It is also an excellent

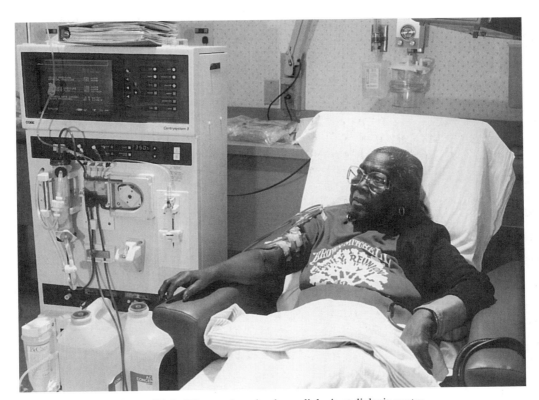

Figure 35–8. Client undergoing hemodialysis at dialysis center.

means to correct excessive fluid-overloaded states such as occur in heart failure.

Hemodialysis is not without side effects. Following a treatment, the client normally feels weak and fatigued, sometimes even too tired to eat. Sudden drops in the blood pressure may cause the client to become weak, dizzy, and nauseated. Cardiac irregularities and angina may occur. Fluid and electrolyte levels drop rapidly and cause the client to feel lethargic and have muscle cramps. Clients are given large amounts of heparin, an anticoagulant used to keep the blood from clotting while it is in the artificial kidney; this may cause bleeding from the puncture sites, gastrointestinal tract, nose, or other sites if injury occurs.

The hemodialysis client requires a surgically placed access site that allows the blood to be removed from the body and replaced back into the body at the time of dialysis. An access is made by joining an artery and a vein together under the skin. There are two kinds of permanent accesses. An arteriovenous graft (A-V graft) uses a piece of special material, usually Gore-Tex, that is sewn to an artery and then attached to a vein. An A-V fistula is made by sewing the vein and the artery together (Fig. 35–9). The graft and

the fistula are both placed in the arm, when possible. Both types of access sites take 1 to 2 weeks to mature once the surgical procedure is completed. This allows the new site to be able to receive the high-pressure blood from the dialyzer following the treatment.

A temporary access is used for clients requiring hemodialysis before the graft or fistula is placed or is usable. This is a special hemodialysis catheter that is placed in the subclavian vein in the neck or the femoral vein in the groin.

Table 35–6. *Care of Blood Access Graft or Fistula*

1. Watch for signs of bleeding or infection at the site.
2. Listen for a bruit at the site by placing the diaphragm of a stethoscope gently on the site. A bruit is a swishing sound made as the blood passes through the access site.
3. Gently palpate the site for a thrill, which is a buzzing or pulsing feeling that indicates good blood flow through the access site.
4. Do not take a blood pressure, use a tourniquet, draw blood, or start any intravenous lines in the affected arm. Injections should be avoided if possible.
5. Many hospitals have the client wear a red arm bracelet to signify that the arm should be protected. A sign above the bed may also be helpful.
6. Teach the client to avoid wearing constrictive clothing or jewelry over the site.
7. Teach the client to avoid prolonged bending or sleeping on the arm with an access.
8. Notify the physician if signs of bleeding or reduced circulation through the access site occur.

Table 35–7. *Nursing Care of the Client Receiving Hemodialysis*

1. Consult with physician about medications to hold before hemodialysis. Some medications such as antihypertensives can be very harmful when they become effective during dialysis and can lower the blood pressure to dangerously low levels. Other medications are water soluble and will be dialyzed out and thus are not effective.
2. Ensure that the client is weighed both before dialysis in the morning and after dialysis to document weight loss as a result of fluid removal.
3. If the client has blood work ordered to be drawn, coordinate this process with the dialysis nurse, who can obtain the blood samples and save the client unnecessary needle sticks.
4. Try to get morning care done early and breakfast given before dialysis. After dialysis clients are often exhausted and need rest.
5. When the client returns from dialysis, assess the access site for bleeding, and make sure the vital signs are stable. Administer medications that were held if not contraindicated and vital signs are stable.
6. Protect the client's dialysis access as outlined in Table 35–6. *No dialysis access site should be utilized for any purpose other than dialysis.*

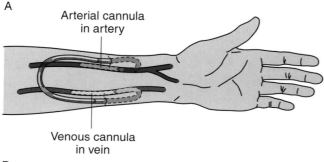

A

Arterial cannula in artery

Venous cannula in vein

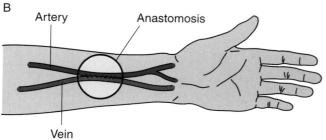

B

Artery   Anastomosis

Vein

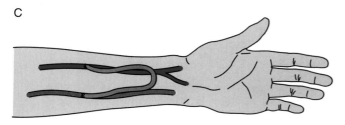

C

Figure 35–9. Hemodialysis access sites. *(A)* Arteriovenous shunt. *(B)* Arteriovenous fistula. *(C)* Arteriovenous vein graft.

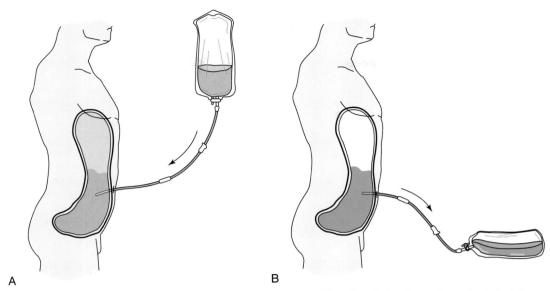

A   B

Figure 35–10. *(A)* Peritoneal dialysis works inside the body. Dialysis solution flows through a tube into the abdominal cavity, where it collects waste products from the blood. *(B)* Periodically, the used dialysis solution is drained from the abdominal cavity, carrying away waste products and excess water from the blood.

Special care of the access site must be taken because this is the client's only way to eliminate waste products. Refer to Table 35–6 for care of a blood access site. It is important that the site be carefully monitored per institution policy to detect any clotting or problems at the site. Early detection of clotting will allow the surgeon an opportunity to save the access by performing a declotting procedure, rather than a total revision.

Refer to Table 35–7 for care of the client during hemodialysis.

Peritoneal Dialysis

Peritoneal dialysis provides continuous dialysis treatment and is done by the client or family in the home. The peritoneal membrane is used as a semipermeable membrane across which excess wastes and fluids move from blood in peritoneal vessels into a dialysate solution that has been instilled into the peritoneal cavity. A peritoneal catheter is placed into the client's abdomen below the waistline. This catheter is used to perform an exchange. The exchange process has three steps: filling, dwell time, and draining.

The fill step involves instilling a bag of sterile dialyzing solution (dialysate) into the client's peritoneal cavity through the catheter. The amount of solution is usually 1500 to 2000 mL. The solution is left to dwell in the abdomen for several hours, allowing time for the waste products

from the blood to pass through the peritoneal membrane into the dialysate solution. See Figure 35–10.

The solution is then drained out of the body and discarded. This process is repeated three or four times a day and is a continuous process for the client. Several different treatment plans use this exchange process; the treatment plan that best suits the client's needs is determined by the client and the dialysis team.

Continuous ambulatory peritoneal dialysis (CAPD) is the most commonly used treatment plan. Usually three exchanges are done during the day and one before bedtime. Other treatment plans allow for the use of a computerized machine called a cycler to regulate the exchanges during sleeping hours. Sometimes medications are added to the dialyzing solutions, such as heparin to prevent clotting of the catheter, insulin for the client with diabetes, or antibiotics if there is infection.

Client and family education is extremely important for peritoneal dialysis to be successful. The client must be taught, and be able to demonstrate that he or she is able, to do a successful exchange. Sterile technique while doing the exchanges is imperative, and the exchanges should be done in a clean environment. A major complication is peritonitis (infection of the peritoneum), which can be life threatening. The major cause of peritonitis is poor technique when connecting the bag of dialyzing solution to the peritoneal catheter. The first sign of peritonitis is usually abdominal pain. Refer to Chapter 31 for additional signs and symptoms of peritonitis. If any symptoms of peritonitis occur, the client must contact the physician immediately so that antibiotic treatment can begin. The client should be

---

peritoneal dialysis: peritoneal—peritoneum + dialysis—the passage of a solute through a membrane

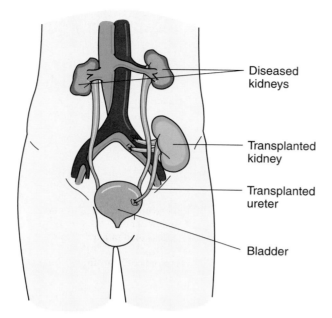

Figure 35–11. A transplanted kidney is placed in the abdomen. The client's kidneys are usually left in place.

Renal Function and Assessment

Because many Vietnamese people believe that the body must be kept intact, even after death, they may object to removal of body parts or organ donation.[6]

Jewish law views organ transplantation from the recipient, the living donor, the cadaver donor, and the dying donor differently.[7] If the recipient's life can be prolonged without considerable risk, transplant is ordained. For a living donor to be approved, the risk to the life of the donor must be considered. One is not obligated to donate a part of himself or herself unless the risk is small. The use of a cadaver for transplant is usually approved if it is saving a life. The nurse may need to assist the Jewish client to obtain a rabbi when making a decision regarding organ donation or transplantation.

taught to wash the exit site (the site where the catheter comes out of the abdomen) daily with soap and water and inspect for any signs of infection.

Dietary education is also important. A dietitian can assist the client in making appropriate choices for adequate calories, protein, and potassium intake. The peritoneal dialysis client generally has fewer dietary and fluid restrictions than the client on hemodialysis, because dialysis is continuous.

KIDNEY TRANSPLANTATION

Another treatment for renal failure is kidney transplantation. A kidney transplant is a procedure in which a donor kidney is placed in the abdomen of a client with chronic renal failure (Fig. 35–11). This healthy transplanted kidney functions as a normal functioning kidney does. The donated kidney can come from a family member, a living-related donor, or a cadaver donor. Tissue and blood types must match for the body's immune system not to reject the donated kidney. Clients receive special drugs to help prevent rejection; currently these drugs must be taken for the rest of the clients' lives, although new treatments are being developed that may replace lifelong drug use. Sometimes even with these drugs, the body will reject the kidney and the client will need to go back on dialysis. See also Cultural Considerations Box 35–5.

NURSING PROCESS

See Nursing Care Plan Box 35–6 for the Client with Renal Failure for a comprehensive summary of nursing care.

 CRITICAL THINKING: Mrs. Jackson

Mrs. Jackson is a 56-year-old woman with a history of type 1 diabetes for 20 years. She is now in chronic renal failure. She is admitted to a medical unit for beginning treatment of renal failure. She has severe edema, oliguria, and cardiac dysrhythmias.

1. What should the nurse assess as part of the morning evaluation of the client's condition?
2. What laboratory tests are essential for the nurse to check?
3. What should the nurse assess related to Mrs. Jackson's understanding of self-care?

Answers at end of chapter.

HOME HEALTH HINTS

- Testing can be done on the client's water to determine the amount of calcium it contains. Excess calcium in the water can lead to kidney stones. If the count is high, the household should be encouraged to switch to bottled water.

- A client on daily weights should be weighed on the same scale each time. For clients whose weight changes are critical to know, encourage the family to buy a scale. Weights should be taken and recorded first thing in the morning, with little or no clothes on.

NURSING CARE PLAN BOX 35–6 FOR THE CLIENT WITH RENAL FAILURE

Fluid volume excess related to kidneys' inability to excrete water

Client Outcomes
Fluid volume will be stable as evidenced by stable weight, absence of edema, lung sounds clear, and blood pressure within client's normal parameters.

Evaluation of Outcomes
Is weight stable? Is edema absent? Are lungs clear? Is blood pressure within client's normal parameters?

Nursing Interventions	Rationale	Evaluation
• Monitor weight daily at same time; report gain of greater than 2 pounds.	Weight gain represents retention of fluid.	Is weight stable? Should physician be notified of change?
• Monitor intake and output.	Monitors degree of fluid retention.	Is output less than intake? Is this a change?
• Assess for and report shortness of breath, tachycardia, crackles in lungs, frothy sputum, heart irregularities, hypotension, cold clammy skin.	These are symptoms of heart failure that may accompany fluid overload.	Are symptoms of heart failure present?
• Watch for new onset of neck vein distention with client's head raised to 30- to 45-degree angle.	Fluid overload causes right-sided heart failure resulting in distended neck veins.	Are neck veins distended? Is this a new finding?
• Monitor vital signs, including orthostatic blood pressure.	Blood pressure changes reflect fluid volume.	Is blood pressure increased?
• Monitor for edema.	Edema is a symptom of fluid overload.	Is edema present? Is this a change?
• Monitor activity tolerance.	Reduced activity tolerance may indicate heart failure related to fluid retention.	Is client's tolerance of activity stable? Worsening?
• Monitor serum protein and albumin levels.	Low serum protein and albumin levels contribute to edema.	Are levels within normal limits?
• Maintain sodium and fluid restrictions as ordered. Develop a plan with specific allotted amounts of fluid at each meal and for medications. Teach client importance of each.	Sodium and fluids cause fluid retention in the client with renal failure.	Does client understand and maintain sodium and fluid restriction?

Activity intolerance related to anemia secondary to impaired synthesis of erythropoietin by the kidneys

Client Outcomes
Client will be able to perform activities important to him or her.

Evaluation of Outcomes
Does client state satisfaction with level of activity tolerance?

Interventions	Rationale	Evaluation
• Assess for pale mucous membranes and skin color, dyspnea, chest pain.	These are signs and symptoms of anemia.	Does client exhibit symptoms of anemia?
• Monitor Hgb, Hct.	Low hemoglobin and hematocrit indicate anemia.	Are Hgb and Hct within normal limits?
• Watch for signs of bleeding.	Bleeding will worsen anemia.	Are signs of bleeding present?
• Administer erythropoietin (Epogen) as ordered. Assist with blood transfusion as necessary.	Erythropoietin stimulates production of red blood cells by bone marrow.	Are Hgb and Hct rising with use of erythropoietin?
• Have client space activities with rest periods.	Rest periods decrease demand for oxygen.	Is client able to tolerate activities with rest periods?

continued

NURSING CARE PLAN BOX 35–6 (continued)

Risk for injury related to bleeding tendency from platelet dysfunction and use of heparin during dialysis, and tendency for gastrointestinal bleeding

Client Outcomes
Client will not experience bleeding. If bleeding occurs, it will be recognized and stopped quickly.

Evaluation of Outcomes
Are signs and symptoms of bleeding absent or recognized and reported quickly?

Interventions	Rationale	Evaluation
• Observe for and report blood in stool or emesis, easy bruising, bleeding from mucous membranes or puncture sites and report immediately if present.	Bleeding must be recognized quickly to prevent complications.	Does client exhibit signs of bleeding?
• Monitor Hgb, Hct, clotting studies, and platelets and report results.	Declining Hgb and Hct indicate blood loss. Declining platelet count or rising clotting times indicate increased risk for bleeding.	Are lab results stable?
• Monitor vital signs.	Falling blood pressure and rising pulse may indicate volume deficit from bleeding.	Are vital signs stable?
• Avoid giving injections if possible.	Injections can cause bleeding into tissue.	Can medications be given by another route?
• If bleeding, apply gentle pressure to site if possible.	Pressure promotes hemostasis.	Does pressure stop bleeding?
• Teach client to prevent injury to self and symptoms of bleeding to report.	Injury can cause bleeding. Understanding of symptoms of bleeding encourages early reporting.	Does client verbalize understanding of instruction?

Risk for infection related to impaired immune system function

Client Outcomes
Client will not develop infection as evidenced by WBCs and temperature within normal limits, no signs and symptoms of infection.

Evaluation of Outcomes
Are WBCs and temperature within normal limits?

Interventions	Rationale	Evaluation
• Monitor for signs and symptoms of infection and report promptly to physician.	Early recognition of infection and prompt treatment help prevent complications.	Does client exhibit symptoms of infection?
• Protect client from any source of infection, including infected roommates, visitors, or nursing staff.	Exposure to pathogens increases risk for infection.	Does anyone in contact with the client have an infection?
• Maintain skin integrity.	Intact skin protects against infection.	Is skin intact?
• Staff and client practice good hand-washing technique.	Hand washing helps control spread of infection.	Is good hand washing being practiced?
• Culture any suspected site of infection as ordered by physician.	A culture identifies pathogens and guides treatment.	Is a culture necessary?
• Consult with physician about influenza and pneumonia vaccines.	Clients with impaired immune function are at risk for influenza and pneumonia.	Has the client been vaccinated?
• Teach client and family signs and symptoms of infection to report to physician.	Early reporting of symptoms allows for prompt initiation of treatment.	Do client and family verbalize understanding of symptoms to report?

continued

NURSING CARE PLAN BOX 35–6 (continued)

Altered nutrition, less than body requirements related to restricted diet, anorexia, nausea, and vomiting, and stomatitis secondary to effect of excessive urea on the gastrointestinal system

Client Outcomes
Client will maintain ideal weight. Serum protein and albumin levels are within normal limits.

Evaluation of Outcomes
Are weight and lab values at desired levels?

Interventions	Rationale	Evaluation
• Monitor weekly weight and serum protein and albumin levels.	Weight and lab results provide information about nutrition status.	Are weight and lab values stable?
• Initiate a calorie count—consult dietitian for assistance.	A calorie count can provide information about the adequacy of the client's diet.	Is client receiving adequate calories?
• Provide frequent oral care.	Oral care enhances appetite.	Does oral care enhance appetite?
• Offer frequent small feedings and dietary supplements.	Smaller feedings are better tolerated and reduce risk of nausea.	Does client tolerate small feedings?
• Offer medications ordered for nausea before meals.	Nausea reduces appetite and must be controlled.	Are antiemetics effective?
• Ensure bowel movement daily or according to client's usual pattern.	Constipation can interfere with appetite.	Are client's bowels functioning normally for him or her?

Risk for injury related to acute confusion, peripheral neuropathy, and hypocalcemia

Client Outcomes
Client will remain alert and oriented as long as possible. Client safety will be maintained. Client will not sustain a fracture.

Evaluation of Outcomes
Is client alert and oriented? If not, is safety maintained? Are fractures avoided?

Interventions	Rationale	Evaluation
• Assess and report decrease in alertness, loss of memory, delirium, seizures, muscle tremors and twitches, and flapping movements of hands.	These are symptoms of uremic encephalopathy and are one reason dialysis may be initiated.	Are symptoms of confusion present?
• Initiate seizure precautions if encephalopathy is present.	The client is at risk for seizures and must be protected.	Are seizure precautions in place?
• Observe for restless legs, numbness, tingling, burning pain in extremities.	These are signs of neuropathy and place client at risk for injury.	Does client exhibit signs of neuropathy?
• Administer medications such as antidepressants and anticonvulsants as ordered.	Antidepressants and anticonvulsants may help the pain of neuropathy.	Do medications help pain?
• Protect from injury and falls.	The client with numbness and pain is at risk for falls and other injuries.	Are measures in place to protect client?
• Observe for and report tetany, seizures, numbness around mouth, bone pain.	These are symptoms of hypocalcemia and calcium loss from bone.	Are symptoms of hypocalcemia present?
• Have client ambulate at least three times daily.	Ambulation prevents calcium mobilization from bones.	Is client ambulating tid?
• Administer phosphate binders and calcium supplements as ordered with meals.	Phosphate binders bind phosphate in diet and aid excretion; calcium supplements raise serum calcium.	Are medications being taken as ordered?
• Move and turn client gently; protect from falls.	Client is at risk for fractures because of calcium loss from bones.	Is client protected from injury?

continued

NURSING CARE PLAN BOX 35–6 (continued)		

Sexual dysfunction related to loss of libido, impotence, amenorrhea, and infertility secondary to a decrease in hormone production and peripheral neuropathy

Client Outcomes
Client expresses satisfaction with sexual function.

Evaluation of Outcomes
Does client express satisfaction with sexual function?

Interventions	*Rationale*	*Evaluation*
• Assess for problems related to sexual function.	The client may not share concerns about sexual functioning unless questioned.	Are problems present?
• Provide opportunity for client to discuss concerns if desired.	Talking about concerns may decrease anxiety.	Does client wish to express concerns?
• Consult with physician for identification of correctable cause of dysfunction.	Sexual dysfunction may have a correctable cause.	Is the cause of dysfunction identifiable and correctable?
• Offer counseling. Include partner as desired by client.	If dysfunction is not correctable, alternatives may be suggested by a licensed counselor.	Is counseling desired and helpful?

Knowledge deficit related to complex treatment regimen for chronic renal failure

Client Outcomes
Client verbalizes understanding of and intent to follow treatment regimen.

Evaluation of Outcomes
Does client verbalize understanding and intent to follow treatment regimen?

Interventions	*Rationale*	*Evaluation*
• Assess client's and family's knowledge of and adherence to treatment regimen.	A baseline assessment provides direction for instruction.	Does client understand and adhere to regimen? Is instruction needed?
• Assist with teaching client use and purpose of medications, fluid restriction, dialysis plan, and renal diet.	The client is ultimately responsible for own self-care and control of blood pressure.	Do client and family demonstrate understanding of the therapeutic regimen?
• Consult renal dietitian, clinical specialist, and social worker as needed.	Specialists in care of the renal client can assist with instruction related to this complex disease and treatment.	Are consultations indicated?

Review Questions

1. Mrs. Clemons has been admitted to the nursing unit with a diagnosis of urinary tract infection. When teaching Mrs. Clemons about her condition, which of the following information is *most* important to share?
   a. Void frequently, void after intercourse
   b. Drink large amounts of citrus juices
   c. Eat large amounts of vegetables
   d. Wash the perineum every 8 hours

2. Which of the following urinalysis results indicates that Mrs. Clemons has a urinary tract infection?
   a. Large amounts of protein
   b. Gross blood
   c. WBCs and bacteria
   d. Large amounts of mucus

3. Mr. Roberts is admitted for treatment of cancer of the bladder. Which of the following is the most common symptom of cancer of the bladder?
   a. Urinary straining
   b. Burning on urination
   c. Urinary retention
   d. Hematuria

4. Mr. Roberts goes to surgery and has an ileal conduit for treatment of his cancer. While changing the pouch at the stoma site, the nurse notes that the stoma is constantly spilling urine. The nurse should
   a. Notify the physician of the constant spillage

b. Recognize that this is a normal occurrence
c. Remove the overflow of urine with a straight catheter
d. Irrigate the stoma with a sterile solution of normal saline

5. Mr. Lasiter is admitted for treatment of renal failure. Which of the following symptoms would indicate chronic renal failure?
a. Weight loss
b. Large urine output
c. Edema
d. Oily skin

6. Mr. Lasiter has a graft inserted into his left arm to provide a blood access for dialysis treatments. Which of the following interventions should be done to determine patency of the graft?
a. Observe the tubing for bright red blood
b. Feel for a brachial pulse on both arms
c. Feel for a thrill over the graft
d. Assess blood pressure in the affected arm

7. Mr. Lasiter asks for a snack in the afternoon. His potassium level remains high. Which of the following foods would be contraindicated?
a. A banana
b. A gelatin desert
c. Clear carbonated beverage
d. A sucker

8. Mr. Lasiter has just returned from his dialysis treatment. Which of the following symptoms would Mr. Lasiter be likely to exhibit?
a. Weight loss
b. Increased blood pressure
c. Polyuria
d. Agitation

ANSWERS TO CRITICAL THINKING

CRITICAL THINKING: Mrs. Milan

1. Sexual intercourse can be a predisposing factor to UTI, especially if the client does not urinate after intercourse.
2. Mrs. Milan should be cautioned to always urinate after intercourse. See also Table 35–1.
3. The urinalysis will show WBCs, bacteria, RBCs, and nitrites.

CRITICAL THINKING: Mr. White

1. Weight, intake and output, blood pressure, lab tests.
2. BUN, serum creatinine, potassium levels.
3. Need to take antihypertensive medications, keep follow-up visits to physician, follow low-sodium diet, fluid restriction if ordered.

CRITICAL THINKING: Mrs. Jackson

1. The nurse should assess Mrs. Jackson's weight and intake and output to monitor fluid balance. A cardiovascular system assessment should be done to see how she is tolerating the dysrhythmia.
2. BUN, serum creatinine, serum potassium, hemoglobin and hematocrit, and blood sugar are monitored.
3. The nurse should assess Mrs. Jackson's understanding of what renal failure is, how it is treated, how to follow the renal diet and fluid restrictions, and the action and importance of medications.

REFERENCES

1. Avorn, J, et al: Reduction of bacteriuria and pyuria after ingestion of cranberry juice. JAMA 271:751, 1994.
2. Haverkorn, MJ, and Mandigers, J: Reduction of bacteriuria and pyuria using cranberry juice (letter). JAMA 272:590, 1994.
3. Curhan, GC, et al: A prospective study of dietary calcium and other nutrients and the risk of symptomatic kidney stones. N Engl J Med 328:833, 1993.
4. Guillermo, T: Health care needs and service delivery for Asian and Pacific Islander Americans: Health policy. In LEAP, the State of Asian Pacific America: Policy Issues to the Year 2020. Asian Pacific Public Policy Institute and Asian American Studies Center, University of California–Los Angeles Press, Los Angeles, 1993.
5. Miranda, E, McBride, M, and Spangler, Z: Filipino Americans. In Purnell, L, and Paulanka, B (eds): Transcultural Health Care: A Culturally Competent Approach. FA Davis, Philadelphia, 1997.
6. Nowak, T, and Nowak, R: Vietnamese Americans. In Purnell, L, and Paulanka, B (eds): Transcultural Health Care: A Culturally Competent Approach. FA Davis, Philadelphia, 1997.
7. Selekman, J: Jewish Americans. In Purnell, L, and Paulanka, B (eds): Transcultural Health Care: A Culturally Competent Approach. FA Davis, Philadelphia, 1997.

BIBLIOGRAPHY

Bakris, GL: Diabetic nephropathy: What you need to know to preserve kidney function. Postgrad Med 93:89, 1993.
Bergus, GR: Urinalysis to diagnose UTI. J Fam Pract 40:601, 1995.
Collings, J, et al: Urinary tract infection rates among incontinent nursing home and community dwelling elderly. Urol Nurs 14:117, 1994.
Dunetz, P: Coordinating care for the dialysis patient. Nursing 27(9):32, 1997.
Erttckson, P: Idiopathic glomerulonephritis: Is it IgA nephropathy? ANNA J 20:127, 1993.
Foxman, B, et al: First-time urinary tract infection and sexual behavior. Epidemiology 6:162, 1995.
Getliffe, KA: The characteristics and management of clients with recurrent blockage of long term urinary catheters. J Adv Nurs 20:140, 1994.
Hampton, BG, and Bryant, RA: Ostomies and Continent Diversions: Nursing Management. Mosby, St Louis, 1992.
Hassey, KA: Effective management of urinary discomfort. Nurse Pract 20:36, 1995.
Klahr, S, et al: The effects of dietary protein restriction and blood pressure control on the progression of chronic renal disease. N Engl J Med 330:877, 1994.

Knox, DM, and Martof, MT: Effects of drug therapy on renal function of healthy older adults. J Gerontol Nurs 21:35, 1995.

Lutz, CA, and Przytulski, KR: Nutrition and Diet Therapy. FA Davis, Philadelphia, 1997.

Maroni, BJ, and Mitch, WE: Role of nutrition in prevention of the progression of renal disease. Annu Rev Nutr 17:435, 1997.

McConnell, E: Managing the patient with acute renal failure. Nursing 22:84, 1992.

Moore, S, et al: Treating bladder cancer, new methods, new management. Am J Nurs 93:32, 1993.

Ouslander, JG: Aging and the lower urinary tract. Am J Med Sci 314:4, 1997.

Razor, BR: Continent urinary reservoirs. Semin Oncol Nurs 9:272, 1993.

Ruth Sahd, LA: Renal calculi. Am J Nurs 95:50, 1995.

Sosa-Guerrero, S, and Gomez, NJ: Dealing with end-stage renal disease. Am J Nurs 97:10, 1997.

Toto, KH: Acute renal failure: A question of location. Am J Nurs 92:44, 1992.

White, MJ, and Mnatt, GE: Early transplantation for clients with diabetic nephropathy. ANNA J 19:457, 1992.

Understanding the Endocrine System

Endocrine System Function and Assessment

36

Paula D. Hopper and Valerie C. Scanlon

Learning Objectives

Upon completion of this chapter, the student will be able to:

1. Identify the glands of the endocrine system.
2. Describe the function of each of the glands and hormones in the endocrine system.
3. List the effects of aging on endocrine system function.
4. Describe nursing assessment of the endocrine system, including health history and physical assessment.
5. Explain the nurse's role when caring for clients undergoing laboratory and diagnostic studies of endocrine function.

Key Words

affect (**AF**-feckt)
exophthalmos (ECKS-off-**THAL**-mus)

Normal Anatomy and Physiology

The endocrine system consists of the endocrine, or ductless, glands, which secrete chemicals called hormones. Unlike other organ systems, the glands of the endocrine system are anatomically separate (Fig. 36–1). Their hormones, however, are involved in all aspects of metabolism: growth, energy production, regulation of fluid and electrolyte balance and pH, resistance to stress, and reproduction. Each hormone is secreted in response to a particular and specific stimulus, is circulated by the blood throughout the body, and exerts its effects on certain target organs or tissues that have receptors for that hormone. The effects of the hormone often will reverse the stimulus and ultimately lead to decreased secretion of the hormone. This is called a negative feedback mechanism; the secretion of many hormones is regulated this way. Some hormones are secreted in response to hormones from other endocrine glands.

PITUITARY GLAND

The pituitary gland is also called the hypophysis; it hangs by a short stalk from the hypothalamus in the brain. The two major parts are the posterior pituitary (neurohypophysis) and anterior pituitary (adenohypophysis).

Posterior Pituitary Gland

The posterior pituitary gland stores antidiuretic hormone (ADH, or sometimes called vasopressin) and oxytocin, which are actually produced by the hypothalamus. Their release is stimulated by nerve impulses from the hypothalamus.

Antidiuretic hormone increases the amount of water reabsorbed by the kidney tubules, which decreases urinary output. The water is reabsorbed back into the blood, thereby maintaining normal blood volume and normal blood pressure. The stimulus for secretion of ADH is a

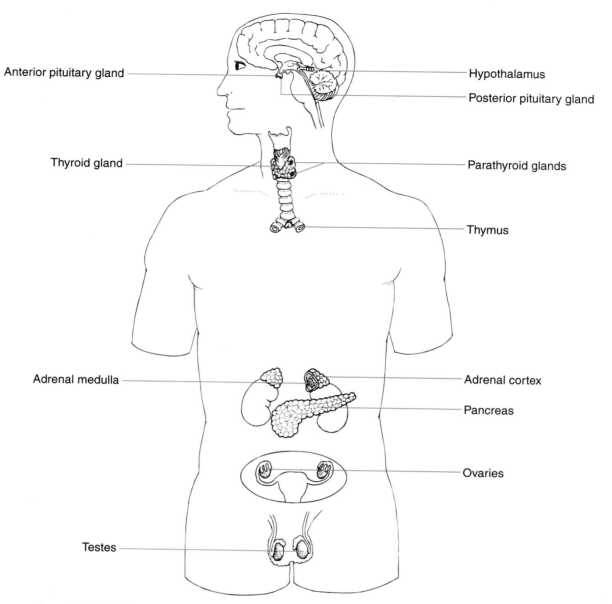

Anterior pituitary gland

Hypothalamus

Posterior pituitary gland

Thyroid gland

Parathyroid glands

Thymus

Adrenal medulla

Adrenal cortex

Pancreas

Ovaries

Testes

Figure 36–1. Glands of the endocrine system. (Modified from Scanlon, VC, and Sanders, T: Essentials of Anatomy and Physiology, ed 2. FA Davis, Philadelphia, 1995, p 219, with permission.) See Plate 8.

decrease in the water content of the body, that is, dehydration. When body water is lost and not replaced, specialized cells in the hypothalamus called osmoreceptors detect the increased salt concentration of body fluids and transmit impulses to the posterior pituitary to secrete ADH to prevent the further loss of water in urine. In cases of great fluid loss, as in severe hemorrhage, the large amount of ADH secreted will cause vasoconstriction, which will also contribute to maintenance of a normal blood pressure.

Oxytocin causes contraction of the smooth muscle in the uterus and mammary glands. At the end of pregnancy, stretching of the cervix generates sensory impulses to the hypothalamus, which then transmits impulses to the posterior pituitary for the release of oxytocin. Oxytocin causes strong contractions of the myometrium to bring about delivery of the baby and the placenta. This is an example of a positive feedback mechanism. The placenta also produces oxytocin, but its precise role in labor and delivery has not yet been determined.

When a baby is breast-fed, the sucking of the baby generates sensory impulses from the mother's nipple to the hypothalamus. The subsequent release of oxytocin causes contraction of the smooth muscle cells around the mammary ducts. This release of milk is sometimes called "milk ejection" or the "milk letdown" reflex.

Anterior Pituitary Gland

The anterior pituitary gland secretes its hormones in response to special releasing hormones from the hypothalamus. The anterior pituitary secretes growth hormone, thyroid-stimulating hormone, adrenocorticotropic hormone, prolactin, follicle-stimulating hormone, and luteinizing hormone.

Growth hormone (GH or somatotropin) increases cell division in those tissues capable of mitosis, which is one of the ways it is involved in growth. It also increases the transport of amino acids into cells and their use in protein synthesis. Growth hormone also increases the release of fat from adipose tissue and the use of fats for energy production; this is important even after growth in height has ceased. The secretion of GH is regulated by growth hormone–releasing hormone (GHRH) and by growth hormone–inhibiting hormone (GHIH or somatostatin), both from the hypothalamus. GHRH is produced during hypoglycemia or when there is a high blood level of amino acids (to be turned into protein). GHIH is secreted during hyperglycemia, when carbohydrates are available for energy production and the mobilization of fat is not necessary.

Thyroid-stimulating hormone (TSH or thyrotropin) has only one target organ: the thyroid gland. TSH stimulates growth of the thyroid and the secretion of two of its hormones, thyroxine (T_4) and triiodothyronine (T_3). The secretion of TSH is stimulated by thyrotropin-releasing hormone (TRH) from the hypothalamus when metabolic rate decreases and there is a need for thyroxine.

Adrenocorticotropic hormone (ACTH) stimulates the secretion of cortisol and related hormones from the adrenal cortex. Corticotropin-releasing hormone (CRH) from the hypothalamus stimulates the release of ACTH. CRH is produced during any type of physiological stress situation, such as injury, disease, exercise, or hypoglycemia.

Prolactin initiates and maintains milk production by the mammary glands. The hypothalamus produces both prolactin-releasing hormone (PRH) and prolactin-inhibiting hormone (PIH); prolactin is not secreted until pregnancy is over and the levels of estrogen and progesterone (from the placenta) have dropped.

Follicle-stimulating hormone (FSH) is a gonadotropic hormone; that is, its target organs are the ovaries or testes. In women, FSH initiates growth of ova in ovarian follicles and secretion of estrogen by the cells of those follicles. In men, FSH initiates sperm production within the seminiferous tubules of the testes. FSH is secreted in response to gonadotropin-releasing hormone (GnRH) from the hypothalamus. Another hormone called inhibin (from the ovaries or testes) decreases the secretion of FSH.

Luteinizing hormone (LH) is another gonadotropic hormone whose secretion is increased by GnRH from the hypothalamus. In women, LH causes ovulation and stimulates the ruptured ovarian follicle to become the corpus luteum and begin secreting progesterone as well as estro-

gen. In men, LH stimulates the secretion of testosterone by the interstitial cells of the testes.

THYROID GLAND

The thyroid gland consists of two lobes connected by a middle piece called the isthmus; the gland is located on the front and sides of the trachea just below the larynx. Three hormones are produced by the thyroid gland. Thyroxine (T_4) and triiodothyronine (T_3) are produced in the thyroid follicles, require iodine (T_4 has four iodine atoms, T_3 has three iodine atoms), and have the same functions. Calcitonin is the third hormone; it is produced by parafollicular cells.

Thyroxine and T_3 regulate normal energy production and protein synthesis. They increase the rate of cell respiration of all food types (carbohydrates, fats, and excess amino acids), which increases the metabolic rate, that is, energy and heat production. They also increase the rate of protein synthesis within cells. These hormones are the most important day-to-day regulators of metabolic rate; their activity is reflected in the functioning of the heart, brain, muscles, and virtually all other organs. They are essential for normal physical growth, mental development, and reproductive maturation.

The direct stimulus for secretion of thyroxine and T_3 is TSH from the anterior pituitary. The sequence of events is as follows: A decrease in metabolic rate (energy production) is detected by the hypothalamus, which secrets TRH. TRH stimulates the anterior pituitary to secrete TSH, which stimulates the thyroid to increase secretion of thyroxine and T_3, which increase energy production to raise the metabolic rate. As the metabolic rate rises, negative feedback decreases the secretion of TRH from the hypothalamus until the metabolic rate drops again.

The third thyroid hormone, calcitonin, has bones as its target and seems to be of greater importance in childhood when bones are growing than in maturity when bone growth has ceased. Calcitonin decreases the reabsorption of calcium and phosphate from the bones to the blood, thereby lowering the blood levels of these minerals as they are retained in bones. This one function of calcitonin has two important results: the maintenance of normal blood levels of calcium and phosphate and the maintenance of a strong, stable bone matrix.

LEARNING TIP

An easy way to remember the function of calcitonin is to remember calci*ton*in *tones* down serum calcium.

The stimulus for secretion of calcitonin is hypercalcemia, a high blood calcium level. When blood calcium level rises, increased calcitonin ensures that no more will be removed from bones until there is a real need for more calcium in the blood.

PARATHYROID GLANDS

There usually are four parathyroid glands, two on the back of each lobe of the thyroid gland. The hormone they produce is called parathyroid hormone (PTH), which is an antagonist to calcitonin for the maintenance of normal blood levels of calcium and phosphate. Besides bone, the target organs of PTH are the small intestine and kidneys.

PTH increases the reabsorption of calcium and phosphate from the bones to the blood, which raises their blood levels. Absorption of calcium and phosphate from food in the small intestine is also increased by PTH through its action of activating vitamin D (calcitriol) in the kidneys. PTH also increases the reabsorption of calcium by the kidneys and the excretion of phosphate (more than is obtained from bones). Therefore the overall effect of PTH is to raise the blood calcium level and lower the blood phosphate level.

Secretion of PTH is stimulated by hypocalcemia, a low blood calcium level, and is inhibited by hypercalcemia. In adults, PTH is probably the most important regulator of blood calcium level. Calcium ions in the blood are essential for normal excitability of neurons and muscle cells and for the process of blood clotting.

ADRENAL GLANDS

The two adrenal (also called suprarenal) glands are located one on top of each kidney. Each adrenal gland consists of an inner adrenal medulla and an outer adrenal cortex.

Adrenal Medulla

The cells of the adrenal medulla are called chromaffin cells. They secrete epinephrine and norepinephrine, which are collectively called catecholamines and are sympathomimetic (mimicking the sympathetic nervous system). Secretion of both hormones is stimulated by sympathetic impulses from the hypothalamus in stressful situations. The functions of the catecholamines mimic and prolong those of the sympathetic nervous system, which enable the individual to respond physiologically to stress situations.

Of the two hormones, epinephrine is secreted in larger amounts (approximately four times that of norepinephrine) and has many effects. It increases heart rate and force of contraction, stimulates vasoconstriction in skin and viscera and vasodilation in skeletal muscles, dilates the bronchioles, decreases peristalsis, stimulates the liver to convert glycogen to glucose, increases the use of fats for energy, and increases the rate of cell respiration. The most significant function of norepinephrine is to cause vasoconstriction in the skin, viscera, and skeletal muscles, thereby raising blood pressure.

Adrenal Cortex

The adrenal cortex secretes three types of steroid hormones: sex hormones, mineralocorticoids, and glucocorticoids. The sex hormones are small amounts of male androgens and even smaller amounts of female estrogens. Their function is not known with certainty, though they may contribute to the growth spurt that often occurs just before puberty and to the libido (sex drive) in adult women.

Aldosterone is the most abundant of the mineralocorticoids, and its target organs are the kidneys. Aldosterone increases the reabsorption of sodium ions and the excretion of potassium ions by the kidney tubules. This means that sodium ions are returned to the blood and potassium ions are eliminated in urine. This function of aldosterone has very important consequences. As sodium ions are reabsorbed, hydrogen ions may be excreted in exchange; this is one mechanism to prevent the accumulation of hydrogen ions that would lead to acidosis. Also as sodium ions are reabsorbed, water and negative ions such as bicarbonate follow and are thus returned to the blood. Although the reabsorption of water is an indirect effect of aldosterone, it is very important for the maintenance of normal blood volume and blood pressure.

Secretion of aldosterone may be stimulated in several ways: low blood level of sodium, high blood level of potassium, or loss of blood or dehydration that lowers blood pressure. Low blood pressure activates the renin-angiotensin mechanism of the kidneys, which culminates in the formation of angiotensin II. One function of angiotensin II is to increase secretion of aldosterone. The hormone called atrial natriuretic peptide (ANP), secreted by the atria of the heart when blood pressure or blood volume rises, seems to inhibit secretion of aldosterone (and renin) and thereby promotes elimination of sodium ions and water by the kidneys.

Cortisol is the most abundant of the glucocorticoids and has many target tissues. Cortisol stimulates the liver to change glucose to glycogen (glycogenesis) for storage. It increases the conversion of excess amino acids to carbohydrates (gluconeogenesis) for energy production and increases the use of fats for energy. By providing these secondary energy sources to most cells, cortisol ensures that whatever glucose is present will be available for the brain (the glucose-sparing effect).

Cortisol also has an anti-inflammatory effect in that it blocks the effects of histamine and stabilizes the lysosomes within cells. Normal cortisol secretion seems to limit the inflammation process to what is useful for tissue repair and to prevent excessive tissue destruction. Excess

Table 36–1 **Review of Endocrine Function**

Hormone	Function(s)	Regulation of Secretion
Hormones of the Posterior Pituitary Gland		
Oxytocin	Promotes contraction of myometrium of uterus (labor)	Nerve impulses from hypothalamus, the result of stretching of cervix or stimulation of nipple
	Promotes release of milk from mammary glands	Secretion from placenta at the end of gestation—stimulus unknown
Antidiuretic Hormone (ADH)	Increases water reabsorption by the kidney tubules (water returns to the blood)	Decreased water content in the body (alcohol inhibits secretion)
Hormones of the Anterior Pituitary Gland		
Growth Hormone (GH)	Increases rate of mitosis Increases amino acid transport into cells Increases rate of protein synthesis Increases use of fats for energy	GHRH (hypothalamus) stimulates secretion GHIH—somatostatin (hypothalamus) inhibits secretion
Thyroid-Stimulating Hormone	Increases secretion of thyroxine and T_3 by thyroid gland	TRH (hypothalamus)
Adrenocorticotropic Hormone (ACTH)	Increases secretion of cortisol by the adrenal cortex	CRH (hypothalamus)
Prolactin	Stimulates milk production by the mammary glands	PRH (hypothalamus) stimulates secretion PIH (hypothalamus) inhibits secretion
Follicle-Stimulating Hormone (FSH)	*In women:* Initiates growth of ova in ovarian follicles Increases secretion of estrogen by follicle cells *In men:* Initiates sperm production in the testes	GnRH (hypothalamus) GnRH (hypothalamus)
Luteinizing Hormone (LH) (ICSH)	*In women:* Causes ovulation Causes the ruptured ovarian follicle to become the corpus luteum Increases secretion of progesterone by the corpus luteum *In men:* Increases secretion of testosterone by the interstitial cells of the testes	GnRH (hypothalamus GnRH (hypothalamus)
Hormones of the Thyroid Gland		
Thyroxine (T_4) and Triiodothyronine (T_3)	Increase energy production from all food types Increase rate of protein synthesis	TSH (anterior pituitary)
Calcitonin	Decreases the reabsorption of calcium and phosphate from bones to blood	Hypercalcemia
Hormones of the Parathyroid Glands		
Parathyroid Hormone (PTH)	Increases the reabsorption of calcium and phosphate from bone to blood Increases absorption of calcium and phosphate by the small intestine Increases the reabsorption of calcium and the excretion of phosphate by the kidneys	Hypocalcemia

continued

Table 36–1 (continued)

Hormone	Function(s)	Regulation of Secretion
	Hormones of the Pancreas	
Glucagon	Increases conversion of glycogen to glucose in the liver Increases the use of excess amino acids and of fats for energy	Hypoglycemia
Insulin	Increases glucose transport into cells and the use of glucose for energy production Increases the conversion of excess glucose to glycogen in the liver and muscles Increases amino acid and fatty acid transport into cells and their use in synthesis reactions	Hyperglycemia
	Hormones of the Adrenal Medulla	
Norepinephrine	Causes vasoconstriction in skin, viscera, skeletal muscles	Sympathetic impulses from the hypothalamus in stress situations
Epinephrine	Increases heart rate and force of contraction Dilates bronchioles Decreases peristalsis Increases conversion of glycogen in glucose in the liver Causes vasodilation in skeletal muscles Causes vasoconstriction in skin and viscera Increases use of fats for energy Increases the rate of cell respiration	
	Hormones of the Adrenal Cortex	
Aldosterone	Increases reabsorption of Na^+ ions by the kidneys to the blood Increases excretion of K^+ ions by the kidneys in urine	Low blood Na^+ level Low blood volume or blood pressure High blood K^+ level
Cortisol	Increases use of fats and excess amino acids for energy Decreases use of glucose for energy (except for the brain) Increases conversion of glucose to glycogen in the liver Anti-inflammatory effect: stabilizes lysosomes and blocks the effects of histamine	ACTH (anterior pituitary) during physiological stress

cortisol has damaging effects, however, in that it decreases the immune response and delays healing of damaged tissue.

The direct stimulus for cortisol secretion is ACTH from the anterior pituitary gland. Cortisol is also a "stress" hormone, and any type of physiological stress (injury, disease, malnutrition) stimulates the hypothalamus to secrete corticotropin-releasing hormone (CRH). CRH increases the se-

cretion of ACTH by the anterior pituitary, which increases cortisol secretion by the adrenal cortex.

PANCREAS

The pancreas is located in the upper left abdominal quadrant and extends from the curve of the duodenum to the spleen. The endocrine portions of the pancreas are called islets of Langerhans (pancreatic islets); they contain alpha cells, which produce glucagon, and beta cells, which produce insulin. Delta cells in the islets secrete somatostatin, which inhibits secretion of both insulin and glucagon.

The functions of glucagon are all concerned with energy production. Glucagon stimulates the liver to change glycogen to glucose (glycogenolysis) and to increase the use of fats and excess amino acids for energy production. The overall effect, therefore, is to raise the blood glucose level and to make all types of food available for cell respiration.

The secretion of glucagon is stimulated by hypoglycemia, a low blood glucose level. Such a state may occur during physiological stress situations such as exercise or simply being between meals.

Insulin increases the transport of glucose from the blood into cells by increasing the permeability of cell membranes to glucose (brain and liver cells, however, are not dependent on insulin for glucose intake). Within cells, glucose is broken down in cell respiration to release energy. The liver and muscles are also stimulated by insulin to change glucose to glycogen (glycogenesis) to be stored for later use. Insulin also enables cells to take in fatty acids and amino acids to use in the synthesis of lipids and proteins (not energy production). Insulin, therefore, decreases blood glucose level by increasing the use of glucose for energy, promoting the storage of excess glucose, and decreasing energy production from other food sources.

Secretion of insulin is stimulated by hyperglycemia, a high blood glucose level. This state occurs after meals, especially those high in carbohydrates. It should be apparent that insulin and glucagon function as antagonists and that normal secretion of both hormones ensures a blood glucose level that fluctuates within normal limits.

See Table 36–1 for a review of endocrine hormone function.

AGING AND THE ENDOCRINE SYSTEM

Most of the endocrine glands decrease their secretions with age, but normal aging usually does not lead to serious hormone deficiencies. There are decreases in adrenal cortical hormones, for example, but the levels are usually sufficient to maintain homeostasis of water, electrolytes, and nutrients. The decreased secretion of growth hormone leads to a decrease in muscle mass and an increase in fat storage. A lower basal metabolic rate is common in elderly people as the thyroid slows its secretion of thyroxine. Although insulin secretion declines somewhat, for most elderly people with a decreased glucose tolerance the cause is a decrease in the cells' sensitivity to insulin. Unless specific pathologies develop, the endocrine system usually continues to function adequately in old age.

Nursing Assessment

HEALTH HISTORY

When performing a health history, a number of questions may be asked to determine whether an endocrine problem

Table 36–2. **Questions Asked during Assessment of the Endocrine System**

Question	Rationale
Have you noticed a change in your energy level?	Lack of energy may be associated with uncontrolled diabetes, hypothyroidism, hyperthyroidism, Addison's disease, or pituitary disorders.
Have you noticed muscle spasms or twitching?	These symptoms may be associated with excessive antidiuretic hormone secretion (SIADH) or calcium depletion resulting from hypoparathyroidism.
Do you have numbness, tingling, or pain in your feet, legs, or hands?	These may be associated with neuropathy resulting from diabetes mellitus. Numbness and tingling may also indicate hypocalcemia related to hypoparathyroidism.
Have you gained or lost weight without trying?	Actual weight gain may be associated with hypothyroidism. Weight gain due to water retention may result from Cushing's syndrome, or SIADH. Weight loss may result from uncontrolled diabetes or hyperthyroidism. Weight loss due to dehydration may be related to Addison's disease.
Have you noticed excessive thirst or urination?	Excessive thirst and urination are classic symptoms of diabetes mellitus and diabetes insipidus.
Do you generally tolerate changes in environmental temperature?	Hypothyroidism can cause cold intolerance. Hyperthyroidism can cause heat intolerance.
Have you noticed a change in your mood or memory?	Mental function may be dull with hypothyroidism. Mood swings may occur with Cushing's syndrome. Agitation or confusion may result from hypoglycemia in a person with diabetes.
Does anyone in your family have a thyroid problem or diabetes?	These may be hereditary.

Table 36–3. **Causes of Abnormal Physical Assessment Findings**

Assessment Finding	Possible Causes
Inappropriate mood or affect	Depressed mood or affect from hypothyroidism
	Nervousness related to hyperthyroidism
	Agitation related to low blood sugar
Weight change	Gain due to decreased metabolic rate in hypothyroidism, fluid excess
	Loss due to increased metabolic rate in hyperthyroidism; uncontrolled diabetes, dehydration
Poor skin turgor	Dehydration due to water loss in Addison's disease, diabetes mellitus, diabetes insipidus
Change in pulse or temperature	Elevated due to increased metabolic rate in hyperthyroidism
	Decreased due to slowed metabolic rate in hypothyroidism
Elevated blood pressure	Increased catecholamine release in pheochromocytoma, or fluid retention in Cushing's syndrome
Decreased blood pressure	Sodium and water loss in Addison's disease
Weak peripheral pulses, dusky lower extremities	Circulatory changes in diabetes mellitus
Tremor	Hyperthyroidism or pheochromocytoma
Exophthalmos (bulging eyes)	Fat deposits and edema behind the eyes in Graves' disease
Fat pads on neck and shoulders ("buffalo hump"), round face	Accumulation of fat in Cushing's syndrome
Enlarged thyroid gland	Excessive stimulation by TSH in hypothyroidism or hyperthyroidism

exists. Frequently, however, the nurse is aware of a history of an endocrine disorder, such as diabetes or hypothyroidism. When a disorder exists or is suspected, a more focused assessment is done. Assessment of individual disorders is provided in Chapters 37 and 38. See Table 36–2 for general questions that can help the nurse identify new problem areas. If the assessment reveals abnormalities, they should be reported to the registered nurse or physician.

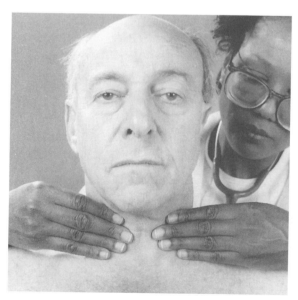

Figure 36–2. Thyroid palpation. (From Morton, PG: Health Assessment in Nursing, ed 2. FA Davis, Philadelphia, 1993, with permission.)

PHYSICAL ASSESSMENT OF THE CLIENT WITH AN ENDOCRINE DISORDER

Physical assessment starts with height, weight, and vital signs. These should always be compared with the client's baseline assessment if available. See Table 36–3 for common causes of physical assessment findings.

INSPECTION

The client is observed for mood and **affect** (emotional tone) throughout the physical assessment. The neck is inspected for thyroid enlargement. Eyes that bulge (**exophthalmos**) are noted. Posture, body fat, and presence of tremor are noted. Skin and hair texture and moisture are observed. The presence of a moonlike face or "buffalo hump" on the upper back is noted. The lower extremities should be observed for color changes that might indicate circulatory impairment. See Table 36–3 for rationale for these observations.

PALPATION

The thyroid gland is the only palpable endocrine gland. The practical nurse may assist the physician or nurse practitioner to palpate the thyroid gland. The physician stands behind or in front of the seated client and palpates the gland while the client swallows a sip of water (Fig. 36–2). The nurse may assist with positioning the client and with providing water, while instructing the client to take a sip of water and hold it in his or her mouth until told to swallow. The thyroid gland should never be palpated in a client with

exophthalmos: exo—outward + ophthalmos—eye

uncontrolled hyperthyroidism, because this may stimulate additional secretion of thyroid hormone.

Peripheral pulses are palpated. The posterior tibial and dorsalis pedis pulses may be diminished in clients with circulatory impairment.

AUSCULTATION AND PERCUSSION

Auscultation and percussion are not usually part of an endocrine assessment.

Diagnostic Tests

HORMONE TESTS

Serum Hormone Levels

Many hormones can be measured from a simple blood test. This is useful in diagnosing hypofunctioning or hyperfunctioning gland states. Some commonly measured hormones include T3 (triiodothyronine), T4 (thyroxine), TSH, GH, and cortisol (see Table 36–4).

Table 36–4. **Common Laboratory Tests**

Test	Normal Values*	Significance
Thyroid Tests		
Thyroid-Stimulating Hormone (TSH)	0.5–5.0 U/mL	↑ in primary hypothyroidism ↓ in primary hyperthyroidism
Triiodothyronine (T₃)	75–195 ng/100 mL	↑ in hyperthyroidism ↓ in hypothyroidism
Thyroxine (T₄)	4–12 μg/100 mL	↑ in hyperthyroidism ↓ in hypothyroidism
Parathyroid Tests		
Parathyroid Hormone (PTH)	<25 pg/mL	↑ in primary hyperparathyroidism ↓ in primary hypoparathyroidism, parathyroid trauma during hyroid surgery
Calcium	8.5–10.5 mg/100 mL	↑ in some cancers, hyperparathyroidism ↓ in hypothyroidism
Pituitary Tests		
Growth Hormone (GH)	<5 ng/mL	↑ in acromegaly ↓ in small stature
Antidiuretic Hormone (ADH)	2.3–3.1 pg/mL	↑ in SIADH ↓ in diabetes insipidus
Urine Specific Gravity	1.003–1.030	↓ in diabetes insipidus — *urine*
Adrenal Tests		
Cortisol	5–25 μg/100 mL	↑ in Cushing's syndrome, stress ↓ in Addison's disease, steroid withdrawal
Vanillylmandelic Acid (VMA) (Urine Test)	0.7–6.8 mg/24 h	↑ in pheochromocytoma — *urine*
Pancreas Tests		
Fasting Blood Sugar (FBS)	70–110 mg/100 mL	↑ in diabetes mellitus, stress, Cushing's syndrome ↓ in hypoglycemia, Addison's disease
Oral Glucose Tolerance Test	Blood glucose returns to normal within 3 h	Any two values over 140 diagnose diabetes mellitus
Two-hour Postprandial Glucose	<120 mg/dL <140 mg/dL in elderly	↑ in diabetes mellitus ↓ in hypoglycemia, gastrointestinal malabsorption
Glycosylated Hemoglobin	4–7%	↑ in poor diabetes control

*All normal values are for a fasting test.

Stimulation Tests

Stimulation tests may also help determine endocrine gland function. For this type of test, a substance is injected to attempt to stimulate a gland. The hormone secreted by that gland is then measured to determine how well it responded to the stimulation. For example, in a TSH stimulation test, TRH is injected. If the pituitary gland responds appropriately, TSH will be secreted. If the thyroid gland responds appropriately to the TSH, T3 and T4 levels will rise. Failure of the TRH to stimulate TSH and thyroid hormone indicates pituitary or thyroid pathology. Further studies might be done to determine the cause.

Suppression Tests

Suppression tests are the opposite of stimulating tests. For this type of test, a substance is injected that is expected to suppress a hormone's release. For example, if dexamethasone (a steroid hormone) is injected, cortisol release is expected to be suppressed via the negative feedback mechanism. If the cortisol level is not suppressed, adrenal cortex dysfunction is suspected.

URINE TESTS

Sometimes it is helpful to measure the amount of hormone or hormone by-product excreted in the urine during a 24-hour period. Examples are cortisol and vanillylmandelic acid, a product of catecholamine metabolism.

To collect a 24-hour urine specimen, it is necessary to obtain a special urine container from the laboratory. It is usually an opaque container that protects the specimen from light and may have preservative in it. Check with the lab to find out whether the specimen needs to be kept on ice during the test and whether the client needs to be on a special diet before or during the test. To keep a specimen on ice, a bath basin is filled with ice and the container is placed in the basin. The ice will need to be refilled every few hours to keep the specimen cold. When initiating the test, the nurse asks the client to urinate and discards the urine. The time of this first discarded voiding is considered the start of the test. Any urine collected from this time forward for 24 hours is saved. At the end of the 24-hour period, the client is again asked to urinate, but this time the urine is saved. The entire collection is then labeled and sent to the lab. The nurse should instruct the client how to do the test, place a sign on the toilet with the start and stop time of the test, and remind all staff to save the urine.

If the client is incontinent or otherwise unable to participate in the test, a catheter may need to be inserted. If the client already has an indwelling catheter, a new bag and tubing should be attached before the start of the test. The lab should be consulted to determine the need for a preservative or ice. Preservative can be added to the catheter bag if necessary. If ice is necessary, the bag should be kept in a basin of ice rather than hanging on the side of the bed. If the specimen must be protected from light, the bag can be covered with dark plastic or foil.

CRITICAL THINKING: Mrs. Trombley

Mrs. Trombley is having a 24-hour urine test done. You begin the test at 0600, and it progresses well until you learn that she got up and voided in the toilet at noon, forgetting to save her urine. What do you do?
Answer at end of chapter.

OTHER LAB TESTS

Some laboratory tests may indirectly reflect the function of an endocrine gland. For example, a serum calcium level helps indicate PTH or calcitonin secretion, and a blood glucose level reflects insulin secretion.

NUCLEAR SCANNING

A thyroid scan may be done to determine the presence of tumors or nodules. For this test, a radioactive material is injected, or radioactive iodine is taken orally. The material is attracted by the thyroid gland. After a specified amount of time, the thyroid gland is scanned with a scintillation camera. The scan will show "hot spots," which are nodules that are not malignant, or "cold spots" (areas that do not take up the radioactivity), which indicate malignancy. Cold spots may then be biopsied to confirm a diagnosis. Because such a small amount of radioactive material is used, there is no risk to the client. The client should be aware that the test takes approximately 30 minutes to complete.

RADIOGRAPHIC TESTS

A computerized tomography (CT) scan or magnetic resonance imaging (MRI) may be done to locate a tumor or identify hypertrophy of a gland.

Review Questions

1. The posterior pituitary gland secretes the following hormone:
   a. Antidiuretic hormone
   b. Thyroid-stimulating hormone
   c. Growth hormone
   d. Luteinizing hormone

2. When the effects of a hormone suppress further secretion of the hormone, which of the following types of feedback has occurred?
   a. Positive feedback
   b. Negative feedback

c. Rhythm feedback
d. Stimulus feedback

3. The functions of thyroxine and T₃ include:
   a. Retention of salt and water
   b. Maintenance of blood sugar
   c. Maintenance of blood pressure
   d. Regulation of energy production

4. Strong bones are maintained by the action of which hormone?
   a. ADH
   b. Insulin
   c. Calcitonin
   d. TRH

5. When collecting a 24-hour urine specimen for hormone measurement, the nurse should do which of the following to begin the test?
   a. Discard the first voided urine
   b. Save the first voided urine
   c. Discard the last voided urine
   d. Save the first and last voided urine

6. When explaining a thyroid scan to a client, which of the following statements is correct?
   a. "You will take a special pill, then an ultrasound will be taken of your neck."
   b. "You will receive an injection of radioactive material, then a special camera will scan your thyroid gland."
   c. "You will be placed into a special machine, and x-rays will be taken of your neck. It may be noisy."
   d. "You will be given a special drink, then magnetic energy is used to visualize the thyroid area."

7. Which of the following values represents a normal fasting blood glucose level?
   a. 5–25 mg/100 mL
   b. 70–110 mg/100 mL
   c. 120–160 mg/100 mL
   d. 200–250 mg/100 mL

8. Which of the following questions by the nurse is appropriate when assessing a client with a thyroid problem?
   a. "Has your weight changed?"
   b. "Have you experienced numbness or tingling?"
   c. "Have you been very thirsty?"
   d. "Have you been having muscle spasms?"

 ANSWER TO CRITICAL THINKING: Mrs. Trombley

The specimen must include all urine for a 24-hour period. Restart the test from 12:00 noon.

BIBLIOGRAPHY

DeCherney, GS: Time for a tune up? Diabetes Forecast, April 1997.

Jarvis, C: Physical Examination and Health Assessment. WB Saunders, Philadelphia, 1992.

Kee, JL: Laboratory and Diagnostic Tests with Nursing Implications, ed 4. Appleton & Lange, Stamford, Conn, 1995.

Morton, PG: Health Assessment in Nursing, ed 2. FA Davis, Philadelphia, 1993.

Watson, J, and Jaffe, MS: Nurse's Manual of Laboratory and Diagnostic Tests, ed 2. FA Davis, Philadelphia, 1995.

Nursing Care of Clients with Endocrine Disorders

37

Paula D. Hopper

Learning Objectives

Upon completion of this chapter, the student will be able to:

1. Identify the disorders caused by variations in the hormones of the pituitary, thyroid, parathyroid, and adrenal glands.

2. Describe the pathophysiology, major signs and symptoms, and complications of selected endocrine disorders.

3. Discuss medical and surgical treatment of the selected endocrine disorders.

4. Use the nursing process to plan care for the client with an endocrine disorder.

Key Words

amenorrhea (ay-MEN-uh-**REE**-ah)

autoimmune (AW-toh-im-**YOON**)

dysphagia (dis-**FAYJ**-ee-ah)

ectopic (eck-**TOP**-ick)

euthyroid (yoo-**THY**-royd)

exophthalmos (ECKS-off-**THAL**-mus)

goiter (**GOY**-ter)

hyperplasia (HIGH-per-**PLAY**-zee-ah)

hypophysectomy (HIGH-pah-fi-**SECK**-tuh-mee)

hypovolemic (HIGH-poh-voh-**LEEM**-ick)

myxedema (MICK-suh-**DEE**-mah)

nephrogenic (NEFF-roh-**JEN**-ick)

nocturia (nock-**TYOO**-ree-ah)

osmolality (ahs-moh-**LAL**-i-tee)

pheochromocytoma (FEE-oh-KROH-moh-sigh-TOH-mah)

polydipsia (PAH-lee-**DIP**-see-ah)

polyuria (PAH-lee-**YOOR**-ee-ah)

psychogenic (SIGH-koh-**JEN**-ick)

tetany (**TET**-uh-nee)

A variety of disorders may be found within the endocrine system. Although the causes vary, the pathophysiology usually involves either too little or too much hormone activity. Insufficient hormone activity may be the result of hypofunction of a gland or insensitivity of the target tissue to a hormone. Excessive hormone activity may be due to a hyperactive gland, **ectopic** hormone production, or self-administration of too much replacement hormone (Table 37–1). If the student can remember the function of each hormone in the body, understanding the problems involved with an altered amount of each hormone becomes easier.

Most endocrine disorders are either primary or secondary. A primary disorder is a problem within the gland that is out of balance. Secondary disorders are caused by problems outside of the gland, such as an imbalance in a tropic hormone, certain drugs, trauma, surgery, or a problem in the feedback mechanism.

LEARNING TIP

If you remember what each hormone does in the body, it will be easier to remember what imbalances of that hormone cause. Most symptoms of hormone hyperactivity are opposite from symptoms of that hormone's hypoactivity.

Pituitary Disorders

Pituitary disorders often involve several hormone imbalances due to general hypopituitarism or hyperpituitarism. For simplicity, imbalances will be considered separately here.

DISORDERS RELATED TO ANTIDIURETIC HORMONE IMBALANCE

Antidiuretic hormone (ADH, also called arginine vasopressin, or AVP) is synthesized in the hypothalamus and stored and secreted by the posterior pituitary. A decrease in ADH activity results in diabetes insipidus (DI). An increase in ADH activity is called syndrome of inappropriate

---

ectopic: ec—away from normal + topic—place

Table 37–1. **Causes of Endocrine Problems**

Insufficient Hormone Activity	Excess Hormone Activity
Gland hypofunction	Gland hyperfunction
Lack of tropic or stimulating hormone	Excess tropic or stimulating hormone
Target tissue insensitivity to hormone	Ectopic hormone production
	Self-administration of too much replacement hormone

antidiuretic hormone (SIADH). Table 37–2 compares DI and SIADH. Note how symptoms of too little ADH (water loss) are opposite from symptoms of too much ADH (water retention).

Diabetes Insipidus

Pathophysiology

ADH is responsible for reabsorption of water by the distal tubules and collecting ducts in the kidneys. If ADH is lacking, adequate reabsorption of water is prevented, leading to diuresis. In **nephrogenic** diabetes insipidus, ADH is present in sufficient amounts, but the kidneys do not respond to it. Clients may urinate from 3 to 15 L per day. This leads to increased serum **osmolality** (concentrated blood) and dehydration. The increased osmolality and decreased blood pressure normally trigger ADH secretion, which then retains water and dilutes the blood; in clients with DI, this does not occur. Increased osmolality also leads to extreme thirst, which usually causes the client to drink enough fluids to maintain fluid balance. In an unconscious client or a client with a defective thirst mechanism, however, dehydration may quickly occur if the problem is not recognized and corrected.

Etiology

The primary causes of diabetes insipidus are tumors or trauma to the pituitary gland. Surgery in the area of the pi-

Table 37–2. **Comparison of Antidiuretic Hormone Disorders**

	Insufficient ADH	Excess ADH
Disorder	Diabetes insipidus	SIADH
Signs and Symptoms	Polyuria, polydipsia, hypernatremia, dehydration	Fluid retention, weight gain, hyponatremia
Usual Treatment	Synthetic ADH replacement	Treat cause
Priority Nursing Diagnoses	Risk for fluid volume deficit	Risk for fluid volume excess

tuitary and certain drugs, such as glucocorticoids or alcohol, may also cause DI. Occasionally the cause is **psychogenic,** with the client drinking large quantities of water in the absence of true disease. Nephrogenic DI is an inherited defect in which the kidneys do not respond to ADH.

Signs and Symptoms

The client with DI urinates frequently (**polyuria**), and nighttime urination (**nocturia**) is present. This results in high serum osmolality and low urine osmolality. Urine specific gravity is decreased (the urine is dilute).

The client experiences extreme thirst (**polydipsia**), and large volumes of water are consumed. Often clients crave ice-cold water. If urine output exceeds fluid intake, dehydration will occur, with characteristic symptoms of hypotension, poor skin turgor, and weakness. **Hypovolemic** shock will occur if fluid balance is not restored. Dehydration and electrolyte imbalances will result in a decrease in level of consciousness and death if the problem is not corrected.

Diagnostic Tests

Diagnosis is based initially on history of risk factors and reported symptoms. Urine specific gravity is less than 1.005 (normal is 1.010–1.025). Figure 37–1 shows use of a uninometer to measure urine specific gravity; this is generally done by the nurse at the bedside. Plasma osmolality is measured. The actual amount of sodium in the blood may be normal, but it appears elevated in relation to the decreased amount of water. Computed tomography (CT) scan or magnetic resonance imaging (MRI) may show a pituitary tumor.

A water deprivation test may be done. For this test, the client is deprived of water for up to 8 hours. Body weight and urine osmolality are tested hourly. If the urine continues to be dilute, even though the client is not drinking and is losing weight due to volume depletion, DI is suspected. In the second stage of the test, the client receives an injection of ADH, with a final urine test done 1 hour later. If the DI is nephrogenic, the kidneys will not respond to the injected ADH.

Medical Treatment

If a pituitary tumor is involved, treatment usually involves removal of the pituitary, or **hypophysectomy.** Medical

---

nephrogenic: nephro—kidney + genic—to produce
psychogenic: psycho—related to the mind + genic—to produce
polyuria: poly—much + uria—urine
nocturia: noc—night + uria—urine
polydipsia: poly—much + dipsia—thirst
hypovolemic: hypo—deficient + vol—volume + emic—blood
hypophysectomy: hypophysis—pituitary + ectomy—surgical removal

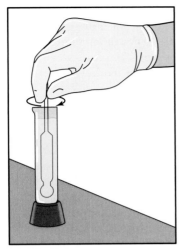 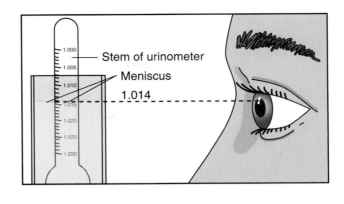

Stem of urinometer

Meniscus

1.014

Figure 37–1. Urimeter and dipstick for measuring urine specific gravity.

treatment of DI involves replacement of ADH. In acute cases, vasopressin, a synthetic form of ADH, is given by the intravenous or subcutaneous route. In clients who require long-term therapy, such as those who have had a hypophysectomy, desmopressin (DDAVP) in the form of a nasal spray is used. Desmopressin's action lasts 18 to 24 hours. Other drugs such as chlorpropamide (Diabinese) stimulate ADH secretion in clients with partial DI. Thiazide diuretics may be ordered to treat nephrogenic DI. Intravenous fluids may be used to replace lost fluids in acute situations.

Nursing Process

ASSESSMENT. When doing a nursing assessment of a client with DI, special attention should be placed on fluid balance. Daily weights are the most reliable method for monitoring the amount of fluid that is being lost. Accurate intake and output is also helpful. Skin turgor will be poor, and mucous membranes will be dry and sticky if the client is becoming dehydrated. Skin integrity is monitored because dehydration increases risk of breakdown. Vital signs are monitored for signs of shock. A dipstick or urimeter is used to measure urine specific gravities. Serum electrolytes and osmolality are monitored as ordered, and level of consciousness is monitored. The client's understanding of his or her disease and treatment are assessed. Once treatment is initiated, the client is observed for fluid overload.

NURSING DIAGNOSIS. Priority nursing diagnoses include fluid volume deficit related to polyuria and knowledge deficit related to self-care of diabetes insipidus.

PLANNING AND IMPLEMENTATION. The client is given oral fluids if the DI is not psychogenic. If the client's thirst mechanism is not intact, the nurse gives fluids hourly. Hypotonic intravenous (IV) fluids such as 0.45 percent saline may be ordered to replace intravascular volume without adding excessive sodium. IV fluids are especially important if the client is unable to take oral fluids. A significant drop in blood pressure and a rising pulse are reported to the registered nurse or physician, because these may be signs of shock. If the client is able, he or she may be involved in maintaining intake and output records.

CLIENT EDUCATION. The nurse teaches the client the basic pathophysiology of his or her disease and how to administer medications and monitor their effectiveness. The client should be taught how to measure urine specific gravity and the significance of results. Signs and symptoms of dehydration and fluid overload are taught. The importance of daily weights is stressed; losses or gains of greater than 2 lb in a day should be reported to the physician. The client is advised to wear identification, such as a Medic Alert bracelet, that identifies the disorder.

EVALUATION. If treatment has been effective, signs of dehydration will be absent, and weight and vital signs will be stable. The client should be able to explain what is happening in his or her disease, symptoms to report, and how to manage self-care.

Syndrome of Inappropriate Antidiuretic Hormone Secretion

Pathophysiology

SIADH results from too much ADH in the body. This causes excess water to be reabsorbed by the kidney tubules and collecting ducts, and the individual becomes fluid overloaded. As fluid builds up in the bloodstream, the osmolality decreases and the blood becomes dilute. Normally, a decreased serum osmolality inhibits release of ADH. In SIADH, however, ADH continues to be released, adding further to the fluid overload.

Etiology

Bronchogenic lung cancer, duodenal cancer, or pancreatic cancer may be ectopic sites of production of an ADH-like substance. Certain drugs, such as tricyclic antidepressants and general anesthetics, may increase ADH secretion. Head trauma or surgery, or a brain tumor affecting pituitary function, may also cause SIADH. It may be a complication of treatment of diabetes insipidus.

Signs and Symptoms

Symptoms of SIADH include symptoms of fluid overload, such as weight gain (usually without edema) and dilutional hyponatremia (Table 37–3). The actual amount of sodium in the blood may be normal, but it appears low because of the diluting effect of the retained fluid. Serum osmolality is less than 275 mOsm/kg. The urine is concentrated because water is not being excreted. Muscle cramps and weakness may occur due to electrolyte imbalance. Because the osmolality of the blood is low, fluid may leak out of the vessels and cause brain swelling. If untreated, this will result in lethargy, seizures, coma, and death.

Diagnostic Tests

Serum and urine sodium levels and osmolality are measured. A water load test may be done, which involves administering a specific amount of water, then measuring blood and urine sodium and osmolality hourly for 6 hours. The client with SIADH retains the water instead of excreting it. Additional testing may be done to diagnose and locate an ADH-secreting tumor.

Medical Treatment

Treatment is aimed at eliminating the cause. If a tumor is secreting ADH, it may be removed. Symptoms may be alleviated by restricting fluids to 800 to 1000 mL per day. Normal or hypertonic saline fluids may be administered in-

travenously to maintain serum sodium level. If the cause is inoperable cancer, drugs such as furosemide (Lasix) and demeclocycline (Declomycin) are used to block the action of ADH in the kidney.

Nursing Process

ASSESSMENT. Fluid overload with hyponatremia is the primary concern for the client with SIADH. To monitor fluid balance, the nurse assesses vital signs, daily weights, intake and output, urine specific gravity, skin turgor, edema, and lung sounds. The client's ability to maintain a fluid restriction is determined. Level of consciousness and neuromuscular function are assessed. Lab tests, including serum sodium level, are monitored as ordered by the physician. Understanding of the disease process and treatment are assessed.

NURSING DIAGNOSES. Priority nursing diagnoses include risk for fluid volume excess and knowledge deficit related to self-care of SIADH.

PLANNING AND IMPLEMENTATION. The nurse explains the importance of maintaining the fluid restriction to the client. Hard candy may help alleviate thirst. Ice chips may also help and are counted as half the volume of fluid; that is, 100 mL of ice chips equal approximately 50 mL of water. Providing calibrated cups can assist the client to maintain the restriction independently, if able. To increase compliance, the client should be allowed to participate in planning the types and times of fluid intake. Fluids high in sodium such as broth, cola, or tomato juice may help correct dilutional hyponatremia. A change in level of consciousness is reported immediately, and the client is monitored for seizures, for which the client is at risk because of increased serum sodium.

CLIENT EDUCATION. The nurse instructs the client to report any weight gain greater than 2 lb in one day, a change in urine output, or acute thirst. Use of Medic Alert or other identification should be encouraged.

EVALUATION. Weight should stabilize at the preillness level once treatment is begun. The serum sodium level should be within normal limits. The client should be able to verbalize the cause of his or her symptoms and demonstrate self-care, including ability to maintain a fluid restriction if necessary.

DISORDERS RELATED TO GROWTH HORMONE IMBALANCE

Growth hormone (GH), also called somatotropin, is responsible for normal growth of bones, cartilage, and soft tissue. GH is synthesized and secreted by the anterior pituitary gland. An excess or deficiency of GH may be related to a more generalized problem with the pituitary gland. Excess GH results in gigantism or acromegaly. A deficit of GH results in dwarfism (Fig. 37–2).

Table 37–3. *Manifestations of Dilutional Hyponatremia*

Bounding pulse
Elevated or normal blood pressure
Muscle weakness
Headache
Personality changes
Nausea
Diarrhea
Convulsions
Coma

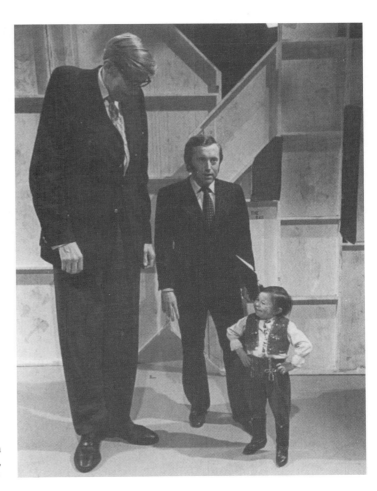

Figure 37–2. Clients with gigantism and dwarfism. (From Tamparo, CD, and Lewis, MA: Diseases of the Human Body, ed 2. FA Davis, Philadelphia, 1995, p 269, with permission.)

Dwarfism

Pathophysiology

Dwarfism, also called short stature, occurs when growth hormone is deficient in childhood. A deficiency of GH does not cause significant symptoms in adults, because growth has already been completed.

Etiology

Growth hormone may be deficient due to a pituitary tumor or failure of the pituitary to develop. It may also be deficient in some cases of neglect or severe emotional stress, causing psychosocial dwarfism. Sometimes the cause is not known. See Cultural Considerations Box 37–1.

Signs and Symptoms

Children may grow to only 3 to 4 feet in height, but they have normal body proportions. Sexual maturation may be slowed, related to involvement of additional pituitary hormones. Dwarfism is sometimes accompanied by mental retardation.

Diagnostic Tests

Growth hormone levels in the blood are measured by a routine laboratory test. A growth hormone stimulation test may be done by measuring GH response to induced hypoglycemia. Radiographic studies help determine the presence of a pituitary tumor.

Medical Treatment

Treatment of dwarfism in a child is administration of growth hormone. In the past, GH was derived from human pituitary glands, so treatment was expensive. Now GH is

CULTURAL CONSIDERATIONS BOX 37–1

Dwarfism, mostly related to a limited gene pool, occurs among Amish communities. Ellis–van Creveld syndrome is prevalent among the Amish of Lancaster County, Pennsylvania.[1] This syndrome is characterized by short stature and an extra digit on each hand, with some individuals having a congenital heart defect and nervous system involvement resulting in a degree of mental handicap.

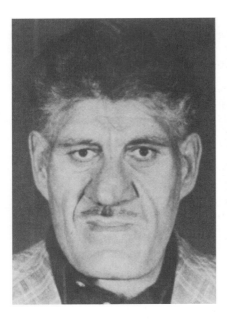
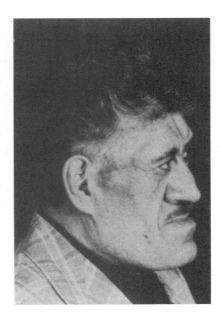

Figure 37–3. Client with acromegaly. (From Tamparo, CD, and Lewis, MA: Diseases of the Human Body, ed 2. FA Davis, Philadelphia, 1995, p 270, with permission.)

made in a laboratory using genetic engineering, and it is more readily available to those who need it. Surgery may be indicated if a tumor is the cause.

Nursing Process

ASSESSMENT. Assessment of the adult with dwarfism includes mental status, ability to cope with the effects of the disorder, and understanding of the treatment plan.

NURSING DIAGNOSIS. Possible priority nursing diagnoses include body image disturbance, ineffective coping, and knowledge deficit. If the adult with dwarfism has accepted and coped well with the condition, diagnosis and treatment by a nurse may not be indicated.

PLANNING AND IMPLEMENTATION. Clients with dwarfism should be approached with an attitude of acceptance and caring. They should be given the opportunity to verbalize their feelings. An occupational therapist may be able to provide techniques to assist the client to adapt to an environment that is geared toward people of average height. Information about support groups may be provided to the client.

EVALUATION. The goal has been achieved if the client is able to express his or her feelings of acceptance of the disorder, demonstrate adaptive techniques, and verbalize understanding of treatment.

 CRITICAL THINKING: Adoption

Three siblings were adopted to a loving home after having been in several foster homes. After a year in their new home, each child suddenly grew 6 to 8 inches. Why might this have happened?
Answer at end of chapter.

Acromegaly

Acromegaly is a rare excess of growth hormone that affects adults, usually in their thirties or forties (Fig. 37–3). If a GH excess occurs in children, the condition is called gigantism.

Pathophysiology

Acromegaly occurs as a result of oversecretion of GH in an adult. Bones increase in size, leading to enlargement of facial features, hands, and feet. Long bones grow in width but not length, because the epiphyseal disks are closed. Subcutaneous connective tissue increases, causing a fleshy appearance. Internal organs and glands enlarge. Fat and carbohydrate metabolism are affected.

Etiology

Acromegaly may be the result of pituitary **hyperplasia,** a benign pituitary tumor, or hypothalamic dysfunction.

Signs and Symptoms

Often the first symptom is a change in hat or shoe size. The nose, jaw, brow, hands, and feet enlarge. The teeth may be displaced, causing difficulty chewing, or dentures may no longer fit. The tongue becomes thick, causing difficulty in speaking and swallowing. Vertebral changes may lead to kyphosis. Visual disturbances may occur due to tumor pressure on the optic nerve. Headaches are a result of tumor pressure on the brain. Diabetes may develop because GH increases blood glucose and causes an increased workload for the pancreas. Osteoporosis and arthritis may occur. Impotence may occur in men, and **amenorrhea** in women.

---

hyperplasia: hyper—excessive + plasia—formation or development

amenorrhea: a—not + men—month + orrhea—flow

With treatment, soft tissues will reduce in size, but bone growth is permanent.

Diagnostic Tests

Serum growth hormone levels are measured. X-rays show abnormal bone growth.

Medical Treatment

Treatment is aimed at the cause. Bromocriptine (Parlodel) may decrease GH levels. Hypophysectomy or radiation may be indicated if a tumor is the cause. If the pituitary is removed, lifelong replacement of thyroid hormone, corticosteroids, and sex hormones is important.

Nursing Process

ASSESSMENT. The nurse caring for the client with acromegaly is concerned with the client's response to the disease. Safety is assessed in relation to impaired eyesight, chewing, and swallowing. Serum glucose levels are monitored for onset of diabetes. Knowledge and acceptance of the disease are assessed. If hypophysectomy is planned, the client is assessed for anxiety related to the surgery, and a preoperative baseline neurological assessment is performed. (See Chapter 45.)

NURSING DIAGNOSIS. Possible nursing diagnoses include body image disturbance, risk for injury related to poor eyesight and **dysphagia,** knowledge deficit, altered comfort, and altered sensory perception. Additional diagnoses will be identified if diabetes or other problems exist.

PLANNING AND IMPLEMENTATION. The client is allowed to verbalize feelings related to the disease. A care plan for safety is implemented if vision or swallowing is disturbed. If pain is present, comfort measures are provided.

CLIENT EDUCATION. The nurse teaches the client and significant others about the disease and treatment. If hypophysectomy was performed, the need for lifelong hormone replacement is stressed.

EVALUATION. The client who is caring for the disease and taking medications properly will have some soft tissues return to normal size. Safety will be maintained. The client should be able to accurately describe self-care requirements.

Care of the Client Undergoing Hypophysectomy

Removal of the pituitary gland is called hypophysectomy. Figure 37–4 shows the transsephenoidal approach to the gland. Some tumors may necessitate removal via a transfrontal craniotomy (entry through the frontal bone of the skull).

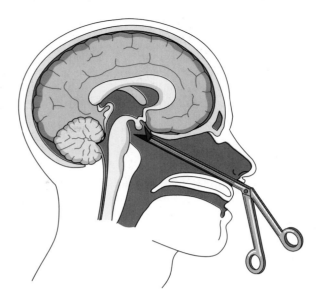

Figure 37–4. Transsphenoidal approach to pituitary gland for hypophysectomy. (Modified from Ignatavicius, Workman, and Mishler: Medical Surgical Nursing. WB Saunders, Philadelphia, 1995, with permission.)

PREOPERATIVE CARE. The nurse ensures that the client understands the physician's explanation of surgery. The client should understand that some symptoms will be relieved, but that bone growth and visual changes may not reverse. The client is prepared for what to expect following surgery. Because coughing is contraindicated, the client is instructed in deep breathing exercises or use of an incentive spirometer.

POSTOPERATIVE CARE. The nurse performs routine neurological assessments to monitor for neurological damage. The nurse also checks urine for specific gravity, because diabetes insipidus may occur following pituitary surgery. If the client has had transsphenoidal surgery, he or she will have nasal packing and a "mustache dressing," which is placed under the nose to collect drips. These are left in place and not removed unless ordered by the physician. The nurse monitors the dressing for signs of cerebrospinal fluid (CSF) leakage. CSF contains glucose, so glucose testing strips can be used to determine if drainage is actually CSF or just nasal discharge. The client should avoid any actions that will increase pressure on the surgical site, such as coughing, sneezing, nose blowing, straining to move bowels, or bending from the waist. The nurse obtains orders for stool softeners and antitussives as needed. Tooth brushing is avoided until the incision line is healed. The client may use floss and mouth rinses. The client will be placed on hormone replacement therapy following hypophysectomy. Pituitary hormones are difficult to replace, so target hormones are generally given. These include thyroid hormone and glucocorticoids. Clients should be instructed in how to administer the hormones, as well as side effects to report.

---

dysphagia: dys—bad + phagia—swallowing

Disorders of the Thyroid Gland

Triiodothyronine (T_3) and thyroxine (T_4) are secreted by the thyroid gland. These hormones may be collectively referred to as thyroid hormone (TH). Deficient secretion of these hormones results in hypothyroidism; excess TH results in hyperthyroidism.

HYPOTHYROIDISM

Hypothyroidism occurs primarily in women 30 to 60 years old. If hypothyroidism occurs in an infant, the result is cretinism. Hypothyroidism that develops in an adult is called myxedema.

Pathophysiology

Primary hypothyroidism occurs when the thyroid gland fails to produce enough TH in the presence of adequate thyroid-stimulating hormone (TSH). The pituitary responds to the low level of TH by producing more TSH. Secondary hypothyroidism is due to low levels of TSH or thyrotropin-releasing hormone (TRH), which fail to stimulate release of TH. Most cases of hypothyroidism are primary (Table 37–4).

Because thyroid hormones are responsible for metabolism, low levels of these hormones result in a slowed metabolic rate, which causes many of the characteristic symptoms of hypothyroidism. Other symptoms are related to **myxedema,** which refers to a nonpitting type of edema that occurs in connective tissues throughout the body.

Etiology

Primary hypothyroidism may be due to a congenital defect, inflammation, iodine deficiency, or thyroidectomy. Hashimoto's thyroiditis is an **autoimmune** disorder that eventually destroys thyroid tissue, leading to hypothyroidism. Secondary hypothyroidism may be due to a pituitary or hypothalamic lesion, or postpartum pituitary necrosis, a rare disorder in which the pituitary destructs following pregnancy and delivery. Peripheral resistance to TH may also occur.

Signs and Symptoms

Manifestations are related primarily to the reduced metabolic rate and include fatigue, weight gain, bradycardia, constipation, mental dullness, cold intolerance, hypoventilation, and dry skin and hair (Table 37–5). Heart failure may occur because of decreased pumping strength of the heart. Altered fat metabolism causes hyperlipidemia. Myxedema causes water retention, with puffiness in the face and around the eye area. Fluid may also accumulate around the heart, causing altered cardiac function.

Table 37–4. *Thyroid Hormone Abnormalities*

	Hyperthyroidism	Hypothyroidism
Primary	TH↑ TSH↓	TH↓ TSH↑
Secondary (Pituitary Cause)	TH↑ TSH↑	TH↓ TSH↓

Complications

If the metabolic rate drops so low as to become life threatening, the result is called myxedema coma. The client becomes hypothermic (with a temperature less than 95°F and has a decreased respiratory rate and blood pressure. Depressed mental function and lethargy may occur. Blood glucose is decreased. Death may occur due to respiratory failure. If the nurse notes changes in mental status or vital signs, the physician should be contacted immediately. Treatment of myxedema coma involves intubation and mechanical ventilation. The client is slowly rewarmed with blankets. Intravenous levothyroxine (Synthroid) is given.

Diagnostic Tests

The T_3 and T_4 levels are low, and TSH may be high or low, depending on the cause. If the pituitary is functioning normally, TSH will be elevated in an attempt to stimulate an increase in TH. Serum cholesterol may be elevated.

Medical Treatment

Hypothyroidism is easily treated with thyroid replacement hormone. Some clients still use TH from animal thyroids. Most clients now take synthetic thyroid hormone (levothyroxine [Synthroid]). Doses are started low and are slowly increased to prevent symptoms of hyperthyroidism or cardiac complications.

Nursing Process

Assessment

The client with hypothyroidism is assessed for symptoms of decreased metabolism, as well as for symptoms of heart failure. The occurrence of weight gain, skin problems, and constipation are noted. The nurse should take care to assess the impact the disease has had on the client's life and ability to perform self-care measures. If the diagnosis is not new, understanding of the treatment regimen and compliance with medication should be assessed.

---

myxedema: myx—mucus + edema—swelling
autoimmune: auto—pertaining to self + immune—exempt

Table 37–5. **Symptoms of Thyroid Disorders**

	Hypothyroidism	Hyperthyroidism
Cardiovascular	Bradycardia, decreased cardiac output, cool skin, cold intolerance	Tachycardia, increased cardiac output, warm skin, heat intolerance
Neurological	Lethargy, slowed movements, memory loss, confusion	Fatigue, restlessness, tremor, insomnia, emotional instability
Pulmonary	Dyspnea, hypoventilation	Dyspnea
Integumentary	Cool, dry skin; brittle, dry hair	Diaphoresis; warm skin; fine, soft hair
Gastrointestinal	Decreased appetite, weight gain, constipation, increased serum lipid levels	Increased appetite, weight loss, frequent stools, decreased serum lipid levels
Reproductive	Decreased libido, impotence	Decreased libido, impotence, amenorrhea

Nursing Diagnosis

Possible nursing diagnoses include activity intolerance related to fatigue, impaired skin integrity, constipation, and altered nutrition related to decreased metabolic rate. Many other diagnoses may also apply depending on the symptoms exhibited by the client.

Planning and Implementation

The nurse assists the client to space rest and activities to prevent fatigue. Care should be taken to protect the skin. Fluids and fiber may be added to the diet to prevent constipation. Dietary adjustments may be needed as treatment begins to be effective and metabolic rate increases.

Client Education

The nurse instructs the client in the importance of consistent use of thyroid replacement medication and regular blood tests to monitor the levels of TH. The client needs to be aware that too much thyroid hormone will cause symptoms of hyperthyroidism. Such symptoms should be reported to the physician immediately.

Evaluation

The client should be able to state correctly how to care for himself or herself. The skin should remain intact, and bowel movements should follow the client's normal preillness pattern. Follow-up TH levels should be normal.

See also Nursing Care Plan Box 37–2 for the Client with Hypothyroidism.

CRITICAL THINKING: Mae

Mae is a 59-year-old woman who is tired all the time and has gained 16 pounds over the past year. Her physician does some blood tests and prescribes levothyroxine PO. Lab results show low T_3 and T_4 and elevated TSH.

1. Why is Mae's TSH elevated?

2. What will happen to Mae's caloric requirements as she begins treatment? Why?
3. Why does the nurse teach Mae to check her pulse?

Answers at end of chapter.

HYPERTHYROIDISM

Hyperthyroidism is most commonly diagnosed in young women. Graves' disease, which is one cause of hyperthyroidism, is more common in young women. Multinodular goiter is more common in older women.

Pathophysiology

Hyperthyroidism results from excessive amounts of circulating thyroid hormone. Primary hyperthyroidism occurs when a problem within the thyroid gland causes excess hormone release. Secondary hyperthyroidism occurs because of excess TSH release from the pituitary or excess TRH from the hypothalamus, which overstimulate the thyroid. Excess thyroid hormone increases the metabolic rate. It is also believed to increase the number of beta-adrenergic receptor sites in the body, which enhances the activity of norepinephrine. The resulting fight or flight response is the cause of many of the symptoms of hyperthyroidism.

Etiology

A variety of disorders may cause hyperthyroidism. Graves' disease is the most common cause. Graves' disease is thought to be an autoimmune disorder, because thyroid-stimulating antibodies are present in the blood of these clients.

Multinodular goiter, in which thyroid nodules secrete excess TH, is sometimes associated with hyperthyroidism. A pituitary tumor may secrete excess TSH, which overstimulates the thyroid gland. A thyroid tumor may secrete TH. Clients taking thyroid hormone for hy-

NURSING CARE PLAN BOX 37–2 FOR THE CLIENT WITH HYPOTHYROIDISM

Activity intolerance related to fatigue

Outcomes
(1) Client reports lessening fatigue after treatment initiated. (2) Client is able to carry out usual activities of daily living (ADL).

Evaluation of Outcomes
(1) Does client report lessening fatigue? (2) Is client able to carry out ADL?

Interventions	Rationale	Evaluation
• Assist client with self-care activities.	Clients with fatigue may have difficulty carrying out activities independently.	Are client's self-care needs being met? Is assistance needed?
• Allow for rest between activities.	Rest periods will enable client to conserve energy for activities.	Does client state rest is adequate?
• Slowly increase client's activities as medication begins to be effective.	As thyroid replacement therapy becomes effective, the client's fatigue will subside.	Does client tolerate increases in activity?

GERIATRIC

• When getting elderly clients up, watch for orthostatic hypotension.	Orthostatic hypotension is common in elderly and may cause falls.	Does client's blood pressure drop when changing positions?

Constipation related to slowed gastrointestinal motility

Outcomes
(1) Soft, formed stool passed at preillness frequency. (2) Client identifies measures to prevent constipation in future.

Evaluation of Outcomes
(1) Are bowels moving according to client's preillness pattern? (2) Does client verbalize measures to prevent constipation?

Interventions	Rationale	Evaluation
• Monitor and record bowel movements.	A record will help determine if a problem exists.	Does record show pattern of bowel movements?
• Help client follow usual preillness pattern (e.g., after morning coffee).	A schedule allows bowel movement to occur before stool becomes hard and dry.	Is client able to identify and implement usual self-care for bowels?
• Increase fluids to eight 8-ounce glasses of water daily if cardiovascular status stable.	Adequate fluid intake helps prevent hard, dry stools.	Does client take adequate fluids?
• Add fiber to diet: fresh fruit, vegetables, bran.	Fiber helps increase the number of bowel movements.	Does client tolerate fiber? Is it effective?
• Encourage regular ambulation.	Activity increases peristalsis.	Is client able to ambulate or engage in other activity?
• Use bedside commode or bathroom rather than bedpan.	The sitting position aids in evacuation.	Is sitting position effective?
• Obtain physician order for stool softener if needed.	Soft stools are passed more easily.	Is stool softener needed? Effective?

continued

NURSING CARE PLAN BOX 37–2 (continued)

Interventions	Rationale	Evaluation
GERIATRIC		
• If the client is impacted, break up stool digitally and gently remove. • Avoid use of enemas	Breaking up stool eases evacuation. Enemas can cause fluid and electrolyte imbalances and can damage mucosa.	Is client impacted? Is digital disimpaction effective? Does client understand need to avoid enemas?

Impaired skin integrity related to dry skin, inactivity

Outcomes
(1) Skin is soft and moist. (2) Skin remains intact.

Evaluation of Outcomes
(1) Is skin soft and moist? (2) Is skin intact?

Interventions	Rationale	Evaluation
• Assess skin daily for breakdown. • Avoid use of soap on dry areas. Try bath oil. • Use nondrying lotion following bath. • Encourage/assist with position changes at least every 2 hours.	Skin lesions are more effectively treated when identified early. Soap is drying to skin. Lotion helps trap moisture in skin. Some lotions contain alcohol, however, which is drying. Changing position enhances circulation to the skin, promoting healing and preventing breakdown.	Is breakdown present? Does use of bath oil help? Does client state relief with use of lotion? Does client change position at least every 2 hours? Are pressure areas prevented?

Altered nutrition, more than requirements, related to decreased metabolic rate

Outcomes
(1) Client will return to preillness weight. (2) Client will verbalize understanding of dietary recommendations.

Evaluation of Outcomes
(1) Is client approaching preillness weight? (2) Is client able to explain dietary recommendations and how they will be implemented?

Interventions	Rationale	Evaluation
• Weigh weekly and record. • Consult dietitian for therapeutic diet until hypothyroidism is controlled. • Encourage regular exercise within limits of fatigue. • Counsel client that weight should normalize once hypothyroidism is controlled.	Weekly weights record progress without the frustration of daily fluctuations. The dietitian can provide food choices for gradual weight loss if necessary. Exercise promotes weight control. Thyroid replacement hormone will increase the metabolic rate, allowing the client to return to normal weight.	Is client losing or maintaining weight? Does client verbalize understanding of and ability to follow diet? Does client verbalize understanding of and ability to follow exercise plan? Does client verbalize understanding of instruction?
GERIATRIC		
• Allow client to help determine acceptable diet modifications.	Older clients may have long-standing dietary habits that are hard to change.	Is client satisfied with weight loss plan?

pothyroidism may take too much. Each of these problems can cause excess circulating TH and symptoms of hyperthyroidism.

Signs and Symptoms

Many signs and symptoms are related to the hypermetabolic state, such as heat intolerance, increased appetite with weight loss, and increased frequency of bowel movements. Nervousness, tremor, tachycardia, and palpitations are due to the increase in sympathetic nervous system activity. Heart failure may occur due to tachycardia and the resulting inefficient pumping of the heart. Emotional lability, warm smooth skin, and muscle weakness may also occur. If treatment is not begun, the client may become manic or psychotic. **Exophthalmos,** which is bulging of the eyes, may occur with Graves' disease (Fig. 37–5). This is due to swelling of the tissues behind the eyes. Thickening of the skin on the anterior legs may also occur in Graves' disease (Table 37–5).

The nurse should be alert to the elderly client, who may not exhibit the typical signs and symptoms of hyperthyroidism. These clients may have heart failure, atrial fibrillation, fatigue, apathy, and depression.

Complications

Thyrotoxic Crisis

Thyrotoxic crisis (also called thyroid storm) is a severe hyperthyroid state that may occur in hyperthyroid individuals who are untreated or who are experiencing another illness or stressor. It may also occur following thyroid surgery in clients who have been inadequately prepared with antithyroid medication. Thyrotoxic crisis may result in death in as little as 2 hours if untreated. Symptoms include tachycardia, high fever, hypertension (with eventual heart failure and hypotension), dehydration, restlessness, and delirium or coma.

If thyrotoxic crisis occurs, treatment is first directed toward relieving the life-threatening symptoms. Acetaminophen is given for the fever. Aspirin is avoided because it binds with the same serum protein as T_4, freeing additional T_4 into the circulation. Intravenous fluids and a cooling blanket may be ordered to cool the client. A beta-adrenergic blocker, such as propranolol, is given for tachycardia. If the client is short of breath due to cardiac dysfunction, oxygen is administered and the head of the bed is elevated. Once symptoms are controlled and the client is safe, the underlying thyroid problem is treated.

Hypothyroidism

Another complication of hyperthyroidism can be hypothyroidism. This may occur as a result of long-term disease or as a result of treatment. Clients with a history of hyperthyroidism should be monitored for recurrent hyperthyroidism or the onset of hypothyroidism.

Diagnostic Tests

Serum levels of T_3 and T_4 are elevated. TSH is low in primary hypothyroidism, or high if the cause is pituitary. A TRH stimulation test may be done. A thyroid scan may be done to locate a tumor.

Medical Treatment

Several medications can be used to treat hyperthyroidism. Propylthiouracil (PTU) and methimazole (Tapazole) inhibit the synthesis of TH. Propranolol (Inderal) is a beta-blocking medication that relieves the sympathetic nervous system symptoms. Radioactive iodine (^{131}I) may be used to destroy a portion of the thyroid gland. Oral iodine suppresses the release of thyroid hormone.

Sometimes medications alone control hyperthyroidism. If this does not occur, surgery is planned. Surgery is the treatment of choice for thyroid cancer. Even if surgery is the treatment chosen, antithyroid medications will be given to calm the thyroid before surgery. They will help slow the heart rate and reduce other symptoms, making surgery safer. Iodine also reduces the vascularity of the thyroid gland, decreasing the risk of bleeding during surgery. Adequate preparation of the client is important, because a **euthyroid** state helps prevent a postoperative thyrotoxic crisis.

Nursing Process

Assessment

The client with hyperthyroidism is monitored closely until normal thyroid activity is restored. Vital signs are monitored, with increases in pulse and blood pressure reported to the physician. Lung sounds are monitored, because crackles may indicate heart failure. Level of anxiety and ability to cope with symptoms are also assessed. Weight and bowel function are monitored. Eyes are assessed for risk for injury due to exophthalmos, and degree of muscle weakness is noted. The nurse should *never* palpate the thyroid gland of a client with hyperthyroidism, because palpation may stimulate release of thyroid hormone.

Nursing Diagnosis

Priority nursing diagnoses include risk for injury related to hypermetabolic state and exophthalmos, hyperthermia, diarrhea, altered nutrition, sleep pattern disturbance, and anxiety.

Planning and Implementation

Vital signs are monitored, and changes are reported to the physician. The client with exophthalmos may benefit from

---

exophthalmos: exo—outward + ophthalmos—eye
euthyroid: eu—normal, healthy + thyroid

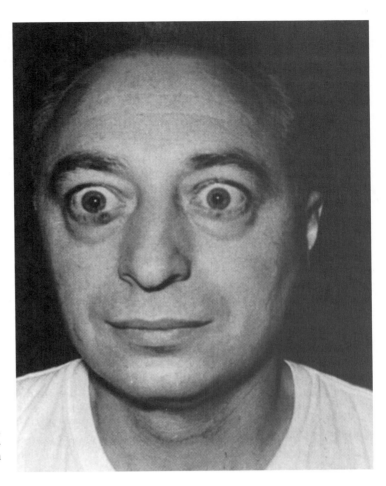

Figure 37–5. Exophthalmos caused by Graves' disease. (From Tamparo, CD, and Lewis, MA: Diseases of the Human Body, ed 2. FA Davis, Philadelphia, 1995, p 275, with permission.)

lubricating eyedrops and dark glasses. The eyes may be gently taped shut with nonallergic tape for sleeping. Elevation of the head of the bed and a low-sodium diet may decrease edema behind the eyes. If routine measures for hyperthermia are ineffective, a cooling blanket may be ordered. Diarrhea may be lessened with a low-fiber diet. A high-calorie diet with six meals a day may be necessary to meet caloric requirements. A restful environment and a mild sleeping aid may assist the client to fall asleep. The nurse assures the client that proper treatment will correct symptoms.

If radioactive iodine is used, it is usually given orally in one dose. If the dose is high, for example for the client with thyroid cancer, the client will be hospitalized. The nurse should limit time spent with the client and maintain a safe distance when providing direct care. The nurse who is pregnant should avoid caring for the client. Urine, vomitus, and other body secretions are contaminated and should be disposed of according to hospital policy. Many hospitals direct nurses to flush the toilet twice following disposal of contaminated material. The radiation safety officer and hospital policy should be consulted for specific precautions.

At home, the client is instructed to avoid close contact with family members for about a week and to use careful hand washing after urinating. Oral contact with others should be avoided, and eating utensils should be washed thoroughly with soap and water.[2] Hospital teaching protocols should be used for specific client teaching. The nurse informs the client that symptoms of hyperthyroidism will subside in about 6 to 8 weeks. In addition, the client should be aware of symptoms of hypothyroidism to be reported, because hypothyroidism may occur up to 15 years after the treatment.

Client Education

The client is taught about his or her disease and symptoms of hyperthyroidism or hypothyroidism to report. The client should also understand how to take antithyroid medication if ordered.

Evaluation

If the plan of care is effective, the client will remain free from complications or injury related to the hypermetabolic state. Eyes will be comfortable and free from injury. Body temperature will be kept within normal limits. Diarrhea will be controlled, and complications of diarrhea such as skin breakdown and dehydration avoided. The client's weight should remain stable. The client should report that he or she is rested on awakening and that anxiety is controlled.

GOITER

Pathophysiology and Etiology

Enlargement of the thyroid gland is called a **goiter.** The thyroid gland may enlarge in response to increased TSH levels. TSH is elevated in response to low TH, iodine deficiency, pregnancy, or viral, genetic, or other conditions. When a goiter is caused by iodine deficiency or other environmental factors, it is called an endemic goiter.

A goiter may be associated with a hyperthyroid, hypothyroid, or euthyroid state. Once the cause of the goiter is removed, the gland usually returns to normal size.

Some foods and medications are goitrogens. These substances interfere with the body's use of iodine, and include such foods as turnips, cabbage, broccoli, horseradish, cauliflower, and carrots. Some goitrogenic medications include propylthiouracil, sulfonamides, lithium, and salicylates. (See Nutrition Notes Box 37–3.)

Signs and Symptoms

The thyroid gland is enlarged, with swelling apparent at the base of the neck (Fig. 37–6). The client may have a full sensation in the neck. If the goiter is large, it may interfere with swallowing or breathing. Symptoms of hypothyroidism or hyperthyroidism may be present.

Diagnostic Tests and Medical Treatment

A thyroid scan shows an enlarged thyroid gland. Serum T_3 and T_4 are measured to determine thyroid function. Treatment is aimed at the cause. If goitrogens are suspect, the

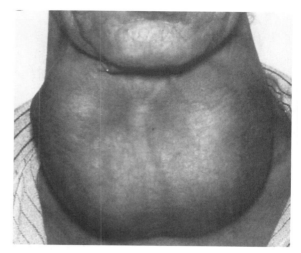

Figure 37–6. Client with goiter. (From Morton, PG: Health Assessment in Nursing, ed 2. FA Davis, Philadelphia, 1993, p 104, with permission.)

client is given a list of foods to be avoided. If iodine deficiency is a problem, it is added to the diet with supplements or iodized salt. A thyroidectomy may be necessary if the gland is interfering with breathing or swallowing.

Nursing Care

The nurse should carefully assess the effect of the goiter on breathing and swallowing. Stridor, a whistling sound, may be heard if the airway is obstructed. Stridor is an ominous sign and should be reported to the physician immediately. If the client experiences difficulty swallowing, the nurse should collaborate with the dietitian to provide soft foods or liquid nutrition. The client should sit upright to eat and swallow twice after each bite.

CANCER OF THE THYROID GLAND

Although thyroid cancer is rare, it is the most common cancer of the endocrine system. Women are affected more often than men. Most tumors of the thyroid gland are not malignant. (See Cultural Considerations Box 37–4.)

NUTRITION NOTES BOX 37–3

Nutrition in Thyroid Disorders

IODINE DEFICIENCY. Inland areas of all continents have iodine-poor soils. People in developing countries with only local food sources are still subject to endemic goiter. Most goitrogens compete with iodide for active transport into thyroid cells but have not been implicated as causing endemic goiter. The antimanic drug lithium inhibits the release of hormones from the thyroid gland. Fortification of salt with iodine has significantly reduced the occurrence of simple goiter in developed countries.

IODINE EXCESS. Food naturally high in iodine are saltwater fish, shellfish, and seaweed. Iodine toxicity has occurred in Japan. Ironically, toxicity produces an "iodine goiter," the same sign as deficiency.

CULTURAL CONSIDERATIONS BOX 37–4

Because of the Chernobyl nuclear disaster in Russia in 1988, Russian immigrants are at exceptionally high risk for developing pituitary, thyroid, and parathyroid disorders and cancers. The proximity of Estonia, Latvia, Lithuania, Poland, and other Eastern European countries to Russia places immigrants and long-term visitors from these countries at risk also. The nurse needs to be alert for endocrine disorders among these populations and assist clients to arrange genetic counseling for those who desire it.

Etiology

Thyroid hyperplasia may lead to thyroid cancer. Other causes include exposure to radiation, iodine deficiency, and prolonged exposure to goitrogens.

Signs and Symptoms

A hard, painless nodule may be palpable on the thyroid gland. Difficulty breathing or swallowing or changes in the voice may occur due to the presence of the tumor near the esophagus and trachea. Most clients with cancer of the thyroid have normal TH levels.

Diagnostic Tests

A thyroid scan shows a "cold" nodule. This is because malignant tumors of the thyroid do not take up the radioactive iodine administered for the scan. A fine-needle aspiration biopsy confirms the diagnosis.

Medical Treatment

A partial or total thyroidectomy may be done. Chemotherapy or radioactive iodine (^{131}I) therapy may also be used, alone or following surgery.

Nursing Care

Nursing care is determined by the symptoms the client is experiencing. See Chapter 10 for care of the client with cancer.

Nursing Care of the Client Undergoing Thyroidectomy

Clients may undergo thyroidectomy for cancer of the thyroid, hyperthyroidism, or a goiter that is causing dyspnea or dysphagia. See Chapter 11 for general care of a client having surgery.

A total thyroidectomy is usually performed if cancer is present. After a total thyroidectomy, lifelong replacement hormone must be taken. A subtotal (partial) thyroidectomy may be done for hyperthyroidism, leaving a portion of the thyroid gland to secrete TH.

Before having a thyroidectomy, the client should be in a euthyroid state. This is accomplished with the use of antithyroid medication. Iodine (SSKI) may also be administered to decrease the size and vascularity of the gland, reducing the risk of bleeding during surgery.

Preoperative Care

Assessment

The client should be assessed for symptoms related to an enlarged thyroid. If difficulty swallowing or breathing is present, appropriate actions should be taken. TH levels are monitored. A drug history is taken. Nutritional status is assessed, and vital signs are monitored. The client's understanding of the procedure and level of anxiety are assessed.

Nursing Diagnosis

Possible diagnoses include anxiety related to impending surgery, knowledge deficit related to surgical procedure, and risk for injury related to surgical procedure.

Planning and Implementation

The nurse reassures the client that he or she will feel relief of symptoms after surgery. The client is allowed to express fears and ask questions. The client is approached slowly and calmly, because the hyperthyroid state increases the client's feelings of anxiety. The nurse reports changes in vital signs, ensures that the client's nutritional needs have been addressed, and verifies that antithyroid drugs have been administered as ordered.

Client Education

The nurse explains what the client may expect before, during, and after surgery (see Chapter 11) and clarifies misconceptions. Before surgery, the client is taught how to perform gentle range of motion exercises of the neck, how to support the neck during position changes, and how to use an incentive spirometer after surgery.

Evaluation

The client will state that anxiety is controlled and that questions related to surgery have been answered. Risk for injury will be minimized by verifying that the client is in a euthyroid state before surgery.

Postoperative Care

Assessment

Vital signs and dressings are monitored every 15 minutes initially, progressing to every 4 hours, as ordered. Decreased blood pressure with increased pulse alert the nurse to the possibility of shock related to blood loss. Tachycardia and fever, along with mental status changes, may indicate thyrotoxic crisis. The back of the neck should be checked for pooling of blood. Due to the location of the surgery, the nurse observes for signs of respiratory distress, including an increase in respiratory rate, dyspnea, or stridor. The nurse asks the client to speak in order to detect hoarseness of the voice, which may indicate trauma to the recurrent laryngeal nerve. The client is monitored for evidence of **tetany.** Any abnormal findings are reported to the physician immediately.

Nursing Diagnosis

Possible diagnoses include risk for injury related to complications and pain related to surgical procedure, risk for altered nutrition, and ineffective airway clearance due to edema at surgical site.

Planning and Implementation

The physician should be notified of changes in vital signs, respiratory distress, or excessive bleeding from the surgical site. A tracheostomy set is kept at the bedside for emergency use if edema causes respiratory obstruction. Semi-Fowler's position helps reduce edema and promotes comfort. Routine interventions to prevent postoperative pain should be implemented. Pillows or sandbags may be used to support the head. The client should be assisted with gentle range of motion exercises, avoiding hyperextension of the neck and subsequent strain on the incision line, and the client is reminded to do coughing and deep breathing exercises every hour. Incentive spirometry is encouraged to assist the client to deep breathe. When the client's swallowing and gag reflexes are intact, clear liquids will be ordered. A dietitian may be consulted to assist the client with potential dietary changes needed following surgery. With correction of metabolic alterations, dietary needs may be significantly altered.

Client Education

The nurse teaches the importance of follow-up care, and how to administer replacement hormone if indicated. The client or significant other is taught how to change the dressing and to report bleeding or signs of infection at the site. Because the threat of thyrotoxic crisis may continue after discharge, the client or significant other should be taught to immediately report unusual irritability, fever, or palpitations.

Evaluation

If the plan has been effective, complications due to surgery will be recognized and reported early. Pain will be prevented or controlled, and the client will demonstrate understanding of dietary modifications.

Complications

Thyrotoxic Crisis

Thyrotoxic crisis may result from manipulation of the thyroid gland during surgery, with the subsequent release of large amounts of thyroid hormone. This is a rare complication since the use of antithyroid drugs before surgery has become routine. For more information on thyrotoxic crisis, see the section on hyperthyroidism earlier in this chapter.

Tetany

Tetany is caused by low calcium levels and is characterized by tingling in the fingers and perioral area (around the mouth), muscle spasms and twitching, and cardiac dysrhythmias. Muscle spasms in the larynx can lead to respiratory obstruction. If the problem is not recognized quickly, death may result. Tetany can occur if the parathyroid glands are accidentally removed during thyroid surgery.

Due to the proximity of the parathyroid glands to the thyroid, it is sometimes difficult to avoid them. In the absence of parathyroid hormone, serum calcium levels drop, and tetany results.

Intravenous calcium gluconate is given to treat acute tetany. To provide temporary relief while medications are being prepared, the nurse has the client breathe into a paper bag. This will cause mild acidosis, which increases ionization of calcium in the blood.

Disorders of the Parathyroid Glands

The parathyroid glands are four small glands that lie behind the thyroid gland. They secrete parathyroid hormone (PTH) in response to low serum calcium levels. PTH raises serum calcium levels by promoting calcium movement from bones to blood and by increasing absorption of dietary calcium. Decreased PTH activity is called hypoparathyroidism. Increased PTH activity is called hyperparathyroidism.

HYPOPARATHYROIDISM

Pathophysiology

A decrease in PTH causes a decrease in bone resorption of calcium. This means that calcium stays in bones instead of being moved into the blood. The result is a decreased serum calcium level, called hypocalcemia. As calcium levels fall, phosphate levels rise.

Etiology

The most common causes of hypoparathyroidism are heredity and the accidental removal of the parathyroid glands during thyroidectomy. Due to the proximity of the glands to the thyroid, it is sometimes difficult to avoid removing them. Hypoparathyroidism also occurs following removal of the parathyroid glands for hyperparathyroidism.

Signs and Symptoms

Calcium plays an important role in nerve cell stability. Hypocalcemia causes neuromuscular irritability. In acute cases, tetany may occur, with numbness and tingling of the fingers and perioral area, muscle spasms, and twitching (Table 37–6). Positive Chvostek's and Trousseau's signs are early signs of tetany (Fig. 37–7).

In chronic hypoparathyroidism, the client is lethargic and experiences muscle spasms. Calcifications may occur in the eyes and brain, leading to psychosis. Convulsions may occur. Death may result from laryngospasm if treatment is not provided.

Table 37–6. **Comparison of Parathyroid Disorders**

	Insufficient PTH	*Excess PTH*
Disorder	Hypoparathyroidism	Hyperparathyroidism
Signs and Symptoms	Hypocalcemia, neuromuscular irritability, tetany	Hypercalcemia, fatigue, pathologic fractures
Usual Treatment	Calcium replacement; high-calcium, low-phosphorus diet	Calcitonin replacement, parathyroidectomy
Priority Nursing Diagnoses	Risk for injury related to tetany	Risk for injury related to bone demineralization

Diagnostic Tests

Chvostek's and Trousseau's signs are present. Laboratory studies show decreased serum calcium and PTH levels.

Medical Treatment

Acute cases of hypoparathyroidism are treated with intravenous calcium gluconate. In addition, rebreathing carbon dioxide by breathing into a paper bag will cause acidosis, which will increase ionization of serum calcium and temporarily raise the calcium level. Long-term treatment includes a high-calcium diet (Table 37–7), with oral calcium and vitamin D supplements. Thiazide diuretics may also be used because they reduce the amount of calcium excreted in the urine.

Nursing Process

Assessment

The client at risk for hypoparathyroidism should be closely monitored for symptoms of tetany. If the nurse suspects tetany, Chvostek's and Trousseau's signs should be checked. Respirations are closely monitored for stridor, a sign of laryngospasm.

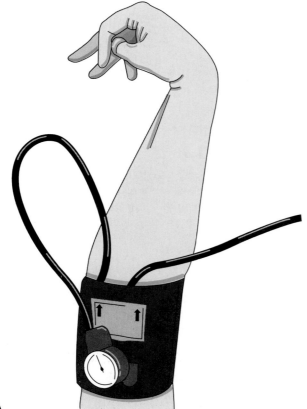

A

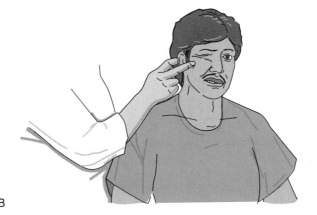

B

Figure 37–7. *(A)* Trousseau's sign seen in hypocalcemia. *(B)* Chvostek's sign seen in hypocalcemia (see page 74.). (Modified from Morton: Health Assessment in Nursing, ed 2. FA Davis, Philadelphia, 1993, p 601, with permission.)

Table 37–7. **Dietary Sources of Calcium**

Milk
Cheeses
Yogurt
Sardines
Oysters
Salmon
Cauliflower
Green leafy vegetables

Nursing Diagnosis

A priority nursing diagnosis is risk for injury related to tetany. In chronic hypoparathyroidism, the client should be assessed for knowledge deficit related to self-care of hypoparathyroidism.

Planning and Implementation

If the client exhibits signs of tetany, the nurse recognizes a potential emergency and notifies the physician immediately. A tracheostomy set, endotracheal tube, and intravenous calcium are kept at the bedside for emergency use. The nurse ensures that the client and significant other have knowledge of home medications and dietary recommendations. A dietitian is consulted if indicated.

Evaluation

Injury is prevented through early recognition and reporting of signs and symptoms of tetany. The client should be able to describe correct treatment for his or her disease.

HYPERPARATHYROIDISM

Pathophysiology

Overactivity of one or more of the parathyroid glands causes an increase in PTH, with a subsequent increase in the serum calcium level (hypercalcemia). This is achieved through movement of calcium out of the bones and into the blood, absorption in the small intestine, and reabsorption by the kidneys. PTH also promotes phosphate excretion by the kidneys.

Etiology

Hyperparathyroidism is usually the result of hyperplasia or a benign tumor of the parathyroid glands, or it may be hereditary. Secondary hyperparathyroidism occurs when the parathyroids secrete excessive PTH in response to low serum calcium levels. Serum calcium may be reduced in kidney disease because of the kidneys' failure to activate vitamin D, which is necessary for absorption of calcium in the small intestine.

Signs and Symptoms

Signs and symptoms of hyperparathyroidism are caused primarily by the increase in serum calcium level, although many clients are asymptomatic. Symptoms include fatigue, depression, confusion, increased urination, anorexia, nausea, vomiting, kidney stones, and cardiac dysrhythmias. The increased serum calcium level also causes gastrin secretion, resulting in abdominal pain and peptic ulcers. Because calcium is being removed from bones, joint pain and pathologic fractures may occur. With severe hypercalcemia, the result may be coma and cardiac arrest.

Diagnostic Tests

Laboratory studies include serum calcium, phosphate, and PTH levels. X-rays may show decreased bone density.

Medical Treatment

The client should be monitored for bone changes and decline in renal function. Hydration with intravenous normal saline lowers the calcium level by dilution. Furosemide (Lasix) is given to increase renal excretion of calcium. Pamidronate (Aredia) or calcitonin may be given to prevent calcium release from bones. Mithramycin may be used to lower serum calcium levels, although its toxicity limits use to two or three doses. If hypercalcemia is severe, or if the client is at risk for bone or kidney complications, surgery to remove the diseased parathyroid glands is performed. If possible, some parathyroid tissue will be left intact to continue to secrete PTH.

Nursing Process

Assessment

The client is assessed for symptoms related to hypercalcemia, including muscle weakness, lethargy, bone pain, anorexia, nausea, vomiting, behavioral changes, and renal insufficiency. Calcium levels are monitored.

Nursing Diagnosis

Nursing diagnoses depend on assessment findings. Risk for injury related to bone demineralization, altered nutrition related to nausea and vomiting, activity intolerance related to fatigue, and altered thought processes related to hypercalcemia are some possible diagnoses.

Planning and Implementation

The client should be protected from injury. Nausea is prevented so nutritional status can be maintained while the underlying problem is being treated. The client is allowed adequate rest periods. Changes in mental status are reported immediately. If surgery is planned, preoperative and postoperative care is similar to that of the client undergoing thyroid surgery.

Evaluation

If the plan is effective, symptoms of hypercalcemia will be recognized and reported quickly, nausea and vomiting will be controlled, and complications and injury will be prevented.

Disorders of the Adrenal Glands

Adrenal disorders may involve the adrenal medulla or the adrenal cortex. Hypersecretion of epinephrine from the adrenal medulla is associated with a rare tumor called a pheochromocytoma. Hyposecretion of epinephrine is rare and generally causes no symptoms. Hypersecretion of cortisol from the adrenal cortex results in Cushing's syndrome. Addison's disease results from hypofunction of the adrenal cortex.

PHEOCHROMOCYTOMA

Pathophysiology

A **pheochromocytoma** is an uncommon tumor that arises from the chromaffin cells of the adrenal medulla. Occasionally, a pheochromocytoma occurs outside the adrenal gland. The tumor autonomously secretes catecholamines (norepinephrine and sometimes epinephrine) in excessive amounts. Ninety percent of pheochromocytomas are benign.

Etiology

The cause of pheochromocytoma is unknown. Ten percent of cases are hereditary.

Signs and Symptoms

Because norepinephrine is the fight or flight hormone, clients with a pheochromocytoma have exaggerated fight or flight symptoms. Manifestations of a pheochromocytoma include hypertension, tachycardia (with heart rate greater than 100), palpitations, diaphoresis, feeling of apprehension, elevated blood glucose, and severe pounding headache. Blood glucose may increase because of catecholamine inhibition of insulin release from the pancreas. The most prominent characteristic, however, is intermittent unstable hypertension. Diastolic pressure may be greater than 115 mm Hg. If hypertension is uncontrolled, the client is at risk for stroke, vision changes, and organ damage. It is

---

pheochromocytoma: pheo—dark + chromo—color + cyt—cell + oma—tumor

estimated that about 0.1 percent of cases of hypertension are caused by a pheochromocytoma.

Diagnostic Tests

Clients with a suspected pheochromocytoma will have a 24-hour urine collection tested for metanephrines and vanillylmandelic acid (VMA). These are end products of catecholamine metabolism. The client should avoid caffeine and medications before the test. If results are elevated, a CT scan or MRI will be done to locate the tumor.

Medical Treatment

Treatment for pheochromocytoma is surgical removal of one or both adrenal glands. However, the client must be stabilized before surgery. Alpha-blocking medications such as phentolamine (Regitine) or phenoxybenzamine (Dibenzyline) will dilate blood vessels to control acute hypertension. Beta-blocking medication may be added to block beta-adrenergic receptors in the heart and lungs, reducing other fight or flight symptoms.

Nursing Care

Clients with pheochromocytoma are at risk for very high blood pressure and related complications. The nurse monitors vital signs closely and reports increases in blood pressure or pulse.

Because of the unstable hypertension and constant fight or flight state, clients are often quite anxious. Stress may precipitate a hypertensive episode. The nurse should approach the client calmly and maintain a quiet environment. The nurse teaches the client how the medications will reduce the symptoms and the importance of avoiding foods and beverages containing caffeine.

If surgery is done to remove the adrenal glands, the client will need to take lifelong replacement corticosteroids.

ADRENOCORTICAL INSUFFICIENCY

Adrenocortical insufficiency (AI) is the insufficient production of the hormones of the adrenal cortex. Primary AI is called Addison's disease.

Pathophysiology

Adrenal insufficiency is associated with reduced levels of cortisol, aldosterone, or both hormones. A deficiency in androgens may exist but usually does not cause symptoms. In primary disease, ACTH levels may be elevated in an attempt to stimulate the adrenal cortex to synthesize more hormone. In secondary disease, deficient ACTH fails to stimulate adrenal steroid synthesis. In most cases, the adrenal glands are atrophied, small, and misshapen and are unable to produce adequate amounts of hormone.

Etiology

Addison's disease is thought to be autoimmune. That is, the gland destroys itself in response to conditions such as tuberculosis, fungal infection, AIDS-related infection, or metastatic cancer. It may also be associated with other autoimmune diseases, such as Hashimoto's thyroiditis. Adrenalectomy also results in adrenal insufficiency.

Secondary AI may be caused by dysfunction of the pituitary or hypothalamus. In addition, prolonged use of corticosteroid drugs may depress ACTH and corticotropin-releasing hormone production, which in turn reduces endogenous (produced by the body) steroids. A client receiving long-term corticosteroid therapy is particularly at risk for AI if the drugs are abruptly discontinued. Because the pituitary has been suppressed for a prolonged period of time, it may take up to a year before ACTH is produced normally again. Therefore, corticosteroid therapy should be slowly tapered, never abruptly discontinued.

Signs and Symptoms

The most significant sign of Addison's disease is hypotension. This is related to the lack of aldosterone. Remember that aldosterone causes sodium and water retention in the kidney and potassium loss. If aldosterone is deficient, sodium and water are lost, and hypotension and tachycardia result. Low cortisol levels cause hypoglycemia, weakness, fatigue, confusion, and psychosis. In primary AI, increased ACTH may cause hyperpigmentation of the skin, causing the client to have a tanned appearance. Anorexia, nausea, and vomiting may also occur, possibly due to electrolyte imbalances.

Complications

If a client is exposed to stress, such as infection, trauma, or psychological stress, the body may be unable to respond normally with secretion of cortisol, and an adrenal crisis may occur. Loss of large amounts of sodium and water and the resulting fluid volume deficit cause profound hypotension, dehydration, and tachycardia. Potassium retention results in cardiac dysrhythmias. Hypoglycemia may be severe. Coma and death result if treatment is not initiated. Treatment of adrenal crisis involves rapidly restoring fluid volume and cortisol levels. Intravenous fluids, glucocorticoids, and mineralocorticoids are administered.

Diagnostic Tests

Serum and urine steroids are measured. These include cortisol, aldosterone, and 17-ketosteroids. Blood glucose is low. Blood urea nitrogen (BUN) and hematocrit may ap-

pear to be elevated due to dehydration. An ACTH stimulation test may help determine whether the adrenal glands are functioning. Serum sodium and potassium levels are monitored.

Medical Treatment

Treatment consists of replacement of glucocorticoids (hydrocortisone) and mineralocorticoids (fludrocortisone). Clients will need hormone replacement therapy for the rest of their lives. Hormones are given in divided doses, with two-thirds of the daily dose given in the morning and one-third in the evening to mimic the body's own diurnal rhythm. During times of stress or illness, doses need to be increased by two to three times the normal dose. The client may also be placed on a high-sodium diet.

Nursing Process

Assessment

The client with Addison's disease should be assessed for understanding of and compliance with the treatment regimen. Daily weights or intake and output help monitor fluid volume. Serum glucose levels and symptoms of hyperkalemia and hyponatremia are monitored. Changes in mental status are noted and reported. If the client is in crisis, vital signs should be monitored closely, and any signs of fluid volume deficit such as orthostatic hypotension or poor skin turgor should be reported to the physician immediately.

Nursing Diagnosis

Priority diagnoses include knowledge deficit related to self-care of Addison's disease and risk for fluid volume deficit.

Planning and Implementation

Nursing actions for the client with adrenal insufficiency primarily involve assessment and education. The nurse notifies the physician if symptoms of fluid volume deficit occur.

Client Education

The nurse teaches the client the importance of hormone replacement. The need to increase medication dosage during stressful times according to the physician's instructions is explained. The nurse helps the client identify his or her causes and symptoms of stress. Medic Alert identification is recommended. If ordered by the physician, the client and significant other are taught how to use an emergency intramuscular hydrocortisone injection kit.

Evaluation

The client and family should be able to describe proper self-care of Addison's disease. If the plan is successful, complications will be prevented, or recognized and reported promptly.

CUSHING'S SYNDROME

Cushing's *disease* is characterized by excess cortisol secretion resulting from secretion of too much adrenocorticotropic hormone (ACTH) by the pituitary. Cushing's *syndrome* refers to symptoms of cortisol excess caused by other factors. See Table 37–8 for a comparison of adrenal insufficiency and Cushing's syndrome.

Pathophysiology

Recall that cortisol, aldosterone, and androgens are the three steroid hormones secreted by the adrenal cortex. Cortisol is essential for survival and is normally secreted in a diurnal rhythm, with levels increasing in the early morning. Secretion is increased during times of stress. In Cushing's syndrome, cortisol is hypersecreted without regard to stress or time of day. When levels of cortisol are very high, effects related to excess aldosterone and androgens are also seen.

LEARNING TIP

An easy way to remember the hormones of the adrenal cortex is to remember "salt, sugar, and sex." Aldosterone promotes salt retention, cortisol affects sugar (carbohydrate) metabolism, and androgens are sex hormones.

Table 37–8. **Comparison of Adrenal Cortex Hormone Imbalances**

	Hypofunction	Hyperfunction
Disorder	Adrenocortical insufficiency, Addison's disease	Cushing's syndrome
Signs and Symptoms	Sodium and water loss, hypotension, hypoglycemia, fatigue	Weight gain, sodium and water retention, hyperglycemia, buffalo hump, moon face
Usual Treatment	Glucocorticoid and mineralocorticoid replacement	Alter steroid therapy schedule; surgery if tumor
Priority Nursing Diagnoses	Risk for fluid volume deficit	Risks for fluid volume excess, glucose intolerance, infection

Etiology

Cushing's disease is caused by the hypersecretion of ACTH by the pituitary. This is most often the result of a pituitary adenoma. Sometimes ACTH is produced by a tumor in the lungs or other organs. The high levels of ACTH cause adrenal hyperplasia, which in turn increases production and release of cortisol.

The most common cause of Cushing's syndrome is prolonged use of glucocorticoid medication for chronic inflammatory disorders such as rheumatoid arthritis, chronic obstructive pulmonary disease, and Crohn's disease.

Signs and Symptoms

Most signs and symptoms of Cushing's syndrome are related to excess cortisol levels. Weight gain, truncal obesity with thin arms and legs, buffalo hump, and moon face result from deposits of adipose tissue at these sites (Fig. 37–8). Cortisol also causes insulin resistance and stimulates gluconeogenesis, which result in glucose intolerance. Some clients develop secondary diabetes. Muscle wasting and thin skin with purple striae occur due to cortisol's catabolic effect on tissues. Catabolic effects on bone lead to osteoporosis, pathologic fractures, and back pain. Because cortisol has anti-inflammatory and immunosuppressive actions, the client is at risk for infection. Hyperpigmentation of the skin may occur. Approximately 50 percent of clients experience mental status changes, from irritability to psychosis (sometimes referred to as steroid psychosis). Sodium and water retention are related to the mineralocorticoid effect. As sodium is retained, potassium is lost in the urine, causing hypokalemia. (See Chapter 5 to review these electrolyte imbalances.) Androgen effects include acne, growth of facial hair, and amenorrhea in women.

Diagnostic Tests

Suspicion of Cushing's syndrome may initially be based on a cushingoid appearance. Plasma and urine cortisol and plasma ACTH are measured. A dexamethasone suppression test may be done.

Medical Treatment

If a pituitary or other ACTH-secreting tumor is present, surgical removal or radiation therapy to the pituitary may be employed. If the adrenals are the primary cause of the problem, radiation or removal of the adrenal gland or glands may be performed. Drugs such as ketoconazole will block production of adrenal steroids.

If the cause of Cushing's syndrome is administration of steroid medication, an every-other-day schedule or once-a-day dosing in the morning may reduce side effects. Often steroids are prescribed as a last resort for chronic disorders that are unresponsive to other treatment. The client and

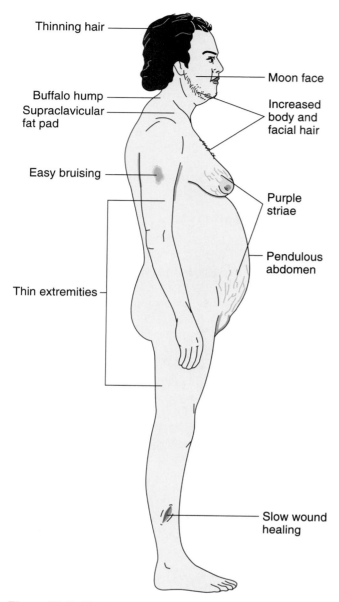

Thinning hair

Buffalo hump

Supraclavicular
fat pad

Easy bruising

Thin extremities

Moon face

Increased
body and
facial hair

Purple
striae

Pendulous
abdomen

Slow wound
healing

Figure 37–8. Physical manifestations seen in Cushing's syndrome.

physician must weigh the risks and benefits of continuing the medication.

Nursing Process

Assessment

The nurse caring for the client with Cushing's disease or syndrome should assess the client's drug history. Vital signs and complications related to fluid and sodium excess are monitored. The lungs are auscultated for crackles, and extremities are assessed for edema. Skin integrity is assessed, and capillary glucose is monitored as ordered by the physician. Signs of infection are monitored.

Nursing Diagnosis

Possible diagnoses include fluid volume excess related to sodium and water retention, risk for impaired skin integrity, risk for infection, and risk for impaired glucose tolerance. Body image disturbance is common due to the cushingoid appearance.

Planning and Implementation

Signs of fluid overload should be reported to the physician. Care should be taken to protect the skin. The client should be protected from infection and instructed to avoid others who are ill. The nurse and other health care workers should use good hand-washing technique. If glucose intolerance occurs, the nurse is prepared to administer insulin, because oral hypoglycemics are not usually effective. If the client is to be on long-term insulin, he or she should be referred to diabetes education classes. A dietitian is consulted for diet counseling.

If surgery is planned, the client is prepared for an adrenalectomy or hypophysectomy, depending on the cause of the disorder.

Evaluation

Complications of fluid overload are recognized and treated early. The skin is intact. The client is free from signs of infection. The client demonstrates skill in self-care of diabetes if indicated.

Nursing Care of the Client Undergoing Adrenalectomy

Preoperative Care

The nurse monitors the client for electrolyte imbalance and hyperglycemia. Abnormalities must be corrected before surgery. To prevent adrenal crisis, glucocorticoids are administered, because removal of the adrenals will cause a sudden drop in adrenal hormones.

Postoperative Care

Following surgery, the client receives routine postoperative care. In addition, the client is closely monitored for changes in fluid and electrolyte balance and adrenal crisis. If a bilateral adrenalectomy is done, the client must take replacement glucocorticoid and mineralocorticoid hormones for the remainder of his or her life. If only one adrenal gland is removed, the remaining gland should eventually produce enough hormone to enable the client to discontinue replacement hormone.

See Table 37–9 for a summary of endocrine disorders.

 CRITICAL THINKING: Mrs. Tercini

Mrs. Tercini is a 62-year-old woman admitted to your unit in addisonian crisis. She is lethargic, with a

Table 37–9. **Summary of Endocrine Problems**

Hormone	Hypofunction	Hyperfunction
Antidiuretic hormone	Diabetes insipidus—water loss	SIADH—water retention
Growth hormone	Dwarfism—short stature	Acromegaly, gigantism—bone and tissue overgrowth
Thyroid hormone	Hypothyroidism—slow metabolism	Hyperthyroidism—increased metabolism
Epinephrine	Rare	Pheochromocytoma—hypertension
Parathyroid hormone	Hypoparathyroidism—low serum calcium, osteoporosis, tetany	Hyperparathyroidism—high calcium, weakness
Cortisol	Addison's disease—sodium and water loss	Cushing's syndrome—sodium and water retention, hyperglycemia; see text

blood pressure of 86/58, pulse 112, and respirations 18. While interviewing her daughter, you learn that Mrs. Tercini has a history of Cushing's syndrome treated with bilateral adrenalectomy 25 years ago. She has been taking fludrocortisone (Florinef) 100 μg and hydrocortisone 200 mg daily ever since. Three days ago she developed the flu.

1. Why is an adrenalectomy done to treat Cushing's syndrome?
2. What is the most effective schedule for Mrs. Tercini's medication?
3. What precipitated this addisonian crisis?
4. Why is Mrs. Tercini's blood pressure low?
5. How could this crisis have been prevented?

Answers at end of chapter.

Review Questions

1. When assessing a client with diabetes insipidus, which of the following findings is expected?
   a. Edema
   b. Polyuria
   c. Heat intolerance
   d. Diarrhea

2. Which of the following expected outcomes is most appropriate for the client with SIADH?
   a. Client will verbalize relief from excessive thirst.
   b. Client will verbalize understanding of importance of increasing fluid intake.
   c. Client's daily weights will be stable.
   d. Client will state pain is relieved.

3. Which action by the nurse is most important following hypophysectomy?
   a. Routine neurological assessment
   b. Encouraging the client to cough and deep breathe
   c. Monitoring for tracheal edema
   d. Strict intake and output

4. Which of the following statements by the client with hypothyroidism indicates to the nurse that the plan of care has been effective?
   a. "I feel so much better now that my energy is returning."
   b. "I'm really glad the diarrhea has stopped."
   c. "I'm so glad I won't have to take medication for very long."
   d. "My fingers aren't tingling any more."

5. Which of the following nursing assessments is most important in the client with hyperthyroidism and risk for thyrotoxic crisis?
   a. Intake and output q2h
   b. Client's understanding of dietary restrictions
   c. Bowel sounds each shift
   d. Frequent vital signs

6. Following a total thyroidectomy, which of the following instructions from the physician will the nurse reinforce?
   a. "You will be taking thyroid replacement hormone for the rest of your life."
   b. "You must weigh yourself daily and report any gain or loss of more than one pound."
   c. "You will need to return to the physician's office for a weekly blood pressure check."
   d. "You will need to restrict your sodium and potassium intake."

7. Which of the following nursing interventions will be most helpful for the client with acute hypertension related to pheochromocytoma?
   a. Offer the client pain medication every 4 hours.
   b. Provide a calm, quiet environment.
   c. Assist the client to elevate the legs.
   d. Encourage increased fluid intake.

8. Which of the following nursing diagnoses is most appropriate for the client with classic symptoms of Cushing's syndrome?
   a. Altered comfort related to heat intolerance
   b. Ineffective airway clearance related to excessive secretions

c. Body image disturbance related to physical changes
d. Constipation related to slowed peristalsis

ANSWERS TO CRITICAL THINKING

CRITICAL THINKING: Adoption

The children's growth hormone secretion was probably suppressed due to psychosocial stress. Once they felt secure in a loving environment, growth hormone levels returned to normal.

CRITICAL THINKING: Mae

1. Mae's TSH is elevated because her pituitary gland is working overtime to try to stimulate the underactive thyroid gland.
2. Mae's metabolism has been slow, so she has been burning fewer calories. When she starts on thyroid replacement hormone, her metabolic rate will return to normal and she will need more calories. Intake of calories should be balanced with the possible need for weight loss.
3. If Mae receives too much thyroid hormone, she will have symptoms of hyperthyroidism, including an increased pulse rate. She should know how to check her pulse and to call her physician if it is elevated.

CRITICAL THINKING: Mrs. Tercini

1. Cushing's syndrome is caused by too much cortisol. The adrenal cortex is responsible for secreting cortisol.
2. Mrs. Tercini should take two-thirds of her daily dose of hydrocortisone and fludrocortisone in the morning and one-third in the evening. This most closely mimics the body's natural corticosteroid secretion.
3. The flu probably triggered this crisis. Illness is a stressor, and normally the body secretes steroids during stress. Because Mrs. Tercini's body is un-able to produce steroids, she experiences symptoms of hypoadrenalism during stressful times.
4. Mrs. Tercini's blood pressure is low because she has insufficient circulating mineralocorticoids. Without aldosterone, sodium and water are lost and blood pressure drops.
5. Mrs. Tercini should have taken extra medication when she became ill.

REFERENCES

McKusick, V, et al: Dwarfism in the Amish. II. Cartilage hair hypoplasia. Bull Johns Hopkins Hosp 116:285, 1965.

Jankowski, CB: Irradiating the thyroid: How to protect yourself and others. Am J Nurs 96:51, 1996.

BIBLIOGRAPHY

Ackley, BJ, and Ladwig, GB: Nursing Diagnosis Handbook: A Guide to Planning Care. Mosby, St Louis, 1995.

Batcheller, J: Disorders of antidiuretic hormone secretion. AACN 3:2, 1992.

Bianco, CM: Diabetes insipidus. Am J Nurs 96:8, 1996.

Deglin, JH, and Vallerand, AH: Davis's Drug Guide for Nurses, ed 4. FA Davis, Philadelphia, 1995.

Hart, JJ: Pheochromocytoma. Am Fam Physician 42:1, 1990.

Isselbacher, KJ, et al: Harrison's Principles of Internal Medicine. McGraw-Hill, New York, 1994, p 2151.

Kessler, CA: An overview of endocrine function and dysfunction. AACN 3:2, 1992.

Lee, L, and Gumowski, J: Adrenocortical insufficiency: A medical emergency. AACN 3:2, 1992.

Lutz, CA, and Przytulski, KR: Nutrition and Diet Therapy. FA Davis, Philadelphia, 1997.

McCance, KL, and Huether, SE: Pathophysiology: The Biologic Basis for Disease in Adults and Children, ed 2. Mosby, St Louis, 1994.

McMorrow, ME: Myxedema coma. Am J Nurs 96:10, 1996.

Patterson, L, and Noroian, E: Diabetes insipidus versus syndrome of inappropriate antidiuretic hormone. Dimen Crit Care Nurs 8:4, 1989.

Spittle, L: Diagnoses in opposition: Thyroid storm and myxedema coma. AACN 3:2, 1992.

Wason, J, and Jaffe, MS: Nurse's Manual of Laboratory and Diagnostic Tests, ed 2. FA Davis, Philadelphia, 1995.

38

Nursing Care of Clients with Disorders of the Endocrine Pancreas

Paula D. Hopper

Learning Objectives

Upon completion of this chapter, the student will be able to:

1. Define diabetes mellitus.
2. Explain the causes, risk factors, and pathophysiology of diabetes mellitus.
3. Differentiate among five types of glucose intolerance.
4. Identify the signs and symptoms of diabetes mellitus and related complications.
5. Describe the diagnostic tests and values used in identifying diabetes mellitus and its complications.
6. Discuss treatment of diabetes mellitus, including diet, exercise, and medication.
7. Provide instruction in survival skills for the client with diabetes mellitus.
8. Describe causes, prevention, and treatment of complications of diabetes mellitus.
9. Use the nursing process to plan care for a client with diabetes mellitus.
10. Discuss care of the client with diabetes mellitus who is undergoing surgery.
11. Define reactive hypoglycemia.
12. Discuss diagnosis and treatment of reactive hypoglycemia.

Key Words

diabetes mellitus (DYE-ah-**BEE**-tis mel-**LYE**-tus)
endogenous (en-**DAH**-jen-us)
gastroparesis (GAS-troh-puh-**REE**-sus)
glycosuria (GLY-kos-**YOO**-ree-ah)
hyperglycemia (HIGH-per-gligh-**SEE**-mee-ah)
hypoglycemia (HIGH-poh-gligh-**SEE**-mee-ah)
ketoacidosis (KEE-toh-ass-i-**DOH**-sis)
Kussmaul's (**KOOS**-mahlz)
nephropathy (ne-**FROP**-uh-thee)
neuropathy (new-**RAH**-puh-thee)

nocturia (nock-**TYOO**-ree-ah)
polydipsia (PAH-lee-**DIP**-see-ah)
polyphagia (PAH-lee-**FAY**-jee-ah)
polyuria (PAH-lee-**YOO**-ree-ah)
retinopathy (RET-i-**NAH**-puh-thee)

Diabetes Mellitus

Diabetes mellitus is a chronic disease of carbohydrate metabolism and, to a lesser degree, fat and protein metabolism. It is characterized by **hyperglycemia** and **glycosuria,** resulting from inadequate production or utilization of insulin. Approximately 8 million people in the United States have been diagnosed with diabetes mellitus. It is estimated that another 8 million have undiagnosed diabetes.[1]

The incidence of diabetes mellitus varies by race and ethnicity. (See Cultural Considerations Box 38–1.)

PATHOPHYSIOLOGY

Body tissues, and the cells that compose them, use glucose for energy. Glucose is a simple sugar provided by foods that are eaten. When carbohydrates are eaten they are broken down into glucose, which is then absorbed into the bloodstream. Carbohydrates provide most of the glucose used by the body; proteins and fats provide smaller amounts of glucose. Glucose is able to enter the cells only with the help of insulin, a hormone produced by the beta cells in the islets of Langerhans of the pancreas (Fig. 38–1). When insulin comes in contact with the cell membrane, it combines with a receptor that allows activation of special glucose transporters in the membrane.

By helping glucose enter the body cells, insulin lowers the blood glucose level. Insulin also helps the body to store excess glucose in the liver, in the form of glycogen. Another hormone, glucagon, is produced by the alpha cells in the islets of Langerhans. Glucagon raises the blood glucose when needed by releasing the stored glucose from the liver. Insulin and glucagon work together to keep the blood glucose at a constant level.

CULTURAL CONSIDERATIONS BOX 38–1

Race or Ethnicity	Prevalence of Diabetes Mellitus
Caucasian	6.2%
Cuban	9.3%
African-American	10.2%
Mexican-American	13.0%
Puerto Rican	13.4%
Japanese-American	13.9%
Pima Indians (Arizona)	27.5%
All Native-Americans	Higher than European-Americans

Source: Diabetes: 1991 Vital Statistics. American Diabetes Association, Alexandria, Va, 1991.

Diabetes results from faulty production of insulin by the beta cells in the pancreas or from inability of the body's cells to use insulin. When glucose is unable to enter body cells, hyperglycemia results.

TYPES AND CAUSES

Type 1 Diabetes Mellitus

Type 1 diabetes (formerly called insulin-dependent diabetes mellitus, or IDDM) is caused by destruction of the beta cells of the pancreas. When the beta cells are destroyed, the pancreas produces no insulin at all. Insulin must be injected in order for the body to use food for energy.

It is believed that the pancreas may attack itself following a viral infection. Almost 85 percent of clients newly diagnosed with type 1 diabetes have islet cell antibodies in their blood. From 10 to 30 percent of type 1 diabetes cases are hereditary (Table 38–1). The client with type 1 diabetes is prone to develop **ketoacidosis** when blood glucose is elevated. When insufficient insulin is available to allow glucose to enter cells, the body breaks down fat to be used for energy. Fat breakdown releases an acid substance called ketones. The buildup of these acids in the blood causes ketoacidosis.

Type 2 Diabetes Mellitus

In type 2 diabetes mellitus (formerly called non-insulin-dependent diabetes mellitus, or NIDDM), some insulin is still made by the pancreas, but in inadequate amounts. Sometimes, the amount of insulin is normal or even high, but the tissues are resistant to it, and hyperglycemia results.

Heredity is responsible for up to 90 percent of cases of type 2 diabetes. Obesity is also a major contributing factor. Often the client with a new diagnosis of type 2 diabetes is obese, relates a family history of diabetes, and has had a recent life stressor such as the death of a family member, illness, or loss of a job. Clients with type 2 diabetes are not prone to developing ketoacidosis, because they usually have some insulin available.

Gestational Diabetes

Gestational diabetes mellitus (GDM) may develop during pregnancy. Gestational diabetes may occur in a woman with the risk factors for type 2 diabetes. The extra metabolic demands of pregnancy trigger the onset of diabetes. Blood glucose usually returns to normal after delivery, but

---

diabetes: passing through

hyperglycemia: hyper—excessive + glyc—glucose + emia—in the blood

glycosuria: glyc—glucose + uria—urine

ketoacidosis: keto—ketones + acid—acidic + osis—condition

A

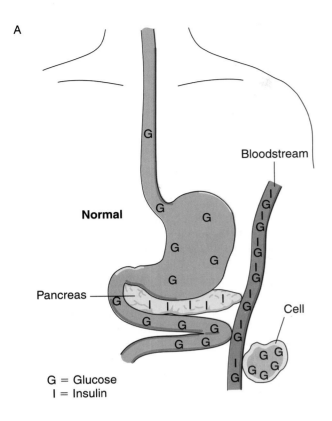

Normal

Pancreas

Bloodstream

Cell

G = Glucose
I = Insulin

B

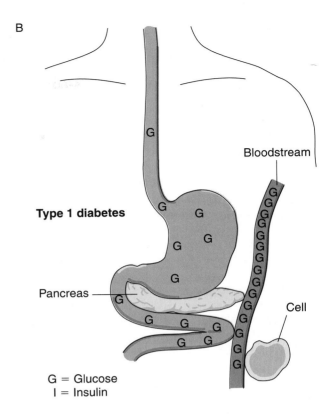

Type 1 diabetes

Pancreas

Bloodstream

Cell

G = Glucose
I = Insulin

C

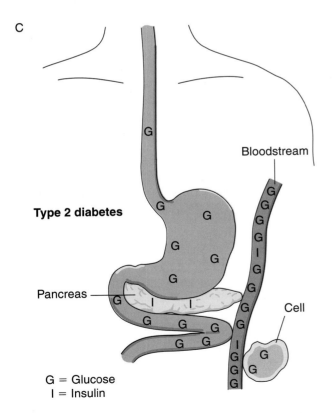

Type 2 diabetes

Pancreas

Bloodstream

Cell

G = Glucose
I = Insulin

Figure 38–1. Maintenance of blood glucose levels. *(A)* Normal physiology: Foods (especially carbohydrates) are broken down into glucose, which is absorbed into the bloodstream for transport to the cells. Insulin, produced by the beta cells of the islets of Langerhans in the pancreas, is needed to "open the door" to the cell, allowing the glucose to enter. *(B)* In type 1 diabetes mellitus, the pancreas does not produce insulin. Because glucose is unable to enter the cells, it builds up in the blood stream, causing hyperglycemia. *(C)* In type 2 diabetes mellitus, insulin production is reduced. Less glucose enters the cell, and hyperglycemia results. In some cases there is enough insulin, but cells are resistant to it.

Table 38–1. *Comparison of Type 1 and Type 2 Diabetes*

	Type 1 (IDDM)	Type 2 (NIDDM)
Onset	Rapid	Slow
Age at onset	Usually < 40	Usually > 40
Risk factors	Virus, autoimmune response, heredity	Heredity, obesity
Body type	Lean	Obese
High blood glucose complication	Ketoacidosis	Hyperosmolar Hyperglycemic Nonketotic syndrome
Treatment	Diet, exercise; must have insulin to survive	Diet, exercise; may need oral hypoglycemics or insulin to control blood glucose level

the mother will have an increased risk for type 2 diabetes in the future. If she is overweight, she should be counseled that weight loss will decrease her risk of developing diabetes. Mothers with GDM require specialized care and should be referred to an expert in this area.

Secondary Diabetes

Secondary diabetes may develop due to another chronic illness such as pancreatitis or cystic fibrosis. It is not true diabetes mellitus, because blood glucose levels usually return to normal when the cause is corrected. Prolonged use of some drugs, most commonly steroids, may also cause secondary diabetes.

Impaired Glucose Tolerance

Impaired glucose tolerance (IGT) is diagnosed when blood glucose levels are above normal but do not meet criteria to diagnose diabetes.

SIGNS AND SYMPTOMS

Classic symptoms of diabetes mellitus include the three P's: **polydipsia** (excessive thirst), **polyuria** (excessive urination), and **polyphagia** (excessive hunger). Because glucose is unable to enter the cells, the cells starve, causing hunger. The large amount of glucose in the blood causes an increase in serum concentration, or osmolality. The renal tubules are unable to reabsorb all the excess glucose that is filtered by the glomeruli, and glycosuria results. Large amounts of body water are required to excrete this glucose, causing polyuria, **nocturia,** and dehydration. The increased osmolality and dehydration cause polydipsia. High blood glucose may also cause fatigue, blurred vision, abdominal pain, and headaches. Ketones may build up in the blood and urine of clients with type 1 diabetes.

DIAGNOSTIC TESTS

Diagnosis is based on blood glucose levels measured by a laboratory. A normal blood glucose level ranges from 60 to 115 mg/dL, although different labs may have slightly different normal values. When the fasting blood glucose (drawn after at least 4 hours without eating) is above 126 mg/dL on two separate occasions, diabetes is diagnosed. Another test to diagnose diabetes is the glucose tolerance test (GTT). A GTT measures blood glucose at intervals after the client drinks a concentrated carbohydrate drink. Diabetes is diagnosed when any two measurements are above 200 mg/dL.

Another useful blood test is the glycohemoglobin test, or HbA1$_c$. Glucose in the blood attaches to hemoglobin in the red blood cells. Red blood cells live about 3 months in the body. When the glucose that is attached to the hemoglobin is measured, it gives an average blood glucose level for the previous 3 months. Results should be from 4 to 7 percent. This is a helpful measurement when blood glucose levels fluctuate and a single measurement would be misleading. It may also assist in determining the degree to which a client is following prescribed treatment.

 CRITICAL THINKING: Mr. McMillan

Mr. McMillan is a 50-year-old client brought into the emergency department with extreme fatigue and dehydration. After the physician sees him, the nurse asks Mr. McMillan some additional questions. Based on the client's answers, the nurse requests that the physician add a glucose level to the lab work. The result is 1400 mg/dL.

1. What questions did the nurse most likely ask?
2. Why was Mr. McMillan fatigued?
3. Why was he dehydrated?

Answers at end of chapter.

TREATMENT

The only cure for diabetes is a pancreas transplant. However, diabetes can be controlled. Treatment begins with diet and exercise. Insulin or oral medication is added as needed. Blood glucose monitoring and education are also important to good diabetes control.

Type 2 diabetes can be prevented or delayed in some cases. In clients with a family history of diabetes, a healthy diet and maintenance of normal weight are advised, along with regular blood glucose screening.

---

polydipsia: poly—many or much + dipsia—thirst
polyuria: poly—many or much + uria—urine
polyphagia: poly—many or much + phagia—to eat
nocturia: noc—by night + uria—urine

NUTRITION NOTES BOX 38-2

Diabetes Mellitus

CARBOHYDRATE REQUIREMENTS. Complex carbohydrates should supply 55 to 60 percent of the day's calories; they are also excellent sources of dietary fiber. Water-soluble fibers found in fruits, oats, barley, and legumes may influence glucose and insulin levels by smoothing out the postprandial glucose curve; they may also help lower plasma lipid levels. About 5 percent of the total carbohydrates may be derived from simple carbohydrates (simple sugars, fruits, some starches, and milk). Foods containing equal amounts of carbohydrate affect blood glucose levels differently. Classification of foods according to this effect is called the glycemic index. Glucose has a high glycemic index, honey has a low glycemic index, and sucrose falls somewhere in between. White bread, potatoes, and corn flakes all have a higher glycemic index than sucrose. Because most meals contain a combination of nutrients, the glycemic index is rarely used in clinical practice except with highly motivated and educated clients.

PROTEIN REQUIREMENTS. The diet should contain 0.8 grams of protein per kilogram of body weight per day; approximately 12 to 20 percent of total calories.

FAT REQUIREMENTS. The diet should contain less than 30 percent of total kilocalories evenly distributed as polyunsaturated, saturated, and monounsaturated fats; cholesterol should be kept to under 300 mg per day.

FOOD AND EXERCISE. Clients with IDDM who exercise and those with NIDDM who engage in nonroutine exercise should monitor their blood glucose levels before, during, and after exercise. If the blood glucose level is greater than 100 milligrams per deciliter and the planned exercise is of short duration and low intensity, usually no additional food is needed. Exercise of long duration and high intensity will generally require more calories. Good choices for exercise snack foods include fruit, starch, and milk exchanges. Exercise is best scheduled 60 to 90 minutes after meals, when the blood glucose level is highest.

APPROACHES TO MEAL PLANNING. Up to 11 different meal planning approaches are available from the American Dietetic Association and the American Diabetes Association. The health educator can select an approach to match the client's interest, motivation, and abilities.

Diet

Because the client with diabetes has a limited amount of insulin, either **endogenous** (from within the body) or injected, it is important to eat an amount of food that will not exceed the insulin's ability to carry it into the cells. The diet should include consistent amounts of carbohydrates, proteins, and fats each day. (See Nutrition Notes Box 38–2.) If a client eats a small amount one day and a large amount the next, the blood glucose will fluctuate, leading to complications. With the more recent availability of blood glucose monitoring at home, it is possible to relax diet restrictions somewhat if the client is willing to test blood glucose frequently and adjust treatment accordingly. This requires in-depth instruction by a diabetes educator or physician.

A variety of diets are available to help control blood glucose, including high-fiber diets, calorie-counting methods, and exchange plans. The nurse should consult a dietitian to assist the client in choosing and learning to follow a diet. Because diabetes increases the risk of high serum cholesterol and triglycerides, all diets limit fat intake. Most diets also encourage the use of complex carbohydrates such as grains, pastas, vegetables, and fruits. Simple sugars, which may cause the blood glucose to rise more rapidly, are limited. The diet should be chosen to fit the client's lifestyle and food preferences. The most commonly prescribed diet is the American Diabetes Association (ADA) diet (Table 38–2). Preferences of ethnic groups should also be considered (Cultural Considerations Box 38–3).

The ADA diet uses a meal plan that is healthy for anyone, so the person with diabetes need not eat meals that are different from the rest of his or her family. The only difference is that portion sizes are measured. The term *meal plan* is often used, because it does not sound as restricting as the word *diet*. The physician, in collaboration with the dietitian, determines the number of calories the client needs each day. The meal plan, based on the chosen calorie amount, prescribes a number of servings from each of the five food groups for each meal, and food choices may be made within each of the food groups.

Exercise

Exercise is an important factor in controlling blood glucose and lipid levels. Exercise lowers blood glucose, both immediately and for approximately 24 hours after the exercise. Insulin is not needed for glucose to enter exercising muscle cells. Exercise also improves blood lipid levels and circulation, which are important for the person with diabetes. Clients are instructed to exercise on a regular basis to keep blood glucose levels stable. A physician or exercise physiologist should be consulted for an individualized exercise plan.

Persons with diabetes should always carry a quick source of sugar when exercising, in case the blood glucose drops too low. They should also be taught to avoid exercising at the time of day when their blood glucose is at its

---

endogenous: endo—within + genous—to produce

Table 38–2. *Sample 1800-Calorie Diabetic Diet*

1800-Cal Meal Plan

	Breakfast	Lunch	Dinner	Hour of Sleep
Milk	1	1	1	
Bread/starch	2	2	2	1
Fruit	1	1	1	
Vegetable		1	1	
Meat	2	2	2	1
Fat	2	2	1	1

Exchange List Examples

Milk Exchange	Amount/Serving
Milk (skim)	1 cup
Milk (2%)	1 cup
Yogurt (plain, low fat)	1 cup

Fruit/Juice Exchange	Amount/Serving
Orange juice	½ cup
Banana	½
Cherries	10 large

Meat/Protein Exchange	Amount/Serving
Egg	1
Poultry	1 oz
Frankfurter	1

Vegetable Exchange	Amount/Serving
Green beans (plain)	1 cup
Mushrooms (plain)	1 cup
Tomato juice	½ cup

Bread/Starch Exchange	Amount/Serving
Hamburger bun (large)	½
Cooked cereal	½ cup
Corn	⅓

Fat Exchange	Amount/Serving
Mayonnaise	1 tsp
Bacon	1 strip
Butter	1 tsp

The exchange lists are based on material in the *Exchange Lists for Meal Planning* prepared by committees of the American Diabetes Association, Inc, and the American Dietetic Association in cooperation with the National Institute of Arthritis, Metabolism, and Digestive Diseases and the National Heart and Lung Institute, National Institutes of Health, Public Health Service, U.S. Department of Health, Education and Welfare. Used with permission.
Source: Adapted from Lutz, CA, and Przytulski, KR: Nutrition and Diet Therapy, ed 2. FA Davis, Philadelphia, 1994, p 508.

CULTURAL CONSIDERATIONS BOX 38–3

The Diabetic Diet

The diabetic diet for ethnic individuals may need a significant adjustment from the American menu. An exchange list of foods for these clients will not be followed because their food choices are different. The client may be labeled noncompliant, when in reality the health care worker has been culturally insensitive.

The nurse can consult the American Diabetes Association in Washington, D.C. (1-800-342-2383) to obtain meal plans for ethnic individuals such as Asians, Hispanics, African-Americans, and Native-Americans.

---

sulin is available, glycogen may be released, further increasing the serum glucose.

Medication

The individual with type 1 diabetes has no endogenous insulin and therefore must inject insulin daily. Insulin cannot be taken by mouth, because it is a protein and is therefore digested. It is generally given subcutaneously, although it may be ordered via the intramuscular or intravenous route in urgent situations. There are several types of insulin and schedules by which it may be given. The type and schedule are determined by the physician, in collaboration with the client, based on his or her lifestyle and willingness to spend time on injections. In general, the more frequent the injections, the better the glucose control.

Insulin injections should be given in a different subcutaneous site each time, to avoid injury to the tissues. A sample rotation chart is shown in Figure 38–2. Because each area absorbs insulin at a slightly different rate, it is advisable to use one area for a week, then move on to the next area. Within that area, each injection should be spaced at least 1 inch from the previous injection. Some experts recommend using only the abdomen in order to provide more uniform absorption.

Most insulin is now synthetically produced in a laboratory and is identical to human insulin. Some clients may still use insulin from beef or pork sources. It is important that the physician include the insulin source in the prescription. The nurse must be careful to check the source when preparing insulin for injection, because insulins from different sources may act slightly differently. Some individuals may be allergic to beef or pork preparations. (See Cultural Considerations Box 38–4.)

Once insulin is injected, a period of time elapses before it begins to lower blood glucose. This time period is called the onset of action. The peak action time occurs when the insulin is working at its hardest and the blood glucose is at its lowest point. It is during this peak time that the client is

lowest point, and to have a protein and carbohydrate snack before exercising if low blood glucose is a problem.

Clients should be cautioned to avoid exercise when their glucose level is at or above 300 mg/dL. If insufficient in-

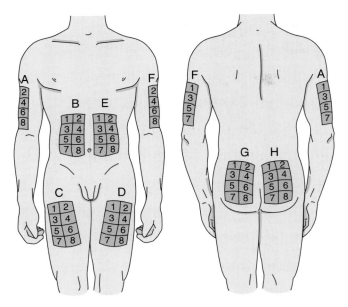

Rotation sites for injection of insulin.

Figure 38–2. Sample insulin rotation chart.

most at risk for an episode of low blood glucose. Duration is the length of time the insulin works before it is used up. Onset, peak, and duration are determined by whether the insulin is short, intermediate, or long-acting (Table 38–3).

It is important for the individual with diabetes and the nurse to be aware of the onset, peak, and duration of any insulin given. This assists in making decisions such as when to exercise and when to be alert to low blood glucose symptoms.

LEARNING TIP

The "Evens and Odds" Rule. To remember the onset, peak, and duration of intermediate-acting insulin, think "evens"—2, 12, and 24 hours. To remember short-acting insulin, think "odds"—1, 3, and 5 hours. These times are not exact, but they are a great memory booster when you need to think fast.

In the past, most clients with diabetes used an injection of an intermediate-acting insulin before breakfast, and possibly a second injection before supper. More clients are now choosing to take more frequent injections of short-acting insulin or a combination of short- and intermediate-acting insulins (Table 38–4) in order to achieve better control. Preset mixtures of intermediate-acting and short-acting insulins are available for clients who have difficulty learning to mix insulins. During times of stress or hospitalization, some clients are placed on sliding scale insulin. This

---

hypoglycemia: hypo—deficient + glyc—glucose + emia—in the blood

---

involves determining the dose of regular (short-acting) insulin based on blood glucose results, usually before meals and at bedtime.

LEARNING TIP

When mixing insulin, remember "clear to cloudy." Always draw up the clear insulin first. This involves injecting air into the cloudy vial first. This is because if the clear is drawn up last, the vial may be contaminated by the cloudy insulin. If cloudy insulin is unknowingly contaminated by clear insulin, the clear will be absorbed and the effect minimal.

The client with type 2 diabetes may be able to control blood glucose levels with diet and exercise alone. If this is not possible, insulin or oral hypoglycemic medication may be prescribed. Oral hypoglycemics are not insulin pills. Many new oral hypoglycemic agents have recently been developed (Table 38–5). Because most oral hypoglycemics depend on at least a partially functioning pancreas, they are not useful for clients with type 1 diabetes.

Older oral hypoglycemic agents, called first-generation drugs, have more side effects, including increased risk of death from cardiovascular disease. Second-generation drugs are more potent and have fewer side effects. A drug approved in late 1994 in the United States is metformin (Glucophage). Metformin increases tissue sensitivity to insulin and suppresses glucose production in the liver, but it does not stimulate insulin release. It therefore reduces blood glucose without risk of **hypoglycemia.** A common side effect of metformin is anorexia, which contributes to weight loss. This may be a desirable effect for many clients, if the anorexia is mild.

Insulin and most oral hypoglycemics should be administered 30 minutes before meals. This allows absorption of the medication before eating. However, care should be taken to prevent passage of more than 30 minutes between medication administration and the meal, because this may result in a hypoglycemic episode.

If blood glucose levels are not controlled with oral hypoglycemic agents, insulin may be necessary for the person with type 2 diabetes. This does *not* mean the person has

Table 38–3. **Onset, Peak, and Duration of Insulins**

	Examples	Onset	Peak	Duration
Very Short Acting	Lispro	15 min	30–90 min	≤5 h
Short Acting	Regular, Semilente	½–1 h	2–5 h	5–8 h
Intermediate Acting	NPH, Lente	1–3 h	6–12 h	18–26 h
Long Acting	Ultralente	4–6 h	14–24 h	26–36 h

type 1 diabetes. Insulin may be necessary to control blood glucose, but it is not necessary to sustain life, as it is for the person with type 1 diabetes.

CRITICAL THINKING: Mrs. Evans

Mrs. Evans is a 60-year-old woman with type 2 diabetes. She is on Lente Insulin every morning.

1. If Mrs. Evans eats her breakfast at 8:00 every morning, what time should she take her insulin?
2. At what time of day should she be alert for symptoms of low blood sugar?

Answers at end of chapter.

Blood and Urine Glucose Monitoring

The ability to test blood glucose levels at home has been a major advance in diabetes care. Blood glucose can be better controlled because of the availability of monitoring at any time, in any place. A variety of blood glucose monitors are on the market at a reasonable price (Fig. 38–3). Most of the cost involved in monitoring is in the test strips that

Table 38–4. **How to Mix Insulin**

1. Assemble equipment: insulins, syringe (be sure it is large enough to hold the entire insulin dose), alcohol swab, physician's order.
2. Check physician's order to confirm correct insulin types and doses of regular (clear) and an intermediate-acting (cloudy) insulin.
3. Roll the bottle of cloudy insulin to mix. Do not shake, because this will cause bubbles.
4. Wipe tops of both vials with alcohol swab.
5. Draw up and inject an amount of air equal to the dose of intermediate-acting insulin into the cloudy vial. Remove syringe from vial.
6. Draw up and inject an amount of air equal to the dose of short-acting insulin into the clear bottle. Leave syringe in vial.
7. Draw up the correct amount of clear insulin. Double-check amount with another nurse if this is the institution's policy.
8. Remove the syringe and insert into the cloudy vial. Carefully draw up the correct amount of insulin. If too much insulin is accidentally drawn into the syringe, the syringe must be discarded and the process repeated. Double-check again with another nurse.

must be used for each test. Health insurance programs will sometimes cover this cost.

Monitoring is generally done before meals and at bedtime for the individual on insulin who wishes to maintain tight control of blood glucose. Less frequent schedules may be prescribed for clients who are unable or unwilling to test four times a day, or for clients not on insulin. Some may test before breakfast and supper, and some may vary testing times from day to day. A few clients who are unable to test at home may have routine laboratory tests done.

The physician should be consulted for desirable blood glucose ranges, because these may differ for each client. For example, a client whose type 2 diabetes is controlled by diet alone may have a goal of 80 to 120 mg/dL. A client who is prone to insulin reactions (hypoglycemia) may have a goal range of 100 to 150 mg/dL. A lower blood glucose for this client may increase the risk of hypoglycemia.

Urine may also be tested for glucose and for ketones. Urine glucose testing was done routinely before the development of blood glucose self-monitoring. A variety of dipsticks and tape products are available for urine testing. When testing urine, the "second voided specimen" technique should be used if the client has not urinated for some time. For this technique, the client empties the bladder, then tests the urine as soon as he or she is able to void again. This avoids testing urine that has been in the bladder for a long period of time. If glucose appears in the urine, the client is warned that the blood glucose is elevated, but the actual level is unknown. It is difficult to base treatment on urine glucose levels.

Urine should be tested for ketones during acute illness or stress, when blood glucose levels are consistently above 300 mg/dL, during pregnancy, or when symptoms of ketoacidosis are present.[2] If ketones are present, the client knows an insulin deficiency is present and should notify the physician. Clients with type 1 diabetes are most at risk for developing ketoacidosis; however, it is wise for the client with type 2 diabetes to test for ketones if risk factors are present.

An important aspect of blood or urine monitoring is the interpretation of results. Monitoring is useless if the results are not used to improve blood glucose control. The client should be instructed to keep a diary of blood glucose levels. Some clients have computer software that graphs results. The client may be taught by a diabetes educator to interpret the trends in the results, or the diary may be taken

Table 38–5. **Oral Hypoglycemic Agents**

Generic Name	Trade Names	Action	Usual Dose	Nursing Considerations
		First-Generation Sulfonylureas		
Tolbutamide	Orinase	Increases insulin secretion	500–2000 mg/day	May cause weight gain; monitor for hypoglycemia
Chlorpropamide	Diabinese	Increases insulin receptor sensitivity	250–500 mg/day	Teach client to avoid alcohol
		Second-Generation Sulfonylureas		
Glipizide	Glucotrol	Increases insulin secretion	2.5–40 mg/day	May cause weight gain; monitor for hypoglycemia
Glyburide	Micronase	Increases insulin receptor sensitivity	2.5–5 mg/day	Teach client to avoid alcohol
	Diabeta Glynase Pres-Tabs		1.5–3 mg/day	
		Other Agents		
Metformin	Glucophage	Increases insulin-stimulated glucose transport in skeletal muscle; reduces production of glucose by liver	500 mg–2.5 g/day	Does not cause hypoglycemia; may cause GI side effects; may enhance weight loss; withhold if client having tests involving iodine
Acarbose	Precose	Reduces the rate of carbohydrate digestion and absorption	25–100 mg before each meal	May cause diarrhea, flatulence, abdominal pain
Troglitazone	Rezulin	Reduces insulin resistance in muscles	200–600 mg/day	Nausea is most common side effect. Regular liver function tests necessary.

on a regular basis to the health care provider for interpretation and adjustment of the treatment plan.

ACUTE COMPLICATIONS OF DIABETES

The individual with diabetes is at risk for a variety of complications. Acute complications related to high and low blood glucose levels are correctable with diligent self-care.

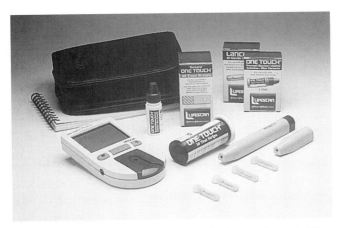

Figure 38–3. Home blood glucose monitoring equipment. (Photograph courtesy of LifeScan Blood Glucose Monitors, Milpitas, Calif.)

High Blood Glucose

When calories eaten exceed insulin available, high blood glucose (hyperglycemia) occurs. The most common cause of hyperglycemia is eating more than the meal plan prescribes. Another major cause is stress. Stress causes the release of counter-regulatory hormones, including epinephrine, cortisol, growth hormone, and glucagon. These hormones all increase the blood glucose level. In a nondiabetic client, this is an adaptive function. However, the client with diabetes is unable to compensate for the increased blood glucose with increased insulin secretion, and hyperglycemia occurs.

Clients must be able to recognize signs and symptoms of high blood glucose and know what to do if they occur (Table 38–6). For many clients, these symptoms are similar to the symptoms they experienced when they were first diagnosed with diabetes. Chronic high blood glucose levels may lead to long-term complications.

Hypoglycemia

Low blood glucose, or hypoglycemia, occurs when there are not enough calories available in relation to circulating insulin. This is sometimes referred to as an insulin reaction. Hypoglycemia is usually defined as a blood glucose

Table 38–6. **Comparison of High and Low Blood Glucose**

	Hyperglycemia	Hypoglycemia
Causes	Overeating Stress Illness Too little insulin or medication	Undereating, skipping a meal Too much insulin or medication Exercise
Symptoms	Polyuria Polydipsia Polyphagia Blurred vision Headache Lethargy Abdominal pain Ketonuria (if type I) Coma	Hunger Sweating Blurred vision Tremor Headache Irritability Confusion Seizures Coma
Treatment	Confirm hyperglycemia with glucose meter; if greater than 300 mg/dL, check urine for ketones and increase fluid intake. Assess cause of hyperglycemia, teach prevention. Return to prescribed treatment plan if applicable. Call physician for medication adjustment if indicated or if blood glucose is >200 mg/dL for 2 days. Call physician if ill or vomiting.	Confirm hypoglycemia with glucose meter (if client is not acutely ill). Administer 15 g fast-acting carbohydrate. Recheck glucose in 15 min; if still low, readminister carbohydrate. Continue checking glucose and administering fast sugar until hypoglycemia subsides; if symptoms worsen, call physician or emergency help. Glucagon subcutaneously or dextrose 50% IV may be administered if ordered. Assess cause of hypoglycemia, teach prevention.

of less than 50 mg/dL, although some clients have symptoms at higher glucose levels. Occasionally, symptoms occur due to a rapid drop in blood glucose, even though the actual glucose level is normal or high. Causes of hypoglycemia may include skipping a meal, exercising more than usual, or accidentally administering too much insulin. An occasional hypoglycemic episode, treated promptly, should not lead to chronic complications. Repeated or extremely low blood glucose levels may cause neurological damage. It is therefore important to teach each client how to prevent and treat low blood sugar.

CRITICAL THINKING: Jeff

Jeff is a 16-year-old who is having trouble with repeated insulin reactions. He says he has not had this trouble before, and it is interfering with his new job. What questions might you ask as you do your assessment?

Answers at end of chapter.

Symptoms of low blood sugar include hunger, sweating, pallor, tremor, palpitations, and headache. These symptoms are caused by activation of the sympathetic nervous system. As hypoglycemia progresses, the brain is deprived of glucose, and neurological symptoms such as irritability, confusion, seizures, and coma may occur.

If the nurse finds a client with symptoms of an altered blood glucose but is unable to identify whether it is high or low, a blood glucose test should be done. However, if the client is exhibiting neurological symptoms, treatment for low blood glucose should be administered immediately. The blood glucose may then be checked and further treatment provided as indicated.

Treatment for low blood glucose is administration of a "fast sugar"—15 g of carbohydrate that will enter the bloodstream quickly. This may be 4 ounces of orange juice, commercially available glucose tablets, or another quickly available source of sugar (Table 38–7). Glucose is rechecked in 15 minutes. If the blood glucose does not return to normal, the procedure should be repeated every 15 minutes until relief occurs. Hypoglycemia should not be overtreated with too much sugar, because this may cause hyperglycemia and rebound hypoglycemia. Many nurses added sugar to orange juice in the past. This is no longer recommended.

If the next meal is more than 1 hour away, the client should follow the treatment with a protein and complex

Table 38–7. **Fast Sugars**

4 oz orange juice
6 oz regular (not diet) soda
Miniature box of raisins
3 glucose tablets
6–8 Life Savers

carbohydrate snack, such as crackers with cheese or peanut butter, or half of a sandwich. If symptoms worsen, the physician should be contacted. Intravenous glucose or subcutaneous glucagon may be given in emergency situations. The nurse should check hospital or agency policy for specific protocol for treating hypoglycemic episodes.

Some elderly clients with poor autonomic nervous system function, or clients taking beta-adrenergic blocking medication (such as propranolol or atenolol), may not feel the symptoms of hypoglycemia. These clients should check glucose levels more frequently and keep the levels in a safe range to prevent hypoglycemic episodes.

Individuals with diabetes should be instructed to keep a fast sugar in their purse or pocket at all times. Fast sugars may also be stored in bedside tables, cars, and desks at work.

Diabetic Ketoacidosis

Diabetic ketoacidosis (DKA) occurs when blood glucose levels become very high and insulin is deficient. This most commonly occurs in individuals with type 1 diabetes. DKA is often the reason a person with undiagnosed type 1 diabetes first seeks help. It may also be the result of stress or illness in a person with previously diagnosed type 1 diabetes. When there is insufficient insulin to allow glucose into cells, the cells starve. The body then breaks down fat to be used for energy. The fat breakdown releases an acid substance called ketones. As ketones build up in the blood, ketoacidosis occurs.

The body attempts to reduce acidosis by deepening respirations, thereby blowing off excess carbon dioxide. (See the section on metabolic acidosis, Chapter 5.) The deep, sighing respiratory pattern is called **Kussmaul's** respirations. The expired air has a fruity odor due to the ketones and may be mistaken for alcohol. Some nurses have likened the odor to Juicy Fruit gum.

With such high blood glucose, and the accompanying polyuria, the body becomes dehydrated very quickly. High blood glucose also causes potassium to leave the cells and accumulate in the blood (hyperkalemia). The combination of dehydration, hyperkalemia, and acidosis causes the client to develop flulike symptoms. The client will lose consciousness and death will occur if the ketoacidosis is not treated.

Treatment includes intravenous (IV) fluids, IV insulin, and blood glucose monitoring. The nurse should watch blood glucose levels closely and notify the physician when the desired level is reached. Glucose should be added to the IV as the blood glucose approaches normal, to avoid hypoglycemia. Potassium should also be monitored, because the potassium level will drop rapidly as it reenters the cells.

Prevention of ketoacidosis involves careful monitoring of blood glucose levels at home. If the blood glucose rises above 300 mg/dL, the client should use a urine dipstick made to detect ketones. If ketones are present, the physician should be notified.

Hyperosmolar, Hyperglycemic, Nonketotic Syndrome

Hyperosmolar, hyperglycemic, nonketotic (HHNK) syndrome occurs primarily in type 2 diabetes, when blood glucose levels are high due to stress or illness. Because the person with type 2 diabetes has some insulin production, cells do not starve, and DKA usually does not occur.

As the blood glucose rises (hyperglycemic), polyuria causes profound dehydration, causing the hyperosmolar (concentrated) state. Blood glucose may rise as high as 1500 mg/dL. Because ketoacidosis is not present, the client usually does not feel physically ill and may delay seeking treatment. Coma and death will occur if HHNK is left untreated.

Treatment includes IV fluids, insulin, and glucose monitoring. HHNK syndrome can be prevented with careful monitoring of glucose levels at home. Clients should be instructed to drink plenty of fluids if blood glucose levels are beginning to rise, especially in times of stress and illness. They should also know when to call their physician with high blood glucose results.

LONG-TERM COMPLICATIONS

Over time, a variety of serious complications may occur in persons with diabetes. These involve the circulatory system, eyes, kidneys, and nerves. The Diabetes Control and Complications Trial (DCCT) showed that individuals who maintain tight control of blood glucose (between 70 and 120 mg/dL) experience 39 to 76 percent fewer long-term complications than individuals who take traditional care of their diabetes.[3] Tight control involves blood glucose testing and insulin injections three or more times a day, or an insulin pump. Unfortunately, even tight control does not guarantee the prevention of all complications.

Circulatory System

Individuals with diabetes develop atherosclerosis and arteriosclerosis faster than the general population. This leads to a higher incidence of strokes, heart attacks, and poor circulation in the feet and legs. The risk of cardiovascular disease and strokes is two to four times more common in persons with diabetes than in the general population.

Diabetes is the leading cause of amputation of the lower extremities. If cuts or sores occur on the feet, the reduced circulation to the area makes healing slow and difficult. Clients should be taught to protect their feet at all times by wearing well-fitting shoes and by washing, drying, and inspecting their feet daily (Table 38–8). If any sores are noted, the client should not delay in seeking treatment. During routine visits to the physician, the client should be sure to remove shoes and socks so the feet can be thoroughly examined. A podiatrist (foot doctor) may be consulted if problems occur.

Table 38–8. **Foot Care Tips**

Wash and dry feet every day. Use warm (not hot) water.

Apply lotion that does not contain alcohol, avoiding areas between toes.

Inspect feet for sores or red areas daily (have a family member help if necessary).

Report any abnormalities immediately.

Wear leather shoes and cotton socks.

Never go barefoot.

Avoid garters and tight socks.

Avoid crossing legs.

Cut toenails to natural shape of nail—not into corners.

See a podiatrist for calluses or problem toenails (avoid "bathroom surgery").

Have feet checked at least once a year, preferably 3–4 times a year, for loss of sensation.

Eyes

Small blood vessels may also become diseased, leading to **retinopathy.** Retinopathy involves damage to the tiny blood vessels that supply the eye. Small hemorrhages occur, which can cause blindness if not corrected. Diabetic retinopathy causes 12,000 to 24,000 new cases of blindness each year.[4] Newer laser surgery techniques may help improve vision after hemorrhages occur. Diabetes is also associated with a high incidence of cataracts. Clients with diabetes should have a yearly eye examination by an ophthalmologist.

Kidneys

Nephropathy is caused by damage to the tiny blood vessels within the kidneys. From 20 to 30 percent of clients with diabetes develop some degree of nephropathy.[5] A primary risk factor for diabetic nephropathy is poor control of blood glucose. If nephropathy occurs, the kidneys are unable to remove waste products and excess fluid from the blood. Diabetes is the leading cause of end-stage renal (kidney) disease. When the kidneys have lost most of their function, clients may have their blood cleansed artificially, by either hemodialysis or peritoneal dialysis, or they may have a kidney transplant.

Clients should be taught the importance of blood glucose control in the prevention or delay of kidney disease. Routine urine tests should be done to check for microalbuminuria (tiny amounts of protein in the urine). If microalbuminuria occurs, a low-protein diet may help delay further development of nephropathy. A trained renal dietitian should work with the client and physician in determining the best diet for the client.

Nerves

Another complication of diabetes is **neuropathy.** Neuropathy is damage to nerves due to chronic hyperglycemia. Neuropathy may cause numbness and pain in the extremi-

ties, impotence in male clients, **gastroparesis** (delayed stomach emptying), and other problems. Numbness in the feet can be especially problematic when combined with poor circulation. It is possible to be unaware of a foot injury, and delayed treatment may mean poor healing. Unfortunately, pain due to neuropathy is difficult to treat with traditional analgesics. Some antidepressant and anticonvulsant drugs may be helpful, or surgery may be necessary.

Infection

Persons with diabetes are prone to infection for several reasons. If injuries occur, healing may be slow due to impaired circulation. There may not be enough blood supply to heal the wound or fight an infection. For the same reason, it may be difficult for IV antibiotics to reach an infected site, and topical antibiotics may be preferable. In the presence of hyperglycemia, white blood cells become sluggish and ineffective, further reducing the body's ability to fight infection.

The incidence of periodontal (gum) disease, caused by bacteria in plaque, is also increased in individuals with diabetes. Clients must be taught to maintain good oral hygiene and make regular visits to the dentist.

 CRITICAL THINKING: Mr. Jones

Mr. Jones is a 54-year-old banker with type 2 diabetes admitted to your unit with a tiny red area on his right heel. His admitting blood glucose is 360 mg/dL. The lesion is so small you wonder what the fuss is about. While doing his assessment, you find that he wore a new pair of shoes to work all day about a month ago and has been avoiding seeing his physician about the resulting red area. He is placed on bed rest and antibiotics, and within 3 days the red area has broken open and has yellow drainage. It takes 6 months to fully heal.

1. List three risk factors for foot problems.
2. Why did the sore take so long to heal?
3. Why was bed rest important?
4. Why might topical antibiotics work better than IV antibiotics?

Answers at end of chapter.

SPECIAL CONSIDERATIONS FOR THE CLIENT UNDERGOING SURGERY

Surgery is a stressor. The counter-regulatory hormones released during surgery cause the blood glucose to rise, even

---

retinopathy: retino—nervous tissue of the eye + pathy—illness
nephropathy: nephro—of the kidney + pathy—illness
neuropathy: neuro—nervous system + pathy—illness
gastroparesis: gastro—stomach + paresis—partial paralysis

if the client has been fasting. Blood glucose should be well controlled before surgery. The physician's orders should be checked for changes in insulin orders. Often clients are placed on intravenous infusions of glucose and insulin during and immediately after surgery. Blood glucose levels should be monitored every 4 to 6 hours or as ordered. Clients should be closely monitored for signs and symptoms of hypoglycemia or hyperglycemia.

Clients who were not previously on insulin may be placed on insulin during surgery and postoperatively. They can generally return to their presurgical treatment plan after the stress of surgery is past.

NURSING PROCESS

Assessment

A complete history and physical assessment should be carried out because diabetes affects every body system. Some areas on which to focus are shown in Table 38–9. It is especially important to assess each client's knowledge of diabetes and its care, so that appropriate teaching can be done.

Nursing Diagnosis

Because diabetes affects so many different areas, nearly any nursing diagnosis may be appropriate. It is important to assess each client as an individual, and choose diagnoses based on assessment findings. A sample care plan is shown for a diagnosis of altered health maintenance, because clients with diabetes must learn to care for themselves in order to maintain their health. The actual presence of the defining characteristics should be confirmed with the client before choosing any nursing diagnosis. (See Nursing Care Plan Box 38–5 for the Client with Diabetes Mellitus.)

Planning and Implementation

Once diagnoses have been identified, planning takes place. This should be done with the client and family. Diabetes affects not only the person with the disease, but the entire family as well. The desired outcome for the plan of care is that the client is knowledgeable about and able to care for his or her disease. The nurse should consult the dietitian, social worker, certified diabetes educator, home care nurse, and other resources as needed.

Unless the client demonstrates complete knowledge, implementation of the care plan should include teaching. As the nurse carries out each phase of the plan, he or she should explain to the client and family what is being done and why. Appointments should be made to sit down with the client and family to discuss new information and allow time for questions. The client should be given ample time to demonstrate any newly learned skills. The nurse should be familiar with hospital policy regarding nursing responsibilities for diabetes education.

Evaluation

The best indicator of the success of a care plan for diabetes is controlled blood glucose levels. Blood glucose and glycohemoglobin levels should be within the negotiated range, without reports of symptoms of hypoglycemia or hyperglycemia. Another important indicator is the client's statement of satisfaction and comfort with the plan and his or her ability to carry it out on a daily basis.

CLIENT EDUCATION

The individual with diabetes must be taught self-care if at all possible. No amount of care from a physician or nurse can replace the self-care required of the person with diabetes. Family or significant other involvement is also important for the success and well-being of the person with diabetes.

If the client is hospitalized at diagnosis, the initial instruction will be done in the hospital. However, with hospital stays becoming shorter, the nurse must not waste any time. As soon as the client is feeling physically well enough to learn, teaching should begin. This is usually the responsibility of the primary or staff registered nurse, although aspects of the instruction may be delegated to the LPN/LVN. Some hospitals have a certified diabetes educa-

Table 38–9. **Assessment of the Client with Diabetes Mellitus**

Acutely Ill Client with Newly Diagnosed Diabetes		Client with Previously Diagnosed Diabetes	
Subjective Data	*Objective Data*	*Subjective Data*	*Objective Data*
• History of current problem • History of stress, illness, virus • Family history of diabetes • Current medications • Other medical or surgical conditions • Knowledge of diabetes care	• Vital signs • Lab values—electrolytes, blood glucose, ketones • Signs of dehydration • Fruity breath • Presence of complications if suspect diabetes was undiagnosed for period of time	• History of diabetes: type, onset, duration, degree of blood glucose control • Knowledge of self-care and degree of compliance • Support systems • History of complications	• Labs: blood glucose level, glycohemoglobin, BUN, creatinine, ketones, cholesterol, triglycerides • Condition of legs and feet; pulses, presence of circulatory or sensation impairment

NURSING CARE PLAN BOX 38–5 FOR THE CLIENT WITH DIABETES MELLITUS

Altered health maintenance related to possible knowledge deficit

Client Outcomes

Blood glucose levels within parameters negotiated with health care provider. Client states satisfaction with understanding of diabetes self-care.

Evaluation of Outcomes

Are blood glucose levels within parameters negotiated? Does client state satisfaction with understanding of diabetes self-care?

Interventions	*Rationale*	*Evaluation*
• Assess knowledge of diabetes self-care. • Assist client to collaborate with health care provider to determine appropriate blood glucose levels and action to be taken if glucose levels are too high or too low.	Teaching should be initiated only if a knowledge deficit exists. Appropriate blood glucose levels are different for each client and should be determined on an individualized basis. The client should know what blood glucose levels require notification of the health care provider.	Does client exhibit knowledge of diabetes self-care? Are blood glucose levels within parameters negotiated with health care provider? Does client state satisfaction with knowledge of diabetes self-care? Does client state appropriate blood glucose levels and action to take if glucose is high or low?
• Assess blood glucose levels before meals and at bedtime, or as ordered by health care provider. Ensure that client knows how to obtain glucose monitor and instruction for home use.	Good blood glucose control depends on knowledge of glucose levels and trends.	Does client demonstrate correct use of glucose monitor or state how monitor and instruction will be obtained?
• Administer insulin or oral hypoglycemic agent 30 minutes before meals (<15 minutes if client is using Lispro). Ensure that meal is begun within 30 minutes of medication. Replace any uneaten foods to prevent hypoglycemia.	The onset of most diabetes medication is about 30 minutes. If more than 30 minutes passes before a meal, the client might experience hypoglycemia.	Does client state correct meal and medication schedule?
• Teach technique for administering insulin if indicated. • Observe for symptoms of hypoglycemia and hyperglycemia and treat as necessary. Teach causes, prevention, recognition, and treatment of hypoglycemia and hyperglycemia.	The client and family should be familiar with the injection procedure. If the client has a good understanding of hypoglycemia and hyperglycemia, most episodes can be prevented. If hypoglycemia or hyperglycemia does occur, prompt treatment is essential to prevent complications.	Does client demonstrate correct injection technique? Does client state causes, prevention, symptoms, and treatment of hypoglycemia?
• Consult with dietitian for diet instruction. • Consult with social worker as needed to arrange follow-up nursing care after discharge. • Provide client with information regarding comprehensive diabetes education after discharge. Remind client that only survival skills have been taught during hospitalization. • Assist client to obtain Medic Alert card or tag that identifies diabetes.	The dietitian is trained to provide in-depth meal plan instruction. Some clients may not have the resources to carry out effective self-care after discharge. Instruction provided in the hospital usually is not comprehensive. Outpatient diabetes classes can provide additional self-care and health promotion information. If the client is ever unresponsive for any reason, the health care provider would need to be aware of diabetes.	Is client able to state plan for obtaining appropriate meals? Does client state availability of adequate resources for self-care at home? Does client state plan for obtaining further diabetes education after discharge? Does client state plan to carry or wear identification at all times?

GERIATRIC

• Assess ability to see and manipulate syringe, glucose monitor, and other equipment. Obtain assistive devices as needed.	The elderly client may have poor eyesight or other sensory deficits.	Is client able to manipulate equipment to safely care for self?

HOME HEATH HINTS

- Some home glucose monitoring devices have a memory that the nurse can access on the visit. It gives the date, time, and blood glucose result. This is a good indication of compliance with self-monitoring performed by client or caregiver.

- The nurse should remember to call the client the day before performing a venipuncture for a fasting blood sugar and remind the client and a family member not to eat after midnight.

- Older clients tend to skip meals.

- The client should be assisted in identifying easy but nutritious meals, such as frozen dinners. Meals-on-wheels is another option.

- Prefilled syringes should be stored in the refrigerator flat or with needles pointing up. This prevents crystals from settling and clogging the needle.

- The client can discard used syringes and needles in a hard plastic container such as a Clorox bottle with a screw top.

- If the client has a visual or dexterity problem, the nurse can suggest getting a syringe magnifier. A pharmacist or occupational therapist may be able to assist with obtaining one.

- The client can use a mirror to look at the bottom of the feet or have a family member examine the client's feet. The client should remove shoes and socks at each physician visit for a thorough foot inspection. Catching a "red spot" early is the goal.

- Due to decreased skin sensation in some diabetics, hot water heaters should be set below 120°F.

---

tor who provides classroom or bedside instruction. The dietitian should be contacted to provide meal plan instruction.

Most hospitals have policies or management plans describing the instruction to be provided by the nurse. Generally this includes "survival skills," which includes the basic information the client will need to survive initially at home. Survival skills include medication administration, glucose monitoring, meal plan basics, and what to do if high or low blood glucose levels occur. A variety of helpful aids are available. Videos may be helpful. Diabetes equipment suppliers provide kits that are full of samples and information. These are a significant help to the nurse. The client should also be advised to purchase a Medic Alert bracelet or necklace.

It is difficult for the nurse to know how to operate and teach glucose monitoring with the wide variety of glucose monitors available. Many drugstores and medical supply stores not only sell the monitors, but also provide training for the client and family. The nurse can obtain this information by calling local medical suppliers or by contacting the diabetes educator.

After discharge, the client is referred to outpatient diabetes classes for further instruction. If classes are unavailable or if the client is unable to leave his or her home, a visiting nurse referral should be made. It is often advisable to have a nurse present for the client's first insulin injection at home.

Because many people with diabetes are elderly, it is important for the nurse to be aware of their special needs. Syringe magnifiers and talking glucose meters are available for those with impaired vision. Family members may be taught to draw up a week's insulin supply for the client. Home meal programs may help ensure an adequate diet. Elderly clients should also have an emergency call system

in their home and regular contact with family members or other support people.

Reactive Hypoglycemia

Reactive hypoglycemia occurs when the blood glucose drops below a normal level, usually below 50 mg/dL. Hypoglycemia is most often a complication of diabetes treatment, but at times it may occur without the presence of diabetes. It may be a warning sign of impending diabetes.

PATHOPHYSIOLOGY

Low blood glucose may occur as an overreaction of the pancreas to eating. The pancreas senses a rising blood glucose, and produces more insulin than is necessary for the use of that glucose. As a result, the blood glucose drops to below normal. Some experts believe that this is a rare condition and that many "hypoglycemic" episodes are due to activation of the sympathetic nervous system for other reasons, without true hypoglycemia.

SIGNS AND SYMPTOMS

Low blood glucose causes release of epinephrine, which in turn causes the blood glucose to rise. Epinephrine release causes a fight or flight reaction, which may produce shaking, sweating, and palpitations. Headache, chills, and confusion may also occur.

DIAGNOSIS

Diagnosis is often based on a 5-hour glucose tolerance test, with below-normal readings between 2 and 5 hours. However, with the availability of home glucose monitors, it is now preferable for clients to monitor blood glucose levels at home. Readings should be taken in the morning on arising, 2 hours after each meal, at bedtime, and during symptoms of hypoglycemia. These results may then be taken to the physician for interpretation.

TREATMENT

Treatment includes frequent small meals and avoidance of fasting. Simple sugars are avoided, because they may aggravate symptoms. A high-protein, low-carbohydrate diet is stressed.

Review Questions

1. Which of the following is a risk factor for type 2 diabetes mellitus?
   a. Cardiovascular disease
   b. Obesity
   c. Age < 40
   d. Smoking

2. In which type of diabetes is insulin totally absent?
   a. Type 1
   b. Type 2
   c. Gestational
   d. IGT

3. Which of the following symptoms is most commonly associated with hyperglycemia?
   a. Tremor
   b. Flank pain
   c. Sweating
   d. Polyuria

4. Protein in the urine is a sign of which long-term complication of diabetes?
   a. Nephropathy
   b. Neuropathy
   c. Retinopathy
   d. Gastroparesis

5. For which of the following blood glucose results would the nurse administer a fast sugar?
   a. 48
   b. 80
   c. 126
   d. 223

6. Which of the following might cause hypoglycemia in the client with diabetes?
   a. Stress
   b. A dish of ice cream
   c. Exercise
   d. A cold or flu

7. Many long-term complications of diabetes are related to damage to the
   a. Bones
   b. Liver
   c. Brain
   d. Blood vessels

8. Which meal plan is best for the client with reactive hypoglycemia?
   a. High-carbohydrate meals
   b. Small, frequent meals
   c. Avoidance of fats and proteins
   d. Three medium to large meals daily

ANSWERS TO CRITICAL THINKING

CRITICAL THINKING: Mr. McMillan

1. Have you been eating or drinking more than usual? Have you been urinating more than usual? Do you get up at night to urinate?
2. Fatigue is caused because the glucose is unable to enter the cells without insulin, so they are starving.
3. He is dehydrated because he is losing excessive amounts of urine as his kidneys excrete extra glucose.

CRITICAL THINKING: Mrs. Evans

1. 7:30 a.m.
2. Midafternoon to just before supper. Although her insulin peaks between 1:30 and 7:30 p.m., her chances of having a hypoglycemic episode are slim once she has eaten her supper.

CRITICAL THINKING: Jeff

What kind of new job is it? Is it more physically strenuous than his previous job? Does it interfere with his usual meal schedule?

CRITICAL THINKING: Mr. Jones

1. Poor circulation, neuropathy, and slow wound healing place Mr. Jones at risk for problems.
2. Circulation to the foot may be poor, and white blood cells are sluggish if the blood glucose is high.
3. Any pressure on the foot while walking may further impair circulation.
4. If circulation to the area is poor, IV antibiotics may not reach the sore.

REFERENCES

1. Reducing the burden of diabetes. Centers for Disease Control and Prevention, CDC Diabetes Home Page, Aug 1997.
2. American Diabetes Association: Tests of glycemia in diabetes. Diabetes Care: Clinical Practice Recommendations, 1997 21(1):67, 1998.

3. The Diabetes Control and Complications Trial Research Group: The effect of intensive treatment of diabetes on the development and progression of long-term complications in insulin-dependent diabetes mellitus. N Engl J Med 329:14, 1993.
4. Reducing the burden of diabetes. Centers for Disease Control and Prevention, CDC Diabetes Home Page, Aug 1997.
5. American Diabetes Association: Diabetic nephropathy. Diabetes Care: Clinical Practice Recommendations, 1997 21(1):50, 1998.

BIBLIOGRAPHY

Ackley, BJ, and Ladwig, GB: Nursing Diagnosis Handbook: A Guide to Planning Care. Mosby, St Louis, 1993, pp 194–195.

Bell, N: Feet first. Diabetes Forecast 50:6, 1997.

Bernstein, G, and Gohdes, D: Reducing lower extremity clinical abnormalities in patients with NIDDM. Clinical Diabetes 12:1, 1994.

Barzilai, N: Clinical use of metformin in the United States. Diabetes Spectrum 8:4, 1995.

Betschart, JM, and Betschart, JE: Periodontal disease and diabetes mellitus. Diabetes Spectrum 10:2, 1997.

Blodgett, J: Metformin—Good news for type 2s. Diabetes Self-Management, March/April 1995.

Borg, WP, Borg, MA, and Tamborlane, WV: The brain and hypoglycemic counterregulation: Insights from hypoglycemic clamp studies. Diabetes Spectrum 10:1, 1997.

Deglin, JH, and Vallerand, AH: Davis's Drug Guide for Nurses, ed 4. FA Davis, Philadelphia, 1995.

Foster, DW, and Rubenstein, AH: Hypoglycemia. In Harrison's Principles of Internal Medicine, ed 12. McGraw-Hill, New York, 1991, pp 1759–1765.

Hirsch, IB: Current concepts in diabetic nephropathy. Clinical Diabetes 12:1, 1994.

Hoyson, PM: Diabetes 2000: Oral medications. RN, 58(5):34, 1995.

Kestel, F: Are you up to date on diabetes medications? Am J Nurs 94:7, 1994.

Lutz, CA, and Przytulski, KR: Nutrition and Diet Therapy. FA Davis, Philadelphia, 1994.

Maffeo, R: Helping families cope with type 1 diabetes. Am J Nurs 97:6, 1997.

Saltiel-Berzin, R: Managing a surgical patient who has diabetes. Nursing 22(4):34, 1992.

Siminerio, LM, and Carroll, PB: Educating secondary diabetes patients. Diabetes Spectrum 7:1, 1994.

White, JR: The pharmacologic management of patients with type 2 diabetes mellitus in the era of new oral agents and insulin analogs. Diabetes Spectrum 9:4, 1996.

Understanding the Reproductive System

Genitourinary and Reproductive System Function and Assessment

Valerie C. Scanlon, Linda Hopper Cook, and Cindy Meredith

Learning Objectives

Upon completion of this chapter, the student will be able to:

1. Identify the structures of the reproductive system.
2. Describe the functions of the reproductive system.
3. List the effects of aging on the reproductive system.
4. Identify information to include in a reproductive system history.
5. Explain the process of breast self-examination and testicular self-examination.
6. State recommendations for routine breast and prostate screening.
7. Briefly explain common tests used to diagnose disorders of the reproductive system.
8. Describe the nurse's role in assisting clients undergoing reproductive system assessments.

Key Words

adnexa (ad-**NECK**-sah)
bimanual (by-**MAN**-yoo-uhl)
circumcised (**SIR**-kuhm-sized)
colposcopy (kul-**POS**-koh-pee)
conization (KOH-ni-**ZAY**-shun)
culdoscopy (kul-**DOS**-koh-pee)
curet (kyoo-**RET**)
cystic (**SIS**-tik)
ectopic (eck-**TOP**-ick)
ejaculation (ee-JAK-yoo-**LAY**-shun)
erection (e-**REK**-shun)
gynecomastia (JIN-e-koh-**MASS**-tee-ah)
hydrocele (**HIGH**-droh-seel)
hypospadias (HIGH-poh-**SPAY**-dee-ahz)
hysterosalpingogram (**HIS**-tur-oh-SAL-pinj-oh-gram)
hysteroscopy (HIS-tur-**AHS**-koh-pee)
insufflation (in-suff-**LAY**-shun)

libido (li-**BEE**-doh)
mammography (mah-**MOG**-rah-fee)
menarche (me-**NAR**-kee)
menopause (**MEN**-oh-pawz)
orgasm (**OR**-gazm)
transillumination (TRANS-i-loo-mi-**NAY**-shun)
varicocele (**VAR**-i-koh-seel)

Review of Normal Anatomy and Physiology

The male and female reproductive systems produce gametes (sperm and egg cells) and ensure the union of gametes in fertilization following sexual intercourse. In women, the uterus provides the site for the developing embryo/fetus until birth.

FEMALE REPRODUCTIVE SYSTEM

The female reproductive system consists of the paired ovaries and fallopian tubes, the single uterus and vagina, and the external genital structures (Fig. 39–1). The mammary glands may be considered accessory organs to the system.

Ovaries

The ovaries are a pair of oval structures about 1.5 inches long on either side of the uterus in the pelvic cavity (Fig. 39–2). The ovarian ligament extends from the medial side of an ovary to the uterine wall, and the broad ligament is a fold of the peritoneum that covers the ovaries. These ligaments help keep the ovaries in place.

The ovaries produce egg cells by the process of meiosis, more specifically called oogenesis, which begins at puberty and ends at menopause, between the ages of 45 and 55. This process is cyclical in that usually one mature ovum is produced every 28 days and is under hormonal control (covered in the section on the menstrual cycle). The follicles of the ovary produce the hormone estrogen, and later, as the corpus luteum, secrete progesterone as well.

Fallopian Tubes

Each fallopian, or uterine, tube is about 4 inches long; the lateral end with its fringelike fimbriae encloses the ovary on its side, and the medial end opens into the uterus. The lining of a fallopian tube is ciliated epithelium; in the wall is smooth muscle. The sweeping of the cilia and the peristaltic contractions of the smooth muscle usually ensure that the ovum (or the zygote after fertilization), which has no means of self-locomotion, will reach the uterus. Fertilization usually takes place within the fallopian tube, and the zygote is swept into the uterus within 4 to 5 days.

Uterus

The uterus is about 3 inches long and 2 inches wide, superior to the urinary bladder and medial to the ovaries in the pelvic cavity. Ligaments help keep the uterus in place, tilted forward over the top of the bladder. During pregnancy the uterus increases greatly in size, contains the placenta to nourish the embryo/fetus, and expels the baby at the end of gestation.

The fundus of the uterus is the upper portion above the entry of the fallopian tubes, and the body is the large central portion. The cervix is the narrow, lower end, which

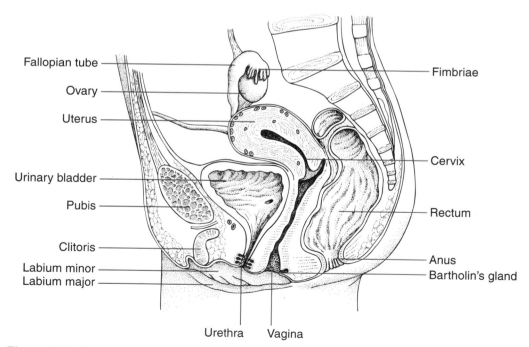

Figure 39–1. Female reproductive system in a midsagittal section. (Modified from Scanlon, VC, Sanders, T: Workbook for Essentials of Anatomy and Physiology, ed 2. FA Davis, Philadelphia, 1995, p 320, with permission.) See Plate 8.

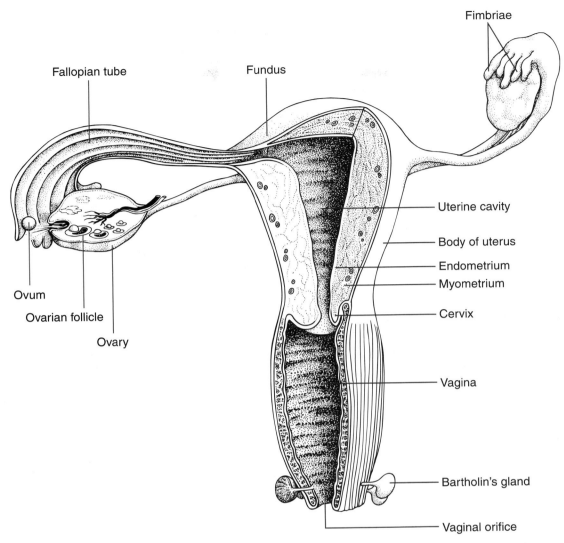

Figure 39–2. Female reproductive system in anterior view and a longitudinal section. (Modified from Scanlon, VC, Sanders, T: Workbook for Essentials of Anatomy and Physiology, ed 2. FA Davis, Philadelphia, 1995, p 322, with permission.)

opens into the vagina. The outermost layer of the uterine wall is the epimetrium, a fold of the peritoneum. The myometrium is the smooth muscle layer; during pregnancy these cells increase in size to accommodate the growing fetus, and they contract for labor and delivery at the end of gestation.

The lining of the uterus is the endometrium, a highly vascular mucous membrane, part of which is lost and regenerated with each menstrual cycle. During pregnancy, the endometrium forms the maternal portion of the placenta.

Vagina

The vagina is a muscular tube about 4 inches long that extends from the cervix to the vaginal orifice in the perineum. It is between the urethra and the rectum. The functions of the vagina are to receive sperm from the penis during sexual intercourse, to serve as the exit for menstrual blood flow, and to serve as the birth canal at the end of pregnancy.

After puberty, the vaginal mucosa is relatively resistant to infection. The normal bacterial flora of the vagina creates an acidic pH that helps inhibit the growth of most pathogens.

External Genitals

Also called the vulva, the female external genital structures are the clitoris, labia majora and minora, and Bartholin's glands. The clitoris is a small mass of erectile tissue anterior to the urethral orifice. Its function is sensory; it responds to sexual stimulation and its vascular sinuses become filled with blood.

The mons pubis is a pad of fat over the pubic bones, covered with skin and pubic hair. Extending posteriorly from the mons are the lateral labia majora and the medial labia minora; these are paired folds of skin. The area between the labia minora is the vestibule; it contains the openings of the urethra and vagina. The labia cover these openings and prevent drying of their mucous membranes. Bartholin's glands, also called vestibular glands, are within the floor of the vestibule; their ducts open into the mucosa at the vaginal orifice. Their secretion keeps the mucosa moist and lubricates the vagina during sexual intercourse.

Mammary Glands

Enclosed within the breasts and surrounded by adipose tissue, the mammary glands produce milk after pregnancy. The milk enters the lactiferous ducts, which converge at the nipple. The skin around the nipple is a pigmented area called the areola. The formation of milk is under hormonal control. During pregnancy, high levels of estrogen and progesterone prepare the glands for milk production. Prolactin from the anterior pituitary causes the actual synthesis of milk after pregnancy. The sucking of the infant on the nipple stimulates the release of oxytocin from the posterior pituitary gland, which in turn stimulates the release of milk.

The Menstrual Cycle

The menstrual cycle depends on follicle-stimulating hormone (FSH) and luteinizing hormone (LH) from the anterior pituitary gland and estrogen and progesterone from the ovaries. These hormones bring about changes in the ovaries and uterus. A cycle may be described in terms of three phases: menstrual phase, follicular phase, and luteal phase.

The menstrual phase involves the loss of the endometrium in menstruation, which may last 2 to 8 days, with an average of 3 to 6 days. At this time, secretion of FSH is increasing, and several ovarian follicles, each with a potential ovum, begin to develop. (See Table 39–1 for a summary of female hormones.)

During the follicular phase, FSH stimulates growth of ovarian follicles and secretion of estrogen by the follicle cells. The secretion of LH is also increasing, but more slowly. FSH and estrogen promote the growth and maturation of the ovum, and estrogen stimulates the growth of blood vessels to regenerate the endometrium. This phase ends with ovulation, when a sharp increase in LH causes rupture of a mature ovarian follicle.

During the luteal phase, LH causes the ruptured follicle to become the corpus luteum, which begins to secrete progesterone in addition to estrogen. Progesterone stimulates further growth of blood vessels in the endometrium and promotes the storage of nutrients such as glycogen. As progesterone secretion increases, LH secretion decreases, and if the ovum is not fertilized, the secretion of progesterone also begins to decrease. Without progesterone, the endometrium cannot be maintained and begins to slough off in menstruation. FSH secretion begins to increase (as estrogen and progesterone decrease), and the cycle begins again. Although an average cycle is 28 days, cycles of 23 to 35 days may also be considered normal.

MALE REPRODUCTIVE SYSTEM

The male reproductive system consists of the testes and a series of ducts and glands. Sperm are produced in the testes and are transported through the reproductive ducts: epididymis, ductus deferens, ejaculatory duct, and urethra (Fig. 39–3). The reproductive glands are the seminal vesi-

Table 39–1. **Female Hormones**

Hormone	Secreted By	Functions
Follicle-Stimulating Hormone (FSH)	Anterior pituitary	Initiates development of ovarian follicles Stimulates secretion of estrogen by follicle cells
Luteinizing Hormone	Anterior pituitary	Causes ovulation Converts the ruptured ovarian follicle into the corpus luteum Stimulates secretion of progesterone by the corpus luteum
Estrogen	Ovary (follicle) Placenta	Promotes maturation of ovarian follicles Promotes growth of blood vessels in the endometrium Initiates development of secondary sex characteristics Promotes growth of duct system of mammary glands
Progesterone	Ovary (corpus luteum) Placenta	Promotes further growth of blood vessels in the endometrium Inhibits contractions of the myometrium during pregnancy Promotes growth of secretory cells of mammary glands
Inhibin	Ovary (corpus luteum)	Decreases secretion of FSH toward end of cycle
Prolactin	Anterior pituitary	Promotes production of milk after birth
Oxytocin	Posterior pituitary	Promotes release of milk

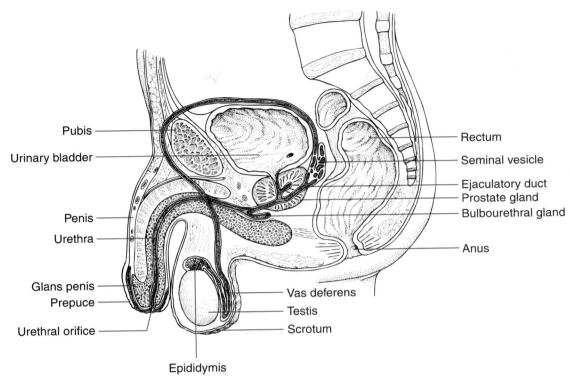

Figure 39–3. Male reproductive system in a midsagittal section. (Modified from Scanlon, VC, Sanders, T: Workbook for Essentials of Anatomy and Physiology, ed 2. FA Davis, Philadelphia, 1995, p 318, with permission.) See Plate 9.

cles, prostate gland, and bulbourethral glands, all of which produce secretions that become part of semen.

Testes

The testes are located in the scrotum between the upper thighs, where the temperature is slightly lower then body temperature, which is necessary for the production of viable sperm. Each testis is about 1.5 inches long and 1 inch wide, and contains the seminiferous tubules in which spermatogenesis (meiosis) takes place. In contrast to oogenesis, once started at puberty, spermatogenesis is a constant rather than cyclical process, and usually continues throughout life. Also in the testes are specialized cells that produce the hormones testosterone and inhibin. Spermatogenesis is initiated by FSH from the anterior pituitary. LH from the anterior pituitary stimulates the secretion of testosterone, which contributes to the maturation of sperm. The secretion of inhibin is stimulated by testosterone; inhibin decreases the secretion of FSH, which helps keep the rate of spermatogenesis fairly constant. The functions of the male hormones are summarized in Table 39–2.

A sperm cell consists of the head, which contains the 23 chromosomes; a flagellum, which provides motility; and the acrosome on the tip of the head, which contains enzymes to digest the membrane of the egg cell. Sperm from all the seminiferous tubules of a testis passes through tubules leading to the epididymis.

Epididymis, Ductus Deferens, and Ejaculatory Ducts

The epididymis is a tube about 20 feet long that is coiled on the posterior side of a testis. Smooth muscle within its wall propels sperm into the ductus deferens.

Table 39–2. **Male Hormones**

Hormone	Secreted By	Functions
Follicle-Stimulating Hormone (FSH)	Anterior pituitary	Initiates production of sperm in the testes
Luteinizing Hormone	Anterior pituitary	Stimulates secretion of testosterone by the testes
Testosterone	Testes	Promotes maturation of sperm Initiates development of male secondary sex characteristics
Inhibin	Testes	Decreases secretion of FSH to maintain a constant rate of spermatogenesis

Also called the vas deferens, the ductus deferens extends from the epididymis in the scrotum through the inguinal canal and into the abdominal cavity. The inguinal canal is an opening in the abdominal wall for the spermatic cord, a connective tissue sheath that contains the ductus deferens, testicular blood vessels, and nerves. Within the abdominal cavity, the ductus deferens extends over the top of the urinary bladder, then down the posterior side to join the ejaculatory duct on its own side.

Each of the two ejaculatory ducts receives sperm from the ductus deferens and the secretion of the seminal vesicle on its own side. Both ejaculatory ducts empty into the urethra.

Seminal Vesicles, Prostate gland, and Bulbourethral Glands

The paired seminal vesicles are posterior to the urinary bladder. Their secretion is alkaline to enhance sperm motility and contains fructose to nourish the sperm. The duct of a seminal vesicle joins the ductus deferens on its side to form the ejaculatory duct.

The prostate gland is a muscular gland that surrounds the first inch of the urethra as it emerges from the urinary bladder. The secretion of the prostate is alkaline and contributes to sperm motility. The smooth muscle of the prostate contracts during ejaculation, the expulsion of semen from the urethra.

The bulbourethral glands are located below the prostate gland and empty into the urethra. Their alkaline secretion coats the interior of the urethra just before ejaculation, which will neutralize any acidic urine that might be present.

The alkaline secretions of the male reproductive glands ensure that sperm will remain viable in the acidic environment of the vagina. The normal bacterial flora of the vagina create an acid pH there, but the pH of semen is about 7.4 and permits sperm to remain motile.

Urethra and Penis

The urethra is the last of the male reproductive ducts, and its longest portion is within the penis. The penis is an external genital organ; its distal end is called the glans penis and is covered with a fold of skin called the prepuce or foreskin. Within the penis are three masses of erectile or cavernous tissue. Each consists of a framework of smooth muscle and connective tissue that contains blood sinuses, which are large, irregular vascular channels.

When blood flow through these sinuses is minimal, the penis is flaccid (soft). Sexual stimulation causes the arteries to the penis to dilate; the sinuses fill with blood, and the penis becomes erect and firm. This is brought about by parasympathetic impulses. The culmination of sexual stimulation is ejaculation, which is brought about by peristalsis of the reproductive ducts and contraction of the prostate gland.

AGING AND THE REPRODUCTIVE SYSTEM

For women there is a definite end to reproductive capability; this is called the menopause and usually occurs between the ages of 45 and 55. Estrogen secretion decreases, and ovulation and menstrual cycles become irregular and finally cease. The decrease in estrogen has other effects as well. Loss of bone matrix may lead to osteoporosis and fractures; an increase in blood cholesterol makes women more likely to develop coronary artery disease; and drying of the vagina mucosa increases susceptibility to vaginal infections.

For most men, testosterone secretion continues throughout life, as does sperm production, although both diminish with advancing age. Perhaps the most common reproductive problem for older men is prostatic hypertrophy, enlargement of the prostate gland. As the urethra is compressed, urination may become difficult. Prostate hypertrophy is usually benign, but cancer of the prostate is one of the more common cancers in elderly men.

Female Assessment

Assessment of women's reproductive health can seem challenging because of the complex relationship of physical and psychosocial factors. Hormones not only affect a multitude of body functions, they also can influence moods and mental functioning. Reproduction involves not only physical processes, but also relationships, role identifications, and self-esteem issues.

NORMAL PHYSIOLOGICAL BASELINES

Knowing normal physiology of the reproductive system is the nurse's best preparation for nursing assessment. Regular, relatively pain-free shedding of an appropriate amount of the lining of the uterus is expected from the teenage years through midlife. Intercourse is normally expected to be pain free, infection free, desired by both partners, and satisfying and to result in pregnancy over a reasonable period of time (unless precautions are taken). Pregnancies are expected to last approximately 40 weeks and to produce a healthy child. Physical and psychological sexual characteristics and function including **libido** are expected to be adequately maintained by hormones. Sexual function, desire, and fertility are expected to change throughout the process of aging. Although individuals may vary somewhat from these expected descriptions, these serve as a baseline for assessment of possible disorders. Chapter 40 further defines specific reproductive system disorders.

Much of what happens with womens' reproductive system disorders occurs inside the body and may not show ex-

libido: sexual desire

ternal signs. Skill in asking appropriate questions, documenting client statements, and describing observations is essential. Descriptions of pain should be thorough and follow the WHAT'S UP format described in Chapter 2. Description of vaginal bleeding or discharge should specify amount, color, and consistency and describe odor (if noticeable). Short quotes of the client's own words to describe change that she has noticed may add valuable information, but the nurse must be careful to use critical thinking skills when interviewing rather than just quoting indiscriminately. Because many signs and symptoms of reproductive system disorders occur in a cyclic fashion, the client may be asked to keep an accurate written record of occurrences, noting times and dates to identify patterns of symptoms.

HISTORY

The nurse is often responsible for recording initial history and physical assessment data. Breast history questions include breast-feeding history, knowledge and practice of breast self-examination, discomforts, and presence of any lumps, thickening, or nipple discharge. Menstrual history questions include age of **menarche** and age of **menopause** (if applicable), length of cycles, length of menses, menstrual regularity, amount of bleeding, presence of clots, discomforts, and measures taken to relieve discomforts.

Obstetrical history includes number of pregnancies, pregnancy outcomes, and complications. These are generally documented using abbreviations of Latin words: G = pregnancies (from the Latin word *gravida*); P = births, whether alive or stillborn (from the Latin word *para*); A = abortions, whether spontaneous or therapeutic (from the Latin word *abortus*); and Roman numerals following the letter to specify the number of each (for example, three pregnancies, twins and one single birth, and one spontaneous abortion are recorded as GIII, PIII, AI). Medical intervention history includes any testing, operations, or treatments done on the reproductive organs and excretory system. Medications the client is taking (for whatever reasons), height-to-weight ratio, and marked changes in weight may also provide significant data for diagnostic and care planning purposes concerning reproductive system disorders.

LEARNING TIP

Remember the word *gravida* by thinking of gravity and that one is heavier when pregnant.

Sexual history questions include whether the client is sexually active, sexual preference, number of partners, history of sexually transmitted disease (STD), knowledge and

---

menarche: men—month + arche—beginning
menopause: men—month + pause—stop

practice of STD risk reduction, history of participation in high-risk sexual activities, birth control knowledge and practice, and level of satisfaction with sexual functioning. Many nurses feel awkward asking these questions, and clients may also feel some uneasiness with this line of questioning. A matter-of-fact attitude, an assurance of confidentiality, and an adequate explanation about why the information is needed tend to encourage client comfort and cooperation.

BREAST ASSESSMENT

Palpation

Palpation is the most important assessment technique for breast examination, because it can be used to identify alterations from normal consistency, to confirm the presence of lumps, and to locate areas of tenderness. Even mammograms do not detect 10 to 15 percent of all lesions that can be found by palpation.[1]

Breast Self-Examination

Self-palpation during breast self-examination (BSE), if done regularly and thoroughly, may be even more sensitive than physician or nurse palpation, because the client becomes so familiar with her own breasts that she is more likely to notice subtle changes that an infrequently visited health practitioner might overlook. BSE is one of the most important health protection skills that nurses can teach to women. The few moments spent monthly on this activity may mean the difference between life and death or comfort and extreme suffering for women.

Client Teaching

BSE should be done regularly once per month. One week after the beginning of the menstrual period is a good time to do BSE because some women's breasts become swollen and feel more lumpy around the beginning of menses. For women who no longer have a regular menstrual period, it is suggested that a certain day such as the first or last of the month be chosen in order to aid memory.

LEARNING TIP

Some women do BSE the day their telephone bill arrives each month, because it is a dependable monthly reminder.

The examination procedure is simple. The client is taught to examine the breasts while standing, lying, and standing in the shower. She first stands in front of a mirror and observes both breasts with arms down at sides, with arms raised, and with hands on hips. She looks for changes in shape, size, skin texture, color, or smoothness. Although most women's breasts are not the same size, marked differences between the breasts or a change in the size of one breast should be checked with a physician. Puckering or dimpling of skin, asymmetrical movement, and different pointing position of the nipples should also be reported to a physician.

The breasts should also be palpated when lying down using the opposite hand to systematically feel all portions of the breast and armpit while making small circular motions as the hand slides over the tissue. The woman first feels using light pressure and then using firmer pressure. She feels for any lumps or changes in thickness of portions of the breast. There is a thick supporting band of tissue at the base of each breast, which is normal, and the ducts and alveoli may feel slightly lumpy. Unusual lumps should be checked by a physician. Although there is debate about whether it is necessary to squeeze the nipple to assess for discharge, the American Cancer Society presently advises that the nipple

be squeezed gently to check for discharge. Palpating the breasts while in the shower also provides another opportunity to feel for the changes mentioned previously, and soap and water allow the hands to glide easily over the surfaces. Whether the breasts are examined in a spiral formation or by following parallel lines moving across and back over the breast is probably insignificant. Women may have been taught either method. It is important to encourage that the examination be methodical and cover all areas of the breast, the tail of Spence, and the axilla (Fig. 39–4).

DIAGNOSTIC TESTS OF THE BREASTS

Ultrasound and Mammography

Further assessment of the breast may be done by several methods. Ultrasound examination is done by bouncing high-frequency sound waves off of the tissues within the

How to do Breast Self-Exam

1. Lie down and put a pillow under your right shoulder. Place your right arm behind your head.

2. Use the finger pads of your three middle fingers on your left hand to feel for lumps or thickening. Your finger pads are the top third of each finger.

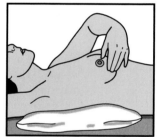

3. Press firmly enough to know how your breast feels. If you're not sure how hard to press, ask your health care provider. Or try to copy the way your health care provider uses the finger pads during a breast exam. Learn what your breast feels like most of the time. A firm ridge in the lower curve of each breast is normal.

4. Move around the breast in a set way. You can choose either the circle (**A**), the up and down (**B**), or the wedge (**C**). Do it the same way every time. It will help you to make sure that you've gone over the entire breast area, and to remember how your breast feels.

5. Now examine your left breast using your right hand finger pads.

6. If you find any changes, see your doctor right away.

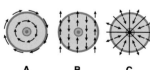

A   B   C

For Added Safety: You should also check your breasts while standing in front of a mirror right after you do your breast self-exam each month. See if there are any changes in the way your breasts look: dimpling of the skin, changes in the nipple, or redness or swelling.

You might also want to do a breast self-exam while you're in the shower. Your soapy hands will glide over wet skin making it easy to check how your breasts feel.

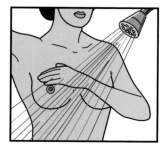

Figure 39–4. Breast self-examination. (Courtesy of the American Cancer Society, copyright 1997.)

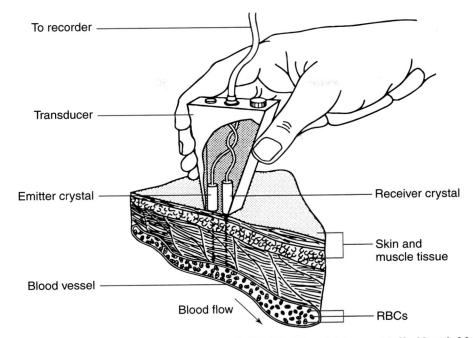

Figure 39–5. Diagnostic testing by using ultrasound. (Modified from Watson and Jaffe: Nurse's Manual of Laboratory and Diagnostic Tests, ed 2. FA Davis, Philadelphia, p 677, with permission.)

breast in order to determine the density of the tissues and to map the breast structures (Fig. 39–5). This is mainly useful for distinguishing fluid-filled (**cystic**) lumps from solid tumors but may also be used to guide a needle for fine-needle aspiration of fluid or core-needle biopsies.

Mammography is a radiographic (x-ray) examination of the breast. A special machine is used that spreads and flattens the breast tissue to a thin layer to more effectively show benign and malignant growths, which might be hidden by breast structures on typical chest x-rays (see Figs. 10–12, 10–13 p. 164). Generally at least two x-rays are taken of each breast with the machine compressing the breast top-to-bottom and side-to-tide to give comparison views of any lumps from more than one angle. If suspicious or unclear spots are seen, additional views may be taken.

The American Cancer Society recommends that women between 20 and 40 years of age do BSE monthly and see their health care provider for a clinical examination at least every 3 years.[2] Women 50 years of age and over are advised to do monthly BSE and to have a yearly clinical breast examination and a mammogram.[2] In a recent controversial move, the American Cancer Society extended the recommendation of yearly clinical examinations and yearly mammograms to women 40 to 49 years of age.[3] Those who experience breast symptoms or have a strong family history of breast cancer may be advised to have more frequent examinations.

cystic: baglike
mammography: mammo—breast + graphy—recording
transillumination: trans—across + illumin—light + ation—process

Client Teaching

Clients should be advised to bathe and not to apply deodorant, powder, or any other substance to the upper body because these may cause false shadows on the test. They should be instructed that if a shadow is seen on a mammogram, further testing will be done to determine the reason for the shadow.

Thermography, Diaphanography, Computed Tomography, and Magnetic Resonance Imaging

There are several other less commonly used methods for diagnosis of breast disorders. Thermography is a method of mapping the breast using photographic paper, which records temperature variations throughout the tissue in different colors. Diaphanography, or **transillumination** of the breast, may also help identify the location of some lumps, but it is very seldom used. Computed tomography (CT) takes very precise x-ray pictures of the breast, layer by layer, as it would look if it were sliced in thin slices. This allows for precise measurement of the position of tumors without the displacement caused by flattening the breast for a mammogram. CT scanning, however, is much more expensive than mammography, so it is not a very practical method to use for general screening of all women to detect possible breast cancers. Magnetic resonance imaging (MRI) uses radio frequency radiation and magnetic fields to map the breast tissue. The equipment needed for this method is very expensive, and it is unavailable in some areas.

Client Teaching

MRI clients should be asked whether they have any metal within their bodies such as orthopedic wires, metal sutures, or artificial joint replacements because heat is generated by the MRI and the procedure may be contraindicated.

Biopsy

If suspicious lumps or lesions are found in the breast by any of these methods, they may be checked using one of the other methods and then further assessed by biopsy. This procedure involves removing a small portion of tissue, fluid, or cells from the breast or lymph nodes for microscopic examination. This may be done by surgically removing a portion of tissue or by aspirating fluid or cells through a needle that is placed into the lump or lesion. Needle biopsies are often done with local anesthetic and may take place in a clinic or physician's office. More extensive biopsies may require a general anesthetic. A frozen section examination may be done in the laboratory by moistening and rapidly freezing a section of tissue, slicing it very thinly, and immediately examining it by microscope. This allows for diagnosis to be made during the course of an operation, so that the client is spared an additional later operation for removal of cancerous tissue.

Nursing Care

As with any surgical intervention, the nurse sets out the sterile equipment and supplies needed for the procedure and ensures that a signed consent has been obtained. Following the biopsy the client is assessed for excessive bleeding and is instructed about signs of impairment of healing processes. It is very important that biopsy samples be clearly labeled, packaged appropriately for transport to laboratory facilities, and delivered promptly. The laboratory should be consulted for information about the transport container and whether a cell fixative is required in the container.

Assessment of the client's psychological condition during breast diagnosis procedures is essential. Few people do not know someone who has had breast cancer. Although breast cancer screening procedures can seem routine to health care workers, they may be a cause of much anxiety for some women and their families. An understanding and calm nurse who can explain the procedures can help the assessment phase to be less traumatic.

ADDITIONAL DIAGNOSTIC TESTS OF THE FEMALE REPRODUCTIVE SYSTEM

There are many tests to assess reproductive system function; this is presently an area of very rapid change. The names of the individual procedures may also vary among institutions or according to particular methods used (for example, a salpingoscopy is also called a falloposcopy, and a laparoscopy is the same thing as a peritoneoscopy). For this reason, this chapter will be limited to general descriptions of categories of medical and surgical assessment procedures rather than attempts to name all tests.

Hormonal Tests

Hormonal tests are commonly used to assess functioning of the endocrine system as it relates to reproduction. They may be used to measure potential fertility, to find reasons for abnormal menses, to assess hormone-producing tumors, and to determine whether treatments to adjust hormone levels have been effective. Several hormones may be tested at any one time. Some hormonal tests are time specific, and the samples can be useless if not gathered within a certain time range.

Nursing Care

The laboratory is consulted for specific instructions for each test. The nurse explains the procedure to the client and supports her. Women who are undergoing hormonal tests may feel embarrassed, worried about their femininity and potential fertility, and depressed because of repeated tests often with little positive result. Some may fear loss of their spouse's love (and perhaps relationship) if they are diagnosed as infertile.

Pelvic Examination

The pelvic examination allows visual inspection of the vagina and cervix, as well as sampling of mucous, discharge, cells, and exudates. Palpation of portions of the reproductive system and some treatments may also be done as part of the procedure.

Nursing Care

Generally, as the nurse sets out the supplies for the examination, explanation of the procedure may be done. Vaginal specula range from tiny virginal sizes to extra large (Fig. 39–6). The appropriate size is related to the size of the woman (or child) and whether she has had children or not. For a small child a nasal speculum may be used. A sterile basin of warm tap water to warm the speculum and a small amount of surgical lubricant should be placed near but not on the speculum (because some tests may be affected by water or lubricant). Two clean gloves for the examiner should be placed nearby, and a light should be adjusted to illuminate the area. Other equipment may be set out according to the tests or treatments that will be carried out during the pelvic examination.

The nurse instructs the client to empty her bladder before the examination. The client is placed (in a gown and without underwear) either on her back with her arms resting down at her sides to aid relaxation of abdominal muscles or in a side-lying position, according to the physician's preference. She is covered with a sheet turned so that there

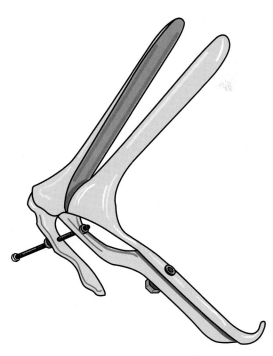

Figure 39–6. Vaginal speculum.

is plenty of room for the legs to spread while the sheet still covers the client on the sides.

Bimanual Palpation

Because much of the reproductive system is not visible even with a speculum, **bimanual** palpation is often done during a pelvic examination. One hand is placed on the abdomen and another gloved hand is inserted deeply into the vagina. The uterus and **adnexa** are moved about between the two hands in order to feel the size, shape, and consistency of the uterus and adnexa and to check for any abnormal growths.

Nursing Care

The nurse explains the procedure and supports the client. Some women may be fearful, embarrassed, or tense and may find the procedure uncomfortable. Active relaxation strategies may decrease discomfort.

 CRITICAL THINKING:
Reproductive Assessment

How might the age of the client change your approach, plans, and teaching for clients who have disorders of the reproductive system? Consider your ap-

---

bimanual: bi—two + manual—hands
adnexa: ad—together + nexa—to tie (usually refers to ovaries and tubes)
conization: coniz—cone-forming + ation—process
curet: scoop

proach, plans, and teaching for each of the following scenarios.

1. A 2-year-old child is brought into the clinic by her mother because she has a foul smell coming from her perineal area and a slight yellowish discharge from her vagina.
2. A 19-year-old woman comes to the doctor's office where you work for renewal of her yearly birth control pill prescription. Your employer enforces regular checks for cervical changes by renewing the prescription only after a Pap smear is done. As you start setting out the Pap smear materials, your client expresses some reluctance to have a Pap smear today because she is so sore already.
3. Your 56-year-old client comes in to "get things checked out" because she hurts every time she and her husband have intercourse.

Answers at end of chapter.

Cytology

Cytology is the study of cells taken as biopsies. There are several ways that cells from the reproductive system may be removed for microscopic examination. During a Papanicolau (Pap) smear one or more small samples of cells are gently scraped away from the surface of the cervical canal using a small wooden spatula or tiny cylindrical brush and then smeared onto microscopic slides for viewing. Cells may also be collected by **conization,** which involves removing a small cone-shaped sample from the cervical canal, or by punch biopsy, which removes a small core of cells. Endometrial biopsies are samples of cells taken from the lining of the uterus by scraping with a small spoon-shaped tool called a **curet,** which is inserted through the cervix. Small biopsies may also be taken by cutting or removing a suspicious lesion. Cells may be observed for changes indicative of hormonal secretion, cellular maturation, or abnormalities such as are seen with viral growths and cancerous or precancerous conditions.

Nursing Care

The nurse adds appropriate sample collection materials and fixatives to the pelvic examination supplies according to the type of cytology being done. For a Pap smear this usually includes one or two clear glass slides labeled with the woman's name, fixative spray, a cytobrush, a wooden cervical spatula, and a transport box for the slides. For larger cell samples a sterile biopsy collection container labeled with the name and site of biopsy and a bottle of fixative solution should be placed close to the pelvic examination supplies. The procedure manual or physician is consulted concerning the types of instruments to put out for biopsies other than Pap smears. Cells die and degrade rapidly once removed from the client, so they must be packaged securely (generally in a preservative solution or sprayed with a fixative) for transport to laboratory facilities.

The client is prepared by explaining the procedure and providing support. The woman may be fearful of cancer or other abnormality. Removal of the sample may cause pain, bleeding, swelling, or later inflammation, so the client is monitored after the procedure and alerted to watch for and report these complications if they occur. The woman's status is documented on the chart, and it is noted that the sample was sent to the laboratory.

Swabs and Smears

Swabs and smears are done to determine which microorganisms are causing disease and to determine which antibiotics should be used.

Nursing Care

The nurse adds sample collection materials, including swabs, slides, and a chlamydia collection kit, to pelvic examination equipment if symptoms of vaginal infection are present. It is important to place samples of discharge into culture media that will support growth—generally clear media for most bacteria and yeasts and charcoal media for gonorrhea, so both types should be set out. Viral swabs require a special collection kit also. Chlamydia samples are especially difficult to transport to laboratories, and special kits are available for this pathogen. Some microorganisms, such as yeasts and trichomonas, can be identified well from smears on slides. Wet mounts are smears of discharge spread onto a slide. These must be taken to the microscope immediately after they are obtained. Sodium chloride and potassium hydroxide are dropped onto individual wet mount slides before they dry in order to aid in identification of some microorganisms. The nurse supports the client, who may be anxious about possible sexually transmitted diseases and effects on relationships.

Sonography

Ultrasound assessment (also called sonography) may be done to determine size, shape, development, and density of structures associated with the female reproductive system, as well as fetal measurements and some types of prenatal diagnoses. This procedure is especially useful for differentiating cysts from solid tumors, as well as locating **ectopic** pregnancies and intrauterine devices. Ultrasound may also be used to guide needles for obtaining samples of fluid or cells. Either external or vaginal transducers may be used to send and receive the signals for this procedure. Vaginal transducers are placed in a plastic sheath before insertion into the vagina. A full bladder may be required for some tests.

Nursing Care

The nurse explains the procedure and supports the client. The pressure of the transducer on the skin may be painful if the underlying structures are inflamed or swollen or if the bladder is very full.

Radiographic Procedures

Several radiographic procedures may be used for diagnosis of reproductive system problems. CT scanning and MRI are used to locate tumors of the reproductive system. Structures of the female reproductive system may also be outlined by taking x-ray pictures of cavities that have been filled with a radiopaque substance. During a **hysterosalpingogram,** dye is injected into the uterus until it comes out of the ends of the fallopian tubes. This test is useful for identifying congenital abnormalities in the shape of the uterus and blockages of the fallopian tubes.

Nursing Care

The nurse prepares the client for this test according to the x-ray department protocol and the physician's orders (this may include a laxative, suppository, or enema). The nurse ensures that the client understands the procedure and that appropriate consents are signed if required. Allergies to iodine and shellfish are assessed, because contrast media may contain iodine. After the procedure, the nurse assesses for nausea, light-headedness, and signs of allergy and promotes comfort, because some cramping may occur. Discharge teaching should include signs of infection and advice that the x-ray dye may stain clothing, so a pad should be worn until any vaginal drainage stops.

Endoscopic Examinations

Several types of endoscopic examinations are done to visually inspect internal areas in order to diagnose (and sometimes treat) reproductive system disorders. The names of the tests vary according to the area inspected, but all of these generally make use of a fiberoptic light and lens system, which is inserted through a tube called a cannula into a small incision. A laparoscopy is done to view the abdominal cavity and is useful for identifying problems such as endometriosis (Fig. 39–7). A salpingoscopy is performed to see the inside of the fallopian tubes and a **hysteroscopy** to see the inside of the uterus. A binocular microscope is used with an endoscope that is introduced through the vagina to closely study lesions of the cervix during a **colposcopy.** During **culdoscopy** an endoscope is introduced through the vagina and into the

---

ectopic: ec—out + top—place + ic—pertaining

hysterosalpingogram: hystero—womb + salpingo—tube + gram—record

hysteroscopy: hystero—womb + scopy—looking

colposcopy: colpo—vagina + scopy—looking

culdoscopy: culdo—cul de sac + scopy—looking

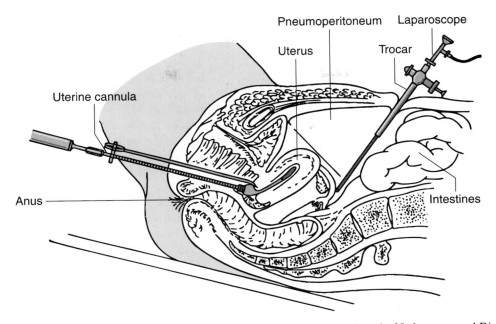

Figure 39–7. Laparoscopy. (Modified from Watson and Jaffe: Nurse's Manual of Laboratory and Diagnostic Tests, ed 2. FA Davis, Philadelphia, p 529, with permission.)

cul-de-sac of Douglas, a cavity behind the uterus (Fig. 39–8).

Nursing Care

Preoperatively, the client is prepared for an endoscopic examination according to institutional protocol. This generally involves asking the client whether she has fasted as instructed, assessing vital signs, recording the time of last voiding, helping the client into the operating room garb, and obtaining a signature on the consent form. General anesthesia may be given for some endoscopic procedures. The nurse explains what to expect and supports the woman. The client may be anxious about possible disorders.

Postoperatively, the nurse promotes comfort. These procedures produce almost no blood loss. The woman may experience pain in the neck, shoulders, and upper back if carbon dioxide (CO_2) gas was used. CO_2 may have been

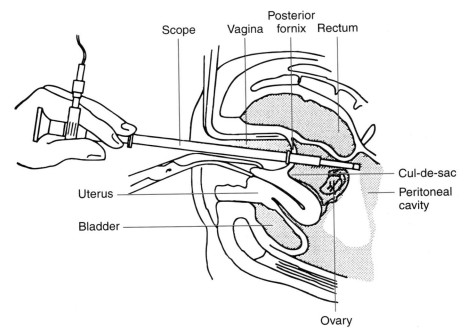

Figure 39–8. Culdoscopy. (Modified from Watson and Jaffe: Nurse's Manual of Laboratory and Diagnostic Tests, ed 2. FA Davis, Philadelphia, p 527, with permission.)

pumped into the body compartment being examined in order to increase the distance between structures so that it is easier for the physician to see to diagnose possible disorders. This is called **insufflation.** The CO_2 remaining after completion of the examination travels to the highest level of the body before being absorbed. Lying flat for a few hours after an endoscopic examination may decrease CO_2 migration discomfort. If incisions were made through the abdominal wall for insertion of the endoscope and for insufflation, these are tiny, and a Band-Aid or small dressing is applied.

Client Teaching

The client is advised to observe the sites for redness, bleeding, or any drainage and to return to the physician promptly if these occur and approximately 1 week later for suture removal (according to physician preference). If the endoscope procedure was done transvaginally, the client is advised to wear a perineal pad until the drainage stops, to report any bright bleeding after the operative day, and to report any fever or foul-smelling discharge.

Further detail about some specific forms of the tests that have been described in this chapter are included with the disorders to which they apply in Chapters 40 and 42.

Male Assessment

As with the female, the male reproductive system is a complex interaction of both physical and psychosocial factors. Unlike women, however, men may find it much more difficult in our society to talk about or admit to having problems related to reproductive health. From toilet training through adulthood men are expected to have behaviors associated with maleness. Unfortunately, by the time some boys reach manhood, their male identity is defined by the successful functioning of their sex organs.

One of the important first steps in obtaining a male reproductive assessment is providing a comfortable, nonjudgmental, confidential atmosphere for discussion. Often this means the nurse must first be knowledgeable and comfortable with sexual issues. Nurses do not hesitate to ask female clients about their menstrual history and should be equally comfortable in asking men about their **erection** or **ejaculation** history. Be open and straightforward with all questions and answers. It may be necessary at times to use more commonly expressed sexual words instead of medical terminology. You will discover that many men do not know the function of their prostate gland or the difference between ejaculation and **orgasm.** Use the assessment as an opportunity to teach men the facts about their own sexual functioning.

HISTORY

There are some basic questions every nurse should ask a male patient during the initial assessment. These include the following:

1. Are you having any problems getting or keeping a useable erection? Additional questions might be whether he can have an erection anytime (with or without a sex partner); if erection problems occur when he is under stress or taking medication; or if he is involved in substance abuse. Does he have erections first thing in the morning or during sleep? If he is able to get an erection, is it straight and firm enough for penetration? Does the erection last long enough for him to reach orgasm?

2. Are you able to ejaculate during orgasm? Questions related to ejaculation may include if there are any painful sensations related to the experience. Does any fluid come out during the ejaculation process, and if so, is it a small, moderate, or large amount, and is it clear, cloudy, or brown in color? (The amount and color may depend on whether he has had recent sexual activity or genitourinary surgery or may indicate a congenital anomaly or infection.)

3. For clients under 40 years old: Do you practice monthly testicular self-examinations? Men under age 40 should be encouraged to perform monthly testicular examinations as a cancer prevention measure.

4. For clients over 40 years old: When was the last time you had a prostate examination? A digital rectal examination (DRE) should be a regular part of a man's routine physical after age 40. Prostate cancer is treatable when detected early.

A more complete male sexual history not only includes information about sexual practices but also medical information. A wide variety of assessment data may affect a man's current and future sexual functioning (Table 39–3).

PHYSICAL EXAMINATION

The physical examination is generally performed by a physician or someone trained in physical assessments. The examination begins with the client's general appearance. He is observed for male patterns of hair growth on the head, face, chest, arms, and legs. Normal male pubic hair pattern is "triangle up," hair growth up towards the umbilicus. The client's height and muscle mass are noted. Men are often over 5 feet 6 inches tall, weight greater than 135 pounds, and shoulders are broader than their hips. The presence of excess breast tissue may indicate **gynecomastia,** an excess of female hormones. Abnormal findings in either hair patterns or muscle mass often indicate a hormone imbalance.

The penis, scrotum, and testes (testicles) are examined by observation and palpation. On observation, the penis is normally flaccid (soft) and hanging down straight. The size can vary greatly and should not be a concern unless it is unusually small (microphallus) or edematous. The left testis

---

insufflation: in—in + suffl—to blow + ation—process
gynecomastia: gyneco—female + mastia—breast

Table 39–3. **Male Sexual Assessment Guidelines**

Subject	Data to Collect	Possible Impact
Medication	Prescribed or over-the-counter medications that affect sexual desire, erection, or ejaculation (refer to Table 41–5)	Loss of sexual desire, erection, ejaculation, orgasm, or fertility
Family History	Any genetically transmitted diseases (e.g., heart problems, hypertension, diabetes), mother's use of DES during pregnancy	High risk for circulation problems that interfere with erections, congenital anomalies of reproductive organs
Personal Habits	Tobacco use, caffeine intake, substance abuse/recreational drugs, steroid use, frequent use of hot tubs, long-distance driving or bike riding	Decreased blood flow to penis, loss of erection; decreased testosterone (male hormone) interferes with erection and fertility; excessive heat decreases sperm production
Personal Health History	Mumps during adolescence, recent infection or fever	Decreased sperm production
Mental Health	Stressful personal problems or job situation, problems with sexual partner, performance anxiety or depression	Decreased sexual desire and ability to have an erection
Circulatory/Respiratory	Heart problems/surgery, high blood pressure, sickle cell disease, lung disease, sleep apnea	Decreased circulation—unable to have usable erection; decreased respiratory—activity intolerance, loss of erection, congenital anomalies of reproductive organs
Gastrointestinal	Liver infection/disease, surgery, bowel problems/surgery	Liver—decreased testosterone and increased estrogen, loss of erection; gastrointestinal/bowel—pain, loss of desire; surgery—loss of blood or nerve flow
Musculoskeletal	Painful joints, back injury/surgery, pelvic/lower back nerve damage	Pain, loss of desire; limited movement/positions, loss of erection, ejaculation, and orgasm
Neurological	Stroke, multiple sclerosis, Parkinson's	Limited movement/positions, loss of sensations, loss of control
Metabolic/Endocrine	Diabetes, obesity, thyroid problems	Diabetes mellitus—circulation problems, retrograde ejaculation, nerve damage; obesity—decreased male hormones, excess female hormones
Genitourinary	Congenital deformity of penis/testicles, prostate problems/surgery, erection/ejaculation problems, sexually transmitted diseases	Difficulty with penetration, erection problems, retrograde ejaculation, infertility
Sexual Practices	Frequency of intercourse (including positions, timing with female ovulation cycle), masturbation, use of lubricants or birth control methods, problems with erectile dysfunction or premature ejaculation	Decrease in quality and quantity of sperm that reach the female egg

will generally hang slightly lower in the scrotum than the right one.

The penis is examined for warts, sores (evidence of sexually transmitted diseases), swelling, curves, or lumps along the shaft. The examiner also makes sure the urethral opening is at the tip of the penis and not on the underside of the shaft (**hypospadias**). If the man is not **circumcised,** the foreskin should be pulled back carefully and the area inspected for signs of inflammation or foul-smelling discharge. The practitioner should be sure to replace the foreskin in the forward position after the examination is completed.

The scrotum and testes are carefully examined and palpated. Both testes should be present and a normal size (approximately 2 cm × 4 cm). The testes are egg shaped and should feel smooth and rubbery when lightly palpated be-

tween the thumb and fingers. The epididymis can be felt along the top edge and posterior section of each testis. The testes and scrotum are palpated for any lumps, cysts, or tumors. If a fluid-filled mass (**hydrocele**) is found, further evaluation should be done. A simple noninvasive test called transillumination is used to determine if the mass is fluid filled or solid. With the room lights out, a flashlight is held behind the scrotum. If the mass is fluid a red glow will appear; if it is solid it will be opaque. The spermatic cord (made up of veins, arteries, lymphatics, nerves, and the vas deferens) is palpated and should feel firm and threadlike. If a condition called a **varicocele** is present, the area feels like a "bag of worms." A varicocele is one of the most common problems associated with male infertility.

The male client is also examined for inguinal hernias by pressing up through the scrotum into each of the inguinal rings while asking him to cough or bear down. Each side is examined separately while he is in the standing position. A hernia feels like a pulsation against the examining fingertips.

In a DRE, the prostate gland is palpated by inserting a gloved, lubricated finger into the rectum while the man is in a knee-chest type of position. The entire posterior lobe of the gland can be felt this way. The gland should feel slightly firm and without any lumps. If the prostate gland feels very hard or soft, enlarged, or contains any lumps, a rectal ultrasound with needle biopsy is often ordered. A very swollen, painful prostate generally indicates that an infection is present. The nurse needs to remind all men over the age of 40 that unless they have had a complete removal of the prostate gland they still need a DRE performed every year. Many men are under the impression that any prostate surgery means the gland has been completely removed. When simple surgery is performed, prostate tissue is left in the body and will begin to regrow over time. This prostatic tissue can become cancerous and needs to be monitored with a yearly DRE.

TESTICULAR SELF-EXAMINATION

All men between the ages of 20 and 40 should do monthly testicular self-examination (TSE) in order to detect any tumors or other changes in the scrotum. See Table 39–4 for instructions that can be used to teach a man how to examine his testicles. Refer also to Figure 39–9.

DIAGNOSTIC TESTS OF THE MALE REPRODUCTIVE SYSTEM

Ultrasound

An ultrasound may be done to diagnose or evaluate a variety of male reproductive or genitourinary problems. A transrectal ultrasound may be done to diagnose prostate cancer.

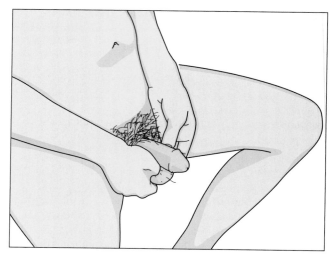

Figure 39–9. Testicular self-examination.

For this procedure, a rectal probe transducer is inserted into the rectum, and sound waves are used to evaluate the prostate gland. An enema may be ordered before the procedure. No special aftercare is necessary.

Pelvic or scrotal ultrasound helps evaluate and locate masses. Ultrasound may also be done to guide the needle during a fine-needle biopsy.

Cystourethroscopy

Cystourethroscopy may be done to evaluate the degree of obstruction by an enlarged prostate gland. For this procedure a Foley catheter is inserted, and a dye is injected into the bladder. X-rays are taken with the dye in the bladder and while voiding after the catheter has been removed.

Nursing Care

The procedure is explained to the client, and possible allergy to dyes is assessed and communicated to the physician as necessary. The client is instructed to void before the procedure. A sedative or analgesic may be ordered to help the client relax during the procedure.

After the procedure, intake and output are measured for 24 hours, and alteration from the client's normal pattern, or absence of urination, are reported to the physician. Fluids are encouraged to promote excretion of the dye.

Laboratory Tests

Prostatic-Specific Antigen

Normal value of prostate-specific antigen (PSA) is less than 4 ng/mL. PSA is a glycoprotein produced by prostate cells. An elevated level indicates prostatic hypertrophy or cancer.

Prostatic Acid Phosphatase

Normal value of prostatic acid phosphatase (PAP) is less than 3 ng/mL. PAP is an enzyme that normally affects me-

Table 39–4. Guidelines for Monthly Testicular Self-Examination

The examination is easiest during or right after a warm shower or bath, when the scrotum is relaxed and the testicles are hanging low. Choose one day a month to always do the examination.

1. Raise the penis up out of the way and look for any difference in size or shape of each side of the scrotum (sac). The left side usually hangs a little lower than the right.
2. Using both hands, hold the scrotum in the palms. Begin, one at a time, to gently roll each testicle between the thumb and first three fingers, feeling for any lumps or hard spots.
3. Identify the parts. The testicles should feel round, smooth, and egg shaped. The epididymis along the top and back side should feel soft and a little bit tender. The spermatic cord is a tube that runs up from the epididymis and usually feels firm, smooth, and movable.
4. See your doctor immediately if you feel any lumps or unusual changes.

tabolism of prostate cancer cells. An elevated level indicates prostate cancer.

Other Tests

If prostate cancer is suspected or diagnosed, additional tests may be done. Acid phosphatase may be elevated in metastatic prostate cancer. Alkaline phosphatase and serum calcium levels may be elevated if metastasis to the bone has occurred.

Tests for Infertility

Various hormone levels may be measured, including FSH, LH, testosterone, and adrenocorticotropic hormone (ACTH) to help determine causes of infertility in male clients.

Semen analysis may be done to provide information about infertility or to evaluate whether a vasectomy has been effective. Semen may be analyzed for sperm count, motility, and shape. Other tests determine whether the semen contains adequate nutrients to support sperm, whether antibodies to the sperm are present, and the ability of the sperm to penetrate an ovum.

Nursing Care

The client is instructed to refrain from ejaculation for 3 days before collecting the semen sample, to avoid altering findings. Generally specimens are collected on three separate occasions over a period of 4 to 6 days. Masturbation and ejaculation directly into a sterile container is recommended to avoid loss of semen. Condoms and lubricants should be avoided. The sample should be taken to the laboratory within 1 hour of collection.

Additional tests of the male reproductive system are discussed in Chapter 41.

Review Questions

1. The male reproductive duct that carries sperm into the abdominal cavity is the
   a. Urethra
   b. Epididymis
   c. Ductus deferens
   d. Ejaculatory duct

2. The site of fertilization is usually the
   b. Ovary
   b. Uterus
   c. Vagina
   d. Fallopian tube

3. According to the American Cancer Society, how often should breast self-examination be done?
   a. Yearly
   b. Monthly
   c. Weekly
   d. Semiannually

4. Which of the following items should NOT be placed out in preparation for a Pap smear?
   a. A syringe
   b. A vaginal speculum
   c. A basin of warm water
   d. A water-soluble lubricant

5. Which of the following techniques is recommended for male clients under the age of 40 to detect prostate cancer early?
   a. Yearly DRE
   b. Monthly STE
   c. Yearly PSA
   d. Bimonthly bimanual examination

6. Anna Brown has just had a laparoscopy to investigate the causes of her infertility. The nurse should instruct her to lie flat in the bed for a few hours for which of the following reasons?
   a. Her blood pressure will be extremely low due to so much blood loss.
   b. She will rip out the stitches in the long incision on her abdomen.
   c. The carbon dioxide left over from the test will travel upward and cause pain.
   d. Her uterus needs to be at the same level as her heart to prevent excessive swelling.

ANSWERS TO CRITICAL THINKING:
Reproductive Assessment

1. Calm fears. Explain simply. Allow parent to stay with the child (if appropriate). Consider whether the child has possibly been abused (if so, evidence needs to be collected and a report filed with the appropriate child protection authorities). Place a nasal speculum out for examination. Place a forceps out for removal of a possible foreign body (not uncommon at this age). Teach that this is a normal part of the body that is to be protected and taken care of.

2. Assess knowledge and maturity. Set out supplies for a Pap smear and for swabs and smears. Teach while getting supplies ready. Explain that vaginal soreness generally needs to be treated and that the doctor must know more about the problem to do so effectively. Explain that inflammations can interfere with Pap smear results, so it may have to be repeated later after treatment. Explain culture and sensitivity testing. Teach about risk reduction and inform that oral contraceptives do not offer a barrier.

3. Try to put the woman at ease through general conversation. Set out supplies for a Pap smear (if needed) and for swabs and smears. Teach while getting supplies ready. Discuss aging and the effects of decreased estrogen in general and specifically on vaginal tissues. Inform that there are sev-

eral ways to deal with the problems resulting from decreased estrogen, such as water-soluble lubricants, vaginal creams, and estrogen patches.

REFERENCES

1. Smith, BL: The breast. In Ryan, KJ, Berkowitz, RS, and Barbieri, RL (eds): Kistner's Gynecology, ed 6. Mosby, St Louis, 1995, p 229.
2. American Cancer Society: Breast Cancer Network [On-line]. Available http://www.cancer.org/health.html, April 5, 1997.
3. CNN interview with Dr. Robert Smith, American Cancer Society. Cable News Network, Atlanta, March 26, 1997.

BIBLIOGRAPHY

Agency for Health Care Policy and Research: Clinical Practice Guidelines, no. 8. AHCPR publication number 94-0582. Benign Prostatic Hyperplasia: Diagnosis and Treatment. US Department of Health and Human Services, Public Health Service, Rockville, Md, 1994.

Carlson, KJ, et al (eds): Primary Care of Women. Mosby, St Louis, 1995.

Fogel, CI, and Woods, NF (eds): Women's Health Care. Sage, Thousand Oaks, Calif, 1995.

Lemcke, DP, et al (eds): Primary Care of Women. Appleton & Lange, Norwalk, Conn, 1995.

Lemone, PM, and Burke, KM (eds): Medical-Surgical Nursing: Critical Thinking in Client Care. Addison-Wesley, Menlo Park, Calif, 1996.

Meredith, CE: Male infertility. In Karlowicz, KA (ed): Urologic Nursing: Principles and Practice. WB Saunders, Philadelphia, 1995.

Meredith, CE: Male genitourinary problems. In Lewis, SM, Collier, IC, and Heitkemper, MM (eds): Medical-Surgical Nursing, ed 4. Mosby, St Louis, 1996.

Phipps, WJ, et al (eds): Medical-Surgical Nursing: Concepts and Clinical Practice. Mosby, St Louis, 1995.

Ryan, KJ, Berkowitz, RS, and Barbieri, RL (eds): Kistner's Gynecology, ed 6. Mosby, St Louis, 1995.

Star, WI, Lommel, LL, and Shannon, MT (eds): Women's Primary Health Care: Protocols for Practice. American Nurses' Association, Washington, DC, 1995.

40

Nursing Care of Women with Reproductive System Disorders

Linda Hopper Cook

Learning Objectives

Upon completion of this chapter, the student will be able to:

1. Define common terms associated with disorders of the reproductive system.
2. Briefly describe the pathophysiology of common female reproductive disorders.
3. Discuss risk factors for development of various reproductive disorders.
4. Outline strategies for risk reduction for various reproductive disorders.
5. Identify client concerns associated with reproductive system disorders.
6. Describe the nurse's role in care of clients with reproductive system disorders.
7. Discuss common treatment options for reproductive system disorders.
8. Plan care for clients with reproductive system disorders using the nursing process.

Key Words

agenesis (ay-**JEN**-uh-sis)
amenorrhea (ay-MEN-uh-**REE**-ah)
anteflexion (AN-tee-**FLECK**-shun)
anteversion (AN-tee-**VER**-zhun)
augmentation (AWG-men-**TAY**-shun)
balanitis (BAL-uh-**NIGH**-tis)
bilateral salpingo-oophorectomy (by-**LAT**-er-uhl sal-PINJ-oh-ah-fuh-**RECK**-tuh-mee)
cautery (**CAW**-tur-ee)
colporrhaphy (kohl-**POOR**-ah-fee)
contraceptive (KON-truh-**SEP**-tiv)
cryotherapy (KRY-oh-**THER**-uh-pee)
culdocentesis (KUL-doh-sen-**TEE**-sis)
culdotomy (kul-**DOT**-uh-mee)
cystocele (**SIS**-toh-seel)
cytolytic (SIGH-toh-**LIT**-ik)
dermoid (**DER**-moyd)
dilation and curettage (DIL-**AY**-shun and kyoor-e-**TAHZH**)
disseminated intravascular coagulation (dis-**SEM**-i-NAY-ted IN-trah-**VAS**-kyoo-lar koh-AG-yoo-**LAY**-shun)
dysmenorrhea (DIS-men-oh-**REE**-ah)
dyspareunia (DIS-puh-**ROO**-nee-ah)
dysplasia (dis-**PLAY**-zee-ah)
ectasia (ek-**TAY**-zee-ah)
endogenous (en-**DAH**-jen-us)
exogenous (ex-**AHJ**-en-us)
fibrinolytic (FIGH-brin-oh-**LIT**-ik)
fibrocystic (FIGH-broh-**SIS**-tik)
gamete (**GAM**-eet)
hypercoagulation (HIGH-per-koh-AG-yoo-**LAY**-shun)
hypermenorrhea (HIGH-per-MEN-oh-**REE**-ah)
hypertrophy (high-**PER**-truh-fee)
hypomenorrhea (HIGH-poh-MEN-oh-**REE**-ah)

hypoplasia (HIGH-poh-**PLAY**-zee-ah)

hysterectomy (HISS-tuh-**RECK**-tuh-mee)

hysterotomy (HISS-tuh-**RAH**-tuh-mee)

imperforate (im-**PER**-foh-rate)

insufflation (in-suff-**LAY**-shun)

in vitro fertilization (in **VEE**-troh FER-ti-li-**ZAY**-shun)

laparotomy (LAP-uh-**RAH**-tuh-mee)

laser ablation (**LAY**-zer uh-**BLAY**-shun)

leiomyoma (LYE-oh-my-**OH**-ma)

mammoplasty (**MAM**-oh-PLAS-tee)

marsupialization (mar-SOO-pee-al-i-**ZAY**-shun)

mastalgia (mass-**TAL**-jee-ah)

mastectomy (mass-**TECK**-tuh-mee)

mastitis (mass-**TIGH**-tis)

mastopexy (**MAS**-toh-PEKS-ee)

menometrorrhagia or metromenorrhagia (MEN-oh-**MET**-roh-**RAY**-jee-ah) (MET-roh-MEN-oh-**RAY**-jee-ah)

menorrhagia (MEN-oh-**RAY**-jee-ah)

metastasis (muh-**TASS**-tuh-sis)

motility (moh-**TIL**-i-tee)

myomectomy (MY-oh-**MECK**-tuh-mee)

neoplasia (NEE-oh-**PLAY**-zee-ah)

oligomenorrhea (AH-li-goh-MEN-uh-**REE**-ah)

osteoporosis (AHS-tee-oh-por-**OH**-sis)

panhysterectomy (PAN-hiss-tuh-**RECK**-tuh-mee)

pedicle (**PED**-i-kuhl)

perimenopausal (PER-ee-MEN-oh-**PAWS**-uhl)

petechiae (pe-**TEE**-kee-ee)

polymenorrhea (PAH-lee-MEN-uh-**REE**-uh)

postcoital (post-**KOH**-i-tal)

rectocele (**RECK**-toh-seel)

retroflexion (RET-roh-**FLECK**-shun)

retrograde (**RET**-roh-grayd)

retroversion (RET-roh-**VER**-zhun)

septa (**SEP**-tuh)

teratoma (ter-uh-**TOH**-muh)

thrombophlebitis (THROM-boh-fle-**BYE**-tis)

vaginosis (VAJ-i-**NOH**-sis)

vasovagal reflex (VAY-zoh-**VAY**-gull **REE**-fleks)

zygote (**ZYE**-goht)

Reproductive system disorders can be frightening, irritating, frustrating, embarrassing, and in some cases fatal. They do not just involve body parts, but may also involve roles, relationships, and sense of identity and purpose in life. Nurses can do a lot to help women who are experiencing disorders of the reproductive system.

Breast Disorders

BENIGN BREAST DISORDERS

Much has been done in recent years to educate the general public concerning breast cancer. It is the second highest cause of cancer death for all ages of American women, and it is estimated that American women have a one in eight chance of developing breast cancer over their lifetime.[1] Heightened awareness of the risks of breast cancer, however, sometimes results in excessive anxiety among women when benign conditions of the breast occur.

Cyclic Breast Discomfort

Pathophysiology and Signs and Symptoms

The most common breast symptoms result from cyclic variations in hormone levels. Breast swelling, tenderness, and sometimes pain (**mastalgia**) can be related to hormone-mediated changes within the breast tissues that prepare them for their potential role in motherhood.

Medical Treatment

If persistent or too severe, these symptoms may be treated with medications that change hormone levels. For most women, however, knowing that the cyclic discomfort is temporary and not the result of a disease process is sufficient to allay fears.

Fibrocystic Breast Changes

Pathophysiology and Signs and Symptoms

Other long-term changes to the breasts are also common and occur in response to hormonal stimulation as a consequence of overresponsiveness of cells. This exaggerated response results in replacement of normal tissue with fibrous tissue, **ectasia** (overdevelopment) of cells, and blockage of ducts so that cysts are formed around the trapped fluid. This makes the breasts feel somewhat hard and lumpy.

Medical Treatment

Generally, no treatment is given. Although **fibrocystic** changes are not cancerous, more frequent mammography or ultrasound may be advised because the fibrocystic changes may make it more difficult to feel early cancerous lumps during breast self-examination (BSE).

---

mastalgia: mast—breast + algia—pain
ectasia: extension

Prevention

Whether caffeine intake contributes to fibrocystic changes is still a matter of debate.

Mastitis

Etiology and Signs and Symptoms

Breast infection with inflammation (**mastitis**) occurs due to injury and introduction of bacteria into the breast. This condition most commonly occurs while breast feeding. The breast becomes swollen, hot, red, and painful and may form an abscess.

Medical and Surgical Treatment

Mastitis may be treated either with antibiotics or, if an abscess forms, by incision and drainage (I&D) of the abscess. The location and type of infection will determine whether breast feeding should be continued or discontinued.

Nursing Care

The nurse may apply a dressing over the I&D site to absorb drainage. Application of warm moist packs may increase the comfort and promote healing for clients with mastitis.

Client Teaching

Client teaching should include instructions to wash hands carefully to prevent the spread of infection and to wear a supportive bra to relieve some of the discomfort.

MALIGNANT BREAST DISORDERS

Etiology

Several risk factors for development of breast cancer have been identified through research.[2] The risk for developing breast cancer increases dramatically with age. Occurrence of breast cancer in one's family or oneself increases the risk of future cancer development. High-fat diets, high alcohol intake, and oral contraceptive medications have all been cited as risk factors.[3] Those who experience either early menarche, late menopause, late first pregnancy, or no pregnancies at all have higher rates of breast cancer. Women who breast feed have somewhat lower rates of breast cancer.[4]

Prevention

Exercising moderation in fat and alcohol consumption and using nonhormonal methods of birth control may be ways of preventing breast cancer. However, there are many factors that we cannot control, so the importance of early detection of breast cancers cannot be overemphasized.[5]

Diagnostic Tests

BSE and clinical breast examinations are important parts of identification of cancer. Cancerous growths tend to be harder, less movable, and more irregularly shaped and tend to have less clearly defined borders than benign growths. The prognosis is good for women who have breast cancers removed in the early stages, but the passage of time can drastically change this prognosis. Teaching and encouraging the regular use of BSE and appropriate use of mammography can save lives (refer to Chapter 39 for BSE instructions and illustration). As mentioned in Chapter 39, sonography, computed tomography (CT) scanning, magnetic resonance imaging (MRI), thermography, diaphanography, and biopsy may all be used to assist in determination of whether tumors of the breast are malignant.

Staging

Once cells have become cancerous, the advancement of the disease is denoted by staging or classification. The spread of cancer cells from a primary tumor by way of the blood and lymph circulation is called **metastasis.** These metastatic cells may then produce secondary cancerous areas in distant lymph nodes or other sites. Breast cancer is categorized according to five stages, ranging from stage 0, in which there is a tumor but no lymph node involvement and no metastasis, to stage IV, in which there is widespread nodal involvement and metastasis.

Medical and Surgical Treatment and Complications

There are five main treatment options for breast cancer: radiation therapy, cytotoxic chemotherapy, hormonal therapy, modification of biological response, and surgery. These options may be used separately or in combination depending on the condition of the client and the advancement of the disease.

The possibility of metastases necessitates drastic treatment of the whole body in many cases to prevent secondary cancer growth at other sites. Both irradiation and cytotoxic chemotherapy generally combat cancer by destroying rapidly reproducing cells. This works well against cancer but also tends to destroy normal body cells that reproduce rapidly, such as hair and the cells lining the mouth, vagina, and gastrointestinal tract. Interventions that help preserve these tissues and maintain ad-

---

mastitis: mast—breast + itis—inflammation
mastectomy: mast—breast + ec—away + tomy—cutting

equate nutrition can promote health during cancer therapy.

Hormonal therapy may be undertaken to deprive cancer cells of hormones that stimulate their growth. Because breast cancer cells are often estrogen sensitive, this may be accomplished by decreasing circulating estrogen levels with drugs or by blocking the use of estrogen by cancer cells as occurs with use of the drug tamoxifen citrate. Interference with estrogen levels, however, may produce menopausal symptoms and increase the risk of osteoporosis and heart disease.

Substances that modify the body's biological responses may be given to intensify positive responses of the body or to decrease negative body responses. The ideal cancer drug would probably be a substance that would stimulate the body to attack cancers and destroy them in much the same way that the body attacks and destroys various substances that could be harmful to the body. Some examples of biological response modifiers are interferons, tumor necrosis factor, interleukins, and immunotherapy formulations. This is an area of much research and is likely to expand greatly over the next few years.

Breast surgeries to remove cancerous tissue can be very disfiguring and have profound effects on the client's self concept. The amount of tissue removed varies depending on the size, nature, and invasiveness of the cancer. A lumpectomy is the surgical removal of just the tumor and a margin of tissue surrounding it. A **mastectomy** is the surgical removal of the breast. A mastectomy may be partial (involving only part of the breast), simple (involving only breast tissue), or radical (involving breast tissue, underlying muscle, and surrounding lymph nodes). In recent years the surgical practice has shifted from mainly radical mastectomies to more breast-conserving surgeries with radiation therapy, with similar survival rates demonstrated. See Nursing Care Plan Box 40–1 for the Mastectomy Client.

Client Teaching

Although some alternative therapies are being used, clients need to be aware that some unethical practitioners are not above using the desperation of incurable clients for their own gain by offering expensive but ineffective treatments. Clients should be especially wary of procedures that can be done only in another country, because this may mean that they would not meet national approval standards for safety and efficacy. The Internet has provided easy access to information from around the world. Some people have gained valuable support and ideas to help them cope with their illnesses and disabilities by this means, but the Internet has no control bodies to ensure that such advice is accurate, ethical, and safe. The client should always be encouraged to check out information with more than one trusted expert on the subject. Cancer research centers and cancer treatment centers generally have people who are willing to answer questions about experimental and alternative therapies.

Nursing Process

Much of the nursing care planning for a mastectomy client is similar to other surgeries (covered in Chapter 11). Particular concerns relevant to the mastectomy client are described in Nursing Care Plan Box 40–1 for the Mastectomy Client.

BREAST MODIFICATION SURGERIES

Mammoplasty is surgical modification of the breast. This may be done to restore a normal shape after removal of cancerous tissues. Many women, however, undergo mammoplasty as an elective surgery to reduce or increase the size or improve the shape of their breasts.

A caring and nonjudgmental attitude about psychosocial concerns that prompt breast modification surgery is essential. Because nurses are very aware of the dangers involved with surgery, concerns about body image may seem to be a trivial reason to voluntarily assume such risks to life and health. However, body image is a very important component of quality of life. Nurses may legitimately feel troubled that current culture seems to overemphasize body shape for women, but clients' informed decisions should be respected if they choose to have this type of surgery.

Breast Reduction

Generally, in breast reduction operations the nipple is separated from the surrounding tissue except for a small section with the blood vessels and nerves that supply it (Fig. 40–1). A large wedge of tissue is removed from the bottom of the breast, the edges are sewn together, and the nipple is reimplanted higher than its previous position. This procedure not only decreases the overall size of the breast, it also corrects excessive sagging—a common problem for women with very large breasts.

Mastopexy

Another procedure that may be done to raise sagging breasts is a **mastopexy,** which involves the removal of some skin and fat and then resuturing so that the breast tissues are held higher on the chest. This may improve the appearance temporarily until tissues stretch again.

Augmentation

Augmentation is a surgery to increase the size of the breasts in which a filler, commonly called an implant, is added to the breast. The implant—either a bag contain-

---

mammoplasty: mamm(o)—breast + plasty—to mold

NURSING CARE PLAN BOX 40-1 FOR THE MASTECTOMY CLIENT

Risk for anxiety related to uncertainty about diagnosis, prognosis, and treatments

Outcomes
Excessive anxiety will not be evident.

Interventions	Rationale	Evaluation
Carry out thorough preoperative teaching about what to expect relative to the surgical experience based on the client's understanding, concerns, and willingness to learn. Support the physician's explanations, answer questions whenever possible, or refer to appropriate knowledgeable sources.	Knowledge dispels unreasonable fears and helps the client to prepare adequately to cope with stressors.	Does the client express satisfaction with amount and type of information? Does the client evidence an adequate understanding of the surgical procedure and changes in condition postoperatively? Do the client's vital signs, verbal, and nonverbal demeanor suggest anxiety?

Risk for ineffective breathing related to pain with chest movement

Outcomes
Effective breathing pattern with clearance of mucous from air passages.

Interventions	Rationale	Evaluation
Medicate to relieve pain as necessary. Encourage deep breathing and coughing each hour. Encourage use of an incentive spirometer each hour when awake.	Pain may inhibit deep breathing efforts. This helps to loosen secretions and to prevent atelectasis, pneumonia, and inadequate oxygenation of tissues.	Does the client evidence pain or guarding during chest movement? Does the chest sound clear? Are skin color and oxygen saturation adequate?

Risk for impaired tissue perfusion and integrity related to damage to blood and lymph vessels and tension at surgical incision site

Outcomes
Incision will heal by primary intention without excessive bleeding or swelling.

Interventions	Rationale	Evaluation
Monitor vital signs, oxygen saturation, and peripheral vascular status according to hospital policy and as necessary. Avoid use of the affected arm for blood pressure, venipunctures, and injections.	Vital signs, oxygen saturation, and peripheral vascular signs reflect circulatory status. Restrictive and invasive procedures might further compromise tissue integrity of the affected arm.	Are vital signs stable and within normal range? Is dressing dry? Is arm protected?
Check for bleeding, amount and color of drainage if a drain device is used, and swelling. Measure circumference of arms daily and compare. Elevate affected arm if swelling occurs. Place items where client may easily reach them.	Excessive bleeding and swelling may further compromise tissue perfusion. Swelling causes an increase in circumference. Gravity aids fluid return to the heart. Excessive movement of the arm may exert tension on incision and increase bleeding.	Does the incisional area look swollen, smooth, or shiny? Is drainage amount and color appropriate? Is the affected arm larger than the unaffected arm? Does elevation prevent swelling? Can the client reach items without abducting the arm over 90 degrees?
Encourage reasonable exercise of the affected arm following postmastectomy exercises that are approved by the institution.	Reasonable exercise promotes circulation, preserves muscle and joint function, and increases self-care ability.	Is the client moving the arm appropriately and gradually increasing range of motion and self-care ability?

continued

NURSING CARE PLAN BOX 40–1 *(continued)*

Risk for ineffective individual coping related to cancer threat and body image disturbance

Outcomes
Client will evidence use of effective coping skills.

Interventions	*Rationale*	*Evaluation*
Maintain an open and trusting therapeutic relationship. Allow grieving to take place. Encourage the client to express feelings and concerns.	Effective communication is based on trust. Loss of a breast disturbs many aspects of body image, and cancer threatens one's sense of security and reasonableness of life.	Is the client talking about concerns? Is the client willing to look at the incision area? How are family members interacting with the client? How is the client responding to family members and friends?
Encourage active problem solving. Help the client remember previous successes in coping and strategies used. Refer to appropriate agencies for further support as needed (e.g., American Cancer Society, Reach for Recovery, local support groups, pastoral counseling).	Active problem solving promotes self-efficacy and combats depression. Memory of prior success can encourage hope for future success. Social support can assist individuals to meet their needs while developing effective coping skills and strategies.	Is grief being expressed? Is the client planning for the future? Is the client taking an active interest in her personal appearance? Does the client have sufficient coping skills or supports available to promote healthy living?

ing saline solution or silicone gel or a transplanted portion of the client's own body tissues from another area—may be inserted under or over the pectoral muscles (Fig. 40–2).

For reconstructive mammoplasty, use of the client's own tissues is generally safer than use of artificial implants, because no foreign material is introduced into the body. For situations in which significant amounts of tissue are needed for reconstruction, a portion of tissue may be moved from one area of the body to another while still maintaining its attachment to the original blood supply. This type of repair is called a **pedicle** (meaning literally "little foot") graft because the graft remains attached to a stalk (containing the blood vessels and nerves) and thus somewhat resembles a little leg with a foot (the graft) attached. Figure 40–3 shows two options for graft repair of a mastectomy—using the latissimus dorsi muscle and overlying tissue on the side of the chest or using the rectus abdominus muscle of the abdomen with its overlying tissue. For both of these procedures, a portion of muscle is separated from its usual attachment. Tissues overlying a part of the muscle are excised and left attached to the muscle. This segment of tissue is then pulled under the skin and superficial layers to an opening made at the mastectomy site. Here it is brought to the surface and attached to reconstruct a breast shape. Tissue also may be removed from the buttock area or the abdomen and grafted onto a mastectomy site without a pedicle.

Complications of Breast Modification Surgeries

Any of these surgeries may be complicated by infection or impaired healing of tissues. The use of silicone implants has been less than satisfactory for many women recently. Some women have experienced hardening of breast tissues and others have developed serious autoimmune disease problems after receiving silicone gel implants. Although it is still uncertain as to whether the implants actually caused all of the problems that were cited, a large proportion of recent breast surgeries have been undertaken to remove previous implants.

Nursing Care

Nurses must carefully assess the healing process when changing dressings, because not all tissues successfully attach at the new site and failure of attachment can require surgical revision. Signs of poor attachment include unnatural color of the incision, graft, or surrounding tissues, swelling, drainage, gaping of incision lines, and sloughing of the graft or edges of the site.

---

pedicle: ped—foot + icle—little

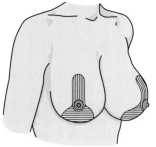

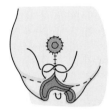
Skin removed

Skin and breast tissue removed

A. Area of skin to be removed   B. Areas marked on breast

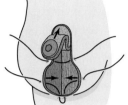

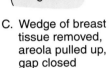

C. Wedge of breast tissue removed, areola pulled up, gap closed

D. Excess tissue removed, skin closed with stitches

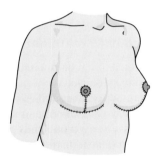

E. Post-operative appearance

Figure 40–1. Breast reduction. (Modified from Love, SM: Dr. Love's Breast Book, ed 2. Addison-Wesley, Menlo Park, Calif, 1995, with permission.)

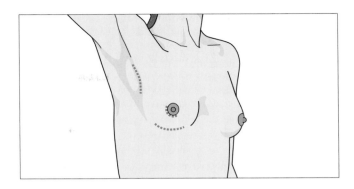

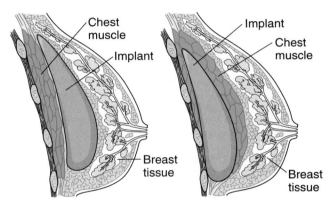
Chest muscle

Implant

Breast tissue

Implant

Chest muscle

Breast tissue

Figure 40–2. Breast implants. *(A)* Implant over muscle. *(B)* Implant under muscle. (Modified from Love, SM: Dr. Love's Breast Book, ed 2. Addison-Wesley, Menlo Park, Calif, 1995, with permission.)

Menstrual Disorders

FLOW AND CYCLE DISORDERS

Etiology

There can be many reasons for menstrual abnormalities. Pregnancy, hormonal imbalances, metabolic imbalances (such as obesity, anorexia nervosa, and loss of too much body fat through excessive exercise), tumors (both benign and malignant), infections, organ diseases (such as liver, kidney, or thyroid disease), blood or bone marrow abnormalities, and the presence of foreign bodies in the uterus (such as intrauterine devices) all can result in abnormal

menses. Menstrual abnormalities can be distressing and can result in anemia, persistent fatigue, and sexual dysfunction. Establishment of a comfortable and open professional relationship with the client is important for communication about these concerns (Table 40–1).

Diagnostic Tests

Appropriate testing to determine the cause(s) of the menstrual abnormalities can involve a thorough medical history and physical examination, swabs of vaginal discharge, a Pap smear, pregnancy testing, urine testing, and extensive blood testing to screen for any of the disorders that may influence the menstrual cycle and flow. Generally physicians test to rule out the most likely causes first and then begin to test for more obscure disorders until the etiology of the menstrual abnormalities is identified. For instance, reproductive hormone levels are likely to be tested before kidney or liver function, unless the latter disorders are evident in the initial history and physical examination.

Medical and Surgical Treatment

Medical treatment of menstrual disorders generally involves manipulation of hormone levels. Surgical treatment

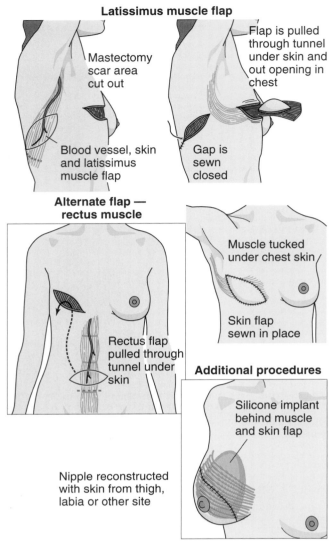

Latissimus muscle flap

Mastectomy scar area cut out

Blood vessel, skin and latissimus muscle flap

Flap is pulled through tunnel under skin and out opening in chest

Gap is sewn closed

Alternate flap — rectus muscle

Rectus flap pulled through tunnel under skin

Muscle tucked under chest skin

Skin flap sewn in place

Additional procedures

Silicone implant behind muscle and skin flap

Nipple reconstructed with skin from thigh, labia or other site

Figure 40–3. Mastectomy reconstruction. (Modified from Love, SM: Dr. Love's Breast Book, ed 2. Addison-Wesley, Menlo Park, Calif, 1995, with permission.)

of menstrual disorders can involve **dilation and curettage** (D&C), **laser ablation** of endometrial tissue, and **hysterectomy.** During D&C the cervix is first dilated, which means that it is opened wider, and then curets—sharp spoonlike instruments—are inserted through the opening and used to scoop out the inner lining of the uterus. Laser ablation involves burning of endometrial tissue with a laser. The burned areas form scar tissue that does not bleed. Hysterectomy is the surgical removal of the uterus and is described more fully later in this chapter.

Nursing Care

Estimation of the amount of blood lost during menses may be difficult because pad counts can vary widely depending on the frequency of pad changes and the portion of the pad that was soaked. The only accurate way to estimate men-

strual flow is by weighing the pads (sealed in a biohazard bag) and then subtracting the weight of the number of original pads. For estimation purposes, 1 g increase in pad weight equals approximately 1 mL of blood loss.

DYSMENORRHEA

Etiology

Painful menstruation, or **dysmenorrhea,** is a common problem of approximately 50 percent of all women, although only about 1 percent of women find the dysmenorrhea to be incapacitating.[6] Primary dysmenorrhea is not pathological and is caused mainly by the action of **endogenous** prostaglandins, which stimulate uterine contractions and result in cramping pain. Secondary dysmenorrhea is caused by some pathology such as endometriosis, pelvic infection, retroversion of the uterus, or tumors.

Diagnostic Tests

For primary dysmenorrhea hormonal tests may be required. For secondary dysmenorrhea, determination of the cause(s) may require laparoscopic examination, biopsies, and various other tests of functioning of the reproductive system.

Medical and Surgical Treatment

Primary dysmenorrhea may be treated with drugs that inhibit prostaglandin synthesis such as aspirin and nonsteroidal anti-inflammatory drugs (NSAIDs). Correction of the causes of secondary dysmenorrhea may be more complicated than for primary dysmenorrhea and may include such measures as hormonal adjustment, dilation and curettage, and other surgical procedures.

Client Teaching

Several nonprescription preparations are available for treatment of dysmenorrhea, but clients should be advised to read the labels carefully, because aspirin and NSAIDs may be bought less expensively as separate drugs and other added drugs such as diuretics may not be necessary. If dysmenorrhea is related to uterine retroversion, assuming a knee-chest position may relieve the discomfort. The sudden development of dysmenorrhea in a woman who previously experienced no discomfort with menses should always be investigated by a physician.

---

dilation and curettage: dilat(e)—to widen + ation—the process of + curet—scoop + tage—doing

laser ablation: laser—light amplification by stimulated emission of radiation + ab—away + lat—to carry + ion—the process

hysterectomy: hyster—womb + ec—away + tomy—cutting

dysmenorrhea: dys—painful + men(o)—month + rrhea—flow

endogenous: endo—within + genous—produced

Table 40–1. **Menstrual Flow Disorders**

Disorder	Description
Amenorrhea	Menses absent for more than 6 months or three of previous cycles
	Called primary amenorrhea when menarche has not occurred by age 17
	Called secondary amenorrhea when menses are absent after menarche
Oligomenorrhea	Menstrual cycles of over 35 days
Hypomenorrhea	Less than the expected amount of menstrual bleeding
Menorrhagia	Passing more than 80 mL of blood per menses
Hypermenorrhea	Lasting longer than 7 days
Polymenorrhea (also called **metrorrhagia**)	More frequently than 21-day intervals
Menometrorrhagia (also called **metromenorrhagia**)	Overly long, heavy, and irregular menses

oligomenorrhea: oligo—little (few) + men(o)—month + rrhea—flow
hypomenorrhea: hypo—little + men(o)—month + rrhea—flow
menorrhagia: men(o)—month + rrhagia—burst forth
hypermenorrhea: hyper—too much + men(o)—month + rrhea—flow
polymenorrhea: poly—many + men(o)—month + rrhea—flow
metrorrhagia: metro—uterus + rrhagia—burst forth
menometrorrhagia: men(o)—month + metro—uterus + rrhagia—burst forth
metromenorrhagia: metro—uterus + men(o)—month + rrhagia—burst forth

PREMENSTRUAL SYNDROME

Signs and Symptoms

Premenstrual syndrome (PMS) is a recurrent problem for many women and involves some or all of the following symptoms: water retention; headaches; discomfort of joints, muscles, and breasts; changes in affect; changes in concentration and coordination; and sensory changes. Only a small number of women find PMS to be serious enough to interfere with work or relationships. Interactions of ovarian hormones, aldosterone, and neurotransmitters such as monoamine oxidase and serotonin, which affect the brain and nervous system, are not well understood, and further research is needed.[7]

Medical Treatment

A variety of drugs have been given to combat PMS with varying degrees of success. Some commonly used PMS medications include drugs that affect prostaglandin production, hormonal balance, and neurotransmitter production and uptake, as well as diuretics and supplements of calcium, magnesium, vitamin E, and vitamin B_6. Clients should be warned, however, that dosages of vitamins should not be increased without professional advice since higher doses of vitamin B_6 than 500 mg/day can cause permanent nerve damage.[8]

Nursing Care

Women who suffer from severe PMS may have been treated as if they are psychologically unbalanced due to the interaction of hormones and neurotransmitters and due to outdated ideas concerning PMS, so an understanding and nonjudgmental attitude is especially important in treatment of these clients.

Client Teaching

Several lifestyle measures seem to help PMS sufferers, including restriction of alcohol, caffeine, nicotine, and simple sugars; participation in regular exercise; and development of stress management skills. The nurse can be helpful to the client by providing educational materials and teaching about self-help strategies for management of this disorder.

ENDOMETRIOSIS

Pathophysiology and Signs and Symptoms

Endometriosis is a condition in which functioning endometrial tissue is located outside of the uterus (Fig. 40–4). There are several theories to explain development of endometriosis. One theory, the coelomic metaplasia theory, suggests that during development certain cells in parts of the body other than the uterus can, in response to certain triggers, differentiate to become endometriotic cells.[9] The most generally accepted explanation, however, is that cells from the uterus can be transported to a distant site either by the blood or lymphatic circulation or through **retrograde** menstruation—a backward leakage of blood and tissue out through the fallopian tubes during the menstrual period.

Endometriotic cells grow in areas of sufficient blood supply—extending into other tissues such as intestinal walls, ovaries, and other abdominal structures. On a cyclic

retrograde: retro—backward + grade—step

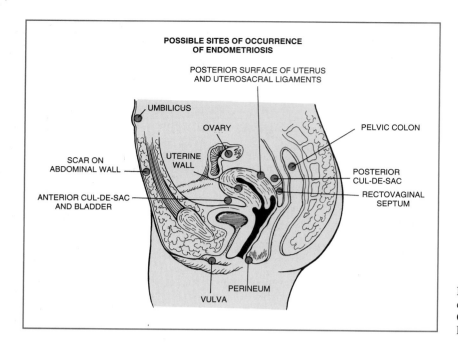

**POSSIBLE SITES OF OCCURRENCE
OF ENDOMETRIOSIS**

Figure 40–4. Possible sites of occurrence of endometriosis. (From Thomas, CL (ed): Taber's Cyclopedic Medical Dictionary, ed 18. FA Davis, Philadelphia, 1997.)

basis, mediated by ovarian hormones, these cells build up and slough in the same manner as endometrial cells inside the uterus. Endometrial cells outside the uterus, however, slough and bleed during menstruation into the enclosed abdominal cavity or into whatever tissues into which they have extended, and this can result in pain, swelling, damage to abdominal organs and structures, scar tissue development, and infertility. Production of complement component 3 and prostaglandins by the ectopic endometrial tissue also contributes to the damage and discomfort experienced by these women because these substances make capillaries more permeable, stimulate other cells that contribute to adhesion development, and cause cramping.

Medical and Surgical Treatment

Surgical intervention may be required to remove seriously affected tissues, especially if scar tissue develops into tight bands, which can cause strangulation of sections of bowel or ureters. Reduction of estrogen and prevention of ovulation either with medications or by surgical removal of the ovaries can be very effective against endometriosis, but loss of fertility and menopausal symptoms, including flushing and osteoporosis, are complications associated with these measures. Analgesics may be required for the pelvic pain associated with endometriosis.

Client Teaching

The severity and persistence of the pain of endometriosis may lead to abuse of pain medication, so teaching clients alternative pain relief strategies such as relaxation exercises and application of heat to the abdomen or back is a very important role for the nurse.

MENOPAUSE

Pathophysiology and Signs and Symptoms

Menopause is the permanent cessation of menstrual cycles due to decreased hormone production. This is a natural process, but it is placed within this section because several uncomfortable symptoms and conditions can occur related to menopause. The time period of gradual decline in hormone production before the permanent end of menses is called the climacteric and may last from months to several years. **Perimenopausal** physical symptoms vary widely and may include erratic menses, atrophy of urogenital tissues with a marked decrease in the amount of natural lubrication and a pH shift toward alkalinity (encouraging yeast overgrowth), and vasomotor instability, resulting in hot flashes and night sweats. Estrogen protects women against several disease processes, so the risk of heart disease and osteoporosis increase with declining estrogen production.

Mental changes may also occur because of the complex interplay of reproductive hormones and neurotransmitters. It is important to acknowledge mental symptoms such as irritability, anxiety, insomnia, and mild depression as a normal part of the hormonal changes in order to reassure perimenopausal women that they are not going crazy.

Medical Treatment

Hormone replacement therapy (HRT) using estrogen can help alleviate perimenopausal symptoms and delay devel-

---

perimenopausal: peri—around + men(o)—month + pausal—stopping

opment of heart disease and osteoporosis, but there are risks involved with HRT. Estrogen given alone can increase the risk of development of endometrial, ovarian, and breast cancers, but if progestins are added, the benefits in reduction of heart disease may outweigh the risks. The most commonly administered medications for menopausal symptoms are conjugated estrogens (such as Premarin), estradiol, and medroxyprogesterone acetate (Provera).

Prevention of osteoporosis begins in early adulthood. Fair-skinned, Caucasian women are at greatest risk of bone loss. Throughout life, adequate intake of calcium and vitamin D, preferably from foods, and regular exercise are recommended to maximize bone mass. At menopause some women may receive estrogen replacement therapy to retard bone loss.

Complications

It is important to note that resumption of vaginal bleeding after menstruation has finally ceased can be a sign of disorder of the cells of the endometrium due to either benign changes such as polyps or malignant changes. Postmenopausal bleeding should be investigated by a physician.

Client Teaching

Clients who are perimenopausal often ask nurses about how to cope effectively with symptoms. Planning ahead for the occurrence of hot flashes helps women cope. For example, dressing in clothing that may be removed or applied in layers for comfort makes adjustment easier. Not allowing hot flashes to interrupt activities is an important strategy, as is engaging in satisfying and calming activities that contribute to a sense of serenity. Treatment of vaginal symptoms with a moisture restorer and lubricant such as Replens or with an estrogen cream can help. Eating a healthy diet that is light on caffeine, sugar, and alcohol also helps women to be more in control of their bodies and minds during this time. Looking forward to new challenges rather than back toward the past also seems to counteract depressive tendencies that may occur with hormonal changes. It is important to remind women who are perimenopausal that they may still be fertile unexpectedly after several months of **amenorrhea**. These women should continue to practice birth control methods until they receive confirmation from their physician of menopausal status if they do not with to conceive.

---

amenorrhea: a—without + men(o)—month + rrhea—flow

vaginosis: vagin—vagina + osis—condition

cytolytic: cyto—cell + lytic—loosening

balanitis: balan—acorn (shape of glans penis) + itis—inflammation

Irritations and Inflammations of the Reproductive Tract

The vulva and the vagina may become irritated for several reasons, and it is sometimes difficult to determine the causative agents. Symptoms are often similar, but there are some differences in the discharge produced in response to the disorders. Sexually transmitted diseases (STDs) are considered separately in Chapter 42, so only non-STD disorders of this type will be included in this chapter (Table 40–2).

Pathophysiology

The normal vaginal environment is a balanced ecosystem with a variety of normal resident microorganisms, which coexist relatively harmoniously. The normal pH is 3.8 to 4.2, which protects against the growth of many pathogenic microorganisms. Lactic acid is produced in the vagina to maintain this acidic environment. Several of the normal resident microorganisms, although usually nonpathogenic, may cause disease if the normal ecological balance is destroyed. Candidiasis, bacterial **vaginosis,** and **cytolytic** vaginitis are all instances of overgrowth of normally resident microorganisms.

Several conditions can predispose clients to development of an overgrowth of resident microbes: poor nutrition (especially diets high in simple sugars), inconsistent control of blood glucose levels with diabetes, stress, pregnancy, marked hormonal fluctuations, pH changes, prolonged overheating of the genital area with little aeration (as happens with sitting still for long periods of time in overly restrictive clothing), and changes in the balance of vaginal flora types because of antibiotic treatment. Clients who have a compromised immune system also may experience frequent overgrowths of resident microbes. Frequently recurring and persistent yeast infections may be one sign of AIDS. Vaginosis can produce irritation and inflammation in the male sexual partner as well and may lead to urethritis, **balanitis,** excoriation, and sores on the penis. If the male partner is not treated also, he may reinfect the woman. For this reason, several types of medication come in "partner packs" so that the woman may give some medication to her partner as well.

Client Teaching

The client is instructed not to douche before the examination visit, so the evidence of the particular microorganism is not washed away, making the diagnosis difficult.

CANDIDIASIS (YEAST OVERGROWTH)

Etiology and Signs and Symptoms

Candidiasis is a common problem for women. It results from the overgrowth of a resident fungus, usually *Candida*

Common Vaginal Irrigations and Inflammations

	Symptoms	Discharge	Treatment
Vaginal Candidiasis	Burning, itching, redness of vulva	White, cottage cheese appearance	Drugs ending in "-azole"
Bacterial Vaginosis	None or vaginal and vulvar irritation	Gray, homogeneous, foul smelling	Metronidazole or clindamycin
Cytolytic Vaginosis	Burning, irritation, pain with intercourse	Nonodorous, thick, white, pasty, or flaking discharge	Alkaline douches containing 1 teaspoon of baking soda per pint of water
Contact Vulvovaginitis	Itching, burning, erythema	Generally no change from normal discharge (though may be increased)	Avoid substances that irritate, take sitz baths, use hydrocortisone cream
Atrophic Vaginitis	Vaginal or vulvar irritation, itching, pain with intercourse	May have little or increased amount, watery yellow or green, may be blood tinged	Estrogen replacement therapy by patch, estrogen vaginal creams, or oral conjugated estrogens (with a progestin)

albicans, although *Candida glabrata* or *Candida tropicalis* may also be involved.[10] This results in a cottage cheese–like discharge accompanied by itching and burning. It may sometimes be mistaken for a urinary tract infection because of the intense burning on urination that can occur due to irritation of the meatus and surrounding tissues.

Prevention

Besides avoiding the risk factors listed previously, some practitioners recommend a diet low in yeasts and sugar for clients who experience recurrent yeast infections.

Diagnostic Tests

Yeast can be rapidly diagnosed from wet mount slides. Yeast are rather large and under a microscope look like tiny tree branches with buds on them. Yeast may also be cultured from a sample of the discharge placed in a culture tube. This, however, takes several days and prolongs the discomfort of the client.

Medical Treatment

Candidiasis is most often treated with medications the names of which end in "-azole" such as miconazole, clotrimazole, butoconazole, and terconazole, which can be applied topically or intravaginally. It may also be treated systemically by oral administration of fluconazole.

BACTERIAL VAGINOSIS

Etiology and Signs and Symptoms

Bacterial vaginosis (BV) is caused by the overgrowth of one resident bacteria called *Gardnerella vaginalis,* which can cause vaginal and vulvar irritation and a fishy-smelling gray discharge.

Diagnostic Tests

This often can be rapidly diagnosed with wet mount slides and pH testing of vaginal discharge. If the wet mount slides show "clue cells" or release a "fishy" odor when potassium hydroxide is dropped onto the slide and if the pH is over 4.5, these results indicate BV.[11] Culture of the discharge is not especially helpful and may delay treatment and prolong the extreme discomfort of the client.

Medical Treatment

Treatment with metronidazole (Flagyl) or clindamycin (for clients intolerant of metronidazole) is effective for most of these infections.

CYTOLYTIC VAGINITIS

Pathophysiology and Etiology

Cytolytic vaginitis results from overgrowth of lactobacilli, which produce so much acid that it causes cell damage to vaginal tissues. Stress and overtreatment with medications for other vaginal infections have been identified as some causes of this problem.

Signs and Symptoms

Women who have cytolytic vaginitis may experience burning, irritation, and pain and may have a nonodorous, thick, white, pasty, or rather dry and flaking discharge.

Diagnostic Tests

Determination of a more acidic than normal vaginal pH with pH indicator tape is a rapid means of diagnosing cytolytic vaginitis. The discharge may also be cultured to identify the microorganisms present, but waiting until the culture results return delays treatment, increases cell damage, and prolongs the discomfort of the client. Thorough investigation of the reason(s) for the overgrowth of lactobacilli should be done by a physician.

Medical Treatment

This may be treated by counteracting the acidity with alkaline douches containing one teaspoon of baking soda per pint of water. Treatment to correct the causative factors also may be required.

CONTACT VAGINITIS

Etiology and Signs and Symptoms

Contact vaginitis (which is also called allergic or irritative vaginitis) can be caused by contact with allergens, foreign substances, or irritating chemicals such as bubble baths and perfumed soaps. This may cause severe enough burning, itching, and erythema (redness) at the vaginal introitus to appear to be a vaginal infection.

Diagnostic Tests

Observation and history questions may be more helpful than diagnostic tests for this disorder. The discharge usually does not appear to be purulent and has no noticeable odor, although it may be more profuse than usual in response to the irritation. Asking questions about any new products that may have been used recently such as deodorant sprays, contraceptive creams, or even perfumed toilet paper may help the client identify the offending substance. Culture of the discharge may be done to rule out other infections, but this condition does not generally grow an abnormal culture.

Medical Treatment

Avoidance of the offending substance is the usual advice. Warm sitz baths or application of a hydrocortisone cream may decrease the discomfort.

ATROPHIC VAGINITIS

Pathophysiology and Signs and Symptoms

Atrophic vaginitis occurs when estrogen levels decrease below the level needed for support of estrogen-sensitive vaginal tissues. This condition most often develops during menopause, although it may also occur with breast feeding, use of some oral contraceptives, and medical treatment for endometriosis. The tissues of the reproductive tract are sensitive to estrogen and proliferate well when sufficient oxygen is present. When the estrogen levels drop, the tissues of the reproductive tract become thin, fragile, and overly sensitive, and the production of lubrication decreases. The protective resident acid-producing microbes that normally populate the vagina decrease, resulting in a more alkaline pH. These changes contribute to discomfort, overgrowth of opportunistic microbes, and increased risk of tissue injury during intercourse.

Diagnostic Tests

A maturation index can be done of cells collected during a vaginal Pap smear to determine whether atrophic cellular changes are present, which indicate this condition. However, this condition is usually diagnosed from history and physical examination findings.

Medical Treatment

Addition of a lubricant may make intercourse more comfortable but does not make the tissues more healthy. Estrogen replacement or application of an estrogen vaginal cream reverses the cellular changes.

Nursing Care

Vaginal inflammations and infections may require local application of medication either in cream, ovule, suppository, or medicated douche form. Depending on the practice laws in the area, the nurse may be applying this for clients who are unable to do this for themselves or teaching clients to self-administer. Remember that anatomically the vagina slopes backward toward the sacrum and is approximately the length of an adult finger (though it can stretch longer). It is easiest to apply vaginal medications when the client is lying down ready to sleep, because medications tend to run out due to gravity when the client stands or sits. Medicated douches may be administered with the client sitting on a bedpan or the toilet. Most vaginal medications come with an applicator that either injects a dose of creamy medication or pushes a firmer, shaped dose of medication off the end of the tube when the plunger is depressed. The nurse should consult instructions supplied with the medication. Clients should be instructed to use all of the medication as instructed and to wear an absorbent pad to prevent possible staining of clothing.

TOXIC SHOCK SYNDROME

Pathophysiology

Toxic shock syndrome (TSS) was first identified in 1978 as a disease primarily associated with tampon use during menstruation, although it can also occur with use of nasal packings and in individuals who are not menstruating and who have no packing in a body cavity. It is caused by a systemic infection with strains of *Staphylococcus aureus,* which produce an epidermal toxin. A similar syndrome has also been identified as resulting from a streptococcal infection.

Prevention

Tampon makers have removed from their product lines the highly absorbent fibers that were most often associated with the syndrome, and occurrences of TSS are now rare. Women can also reduce their risk of developing TSS by substituting sanitary pads for tampons at least part of the time, changing tampons every 4 hours, washing hands carefully before vaginal insertion of anything, not leaving female barrier contraceptives in place for longer than required for conception control, and not using tampons or female barrier contraceptives in the first 12 weeks after a birth.

Signs and Symptoms

Individuals with TSS have shown a sudden high fever with sore throat, headache, dizziness, and confusion. Skin involvement may include redness of the palms and soles of the feet, skin rashes, blisters, and **petechiae** followed by peeling of the skin. Muscle weakness, muscle pain, and gastrointestinal upsets also have been reported.

Complications

The effect of the toxin on the liver, kidneys, and circulatory system makes this a life-threatening condition.

Client Teaching

All menstruating women should be taught measures to prevent TSS. They should also be taught to recognize symptoms of TSS, because early identification and treatment with antibiotics and circulatory support can save lives.

Disorders Related to the Development of the Genital Organs

Pathophysiology

Several types of congenital malformations of the genital organs may affect the health of female clients. These defects may be caused by genetic factors or by environmental factors during pregnancy. These may require medical or surgical treatment at some point in life. **Agenesis** of structures means that they never developed. **Hypoplasia** of reproductive tract portions means that they are underdeveloped. **Imperforate** means that expected openings do not exist. Blind pouches exist where cavities should meet but do not. The uterus can form in several different configurations, including a double uterus.

Signs and Symptoms

Many malformations are discovered during childhood or early adolescence, but some are identified when clients seek medical help because of dysmenorrhea, **dyspareunia** (pain with intercourse), infertility, or repeated spontaneous abortions.

Diagnostic Tests

Such procedures as ultrasonography, hysterosalpingography, CT scanning, MRI, and endoscopic examinations may be used to determine the type and extent of developmental defects.

Surgical Treatment

Some of the defects can be repaired surgically, but others cannot. Depending on the type and location of the defect(s), surgeries may be done by endoscopy or by surgical incision.

Nursing Care

Clients who have these problems may struggle with self-esteem issues, for example feeling that they are somehow incomplete or have been cheated of something they desire. The understanding nurse should clearly show that he or she is willing to listen if and when the client wishes to talk while allowing the woman as much privacy as she desires.

Displacement Disorders

Pathophysiology

The pelvic organs are suspended within the pelvis by ligaments and supported by muscles and fascia. The pubococcygeal muscle runs from the pubis to the coccyx and supplies support from below. Pregnancies (especially producing large babies) and rapid or traumatic deliveries may result in stretching and injury of the supporting structures, which can cause displacement of the uterus, vagina, bladder, or bowel from their normal positions. The observation that some children have defective muscle support of the pelvic organs and that prolapse is more prevalent in some families seems to suggest that congenital defects and genetic inheritance may also influence displacement disorders even without pregnancy. Scarring from sexually transmitted diseases also may cause some displacement of the pelvic organs. Aging generally increases the problem be-

---

petechiae: flea bites (used for tiny skin discolorations caused by bleeding)
agenesis: a—without + genesis—production
hypoplasia: hypo—little + shape (or form)
imperforate: im—not + perforate—pierced
dyspareunia: dys—painful or abnormal + pareunia—mating

cause the effects of gravity over time contribute to stretching and lower estrogen levels weaken estrogen-dependent supportive tissues. Obesity and lack of exercise also worsen these problems.

Prevention and Client Education

Dietary moderation to avoid obesity can help somewhat to prevent displacement disorders. Avoidance of STDs also can prevent some of these problems. Keeping the muscles in good condition is an important activity that women can do for themselves. Kegel exercises strengthen the pubococcygeal muscle, which helps support the organs in the pelvic cavity. There are several variations of such exercises taught today. The important idea is that the appropriate muscles are exercised adequately to strengthen and build up ability to control muscle contractions. The nurse can provide the following instructions for the client:

1. To find the pubococcygeal muscle, tighten while urinating enough to stop the urine flow. The muscles that stop urinary flow are the same muscles that provide support.
2. Squeeze the muscle tightly and hold for 6 to 10 seconds totally relaxing the muscle afterwards, repeating this maneuver 12 to 24 times per day.
3. Practice controlling the muscle contraction by slowly contracting the muscle more and more as if moving the pelvic floor upward very slowly and then downward very slowly. Repeat this maneuver 10 times per day.
4. These exercises can be done anywhere and are not evident to anyone watching. Perhaps doing Kegel exercises while waiting in lines would be a health-promoting use of otherwise wasted time. Another suggestion is to plan specific times of day or activities that would include Kegel exercises in order to regularly exercise the pubococcygeal muscle.

Medical Treatment

A *pessary* is a supportive (usually ring-shaped) device that is placed in the proximal end of the vagina to help support the pelvic organs. These are usually removed daily at bedtime for cleaning, but some types are designed to remain in the vagina for months at a time. When pessary use is begun, it is important that the woman re-

turn to the physician for a recheck after an initial period of use to determine whether the pessary is causing pressure damage to the vaginal tissues. Because the pessary is a foreign object in the vagina, increased vaginal discharge may be expected, but the discharge should not be pink, bloody, or purulent.

CYSTOCELE

Etiology and Signs and Symptoms

Cystocele occurs when the bladder sags into the vaginal space (Fig. 40–5). A feeling of pelvic pressure and stress incontinence are common with this condition.

Medical and Surgical Treatment

Kegel exercises or the use of a pessary may help this condition. If these measures are ineffective, anterior **colporrhaphy,** which is a surgical repair of the anterior portion of the vagina, may be necessary to correct this problem. Another possible surgical treatment involves resuspending the bladder.

RECTOCELE

Etiology and Signs and Symptoms

Rectocele occurs when a portion of the rectum sags into the vagina (Fig. 40–5). A feeling of pelvic pressure, as well as fecal incontinence, constipation, and hemorrhoids may result.

Medical and Surgical Treatment

Kegel exercises may help strengthen the supporting muscles. The client should maintain bowel regularity with a high-fiber diet in order to avoid further discomfort and sagging from bowel overdistention. Posterior colporrhaphy may be necessary to correct this problem.

UTERINE POSITION DISORDERS

Pathophysiology

The most common variations of position of the uterus are **anteversion, anteflexion, retroversion,** and **retroflexion** (Fig. 40–6). In anteversion the uterus lies too far forward and in retroversion it lies too far backward. In anteflexion the upper portion of the uterus bends forward and in retroflexion it bends backward.

Signs and Symptoms

Symptoms that may result from these uterine displacements are painful menstruation and intercourse, infertility, and repeated spontaneous abortion.

---

cystocele: cysto—bag (bladder) + cele—hernia
colporrhaphy: colpo—vagina + rrhaphy—suture
rectocele: recto—rectum + cele—hernia
anteversion: ante—front + version—turning
anteflexion: ante—front + flexion—bending
retroversion: retro—back + version—turning
retroflexion: retro—back + flexion—bending

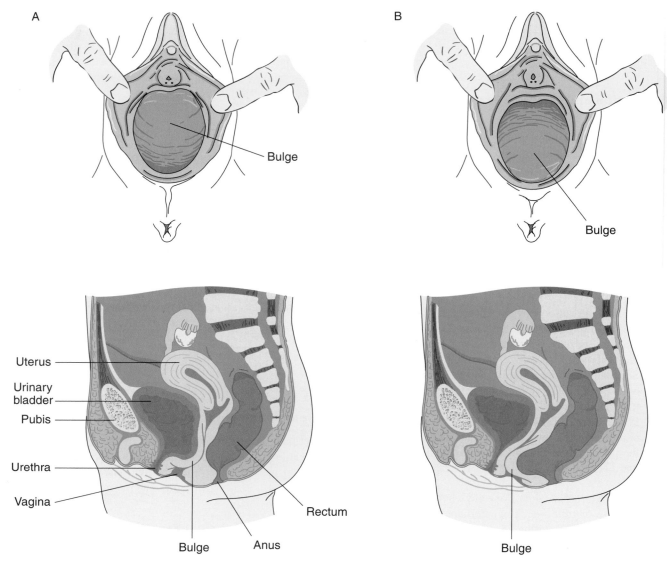

A

B

Bulge

Bulge

Uterus

Urinary bladder

Pubis

Urethra

Vagina

Rectum

Bulge   Anus

Bulge

Figure 40–5. *(A)* Cystocele. *(B)* Rectocele.

Medical Treatment

A pessary may correct some positional problems. If infertility or recurrent spontaneous abortion is involved or the condition is very painful, surgery to correct the condition may be undertaken.

UTERINE PROLAPSE

Pathophysiology

Uterine prolapse occurs when the uterus sags into the vagina (Fig. 40–7). The amount of sagging can vary and may increase over time due to the effects of gravity. In first-degree prolapse, less than half of the uterus sags into the vagina. In second-degree prolapse, the entire uterus sags into the vagina. In third-degree prolapse, the entire uterus sags outside of the body, turning the vagina inside out.

Signs and Symptoms

Uterine prolapse can be very uncomfortable, resulting in back pain, pelvic pain, pain with intercourse (or inability to have intercourse), urinary incontinence, constipation, and the development of hemorrhoids. The pressure on the uterus also may compromise circulation, resulting in tissue necrosis.

Medical and Surgical Treatment

Some of the more minor uterine displacements may be treated with use of a pessary. Kegel exercises may be more effective in prevention of uterine prolapse than in treatment because once the tissues become stretched sufficiently for the uterus to sag into the vagina, the continued weight of the uterus prevents the muscles from contracting well. Surgery will probably be required to correct this

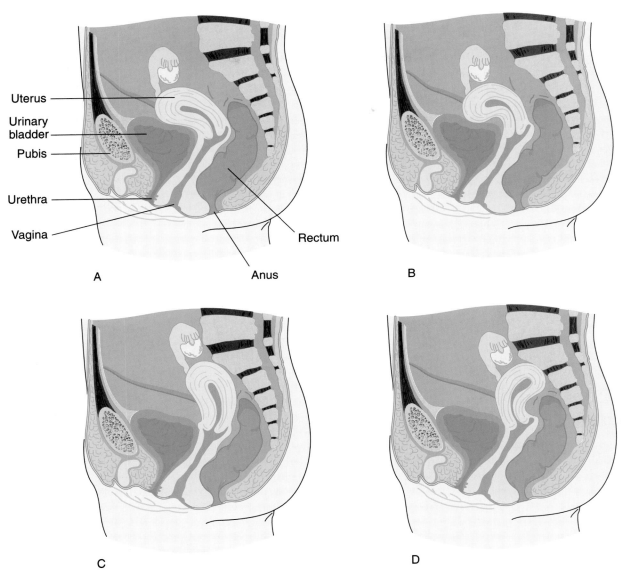

Figure 40–6. Uterine positions. *(A)* Anteversion. *(B)* Anteflexion. *(C)* Retroversion. *(D)* Retroflexion.

problem. Although the uterus may be resuspended by shortening the muscles and fascia, hysterectomy is the more common treatment unless further childbearing is desired.

Fertility Disorders

Infertility is a complicated problem that must be considered according to the causative factors. Rein and Schiff[12] rank the causes of infertility as follows: male problems 35 percent, ovulation problems 20 percent, tubal problems 20 percent, cervical problems 5 percent, endometriosis 10 percent, and unexplained problems 10 percent. They estimate that 25 to 35 percent of infertile couples have multiple reproductive problems.[12]

MALE REPRODUCTIVE DISORDERS

Pathophysiology

This section is mentioned briefly here because infertility of male partners affects female clients who desire to conceive also (see Chapter 41 for greater detail). Male reproductive problems may be caused by anatomical abnormalities, hormonal factors, genetic defects, inflammatory conditions, immune system problems, difficulties with sexual function or technique, or **exogenous** influences such as drug use, radiation or chemical exposure, trauma, and excessive testic-

---

exogenous: ex(o)—outside + genous—produced

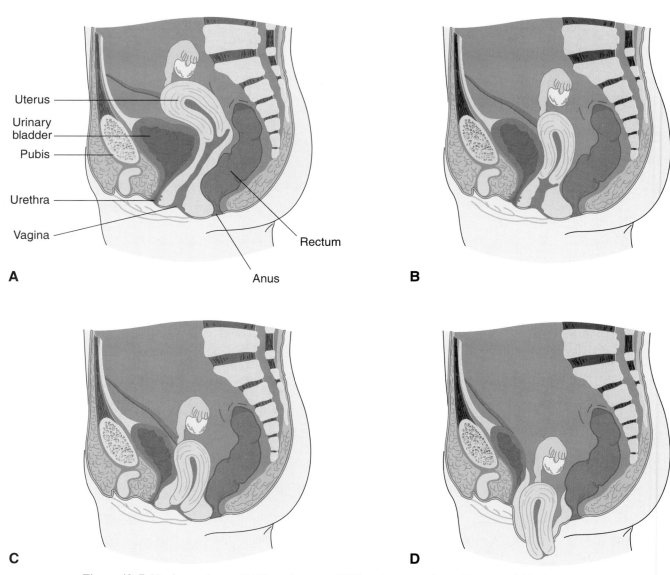

Uterus
Urinary bladder
Pubis
Urethra
Vagina
Rectum
Anus

A

B

C

D

Figure 40–7. Uterine prolapse. *(A)* Normal uterus. *(B)* First-degree prolapse: Descent within the vagina. *(C)* Second-degree prolapse: The cervix protrudes through the introitus. *(D)* Third-degree prolapse: The vagina is completely everted.

ular temperatures (as may occur with prolonged hot tub use and too tight clothing).

Diagnostic Tests

Semen analysis is the primary test for evaluation of male factors. The numbers, condition, and movement of the sperm and the composition of the seminal fluid are all evaluated using various test methods.

OVULATION DISORDERS

Pathophysiology

Ovulation problems may be caused by anatomical and physiological abnormalities of the ovaries or hormonal

balance problems related to the hypothalamus, thyroid, or adrenal glands.

Diagnostic Tests

Some tests related to ovulation are basal body temperature charting, midluteal serum progesterone (MSP) levels determination, luteinizing hormone (LH) levels determination, ultrasound monitoring of a follicle, and endometrial biopsy.

The nurse may teach the client to keep a record of her oral temperatures taken regularly each morning on awakening and before any activity. A basal thermometer with very precise measurement of temperatures should be used, and day 1 of the chart should be the first day of her menses.

Changing levels of hormones result in slight changes in body temperature, which can be used to identify when ovulation seems to be occurring. Because the pattern may vary for many reasons, it is best to explain that it may take a few months of recording to clearly identify her own pattern. The temperature charts may be helpful as well for determination of times for measuring hormone levels to avoid excessive cost for repeated blood tests.

Repeated ultrasound monitoring of a follicle over a period of several days may demonstrate the growth of a follicle and the subsequent marked shrinkage of the follicle after rupture or may show evidence of an ovarian disease in which the oocyte becomes trapped in the follicle. Levels of MSP and LH may be determined by blood tests or in the case of LH by urine tests.

Endometrial biopsy may be done during a pelvic examination 2 or 3 days before the menses is expected to occur. A pregnancy test should be done before this procedure to avoid interfering with a pregnancy. The woman may receive a pain medication and a paracervical block for the procedure. Epinephrine, a tourniquet, and a syringe should be kept handy for injection if a **vasovagal reflex** occurs during the procedure. Vasovagal reflex is a reflex stimulation of the vagal nerve that can happen when the cervix, larynx, or trachea is manipulated. It results in slowing of the heart rate and decreased cardiac output.

TUBAL DISORDERS

Pathophysiology

Tubal problems may result from obstruction of the fallopian tubes due to anatomical variations, scarring, or adhesions. Sexually transmitted diseases, endometriosis, prior surgical procedures, and inflammatory processes involving other abdominal tissues can contribute to tubal problems.

Diagnostic Tests

Hysterosalpingography and salpingoscopy (described in Chapter 39) may be useful for identifying tubal obstructions.

Surgical Treatment

Endoscopic surgery can repair some tubal defects and obstructions.

---

vasovagal reflex: vaso—vessel + vagal—vagus nerve + re—back + flex—bend

postcoital: post—after + coital—pertaining to intercourse

motility: motil(e)—moving often + ity—condition of

in vitro fertilization: in—inside + vitro—glass + fertiliz—fruitful + ation—process

UTERINE DISORDERS

Pathophysiology

Uterine problems are a relatively uncommon cause of infertility. Abnormalities in shape and blockages within the uterus can cause the loss of pregnancies before maturity of the fetus. Menstrual disorders especially involving the endometrium can also affect the ability to produce a viable infant.

Diagnostic Tests

Hysterosalpingography and hysteroscopy (described in Chapter 39) can be used to assess for internal abnormalities of the uterus. Ancillary tools can be introduced through the endoscope to take tissue samples and perform minor surgical procedures if necessary.

Diagnostic Tests for Other Sources of Infertility

Laparoscopic examination is often used to determine other causes of infertility. A **postcoital** test (PCT) can be used to determine whether the environment is conducive to fertilization. For this test the couple is instructed to have intercourse when the luteinizing hormone and estrogen levels are high, and then a specimen of cervical mucus is taken from the woman 2 to 12 hours afterward.

Medical and Surgical Treatment of Infertility

Treatment of infertility is designed to ensure that an adequate amount of sperm and an ovum can be in close proximity in the most conducive environment for fertilization to occur. Removal of barriers such as scar tissue may be facilitated by surgery.

Depending on the results of the PCT, adjustments of environmental factors may involve such actions as sperm washing to avoid destructive antigen-antibody responses, changing the pH of the seminal fluid to encourage sperm **motility,** or treating the female partner to prevent substances in her genital tract fluids from disabling the sperm. The number of sperm or ova available may be increased through use of such fertility drugs as clomiphene citrate or various hormone preparations. Medical infertility treatments are quite complicated and change from time to time due to ongoing research. In-depth coverage of these treatments is beyond the scope or focus of this book.

Various methods may be used to bring the gametes into close proximity. If the problem involves inability to get the sperm close enough to the ovum (as may happen with ejaculatory problems), the physician may place a semen sample from the male partner closer to the ovum via a small catheter. **In vitro fertilization** (IVF) involves bringing ova and sperm together outside of the bodies of the participants. Ova may be harvested after hormonal preparation of the woman using a long needle inserted through the vagina and into an ovary. Sperm may be obtained through masturbation; intercourse with a nonlubricated, nonspermicidal condom; or electrical stimulation of ejaculation for clients with spinal cord injuries.

For those whose sperm is unable to successfully penetrate the ovum, procedures involving gamete micromanipulation may be done. Under a microscope an ovum from the female partner is partially opened by removing a portion of the outer covering to facilitate sperm penetration, or sperm may be injected into the ovum. This fertilized ovum is then reinserted into the woman's body.

When measures to improve the chances of conception using the partners' own **gametes** are unsuccessful, gametes from donors may be utilized. Artificial insemination by injecting another man's sperm into the genital tract of the female client is the simplest of the donor procedures. Ova also may be harvested from a donor woman and used for in vitro fertilization using the male partner's sperm if possible. Both of these procedures allow for genetic inheritance from one member of the couple. If genetic inheritance is not possible or desirable (as with familial disease carriers), both donor sperm and ova may be used for in vitro fertilization with the resulting embryos being transferred into the female client. Surrogacy is a situation in which an embryo from one couple is placed into a "host" mother for growth of a baby for the couple and is a topic of much ethical debate.

Nursing Care

Clients who are undergoing fertility testing and treatment may experience many upsetting and distressing feelings. Feelings of inadequacy, frustration, depression, and anger are common. If the infertility was caused by something the client perceives as avoidable, such as sexually transmitted disease, guilt feelings may add to the psychological discomfort. Any or all of the previously described tests may be completed and some repeated many times without identification of reasons for the infertility, resulting in feelings that hopes are dashed repeatedly. Some clients cling to the hope that new tests and treatments are being developed which may help them, while others feel that they are being used as a "guinea pig" for development of new strategies. The beginning of menses may signal a time of mourning for these couples. Depression is the outcome for approximately 20 percent of the women who experience a failed IVF attempt. Strained relationships may develop between marriage partners, especially if there is disagreement about the value of testing or the importance of having children. The testing and treatment can be expensive, time-consuming, painful, and sometimes dangerous with no guarantee that a child will result from the efforts.

Nurses who work with infertile clients during testing and treatment procedures need to be especially understanding and to offer a listening ear while being careful not to give advice about testing or treatment modalities. There are many ongoing debates among researchers and practitioners as to the value of particular test procedures; consequently, assessment strategies may vary widely from one physician to another. Encourage open communication among the client, the physician, and the client's spouse, and encourage decision making that is informed and based on the client's values.

There are many varieties of assistive reproductive technology available, and the number is growing steadily as new ways are identified to increase the likelihood of producing viable children. Most of the procedures are called by acronyms that are names developed by using first letters of each of the descriptive terms of the procedure. For example, GIFT means gamete intrafallopian transfer, or, in simpler terms, putting the gametes together in the fallopian tube so that fertilization can easily take place and the **zygote** can then travel into the uterus for implantation. Acronyms can be very useful rather than saying or writing the names out fully; however, the use of too many acronyms can be confusing. Most nurses probably will not need to know all of the acronyms associated with infertility treatments unless they happen to be working in a gynecologist's office or infertility clinic. Knowing that words written all in capital letters are generally acronyms, however, is the first step to understanding many medical and surgical procedures.

Contraception

Contraceptive education is an area in which nurses can contribute greatly to the overall health and quality of life for women and families. There are many different types of birth control available at the present time, and several additional types are in developmental and testing stages. Because there can be many differences among particular forms of the same category of contraceptive agents, this portion of the text will remain rather general. Knowledge of how the different types of contraceptives work can assist the nurse in answering client questions or helping clients find additional information. This chapter is not intended to be a substitute for information found in manufacturers' circulars and educational material supplied with their products. No numerical statements of effectiveness are included in this section, because several different sets of

---

gamete: Greek word for marriage partner—sperm or ovum
zygote: union or fusion—ovum and sperm joined together
contraceptive: contra—against + ceptive—taking in (conceiving)

statistics are currently being used. It seems likely that as products improve, hormone dosages are changed, or more data comes in from users, the numbers will be adjusted. The content presentation order in this chapter, however, is intended to follow a general trend from most effective methods to least effective methods (with the exception that experimental methods are included near the end of this section regardless of their efficacy). The wisest course for the nurse working in this area would be to consult his or her employer for a current comparison list of the relative effectiveness of the various methods.

For some clients the distinction of whether the birth control method actually prevents conception or only interferes with implantation or maintenance of a pregnancy is a very important factor in their decision of which method to choose. If they believe life begins at conception, any action other than prevention of conception would be considered equivalent to abortion (Fig. 40–8).

ORAL CONTRACEPTIVES

Actions

Oral contraceptive (OC) medications are among the most widely used forms of birth control in North America. Most contain an estrogen and a progestin in combination, although some (minipills) contain only a progestin. Some work to prevent conception by inhibiting ovulation or changing the environment of the reproductive tract so that activity of the sperm is inhibited. Others do not prevent conception, but make implantation less likely and hasten the breakdown of the corpus luteum so that pregnancy-sustaining hormones are not produced. The dosages of hormones in these preparations vary, and side effects and adverse effects increase with higher levels of hormones.

Oral contraceptives may also be used in some instances to regulate irregular menses and to decrease dysmenorrhea. Although some authors have suggested that oral contraceptive agents may offer some protection against some sexually transmitted diseases, these assumptions are based on statistical rates of STDs among OC users and may be affected by many factors other than actual medication effects. One possible explanation for the statistical results might be that people who are motivated enough and health-conscious enough to take OCs regularly might be more careful about risks of contracting STDs than people who choose other methods because they require less effort and motivation. The cellular changes of the cervix seen with OC use may actually make women more vulnerable to human papillomavirus, human immunodeficiency virus, and chlamydia infections. Unless some specific mechanism of prevention is demonstrated by research, it seems irresponsible to suggest that oral contraceptives offer any protection against anything other than pregnancy. Therefore women should still be advised about the risks of

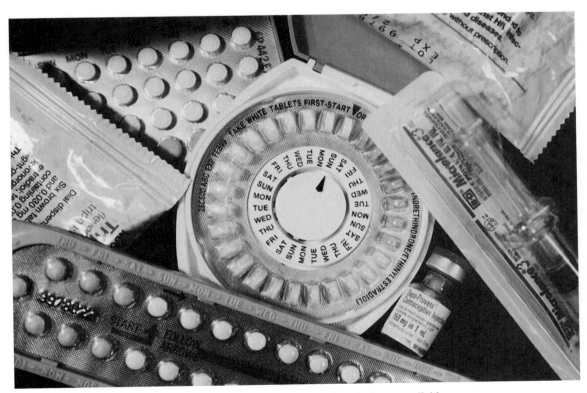

Figure 40–8. A variety of birth control methods are available.

contracting sexually transmitted diseases while on OC medication.

Advantages and Disadvantages

Oral contraceptives are very effective. Improvement of dysmenorrhea, increased regularity of menses, and decrease in menstrual flow may occur; however, some women experience menstrual changes such as amenorrhea, irregular or prolonged menses, and intermenstrual spotting. Oral contraceptive agents require a great deal of commitment because irregular use decreases effectiveness. To encourage regular use, some companies include unmedicated pills in the package to be taken during the time of hormone cessation for menses so that the woman only has to remember to take a pill every day. Dispensers with the days of the week printed by each pill also encourage regular use.

Side Effects and Risks

Some women experience side effects such as acne, fluid retention, headaches, breast swelling and discomfort, midcycle bleeding, and sometimes depression. Oral contraceptive use also has some risks. Higher rates of blood clot formation, strokes, high blood pressure, and heart attacks and worsening of diabetes have been documented with OC use, although the lower-dosage preparations prescribed in recent years have much lower risks than the earlier higher-dosage preparations. Women who smoke or have diabetes, high blood pressure, heart disease, or a history of **thrombophlebitis** should probably be advised to use some other form of contraception. Conflicting research results exist about whether oral contraceptive use increases cervical cancer risk, although one group of authors cites a doubling of the incidence of cervical **dysplasia** (cell changes that may become cancerous) among OC users.[13] Women should definitely be advised to have regular yearly (or more frequent if abnormalities develop) Pap smears while taking OC medication. Many other medications can alter the effectiveness of oral contraceptive agents, and women should be warned always to alert physicians and pharmacists that they are on an oral contraceptive whenever a new medication is to be started or a regular medication is discontinued.

Use of OCs for more than 2 or 3 years increases the risk of vitamin B_6 deficiency. These women, as well as infants of women who took OCs for more than 30 months before conception, should be monitored for deficiencies.

CONTRACEPTIVE IMPLANTS

Actions

Implants recently have been introduced for general contraceptive use. These act similarly to the progestin-only minipills but have the advantage of providing rapid and continued contraceptive effects for up to 5 years.[14] This is done by surgically implanting several small silastic tubes through a small incision under the skin of the upper arm. These tubes slowly release medication (such as levonorgestrel).

Advantages and Disadvantages

Long-term contraceptive effect without having to remember to take daily medication is the main advantage of this type of contraceptive. Improvement of dysmenorrhea and decrease in menstrual flow may occur with use of implants; however, some women experience menstrual changes such as amenorrhea, irregular or prolonged menses, and breakthrough bleeding (especially in the first year of use). Women over 30 years of age may experience some delay of fertility after removal of the implants.[15]

Side Effects and Contraindications

Acne, breast swelling, and headaches are associated with implant use, but improve over time for some women. Contraindications are similar to those for oral contraceptives, and women with history of jaundice or liver disease should also be advised to use some other method of birth control.

Client Teaching

Instruct the client to return to the physician if redness, swelling, or inflammation occurs at the insertion site.

DEPOT MEDICATIONS

Actions

Depot medications are injectable chemicals in a slow-release substance that, once administered, continue to release the medication for a long period of time. Medroxyprogesterone and norethindrone exanthane are two types of contraceptive agents available as depot intramuscular injections that are effective for 3 months. Some other forms of depot contraceptives require monthly injections.

Advantages and Disadvantages

The main advantage is that there is no requirement to take medication daily. One disadvantage is that the medication is not immediately effective, so users should be advised to practice another method of birth control also for the first 2 weeks after the initial injection. Another disadvantage is

---

thrombophlebitis: thrombo—clot + phleb—vein + itis—inflammation

dysplasia: dys—painful or abnormal + plasia—shape or form

that fertility may not return for several months to 1 year after cessation of the injections.

Side Effects and Risks

Alterations in menstrual flow, especially amenorrhea, are the most commonly noted side effects. Other side effects and risks are similar to those encountered with oral contraceptive use.

BARRIER METHODS

Barrier methods of birth control are less effective than most of the previously mentioned methods. Barriers are intended to prevent sperm from reaching the ovum. There are several forms of barrier contraceptives. Effectiveness of all of the barrier methods may be increased by use of a spermicidal preparation with them. Spermicidal preparations may be purchased without a prescription in pharmacies.

Condoms

Condoms are intended for one use only and then should be discarded into a waste receptacle. They should be stored in a cool dry place before use, and should not be stored tightly pressed, because heat and continued pressure can weaken them. Storage in a wallet or glove compartment is not advisable. Petroleum-based substances, such as Vaseline, can also weaken condoms, so use of water-soluble lubricants (preferably spermicides) should be advised.

Advantages and Disadvantages of Male Condoms

Male condoms have long been used for contraception because they are a relatively inexpensive, totally reversible method of contraception that men can initiate at the time of intercourse. They provide some barrier protection against transmission of sexually transmitted disease organisms as well. A recent electron microscope study of a sample of nonlubricated latex condoms, however, found that the majority of those viewed had surface abnormalities, including cracking and melted areas.[16] Clients should be educated about risks involved with intercourse and should be informed that barrier methods do not absolutely prevent transmission of STDs, especially those which may be transmitted in areas not covered by the barrier. The main disadvantages of condom use are interruption of foreplay for application, decreased sensation, and the possibility of slippage or breakage during intercourse. These disadvantages may be overcome by incorporating application of the condom by the female partner as a part of foreplay; using thinner, lubricated, or textured condoms to increase sensation; and using the correct size condom with a reservoir or applied with approximately ½ inch at the tip of the condom loose enough to serve as a reservoir for the semen (Fig. 40–9).

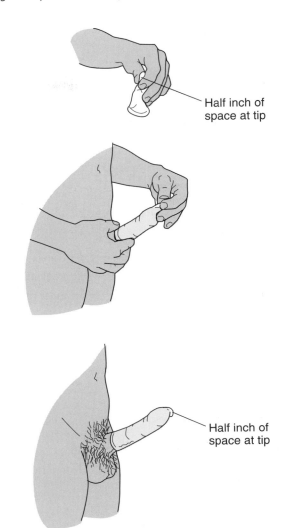

Figure 40–9. Correct application of a condom.

Advantages and Disadvantages of Female Condoms

Female condoms are a more recent innovation that allows female initiation of contraception as well as some barrier protection against infection with sexually transmitted diseases. Coverage of the labia by the condom may provide more of a barrier than male condoms (Fig. 40–10). Disadvantages are the expense for the purchase, decreased sensation, necessity to apply before intercourse, and possibility of flaws in the condom material. As of the writing of this book, there had been relatively little research on this type of condom to identify other possible advantages or disadvantages.

Diaphragms, Cervical Caps, and Sponges

Actions

Diaphragms, cervical caps, and sponges all work in the same manner by blocking the entry of sperm through the

A

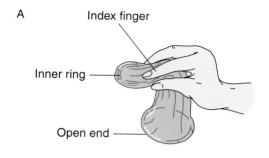

Index finger

Inner ring

Open end

B

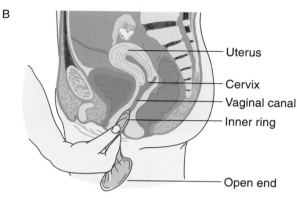

Uterus

Cervix

Vaginal canal

Inner ring

Open end

C

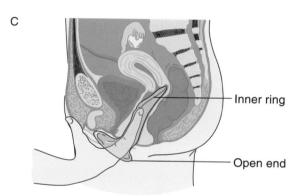

Inner ring

Open end

D

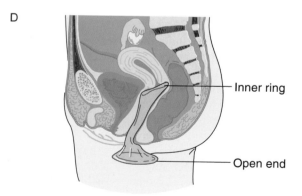

Inner ring

Open end

Figure 40–10. Female condom application. *(A)* Inner ring is squeezed for insertion. *(B)* Sheath is inserted similar to a tampon. *(C)* Inner ring is pushed up as far as it can go with index finger. *(D)* Condom in place.

cervix. The barrier effect is enhanced by a spermicide. The sponge comes presaturated with a spermicide and generally needs to be moistened slightly with water and inserted with the indentation toward the cervix. The diaphragm and cervical cap require application of spermicide to the edges and a small amount in the cup before application. A new form of barrier device called Lea's Shield may offer improvements over the traditional diaphragm because it has a loop for ease of removal, fits closer to the cervix with less pressure exerted toward the urethra, and needs less spermicide than a traditional diaphragm.[17]

Advantages and Disadvantages

All of these methods are relatively inexpensive, are female initiated, and work without systemic medication. Diaphragms and cervical caps require initial fitting and a prescription to buy them, may need to be refitted after childbirths and the loss or gaining of weight, and can last for years. These devices should be replaced periodically as the manufacturer recommends or whenever there is any evidence of hardening, cracking, or thin spots. They need to be washed with soap and water, dried, and stored in a case away from heat and sunlight between uses. Sponges do not require fitting, but they are more expensive than the other two methods and are used only once.

Women and their partners may experience irritation or allergic reaction in response to the spermicide or the material of the contraceptive device, which would require changing birth control methods. All of these methods require that the device be inserted before intercourse and left in place for several hours after intercourse (see package insert for recommendations). An increase in incidence of urinary tract infection has been reported with use of the diaphragm, and risk of toxic shock syndrome increases with prolonged uninterrupted use of cervical barriers. Adequate fluid intake, voiding shortly after intercourse, and removal of the device when 8 hours have passed since intercourse all help prevent these potential problems. If urinary tract infections are recurrent using the diaphragm, changing to a cervical cap may decrease the occurrence because there is less pressure against the bladder side of the vagina.

SPERMICIDES

Actions

Spermicidal agents also may be used by themselves, although use in combination with a barrier method is much more effective. They come in a variety of forms such as creams, gels, foams, and suppositories, which kill or disable sperm so that fertilization does not occur.

Advantages and Disadvantages

Spermicidal preparations are relatively inexpensive and can be female initiated. They do not produce systemic effects, and no hormones are involved. They are less effective alone than the previously described methods. Spermicides require application before each act of intercourse and are considered by some clients to be somewhat messy. Most of them contain the same ingredient—nonoxynol 9. If genital irritation or a rash occurs with use of spermicides, the client should read the labels carefully because another brand may contain the same ingredient.

INTRAUTERINE DEVICES

Actions

The presence of a foreign object in the uterus is thought to alter the environment so that implantation is less likely to occur. Intrauterine devices (IUDs) are generally made of some form of plastic and may contain copper wire or a supply of a progestin. Slow release of a progestin or copper into the system may further alter the environment so that fertilization is hindered.

Advantages and Disadvantages

The main advantage of use of an IUD is continued contraception without the necessity of remembering to take medication and without the side effects associated with medications. The disadvantages are changes in menstrual bleeding (especially increases in bleeding), cramping, and increased risk of pelvic inflammatory disease. Rarely an IUD has caused a uterine perforation. IUDs are contraindicated for women who have never been pregnant, those with uterine abnormalities, and those who have a history of anemia or heavy menstrual flow. Expulsion or displacement of the IUD can occur, so women should be taught to feel for the string before intercourse.

Insertion Procedure

Insertion of an IUD is generally done as a physician's office procedure with a nurse assisting. This is done usually during the first 7 days of the menstrual cycle because the cervix is generally slightly dilated at this time. The IUD is generally inserted into the vagina through a tube, which temporarily holds the IUD flat or folded so that it requires less room for insertion. When the IUD is pushed out of the end of the tube it springs into a shape that helps keep it inside the uterus. One potential danger associated with IUD insertion is vasovagal reflex stimulation (previously described in association with endometrial biopsy). The role of the nurse may include periodic assessment of the pulse or blood pressure during the procedure. Epinephrine

should be kept handy for injection if the heart rate becomes too slow.

NATURAL FAMILY PLANNING

Actions

Periodic abstinence, or natural family planning, is less effective than the previously described methods. It is a method by which couples control their fertility by restricting intercourse to "safe periods" in which risk of conception is low. Many signs may be assessed to determine "safe" days, including temperature changes, cervical consistency and mucus changes, calendar timing, and awareness of symptoms of fertility.

Slight body temperature changes can indicate ovulation. During the first half of the menstrual cycle the temperature remains low with a marked drop just before ovulation occurs. With ovulation the temperature rises and stays higher for the last half of the cycle. Women who use this assessment method should use a basal body temperature thermometer because the expanded scale allows for more precise readings than a standard fever thermometer. The temperature should be taken orally before getting out of bed each morning and recorded on a chart.

Cervical consistency and mucus changes may also help pinpoint ovulation. As hormone levels change, the consistency of cervical mucus changes. As ovulation approaches, there is an increase in the amount of mucus and the mucus becomes more clear, thin, slippery, and stretchable than at other times of the month. Around the time of ovulation the cervix becomes softer to touch and more open than at other times of the cycle.

Following the calendar can work fairly well if the woman is very regular with menstrual periods, but becoming aware of her pattern may take time. Symptoms such as breast tenderness and midcycle discomfort (mittelschmerz) may also help identify ovulation. Users of this method should be advised to abstain for approximately 3 days before ovulation and 3 to 4 days after, because the sperm and ovum can survive for a long period of time in the female genital tract.

Advantages and Disadvantages

The advantages of this method are that it is inexpensive, it requires no medication, and it is the only birth control method presently approved by the Catholic Church. The disadvantages are that it requires the cooperation of both partners and may interfere with spontaneity of sexual expression. It is generally not very effective as a means of birth control. It may be difficult to be accurate about ovulation times because infectious and inflammatory processes may affect temperature readings, infections and feminine hygiene products may affect cervical mucus, and irregularity of flow and symptoms may make prediction difficult.

COITUS INTERRUPTUS

Actions

This method involves removal of the penis from the vagina before ejaculation occurs.

Advantages and Disadvantages

Although this method requires no expense or preparation, it is not very effective. Excellent control of ejaculation is required for this method to be effective, and even the small amount of sperm that may be present in preejaculatory fluid may result in pregnancy.

POSTCOITAL DOUCHING

Actions

The intended purpose of this procedure is to wash sperm out of the reproductive tract or to kill or immobilize sperm that the douche solution contacts.

Advantages and Disadvantages

Although this is relatively inexpensive and female initiated, it is not a very effective method. Sperm move very rapidly once deposited in the vagina, and douching may actually push the sperm upward.

BREAST FEEDING

Actions

Breast feeding is sometimes used as a method of birth control because the high blood levels of prolactin that occur with breast feeding may prevent ovulation.

Advantages and Disadvantages

Although this method costs nothing, it is not a very effective method. Prolactin levels can vary widely, and ovulation may resume at any time without any noticeable signs.

ONGOING RESEARCH: FUTURE POSSIBILITIES FOR CONTRACEPTIVE CHOICES

Several contraceptive agents are presently under investigation. An estrogen-progestogen contraceptive ring, which is inserted into the vagina much in the manner of a dia-

phragm, has been well accepted in clinical trials.[18] This method requires the user to insert it once, leave it in for 3 weeks, and then remove it for 1 week. Not having to remember daily medication can be an advantage, but failing to remove it at the right time may disrupt the regularity of the menstrual cycles.

A single contraceptive implant containing nomogestral acetate (Uniplant) implanted under the skin of the upper arm or gluteal region has been tested in clinical trials and found to be effective for 1 year. This method, however, will probably be further refined before it is available to the general public, because 44 percent of the women using it in trials had changes in their menstrual cycles.[19]

An IUD with a reservoir that slowly releases levonorgestrel has been subjected to clinical trials in Scandinavia and the United Kingdom with promising results for contraception and for reduction of menorrhagia.[20] This IUD offers the same benefits as both IUDs and oral contraceptive medications without the necessity of taking oral medication.

Many researchers have tried to develop effective and reversible male contraceptives. A plant called Tripterygium is being investigated because it yields substances that, when taken orally by men, can limit the fertility of their sperm.[21] The active ingredients of Tripterygium, however, also suppresses immunity somewhat, so further investigation is necessary. A reversible injection procedure that blocks the seminal vas deferens has been used for a large number of men in China and may offer another form of contraception that requires no motivation to take regular medication and yet does not permanently stop fertility.[22]

Much research is also being done to develop effective and reversible birth control vaccines. The goal of these efforts is to cause an immune response to occur at some vital point in the process of conception. Researchers have aimed at many different points in the process, so there are wide variety of vaccines presently being tested both for men and for women.[23] One advantage of this method would be that little motivation is required to maintain contraception once the vaccine is given. Some disadvantages are that there may be no personal awareness when the immunity is decreasing, there may be unknown long-term repercussions of stimulating the body to respond with immunity to "self," and governments could use this means to control populations as a public health measure without the consent of the people.[24] Another frightening possibility is that with further removal of the threat of pregnancy even fewer people will use barrier methods and STDs will increase even more dramatically.

CRITICAL THINKING: Jessica

You have just observed a client who looks to be about 13 years old announce loudly at the clinic reception desk that she is "ready to be a responsible adult" and would like some birth control.

1. What information needs to be gathered from her?
2. What do you think she needs to know?
3. How can contraceptive teaching capitalize on her desire to be a responsible adult?

Answers at end of chapter.

STERILIZATION

Actions

Permanent sterilization can be accomplished by either interrupting the fallopian tubes or vas deferens in some manner or removing the uterus and suturing the proximal end of the vagina closed. Tubal interruption may be done by tying a suture or placing a ring or clip around each fallopian tube, by coagulating a section of the tubes, or by surgically removing a portion of the tube and suturing the ends. These procedures are usually done by laparoscope.

Advantages and Disadvantages

Although this method is not absolutely certain to be permanent, the failure rate is only about 2 per 1000 operations. Tubal repair is sometimes requested at a later date in order to reestablish fertility. This requires microsurgery with anesthesia and has a poor success rate. Clients should be advised about the complications of reversal by their physician before they sign a consent for sterilization. If the client seems uncertain about the wish to cease childbearing, the physician should be notified.

Pregnancy Termination

Abortion is a difficult topic to consider. Discussions about it are often highly charged with emotion. Both pro-life and pro-choice advocates argue on the basis of human rights—the former based on supposed rights of the fetus and the latter on supposed rights of the mother because of the humanity of each party. There are very few people on either side of the philosophical argument, however, who would describe abortion as a healthy medical intervention. When the shouting about rights is over, abortion is more likely to be seen as a sad and wasteful solution to a problematic situation. There are instances in which carrying a pregnancy to term threatens the life of the mother. There are also many more instances in which a pregnancy is inconvenient or undesired. Although discussion of the ethical issues surrounding abortion is encouraged, it is beyond the scope of this book to satisfactorily address all of the issues. (See Ethical Considerations Box 40–2.)

ETHICAL CONSIDERATIONS BOX 40-2

Ethical Issues of Abortion

The famous case of *Roe v. Wade* (1973) changed the legal status of therapeutic abortion in the United States but added a great deal of confusion to its ethical and moral status. A careful reading of the *Roe v. Wade* decision reveals that the court made no decision about ethics or morality of elective (therapeutic) abortion. Rather, the court said that, according to the U.S. Constitution, all people, including women, have a right to determine what they can do with their bodies (right to self-determination), and that right, incidentally, included the termination of a pregnancy. This point of right to self-determination or freedom of choice has become the central issue of the pro-abortion groups.

The anti-abortion (pro-life) faction believes that abortion is fundamentally a killing act. They hold to the belief that the only outcome of all therapeutic abortions is the death of the fetus. A critical issue in the debate concerns when the fetus is considered to be a human being. The pro-life groups believe that because all the required genetic material and genetic codes to produce an individual are present at this time, a unique individual human being exists at the moment of conception. The pro-abortion proponents argue that this mass of developing cells is not a human being, but rather a type of tissue, much like a tumor. The pro-abortion proponents argue that the fetus is not really human until it reaches the point of development where it can live outside the mother's body (i.e., the age of viability). Abortion represents a basic conflict of rights.

THE NURSE'S RIGHTS AND RESPONSIBILITIES RELATED TO ABORTION

Ethically, an individual nurse should not be required to assist in any treatment which demands that he or she act in a way that contradicts personal moral beliefs—this would violate the nurse's rights. However, there is also an ethical duty to provide care to clients for whom the nurse is responsible. Therefore it is wise for nurses who have moral objections to abortion to carefully choose their work setting. For example, choosing to work in day surgery in a hospital that performs abortions and refusing to care for abortion clients is not a legitimate option. One way that nurses can positively influence the abortion situation is by teaching about family planning (which may lower the frequency of requests for abortions). Another way might be to assist and promote agencies that help pregnant women to have viable alternatives to abortion.

METHODS OF ABORTION

Several methods of abortion are available. The method is determined primarily by the length of the gestation and the goal of inflicting as little trauma to the mother's reproductive system as possible while still inducing pregnancy loss. The allowable time periods for the different abortion methods and the allowable reasons for legal abortion vary according to the laws of the state, province, or country.

Chemical Agents

The "morning after pill" treatment consists of postcoital administration of sufficient estrogen or an estrogen/progestin combination to cause sudden sloughing of the endometrial lining of the uterus to prevent implantation of a possibly fertilized ovum. For this to be effective, the initial dose should be given within 72 hours of the intercourse. This treatment is used in case of unexpected unprotected sexual intercourse (as with sexual assault) or unexpected risk of conception (as with condom failure) but should not be assumed to be a casual method of birth control. Nausea and cramping may accompany the shedding of the uterine lining. This method requires no advance planning before intercourse and can be abused as a casual form of birth control. These clients may need education about appropriate birth control methods.

Another example of postcoital contraception is the drug RU 486, which is a progestin antagonist. It prevents the binding of progestins at their receptors resulting in a chemically induced abortion up to the tenth week of pregnancy. There is much debate about whether this drug should be used at all or within specific guidelines. Nausea and cramping may accompany expulsion of uterine contents.

Abortion Methods for Early Pregnancy

Early in the pregnancy (during approximately the first 13 weeks) there are three primary means of pregnancy termination—menstrual extraction, vacuum aspiration, and D&C. Menstrual extraction is removal of the endometrial lining by manual suction and can be done only during the first 7 weeks following the last menstrual period (LMP). This can be done without anesthesia and without cervical dilation by inserting a small cannula into the cervix and aspirating with a large syringe. Vacuum aspiration is a similar process that is used from confirmation of pregnancy through the first 13 weeks. It requires cervical dilation and is generally done with local anesthesia. The client returns home 1 to 4 hours after the procedure. D&C may also be used during the first 13 weeks. In this procedure the uterine contents are scraped away rather than being removed by suction.

Abortion Methods for Later Pregnancy

During the second trimester the fetus is much larger, so more dilation is required. A dilation and evacuation (D&E) may be performed, in much the same manner as a D&C. Generally dried laminaria (a type of seaweed) or some other absorbent substance is placed inside the cervical canal. This absorbs fluid and swells, thus gradually dilating the cervix. Prostaglandin may be administered either by suppository into the vagina or by injection into the amniotic sac; this usually induces uterine contractions and results in delivery a few hours later. Unfortunately, a live fetus may be born by this method who is too premature to survive for very long and yet who continues to breathe for a time until he or she dies.

An induction with either a saline or urea injection may be used for pregnancies beyond 16 weeks. A portion of amniotic fluid is removed and replaced with concentrated saline or urea solution, which kills the fetus and stimulates contractions. Sometimes saline and prostaglandins are used in combination to terminate a pregnancy. **Hysterotomy** involves removal of the uterine contents through an abdominal incision in the same manner as a cesarean section. This procedure is rarely done for pregnancy termination.

Risks and Complications

Abortion involves risks. Some are the same risks inherent in childbirth, such as possible hemorrhage or introduction of infection, but there are additional risks related to interruption of natural processes and the aggressiveness with which the products of conception are removed during abortion. During an uncomplicated childbirth the uterine lining is not scraped or forcefully emptied by suction. Natural hormonal preparation for term childbirth contributes to uterine contraction after the birth, which decreases blood loss, but no such preparation occurs for abortion. Artificial dilation of the cervix may cause injury, as may introduction of the instruments used for abortion. Injured tissues are more likely to become sites for growth of microorganisms than are intact tissues. Finally, the possibility of infertility as a result of complications related to abortion, although relatively uncommon, is a risk.

Some possible physical complications following therapeutic abortion are injuries to the uterus or cervix, excessive bleeding, infection, retention of some products of conception, and possible failure of abortion. Rarely, second trimester abortions can be complicated by amniotic fluid embolism, in which amniotic fluid is absorbed into the uterine circulation because of disruption of placental at-

hysterotomy: hystero—womb + tomy—cutting

tachments with instruments. Amniotic fluid in the mother's circulatory system can result in circulatory collapse and **disseminated intravascular coagulation** (DIC). DIC is a serious derangement of the body's blood clotting controls. Clotting mechanisms are overstimulated so that the blood begins to form clots in vessels all over the body. In response to this **hypercoagulation, fibrinolytic** mechanisms are overstimulated and the client may suffer severe and widespread bleeding. Treatment of this disorder is very difficult because the normal mechanisms for both sides of this clotting/clot dissolving equation are hypersensitive. Approximately 85 percent of the women who suffer from DIC die from the condition.[25]

Therapeutic Abortion for Ectopic Pregnancy

Ectopic pregnancy generally requires surgical termination either by laparoscopy or **laparotomy.** An ectopic pregnancy is any implantation of a fertilized ovum other than in the uterus. Some reasons for ectopic implantation are an abnormally shaped uterus or fallopian tubes that are obstructed due to abnormal development or scarring from STDs or other inflammatory processes.

Therapeutic Abortion for Prenatal Abnormalities

Development of a wide variety of prenatal testing methods has introduced the possibility of knowing many things about a baby before birth. Prenatal testing may be done using ultrasound, samples of fluid taken from the amniotic sac or the placental villi, or blood samples from the mother. From these tests, several genetic diseases and congenital deformities can be identified. After anomalies are diagnosed, some clients choose to abort the baby. This is a very difficult decision to consider even in instances in which the baby has a fatal defect that will not allow it to live outside of the uterus. Information about alternatives to abortion and possible treatments for their child are very important for clients who have a serious prenatal diagnosis. No one should feel pressured to abort. Abortion because of fetal

---

disseminated intravascular coagulation: dis—far from + seminated—planted + intra—within + vascular—little vessel + coagul—clot + ation—process

hypercoagulation: hyper—too much + coagul—clot + ation—process

fibrinolytic: fibrin(o)—fiber + lytic—loosening

laparotomy: lapar(o)—abdominal wall + tomy—cutting

leiomyoma: leio—smooth + myom(a)—fibroid

myomectomy: myom(a)—fibroid + ec—away + tomy—cutting

---

abnormality may result in much grieving for the client and her family.

Nursing Care

Aftercare is very important. These clients rarely stay overnight, and complications may occur after they are discharged. They should be carefully assessed after the procedure for excessive bleeding, and vital signs should be assessed. They should be instructed that bleeding should not exceed that of a heavy period, that the passage of clots larger than a quarter may be a sign of complications, and that the discharge should not become foul smelling. They should be instructed as to what phone number they should call if fever, chills, excessive bleeding, or any signs of infection occur. The client should be advised to abstain from sexual intercourse for the period of time specified by her physician (usually about 3 weeks). A grief response may occur after a pregnancy termination even if the baby was definitely unwanted and the client does not have strong beliefs against abortion. Loss and trauma have occurred in any case, and reorganization of the self takes time. Psychological follow-up of women after abortion is very important, and a counseling referral may be made. Birth control teaching may also be required.

Tumors of the Cervix, Uterus, and Ovaries

BENIGN GROWTHS

Fibroid Tumors

Pathophysiology

Fibroid tumors or **leiomyoma** (singular form is leiomyomata) are benign tumors made up of endometrial cells that have implanted on or within the walls of the uterus. These can grow very large and may cause pain or menstrual disorders, exert pressure on the bladder or bowel, cause necrosis because of pressure on the blood supply to tissues, and interfere with fertility.

Medical and Surgical Treatment

Because fibroids are estrogen sensitive, medical treatment may involve hormone suppression. Surgical treatment may involve **myomectomy** or hysterectomy. Myomectomy is removal of only the fibroid tumor and may be chosen in order to preserve fertility. Myomectomy may be done surgically through an abdominal or vaginal incision or with a laser introduced through a laparoscope. Hysterectomy may be necessary for very large fibroids or those that cause severe bleeding or discomfort.

Polyps

Pathophysiology

Polyps are benign growths. They may occur inside the uterus or on the cervix and may bleed after intercourse or between menstrual cycles. These are generally teardrop shaped and are attached by a stalk. Polyps develop most often after the age of 40.

Medical and Surgical Treatment

Polyps are generally removed vaginally or transcervically by separating the stalk from the uterus and then stopping the bleeding by use of chemical, electrical, or laser **cautery.** Removal of polyps in the vagina is generally done without anesthetic in a physician's office. Removal of polyps transcervically requires cervical dilation and is more likely to be done in a hospital with anesthesia.

Reproductive System Cysts

Pathophysiology

Several types of cysts may affect women's health. Cysts of the ovaries may develop associated with incomplete ovulation, **hypertrophy** of the corpus luteum after ovulation, or inflammation of the ovary. Most ovarian cysts spontaneously shrink eventually and merely cause discomfort for a period of time. Chocolate cysts are formed when endometrial cells bleed into an enclosed space, as occurs with endometriosis. These are called chocolate cysts because they are filled with old blood, which has become chocolate colored. Cystadenomas are benign growths that can sometimes undergo cellular transformation and become cancerous. Any pelvic mass in a postmenopausal woman has a high potential for malignancy.

Medical and Surgical Treatment

Most cysts are not surgically removed, but excessive size, interference with fertility, and high cancer potential may make needle drainage, biopsy, laparoscopic surgery, or laparotomy advisable.

Nursing Care

Heat application to the abdomen or back may help promote comfort.

Bartholin Cysts

Etiology

Bartholin cysts are actually infected or obstructed Bartholin glands at either side of the vaginal opening.

Signs and Symptoms

Excessive swelling of the Bartholin glands results in pain with sitting and with intercourse.

Surgical Treatment

Incision and drainage may alleviate the discomfort. If Bartholin cyst formation occurs frequently, **marsupialization**—the surgical formation of a pouch around an opening made into a gland to facilitate drainage—may be necessary.

Nursing Care

Sitz baths may be ordered to cleanse the area and to promote comfort and healing.

Dermoid Cysts

Pathophysiology

Rarely, a **dermoid** cyst (also called a cystic **teratoma**) may develop from a germinal cell of an ovary. This cell divides and differentiates into various tissue types such as skin, teeth, bones, hair, and even extremities in a disordered arrangement. This type of cyst may grow quite large and may occur on both ovaries at the same time.

Medical and Surgical Treatment

Dermoid cysts are removed by laparoscopy or laparotomy. If the cyst contained glandular tissue that was secreting hormones, adjustment of hormone levels to normal may take some time. Although most teratomas are benign, some are malignant, especially in postmenopausal women, so a biopsy is generally done on the tissue.

Nursing Care

Growth of a dermoid can be a frightening experience for a woman. Reassurance that this is merely a disordered group of cells identical to the other cells in her body, rather than a monster or deformed baby, is important.

MALIGNANT DISORDERS

It is sometimes difficult to distinguish benign growths from malignant growths without biopsy results, and some benign growths can become cancerous. Malignancies can occur in all parts of the reproductive system and can occur at all ages. Although reproductive system cancers are more

---

cautery: branding iron

hypertrophy: hyper—too much + trophy—nourishment (growth)

marsupialization: marsupial—pouch + ization—process of making

dermoid: derm—skin + oid—form

teratoma: terat—monster + oma—growth

common in older age groups, ovarian tumors can occur even in young children, and endodermal sinus tumors and embryonal rhabdomyosarcomas can occur in infants less than 2 years of age. Children of women who were given diethylstilbestrol (DES) in the 1940s to prevent premature delivery in high-risk pregnancies have experienced a high incidence of developmental defects and cancers of the reproductive organs.

Many different types of genital cancer are possible, and discussion of every type in detail is beyond the focus of this book. This section will present a general overview of the most common concepts. Cancerous changes often can be observed or noticed, and if investigated and treated early enough, cure is often complete.

LEARNING TIP

Three "**C**" changes that may indicate cancer are changes in **c**olor, **c**ontour, and **c**onsistency.

Vulvar Cancer

Signs and Symptoms

For visible portions of the reproductive system such as the vulva, alertness to changes can result in early diagnosis and requirement of less drastic treatment with more positive results. Persistent itching of the vulva or appearance of white or red patches, rough areas, skin ulcers, or wartlike growths on the vulva should not be ignored; these can be signs of precancerous or cancerous changes.

Risk Factors and Prevention

Risk factors for development of vulvar cancer are an STD of any type, precancerous or cancerous changes of the anus or any of the genitalia, immune system depression, and smoking. Prevention involves avoiding sexually transmitted diseases, not smoking, and having regular Pap smears and physical examinations.

Diagnostic Tests

Biopsy is the main method of diagnosing vulvar cancer.

Medical and Surgical Treatment

Vulvar cancer if discovered early may require removal or destruction of cancerous cells. If not diagnosed early, it may require surgical removal of the entire vulva and associated lymph nodes (a radical vulvectomy) with subsequent skin grafting from other areas of the body for repair.

---

neoplasia: neo—new + plasia—shape or form
cryotherapy: cryo—cold + therapy—treatment

Cervical Cancer

Pathophysiology

Cervical intraepithelial **neoplasia** (CIN) cellular changes are ranked by the amount of dysplasia or disorderedness of the cells. Cells that evidence dysplasia are generally less differentiated or less ordered than expected for their cell type. Ranking systems vary, but Pap smear results are usually presented in categories that range from no atypical cells seen to invasive cancer evident.

Risk Factors and Prevention

Some identified risk factors for development of cervical cancer include starting sexual activity at an early age, having multiple sexual partners, having several pregnancies, smoking, and being infected with human papillomavirus or herpes simplex virus 2 (HSV2). Use of OCs for several years may also increase a woman's risk of developing cervical cancer, although part of the difference in incidence may be because of the protection against STDs that barrier methods offer and that OCs do not provide.

Avoiding the risk factors is the best means of prevention; however, early diagnosis and treatment can prevent invasive cancer and metastasis. Regular Pap smears can mean the difference between life and death. Research is ongoing to develop a vaccine against human papillomavirus, which causes many cases of cervical cancer.[26]

Symptoms

Although some women experience slight spotting or a serosanguineous discharge with cervical cancer, many are asymptomatic until the cancer is widespread.

Diagnostic Tests for Cervical Cancer

Pap smears are the best method of screening for cervical cancer that we have presently. This procedure has significantly reduced the incidence of invasive cervical cancer over the years since its introduction, because cellular changes can be identified early enough for treatment before the cells become cancerous. Classification of abnormal Pap smears is done according to the amount of cellular changes and invasiveness of the abnormal tissues.

Recommendations for frequency of screening also vary, but most recommend that Pap smears begin at either 18 years of age or with the start of sexual activity and be done at first yearly unless abnormalities develop. After a period of normal Pap smears, some physicians advocate longer intervals for low-risk individuals.

Medical and Surgical Treatment

Treatments for preinvasive neoplasia include **cryotherapy** (freezing), laser therapy (burning), or surgical removal of the involved area with a loop excision instrument or by conization (Fig. 40–11). All of these procedures are done through the vagina, so there are no

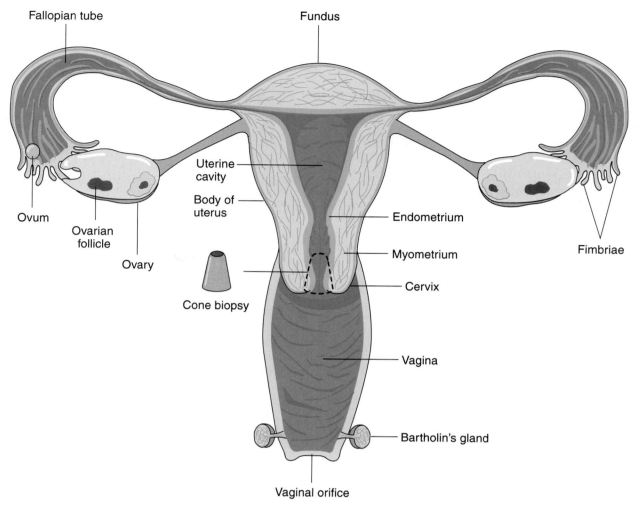

Figure 40–11. Conization.

external incisions. After any of these treatments the client is advised not to douche, use tampons, or have intercourse for approximately 2 weeks to allow for healing to take place. She should be advised to report immediately if fever or bloody or foul discharge occurs. For invasive cancers, hysterectomy or radiation implant or chemotherapy may be undertaken.

Endometrial Cancer

Etiology

Endometrial cancer is the most common type of uterine cancer. Most develop in response to relative estrogen excess.

Signs and Symptoms

Abrupt changes in bleeding patterns, especially bleeding in a menopausal woman, may indicate endometrial cancer development.

Risk Factors and Prevention

Risk factors include obesity, perimenopausal status, estrogen replacement therapy, genetic factors, and perhaps alcohol consumption. Endometrial cancer results from an excess of estrogen. Obesity results in increased estrogen production that is not balanced by progestins. Estrogen levels can vary widely in the perimenopausal time period. Estrogen replacement therapy for menopausal symptoms without the addition of progestins also has been associated with an increase in endometrial cancer, but addition of a progestin may decrease the risk of endometrial cancer to less than that of untreated women. Whether alcohol consumption increases the risk of endometrial cancer by interfering with estrogen metabolism is still a matter of debate. Some endometrial cancer, however, is unexplained by any presently known risk factors.

Avoidance of the risk factors and moderation in diet and alcohol consumption may help prevent this disorder.

Prompt medical investigation of changes in menstrual patterns, especially in the perimenopausal and menopausal age group, may prevent the spread of cancer to other areas.

Diagnostic Tests

Diagnosis is generally done by endometrial biopsy, but MRI may be used to evaluate invasiveness and involvement of lymph nodes.

Medical and Surgical Treatment

Depending on the stage of endometrial cancer and metastasis, hysterectomy, radiation, or chemotherapy may be used.

Ovarian Cancer

Pathophysiology and Signs and Symptoms

Ovarian cancer is the fifth leading cause of cancer death among American women.[27] Much of the reason that this occurs is that the cellular changes that occur when ovarian cells become cancerous may cause no symptoms until the cancer is quite advanced. We know little about what prompts these cells to undergo malignant changes.

Risk Factors

Risk factors are not definitely identified, but some proposed factors include low fertility and number of children, late menopause, a family history of reproductive or colon cancers, contact of talc on the perineum, mumps as a child, and a diet rich in animal fats. Contrary to most other types of reproductive system cancer, use of hormonal contraception may help prevent this, because less ovulation occurs in the lifetime.

Diagnostic Tests

Identification of abnormal growths on the ovaries may begin with bimanual examination, so it is important for women, especially in the older age groups, to continue to have regular pelvic examinations even if they are not sexually active. Various blood tests measuring tumor marker substances, ultrasonography, CT scanning, and MRI may also be used to assist in diagnosis.

Medical and Surgical Treatment

Treatment may involve surgery (by laparoscopy or laparotomy). The ovaries may be removed to prevent the disease in women who have a high familial risk or to remove cancerous tissues. Radiation and combination chemotherapy may also be used.

Nursing Care of Clients with Malignant Disorders

Radiation therapy for cancers of the reproductive system may involve placing radioactive implants into the patient's body for 24 to 72 hours. The nurse should avoid prolonged contact with the client and should perform care in a manner that keeps as much of the client's body between the nurse and the implant as possible (e.g., for cervical implants the nurse stands at the head of the bed rather than at the foot of the bed). The nurse should also help the client avoid inappropriate radiation of other body parts by maintaining patency of a urinary catheter to avoid unnecessary exposure of the bladder to radiation. Institutional guidelines for radiation precautions are followed. Pregnant nurses should not give care to clients with radioactive implants. A foul vaginal discharge is expected after radiation by implant because of tissue destruction caused by the radiation.

Chemotherapy treatments often cause severe nausea, as well as anorexia and sores of the mouth, vagina, and anus. The client may find it easier not to eat or drink. Supplying antiemetic medications before meals and as needed, giving good mouth care and good perineal care, helping the client to select foods and drinks that she likes, and assisting the client to take small frequent feedings can improve nutritional status during chemotherapy. (See also Chapter 10.)

Gynecological Surgery

ENDOSCOPIC SURGERIES

Many of the surgeries performed on the reproductive system may be done using an endoscope. The scopes used contain not only magnifying lenses and a light source, but may also include tiny tools for performing surgery, for removal of small areas of diseased tissue and samples, for suction, and for cauterization of bleeding vessels. Because endoscopic surgeries require tiny incisions (usually less than 1 inch long), there is less tissue disruption and very little bleeding when compared with traditional surgical techniques. Smaller incisions also present less risk of infection than traditional methods, and recuperation is generally more rapid with fewer complications. Overall, the danger to the client is generally low for endoscopic surgeries; however, not all surgical situations may be satisfactorily handled in this way. The size of the cannula restricts the size of tissues that can be removed, unless they can be divided into smaller sections and then pulled out through the cannula. If affected areas are very widespread, the scope may not be able to reach all sites. Traditional surgery still may have to be done when endoscopic surgery has been ineffective, and this can be frustrating to clients. Information gained through the prior endoscopic surgery may decrease the time required for the traditional surgery.

Laparoscopies are the most common type of endoscopic surgical procedure employed for women's reproductive system surgeries. This method can be used for access to the abdominal cavity and the anterior portions of the reproductive organs. Tubal ligations, tubal repairs, removal of ectopic pregnancy implantations, removal of small tumors, removal of endometriotic sections of tissue, and aspiration of fluid-filled cysts can all be done by this method.

Culdoscopies may be done to access the area at the back of the uterus. A **culdotomy,** which is an incision into the upper posterior portion of the vagina, is necessary to insert the cannula. A **culdocentesis,** which is the removal of fluid from the cul de sac of Douglas, may be done during a culdoscopy. Aftercare is much the same as for laparoscopy, although the client should be informed that a small amount of vaginal spotting may be expected due to the incision, but heavy, purulent, or foul-smelling discharge could indicate infection.

Colposcopies are generally used to treat problems of the cervix. The binocular microscope attached to the scope cannula, which is introduced into the vagina, allows the physician to examine dysplastic cells while they are still in their normal place and to treat cervical dysplasia as previously described. Hysteroscopy may be used to treat problems within the uterus. Removal of polyps and other growths, modification of congenital malformations such as **septa** (walls of tissue where there should be none), and laser ablation of endometrial tissue may all be done during hysteroscopy. If the endoscope is inserted further into the fallopian tubes to perform a salpingoscopy, blockages of the tubes may be opened surgically or with laser treatment.

Nursing Care

Postoperative care involves careful assessment for signs of possible excessive internal bleeding, including checks of vital signs, skin color and temperature, and pain. Measures to reduce the discomfort produced by residual CO_2 from **insufflation** may include instruction to lie flat for a few hours, massaging of the back and shoulders, and administration of pain medication. Instruction about possible danger signs, any medications, and when and where to go for suture removal complete the discharge teaching.

HYSTERECTOMY

Removal of the uterus (hysterectomy) may be done for a variety of reasons, including abnormally heavy or painful menstruation, large fibroids or other benign tumors, severe

---

NUTRITION NOTES BOX 40-4

To prevent neural tube defects in infants, the U.S. Public Health Service recommends that all women who might become pregnant consume 0.4 mg (400 μg) of folic acid daily. Neural tube defects include anencephaly, meningoencephalocele, spina bifida, and meningocele. Most experts believe these neural tube defects occur in the first 4 weeks of gestation, before many women realize they are pregnant. Consequently, to increase likelihood of adequate folic acid intake, for the first time since 1943 the Food and Drug Administration has issued a fortification order. Beginning January 1, 1998, specified amounts of folic acid will be added to all enriched foods in an attempt to reduce the occurrence of these defects. Even so, the woman must eat the enriched foods as part of a balanced diet, including liberal amounts of green leafy vegetables, to obtain the desired result.

---

uterine prolapse, and cancer of the uterus. It should not be done merely as a sterilization procedure, because the risks involved in hysterectomy surgery are much greater than risks associated with tubal ligation. The surgery is usually performed through an abdominal incision, but it may be done vaginally in some cases. The vagina is left intact except for suturing of the proximal end, which had been attached to the uterus, forming a blind pouch. Although less vaginal lubrication is present after hysterectomy, nerve routes are maintained and satisfactory sexual intercourse is an expected outcome.

The uterus alone may be removed, or in some cases the tubes and ovaries may also be removed—a procedure called total abdominal hysterectomy with **bilateral salpingo-oophorectomy** (TAH-BSO) or **panhysterectomy.** If the ovaries are removed, the woman undergoes immediate menopause and may suffer from any of the symptoms associated with menopause. Because removal of the ovaries is usually done due to the presence of estrogen-dependent cancer, estrogen replacement is not usually feasible in these cases, and extra care, comfort, and explanation from nurses are very necessary. (See Nursing Care Plan Box 40–3 for the Hysterectomy Client.)

---

culdotomy: culdo—cul de sac + tomy—cutting
culdocentesis: culdo—cul de sac + centesis—puncturing
septa: walls
bilateral salpingo-oophorectomy: bi—two + lateral—sided + salpingo—tubal + oophor—ovary + ec—from + tomy—cutting
panhysterectomy: pan—all + hyster—uterus + ec—from + tomy—cutting

NURSING CARE PLAN BOX 40–3 FOR THE HYSTERECTOMY CLIENT

Risk for anxiety related to uncertainty about the surgery and resulting body changes

Outcomes
Excessive anxiety will not be evident.

Interventions	Rationale	Evaluation
Carry out thorough individualized preoperative teaching about what to expect relative to the surgery and resulting body changes. Support the physician's explanations, answer questions when possible, or refer to an appropriate source.	Knowledge dispels unreasonable fears and helps the client to prepare adequately to cope with stressors.	Does the client express satisfaction with amount and type of information? Does the client evidence an adequate understanding of the surgical procedures and changes in condition postoperatively? Do the client's vital signs, verbal, and nonverbal demeanor suggest anxiety?

Risk for impaired tissue integrity related to surgical incision and removal of the uterus (and possibly the ovaries)

Outcomes
Incision(s) will heal by primary intention without excessive bleeding.

Interventions	Rationale	Evaluation
Monitor vital signs and oxygen saturation according to hospital policy and as necessary.	Vital signs and oxygen saturation reflect tissue perfusion status.	Are vital signs stable and within normal range?
Check for bleeding or other discharge on the perineal pad and on the abdominal dressing (if applicable).	Excessive bleeding may compromise tissue perfusion and slow healing. Vaginal discharge gives clues to healing of incision at the proximal end of the vagina.	Is the pad or dressing dry? Is the discharge foul smelling?
Assess wound healing twice a day (bid) and report any evidence of infection or inadequate healing promptly.	Early treatment of inadequate wound healing decreases postoperative complications.	Is the incisional area swollen, reddened, or draining purulent material?

Risk for altered urinary elimination related to manipulation of the bladder and ureters during surgery, anticholinergic drugs, fluid intake changes, and fear of pain

Outcomes
The client will have adequate urinary output without difficulty.

Interventions	Rationale	Evaluation
Assess urinary output after surgery. Report if less than 30 mL/h or unable to void.	Inadequate urinary output can be an evidence of dehydration, low glomerular perfusion, kidney dysfunction, damage to a ureter, or urinary retention. Urinary retention can cause damage to the kidneys, ureters, and bladder.	Is the output adequate? Is the client able to void without discomfort?
Assess bladder fullness using Doppler monitoring or the scratch text (listening with a stethoscope, lightly scratch the abdomen as you move downward from the xiphoid until you hear a change in sound indicating the top of the bladder).	Scratch test and Doppler monitoring cause less discomfort and pressure to an abdominal incision area.	Does the client feel she is emptying fully when voiding? Does the Doppler indicate residual urine after voiding? Where is the level of sound change with the scratch test?

continued

NURSING CARE PLAN BOX 40–3 (continued)

Interventions	Rationale	Evaluation
Medicate for pain on a fixed schedule for the operative day and first postoperative day (unless the client declines pain medication).	Maintenance of a consistent blood level of medication in the immediate postoperative period provides relief of pain and promotes voiding without fear of discomfort.	Does the client state that she is comfortable?

Risk for constipation and gas related to manipulation of the bowel during surgery, opioid analgesics and anticholinergic drugs, diet changes, less exercise than usual, and fear of pain when passing stool

Outcomes
The client will pass adequate soft formed stool without excessive gas discomfort by third postoperative day.

Interventions	Rationale	Evaluation
Assess for active bowel sounds in all four abdominal quadrants before giving anything orally.	Manipulation of the bowel during surgery or anesthetics and other medications may interfere with bowel function.	Are the bowel sounds sluggish, active, or hyperactive? Are they present in all four quadrants?
Encourage high fluid intake, and graduate the diet toward a high-fiber, regular diet as soon as the client is able to tolerate it (or doctor's orders prescribe).	Adequate fluid and fiber in the diet softens the stool for easy passage.	Is the client drinking well? Is the client ready for more normal foods, as well as liquids?
Encourage adequate exercise.	Reasonable exercise promotes peristalsis and relieves gas discomfort.	Has the client dangled at the bedside the day of surgery and then walked increasing amounts each day following?
Control pain with analgesics, especially before administering a suppository or enema.	The presence of pain may inhibit defecation.	Is the client passing intestinal gas without difficulty? Does the client express satisfaction with pain control?
Give stool softeners, laxatives, suppositories, or enemas as ordered (check bowel protocol or standing orders).	Soft stool is easier to pass.	Has the client passed a soft formed stool by the third day after surgery?

Risk for ineffective individual coping related to body image disturbance (and hormonal disturbance if ovaries were also removed)

Outcomes
Client will evidence use of effective coping skills.

Interventions	Rationale	Evaluation
Maintain an open and trusting therapeutic relationship.	Effective communication is based on trust.	Is the client talking about concerns?
Allow grieving to take place (tears are not uncommon after this surgery).	Loss of the reproductive function and role disturbs many aspects of body image.	Is healthy grief being expressed?
Encourage the client to express feelings and concerns.	Memory of prior successes can strengthen resolve to cope effectively again.	Does the client recount any prior successes?
Help the client remember previous changes in her life with which she has coped well.		
Encourage self-care as much as is feasible.	Self-care promotes feelings of self-assurance and combats depression.	Is the client taking an active interest in her personal appearance?
Refer to appropriate agencies for further support as needed (e.g., American Cancer Society or local cancer support agency if the surgery was done because of cancer).	Social support can assist individuals to meet their needs while developing effective coping skills and strategies.	Is the client planning realistically for discharge? Does the client evidence sufficient coping skills or have supports available to continue the healing process at home?

Review Questions

1. Which of the following is the *least* effective form of contraception?
   a. Douching
   b. Condom with spermicide
   c. Diaphragm with spermicide
   d. Oral contraceptive medication

Match the following surgical procedures with their descriptions.

2. Laser ablation
3. Marsupialization
4. Panhysterectomy
5. Dilation and curettage
6. Bilateral salpingo-oophorectomy

   a. Destruction of tissue by burning it with a laser
   b. Opening of the cervix and removal of uterine contents
   c. Removal of both of the fallopian tubes and both ovaries
   d. Removal of the entire uterus, fallopian tubes, and ovaries
   e. Surgical formation of a pouch around an opening made into a Bartholin gland to facilitate drainage

7. Why should male partners be treated for yeast along with the affected woman?
   a. To prevent cancer
   b. To prevent infertility
   c. To avoid reinfecting her after treatment
   d. To avoid becoming infected with the yeast himself

8. Which response by the nurse is most appropriate when a 60-year-old neighbor, Maria Gonzalez, who has been menopausal for several years, asks what could be wrong because she has begun having vaginal bleeding again?
   a. "Ignore it—it is perfectly normal."
   b. "I guess you were not really menopausal yet."
   c. "You should see a doctor to have that checked as soon as possible."
   d. "Give it time—most problems go away if they are given enough time."

9. If a mastectomy client has a Hemovac drain in place postoperatively, nursing actions should include which of the following?
   a. No action is necessary.
   b. Stop the drain by clamping it.
   c. Empty the bag as ordered and note the amount and color of drainage.
   d. Leave the drainage in the bag until the Hemovac is removed from the client.

10. Primary dysmenorrhea is treated by blocking prostaglandin synthesis with:

   a. Vitamins
   b. Antacids
   c. Morphine
   d. Nonsteroidal anti-inflammatory drugs

ANSWERS TO CRITICAL THINKING: Jessica

1. Some important information from her would include her true age (laws vary concerning birth control for minors), her intentions, her family situation, whether she is already sexually active, and what information she wants.

2. She needs to know that being sexually active involves more risks than just pregnancy. Discussion of STDs is vital. Discussion of violence, potential for abuse, and psychological suffering, which may accompany early sexual activity, may also be important. The choices of birth control should be explained, including the risks, effectiveness, disadvantages, and advantages of each method.

3. While focusing on her desire to be a responsible adult is an admirable attitude, potential scenarios can be presented for her "responsible" consideration, such as the following: What would she do if contraceptive failure resulted in a pregnancy? How would she feel if she contracted an incurable or permanently damaging sexually transmitted disease? How would she react now to being "dumped" by someone she cares for who is less responsible and mature? Asking about her goals and plans in life may be very significant. Counseling that evidences concern for the individual at this stage may do a lot to postpone sexual activity until the client is more mature. It is important for her to realize that choosing to delay sexual activity at this time may be the most responsible and health-promoting life decision she might make.

REFERENCES

1. Parker, SL, et al: Cancer statistics 1996. CA Cancer J Clin 65:5, 1996.
2. Bilmoria, MM, and Morrow, M: The woman at increased risk for breast cancer; Evaluation and management strategies. CA Cancer J Clin 45:263, 1995.
3. Kuter, I: Breast cancer. In Lemcke, DP, et al (eds): Primary Care of Women. Appleton & Lange, Norwalk, Conn, 1995, pp 194–195.
4. Newcomb, PA, et al: Lactation and a reduced risk of premenopausal breast cancer (abstract). N Engl J Med 330:81, 1994.
5. Kuter, I: Breast cancer. In Lemcke, DP, et al (eds): Primary Care of women. Appleton & Lange, Norwalk, Conn, 1995, pp 194–195.
6. Barbieri, RL, and Ryan, DK: The menstrual cycle. In Ryan, KJ, Berkowitz, RS, and Barbieri, RL (eds): Kistner's Gynecology, ed 6. Mosby, St Louis, 1995, p 44.
7. Lemone, PM, and Burke, KM (eds): Medical Surgical Nursing: Critical Thinking in Client Care. Addison-Wesley, Menlo Park, Calif, 1996, p 1991.
8. Taylor, D: Perimenstrual symptoms and premenstrual syndrome. In Star, WI, Lommel, LL, and Shannon, MT (eds): Women's Primary

Health Care: Protocols for Practice. American Nurses' Association, Washington, DC, 1995, pp 141–157.

9. Isaacson, KB: Endometriosis. In Carlson, KJ, et al (eds): Primary Care of Women. Mosby, St Louis, 1995, pp 234–239.

10. Star, WL: Bacterial vaginosis. In Star, WI, Lommel, LL, and Shannon, MT (eds): Women's Primary Health Care: Protocols for Practice. American Nurses' Association, Washington, DC, 1995, p 214.

11. Bengtson, JM: The vagina. In Ryan, KJ, Berkowitz, RS, and Barbieri, RL (eds): Kistner's Gynecology, ed 6. Mosby, St Louis, 1995, pp 85–86.

12. Rein, MS, and Schiff, I: Evaluation of the infertile couple. In Ryan, KJ, Berkowitz, RS, and Barbieri, RL (eds): Kistner's Gynecology, ed 6. Mosby, St Louis, 1995, p 279.

13. Osathanondh, R, Stelluto, MR, and Carlson, KJ: Contraception. In Carlson, KJ, et al (eds): Primary Care of Women. Mosby, St Louis, 1995, p 203.

14. Letterie, GS, and Royce R: Contraception. In Lemcke, DP, et al (eds): Primary Care of Women. Appleton & Lange, Norwalk, Conn, 1995, p 488.

15. Buckshee, K, et al: Return of fertility following discontinuation of Norplant-II subdermal implants. Contraception 51:237, 1995.

16. Rosenweig, BA, Even, A, and Budnick, LE: Observations of scanning electron microscopy detected abnormalities of non-lubricated latex condoms. Contraception 53:49, 1996.

17. Archer, DF, et al: Lea's Shield: A phase I postcoital study of a new contraceptive barrier device. Contraception 52:167, 1995.

18. Weisberg, E, et al: The acceptability of a combined oestrogen/progestogen contraceptive vaginal ring. Contraception 51:39, 1995.

19. Coutinho, EM, et al: Multicenter clinical trial on the efficacy and acceptability of a single contraceptive implant of nomogestrol acetate, Uniplant. Contraception 53:121, 1996.

20. Luukkainen, T, and Toivonen, J: Levonorgestrel-releasing IUD as a method of contraception with therapeutic properties. Contraception 52:269, 1995.

21. Zhen, QS, and Wei, ZJ: Recent progress in research on Tripterygium: A male antifertility plant. Contraception 51:121.

22. Yi, Q, et al: The change of carnitine content in seminal plasma after reversible injection occlusion of vas deferens. Contraception 51:261, 1995.

23. Alexander, NJ, and Bialy, G: Contraceptive vaccine development (abstract). Reprod Fertil Dev 6(3):273, 1994.

24. Schrater, AF: Immunization to regulate fertility: Biological and cultural frameworks (abstract). Soc Sci Med 41(5):657, 1995.

25. Aboulafia, DM: Hematologic complications of pregnancy. In Lemcke, DP, et al (eds): Primary Care of Women. Appleton & Lange, Norwalk, Conn, 1995, pp 370–381.

26. Ressing, ME, et al: Occasional memory cytotoxic T-cell responses of patients with human papillomavirus type 16–positive cervical lesions against a human leucocyte antigen A*0201-restricted E7-encoded epitope. Cancer Res 56:582, 1996.

27. Parker, SL, et al: Cancer statistics, 1996. CA Cancer J Clin 65:5, 1996.

BIBLIOGRAPHY

Albaugh, B, and Gettrust, KV: Plans of Care for Specialty Practice: Surgical Nursing: Delmar, Albany, NY, 1994.

Anderson, KN, Anderson, L, and Glanze, WD (eds): Mosby's Medical, Nursing and Allied Health Dictionary, ed 4. Mosby, St Louis, 1994.

Bassol, S, et al: A comparative study on the return to ovulation following chronic use of once-a-month injectable contraceptives. Contraception 51:307, 1995.

Bengston, JM: The vagina. In Ryan, KJ, Berkowitz, RS, and Barbieri, RL (eds): Kistner's Gynecology, ed 6. Mosby, St Louis, 1995.

Bobak, IM, et al (eds): Maternity Nursing, ed 4. Mosby, St Louis, 1995.

Carlson, KJ, et al (eds): Primary Care of Women. Mosby, St Louis, 1995.

Cashion, K, and Johnston, CLA: Nursing Care during the Postpartum Period. In Bobak, IM, et al (eds): Maternity Nursing, ed 4. Mosby, St Louis, 1995.

Fischer, RA, and Ravnikar, VA: Infertility. In Carlson, KJ, et al (eds): Primary Care of Women. Mosby, St Louis, 1995.

Fogel, CI, and Woods, NF (eds): Women's Health Care. Sage, Thousand Oaks, Calif, 1995.

Genuis, SJ, and Genuis, SK: Adolescent sexual involvement: Time for primary prevention. Lancet 35(8944):240, 1995.

Hornstein, MD, and Barbieri, RL: Endometriosis. In Ryan, KJ, Berkowitz, RS, and Barbieri, RL (eds): Kistner's Gynecology, ed 6. Mosby, St Louis, 1995.

Isaacson, KB: Endometriosis. In Carlson, KJ, et al (eds): Primary Care of Women. Mosby, St Louis, 1995.

Katz, ME, and Osathanondh, R: Abortion. In Carlson, KJ, et al (eds): Primary Care of Women. Mosby, St Louis, 1995.

Ketchum, KM, and Ritchie, DJ: Antifungal drugs. In Pinnell, NL (ed): Nursing Pharmacology. WB Saunders, Philadelphia, 1996.

Klock, SC: Psychosomatic issues in obstetrics and gynecology. In Ryan, KJ, Berkowitz, RS, and Barbieri, RL (eds): Kistner's Gynecology, ed 6. Mosby, St Louis, 1995.

Lehne, RA, et al: Pharmacology for Nursing Care, ed 2. WB Saunders, Philadelphia, 1994.

Lemcke, DP, et al (eds): Primary Care of Women. Appleton & Lange, Norwalk, Conn, 1995.

Lemone, PM, and Burke, KM (eds): Medical Surgical Nursing: Critical Thinking in Client Care. Addison-Wesley, Menlo Park, Calif, 1996.

Lethbridge, DJ: Unwanted pregnancy. In Fogel, CI, and Woods, NF (eds): Women's Health Care. Sage, Thousand Oaks, Calif, 1995.

Letterie, GS, and Royce, R: Contraception. In Lemcke, DP, et al (eds): Primary Care of Women. Appleton & Lange, Norwalk, Conn, 1995.

Lommel, LL: Breast disorders. In Star, WI, Lommel, LL, and Shannon, MT (eds): Women's Primary Health Care: Protocols for Practice. American Nurses' Association, Washington, DC, 1995.

Love, SM: Dr. Susan Love's Breast Book. Addison-Wesley, Reading, Mass, 1995.

Monif, GRG, et al: Infectious Diseases in Obstetrics and Gynecology. IDI, Omaha, Neb, 1993.

Moore, MP, and Kinne, DW: The surgical management of primary invasive breast cancer. CA Cancer J Clin 45:280, 1995.

Murch, M: Nonsteroidal antiinflammatory drugs. In Pinell, NL (ed): Nursing Pharmacology. WB Saunders, Philadelphia, 1996.

Murtz, HG: Cervical cancer screening and management of the abnormal Papanicolau smear. In Lemcke, DP, et al (eds): Primary Care of Women. Appleton & Lange, Norwalk, Conn, 1995.

Muto, MG, and Friedman, AJ: The uterine corpus. In Ryan, KJ, Berkowitz, RS, and Barbieri, RL (eds): Kistner's Gynecology, ed 6. Mosby, St Louis, 1995.

Nettles-Carlson, B: Problems of the breast. In Fogel, CI, and Woods, NF (eds): Women's Health Care. Sage, Thousand Oaks, Calif, 1995.

Nichols, DH, and Brubaker, L: Incontinence and genital prolapse. In Carlson, KJ, et al (eds): Primary Care of Women. Mosby, St Louis, 1995.

Osathanondh, R: Conception control. In Ryan, KJ, Berkowitz, RS, and Barbieri, RL (eds): Kistner's Gynecology, ed 6. Mosby, St Louis, 1995.

Osathanondh, R, Stelluto, MR, and Carlson, KJ: Contraception. In Carlson, KJ, et al (eds): Primary Care of Women. Mosby, St Louis, 1995.

Phipps, WJ, et al (eds): Medical Surgical Nursing: Concepts and Clinical Practice. Mosby, St Louis, 1995.

Pillitteri, A: Maternal-Child Nursing. JB Lippincott, Philadelphia, 1995.

Rice, LW, and Barbieri, RL: The ovary. In Ryan, KJ, Berkowitz, RS, and Barbieri, RL (eds): Kistner's Gynecology, ed 6. Mosby, St Louis, 1995.

Robinson, KM, and McCance, KL: Alterations of the reproductive systems including sexually transmitted disease. In Huether, SE, and McCance, KL (eds): Understanding Pathophysiology. Mosby, St Louis, 1996.

Ryan, KJ, Berkowitz, RS, and Barbieri, RL (eds): Kistner's Gynecology, ed 6. Mosby, St Louis, 1995.

Scura, KW, and Whipple, B: How to provide better care of the post-menopausal woman. Am J Nurs 4:36, 1997.

Shannon, M: Toxic shock syndrome. In Star, WI, Lommel, LL, and Shannon, MT (eds): Women's Primary Health Care: Protocols for Practice. American Nurses' Association, Washington, DC, 1995.

Sherwen, LN, Scoloveno, MA, and Weingarten, CT: Nursing Care of the Childbearing Family, ed 2. Appleton & Lange, Norwalk, Conn, 1995.

Sillman, FH, and Muto, MG: The vulva. In Ryan, KJ, Berkowitz, RS, and Barbieri, RL (eds): Kistner's Gynecology, ed 6. Mosby, St Louis, 1995.

Smith, BL: The breast. In Ryan, KJ, Berkowitz, RS, and Barbieri, RL (eds): Kistner's Gynecology, ed 6. Mosby, St Louis, 1995.

Star, WI, Lommel, LL, and Shannon, MT (eds): Women's Primary Health Care: Protocols for Practice. American Nurses' Association, Washington, DC, 1995.

Taylor, D: Perimenstrual symptoms and premenstrual syndrome. In Star, WI, Lommel, LL, and Shannon, MT (eds): Women's Primary Health Care: Protocols for Practice. American Nurses' Association, Washington, DC, 1995.

Thompson, ED (ed): Maternity and Pediatric Nursing, ed 2. WB Saunders, Philadelphia, 1995.

Tuomala, R: Gynecologic infections: In Ryan, KJ, Berkowitz, RS, and Barbieri, RL (eds): Kistner's Gynecology, ed 6. Mosby, St Louis, 1995.

Viamontes, CM, Gerber, WR, and Thomure, MF: Drugs affecting the female reproductive system. In Pinnell, NL (ed): Nursing Pharmacology. WB Saunders, Philadelphia, 1996.

Wakamatsu, MM: Vaginitis. In Carlson, KJ, et al (eds): Primary Care of Women. Mosby, St Louis, 1995.

Walsh, BW: Menopause. In Ryan, KJ, Berkowitz, RS, and Barbieri, RL (eds): Kistner's Gynecology, ed 6. Mosby, St Louis, 1995.

Wertheim, I, Soto-Wright, VJ, and Goodman, HM: Gynecologic cancers. In Carlson, KJ, et al (eds): Primary Care of Women. Mosby, St Louis, 1995.

Weseman, LM: Clomiphene citrate. Some fertility drugs can cause multiple births. In Star, WI, Lommel, LL, and Shannon, MT (eds): Women's Primary Health Care: Protocols for Practice. American Nurses' Association, Washington, DC, 1995.

41

Nursing Care of Male Clients with Genitourinary Disorders

Cindy Meredith

Learning Objectives

Upon completion of this chapter, the student will be able to:

1. Identify pathophysiology associated with male genitourinary and reproductive disorders.
2. Recognize signs and symptoms of prostate problems.
3. Describe treatment options for benign and cancerous enlargements of the prostate.
4. Discuss disorders of the penis that may interfere with normal function.
5. Identify disorders of the testes and their impact on sexual function.
6. Recognize physical and emotional causes of erectile dysfunction.
7. Discuss medical, surgical, and psychological treatment options for erectile function.
8. Explain the nurse's role in helping men cope with the loss of sexual function.
9. Recognize male factors that interfere with fertility.
10. Describe treatment options for male infertility.

Key Words

cryptorchidism (kript-**OR**-ki-dizm)
dysuria (dis-**YOO**-ree-ah)
epididymitis (EP-i-DID-i-**MY**-tis)
erectile dysfunction (e-**RECK**-tile dis-**FUNCK**-shun)
hematuria (HEM-uh-**TYOOR**-ee-ah)
hydrocele (**HIGH**-droh-seel)
hydronephrosis (HIGH-droh-ne-**FROH**-sis)
hyperplasia (HIGH-per-**PLAY**-zee-ah)
nocturia (nock-**TYOO**-ree-ah)
orchiectomy (or-ki-**EK**-toh-mee)
orchitis (or-**KIGH**-tis)
orgasm (**OR**-gazm)
paraphimosis (PAR-uh-figh-**MOH**-sis)
Peyronie's (pay-roh-**NEZ**)

phimosis (figh-**MOH**-sis)
priapism (**PRY**-uh-pizm)
prostatectomy (PRAHS-tah-**TEK**-tuh-mee)
prostatitis (PRAHS-tuh-**TIGH**-tis)
reflux (**REE**-fluks)
retrograde (**RET**-troh-grayd)
suprapubic (SOO-pruh-**PEW**-bik)
tamponade (TAM-pon-**AYD**)
urodynamic (YOO-roh-dye-**NAM**-ik)
urosepsis (YOO-roh-**SEP**-sis)
varicocele (**VAR**-i-koh-seel)
vasectomy (va-**SEK**-tuh-mee)

Problems affecting the male genitals and urinary system are generally difficult areas for both the client and the nurse to deal with due to the sexual nature of the male anatomy. Unfortunately our society does not encourage men to seek medical care or talk about problems related to the male genitals. It is important to realize that sexuality is a natural part of each of us as human beings and should not be avoided when we provide care to clients. Very often the nurse is in an ideal position to provide important sexual health care teaching to clients. If the client is approached in a confident, confidential manner, it can be a positive learning experience for both the client and the nurse.

Prostate Disorders

The prostate gland sits at the base of the bladder and wraps around the upper part of the male urethra like a donut. It is traditionally divided into lobes: the anterior, posterior, median, and lateral lobes. The primary purpose of the prostate is to provide alkaline secretions to semen and aid in ejaculation. It does not contain any hormones; however, many men fear that prostate problems and treatment will cause problems with their erections or their "nature" (sexual activities).

PROSTATITIS

Pathophysiology

Prostatitis, or inflammation of the prostate gland, can occur any time after puberty. The problem may be chronic or a single, acute episode. The inflammation causes the prostate gland to swell resulting in pain, especially when standing. It eventually may lead to difficulty in passing urine due to an inward squeezing of the urethra causing a mild obstruction.

Etiology

There are three basic types of prostatitis: (1) acute bacterial, (2) chronic bacterial, and (3) nonbacterial. Bacterial prostatitis is most common in older men. It results in edema and inflammation of all or part of the prostate gland.

The bacteria primarily responsible for the infection are gram-negative organisms such as *Escherichia coli;* however, gram-positive and gonococcal bacteria may also play a part. The prostate gland may become infected by (1) bacteria ascending the urethra, (2) infected bladder urine **reflux**ing into the prostatic ducts, (3) bacteria in the blood or lymph supply to the gland, or (4) surgical instrumentation or other forms of urethral trauma.

Prevention

Ways to prevent prostatitis are regular and complete emptying of the bladder to prevent urinary tract infection (UTI), avoiding excess alcohol (more than 2 to 3 oz/day—alcohol is a bladder irritant), and avoiding certain high-risk sexual practices. Avoiding contamination of the urinary tract and factors that produce congestion of the prostate gland are the best preventive measures.

Signs and Symptoms

The most common symptoms are the same ones that occur with any UTI: complaints of urgency, frequency, hesitancy, and **dysuria.** Because of the location and role of the prostate gland, the client may complain of low back, perineal, and postejaculation pain; he may also have a fever and chills.

Complications

One complication of acute bacterial prostatitis is urinary retention. If the prostate is extremely swollen it prevents complete bladder emptying. For most men, the most troublesome complication may be a temporary problem with erections. Ascending infections, prostatic abscess, epididymitis, and prostatic calculi (stones) are some of the more serious or rare complications of prostatitis.

Diagnostic Tests

The first test performed is a careful, gentle, digital rectal examination (DRE) of the prostate. The prostate gland is examined by the physician by insertion of a gloved finger into the rectum. The examiner may find a warm, irregular, swollen, painful prostate gland. A urine culture will generally be positive for bacteria. The examiner may also gently massage the prostate gland and order an expressed prostate secretion (EPS) test that will reveal bacteria and a large number of white blood cells.

Medical Treatment

Acute bacterial prostatitis is usually treated medically with antibiotic therapy. The preferred treatment is trimethoprim and sulfamethoxazole (Bactrim, Septra) for 30 days. Antibiotics that are used for chronic or nonbacterial prostatitis include carbenicillin (Geopen), erythromycin (Erythrocin), nitrofurantoin (Macrodantin), and tetracycline (Vibramycin).

Other forms of treatment may include anti-inflammatory agents, warm sitz baths, prostatic massage, and diet changes that will decrease spicy foods and alcohol. In

---

prostatitis: prostat—prostate gland + itis—inflammation
dysuria: dys—painful + uria—urination
nocturia: noc—night + uria—urination

some cases prostate surgery is necessary to remove the obstruction.

Nursing Process

Assessment

Assessment should begin by asking the client to describe signs and symptoms that would indicate evidence of a UTI, such as sudden fever, chills, complaints of urgency, frequency, hesitancy, dysuria, and **nocturia.** In addition, the client may have complaints of pain in the lower back, in the perineum, or after ejaculating. The nurse asks if the client has ever had a UTI or prostate infection in the past. Care must be taken to assess urinary retention due to obstruction. The nurse obtains a urine culture and assists with collection of the EPS specimen, if requested, as part of the client assessment.

Nursing Diagnosis

The nursing diagnoses for clients with prostatitis may include altered health maintenance: knowledge deficit related to causes, treatment, and prevention of prostatitis, particularly for those with their first acute episode. Due to the alteration in comfort a diagnosis related to pain should be included. Because the prostate gland is so closely associated with sexual activity, a diagnosis of anxiety related to

sexual concerns should be considered for most clients. Refer to Nursing Care Plan Box 41–1 for the Client with Prostatitis.

Planning

Because of the nature of prostatitis and its accompanying discomfort, the client's sexual partner is often included in the plan of care. If the bacteria causing the problem is a sexually transmitted organism such as chlamydia or gonococcus, both partners should be treated with antibiotics; sexual intercourse should be avoided during treatment. Scheduled medications and frequent sitz baths may require adjustments in work or normal routines. If a urinary catheter is required, proper catheter care and monitoring of fluid intake and output every 8 hours are done.

Interventions

Special care should be taken to maintain privacy and sensitivity in discussing treatment with the client. The nurse needs to emphasize the preventive measures that would help the client avoid future infection. An area of special concern is reinfection due to not taking antibiotics until the medicine is completely gone. Many clients take antibiotics only until the symptoms disappear and should be reminded to carefully follow directions for taking their medications.

NURSING CARE PLAN BOX 41–1 FOR THE CLIENT WITH PROSTATITIS

Alteration in urinary elimination related to inflammation and irritation of the prostate gland

Client Outcomes
(1) Client implements measures to eliminate signs and symptoms of prostatitis. (2) Client verbalizes the importance of completing antibiotic treatment.

Evaluation of Outcomes
(1) Are signs and symptoms relieved? (2) Does client verbalize importance of completing antibiotic treatment?

Interventions	Rationale	Evaluation
• Assess for presence of fever, chills, urinary urgency, frequency, dysuria, nocturia.	These are symptoms of prostatitis.	Does client have symptoms of prostatitis?
• Assist client with warm sitz bath.	Warm water to the perineal area will increase circulation and decrease inflammation.	Does the client report a lessening of symptoms?
• Encourage an increase in noncaffeine, nonalcoholic fluids to 2500 to 3000 mL/day.	Caffeine, alcohol are irritants to be avoided.	Is the client drinking enough to "flush" the system?
• Teach client to empty bladder every 2 to 3 hours.	Frequent emptying decreases bladder bacteria counts.	Is the client voiding 30 to 40 mL/h?
• Administer antibiotics as prescribed. Teach client to continue prescription until it is completed.	Antibiotics treat infection. The entire prescription must be taken in order to prevent reinfection.	Is the client taking the antibiotic as prescribed?

Evaluation

A clean urine culture with complete disappearance of signs and symptoms of prostatitis is the desired outcome. Prevention of chronic prostatitis can generally be achieved with client education.

Client Education

The nurse plays a key role in helping the client understand the causes, prevention, and treatment of prostatitis. The client should be taught about risk factors such as indwelling urinary catheters, poor hygiene or sexual practices, excessive intake of bladder irritants, ignoring signs and symptoms of UTIs, or poor compliance with the antibiotic treatment plan.

The client should be encouraged to wash his hands and sitz bath equipment before and after each treatment. Fluids such as water and cranberry juice should be encouraged up to 2500 to 3000 mL per day, unless contraindicated. Bladder irritants in the form of caffeine products (such as coffee, tea, cola, and chocolate), citrus juices, and alcohol should be taken in very limited amounts. The client is encouraged to empty his bladder every 2 to 3 hours whether or not he feels the urge to urinate.

The client should be encouraged to discuss possible complications and questions about sexual practices with his physician. In some cases, sexual intercourse is encouraged as a means of relieving prostatic congestion; in other situations it may be contraindicated.

BENIGN PROSTATIC HYPERPLASIA

Enlargement of the prostate gland is a normal process in older men. It begins at about age 50 and happens in 75 percent of men over the age of 70. Benign prostatic **hyperplasia** (BPH) is a nonmalignant growth of the prostate that gradually causes urinary obstruction. According to current studies, BPH does not increase a man's risk of developing cancer of the prostate.

Pathophysiology

There is a slow increase in the number of cells in the prostate gland, generally the results of aging and the male hormone dihydrotestosterone. As the size of the prostate gland increases it begins to compress or squeeze the urethra shut. The narrowing of the urethra means the bladder must work harder to expel the urine. More effort and a longer time is required to empty the bladder. Eventually the narrowing causes an obstruction and may lead to urinary retention or eventually distention of the kidney with urine (**hydronephrosis**).

It is the *location* of the enlargement, not the amount, that causes the problem. A small growth in the prostate gland closest to the urethra may cause more problems with urina-

tion than a growth the size of an orange in the outer portion of the gland.

Etiology

There is no known cause of BPH other than normal aging. Some men think they may have caused the problem by certain sexual practices; however, there is no scientific proof at this time. Some factors that are being investigated in research studies are high-fat diet, ethnic background, and lifestyle issues.

Prevention

Because there is no known cause, there is no known method to prevent enlargement of the prostate gland. There are many new treatments that are aimed at slowing down the enlargement process, but none so far that can prevent the normal changes associated with aging.

Signs and Symptoms

The symptoms of BPH are usually identified in two ways (Table 41–1). A prostate symptom index score sheet has been developed, and physicians are being encouraged to ask their older clients to take the test as a way of assessing the seriousness of their symptoms and deciding treatment options.

Complications

When BPH is untreated and obstruction is prolonged, several serious complications may occur. Urine that sits in the bladder for too long can (1) back up into the kidneys and cause hydronephrosis, renal insufficiency, or **urosepsis** or (2) damage the bladder walls, lead to bladder dysfunction, recurrent UTIs, or calculi (stones).

Diagnostic Tests

The first step is a medical history including specific questions about the client's symptoms. A DRE of the prostate is then conducted by the physician to assess for enlargement and whether the gland is hard, lumpy, or "boggy." A urinalysis is done to look for evidence of white blood cells or **hematuria,** which would indicate infection or inflammation. The physician may also request blood tests to look at the blood urea nitrogen (BUN) and serum creatinine level

---

hyperplasia: hyper—excessive + plasia—formation
hydronephrosis: hydro—water + nephr—kidney + osis—condition
urosepsis: uro—urine + sepsis—systemic infection
hematuria: hemat—blood + uria—in the urine

Table 41–1. Symptoms of Benign Prostatic Hyperplasia

Symptoms Related to Obstruction

1. Decrease in size and force of urinary stream
2. Difficulty in starting stream or pushing to start
3. Dribbling at the end of urinating
4. Interrupted stream, starting and stopping of stream
5. Urinary retention—feeling bladder is not empty
6. Overflow incontinence—leaking urine

Symptoms Related to Irritation

1. Nocturia
2. Dysuria
3. Urgency

for kidney function. In addition a test for prostate-specific antigen (PSA), a possible indicator of prostate cancer, may be ordered if cancer is suspected.

The second level of diagnostic testing may include **urodynamic** flow studies to determine bladder function, transrectal ultrasound of the prostate with or without a biopsy, and cystoscopy (for surgical candidates).

Medical Treatment

If the client has no symptoms or only mild ones the most current medical approach is "watchful waiting." The physician watches for any increase in symptoms or signs that the urethra is becoming obstructed. Treatment of symptoms may include use of a catheter (indwelling or intermittent), encouraging oral fluids, and antibiotics for UTI.

Conservative medical treatment now includes the use of medication to either relax the smooth muscles of the prostate and bladder neck or block the male hormone to prevent or shrink tissue growth. Alpha blockers are medications that relax the smooth muscles and include prazosin (Minipress), terazosin (Hytrin), and doxazosin (Cardura). These medications are also used to treat high blood pressure, and clients need to work closely with their physicians to avoid overdose or the negative side effects of postural hypotension. The most commonly used medication to block the action of the male hormone in the prostate gland is called finasteride (Proscar). All of these medications must be taken on a long-term, continuous basis to achieve results. Conservative measures are used initially unless there are recurring infections, repeated gross hematuria, bladder or kidney damage, evidence of cancer, or unsatisfactory lifestyle changes.

urodynamic: uro—urine + dynamic—force

Nonsurgical invasive treatments, some of which are experimental, are available in some areas of the country in addition to surgical options (Table 41–2).

Surgical Treatment

Transurethral Resection of the Prostate

Over the past 50 years, transurethral resection of the prostate (TURP) has been the surgical treatment used most often to relieve obstruction caused by an enlarged prostate (Fig. 41–1). The client is given anesthesia and the surgery is performed using an instrument called a resectoscope. The resectoscope is put into the urethra and the prostate gland is "chipped" away a piece at a time. Special surgical instruments are now being used that will "vaporize" or "microwave" the pieces and cut down on the amount of bleeding during surgery. During routine TURP the "chips" are flushed out using an irrigating solution and are sent to the lab to be analyzed for possible evidence of cancer. The prostate gland is not completely removed but peeled away like the rind of an orange. The prostate tissue that is left will eventually grow back and can cause obstruction again at a later time. Clients need to be reminded to continue having yearly prostate exams.

Table 41–2. Invasive Treatments for Benign Prostatic Hyperplasia

Nonsurgical (Experimental) Options	Method
Transurethral microwave antenna (TUMA)	Heat applied directly to gland
Prostatic balloon	Dilates the urethra by stretching or compressing
Prostatic stents	Device placed to open passage for urine flow
Transurethral Options	**Method**
Transurethral incision of the prostate (TUIP)	Surgical incisions made into gland to relieve obstruction
Transurethral ultrasound-guided laser-induced prostatectomy (TULIP)	Laser incisions made to relieve obstructions
Transurethral resection of the prostate (TURP)	Resectoscope removes small pieces of tissue
Open Prostatectomy	**Method**
Suprapubic resection	Abdominal incision, scooping out of gland through the bladder
Retropubic resection	Abdominal incision, scooping out of gland through prostate capsule
Perineal resection	Incision between scrotum and anus, removal of gland and low pelvic mass

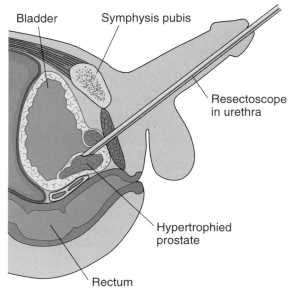

Figure 41–1. Transurethral resection of the prostate.

As the tissue is removed during TURP, bleeding occurs. A Foley catheter is left in place with 30 to 60 mL of sterile water inflating the balloon. The balloon is overfilled and secured to the leg or abdomen in order to **tamponade** (compress) the prostate area to stop the bleeding. Irrigation solution generally flows continuously; manual irrigation may be done for the first 24 hours to help maintain catheter patency by removing clots and chips. The physician will remove the Foley catheter after the danger of hemorrhage has passed.

Complications associated with prostate surgery depend on the type of procedure performed. The main medical complications include clot formation, bladder spasms, and infection. Less common complications may be urinary incontinence, hemorrhage, and erectile dysfunction. (See Nursing Care Plan Box 41–2.)

Retrograde ejaculation is a common side effect of prostate surgery. When any of the prostate gland is removed, there is a decrease in the amount of semen produced and a part of the ejaculatory ducts may be removed. The result is less semen to be pushed to the outside of the body and instead it "falls back" into the bladder. This causes no harm to the man, who will simply pass the semen out the next time he urinates.

It is important to understand that erection, ejaculation, and **orgasm** are all separate actions. Erection means the penis becomes hard; ejaculation is the release of semen; and orgasm is felt as pulsations along the urethra. Unless additional problems are present, the client will continue to have erections and orgasmic sensations but decreased or no ejaculation.

Open Prostatectomy

When the prostate gland is very large and causing obstruction, surgery called an open **prostatectomy** is performed (Fig. 41–2). In the suprapubic approach, an incision is made through the lower abdomen into the bladder. The gland is then removed, and the urethra is reattached to the bladder. The retropubic approach is very similar except there is no incision into the bladder. A perineal prostectomy procedure is rarely done due to the increased risk of contamination of the incision (close to the rectum), urinary incontinence, erectile dysfunction, or injury to the rectum.

An open prostatectomy means a longer hospital stay compared with the other BPH surgeries. A suprapubic catheter and care for an abdominal incision increase the length of stay and the risk for complications. Follow-up home care for wound dressing changes and catheter care is an important aspect of nursing interventions for these clients.

Nursing Process

Assessment

The nurse begins by asking the client if he has ever had treatment or surgery for prostate trouble. Amount and type of fluid intake per day are assessed and whether the client has noticed any of the symptoms of BPH.

Nursing Diagnosis

The nursing diagnoses for clients with mild or no symptoms are directed at knowledge deficits related to prevention of UTIs, knowing when to report an increase in symptoms to the physician, and taking medication exactly as the physician orders. For clients scheduled for prostate surgery, the preoperative nursing diagnoses might include the following:

- Altered health maintenance related to insufficient knowledge of condition, surgery, and postsurgical activities
- Self-concept disturbance related to loss of normal urination
- Anxiety related to insufficient knowledge of preoperative and postoperative routines and sensations
- Alteration in comfort: acute/chronic pain related to urinary retention
- Sleep pattern disturbance related to frequency of urination

Nursing care for TURP clients follows standard guidelines for routine care. (See Nursing Care Plan Box 41–2.) In addition each client may experience individual responses and needs. Individualized care plans are often needed, because the majority of these clients are elderly

---

retrograde: retro—backward + grade—step
prostatectomy: prostat—prostate gland + ectomy—excision

NURSING CARE PLAN BOX 41-2
FOR THE POSTSURGICAL CLIENT HAVING TRANSURETHRAL RESECTION OF THE PROSTATE FOR BENIGN PROSTATIC HYPERPLASIA

Altered comfort: acute pain related to bladder spasms, obstruction, or surgical process

Client Outcomes
(1) Client states pain has decreased. (2) Client identifies at least two comfort measures.

Evaluation of Outcomes
(1) Does client state that pain is decreased? (2) Is client able to identify at least two measures that will help relieve pain?

Interventions	Rationale	Evaluation
• Monitor pain every 2 to 4 hours using a pain scale for first 48 hours. • Monitor for signs of bladder spasm, such as facial grimaces, irrigation solution does not flow into bladder, urinating around catheter, multiple clots.	A pain scale is a more accurate measure of pain. Relief of spasms will promote comfort, rest, and healing.	Does the client verbalize the pain as increasing or decreasing on the scale? Is the number of spasms increasing or decreasing?
• Give prescribed medication (analgesics, antispasmodics) and monitor response. • Irrigate catheter as ordered.	Medications relieve symptoms. Removal of clots reduces spasms and pain.	Does the client state relief when medications are given? Does the irrigating solution go in and out easily? Are clots being removed?
• Teach relaxation, deep breathing techniques.	Relaxation will calm the spasms and relieve pain.	Is the client able to relax?

Urge incontinence related to poor sphincter control

Client Outcomes
(1) Client identifies at least two methods to achieve dryness. (2) Client verbalizes satisfactory control of dribbling.

Evaluation of Outcomes
(1) Does client identify ways to prevent incontinence? Do they help? (2) Does client verbalize satisfaction with outcome?

Interventions	Rationale	Evaluation
• Teach Kegel (pelvic floor) exercises (see Chapter 40)—to be practiced every time client urinates and throughout the day.	Strengthens muscle tone to hold urine after catheter is removed.	Is client able to start and stop his urine stream?
• Discuss use of condom catheter or penile pads. • Instruct client to continue drinking 2000 to 4000 mL of noncaffeine, nonalcohol beverages each day.	Specific urine control devices are available for men. Adequate nonirritating fluid intake is important for healing and preventing UTI.	Does client indicate an informed choice of incontinence products? Does client drink adequate fluids even though he dribbles?
• Encourage client to discuss long-term (>6 months) incontinence problems with physician. National incontinence support groups are available.	Client may need to learn self-catheterization or try medication.	Does client verbalize understanding of what to do if incontinence continues?

continued

NURSING CARE PLAN BOX 41–2 (continued)

Ineffective management of therapeutic regimen related to lack of knowledge of postoperative restrictions and care

Outcomes
(1) Client avoids activities that increase intra-abdominal pressure resulting in excessive bleeding. (2) Client verbalizes understanding of how to prevent postoperative infection.

Evaluation of Outcomes
(1) Does client verbalize understanding of how to prevent bleeding? (2) Is infection prevented?

Interventions	Rationale	Evaluation
• Teach client to avoid lifting heavy objects (>10 lb), stair climbing, driving, strenuous exercise, constipation, straining during bowel movements, and sexual activities until approved by physician (about 6 weeks).	Increased abdominal pressure can cause healing tissue to break apart in the prostate capsule, and excessive bleeding will occur.	Is client able to identify activities that would cause risk for excessive bleeding?
• Instruct client on proper catheter care using verbal, written, and demonstration techniques (many are sent home before catheter is removed). Include the following information: • Keep catheter bag secured to abdomen or thigh and below the bladder. • Wash catheter/meatal junction with soap and water once daily. • Use clean technique to change from leg bag to night drainage bag. • Report signs and symptoms of UTI to physician immediately. • Encourage oral fluids.	Urinary tract infections are extremely dangerous and can cause death following genitourinary surgery in an elderly client.	Can the client give a return demonstration of proper catheter care? Is client free from signs and symptoms of infection?

Anxiety related to concerns over loss of sexual functioning

Outcome
(1) Client verbalizes normal sexual changes that happen after prostate surgery. (2) Client identifies support systems if needed.

Interventions	Rationale	Evaluation
• Explain to client that he will probably have retrograde ejaculation into the bladder after surgery. It is not harmful and the semen will come out when he urinates.	Removal of the prostate gland results in retrograde ejaculation.	Does client understand what will happen when he ejaculates?
• Instruct client to talk with his urologist if erection problems occur.	Urologists who specialize in treatment of erectile dysfunction can be helpful.	Is the client aware of local support services?

and have secondary medical problems such as cardiovascular disease.

Planning

Planning should include use of educational materials to discuss the expected surgical outcomes with both the client and his family whenever possible. It is important that they know about bladder spasm sensations and that the treatment option may be a belladonna and opium (B&O) suppository. Very often if the nurse asks the client if he wants a suppository for pain, the answer will be no, because he does not realize it is not for his bowels but to relieve the spasms.

Seeing the catheter drainage bag filled with bloody drainage may also be very upsetting to a client or his family. Tell them it is normal to have this type of drainage and

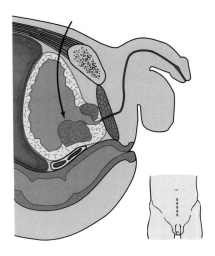

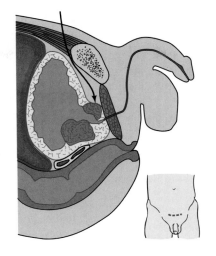

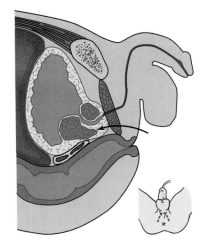

A. Suprapubic prostatectomy   B. Retropubic prostatectomy   C. Perineal prostatectomy

Figure 41–2. *(A)* Suprapubic prostatectomy. *(B)* Retropubic prostatectomy. *(C)* Perineal prostatectomy.

that what they see is actually a little blood mixed with a large amount of irrigating solution. It is important for the nurse to closely monitor the urinary output in terms of amount, color, and presence of clots at least every hour for the first 24 to 48 hours postoperatively. Careful monitoring and documentation of vital signs and fluid intake and output can help prevent major complications.

Interventions

Special care should be taken to control bladder spasms, prevent excessive bleeding, and prevent infection. Clients should be encouraged to ask for pain medication before it becomes too severe. Often men are reluctant to ask for pain medication, so it is important to monitor closely for evidence of pain. Routinely offer the client pain medication if he does not ask on his own.

Ambulation and other activity levels should be limited and can be closely monitored based on the characteristics of the drainage in the catheter bag. If the drainage is bright red or has large clots, the client should be encouraged to lie down in bed until the color lightens and the clots are diminished. Interventions on the part of the nurse to clear the catheter require increasing either the continuous or manual irrigation process.

The risk for catheter-induced infections is very high unless sterile technique is used when the catheter is opened for irrigation. If the client is being discharged home with a catheter, careful written instructions regarding catheter care and the need for increased fluid intake to prevent UTI are an important part of discharge planning. Clients are routinely placed on antibiotics during the operation and sometimes postoperatively to prevent infections.

Evaluation

A client should be discharged home with a minimum of bladder discomfort, light pink to clear urine, and no evidence of UTI. Home care nursing may be required if the client lives alone or does not have the capacity to provide for meals, toileting, or transportation for the follow-up visit.

Client Education

Prevention of complications such as postoperative bleeding and infections are critical to these clients' recovery. They should be encouraged to drink up to 2500 mL/day (unless contraindicated by other medical conditions) of water, noncitrus juices (prune juice to prevent straining from constipation and cranberry juice to prevent UTI), and other noncaffeine, nonalcoholic beverages. Activities should be limited to short periods of sitting or walking followed by rest. Climbing stairs should be limited to once a day, which may mean keeping a urinal handy if a bathroom is unavailable on the level where the kitchen and television are located. The client should not drive or engage in sexual intercourse until after he is given the final checkup with his physician (usually 4 to 6 weeks). Heavy lifting must also be avoided during this time (limited to 10 lb or under).

> **CRITICAL THINKING: Mr. Atkinson**
>
> Mr. Atkinson is a 68-year-old African-American farmer with an enlarged prostate. He lives on a 75-acre farm with his wife and one son. He is scheduled for a TURP the beginning of March.
>
> 1. What postoperative instructions should he be given in light of his occupation?
> 2. What should you tell him if he asks about how the surgery will affect his "nature" (sexual activities)?
>
> *Answers at end of chapter.*

CANCER OF THE PROSTATE

Cancer of the prostate is the second most common cause of cancer death in American men over 60 years of age. Chances are unless a cause other than age is found, the numbers will continue to increase in the years to come due to more men living longer.

Pathophysiology

Prostate cancer depends on testosterone to grow. The cancer cells are usually slow growing and begin in the posterior (back) or lateral (side) part of the gland. The cancer spreads by one of three routes. If it spreads by local invasion it will move into the bladder, seminal vesicles, or peritoneum. The cancer may also spread through the lymph system to the pelvic nodes and may travel as far as the supraclavicular nodes. The third route is through the vascular system to bone, lung, and liver. Prostate cancer is staged or graded based on the growth or spread.

Etiology

Age is the primary risk factor. Prostate cancer is found most often in men over the age of 65 years and is rare in men under the age of 40 years. Other risk factors are higher levels of testosterone, high-fat diet, and immediate family history.

Prostate cancer is the highest in the world in African-American men and lowest in Japanese men. Occupational exposure to cadmium (e.g., welding, electroplating, alkaline battery manufacturing) has been identified as an added risk factor.

Signs and Symptoms

Symptoms are rare in the early stage (stage A) of prostate cancer. Later stages (stages B and C) include symptoms of urinary obstruction, hematuria, and urinary retention. In the advanced (metastatic) stage (stage D), symptoms may be bone pain in the back or hip, anemia, weakness, weight loss, and overall tiredness.

Complications

Early complications of prostate cancer are related to bladder problems, such as difficulty in urinating, and bladder or kidney infection. As the cancer metastasizes the client may develop problems such as pain, bone fractures, weight loss, depression, and eventual death if treatment is not successful.

Diagnostic Tests

A routine digital rectal examination (DRE) of the prostate is the first test; often the examiner finds a hard lump or hardened lobe. A blood test looking for high levels of prostate-specific antigen (PSA) or prostatic acid phosphatase (PAP) is done to detect prostate cancer. When there is a palpable tumor, the physician may order a transrectal ultrasound and biopsy to help confirm the diagnosis. Bone scans and other tests may be ordered to determine if the cancer has spread outside of the prostate gland.

Medical Treatment

Prostate cancer in stage A may be treated with (1) testosterone-suppressing medications such as leuprolide (Lupron) or goserelin (Zoladex), (2) surgery such as TURP or open prostatectomy, or (3) a combination of medication and radiation therapy. In stage B and C the treatment is usually a radical prostatectomy, radiation therapy, or implanting radioactive seeds into the prostate. In stage D prostate cancer treatment involves relief of symptoms or blocking testosterone by (1) bilateral **orchiectomy,** (2) estrogen therapy (DES), (3) antiandrogen (flutamide [Eulexin]), or (4) agents such as leuprolide (Lupron) and goserelin (Zoladex). Sometimes chemotherapy is used to help relieve symptoms from the cancer spread.

Radical Prostatectomy

The radical prostatectomy procedure is generally reserved for clients with cancer of the prostate or when the gland is too large to resect using the TURP method.

The client returns from surgery with a large indwelling catheter in the urethra and may also have a **suprapubic** catheter. Often there will be a Penrose or sump drain in place to remove fluids from the abdominal cavity and allow the wound to heal from the inside outward. Special care must be taken to keep the incision and drain sites clean and dry. Dressings should be changed according to institution policy using sterile technique.

There are more complications associated with radical prostatectomy than any other treatment option. The major complications are hemorrhage, infection, loss of urinary control, and erectile dysfunction.

Client Education

All men over the age of 40 years should be encouraged to have a yearly DRE of the prostate. Prevention and early detection are the best ways to fight prostate cancer.

Penile Disorders

Problems of the penis, aside from sexually transmitted diseases, are fairly rare but may cause great concern and

---

orchiectomy: orchi—testes + ectomy—excision
suprapubic: supra—above + pubic—pubic bone

worry for the client. Most men have difficulty seeking help for a "private" problem. The nurse must be sensitive when assessing or providing care for these clients.

PEYRONIE'S DISEASE

Peyronie's disease often gives the penis a curved or crooked look when it is erect. Fibrous bands or plaques form mainly on the dorsal (top) part of the layer of tissue that surrounds one of the corpora cavernosa of the penis. The plaque may be caused by injury or inflammation of the penile tissue, or it may come and go spontaneously. If the plaque is thick enough, it can cause curvature, painful erection, difficulty in vaginal penetration, and erectile dysfunction. When conservative treatments such as vitamin E, steroids, or ultrasound do not work, surgery may be needed to remove the plaque. Clients need to be reassured that the problem is not life threatening and can be treated.

PRIAPISM

Priapism is a painful erection that lasts too long. Any time an erection lasts for longer than 4 to 6 hours it can become a medical emergency. The small veins in the corpora cavernosa spasm so the blood cannot drain back out of the penis as it should. When the blood cannot drain out, the tissue of the penis does not get oxygen and there can be permanent tissue damage. There may be a complete loss of erection ability after the priapism episode. Prolonged priapism can also prevent the client from passing urine, which can lead to painful bladder and kidney problems. Some causes of priapism are prolonged sexual activity, sickle cell anemia, leukemia, widespread cancer, spinal cord injury or tumors, and use of crack cocaine or certain other drugs. Treatment in the emergency department may include ice packs, sedatives, analgesics, injection of medications directly into the penis to relax the vein spasms, needle aspiration, and irrigation of the corpora. If all else fails surgery is done to drain the blood out of the penis.

PHIMOSIS AND PARAPHIMOSIS

Phimosis is the term used to describe a condition in which the foreskin of an uncircumcised male becomes so tight it is difficult or impossible to pull back away from the head of the penis. It may make it impossible to clean the area underneath. Smegma, a cottage cheese–like secretion made by the glands of the foreskin, becomes trapped under the foreskin and is an excellent place for the growth of bacterial and yeast infections. Treatment usually begins with antibiotics and warm soaks to the area. The physician may then cut a small slit in the foreskin to relieve the pressure

and treat the infection. A full circumcision may be recommended to the client if the problem continues or if a condom catheter is necessary for urine drainage. Phimosis is generally prevented by teaching uncircumcised males to pull the foreskin back carefully, wash with mild soap and water daily, and replace the foreskin to its normal position.

Paraphimosis occurs when the uncircumcised foreskin is pulled back, during intercourse or bathing, and not immediately replaced in a forward position. This causes constriction of the dorsal veins, which leads to edema and pain. Moderate to severe paraphimosis is a medical emergency and requires immediate care by a physician. The longer the problem continues, the greater the risk of circulation problems and possible gangrene. Again, prevention through daily cleaning and replacing the foreskin in its normal place is important.

CANCER OF THE PENIS

Cancer of the penis is a rare skin cancer in the United States and is usually found only in men who were not circumcised as babies. The tumor looks like a small, round, raised wart and may even be mistaken for a venereal wart. It is one form of cancer that may be spread to the sex partner. Several research studies have found a link between cancer of the penis and cancer of the uterine cervix. Cancer of the penis may be treated with minor surgery such as a circumcision or laser removal of the growth. If the cancer has spread the treatment may mean cutting away part or all of the penis or radiation or chemotherapy. Finding and treating any wartlike tumor in its earliest stages is an important part of client education.

Testicular Disorders

CRYPTORCHIDISM

Cryptorchidism (undescended testes) is a congenital condition in which a baby boy is born with either one or both of his testes not in the scrotum. The testes normally drop down (descend) into the scrotum in the last 1 to 2 months before the boy is born. Many times the testes will descend into the scrotum on their own by 2 years of age. If they do not descend by the age of 2, surgery should be done to correct the problem. Testes that are not brought down into the scrotum will decrease a man's chances of producing a child. This is usually due to excessive body heat damaging sperm production in the testes. Studies have shown that the chances of testicular cancer are also higher if the condition is not corrected before the child reaches his teen years. If normal male sex characteristics do not develop during puberty because the testosterone level is too low, extra testosterone medication may be given. Testosterone can be administered in the form of a daily pill or long term by injection or patch.

---

cryptorchidism: crypt—hidden + orchid—testis + ism—condition

HYDROCELE

A **hydrocele** is a collection of fluid in the scrotal sac. Hydroceles are not dangerous and generally do not cause any pain. The cause is not really known and it can happen at any time during the male lifetime. No treatment is necessary unless it is so large that it causes discomfort, causes embarrassment, or is a threat to the blood supply to the testes. If treatment is needed, the physician will aspirate or surgically drain the fluid.

VARICOCELE

A **varicocele** is a condition sometimes called varicose veins of the scrotum. The main blood supply to the testes travels along the spermatic cord. The veins become dilated, and when the man is standing the area in the scrotum begins to feel like a "bag of worms." The client may complain of a pulling sensation, a dull ache, or scrotal pain. The sensations are most often felt when standing up. Most varicoceles occur on the left side because of the way the scrotal vein enters at a sharp angle from the left renal vein.

A varicocele is often not discovered until a couple try to have a baby and are unable to conceive. It is believed that the varicose veins may increase the temperature of the testes and cause damage to the sperm. The most successful treatment is surgical repair of the varicose veins.

EPIDIDYMITIS

The epididymis is a small tube along the back of the testes where sperm is matured for its last 10 to 12 days before it is ready to be ejaculated. **Epididymitis** is inflammation or infection of the epididymis that may be caused by bacteria, viruses, parasites, chemicals, or trauma. Epididymitis may be facilitated by sexual or nonsexual contact, a complication of some urological procedures, or reflux (backflow) of urine. The problem may also be associated with prostate infections and is usually painful with the scrotal skin being tender, red, and warm to the touch.

Epididymitis is treated with antibiotics, involving the partner if it was sexually transmitted. Depending on how severe the pain is, the client may be placed on bed rest with the scrotum elevated, possibly on ice packs, and also given analgesics. The pain and tenderness usually go away in about a week although the swelling may last for several weeks. Complications may include chronic epididymitis, abscess formation, or sterility.

ORCHITIS

Orchitis is a rare inflammation or infection of the testes. The problem may be caused by trauma or surgical procedures, chemical substances, infection from epididymitis, a UTI, or systemic diseases such as influenza, infectious mononucleosis, tuberculosis, gout, pneumonia, or mumps (after puberty). The client will have swollen, extremely tender testes, red scrotal skin, and a fever. Interventions are basically the same as for epididymitis and include bed rest, scrotal support, antibiotics, and medication to relieve pain and fever. Complications such as sterility from mumps orchitis can be prevented by giving boys the mumps vaccine at an early age.

CANCER OF THE TESTES

Pathophysiology and Etiology

Cancer of the testes is the most common solid tumor in men 15 to 40 years of age and peaks between 20 and 34 years of age. The etiology of testicular cancer is unknown. Some of the known risk factors are cryptorchidism, family history, mother's use of diethylstilbestrol (DES, an estrogen preparation once used to prevent spontaneous abortion) while pregnant, Caucasian, and high socioeconomic status. The tumors are mostly a germ cell type of cancer formed during normal embryo development.

Prevention

The best prevention is monthly testicular self-examination (TSE). The procedure is simple and easy to learn, and should be taught to males between the ages of 15 and 40. See Chapter 39 for instructions on TSE.

Signs and Symptoms

Early warning signs of cancer may include a small painless lump on the side or front of the testes. The client may also notice that the scrotum is swollen and feels heavy. Late symptoms of back pain, shortness of breath, difficulty swallowing, breast enlargement, and changes in vision or mental status indicate metastasis of the cancer.

Complications

Emotional complications can range from fear of cancer and death to feelings of loss of masculine body image and sexual function. Physical complications may involve dealing with pain and the effects of metastasis to areas such as the lungs, abdomen, or lymph nodes. Other, less common areas of cancer spread are the liver, brain, and bone. Treatments such as surgery, chemotherapy, and radiation therapy can all have negative side effects on the client and require special care.

---

hydrocele: hydro—water + cele—swelling
varicocele: varico—vein + cele—swelling
epididymitis: epi—upon + didym—testis + itis—inflammation
orchitis: orch—testis + itis—inflammation

Diagnostic Tests

When a tumor is found, several laboratory and radiographic tests are done. An ultrasound of the testes is done first. If the test shows cancer, a chest x-ray is done to look for spread to the lungs. A scan of the lymph nodes, liver, brain, and bones may also be ordered. Blood is drawn to look for what are called tumor markers. An example of a tumor marker for testicular cancer is β human chorionic gonadotropin (β hCG). An exploration, biopsy, and removal of the testes is done to decide the stage of the tumor.

Testicular tumors may be staged or classified in several ways. The simplest way to stage a testicular tumor is as follows:

Stage I: tumor only in the testes
Stage II: tumor spread to groin lymph nodes
Stage III: tumor spread past lymph nodes, usually to the lungs

Medical Treatment

Intervention depends on the stage of the cancer. All treatment begins with complete removal of the cancerous testes, spermatic cord, and local lymph nodes. Stage I tumor treatment then includes radiation to the groin area lymph nodes. Treatment for stage II involves chemotherapy. Stage III or metastatic cancer is treated with both radiation and chemotherapy. If the cancer is found in the beginning stages the chances for complete recovery are about 75 percent. All clients should have regular follow-up testing.

Nursing Care

Nursing care is directed first at prevention, by teaching young men to practice monthly testicular self-examination and to see their physician if they notice any changes. If a diagnosis of cancer has been made, the nurse supports the client emotionally. If the client wants to have children he should be encouraged to make deposits in a sperm bank before any surgery or treatment is started. The client and his partner may have many questions about sexual activities as they go through treatment. They should be encouraged to talk with their physician or a sex therapist about ways to express love and tenderness toward one another. Helping the client deal with pain and the side effects of chemotherapy or radiation therapy are also important nursing interventions for these clients.

CRITICAL THINKING: Mr. Cunningham

Mr. Cunningham is a 23-year-old white college student engaged to be married next spring. While taking a shower one day he discovers a lump on his left testes.

1. What should he do?
2. If it is cancer of the testes, what are the treatment options?
3. How can the nurse help Mr. Cunningham cope with the diagnosis?

Answers at end of chapter.

Sexual Functioning

VASECTOMY

A **vasectomy** is the surgical cutting and sealing off of the vas deferens to prevent sperm from reaching the outside of the body. This 15- to 30-minute surgery is performed most often as a permanent birth control method but may also be performed on some men during prostate gland removal. The male client should carefully discuss the surgery with his physician so there is a clear understanding of the results following the procedure.

The testes will continue to produce the male hormone testosterone and sperm. The prostate gland along with the seminal vesicles will still ejaculate semen, but the semen will not contain sperm. There should be no major change in the way the ejaculate looks or feels following the procedure. The client should be encouraged to continue using another birth control method for about 6 weeks after surgery to be sure there are no sperm left in the tract above the surgical site. The sperm will continue to be produced in the testes but will be absorbed by the body.

There are times when the man may decide he wants to have more children and asks to have the vasectomy "undone." The surgical procedure to reverse a vasectomy is called a vasovasotomy. Using microscopic instruments, the surgeon reconnects the two pieces of the vas deferens. During the surgery the physician will generally try to determine whether the testes are still producing good sperm. If the vasectomy was done less than 10 years before, the fertility success rate is higher. A vasovasotomy is generally not an option if the vasectomy procedure was more than 10 years old.

IMPOTENCE/ERECTILE DYSFUNCTION

Problems with getting or keeping an erection can happen at any age and have been a concern of men and their partners for centuries. It is a unique problem because it affects not only the client but his sex partner as well. Most men experience a temporary erection problem at some time during their life. It is often caused by stress, illness, fatigue, or an excessive use of alcohol or drugs. When the problem becomes persistent, as it does for over 20 million men in the United States, it is time to seek medical help.

---

vasectomy: vas—vas deferens + ectomy—excision

Before the 1980s, 90 percent of men who went to their physicians for help were told the problem was emotional, not physical. Through improved testing methods it is now believed that 80 to 90 percent of erection problems have a physical cause.

Pathophysiology

The term *impotence* means powerlessness. It is being replaced with the more accurate term **erectile dysfunction,** which describes a physical condition. Erectile dysfunction means that a man cannot get or keep a usable erection, one that is firm enough and long-lasting enough for satisfactory sexual intercourse. In order for a man to have a usable erection, several conditions must be met.

1. *Circulatory system.* The blood supply coming into the penis from the arteries must be sufficient to fill the corpora cavernosa (spongy erectile tissue inside the penis) causing the penis to become rigid. The diameter of these vessels is about the size of pencil lead. The veins in the penis must then be able to constrict (narrow down) to trap the blood in the corporal bodies in order to keep the penis erect. The most common cause of erectile dysfunction is failure in the circulatory system.
2. *Nervous system.* Both the sympathetic and parasympathetic nerves are involved in the erection, ejaculation, orgasm, and resting phases of the penile response cycle. There are many nerve receptors and transmitters in the spinal cord and the penis that must be intact for a usable erection. Spinal cord injuries are the most common neurological cause of erection problems. The remarkable fact about spinal cord injuries is that higher cord injuries (cervical or thoracic) have less negative impact on erections than those in the lumbar or sacral area.
3. *Hormonal system.* There are three basic male hormones involved with an erection. The most important hormone, testosterone (normal level between 350 and 1000 ng/dL), affects a man's sex drive and desire. The testosterone level is highest when a man is in his late teens and begins to decline in middle age. Luteinizing hormone (LH, 5 to 18 mL U/mL) stimulates the production of testosterone, and prolactin (<15 ng/mL) in large amounts may block testosterone.
4. *Limbic system.* This is the center in the brain that affects how we feel emotionally. It works with our five senses to stimulate the desire for sex.

All of these systems can be influenced by physical, emotional, and chemical factors. A good assessment is important to determine the cause of erectile dysfunction.

Etiology

The psychological causes of erectile dysfunction usually come from stress or anxiety. Marital problems, financial worries, job frustration, or even fear of not being able to perform due to an isolated incidence of erection problems may lead to sexual dysfunction.

Even when the cause is physical, there are psychological (emotional) side effects. Fear of failure, ridicule, or rejection by the partner will lead to a lack of self-esteem or self-confidence.

The list of physical causes is long because it includes anything that may interfere with the flow of blood, the nerve supply, the balance of hormones, or the effects of emotions (Table 41–3). There are many medications and chemicals that can interfere with desire, blood supply, or nerve transmission and cause problems with erections (Table 41–4). The most common types of medications that cause problems are high blood pressure and cardiovascular medications.

Diagnostic Tests

Assessment of erectile dysfunction has now been divided into primary and secondary diagnostic studies according to guidelines developed by the National Institutes of Health. The first step begins with a careful history that is especially designed to focus on the medical-surgical history, medica-

Table 41–3. **Causes of Erectile Dysfunction**

Psychogenic	Surgical	Vascular	Cardiorespiratory	Neurologic
Excessive stress in family, work or interpersonal relationships, depression, fatigue, and fear of failure to perform	Coronary artery bypass Abdominal-perineal resection Cystectomy Radical prostatectomy Pelvic lymphadenectomy Renal transplant Sympathectomy TURP	Aortic aneurysm Arteriosclerosis Aortofemoral bypass Cerebrovascular disease/accident Pelvic steal syndrome Venous leak Hypertension	Angina pectoris Myocardial infarction COPD Coronary insufficiency Congestive heart failure	Electroshock therapy Multiple sclerosis Parkinson's disease Cerebral palsy Myasthenia gravis Peripheral neuropathy Sympathectomy Tumors/transection of spinal cord Trauma to spinal cord Head injuries Spina bifida

Table 41–4. Medications Contributing to Erectile Dysfunction

Antianxiety agents	Glucocorticoids
Antidepressants	H₂ antagonists
Antihistamines	Major tranquilizers
Antineoplastic agents	Muscle relaxants
Blood-pressure medications	Commonly abused drugs
ACE inhibitors	Alcohol
Beta-blocking agents	Amphetamines
Others	Barbiturates
Diuretics	Caffeine
Drugs for Parkinson's disease	Cocaine
Estrogens	Marijuana
	Nicotine
	Opiates

Note: Not all drugs in a category cause erectile dysfunction.

tions including any substance abuse, lifestyle patterns, and a sexual history. The main areas to investigate are those that indicate vascular, neurological, endocrine, and psychological factors. A physical exam looks for evidence of abnormal genital disorders, hormonal imbalance (such as hair patterns or enlarged breasts), surgical interventions, decreased circulation, or lack of nerve sensations. Blood is taken to look at glucose levels; testosterone; evidence of liver, heart, or kidney disorders; signs of infection; or blood disorders. The physician may also order specific blood tests if other problems exist that may have an impact on erections. Some physicians are also using intracorporeal injection of vasoactive medications that can create an erection, in order to test the blood flow in the penis. A psychological evaluation is recommended to rule out any serious issues in the sexual relationship or emotional problems that may contribute to erectile dysfunction or affect the treatment outcome.

Secondary level of testing may involve the use of sophisticated vascular flow studies to locate areas where either the blood vessels are narrowed or the veins allow the blood to drain out of the penis too rapidly. Another area of testing may be related to sleep tumescence and apnea studies. These studies are based on the physiological process of erections during rapid eye movement (REM) sleep. A "normal" man will have erections every 60 to 70 minutes while he sleeps. Due to the expense of vascular flow studies and sleep studies, they are utilized on a limited basis.

Medical Treatment

One of the most important treatment options begins with the couple being able to share intimate communication. No matter what may be causing the problem, if the client and his partner are not touching, talking, and sharing feelings with one another, any treatment option is going to have limited success.

When the problem has clearly been identified as psychological, counseling therapy for the client and partner is the treatment of choice. If long-term therapy has been tried and had only limited success, the addition of oral medication or even intracorporeal injection therapy may be added to provide a boost in confidence and self-esteem. Medical treatment for physical erection problems begins with conservative, nonsurgical treatment and then may progress to surgical options if necessary.

Medication Changes

Sometimes all that is needed to correct the problem is a change in medication the client is taking. There are many prescription, over-the-counter, and street drugs that can cause erection problems (Table 41–4). It is important for the client to talk with the physician *first* before discontinuing *any* medication. Some men have been known to stop taking their blood pressure medication and risk a stroke or heart attack because the medication interfered with their sexual activity.

Hormone Treatment

If the testosterone level is low, and it is not due to a pituitary tumor or thyroid problem, replacement hormone may be needed. The physician should first examine the client very carefully for any evidence of prostate cancer, because testosterone treatment would cause the cancer to grow and spread. Testosterone treatment works best when it is given by intramuscular (IM) injections. It may take several weeks to raise the hormone level high enough to see any benefits. If after about 6 to 8 weeks of treatment there is no increase in the number or quality of erections, a different treatment should be tried.

Yohimbine

Most men are looking for a magic pill or potion to correct the problem. Some physicians will prescribe a pill called yohimbine (Yocon, Yohimex), which is thought to be a mild aphrodisiac and vasodilator. Whether it really has the ability to increase blood flow or is simply a placebo has not been determined. In borderline cases where the cause may be psychological or a mild physical one, the medication may be helpful in restoring confidence and erections.

Intracorporeal Medications

The use of a vasoactive medicine is the latest nonsurgical treatment option. The medication (papaverine, prostaglandin E, phentolamine, or sildenafil) causes the arterioles and cavernous tissue to relax, allowing more blood to flow in and lowering peripheral resistance, trapping blood in the cavernous bodies to maintain the erection. There are now four methods of administering the medication: direct injection into the corporeal bodies, transurethral suppository-pellet, transdermal patch, and pill form.

INJECTION METHOD. After careful evaluation, the client or his partner is taught how to inject the medication into the penis using a 26- or 27-gauge needle on a tuberculosis syringe or a prefilled autoinjector. The injections are nearly painless and produce a natural erection in 10 to 15 minutes. The erection may last 1 to 2 hours, and clients are generally limited to a maximum of 3 injections per week. The dosage is regulated on an individual basis. The most serious side effect is priapism, which requires immediate reversal in a physician's office or emergency room. When the client is taught and monitored carefully the risk of complications is minimal.

TRANSURETHRAL SUPPOSITORY. The client is instructed to urinate first in order to disperse the medicated pellet and help promote absorption of the medication. A tiny pellet (microsuppository) is inserted into the urethra using a specialized single-dose applicator. The medication usually begins to work in 5 to 10 minutes, and the effects last for approximately 30 to 60 minutes. The most common side effect has been pain in the penis when high dosages were used.

TRANSDERMAL PATCH. A skin patch containing the vasoactive medication may be applied to the penis. Special care must be taken with some forms so that the partner does not absorb the medication. This can be prevented by having the male wear a condom over the patch.

ORAL PILL. The latest development has been the use of oral vasoactive medications. The most widely prescribed pill currently is sildenafil (Viagra). The pill is usually taken 30 to 60 minutes before sexual intercourse. It provides an easy way to administer the medication and has a success rate of between 40 and 80 percent, depending on the cause of the problem. Men using nitrate medication (antianginal agents) should avoid using the pill because it is vasoactive. It can also cause abnormal visual problems for some men.

Other Nonsurgical Treatments

Sexual Devices and Techniques

There are a wide variety of sexual aids such as vibrators and dildos (hollow penis) that may be an alternative for clients who do not want or cannot afford expensive medical treatment. They should be encouraged to talk with a physician or qualified sex therapist before trying these alternatives.

Suction devices are another nonsurgical treatment option. This is an external cylinder vacuum device that fits over the penis and draws the blood up into the corporeal bodies, causing an erection. A penile ring is then slipped onto the base of the penis. Once the cylinder is removed, sexual intercourse can begin. Special care must be taken to remove the penile ring within 15 to 20 minutes to prevent tissue damage. The suction device may be used alone or with intracorporeal injection therapy for clients who have difficulty keeping an erection. The companies that manufacture the suction devices provide free videotapes and written client instruction booklets.

Surgical Treatments

Penile Implants (Prosthesis)

Penile implants are a pair of solid or fluid-filled chambers that are surgically placed into the corporeal bodies in the penis to produce an erection. This treatment option has been used successfully for over 25 years. There are two basic types of implants—noninflatable and inflatable (Fig. 41–3). The noninflatable type is economical, is able to be surgically implanted in less than an hour, and provides firmness for penetration. The inflatable device contains a sterile saline solution that fills the cylinders using a manual pumping action. When activated, the inflatable implant provides both firmness and an increase in diameter of the penis. Although the inflatable device is more expensive and has a greater risk of mechanical failure, it provides a more natural appearing and functioning erection than the noninflatable implant.

Penile implants are considered secondary treatment options because they have a risk of complications such as mechanical failure, infection, and erosion. Clients at greatest risk for complications are those with uncontrolled diabetes and those with severe circulation problems. Clients should be taught that an implant will not restore ejaculation or orgasm if these functions have been lost before the surgery. Surgery recovery time varies from 4 to 6 weeks; the client must receive approval from the physician before having sexual intercourse.

Vascular Surgery

If a younger client (<35 years) has an erection problem due to poor blood flow into the penis or from blood leaking out of the penis rapidly causing the loss of the erection, corrective surgery may be performed. A bypass graft may be done to increase the blood flow into the penis or go around a blockage (e.g., Peyronie's disease). If the blood leaves the corporeal bodies too fast, a procedure to ligate (tie off) the leaking veins may be successful. Neither surgery works well in older men because the bypass graft rapidly becomes obstructed and the natural tendency of the older body is to form collateral circulation around the veins that are tied off.

Nursing Process

Assessment

Before the assessment begins it is important to provide privacy and ensure confidentiality. A complete sexual history, often conducted by a nurse, is taken with special focus on factors related to the circulatory, nervous, and endocrine systems. The questions will cover (1) medical problems; (2) surgical treatments that might interfere with blood flow or nerve supply to the groin or spine; (3) genitourinary problems; (4) a complete list of medications, including over-the-counter drugs and any evidence of substance abuse; (5) general lifestyle patterns, including stress fac-

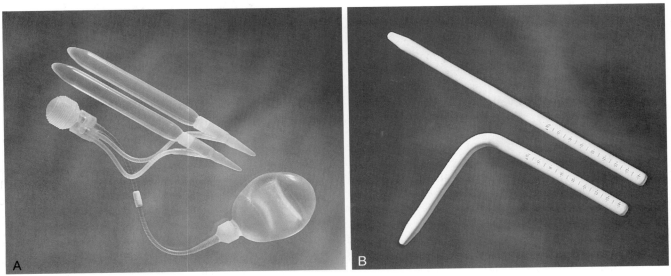

Figure 41–3. Penile implants. *(A)* Inflatable penile implant. Inflatable cylinders are implanted in the penis, the small hydraulic pump in the scrotum, and the fluid-filled reservoir in the lower abdomen. Sterile radiopaque saline from the reservoir fills the cylinders to provide an erection. (Alpha-1 implant photo courtesy of Mentor Urology.) *(B)* Malleable penile implant. Malleable rods are implanted into the penis. The penis is always firm, but the rods can be bent close to the body when erection is not desired. (Acu-Form implant photo courtesy of Mentor Urology.)

tors, depression, and excessive use of caffeine or nicotine (causing vasoconstriction); and (6) sexual patterns and practices. A physical exam is performed by the physician to assess for any evidence of congenital deformities, hormonal imbalance, decreased circulation, or nerve damage. Throughout the assessment process it is important to observe for any signs of psychological or emotional distress.

Nursing Diagnosis

Due to the nature of the problem, it is important to recognize nursing concerns related to anxiety, fear, powerlessness, knowledge deficit, and issues related to altered role function or family dynamics. The present nursing diagnosis label of altered sexual functioning is very broad and does not focus on specific aspects of male erectile dysfunction.

Planning

Planning generally involves not only the male client but also his sexual partner. Treatment success rates are much higher when the support person is included in the decision-making process.

Unrealistic expectations are common in the beginning period of restoration. The client must be encouraged to communicate with his partner through both talk and touch. Restoration of an erection will not repair a bad relationship, and often counseling is an important part of the treatment plan.

Implementation

Special care should be taken in selecting the treatment option that will work best for the client and his partner. They should be encouraged to ask questions of their physician and other health care professionals involved in their care. Where available, support groups that are focused on men and their partners have provided excellent resources and information on treatment options. Conservative treatment options should be tried first, with surgical interventions reserved as a last resort. Nursing care focuses both on the emotional and physical discomfort associated with the diagnosis and treatment options.

Evaluation

The best indicator of a positive outcome is restoration of erectile function with a verbal account of satisfaction. Sometimes the physical problem is easier to correct than the emotional scars that the problem has created. It is important to evaluate both the physiological and emotional outcomes of treatment.

Client Education

The nurse plays an important role in public education related to erectile dysfunction. Men need to know that they are not alone with their problem. More than 20 million men in the United States experience ongoing problems with erections. The majority of the causes are physical, and help is available through physicians and nurses who specialize in treating erectile dysfunction.

Treatment may be as simple as a change in lifestyle or in medication. Men need to be encouraged to seek help from appropriate health care providers and recognize that erectile dysfunction is a treatable condition with positive outcomes.

INFERTILITY

A growing number of couples in the United States are having difficulty conceiving a child. Several factors can interfere with a man's ability to father a child.

Physiology

Eight fundamental male physiological factors are necessary for normal conception to occur: (1) proper endocrine function between the hypothalamus, pituitary gland, and testes; (2) at least one testes that will produce quality sperm; (3) an epididymis or storage place to mature the sperm; (4) a duct system to transport sperm from the testes to the outside of the body; (5) glands that secrete the right type and amount of seminal fluid that will nurture and transport the sperm; (6) an intact nervous system that helps provide an erection and ejaculation; (7) semen that meets the following criteria: volume 1.5 to 5.0 mL, a concentration of over 20 million sperm/mL, 50 to 60 percent of the sperm are classified as grade 2 mobility, 60 to 80 percent have a normal shape, the pH is between 7.2 and 7.8, there is a small amount of fructose (sugar—food supply), and the sperm/semen first coagulate and then liquefy; and (8) a basic knowledge of sexual practices along with a willing partner.

Etiology

The factors related to infertility are divided into three general categories: pretesticular, testicular, and posttesticular.

Pretesticular (Endocrine) Factors

The first factor involves the proper functioning of the hypothalamus, the pituitary gland, and the testes. These endocrine functions are very complex and a rare (3%) cause of infertility. Examples of endocrine causes might be pituitary or adrenal tumors, thyroid problems, or uncontrolled diabetes.

Testicular Factors

The two most common causes of male infertility are a varicocele (40 to 50%) and idiopathic causes (40%). It is believed that a varicocele lowers sperm count by raising the blood flow and the temperature in the testes. Sperm cannot live if the temperature is too high or too low.

Congenital anomalies such as Klinefelter's syndrome (a chromosome defect) or cryptorchidism result in absent or damaged testes. Failure of a part of the male reproductive system to develop due to the mother's use of DES or other drugs during pregnancy may also result in fertility problems.

Certain disease or inflammatory processes may cause damage to the storage area (epididymitis) or to the testes themselves (mumps orchitis). Any high fever or viral infection can interfere with the production of sperm for up to 3 months.

Medications, radiation, substance abuse, environmental hazards, and lifestyle practices have all been identified as possible factors that can interfere with spermatogenesis (sperm production). Medications such as cimetidine (Tagamet), sulfasalazine (Azulfidine), anabolic steroids (testosterone), anticancer drugs (Cytoxan, methotrexate), recreational drugs (cocaine, marijuana), and antihypertensives (methyldopa) have all been identified as possible causes of infertility. Radiation damage, whether as treatment for cancer or job related, tends to depend on the dosage received. A small amount of radiation will cause temporary loss of sperm. Permanent sterility happens with large doses or prolonged treatment. The relation between use of cocaine and marijuana and infertility has been documented in several articles, but there is no clear indication of the amount or length of time it takes for these substances to cause infertility problems. Environmental hazards such as pesticides, Agent Orange, and lead poisoning have been listed and are still under investigation. Excessive use of hot tubs and saunas, wearing of tight jeans, and long haul truck driving have all been identified as raising the temperature level in the scrotum to the point that the sperm production is decreased.

Posttesticular Factors

The most common factor in posttesticular infertility is the result of surgery or injury along the pathway from the testes to the outside of the man's body. Examples of surgical causes are vasectomy, bladder neck reconstruction, pelvic lymph node removal, or any surgery that causes retrograde ejaculation. Congenital anomalies and various types of infections may also cause infertility problems.

Prevention

Prevention involves possible lifestyle changes to avoid excessive heat to the scrotum, substance abuse, exposure to toxins, or environmental hazards. Problems related to medication or infections should be discussed with the physician.

Signs and Symptoms

A couple is considered infertile if they have been unsuccessful at becoming pregnant after at least 1 year of uninterrupted attempts. If pregnancy has occurred during the year but there was no delivery, the problem is generally considered a female rather than a male factor.

Diagnostic Tests

Diagnosis begins with a detailed history and physical exam that looks for known male causes of infertility.

History

Sexual Practices

Assessment includes frequency of intercourse, positions, timing (according to ovulation cycle), use of contraceptives, problems with premature ejaculation, or erection problems.

Lifestyle Practices

Weight lifting or use of steroids, hot tubs, or saunas; tight jeans; use of nicotine, caffeine, alcohol, or marijuana; and the strength of desire for children on the part of the man are all assessed.

Occupation

High stress, long periods of sitting, and exposure to environmental toxins are determined.

Medical-Surgical History

Assessment includes any sexually transmitted viruses or diseases, endocrine problems, congenital urinary problems, serious illnesses or groin injuries, cancer, or treatment with chemotherapy or radiation.

Physical Examination

The nurse observes for normal hair pattern and growth, muscle development, size of testes, and any evidence of a varicocele or hydrocele.

Diagnostic Tests

A semen analysis is done after collecting several specimens following a special collection technique. It is analyzed to see if it contains the right amount and type of healthy sperm needed for a pregnancy. There are several other tests that may be done, depending on the level of desire and the financial resources of the couple. Many insurance companies do not pay for the tests or treatment options for infertility.

Medical Treatment

Treatment may be as simple as making a change in sexual or lifestyle practices. If the couple is able to handle the emotional and financial strain they may try male surgery to correct a varicocele or a variety of in vitro fertilization procedures. The success rates for in vitro fertilization range from 8 to 60 percent and generally cost several thousand dollars each time an attempt is made. Another possible option that should be presented to the couple is adoption.

The nurse plays an important role in the emotional support a couple needs during infertility studies. It is important that the couple feel comfortable in communicating their feelings and frustrations with one another and their

physician. The nurse may need to be the communication link for explaining various tests and cost factors and in discussing how long the couple may want to continue trying the various treatment options. It may also help them to talk with other couples or attend a support group designed for couples experiencing infertility.

Review Questions

1. Which test is encouraged annually for every man over the age of 40 years?
   a. Prostate ultrasound
   b. Serum creatinine
   c. Rectal exam
   d. Acid phosphatase

2. Which of the following is the greatest risk factor for prostate cancer?
   a. Smoking
   b. Aging
   c. Drugs
   d. STDs

3. Which of the following is the most commonly used surgical treatment for BPH?
   a. TUIP
   b. TUMA
   c. TURP
   d. TULIP

4. The most common cause of erectile dysfunction is
   a. Endocrine problems
   b. Circulatory problems
   c. Excessive stress
   d. Excessive alcohol use

 ANSWERS TO CRITICAL THINKING

CRITICAL THINKING: Mr. Atkinson

1. Mr. Atkinson should be instructed not to lift anything over 10 pounds for the first 6 weeks, and he will not be able to plow or drive for the first 6 weeks. It will be important that his son understand the limitations for his father and how important it will be for him to help out with the farm chores.

2. Mr. Atkinson will notice a change in his ejaculation (either very little or none at all). If he could get an erection before surgery, his chances are very good that he will continue to be able to have intercourse; however, he will not ejaculate.

CRITICAL THINKING: Mr. Cunningham

1. Mr. Cunningham should be encouraged to see his physician immediately for an evaluation to rule out cancer of the testes.

2. Depending on the stage of the cancer, he will have the cancerous testes, cord, and lymph nodes removed. He may also need chemotherapy or radiation treatments as well.

3. Mr. Cunningham should be encouraged to make deposits at a certified sperm bank before any treatments. It will also be important to include his future wife and his family in the decision-making process and encourage them to share their feelings and concerns with one another. Cancer support groups may also be helpful to Mr. Cunningham.

REFERENCE

1. Meredith, CE: Erectile dysfunction. In Karlowicz, KA (ed): Urologic Nursing: Principles and Practice. WB Saunders, Philadelphia, 1995, pp 332–357.

BIBLIOGRAPHY

American Cancer Society: Cancer Facts and Figures. Atlanta, 1995.

Barry, MJ, et al: A nationwide survey of practicing urologists: Current management of benign prostatic hyperplasia and clinically localized prostate cancer. J Urol 158:2, 1997.

Campo, B, et al: Transurethral needle ablation (TUNA) of the prostate: A clinical and urodynamic evaluation. Urology 49:6, 1997.

Carpenito, LJ: Nursing Diagnosis: Application to Clinical Practice, ed 6. JB Lippincott, Philadelphia, 1995.

Clinical Practice Guidelines: Benign Prostatic Hyperplasia: Diagnosis and Treatment. US Department of Health and Human Services, Rockville, Md, 1994.

Davison, BJ, and Degner, LF: Empowerment of men newly diagnosed with prostate cancer. Cancer Nurs 20:3, 1997.

Greiner, KA, and Weigel, JW: Erectile dysfunction. Am Fam Physician 54:5, 1996.

Held, JL, et al: Cancer of the prostate: Treatment and nursing implications. Oncol Nurs Forum 21:1517, 1994.

Howards, SS: Treatment of male infertility. N Engl J Med 332:312, 1995.

Jakobsson, L, Hallberg, IR, and Loven, L: Met and unmet nursing care needs in men with prostate cancer. An explorative study. Part II. Eur J Cancer Care 6:2, 1997.

Kim, ED, and Lipshultz, LI: Advances in the treatment of organic erectile dysfunction. Hosp Pract 32:4, 1997.

Klimaszewski, AD, and Karlowicz, KA: Cancer of the male genitalia. In Karlowicz, KA (ed): Urologic Nursing: Principles and Practice. WB Saunders, Philadelphia, 1995, pp 271–308.

LaFollette, SS, and Reilly, NJ: Cancer of the prostate. In Meredith, CE, and Karlowicz, KA (eds): Urologic Nursing: A Study Guide. Society of Urologic Nurses and Associates, Pitman, NJ, 1995, pp 114–117.

Meredith, CE: Erectile dysfunction. In Meredith, CE, and Karlowicz, KA (eds): Urologic Nursing: A Study Guide. Society of Urologic Nurses and Associates, Pitman, NJ, 1995, pp 137–141.

Meredith, CE: Male infertility. In Karlowicz, KA (ed): Urologic Nursing: Principles and Practice. WB Saunders, Philadelphia, 1995, pp 360–372.

Meredith, CE: Male infertility. In Meredith, CE, and Karlowicz, KA (eds): Urologic Nursing: A Study Guide. Society of Urologic Nurses and Associates, Pitman, NJ, 1995, pp 145–148.

Meredith, CE: Male genitourinary problems. In Lewis, SM, Collier, IC, and Heitkemper, MM (eds): Medical-Surgical Nursing, ed 4. Mosby, St Louis, 1996, pp 1626–1651.

Montague, DK, et al: Clinical guidelines panel on erectile dysfunction: Summary report on the treatment of organic erectile dysfunction. The American Urological Association. J Urol 156:6, 1996.

National Institutes of Health: Impotence, NIH consensus statement. National Institutes of Health, Bethesda, Md, 1992.

Padma-Nathan, H, et al: Treatment of men with erectile dysfunction with transurethral alprostadil. Medicated Urethral System for Erection (MUSE) Study Group. N Engl J Med 336:1, 1997.

Powell, IJ, et al: Outcome of African American men screened for prostate cancer: The Detroit Education and Early Detection Study. J Urol 158:1, 1997.

Ramsey, EW, Miller, PD, and Parsons, K: A novel trans-urethral microwave thermal ablation system to treat benign prostatic hyperplasia: Results of a prospective multicenter clinical trial. J Urol 158:1, 1997.

Riley, AJ, and Athanasiadis, L: Impotence and its non-surgical management. Br J Clin Pract 51:2, 1997.

Rosen, RC, et al: The International Index of Erectile Function (IIEF): A multidimensional scale for assessment of erectile dysfunction. Urology 49:6, 1997.

Soderdahl, DW, Thrasher, JB, and Hansberry, KL: Intracavernosal drug-induced erection therapy versus external vacuum devices in the treatment of erectile dysfunction. Br J Urol 79:6, 1997.

Sundaram, CP, et al: Long-term follow-up of patients receiving injection therapy for erectile dysfunction. Urology 49:6, 1997.

Razanauzskas, M, and Hoebler, L: Treating prostate cancer with cryosurgery. Nursing 24(11):66, 1994.

Reilly, NJ: Benign prostatic hyperplasia. In Meredith, CE, and Karlowicz, KA (eds): Urologic Nursing: A Study Guide. Society of Urologic Nurses and Associates, Pitman, NJ, 1995, pp 55–58.

Nursing Care of Clients with Sexually Transmitted Diseases

Linda Hopper Cook

Learning Objectives

Upon completion of this chapter, the student will be able to:

1. Define common terms associated with sexually transmitted diseases (STDs).
2. Briefly describe the pathophysiology of STDs for clients, their sexual partners, and unborn babies of women who have STDs.
3. Discuss risk factors for development of STDs.
4. Outline strategies for risk reduction.
5. Identify client concerns associated with various STDs.
6. Describe the nurse's role in care of clients who have (or are at high risk for) STDs.
7. Discuss common treatments for STDs.
8. Use the nursing process to plan care for clients who have STDs.
9. Identify some myths about sex and STDs and present scientifically correct information.

Key Words

autologous vaccine (aw-**TAHL**-ah-gus **VACK**-seen)

chancre (**SHANK**-er)

condylomata acuminatum (KON-di-**LOH**-ma-tah ah-**KYOOM**-in-**AH**-tah)

condylomatous (KON-di-**LOH**-ma-tus)

conjunctivitis (kon-JUNK-ti-**VIGH**-tis)

cytotoxic (SIGH-toh-**TOCK**-sick)

electrocautery (ee-LECK-troh-**CAW**-tur-ee)

electrocoagulated (ee-LECK-troh-coh-**AG**-yoo-LAY-ted)

endometritis (EN-doh-me-**TRY**-tis)

enteritis (en-ter-**EYE**-tis)

epidemiological (EP-i-DEE-me-ah-**LAHJ**-i-kuhl)

gummas (**GUM**-ahs)

hepatosplenomegaly (he-PA-toh-SPLE-noh-**MEG**-ah-lee)

herpetic (her-**PET**-ick)

interferons (IN-ter-**FEER**-ons)

lymphadenopathy (lim-FAD-e-**NAH**-puh-thee)

mucopurulent cervicitis (MYOO-koh-**PYOOR**-uh-lent SIR-vi-**SIGH**-tis)

ophthalmia neonatorum (ahf-**THAL**-mee-ah NEE-oh-nuh-**TOR**-uhm)

perinatal (PAIR-ee-**NAY**-tuhl)

proctitis (prock-**TIGH**-tis)

puerperal (pyoo-**ER**-per-uhl)

sacral radiculopathy (**SAY**-krul ra-DICK-yoo-**LAH**-puh-thee)

salpingitis (SAL-pin-**JIGH**-tis)

serological (SEAR-uh-**LAJ**-ick-uhl)

urethritis (YOO-ree-**THRIGH**-tis)

verrucous (ve-**ROO**-kus)

vesicular (ve-**SICK**-yoo-ler)

Sexually transmitted diseases (STDs), also referred to as venereal disease (VD), are defined as any infections that can be transmitted through intimate contact with the genitals, mouth, or rectum of another individual. Some of the causative organisms may be spread by other routes such as contact with blood or body fluids as well as by sexual activity. The nurse's best protection against contracting diseases that may be transmitted by contact with blood and body fluids from clients is the strict practice of universal precautions.

Physically STDs may cause tremendous suffering through pain, scarring of genitourinary structures, damage to other body organs, infertility, birth defects, nervous system damage, development of cancer, and even death of the infected adults and sometimes their children. Psychologically and socially these diseases also have profound effects on people, families, and relationships. A psychological "herpes syndrome" involving depression, loss of self-esteem, feelings of shame, and avoidance of intimacy has been documented in both medical and lay literature. Guilt over passing on an incurable disease to a loved one or feelings of betrayal because of being infected as a result of someone else's promiscuity are only part of the emotional consequences of STDs.

Changing sexual mores have been associated with increasing incidence of almost all types of sexually transmitted diseases, including some previously rare disease manifestations related to anal intercourse. Coexistence of more than one STD in an individual is also being seen more often by health care workers. Although there are over 50 diseases and syndromes associated with sexually transmitted diseases, only the more common diseases, syndromes, and causative agents will be discussed in this text. Descriptions of symptoms, diagnostic techniques, and treatment regimens vary for different areas. Availability of equipment for diagnosis, experience with clients who are atypical or antibiotic resistant, and physician preferences are responsible for much of the variety that is documented in the literature. As an introduction for practical nurses, general overviews are presented. Attempts have been made to present consensus from a wide variety of the available health care literature.

Pathophysiology of Disorders and Syndromes Related to Sexually Transmitted Diseases

Vulvovaginitis is an inflammation of the vulva and vagina that can produce either no noticeable symptoms or may cause redness, itching, burning, excoriation, pain, swelling of the vagina and labia, and a discharge. This type of inflammation can result from a variety of sexually transmitted and nonsexually transmitted infectious agents, and the smell, consistency, and color of the discharge varies with the different microbes involved. Nonsexually transmitted vaginitis, vulvovaginitis, and vaginosis are described in Chapter 40. Some microorganisms may be acquired either by sexual or nonsexual routes, so they will also be mentioned in this chapter. Bartholin's gland abscesses may be caused by nonsexual infection as well as by STDs from microorganisms such as *Neisseria gonorrhoeae* and *Chlamydia trachomatis*.

Urethritis can also be caused by sexually transmitted and nonsexually transmitted microorganisms. A urethritis syndrome involves inflammation of the urethra, prostate, and epididymis of men. The infected men generally experience difficult, painful, and frequent urination and a urethral discharge, which may be clear, cloudy, or yellow. Partners of men with urethritis may also suffer from urethritis, but they may also develop **mucopurulent cervicitis** (MPC) and a variety of other manifestations of infection dependent on the type of organism transmitted during sexual contact. Some of the causative agents for urethritis include *Neisseria gonorrhoeae, Chlamydia trachomatis, Ureaplasma urealyticum, Trichomonas vaginalis, Candida albicans,* and herpes simplex. Often this disease category is divided into gonococcal urethritis (GU) and nongonococcal urethritis (NGU).

Mucopurulent cervicitis (MPC) is an inflammation of the cervix that may produce a mucopurulent yellow exudate on the cervix or may have no noticeable symptoms. Development of MPC in pregnancy can result in **conjunctivitis** and pneumonia in newborn babies, as well as **puerperal** fever of the mother. MPC can be caused by such organisms as *Chlamydia trachomatis, Neisseria gonorrhoeae, Trichomonas vaginalis, Candida albicans,* and herpes simplex.

MPC may spread to become pelvic inflammatory disease (PID) and become chronic involving the lining of the uterus (**endometritis**) and the fallopian tubes (**salpingitis**), resulting in scarring, infertility, and increased risk of ectopic pregnancy (because scar tissue may prevent the fertilized ovum from entering and implanting in the uterus). Two of the most common causative agents of PID are *Chlamydia trachomatis* and *Neisseria gonorrhoeae*, often in combination, which requires treatment for both.

---

urethritis: ureth—urethra + itis—inflammation

mucopurulent cervicitis: muco—involving mucous + purulent—involving pus + cervic—cervix + itis—inflammation

conjunctivitis: conjunctiv(a)—lining of the eyelids and sclera of the eye + itis—inflammation

puerperal: childbirth

endometritis: endo—inside + metr—womb + itis—inflammation

salpingitis salping—tube + itis—infection

proctitis: proct—anus + itis—inflammation

Proctitis is inflammation of the rectum and anus due to infection. Not all proctitis is caused by STDs, but STDs can cause proctitis. This is especially prevalent among those who practice anal intercourse—both heterosexual and homosexual. **Enteritis,** which is inflammation of the lining of the intestine, may occur due to contamination during anal intercourse. Infection with *Campylobacter, Shigella,* and *Giardia lamblia* can be a problem for homosexual men. Care of clients who have gastrointestinal disorders is discussed in Unit VII.

Genital ulcers are formed when papules or macules erode and leave often painful raw pitted or excoriated areas on or around the genitals. Not all genital ulcers are caused by STDs—injury, some non-STD viruses, some types of drug reactions, radiation, and some forms of cancer can also produce genital ulcers. However, several STDs can produce genital ulcers, including syphilis, herpes, chlamydia, chancroid, granuloma inguinale, and human immunodeficiency virus (HIV). The presence of genital ulcers from one type of disease may increase the risk of infection with other STDs during sexual activity, because the open areas present an easy portal of entry for infectious organisms.

Cellular changes can also be caused by STDs, including **condylomatous** (wartlike) growth and dysplasia or neoplasia, which may result in precancerous or cancerous conditions. Herpes viruses, HIV, and human papillomavirus (HPV) have all been linked to the development of cancer.

Chlamydia

ETIOLOGY AND SIGNS AND SYMPTOMS

Chlamydia is the most common STD in the United States.[1] It can be transmitted sexually and by contact with blood and body fluids. There are several serotypes of the bacteria *Chlamydia trachomatis.* Chlamydia is often asymptomatic in women, but urethritis, MPC, and conjunctivitis may result from this infection. Fitz-Hugh–Curtis syndrome, a surface inflammation of the liver, can be caused by *Chlamydia trachomatis.* This inflammation may cause nausea, vomiting, and sharp pain at the base of the ribs that sometimes refers to the right shoulder and arm. From 25 to 50 percent of cases of PID can be attributed to chlamydia; this can increase risk of infertility by 10 to 20 percent and risk of ectopic pregnancy by 700 percent.[2] Chlamydia infection can be passed from mother to baby during birth, resulting in conjunctivitis and neonatal pneumonia.

Lymphogranuloma venereum (LGV) is also caused by some serotypes of *Chlamydia trachomatis* but is more commonly seen in tropical climates or among people who emigrated from these areas. This disease also causes urethritis and proctitis, and it inflames lymph nodes that drain the pelvic area, resulting in draining sores and fistula development. Scarring from this disease can complicate vaginal deliveries.

DIAGNOSTIC TESTS

Diagnosis is made presently by cell culture and by two antigen tests. Culture is difficult and expensive and generally requires 2 to 6 days for results to be available, depending on the availability of a fluorescence microscope. Samples for culture are generally gathered in a special collection tube for sending to a laboratory for microscopic examination. Because this disease is so common, the nurse is wise to set out an unopened chlamydia collection kit within easy reach of the physician for each pelvic examination.

MEDICAL TREATMENT

Tetracyclines, erythromycins, azithromycin, and sulfonamides may be given to treat chlamydia in nonpregnant clients, but tetracyclines are contraindicated for pregnant women. Fluoroquinolones (such as ofloxacin) may also be used to combat chlamydia, but these drugs are contraindicated during pregnancy and for clients under 18 years of age. Clindamycin may be given during pregnancy.[3] Eyedrops of tetracycline or erythromycin may be given shortly after birth for the prevention of conjunctivitis. Institutional policies and state regulations determine the type of eyedrops to be used and whether administration of the drops requires specific consent of the parents.

Gonorrhea

ETIOLOGY AND SIGNS AND SYMPTOMS

The bacteria *Neisseria gonorrhoeae* causes a variety of symptoms identified as gonorrhea. This microorganism may be transmitted vaginally, rectally, orally, and through contact with blood and body fluids. Men who contract the disease may have no noticeable genitourinary symptoms or may have urethritis with a yellow urethral discharge. Women who have gonorrhea may have either no noticeable symptoms or have a sore throat, MPC, urethritis, or abnormal menstrual symptoms such as bleeding between periods. From 20 to 40 percent of cases of PID are caused by gonorrhea. Intercourse with an infected partner during menstruation may be especially risky for development of PID, because removal of the cervical mucous barrier can promote the growth of the gonococcus in the higher reproductive tract. Gonorrhea can also cause Fitz-Hugh–Curtis

---

enteritis: enter—intestinal + itis—inflammation
condylomatous: condyl—rounded projection + oma(t)—growth + ous—like

syndrome. Fever, nausea, vomiting, and lower abdominal pain may be present. Gonorrhea may also infect the throat and the rectum and may cause disseminated (scattered or widespread) gonococcal infection resulting in inflammation of the joints, skin, meninges, and the lining of the heart.

Newborns born to mothers who have gonorrhea can develop **ophthalmia neonatorum,** which involves inflammation of the conjunctiva and deeper parts of the eye and can result in blindness. The newborn may also experience disease at other sites of infection with gonorrhea at birth. Abscesses may develop where fetal scalp monitors were attached during labor, and infection of the nose, lungs, and rectum may occur.

DIAGNOSTIC TESTS

Diagnosis is done by microscopic examination of smears and cultures of the discharge.

MEDICAL TREATMENT

Development of antibiotic resistance by *Neisseria gonorrhoeae* is making treatment more complicated. Presently recommended treatment may involve drugs such as cefixime, ciprofloxacin, or ofloxacin. There is some debate about the effectiveness of using spectinomycin for highly resistant strains.[4] Development of ophthalmia neonatorum may be prevented by use of special eye medications for the newborn at birth. Institutional policies and state regulations determine the type of eyedrops to be used and whether administration of the drops requires specific consent of the parents.

Syphilis

ETIOLOGY AND SIGNS AND SYMPTOMS

Syphilis is an ancient disease that has not disappeared, although it is overshadowed by more commonly occurring diseases such as chlamydia. From 40,000 to 50,000 new cases per year are diagnosed in the United States—the largest number of cases since 1949.[5] The primary stage of syphilis begins with the entry of the *Treponema pallidum* spirochete through the skin or mucous membranes. Between 3 and 90 days later a papule develops at the site of entry; this sloughs off leaving a painless, red ulcerated area called a **chancre** (Fig. 42–1). Chancres may also develop in other areas of the body at this time. Chancre formation is generally the only symptom of this stage of syphilis. The chancre eventually heals, but the spirochete remains active in the infected individual and can be passed on to others. Secondary syphilis begins 2 to 8 weeks later and affects the body more generally, causing such problems as flulike symptoms, joint pain, hair loss, skin rashes, mouth sores,

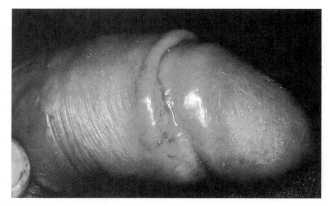

Figure 42–1. Syphilis chancre. (From Lemone, P, and Burke, KM: Medical-Surgical Nursing: Critical Thinking in Client Care. Addison-Wesley, Menlo Park, Calif, 1996, p 2069, with permission.)

and condylomatous growths in moist areas of the body. Serious damage can occur if syphilis is untreated in the early stages. The disease may not progress to the tertiary (or late) stage for 3 to 15 years. At this stage it can involve any organ system of the body. In the tertiary stage the spirochete may form **gummas,** which are tumors of a rubbery consistency that can break down and ulcerate leaving holes in body tissues. These gummas may damage the heart, circulatory system, and nervous system. Ulceration of gummas may destroy areas of vital tissue and lead to mental and physical disability or early death.

Syphilis can be passed on to the unborn children of women who carry the spirochete resulting in **hepatosplenomegaly,** increase in bilirubin, destruction of red blood cells, and **lymphadenopathy.** If left untreated, syphilis in pregnancy may cause lesions in various organs of the unborn baby and result in higher rates of spontaneous abortion, stillbirth, and premature births.

DIAGNOSTIC TESTS

Several tests for syphilis exist. The organism is difficult to grow in culture and is so tiny that it cannot be seen with a light microscope. Dark-field microscopy of material from a chancre may show the organism but may also be negative in spite of definite symptoms of systemic syphilis infection. **Serological** (blood) tests are categorized as non-

---

ophthalmia neonatorum: ophthalmia—eye disease + neonatorum—of the newborn

gummas: from the word meaning rubber—rubbery tumors

hepatosplenomegaly: hepato—liver + spleno—spleen + megaly—enlargement

lymphadenopathy: lymph—lymph + adeno—node + pathy—disorder

serological: sero—blood + logic—science

treponemal and treponemal. Nontreponemal tests include the Venereal Disease Research Laboratory (VDRL) test, the rapid plasma reagin (RPR) test, and the automated reagin test (ART). These tests indirectly check for syphilis by detecting the presence of antibodies that the body forms in response to treponema and, unfortunately, in response to some other disorders, so false-positive results can occur. Treponemal tests are much more specific for syphilis but, unfortunately, can remain positive long after the disease has been effectively treated, so a combination of testing methods may be used to determine whether a client truly has syphilis. Diagnosis of neurosyphilis is even more difficult because some testing of cerebrospinal fluid may result in false-negative tests. Further research is needed to improve test methods for this disease. Molecular amplification techniques are improving the accuracy of diagnosis in this disease.

MEDICAL TREATMENT

Penicillins may be used to treat syphilis of nonpregnant, pregnant, and newborn clients. For those who are allergic to penicillin, desensitization treatments may be tried. Azithromycin and ceftriaxone have shown promising results for those who are allergic to penicillin, but large-scale controlled trials are lacking at the time of the writing of this book.[6]

Trichomonas

SIGNS AND SYMPTOMS

Trichomonas is generally a sexually transmitted disease, but it may be transmitted through nonsexual contact with infected articles, because it can survive for quite a long time outside of the body.[7] Most people carrying the microorganism *Trichomonas vaginalis* are asymptomatic and may remain so for years. Changes in vaginal or urethral conditions may encourage an outbreak of the disease. Increase in pH from a decrease in acid-producing resident bacteria, injuries to the vaginal tissues, and development of lesions from some other STDs or from some forms of cancer may activate the organism. Large amounts of frothy, foul-smelling, creamy to green color discharge, redness, swelling, itching, and burning of the genital area, as well as pain with intercourse and voiding, may be seen with this disease.

DIAGNOSTIC TESTS

Trichomonas can be rapidly diagnosed because the organism is so large and distinctively shaped. The organisms can be easily seen on wet mount slides of the discharge. They can be easily identified with a microscope because of their flagellae—whiplike protuberances. *Trichomonas* may produce abnormal Pap smear readings, which require that more frequent Pap smears be done to provide adequate surveillance of cellular changes.

MEDICAL TREATMENT

The drug treatment of choice is metronidazole, except for the first trimester of pregnancy, during which a clindamycin 2 percent vaginal cream is recommended. Some strains of *Trichomonas* may exhibit resistance but generally succumb to much higher doses of the drug. Because some people carry the organism without symptoms, sexual partners should probably be treated regardless of whether they show the symptoms.

Herpes

ETIOLOGY AND SIGNS AND SYMPTOMS

Herpes genitalis is caused by infection with the herpes simplex viruses, types 1 and 2 (HSV1 and HSV2). Herpes viruses have an affinity for tissues of the skin and nervous system. The viruses can lie dormant in nervous system tissues and then reactivate periodically when the body undergoes stress, fever, or immune system compromise. HSV1 is the causative agent for commonly seen "fever blisters" of the mouth and can cause genital lesions as well. HSV2 causes a more severe genital version of this disorder. The disease pattern is generally one of **vesicular** outbreaks interspersed with asymptomatic latent periods during which the virus may still be transmitted to others. Both men and women can develop **herpetic** blisters on the genitalia that spontaneously rupture, producing ulceration of the underlying skin tissues, which can be quite painful (Fig. 42–2). Some clients infected with HSV, however, may show no noticeable symptoms and yet transmit the disease.

Initial infection with herpes may produce a flulike condition. Urethritis, cystitis, and MPC with a vaginal discharge may also result from herpes infection. Infection of the spinal nerve roots by HSV may result in **sacral radiculopathy** in which the sacral spinal nerves are damaged resulting in retention of urine and feces. Herpes can also have serious systemic effects for both men and women through development of a disseminated (scattered or widespread) herpetic infection resulting in inflammation of the spinal cord, meninges, nerve pathways, and lymph nodes. Urethral strictures and increased risk for development of cervical cancer in women are also consequences of herpes infections.

---

vesicular: vesicul—blister + ar—type
herpetic: herpet—herpes + ic—pertaining to
sacral radiculopathy: sacral—sacrum + radiculo—root + pathy—disorder, disease

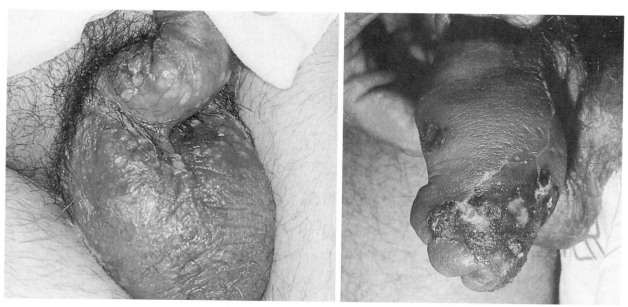

Figure 42–2. Herpes lesions. (From Lemone, P, and Burke, KM: Medical-Surgical Nursing: Critical Thinking in Client Care. Addison-Wesley, Menlo Park, Calif, 1996, p 2073, with permission.)

The virus may be transmitted from a mother to her child during pregnancy, during delivery, and by breast feeding. It is estimated that one in five of all pregnant women carry herpes.[8] Most of the babies born to mothers with herpes do not develop herpetic disease; however, in cases where transmission occurs, the involvement may range from infection of the baby's skin, eyes, mucous membranes, and nervous system to death from disseminated herpes infection. The risk of transmission may be increased by active lesions or asymptomatic viral shedding at the time of delivery.

DIAGNOSTIC TESTS

Testing for HSV requires special viral collection kits for swabbed or scraped specimens from lesions. Blood tests may also be done, but the sensitivity to distinguish whether the infection is due to HSV1 or HSV2 in serological testing is not very precise.

MEDICAL TREATMENT

There is presently no known cure for herpes infection, although antiviral medications such as acyclovir may be given to decrease the severity of symptoms. Acyclovir may also be given during pregnancy to decrease the severity of the mother's HSV activity, which may reduce the risk of transmission to the baby. Cesarean section delivery may also decrease the risk of transmission of the disease from the mother to the baby if there are active, open lesions around the time of delivery.

See also Nursing Care Plan Box 42–1 for the Client with Genital Herpes.

Cytomegalovirus

ETIOLOGY AND SIGNS AND SYMPTOMS

Cytomegalovirus (CMV), another herpes virus, although not considered to be a classic STD, can also be transmitted sexually and by breast milk. CMV infection in a pregnant woman can cause birth defects in every organ system of the developing fetus and may cause some early spontaneous abortions and fetal deaths. The mother's disease process related to cytomegalovirus infection can be a mononucleosis-like episode with fever, fatigue, and swollen lymph nodes.

DIAGNOSTIC TESTS

Diagnosis is made by antibody-specific blood tests of the mother, by examination of sloughed kidney cells in a urine sample from the baby, or by a careful examination of the placenta.

MEDICAL AND SURGICAL TREATMENT

At the time of writing of this book there is no known cure for CMV infection, but antiviral medications, such as acyclovir, may be given to decrease viral activity. Infected infants can shed viral material and infect others, so may have to be treated with isolation precautions. Women who have a known case of active CMV infection during pregnancy may be offered therapeutic abortion because of the severity of the disease for the developing fetus.

NURSING CARE PLAN BOX 42–1 FOR THE CLIENT WITH GENITAL HERPES

Pain related to inflammation, skin lesions

Client Outcomes
The client will express pain relief and will rest and move well.

Evaluation of Outcome
Does client state relief of pain?

Interventions	Rationale	Evaluation
Assess pain using the WHAT'S UP? format.	Assessment of the characteristics of the pain will assist the nurse in providing appropriate relief measures.	Can the client describe the pain characteristics?
Recommend pain relief measures appropriate to the type and location of the pain (both alternative measures, such as heat, ice, and change of position, and medication may be offered).	Not all types of pain respond well to the same treatment.	Does the client express satisfactory relief of pain? Does the client move and rest without evidence of pain?
Document results of pain relief measures.	Documentation alerts other caregivers about what works and does not work, thus providing more consistent, effective pain relief.	Have you gained sufficient information from the client to document results?
Instruct the client about self-care for pain and STD treatment at home.	Most STDs are treated at home.	Does client verbalize understanding of self-care measures?

Risk for transmission of infection to others related to lack of knowledge about transmission, symptoms, and treatment

Client Outcome
Client will verbalize understanding of measures to prevent transmission to others.

Evaluation of Outcome
Does client verbalize understanding of transmission prevention? Does client practice preventive behaviors?

Interventions	Rationale	Evaluation
Assess client's understanding of transmission, symptoms, complications, and treatment of STDs.	New instruction should be based on client's previous knowledge.	Is client's current understanding accurate? What teaching is necessary?
Assess whether the client is engaging in high-risk behaviors.	If the client is continuing to engage in high-risk behaviors, the risk for infection of others is high.	Is the client protecting self and others appropriately?
Use universal precautions and strict aseptic technique for *all* procedures involving blood and body fluids.	The health team, in addition to other client contacts, must be protected.	Are universal precautions observed?
Instruct client in appropriate strategies to reduce risk of infecting others: • Abstinence • Monogamy (if no active infection) • Use of barrier methods and spermicides • Adherence to treatment regimen	These measures may help prevent transmission of infection to others.	Does the client verbalize understanding of methods to prevent transmission, and intent to practice them?
Teach client signs and symptoms of STDs to report immediately.	Prompt treatment of client and partners further reduces risk of transmission of infection.	Does client verbalize understanding of signs and symptoms to report?

continued

NURSING CARE PLAN BOX 42–1 (continued)

Fear related to diagnosis of an incurable illness and effects on sexual relationships and reproduction

Client Outcome
Client will verbalize realistic and accurate information about disease process and relate control of excessive fear

Evaluation of Outcome
Does client relate accurate knowledge? Is fear manageable?

Interventions	Rationale	Evaluation
Assess client's fears.	Fear is a normal response and may be appropriate.	What does client fear?
If fear is based on misconceptions, provide factual information.	When fear is based on misconceptions, they should be corrected.	Are fears based on factual information?
Allow client to verbalize feelings. Be empathetic, but do not offer false hope.	Sharing fears may help client gain insight into dealing with them.	Is client able to verbalize feelings?
Explain all procedures and treatments.	Unfamiliar procedures or treatments may contribute to fear.	Does client understand procedures and treatments?
Help client identify support systems and coping strategies that have worked in the past.	Methods that have worked for the client before are likely to be helpful again.	Does the client have effective coping skills and support systems?

Genital Warts

SIGNS AND SYMPTOMS

Condylomata acuminatum (genital warts) are the most common sexually transmitted viral disease, and the incidence is increasing very rapidly. Infection with human papillomavirus (HPV) produces the condylomata—soft, raised, **verrucous** fleshy tumors, which may also have fingerlike projections (Fig. 42–3). However, some people who are infected and can transmit the infection may have no noticeable symptoms. There are over 60 known types of HPV identified, and several of the types of the virus have been closely linked to development of cancers of the reproductive organs and anus in both males and females. There may be a long latent period of as much as 3 years' duration from the time of exposure to development of the warts.

HPV can be passed on from a pregnant woman to her fetus resulting in the growth of genital warts on the baby, HPV infection of the baby's respiratory tract, and a possible increased risk of cancer development. HPV infection during pregnancy can cause particularly difficult problems. Genital warts tend to grow more rapidly in pregnant women and to bleed more easily with injury than in nonpregnant women.

DIAGNOSTIC TESTS

Diagnosis may be made by applying dilute acetic acid (vinegar) to the skin of the external genital area, vagina, cervix, and anus and then closely examining with a colposcope the areas that turn a lighter color. Biopsies of the suspicious areas can be sent for further study of the cells to determine the DNA type of the papillomavirus. The virus is difficult to culture, but molecular amplification seems hopeful as a way to improve accuracy of diagnosis and DNA identification of the strain of HPV. Other tests to diagnose HPV include an antigen test and the Southern and dot blot tests, which use radioactive probes. Cancerous changes stimulated by this virus may be identified on Pap smears.

MEDICAL TREATMENT

There is presently no known cure for infection with papillomavirus. The warts may be treated by freezing, burning, or chemically destroying them, or by manipulation of the client's immune system to attack the virus. Cryotherapy (freezing) of the warts may be done by touching each wart with a cryoprobe or a liquid nitrogen–soaked swab. Warts may also be burned or **electrocoagulated** with an **electrocautery** or a laser. The heat generated within the wart

---

condylomata acuminatum: condyl—rounded projection + oma—growth + ta—pluralizes the word (singular form is condyloma) + acuminatum—specifies genital type of growths

verrucous: verruc—wart + ous—like

electrocoagulate: electro—electrical + coagul—curdled or hardened + ated—process completed

electrocautery: electro—electrical + cautery—branding iron

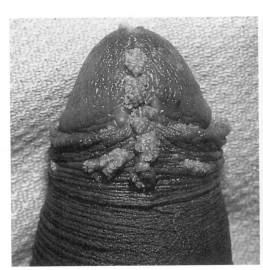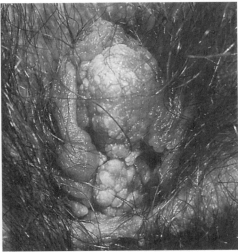

Figure 42–3. Condylomata (genital warts). (From Lemone, P, and Burke, KM: Medical-Surgical Nursing: Critical Thinking in Client Care. Addison-Wesley, Menlo Park, Calif, 1996, p 2079, with permission.)

causes the proteins to coagulate, resulting in death of the wart tissue. Podofilox, podophyllin, trichloroacetic acid (TCA), and 5-fluorouracil (5-FU) are some of the chemical agents that may be applied topically to the warts. Many of the treatment options are not appropriate for use during pregnancy due to their **cytotoxic** effects, which might damage the fetus, but cryosurgery and laser destruction of the wart tissue may be done during pregnancy. All of the wart treatments may require multiple applications and generally result in a lot of discomfort as the warts degenerate, ulcerate, and slough over a long time period.

Various types of immunotherapy have been used against HPV. **Interferons** are proteins produced by the body that can inhibit viral growth. Several types of interferon have been used to combat HPV. These substances may be applied topically, injected into the condyloma, or administered systemically. Interferons, however, can produce side effects of flulike symptoms, a drop in the number of white blood cells, and changes in liver function. Systemic interferon treatment, however, may offer the advantage of being able to attack warts all over the body at the same time, rather than individually as with topical treatments, thus speeding the process of treatment. **Autologous vaccine** treatments and dinitrochlorobenzene (DNCB) hypersensitivity induction treatments are two methods being used experimentally to encourage the body to attack the warts.[9] In the former method, a vaccine is made from wart tissue;

when injected on a weekly basis, the vaccine is intended to stimulate the body's own immune responses to destroy warts. The latter method relies on stimulating a DNCB allergy in the client and then applying DNCB to the warts, resulting in destruction of the wart by the body's own defense system. One of the most significant difficulties with HPV treatments is that widespread destruction of tissue in the most sensitive areas of the body can cause severe discomfort. More conservative treatments, however, may not keep pace with the growth of new warts.

HOME CARE

Clients who have genital warts (condylomata acuminatum) burned off will need to have burns cared for at home. If the burns (there may be multiple areas treated) are near the urethra or rectum, the client may need a Foley catheter inserted to avoid contamination. Also, the client is instructed to increase dietary roughage and fluids to prevent constipation. The physician is consulted for orders on care of burns. Sterile technique is used for dressing changes. The client is premedicated for pain control if necessary.

Hepatitis B

ETIOLOGY AND SIGNS AND SYMPTOMS

There are several main types of hepatitis viruses, but this portion will deal only with hepatitis B virus (HBV), which is generally considered within the STD category because it can be transmitted through sexual contact with blood and body fluids. Early signs of hepatitis are loss of appetite, rashes, malaise, muscle and joint pain, headaches, nausea, and vom-

---

cytotoxic: cyto—cell + toxic—poison
interferons: inter—between + fer (from Latin *ferire*)—to strike + ons—agents
autologous vaccine: auto—self + logous—source + vaccine

iting. As the liver is affected more by the virus, the urine may darken and the stool color lighten (due to changes in bile excretion), liver enzymes may rise, and jaundice may appear. Enlargement of the spleen, enlargement and tenderness of the liver, necrosis of liver cells, cirrhosis, coma, and death may follow if the disease is severe. Chronic asymptomatic carrier status may follow hepatitis virus infection.

During pregnancy, hepatitis B virus may be transmitted to the unborn baby, which can result in acute hepatitis and the possibility of becoming a chronic carrier of HBV.

DIAGNOSTIC TESTS

Diagnosis of hepatitis is generally made using a variety of blood tests based on antigen and antibody responses.

MEDICAL TREATMENT

Supportive medical care with avoidance of drugs that require liver metabolism may help the client through the active stage of the disease. Treatment of the disease may involve injection of serum immune globulins to confer passive immunity. It is recommended that all babies of HBV-positive mothers receive a 0.5 mL dose of HBV immune globulin less than 12 hours after birth and then be immunized with HBV vaccine 1 week, 1 month, and 6 months after birth.[10] See Chapter 33 for more information.

PREVENTION

Prevention is better than treatment and may be accomplished using HBV vaccine. This is especially recommended for health care workers who come in contact with blood and body fluids.

Human Immunodeficiency Virus

ETIOLOGY AND SIGNS AND SYMPTOMS

HIV, the causative agent for acquired immunodeficiency syndrome (AIDS), can be transmitted through sexual contact and by exchange of blood and body fluids. The agent is a retrovirus that binds to the surface of cells and inserts viral genetic material into the cells for replication. The initial infection often is asymptomatic or similar to a mild case of mononucleosis with perhaps a rash as well. The virus may remain dormant in the body of a carrier for many years before symptoms occur. Several more years may pass before changes in the immune system caused by the virus result in the symptoms of full-blown AIDS. Opportunistic diseases (diseases caused by normally present pathogens which take advantage of the client's immune deficient state) such as *Pneumocystis carinii* pneumonia, fungal overgrowth, Kaposi's sarcoma, and cervical cancer develop as the body's

immune system becomes ineffective because of damage by the virus. Latent diseases such as tuberculosis, syphilis, and toxoplasmosis may be reactivated as the immune system is damaged. Psychiatric changes may be seen. An AIDS dementia complex (ADC) has been documented involving behavioral, reasoning, and motor control changes.

HIV may be passed from a pregnant mother to her fetus with disastrous effects. The baby born with HIV infection seldom lives more than 3 years, because the baby's immune system is unable to fight infections.

DIAGNOSTIC TESTS

Serological testing for HIV cannot test directly for the presence of the virus because it can lie dormant within cells for long periods of time. Tests for antibodies, however, such as the enzyme-linked immunosorbent assay (ELISA) and Western blot test can provide evidence of HIV once seroconversion to HIV-positive status has occurred. Additional tests may be done to monitor the progress of the disease, for example CD4 cell readings for evidence of the immune system functioning, Pap smears to check for cervical cancer (which is more common in immune-compromised individuals), and tests for diseases that might become active in the immunocompromised host, such as tuberculosis, gonorrhea, syphilis, and toxoplasmosis.

MEDICAL AND SURGICAL TREATMENT

Studies are ongoing to find ways to combat this catastrophic disease. At the present time there is no cure. Treatment is aimed at either improving the body's immune functioning or preventing replication of the virus. Giving the client new bone marrow, white blood cells, interleukin 2, and interferon are all examples of attempts to improve immune function. Zidovudine (AZT), dideoxyinosine (ddI), dideoxycytidine (ddC), and staduvidine are considered to be effective agents in slowing the growth of the virus in adults; AZT has also shown hopeful results in decreasing the risk of prenatal transmission of the virus. Research is also being conducted to develop a vaccine against HIV, but efforts have not been hopeful thus far because the virus can mutate readily. Up to 30 or 40 different versions of the virus may be present in an individual as the disease progresses.

See Chapter 53 for a more complete discussion of HIV. See also Ethical Considerations Box 42–2.

Genital Parasites

ETIOLOGY AND SIGNS AND SYMPTOMS

Genital parasites are not a true STD, but they may be transmitted during close body contact. The two most commonly

ETHICAL CONSIDERATIONS BOX 42–2

Ethical Issues Surrounding HIV

There are several ethical issues underlying the controversy surrounding AIDS. The right to privacy is often one of the first issues mentioned. Many diseases, such as tuberculosis, gonorrhea, syphilis, or hepatitis, that are highly contagious and sometimes fatal, must be reported to public health officials. Although there is a general requirement to report infection with HIV/AIDS to the Centers for Disease Control and Prevention (CDC), many states have strict laws regarding the confidentiality of the diagnosis. Revealing the diagnosis of HIV/AIDS brings the possibility of a lawsuit against the health care provider or institution.

It is important to remember that the right to privacy is not an absolute right. If the right to privacy can be violated when the public welfare is at stake with other contagious diseases, does not AIDS represent the same type of threat? It seems to be unjust to ask health care providers to care for clients with this disease without knowing that the client has it. On the other hand, do clients have a right to know that a health care provider is infected with HIV/AIDS?

Another important ethical issue is the right to care. Can a nurse refuse to care for an AIDS client? Obviously, a fundamental right of being a client is to receive care, and a fundamental obligation of a nurse is to provide care. The first statement of the American Nurses' Association (ANA) Nurses Code of Ethics states that a nurse must provide care unrestricted by any considerations. Surely there are some exceptions, for example if the nurse is pregnant, is receiving chemotherapy, or has other immunity problems. But in most situations, the nurse would be obligated to provide the best nursing care possible for all clients, including those with AIDS.

What about the tremendous cost involved in treating individuals who have AIDS? Recent studies estimate that the medical cost of treating an AIDS client from the time of diagnosis to the time of death will be in the neighborhood of $750,000 per client. In the face of this crisis, governmental agencies, who bear the brunt of paying for AIDS treatment, will have to make some hard decisions concerning this issue. With more than 1 million people already infected with this disease, the cost to society is astronomical. Nurses have the obligation to care for all clients, but are physicians, hospitals, or governmental agencies also held to this same precept? Is the right to health care really a privilege?

seen parasites are pubic lice (*Phthirus pubis,* commonly called "crabs" because of the shape of the lice) and scabies (*Sarcoptes scabiei*). These parasites cause itching, redness, and for scabies tracks under the skin where the females burrow to lay their eggs.

DIAGNOSTIC TESTS

Direct visual or magnified view of the parasites aids in diagnosis.

MEDICAL TREATMENT

Parasites are treated with topical insecticides such as lindane or permethrin. The nurse should refer to package inserts for application instructions and precautions to avoid reinfection.

Pediatric Sexually Transmitted Diseases

Not all STD clients are adults. Unfortunately childhood sexual abuse does occur. The nurse may play a very important role in providing explanations in simple terms for procedures and in comforting and supporting the child. Fortunately, not all STDs grow well in immature genital tracts. However, chlamydia, syphilis, herpes, and genital warts are sometimes seen in young children. It is very important that child sexual abuse be reported and investigated. For this to occur effectively evidence must be gathered. The physician may request an evidence kit from the local police for use during the examination. Accusations of sexual abuse have sometimes been wrongly filed and have produced a lot of trauma to children. Some forms of STDs may have been transmitted at or before birth and later have presented symptoms. It is probably wisest to report suspicions with documentation of evidence to a supervisor if the client is seen in a health care setting. In the community, child welfare agencies may be contacted. Depending on the state, province, or country, the nurse may be required by law to report directly to a child protection agency any suspicion of child abuse. Children who frequently scratch their genital areas or who have a foul smell emanating from the genital area may be victims of sexual abuse or may have put a foreign object into the vagina. Examination of a small child may be done with a nasal speculum rather than a vaginal speculum. Further content on care and examination of children is addressed in pediatrics texts.

Older clients may also have an STD. See Gerontological Issues Box 42–3.

GERONTOLOGICAL ISSUES BOX 42-3

Older adults remain sexually active even though society often views them as asexual. The nurse should not assume that because an older adult is single or widowed he or she is not sexually active. Older adults who have enjoyed active and fulfilling sex lives with a spouse or partner will seek that in new relationships. Older adults who engage in high-risk sexual behaviors (multiple partners, genital-anal sex, no use of barriers during sexual intercourse) will also be at risk for sexually transmitted diseases.

Reporting of Sexually Transmitted Diseases

Nurses may also facilitate the reporting and public health follow-up of STDs by filling in client information on the STD reporting form and placing the form into the client's chart for completion by the physician. The requirements for reporting STDs may vary for different states, provinces, and countries. In some areas, laboratories are also required to submit a report form for positive reportable STD tests. Laboratory reports that are not followed by a physician's report may result in investigation of the situation by an STD investigator. Generally the report form has spaces for listing of sexual contacts who should be notified of possible STD exposure. Depending on the laws of the state, province, or country, the client may notify contacts or have the physician do so, or contacts may be notified by a public health authority that they have been listed as a sexual contact by an anonymous person who has tested positive for a particular STD.

Nursing Process: Persons Who Have Sexually Transmitted Diseases

STDs are usually diagnosed and treated in physician's offices and clinics. Hospitalization related to STDs generally occurs only in conjunction with infertility investigations, **perinatal** difficulties caused by STDs, or serious long-term complications resulting from STDs, such as AIDS. If the complication is, for instance, meningitis caused by a herpes virus, the plan of care would be very similar to the plan for any other type of meningitis with the consideration that psychosocial concerns may differ

somewhat because of the source of the infection. The nurse's role in the care of clients with STDs includes observation and documentation of signs and symptoms, providing education, and client support during times of diagnosis and treatment.

ASSESSMENT

Sometimes clients visit clinics or physician's offices for stated reasons other than STDs, yet their real concern is an STD. A female client may state that she needs a Pap smear, when her real concern is the possibility of STDs. After the client has been placed in an examining room, asking the date of the last Pap smear and whether she is presently experiencing any irritation, pain, or unusual growths or discharges in her private areas may clarify the request without being considered too intrusive. Explaining to the client the need to know what examination supplies to set out for the physician may further help put the client at ease. Some people misunderstand the purpose of Pap smears and believe that any problems of the reproductive organs can be diagnosed through this test. If appropriate questioning does not determine the real needs of the client, she may believe that she has received testing that in reality was not done. If she is asymptomatic by visual inspection and does not tell the physician about her concerns, a Pap smear may be all that is done. Furthermore, the results for Pap smears that are done when there is an active infection may read "inflammatory changes present, repeat Pap smear after resolution of the inflammation." Although this may eventually alert the physician that there was an infection at the time of the Pap smear, the infective agent is not identified, another pelvic examination will probably be required, and the diagnosis is delayed needlessly (during which time the infection may have been transmitted to others). Similar concerns exist for the male client.

If an STD is diagnosed, it is important to ask the client about date of exposure and recent sexual contacts that may need to be notified. Discharge, rashes, or other lesions should be examined and documented. Universal precautions should be observed during the examination and all subsequent care, to protect the health team and other clients.

NURSING DIAGNOSIS

Nursing diagnoses that may be identified for the client with an STD include the following:

- Pain related to inflammation or skin lesions
- Risk for transmission of infection to others

---

perinatal: peri—around + natal—birth

- Altered sexuality pattern related to illness and risk for transmission
- Fear related to diagnosis, possible incurable illness

PLANNING

The plan of care should include measures to increase client comfort, instruction on safer sex practices and how to prevent transmission of the disease, and identification of coping behaviors that help reduce fear.

IMPLEMENTATION AND CLIENT EDUCATION

Because the majority of STD treatment takes place in outpatient settings, intervention focuses on client education. The client is advised that pain will subside with effective treatment of the infection. The nurse ensures that the client understands self-administration of analgesics and other prescribed treatments, as well as signs of possible complications to report.

Nurses may be expected to set out supplies for pelvic examinations and to be present during the examination as a chaperon or client support person. Some client teaching may take place as the supplies are readied. Explanation of what to expect during the examination and collection of test samples may help decrease client anxiety. Information about possible risk reduction strategies may also be needed. Pamphlets or other reading materials may be available to provide to the client. The nurse should clarify with the employer the type and depth of information clients should be given so that teaching is not duplicated, confused, or omitted.

It has been said that the only sure prevention of sexually transmitted diseases is abstinence. Lifelong monogamy of both sexual partners in a relationship would prevent a lot of suffering. Clients should be made aware that having a sexual relationship with someone is the **epidemiological** equivalent of engaging in sexual activity with all of that person's previous partners as well. Ignorance of the serious repercussions of some STDs may explain some of the apathy surrounding risk reduction.

Many myths about sexual activity are sincerely believed by some clients (Table 42–1). The nurse must assess the client's beliefs and correct misconceptions. It is vitally important for clients to know the sexual and lifestyle history of any potential partner before sexual activity has occurred and before emotional issues may cloud judgment. Development of a healthy relationship in which honest communication can occur generally takes time and effort.

When teaching clients, the terms *safe sex* and *STD prevention* are misnomers. Nurses should more accurately refer to information about barrier methods as "safer sex" practices, which may decrease the risk of (but not absolutely prevent) transmission of STDs (Table 42–2).

One of the most common contributing factors for infection with an STD is the consumption of alcohol or other psychoactive drugs. Clients should be advised that reduction of inhibitions and changes in judgment may result in unintended sexual encounters, which can transmit STDs. Avoiding or limiting alcohol and other drug consumption when with potential partners could do a lot to prevent STD infection from occurring.

For those who choose to be sexually active with more than one person (or with a person who has been sexually active with others) and for those who choose to practice high-risk behaviors, barrier protection may decrease the chances of developing an STD. Information on how to use barrier methods effectively is essential. The nurse should also ensure that the client has access to these methods.

Finally, the client is allowed to discuss fears related to the STD and possible consequences. The nurse ensures that the client has accurate information about the STD and that the client has the knowledge and resources to carry out prescribed treatment.

EVALUATION

Goals have been met if the client:

- States pain is controlled
- Verbalizes understanding of and intent to follow recommendations for prevention of infection transmission
- Describes safer sexual practices
- Relates accurate information and reduction in fear

CRITICAL THINKING: Stephanie

As you seat a young woman in an examining room of the clinic where you work, she comments, "I am new to this area and I've heard that there are three guys in this town who have AIDS and are spreading it around. Is that true?"

1. What are some concerns this question might reflect?
2. You find out that she knows very little about AIDS. List in outline form a teaching plan that would include the information that is important for her to know about HIV and AIDS.

Answers at end of chapter.

---

epidemiological: epi—on or upon + demio—people + logical— pertaining to science

text continues on page 866

Table 42–1. **Common Myths about Sexually Transmitted Diseases**

Myth	Factual Data
People who have STDs are easily identifiable.	Inspection of the potential partner's genitals before sexual activity may decrease the risk (if one does not participate in sexual activity with a person who has visible lesions), *but . . .* • Not all people who are infected have visible symptoms. • There is no standard personality or physical profile for people who can be infected with STDs—*anyone* can be infected.
Avoiding persons who have a history of casual sex, intravenous drug use, homosexual activity, bisexual activity, or a previous sexual relationship with persons who engage in these high-risk practices effectively protects one from infection with STDs.	Avoiding people with these types of history may decrease risk, *but . . .* • Not everyone is honest when responding to questions about sexual history. • Not everyone is aware of their previous partners' histories or the histories of others with whom their previous partners have had sexual relationships. • Asking these kinds of questions is difficult and may be postponed at times until emotional factors complicate such communication.
STDs never happen the first time. Intact genital skin is impervious to the germs (and gentle sexual activity does no harm).	Only one contact with one microorganism is necessary for infection. Intact skin is the body's first line of defense, *but . . .* • Some microorganisms can be transmitted without a noticeable tissue injury. • Minor injuries can occur during many types of sexual activity, including vaginal intercourse.
Condoms prevent the spread of all STDs.	Condoms can greatly decrease the risk of STDs, *but . . .* • Condoms can have tiny channels in the rubber (or other elastic material), which can allow microorganisms to pass through. • Condoms can break, slip off, or be applied improperly. • Petroleum-based lubricants may weaken latex condoms. • Condoms do not provide a barrier for any area other than the penis and most of the vagina (or anus). Some STDs may still be transmitted by contact of surrounding uncovered tissues.
The female condom prevents all transmission of STDs.	It does cover more surface area, but it may have similar problems to male condoms (see above). There is not much research data available yet on this barrier method.
Manual, oral, and anal stimulation cannot transmit STDs.	Contact of hands to genitals can allow for transmission of microorganisms through breaks in the skin. Oral sex can transmit some STD-causing microorganisms. Anal intercourse is a very high-risk activity for transmission of STDs because anal tissues are easily injured and the gastrointestinal tract can be a reservoir for many microorganisms.
Nonoxynol 9 spermicide kills all STD germs.	Nonoxynol 9 can reduce the risk of transmission of STDs, *but . . .* • Nonoxynol 9 is *not* guaranteed to kill all microorganisms.
People get AIDS only by homosexual sexual activity or by blood transfusion. A woman cannot transmit HIV to a man. A man cannot transmit HIV to a woman.	Homosexual activity may result in a higher incidence of transmission of human immunodeficiency virus, *but . . .* • HIV can be transmitted during heterosexual activity. • The gender of the individual does not protect him or her from being infected with HIV.
Sexual activity during menstruation is less likely to result in STDs.	Sexual activity during menstruation is more likely to result in transmission of some microorganisms that cause STDs because of the vulnerability of the lining of the uterus due to sloughing of the outer layers of cells and because blood and cellular debris may serve as a nutritious medium for growth of microorganisms.
Lesbian sexual activity cannot transmit STDs.	Transmission of microorganisms can occur by contact with mouth, anal, or genital tissues or fomites (inanimate objects, such as vibrators and other sex paraphernalia) that have been contaminated with microorganisms from an infected individual—regardless of the original source of the infection.
Individuals who have not been infected after sexual activity with several people are naturally immune to STDs. Those who have had an STD and have been cured of it by taking medicine are now immune to that disease.	There is no known natural immunity to STDs. The individual may not yet have contacted someone with an active STD. Infection that has been eradicated by medication does not confer immunity.

continued

Table 42–1. (continued)

Myth	Factual Data
People can be certified free of all STDs by having a blood test and taking a simple medication if an infection is present.	Testing of those who suspect they may have contracted an STD and treatment (if possible) may decrease the spread of STDs, *but . . .* • No one test identifies all STDs. Some are identified by examination, and not all infected people show symptoms. • Some STDs do not show positive test results for long periods of time yet may be transmitted by the individual while the tests are still negative. • People may be infected with more than one causative agent at a time and each must be treated (if possible). One STD may obscure the symptoms of other concurrent STDs so that one or more types may go unnoticed and untreated or may not be evident until other STDs have been treated. • There are no known cures for some STDs.
Oral contraceptive (OC) pills give protection against STDs.	OC preparations are *not* an antibiotic—they provide only some protection against conception. Use of a barrier method with spermicide along with the OC can decrease risk of STDs as well as pregnancy.

Table 42–2. **Information about Barrier Methods for Safer Sex**

Barrier	Related Information
Male condoms	Latex condoms are less likely to break during intercourse than other types. Lubrication decreases the chances of breakage during use, but only water-soluble lubricants should be used, because substances such as petroleum jelly (Vaseline) may weaken the condom. Condoms should never be inflated to test them, because this can weaken them. Condoms should be applied only when the penis is erect. Either condoms with a reservoir tip or regular condoms that have been applied while holding approximately ½ inch of the closed end flat between the fingertips allow room for expansion by the ejaculate without creating excessive pressure, which might break the condom. The penis should be withdrawn after ejaculation before the erection begins to subside while holding the top of the condom securely around the penis to avoid spillage. Condoms should never be reused and should be discarded properly after use so that others will not come in contact with the contents.
Female condoms	Female condoms should be applied before any penetration occurs (even preejaculation fluid can contain microorganisms). Lubrication decreases the chances of breakage during use, but only water-soluble lubricants should be used, because substances such as petroleum jelly may weaken the condom. Female condoms should never be reused and should be discarded properly after use so that others will not come in contact with the contents.
Cervical caps or diaphragms	These may provide some protection for the cervix only. They are not effective barriers against STD infection.
Rubber gloves, rubber dental dams, split (opened) male condoms	These may provide some barrier protection for manual and oral sexual activity. Although some groups suggest that male condoms may be split down one side and opened or rubber dental dam material may be taped over areas that have lesions to avoid direct contact with blood and body fluid, especially during sadomasochistic sexual activity, this *very high-risk behavior* is not recommended.
Double condoms	Anal intercourse is a *very high-risk activity* for transmission of many types of STDs, as well as many intestinal organisms, and is not recommended. Homosexual networks advise wearing double condoms and using water-soluble lubricants, preferably containing nonoxynol 9, to decrease risk somewhat if engaging in this type of sexual activity.

Conclusion

Neighbors, friends, or family members may seek information from nurses because they know nurses have health expertise. Such questions may be stated in indirect terms, such as, "I have a friend who is having a problem . . ." It is often wisest to identify broad areas of information that people seem to be seeking without going into perhaps embarrassing details. Suggesting that the concerned person see a physician or contact the local STD clinic for further investigation or information is wise. Emphasis on some serious consequences of untreated STDs and the impossibility of effective self-treatment further underscores the necessity of medical follow-up. If the person wishes to know what to expect from such a visit, a general overview of some interview questions, pelvic examination, swab and smear collection, and a statement about the necessity to test for several possible organisms by various means is a good introduction. The nurse should avoid stating that there is no cure for a particular type of STD, because research is ongoing and sometimes cures are developed and tested before the general medical community becomes aware of them.

STD diagnosis is a complicated process. Individual pathogens may affect the body in a wide variety of ways, and infection with more than one pathogen may further complicate the picture. Some signs and symptoms that are seen with STDs may also be caused by nonsexually transmitted infection or overgrowth of the body's resident microorganisms. General awareness of common signs and symptoms of STDs, however, is important for nurses. Some clients admitted for other diagnoses may be unaware that they have STDs as well. Nurses are often the ones who bathe and given perineal care to clients. Unusual discharges, redness, blisters, swollen areas, ulcers, and evidence of parasites in the genital area may be observed during client care. STD awareness can sensitize the nurse to the possible significance of client complaints such as descriptions of persistent pelvic pain, dysuria, discharges, and rectal soreness. Such problems should be accurately documented and reported so that further investigation and possible treatment can take place.

One of the most important ways a nurse can help those who experience STDs is by being kind, polite, nonjudgmental, and sensitive to the client's communication. Keeping the arms crossed over the chest or other closed postures may be interpreted as evidence of a judgmental attitude, regardless of the nurse's feelings. Maintaining an open posture and eye contact that is appropriate for the client's culture relays a sense of openness and willingness to talk and preserves the possibility of continuing health promotion with these individuals in the future.

Review Questions

1. Medication may be put in newborns' eyes to protect them against which of the following disorders?
   a. Hepatosplenomegaly
   b. Neonatal pneumonia
   c. Ophthalmia neonatorum
   d. Becoming a chronic carrier of HBV

2. Which of the following pathogens causes syphilis?
   a. *Treponema pallidum*
   b. *Chlamydia trachomatis*
   c. Human papillomavirus
   d. Human immunodeficiency virus

3. Which of the following pathogens causes genital warts?
   a. *Sarcoptes scabiei*
   b. Hepatitis A and B
   c. *Chlamydia trachomatis*
   d. Human papillomavirus

4. Which of the following has been linked to cancerous changes in cervical cells?
   a. Syphilis
   b. Gonorrhea
   c. Chlamydia
   d. Human papillomavirus

5. Serological tests for STDs are tests of which substance?
   a. Urine
   b. Blood
   c. Urethral discharge
   d. Scrapings of ulcer material

6. Which is the *least* accurate term for nurses to use when teaching clients about STD prevention?
   a. Safe sex strategies
   b. Safer sex strategies
   c. Risk reduction strategies

7. What is *least* likely to be a client concern when coming for diagnosis and treatment of an STD?
   a. Possible effects on relationships
   b. Possible effects on future fertility
   c. Possible effects on STD statistics
   d. Possible effects on unborn children

8. Which of the following statements about STDs is true?
   a. Avoiding prostitutes will prevent all STDs.
   b. Being symptom free means that one is STD free.
   c. Your partner's past sexual encounters can give you an STD.
   d. Having intercourse with only one person will prevent all STDs.

9. What is the worst possible outcome of an STD?
   a. Pain
   b. Death
   c. Scarring
   d. Infertility

 ANSWERS TO CRITICAL THINKING

CRITICAL THINKING: Stephanie

1. Concerns might include (a) a wish to speak with a health care worker; (b) uncertainty about whether

client information will be kept confidential; (c) fear that she might have become infected through heterosexual contact; (d) a desire to protect herself by avoiding those who have this problem; and (e) a desire for information about HIV and its transmission routes.

2. The teaching plan might include information about (a) the virus and the progression from HIV infection to AIDS; (b) signs and symptoms; (c) means of transmission; (d) strategies for risk reduction; (e) treatments and research; and (f) rights and responsibilities of those who have the disease.

REFERENCES

1. Felsenstein, D: Sexually transmitted disease. In Carlson, KJ, et al (eds): Primary Care of Women. Mosby, St Louis, 1995, p 118.
2. Felsenstein, D: Sexually transmitted disease. In Carlson, KJ, et al (eds): Primary Care of Women. Mosby, St Louis, 1995, p 119.
3. Levine, WC, et al: Development of sexually transmitted diseases treatment guidelines, 1993. Sex Transm Dis 21(2):S99, 1994.
4. Monif, GRG, et al (eds): Infectious Diseases in Obstetrics and Gynecology. IDI, Omaha, Nebr, 1993, p 189.
5. Felsenstein, D: Sexually transmitted disease. In Carlson, KJ, et al (eds): Primary Care of Women. Mosby, St Louis, 1995, p 121.
6. Levine, WC, et al: Development of sexually transmitted diseases treatment guidelines, 1993. Sex Transm Dis 21(2):S98, 1994.
7. Bard, DS, and Monif, GRG: *Trichomonas vaginalis.* In Monif, GRG, et al (eds): Infectious Diseases in Obstetrics and Gynecology. IDI, Omaha, Nebr, 1993, p 354.
8. Eisenstat, SA: Infectious exposure and immunization during pregnancy. In Carlson, KJ, et al (eds): Primary Care of Women. Mosby, St Louis, 1995, p 331.
9. Gall, S: Human genital papillomavirus infection. In Monif, GRG, et al (eds): Infectious Diseases in Obstetrics and Gynecology. IDI, Omaha, Nebr, 1993, p 108.
10. Eisenstat, SA: Infectious exposure and immunization during pregnancy. In Carlson, KJ, et al (eds): Primary Care of Women. Mosby, St Louis, 1995, p 332.

BIBLIOGRAPHY

Albaugh, B, and Gettrust, KV: Plans of Care for Specialty Practice: Surgical Nursing. Delmar, Albany, NY, 1994.

Anderson, C: Childhood sexually transmitted diseases: One consequence of sexual abuse. Public Health Nurs 12:1, 1995.

Carlson, KJ, et al (eds): Primary Care of Women. Mosby, St Louis, 1995, pp 106–125.

Eisenstat, SA: Infectious exposure and immunization during pregnancy. In Carlson, KJ, et al (eds): Primary Care of Women. Mosby, St Louis, 1995.

Felsenstein, D: Sexually transmitted disease. In Carlson, KJ, et al (eds): Primary Care of Women. Mosby, St Louis, 1995.

Fogel, CI, and Woods, NF (eds): Women's Health Care. Sage, Thousand Oaks, Calif, 1995, pp 572–609.

Gall, S: Human genital papillomavirus infection. In Monif, GRG, et al (eds): Infectious Diseases in Obstetrics and Gynecology. IDI, Omaha, Nebr, 1993.

Kazanjian, PH, and Eisenstat, SA: Human immunodeficiency virus. In Carlson, KJ, et al (eds): Primary Care of Women. Mosby, St Louis, 1995.

Kottman, LM: Pelvic inflammatory disease: Clinical overview. JOGNN, 24:8, 1995.

Koziel, MJ: Immunology of viral hepatitis. Am J Med 100(1):98, 1996.

Lehne, RA, et al: Pharmacology for Nursing Care, ed 2. WB Saunders, Philadelphia, 1994.

Lemcke, DP, et al (eds): Primary Care of Women. Appleton & Lange, Norwalk, Conn, 1995, pp 331–347.

Lemone, PM, and Burke, KM (eds): Medical Surgical Nursing: Critical Thinking in Client Care. Addison-Wesley, Menlo Park, Calif, 1996, pp 227–237.

Levine, WC, et al: Development of sexually transmitted diseases treatment guidelines, 1993. Sex Transm Dis 21(2):519, 1994.

McKinney, ES: Nursing care of women with complications during pregnancy. In Thompson, ED (ed): Maternity and Pediatric Nursing, ed 2. WB Saunders, Philadelphia, 1995.

Milburn, A, and Brewer, K: Sexually transmitted diseases. In O'Hara, MW, et al (eds): Psychological Aspects of Women's Health. Springer, New York, 1995.

Monif, GRG, et al (eds): Infectious Diseases in Obstetrics and Gynecology. IDI, Omaha, Nebr, 1993.

Phipps, WJ, et al (eds): Medical Surgical Nursing: Concepts and Clinical Practice. Mosby, St Louis, 1995, pp 1854–1878.

Quinn, TC: Recent advances in diagnosis of sexually transmitted diseases. Sex Transm Dis 21(2):96, 1994.

Rote, NS, Huether, SE, and McCance, KL: Hypersensitivities, infection and immunodeficiencies. In Huether, SE, and McCance (eds): Understanding Pathophysiology. Mosby, St Louis, 1996.

Ryan, KJ, Berkowitz, RS, and Barbieri, RL (eds): Kistner's Gynecology, ed 6. Mosby, St Louis, 1995, pp 496–531.

Sharts-Hopko, NC: Sexually transmitted diseases in women: What you need to know. Am J Nurs 4:46, 1997.

Sherwen, LN, Scoloveno, MA, and Weingarten, CT: Nursing Care of the Childbearing Family, ed 2. Appleton & Lange, Norwalk, Conn, 1995, pp 171–185.

Star, WI, Lommel, LL, and Shannon, MT (eds): Women's Primary Health Care: Protocols for Practice. American Nurses' Association, Washington, DC, 1995, pp 12-204, 13-3–13-16.

Thompson, ED (ed): Maternity and Pediatric Nursing, ed 2. WB Saunders, Philadelphia, 1995, pp 107–120.

Understanding the Musculoskeletal System

Musculoskeletal Function and Assessment

43

Donna D. Ignatavicius and Valerie C. Scanlon

Learning Objectives

Upon completion of this chapter, the student will be able to:

1. Describe the structure and function of the musculoskeletal system.
2. Identify major changes in the musculoskeletal system related to the aging process.
3. Discuss the importance of inspection, palpation, and determining mobility in a client with a musculoskeletal problem.
4. Describe the technique for performing a neurovascular assessment.
5. Discuss potential psychosocial problems that the nurse should assess when caring for clients with musculoskeletal problems.
6. Identify the major diagnostic tests used for clients with musculoskeletal problems and the associated nursing implications for each test.

Key Words

arthroscopy (ar-**THROW**-scop-ee)
articular (ar-**TIK**-yoo-lar)
bone (BOWN)
bursae (**BURR**-sah)
crepitation (crep-i-**TAY**-shun)
joint (JOYNT)
muscle (**MUSS**-uhl)
synovitis (sin-oh-**VIGH**-tis)
vertebrae (**VER**-te-bray)

Review of Normal Anatomy and Physiology

The skeletal and muscular systems may be considered one system because they work together to enable the body to move. The skeleton is the framework that supports the body and to which the voluntary **muscles** are attached. The skeletal framework includes the **joints** or articulations between **bones.** Contraction of a muscle pulls a bone and changes the angle of a joint. It is important to remember, however, that movement would not be possible without the proper functioning of the nervous, cardiovascular, and respiratory systems. Voluntary muscles require nerve impulses to contract, a continuous supply of blood provided by the circulatory system, and the oxygen provided by the respiratory system. See Cultural Considerations Box 43–1.

Skeletal System Tissues and Their Functions

The tissues that make up the skeletal system are bone tissue; cartilage, which covers most joint surfaces; and fibrous connective tissue, which forms the ligaments that connect one bone to another and is also part of the structure of joints. The tissues of the muscular system are skeletal (also called striated or voluntary) muscle; fibrous connective tissue, which forms the tendons that connect muscle to bone; and the fasciae, the strong membranes that enclose individual muscles.

Besides its role in movement, the skeleton has other functions. It protects organs from mechanical injury. For example the brain is protected by the skull and the heart and lungs are protected by the rib cage. Flat and irregular bones contain and protect the red bone marrow, one of the hematopoietic (blood-forming) tissues. The bones are also a storage site for excess calcium, which may be removed from bones to maintain a normal blood calcium level. Calcium in the blood is necessary for blood clotting and for the proper functioning of nerves and muscles.

Among the Chinese, the ulnar bone is longer than the radius, hip measurements are significantly smaller than Caucasians, and bone density is less.

African-Americans and European-Americans are taller than Native-Americans, followed by Mexican-Americans, who are taller than Asian-Americans. Children and adults from higher socioeconomic backgrounds are taller than their racial cohort group from lower socioeconomic backgrounds. Thus an adequate diet early in childhood affects the overall height of all ethnic and racial groups.

African-Americans have longer legs in comparison with European-Americans and Mexican-Americans. Thus their sitting/standing height ratio is greater.[1] Chairs may need to be adapted for more comfortable seating.

African-Americans have more muscle mass than do European-Americans. Women's bones are less dense than men's. Black women have denser bones than European-Americans, Asian-Americans, and Native-Americans. African-American women have a bone density similar to that of white men. Thus osteoporosis is less common among African-Americans.

The number of vertebrae varies from 23 to 25. Women more frequently have 23, and Eskimo and Native-Americans more frequently have 25.[1] This normal variant has no clinical significance.

Although the primary function of the muscular system is to move the skeleton, the voluntary muscles collectively contribute significantly to the heat production that maintains normal body temperature. Heat is one of the energy products of cell respiration, the process that produces adenosine triphosphate (ATP), the direct energy source for muscle contraction.

BONE TISSUE AND GROWTH OF BONE

Bone tissue is composed of bone cells, called osteocytes, within a strong nonliving matrix made of calcium salts and the protein collagen. In compact bone the osteocytes and matrix are in precise arrangements called haversian systems. Compact bone is very dense and to the unaided eye appears solid. In spongy bone the arrangement of cells and matrix is less precise, giving the bone a spongy appearance. Compact bone forms the diaphyses (shafts) of the long bones of the extremities and covers the spongy bone that forms the bulk of short, flat, and irregular bones.

A living bone is covered by a fibrous connective tissue membrane called the periosteum, which is the anchor for tendons and ligaments because the collagen fibers of all these structures merge to form connections of great strength. This membrane also contains the blood vessels that enter the bone itself (most bone has a very good blood supply) and bone-producing cells called osteoblasts that are activated to initiate repair when bone is damaged.

The growth of bone from fetal life until final adult height is attained depends on many factors. Proper nutrition provides the raw material to produce bone matrix: calcium, phosphorous, and protein. Vitamin D is essential for the efficient absorption of calcium and phosphorous from food in the small intestine. Vitamins A and C do not become part of bone but are needed for enzymes involved in the production of bone matrix (a process called calcification or ossification). Hormones directly necessary for growth include growth hormone (GH) from the anterior pituitary gland, thyroxine from the thyroid gland, and insulin from the pancreas. Growth hormone increases mitosis and protein synthesis in growing bones; thyroxine also increases protein synthesis, as well as increasing energy production from food. Insulin is essential for the efficient use of glucose to provide energy. If a child is lacking any of these hormones, growth will be much slower and the child will not reach his or her genetic potential for height.

Bone is not a static tissue, even when growth in height has ceased. There is a constant removal and replacement of calcium and phosphate (usually the rates are equal) to maintain normal blood levels of these minerals. Parathyroid hormone secreted by the parathyroid glands increases the removal of calcium and phosphate from bones; the hormone calcitonin from the thyroid gland promotes the retention of calcium in bones, although its greatest effects may be during childhood.

Osteoblasts produce bone matrix during normal growth, to replace matrix lost during normal turnover and to repair fractures. Other cells called osteoclasts reabsorb bone matrix when more calcium is needed in the blood and during normal growth and fracture repair when excess bone must be removed as bones change shape.

The sex hormones, estrogen from the ovaries or testosterone from the testes, are important for the retention of calcium in adult bones. For women after menopause, more calcium may be removed from bones than is replaced, leading to a thinning of bone tissue and the possibility of spontaneous fractures.

STRUCTURE OF THE SKELETON

The 206 bones of the human skeleton are in two divisions: the axial skeleton and the appendicular skeleton. The axial skeleton consists of the skull, vertebral column, and rib cage; all are flat or irregular bones and contain red bone marrow. The appendicular skeleton consists of the bones of the arms and legs and the shoulder and pelvic girdles, which attach the extremities to the axial skeleton (Fig. 43–1).

The long bones of the limbs are those of the arm, forearm, hand, and fingers and those of the thigh, leg, foot, and toes. All long bones have the same general structure: a central diaphysis or shaft with two ends called epiphyses. The

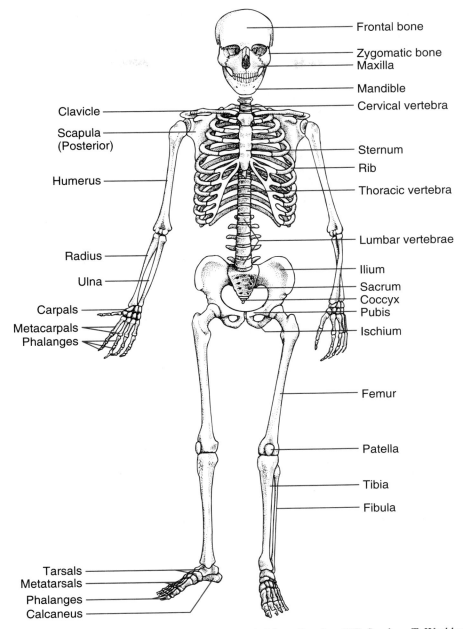

Figure 43–1. The full skeleton in anterior view. (Modified from Scanlon, VC, Sanders, T: Workbook for Essentials of Anatomy and Physiology, ed 2. FA Davis, Philadelphia, 1995, p 74, with permission.) See Plate 9.

diaphyses of long bones contain yellow bone marrow, which is mostly fat, that is, stored energy. The bones of the wrist and ankle are short bones, and those of the shoulder and pelvic girdles are considered flat bones. These bones also contain red bone marrow.

SKULL

The skull consists of 8 cranial bones and 14 facial bones and also contains the 3 auditory bones found in each middle ear cavity. The cranial bones that enclose and protect the brain are the frontal, two parietal, two temporal, occipi-

tal, sphenoid, and ethmoid (Fig. 43–2). All the joints between cranial bones and those between most of the facial bones are immovable joints called sutures. The mandible is the only movable facial bone; the temporomandibular joint is a condyloid joint (Table 43–1). The maxillae are the upper jaw bones, which also form the front of the hard palate. The rest of the facial bones are shown in Fig. 43–2.

VERTEBRAL COLUMN

The vertebral column (or spinal column) is made of individual bones called **vertebrae** (see Fig. 43–1). From top to

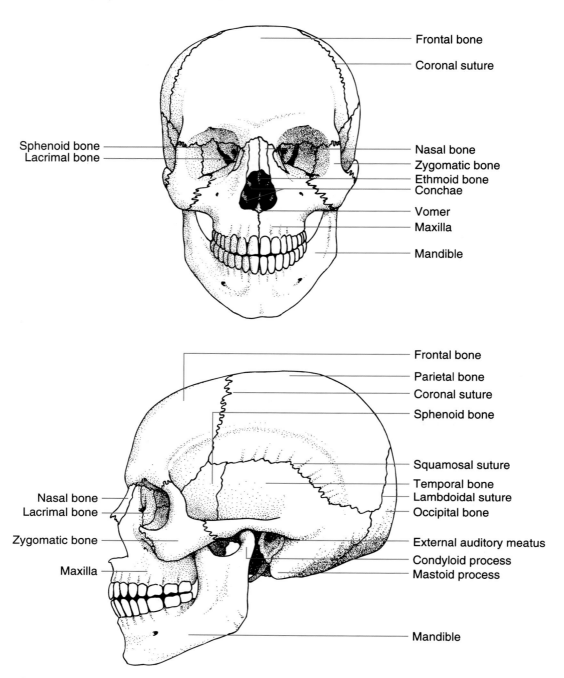

Figure 43–2. Anterior (*upper*) and left lateral (*lower*) views of the skull. (Modified from Scanlon, VC, Sanders, T: Workbook for Essentials of Anatomy and Physiology, ed 2. FA Davis, Philadelphia, 1995, p 75, with permission.) See Plate 10.

bottom there are 7 cervical, 12 thoracic, 5 lumbar, 5 sacral fused into 1 sacrum, and 4 or 5 coccygeal vertebrae fused into one coccyx.

The first cervical vertebra is the atlas, which articulates with the occipital bone of the skull and forms a pivot joint with the axis, the second cervical vertebra. The thoracic vertebrae articulate with the posterior ends of the ribs. The lumbar vertebrae are the largest and strongest. The sacrum permits the articulation of the two hip bones, the sacroiliac joints. The coccyx is the remnant of tail vertebrae, and some muscles of the perineum are attached to it.

The vertebrae as a unit form a flexible backbone that supports the trunk and head and contains and protects the spinal cord. The joints between vertebrae are symphysis joints in which a disk of fibrous cartilage serves as a cushion and permits slight movement.

Table 43–1. *Joints of the Appendicular Skeleton*

Type of Joint and Description	Examples
Symphysis—disk of fibrous cartilage between bones	Between vertebrae Between pubic bones
Ball and socket—movement in all planes	Scapula and humerus (shoulder) Pelvic bone and femur (hip)
Hinge—movement in one plane	Humerus and ulna (elbow) Femur and tibia (knee) Between phalanges (fingers and toes)
Condyloid—a hinge with some lateral movement	Temporal bone and mandible (lower jaw)
Pivot—rotation	Atlas and axis (neck) Radius and ulna (distal to elbow)
Gliding—side-to-side movement	Between carpals (wrist)
Saddle—movement in several planes	Carpometacarpal of thumb

RIB CAGE

The rib cage consists of the 12 pairs of ribs and the sternum, or breastbone. All the ribs articulate posteriorly with the thoracic vertebrae. The seven pairs of true ribs articulate directly with the sternum by means of costal cartilages; the three pairs of false ribs articulate indirectly with the sternum, and the two pairs of floating ribs do not articulate with the sternum at all.

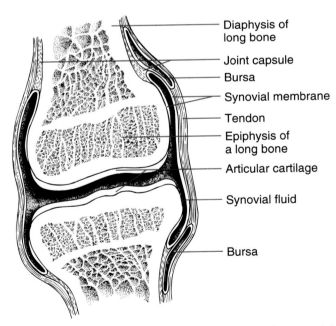

- Diaphysis of long bone
- Joint capsule
- Bursa
- Synovial membrane
- Tendon
- Epiphysis of a long bone
- Articular cartilage
- Synovial fluid
- Bursa

Figure 43–3. Longitudinal section through a typical synovial joint. (Modified from Scanlon, VC, Sanders, T: Workbook for Essentials of Anatomy and Physiology, ed 2. FA Davis, Philadelphia, 1995, p 85, with permission.)

The rib cage protects the heart and lungs, as well as upper abdominal organs such as the liver and spleen, from mechanical injury. During breathing, the flexible rib cage is pulled upward and outward by the external intercostal muscles to expand the chest cavity and bring about inhalation.

APPENDICULAR SKELETON

The bones of the appendicular skeleton are shown in Fig. 43–1. The important joints of the appendicular skeleton are summarized in Table 43–1.

STRUCTURE OF SYNOVIAL JOINTS

All freely movable joints (this excludes sutures and symphyses) are synovial joints in that they share similarities of structure (Fig. 43–3). On the joint surface of each bone is the **articular** cartilage, which provides a smooth surface. The joint capsule is similar to a sleeve. It is made of fibrous connective tissue and forms a strong sheath that encloses the joint. Lining the joint capsule is the synovial membrane, which secrets synovial fluid into the joint cavity. Synovial fluid prevents friction as the bones move.

Many synovial joints also have **bursae,** which are small sacs of synovial fluid between the joint and the tendons that cross over the joint. Bursae permit the tendons to slide easily as the joint moves.

Muscle Structure and Arrangements

One muscle is made of thousands of muscle cells (fibers), which are specialized for contraction. When a muscle contracts it shortens and pulls on a bone. Each muscle fiber receives its own motor nerve ending, and the number of fibers that contract will depend on the job the muscle has to do. Muscles are anchored to bones by tendons, which are made of fibrous connective tissue. A muscle usually has at least two tendons, each attached to a different bone. The more stationary attachment of the muscle is its origin; the more movable attachment is the insertion. The muscle itself crosses the joint formed by the two bones to which it is attached, and when the muscle contracts it pulls on the insertion and moves the bone in a specific direction.

The more than 600 muscles in the body are arranged so as to bring about a variety of movements. The two general types of arrangements are the opposing antagonists and the cooperative synergists.

Antagonistic muscles have opposite functions; such arrangements are necessary because muscles can only pull, not push. If the biceps brachii, for example, flexes the forearm, an antagonist, the triceps brachii, is needed to extend the forearm. Other examples of antagonists (Fig. 43–4) are

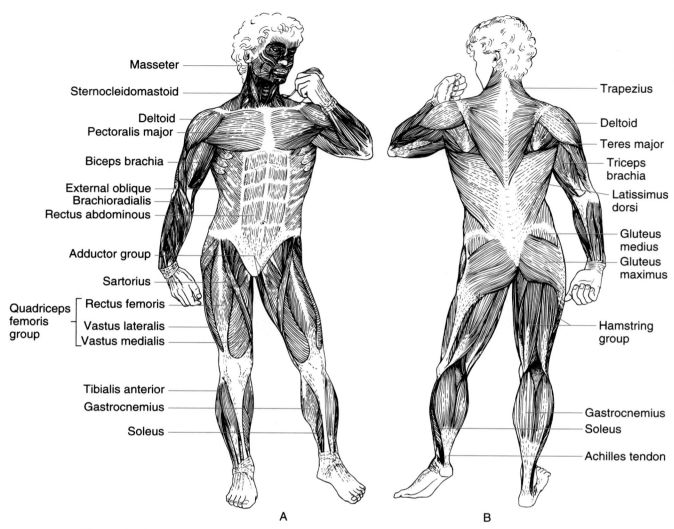

Figure 43–4. Major muscles. *(A)* Anterior view. *(B)* Posterior view. (Modified from Scanlon, VC, Sanders, T: Workbook for Essentials of Anatomy and Physiology, ed 2. FA Davis, Philadelphia, 1995, pp 100–101, with permission.) See Plate 11.

the quadriceps femoris and hamstring groups, the pectoralis major and the latissimus dorsi, and the tibialis anterior and gastrocnemius.

Synergistic muscles have similar functions or work together to perform a particular function. The brachioradialis is a synergist to the biceps brachii for flexion of the forearm; the sartorius is a synergist to the quadriceps group for flexion of the thigh. Synergists are necessary to provide slight differences in angles when joints are moved.

Role of the Nervous system

Skeletal muscles are voluntary muscles in that nerve impulses are essential to cause contraction. Such nerve impulses originate in the motor areas of the frontal lobes of the cerebral cortex. The coordination of voluntary movement is a function of the cerebellum. The cerebellum also regulates muscle tone, the state of slight contraction usually present in muscles. Good muscle tone is important for posture and for good coordination.

NEUROMUSCULAR JUNCTION

Each of the thousands of muscle fibers in a muscle has its own motor nerve ending; the neuromuscular junction is the termination of the motor neuron on the muscle fiber (Fig. 43–5). The axon terminal is the enlarged tip of the motor neuron. It contains sacs of the neurotransmitter acetylcholine. The membrane of the muscle fiber, called the sarcolemma, contains receptor sites for acetylcholine and also the inactivator cholinesterase. The synaptic cleft is the small space between the axon terminal and the sarcolemma.

When a nerve impulse arrives at the axon terminal, it causes the release of acetylcholine, which diffuses across

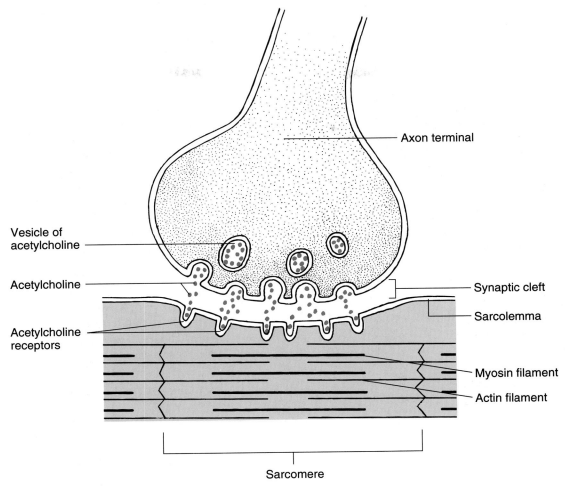

Figure 43–5. Neuromuscular junction and sarcomeres. (Modified from Scanlon, VC, Sanders, T: Workbook for Essentials of Anatomy and Physiology, ed 2. FA Davis, Philadelphia, 1995, p 97, with permission.)

the synaptic cleft and bonds to the acetylcholine receptors on the sarcolemma. This makes the sarcolemma very permeable to sodium ions, which rush into the cell and generate an electrical impulse (an action potential) along the entire sarcolemma. This electrical change triggers a series of reactions in the internal units of contraction called sarcomeres. Put very simply, filaments of the protein myosin pull on filaments of another protein called actin, and the sarcomere shortens. All of the thousands of sarcomeres in a muscle fiber shorten, and the entire cell contracts. If a muscle has little work to do, few of its many muscle fibers will contract, but if the muscle has more work to do, more of its muscle fibers will contract.

Aging and the Musculoskeletal System

The amount of calcium in bones is dependent on several factors. Good nutrition is certainly one, but age is another,

especially for women. One function of estrogen or testosterone is the maintenance of a strong bone matrix. For women after menopause, bone matrix loses more calcium than is replaced. Weight-bearing joints are also subject to damage after many years. Often the articular cartilage wears down and becomes rough, leading to pain and stiffness.

Muscle strength declines with age as the process of protein synthesis decreases. Such loss of strength need not be drastic, however, and even aging muscles benefit from regular exercise.

Nursing Assessment of the Musculoskeletal System

Unlike other body systems, nursing assessment of the client with a musculoskeletal health problem is limited by the structure of the body system. The initial assessment begins with a history and then proceeds to a physical and psychosocial assessment. Frequent neurovascular assessments may be needed if there is a risk of circulation impairment, for example, if the client has a fracture or musculoskeletal surgery (Table 43–2).

SUBJECTIVE DATA

History

The initial assessment begins with a client history. The nurse gathers information about the client's musculoskeletal problems. Often, the client reports pain or related stiffness and tenderness. The pain may be acute or chronic. The P-Q-R-S-T model can be used to assess the client's pain:

P—Provoking incident? (Did a certain incident or event cause the pain?)

Q—Quality of pain? (What does the pain feel like? For example, is it burning, throbbing, or stabbing?)

R—Region, radiation, and relief? (Where is the pain? Does the pain move? Does anything help relieve the pain?)

S—Severity of pain? (How severe is the pain? See Chapter 9 for a discussion of pain rating.)

T—Time? (How long does the pain last? When does it occur? Is it worse at night or during the day?)

Physical Assessment

Three areas of musculoskeletal assessment are important—inspection, palpation, and mobility. If the client is able to walk, the nurse assesses the client's posture and gait, noting poor posture or limping. Spinal deformities are especially significant because they can compromise breathing and balance. Other gross deformities, such as unequal limbs or malalignment, are recorded. The joints and muscles of the arms, hands, legs, and feet are inspected for deformity, redness, swelling, or **crepitation** (grating sound as joint or bone moves).

After inspection, the nurse palpates areas of swelling or redness, or areas where the client reported pain. For exam-

ple, reddened joints should be palpated for **synovitis** (swollen synovial tissue within the joint) or the presence of bony nodes. In some cases, joints and muscles may seem healthy but are tender when palpated.

After inspection and palpation, the nurse assesses joint mobility. The client should have sufficient range of motion to independently perform activities of daily living. The nurse pays particular attention to the hands and observes movement in finger joints. For a quick and easy assessment of range of motion in the hands, the nurse asks the client to touch each finger, one by one, to the thumb, and then to make a fist.

Muscle strength should also be evaluated. The client can grip the nurse's hand or squeeze a sphygmomanometer bulb to check grip strength. Pushing an extremity against the nurse's hand provides a general indication of muscle strength. More specific evaluation is performed by a physical therapist (PT) or occupational therapist (OT). Using a scale of 0 to 5 (0 = paralysis and 5 = moving a muscle against resistance) the PT or OT measures the strength of each muscle group and rates it as a fraction. For example, 5/5 means that the client reached a 5 out of 5 possible on the muscle strength scale.

Psychosocial Assessment

Deformity from arthritis or other musculoskeletal disorder can affect a client's body image and self-concept. Clients often avoid social events and tend to withdraw from people. Chronic pain may also keep the client from socializing or from working. Many work days are lost as a result of both acute and chronic musculoskeletal problems.

Clients may experience a tremendous amount of stress from the pain, loss of income, and withdrawal from friends and family. The nurse assesses the client's ability to cope, asking what coping strategies have been used in the past for other life stressors. Support systems for the client need to be identified, especially spiritual and social systems.

CRITICAL THINKING: Mr. Smith

Mr. Smith, 80, is brought to the emergency department with a left fractured hip. He is positioned for comfort while the nurse collects data.

1. What information should the nurse obtain in Mr. Smith's history?
2. What areas should be assessed in Mr. Smith's physical examination?

Answers at end of chapter.

Table 43–2. **Neurovascular Assessment**

Assess for:	Note and Report:
Color	Pallor, cyanosis, redness, or discoloration
Temperature	Unusual coolness or warmth
Pain	Pain that is worse on passive motion, pain that no longer responds to analgesics
Movement	Inability to move
Sensation	Inability to feel or tingling
Pulses	Diminished or no distal pulses
Capillary refill	Nailbed that does not blanch in 3–5 seconds

synovitis: synovia—joint + itis—inflammation

Diagnostic Tests

Diagnosis of musculoskeletal problems is assisted by laboratory tests, x-rays, and other nonradiological tests. Specific tests for clients with connective tissue diseases are described in Chapter 44.

LABORATORY TESTS

Serum Calcium and Phosphorus

Bone disorders often cause changes in calcium and phosphorus (or phosphate) levels. When a person is healthy, calcium and phosphorus have an inverse relationship. This means that when serum calcium increases, serum phosphorus decreases, and vice versa. Some disorders, however, cause an increase in both values or a decrease in both values. Calcium and phosphorus levels are also abnormal when the parathyroid glands are not functioning properly.

Serum calcium tends to decrease in clients with osteoporosis or in people who consume inadequate amounts of calcium in their diets. Serum calcium levels increase in clients with bone cancer, particularly those with metastatic disease.

Alkaline Phosphatase

Alkaline phosphatase (ALP) is an enzyme that increases when bone or liver tissue is damaged. In metabolic bone diseases and bone cancer, ALP increases to reflect osteoblast (bone-forming cell) activity.

Serum Muscle Enzymes

When muscle tissue is damaged, a number of serum enzymes are released into the bloodstream, including skeletal muscle creatine kinase (CK-MM [CK_3]), aldolase (ALD), aspartate aminotransferase (AST), and lactate dehydrogenase (LDH). These enzymes increase in certain muscle diseases such as polymyositis and dermatomyositis.

RADIOGRAPHICAL TESTS

Standard X-Rays

The skeleton and surrounding tissues can easily be seen on standard x-rays (Fig. 43–6). An x-ray can determine bone density (although not as well as some other tests for this), alignment, swelling, and intactness.

Although there is no special nursing care associated with x-rays, the nurse should inform the elderly client or clients with pain that when they lie on the x-ray table it will be cold and hard.

Computed Tomography

Tomograms are x-rays that produce slices of tissue for clearer imaging focus of a particular part of the bone. Com-

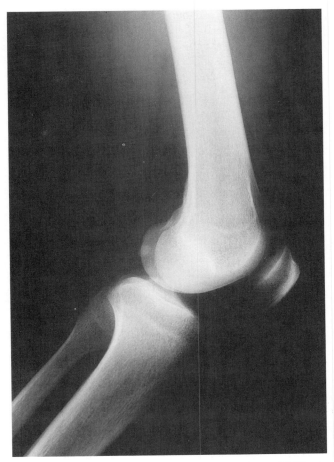

Figure 43–6. A lateral x-ray of a normal knee. (From McKinnis, LN: Fundamentals of Orthopedic Radiology. FA Davis, Philadelphia, 1997, p 255, with permission.)

puted tomography (CT) is especially helpful for diagnosing problems of the joints or vertebral column (Fig. 43–7). It may be used with or without a contrast medium (similar to a dye), which is given orally or intravenously. If a contrast medium is used, the nurse checks that the client is not allergic to iodine or shellfish. The client should be given nothing by mouth (NPO) for at least 4 hours before the test.

The nurse teaches the client that he or she must lie still for 30 minutes or longer during the test while encased in a machine. Reports of claustrophobia and annoying clicking sounds made by the scanner while it is rotating are common.

Arthrography

An x-ray of any synovial joint can be performed for clients with suspected joint trauma. The most common joints tested are the knee and shoulder. For this test, a contrast medium is injected into the joint to help visualize the soft tissues.

The nurse informs the client that the test may be temporarily uncomfortable while the contrast medium is injected. After the procedure, the joint is usually swollen for

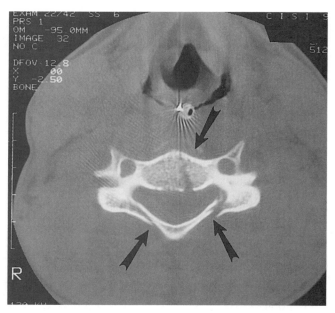

Figure 43–7. Computer tomography scan of fifth cervical vertebra showing a burst fracture of the vertebral body *(top arrow)* and both laminae *(bottom arrows)*. (From McKinnis, LN: Fundamentals of Orthopedic Radiology. FA Davis, Philadelphia, 1997, p 23, with permission.)

several days. Ice and elevation help diminish swelling. Strenuous physical activity should be avoided for 12 to 24 hours.

OTHER DIAGNOSTIC TESTS

Magnetic Resonance Imaging

Magnetic resonance imaging (MRI), with or without contrast media, is a commonly performed test to diagnose

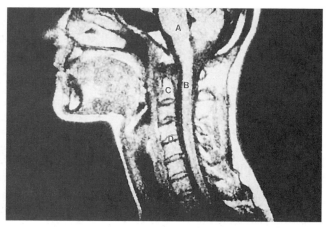

Figure 43–8. Magnetic resonance image of a normal cervical spine. *(A)* Cerebellum. *(B)* Spinal cord. *(C)* Marrow of C2 vertebral body. *(D)* C4-5 intervertebral disk. (From McKinnis, LN: Fundamentals of Orthopedic Radiology. FA Davis, Philadelphia, 1997, p 26, with permission.)

musculoskeletal problems, especially those involving soft tissue (Fig. 43–8). MRI is more accurate than CT for diagnosing many problems of the vertebral column. If the client has had previous spinal surgery, a contrast medium is used.

The image is produced by the interaction of the magnetic fields and radio waves. For very large clients or those who are claustrophobic, the open MRI offers a comfortable alternative to the traditional machine.

The nurse or radiological technician ensures that the client removes all metal objects. Pacemakers, surgical clips, and any other internal metal in the client are contraindications for MRI (Table 43–3).

Nuclear Medicine Scans

Several tests are performed using radioactive material to help visualize bone and other tissues. A bone scan allows visualization of the entire skeleton, if desired (Fig. 43–9). It is used primarily for detecting metastatic bone disease, osteomyelitis (bone infection), and unexplained bone pain. Advances in MRI have decreased the use of bone scans.

A nuclear medicine physician or technician injects the client with technetium, a radioactive substance. As a bone-seeking material, it migrates to bone tissue. The client is reassured that the substance is not harmful in any way.

For an accurate test, the client must be able to lie still for 30 to 60 minutes during scanning. Clients who are elderly, restless, agitated, or in pain may therefore find this test uncomfortable. The physician looks for "hot spots," indicating areas where the radioactive substance is concentrated. These hot spots indicate abnormal bone metabolism, a sign of bone disease.

LEARNING TIP

Hot spots are created because increased circulation occurs in abnormal bone areas, resulting in increased amounts of the radioactive substance being transported to the abnormal area. This produces a hot spot.

Gallium/Thallium Scans

A gallium or thallium scan is similar to a bone scan but is more specific and sensitive as a diagnostic test. Gallium migrates to bone, brain, and breast tissue and is therefore used to diagnose problems in these tissues as well.

Thallium is better for detecting osteosarcoma than gallium. Traditionally used for heart problems, especially myocardial damage, thallium is now used for evaluation of bone cancers. Like the bone scan, these scans are not harmful to the client.

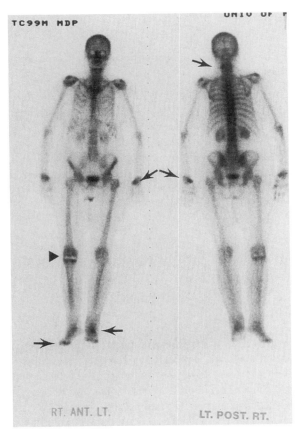

Figure 43–9. Bone scan of whole skeleton in client with degenerative joint disease. Arrows show abnormal areas with increased uptake. Total knee prosthesis is shown at arrowhead. (From Richardson, JK, and Iglarsh, ZA: Clinical Orthopaedic Physical Therapy. WB Saunders, Philadelphia, 1994, p 646, with permission.)

Arthroscopy

An arthroscope is a tubular instrument that allows the surgeon to look directly into a joint. The knee and shoulder are the joints most often evaluated.

Because **arthroscopy** is an invasive procedure performed under local or light general anesthesia, the client is treated as a surgical candidate. The procedure is done on an ambulatory basis in same-day surgery settings.

For the knee, the surgeon makes several very small incisions and inserts the scope to visualize the soft tissues from several angles. The knee joint is flexed and irrigated during the procedure. If the surgeon discovers a tear or other soft tissue damage, he or she usually repairs the injury through the scope using special instrumentation. After the procedure, a bulky dressing wrapped with an elastic bandage is typically applied, depending on the surgeon and nature of the procedure.

---

arthroscopy: arthron—joint + skopein—to examine

Table 43–3. **The Client Preparing for Magnetic Resonance Imaging**

- Is the client pregnant?
- Does the client have magnetic metal fragments or implants, such as an aneurysm clip?
- If the client has an IV catheter, can it be converted to a saline lock temporarily?
- Is the client claustrophobic?
- Does the client have a pacemaker or electronic implant?
- Can the client be without supplemental oxygen for an hour?
- Can the client tolerate the supine position for 20–30 min?
- Can the client lie still for 20–30 min?
- Does the client need life support equipment?
- Can the client communicate clearly and understand verbal communication?

(From Ignatavicius, DD, Workman, ML, and Mishler, MA: Medical-Surgical Nursing: A Nursing Process Approach, ed 2. WB Saunders, Philadelphia, 1995, Chart 49–3, with permission.)

The nurse in the postanesthesia care unit (PACU) assesses neurovascular status of the surgical foot and leg frequently (see Table 43–2). If the client had a diagnostic arthroscopy and no surgical repair, the PACU nurse encourages the client to exercise the leg, including straight-leg raises. A mild analgesic usually relieves pain, and the client returns to regular activities within the next 24 to 48 hours. However, if surgery was performed, the client may have activity restriction and need a stronger analgesic, such as oxycodone with acetaminophen (Tylox, Percocet).

Although complications are not common, the nurse monitors and teaches the client to monitor the following:

- Thrombophlebitis (blood clot and vein inflammation)
- Infection
- Increased joint pain
- Hypothermia (decreased body temperature that can occur within a few hours after the procedure)

If the client had surgery, the client returns to the physician's office in about a week to check for complications and progress. The client may need crutches for the first week to limit weight bearing, depending on the surgical procedure performed.

Bone or Muscle Biopsy

Bone or muscle tissue can be surgically extracted for microscopic examination. This invasive test may confirm cancer or infection (bone biopsy) or inflammation or damage (muscle biopsy). Two techniques are used to retrieve tissue: needle (closed) or incisional (open) biopsy.

A closed biopsy can be performed in the client's room or special procedures area. After local or general anesthesia, the physician inserts a long needle into the tissue for extraction of a sample.

The open biopsy is performed in the operating suite under general anesthesia. A small incision is made and a sec-

HOME HEALTH HINTS

- Clients are considered homebound if (1) they are bed-bound or require the maximum assistance to ambulate while using a walker or to transfer; (2) they can ambulate with only moderate assistance while using a cane to negotiate uneven surfaces; or (3) they can leave home only for periods of relatively short duration or for need of medical treatment.

- When testing strength, extend two or three fingers (with no rings on them) and ask the client to squeeze the fingers.

- Observe clients moving around a room or bed. If they are clumsy or have involuntary movement, make efforts during that visit and subsequent visits to protect them from potential injury. Research has shown that pain or fear of falling may prevent a client from moving and functioning to maximum potential.

- Encourage clients to wear flat, sturdy, rubber-soled shoes to prevent slipping, tripping, or turning an ankle.

- Use sand or cat box filler on icy steps to increase traction, preventing slips and falls.

- Clients who use walkers can get pressure ulcers on their palms. One way to relieve the pressure is to wear padded cycling gloves that leave the fingers free.

tion of bone or muscle is removed. A sterile pressure dressing is applied because bone is very vascular.

The nurse inspects the biopsy site for bleeding, swelling, and hematoma formation. Increased pain that is unresponsive to analgesic medication may indicate bleeding in the soft tissue. The area is not moved for 8 to 12 hours to prevent bleeding. Vital signs and neurovascular assessments are monitored (see Table 43–2).

Ultrasonography

Sound waves are used to detect osteomyelitis (bone infection), soft tissue disorders, traumatic joint injuries, and surgical hardware placement. For this noninvasive procedure, the technician first applies a jellylike conducting substance over the area to be tested. A metal probe is moved over the area while a machine records the images. No special client instructions are needed for this test.

Review Questions

1. Which one of the following bones of the skull is not directly involved in protecting the brain?
   a. Temporal
   b. Occipital
   c. Sphenoid
   d. Zygomatic

2. Which one of the following joints is an immovable joint?
   a. Hinge
   b. Pivot
   c. Suture
   d. Ball and socket

3. In a synovial joint, a smooth surface on the ends of the bones is provided by which one of the following?
   a. Articular cartilage
   b. Synovial membrane
   c. Bursae
   d. Joint capsule

4. Which one of the following is the function of synovial fluid in joints?
   a. Exchange nutrients
   b. Prevent friction
   c. Absorb water
   d. Wear away rough surfaces

5. When a muscle contracts, which one of the following occurs?
   a. Lengthens and pulls a bone
   b. Shortens and pushes a bone
   c. Lengthens and pushes a bone
   d. Shortens and pulls a bone

6. Which one of the following is included in neurovascular checks of the lower extremities?
   a. Level of consciousness
   b. Pupil reaction
   c. Femoral pulses
   d. Orientation

7. When the nurse is evaluating discharge teaching knowledge regarding activity for a client who had an arthroscopy, the nurse would document understanding if which one of the following statements is made by the client?
   a. "I can return to my construction job in the morning."
   b. "I should exercise my right knee every 2 hours."
   c. "I will immobilize my left leg for 12 hours."
   d. "I will rest my right leg for 48 hours."

ANSWERS TO CRITICAL THINKING

CRITICAL THINKING: Mr. Smith

1. Allergies, how and when injury occurred, previous surgeries, medications, medical history.
2. Left leg compared with right leg: limb length, deformity, pain, loss of range of motion, edema, ecchymosis; neurovascular checks: movement, sensation (numbness/tingling); presence of pulses, skin temperature, color, capillary refill.

REFERENCE

1. Seidel, H, et al: Mosby's Guide to Physical Examination, ed 3. Mosby, St Louis, 1995.

BIBLIOGRAPHY

Bates, BB: A Guide to Physical Examination and History Taking. WB Saunders, Philadelphia, 1995.

Ignatavicius, DD, Workman, ML, and Mishler, MA: Medical-Surgical Nursing: A Nursing Process Approach, ed 2. WB Saunders, Philadelphia, 1995.

Jarvis, C: Physical Examination and Health Assessment, ed 2. WB Saunders, Philadelphia, 1997.

McKinnis, LN: Fundamentals of Orthopedic Radiology. FA Davis, Philadelphia, 1997.

Neal, L: Basic musculoskeletal assessment: Tips for the home health nurse. Home Healthc Nurse 15(4):227, 1997.

Patel, PR, and Lauerman, WC: The use of magnetic resonance imaging in the diagnosis of lumbar disc disease. Orthop Nurs 16(1):59, 1997.

Nursing Care of Clients with Musculoskeletal and Connective Tissue Disorders

Donna D. Ignatavicius

Learning Objectives

Upon completion of this chapter, the student will be able to:

1. Differentiate between the care for osteoarthritis and rheumatoid arthritis.
2. Describe the pathophysiology and treatment for gout.
3. Discuss nursing care for the client with systemic lupus erythematosus, progressive systemic sclerosis, and polymyositis.
4. Plan care for the client undergoing a total joint replacement.
5. Provide client education for a client with a lower extremity amputation and prosthesis.
6. Define sprain and strain injuries.
7. Identify the signs and symptoms of fractures.
8. Describe the nursing care associated with casts and traction.
9. Plan care for a client with a fractured hip.
10. Discuss the common causes of osteomyelitis.
11. List risk factors for the development of osteoporosis.
12. Identify the signs and symptoms that may be seen in clients with Paget's disease.
13. Explain the characteristics and treatment for clients with primary and metastatic bone tumors.

Key Words

arthritis (ar-**THRYE**-tis)
arthrocentesis (AR-throw-cen-**TEE**-sis)
arthroplasty (**AR**-throw-PLAS-te)
avascular necrosis (a-**VAS**-kue-lar ne-**KROW**-sis)
fasciotomy (fash-e-**OTT**-oh-me)
hemipelvectomy (hem-e-pell-**VEC**-toe-me)
hyperuricemia (HIGH-per-yoor-a-**SEE**-me-ah)
osteomyelitis (AHS-tee-oh-my-**LIGHT**-tis)

osteosarcoma (AHS-tee-oh-sar-**KOH**-mah)
polymyositis (PAH-lee-my-oh-**SIGH**-tis)
replantation (re-plan-**TAY**-shun)
scleroderma (SKLER-ah-**DER**-ma)
synovitis (sin-oh-**VIGH**-tis)
vasculitis (VAS-kue-**LIGH**-tis)

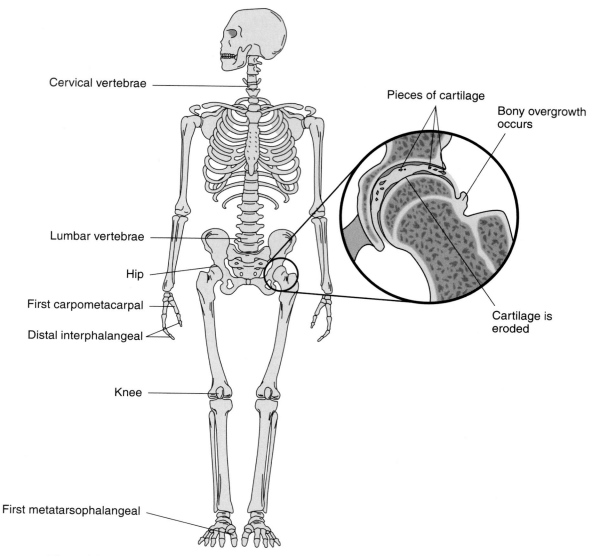

Figure 44–1. Common joints affected by osteoarthritis and the changes that result within the joint.

Connective Tissue Disorders

Connective tissue disorders (CTDs) comprise a group of over 100 diseases in which the major signs and symptoms result from joint involvement. Some CTDs affect only one part of the body; others affect many body organs and systems. Several of the most common disorders are discussed here, including osteoarthritis, gout, rheumatoid **arthritis,** systemic lupus erythematosus, progressive systemic sclerosis, and polymyositis.

OSTEOARTHRITIS

Osteoarthritis (OA) is the most common type of connective tissue disorder, affecting more than 20 million people in the United States. The term *arthritis* means inflammation of the joint, but OA is *not* a primary inflammatory process.

Therefore some health care providers may refer to this disorder as degenerative joint disease (DJD). This term better reflects its pathophysiology.

Pathophysiology

Osteoarthritis occurs when the articular cartilage and bone ends of joints slowly deteriorate. The joint space narrows and bone spurs develop. The joint may become somewhat inflamed, but this repair process is not able to overcome the rapid loss of cartilage and bone. Eventually, joint deformities, pain, and immobility result in the client's functional decline. Weight-bearing joints (hips and knees), hands, and the vertebral column are most often affected (Fig. 44–1).

---

arthritis: arthron—joint + itis—inflammation

Causes and Types

The most common type of OA is primary (idiopathic) osteoarthritis. In this type, the cause of the disorder has not been identified; however, several risk factors are known. Aging, obesity, and physical activities that create mechanical stress on joints are major risks. Each of these factors causes prolonged or excessive "wear and tear" on synovial joints. Almost everyone over 60 years of age has some degree of symptomatic joint degeneration. Native-Americans are affected more often than other groups, but the reason for this has not been found.

Clients with secondary osteoarthritis develop their joint degeneration as a result of trauma, sepsis, congenital anomalies, certain metabolic diseases (such as Paget's disease), or systemic inflammatory connective tissue disorders such as rheumatoid arthritis.

Signs and Symptoms

The client usually seeks medical attention when joint pain and stiffness become severe or the client has problems with everyday activities. One or more joints may be affected. Joint pain intensifies after physical activity but lessens following rest. If the vertebral column is involved, the client complains of radiating pain and muscle spasms in the affected extremity.

About half of clients with OA have bony nodes on the joints of their fingers, called Heberden's and Bouchard's nodes. Women tend to have them more often than men, and they may or may not be painful. The nodes have a familial tendency and are often a cosmetic concern to female clients.

Diagnostic Tests

X-rays are very useful in outlining joint structure and detecting bone changes. A computed tomography (CT) or magnetic resonance imaging (MRI) scan may be used to diagnose vertebral joint involvement.

CRITICAL THINKING: Mr. Dennis

Mr. Dennis is a 59-year-old, overweight carpenter who visits his physician with complaints of knee and wrist pain. He has noticed that it is becoming increasingly difficult to climb a ladder or use a hammer. The physician suspects osteoarthritis.

1. What questions would the physician most likely ask Mr. Dennis?
2. What risk factor(s) does he have?
3. What other signs and symptoms might he have?

Answers at end of chapter.

Treatment

Management of clients with OA centers on pain control, which is accomplished by drug therapy and other pain relief measures. An interdisciplinary approach is needed to prevent decreased mobility and preserve joint function.

Medication

Although not used alone, drug therapy to reduce pain is common for clients with OA. The most typically used drugs are nonsteroidal anti-inflammatory drugs (NSAIDs) (Table 44–1). These drugs have analgesic and anti-inflammatory effects, but may cause side effects if not carefully monitored. Common side effects include gastrointestinal distress, bleeding tendencies, and sodium and fluid retention. Elderly clients receiving NSAIDs on a routine basis should be carefully monitored for congestive heart failure or high blood pressure as a result of fluid retention.

Other commonly prescribed drugs are acetaminophen (Tylenol) and muscle relaxants, such as cyclobenzaprine HCl (Flexeril), if the client experiences muscle spasms with vertebral spine involvement.

Rest and Exercise

Joint pain tends to decrease in clients with OA when they rest. Rest must be balanced with exercise, though, to prevent muscle atrophy from disuse. A severely inflamed joint may be splinted by the occupational or physical therapist to promote rest to a selected joint.

Joints should always be placed in their functional position, that is, a position that will not lead to contractures. For example, only a small pillow should be placed under the head to prevent excessive neck flexion.

Heat and Cold

The client with OA usually prefers heat therapy unless the joint is acutely inflamed. Hot packs, warm compresses, warm showers, moist heating pads, and paraffin dips provide sources of heat for the client.

Table 44–1. **Common Drugs Used for Connective Tissue Diseases**

Salicylates (aspirin, Ecotrin)
Nonsteroidal anti-inflammatory drugs
- Naproxen (Naprosyn)
- Flurbiprofen (Ansaid)
- Piroxicam (Feldene)
- Diclofenac (Voltaren)
Methotrexate (Mexate)
Gold salts (auranofin [Ridaura])
Plaquenil Sulfate
D-penicillamine (Cuprimine)
Prednisone (Deltasone)
Azathioprine (Imuran)
Cyclophosphamide (Cytoxan)

Diet

There is no arthritis diet that cures or reverses osteoarthritis. The obese or overweight client needs to lose weight to decrease stress, and therefore pain, on weight-bearing joints.

Complementary Therapies

In the United States, the popularity of complementary or alternative therapies to reduce pain and stress has grown tremendously. Many people spend out-of-pocket money for imagery, music therapy, acupressure, acupuncture, and other holistic modalities to foster the mind-body-spirit connection. Clients with arthritis also seek these interventions, especially when traditional treatments fail.

Surgery

If the client's pain is not successfully managed, a total joint replacement (TJR) may be indicated. A TJR is the most common type of **arthroplasty** that is performed, and it is discussed in detail later in this chapter under Musculoskeletal Surgery.

Nursing Process

Assessment

The nurse assesses the client's complaint of pain and observes the joints for signs of inflammation or deformity. After pain management modalities are implemented, it is especially important to note the client's response to these interventions.

Nursing Diagnosis

The primary nursing diagnoses for the client with OA include but are not limited to the following:

- Chronic pain
- Body image disturbance
- Self-care deficit
- Impaired physical mobility

Planning

The nurse collaborates with the interdisciplinary health team, especially the physical or occupational therapist, to meet the goals of pain management and improved mobility. For clients who need weight reduction, the dietitian is an important resource. The social worker, discharge planner, or case manager can help make arrangements for home care if needed. A home care aide may be necessary to help the client with activities of daily living (ADL) and mobility.

Implementation

The case manager coordinates the activities of the health care team. A vital function of each member is health teaching.

Table 44–2. Energy Conservation for the Client with Arthritis

- Balance activity with rest. Take one or two naps each day.
- Pace yourself; do not plan too much for one day.
- Set priorities. Determine which activities are most important, and do them first.
- Delegate responsibility and tasks to your family and friends.
- Plan ahead to prevent last-minute rushing and stress.
- Learn your own activity tolerance and do not exceed it.

(From Ignatavicius, DD, Workman, ML, and Mishler, MA: Medical-Surgical Nursing: A Nursing Process Approach, ed 2. WB Saunders, Philadelphia, 1995, with permission.)

Evaluation

The best indicator of whether the plan of care was successful for the client with OA is the client's report of pain. If pain subsides or decreases, the plan was successful. If the pain worsens, surgery may be needed. Another important outcome is the client's satisfaction with his or her ability to function every day.

Client Education

The client with osteoarthritis is seldom admitted to the hospital for OA unless surgery is scheduled. However, many clients with OA are admitted for other reasons, and their arthritis needs must also be considered in the comprehensive plan of care. Most clients residing in nursing homes also have osteoarthritis, which can affect their participation in recreational activities, as well as their ADL.

In any setting, including the home, clients can be taught ways to protect their joints and conserve energy. Nurses need to teach clients and their families how to promote health. Table 44–2 lists tips for joint protection and energy conservation.

RHEUMATOID ARTHRITIS

Rheumatoid arthritis (RA) is a chronic, progressive, systemic inflammatory disease that destroys synovial joints and other connective tissues, including major organs. It affects women three times more often than men, and Native-Americans, especially Pima Indians, more often than other ethnic groups. The typical age of onset is the young to middle-aged woman.

Pathophysiology

Inflammatory cells and chemicals cause **synovitis,** an inflammation of the synovium (lining within the joint capsule). As the inflammation progresses, the synovium becomes thick and fluid accumulation causes joint swelling

---

arthroplasty: arthro—joint + plasty—creation of
synovitis: synovia—synovial fluid or tissue + itis—inflammation

and pain (Fig. 44–2). A destructive pannus consisting of vascular granulation tissue erodes the joint cartilage and eventually destroys bone. Joint deformity and bone loss are common in late RA.

Synovial joints are not the only connective tissues involved in RA. Any connective tissue may be affected, including blood vessels, nerves, kidneys, pericardium, lungs, and subcutaneous tissue. The result of body system involvement is malfunction or failure of the organ or system. Death can occur if the disease does not respond to treatment.

Many clients experience spontaneous remissions and exacerbations of RA. The symptoms of the disease may disappear without treatment for months or years. Then the disease may exacerbate ("flare up") just as unpredictably. Exacerbations usually occur when the client experiences physical or emotional stress, such as surgery or infection.

Causes and Types

Rheumatoid arthritis can occur at any age. When affecting children, the disease is sometimes called juvenile RA. At any age, the exact cause of RA is unknown. It is probably an autoimmune disease, meaning that unusual antibodies (rheumatoid factor) develop against normal antibodies in the body, forming antibody complexes. These complexes lodge in synovium and other connective tissues, causing local and systemic inflammation.

The origin of the rheumatoid factor is not clear, but a genetic predisposition is likely. RA affects people with a family history of the disease two to three times more often than the rest of the population.

Signs and Symptoms

Signs and symptoms vary because the disease progresses in different patterns and rates from person to person. In general, the signs and symptoms can be divided into early and late manifestations (Table 44–3).

Table 44–3. Key Features of Rheumatoid Arthritis

Early Manifestations

Joint
• Inflammation

Systemic
• Low-grade fever
• Fatigue
• Weakness
• Anorexia
• Paresthesias

Late Manifestations

Joint
• Deformities, e.g., swan neck or ulnar deviation
• Moderate to severe pain and morning stiffness

Systemic
• Osteoporosis
• Severe fatigue
• Anemia
• Weight loss
• Subcutaneous nodules
• Peripheral neuropathy
• Vasculitis
• Pericarditis
• Fibrotic lung disease
• Sjögren's syndrome
• Renal disease

(From Ignatavicius, DD, Workman, ML, and Mishler, MA: Medical-Surgical Nursing: A Nursing Process Approach, ed 2. WB Saunders, Philadelphia, 1995, with permission.)

The typical pattern of joint inflammation is bilateral and symmetrical. The disease usually begins in the upper extremities and progresses to other joints over many years (Fig. 44–3). Affected joints are slightly reddened, warm, swollen, stiff, and painful. The client with RA often has difficulty moving for over 30 minutes after resting, sometimes referred to as morning stiffness. Activity decreases pain and stiffness.

Because RA is systemic, the client may have a low-grade fever, weakness, fatigue, anorexia, and a mild weight loss. As the disease worsens, major organs or body systems are affected. Joint deformities occur as a late symptom, and secondary osteoporosis (bone loss) can lead to fractures.

Several associated syndromes are seen in some clients with rheumatoid arthritis. For example, Sjögren's syndrome is an inflammation of tear ducts (causing dry eyes) and salivary glands (causing dry mouth). Felty's syndrome is less common and is characterized by an enlarged liver and spleen and leukopenia (decreased white blood cell count).

Diagnosis

No single diagnostic test confirms RA, but several laboratory tests help support the diagnosis. An increase in white blood cells and platelets is typical, unless the client has Felty's syndrome. A group of immunological tests are usu-

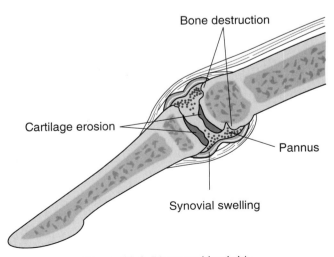

Figure 44–2. Rheumatoid arthritis.

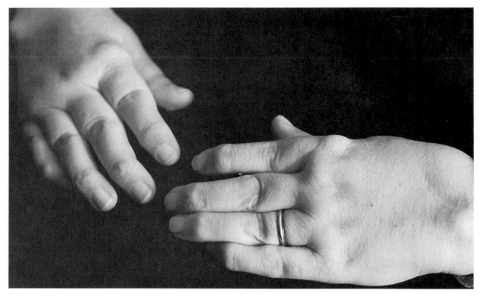

Figure 44–3. Joint abnormalities in hands of client with rheumatoid arthritis.

ally performed, and typical findings for clients with RA include the following:

- Positive Rose or latex agglutination titer (presence of rheumatoid factor)
- Positive antinuclear antibody test (presence of abnormal antibodies)
- Increased erythrocyte sedimentation rate (ESR), indicating systemic inflammation

The ESR is also obtained to evaluate the effectiveness of treatment. If the disease responds to treatment, the ESR decreases. The higher the ESR, the more active the disease process.

LEARNING TIP

The erythrocyte sedimentation rate is a general screening test for inflammation. It measures the amount of time it takes red blood cells to settle to the bottom of a test tube. In the presence of inflammation, red blood cells settle faster in the tube. Therefore the ESR increases with the presence of inflammation.

X-ray and MRI detect joint damage and bone loss, especially in the vertebral column. A bone or joint scan assesses the extent of joint involvement throughout the body. For some clients, an **arthrocentesis** may be performed in which fluid is aspirated from a swollen joint and analyzed in the laboratory.

Medical Treatment

Like the client with osteoarthritis, the client with RA experiences chronic joint pain. Pain can interfere with mobility or the ability to perform activities of daily living. Drug therapy is often needed to relieve or reduce pain, as well as slow the progression of the disease.

Medication

Numerous medications are available for clients with RA. Most of them have analgesic and anti-inflammatory properties (see Table 44–1).

Salicylates in high doses, such as aspirin, and NSAIDs, such as ibuprofen (Motrin), are commonly prescribed for arthritic pain and inflammation. Although these drugs do not slow the disease process, they are often effective for pain control. Gold therapy, either orally or intramuscularly, low-dose methotrexate (MTX), and prednisone are remittive agents that may be administered to induce disease remission. Many of these medications have potentially serious side effects that must be monitored carefully.

Heat and Cold

Heat applications or hot showers help decrease joint stiffness and make exercise easier for the client. For acutely inflamed, or "hot," joints, cold applications are preferred. As for clients with osteoarthritis, a program that balances rest and exercise is most beneficial for the client.

Surgery

If nonsurgical approaches are not effective in relieving arthritic pain, the client may have a total joint replacement (discussed later). In general clients with RA who have sur-

---

arthrocentesis: arthro—joint + centesis—puncture of a cavity gery are not as successful when compared with clients with osteoarthritis. The presence of a systemic disease predisposes clients with RA to more postoperative complications.

Nursing Process

Assessment

A thorough history and physical assessment is needed for the client with RA because the disease can involve every system of the body. In addition to assessing the physical signs and symptoms, the nurse assesses the client for psychosocial, functional, and vocational needs.

Body changes due to joint deformity may lead to poor self-esteem and body image. Clients may feel helpless as they lose control over a disease process that is affecting many parts of the body. Chronic pain and suffering negatively affect the quality of one's life, and the client may experience depression.

After 15 or so years of having the disease, fewer than half of RA clients are totally independent in their activities of daily living. These limitations may place a burden on family members, who must be included in the care of the client with RA.

Many clients with the disease are young or middle aged. RA can impair their ability to work, depending on the type of job they have. Chronic fatigue requires frequent rest periods that may not fit into a day's work schedule. The health care team assesses the client's work skills to determine the need for changes in the workplace or a need to train for a new type of work.

Nursing Diagnosis

The nursing diagnoses depend on the severity of the disorder and whether organ or systems are involved. All clients with RA typically experience but are not limited to the following:

- Chronic pain
- Body image disturbance
- Fatigue
- Self-care deficit
- Impaired physical mobility

Planning

The plan of care for the client with RA must be interdisciplinary, involving many members of the health team. For most clients, the physical therapist, occupational therapist, and social worker or case manager are vital in successfully meeting client outcomes and improving quality of life. Family and significant others should be an integral part of the planning process.

Implementation

Each client's treatment plan is individualized to meet his or her needs. The nurse's major intervention is client teaching to reinforce the treatment plan, as well as ensure that the interdisciplinary plan of care is carried out.

Evaluation

The expected outcomes for the client are relief of pain and disease remission. Medications are adjusted to control pain, as well as to decrease the inflammatory process. ESR is used as an indicator of how well the treatment plan worked because its value decreases as inflammation subsides.

CRITICAL THINKING: Mrs. Summers

Mrs. Summers is a 48-year-old nurse who has had upper extremity joint pain and swelling for about 4 years. She was recently diagnosed with RA but has no systemic involvement other than extreme fatigue at this time. She is concerned that she will have to give up providing direct client care on a busy medical unit in the local hospital.

1. What questions might you ask her at this time about her illness?
2. What should you teach her about pain management?

Answers at end of chapter.

Client Education

The client with RA needs extensive client education regarding the disease process, medication management, and the comprehensive plan of care. Many fads and myths published in popular tabloids are available, and some publicized "cures" can actually be harmful to the client.

The nurse, in collaboration with the health team members, may need to help the client plan a daily schedule that balances rest and exercise (see Table 44–2). Child care responsibilities and other day-to-day activities need to be decided. A vocational counselor may be necessary for job training if the client needs to pursue a different occupation. Clients who are unable to work may be able to qualify for disability benefits through the Social Security program.

The nurse informs the client about community resources, such as the local chapter of the Arthritis Foundation. This organization provides support groups, information, and other resources for clients with RA and other types of connective tissue disorders.

GOUT

Gout, sometimes referred to as gouty arthritis, is also a systemic connective tissue disorder, but it can be easily treated. Men, especially middle-aged and older men, are affected more than women. Clients with gout are seldom hospitalized for their disease.

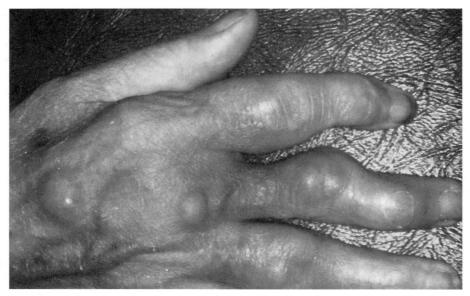

Figure 44–4. Gout: subcutaneous nontender lesions near joints. (From Goldsmith, LA, et al: Adult and Pediatric Dermatology. FA Davis, Philadelphia, 1997, p 405, with permission.) See Plate 19.

Pathophysiology

Gout is a systemic disease in which urate crystals, formed from excessive uric acid, deposit in joints and other connective tissues, causing severe inflammation. Uric acid is a waste product from the breakdown of proteins (purines) in the body. Most clients experience four phases of the disease. In the asymptomatic phase, the client is unaware that the serum uric acid level is elevated, also called **hyperuricemia.** The first "attack" of gout begins the second, or acute, phase. The client unexpectedly has severe pain and inflammation in one or more small joints, usually the great toe. The client typically sees a physician or other health care provider for treatment. If not, the inflammation tends to completely resolve in several days. Months or years may occur between attacks. This period of time is known as the intercurrent phase. The client has no signs or symptoms between episodes of joint inflammation. After several attacks, the client begins the chronic phase. Urate deposits may appear under the skin (tophi) or within the kidneys or urinary system causing stone (calculi) formation (Fig. 44–4). Care of clients with renal or urinary stones is found in Chapter 35.

Causes and Types

The causes and types of gout are well known. Primary gout is the most common type and is caused by an inherited problem with purine metabolism. Uric acid production from the breakdown of purines is greater than the kidneys' ability to excrete it. Therefore the amount of uric acid in the blood increases. About 25 percent of clients have a family history of primary gout.

Clients with secondary gout also experience hyperuricemia, but the increase is the result of another health problem, such as renal insufficiency, or medications, such as diuretic therapy and certain chemotherapeutic agents.

Signs and Symptoms

Acute Gout

Clients with acute gout have one or more severely inflamed joints, usually small joints. The joint is swollen, red, hot, and usually too painful to be touched.

Chronic Gout

Clients with chronic gout may not have obvious signs and symptoms. Tophi, small urate deposits under the skin, are not commonly seen today because management of clients with gout has improved. If they are present, they tend to appear on the outer ear most often. Renal stones develop in about 20 percent of clients with gout. Various diagnostic tests may be needed to determine stone formation.

Diagnostic Tests

Diagnosis of gout is based on the serum uric acid level, which should be below 8 mg/dL. Urinary uric acid levels may also be assessed. To determine if kidney damage has occurred, renal function tests such as blood urea nitrogen

---

hyperuricemia: hyper—excessive + uric—uric acid + emia—in blood

(BUN) and serum creatinine are evaluated. X-rays of the kidney determine the presence of calculi.

Treatment

Medication

The treatment of secondary gout is management or removal of the underlying cause. Drug therapy is the first-line treatment for primary gout. When the client has an acute gout episode, the physician usually prescribes either an NSAID or colchicine, which interferes with the white blood cell (WBC) inflammatory response to urate crystals. The client takes these medications until joint inflammation subsides or until severe diarrhea occurs (a side effect of colchicine).

Allopurinol (Zyloprim) is the preferred drug for chronic gout. Allopurinol works by decreasing the production of uric acid and therefore takes several weeks to be effective. The client must take it every day to keep the uric acid level within the normal range. Probenecid (Benemid) may also be used temporarily to increase renal excretion of uric acid. The client's serum uric acid level is monitored periodically.

Diet

There is no special therapeutic diet for clients with gout; however, certain foods should be avoided or consumed in moderation (Table 44–4). The client should be instructed to avoid all forms of aspirin and diuretics because they can cause an attack. Increasing daily fluid intake is also important to help prevent kidney stones.

SYSTEMIC LUPUS ERYTHEMATOSUS

The word lupus comes from the Latin word for wolf to reflect the masklike appearance that clients have when they have a lupus facial rash. The rash is red, and thus the word erythematosus, meaning reddened, was added to describe the disease.

Most clients with lupus have the systemic type, but a small percentage have the type that affects only the skin, a condition called discoid lupus erythematosus. Discoid lupus is not life threatening; systemic lupus erythematosus (SLE) can be life threatening because it is a progressive, systemic inflammatory disease that can cause major body organ and system failure. Although this definition seems similar to the definition of rheumatoid arthritis, one distinct difference exists. Clients with SLE typically have more body organ development earlier in their disease than do clients with RA.

Pathophysiology

SLE is thought to be an autoimmune disease characterized by spontaneous remissions and exacerbations, much like rheumatoid arthritis. Abnormal antibodies are produced that react with the client's healthy connective tissues. The immune complexes that result lodge in the blood and organs of the client, leading to inflammation, damage, and possibly death. The cause of SLE is unknown, but it tends to run in families. Identified chromosomal markers indicate a genetic link.

The mortality rate for clients with the disease has improved greatly over the past 30 years. The leading causes of death are kidney failure, heart failure, and central nervous system involvement. Lupus most often affects women between the ages of 15 and 40 at a rate 8 to 10 times more often than for men. African-American women are at a greater risk for the disease than women of other racial or ethnic backgrounds.

Signs and Symptoms

Unfortunately there is no classic textbook description of clients with SLE. Some clients have a very mild form of the disease in which the skin and joints are affected. Others have devastating signs and symptoms when the disease affects multiple body systems at the same time.

The classic feature of lupus is the characteristic butterfly rash (Fig. 44–5). A raised, reddened rash over the bridge of the nose that extends to both cheeks is seen. The rash is usually dry and may itch. Only half of clients with lupus have the facial rash. Others have discoid (coinlike) skin lesions on other parts of the body. The rash tends to worsen during an exacerbation, which can be triggered by sun or ultraviolet light exposure, or by physical stressors, such as pregnancy or infection. The client experiences fever when a flare-up of the disease occurs. Table 44–5 lists other possible signs and symptoms of SLE.

Diagnostic Tests

Skin lesions can be biopsied and examined microscopically for signs of inflammation. Clients with suspected SLE are evaluated using the same immunologically based laboratory tests that are used to assess clients with rheumatoid arthritis. These tests include erythrocyte sedimentation

Table 44–4. **Health Promotion for Clients with Gout**

- Avoid high-purine (protein) foods, such as organ meats, shellfish, and oily fish (e.g., sardines).
- Avoid alcohol.
- Drink plenty of fluids, especially water.
- Avoid all forms of aspirin and drugs containing aspirin.
- Avoid diuretics.
- Avoid excessive physical or emotional stress.

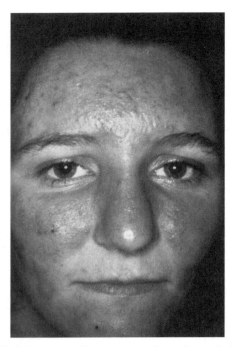

Figure 44–5. Lupus erythematosus: red papules and plaques in butterfly pattern on face. (From Goldsmith, LA, et al: Adult and Pediatric Dermatology. FA Davis, Philadelphia, 1997, p 230, with permission.) See Plate 19.

rate (to detect systemic inflammation) and antinuclear antibody titers (to detect the presence of abnormal antibodies, sometimes called LE cells). Although no laboratory test confirms a diagnosis of lupus, the results of the immunological tests may support the diagnosis.

Treatment

Treatment of SLE focuses on decreasing inflammation and preventing life-threatening organ damage. Many clients are placed on medications for this purpose.

Medication

Topical cortisone preparations may help reduce skin inflammation and promote fading of skin lesions. For some clients with discoid or systemic lupus, the antimalarial drug hydroxychloroquine (Plaquenil) may be prescribed (see Table 44–1).

Clients who experience joint inflammation are usually placed on an NSAID. Clients with organ or major body system involvement are given more potent drugs that suppress the immune process, including oral steroids such as prednisone or chemotherapeutic agents such as azathioprine (Imuran). These drugs have serious side effects, and clients receiving them are monitored very carefully. In addition to monitoring for a variety of side effects, clients must be taught to avoid people with infections because they are immunocompromised while taking any of these medications.

Table 44–5. Key Features of Systemic Lupus Erythematosus (SLE) and Progressive Systemic Sclerosis (PSS)

SLE	PSS
Skin Manifestations	
• Inflamed, red rash	• Inflamed
• Discoid lesions	• Fibrotic
	• Sclerotic
	• Edematous
Renal Manifestations	
• Nephritis	• Renal failure
Cardiovascular Manifestations	
• Pericarditis	• Myocardial fibrosis
• Raynaud's phenomenon	• Raynaud's phenomenon
Pulmonary Manifestations	
• Pleural effusions	• Interstitial fibrosis
Neurological Manifestations	
• CNS lupus	• Not common
Gastrointestinal Manifestations	
• Abdominal pain	• Esophagitis
	• Ulcers
Musculoskeletal Manifestations	
• Joint inflammation	• Joint inflammation
• Myositis	• Myositis
Other Manifestations	
• Fever	• Fever
• Fatigue	• Fatigue
• Anorexia	• Anorexia
• Vasculitis	• Vasculitis

(From Ignatavicius, DD, Workman, ML, and Mishler, MA: Medical-Surgical Nursing: A Nursing Process Approach, ed 2. WB Saunders, Philadelphia, 1995, with permission.)

Nursing Process

Assessment

The nurse assesses the client to determine the extent and severity of signs and symptoms, such as pain, fatigue, skin lesions, and fever. The plan of care for the client is individualized because every client with SLE is unique.

Nursing Diagnosis

The nursing diagnoses are derived from the assessment. Most clients with lupus have but are not limited to the following:

- Impaired skin integrity
- Chronic pain
- Fatigue
- Body image disturbance

Other nursing diagnoses depend on the extent of organ involvement.

Planning

The nurse collaborates with other health care team members as needed to promote or maintain function. If joints are involved, the client may benefit from physical therapy for exercise. The nurse identifies coping strategies that the client has used in the past and relies on those strategies in mutual care planning with the client and family. Young clients are often concerned about issues related to sexuality, pregnancy, and child rearing. These lifestyle concerns must be addressed with the appropriate health care professional.

Implementation

One of the most important roles for the nurse is coordination of care and client education. The health of the client with SLE can vary from seemingly healthy to severely ill in a critical care unit. These extremes can cause anxiety and concern about whether the client may die from disease complications. The nurse offers emotional support to both the client and family or significant other.

Evaluation

The expected outcome of care is that the client can function daily without severe pain or fatigue and can avoid exacerbations of the disease.

Client Education

The nurse teaches the client about skin care and ways to prevent disease exacerbations. The client should avoid prolonged exposure to sunlight or other forms of ultraviolet light. These rays can precipitate a flare-up of the illness. In addition, the nurse teaches the client how to care for the skin using mild soap and nondrying substances. Table 44–6 lists guidelines for client education and health promotion for the client with lupus.

The Arthritis Foundation and the Lupus Foundation are national organizations that can provide information, assistance, and community support groups for clients diagnosed with lupus.

PROGRESSIVE SYSTEMIC SCLEROSIS

Progressive systemic sclerosis (PSS), formerly called systemic **scleroderma,** is similar to systemic lupus erythematosus in that it can affect multiple body organs and other connective tissues. PSS is not as common as lupus but has a higher mortality rate.

Pathophysiology

PSS is characterized by inflammation that develops into fibrosis (scarring) and then sclerosis (hardening) of tissues.

---

scleroderma: sclero—hardening + derma—skin

Table 44–6. ***Skin Protection and Care for Clients with Lupus Erythematosus***

- Cleanse skin with a mild soap such as Ivory.
- Dry skin thoroughly by patting rather than rubbing.
- Apply lotion liberally to dry skin areas.
- Avoid powder and other drying agents, such as rubbing alcohol.
- Use cosmetics that contain moisturizers.
- Avoid direct sunlight and any other type of ultraviolet lighting (including tanning beds).
- Wear a large-brimmed hat, long sleeves, and long pants when in the sun.
- Use a sun-blocking agent with at least a sunburn protection factor (SPF) of 30.
- Inspect skin daily for open areas and rashes.

(From Ignatavicius, DD, Workman, ML, and Mishler, MA: Medical-Surgical Nursing: A Nursing Process Approach, ed 2. WB Saunders, Philadelphia, 1995, with permission.)

Little is known about the cause of this disease, but autoimmunity is likely. Like some of the other systemic connective tissue diseases, abnormal antibodies damage healthy tissue.

PSS affects women three to four times more often than men, usually between 30 and 50 years of age. The disease tends to progress very rapidly and does not respond well to treatment. Spontaneous remissions and exacerbations can occur.

Signs and Symptoms

Although arthritis and fatigue are commonly seen, the most obvious sign of PSS is scleroderma, which is manifested at first by pitting edema, starting in the upper extremities. The skin is taut, shiny, and without wrinkles. If occurring as part of the systemic form of the disease (progressive systemic sclerosis), the swelling is replaced by tightening, hardening, and thickening of skin tissue. The skin then loses its elasticity, range of motion is decreased, and skin ulcers may appear. As the disease progresses, the client loses range of motion and becomes contracted.

The same pathophysiological process affects certain body systems, especially the kidneys, lungs, heart, and gastrointestinal tract. If any of these systems is affected, the corresponding signs and symptoms are present. For example, gastrointestinal tract involvement usually manifests as esophagitis, dysphagia (difficulty swallowing), and decreased intestinal peristalsis caused by decreased smooth muscle elasticity.

The prognosis is thought to be worse when the client has the CREST syndrome, a group of signs and symptoms occurring at the same time:

- **C**alcinosis (calcium deposits)
- **R**aynaud's phenomenon (severe vasospasms of the small vessels in the hands and feet)
- **E**sophageal dysmotility (decreased activity)

- **S**clerodactyly (scleroderma of the finger digits)
- **T**elangietasias (spiderlike skin lesions)

Diagnosis

Laboratory or other diagnostic testing is not very helpful in diagnosing this condition.

Treatment

The goal of medical management is to slow the progression of the disease. Systemic steroids, such as prednisone, and immunosuppressant drugs are used in large doses and in combination during a flare-up of PSS.

Other care approaches are directed toward symptom management. Skin protective measures can help minimize the chance of ulcerations or irritation (see Table 44–6). For example, the nurse teaches the client to use mild soaps and lotions to moisturize the skin.

If the client has esophageal involvement, small, frequent, bland meals are better tolerated than large, spicy ones. Medications to treat esophageal reflux, such as antacids and histamine blockers, may be prescribed.

Clients who have Raynaud's phenomenon or other type of **vasculitis** usually experience severe pain when small blood vessels constrict. They may also have painful joints. Pain management is a priority in the care of clients with PSS. A bed cradle or footboard keeps bed covers away from skin. Socks and gloves may keep the fingers and toes warm, thus diminishing pain.

Rehabilitative therapy may be needed to help the client be as independent as possible with activities of daily living and mobility. The nurse collaborates with other members of the interdisciplinary team to individualize care.

POLYMYOSITIS

Polymyositis is a diffuse inflammation of skeletal muscle that results in weakness and atrophy. When a rash is present with muscle inflammation, the disease is called dermatomyositis. Like most systemic connective tissue diseases, the exact cause is unknown, but it is thought to be autoimmune. The disease progresses and remissions and exacerbations are common. Women are affected more than men, especially in their middle-age years.

The shoulder and pelvic girdle muscles (proximal muscles) are most commonly affected. The client also has arthritis, fatigue, and possibly Raynaud's phenomenon (spasms and constriction of small vessels in the hands and feet). Clients with dermatomyositis also have the classic heliotrope (lilac) rash and periorbital (around the eyes) swelling. Malignant tumors occur in clients with these diseases more often than the rest of the population.

Clients are treated symptomatically, using an interdisciplinary approach, to maintain optimum function. The drug of choice is high doses of prednisone.

MUSCULAR DYSTROPHY

Muscular dystrophy (MD) is diagnosed in childhood, so it is primarily seen in children. However, individuals with muscular dystrophy are now living longer into adulthood due to treatment advances.

Pathophysiology and Etiology

Muscular dystrophy has a genetic origin. However, the exact cause is unknown. Skeletal (voluntary) muscle fibers degenerate and atrophy. This loss of muscle tissue results in muscle weakness and wasting. Muscle tissue is replaced by connective tissue. These changes in muscle tissue result in increasing disability and deformity. Length of life after diagnosis depends on the type of MD.

Signs and Symptoms

Signs and symptoms become apparent in childhood. Difficulty walking and muscle weakness in the arms, legs, and trunk are indicators of MD. Individuals with MD may have difficulty raising their arms above their heads or climbing stairs.

Diagnosis

An increase in serum creatinine phosphokinase due to muscle atrophy will be present in MD. Electromyography (EMG) and muscle biopsy can be used for diagnosis.

Medical Treatment

Goals include supportive care and prevention of complications. Keeping the client as active as possible is a priority in the planning of care. Exercise programs (range of motion, physical therapy) help prevent muscle tightness, contractures, and atrophy. Splints and braces provide support during ADL. Surgery may be done to correct deformities.

Nursing Process

Assessment

The nurse needs to assess for muscle weakness, what areas of the body are affected, and the severity of the weaknesses. Asking the client and family what activities can be done with and without assistance helps determine the plan of care.

Planning

The client and family should be involved in all aspects of care. The goal for impaired physical mobility is to maintain activity or use adaptive equipment. The goal for ineffective

---

vasculitis: vascul—blood vessel + itis—inflammation
polymyositis: poly—many + myo—muscle + itis—inflammation

breathing pattern is to maintain arterial blood gases within normal limits.

Nursing Diagnosis

Priority diagnoses are impaired physical mobility related to muscle weakness and ineffective breathing pattern related to muscle weakness.

Implementation

Providing assistive devices (braces, splints, wheelchair) increases mobility. Range of motion (ROM) exercises and other physical therapy prevent contractures and improve muscle strength. Encouraging the client to do as much as possible increases independence and helps maintain muscle function. Respiratory rate and effort should be monitored every 4 hours. Measures to prevent skin breakdown need to be instituted, such as frequent turning or repositioning and teaching clients to shift their weight if able every 15 minutes while sitting or lying.

Client Education

The client and family need to understand the importance of physical therapy in maintaining function and preventing complications. National organizations and support groups provide information, resources, and emotional support. Family members need to encourage the client to have activity and rest periods. As with any neuromuscular condition, the client needs to avoid exposure to the cold and persons with infections.

Evaluation

The client's goals are met if the client maintains muscle function and desired level of activity; no evidence of skin breakdown, contractures, or injury is present; and the client maintains or improves pulmonary status.

Musculoskeletal Surgery

Some health problems cannot be managed conservatively and require surgery. Other disorders are initially treated medically but may need surgery if treatment is unsuccessful. The most common surgeries are discussed here.

TOTAL JOINT REPLACEMENT

Total joint replacement is most often performed for clients who have some type of connective tissue disease in which their joints become severely deteriorated. TJR may also be done for clients on chronic steroid therapy, such as clients with systemic lupus erythematosus or asthma. Long-term use of steroids can cause **avascular necrosis** (AVN), a condition in which bone tissue dies (usually the femoral head)

as a result of impaired blood supply. Advanced AVN is very painful and usually does not respond to conservative pain relief measures. The primary goal of total joint replacement is to relieve severe chronic pain when no other treatment is successful.

The most common surgeries are the total hip replacement (THR) and total knee replacement (TKR), although any synovial joint can be replaced. The replacement devices, sometimes referred to as prostheses, are made of metal, ceramic, plastic, or a combination of these materials. Some prostheses are held in place by cement. Others are secured by the client's bone as it grafts and connects to the prosthesis.

Total Hip Replacement

A total hip replacement is a two-piece device consisting of an acetabular cup that is inserted into the pelvic acetabulum and a femoral component that is inserted into the femur to replace the femoral head and neck (Fig. 44–6). The average life span of a cemented THR is about 10 years. Noncemented prostheses used in younger clients may last longer.

Preoperative Care

Total joint surgery is an elective procedure and scheduled far enough in advance to allow ample time for preoperative teaching and screening. Depending on the client's health insurance, a case manager may be assigned to assess the client's needs and support systems that are available postoperatively. Some insurers will not approve the surgery if the client does not have a caregiver who can assist the client after surgery.

In the orthopedic surgeon's office, the client is taught about the surgery and what to expect postoperatively. Some clients are scheduled to meet with the physical therapist to learn ambulation with a walker or crutches and postoperative exercises. Some institutions have total joint education programs, which are a series of educational sessions designed to make the recovery process smoother and more effective for the client.

Depending on the amount of blood loss during surgery, some clients receive postoperative blood transfusions. Because total joint surgery is an elective procedure, the client may opt for autologous blood transfusions. The client donates blood before surgery that is available for reinfusion postoperatively, if needed. This predeposit blood donation is cost-effective and reassures clients who are concerned about receiving blood from other donors.

Clients are admitted to the hospital the morning of surgery and are usually transferred to a surgical or medical-surgical unit after recovery in the postanesthesia care unit (PACU). The client's length of stay on this unit varies from 3 to 5 days, depending on the client's age and progress.

Postoperative Care

In addition to providing the general postoperative care that all clients undergoing general or epidural anesthesia re-

---

avascular necrosis: a—without + vascular—blood + necrosis—death

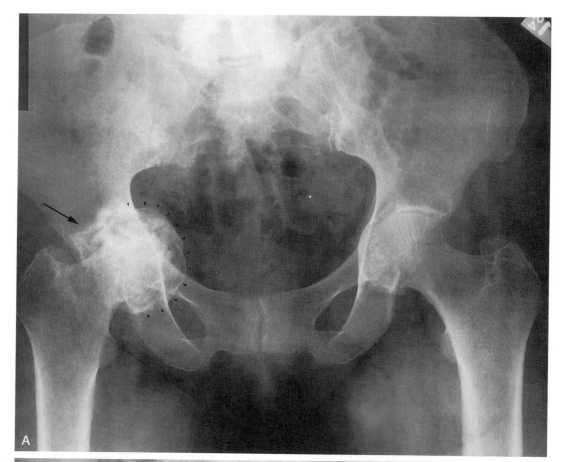

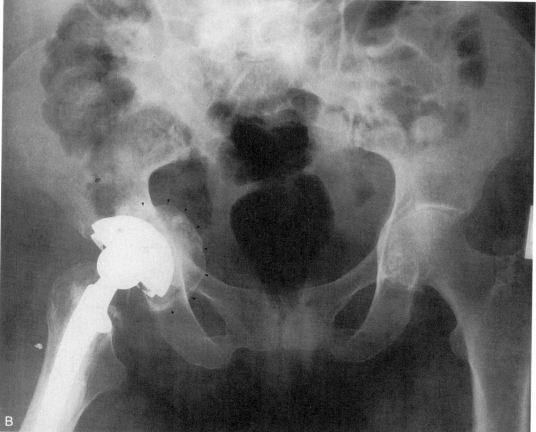

Figure 44–6. *(A)* Client with arthritis of right hip. *(B)* Total hip arthroplasty of arthritic right hip. (From McKinnis, LN: Fundamentals of Orthopedic Radiology. FA Davis, Philadelphia, 1997, with permission.)

quire (see Chapter 11), the nurse plans and implements interventions to help prevent common complications of THR.

HIP DISLOCATION. The most common postoperative complication for the client having a THR is subluxation (partial dislocation) or total dislocation. Dislocation occurs when the femoral component becomes dislodged from the acetabular cup. The client experiences increased hip pain, shortening of the surgical leg, and possibly surgical leg rotation. If any of these signs and symptoms occur, the nurse notifies the surgeon immediately and keeps the client in bed. Under anesthesia, the surgeon manipulates the hip back into alignment and immobilizes the leg until healing occurs.

Prevention of dislocation is a major nursing responsibility. Correct positioning of the surgical leg is critical. The primary goals are to prevent hip adduction (across the body's midline) and hyperflexion (bending forward more than 90 degrees). To accomplish these goals, the nurse initially places the client returning from PACU in a supine position with the head slightly elevated. A trapezoid-shaped abduction pillow, splint, wedge, or regular bed pillows may be used between the legs to prevent adduction (Fig. 44–7). The client is turned with pillow(s) in place between the legs. Turning the client to either side is acceptable as long as hip adduction is avoided unless the surgeon specifies which direction to turn the client.

To prevent hyperflexion, some surgeons initially allow the client to sit at no more than a 60-degree angle in a reclining chair. The client's position is progressed to 90 degrees, the maximum allowed to prevent hyperflexion (Fig. 44–8).

SKIN BREAKDOWN. Because most clients having total joint replacements are elderly, skin breakdown is a major concern as part of postoperative care. Turning the client at least every 2 hours and keeping the heels off the bed are the key nursing interventions to prevent pressure ulcers. Heels and the sacrum are very vulnerable and can break down in 24 hours. A reddened area that does not blanch is a stage 1 pressure ulcer and must be treated aggressively to prevent progression to other stages.

For clients who are incontinent, the nurse and staff must keep the client clean and dry. Toileting the client every 2 hours, using a protective barrier cream, and avoiding the use of diapers also help prevent skin problems related to incontinence. Table 44–7 describes other nursing interventions that meet the special needs of elderly postoperative clients.

INFECTION. Any surgical client is at risk of wound infection. The surgeon orders an intravenous antibiotic to be used prophylactically (for prevention) during surgery, and may continue antibiotics for 24 hours postoperatively.

Once the initial surgical dressing is removed by the surgeon, the nurse observes the incision frequently for signs and symptoms of infection. Temperature is monitored carefully. An elderly client may not experience a fever but may appear confused instead.

Infection may not occur during the client's hospital stay but can occur 1 or more years later. If this late infection does not respond to antibiotics, the prosthesis may be removed and replaced. Antibiotics are often inserted directly into the wound during surgery as beads, as part of the cement mixture, and as the irrigating solution to prevent infection.

BLEEDING. Like any surgical wound, some bleeding is expected. The client has at least one surgical drain that is emptied every 8 to 12 hours for the first day or two. On the second or third postoperative day, the client's hemoglobin and hematocrit may decrease to the point that blood transfusion is needed. The client may receive the preoperatively donated autologous blood or may receive salvaged operative or postoperative blood. Using a cell saver during surgery, about 50 percent of blood that is lost can be recovered and saved for reinfusion into the same client. Postoperatively, blood can be replaced by collecting shed blood via suction into a reservoir, then filtering and reinfusing it within 6 hours of collection.

NEUROVASCULAR COMPROMISE. For any musculoskeletal surgery or injury, frequent neurovascular assessments or

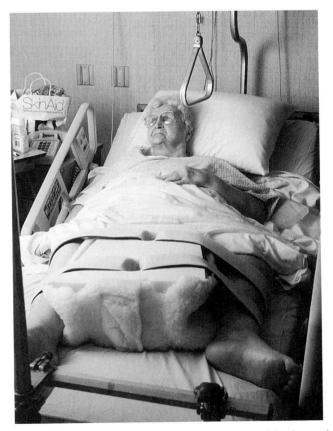

Figure 44–7. Abductor pillow is used to prevent adduction and hip dislocation.

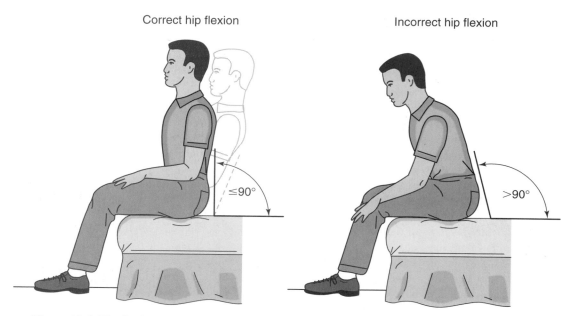

Correct hip flexion · ≤90° · Incorrect hip flexion · >90°

Figure 44–8. Hip flexion after total hip replacement should be 90 degrees or less to prevent dislocation.

checks, also called "circ checks," are performed when vital signs are assessed. The procedure and significance of these assessments are described in Chapter 43.

PAIN. Total joint replacements are performed to relieve pain. Some clients report that they have less pain postoperatively than they had before surgery. Initially pain is typically managed by epidural analgesia, patient-controlled analgesia (PCA), or injections with meperidine (Demerol) or morphine. After the first postoperative day, the client

Table 44–7. *Total Hip Replacement*

- Use an abduction pillow or splint to prevent adduction after surgery if the client is very restless or has an altered mental state.
- Keep the client's heels off of the bed to prevent pressure sores.
- Do not rely on fever as a sign of infection; elderly clients often have infection without fever. Decreasing mental status typically occurs when the client has an infection.
- When assisting the client out of bed, move the client slowly to prevent orthostatic (postural) hypotension.
- Encourage the client to deep breathe and cough, and use the incentive spirometer every 2 hours to prevent atelectasis and pneumonia.
- As soon as permitted, get the client out of bed to prevent complications of immobility.
- Anticipate the client's need for pain medication, especially if the client is unable to verbalize the need for pain control.
- Expect a temporary change in mental state immediately after surgery as a result of the anesthesia and unfamiliar sensory stimuli. Reorient the client frequently.

(From Ignatavicius, DD, Workman, ML, and Mishler, MA: Medical-Surgical Nursing: A Nursing Process Approach, ed 2. WB Saunders, Philadelphia, 1995, with permission.)

usually progresses to oral opioid analgesia with a drug such as Percocet.

AMBULATION. Care for the client having a THR is interdisciplinary. The client usually gets out of bed in a chair the night of surgery or early the next day. The nurse ensures that the client does not adduct or hyperflex the surgical hip during transfer to the chair. The chair should have a straight back and be high enough to prevent excessive flexion. The toilet seat should also be raised for the same purpose. Permitted amounts of weight bearing depend on the type of prosthesis that is used. In general, weight bearing to tolerance or full weight bearing (FWB) is used for cemented prostheses. If an uncemented device is used, the client may be restricted to toe-touch or partial weight bearing (PWB).

Early ambulation helps prevent postoperative complications such as atelectasis and deep vein thrombi. The physical therapist works with the client for ambulation with a walker or crutches. Crutches are reserved for young clients. After 4 to 6 weeks, the client is progressed to a cane. When the limp disappears, the client does not need an ambulatory device.

THROMBOEMBOLIC (TE) COMPLICATIONS. Clients having hip surgery are the highest-risk group for deep vein thrombosis or pulmonary embolus. Elderly clients are especially at risk due to compromised circulation from aging. Obese clients and those with a history of TE problems are also at an exceptionally high risk for potentially fatal problems.

Thigh-high elastic stockings, such as TED stockings, and sequential compression devices (SCDs) may be used while the client is hospitalized (see Chapter 11). The surgeon orders an anticoagulant medication to help prevent clot formation, including subcutaneous low-molecular-weight heparin, enoxaparin (Lovenox), or warfarin (Coumadin). The amount of these drugs ordered each day is determined by their coagulation studies. Partial thromboplastin times are monitored for heparin. Prothrombin time and international normalized ratio (INR) are monitored when giving warfarin.

LEARNING TIP

When giving enoxaparin (Lovenox), follow manufacturer's instructions for administration. The air bubble should not be removed from the prefilled syringe before administration.

Because most deep vein thrombi (DVT) occur in the lower extremities, leg exercises are started in the immediate postoperative period and continued until the client is fully ambulatory. The physical therapist teaches the client how to perform heel-pumping exercises, foot circles, and straight-leg raises (SLRs). The client also performs quadriceps-setting exercises ("quad sets") by straightening the legs and pushing the back of the knees toward the bed. The nurse reminds the client to do several sets of these exercises each day to improve muscle tone and to help prevent leg clots.

SELF-CARE. Due to restrictions in hip flexion, clients are unable to bend forward to tie shoes or don pants. The occupational therapist provides adaptive or assistive devices, such as dressing sticks and long-handled shoe horns to assist the client in being independent in activities of daily living.

If the client is medically stable, he or she is discharged to home for rehabilitation or to a subacute care unit, rehabilitation unit, or nursing home for short-term rehabilitation, lasting a week or less. The rehabilitation program that began in the hospital continues after discharge until the client is independent in ambulation and self-care.

Before hospital discharge, the interdisciplinary team provides client education for home care, including hip pre-

---

HOME HEALTH HINTS

- A client on crutches can use the crutch to prop a casted leg or foot for extremity elevation.
- Peak incidence of DVT after hip or knee surgery is highest by the fifth postoperative day with that risk persisting for up to 12 weeks. Therefore it is imperative that the home health nurse be alert for signs of DVT: pain, warmth, redness, edema, Homans' sign, and client protective behavior of the affected leg.

Table 44–8. *Education for Total Hip Replacement*

Hip Precautions
- Do not sit or stand for prolonged periods.
- Do not cross legs beyond midline of body.
- Do not bend hips more than 90 degrees.
- Use an ambulatory aid, such as a walker, when walking.
- Use assistive/adaptive devices for dressing, such as for putting on shoes and socks.
- Resume sexual intercourse as usual, but when doing so, use the hip precautions learned in the hospital.

(From Ignatavicius, DD, Workman, ML, and Mishler, MA: Medical-Surgical Nursing: A Nursing Process Approach, ed 2. WB Saunders, Philadelphia, 1995, with permission.)

---

cautions that need to be used until the surgeon reevaluates the client at the 6- to 8-week follow-up visit (Table 44–8).

Total Knee Replacement

The knee is the second most commonly replaced joint. Compared with the hip, it is a much more complicated joint and requires three components for replacement: a femoral component, a tibial component, and a patellar button (Fig. 44–9).

The care for the client with a TKR is very similar to that required for a client with a hip replacement. Although pre-

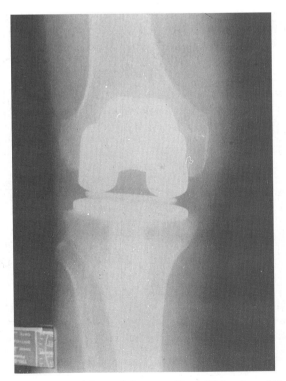

Figure 44–9. Knee joint replacement. (From Richardson, JK, and Iglarsh, ZA: Clinical Orthopaedic Physical Therapy. WB Saunders, Philadelphia, 1994, p 651, with permission.)

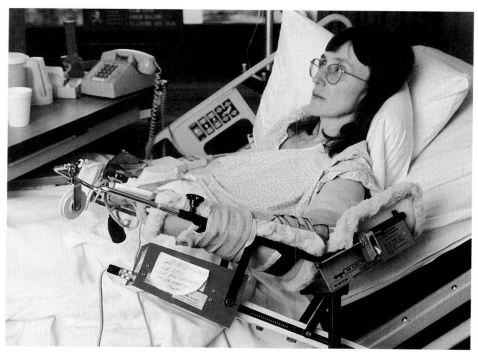

Figure 44–10. A continuous passive motion (CPM) machine is used following knee or elbow (as shown here) joint replacement to increase joint mobility and enhance recovery. The CPM machine slowly moves along the track at the set degree of flexion and speed.

cautions to prevent dislocation are not applicable for the client with a knee replacement, other medical complications described for the THR may be seen in the TKR client.

Most surgeons order a continuous passive motion machine (CPM) for the surgical leg. This motorized machine has a flexible extremity (for either the leg or arm) rest that glides back and forth on a track (Fig. 44–10). The CPM is set at the degree of flexion and speed ordered by the physician. It is applied by the nurse, physical therapist, or technician and is usually begun in the PACU. It is used either intermittently up to 8 to 12 hours a day or continuously while the client is in bed. The purpose of the machine is to keep the knee joint mobile. Nursing care associated with the use of the machine is summarized in Table 44–9.

Amputation

Simply defined, an amputation is the removal of a body part, which can be as limited as removing part of a finger or as devastating as removing nearly half of the body. Amputations may be surgical due to disease or traumatic due to an accident. Surgical amputations are the most common type and are most often scheduled as elective surgery.

Surgical Amputations

The main indication for surgical amputations is ischemia from peripheral vascular disease in the elderly. The rate of lower extremity amputation is much greater in the diabetic client than in the nondiabetic client (see discussion of diabetes in Chapter 38). Surgical amputations may also be done for bone tumors, thermal injuries (frostbite), congenital problems, or infections.

Traumatic Amputations

Traumatic amputations occur from accidents, often in young and middle-age adults. Industrial machinery, motor vehicles, lawn mowers, chain saws, and snow blowers are common causes of accidental amputation.

Table 44–9. *The Client Using a Continuous Passive Motion (CPM) Machine*

- Ensure that the machine is well padded with sheepskin or other similar material.
- Check the cycle and range-of-motion settings at least once per shift (every 8 hours).
- Ensure that the joint being moved is properly positioned on the machine.
- If the client is confused, place the controls to the machine out of the client's reach.
- Assess the client's response to the machine.
- Turn off the machine while the client is having a meal in bed.
- When the machine is not in use, do not store it on the floor.

(From Ignatavicius, DD, Workman, ML, and Mishler, MA: Medical-Surgical Nursing: A Nursing Process Approach, ed 2. WB Saunders, Philadelphia, 1995, with permission.)

Because the amputated part in these clients is usually healthy, attempts at **replantation** may be made. One of the most common replantations is one or more fingers. The current recommendation for prehospital care of the severed part is to wrap it in a cool, slightly moist cloth and place it in a sealed plastic bag. The bag may be submerged in cold water until the part is carried to the hospital.

The surgical procedure is performed by specialists who operate using a microscope. Nerves, vessels, and muscle must be reattached. These procedures are generally performed at large tertiary care centers that have specialty practitioners and equipment for replantation.

Levels of Amputation

The most common surgical amputation is part of the lower extremity (LE). The loss of any or all of the small toes presents little problem. However, the loss of the great toe is more important because balance and gait are affected. Midfoot amputations are preferred over below-the-knee (BKA) amputations for peripheral vascular disease (PVD). For the Syme amputation, the surgeon removes most of the foot but leaves the ankle intact for ambulation and weight bearing.

If the lower leg is amputated, a BKA is preferred over an above-the-knee (AKA) amputation to preserve joint function. The higher the level of amputation, the more energy is required for ambulation. Hip disarticulation (removal through the hip joint) and **hemipelvectomy** (removal through part of the pelvis) are reserved for young clients who have cancer or severe trauma. Rarely, a hemicorporectomy (hemipelvectomy plus a translumbar amputation) is performed as a last resort for young clients with cancer. This radical surgery removes nearly half of the body and requires both bowel and urinary diversion surgeries (ostomies) as well.

Upper extremity (UE) amputations are usually more significant than LE amputations and result more often from trauma. The arms and hands are necessary for performing activities of daily living. Early replacement with a prosthesis is crucial for the client with a UE amputation.

Preoperative Care

Clients who are scheduled for elective amputations have the advantage of time for preoperative teaching, prosthesis fitting, and adjustment to the loss of part of their bodies. Preoperative teaching is started in the surgeon's office. Postoperative and rehabilitative care are reviewed with the client and family or significant other.

Preoperatively, the client should be referred to a certified prosthetist-orthotist (CPO) to begin plans for replacing the removed body part with a prosthesis. When the client is fitted for an LE prosthesis, he or she needs to bring a sturdy pair of shoes that will be worn with the prosthetic device.

Body image disturbance is a common nursing diagnosis for the client having an amputation. If possible, it is helpful for the preoperative client to meet with a rehabilitated amputee. The nurse assesses the client's reaction to having an amputation with the expectation that the client will experience many of the stages of loss and grieving. Support systems and coping mechanisms are identified that can help the client through the surgery and postoperative period.

Postoperative Care

In addition to the general postoperative care described in Chapter 11, the nurse plans and implements interventions to help prevent postoperative complications.

HEMORRHAGE. When a client loses part of the body, either by surgery or trauma, blood vessels are severed or damaged. The client returns from surgery with a large pressure dressing that is secured with an elastic wrap. The nurse assesses the closest proximal pulse between the heart and the amputated body part for strength and compares findings with the nonsurgical extremity. The nurse assesses the bulky dressing for bloody drainage. If blood is on the dressing when the client is admitted to the PACU or the surgical unit, the nurse circles, dates, and times the drainage. The area is closely monitored for enlargement. If bleeding continues, the surgeon is notified immediately. A tourniquet should be readily available in the event that severe hemorrhage occurs.

After the dressing is removed, the nurse observes for adequate perfusion to the skin flap at the end of the residual limb, sometimes called the "stump." The skin should be pink in a light-skinned client and not discolored (lighter or darker than other skin pigmentation) in a dark-skinned client. The residual limb should be warm but not hot.

INFECTION. Infection of the wound can be problematic, especially if the infection enters the bone, a condition referred to as osteomyelitis (see discussion later in chapter). The nurse inspects the wound for intense redness or drainage. Temperature is monitored for an elevation, which could indicate a wound or other type of infection.

PAIN. In addition to the usual incisional pain that is expected following a surgical procedure, phantom limb pain (PLP) occurs in as many as 80 percent of all amputees. The client complains of severe pain in the removed body part. The pain may be described as either intense burning, a crushing sensation, or cramping. This type of pain is not common in clients who have traumatic amputations.

PLP can be triggered by touching the residual limb, feeling fatigued, or experiencing emotional stress. Although it occurs most often in the immediate postoperative period,

---

replantation: re—again + plant—to plant + tion—process
hemipelvectomy: hemi—half + pelv—pelvis + ectomy—removal of

PLP may occur at any time during the first postoperative year. The cause of PLP is not clear.

The nurse never doubts that the client is experiencing pain in the removed body part. Instead the pain is treated aggressively with medications and complementary therapies. The surgeon prescribes medication based on the type of pain sensation the client experiences. For example, anticonvulsants, such as phenytoin (Dilantin), are used for knifelike pain. Beta-blocking agents, such as propranolol (Inderal) are appropriate for burning sensations. To complement traditional therapy, a number of therapies may be useful, including biofeedback, massage, imagery, hypnosis, and distraction.

MOBILITY AND AMBULATION. To reduce surgical swelling, the residual limb may be placed on a pillow for 24 hours or less. Continued use of a pillow for elevation can lead to flexion contractures, especially for clients with a BKA or an AKA. If the hip becomes contracted, using a prosthesis will not be possible because the client will not be able to walk. The nurse checks the limb periodically to ensure that it lies completely flat on the bed. The client should avoid positions of flexion such as sitting for long periods of time. If the client is able, lying prone (on stomach) for 30 minutes four times daily helps prevent contracture development.

Postoperative care of the client experiencing an amputation is interdisciplinary, often requiring an extensive rehabilitation program in a subacute unit, nursing home, or ambulatory basis. The physical therapist teaches the client muscle-strengthening exercises that will help with ambulation and transfers, as well as prevent flexion contractures. A trapeze and overhead frame aids in strengthening the upper extremities and helps the client move around in the bed.

PROSTHESIS. The residual limb must be prepared for wearing the prosthesis. A temporary prosthesis may be worn until the swelling subsides.

The residual limb is wrapped at least every 8 hours using an elastic wrap in a figure-of-eight fashion (Fig. 44–11). The nurse begins with the most distal portion and proceeds proximally until the bandage is secured to the most proximal joint. The bandage should be tighter at the distal end.

The prosthesis requires special care and attention. Table 44–10 summarizes discharge teaching for the amputee with a prosthesis.

LIFESTYLE ADAPTATION. The client may feel that life will be markedly changed as a result of the amputation. With the technological advances in prostheses, most clients who worked before surgery are able to return to their jobs after surgery. If the discharge planner or case manager thinks it is needed, a job analysis may be conducted by a vocational analyst or specialized case manager. Many clients with amputations are able to bowl, ski, hike, and do

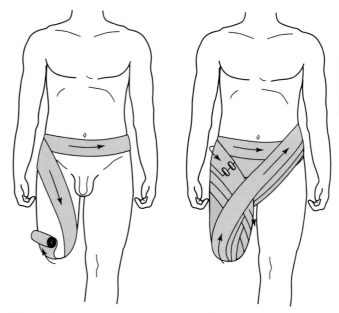

Figure 44–11. Application of elastic wraps on an above-the-knee amputation helps mold the stump for a prosthesis.

all the recreational hobbies that they were able to do before surgery.

A supportive family or significant other is vital to help the client adjust to body image change. The nurse considers the need for a sexual counselor or psychologist if indicated. For any client with an amputation, the nurse also helps the client set realistic expectations and to take one day at a time.

For the client who is not a candidate for a prosthesis, home adaptations for a wheelchair may be needed. The client must have access to toileting facilities and areas necessary for self-care. Structural changes in the living environment may be necessary before the client can be discharged from rehabilitation.

Table 44–10. *Client Education for Prosthesis Care*

- Have a wooden prosthesis refinished at least every 6 months.
- Clean the prosthesis socket with mild soap and water and dry it completely.
- Replace worn inserts and liners when they become too soiled to clean adequately.
- Check all mechanical parts such as bolts periodically for unusual sounds or movement.
- Grease the mechanical parts as instructed by prosthetist.
- Use garters to keep socks or stockings in place.
- Replace shoes when they wear out with new ones of the same height and type.

(From Ignatavicius, DD, Workman, ML, and Mishler, MA: Medical-Surgical Nursing: A Nursing Process Approach, ed 2. WB Saunders, Philadelphia, 1995, with permission.)

A small percentage of amputees return to their nursing home environment without prostheses. These clients need rehabilitation to ensure that they can be as independent as possible.

Bone and Soft Tissue Disorders

The musculoskeletal system is the second largest system in the body. A variety of injuries and diseases can affect bone, soft tissue, or both. The most common problems are discussed in this section.

STRAINS

A strain is a soft tissue injury that occurs when a muscle or tendon is excessively stretched. Causes of strains include falls, excessive exercise, and lifting heavy items without using proper body mechanics. Back and ankle injuries are common. Strains can be mild, moderate, or severe. A mild strain causes minimal inflammation; swelling and tenderness are present. A moderate strain involves partial tearing of the muscle or tendon fibers. Pain and inability to move the affected body part result. The most severe strain occurs when a muscle or tendon is ruptured with separation of muscle from muscle, tendon from muscle, or tendon from bone. Severe pain and disability result from this injury.

Immediately after a strain, ice should be applied to decrease pain, swelling, and inflammation. Once inflammation subsides, heat application brings increased blood flow to the injured area for healing. Activity is limited until the soft tissue heals, and anti-inflammatory drugs are prescribed. Muscle relaxants may be used for muscle pulls as well. For more severe strains, surgery to repair the tear or rupture may be needed. These procedures are done on an ambulatory, same-day surgery basis.

SPRAINS

A sprain is excessive stretching of one or more ligaments that usually results from twisting movements during a sports activity, exercise, or fall. Like strains, sprains also vary in severity. A mild sprain involves tearing of just a few ligament fibers and causes tenderness. In a moderate sprain, more fibers are torn but the stability of the joint is not affected. A moderate sprain is uncomfortable, especially with activity. A severe sprain causes instability of the joint and usually requires surgical intervention for tissue repair or grafting. Pain and inflammation prevent mobility.

For mild sprains, rest, ice applications, and a compression (elastic) bandage are used for several days until swelling and pain diminish. Anti-inflammatory drugs are also used to decrease inflammation and control pain. Moderate sprains may need immobilization with a brace or cast until healing occurs.

CARPAL TUNNEL SYNDROME

Pathophysiology

Carpal tunnel syndrome results in the compression of the median nerve within the carpal tunnel when swelling in the tunnel occurs. This swelling can result from edema, trauma, rheumatoid arthritis, or repetitive hand movements as used in some occupations such as typing or cash register operation.

Signs and Symptoms

Carpal tunnel syndrome usually results in slow-onset hand pain and numbness. Painful tingling may also be present. Eventually, fine motor deficits and then muscle weakness may develop.

Diagnosis

Diagnosis is often made based on signs and symptoms along with the client's history. A positive Phalen's sign is often present, which is the occurrence of numbness with wrist flexion. EMG can also be used to detect nerve abnormalities.

Medical Management

Medical treatment focuses on relieving the inflammation and resting the wrist. A splint is often ordered for the client to wear. Medications to reduce pain and inflammation are ordered such as aspirin and nonsteroidal anti-inflammatory medications. Cortisone may be injected into the carpal tunnel.

For some clients surgery may be necessary. An open incision or endoscopy can be used. The median nerve is released from compression during the surgery.

Nursing Management

The nurse educates the client on methods to prevent carpal tunnel syndrome, provides pain relief as ordered, and if surgery is performed, provides routine preoperative and postoperative care. Postoperatively the client elevates the hand and may have a splint ordered for up to 2 weeks. Lifting is restricted for several weeks. The client is taught neurovascular compromise signs and symptoms to report such as numbness and tingling, coolness, lack of pulse, pale skin or nailbeds, or limited movement. Family assistance with activities of daily living may be required by the client.

FRACTURES

A fracture is a break in a bone and can occur at any age and in any bone. Some fractures are minor and are treated on an ambulatory basis; others are more complex and require surgical intervention with hospitalization and rehabilitation.

Pathophysiology

Bone is a very dynamic, changing tissue. When it is broken, the body immediately begins to repair the injury (Fig. 44–12). For an adult, within 48 to 72 hours after the injury, a hematoma (blood clot) forms at the fracture site because bone has a rich blood supply. Various cells to begin the healing process are attracted to the damaged bone. In about a week or so, a nonbony union called callus develops and can be seen on x-ray. As healing continues, osteoclasts (bone-destroying cells) resorb the necrotic bone and osteoblasts (bone-building cells) make new bone as a replacement. This process is sometimes referred to as bone remodeling. Young, healthy adult bone completely heals in about 6 weeks. An older person takes longer to heal; a child heals more quickly.

Causes and Types

The major reason for a fracture is trauma, from either a fall or a motor vehicle accident. Bone disease, such as osteoporosis and metastatic bone cancer, and malnutrition can lead to fractures as well. Fractures resulting from any of these diseases are referred to as pathological fractures. One of the most common types of fractures is the hip fracture, which occurs in middle-aged and elderly women who have osteoporosis (irreversible bone loss), a condition discussed later in this chapter.

Fractures can be classified by type in several ways—by the extent of the fracture, the extent of the associated soft tissue damage, or the configuration of the bone after it breaks. A fracture that is complete breaks the bone into two separate pieces, also called a displaced fracture. An incomplete fracture does not divide the bone into two pieces; it may also be referred to as a nondisplaced fracture. Complete fractures are more life threatening because sharp bone fragments can sever blood vessels and nerves.

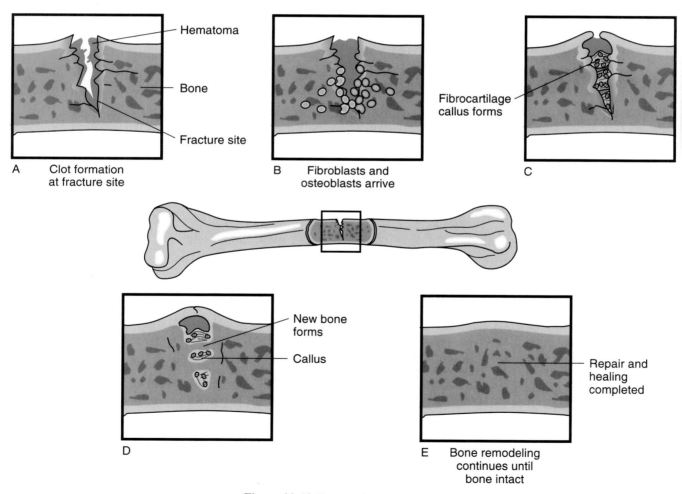

Figure 44–12. Fracture healing phases.

A fracture may also be classified as open or closed. In an open (or compound) fracture, the bone breaks the skin. A closed fracture does not disrupt the skin. Open fractures are more likely to become infected than closed fractures.

Another way to describe fractures is by the way that the bone breaks, for example, in a spiral or oblique fashion (Fig. 44–13). These fractures may be open or closed, complete or incomplete.

Signs and Symptoms

This section focuses on fractures of upper and lower extremities. Signs and symptoms of skull or vertebral frac-

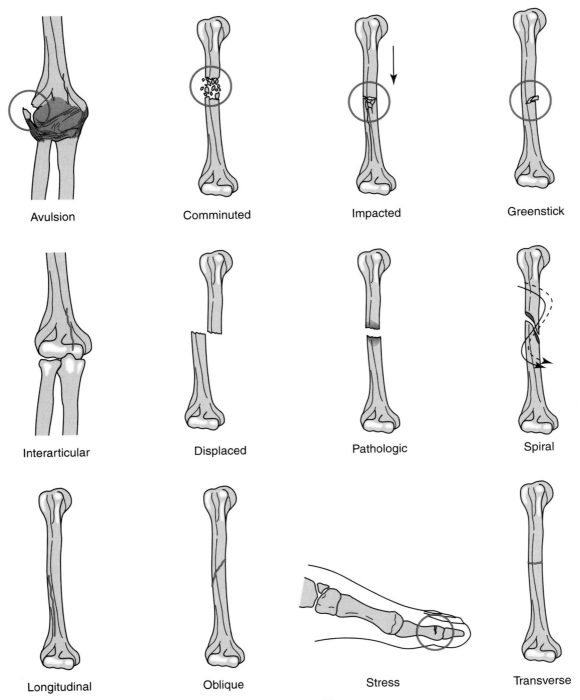

Figure 44–13. Types of fractures.

tures are described in Chapter 46. If the client sustains a hairline (microscopic) fracture, the signs and symptoms are not readily observable. The client may complain of tenderness or more severe pain when moving the affected part of the body. The elderly client with a hip fracture usually complains of pain either in the groin area (the hip is a deep joint) or at the back of the knee (referred pain).

In addition to pain, clients with more complex fractures experience limb rotation or deformity and shortening of the limb (if a limb bone is broken). Range of motion is decreased. If the affected part is moved, a continuous grating sound (crepitation) caused by bone fragments may be heard. The extremity should not be moved if crepitation is present.

The nurse also inspects the skin for intactness. A client with a closed fracture may have ecchymoses (bruising) over the fractured bone from bleeding into the soft underlying tissue. Ecchymosis may not develop for several days after the injury. Swelling may also be present and can impair blood flow, causing marked neurovascular compromise. In an open fracture, one or more bone ends pierce the skin, causing a wound.

Diagnostic Tests

An x-ray usually visualizes bone fractures, showing bone malalignment or disruption. Computed tomography may be needed to help detect fractures of complex areas, such as the hip and pelvis. Magnetic resonance imaging is useful in determining the extent of associated soft tissue damage.

For clients experiencing moderate to severe bleeding, a hemoglobin and hematocrit level is obtained. If extensive soft tissue damage is present, the ESR is usually elevated, indicating the expected inflammatory response.

Emergency Treatment

A client with a suspected fracture often has injuries elsewhere in the body. The nurse or other first-line caregiver assesses the client for respiratory distress, bleeding, and head and spine injury. If any of these problems occur, emergency treatment is provided before concern is given to extremity or other fractures.

The treatment of fractures depends on the type and extent of the injury. Emergency treatment is essential to prevent possible life-threatening complications. Table 44–11 describes the emergency interventions for the client with an extremity fracture.

LEARNING TIP

For emergency care of a suspected fracture: Splint it as it lies!

Fracture Management

The two goals of fracture management are reduction, or realignment of bone ends, and immobilization of the fractured bone with bandages, casts, traction, or a fixation device. These interventions prevent further injury, reduce pain, and promote healing.

Closed Reduction

Closed reduction is the most common treatment for simple fractures. While applying a manual pull on the bone, the physician manipulates the bone ends into realignment. Analgesia is typically used before the procedure. An x-ray is done to confirm that the bone ends are aligned before the area is immobilized.

Bandages and Splints

For some areas of the body, such as the clavicle or wrist, an elastic or a muslin bandage or a splint may be used to immobilize the bone during the healing phase. The nurse performs neurovascular assessments to ensure adequate blood flow to the area. Chapter 43 describes this assessment in detail.

Casts

For more extensive fractures or for weight-bearing areas, a more rigid and durable cast is used for immobilization. Casts allow early mobility and decrease pain for reduced fractures or for deformities, such as flexion contractures. When bone healing is complete, the cast is removed.

Several types of materials are used for casts, including the traditional plaster of paris (anhydrous calcium sulfate) and a variety of synthetic products such as fiberglass. The plaster cast is used for large casts and for weight-bearing areas. The cast feels hot when applied but soon becomes damp and cool, taking anywhere from 24 to 72 hours to completely dry. The cast is dry when it feels hard and firm,

---

Table 44–11. ***Emergency Care of the Client with an Extremity Fracture***

1. Remove the client's clothing (cut, if necessary) to inspect the affected area.
2. Apply direct pressure on the area if there is bleeding and pressure over the proximal artery nearest the fracture.
3. Keep the client warm and in a supine position.
4. Check the neurovascular status of the area distal to the extremity: temperature, color, sensation, movement, and capillary refill. Compare affected and unaffected limbs.
5. Immobilize the extremity by splinting; include joints above and below the fracture site.
6. Cover the affected area with a clean cloth (e.g., a handkerchief).

(From Ignatavicius, DD, Workman, ML, and Mishler, MA: Medical-Surgical Nursing: A Nursing Process Approach, ed 2. WB Saunders, Philadelphia, 1995, with permission.)

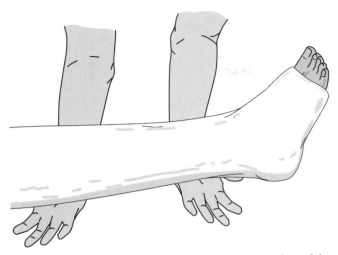

Figure 44–14. A wet plaster cast is moved with the palms of the hand to prevent making indentations in the plaster that could become pressure points.

is odorless, and is shiny white. The nurse keeps the wet cast open to air to aid in drying. A wet cast should be handled with the palms of the hand ("palming the cast") to prevent indentations or a change in the shape of the cast (Fig. 44–14). A synthetic material cast takes only minutes to dry.

A casted limb is elevated for about 24 hours, and ice is applied to reduce swelling. The nurse assesses the cast for dryness, tightness, drainage, and odor. If the cast becomes too tight, the physician orders it to be cut (bivalved) with a cast cutter to relieve pressure and prevent pressure necrosis of the underlying skin (Fig. 44–15). If a wound is present or an odor is detected, the physician cuts a window opening into the cast to treat the underlying skin problem, often an infected area. The cast window should always be taped in place when wound care is not being provided to prevent the skin from "popping up" through the window and devel-

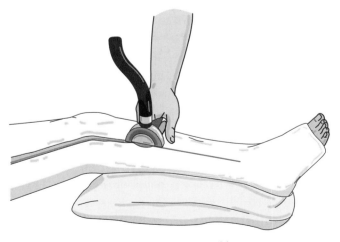

Figure 44–15. Bivalving a cast with a cast saw.

Table 44–12. **The Client with a Cast**

1. Monitor the neurovascular status of the casted extremity every 1–2 hr for the first 24 hr and every 4 hr thereafter.
   a. Perform a circulation check, as described in Ch. 43.
   b. Ask the client if the cast feels too tight.
   c. Have the cast cutter available.
2. Maintain integrity of the cast.
   a. Turn the client every 1–2 hr.
   b. Use the palms of the hands when handling a wet cast.
   c. Do not turn the client by holding on to the abductor bar (e.g., hip spica).
   d. Do not cover a wet cast or place it on a plastic-coated pillow.
   e. Protect other parts from irritation caused by the rough surface of a cast made from synthetics.
   f. Keep set plaster cast dry during bathing by covering it completely with plastic (also, tuck plastic into the ends to prevent water seepage under the cast).
   g. Immerse a synthetic cast in water during bathing, if permitted.
   h. Clean a soiled plaster cast with mild detergent and a damp cloth as necessary.
   i. Inspect the cast when performing circulation checks for crumbling and cracking.
3. Maintain skin integrity.
   a. Examine the skin around the cast edges for redness and irritation.
   b. Trim the edges of the cast to prevent roughness.
   c. Petal the edge with 1- to 2-inch adhesive strips if stockinette edging is not used.
   d. Do not use lotions or powder on the skin around the cast.
   e. Teach the client not to place foreign objects inside the cast (e.g., wire hanger to scratch under the cast).
   f. Smell the cast for foul odor and palpate for hot areas every shift.
   g. Inspect the cast for an increase in drainage every shift.

(From Ignatavicius, DD, Workman, ML, and Mishler, MA: Medical-Surgical Nursing: A Nursing Process Approach, ed 2. WB Saunders, Philadelphia, 1995, with permission.)

oping pressure points and ischemia. Table 44–12 lists important nursing interventions when caring for a client who has a cast.

Traction

Casts can be worn in or out of a hospital setting, but traction for fracture treatment usually requires that the client be hospitalized. As a general definition, traction is the application of a pulling force to a part of the body to provide fracture reduction, alignment, or pain relief.

Traction is classified as either continuous or intermittent. Continuous traction is required for fracture management; intermittent traction, although not commonly used, may be applied for clients experiencing muscle spasm. Most traction is either the "skin" or skeletal type. Skin traction typically involves the use of a Velcro boot (Buck's traction), sling (Russell's traction—knee sling), belt (pelvic), or halter, which is secured around a part of the body (Fig. 44–16). This type of traction does not promote

A

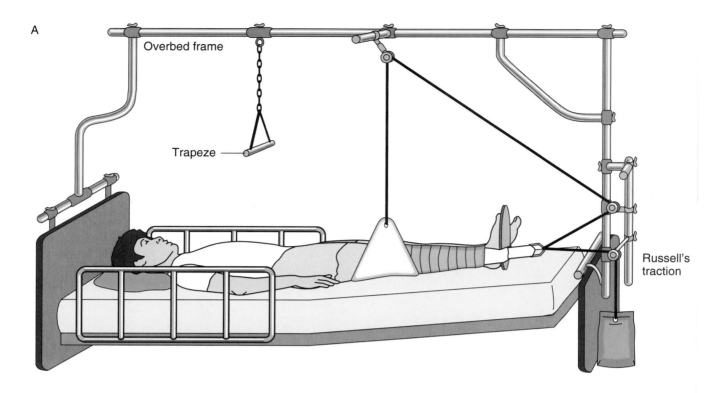

Overbed frame

Trapeze

Russell's traction

B

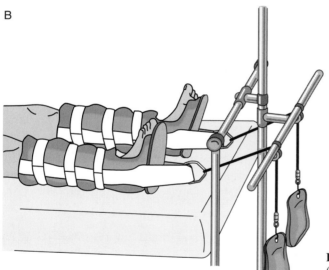

Figure 44–16. Types of skin traction. *(A)* Russell's traction. *(B)* Buck's (boot) traction.

bone alignment or healing, but is used instead for relief of painful muscle spasms that often accompany fractures. Buck's traction is indicated for clients with hip fractures. The weight applied is between 5 and 10 pounds. Skeletal traction involves the use of pins (Steinmann), screws, wires (Kirschner), or tongs (Gardner-Wells, Crutchfield), which are surgically inserted into the bone for the purpose of alignment while the fracture heals (Fig. 44–17). From 20 to 40 pounds of weight are usually applied for skeletal traction, depending on the physician's order.

Balanced suspension maintains the traction while allowing the client some mobility in bed. A Thomas (or T) splint with Pearson's attachment can be used to provide balanced suspension for the lower extremity. The client's leg rests on the suspended sheepskin-covered splint.

The role of the nurse in caring for the client in traction includes frequently monitoring neurovascular status for impaired blood flow, checking the equipment to ensure proper functioning, and monitoring skin condition for pressure points or irritation from equipment. Traction must be

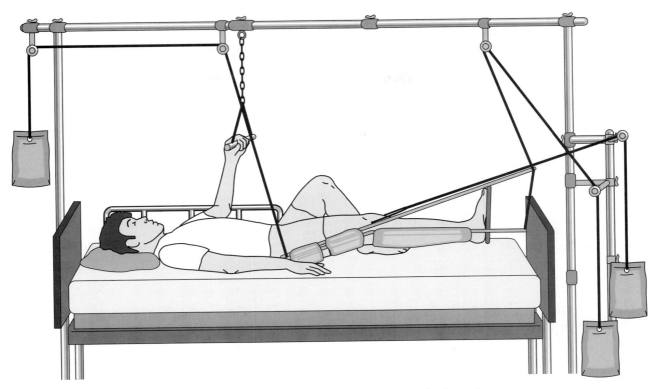

Figure 44–17. Balanced suspension and skeletal traction for femur fracture.

maintained at all times for fractures. All knots, ropes, weights, and pulleys are inspected every 8 to 12 hours for any loosening and intactness. Weights should never touch the floor, be removed, or be lifted. The client's feet should not rest against the end of the bed. Assistance should be obtained to reposition the client in bed, especially with heavy weights in use.

For clients in skeletal traction, pin sites are observed for redness and drainage. Clear, odorless drainage is expected. Some agencies or physicians advocate special solutions or ointments for the skin around the pins (pin care). Others recommend no cleaning to maintain skin integrity. The nurse follows the agency's policy or physician's order for pin care.

Clients who have traction are immobilized for an extended period of time and often experience problems associated with immobility. For example, pressure ulcers on heels are common among elderly clients in traction.

CRITICAL THINKING: Mrs. Brown

Mrs. Brown, a long-time resident of Happy Hills Nursing Home, fell in the day room and sustained a fractured hip. She was rushed to the local community hospital, where she was diagnosed as having a nondisplaced femoral neck (hip) fracture. Her physician ordered 5 pounds of Buck's traction. Mrs.

Brown is restless and picking at her bedcovers when you assess her at the beginning of your shift.

1. What is the purpose of Buck's traction for Mrs. Brown?
2. What are your nursing responsibilities while caring for Mrs. Brown?
3. What might explain her restlessness?

Answers at end of chapter.

Open Reduction with Internal Fixation

An open reduction with internal fixation (ORIF) is a treatment reserved for clients who cannot be managed by casts or traction. One of the most common indications for this surgical procedure is fractured hips. Fractures of the hip involve the proximal femur and affect the elderly more than any other age group. ORIF of the hip allows early mobilization while the bone is healing.

As the name implies, the bone ends are realigned (reduced) by direct visualization through a surgical incision. The bone ends are held in place with metal hardware or prosthesis (femoral component similar to that for total joint replacement) as the internal fixation device (Fig. 44–18). For hip surgery, the IF device is not removed after the fracture heals. For ankle or long bone surgery, the hardware may need to be removed after healing to pre-

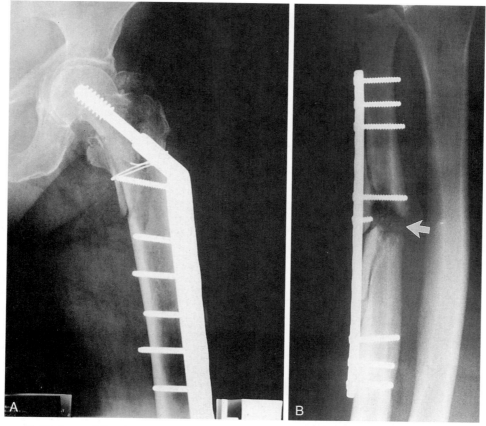

Figure 44–18. Internal fixation. *(A)* Intertrochanteric fracture of the hip with fracture fixation via a side plate and screw combination device. *(B)* Side plate and screw fixation of radial fracture. (From McKinnis, LN: Fundamentals of Orthopedic Radiology. FA Davis, Philadelphia, 1997, with permission.)

vent it from loosening over time. See Nursing Care Plan Box 44–1.

External Fixation

An alternative treatment for some fractures is external fixation. After the fracture is reduced, the physician surgically inserts pins into the bone, which are held in place by an external metal frame to prevent bone movement (Fig. 44–19). External fixation is ideal for the client who has an open fracture with soft tissue damage that can be treated at the same time. Like skeletal traction, the client with this device is at risk for pin site infection. Pin care may or may not be required, but pin sites are observed frequently for signs and symptoms of infection.

Nonunion Modalities

Although most bones heal properly with the correct treatment, some clients experience malunion (malalignment of healed bone) or nonunion (delayed or no healing). A number of variables influence how a bone heals, including age, nutritional status, and the presence of other diseases that alter the healing process, such as diabetes mellitus.

Several methods for treating nonunion are available, including electrical bone stimulation and bone grafting. For selected clients, bone stimulation may be effective in promoting healing; the exact mechanism of action is not known. Bone grafting involves adding packed bone to the fracture site in an attempt to facilitate healing.

The newest advance in fracture healing methods is low-intensity pulsed ultrasound (also called Exogen therapy). Ultrasound treatment has provided excellent results for slow-healing fractures, as well as for fresh fractures. The client applies the treatment for about 20 minutes each day.

Complications of Fractures

The nurse monitors for possible complications and implements interventions to prevent their occurrence when possible. The most common complications include hemorrhage, infection, and thromboembolitic complications. These problems are discussed in more detail in other parts of this text. Although they do not occur often, acute compartment syndrome and fat embolism syndrome are life-threatening complications seen with fractures.

Hemorrhage

Bone is very vascular, and damage or surgery to bone can cause bleeding. The nurse assesses for bleeding and moni-

NURSING CARE PLAN BOX 44–1 FOR THE CLIENT AFTER OPEN REDUCTION WITH INTERNAL FIXATION (ORIF) OF THE HIP

Pain related to surgical wound

Client Outcome
Client states that pain is relieved at satisfactory level.

Evaluation of Outcome
Does client state that pain is absent or at tolerable level?

Intervention	*Rationale*	*Evaluation*
• Give pain medication as needed; anticipate need for pain medication. • Give pain medication before session with physical therapist. • Use fracture bedpan. • Use nondrug pain relief measures, such as music and relaxation.	Pain medication relieves pain, especially if given before pain is severe. Increased activity can cause pain. Fracture bedpans are more comfortable and easier to position for clients. Analgesic therapy is enhanced with complementary pain relief measures.	Does client state pain is relieved? Is client restless or agitated during physical therapy? Is client able to use fracture pan with comfort? Does client report pain relief is enhanced with music or relaxation?

Risk for infection related to skin integrity impairment

Client Outcome
Client will not develop an infection.

Evaluation of Outcome
Does client remain free from infection?

Intervention	*Rationale*	*Evaluation*
• Inspect dressing/wound for signs and symptoms of infection. • Monitor color of and measure wound drainage. • Monitor vital signs frequently.	Infection signs and symptoms are warmth, redness, drainage, pain. Wound drainage color and amount can indicate severity of infection. Elevated vital signs can indicate infection.	Is surgical wound infected? Does wound have purulent, large drainage? Are vital signs within baseline findings?

Impaired physical mobility related to hip precautions and surgical pain

Client Outcome
Client will maintain desired level of activity.

Evaluation of Outcome
Does client maintain activity desired?

Intervention	*Rationale*	*Evaluation*
• Reinforce transfer and ambulation techniques. • Place overhead frame and trapeze on bed; teach client how to use it.	Activity is restricted due to hip precautions and weight-bearing limitations. Client mobility is increased and pain decreased with use of trapeze for movement.	Does client transfer and ambulate as instructed by physical therapist? Does client use overhead frame and trapeze for movement in bed with less pain?

continued

NURSING CARE PLAN BOX 44–1 (continued)

Intervention	Rationale	Evaluation
• Assess the client for and take measures to prevent complications of immobility: turn client every 2 hours and check skin; keep heels off of bed; teach client to deep breathe and cough q2h; also teach use of incentive spirometer. • Apply thigh-high elastic stockings. • Give anticoagulants as ordered. • Get client out of bed as soon as possible. • Ambulate client as early as possible. • Remind client to practice leg exercises.	Immobility complications can occur if preventive measures are not used.	Does client experience complications of immobility?

tors vital signs carefully. Hypovolemic shock may result from severe hemorrhage.

Infection

Trauma predisposes the body to infection, especially when the skin, the body's first line of defense, is disrupted. Wound infections, pin site infections, and osteomyelitis (bone infection) are common. Hospital-acquired infections, such as pneumonia or urinary tract infection, occur in elderly clients who are immobilized for extensive periods of time while their fractures heal.

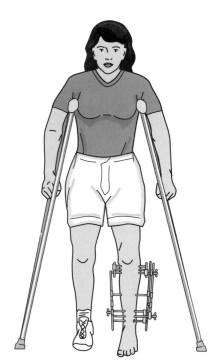

Figure 44–19. External fixation for complex fractures and wound care.

Thromboembolic Complications

Deep vein thrombosis or pulmonary embolus (PE) also develop in clients who are immobile because of trauma or surgery. Thromboembolic (TE) complications are the most common problems of lower extremity surgery or trauma and the most fatal complication of musculoskeletal surgery, particularly in the elderly. Leg exercises and early ambulation help prevent these problems.

Acute Compartment Syndrome

Compartments are sheaths of fibrous tissue that support and partition nerves, muscles, and blood vessels, primarily in the extremities (Fig. 44–20). There are several compartments within each extremity. Acute compartment syndrome (ACS) is a serious problem in which the pressure within one or more extremity compartments increases, causing massive circulation impairment to the area. Pressure can increase from tissue swelling or from compression due to an external device such as a cast or bulky dressing. The early symptom of ACS is the client's report of severe, increasing pain that is not relieved with narcotics and occurs more on active movement than passive movement. Decreased sensation follows before ischemia becomes severe. In severe ACS, the client has the six P's, which are late symptoms:

- Pulselessness
- Paresthesia (painful tingling)
- Paralysis
- Pallor
- Pain (severe and unrelenting)
- Poikilothermia (temperature matches enviroment)

Relief of pressure is the goal. It may be accomplished by removing the source of pressure, such as bivalving a cast, or by performing a **fasciotomy,** which is an incision into

fasciotomy: fascia—fibrous tissue + otomy—opening into

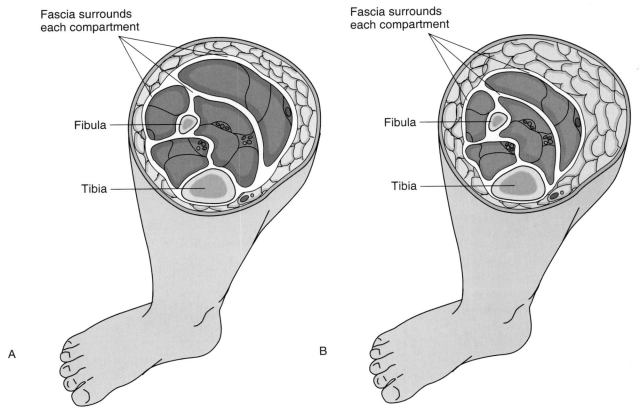

Figure 44–20. *(A)* Lower leg compartments. Each compartment contains muscles, an artery, a vein, and a nerve. *(B)* Compartment syndrome. Increased pressure in a compartment compresses structures within the compartment.

the fascia that encloses the compartment. This incision allows the compartment tissue room to expand and relieves the pressure. If more than one compartment has increased pressure, multiple fasciotomies are required. These surgical wounds remain open until the pressure decreases. Then they are closed and may require skin grafting. If this condition continues without pressure relief, tissue necrosis, infection, extremity contracture, or renal failure may result. Renal failure is a potentially fatal complication of ACS.

Fat Embolism Syndrome

Fat embolism syndrome (FES) is another serious complication in which small fat globules are released from yellow bone marrow into the bloodstream. The globules then travel to the lung fields, causing respiratory distress. This process most often occurs when long bones are fractured or when the client has multiple fractures. The elderly client with a fractured hip is also at a high risk for FES.

The earliest manifestation of FES is altered mental status resulting from a low arterial oxygen level. The client then experiences tachycardia, tachypnea, fever, high blood pressure, and severe respiratory distress. Most clients also have a measles-like rash, called petechiae, over the upper body. Even when aggressively treated, clients with FES often die from the pulmonary edema that typically develops.

The nurse notes the early signs and symptoms and reports them to the physician immediately.

Nursing Process

Caring for the client with a fracture may require an interdisciplinary approach, especially for complex or multiple fractures. The nurse coordinates care with other health team members.

Assessment

The most important aspect of assessment for the client with a fracture is frequent monitoring of neurovascular status distal to the fracture site. As mentioned earlier, acute compartment syndrome is a potentially limb or life-threatening complication that results when blood flow is impaired. Chapter 43 describes the procedure for this assessment and its significance.

Pain is assessed and managed by both medications and complementary therapies, such as imagery. Bone pain can be very excruciating and must be treated aggressively. For the client who cannot ask for pain medication, particularly the confused elderly client with a hip fracture, the nurse looks for nonverbal indicators, including restlessness and behavioral problems such as screaming. The nurse anticipates the client's need for medication to keep the client comfortable.

Nursing Diagnosis

The common nursing diagnoses for the client with a fracture may include the following:

- Pain
- Risk for neurovascular dysfunction
- Impaired physical mobility
- Risk for infection

Planning

The plan of care is derived from the nursing diagnoses and risk for medical complications. Clients with uncomplicated fractures are discharged directly from the clinic or emergency department. Clients with multiple or more complex fractures, especially involving soft tissue injury, are admitted to the hospital for care. To ensure continuity of care, the discharge planner, social worker, and case manager are involved from the time of admission through the continuing care phase.

Implementation

The most common fracture that leads to hospitalization is the hip fracture. Nursing Care Plan Box 44–1 highlights the most important aspects of care for the client with a fractured hip.

Evaluation

The expected outcomes for the client are relief of pain and healing without complications. The interdisciplinary team evaluates care to ensure that it is directed toward meeting these outcomes.

Client Education

If the client is casted, the nurse reviews the appropriate instructions for cast care, as discussed earlier. Health teaching is also important for care of the extremity after cast removal (Table 44–13). The client may also have a wound that will be managed at home. The nurse teaches the client and caregiver how to assess and dress the wound and when to report changes such as signs and symptoms of infection.

Nutritional education is also essential. The body needs adequate protein, calories, and vitamins for healing to occur. Unless otherwise contraindicated, milkshakes and instant breakfast preparations are good sources of additional protein and calories, as well as a source of calcium.

OSTEOMYELITIS

Osteomyelitis is an infection of bone that can be either acute or chronic. A bone infection lasting less than 4 weeks is considered acute; one that lasts more than 4 weeks is chronic.

Table 44–13. ***Care of the Extremity After Cast Removal***

- Remove scaly, dead skin carefully by soaking—do not scrub.
- Move the extremity carefully. Expect discomfort, weakness, and decreased range of motion.
- Support the extremity with pillows or your orthotic device until strength and movement return.
- Exercise slowly as instructed by your physical therapist.
- Wear support stockings or elastic bandages to prevent swelling (for lower extremity).

(From Ignatavicius, DD, Workman, ML, and Mishler, MA: Medical-Surgical Nursing: A Nursing Process Approach, ed 2. WB Saunders, Philadelphia, 1995, with permission.)

Pathophysiology

Regardless of type, osteomyelitis results from invasion of bacteria into bone and surrounding soft tissues. Inflammation occurs, followed by ischemia (decreased blood flow) (Fig. 44–21). Bone tissue then becomes necrotic (dies), which retards healing and causes more infection, often as a bone abscess.

Pathogens enter bone in several ways. Direct inoculation means that an injury to the body allows the offending microbes direct access to bone tissue. An open fracture is an example of that process. Contiguous spread occurs when surrounding soft tissue becomes infected. An example is the client with cellulitis whose infection then spreads to underlying bone. In hematogenous spread, an infection beginning in another part of the body migrates to bone. For instance, a client with a total hip replacement may get osteomyelitis from a urinary tract infection.

Causes and Types

Penetrating trauma leads to acute osteomyelitis by direct inoculation. The most common pathogen is *Pseudomonas aeruginosa*. The leading cause of contiguous spread is the client with diabetes mellitus or peripheral vascular disease who has a slow-healing foot ulcer. Multiple organisms may be present in the wound and subsequently the bone. Hematogenous spread results from bacteremia (infection of the blood), underlying disease, or nonpenetrating trauma. Long-term intravenous catheters are primary sources of infection.

Signs and Symptoms

The client with acute osteomyelitis has fever, as well as local signs of inflammation—tenderness, redness, heat, pain, and swelling. Pain may be the only apparent complaint. Ul-

---

osteomyelitis: osteo—bone + myel—bone marrow + itis—inflammation

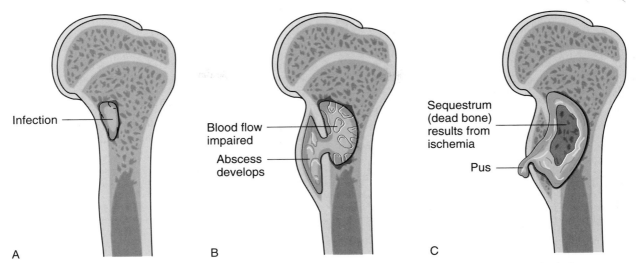

Figure 44–21. Sequence of osteomyelitis development. *(A)* Infection begins. *(B)* Blood flow is blocked in the area of infection. An abscess with pus forms. *(C)* Bone dies within the infection site, and pus formation continues.

ceration, drainage, and localized pain are typical signs and symptoms of chronic osteomyelitis.

Diagnostic Tests

The client with osteomyelitis typically has an elevated leukocyte (white blood cell) count, an elevated erythrocyte sedimentation rate, and positive bone biopsy for infection. Some clients also have a positive blood culture.

Treatment

Long-term antibiotic therapy is the treatment of choice for clients with bone infection. Infection in bone tissue is difficult to resolve and may require weeks to months of medication. Clients often administer their intravenous antibiotics at home rather than stay in a costly hospital bed. Central venous access devices, such as Hickman catheters, are used for intravenous drug administration. The nurse teaches the client and caregiver about the side effects, toxicity, interactions, and precautions for antibiotic therapy. A home care nurse may be needed to assist the client.

If a soft tissue wound is present, it may need irrigations and dressing changes that must be taught to the client and family or significant other. The nurse teaches the client about the importance of hand washing and how to avoid the spread of pathogens. Some clients are placed on Standard Precautions or other isolation precautions, depending on the offending organism(s).

Antibiotic therapy alone may not resolve the infection. Clients with chronic osteomyelitis may require surgery to remove necrotic bone tissue or replace it with healthy bone tissue. Amputations are reserved for clients who have massive infections that have not responded to one of the conventional treatments.

OSTEOPOROSIS

Osteoporosis is a common metabolic disorder in which the bone loses its density, resulting in fragile bones and possibly resulting in fractures. The wrist, hip, and vertebral column are most frequently involved.

Pathophysiology

Bone is a very dynamic tissue, constantly building new tissue and resorbing (breaking down) old tissue. Bone density (mass) peaks between 30 and 35 years of age. After these peak years, the rate of bone breakdown exceeds the rate of bone building. The result is irreversible bone loss that worsens with aging. Trabecular (cancellous) bone is lost first, followed by a loss of cortical (compact) bone. As a result, more than 1.5 million fractures occur each year in people over 45 years of age. Hip fractures are among the most common, accounting for over 250,000 per year. The mortality rate for hip fractures is about 50 percent during the first year after the fracture.

Cause and Types

Osteoporosis is either primary or secondary. Primary osteoporosis is the most common and is not associated with another disease or health problem. Risk factors for primary osteoporosis include the following:

- Caucasian postmenopausal woman (less estrogen available to protect bone)
- Sedentary lifestyle
- Decreased calcium intake
- Lack of vitamin D (to absorb calcium)
- Excessive alcohol consumption
- Cigarette smoking

- Excessive caffeine intake
- Petite body build

Secondary osteoporosis results from an associated medical condition, such as hyperparathyroidism, long-term drug therapy, especially steroids, and prolonged immobility, such as that seen with clients who have a spinal cord injury.

Signs and Symptoms

Most women do not realize they have osteoporosis until they fracture a bone. During the late middle years, the classic "dowager's hump," or kyphosis of the spine, is usually present. The client's height decreases and back pain may be present. The client may be embarrassed by the change in body image and may have curtailed social activities. Some clients have difficulty finding clothes that fit comfortably.

Diagnostic Tests

X-ray of the bone is not helpful in diagnosing bone loss in its early stages. Computed tomography and quantitative CT detect early spine changes and measure bone density. One of the newest tests is dual-energy x-ray absorptiometry (DXA), which is used as a screening tool to measure bone mineral content. This test is noninvasive and is becoming more readily accessible.

Serum calcium and vitamin D levels may be decreased, and serum phosphorus may be increased. With severe bone loss, alkaline phosphatase levels may be elevated, confirming bone damage.

Treatment

The cornerstone of treatment for osteoporosis is medication and avoidance of modifiable risk factors to prevent bone loss.

Medication

Medication may be used for prevention or treatment purposes. The current drugs of choice are estrogen, calcium supplements, vitamin D, and alendronate (Fosamax).

Estrogen replacement is helpful because estrogen prevents bone loss. It may be given orally or worn as a topical patch. Although the drug has been associated with cervical cancer, the benefit of estrogen outweighs its risk for many women.

Calcium is also important to prevent bone loss. If serum calcium falls below normal levels, the parathyroid glands stimulate the bone to release calcium into the bloodstream. The result is demineralized bone. Therefore calcium supplements are an important aspect of treatment. The nurse teaches the client to drink plenty of fluids to prevent calcium-based urinary stones. Vitamin D supplementation may also be necessary for clients who have inadequate sunlight exposure or who cannot metabolize vitamin D.

Alendronate is one of the newest drugs used to prevent or slow the progress of osteoporosis. It is classified as a bone resorption inhibitor, preventing the breakdown of bone. Although side effects are not common, serious cases of esophagitis and esophageal ulcers have been reported. Therefore the nurse teaches the client to take the drug early in the morning and follow it with a full glass of water. The client should not lie down for at least 1 hour after taking the drug.

The newest drug class for osteoporosis is the selective estrogen receptor modulator (SERM). Although not yet approved for general use at this time, raloxifene (Evista), one of the most promising SERMs, increases bone mass 2 to 3 percent each year. These drugs are designed to mimic estrogen in some parts of the body while blocking its effects elsewhere.

Other drugs that may be used include testosterone (a bone-building hormone), calcitonin, and sodium fluoride. All of these medications have major disadvantages and are consequently not commonly given. Any drug used to prevent or control osteoporosis must be administered under the supervision of a physician, including calcium and vitamin D supplements.

Diet

Increasing calcium and fluids in the diet are the main dietary considerations for women. The nurse teaches clients what foods are high in calcium, such as dairy products and dark green, leafy vegetables. If the client consumes excessive caffeine or alcohol, the nurse teaches about the need to avoid these substances. The National Osteoporosis Foundation can provide information and literature to clients and their families about diet and other aspects of treatment and prevention.

Exercise

Weight-bearing exercise, especially walking, stimulates bone building. The client should wear well-supporting, nonskid shoes at all times and avoid uneven surfaces that could contribute to falls.

Fall Prevention

Osteoporotic bone may cause a pathological fracture in which the hip breaks before the fall. For other clients, a fall can cause a hip or other fracture. Therefore, falls prevention programs in hospitals and nursing homes are very important.

In collaboration with the physical or occupational therapist, case manager, or discharge planner, the nurse assesses the client's home environment. The client and family are taught how to create a hazard-free environment, such as avoiding scatter rugs and slippery floors. Walking paths in the home must be kept free of clutter to prevent falls. If needed, a walker or cane provides additional support.

PAGET'S DISEASE

Paget's disease, also called osteitis deformans, is a metabolic bone disease in which increased bone loss results in large, disorganized bone deposits throughout the body. It is primarily a disease of the elderly.

Pathophysiology

Three phases of the disorder have been described: active, mixed, and inactive. A prolific increase in osteoclasts (cells that break down bone) causes massive bone deformity and destruction. Osteoblasts (bone-building cells) then react to form new bone. However, the result is disorganized in structure. Finally, when osteoblastic activity exceeds the osteoclastic activity, the inactive phase occurs. The newly formed bone becomes sclerotic with increased vascularity.

Paget's disease can affect one or multiple bones. The most common areas involved are the femur, skull, vertebrae, and pelvis.

Causes and Types

The exact cause of this disease is not known, but it tends to run in families. Paget's disease may be the result of a latent viral infection contracted in young adulthood. It is more common in Europe than in the United States.

Signs and Symptoms

Most clients with Paget's disease have no obvious symptoms, particularly when the disorder is confined to one bone. For clients with more severe disease, signs and symptoms are varied and potentially fatal. Table 44–14 lists the key features of this disease.

Diagnostic Tests

Diagnosis may be made solely on x-ray findings. X-rays of pagetic bone show punched-out areas indicating increased bone resorption. The overall mass of bone may be enlarged, depending on the phase of the disorder. Deformities, fractures, and arthritic changes are not uncommon.

The primary laboratory findings are an increased alkaline phosphatase (ALP) and an increase in urinary hydroxyproline. ALP reflects bone damage. Urinary hydroxyproline indicates an increase in bone turnover. The higher the level, the more severe the disease. Calcium levels in both blood and urine are elevated as damaged bone releases calcium into the bloodstream.

Treatment

Nonsurgical management is employed to relieve pain and promote a reasonable quality of life for the client. For mild disease, NSAIDs are given.

Table 44–14. *Key Features of Paget's Disease of the Bone*

Musculoskeletal Manifestations
- Bone and joint pain (may be in a single bone) that is aching, poorly described, and aggravated by walking.
- Low back and sciatic nerve pain
- Bowing of long bones
- Loss of normal spinal curvature
- Enlarged, thick skull
- Pathological fractures
- Osteogenic sarcoma

Skin Manifestations
- Flushed, warm skin

Other Manifestations
- Apathy, lethargy, fatigue
- Hyperparathyroidism
- Gout
- Urinary or renal stones
- Heart failure from fluid overload

(From Ignatavicius, DD, Workman, ML, and Mishler, MA: Medical-Surgical Nursing: A Nursing Process Approach, ed 2. WB Saunders, Philadelphia, 1995, with permission.)

Medication

The purpose of drug therapy for the client with Paget's disease is to relieve pain and decrease bone loss. Calcitonin (Calcimar) is a thyroid hormone that is often effective in initiating a remission of the disease. It appears to decrease bone loss while decreasing pain. If effective, the ALP level decreases. The usual duration of therapy is 6 months followed by 6 months of etidronate disodium (Didronel). Its action is similar to that of calcitonin, and it must be taken on an empty stomach.

Plicamycin (mithramycin, Mithracin) is a potent anticancer drug and antibiotic that is reserved for clients with severe hypercalcemia or severe disease with neurological involvement. This drug suppresses both osteoclastic and osteoblastic activity within days, but it has serious adverse effects. As with all drugs, the nurse observes for toxic effects such as liver and kidney failure. Platelet count is monitored because the drug can decrease platelet production. When liver enzymes become too high, the drug is temporarily discontinued until they return to baseline.

Alendronate (Fosamax) is a new drug that is a bone resorption inhibitor and calcium regulator. Intravenous dosing for 5 days may initiate a disease remission.

Other Treatment

Additional management for Paget's disease depends on the clinical manifestations. For example, if the client has osteogenic sarcoma, the appropriate treatment for bone tumors is initiated.

BONE CANCER

Bone tumors may be benign or malignant. Malignant tumors may be either primary or metastatic, originating from another location and migrating to bone. Primary bone tumors tend to develop in people under 30 years of age and account for only a small percentage of bone cancers. Metastatic lesions are much more common and most often affect the elderly.

Pathophysiology

The pathophysiology depends on the type of bone cancer. The cause of bone cancer is not known.

Primary Malignant Tumors

Osteosarcoma, or osteogenic sarcoma, is the most common primary malignant bone tumor. It is a fairly large tumor that typically metastasizes to the lung within 2 years of diagnosis and treatment. More than 50 percent of osteosarcomas occur in the distal femur in young men. Older clients with Paget's disease may also develop these lesions.

Ewing's sarcoma is the most malignant. In addition to local pain and swelling, systemic signs and symptoms, including low-grade fever, leukocytosis, and anemia, are common. The pelvis and lower extremity are most often affected in children and young men.

Clients with a chrondrosarcoma have a better prognosis than those with the previously described types of bone cancer. This type of cancer occurs in middle-aged and older people.

Metastatic Bone Disease

Primary malignant tumors that occur in the prostate, breast, lung, and thyroid gland are called bone-seeking cancers because they migrate to bone more than any other primary cancer. Multiple bone sites are typically seen. Pathological fractures and severe pain are major concerns in managing metastatic disease.

Signs and Symptoms

Primary tumors cause local swelling and pain at the site. A tender, palpable mass is often present. Metastatic disease is not as visible, but the client complains of diffuse severe pain, eventually leading to marked disability.

Diagnostic Tests

Diagnosis of bone cancer is made by x-ray, computed tomography, bone scan, or bone biopsy. Chapter 43 discusses these tests in detail.

The client with metastatic disease has an elevated ALP level and possibly an elevated erythrocyte sedimentation rate, indicating secondary tissue inflammation.

Treatment

Management of bone cancer depends on the type and extent of the tumor. The treatment of primary bone tumors is usually surgery, often combined with chemotherapy or radiation. The surgeon attempts to salvage the limb and performs a resection of the tumor. For clients with Ewing's sarcoma or early osteosarcoma, external radiation may be the treatment of choice to reduce tumor size and pain.

Care of the postoperative client is similar to that for any client undergoing musculoskeletal surgery. Monitoring neurovascular status of the operative limb is a vital nursing intervention (see Chapter 43). Other general postoperative care is discussed in Chapter 11.

For metastatic bone disease, surgery is not appropriate. External radiation is given primarily for palliation. The radiation is directed toward the most painful sites in an attempt to shrink them and provide more comfort for the client.

Nursing care for the client with bone cancer is not unlike that for clients with any other type of cancer. The nurse helps the client adjust to the diagnosis and refers the client to resources such as the American Cancer Society and its various support groups. Chapter 10 describes the nursing care associated with chemotherapy and radiation therapy.

Review Questions

1. Wilma has been diagnosed with rheumatoid arthritis. Which of the following symptoms would the nurse most likely be told was the first symptom that caused Wilma to seek health care?
   a. Fatigue
   b. Stiff, sore joints
   c. Shortness of breath
   d. Crepitation

2. Bill has osteoporosis and is scheduled for a right total hip replacement. Bill's preoperative teaching for postoperative leg positioning will include which of the following?
   a. Maintain legs in adduction
   b. Maintain legs in abduction
   c. Maintain internal leg rotation
   d. Maintain more than 90-degree hip flexion

3. Bernie is being seen for gout. Which of the following medications would be helpful in treating Bernie's gout?
   a. Allopurinol
   b. Calcitonin
   c. Dilantin
   d. Lasix

---

osteosarcoma: osteo—bone + sarco—flesh + oma—tumor

4. Sarah has systemic lupus erythematosus. Which of the following would be a priority nursing diagnosis?
   a. Impaired swallowing
   b. Impaired physical mobility
   c. Risk for aspiration
   d. Body image disturbance

5. Lou fractured his hip and is scheduled for surgery. He is placed in Buck's (boot) traction. Which one of the following is the primary purpose for placing Lou in Buck's traction?
   a. Reduce muscle spasms
   b. Maintain bed rest
   c. Prevent leg adduction
   d. Prevent leg abduction

6. Randy has a 36-hour-old fractured femur and is in traction. He had morphine 10 mg IM 2 hours ago. He reports severe unrelieved pain. Which one of the following actions would be most appropriate for the nurse to take?
   a. Give pain medication
   b. Adjust the traction
   c. Assess pulse oximeter
   d. Notify client's physician

7. Jeff is in skeletal traction. Which one of the following is an example of skeletal traction?
   a. Russell's traction
   b. Buck's traction
   c. Boot traction
   d. Kirschner wire

8. Trent sustains a closed fracture of his left tibia and is placed in a long-leg plaster cast that is damp. Which one of the following actions should the nurse take to facilitate cast drying?
   a. Cover cast with blankets to provide extra warmth
   b. Turn patient every 2 hours
   c. Increase room temperature to 80°F
   d. Dry cast with blow dryer, applying heat every 30 minutes

9. Margaret is postmenopausal, has lost 2 inches of height, is thin, and has never exercised regularly. She has osteoporosis. Which one of the following interventions should be included in Margaret's plan of care to prevent further bone loss?
   a. Decrease participation in ADL
   b. Decrease weight-bearing activities
   c. Encourage regular exercise
   d. Encourage weight gain

10. Ray is scheduled for a below-the-knee amputation (BKA). Which one of the following actions is a priority for the nurse to take before Ray's admittance to his postoperative room after surgery?
    a. Change the bed linen
    b. Place a tourniquet in the room
    c. Pad the siderails
    d. Place scissors in the room

11. Mary has Paget's disease. A priority nursing diagnosis for Mary would include which one of the following?
    a. Pain
    b. Knowledge deficit
    c. Fluid volume excess
    d. Fluid volume deficit

12. Which one of the following is a common sign or symptom of chronic osteomyelitis?
    a. Positive Homans' sign
    b. Palpable vein
    c. Ulceration
    d. Phantom pain

ANSWERS TO CRITICAL THINKING

CRITICAL THINKING: Mr. Dennis

1. Ask the client the following questions:
   - "What is your typical day on the job like?"
   - "Do certain activities increase joint pain?"
   - "When is your pain worse—after activity or after rest?"
   - "How long have you experienced joint pain?"
2. Risk factors include that he is overweight, is in late middle age, and has a physically demanding job.
3. Other signs and symptoms include bony nodules on his fingers (such as Heberden's nodes) and secondary inflammation causing joint swelling.

CRITICAL THINKING: Mrs. Summers

1. Ask Mrs. Summers about the following:
   - The nature of her pain
   - If it is worse after activity or rest
   - If she experiences joint stiffness and, if so, when
2. Teach her to do the following:
   - Balance rest with exercise
   - Use ice for very hot, swollen joints
   - Use heat to decrease stiffness

CRITICAL THINKING: Mrs. Brown

1. To reduce muscle spasms that often accompany fractures.
2. Nursing responsibilities include the following:
   - Check neurovascular status frequently.
   - Check equipment, including rope, pulleys, knots, and weights.
   - Do not allow the weights to rest on the floor.
   - Assess client's skin often for areas of potential breakdown.
3. Her restlessness is most likely due to pain. She may be unable to state that she is in pain, and the

nurse uses behaviors such as restlessness and other nonverbal cues to evaluate her need for pain management modalities.

BIBLIOGRAPHY

Ashworth, L: Can alendronate help my osteoporosis? Home Care Provider 2(1):37, 1997.

Crutchfield, J, Zimmerman, L, Nieveen, J, et al: Preoperative and postoperative pain in total knee replacement. Orthop Nurs 15(2):65, 1996.

Department of Health and Human Services: Healthy People 2000. Department of Health and Human Services, Rockville, Md, 1990.

Gio-Fitman, J: The role of psychological stress in rheumatoid arthritis. Medsurg Nurs 5:422, 1996.

Hunt, AH: The relationship between height change and bone mineral density. Orthop Nurs 15(3):57, 1996.

Ignatavicius, DD, Workman, ML, and Mishler, MA: Medical-Surgical Nursing: A Nursing Process Approach, ed 2. WB Saunders, Philadelphia, 1995.

Kessenich, CR, and Rosen, CJ: Vitamin D and bone status in elderly women. Orthop Nurs 15(3):67, 1996.

Maher, AB, Salmond, SW, and Pellino, TA: Orthopaedic Nursing. WB Saunders, Philadelphia, 1994.

Matteson, MA, McConnell, ES, and Linton, AD: Gerontological Nursing, ed 2. WB Saunders, Philadelphia, 1997.

National Osteoporosis Foundation: Position Paper: Current Perspective on Diagnosis, Prevention, and Treatment of Osteoporosis. National Osteoporosis Foundation, Washington, DC, 1995.

Ulak, LJ: Special considerations for SLE patients. Medsurg Nurs 4(2):146, 1995.

Wetherbee, LL: Caring for the client with rheumatoid arthritis. Home Healthc Nurse 12(1):13, 1994.

Understanding the Nervous System

45

Neurological Function, Assessment, and Therapeutic Measures

Sally Schnell

Learning Objectives

Upon completion of this chapter, the student will be able to:

1. Describe the structure of the central and peripheral portions of the nervous system.
2. Explain how the nervous system controls body functions.
3. List the effects of aging on nervous system function.
4. Identify signs and symptoms of increased intracranial pressure.
5. Explain the Monro-Kellie doctrine.
6. Identify the rationale for performing a baseline neurological examination on all clients.
7. Describe the components of a baseline neurological examination.
8. Identify changes in the client's neurological function that warrant immediate notification of the physician.
9. Assess level of consciousness using the Glasgow Coma Scale.
10. Modify the neurological examination for use with aphasic clients.
11. Identify neurological deficits that may affect client safety.
12. Identify client neurological deficits that should be communicated to ancillary personnel who interact with the client.
13. Explain the nurse's role when caring for clients undergoing diagnostic tests for nervous system dysfunction.
14. Use findings from the neurological examination to plan safe care.
15. Describe nursing care of clients with selected neurological deficits.

Key Words

anisocoria (an-i-soh-**KOH**-ree-ah)
aphasia (ah-**FAY**-zee-ah)
cerebrovascular (SER-ee-broh-**VAS**-kyoo-lur)
contractures (kon-**TRAK**-churs)
decerebrate (dee-**SER**-e-brayt)
decorticate (dee-**KOR**-ti-kayt)
dysarthria (dis-**AR**-three-ah)
dysphagia (dis-**FAYJ**-ee-ah)
electroencephalogram (ee-LEK-troh-en-**SEFF**-uh-loh-gram)
hemiparesis (hem-ee-puh-**REE**-sis)
intraparenchymal (IN-trah-PAIR-en-**KYE**-mul)
myelogram (**MY**-e-loh-gram)
neuropathy (new-**RAH**-puh-thee)
nystagmus (nis-**TAG**-muss)
paresis (puh-**REE**-sis)
paresthesia (PAR-es-**THEE**-zee-ah)
radiculopathy (ra-DIK-yoo-**LAH**-puh-thee)
subarachnoid (SUB-uh-**RAK**-noyd)

Review of Normal Anatomy and Physiology

The nervous system is one of the body's control systems; by means of electrochemical impulses we are able to detect changes and feel sensations, initiate appropriate responses to changes, and organize and store information for future use. Some of this is conscious activity, but much of it is reflex in nature and happens without our awareness.

The nervous system has two divisions. The central nervous system (CNS) consists of the brain and spinal cord.

The peripheral nervous system (PNS) consists of cranial nerves and spinal nerves, which include the nerves of the autonomic nervous system (ANS).

NERVE TISSUE

Nerve tissue consists of neurons and specialized supporting cells. There are many kinds of neurons (nerve cells or nerve fibers), but they all have the same general structure (Fig. 45–1). The cell body contains the nucleus and is essential for the continued life of the neuron. All neuron cell bodies are found in the brain or spinal cord or within the

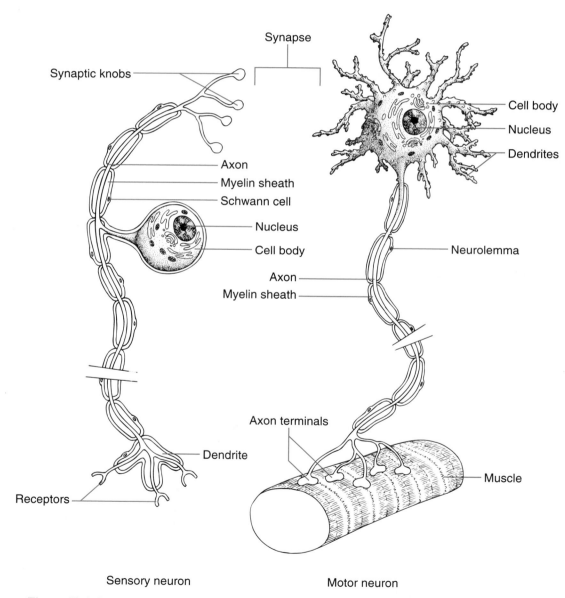

Sensory neuron   Motor neuron

Figure 45–1. Structure of sensory and motor neurons. (Modified from Scanlon, VC, Sanders, T: Workbook for Essentials of Anatomy and Physiology, ed 2. FA Davis, Philadelphia, 1995, p 109, with permission.)

trunk of the body; in these locations they are protected by bone. A neuron may have one to many dendrites, which are extensions that carry impulses toward the cell body. A neuron has one axon that transmits impulses away from the cell body. It is the cell membrane of the dendrites, cell body, and axon that carries the electrical nerve impulse.

In the peripheral nervous system, axons and dendrites are wrapped in specialized cells called Schwann cells. The concentric layers of cell membrane of a Schwann cell form the myelin sheath. Myelin is a phospholipid that electrically insulates neurons from one another. The spaces between adjacent Schwann cells are called nodes of Ranvier (neurofibril nodes); only these parts of the neuron cell membrane depolarize when an electrical impulse is transmitted, which makes impulse conduction rapid. The nuclei and cytoplasm of Schwann cells are outside the myelin sheath and form the neurolemma. If a peripheral nerve is severed and reattached, the individual axons and dendrites may regrow through the tunnels provided by the neurolemma. Growth factors produced by the Schwann cells are also believed to contribute to such regeneration.

In the central nervous system, the myelin sheaths (but not a neurolemma) are formed by oligodendrocytes, one of the neuroglia, the specialized cells found only in the brain and spinal cord. See Table 45–1 for the names and functions of the other neuroglial cells.

Synapses

When the axon of a neuron must transmit an impulse to the dendrite or cell body of another neuron, the impulse must cross a small gap called a synapse. An electrical impulse is incapable of crossing this microscopic space, and at synapses impulse transmission becomes chemical. The

Table 45–1. **Neuroglia**

Name	Function
Oligodendrocytes	Produce the myelin sheath to electrically insulate neurons of the CNS
Microglia	Capable of movement and phagocytosis of pathogens and damaged tissue
Astrocytes	Contribute to the blood-brain barrier, which prevents potentially toxic waste products in the blood from diffusing out into brain tissue; disadvantage: some useful medications cannot cross it, which becomes important during brain infection, inflammation, or other disease
Ependyma	Line the ventricles of the brain; many of the cells are ciliated; involved in the circulation of cerebrospinal fluid

end of the axon (the presynaptic neuron) is called the synaptic knob and contains a chemical neurotransmitter that is released into the synapse by the arrival of the electrical impulse. The neurotransmitter diffuses across the synapse and combines with specific receptor sites on the postsynaptic membrane (Fig. 45–2). At excitatory synapses, the neurotransmitter makes the postsynaptic membrane more permeable to sodium ions, which rush into the cell, initiating an electrical impulse on the membrane of the postsynaptic neuron. The neurotransmitter is then inactivated to prevent continuous impulses. For example, the neurotransmitter acetylcholine is inactivated by the chemical called cholinesterase; each transmitter has its own specific inactivator.

Some synapses are inhibitory synapses in that the neurotransmitter makes the postsynaptic membrane more permeable to potassium ions, which leave the cell and make the membrane resistant to the electrical change required for an impulse. Thus the electrical impulse is stopped. Inhibitory synapses are important for such things as slowing the heart rate or balancing the excitatory impulses transmitted to skeletal muscles, which prevents excessive contraction and is important for coordination.

At synapses, impulse transmission is one-way only because the neurotransmitter is released only by the presynaptic neuron; the impulse cannot go backwards. This is important for the normal activity of the functional types of neurons. The relative complexity of synapses also makes them a potential target for the actions of medications.

TYPES OF NEURONS

A useful classification of neurons is a functional one; a neuron is either a sensory neuron, a motor neuron, or an interneuron. Sensory (afferent) neurons transmit impulses from receptors to the central nervous system. Receptors are specialized to detect external or internal changes and then generate electrical impulses. Sensory neurons from receptors in the skin, skeletal muscles, and joints are called somatic; those from receptors in internal organs are called visceral sensory neurons.

Motor (efferent) neurons transmit impulses from the central nervous system to effectors, that is, muscles and glands. Motor neurons to skeletal muscle are called somatic; those to smooth muscle, cardiac muscle, and glands are called visceral. Sensory and motor neurons make up the peripheral nervous system. Visceral motor neurons form the autonomic nervous system, a specialized part of the PNS.

Interneurons (or association neurons) are found entirely within the central nervous system. Each is specialized to transmit sensory or motor impulses or to integrate these functions. Such integration would be involved in thinking and learning.

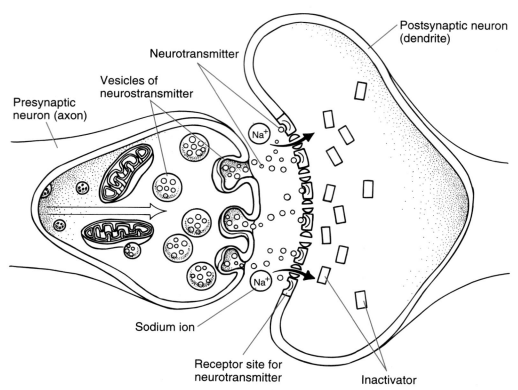

Figure 45–2. Structure of a synapse and the effect of a neurotransmitter such as acetylcholine. (Modified from Scanlon, VC, Sanders, T: Workbook for Essentials of Anatomy and Physiology, ed 2. FA Davis, Philadelphia, 1995, p 110, with permission.)

NERVES AND NERVE TRACTS

A nerve is a group of peripheral axons, dendrites, or both, with blood vessels and connective tissue. Most peripheral nerves are mixed, that is, they contain both sensory and motor neurons. An example of a purely sensory nerve is the optic nerve for vision; the autonomic nerves are purely motor nerves.

A nerve tract is a group of neurons within the central nervous system; such tracts are often called white matter because the myelin sheaths of the individual neurons are white. A nerve tract within the spinal cord carries either sensory or motor impulses; those within the brain may have either sensory or motor or integrative functions.

NERVE IMPULSE

A nerve impulse, which may also be called an action potential, is an electrical change brought about by the movement of ions across the neuron cell membrane. When a neuron is not carrying an impulse it is in a state of polarization with a positive charge outside the membrane and a relatively negative charge inside the membrane. Sodium ions are more abundant outside the cell, and potassium and negative ions are more abundant inside the cell. A stimulus makes the membrane very permeable to sodium ions, which rush into the cell, making the inside positive and the outside rela-

tively negative. This reversal of charges is called depolarization and spreads from the point of the stimulus along the entire neuron membrane.

Immediately following depolarization, the membrane becomes very permeable to potassium ions, which rush out of the cell. This is called repolarization and restores the positive charge outside and the negative charge inside. The sodium and potassium pumps return the sodium ions back outside and the potassium ions inside, and the neuron is polarized again and ready to respond to another stimulus. A neuron is capable of transmitting hundreds of impulses per second, and at great speed, many meters per second.

SPINAL CORD

The spinal cord transmits impulses to and from the brain and is the integrating center for the spinal cord reflexes. The spinal cord is within the vertebral canal formed by the vertebrae, and extends from the foramen magnum of the occipital bone to the disk between the first and second lumbar vertebrae. The spinal nerves emerge from the intervertebral foramina.

In cross section the spinal cord is round or oval; internally is an H-shaped mass of gray matter surrounded by white matter (Fig. 45–3). The gray matter is the cell bodies of motor neurons and interneurons. The white matter is

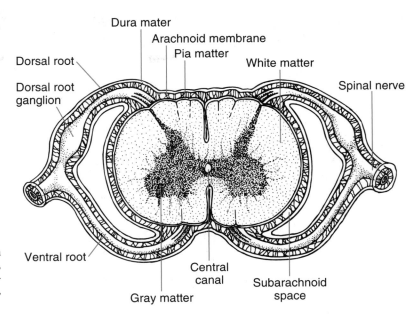

Figure 45–3. Spinal cord in cross section, with nerve roots and meninges. (Modified from Scanlon, VC, Sanders, T: Workbook for Essentials of Anatomy and Physiology, ed 2. FA Davis, Philadelphia, 1995, p 119, with permission.) See Plate 12.

the myelinated axons and dendrites of the interneurons. These nerve fibers are arranged in tracts based on their functions; ascending tracts transmit sensory impulses to the brain, and descending tracts transmit motor impulses from the brain to motor neurons. The central canal of the spinal cord is a small tunnel that is continuous with the ventricles of the brain; it contains cerebrospinal fluid (CSF).

Spinal Nerves

There are 31 pairs of spinal nerves, named according to their respective vertebrae: 8 cervical pairs, 12 thoracic pairs, 5 lumbar pairs, 5 sacral pairs, and 1 very small coccygeal pair. These nerves are often referred to by letter and number: the second cervical nerve is C2, the tenth thoracic is T10, and so on.

In general, the cervical nerves supply the back of the head; the neck, shoulders, and arms; and the diaphragm (the phrenic nerves). The first thoracic nerve also contributes to nerves in the arms. The remaining thoracic nerves supply the trunk of the body. The lumbar and sacral nerves supply the hips, pelvic cavity, and legs. The small coccygeal pair (Co1) supplies the area around the coccyx.

Each spinal nerve has two roots, which are neurons entering or leaving the spinal cord. The dorsal root is made of sensory neurons that carry impulses into the spinal cord. The dorsal root ganglion is an enlargement of this root that contains the cell bodies of these sensory neurons. The ventral root is the motor root; it is made of motor neurons that carry impulses from the spinal cord to muscles or glands (their cell bodies are in the gray matter of the spinal cord). When the two roots merge, the nerve thus formed is a mixed nerve.

SPINAL CORD REFLEXES

A reflex is an involuntary response to a stimulus, an automatic reaction triggered by a specific change. Spinal cord reflexes are those that do not depend directly on the brain, although the brain may inhibit or enhance them.

Reflex Arc

A reflex arc is the pathway nerve impulses travel when a reflex is elicited. There are five parts:

1. Receptors detect a change (the stimulus) and generate impulses.
2. Sensory neurons transmit impulses from receptors to the CNS.
3. Central nervous system contains one or more synapses and the interneurons that may be part of the pathway.
4. Motor neurons transmit impulses from the CNS to an effector.
5. Effector performs its characteristic action.

The spinal cord reflexes include stretch reflexes and flexor reflexes. In a stretch reflex, a muscle that is stretched will automatically contract; an example is the familiar patellar or knee-jerk reflex, but all skeletal muscles have such a reflex. The purpose of these reflexes is to keep us upright (because gravity exerts a constant pull on the body) without our having to think about it. Flexor reflexes may also be called withdrawal reflexes; the stimulus is something painful and the response is to pull away from it. Again, this occurs without the need for conscious thought; the brain is not directly involved.

The clinical testing of certain spinal cord reflexes provides a way to assess the functioning of their reflex arcs. If the patellar reflex, for example, were absent, the problem might be in the quadriceps femoris muscle, the femoral nerve, or in the spinal cord itself. If the reflex is present, however, it indicates that all parts of the reflex arc are functioning normally.

BRAIN

The brain consists of many parts, which function as an integrated whole. The major parts are the medulla, pons, and midbrain (the brain stem), the cerebellum, the hypothalamus and thalamus, and the cerebrum (Fig. 45–4).

Ventricles

The ventricles are four cavities within the brain: two lateral ventricles within the cerebral hemispheres, the third ventricle within the thalamus and hypothalamus, and the fourth ventricle between the medulla and cerebellum. Each ventricle contains a capillary network called a choroid plexus, which forms cerebrospinal fluid (the tissue fluid of the CNS) from blood plasma.

Medulla

The medulla is anterior to the cerebellum, extends from the spinal cord to the pons, and regulates our most vital functions. Within the medulla are cardiac centers that regulate heart rate, respiratory centers that regulate breathing, and vasomotor centers that regulate the diameter of blood vessels and, thereby, blood pressure. Also in the medulla are reflex centers for coughing, sneezing, swallowing, and vomiting.

Pons

The pons is anterior to the upper portion of the medulla. Within the pons are two respiratory centers that work with those in the medulla to produce a normal breathing rhythm.

Midbrain

The midbrain extends from the pons to the hypothalamus and encloses the cerebral aqueduct, a tunnel that connects the third and fourth ventricles. Primarily a reflex center, the midbrain regulates visual reflexes (coordinated movement of the eyes), auditory reflexes (turning the ear to a sound), and righting reflexes that keep the head upright and contribute to balance.

Cerebellum

The cerebellum is posterior to the medulla and pons, separated from them by the fourth ventricle; it is overlapped by the occipital lobes of the cerebrum. The functions of the cerebellum are concerned with the involuntary aspects of voluntary movement: coordination, regulation of muscle tone, the appropriate trajectory and endpoint of movements, and the maintenance of posture and balance or equilibrium. For the maintenance of balance, the cerebellum (and midbrain) uses sensory information provided by the

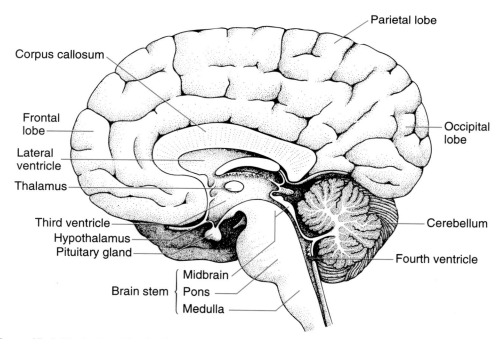

Figure 45–4. The brain midsagittal section; medial surface of the right cerebral hemisphere. (Modified from Scanlon, VC, Sanders, T: Workbook for Essentials of Anatomy and Physiology, ed 2. FA Davis, Philadelphia, 1995, p 116, with permission.) See Plate 12.

receptors in the inner ear that detect movement and changes in position of the head.

Hypothalamus

The hypothalamus is located above the pituitary gland and below the thalamus; it has many diverse functions.

1. Production of antidiuretic hormone (ADH) and oxytocin; these hormones are then stored in the posterior pituitary gland. ADH increases the reabsorption of water by the kidneys and thus helps maintain blood volume. Oxytocin causes contractions of the myometrium of the uterus to bring about labor and delivery.
2. Production of releasing hormones that stimulate secretion of the hormones of the anterior pituitary gland. An example is growth hormone–releasing hormone (GHRH), which stimulates the anterior pituitary to secrete growth hormone.
3. Regulation of body temperature by promoting responses such as shivering in a cold environment or sweating in a warm environment.
4. Regulation of food intake; the hypothalamus is believed to respond to changes in blood nutrient levels. Low blood nutrient levels bring on a feeling of hunger and eating, which raises blood nutrient levels and brings about a feeling of satiety or fullness, and eating ceases.
5. Integration of the functioning of the autonomic nervous system, which will be covered in a later section.
6. Stimulation of visceral responses in emotional situations, such as increased heart rate when angry or afraid. The neurological basis of emotions is not well understood, but the hypothalamus brings about bodily changes by way of the autonomic nervous system.

Thalamus

The thalamus is above the hypothalamus and below the cerebrum; its functions are concerned with sensation. Sensory pathways (except olfactory ones) to the brain converge in the thalamus, which begins to integrate sensations, which in turn permits more rapid interpretation by the cerebrum. The thalamus is also capable of suppressing unimportant sensations, permitting the cerebrum to concentrate without the distraction of minor sensations.

Cerebrum

The two cerebral hemispheres form the largest part of the human brain. The right and left hemispheres are connected by the corpus callosum, a band of about 200 million nerve fibers that allows each hemisphere to know what is going on in the other.

The cerebral cortex is the surface of the cerebrum; it is gray matter that consists of the cell bodies of neurons. The cerebral cortex is folded extensively into convolutions (or gyri) that permit more space for neurons. The grooves between the folds are called fissures or sulci. Interior to the gray matter is white matter, myelinated axons and dendrites that connect the parts of the cerebral cortex to one another, and the cerebrum to other parts of the brain. The cerebral cortex is divided into lobes that have been extensively mapped as to their functions.

The frontal lobes contain the motor areas that generate the impulses that bring about voluntary movement. Each motor area controls movement on the opposite side of the body. Also in the frontal lobe, usually only the left lobe, is the Broca's motor speech area, which controls the movements involved in speaking.

The parietal lobes contain the general sensory areas for the cutaneous senses and conscious muscle sense. This is where these sensations are felt and interpreted.

The temporal lobes contain sensory areas for hearing, smell, and taste. Also in the temporal and parietal lobes, usually only on the left side, are speech areas involved in the thought that precedes speech.

The occipital lobes contain the visual areas that receive impulses from the retinas of the eyes; they "see" and interpret what is being seen.

In all lobes of the cerebral cortex are association areas that enable us to learn, remember, and think, and probably give us our individual personalities. These have not yet been as precisely mapped as the sensory and motor areas.

Deep within the white matter of the cerebral hemispheres are masses of gray matter called the basal ganglia. Their functions are concerned with certain subconscious aspects of voluntary movement: regulation of muscle tone, inhibiting tremor, and the use of accessory movements such as gestures when speaking.

MENINGES AND CEREBROSPINAL FLUID

The meninges are the three layers of connective tissue that cover the central nervous system. The outermost is the dura mater, made of thick fibrous connective tissue. The middle layer is called the arachnoid membrane, which has a web-like appearance, and the inner layer is the pia mater, very thin connective tissue on the surface of the brain and spinal cord. Between the arachnoid membrane and the pia mater is the subarachnoid space, which contains cerebrospinal fluid.

Each of the four ventricles of the brain contains a choroid plexus, a capillary network that forms cerebrospinal fluid from blood plasma. This is a continuous process, and the cerebrospinal fluid then circulates from the ventricles to the central canal of the spinal cord and to the subarachnoid spaces around the brain and spinal cord. From the cranial subarachnoid space, cerebrospinal fluid is reabsorbed back to the blood through arachnoid villi that project into the cranial venous sinuses, large veins between the two layers of the cranial dura mater. The rate of reabsorption usually equals the rate of production.

As the tissue fluid of the CNS, cerebrospinal fluid permits the exchanges of nutrients and wastes between the blood and CNS neurons. It also acts as a cushion or shock absorber for the CNS. The pressure and constituents of cerebrospinal fluid may be determined by means of a lumbar puncture (spinal tap) and may be helpful in the diagnosis of diseases such as meningitis.

CRANIAL NERVES

The 12 pairs of cranial nerves emerge from the brain stem or other parts of the brain; some are purely sensory nerves, whereas others are mixed nerves. The impulses for sight, smell, hearing, taste, and equilibrium are all carried by cranial nerves to their respective sensory areas in the brain. Other cranial nerves carry motor impulses to muscles of the face or to glands. The functions of all the cranial nerves are summarized in Table 45–2.

AUTONOMIC NERVOUS SYSTEM

The ANS is part of the peripheral nervous system in that it consists of the motor portions of some cranial and spinal nerves. These are the visceral motor neurons to visceral effectors, that is, smooth muscle, cardiac muscle, and glands. The ANS has two divisions, sympathetic and parasympathetic; often they function in opposition to each other, and their activity is integrated by the hypothalamus.

An autonomic nerve pathway from the CNS to a visceral effector consists of two motor neurons that synapse in a ganglion outside the CNS (Fig. 45–5). The first neuron is called the preganglionic neuron, from the CNS to the ganglion. The second neuron is called the postganglionic neuron, from the ganglion to the visceral effector. The ganglia are actually the cell bodies of the postganglionic neurons.

Sympathetic Division

The cell bodies of the sympathetic preganglionic neurons are in the thoracic and some of the lumbar segments of the spinal cord. The axons of these neurons extend to the sympathetic ganglia, most of which are in two chains just outside the spinal column. Within the ganglia are the synapses between the preganglionic and postganglionic neurons; the axons of the postganglionic neurons then go to the visceral effectors. One preganglionic neuron often synapses with many postganglionic neurons to many effectors; this permits widespread responses in many organs.

The sympathetic division is dominant in stressful situations such as fear, anger, anxiety, and exercise, and the responses it brings about involve preparedness for physical activity, whether or not it is actually needed. (Table 45–3 summarizes both ANS divisions.) The heart rate increases, vasodilation in skeletal muscles supplies them with more oxygen, the bronchioles dilate to take in more air, and the liver changes glycogen to glucose to provide energy. Relatively unimportant activities such as digestion are slowed, and vasoconstriction in the skin and viscera permits greater blood flow to more vital organs such as the brain, heart, and muscles.

The neurotransmitters of the sympathetic division are acetylcholine and norepinephrine. Acetylcholine is released by sympathetic preganglionic neurons; its inactivator is cholinesterase. Norepinephrine is released by most sympathetic postganglionic neurons at the synapses with the effector cells; its inactivator is catechol *O*-methyltransferase.

Parasympathetic Division

The cell bodies of the parasympathetic preganglionic neurons are in the brain stem and the sacral segments of the spinal cord. The axons of these neurons are in cranial nerve pairs 3, 7, 9, and 10 and in some sacral nerves, and they extend to the parasympathetic ganglia. These ganglia are very close to or actually in the visceral effector and contain the postganglionic cell bodies, with very short axons to the cells of the visceral effector. One preganglionic neuron

Table 45–2. **Cranial Nerves***

Number	Name	Function
I	Olfactory	Sense of smell
II	Optic	Sense of sight
III	Oculomotor	Movement of eyeball; constriction of pupil for bright light or near vision
IV	Trochlear	Movement of eyeball
V	Trigeminal	Sensation in face, scalp, and teeth; contraction of chewing muscles
VI	Abducens	Movement of eyeball
VII	Facial	Sense of taste; contraction of facial muscles; secretion of saliva
VIII	Acoustic	Sense of hearing; sense of equilibrium
IX	Glossopharyngeal	Sense of taste; secretion of saliva; sensory for cardiac, respiratory, and blood pressure reflexes; contraction of pharynx
X	Vagus	Sensory in cardiac, respiratory, and blood pressure reflexes; sensory and motor to larynx (speaking); decreases heart rate; contraction of alimentary tube (peristalsis); increases digestive secretions
XI	Accessory	Contraction of neck and shoulder muscles; motor to larynx (speaking)
XII	Hypoglossal	Movement of the tongue

*See Plate 13.

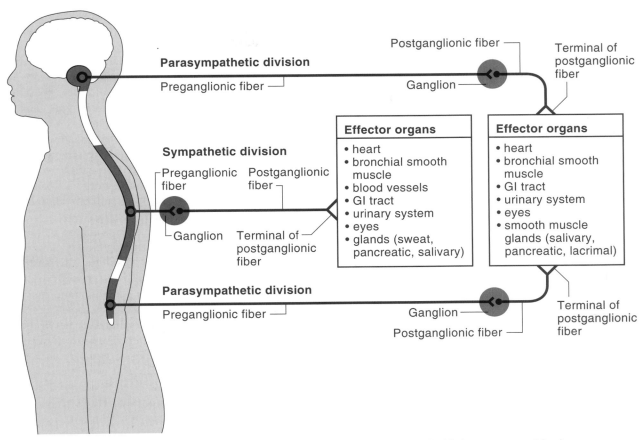

Figure 45–5. Autonomic nervous system. (Modified from Morton, PG: Health Assessment on Nursing, ed 2. Springhouse, Springhouse, Pa, p 467, with permission.)

synapses with just a few postganglionic neurons to only one effector. This permits very localized responses.

The parasympathetic division dominates during relaxed, nonstressful situations to promote normal functioning of several organ systems. Digestion will proceed normally, with increased secretions and peristalsis; defecation and urination may occur, and the heart will beat at a normal resting rate (see Table 45–3).

Table 45–3. **Functions of the Autonomic Nervous System**

Organ	Sympathetic Response	Parasympathetic Response
Heart (cardiac muscle)	Increase rate	Decrease rate (to normal)
Bronchioles (smooth muscle)	Dilate	Constrict (to normal)
Iris (smooth muscle)	Pupil dilates	Pupil constricts (to normal)
Salivary glands	Decrease secretion	Increase secretion (to normal)
Stomach and intestines (smooth muscle)	Decrease peristalsis	Increase peristalsis for normal digestion
Stomach and intestines (glands)	Decrease secretion	Increase secretion for normal digestion
Internal anal sphincter	Contracts to prevent defecation	Relaxes to permit defecation
Urinary bladder (smooth muscle)	Relaxes to prevent urination	Contracts for normal urination
Internal urethral sphincter	Contracts to prevent urination	Relaxes to permit urination
Liver	Changes glycogen to glucose	None
Sweat glands	Increase secretion	None
Blood vessels in skin and viscera (smooth muscle)	Constrict	None
Blood vessels in skeletal muscle (smooth muscle)	Dilate	None
Adrenal glands	Increase secretion of epinephrine and nor-epinephrine	None

Acetylcholine is the neurotransmitter at all parasympathetic synapses, both preganglionic and postganglionic; it is inactivated by cholinesterase.

AGING AND THE NERVOUS SYSTEM

With age the brain loses neurons, but this is only a small percentage of the total and is not the usual cause of mental impairment in the elderly; far more common causes are depression, malnutrition, hypotension, and the side effects of medications. Some forgetfulness is to be expected, however, as is a decreased ability for problem solving. Voluntary movements become slower, as do reflexes and reaction time.

Assessment of the Neurological System

INCREASED INTRACRANIAL PRESSURE PATHOPHYSIOLOGY AND MONITORING

Any client with intracranial pathology is potentially at risk for increased intracranial pressure (ICP). Common etiologies include brain trauma, intracranial hemorrhage, and brain tumors. Prompt detection of changes in neurological status indicating increased intracranial pressure allows intervention aimed at preventing permanent brain damage.

The Monro-Kellie doctrine states that the skull is a rigid compartment containing three components: brain tissue, blood, and cerebrospinal fluid. If an increase in one component is not accompanied by a decrease in one or both of the other components, the result is increased intracranial pressure. The consequences of increased ICP depend on the degree of elevation and the speed with which the ICP increases. Clients with slow-growing tumors may have significantly increased intracranial pressure before they develop symptoms. Conversely, clients with a subarachnoid hemorrhage may sustain a sudden sharp increase in intracranial pressure.

The normally functioning body has several methods of compensating for increased intracranial pressure. Cerebrospinal fluid can be shunted into the spinal subarachnoid space. Hyperventilation may trigger constriction of cerebral blood vessels, decreasing the amount of blood within the cranial vault. These compensatory mechanisms are temporary and not particularly effective if the increase in ICP is sudden and severe.

Increased ICP may first be manifested by a decrease in level of consciousness as cerebral cortex function is impaired. If not intubated, the client may hyperventilate, causing vasoconstriction as the body attempts to compensate. As the pressure increases the oculomotor nerve may be compressed on the side of the pathology. Compression of the outermost fibers of the oculomotor nerve results in diminished reactivity and dilation of the pupil. As the fibers become increasingly compressed the pupil stops reacting to light. If the compression continues both pupils become fixed and dilated.

Vital sign changes are a *late* sign of increasing intracranial pressure. Cushing's response is characterized by bradycardia and increasing systolic blood pressure while diastolic blood pressure remains the same, resulting in widening pulse pressure (Fig. 45–6). By the time these symptoms appear the intracranial pressure is significantly increased and interventions may not be successful.

Intracranial monitoring is indicated when the client demonstrates unequal pupils. Other reasons for monitoring

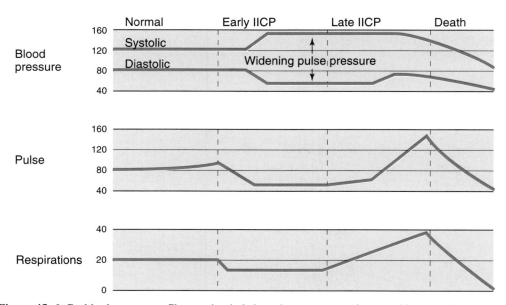

Figure 45–6. Cushing's response. Changes in vital signs that accompany increased intracranial pressure.

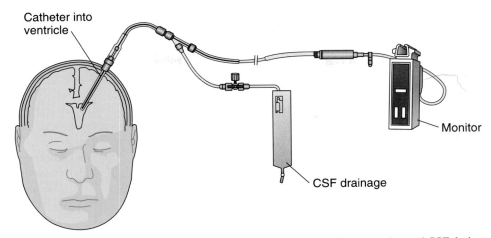

Figure 45–7. Ventricular drain. A catheter into the ventricle allows ICP monitoring and CSF drainage.

include a computerized tomography (CT) scan demonstrating midline shift and the decision to use neuromuscular blocking agents and sedatives. The most common methods of monitoring ICP in adults are external ventricular drain, subarachnoid bolt, and **intraparenchymal** monitor. All three methods involve anesthetizing the scalp and drilling a burr hole in the skull. Clients who are restless or agitated may require sedation in order for the procedure to be completed safely. Informed consent must be obtained, but in some emergent cases the monitor will be inserted without consent.

Placement of a catheter into one of the lateral ventricles is referred to as external ventricular drainage (Fig. 45–7). Drainage of cerebrospinal fluid reduces intracranial pressure, which can be therapeutic, as well as a way of monitoring pressure. Disadvantages to this method include difficulty in locating the ventricle for insertion of the catheter and clotting of the catheter by blood in cerebrospinal fluid.

A subarachnoid bolt is tightly screwed into the burr hole after the dura has been punctured, to allow communication with the subarachnoid space (Fig. 45–8). The advantage to a subarachnoid bolt is ease of placement. Disadvantages include occlusion of the sensor portion of the bolt with brain tissue and inability to drain CSF. An intraparenchymal monitor is placed directly into brain tissue. Some physicians believe that this most accurately reflects the actual situation within the skull. These monitors cannot be used to drain CSF and may become occluded by brain tissue.

Clients with ICP monitors are cared for in an intensive care unit (ICU) and require aggressive nursing care to prevent complications. These clients are frequently mechanically ventilated and may be pharmacologically paralyzed and sedated. They may be completely dependent for all care. In addition to meeting the client's physiological needs and preventing complications, the nurse must provide education and emotional support to the significant others. Clients who require intracranial pressure monitoring are seriously ill, and their significant others need frequent honest communication regarding the clinical situation and prognosis.

NURSING ASSESSMENT

The focus of the nursing neurological examination is to establish the present function of the client's neurological system and to detect changes from previous assessments. A complete neurological examination, intended to determine the existence of neurological disease, is typically performed by a physician. A baseline neurological assessment should be performed on every client admission. In addition to giving valuable information about the current functioning of the client's neurological system the assessment provides a basis for comparison. This is especially important if the client has chronic neurological deficits on admission. One example is a client, admitted for placement of a prosthetic hip, who has had a previous **cerebrovascular** accident resulting in **paresis** of the right arm. A complete neurological assessment would document that the right arm is weaker than the left. If during the postoperative course the assessment demonstrates that both arms are equal in strength, the client would be evaluated for possible causes of weakening of the left arm.

The results of the baseline assessment are invaluable in planning and implementing safe care. For example, clients who give a history of seizure activity need careful monitoring, and all staff members who interact with such clients should be aware of how to respond to a seizure. Clients with **dysphagia** (difficulty swallowing) may need to have restrictions placed on the types of food or fluids they may have. This information must be consistently communicated to all staff who are involved in the client's care.

---

intraparenchymal: intra—within + parenchymal—pertaining to brain tissue
dysphagia: dys—difficult + phagia—eating

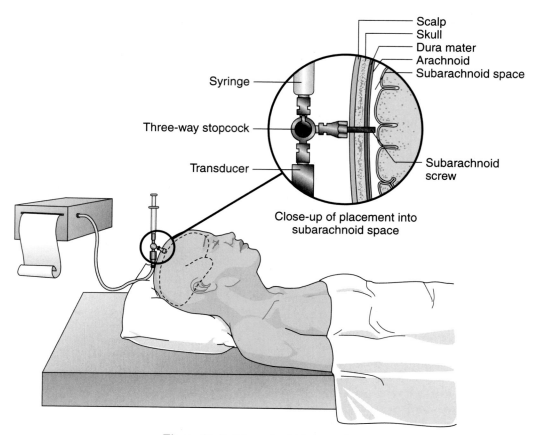

Scalp
Skull
Dura mater
Arachnoid
Subarachnoid space

Syringe

Three-way stopcock

Transducer

Subarachnoid screw

Close-up of placement into subarachnoid space

Figure 45–8. Subarachnoid bolt monitor.

The client's admitting diagnosis, the presence of any chronic neurological disorders, and the current functioning of the client's neurological system all influence how often neurological assessments should be done. Physician orders for neurological assessments may vary from every 15 minutes for an acutely ill postoperative client to every 8 hours for a client who is close to being discharged. It is always appropriate for a nurse to assess a client more often than ordered, based on observed changes in the client's condition, and to communicate the findings of those assessments to the physician. The changes noted while assessing the client may indicate changes in the central nervous system. Rapid detection and intervention may mean the difference between life and death for the client.

Health History

The nurse obtains a history of the client's general health and then focuses on the neurological symptoms. Symptoms of neurological disorders vary in type, location, and intensity. It is important to remember that some neurological disorders may affect the client's ability to think, remember, speak, or interpret stimuli. It may be necessary to question significant others about duration and severity of symptoms. Some clients may not be able to recognize their own neurological deficits. In these cases the significant other usually initiates contact with the health care system and provides the medical and social history.

All symptoms should be assessed individually using the WHAT'S UP? acronym:

WHERE IS IT? In addition to location of the symptom ask whether the sensation radiates, indicating the possibility of a **radiculopathy,** or occurs in the same location on the other side of the body. The client may focus on the most intense symptoms and not realize until asked that the symptom also occurs on the other side of the body.

HOW DOES IT FEEL? Painful, achy, tingly, or numb are some of the adjectives used to describe the sensation associated with neurological disorders. Clients may use phrases such as "pins and needles in my arm" or "it feels like my leg is asleep" to describe **paresthesia.** Nerve pain may be described as "shooting or burning" in nature. Clients who suffer from vascular anomalies or **subarachnoid** hemorrhage may complain of throbbing headaches.

---

radiculopathy: radiculo—spinal nerve root + pathy—disorder or disease
paresthesia: para—beside + asthesia—sensations
subarachnoid: sub—below + arachnoid—middle layer of the meninges

AGGRAVATING OR ALLEVIATING FACTORS. Does exercise or fatigue make it worse? Clients may relate that paresis or tremors are more pronounced if they are fatigued. Does rest help? Does application of ice or heat help to make the symptoms worse? Do changes in the weather have an impact? Clients with multiple sclerosis may have exacerbations of symptoms in hot weather. Some clients with back or neck pain experience more pain when the weather is cold or rainy.

TIMING. How long has the client had symptoms? Have the symptoms changed? Is the symptom becoming more intense? Has it moved or spread to another part of the body? Clients with multiple sclerosis may experience symptoms that change location or intensity. Are particular times of the day worse? Clients with back or neck pain may complain of stiffness in the morning or increased pain after finishing work.

SEVERITY. How severe is the symptom on a scale of 0 to 10? Also ask how the symptom affects the client's lifestyle, job, and activities of daily living (ADL). Clients with muscular weakness may have difficulty climbing stairs or getting in and out of the bathtub. Elderly clients in particular may be severely compromised by relatively mild deficits. Clients with spinal stenosis may be relatively pain free when sitting or lying down but are unable to stand up and walk long enough to shop for groceries or clean their house.

USEFUL OTHER DATA. Is the client on any medication? Some medication may cause memory impairments, balance difficulties, or headaches. Does the client have any other illnesses? Pain in the leg may be caused by compression of a spinal nerve root (radiculopathy), but it could also be a complication of diabetes or alcoholism (**neuropathy**). This is an example of the importance of asking if symptoms exist on the other side. It is unusual for a client to have bilateral radiculopathies, but bilateral neuropathies are not uncommon.

PATIENT'S PERCEPTION. In addition to asking about impact on activities of daily living and job requirements, ask the client about how symptoms affect personal relationships and family obligations. Clients may need encouragement to discuss the impact of **hemiparesis** on sexual function or the effect of memory impairment on parenting. Clients with cognitive deficits may fear that they have Alzheimer's disease or are "going crazy." It is also important to assess the impact of the disorder on the client's significant others, especially if they are also the client's caregivers.

In addition to using these questions, the nurse observes the client during the health history. Is he or she shifting positions and exhibiting signs of discomfort? Is the client able to change position and move about easily? Is he or she able to carry on a coherent conversation?

Physical Assessment

Glasgow Coma Scale

Many health care institutions use the Glasgow Coma Scale (GCS) to assess level of consciousness (LOC) and document the findings (Table 45–4). In use since the 1970s, this relatively objective scale provides caregivers with a concrete way to compare their assessment findings with those of other caregivers. Each section of the scale assesses level of consciousness via a different means. The level of consciousness should be the first thing assessed during a neurological examination because the information obtained can be used to modify the remainder of the examination if necessary. The nurse should remember that a decrease in the level of consciousness can be caused by hypoxia, hypoglycemia, intoxication, or other problems, as well as dysfunction of the neurological system.

The first section of the GCS evaluates the stimulus needed to get clients to open their eyes. Individuals with normal neurological function open their eyes spontaneously (score of 4). People with mildly decreased LOC will require verbal stimuli, such as calling out the client's name or asking the client to open his or her eyes (score of 3). The nurse should not confuse this response with clients who

Table 45–4. **Glasgow Coma Scale**

Eye Opening	
Spontaneous	4
To verbal stimulus	3
To painful stimulus	2
No response	1

Verbal Response	
Spontaneous	5
Confused conversation	4
Inappropriate words	3
Incomprehensible sounds	2
No response	1

Motor Response	
Obeys commands	6
Localizes pain	5
Withdraws from pain	4
Abnormal flexion	3
Abnormal extension	2
No response	1

---

neuropathy: neuro—pertaining to a nerve + pathy—disorder

hemiparesis: hemi—divided in half on a vertical plane + paresis—weakness

open their eyes to any loud noise. That is a reflex and indicates a lower level of consciousness. One way to differentiate is to call the client by another person's name; if the client opens his or her eyes, it does not count as "opens eyes to voice." A lower level of consciousness is indicated by eye opening in response to painful stimuli (score of 2). Pressure on the nail bed or trapezius muscle are two common ways of providing a painful stimulus. Care must be taken not to damage or bruise the skin or underlying tissue. Only enough pressure to elicit a response should be used. If no response is noted, the client receives a score of 1 for this section of the GCS.

Some clients may be unable to open their eyes due to facial trauma or swelling. This should be recorded as C, indicating eyes closed, rather than 1 for no response. Physical inability to open the eyes does not indicate a decreased level of consciousness.

The second section of the GCS addresses verbal response to the examiner. Orientation refers to the client's cognitive awareness. Clients are frequently referred to as being oriented to person, place, and time, or "oriented × 3." Some clinicians include a fourth category, situation, indicating whether the client understands what is happening to her or him. A client who is fully oriented receives a score of 4 on the GCS. Assessment of orientation should not be superficial. Typical questions include "What is your name? Where are you? What is the date?" Clients may be able to recall the name of the hospital and the date but have no idea why they are in the hospital. If the client is unable to speak because of a stroke (expressive **aphasia**) the condition does not rule out the possibility that the client is oriented. Give expressively aphasic clients yes-or-no questions such as "Are you in a grocery store? Are you in a bowling alley? Are you in a hospital?" and "Is the month June? Is it September?" Clients who are unable to understand what is being said to them are referred to as receptively aphasic. These clients may be able to match a spoken name with a picture of a family member.

Confusion and *disorientation* are terms that are sometimes used interchangeably. If the client is confused it is helpful to determine the extent of the confusion. Clients who have been in a hospital or long-term care facility for an extended period of time may lose track of the date but still be oriented to person and place. A client who can tell the nurse the year and who is president, but not the precise date, is less confused than someone who thinks it is 1945 and Franklin Roosevelt is president. Clients who are disoriented should have the correct information reinforced to them frequently. A calendar in an easily visible place, telling clients about current events in the family, and telling clients the date and why they are in the hospital or long-term care facility all reinforce orientation. Clients with short-term memory deficits may understand the information they are told but be unable to retain it long enough to use it.

A score of 3 is given to those clients who are not able to carry on a conversation but are limited to using words inappropriately. This includes those clients who spontaneously call out words that do not have meaning in that situation or who merely call out profanities at random. Incomprehensible sounds are those vocalizations that are not recognizable as words, and these clients are given a score of 2. Again, a score of 1 is given for no response. Clients who are intubated or have a tracheostomy should not automatically be scored as having no response. Head nodding, mouthing words, or using a picture board are all ways that allow for intubated clients to respond to questions and have their orientation status assessed.

Typically, motor response is scored based on the best arm function that can be elicited. For some clients this part of the examination must be modified. A client who is paralyzed may be able only to blink. If the client can blink on command that is scored as "6, obeys command." Clients may be unable to use their arms but have voluntary movement of their legs. If these clients follow commands with their legs they would receive a score of 6.

Localizing pain indicates that the client has an adequate level of consciousness to recognize where the pain is coming from and to attempt to push it away. An example is the client who pushes against the examiner's hand when pressure is applied to the client's nail bed. The ability to localize pain is scored as a 5. Withdrawal from pain indicates less function of the cerebral cortex. In this case the client is able to recognize the source of the painful stimuli but withdraws from it instead of trying to push the source away. This withdrawal is rated as a 4. Abnormal flexion posturing, characterized by flexion of the arms at the elbow, bringing the hands up toward the chest with the legs extended (**decorticate** posturing), indicates significant impairment of the cerebral functioning. A score of 3 is given to clients who exhibit abnormal flexion posturing (Fig. 45–9). Abnormal extension posturing, or **decerebrate** posturing, indicates damage in the area of the brain stem. In this case, both the upper and lower extremities are extended and the arms are internally rotated. Abnormal extension posturing is scored as a 2. As with the other categories, no response is rated as 1.

The total possible score on the GCS ranges from 3 to 15 with a score of 3 indicating profound coma and 15 indicating normal function. When used to score the effects of a head injury a score of 13 or 14 indicates mild head injury, 9 to 12 indicates moderate injury, and any score of 8 or below indicates a severe head injury. For all of the categories of the GCS, the type of painful stimuli required to elicit a response should be documented. Deterioration in the client's condition (i.e., a lowering of the GCS score) should be reported to the physician promptly. Changes in

---

aphasia: a—absence + phasia—speech

A. Decorticate posturing

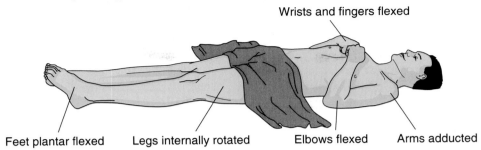

Wrists and fingers flexed

Feet plantar flexed   Legs internally rotated   Elbows flexed   Arms adducted

B. Decerebrate posturing

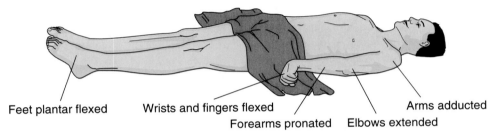

Feet plantar flexed   Wrists and fingers flexed   Arms adducted
Forearms pronated   Elbows extended

Figure 45–9. Abnormal posturing.

GCS are often used as an indication of the need for intracranial pressure monitoring.

Assessment of the Eyes

Assessment of pupillary response is an important part of the recurrent neurological assessment, as well as the cranial nerve evaluation. The size of the pupils at rest is documented. Many institutions use a millimeter gauge for measuring pupils. This allows an objective description of the size. If the client's pupils are unusually large or small, the nurse should determine if the client has had any eyedrops instilled or has taken any medications that might affect the size of the pupils. Approximately 17 percent of individuals have unequal pupils (**anisocoria**) without any underlying pathology. If the client's pupils are unequal in size, without a correlating diagnosis or symptoms, ask the client or his or her significant others if this is the client's normal state. Development of unequal pupils in a client who previously had equal pupils is an emergency and should be reported to the physician immediately. Any deviation from the normal round shape of the pupils is documented.

Once the resting size of the pupils has been noted the next step is to assess their response to light. In a darkened room, a light source is directed at the pupil from the lateral aspect of the eye. This allows the examiner to see the consensual response. A consensual response means that when one pupil is exposed to direct light the other pupil also constricts. Absence of a consensual response may indicate pathology in the area of the optic chiasm. Typically, the speed of light reaction is rated as brisk, sluggish, or absent. Differences in the speed or size of constriction between the two pupils should be reported to the physician.

Accommodation refers to the client's ability to focus on an object as it moves closer to her or him. The examiner asks the client to watch the examiner's finger as the examiner holds it about 18 inches in front of the client's face. As the examiner moves the finger toward the client's face, the client's eyes should turn toward the midline and the pupils should constrict. It is important to remember that only clients who can follow commands can be assessed for accommodation.

The eyes are evaluated for limitations in range of motion and for smoothness and coordination of movements. Eyes that move in the same direction in a coordinated manner are said to have a conjugate gaze. Conversely, a dysconjugate gaze refers to movement of the eyes in different directions. Some clients may be unable to move one or both eyes in a specific direction; this is called opthalmoplegia. It is often documented as limited extraocular movements. The nurse should always document what the limitation is; for example, "Client is unable to look laterally with left

---

anisocoria: aniso—unequal + coria—pupil

eye." This allows colleagues to compare their findings with the nurse's and detect any changes.

Nystagmus is involuntary movements of the eyes. Nystagmus varies in the speed of the movement and the direction. Horizontal nystagmus is the most commonly seen type. Common causes of nystagmus are Dilantin toxicity and injury to the brain stem.

Assessment of Muscle Function

Following assessment of level of consciousness and pupillary response the evaluation focuses on muscle function. Muscle groups are compared for symmetry of size and strength. Compression of a specific nerve root may cause atrophy and weakness of the corresponding muscle (e.g., C5-6 compression leading to atrophy and weakness of the biceps).

The nurse systematically assesses muscle groups in the upper extremities and then the lower extremities, comparing right to left. The individual's age and general physical condition should be kept in mind when evaluating muscle strength. One would not expect the same amount of strength from a 75-year-old woman as from a 20-year-old man. If the client has chronic neurological deficits, ask if the results of the assessment are different from his or her usual functioning.

Many health care providers use a 5-point scale to document muscle strength. A score of 5 indicates a client who is able to move the extremity against gravity and the resistance of the examiner, displaying normal muscle strength. If the examiner is able to provide more resistance than the client can overcome with active movement, the score is 4. If the client is able to move the extremity only against gravity, but not resistance, the score is 3. If gravity must be eliminated by having the examiner support the extremity in order for the client to move the extremity, the score is 2. A score of 1 is given if there is no active movement of the extremity, but a minimum muscular contraction can be palpated. If the examiner is unable to detect any muscular function, a score of 0 is given.

To test the deltoids the nurse asks the client to raise the arms at the shoulder. The nurse has the client resist as the nurse pushes down on the upper arms. The biceps are tested by having the client flex the arm at the elbow and bring the palm toward the face. The nurse has the client resist as the nurse attempts to straighten the arm by pulling on the forearm. The nurse can tell the client to "make a muscle." With the arm similarly flexed, the nurse asks the client to straighten the arm while the nurse resists the movement.

Hand grasps are tested by having the client squeeze the nurse's fingers. If the client does not release the grasp when told to, it is a reflex grasp, not a response to command. A reflex palmar grasp may indicate frontal lobe pathology.

Assess the client for arm drift by asking the client to hold both arms straight in front with the palms upward while keeping the eyes closed. A downward drift of the arm, or rotation so that the palm is down, indicates impairment of the opposite side of the brain. Arm drift may be apparent before differences in muscle strength can be detected.

Assessment of leg muscle strength begins with the iliopsoas muscle. The nurse places his or her hand on the client's thigh and asks the client to raise the leg, flexing at the hip. Hip adductors are tested by having the client bring his or her legs together against the examiner's hands. The hip abductors and gluteus medius and minimus are tested by having the client move the legs apart against resistance. Hip extension by the gluteus maximus is tested by placing the hand under the thigh and having the client push down with the leg. The quadriceps femoris extends the knee and is tested by having the client attempt to straighten the leg at the knee. The hamstrings are responsible for knee flexion and are evaluated by having the client attempt to keep the heel of the foot against the bed or chair rung. Dorsiflexion is tested by having the client pull the toes toward the head. Plantar flexion is tested by having the client push against the examiner's hand with the ball of the foot.

Babinski's reflex is tested by stroking the sole of the foot. Normal response is flexion of the great toe. If the great toe extends and the other toes fan out, neurological dysfunction should be suspected if the client is over 6 months old. Deep tendon reflexes are not usually part of the nursing neurological assessment. The client's gait should be assessed, not only to detect any neurological dysfunction but to assess ability to ambulate safely. Clients who stagger, weave, or bump into objects may need assistance when out of bed.

Assessment of Cranial Nerves

The cranial nerves are usually not examined in depth during routine bedside neurological assessments. The following recommendations assume a client who is able to cooperate with the examiner and are intended to give a superficial assessment of cranial nerve function. The olfactory nerve can be tested by asking the client to identify common scents such as coffee or cinnamon. The optic nerve can be assessed by asking the client to read something, identify a picture, or tell the examiner how many fingers are being held up. Check the pupils for consensual reaction to light, indicating function of the oculomotor nerve. The examiner evaluates extraocular movements by asking the client to follow the examiner's finger while it is moved in front of the client's eyes. Extraocular movements are controlled by the oculomotor, trochlear, and abducen nerves. Lightly touching different parts of the face with a tissue tests the trigeminal nerve for decreased sensation. Evaluate the face for symmetry at rest and during movement. Ask the client to frown, smile broadly, and wrinkle the forehead, all of which test the facial nerve. Conversing with the client gives a basic evaluation of the auditory portion of the acoustic nerve. Dysfunction of the acoustic nerve may also cause difficulties with balance, which may be observed as the client ambulates. Typically the glossopharyngeal and vagus nerves are tested together by assessing the gag reflex and by asking the client to say "Ah." The spinal accessory nerve is assessed by asking the client to shrug the shoulders against resistance. Ask the client to stick out the tongue and move it from side to side. Evaluate for symmetry of size and movement as an indication of function of the hypoglossal nerve.

LEARNING TIP

The cranial nerves are easier to remember when a mnemonic device is used:

On	Olfactory
Old	Optic
Olympus'	Oculomotor
Towering	Trochlear
Top	Trigeminal
A	Abducens
Finn	Facial
And	Acoustic
German	Glossopharyngeal
Viewed	Vagal
Some	Spinal accessory
Hops	Hypoglossal

In all cases the findings of the neurological examination should be correlated with the remainder of the assessment findings. A decreased level of consciousness, coupled with a decreased O_2 saturation on pulse oximetry, would point to hypoxia as an etiology. Correlation of vital signs with neurological signs is particularly important. Bradycardia, increasing systolic blood pressure, and widening pulse pressure, commonly referred to as Cushing's response, is a late indication of increasing intracranial pressure. These findings, in conjunction with a unilateral dilated pupil, may indicate impending herniation of the brain (discussed further in Chapter 46).

CRITICAL THINKING: Tim Thompson

The nurse is caring for Tim, a 78-year-old gentleman admitted with heart problems. As the nurse enters his room with his afternoon medications, the nurse finds him confused. He thinks he is at home in 1968 and does not understand who the nurse is or why the nurse is there. He recognizes his wife, who is at his bedside, and knows his own name.

1. How would the nurse describe his mental status?
2. What additional data does the nurse need to decide how to proceed?
3. What may have contributed to his confusion?

Answers at end of chapter.

Diagnostic Tests

LABORATORY TESTS

Specific diagnostic blood tests do not exist for neurological disorders. Measurement of erythrocyte sedimentation rate (ESR) and white blood cell count (WBC) may indicate an infection, such as meningitis. Hormone levels, such as prolactin or cortisol, may indicate dysfunction of the pituitary gland related to a brain tumor.

LUMBAR PUNCTURE

Cerebrospinal fluid may be obtained via lumbar puncture and evaluated for glucose and protein levels, presence of bacteria and white blood cells, levels of immunoglobulin, and culture and sensitivity. Cerebrospinal fluid samples should be sent to the lab immediately following the procedure.

LEARNING TIP

The idea of a needle being introduced into the spinal canal is frightening to many people. Give simple, clear directions to the client; help the client maintain his or her position; and provide emotional support.

Typically the lumbar puncture needle is placed at the level of L3-4 or L4-5 in an adult. Because the spinal cord ends at the L1 level, this placement prevents damage to the cord by the needle.

Nursing Care

The client is asked to lie on his or her side with his or her back as close to the edge of the bed as possible. Depending on the client's condition, the nurse may need to help the client flex his or her knees up to the chest (Fig. 45–10). This position maximizes the space between the vertebrae, which makes it easier for the physician to insert the needle. An alternative position is to have the client sit with the back perpendicular to the edge of the bed. Leaning over a bedside table may help the client maintain the position.

After the lumbar puncture is completed, instruct the client to remain on bed rest with the head of the bed flat for 6 to 8 hours, or as long as ordered by the physician, and to increase oral intake of fluids. Keeping the head flat decreases the likelihood of leakage of cerebrospinal fluid from the puncture site. Increasing fluid intake promotes replacement of the fluid that was removed. Check the puncture site for leakage of cerebrospinal fluid and report any leakage to the physician. Assess the client for headache, a common complaint following lumbar puncture. If necessary, obtain an order for analgesia.

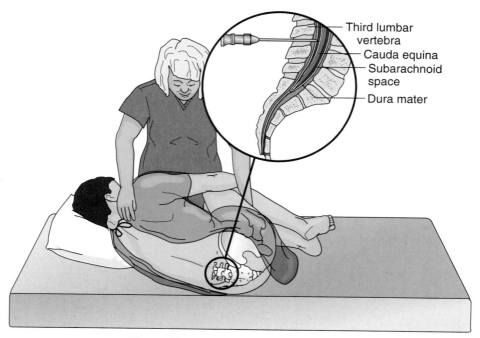

Third lumbar vertebra
Cauda equina
Subarachnoid space
Dura mater

Figure 45–10. Position for lumbar puncture.

X-RAYS

Spinal x-rays are done to determine the status of individual vertebrae and their relationship to one another. If the client experiences pain with certain movements, the client may be asked to flex and extend the area of the spine being examined while the x-rays are taken. This allows detection of abnormal movement of the vertebrae. If the client has possibly sustained trauma to the spine, particularly the cervical spine, x-rays are performed before immobilizing devices are removed. Skull x-rays may be done to detect skull fractures or foreign bodies.

Computerized Tomography

A CT scan is commonly the test ordered if the client initially consults a general practitioner. CT scans for the purpose of diagnosing neurological disorders can be performed on the brain or the spine. Some of the disorders that can be detected by CT are tumors, skull fractures, and abscesses. The scan may be performed with or without radiopaque contrast material to enhance the clarity of the images that are recorded. If contrast material is used, a series of images is filmed, and then the contrast material is given intravenously and another series of images is filmed. The client should be questioned about any allergies to contrast material, iodine, or shellfish. The blood urea nitrogen (BUN) and creatinine levels should be checked before administration of contrast material because it is excreted through the kidneys. Clients with elevated BUN and creatinine or known renal disease may be unable to tolerate the contrast material. Contrast material is most commonly used if a tumor is suspected or following surgery in the area to be scanned.

CT scans are commonly used in emergency evaluations because they can be done quickly, an important consideration if the client is ventilated or unstable.

During the CT scan the client must lie still on a moveable table. Noncontrast scans take approximately 10 minutes; contrast scans take between 20 and 30 minutes. Clients who are receiving dye should be warned that they may feel a sensation of warmth; nausea, diaphoresis, itching, and difficulty breathing may indicate allergy to the dye and should be reported immediately to the physician. Sedation may be required for clients who are agitated or disoriented. Clients who are in pain may require pain medication before the examination.

Magnetic Resonance Image

Magnetic resonance imaging (MRI) gives a more detailed image of soft tissue than a CT scan. It is not as useful when looking for bony abnormalities. MRI is a longer procedure and commonly requires transportation to distant areas of the hospital, which may be problematic for unstable, disoriented, or ventilated clients. As with a CT scan the MRI can be done with or without contrast material.

Due to the magnetic fields being used there are restrictions placed on clients undergoing an MRI and the health care personnel who work within the MRI facility. Individuals with pacemakers or any type of metallic prosthesis are not able to undergo MRI or be in the room when one is performed. This is because the magnetic field is so strong that it could dislodge the prosthesis or pacemaker. Individuals who may have accidentally acquired metallic foreign bodies (e.g., metal slivers in the eye or shrapnel that was not removed) may need an x-ray to determine the presence or absence of such objects. Carefully question clients or their significant others regarding any possible contraindications. MRI is commonly used when herniated intravertebral disks are suspected. It may be difficult for the client to lie in one position for a prolonged period of time. Assessment of the client's need for pain medication should be done before the procedure. Use of pillows for positioning may improve comfort. The narrow, tunnel-like structure of the MRI unit causes claustrophobia in some clients. Some clients may require use of medications or open MRI units. Encourage the use of deep breathing, guided imagery, and other relaxation techniques. Some facilities have the capability to perform magnetic resonance angiograms (MRA). This test allows visualization of blood vessels and assessment of blood flow without being as invasive as a traditional angiogram.

Angiogram

This x-ray study of blood vessels is used when an abnormality of cerebral or spinal blood vessels is suspected or to obtain information about blood supply to a tumor. Following injection of a local anesthetic a catheter is inserted through the femoral artery and advanced until contrast material can be injected into the cerebral vessels. Information is obtained about the structure of specific vessels, as well as overall circulation of the area.

Nursing Care

Before an angiogram the client receives a clear liquid diet and has an intravenous needle in place. The BUN and creatinine levels are evaluated because the contrast material is excreted through the kidneys. Potential for bleeding is assessed by prothrombin time and partial thromboplastin time tests, as a puncture is being made in a large artery. Typically, the client will receive some type of sedation before being transported to the angiography suite. During the injection of the contrast material the client may complain of severe heat sensations and a metallic taste in the mouth. The client must lie still while the x-rays are being taken and so should be told about the sensations he or she may experience. If the client is disoriented or agitated, he or she may require sedation in order to complete the test.

Following the procedure pressure is maintained on the catheter insertion site to prevent bleeding or hematoma formation. After returning from the test the client is kept flat in bed for 6 to 8 hours to prevent bleeding from the insertion site. The client may turn from side to side but must keep the affected leg straight. In addition to assessing vital signs the nurse evaluates the catheter insertion site and the presence and quality of the popliteal and pedal pulses in the affected leg. Decrease or loss of the pedal pulse may indicate a clot in the femoral artery and should be reported to the physician immediately. Clients should be encouraged to increase oral intake in addition to the IV fluids that are administered to aid in the excretion of the contrast material.

Myelogram

A **myelogram** is an x-ray examination of the spinal canal and its contents. Following a lumbar puncture cerebrospinal fluid is removed and sent for laboratory analysis. Then contrast material is injected into the subarachnoid space. The client is moved into various positions and x-rays are taken. Compression of nerve roots, herniation of intravertebral disks, and blockage of cerebrospinal fluid circulation may all be detected by myelogram.

Nursing Care

Following the procedure the client is kept on bed rest with the head elevated. This lessens the possibility of the contrast material getting into the cerebral cerebrospinal fluid circulation. The contrast material used for myelograms can lower the seizure threshold in some clients. Any client with a known seizure disorder should have serum levels of his or her anticonvulsants evaluated and be carefully observed for signs of seizures.

Because of their invasive nature, a separate informed consent form is normally required for angiogram, lumbar puncture, and myelogram. The physician performing the test will explain the risks, benefits, and possible complications of the examination. Clients who need these diagnostic procedures, particularly lumbar puncture and angiogram, may have cognitive deficits, therefore consent may need to be obtained from the legal next of kin.

ELECTROENCEPHALOGRAM

Evaluation of the electrical activity of the brain is obtained through an **electroencephalogram** (EEG). Electrodes are attached to the scalp by adhesive. Electrical activity is transmitted through the electrodes to a tracing. Analysis of the tracing can identify areas of abnormality, such as seizure focus or areas of slowing.

Nursing Care

Before the test make sure that the client's hair is clean and dry. The physician may write orders to withhold any sedatives to prevent interference with the EEG, and clients may be weaned from their anticonvulsants if the goal of the test is to identify the seizure focus during a seizure. These clients must be very carefully monitored and protected from harm. Typically they will undergo videotaping while the EEG is performed.

---

myelogram: myelo—referring to the spinal cord + gram—picture

electroencephalogram: electro—electrical activity + encephalo—referring to the brain + gram—picture

Therapeutic Measures

POSITIONING

Clients who have pain may need help in changing positions and ambulating. Use of heat, cold, or analgesics may allow the patient to be more independent in mobility. Clients with paresis, paralysis, or paresthesias may be partially or completely dependent in positioning. Care should be taken to maintain the body in functional positions when routine position changes are made. If the client experiences sensory loss, the person assisting with position changes must ensure that no part of the body is inadvertently compressed (e.g., a hand caught under a hip or the scrotum compressed between the legs). Collaboration with the physical therapist may yield positioning techniques that maximize the chance of useful recovery.

Contractures and footdrop are complications that are often associated with neurological disorders. Contractures are permanent muscle contractions with fibrosis of connective tissue that occurs from lack of use of a muscle or muscle group. They cause permanent deformities and prevent normal functioning of the affected part. Footdrop occurs when the feet are not supported in a functional position and become contracted in a position of plantar flexion (Fig. 45–11). Some of the interventions used to prevent footdrop are foot boards, high-top tennis shoes, and splints. Splints are commonly used to prevent contractures of the upper and lower extremities. If splints are used, the client must be evaluated for discomfort and skin breakdown at the splint site.

Mobilization should be begun as soon as the client is medically stable. Initially this may involve the use of a cardiac chair if the client is unable to bear weight. Transfer of the client to a bedside chair or use of ambulation aids may require a multidisciplinary approach. The nurse must recognize any physical or cognitive deficits that may affect safety and adjust the environment to protect the client. This includes communicating any safety concerns to unlicensed personnel who interact with the client.

ACTIVITIES OF DAILY LIVING

The effects of neurological disorders on activities of daily living (ADL) may range from an inconvenience to complete dependence. Clients may have trouble bending over to put on their shoes and socks, lifting a full cooking pot, or caring for an infant. A high-level quadriplegic may be completely unable to perform ADL but can be taught to direct his or her own personal care. Clients should be encouraged to use strategies taught in occupational or physical therapy.

Assessment should include a discussion of the strategies the client normally uses to accomplish ADL. Every attempt should be made to continue to use these strategies. This is particularly true if the client is admitted to a long-term care facility. Clients who have normal cognitive function should be included in care planning and encouraged to work collaboratively with caregivers. If the strategies the client uses during ADL must be changed, the rationale for the changes should be explained to the client and significant others. An example would be if the client was using a transfer technique that was unsafe for the client or caregivers. If clients have impaired cognitive function, try to maintain a specific routine that is as close to their normal environment as possible. By normalizing their routines the nurse may help clients adapt to a change in environment and maximize their ability to function.

COMMUNICATION

The communication problems associated with neurological disorders have a variety of etiologies. Some neurological disorders cause difficulty speaking (**dysarthria**). Dysfunction of the lips, tongue, or jaw makes speech difficult or impossible to understand. When dysarthric individuals know what they want to say but cannot be understood, the frustration level is very high. This frustration is compounded if the clients are treated as if they have cognitive deficits merely because they have difficulty communicating.

Clients who have had a stroke can experience different types of aphasia. Expressive aphasia is difficulty or inability to verbally communicate with others. The client may be able to speak in sentences but inappropriately substitutes words—for example, "The sky is dish." Word finding difficulty is another type of expressive aphasia. These clients

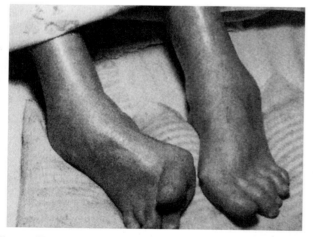

Figure 45–11. Contractures, footdrop. (Reproduced by permission. Assisting in Long Term Care, 3E, by Hegner. Delmar Publishers, Albany, New York. Copyright 1998.)

---

dysarthria: dys—dysfunctional + arthria—movement of the joints used in speech

may tell you "I want a . . ." and then be unable to complete the sentence. In severe cases of aphasia the client may say sounds that resemble words or may only utter sounds. For individuals with no intelligible speech, or word-finding difficulty, a picture board with commonly used items may facilitate communication. Keep in mind that clients with expressive aphasia may answer yes to all questions, rather than just those where yes is correct. The same is true of answering no. This is one example why a nurse should never ask a client "Are you Mrs. Gonzalez?" An aphasic client may say yes even if that is not her name. Instead, ask the client to state her name. If she cannot state her name, check her identification band.

For clients who substitute words, simply correct the substitution and continue the conversation. Clients with expressive aphasia are often very aware of, and frustrated by, their difficulty in communicating. Give them time to try to express themselves. If the nurse cannot understand them, the nurse should offer possibilities based on the situation. If the client is sitting in the chair, ask if he or she wants to go back to bed or wants to use the bathroom. If the client is restless, ask if he or she is in pain.

Some clients use the same word in response to all questions, and for some clients that word is a profanity. This is very difficult for significant others to deal with, particularly if swearing is not something the client normally did. Make it clear to the family that you understand that this behavior is part of the client's illness.

Receptive aphasia affects the client's ability to understand spoken language. Again, the severity of the aphasia varies. Some clients may understand simple directions such as "sit down" or "squeeze my fingers." In other cases the nurse may need to pantomime the action the nurse wants the client to perform, such as showing the client pills and then mimicking taking the pills and drinking water.

LEARNING TIP

If the client has receptive aphasia, assume that he or she will not understand or follow safety instructions, such as "Do not stand up until I get back." Even going to the bathroom to get a towel can give a client enough time to try to stand up and subsequently fall.

NUTRITION

Alterations in ability to maintain an adequate nutritional intake can have many causes. The level of consciousness may be depressed enough that the client does not recognize that she or he is hungry or thirsty. Decreased level of consciousness or cranial nerve dysfunction may impair the client's ability to swallow safely. Severe weakness may limit the client's ability to take in enough food to meet the body's requirements. These conditions are frequently com-

pounded by the increased metabolic rate that accompanies neurological injury or illness.

If there is any question of the client's ability to swallow, a swallowing evaluation should be performed by a speech therapist. Food coloring can be added to food or fluids and the client watched until the food is swallowed. If respiratory secretions are the same color as the food coloring, the client has aspirated and is not able to safely swallow the food or fluid. Some institutions use a radiological examination to evaluate the ability to swallow. A small amount of barium is added to the food or fluid and fluoroscopy is used while the client swallows. This allows visualization of the path of the food or fluid. Clients with swallowing difficulty (dysphagia) may have better success with foods rather than fluids, particularly thin fluids. Fluids may be thickened with special thickening agents to allow easier swallowing. All clients should be positioned as upright as possible while eating or drinking.

If weakness or fatigue is the cause of decreased nutritional intake, several modifications are possible. Serving small portions of food frequently can increase intake. Using high-protein, high-calorie foods and supplements increases the nutritional content of small amounts of foods.

For clients who are unable to swallow, or who cannot swallow enough food, enteral tube feedings may be required. If enteral feedings are anticipated to be for a short duration, a nasogastric tube may be used. The disadvantages of nasogastric tubes include impairment of the integrity of nasal skin and the risk of aspiration. The risk of aspiration in neurologically impaired clients who have cognitive impairments is increased because these clients may pull out the nasogastric tube because they do not understand its purpose. If long-term enteral feedings are anticipated, a gastrostomy tube may be placed directly through the abdominal wall into the stomach. This feeding method has the advantage of eliminating the risks of aspiration and nasal skin breakdown.

Review Questions

1. Neurons that carry impulses from the CNS to effectors are called
   a. Mixed
   b. Motor
   c. Afferent
   d. Sensory

2. Which of the following is *not* a sympathetic response?
   a. Decreased peristalsis
   b. Dilation of the bronchioles
   c. Decreased heart rate
   d. Secretion of epinephrine

3. Symptoms of increasing intracranial pressure include
   a. Constricted pupils
   b. Decreasing level of consciousness

c. Narrowing pulse pressure

d. Bradypnea

4. When the nurse shines a light in Joe's left pupil, both of his pupils constrict. What type of response is this?

a. Direct

b. Abnormal

c. Accommodation

d. Consensual

5. Which of the following actions by the nurse is the best way to determine if a client with expressive aphasia is oriented?

a. Ask yes-or-no questions

b. Ask the client to name the family member in the room

c. Ask the client who the current president is

d. Have the client count backward from 10

6. Asking the client to stick out his or her tongue evaluates the function of which cranial nerve?

a. IV—trochlear

b. V—trigeminal

c. IX—glossopharyngeal

d. XII—hypoglossal

7. The client with dysphagia should avoid which of the following foods?

a. Dry breads

b. Meats

c. Thin fluids

d. Ice cream

8. Which of the following nursing interventions can help prevent footdrop?

a. Positioning the client in the left lateral position

b. Providing daily foot massage

c. Using high-top tennis shoes

d. Maintaining an upright position as much as possible

9. Which of the following activities should be encouraged when a client returns from a CT scan using a contrast medium?

a. Ambulation

b. Drinking fluids

c. Turning side to side

d. Coughing and deep breathing

10. Following a lumbar puncture, the client should follow which activity orders?

a. Bed rest for 6 to 8 hours

b. Ambulate at least every 3 hours

c. Maintain a high Fowler's position for 2 hours

d. No restrictions are necessary

ANSWERS TO CRITICAL THINKING:
Tim Thompson

1. He is alert but confused, oriented to person only.

2. The nurse should ask his wife if this has ever happened before; check his medical history for any disorders that may contribute to neurological dysfunction; do a quick neurological assessment to determine if any additional deficits exist; check vital signs and pulse oximetry, if available; and notify the physician immediately if the symptoms are a new finding.

3. Some possible explanations to explore include hypoxemia, stroke, worsening heart problems causing inadequate flow of blood to the brain, hypoglycemia, or even confusion related to a sudden transition from home to an unfamiliar environment.

BIBLIOGRAPHY

Beveridge, DL: Back to basics. Axon 17:1, 1995.

Hickey, JV: The Clinical Practice of Neurological and Neurosurgical Nursing, ed 4. JB Lippincott, Philadelphia, 1997.

Ditunno, JF, Graziani, V, and Tessler, A: Neurological assessment in spinal cord injury. Advances in Neurology 72:325, 1997.

Mitrushina, M, and Statz, P: Reliability and validity of the Mini-Mental State Exam in neurologically intact elderly. J Clin Psychol 47:4, 1991.

Shpritz, DW: Understanding neurological assessment. J Post Anesth Nurs 10:4, 1995.

Stewart, N: Neurological observations. Prof Nurse 11:6, 1996.

Wooten, C: The top 10 ways to detect deteriorating central neurological status. J Trauma Nurs 3:1, 1996.

Nursing Care of Clients with Central Nervous System Disorders

Sally Schnell

46

Learning Objectives

Upon completion of this chapter, the student will be able to:

1. Explain the causes, risk factors, and pathophysiology of inflammatory and infectious disorders of the central nervous system.
2. Use the nursing process to plan care for a client with an inflammatory or infectious disorder of the central nervous system.
3. Explain the causes, risk factors, and pathophysiology of cerebrovascular disorders.
4. Identify the signs and symptoms of cerebrovascular disorders.
5. Discuss treatment of cerebrovascular disorders, including surgery, medication, and rehabilitation.
6. Use the nursing process to plan care for the client with a cerebrovascular disorder.
7. Differentiate between a seizure and epilepsy.
8. Use the nursing process to plan care for the client with a seizure disorder.
9. Discuss nursing care of the client with a traumatic brain injury.
10. Identify signs and symptoms of brain tumors.
11. Discuss nursing care of the client undergoing intracranial surgery.
12. Identify the signs and symptoms of herniated spinal disks.
13. Discuss nursing care of the client undergoing surgery for a herniated disc.
14. Explain the causes and pathophysiology of spinal cord injuries.
15. Use the nursing process to plan care for a client with a spinal cord injury.
16. Describe the pathophysiology associated with degenerative neuromuscular disorders.
17. Recognize safety risks associated with degenerative neuromuscular disorders and plan care to minimize those risks.
18. Recognize the impact of degenerative neuromuscular disorders on the client and significant others and plan holistic care.
19. Describe the pathophysiology and progression of symptoms seen in clients with Alzheimer's disease.
20. Assist significant others in realistically planning care for the client with Alzheimer's disease.

Key Words

akinesia (A-ki-**NEE**-zee-uh)
ataxia (ah-**TAK**-see-ah)
bradykinesia (BRAY-dee-kin-**EE**-zee-ah)
burr hole (BERR HOHLE)
contracture (kon-**TRAK**-chur)
contralateral (KON-truh-**LAT**-er-uhl)
craniectomy (KRAY-nee-**EK**-tuh-mee)
cranioplasty (**KRAY**-nee-oh-plas-tee)
craniotomy (KRAY-nee-**AHT**-oh-mee)
dementia (dee-**MEN**-cha)
dysreflexia (DIS-re-**FLEK**-see-ah)
encephalitis (EN-seff-uh-**LYE**-tis)
encephalopathy (en-SEFF-uh-**LAHP**-ah-thee)
endarterectomy (end-AR-tur-**ECK**-tuh-mee)
epidural (EP-i-**DUHR**-uhl)
flaccid (**FLA**-sid)
hemiparesis (hem-ee-puh-**REE**-sis)
hemiplegia (hem-ee-**PLEE**-jee-ah)
hydrocephalus (HIGH-droh-**SEF**-uh-luhs)
ipsilateral (IP-si-**LAT**-er-uhl)
laminectomy (LAM-i-**NEK**-toh-mee)
meningitis (MEN-in-**JIGH**-tis)
nuchal rigidity (**NEW**-kuhl re-**JID**-i-tee)
paraplegic (PAR-ah-**PLEE**-jik)
paresthesia (PAR-es-**THEE**-zee-ah)

persistent vegetative state (per-**SISS**-tent **VEJ**-uh-tay-tiv STAYT)

photophobia (FOH-tuh-**FOH**-bee-ah)

postictal (pohst-**IK**-tuhl)

prodrome (**PROH**-drohm)

quadriplegic (KWA-dri-**PLEE**-jik)

subdural (sub-**DUHR**-uhl

thrombolytic (throm-boh-**LIT**-ik)

turbid (**TER**-bid)

Disorders of the central nervous system (CNS) include problems originating in the brain and spinal cord. Because the CNS is the control center for the entire body, disorders in this system can cause symptoms in any part of the body, which can range from pain to paralysis, confusion, and coma. This chapter will present nursing care of clients with these disorders.

Central Nervous System Infections

Infectious agents may enter the central nervous system via a variety of routes (Table 46–1). Anything that depresses the client's immune system, such as steroid administration, chemotherapy, radiation therapy, and malnutrition, can make the client more vulnerable to infection.

MENINGITIS

Meningitis is a purulent infection, caused by bacteria or virus invasion of the pia mater, arachnoid, and subarachnoid space surrounding the brain and spinal cord. The membranes react to the infection with an inflammatory response. Bacterial meningitis is more common than viral. Occasionally, meningitis is caused by a noninfectious irritant, such as dye from a myelogram.

Table 46–1. **Routes of Entry for Central Nervous System Infections**

Route of Entry	Examples
Bloodstream	Insect bite
	Otitis media
Direct extension	Fracture of frontal or facial bones
Cerebrospinal fluid	Dural tear
	Poor sterile technique
Nose or mouth	Meningococcus meningitis
In utero	Contamination of amniotic fluid
	Rubella
	Vaginal infection

Table 46–2. **Cranial Nerves Affected by Meningitis**

Cranial Nerve Affected	Manifestation
III, IV, VI	Ocular palsies
	Unequal and sluggishly reactive pupils
VII	Facial weakness
VIII	Deafness and vertigo

Pathophysiology and Etiology

The most common organisms causing meningitis include meningococcus, pneumococcus, and *Haemophilus influenzae*. The infection generally begins in another area such as an upper respiratory infection, which enters the blood and invades the CNS, especially if the immune system is not functioning effectively. Bacterial invasion leads to a rapidly increased blood supply to the meninges with massive neutrophil migration. The neutrophils then engulf the bacteria and disintegrate, causing purulent material to form. Exudate from tissue destruction also contributes to this purulent material. The purulent material causes the meninges to become inflamed, and intracranial pressure increases. Cranial nerve function may be transiently or permanently affected by meningitis. Some of the effects are listed in Table 46–2.

A common endocrine disorder associated with meningitis is a cycle of increased intracranial pressure leading to excessive release of antidiuretic hormone (ADH). ADH acts by inhibiting urination. This in turn leads to water retention, oliguria (reduced urination), hypervolemia (excess blood volume), hyponatremia (low serum sodium), and further increases in intracranial pressure.

Prevention

Vaccines are available against *H. influenzae* and *Streptococcus pneumoniae*. Other vaccines are being developed.

Signs and Symptoms

The initial symptom of meningitis is a severe headache, caused by tension on blood vessels and irritation of the pain-sensitive dura mater. Fever is commonly 101°F to 103°F or higher. If the meningitis is not resolved, pressure on the brainstem may elevate the temperature to 105°F or higher during the terminal phase. **Photophobia** may be present. The client with meningococcal meningitis has a petechial rash on the skin and mucous membranes.

meningitis: mening—membranous covering of the brain + itis—inflammation

photophobia: photo—light + phobia—fear or intolerance

A

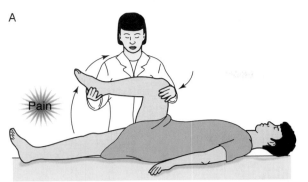

B

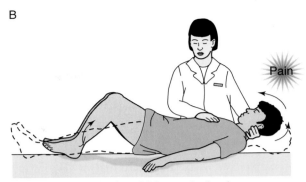

Figure 46–1. *(A)* Kernig's sign. *(B)* Brudzinski's sign. (Modified from Black and Matassarin-Jacobs: Medical-Surgical Nursing: Clinical Management for Continuity of Care, ed 5. WB Saunders, Philadelphia, p 857, with permission.)

Nuchal rigidity (pain and stiffness when the neck is moved) is caused by spasm of the extensor muscles of the neck. Kernig's sign and Brudzinski's sign are frequently seen in clients suffering from meningitis. Both signs are caused by inflammation of the meninges and spinal nerve roots. Brudzinski's sign is positive when flexion of the client's neck causes the hips and knees to flex. To elicit Kernig's sign the examiner flexes the client's hip to 90 degrees and tries to extend the client's knee. The sign is positive if the client experiences pain and spasm of the hamstring (Fig. 46–1). The nausea and vomiting associated with meningitis are caused by direct irritation of brain tissue and by increased intracranial pressure (ICP).

Encephalopathy refers to the mental status changes seen in clients with meningitis. These are manifested as short attention span, poor memory, disorientation, difficulty following commands, and a tendency to misinterpret environmental stimuli. Late signs of meningitis include lethargy and seizures.

Acute Complications of Meningitis

Hydrocephalus can occur when purulent material interferes with circulation and reabsorption of cerebrospinal fluid. The client may begin to improve following the initiation of treatment and then experience neurological deterioration as hydrocephalus develops. Careful and frequent neurological assessments allow for the detection of subtle changes.

Irritation of the cerebral cortex makes clients prone to seizures. Seizure precautions should be in place for all clients with meningitis. These include padded bed side rails and ready availability of suction and an oral airway. The oral airway should be used only if the client's mouth is

open. *Never* attempt to insert something into the mouth of a seizing client if the jaws are clenched. See also Table 46–3.

As with all clients with neurological disorders, frequent assessment of respiratory function is necessary. Inflammation and edema may place pressure on the respiratory center and result in hypoxia. Hypoxia causes vasodilation, which increases intracranial pressure. If the client experiences significant neurological and respiratory impairment, intubation and mechanical ventilation may be necessary.

Long-Term Complications

Resolution of meningitis depends on how quickly and effectively the disease is treated. Some individuals experi-

Table 46–3. **Interventions for Seizures**

Seizure Precautions
• Pad side rails of hospital bed with commercial pads or bath blankets folded over and pinned in place.
• Keep call light within reach.
• Assist client when ambulating.
• Keep suction and oral airway at bedside.

Nursing Care during a Seizure
• Stay with client.
• Do not restrain client.
• Protect from injury (move nearby objects, place pillow under head).
• Loosen tight clothing.
• Turn to side when able to prevent occlusion of airway or aspiration.
• Suction if needed.
• Monitor vital signs when able.
• Be prepared to assist with breathing if necessary.
• Observe and document progression of symptoms.

---

encephalopathy: encephalo—brain + pathy—illness

hydrocephalus: hydro—water + cephalus—head

ence no lasting effects. Other clients have permanent neurological deficits. Cranial nerve damage may leave the client blind or deaf. Seizures may continue to occur even after the acute phase of the illness has passed. Cognitive deficits ranging from memory impairment to profound learning disabilities may occur.

Diagnostic Tests

A lumbar puncture is the most informative diagnostic test for a client with suspected meningitis (see Chapter 45). Viral meningitis is characterized by clear cerebrospinal fluid with normal glucose level and normal or slightly increased protein level. There are no bacteria seen, but white blood cell count is usually increased. In contrast, the cerebrospinal fluid of an individual with bacterial meningitis is **turbid** or cloudy, due to the massive number of white blood cells. Bacteria are identified on the Gram stain and culture. The bacteria utilize the glucose normally found in cerebrospinal fluid (CSF), thereby lowering the glucose level. The amount of protein in the cerebrospinal fluid is elevated.

Medical Treatment

Meningitis can be fatal if not promptly treated. Broad-spectrum antibiotics are administered intravenously. After a culture and sensitivity is done on CSF the antibiotic may be changed. Antibiotics are not effective in the treatment of viral meningitis.

Symptom management is the same for viral or bacterial meningitis. Antipyretics such as acetaminophen are used to control the fever. Cooling blankets may also be utilized. Care should be taken to avoid cooling the client too much and causing shivering, because this increases the metabolic demand for oxygen and glucose. A quiet, dark environment lessens the stimulation to a client who has a headache or photophobia (sensitivity to light) and who may be agitated, disoriented, or at risk for seizures.

Pain medications are given to lessen the head and neck pain. Opioids are rarely used because of the risk of masking neurological changes. Codeine products are preferred because they are less sedating than other opioids and do not affect pupil response. Nausea and vomiting are controlled by administering antiemetic medications. The client with meningococcal meningitis should be placed in isolation, because it can be transmitted to others.

Clients may become agitated and attempt to leave the hospital because they do not comprehend or remember how ill they are. An important aspect of nursing care focuses on keeping clients from harming themselves. It is very upsetting to families to see a loved one acting agitated or disoriented. The nurse can teach the family about symptoms and treatment goals for the client.

ENCEPHALITIS

Pathophysiology

Encephalitis is inflammation of brain tissue. Nerve cell damage, edema, and necrosis cause neurological findings localized to the specific areas of the brain affected. Hemorrhage may occur in some types of encephalitis. Increased intracranial pressure may lead to herniation of the brain (see Fig. 46–8).

Etiology

Viruses are the most common cause of encephalitis. They may be specifically related to a particular time of year or geographic location. Some viruses are carried by ticks or mosquitoes. Others are systemic viral infections such as infectious mononucleosis or mumps that spread to the brain. Parasites, toxic substances, bacteria, vaccines, and fungi are other potential causes of encephalitis.

Herpes simplex is the most common non–insect-borne virus to cause encephalitis. The majority of individuals harbor herpes simplex virus type 1 in a dormant state. This is the virus responsible for cold sores on the oral mucous membranes. Infectious diseases, fever, and emotional stress are possible reasons for the virus becoming active, but the exact mechanism is not known.

Signs and Symptoms

As with meningitis, headache and fever are common presenting symptoms. The client may also complain of nausea and vomiting and general malaise. These symptoms usually develop over a period of several days.

The viruses cause nuchal rigidity, confusion, decreased level of consciousness, seizures, sensitivity to light, **ataxia,** and tremors. The client may have **hemiparesis** and exhibit abnormal deep tendon reflexes.

The client with herpes encephalitis develops edema and necrosis (sometimes associated with hemorrhage), most commonly in the temporal lobes. This significant cerebral edema causes increased ICP and can lead to herniation. If the client becomes comatose before treatment is begun, the mortality rate may be as high as 70 to 80 percent. The first 72 hours, when cerebral edema is worst, is the most likely time for death to occur.

Long-Term Complications of Encephalitis

Clients who have had encephalitis are frequently left with cognitive disabilities and personality changes. Ongoing seizures, motor deficits, and blindness may also occur. De-

---

encephalitis: encephalo—brain + itis—inflammation
hemiparesis: hemi—one side + paresis—partial paralysis

terioration in cognition and personality control are particularly stressful for significant others. The client's behavioral control is a major factor in determining discharge plans. The nurse needs to help significant others to realistically assess the client's functional level and the family's ability to care for the client. In-home care, outpatient therapy, and adult day care are options to explore. For some severely impaired individuals, custodial care may be the only feasible and safe discharge option.

Diagnostic Tests

Computed tomography (CT) scan, lumbar puncture to obtain cerebrospinal fluid, and electroencephalogram (EEG) are used to diagnose encephalitis. Cerebrospinal fluid analysis typically reveals increased white blood cell count and protein level and normal glucose levels. Breakdown of blood after cerebral hemorrhage results in a yellow CSF color.

Treatment

No treatment is currently available for insect-borne encephalitis. Careful neurological assessment and a symptomatic approach to care help prevent complications and improve survival. Medications to reduce pain and fever and anticonvulsant medication are frequently administered. Significant others need emotional support and ongoing teaching.

Acyclovir (Zovirax) is given intravenously to treat herpes simplex encephalitis. Therapy should be instituted as soon as possible after diagnosis. The most favorable outcomes are noted when acyclovir is administered before the Glasgow Coma Score is below 10. Even with prompt treatment only 38 percent of clients with herpes simplex encephalitis regain normal function.

POLIOMYELITIS/POST-POLIO SYNDROME

Poliomyelitis is a viral infection characterized by impairment of muscle function. The effects may be transient or permanent and vary from no impairment to paralysis. The incidence of poliomyelitis in the Western Hemisphere is almost zero due to successful mass immunization programs. However, individuals who had polio as children are now entering the health care system with post-polio syndrome.

Pathophysiology and Etiology

The poliomyelitis virus is found in the feces and oral or nasal secretions of infected individuals. The disease is spread through contact with these secretions. Once infection takes place the virus attacks the spinal cord, affecting the motor cells of the anterior horn. This results in muscle weakness or paralysis. Sensation is not affected, therefore these clients do experience pain.

Signs and Symptoms

Symptoms of initial infection include flulike manifestations such as fever, sore throat, headache, nausea and vomiting, and sometimes neck stiffness. Permanent paralysis, contractures, and deformities may result.

Treatment

There is no cure for poliomyelitis. Treatment is supportive in nature. Depending on the amount of paralysis the client may be completely dependent. If paralysis of the respiratory muscles occurs, the client will require mechanical ventilation. Intensive rehabilitation is typically needed after the acute phase of the illness.

Long-Term Complications

Post-polio syndrome occurs in approximately 20 to 80 percent of poliomyelitis survivors. These clients develop new or recurrent symptoms 10 to 30 years after the initial illness. Respiratory impairment, fatigue, muscle weakness, pain, and cold intolerance are the most commonly identified complaints. Not all poliomyelitis survivors develop this syndrome. Those at higher risk are the clients who made a rapid recovery after the initial illness, those who were over 10 years old when they first became ill, women, and those with more extensive physical disability.

Among the etiological theories of post-polio syndrome are the long-term effects of compensating for disabilities and stress. It is believed that collateral reinnervation is responsible for recovery of function following the acute illness. Failure of this reinnervation as the client ages may account for the return of muscle weakness. Fatigue and pain may be correlated to the ongoing stress imposed on the neurological and psychological systems by chronically coping with a disability. When the normal aging process is superimposed, the previously impaired nervous system can no longer compensate. No specific cause for post-polio syndrome has been identified. A combination of factors is most likely involved.

Development of post-polio syndrome is very physically and psychologically difficult for clients to deal with. These individuals have typically worked very hard to overcome their disabilities and maximize their functional level. They may also have worked very hard to put the initial illness experience behind them. Now they are faced with not only the normal aging process but additional threats to their physical and psychological integrity. To a disabled person even a small change in strength or mobility may mean the difference between independence and having to rely on others for assistance.

A structured regimen of rest and non–fatigue-producing exercise helps maximize muscle strength and day-to-day functioning. This can be very difficult for those individuals who believe that if they work hard enough they can overcome their symptoms. Referral to a support group of other people with post-polio syndrome may be helpful.

Nursing Process: The Client with an Infectious or Inflammatory Neurological Disorder

Assessment

A complete history should be obtained from the client, if feasible, and from significant others. Particular attention is paid to exposure to risk factors and symptoms of generalized malaise. The physical assessment must include all body systems because neurological impairment affects the entire person. Following the initial assessment, serial neurological assessments continue to be important to detect and report changes promptly. Pupil response and vital signs are monitored for signs of increased intracranial pressure (Table 46–4). Headache is monitored on a pain scale. The Glasgow Coma Scale presented in Chapter 45 is a valuable tool to monitor level of consciousness.

Nursing Diagnosis

Possible nursing diagnoses for the client with a central nervous system infection include the following:

- Decreased adaptive capacity: intracranial related to infectious or inflammatory process
- Pain related to headache and nuchal rigidity
- Hyperthermia related to infectious process
- Risk for injury related to seizures or falls
- Sensory-perceptual alterations related to cranial nerve involvement
- Impaired physical mobility related to long-term complications of disease

Planning

The nurse must plan to meet the physical needs of the client as well as the emotional needs of the client and significant others during the acute phase of illness. Whenever possible, the goal is to support the client and prevent long-term complications. This requires careful monitoring and timely reporting of changes in neurological status.

Table 46–4. *Signs and Symptoms of Increased Intracranial Pressure*

Vomiting
Headache
Dilated pupil on affected side
Hemiparesis or hemiplegia
Decorticate then decerebrate posturing
Decreasing level of consciousness
Increasing systolic blood pressure
Increasing then decreasing pulse rate
Rising temperature

Implementation

DECREASED ADAPTIVE CAPACITY. This refers to the client's inability to maintain normal intracranial pressure. Measures such as avoiding the Valsalva's maneuver during bowel movements and avoiding flexion of the neck when positioning the client help prevent increases in ICP. The client with increased intracranial pressure is usually cared for in an intensive care setting, and the LPN-LVN collaborates with the registered nurse in implementing care. See Table 46–5 and Chapter 45 for additional information.

PAIN. Headache and other alterations in comfort are difficult to treat. Opioid analgesics (with the possible exception of codeine) are usually avoided because they mask neurological symptoms and make detection of changes difficult. If they are used, the client is monitored carefully for changes in level of consciousness or other neurological changes. The client is assisted to whatever position is most comfortable. A dark, quiet room with few distractions may also reduce headache.

HYPERTHERMIA. Control of fever with acetaminophen or aspirin is important because a high temperature can increase the risk for seizures. A cooling mattress and tepid sponge baths may be necessary, but are uncomfortable for the client. Comfort can be increased and shivering reduced by cooling the client gradually and wrapping extremities in bath blankets during cooling mattress therapy.

Table 46–5. *Interventions to Prevent Increased Intracranial Pressure*

Action	Rationale
Keep head of bed elevated 30 degrees unless contraindicated.	Head elevation reduces ICP in some clients.
Avoid flexing the neck; keep head and neck in midline position.	Neck flexion may obstruct venous outflow.
Administer antiemetics or antitussives as necessary to prevent vomiting and cough.	Coughing and vomiting can increase ICP.
Administer stool softeners.	Straining for bowel movement can increase ICP.
Minimize suctioning. If absolutely necessary, oxygenate first and limit suction passes to one or two.	Suctioning can increase ICP.
Avoid hip flexion.	Hip flexion can increase intraabdominal and thoracic pressure, which can increase ICP.
Prevent unnecessary noise and startling the client.	Noxious stimuli can increase ICP in some clients.
Space care activities to provide rest between each disturbance.	Clustering care activities may increase ICP.

RISK FOR INJURY. Client safety is maintained with seizure precautions (see the section on seizures, later in this chapter), use of side rails, and reminders not to get up without help if indicated. Having a family member stay with the client can help the client feel more secure and prevent falls if the client's ability to remember instructions is impaired.

SENSORY-PERCEPTUAL ALTERATIONS. Sensory problems can increase risk of injury. The client is monitored closely for changes in level of consciousness. See Chapters 48 and 49 for specific interventions for clients with sensory problems.

IMPAIRED PHYSICAL MOBILITY. Physical mobility should be maintained as much as possible. The client should be encouraged to move and turn in bed and ambulate when able. Long-term mobility problems such as hemiparesis may be reduced with the help of a physical therapy consultation. Measures to prevent impaired skin integrity should be implemented.

Evaluation

Successful nursing management of a client with an infectious or inflammatory neurological disorder is evidenced by a client with no preventable complications such as pressure ulcers or contractures. This increases the possibility that the client with a neurological deficit will benefit from rehabilitation and improve his or her level of functioning.

Client Education

The nature and focus of teaching depends on the client's level of consciousness and cognitive status. When appropriate, both the client and significant others should be included in the education process. If the client is not able to participate, the significant others become the focus of the nurse's teaching.

Describing the brain as in control of bodily functions may help significant others to understand some of the symptoms of neurological disorders. The spinal cord can be compared to a telephone cord, with hundreds of tiny individual wires (nerves) making up the cord. The specific wires affected by disease determine the symptoms the client will experience.

CRITICAL THINKING: Mr. Chung

Mr. Chung is an 18-year-old Asian college student. He comes to the emergency department complaining of headache, stiff neck, and fever. On physical assessment you notice a petechial rash on his legs and torso. The physician diagnoses meningococcal meningitis.

1. What tests are likely to be performed?
2. How should patient education be planned for Mr. Chung?
3. What infection control practices should be instituted?
4. What comfort measures could be offered to Mr. Chung?
5. What concerns do you have about how Mr. Chung contracted his illness?

Answers at end of chapter.

Headaches

As mentioned throughout this chapter, headache is a common symptom of neurological disorders. However, most headaches are transient events and do not indicate serious pathology. If headaches are recurrent, persistent, or increasing in severity, the client should undergo a neurological evaluation.

Because the causes, signs and symptoms, pathophysiology, and treatment of headaches vary based on the type of headache experienced, these subjects will be discussed separately for each type of headache.

TYPES OF HEADACHES

Tension or Muscle Contraction Headaches

Persistent contraction of the scalp, facial, cervical, and upper thoracic muscles can cause tension headaches. A cycle of muscle tension, muscle tenderness, and further muscle tension is established. This cycle may or may not be associated with vasodilation of cerebral arteries. Headaches of this type may be associated with premenstrual syndrome or psychosocial stressors such as anxiety, emotional distress, or depression. Symptoms typically develop gradually. Radiation of pain to the crown of the head and base of the skull, with variations in location and intensity, is common. *Pressure, aching, steady,* and *tight* are some of the adjectives used to describe the pain of tension headaches.

Care must be taken to thoroughly rule out physical causes before attributing the headache to psychosocial origins. Symptom management may include the use of relaxation techniques, massage of the affected muscles, rest, localized heat application, nonnarcotic analgesics, and appropriate counseling.

Migraine Headaches

A number of theories have been proposed to explain migraine headaches. It is believed that cerebral vasoconstriction followed by vasodilation is a major factor. This response may be triggered by the trigeminal nerve, which in turn stimulates release of substance P, a pain transmitter, into the vessels. Serotonin is another neurotransmitter that may play a role in migraine pain. The tendency to develop

954 UNIT 13—Understanding the Nervous System

migraine headaches is often hereditary. Migraine episodes can be triggered by a variety of factors, including noise, bright light, alcohol, and stress. Some clients can identify specific foods that trigger the headache.

Symptoms include a **prodromal** period, in which the client may experience several hours to days of changes in mood and appetite, drowsiness, or frequent yawning. Some clients experience additional neurological symptoms such as visual changes, immediately before the pain begins. Many clients report seeing flashing lights. The headache that follows is usually on one side, is often accompanied by nausea and sometimes vomiting, and may last for hours to days. Commonly used descriptors of migraine pain include *throbbing, boring, viselike,* and *pounding.* It is usually on one side of the head. Noise and light tend to exacerbate the headache, leading the client to rest in a dark, quiet environment.

Treatment of migraine may be prophylactic or directed at an acute episode. Prophylactic treatment is usually reserved for those clients experiencing one or more headaches per week. Dietary restrictions may be helpful if precipitating foods or beverages can be identified. Nifedipine, a calcium channel blocker, amitriptyline, a tricyclic antidepressant, and propanolol, a beta-adrenergic blocker, are prophylactic treatments that may be used for migraine headaches. Propanolol and nifedipine should be used cautiously because of the potential for lowering blood pressure (BP). This is particularly true of young, slender females, who may normally have a low BP. Amitriptyline may cause drowsiness, dry mouth, and weight gain. None of these medications should be stopped abruptly after long-term use.

Several types of medications are available to treat the acute migraine headache. Ergot (Cafergot) is a vasoconstrictor; it is effective only if taken before the vessel walls become edematous, usually within 30 to 60 minutes of headache onset. Sumitriptan (Imitrex) is the newest medication available for migraine relief. This drug works at the serotonin receptor sites and has a vasoconstricting action. It has been demonstrated to be effective in both intramuscular and oral forms. The potentially additive nature of multidrug medications and opioids requires careful monitoring of clients using them. Clients must be educated regarding proper use of the medication, potential side effects, and consequences of misuse.

Cluster Headaches

Vascular disturbance, stress, anxiety, and emotional distress are all proposed causes of cluster headache. As indicated by the name, these headaches tend to occur in clusters over a time span of several days to weeks. Months or even years may pass between episodes. Alcohol consumption may worsen the episodes.

The client may state that the headache begins suddenly, typically at the same time of night. *Throbbing* and *excruci-*

ating are frequently the adjectives used by the client. The headache tends to be unilateral, affecting the nose, eye, and forehead. A bloodshot, teary appearance of the affected eye is common.

Due to the brief nature of cluster headaches, treatment is difficult. A quiet, dark environment and cold compresses may lessen the intensity of the pain. Nonsteroidal anti-inflammatory drugs (NSAIDs) or tricyclic antidepressants may be prescribed.

DIAGNOSIS

Most headaches are diagnosed based on the client's history and symptoms, after other causes have been ruled out. Magnetic resonance imaging (MRI), CT, or other testing may be done to make sure that a brain tumor or other structural problem is not causing the headaches.

NURSING CARE

Assessment

The WHAT'S UP mnemonic is particularly useful in helping the client provide useful information regarding the headache.

W—Where is the pain? Does it remain in one place or radiate to other areas of the head? Does the headache consistently start in one place?

H—How does the headache feel? Throbbing, steady, dull, bandlike, other qualities?

A—Aggravating or alleviating factors should be assessed. Some aggravating factors include red wine, caffeine, chocolate, and foods containing nitrates. Others include particular stages of the menstrual cycle, emotional stress, and tension. Alleviating factors might include lying down in a dark room, cold compresses, and over-the-counter medications.

T—Timing may be a factor for a client who experiences headaches just before or during her menstrual period. For other clients there may be no predictive timing. Also ask how long the headache lasted.

S—Ask the client to rate the severity on a scale of 1 to 10. Is the severity consistent or does it vary from headache to headache?

U—Ask the client about associated symptoms such as nausea, vomiting, or bloodshot eyes.

P—Obtain the client's perception of the headache. Does it interfere with the client's life? If so, how? Has the client had a previous evaluation of headaches?

Client Education

The first step in client education is to help the client identify and reduce or eliminate aggravating factors. This can be accomplished by keeping a headache diary for a period of time, recording the time of day the headache occurs, foods eaten or other aggravating factors, description of the pain, identification of associated symptoms such as nausea or visual disturbances, and other factors related to headache symptoms. This can help the client lessen the frequency and intensity of attacks and provides a sense of control over his or her illness. Similarly, encouraging the client to use alleviating techniques such as biofeedback or stress reduction helps the client participate in the treatment of the headache. Relaxation exercises or warm moist compresses may be helpful for tension headaches. A dark room and rest are essential during a migraine headache.

Education regarding medications, appropriate dosage, expected action, side effects, and consequences of misuse is essential. Depending on the client's learning ability and interest, information may be given orally or in written format. Drawings, diagrams, and commercially prepared drug information are potential teaching aids.

Cerebrovascular Disorders

TRANSIENT ISCHEMIC ATTACK

Transient ischemic attack (TIA) is a temporary impairment of the cerebral circulation causing neurological impairment. It is characterized by focal neurological deficits, typically minutes to hours in duration. Symptoms resolve completely within 24 hours. Symptoms that last longer than 24 hours but do not cause permanent neurological changes are called reversible ischemic neurological deficits (RIND).

Pathophysiology

Cerebral function is dependent on oxygen and glucose delivery to neurons. Interruption of blood flow to the brain deprives neurons of needed glucose and oxygen. The particular vessel or vessels involved determine the area of the brain affected and therefore the symptoms observed. The duration of ischemia determines whether the symptoms are transient or permanent. A transient ischemic attack may be a warning of an impending cerebrovascular accident.

Etiology

Atherosclerosis resulting in narrowing of arterial diameter is the most common cause of a transient ischemic attack. Although any vessel may be involved, the bifurcation of the common carotid artery into the internal and external branches is the most common location for cerebral occlusion. Emboli may lodge in cerebral vessels, resulting in occlusion, ischemia, and infarct. Emboli may break off of arterial plaque or be released into the circulation during atrial fibrillation.

Signs and Symptoms

Symptoms depend on the area of the brain affected. Common symptoms include visual disturbances, difficulty with speech, weakness or paralysis on one side of the body, and transient confusion. They subside within 24 hours. See Table 46–6 for the symptoms associated with occlusion of specific arteries.

Diagnostic Tests

Carotid Doppler testing can determine if stenosis of the carotid arteries exists. This noninvasive test involves bouncing sound waves off of the carotid arteries to determine the velocity and turbulence of blood flow.

Clients may undergo an echocardiogram to determine the presence of heart disease that may increase risk of thrombus formation. CT scan or MRI may be used to assess for previous, possibly asymptomatic, infarctions. A cerebral angiogram may be done to determine the patency of cerebral vessels and the status of any collateral circulation. Refer to Chapter 45 for a description of this examination.

Treatment

Medical Management

Medical management focuses on controlling the cause of the transient ischemic attack. Medications are used to control atrial fibrillation or hypertension. Warfarin (Coumadin) may be prescribed for clients prone to clot development. Education regarding safety precautions is essential for these clients. They should be instructed to use electric razors to minimize nicks and to be careful to avoid

Table 46–6. **Symptoms of Cerebrovascular Accident According to Artery Affected**

	Hemiparesis	Dysphasia	Visual Changes	Altered Level of Consciousness	Ataxia
Carotid	X	X	X	X	
Middle cerebral	X	X	X	X	
Vertebrobasilar			X		X

any injury that might cause bleeding. The possible development of a cerebral hematoma following a fall or blow to the head must be stressed to the client and significant others.

Antiplatelet drugs such as ticlopidine (Ticlid) or aspirin are often prescribed for clients experiencing transient ischemic attacks. Decreasing platelet aggregation lessens the likelihood of thrombus formation. If aspirin is prescribed for its antiplatelet properties, the client should be instructed not to use aspirin or products containing aspirin for pain relief. Because ticlopidine is metabolized by the liver it may elevate liver enzymes, and regular blood tests are required.

Surgical Management

If carotid stenosis of greater than 70 percent is detected, a carotid **endarterectomy** may be performed. During this surgical procedure, the carotid artery is opened and the plaque removed. Nursing care focuses on careful neurological assessment for signs of deterioration related to ischemia. The incision is monitored for hematoma development and bleeding. Development of a hematoma can compromise the client's airway. Bleeding at the suture line, particularly of bright red blood, may indicate failure of the sutures. This emergency situation requires prompt response to prevent massive blood loss. Balloon angioplasty for carotid stenosis is being investigated as a potential treatment in large facilities.

Acute Complications

By definition, a transient ischemic attack is an event that results in no permanent neurological deficit. However, clients can experience complications from events that occur during a transient ischemic attack. Falls may result in broken bones, abrasions and lacerations, or cerebral hematomas, particularly if the client is on anticoagulants. Motor vehicle accidents may occur if the client experiences visual or cognitive impairments. Hemiparesis can cause clients to burn or cut themselves if cooking or operating power tools. There are no long-term complications of transient ischemic attacks.

CEREBROVASCULAR ACCIDENT (BRAIN ATTACK, STROKE)

Cerebrovascular accident (CVA, or stroke) is the infarction of brain tissue due to the disruption of blood flow to the brain. It is characterized by focal neurological deficits specific to the area of the brain involved. Although CVAs are most frequently associated with elderly clients, they affect approximately 500,000 individuals of all ages each year. A newer term for CVA is *brain attack*. This reminds us that like a heart attack, a CVA is an urgent condition that can be treated if medical care is sought immediately. Exciting new treatment developments may now allow clients to be deficit free if help is sought in time.

Pathophysiology

Infarction of brain tissue happens when there is inadequate blood flow to an area of the brain. When blood flow is severely compromised, or absent, the oxygen and glucose needed to meet the brain's metabolic needs are not available. The brain has no capability to store oxygen or glucose, so it relies on a constant supply of these nutrients. If the supply of oxygen and glucose is stopped, the brain tissue dies. In contrast to TIA, a brain attack can cause permanent damage if it is not reversed with timely treatment.

Causes and Types

A brain attack can either be ischemic (from deficient blood supply to the brain) or hemorrhagic (from bleeding into the brain). An ischemic brain attack is either thrombotic or embolic. Thrombosis or atherosclerosis can narrow or completely occlude a vessel. People with diabetes and hypertension have an increased risk for atherosclerosis and stroke. Emboli can lodge in a cerebral vessel, stopping the blood flow to that area of the brain. Emboli can occur as a result of endocarditis, atrial fibrillation, or valvular disease, but can be dissolved with thrombolytic medication if treatment is sought quickly.

Rupture of a cerebral blood vessel can result in a hemorrhagic brain attack. The most common cause of an intracerebral hemorrhage is poorly controlled hypertension. These hemorrhages tend to occur deep within the brain tissue. This type of infarct has the slowest rate of recovery and the highest probability of leaving the client with extensive neurological deficits. There is no medication to reverse the effects of this type of brain attack.

The most common etiology of brain attack in younger clients is illicit drug usage. PCP, crack, cocaine, amphetamines, and heroin have all been associated with cerebrovascular accident from subarachnoid or intracerebral hemorrhage, because these drugs raise the blood pressure and increase pressure within the cerebral vessels.

Prevention

Incidence of CVA can be lessened by reduction of risk factors. Risk factors include hypertension, smoking, atherosclerosis, diabetes, and cardiac problems that cause emboli to form. Keeping hypertension and diabetes controlled can go a long way in preventing strokes. Emboli can be pre-

---

endarterectomy: endo—inside + arter—artery + ectomy—surgical removal of vented with warfarin (Coumadin) in individuals with high risk. Aspirin or ticlopidine (Ticlid) may also be used. If atherosclerosis is a concern, a carotid endarterectomy may be done.

It is important to educate all clients about new treatments for stroke and the potential for reversal of symptoms with the use of thrombolytic agents. Clients must be aware of symptoms of stroke, and the importance of emergency treatment to maximize the potential for prevention of neurological deficits. Too often clients ignore early symptoms or delay calling for help. This delay can mean the difference between leading a normal life and permanent disability.

Signs and Symptoms

As with transient ischemic attacks, the signs and symptoms of a cerebrovascular accident relate to the specific vessel involved (see Table 46–6). There are some symptoms common to cerebrovascular accidents of different etiologies. These may include changes in level of consciousness, fever, headache, vomiting, and seizures. Other common symptoms include numbness, weakness, or paralysis of one side of the face and one arm or leg; trouble understanding language or speaking coherently; vision changes; and impaired coordination or balance. Additional short-term and long-term manifestations are discussed below.

Short-Term Effects

NEUROLOGICAL DETERIORATION. Clients suffering from a brain attack develop increased intracranial pressure, which further adds to brain damage. Clients are also vulnerable to repeat cerebrovascular accidents. Careful serial neurological assessments are needed to promptly detect and report changes.

RESPIRATORY COMPROMISE. Respiratory compromise may occur related to an increase in intracranial pressure. Clients with cerebrovascular accident are prone to aspiration because of decreased level of consciousness or impaired swallowing ability. Clients should be suctioned as needed to keep the airway clear. If the client vomits, he or she should be turned to the side to lessen the risk of aspiration. Oral feedings should be begun carefully and progressed slowly only after the client is alert and able to swallow safely.

Long-Term Effects

MOTOR FUNCTION. The side of the body opposite the side of the cerebral infarct is affected, because nerve fibers cross over as they pass from the brain to the spinal cord (Fig. 46–2). The affected extremities may be weak or to-

tally paralyzed (**hemiplegia**). An extremity that has no muscle tone or movement at all is called **flaccid.** Depending on the artery affected, the arm may be weaker than the leg or vice versa. These clients are particularly prone to **contractures,** which cause permanent immobility of a muscle or joint from fibrosis of connective tissue. Adaptation or assistance with activities of daily living (ADL) will be required. Sensory changes may prevent the client from being aware of injuries to the affected side. Clients should be mobilized within 24 to 48 hours if possible to prevent complications of immobility. Physical and occupational therapy are provided to maximize functioning, and the client must be taught to deliberately be aware of and protect the involved limbs.

Motor involvement often affects swallowing, control of urination, and bowel function. Difficulty swallowing (dysphagia) is a major problem for clients after a stroke and can cause aspiration pneumonia, which can lead to death.

APHASIA. If the infarct is on the dominant side of the brain, the speech center will probably be affected. Aphasia may be expressive, receptive, or global. Persons with expressive aphasia know what they want to say but are unable to speak in a way that can be understood. They may be able to say words but are not able to form coherent speech, such as the client who picks up a fork but calls it a comb. A client with receptive aphasia does not understand what is said to him or her. In this situation it is easy to attempt to speak louder to try to help the client understand. The nurse must remember that it is not the client's hearing that is affected. Global aphasia is a combination of expressive and receptive disturbance.

EMOTIONAL LABILITY. Emotional lability or instability is a common consequence of cerebrovascular accident. Clients may move rapidly from profound sadness to an almost euphoric state and back again. Laughing or crying may have no relationship to the client's situation at any given moment. Families can be upset by this behavior, because they do not understand why a once happy person is now crying all the time, or why the client laughs inappropriately. The nurse can help by explaining that these responses probably do not reflect how the client is feeling, but rather are a manifestation of the stroke damage.

IMPAIRED JUDGMENT. Clients who have had a CVA, particularly those with right-sided lesions, present safety risks. Clients may have poor understanding of their own limitations and believe that they are capable of performing tasks they did before the cerebrovascular accident. Precautions must be taken to prevent the client from injury.

If the frontal lobes are involved, learned social behaviors may be lost. The client may undress in public, use profanity, or make inappropriate sexual advances. These behaviors are extremely difficult for significant others to cope with. Education and emotional support of the signifi-

---

hemiplegia: hemi—one side + plegic—paralysis

Left-side infarct

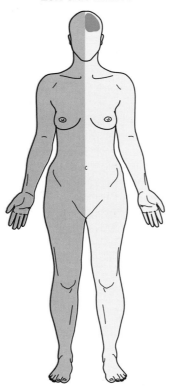

Right-sided weakness or paralysis
Aphasia (in left–brain-dominant clients)
Depression related to disability common

Right-side infarct

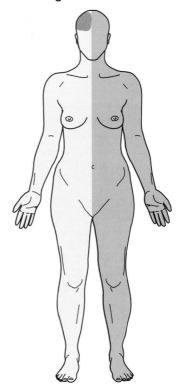

Left-sided weakness or paralysis
Impaired judgement/safety risk
Unilateral neglect more common
Indifferent to disability

Figure 46–2. The side opposite the infarct is affected in a brain attack.

cant others are essential. Allowing them to vent their frustration and anger may facilitate coping. Distracting the client from inappropriate behavior may help. The client should never be reprimanded or punished, because he or she no longer has the cognitive ability to control the behaviors.

UNILATERAL NEGLECT. This phenomenon is seen predominantly in clients who have right hemisphere infarcts. These individuals do not acknowledge the left side of their environment. In severe cases the client may forget to dress the left side of the body. Initially, the nurse approaches these clients from the right side. Essential items such as the call light and telephone are placed on the client's right side. The bed should be positioned so that the client's right side is toward the door. Gradually the health team can begin teaching the client to focus on the left side. This involves teaching the client to purposefully check where the left limbs are positioned and to look for safety risks. The client can learn to turn his or her head and scan the environment. Clients may need reminders to turn their

plates during meals to recognize the food on the left side of the plate.

HOMONYMOUS HEMIANOPSIA. Some clients experience a loss of visual field in the same side of each eye. This is called homonymous hemianopsia, and it can cause the client to ignore one side of a dinner tray or neglect to care for one side of the body.

LEARNING TIP

When preparing a room for a client following a stroke, the caretaker should choose a room in which the client can have the unaffected side toward the door if at all possible.

Diagnostic Tests

A CT scan can help determine the size and location of the infarct and whether the cause is hemorrhagic or occlusion of the artery. An EEG, arteriography, or MRI may be done. If an embolism is suspected, cardiac tests may be done to determine the source.

Treatment

Medical Management

Thrombolytic therapy is a recent development in the treatment of ischemic brain attack. Intracerebral hemorrhage must be ruled out before thrombolytic therapy is instituted. The goal of thrombolytic agents is to actually break down the thrombus causing the ischemia, which can potentially prevent or completely reverse the symptoms of stroke. Plasmin is the enzyme that causes thrombi to break down. Thrombolytic agents accomplish thrombus lysis by causing the conversion of plasminogen to plasmin. The three most commonly used thrombolytic agents are streptokinase, urokinase, and tissue-type plasminogen activator (tPA). Cerebral hemorrhage is a major complication of thrombolytic therapy. Clients treated effectively with thrombolytic therapy may be able to leave the hospital within 1 or 2 days, with no residual effects.

To be effective, thrombolytic therapy must be administered within 3 hours of the onset of symptoms. This time frame has clear implications for nurses. Clients in the emergency department with neurological symptoms must be assessed and stabilized promptly. A CT scan and, if an ischemic cause is suspected, an angiogram are performed quickly. Some people may be surprised to learn that there are treatments available for brain attack. Due to the time constraints, individuals may be asked to make treatment decisions before other family members are able to arrive. This places a significant burden on people who are already experiencing stress. The nurse can help ease this burden by explaining the time factor, repeating information as needed, and ensuring that the individuals involved have the opportunity to ask questions.

LEARNING TIP

Time is brain. This means the faster the stroke victim receives treatment, the more brain may be saved.

Management of the airway and control of hypertension if present are vital for the client. Care is taken not to lower the blood pressure too quickly or too far. If the client has long-standing hypertension, lowering the blood pressure to a "normal" level may actually cause further ischemia. Current recommendations are to not lower blood pressure

---

thrombolytic: thrombo—clot + lytic—causing breakdown
craniotomy: crani—skull + otomy—surgical opening

---

more than 10 percent from baseline at one time. Vasoactive drugs must be used carefully and blood pressure monitored frequently. If the client experiences neurological deterioration the physician may adjust treatment to increase the blood pressure. Some physicians believe that the blood pressure should not be lowered because chronically hypertensive clients require a higher BP to maintain adequate cerebral perfusion. As soon as the client is stabilized, a CT scan is performed to identify any cerebral hemorrhage. Further treatment is dependent on the presence or absence of hemorrhage.

If a cerebrovascular accident is caused by an embolism, anticoagulants may be prescribed. Treatment begins with intravenous heparin sodium. When the clotting studies reach a therapeutic level, oral warfarin (Coumadin) is begun. The infusion rate of the heparin is gradually decreased and then stopped while clotting tests are monitored. Clients will need monitoring of the prothrombin time (PT) and international normalized ratio (INR), and adjustment of warfarin dosage as long as they are on warfarin. These clients must be instructed to inform all health care providers, including dentists, that they are taking warfarin. The warfarin dosage will need to be adjusted before any invasive procedures are performed. Antiplatelet drugs may be used to lessen platelet aggregation.

Surgical Management

Surgical treatment to prevent a cerebrovascular accident was discussed earlier in the section on transient ischemic attacks. Occasionally a **craniotomy** is performed to remove an embolus or thrombus. This surgery must be performed within a few hours of the ischemic event if there is to be any possibility of preventing permanent neurological deficits.

Nursing Care

See Nursing Process: The Client with a Cerebrovascular Disorder. Also see Clinical Pathway Box 46–1. A clinical pathway (also called a care map or critical path) is a guideline that helps coordinate and direct the care of the client. It is part of a managed care system, as described in Chapter 1.

CEREBRAL ANEURYSM/SUBARACHNOID HEMORRHAGE

A cerebral aneurysm is a weakness in the wall of an artery. It may be congenital, traumatic, or the result of disease. If the aneurysm ruptures, a subarachnoid hemorrhage results. It is unknown what causes the formation of congenital aneurysms or what causes them to rupture. Unruptured aneurysms are typically asymptomatic. The exception to this is very large aneurysms that can cause symptoms simi-

text continues on page 963

CLINICAL PATHWAY BOX 46–1 CEREBRAL THROMBOSIS, COMPLETED STROKE IN A PATIENT WHO IS *NOT* INDEPENDENT IN AMBULATION

DRG: 014 ICD.9 434.0, 434.9
LOS: 2 days

Patient Problem	Emergent/Direct	Day 1	Goals Day 2	Day 3/Discharge
1. Knowledge deficit A. Disease process	Client/family can describe his/her disease process as outlined in the client language pathway booklet.	Client/family can describe his/her disease process as outlined in the client language pathway booklet.	Client/family can describe his/her disease process as outlined in the client language pathway booklet. Client/family state area of stroke and residual effects.	Client/family state signs and symptoms of CVA. Client/family state client's specific risk factors.
B. Hospitalization	Client/family states expected plan of care and projected LOS as stated in the Client language pathway booklet.	Client participates in his/her care as outlined in the client language pathway booklet.	Client participates in their care as outlined in the client language pathway booklet.	Client participates in his/her care as outlined in the client language pathway booklet. Client/family can state discharge meds, including side effects and interactions, symptoms to report to the physician, activity level, and next doctor's appointment.
2. Discharge Planning	Client/family participate in identification of discharge needs.	Client/family participate in identification of discharge needs. Client/family participate in evaluation of family support abilities and possible rehabilitation placement needs.	Client/family identify 1st and 2nd choice for placement as necessary. Client/family agree to proposed discharge plan.	Family verifies transfer plan as necessary. Client has met all discharge goals.
3. Potential complications A. Altered level of consciousness	Client participates in baseline assessment.	Client participates in baseline assessment.		
B. Obstructed airway	Client will maintain an airway. Client will maintain effective airway clearance.	Client will maintain effective airway clearance.		
C. Loss of language function	Client participates in baseline assessment.	Client participates in speech/language evaluation.		
D. Loss of functional mobility	Client participates in baseline assessment.	Client participates in PT/OT evaluations and performs bed mobility with assistance of 2 persons.		
E. Loss of visual/ perceptual function	Client participates in baseline assessment.	Client participates in baseline assessment.		

continued

CLINICAL PATHWAY BOX 46–1 *(continued)*

Patient Problem			Goals	
	Emergent/Direct	*Day 1*	*Day 2*	*Day 3/Discharge*
F. Loss of bowel and bladder function	Client/family participate in baseline assessment.	Client/family participate in baseline assessment.		
4. Safety	Client will remain free from injury. Client's skin integrity will be maintained. Client will remain free from shoulder sublaxation.	Client will remain free from injury. Client's skin integrity will be maintained.	Client will remain free from injury. Client's skin integrity will be maintained.	Client will remain free from injury. Client's skin integrity will be maintained.
5. Medication maintenance	Client/family identify current medication regimen.	Client's maintenance medications will be maintained.	Client's maintenance medications will be maintained.	Client's maintenance medications will be maintained.

Plan

Consults	Finance/benefits verified including coverage of posthospital needs. Notify case manager. Consider neurology consult	Notify Physical Therapy. Notify Occupational Therapy. Notify Speech Pathology. Notify Social Work. Refer client to smoking cessation counselor if client is a smoker.		
Tests	CBC ECG PT SMA7 U/A PTT CT scan of head. Echocardiogram.	Carotid duplex scan. Consider MRI. Consider EEG. Consider 24 hr holter monitor. ESR, ANA, lipid profile.		Consider repeat CT scan of head at f72 hr if the first CT scan was negative.
Activity	Bed rest.	Bed mobility HOB ↑30°. Maintain body alignment.	Bed mobility HOB ↑30°. OOB bid 60 min.	Bed mobility HOB ↑30°. OOB tid 30–60 min.
Assessment	Physiological Monitoring Protocol. IV Therapy Protocol Fall Prevention Protocol. O_2 Therapy Protocol. Neuro checks every 2 hr × 8 hr then every 4 hr × 24 hr then as per protocol. Bowel/bladder assessment.	Physiological Monitoring Protocol. IV Therapy Protocol. Fall Prevention Protocol. O_2 Therapy Protocol. Neuro checks per protocol. PT assessment for motor/balance deficits. OT assessment for visual/perceptive, ADL deficits. Speech assessment for language, swallowing, cognitive deficit. Social Work assessment for placement. Skin integrity protocol.	Physiological Monitoring Protocol. IV Therapy Protocol. Fall Prevention Protocol. O_2 Therapy Protocol. Neuro checks per protocol.	Physiological Monitoring Protocol. IV Therapy Protocol. Fall Prevention Protocol. O_2 Therapy Protocol. Neuro checks per protocol.

continued

CLINICAL PATHWAY BOX 46–1 (continued)

Plan

Treatments	IV. O_2 (titrate to maintain SaO_2 >92%). Foley catheter to straight drainage.	IV. O_2 (titrate to maintain SaO_2 >92%). Foley catheter to straight drainage. PT/OT/SLP treatment. Order UE/LE splints as necessary. Suction secretions prn.	IV. O_2 (titrate to maintain SaO_2 >92%). Foley catheter to straight drainage. PT/OT/SLP treatments. D/C foley catheter. Order UE/LE splints as necessary. Suction secretions prn.	D/C IV. If client's SaO_2 ≥92% on room air d/c O_2. Suction secretions prn.
Medications	Current medication history. Antiplatelet treatment.	Antiplatelet treatment.	Antiplatelet treatment.	Antiplatelet treatment.
Nutrition	NPO.	Liquid diet. Advance as tolerated.		
Discharge planning	Assessment of family support system. Admit to Med-Surg floor.	Continued assessment of discharge needs. Evaluate for transfer to lower level of care. *Plan discharge based on criteria: <1° of active participation = home health care/nursing home; 1–3° subacute; 3+° inpatient rehab.	Continued assessment of discharge needs. Evaluate for transfer to lower level of care. Provide adaptive/assistive equipment as necessary. If client is unable to speak, establish alternative method of communication, e.g., letterboard.	Discharge to acute rehabilitation facility or skilled nursing facility.
Education	Orient client/family to unit. Teach client/family about disease process. Review client language pathway booklet specifying projected LOS and plan of care.	Include anticoagulant teaching, if necessary. Teach client/family about disease process. Review client language pathway booklet specifying goals for the day and progress toward discharge. Instruct client/family in discharge meds, including side effects and interactions. Teach client/family area of stroke and residual effects.	Educate client/family in UE/LE splint use. Teach client/family about disease process. Teach client/family signs and symptoms of stroke. Teach client/family client's specific risk factors. Teach client use of compensatory strategies.	Emphasize "reasons to call physician" as presented in the client language pathway booklet.
Psychosocial	Provide emotional support to client/family. Explain all procedures to client/family. Identify spokesperson.	Provide emotional support to client/family. Explain all procedures to client/family.	Provide emotional support to client/family. Explain all procedures to client/family.	Provide emotional support to client/family. Explain all procedures to client/family.

Additional protocols

Inclusion criteria: CT excluded hemorrhage
Hemiparesis
No cognitive impairment
Unimpaired swallowing

*Criteria: Rehab. d/c planning:
- moderate to complete med. stability
- 1+ persistent disabilities (mobility, ADL, swallowing, B/B control, cognition, communication, pain mgt., psycho-emot. functional)
- able to learn
- adequate physical endurance for at least 1° day to participate in rehab.

INITIALS	SIGNATURE/TITLE	DATE/TIME	INITIALS	SIGNATURE/TITLE	DATE/TIME

lar to brain tumors. Aneurysms often affect young, otherwise healthy adults.

Pathophysiology and Etiology

Aneurysms can occur in any of the cerebral arteries. Eighty percent of cerebral aneurysms occur in the circle of Willis. The most common site is at the bifurcation of an artery. It is theorized that increased turbulence at the bifurcation causes an outpouching of a congenitally weak arterial wall.

Subarachnoid hemorrhage is the collection of blood beneath the arachnoid mater following aneurysm rupture. Rupture of an arteriovenous malformation (Fig. 46–3) or head trauma may also result in subarachnoid hemorrhage. The presence of blood outside of the blood vessels is very irritating to brain tissue. It is believed that irritation from blood breakdown is the major cause of vasospasm, a common complication of subarachnoid hemorrhage.

It is unclear what causes an aneurysm to rupture at a given time. Some individuals experience a subarachnoid hemorrhage while performing the Valsalva's maneuver, engaging in sexual activity, or physically exerting themselves. For other clients the aneurysm ruptures during a quiet, nonactive period. If the aneurysm rupture is associated with a particular activity the client may be very frightened of engaging in that activity again. This may have a negative effect on the client's interpersonal relationships if the associated activity was sexual in nature. The client's partner may feel guilty or responsible for the hemorrhage. Emotional support and confidentiality regarding associated events help both the client and significant other.

Signs and Symptoms

Some clients experience a small hemorrhage before diagnosis of subarachnoid hemorrhage. This leakage of blood may cause a mild headache, vomiting, or disorientation. The symptoms may be attributed to a flulike syndrome. Clients may dismiss the symptoms and not seek medical care.

The most common presentation of rupture of an aneurysm is sudden onset of severe headaches. Typically clients state, "I have never had a headache this bad in my life." Clients may hold their heads and moan or cry in pain. Sensitivity to light is a common finding. This may make clients very reluctant to cooperate with pupil checks.

Level of consciousness varies based on the severity of the hemorrhage. Clients may be alert and coherent, may lose consciousness immediately, or may gradually become less responsive. The decreased level of consciousness is caused by increased ICP and impairment of cerebral blood flow. Clients may experience generalized seizures.

Blood in the subarachnoid space causes meningeal irritation. The client may complain of nuchal rigidity. The most commonly affected cranial nerves are III and VI. This is manifested as an enlarged pupil or dysconjugate gaze. Motor dysfunction may involve one or both limbs on the side opposite the hemorrhage.

Diagnostic Tests

Clients with subarachnoid hemorrhage almost always come to the emergency department rather than seeking care from routine health care providers, due to the severe nature of the symptoms. A CT scan is done to identify the

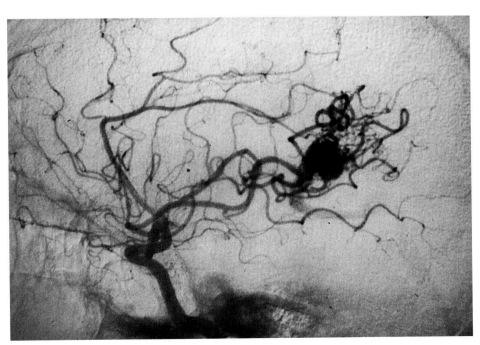

Figure 46–3. Arteriovenous malformation. Note tangled vessels.

presence and location of a hemorrhage. Precise diagnosis of an aneurysm requires a cerebral angiogram. The contrast material will fill the aneurysm if one exists. For a client with a severe headache and facing a life-threatening illness, this test can be very frightening. If the client's neurological status does not allow him or her to cooperate, sedation may be required before and during the examination.

Treatment

Surgical Management

There is no cure for subarachnoid hemorrhage. Treatment consists of correcting the cause of the hemorrhage if possible. Preventing or managing complications and providing supportive care are important aspects of nursing care. Definitive treatment of the aneurysm involves performing a craniotomy and exposing the aneurysm. If the aneurysm has a neck (berry aneurysm), it is identified and clamped with a metal clip (Fig. 46–4). An aneurysm without a neck may be wrapped with very fine sterile muslin. This provides stability to the aneurysm walls, lessening the chance of rupture. In some situations it is possible to clamp the artery on either side of the aneurysm, removing that portion of the vessel, and the aneurysm, from the circulation.

Medical Management

Nonsurgical intervention may be provided for aneurysms that are inoperable due to size, configuration, or the client's medical status. A foreign material such as a tiny metallic coil or fibrin glue may be introduced into the aneurysm. A thrombus develops around the foreign body, and hopefully occludes the aneurysm. The goal is to fill the aneurysm enough to prevent blood flowing into it, without causing rupture.

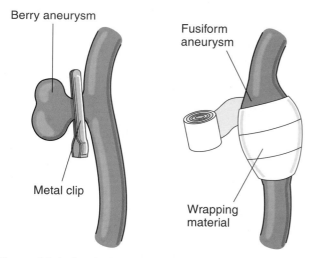

Figure 46–4. Surgical management of aneurysms. (Modified from Lewis, SM, Collier, IC, and Heitkemper, MM: Medical-Surgical Nursing: Assessment and Management of Clinical Problems, ed 4. Mosby, St Louis, p 1732, with permission.)

Clients experiencing a subarachnoid hemorrhage are cared for in an intensive care unit (ICU) setting. They typically have an arterial line and a central venous pressure monitoring catheter. The blood pressure is carefully monitored, because high pressures increase the risk of rerupture of the aneurysm and low pressures may be associated with ischemia. Values outside parameters identified by the physician are reported. Typically the systolic BP is kept between 120 and 160. Vasoactive drugs may be required to maintain BP within the prescribed parameters.

Acute Complications

Rebleeding

Recurrent rupture of cerebral aneurysm carries a significant morbidity and mortality rate. Clients are at risk for rebleeding until the aneurysm is surgically repaired. If the aneurysm is wrapped or embolized, there is a risk of rebleeding, but it is much less than if the aneurysm is left untreated.

Hydrocephalus

Blood within the ventricular system interferes with the circulation, and reabsorption of CSF and hydrocephalus may develop. Early in the course of subarachnoid hemorrhage an external ventricular drain may be used to treat hydrocephalus (discussed in Chapter 45).

Approximately 25 percent of clients with subarachnoid hemorrhage require placement of a ventriculoperitoneal shunt to treat their hydrocephalus (Fig. 46–5). This surgical procedure involves placement of a ventricular catheter (as described in Chapter 45). This catheter is then connected to a valve, which regulates the rate of cerebrospinal fluid drainage. Another catheter connects to the valve and is passed down to the peritoneal cavity. The cerebrospinal fluid drains out of the peritoneal catheter and is absorbed into the peritoneal cavity.

Vasospasm

Vasospasm is responsible for the majority of long-term complications of subarachnoid hemorrhage. Vasospasm is the narrowing of a blood vessel diameter. Although it typically begins in the vessel giving rise to the aneurysm, vasospasm may spread to other vessels. This explains why the ischemia or infarct caused by vasospasm can be so widespread and devastating.

The long-term complications of subarachnoid hemorrhage are similar to those of cerebrovascular accident.

Nursing Process: The Client with a Cerebrovascular Disorder

Assessment

Clients with cerebrovascular disorders require careful serial assessments of their neurological status, as described in

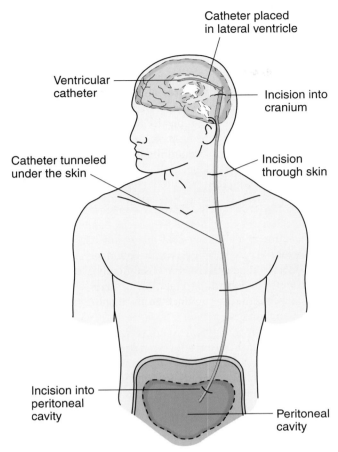

Figure 46–5. A ventriculoperitoneal shunt drains cerebrospinal fluid into the peritoneal cavity. (Modified from Black and Matassarin-Jacobs: Medical-Surgical Nursing: Clinical Management for Continuity of Care, ed 5. WB Saunders, Philadelphia, p 783, with permission.)

Chapter 45. Subtle changes in orientation, level of consciousness, or motor strength may indicate ischemia or increasing intracranial pressure. By detecting and reporting such changes quickly the nurse improves the likelihood of a successful outcome for the client. In addition to assessing for changes in status, the client's ability to use the call light should be determined. Swallowing ability should be assessed before offering food or drink to prevent aspiration. This may involve radiological swallowing studies. The client should not be fed if swallowing ability is in question. Ability to move and need for assistance with turning in bed should be determined. The client and family can also provide information about the client's previous level of functioning.

Nursing Diagnosis

Possible nursing diagnoses during the acute phase of illness include the following:

- Altered tissue perfusion related to increased ICP
- Risk for injury related to seizure or repeat CVA

- Altered nutrition related to impaired swallowing, motor deficits
- Impaired mobility related to neurological deficits
- Impaired communication related to aphasia
- Knowledge deficit related to new diagnosis and treatment
- Risk for caregiver role strain related to new responsibilities

Planning

Goals during the acute phase of the CVA include prevention of complications and recurrent CVA. Discharge planning should be initiated as soon as possible after admission, though it may be difficult to anticipate needs until the extent of the client's deficits are known. Most clients will require some rehabilitation in order to reach an optimal level of function. Consultation with the client, significant others, and the social worker or discharge planner should be ongoing.

Implementation

ALTERED TISSUE PERFUSION. Clients are at risk for increased intracranial pressure following a CVA. The client in intensive care may have an intracranial pressure monitor. Any activities or interventions that increase ICP should be avoided, such as repeated suctioning, coughing, and vigorous turning. See Table 46–5.

RISK FOR INJURY. Precautions should be taken to prevent injury in the event of a seizure (see Table 46–3). If the client has had a seizure, anticonvulsant medications may be ordered. Clients who have had a CVA are also at risk for a repeat CVA. Changes in neurological status should be reported immediately to the physician.

Clients are also at risk for falls because of motor and sensory deficits and impaired judgment. Clients should be assisted with transfers and ambulation. Because many falls occur as clients are attempting to get up to use the bathroom, assisting the client to the bathroom or bedside commode on a routine basis can help. Care should be taken to keep the client's path unobstructed. Family members should be instructed in fall prevention if the client will be going home.

ALTERED NUTRITION. If the client has difficulty swallowing or is unable to self-feed, altered nutrition will be a concern. The physician may order a swallowing study to determine the extent of the problem. A speech-language pathologist assesses the client and makes recommendations for safe swallowing techniques. Measures to prevent aspiration generally include staying with the client during meals, having the client in a chair or high Fowler's position for meals, avoiding straws, using a thickening agent for thin liquids, and having the client swallow twice after each bite. The nurse should check the client's mouth after each bite, because clients may pocket food on the affected side of the mouth. See Nutrition Notes Box 46–2 for additional interventions. Some clients may require a feeding tube. Advance directives should be consulted before a feeding tube is placed.

IMPAIRED MOBILITY. The client with hemiplegia will have difficulty turning or repositioning. If the client has sensory deficits, pain or pressure will not be noticed, and injury may occur. Careful and frequent repositioning by the nurse is essential to prevent skin, respiratory, and musculoskeletal complications. Pillows can be used to maintain the body in good alignment and promote comfort. Skin should be inspected each time the client is repositioned. Range-of-motion exercises should be begun within 24 hours of admission to help prevent contractures. Splints may be used for some clients to maintain a functional position of extremities. Some clients experience injury to the shoulder of an affected arm. Care should be taken to support the arm on pillows when it is in a dependent position. A physical therapist can be consulted to assess the client and make specific recommendations related to mobility.

IMPAIRED COMMUNICATION. Aphasia can cause great frustration to the client, family, and caregivers. Care depends on whether the aphasia is receptive or expressive. If the nurse has determined that the client's responses are valid, asking yes/no questions may be helpful. Gestures and visual aids may be tried. The nurse can contact a speech or occupational therapist to acquire a picture board for the client. This board has pictures on it that the client can point to, such as a glass of water, tissue, toilet, hungry, too hot, and others (Fig. 46–6). Some clients can relearn language skills with the help of a speech therapist. It is important for the nurse to continue to speak to the client, because he or she may understand what is being said but may be unable to respond.

KNOWLEDGE DEFICIT. The client and significant other are likely to be very frightened of what is happening. Correct information about what a CVA is, tests and procedures, and rationale for care activities will help reduce anxiety. Information should be presented in small amounts and as simply as possible. Orientation to the ICU or other setting and the constant monitoring provided helps reassure the client and significant others that he or she is receiving competent care. If the client is unable to communicate, the nurse must not assume that he or she cannot hear and understand. Every effort should be made to speak to the client and to keep conversation appropriate when it is within the client's range of hearing.

RISK FOR CAREGIVER ROLE STRAIN. Cerebrovascular accidents, even those that leave relatively mild residual effects, have a significant impact on psychosocial functioning. Clients and their significant others may experience changes in roles, responsibilities, finances, and intimacy. Significant others should be encouraged to assess how the client's functional level will affect their lives. Encourage them to identify support systems and make use of community resources (Table 46–7). Assumption of roles or responsibilities previously fulfilled by the client may be very stressful to significant others. The nurse and social worker can help them identify priorities and plan ways of adapting to change.

Evaluation

As with all neurological disorders, the goal is to return the client to his or her previous level of functioning. If this is not feasible, success is measured in the client's lack of preventable complications and readiness for rehabilitation.

Rehabilitation

If the client is able to tolerate intensive therapy, discharge from the hospital may be to a rehabilitation center. With rehabilitation, most clients can learn to walk, some with a walker or cane. Speech therapy can help the client learn to communicate. Many clients can learn to take care of themselves. Some may be able to drive again and even have a job.

NUTRITION NOTES BOX 46-2

Nutritional Concerns with Swallowing Disorders

Suggested approaches for persons with difficulty swallowing:

- Eat slowly.
- Avoid distractions while eating.
- Do not talk while eating.
- Sit up straight while eating.
- Use a regular teaspoon, taking only one-half teaspoonful at a time.
- Swallow completely between bites or sips.

Possible nursing interventions to aid a person with a swallowing disorder:

- Serve foods that require minimal chewing.
- Remove loose dentures.
- Position the head correctly. A speech therapist can help determine the optimal head position. A hemiplegic client often benefits from turning the head toward the weak side.
- When spoon-feeding a hemiplegic client, place the food on the unaffected side of the tongue.
- Consult a dietitian concerning appropriate textures. Often thicker substances help the client to better manage liquids. Although baby cereal can be an effective thickener, on a psychological basis it may be rejected by the client in favor of a commercial thickener.

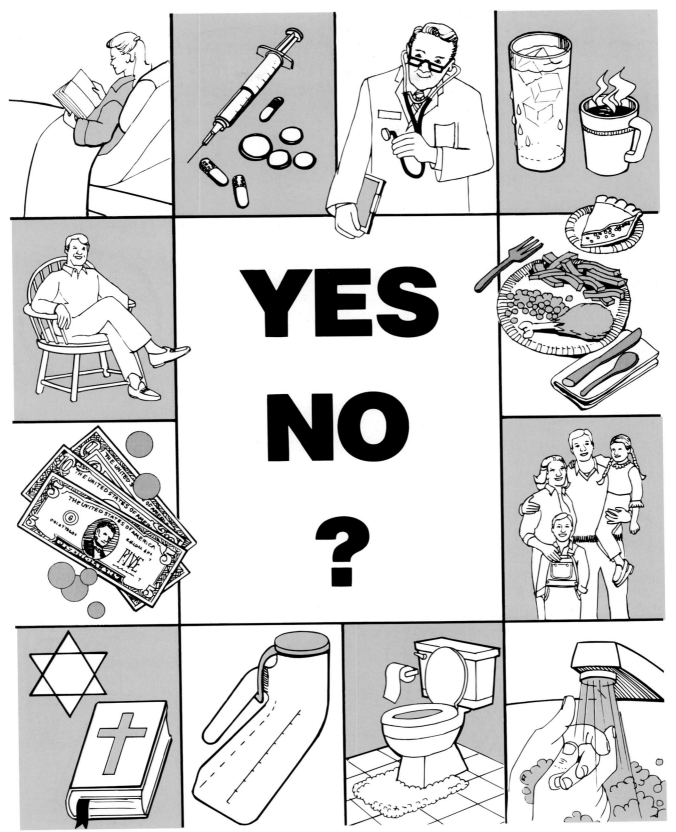

Figure 46–6. Picture board. (From the *Visiboard*™ (© 1987). Stow, Ohio: Interactive Therapeutics, Inc. Reprinted with permission.)

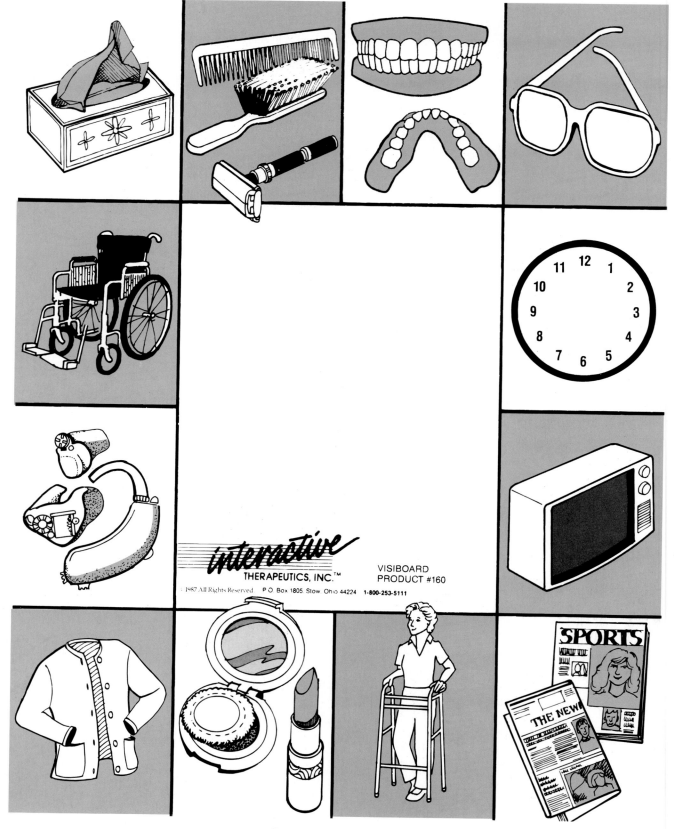

Figure 46–6. *(continued)*

Table 46–7. **Resources for Neurological Disorders**

Parkinson's disease	National Parkinson Foundation, Inc 1501 N.W. 9th Avenue/Bob Hope Road Miami, FL 33136 (800) 327-4545 http://www.parkinson.org
Huntington's disease	Huntington's Disease Society of America (HDSA) 140 W. 22nd Street New York, NY 10011 (212) 242-1968 http://www.kumc.edu/hospital/huntingons/
Alzheimer's disease	Alzheimer's Association (800) 272-3900 http://www.alz.org
Epilepsy	Epilepsy Foundation of America 4351 Garden City Drive Landover, MD 20785 (301) 459-3700 (800) 332-1000 http://neurosurgery.mgh.harvard.edu/ep-resrc.htm#EFA
Traumatic brain injury	National Resource Center for Traumatic Brain Injury P.O. Box 980542 Richmond, VA 23298-0542 (804) 828-9055 http://www.neuro.pmr.vcu.edu/search.htm Brain Injury Association, Inc. 105 N. Alfred Street Alexandria, VA 22314 (703) 236-6000 http://www.biausa.org/
Spinal cord injury	American Paralysis Association http://www.apacure.com/ Spinal Cord Injury Information Network http://www.spinalcord.uab.edu/
Stroke	American Heart Association Stroke Connection (800) 553-6321 (800) AHA-USA1 National Institute of Neurological Disorders and Stroke National Institutes of Health Bethesda, MD 20892 National Stroke Association http://www.stroke.org

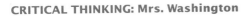

CRITICAL THINKING: Mrs. Washington

Mrs. Washington is a 68-year-old African-American retired office worker. She was admitted to your unit following a right-sided intracerebral hemorrhage. Her daughter states that Mrs. Washington has taken antihypertensive medication for the last 20 years. However, she states that her mother has been "forgetful" lately and there are five more pills in the medicine bottle than expected. On admission Mrs. Washington is oriented only to person and has hemiparesis.

1. What may have precipitated Mrs. Washington's CVA?
2. On which side are Mrs. Washington's extremities affected?
3. List two safety concerns and strategies to promote client safety.
4. List at least two educational needs for Mrs. Washington and her daughter.

Answers at end of chapter.

Seizure Disorders

Epilepsy is a chronic neurological disorder characterized by recurrent seizure activity. A seizure is defined as an abnormal electrical discharge within the neuronal structure of the brain. A seizure may be a symptom of epilepsy or of other neurological disorders such as a brain tumor or brain attack.

PATHOPHYSIOLOGY

The normal stability of the neuron cell membrane is impaired in individuals with epilepsy. This instability allows for abnormal electrical discharges to occur. These discharges cause the characteristic symptoms seen during a seizure.

Seizures can be classified as partial or generalized. Partial seizures begin on one side of the cerebral cortex. In some cases the electrical discharge spreads to the other hemisphere and the seizure becomes generalized. Generalized seizures are characterized by involvement of both cerebral hemispheres.

ETIOLOGY

Epilepsy may be acquired or idiopathic. Causes of acquired epilepsy include traumatic brain injury and anoxic events. No cause has been identified for idiopathic epilepsy. The most common time for idiopathic epilepsy to begin is before the age of 20. New-onset seizures after this age are most commonly due to an underlying neurological disorder.

SIGNS AND SYMPTOMS

Symptoms of seizure activity correlate with the area of the brain where the seizure begins. Some clients experience an aura or sensation that warns the client that a seizure is about to occur. An aura may be a visual distortion, a noxious odor, or an unusual sound. Clients who experience an aura may have enough time to sit or lie down before the seizure starts, thereby minimizing the chance of injury.

Partial Seizures

Repetitive, purposeless behaviors, called automatisms, are the classic symptom of this type of seizures. The client appears to be in a dreamlike state while picking at his or her clothing, chewing, or smacking his or her lips. Clients may be labeled as mentally ill, particularly if automatisms include unacceptable social behaviors such as spitting or fondling themselves. Clients are not aware of their behavior or that it is inappropriate. If the client does not lose consciousness, the seizure is labeled as simple partial, and usually lasts less than 1 minute. Older terms for simple partial seizures include jacksonian and focal motor. If consciousness is lost, it is called a complex partial seizure or psychomotor seizure. It may last from 2 to 15 minutes.

Partial seizures arising from the parietal lobe may cause paresthesias on the side of the body opposite the seizure focus. Visual disturbances are seen if the occipital lobe is the originating site. Involvement of the motor cortex results in involuntary movements of the opposite side of the body. Typically movements begin in the arm and hand and may spread to the leg and face.

Generalized Seizures

Generalized seizures affect the entire brain. Two types of generalized seizures are absence seizures and tonic-clonic seizures. Absence seizures, sometimes referred to as petit mal seizures, occur most often in children and are manifested by a period of staring that lasts several seconds.

Tonic-clonic seizures are what most laypeople envision when they think of seizures. They are sometimes called grand mal seizures or convulsions. Tonic-clonic seizures follow a typical progression. Aura and loss of consciousness may or may not occur. The tonic phase, lasting 30 to 60 seconds, is characterized by rigidity, causing the client to fall if not lying down. The pupils are fixed and dilated, the hands and jaws are clenched, and the client may temporarily stop breathing. The clonic phase is signaled by contraction and relaxation of all muscles in a jerky, rhythmic fashion. The extremities may move forcefully, causing injury if the client strikes furniture or walls. The client is often incontinent. Biting the lips or tongue may cause bleeding. An oral airway can be used to prevent self-injury if the client's mouth is open. *Never* attempt to force an airway, or anything else, into the client's mouth if the jaws are clenched.

Postictal refers to the recovery period after a seizure. Following a partial seizure the postictal phase may be no more than a few minutes of disorientation. Clients who experience a generalized seizure may sleep deeply for 30 minutes to several hours. Following this deep sleep, clients may complain of headache, confusion, and fatigue. Clients may realize that they had a seizure but not remember the event itself.

DIAGNOSTIC TESTS

An EEG is the most useful test for evaluating seizures. An EEG can determine where in the brain the seizures start, the frequency and duration of seizures, and the presence of subclinical (asymptomatic) seizures. Sleep deprivation and flashing light stimulation may be used to evaluate the seizure threshold. See Chapter 45 for more information on EEG.

TREATMENT

If an underlying cause for the seizure is identified, treatment focuses on correcting the cause. If no cause is found or if the seizures continue despite treatment of concurrent disorders, treatment focuses on the seizure activity.

Medical Management

Numerous anticonvulsant medications are available, each with specific actions, therapeutic ranges, and potential side

---

postictal: post—after + ictal—seizure

effects (Table 46–8). Typically the client is started on one drug and the dosage is increased until therapeutic levels are attained or side effects become troublesome. If seizures are not controlled on a single drug, another medication is added. Anticonvulsant therapy requires periodic blood tests to monitor serum levels and kidney and liver function. If seizures continue despite anticonvulsant therapy, surgical intervention may be considered.

Surgical Management

The success of surgical intervention for epilepsy depends on identification of an epileptic focus within nonvital brain tissue. If no focus is identified or if it is in a vital area such as the motor cortex or speech center, surgery is not feasible. The surgeon attempts to resect the area affected to prevent spread of seizure activity. In some cases, seizures may be cured, but in others the goal is to reduce the frequency or severity of the seizures.

The preoperative assessment for epilepsy surgery is an extensive multistage process. Thorough assessment and teaching are essential. In order to adequately identify seizure foci the client is weaned off of anticonvulsant therapy. Increasing the frequency of seizures is anxiety provoking to clients and significant others.

Emergency Care

The prime objective in caring for a client experiencing a seizure is to prevent injury. Side rails should be padded to prevent injury if the client strikes his or her extremities against them. If the client falls to the floor, move furniture out of the way. A pillow should be placed under the client's head to prevent striking it on the floor. If possible, turn the client on his or her side to prevent aspiration if vomiting occurs. An oral airway and suction should be readily available. The individual should not be restrained, because this may increase the risk of injury. Observe and document eye deviation, incontinence, which part of the body was first involved, and progression of the seizure.

Status Epilepticus

Status epilepticus is characterized by at least 30 minutes of repetitive seizure activity without a return to consciousness. This is a medical emergency and requires prompt intervention to prevent irreversible neurological damage. Abrupt cessation of anticonvulsant therapy is the usual cause of status epilepticus.

Seizure activity precipitates a significant increase in the brain's need for glucose and oxygen. This metabolic demand is even greater during status epilepticus. Irreversible neuronal damage may occur if cerebral metabolic needs cannot be fulfilled. Adequate oxygenation must be maintained, if necessary by intubating and mechanically ventilating the client. These clients are also at significant risk for aspiration.

Intravenous diazepam (Valium) or lorazepam (Ativan) are given to stop the seizures. Because both of these drugs may cause respiratory depression, careful airway management is required. After obtaining serum drug levels, anticonvulsant therapy is adjusted to achieve therapeutic levels.

If seizures remain resistant to treatment, a barbiturate coma may be induced with intravenous pentobarbital. The last line of treatment for status epilepticus is general anesthesia or pharmacological paralysis. Both of these therapies require intubation, mechanical ventilation, and management in an ICU setting. Continuous EEG monitoring is used to verify that the seizures have actually stopped. A client treated with neuromuscular blockade drugs may still be seizing but have no visible manifestations.

NURSING MANAGEMENT

Assessment

The nurse does a general neurological assessment of the client with a history of seizures. Type of seizure manifestations and occurrence of an aura are determined. The client's knowledge of the disease and its treatment are assessed. It is important to assess whether the client has the resources to purchase prescribed anticonvulsant medica-

Table 46–8. **Anticonvulsant Medications**

Medication	Action	Side Effects/Comments
Phenytoin (Dilantin)	Limits seizure propagation; may also be used for some cardiac dysrhythmias and some types of nerve pain	May cause gingival hyperplasia, nausea, ataxia, rash; regular dental care essential; therapeutic level is 10–20 µg/mL
Phenobarbital (Luminal)	CNS depressant; raises seizure threshold	Causes drowsiness; often given with phenytoin
Carbamazepine (Tegretol)	Decreases synaptic transmission in CNS; may be used for some types of neuralgias	Common side effects: drowsiness and ataxia; used if other drugs ineffective; therapeutic level 6–12 µg/mL
Valproic acid (Depakote)	Increases GABA, an inhibitory neurotransmitter in CNS	Causes GI upset, nausea, vomiting; therapeutic level 50–100 µg/mL
Clonazepam (Klonapin)	CNS sedative; may also be used for neuralgia or restless leg syndrome	Side effects: drowsiness, ataxia, changes in behavior; therapeutic level 20–80 ng/ml

tions and whether the medication regimen is adhered to. Drug levels may help determine degree of compliance with therapy.

Nursing Diagnosis

Priority nursing diagnoses for the client at risk for seizures include the following:

- Risk for injury related to seizure activity
- Risk for ineffective management of therapeutic regimen related to complex regimen and possible lack of resources
- Anxiety related to risk for seizures
- Altered role performance related to possible disabling disorder

Planning

The goal is for the client and significant others to be able to manage the treatment effectively in order to prevent seizures. If seizures occur, the goal is to prevent injury.

Implementation

Risk for Injury

The client is instructed to recognize his or her aura and to get to safety if it occurs. This may mean lying down away from furniture or other objects that may cause harm. For the client admitted to a health care institution, seizure precautions are instituted. If a seizure does occur, the client's safety is maintained. See Table 46–3 for precautions and interventions for seizures. All clients are encouraged to wear Medic Alert or other identification to alert others to the presence of seizure disorder.

Some clients can identify conditions that trigger seizures. Hypoglycemia, hypoxia, and hyponatremia are all potential triggers of hypersensitive neurons. The nurse teaches the client the importance of a consistent schedule of eating and sleeping.

Risk for Ineffective Management of Therapeutic Regimen

Clients with seizures may have several medications to take, several times each day. This makes compliance difficult at best. Medication teaching is vital. Clients need to understand dosing, potential side effects, possible interactions with alcohol and other medications, and the importance of regular blood tests. If finances are a concern, the client may be unable to obtain prescriptions. Clients must understand the risk for seizures and status epilepticus if medications are stopped abruptly. The nurse or social worker can help the client apply for assistance to pay for medications if necessary. See Ethical Considerations Box 46–3.

ETHICAL CONSIDERATIONS BOX 46-3

Public Safety vs. Confidentiality

Susan, a 31-year-old mother of two, is brought into the emergency department (ED) following a tonic-clonic type of seizure at a shopping mall. Susan is known to the emergency department nurses because she has been treated several times for seizures due to her failure to take her antiseizure medications. She says the medications make her feel "dopey" and tired all the time and she hates the way she feels.

Recently, Susan has started driving one of her children and four other children to school in the neighborhood car pool 1 day a week. She also drives 62 miles one way on the interstate twice a week to visit her aging mother in a nursing home in a different city. The nurse caring for Susan this way in the ED knows that the state licensing laws require that an individual with uncontrolled seizures must report the fact to the department of motor vehicles and is usually ineligible for a driver's license. When the nurse mentions that she is going to have to report the seizure, Susan begs her not to report it. She would have no way of getting her children to school or visiting her mother. She assures the nurse that she will take her medication no matter how it makes her feel. The nurse debates whether the public's right to safety always outweighs the client's right to confidentiality. What if Susan does take her medication and has no more seizures? What decision should the nurse make?

Anxiety

Epilepsy is a chronic disorder with significant impact on lifestyle. Clients may be ashamed to acknowledge their condition and may try to hide it from others. Providing the client with current, accurate information and helping him or her identify coping strategies can maximize independence. Support groups may also be helpful.

Altered Role Performance

Finances can be a major concern to these clients. Some clients with epilepsy experience hiring discrimination, or they may not qualify for some jobs in which safety is a concern. Remind clients that falsifying information on job applications may be grounds for dismissal. Refusal of health insurance coverage can create financial hardships for clients on long-term medications. Most clients whose seizures are controlled can work and lead productive lives. The nurse can help clients explore options for financial assistance if necessary.

Clients with poorly controlled seizures should not operate motor vehicles. In our society a driver's license is a sign of adulthood and independence, and clients who cannot drive may experience lowered self-esteem. Job opportunities may be limited for clients who depend on public transportation. Encourage the client to obtain a state identification card. This can be used in place of a driver's license for identification.

Clients may limit interpersonal relationships out of fear of having a seizure. The involuntary movements, sounds, and possible incontinence that occur with seizures are embarrassing to clients and can be frightening to laypeople. Role playing may help the client determine when and how to confide in others.

Evaluation

Successful care of a client with epilepsy is manifested by a decrease in seizures to the lowest possible frequency. Client verbalization of understanding of needed lifestyle changes is another indication of success. Clients should be able to state measures to prevent injury if a seizure should occur and should verbalize understanding of all medications and their administration schedules. Therapeutic drug levels may be measured to evaluate compliance with the medication regimen.

Traumatic Brain Injury

Traumatic brain injury (TBI) is a major cause of death and disability in adults. Young males make up a large proportion of brain injury victims. The use of alcohol and illicit drugs is frequently associated with brain injury.

PATHOPHYSIOLOGY

Traumatic brain injury is a complex phenomenon with results ranging from no detectable effect to **persistent vegetative state** (see Ethical Considerations Box 46–4). Trauma can result in hemorrhage, contusion or laceration of the brain, and damage at the cellular level. In addition to the primary insult, the brain injury may be compounded by cerebral edema, hyperemia, or hydrocephalus.

ETIOLOGY

Motor vehicle accidents account for the largest percentage of traumatic brain injuries. Violent assaults are increasing in frequency and may be accompanied by penetrating brain injuries. Falls and sports-related injuries are also common causes of TBI.

The brain is susceptible to several types of injury. *Acceleration injury* is the term used to describe a moving object hitting a stationary head. An example of this type of injury is a client who is hit in the head with a baseball bat. A *deceleration injury* refers to the head being in motion and

striking a stationary surface. This type of injury is seen in clients who trip and fall, hitting their head on furniture or the floor.

A combination of *acceleration-deceleration injury* occurs when the stationary head is hit by a mobile object and the head then strikes a stationary surface. A soccer player who sustains a blow to the head and then hits the ground with his or her head may sustain an acceleration-deceleration injury.

Rotational injuries have the potential to cause shearing damage to the brain, as well as laceration and contusions. Rotational injuries may be caused by a direct blow to the head or during a motor vehicle accident in which the vehicle is struck from the side. Twisting of the brain stem can damage the reticular activating system, causing loss of consciousness. Movement of the brain within the skull may result in bruising or tearing of brain tissue where it comes in contact with the inside of the skull.

TYPES OF BRAIN INJURY AND SIGNS AND SYMPTOMS

Concussion

Cerebral concussion is considered a mild brain injury. If there is a loss of consciousness it is for 5 minutes or less. Concussion is characterized by headache, dizziness, or nausea and vomiting. The client may complain of amnesia of events before or after the trauma. On clinical examination there is no skull or dura injury and no abnormality detected on CT or MRI.

Contusion

Cerebral contusion is characterized by bruising of brain tissue, possibly accompanied by hemorrhage. There may be multiple areas of contusion, depending on the causative mechanism. Severe contusions can result in diffuse axonal injury. The symptoms of a cerebral contusion depend on the area of the brain involved.

Brain stem contusions affect level of consciousness. The decreased level of consciousness may be transient or permanent. Respirations, pupil reaction, eye movement, and motor response to stimuli may also be affected. The autonomic nervous system may be affected by edema or by hypothalamic injury, causing rapid heart rate and respiratory rate, fever, and diaphoresis.

Hematoma

Subdural hematomas are classified as acute or chronic based on the time interval between injury and onset of symptoms. Acute subdural hematoma is characterized by appearance of symptoms within 24 hours following injury. The bleeding is typically venous in nature and accumulates between the dura and arachnoid membranes (Fig. 46–7).

---

subdural: sub—below + dura—dura mater

ETHICAL CONSIDERATIONS BOX 46-4

Persistent Vegetative State

Persistent vegetative state (PVS) describes a condition in which a client is awake but shows no awareness of self or environment and has no voluntary movements, emotional responses, or cognitive ability. Unlike brain death, clients in PVS do have reflex responses, brain stem activity, eye movements, and cycles of sleep and wakefulness. Medical science is not sure what causes PVS, has no specific tests or criteria to diagnose it, and finds similar symptoms in conditions such as coma, dementia, and unconsciousness.

Clients who have PVS have about a 50-50 chance of regaining some degree of normal functioning and may live, with artificial hydration and nutrition, for over 5 years in this state. The age ranges of the 5000 to 10,000 PVS clients in the United States is from very young to very old. Many are institutionalized in long-term care facilities, but an increasing number are cared for at home by family members with the assistance of home health care nurses. The cost of maintaining one of these clients for 1 year is estimated at almost $100,000.

Some medical experts have suggested that the definition of brain death be expanded to include clients who have PVS. They argue that loss of the higher brain functions, especially of the cerebral cortex as is seen in PVS, should serve as the legal definition of death. By expanding this definition of brain death, clients in PVS could be allowed to die by the withdrawal of IV fluids and tube feedings, thereby saving the health care system almost 1 billion dollars per year. In today's health care system, even without this expanded definition of death, many clients with PVS are allowed to die through dehydration, starvation, or both. The cases of Nancy Cruzan and Christine Busalacchi demonstrate the court's willingness to withdraw artificial nutrition and hydration if the likelihood of recovery is nonexistent.

Yet many ethical questions persist. Nurses, as the health care providers most immediately involved with the care of PVS clients, and directly responsible for the withholding of fluids and feedings, are placed in a particularly sensitive ethical position. If PVS clients are indeed alive, nurses have a strong ethical obligation to provide the same type of care as they would for any other client. The ethical obligations become even more complicated if PVS clients are considered to be dead.

Strictly speaking, clients who are dead have no rights, therefore there are basically no obligations on the part of the health care provider. Yet, PVS clients do breathe, do have a heartbeat, and can absorb nutrients and fluids. In addition, these clients may have expressed some wishes or desires about treatment to be given or not given if they were ever to become unable to make decisions about their care. These wishes may be expressed in the formal manner of a living will, but they may also take the form of a designated decision maker (durable power of attorney) or an informal declaration to a relative. Often living wills do not cover situations such as PVS and may not be an accurate indication of the client's wish to die, particularly if there is a chance the client may recover.

The ethical principle of beneficence (doing good for the client) must take over in situations where the expressed wishes of the client are not clearly known. In these situations, nurses have the ethical and legal duty to care for clients and assume that their desire is to obtain the treatments necessary to live. Nurses are obligated to care for these clients until ordered to stop either by the clients themselves or by a person authorized to speak for them. The most serious ethical dilemma arises when the person ordering the care stopped does not have the legal authority to make that decision.

Nurses have a general prohibition against participating in executions. The key issue is whether withholding liquids and nutrition from clients is a form of execution. The nursing code of ethics is rooted in the belief of respect for persons, the noninfliction of harm, and faithfulness to the clients being cared for. Yet nurses are not required to prolong life (or death) at all costs, particularly in the case of obviously terminal clients. An ethical dilemma arises for many nurses because PVS clients are not necessarily terminal and because fluids and nutrition are not really death-prolonging treatments.

Like many ethical issues, the care and destiny of PVS clients has no perfect solution. Although the courts have attempted to deal with this dilemma, the decisions made have been inconsistent. Some states have enacted "conscience clauses" in their nurse practice acts that would allow nurses to refuse to participate in procedures that would lead to the death of PVS clients. Although conscience clauses demonstrate legislative concern for nursing's ethics and morals, they may open the door to lawsuits against nurses for participating in death-causing procedures because nurses can no longer claim that they had no choice. In any case, nurses need to carefully consider how and when they participate in withholding care to nondying patients.

Approximately 24 percent of clients who sustain a severe brain injury develop an acute subdural hematoma. Damage to the brain tissue itself may cause an altered level of consciousness. Therefore it can be difficult to recognize a subdural hematoma based only on clinical examination. As the subdural hematoma increases in size, the client may exhibit one-sided paralysis of extraocular movement, extremity weakness, or dilation of the pupil. Level of consciousness may deteriorate further as ICP increases.

Elderly and alcoholic individuals are particularly prone to chronic subdural hematomas. Atrophy of the brain, common in these populations, stretches the veins between the brain and the dura. A seemingly minor fall or blow to the head can cause these stretched veins to rupture and bleed.

A

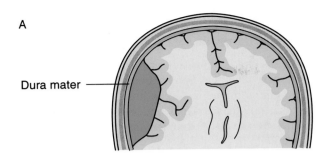

Dura mater —

B

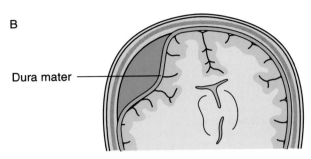

Dura mater —

Figure 46–7. *(A)* A subdural hematoma is usually venous and forms between the dura and the arachnoid membranes. *(B)* An epidural hematoma is usually from an arterial bleed and forms between the dura mater and the skull.

Often there are no other injuries associated with the trauma. Because a chronic subdural hematoma can develop weeks to months after the injury, the client may not remember an injury occurring.

The client with a chronic subdural hematoma may be forgetful, lethargic, or irritable or may complain of a headache. If the hematoma persists or increases in size, the client may develop hemiparesis and pupillary changes. The client or significant other may not associate the symptoms with a previous injury and therefore may delay seeking medical care.

Approximately 10 percent of clients with severe brain injuries develop **epidural** hematomas. This collection of blood between the dura mater and skull is usually arterial in nature and is often associated with skull fracture (see Fig. 46–7). Arterial bleeding can cause the hematoma to become large very quickly. Clients with epidural hematoma typically exhibit a progressive course of symptoms. The client loses consciousness directly after the injury; he or she then regains consciousness and is coherent for a brief period. The client then develops a dilated pupil and paralyzed extraocular muscles on the side of the hematoma and becomes less responsive. If there is no intervention, the client becomes unresponsive. Seizures or hemiparesis may occur. Once the client exhibits symptoms the deterioration may be very rapid. Airway management and control

---

epidural: epi—above + dural—pertaining to the dura

of ICP needs to be instituted immediately. If ICP is not controlled the client will die.

DIAGNOSTIC TESTS

CT scan is usually the first imaging test performed on the brain-injured client. It is faster and more accessible than MRI. This is particularly important for unstable clients or those with multiple injuries. It is easier to identify skull fractures on CT than on MRI. MRI may be used later to identify damage to the brain tissue.

Neuropsychological testing can be useful in assessing the client's cognitive function. This information helps direct rehabilitation placement, discharge planning, and return to work or school. Neuropsychological testing identifies problems with memory, judgment, learning, and comprehension. Compensation strategies can be suggested to the client and significant others based on the results.

TREATMENT

Surgical Management

Surgical treatment of hematomas is discussed under intracranial surgery later in this chapter.

Medical Management

Medical management of TBI involves control of intracranial pressure and support of body functions. Brain-injured clients may be partially or completely dependent for maintenance of respiration, nutrition, elimination, movement, and skin integrity.

A variety of techniques are used to control intracranial pressure in the client with moderate or severe brain injury. The first step is to insert an intracranial pressure monitor to allow determination of the intracranial pressure. Refer to Chapter 45 for further information.

If intracranial pressure remains elevated despite drainage of cerebrospinal fluid, the next step is use of an osmotic diuretic. The most commonly used drug is intravenous mannitol (Osmitrol). Mannitol utilizes osmosis to pull fluid into the intravascular space and eliminate it via the renal system. Serum osmolarity and electrolytes must be carefully monitored when mannitol is being administered. Some clients experience a rebound increase in intracranial pressure after the mannitol wears off.

Mechanical hyperventilation is the next step if the client is still experiencing increased intracranial pressure. Hyperventilation is effective in lowering intracranial pressure because it causes vasoconstriction. This allows less blood into the cranium, thereby lowering intracranial pressure. Research has demonstrated, however, that aggressive hyperventilation, particularly within the first 24 hours after injury, may induce ischemia in the already compromised brain. Therefore hyperventilation is now reserved for increased intracranial pressure that does not respond to other treatments.

High-dose barbiturate therapy may be used to induce a therapeutic coma, which reduces the metabolic needs of the brain during the acute phase following injury. These clients are completely dependent for all their needs and care. They will be mechanically ventilated and cared for in an ICU setting. Vasopressors may be required to maintain blood pressure, and the client's temperature should be kept as normal as possible.

If none of these interventions is successful, the client may experience uncontrolled edema or herniation of brain tissue (Fig. 46–8). Herniation is displacement of brain tissue out of its normal anatomical location. This displacement prevents function of the herniated tissue and places pressure on other vital structures, most commonly the brain stem. Herniation usually results in brain death.

Clients who experience brain death may be suitable candidates for organ donation. For some significant others the opportunity to donate their loved one's organs provides some sense of purpose in the death.

ACUTE COMPLICATIONS OF TBI

Diabetes Insipidus

Edema or direct injury affects the posterior portion of the pituitary gland or hypothalamus. Inadequate release of antidiuretic hormone results in polyuria and, if the client is awake, polydipsia. Fluid replacement and intravenous vasopressin are used to maintain fluid and electrolyte balance.

Acute Hydrocephalus

Cerebral edema can interfere with cerebrospinal fluid circulation, causing hydrocephalus. Initial treatment is with an external ventricular drain, followed by a ventriculoperitoneal shunt if necessary.

Labile Vital Signs

Direct trauma to or pressure on the brain stem can cause fluctuations in blood pressure, cardiac rhythm, or respiratory pattern. Treatment is aimed at control of intracranial pressure.

LONG-TERM COMPLICATIONS

Posttraumatic Syndrome

Clients who sustain a concussion may experience ongoing, somewhat vague symptoms. These individuals complain of headache, fatigue, difficulty concentrating, depression, or memory impairment. Symptoms may be severe enough to interfere with work, school, and interpersonal relationships. Neuropsychological testing may provide objective evidence of cognitive dysfunction and establish the need for cognitive rehabilitation. Symptoms may take 3 to 12 months to resolve.

Cognitive and Personality Changes

Alterations in personality and cognition may be the most difficult long-term complication for clients and significant others to adjust to. The client may have significant short-term memory impairment. This limits his or her ability to learn new information and may interfere with ability to function at work or school. Impaired judgment can make the client a safety risk to self or others. It also affects social functioning.

Emotional lability, loss of social inhibitions, and personality changes may occur. These consequences of traumatic brain injury have a profound effect on the client and significant others. Spouses may state, "This is not the person I married." If behavior is violent, bizarre, or profane, children may be unwilling to bring their friends home and may become socially isolated. Young children, in particular, have difficulty understanding why the parent is behaving so differently. Disintegration of relationships is not uncommon following traumatic brain injury.

A

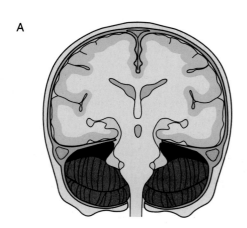

B

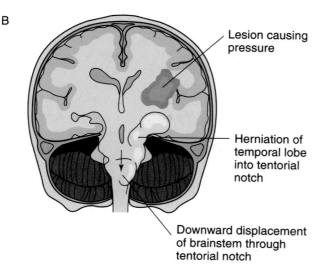

Lesion causing pressure

Herniation of temporal lobe into tentorial notch

Downward displacement of brainstem through tentorial notch

Figure 46–8. Herniation of the brain. *(A)* Normal brain. *(B)* Herniation of brain tissue into tentorial notch.

Neuropsychological testing objectively identifies problems. These deficits can then be addressed with cognitive rehabilitation. Individual and family counseling may be of benefit. Support groups for clients and significant others are often very helpful (see Table 46–7).

Motor and speech impairment are additional possible long-term complications of traumatic brain injury. Intensive rehabilitation provides the best opportunity for maximizing recovery.

NURSING PROCESS: THE CLIENT WITH TRAUMATIC BRAIN INJURY

Assessment

After stabilization in the emergency department, care of the client with TBI will be in the intensive care setting, where ICP can be carefully monitored. Neurological status is assessed frequently, including Glasgow Coma Scale, pupil responses, muscle strength, and vital signs. See Table 46–4 for signs of increased ICP. Once the client is stabilized, neurological damage is assessed. Identification of deficits guides nursing care. Assessment of discharge needs should also begin as soon as possible. The client may require extensive rehabilitation, and early referral may speed transfer to an appropriate facility.

Nursing Diagnosis

The client with TBI may have many nursing problems. Common diagnoses include the following:

- Altered tissue perfusion related to increased intracranial pressure
- Ineffective breathing pattern related to pressure on respiratory center
- Impaired airway clearance related to reduced cough reflex, decreased level of consciousness (LOC)
- Pain related to tissue damage
- Impaired physical mobility related to decreased LOC
- Self-care deficit related to decreased LOC
- Sensory-perceptual alterations related to cranial nerve damage
- Risk for injury related to decreased LOC, risk for seizures
- Altered thought processes related to decreased LOC, brain damage
- Altered role function related to long-term effects of injury

Planning

The goals of care are to prevent further injury or complications while the client stabilizes and then to provide rehabilitation in order to maximize functioning. Assessment and rapid reporting of changes is an important intervention in maximizing recovery potential.

Implementation

Altered Cerebral Tissue Perfusion

If assessment reveals signs of increased ICP, the physician is notified. See Table 46–5 for interventions to prevent increased ICP.

Ineffective Breathing Pattern

Respiratory rate and depth are closely monitored. Arterial blood gases help determine effectiveness of respiration. Mechanical ventilation may be necessary.

Ineffective Airway Clearance

Monitor airway and breath sounds. If the client is unable to cough effectively, suctioning may be necessary. Suction passes should be limited to one or two at a time, to prevent increased ICP.

Pain

The only sign of pain in the unconscious client may be restlessness or a change in vital signs. Opioids are avoided because they further depress LOC and may mask changes in neurological status. Codeine may be ordered, because it has less effect on LOC and pupils.

Impaired Physical Mobility

Mobility is maintained with range-of-motion exercises at least three times a day and position changes every 1 to 2 hours (if ICP is not elevated). Skin is monitored closely for breakdown. The client is positioned in functional body alignment to prevent contractures that can interfere with function after recovery. Physical and occupational therapy can be instituted once the client is stable.

Self-Care Deficit

Initially, the client may be totally dependent for routine care. Activities should be spaced to allow for rest, because clustered activities may increase ICP. Bowel and bladder function must be monitored. A bowel program may be necessary to maintain regular bowel movements. An indwelling catheter may be used immediately following the injury to monitor fluid balance. Catheters are avoided long term, however, because of risk of infection.

Sensory-Perceptual Alterations

The client may not have a normal corneal reflex and may not be able to protect his or her eyes. Lubricating eyedrops and taping the eyes shut help protect the eyes. See Chapters 48 and 49 for interventions for specific sensory problems.

Risk for Injury

If the client is at risk for injury, routine safety precautions are instituted. Seizure precautions are instituted (see Table 46–3).

Altered Thought Processes

Confusion increases risk for injury. The confused client is reoriented as needed. A calendar, clock, family photos, and other familiar items in the client's room may help promote orientation. The nurse may wish to ask a family member or significant other to stay with the client to prevent the need for restraints to maintain safety.

Altered Role Function

The effects of a head injury can have a profound impact on the client and family. The nurse provides emotional support. The entire health team is needed to coordinate discharge to a safe environment. A social work consult can help assess specific needs and identify resources for physical care and financial assistance if necessary.

Evaluation

The plan of care has been successful if the client shows no unexpected worsening of neurological function and injuries and complications are prevented. The airway is clear. The client is kept comfortable, and self-care needs are met.

Rehabilitation

Once the client is stabilized, evaluation for discharge to a rehabilitation facility is done. The client must be able to physically tolerate the rehabilitation program. He or she will be taught to function as independently as possible. The family must be prepared for changes in the client's ability to function and possible changes in personality. It may take months to years before the client reaches his or her maximum potential. In some cases of severe brain damage or continued comatose state, rehabilitation is not feasible, and the client will be discharged to home or a long-term facility for custodial care.

Brain Tumors

Brain tumors are neoplastic growths of the brain or meninges. They may be characterized by vague symptoms such as headache or visual changes or by focal neurological deficits such as hemiparesis or seizures.

PATHOPHYSIOLOGY AND ETIOLOGY

Brain tumors cause symptoms by either compressing or infiltrating brain tissue. Tumors may arise from central nervous system cells or may metastasize from other locations in the body. Primary brain tumors rarely metastasize. If they do metastasize, it is to the spine.

There is no established cause for primary brain tumors. It is unclear what causes the cells to begin reproducing in an uncontrolled fashion. Brain tumors can be classified in several different ways. The traditional distinction of be-

nign and malignant is less applicable when discussing brain tumors. A benign tumor in the brain stem may be fatal while a malignant tumor in the frontal lobe may not be fatal. Location of the tumor can be just as important a factor in outcome as the cell type.

Primary tumors are those arising from cells of the central nervous system. From 80 to 90 percent of brain tumors are primary in nature. Secondary tumors are those that metastasize from primary malignancies elsewhere in the body (Fig. 46–9). Intra-axial tumors refer to those tumors that arise from the glial cells within the cerebrum, cerebellum, or brain stem. These tumors infiltrate and invade brain tissue itself. Extra-axial tumors arise from the skull, meninges, pituitary gland, or cranial nerves. These tumors have a compressive effect on the brain.

Approximately 10 to 20 percent of all brain tumors are metastatic from a primary malignancy elsewhere in the body. These tumors commonly spread via the arterial system. If untreated, these tumors cause increased intracranial pressure. This may be the cause of the client's death, rather than the primary malignancy.

SIGNS AND SYMPTOMS

The symptoms of a brain tumor are directly related to the location of the tumor within the brain and to the rate of growth. Slow-growing types of tumors such as meningiomas (a tumor arising from the meninges, Fig. 46–10) can get to be quite large before becoming symptomatic. Conversely, glioblastoma multiforme or metastatic tumors may abruptly cause seizures or hemiparesis. Other types of tumors include oligodendroglioma, astrocytoma, and acoustic neuroma. The suffix -oma refers to tumor. The prefix denotes the type of cell the tumor arose from.

Symptoms can include seizures, motor and sensory deficits, headaches, and visual disturbances. If the pituitary gland is involved, additional symptoms such as abnormal growth or fluid volume changes are related to changes in hormone secretion.

LEARNING TIP

The phrase "P.T. Barnum loves kids" can be used to help remember the locations of tumors that most commonly metastasize to the brain:

P	Prostate
T	Thyroid
Barnum	Breast
Loves	Liver
Kids	Kidney

DIAGNOSTIC TESTS

MRI gives the clearest images of a brain tumor. Many health care providers order a CT scan first because it is

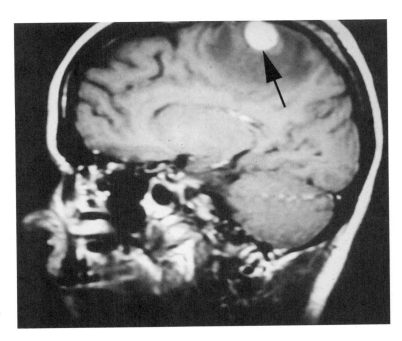

Figure 46–9. Metastatic brain tumor. This client's primary cancer was in the lung.

cheaper. If the tumor appears to be very vascular or in close proximity to major blood vessels, an angiogram may be performed. It is now possible to do magnetic resonance angiograms. This involves the intravenous administration of contrast material and is much less invasive than a traditional angiogram. If the tumor is in the region of the pituitary gland, serum hormone levels are evaluated.

TREATMENT

Surgical treatment involves removal of the tumor or as much of the tumor as possible. Care of the client undergoing intracranial surgery is discussed later in this chapter.

Medical Management

Medical treatment consists of controlling symptoms and administering additional therapies. Clients who have a seizure will be placed on anticonvulsants. If significant cerebral edema is noted on the CT or MRI, or if the client is suffering from headaches, dexamethasone (Decadron) may be prescribed to lessen the edema. Typically, these clients do not require narcotics for pain relief.

Radiation Therapy

External beam radiation therapy is standard treatment for many brain tumor clients. The therapy is typically given 5 days a week for 6 weeks. Some clinicians use a hyperfractionated schedule, in which the client has therapy twice a day for less time. Brachytherapy is a means of delivering radiation therapy directly to the tumor. Small catheters are implanted in the tumor and then tiny radioactive particles are inserted into the catheters. The treatment typically takes 3 to 5 days. During this time the client is confined to a private room, and interaction with visitors and staff is kept to a minimum due to radioactivity. This therapy is not appropriate for confused individuals because they may not be able to cooperate with restrictions.

Stereotactic radiosurgery is a technique that utilizes small amounts of radiation directed at the tumor from different angles. A metal frame is affixed to the client's skull, and the tumor is visualized within the framework on a CT

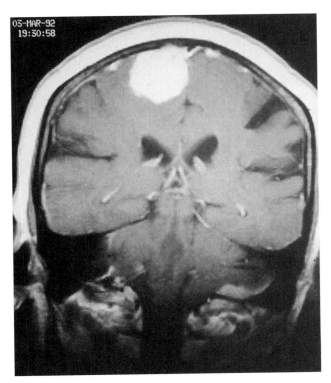

Figure 46–10. Meningioma.

or MRI. A computer plan is generated to direct the radiation. Because multiple small sources are used, the normal brain tissue receives very little radiation while the majority of the radiation accumulates in the tumor.

Chemotherapy

The blood-brain barrier is a protective mechanism that prevents many injurious substances from reaching brain tissue. Unfortunately, it is also very effective in preventing chemotherapeutic agents from reaching the brain. In order to penetrate the blood-brain barrier, very large doses of chemotherapy may be required. These doses may not be well tolerated by other systems of the body. New treatments are currently being investigated. Some clinicians place chemotherapeutic substances in the cavity left by surgical resection. Others disrupt the blood-brain barrier with mannitol and then deliver intra-arterial chemotherapy under general anesthesia. Gene therapy is being used in an effort to kill malignant cells.

Complementary Therapies

The rate of success for treatment of brain tumors is not as high as treatment of other neoplasms. Clients may be drawn to nontraditional therapies both as cures and for treatment of symptoms. Encourage clients to look at each option in a rationale manner. Some questions they should ask themselves include the following:

- Will this interfere with any of my other treatments or medications?
- What is the cost?
- What are the side effects?
- Is there any objective information available?
- What does my physician think of this?

ACUTE AND LONG-TERM COMPLICATIONS

It is difficult to distinguish between symptoms of a brain tumor and complications of treatment. Seizures, headaches, memory impairment, cognitive changes, and ataxia may be symptoms of the tumor or the result of surgery or radiation therapy. Clients may experience hemiparesis or aphasia following surgery. If the tumor continues to grow despite treatment, the client will experience further decline in function. Gradually the client becomes more lethargic and unresponsive. Once the client becomes comatose, death occurs within a matter of days, particularly if artificial nutrition and hydration are not administered.

NURSING CARE

Nursing care depends on the treatment planned for the client. Nursing process for the client with a brain tumor

and nursing process for the client undergoing intracranial surgery are both presented below.

NURSING PROCESS: THE CLIENT WITH A BRAIN TUMOR

Assessment

The nurse does routine neurological assessment to determine level of functioning and presence of neurological deficits such as vision changes, movement problems, altered thought processes, or changes in level of consciousness. A pain assessment is done using the WHAT'S UP? format presented in Chapter 2. Asking the client open-ended questions about how he or she is coping with the diagnosis may help open up communication about fears and grieving.

Nursing Diagnosis

Nursing diagnoses are based on actual problems the client is experiencing. Possible diagnoses include the following:

- Altered thought processes related to involvement of brain tissue
- Self-care deficit related to impaired mobility
- Pain related to cerebral edema
- Sensory-perceptual alterations related to cranial nerve involvement
- Risk for injury related to seizures or neurological deficits
- Anticipatory grieving related to potential loss of function and death

Planning

The client who is not anticipating surgery or curative treatment is assisted to function as effectively as possible for as long as possible. The plan of care includes measures to maintain safety, whether in the home or in a health care setting. The client is assisted to express feelings and plan for end-of-life care.

Implementation

Altered Thought Processes

If the client is disoriented, routine precautions are implemented to keep the client safe. The client is reoriented as needed. The use of calendars, clocks, and familiar furnishings may help the client reorient. A sudden worsening in thought processes should be reported to the RN or physician immediately. The cause may be reversible.

Self-Care Deficit

The client may be unable to care for himself or herself because of altered thought processes or mobility problems. The nurse provides assistance as needed, while encouraging the client to maintain as much independence as possible. If the client becomes totally dependent, a long-term care facility may become necessary.

Pain

If the client experiences headaches or other discomforts, pain medication is provided. Nonnarcotic medications are preferred because they do not alter the level of consciousness. If these are not effective, codeine preparations, which have a minimal effect on LOC, may be used.

Sensory-Perceptual Alterations

Alterations in sensations can take on a variety of forms, including changes in vision, hearing, and paresthesia. See Chapters 48 and 49 for interventions for clients with sensory deficits. Care must be taken to protect the client's skin if tactile sensation is reduced. Assist the client out of bed and into a different environment to help prevent sensory deprivation. Remember to provide sensory stimulation such as conversation, radio, and television if tolerated and enjoyed by the client.

Risk for Injury

In addition to routine safety precautions, the client is protected from injury that may occur as a result of seizures. Seizure precautions are listed in Table 46–3.

Anticipatory Grieving

Both the family and client may be grieving loss of function, as well as a terminal prognosis. Clients and their significant others will require emotional support to face the challenges presented by the diagnosis of brain tumor. They must make decisions regarding treatment at the same time that they may be facing a deterioration in function. How aggressively to pursue treatment and when to change the focus from treatment to palliation are questions that confront these individuals. Clients should be encouraged to organize their personal affairs and make their decisions known while they are still able. Referral to a support group, social worker, or pastoral care person may be beneficial.

Evaluation

An effective plan will result in a client who is safe and comfortable. The client and significant others will be able to express feelings and have the support necessary to plan and carry out necessary care.

Intracranial Surgery

The primary purpose of intracranial surgery is to remove a mass lesion. These types of lesions include hematomas, tumors, arteriovenous malformations, and occasionally contused brain tissue. Other indications for surgery include elevation of a depressed skull fracture, removal of a foreign body, debridement of wounds, or resection of a seizure focus. Craniotomy refers to any surgical opening in the skull. A **burr hole** is an opening into the cranium made with a drill. **Craniecteomy** is the term used to describe removal of part of the cranial bone. **Cranioplasty** refers to repair of bone or use of a prosthesis to replace bone following surgery.

The goal of intracranial tumor surgery is gross total resection of the tumor. This involves removal of all visible tumor, called debulking. Even with the use of the operative microscope there may be viable tumor cells left behind. It is these cells that give rise to recurrence. If all the tumor cannot be removed, the surgeon will debulk as much as possible. By debulking the tumor the surgeon reduces the amount of neoplasm, thereby giving radiation therapy or chemotherapy less of a burden to combat. In some cases it is not feasible to attempt more than a biopsy of the tumor. Location of the tumor or the client's age or medical condition may not allow the client to tolerate a full craniotomy. The biopsy may be done under local or general anesthesia depending on the client's condition. The goal of a biopsy is to obtain tissue that will allow pathological diagnosis of the tumor. The diagnosis will then guide any further treatment.

Intracranial surgery is usually performed under general anesthesia. Occasionally a procedure will require that the client be awake and cooperative.

PREOPERATIVE CARE

Preoperative care of the client undergoing intracranial surgery is similar to that of clients having other surgeries (see Chapter 11). The client will undergo a lab workup and anesthesia evaluation. If the client has cognitive impairments it is important that a significant other be available to provide information.

Client education is important preoperatively. The extent of education depends on the client's ability to absorb new information. This is influenced by the disease process, cognitive functioning, anxiety, and educational level. Significant others are involved as needed. Information about the disease process and surgery are provided by the surgeon. The nurse plays an important role in reinforcing and clarifying the information presented.

Anxiety is also a significant concern before surgery. The client is anticipating serious surgery, as well as a possibly unknown outcome. The nurse must allow time for the client and significant others to express their fears and ask questions. Honest and accurate information should be provided.

Significant others should be prepared for how the client will look after surgery. A preoperative visit to the intensive care unit may help prevent some anxiety postoperatively. Significant others should be accompanied on this visit by a knowledgeable nurse who can explain what they are seeing.

Surgery may last 2 hours for a biopsy to 12 hours or longer for more intricate procedures. Clients and significant others should be prepared for the idea that some or all of the client's hair will be shaved off. Some people prefer to have all their hair shaved rather than just part. The client should be prepared to see his or her face swollen after surgery, particularly around the eyes. The periorbital region may be bruised. Many clients wish to wear a scarf or scrub cap after the dressing is removed.

POSTOPERATIVE CARE

Assessment

Following intracranial surgery the nurse does frequent neurological assessments in addition to routine postoperative monitoring. Clients should have their neurological status assessed every hour for the first 24 hours or as ordered by the physician. Any deterioration in status should be immediately reported to the physician. Many clients will undergo a CT scan within the first 24 hours following surgery to assess cerebral edema.

Nursing Diagnosis

The client is at risk for the following nursing diagnoses:

- Altered cerebral tissue perfusion related to edema of the operative site
- Pain related to surgical procedure
- Risk for infection related to surgical procedure
- Impaired physical mobility related to motor deficits
- Body image disturbance related to changes in appearance or function
- Knowledge deficit related to change in treatment regimen following surgery

Planning

The primary goal following intracranial surgery is prevention of complications. Once the client is stabilized, goals can change to longer-term outcomes such as acceptance of changes in body image and understanding of self-care following discharge. If the client has severe deficits following surgery, rehabilitation or long-term care may become necessary. A social work consult can help with planning for this transition.

Implementation

Risk for Altered Cerebral Tissue Perfusion

Clients who have undergone intracranial surgery will be placed in an intensive care unit postoperatively. They are typically positioned with the head of the bed at 30 degrees or higher to promote venous drainage and minimize increases in intracranial pressure. The exception to this is clients who have had a chronic subdural hematoma re-

moved, who must remain flat. Clients may turn from side to side or lie on their back. The client should be encouraged not to lie on the operative side. Seizure precautions are instituted because the client is at risk for seizures.

The client may have an intracranial monitor in place following surgery to monitor intracranial pressure. Some clients may also have central venous pressure catheters or pulmonary artery catheters. Urinary catheters are used during the immediate postoperative period to accurately monitor fluid balance.

Dressings should be monitored for drainage. Drainage that is blood tinged in the center with a yellowish ring around it may be CSF leakage. A suspected CSF leak should be reported to the RN or physician immediately.

Pain

Intramuscular codeine or oral acetaminophen with codeine (Tylenol with Codeine No. 3) are the pain medications of choice for clients after intracranial surgery. These medications provide pain relief without causing sedation, which can interfere with the neurological assessment. Opioids are not used because they depress respirations and can mask signs of increasing intracranial pressure. Most clients complain of a headache postoperatively, but not severe pain.

Risk for Infection

As with any surgery, a break in the integrity of the skin (and in this case, skull) creates a risk for entry of pathogenic organisms. Infection following craniotomy can be deadly. All care of the incision, dressing, and monitoring equipment sites should be done using strict aseptic technique. Any signs of infection should be reported immediately.

Impaired Physical Mobility

Some clients will have residual effects from the tumor or other pathology or from the surgery. These can range from weakness and paresthesias to paralysis. To prevent contractures and skin breakdown, the client should be turned every 1 to 2 hours after surgery and avoid lying on the operative site unless specifically permitted by the surgeon. Careful positioning in correct body alignment will also help prevent contractures or other injuries. High-top tennis shoes, trochanter rolls, and slings can be used to keep the body in alignment. Range-of-motion exercises and physical therapy are initiated when permitted by the surgeon. An occupational therapist may also be able to assist the client in learning to perform ADL with a new disability.

Body Image Disturbance

The client will have a shaved or partially shaved head after surgery. In addition, depending on the outcome of surgery, residual motor or sensory deficits may be present. The client should be allowed to express his or her feelings if desired. The nurse should portray an accepting attitude. A turban, scarf, or hat may help conceal a shaved head.

Knowledge Deficit

If the client will be discharged home, discuss any activity restrictions, particularly driving. Evaluate the client's understanding of the medication regimen and wound care. Have the client and significant others verbalize the signs of infection or other possible complications to report.

Evaluation

Interventions have been effective if infection and other complications have been prevented and the client states that pain is controlled. The client should be able to look in the mirror and begin to show evidence of acceptance of changes in body image. The client and significant others should be able to describe appropriate follow-up care.

CRITICAL THINKING: Mr. Esposito

Mr. Esposito is a 24-year-old white male who was involved in a motor vehicle accident. His blood alcohol level was 0.24. Mr. Esposito has no preexisting medical problems. Emergency medical services personnel report that Mr. Esposito was unconscious on their arrival at the scene and then became alert and combative. His CT scan shows a left-sided epidural hematoma. Mr. Esposito is admitted to your unit for observation.

1. What symptoms would you expect to see if Mr. Esposito's hematoma increases in size?
2. What emergency preparations should you have ready?
3. What psychosocial assessments would you do?

Answers at end of chapter.

Spinal Disorders

HERNIATED DISKS

Herniated intravertebral disks are a common health problem. They are characterized by pain and paresthesias that follow a radicular (nerve path) pattern. It is not uncommon for clients to have more than one herniated disk or to have herniated disks in different areas of the spine.

Pathophysiology

When the disk between two vertebrae herniates, it moves out of its normal anatomical position. In most cases the annulus fibrosus, the touch outer ring of the disk, tears. This allows escape of the nucleus pulposus, the soft inner portion of the disk. Displacement of the disk compresses one or more nerve roots, causing the characteristic symptoms (Fig. 46–11).

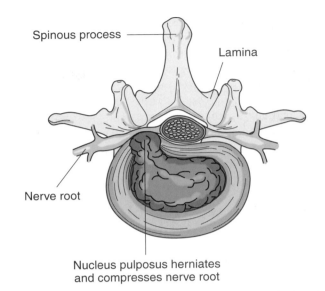

Figure 46–11. A herniated disk places pressure on a spinal nerve root.

Etiology

In some cases a specific event can be correlated with a herniated disk. The client may describe a fall, lifting a heavy object, or a motor vehicle crash. In other instances, the client cannot identify a triggering incident.

Signs and Symptoms

Cervical disk herniation causes pain and muscle spasm in the neck. The client may exhibit decreased range of motion secondary to pain. Hand and arm pain is unilateral (one sided) and follows the distribution of the spinal nerve root. Clients often complain of numbness or tingling in the extremity. Asymmetric weakness and atrophy of specific muscle groups may be detected. If weakness involves the entire extremity it is unlikely that disk herniation is the etiology. The severity of the pain or paresthesia does not correlate directly with the severity of the nerve compression. However, weakness and atrophy are indicators of significant nerve compression.

Thoracic herniated disks are not very common. This portion of the spine is the least mobile, therefore less stress is exerted on the disk. Clients with herniated thoracic disks may complain of pain in the back. It is uncommon to detect muscular weakness.

A herniated lumbar disk is typically characterized by low back pain, pain radiating down one leg, paresthesias, and weakness. The client may limp on the affected leg or may have difficulty walking on his or her heels or toes. Muscle spasm is often present. Pain and muscle spasm may limit the client's range of motion. Depending on the disk affected, the knee or ankle deep tendon reflex may be decreased or absent. A severely herniated lumbar 5–sacral 1 disk may affect bowel or bladder continence.

This is an emergency situation and should be reported immediately.

The WHAT'S UP mnemonic can be used to assess symptoms of herniated disks at any level:

W—Where is the pain? Does it radiate into an extremity? In what distribution?

H—How does it feel? Sharp, stabbing, burning?

A—Do certain positions or activities alleviate or aggravate the pain? Holding the affected arm above the head may alleviate cervical pain. Sitting places pressure on disks and aggravates lumbar pain. Lying down may relieve it.

T—Is there a correlation between time and pain? Some clients have more pain at the end of the day. Is the pain constant?

S—Ask the client to rate the severity of the pain on a scale of 1 to 10. Which is the most painful, the spine or the extremity?

U—Ask the client to identify associated symptoms such as numbness, tingling, or weakness.

P—What is the client's perception of the pain? Is it interfering with work or other aspects of the client's life?

Diagnostic Tests

An MRI will detect herniation of a disk and compression or abnormality of the spinal cord. If the client has previously had surgery in the area of the suspected herniation, the MRI is done with and without contrast to differentiate between scar tissue and herniated disk.

If the client cannot tolerate MRI, or if the MRI does not provide enough information, a myelogram will be done. Refer to Chapter 45 for a description of both tests.

Treatment

Most clinicians and clients prefer to try conservative therapy before performing surgery for a herniated disk.

Medical Management

REST. In the past bed rest was advised as part of conservative management. The current recommendation is 1 or 2 days of bed rest, followed by a careful, gradual increase in activity.

PHYSICAL THERAPY. Physical therapy can be very useful for some clients. A gradually progressive course of exercise strengthens the muscles. This is particularly important in the lumbar spine, where the muscles help stabilize the spine. Techniques such as ultrasound, heat, ice, and deep massage can decrease muscle spasm and allow for increased range of motion. Instructions in proper body mechanics and strategies for avoiding reinjury are an important component of physical therapy.

A transcutaneous electrical nerve stimulator (TENS) is a noninvasive pain-relief technique. Small electrodes are placed on the skin around the area of the pain. The device then transmits a low-voltage electrical current through the skin. The client feels a tingling or buzzing sensation, which may block the pain impulses. The physical therapist shows the client where to place the electrodes and how to operate the unit. The client decides when to use it and at what settings. This allows the client to actively participate in his or her care and have some control over his or her pain level.

TRACTION. Cervical traction is a noninvasive technique sometimes used by physical therapists for clients with herniated cervical disks. The client's head is placed in a halter-like device. A series of ropes and pulleys connect the halter to a weight. This gently pulls the head away from the shoulders. The rationale is that this traction will slightly separate the vertebral bodies and may allow the disk to return to its proper position. If it is effective in relieving the client's pain, cervical traction may be done at home on an as-needed basis. If it increases the client's pain the traction is discontinued immediately. Lumbar traction is not particularly effective because the lumbar paraspinal muscles are very large and strong. The amount of traction needed to overcome the muscular resistance can cause injury.

MEDICATION. Muscle relaxants are frequently prescribed for clients who are experiencing spasm. These medications decrease pain by decreasing the spasm, helping the client increase range of motion and activity. Muscle spasm is actually a protective mechanism. Muscles tighten and become painful, causing the client to limit movement. This lessens the chance that the disk will be further injured. However, chronic spasm can cause tearing and scarring of the muscles. It is hard to predict which muscle relaxant will be most effective for a given client. Clients should be warned that drowsiness is a common side effect of muscle relaxants. They should be cautioned against driving or operating machinery until they determine how well they tolerate the medication. Diazepam (Valium) is a very effective muscle relaxant; however, it has a strong potential for addiction. Therefore it is usually used only if muscle spasm cannot be adequately treated with other medications.

Inflammation of the nerve root is caused by compression and irritation from the herniated disk. Nonsteroidal anti-inflammatory drugs (NSAIDs) can be very effective in reducing this inflammation, but there is no way of predicting response to a given drug. It may be necessary for the client to try several nonsteroidal drugs before an effective one is found. Because several of these drugs are now available without prescription, the client should be cautioned not to use a nonprescription NSAID at the same time as a prescription NSAID. Clients should be instructed to report any stomach upset to the clinician, because NSAIDs have the potential to cause gastric bleeding. Occasionally, oral steroids will be used on a short-term basis. A rapidly tapering dose of steroid over 1 week is often used. This is used for clients with severe inflammation that does not respond to other treatments. Warn the client about gastric upset. Steroids may cause elevated serum glucose levels. Instruct the diabetic client to monitor glucose levels closely and consult his or her physician if the levels are outside his or her normal parameters.

Epidural injections are an option for clients who are unable or do not wish to have surgery. A mixture of medications, typically a steroid, long-acting anesthetic, and long-acting pain reliever, is injected into the epidural space. The anesthetic provides immediate relief while the steroid reduces swelling for a longer-lasting effect. If relief is obtained the injection can be repeated every 3 to 4 months.

The use of pain medication is a subject of concern in the treatment of clients with herniated disks. Opioids may be appropriate for short-term use. This includes clients who are trying conservative therapy or those who are not able to have surgery immediately. If surgery is not an option or is not successful, the condition may be a chronic source of pain. In that circumstance, the physician is unlikely to prescribe ongoing opioids. The client, on the other hand, may wish to continue using opioids because they provide substantial pain relief. The physician and client must discuss the potential complications of long-term opioid use such as constipation, tolerance, and dependence. They should not be taken at the same time as alcohol.

Surgical Management

Several types of surgery can be done. A **laminectomy** removes one of the laminae, the flat pieces of bone on each side of a vertebra. This may be done to relieve pressure or to gain access for removal of a herniated disk. A diskectomy removes the entire disk. A spinal fusion uses a bone graft to fuse two vertebrae together if the area is unstable. Surgery may be done through a microscope for less scarring and better recovery. Most clients are discharged within 24 hours of surgery. This is in contrast to several weeks in the hospital on bed rest in the recent past.

A diskectomy is generally done for a herniated cervical disk. This can be accomplished via an anterior or posterior approach. Most surgeons use the anterior approach for cervical herniations, because the muscles in the front of the neck are much smaller and more moveable than those in the back of the neck. Therefore there is less pain and muscle spasm following surgery. It is also safer than the posterior approach, which involves more maneuvering around the spinal cord.

Most surgeons replace the disk with bone or another material. This prevents collapse of the disk space and creates a spinal fusion. If bone is used it may be harvested from the client's iliac crest or donated from a cadaver. Mobility of the spine is lost in the area of a fusion. Spinal fusions may also be done to correct instability of the spine from other causes such as scoliosis or degenerative disorders.

A posterior approach is utilized for a herniated lumbar disk. Typically the vertical incision is 1 to 2 inches long. It

---

laminectomy: lamin—a posterior portion of the vertebra + ectomy—surgical removal of

is necessary to pull some of the muscle away from the bone, which accounts for some of the postoperative pain that clients experience. A laminectomy is done, and the herniated portion of the disk is resected. The remainder of the disk continues to provide a cushion between the intravertebral bodies. The surgeon removes any free fragments and any disk material that appears unstable.

Percutaneous diskectomy involves insertion of a large needle into the disk under local anesthesia to aspirate herniated disk material. This technique is not used for severely herniated disks. Laser disk surgery may be used to disintegrate the herniated tissue. Laparoscopic techniques may also be used.

Complications after Surgery

Hemorrhage

As with any surgery, intraoperative hemorrhage is possible. It is not common in disk surgery. If a postoperative hemorrhage occurs in a client who has had an anterior cervical diskectomy, the airway may become occluded. The client is monitored for bleeding from the incision and respiratory distress.

Nerve Root Damage

If the nerve root is severed during surgery the client will have loss of motor and sensory function in that distribution. This may result in decreased use of the extremity. If the nerve root is damaged or excessive scarring occurs, the client may experience pain, weakness, or paresthesias. In some cases, physical therapy and nonsteroidal anti-inflammatory drugs may be effective in improving function and lessening pain.

Reherniation

Lumbar disks may reherniate. This can occur anywhere from 1 week to several years after the initial surgery. If the reherniation occurs within a few weeks to months after the first surgery, the client usually undergoes another microdiskectomy. Reherniation of the cervical disk does not occur because the entire disk is removed.

Herniation of Another Disk

Fusion of the cervical spine results in loss of movement at that motion segment. This can place increased stress on the disks above and below the fusion. This may increase the risk of another herniated disk, especially if the client already has degeneration of other disks. The client should be instructed to maintain an exercise program and to frequently move the spine through range-of-motion exercises.

SPINAL STENOSIS

Spinal stenosis is a condition in which the spinal canal is compressing the spinal cord (Fig. 46–12). Arthritis is a major cause of spinal stenosis. The facet joints of the spine become inflamed and enlarged, narrowing the diameter of the spinal canal and compressing the spinal cord. Clients may complain of pain and weakness. Compression of the cervical portion of the spinal cord may result in hyperreflexia and weakness of the legs and arms.

A laminectomy may be done to relieve pressure on the spinal cord. The size of the incision depends on the number of vertebrae involved. Clients are typically in the hospital for 4 or 5 days. These clients are often elderly and may have concurrent illnesses. They may require inpatient rehabilitation before returning to their homes.

NURSING PROCESS:
THE CLIENT HAVING SPINAL SURGERY

Preoperative Care

Routine preoperative care is appropriate for the client undergoing spinal surgery. In addition to routine teaching, the client is instructed in how to logroll following surgery. This procedure involves keeping the body in alignment and rolling as a unit, without twisting the spine, to prevent injury to the operative site.

Postoperative Care

Assessment

In addition to routine postoperative assessment, the extremities are monitored for changes in circulation, movement,

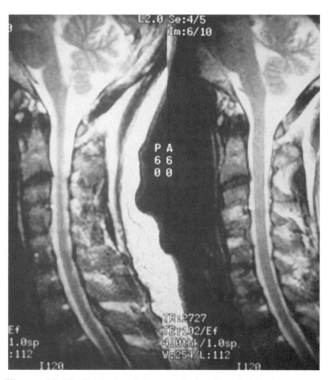

Figure 46–12. Stenosis of the cervical spine *(left)*. Compare to normal spinal column *(right)*.

and sensation. Circulation is checked by the color, warmth, and presence of pulses in the extremity. Movement is assessed by asking the client to move the extremity. Sensation is assessed by gently touching the client's extremity and asking if feeling is present. Any changes are reported immediately to the physician because this may indicate nerve or circulatory damage. Pain is assessed. The pain that necessitated surgery should be relieved, but the client may still have muscle and incisional pain. The client should be reassured that it will gradually subside. The surgical dressing and drain if present are monitored for CSF drainage or bleeding. If bone was taken from a separate donor site, this site must also be monitored. Intake and output are measured to ensure that the client is able to void. The physician is notified if the client had difficulty voiding.

Nursing Diagnosis

Possible postoperative diagnoses include the following:

- Pain related to surgical procedure
- Risk for impaired physical mobility related to neuromuscular impairment
- Risk for altered urinary elimination related to effects of surgery
- Risk for injury related to immobility and neuromuscular impairment

Planning

Goals of nursing are to keep the client safe and free from injury or complications and free of pain. Gradual return to normal physical activity is expected.

Implementation

If a local anesthetic was injected into the surgical site during surgery, the client may not have pain postoperatively. Muscle relaxants, analgesics, and NSAIDs are given as ordered. The client is positioned in bed in correct body alignment and may have orders to be kept flat for 6 to 8 hours. A pillow between the legs when side lying promotes alignment and comfort. The client is assisted to logroll to get out of bed and ambulate on the first postoperative day. If a spinal fusion has been done, the fused area of the spine will be immobile. The client with a cervical laminectomy may have a soft cervical collar for neck support. Clients may have difficulty voiding following lumbar surgery because of anesthesia, immobility, or occasionally because of nerve damage related to surgery. Getting up to go to the bathroom (or standing for men) and running water should promote bladder emptying. If difficulty urinating occurs, the physician should be contacted for an order for intermittent catheterization until the problem resolves. Most clients go home within 24 to 48 hours of surgery.

Evaluation

The client is expected to be free of complications and pain, be able to urinate, be able to move all extremities, and return gradually to preillness activity.

Spinal Cord Injuries

Injuries to the spinal cord affect people of all ages but take their greatest toll on young people. These injuries are characterized by decrease or loss of sensory and motor function below the level of the injury.

PATHOPHYSIOLOGY

The spinal cord is made up of nerve fibers that allow communication between the brain and the rest of the body. Damage to the spinal cord results in interference with this communication process. Damage may be caused by bruising, tearing, cutting, or bleeding into the cord. The damage may be caused by external forces or by fragments of fractured bone.

CAUSES AND TYPES

The causes of spinal cord injury are similar to those of traumatic brain injury. It is not uncommon for a client to have both a spinal cord injury and traumatic brain injury. Motor vehicle crashes, falls, and sports-related injuries are common causes. Diving into shallow water is frequently the cause of cervical cord injury. Assaults may cause cord injury if a knife or bullet penetrates the spinal cord.

Spinal cord injuries may be classified by location or by degree of damage to the cord. A complete spinal cord injury means that there is no motor or sensory function below the level of the injury. An incomplete lesion means that there is some function remaining. This does not necessarily mean that the remaining function will be useful to the client. Some clients find that having areas where sensation is intact may be more painful than useful.

The cervical and lumbar portions of the spine are injured more often than the thoracic or sacral segments. This is because the cervical and lumbar areas are the most mobile portions of the spine.

SIGNS AND SYMPTOMS

Cervical Injuries

Cervical cord injuries can affect all four extremities, causing paralysis and **paresthesias,** impaired respiration, and loss of bowel and bladder control. Paralysis of all four extremities is called **quadriplegia;** weakness of all extremities is called **quadriparesis.** If the injury is at C3 or above,

the injury is usually fatal because muscles used for breathing are paralyzed. An injury at the fourth or fifth cervical vertebrae will affect breathing and may necessitate some type of ventilatory support. These clients typically need long-term assistance with activities of daily living (Fig. 46–13).

Thoracic/Lumbar Injuries

Thoracic and lumbar injuries affect the legs, bowel, and bladder. Paralysis of the legs is called **paraplegia;** weakness of the legs is called **paraparesis.** Sacral injuries affect bowel and bladder continence and may affect foot function. Individuals with thoracic, lumbar, and sacral injuries can usually learn to perform activities of daily living independently.

Spinal Shock

Spinal cord injury has a profound effect on the autonomic nervous system. Immediately following injury the cord below the injury stops functioning completely. This causes a disruption of the sympathetic nervous system, resulting in vasodilation, hypotension, and bradycardia (neurogenic shock or spinal shock). Dilation of the blood vessels allows more blood flow just beneath the skin. This blood cools and is circulated throughout the body, causing hypothermia. Keep the client covered as much as possible but avoid overheating. This may last from a week to many weeks in some clients.

COMPLICATIONS

Infection

Impaired respiratory effort, decreased cough, mechanical ventilation, and immobility all predispose the cervical cord–injured client to pneumonia. Catheterization, whether indwelling or intermittent, places clients at risk for urinary tract infection.

Deep Vein Thrombosis

Lack of movement in the legs inhibits normal blood circulation. Compression stockings, sequential compression devices, and subcutaneous heparin may be used separately or together to reduce the risk of deep vein thrombosis.

Orthostatic Hypotension

Spinal cord–injured clients no longer have muscular function in their legs to promote venous return to the heart. They also have impaired vasoconstriction. This leads to pooling of the blood in the legs when the client moves from

---

paresthesia: para—beside + esthesia—sensation
quadriplegia: quad—four + plegic—paralysis
quadriparesis: quad—four + paresis—partial paralysis
paraplegia: para—beside + plegia—paralysis
paraparesis: para—beside + paresis—partial paralysis

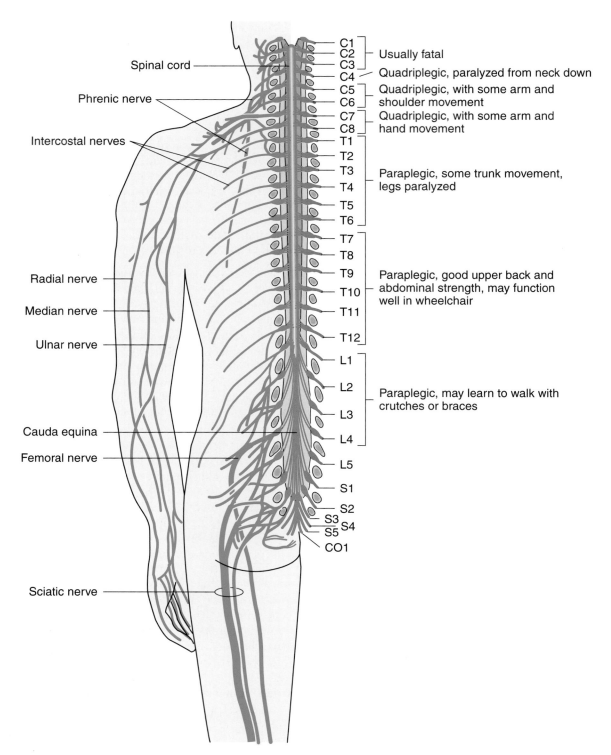

Figure 46–13. Spinal cord injury—quad versus para. (Modified from Scanlon, VC, Sanders, T: Workbook for Essentials of Anatomy and Physiology, ed 2. FA Davis, Philadelphia, 1995, p 167, with permission.)

a supine to a sitting position. If the movement is sudden the client may faint. Gradual elevation of the head, use of elastic stockings, and a reclining wheelchair help lessen this response.

Skin Breakdown

Clients or their caregivers must be diligent about relieving pressure on the skin by position changes and cushioning of bony prominences. Development of pressure ulcers can lead to infection and loss of skin, muscle, or bone. Treatment of pressure ulcers is time consuming and expensive and may interfere with work or school.

Renal Complications

Urinary tract infections are an ongoing concern to spinal cord–injured clients. Both urinary reflux and untreated urinary tract infections can cause permanent damage to the kidneys.

Depression and Substance Abuse

Clients with spinal cord injury have a higher than average incidence of depression and substance abuse. Both of these factors can interfere with the client's ability to care for himself or herself. Individual or family counseling may be helpful. Some rehabilitation centers have support groups for spinal cord–injured clients.

Autonomic Dysreflexia

This life-threatening complication occurs in clients with injuries above the T6 level. The spinal cord injury impairs the normal equilibrium between the sympathetic and parasympathetic autonomic nervous system. Some type of noxious stimuli below the spinal cord injury causes activation of the sympathetic system. This response continues unchecked because the parasympathetic responses cannot descend past the spinal cord injury.

Common causes of autonomic **dysreflexia** are bowel impaction, bladder distention, urinary tract infection, ingrown toenails, pressure ulcers, and labor. Stimulation of the sympathetic nervous system results in cool, pale skin, gooseflesh, and vasoconstriction seen below the level of the injury. Blood pressure may rise to 300 mm Hg systolic. The parasympathetic response results in vasodilation, causing flushing and diaphoresis above the lesion, and bradycardia as low as 30 beats per minute. The client complains of a pounding headache and nasal congestion secondary to the dilated blood vessels.

---

dysreflexia: dys—abnormal + reflexia—reflex activity

DIAGNOSTIC TESTS

Plain x-rays are done to identify fractures or displacement of vertebrae. A CT scan is also useful for identifying fractures. MRI may demonstrate lesions within the cord.

TREATMENT

Clients with spinal cord injuries typically are brought to the emergency department. They should be kept immobilized until they are assessed by the physician. If injury to the spinal cord is detected, the client will need to remain immobilized.

Medical Management

Emergency management involves careful monitoring of vital signs and airway and keeping the client immobilized. Intubation and mechanical ventilation may be necessary. Intravenous normal saline may be used for fluid replacement. The physician does not rely on fluid administration alone to correct hypotension. It is possible to administer enough fluid to cause pulmonary edema and not correct the hypotension. Vasoactive drugs may be required. Various medications to reduce the extent of injury, including intravenous methylprednisolone, are currently being researched.

Respiratory Management

Clients with injuries above C4–5 will have some degree of respiratory impairment. The client may require a tracheostomy and continuous mechanical ventilation or require a ventilator only at night or when fatigued. Some clients are able to breathe by using a phrenic nerve stimulator. This device, similar to a pacemaker, artificially stimulates the phrenic nerve, causing the diaphragm to move. These clients use a mechanical ventilator at night. This lessens the stress on the phrenic nerve and removes the risk of the system failing while the client is asleep.

Clients may be breathing independently when they first arrive in the emergency department and then experience respiratory compromise as the spinal cord becomes edematous. Edema can compress the spinal cord above the lesion, leading to symptoms at a higher level. This deterioration is usually temporary. Fatigue of the accessory muscles may also cause respiratory compromise. The intercostal muscles are not normally of major importance in respiration. However, if the diaphragm is paralyzed, the intercostal muscles become very important. As these muscles fatigue, the client's breathing becomes shallow and rapid. Elective intubation and mechanical ventilation protect the client from expending huge amounts of energy trying to breathe. Feeling their breathing becoming more labored is terrifying to these clients, and they need to be reassured that it is probably a temporary setback. As the edema recedes and the accessory muscles become stronger, they will be weaned from the ventilator.

Gastrointestinal Management

Absence of bowel sounds is a common finding on examination. Oral or enteral feedings are not started until bowel function resumes. The metabolic needs of the clients are influenced by the work of breathing and the extent of other injuries. If positioning or paralytic ileus preclude oral or enteral feedings, hyperalimentation is begun.

Genitourinary Management

An indwelling urinary catheter is placed to prevent bladder distention and protect skin integrity until spinal shock resolves. Once it is determined what degree of hand function the client will have, a bladder management program is devised.

Immobilization

The cervical spine may be immobilized with skeletal traction such as Crutchfield or Gardner-Wells tongs (Fig. 46–14). Some clients have a halo brace, a device that attaches to the skull with four small pins. The skull ring attaches to a rigid plastic vest by four poles (Fig. 46–15). This device keeps the head and neck immobile while fusion and healing take place. The advantage over traction is that the client is not confined to bed.

Surgical Management

The goal of surgery following spinal cord injury is to stabilize the bony elements of the spine and relieve pressure on the spinal cord. Surgery may or may not improve functional outcome.

Stabilization of the spine allows for earlier mobilization of the client. This decreases the risk of complications from immobility and quickens the transition to rehabilitation. Clients who have been in cervical traction before surgery may be placed in a halo brace postoperatively.

Unstable thoracic and lumbar fractures may also be treated with surgical implantation of rods to stabilize the spine. It is more difficult to stabilize these areas in the postoperative recovery period. Clients may wear a supportive corset, a rigid brace, or occasionally a body cast to supplement the support provided by the internal fixation devices.

NURSING PROCESS

Assessment

Clients with spinal cord injury need ongoing evaluation of all body systems. Frequent neurological and respiratory assessments are done. Early assessment of the client's support system can help with discharge and rehabilitation planning.

Nursing Diagnosis

Possible nursing diagnoses include the following:

- Impaired physical mobility related to injury
- Altered urinary elimination related to nerve damage
- Constipation related to immobility and nerve damage
- Self-care deficit related to paralysis

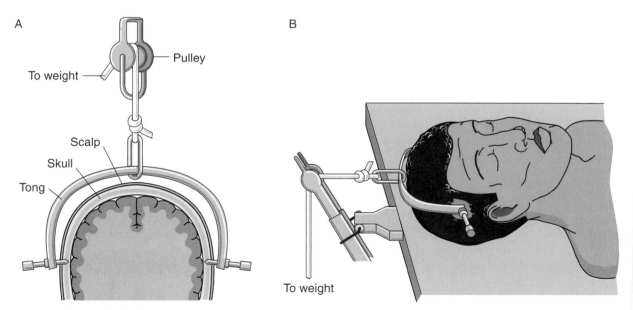

Figure 46–14. Skeletal traction for cervical injuries. *(A)* Crutchfield tongs. *(B)* Gardner-Wells tongs. (Modified from Black and Matassarin-Jacobs: Medical-Surgical Nursing: Clinical Management for Continuity of Care, ed 4. WB Saunders, Philadelphia, p 799, with permission.)

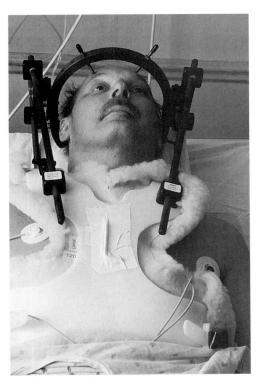

Figure 46–15. Halo brace.

- Ineffective coping related to life crisis
- Risk for dysreflexia related to stimuli below level of injury
- Risk for ineffective airway clearance related to ineffective cough and decreased muscle control
- Risk for impaired skin integrity related to immobility and possible paresthesias
- Risk for sexual dysfunction related to autonomic nervous system dysfunction
- Risk for altered role performance related to effects of injury

Planning

Initial goals for the client include maintenance of safety and prevention of complications. Long-term goals include rehabilitation and maximizing remaining function.

Implementation

Impaired Mobility

Range-of-motion exercises help prevent contractures. Regular turning and repositioning help prevent respiratory and other complications. Some clients are placed on special beds (such as the Roto-Rest bed) that move the client frequently without the need for turning. Splints may be used to maintain functional positioning of extremities. This may include the use of high-top tennis shoes to prevent foot-

drop. If the client is ambulatory he or she should not walk alone initially. Special care should be provided when ambulating the client with a halo brace. The halo brace alters the client's center of gravity and requires an adjustment of the client's sense of balance. Falling while in the halo brace can cause further injury to the spinal cord.

Altered Urinary Elimination

Male clients may use an external, condom type of catheter if the bladder empties reflexively when full. If the bladder does not empty reflexively or if the client does not wish to wear a leg bag to collect urine, the physician may order intermittent catheterization. Clean technique is used to intermittently insert a catheter and empty the bladder (see Chapter 34). Male clients with good hand function can be taught to catheterize themselves. Clients with poor hand function may depend on a caregiver to perform intermittent catheterization or use an indwelling catheter.

Female clients with good hand function may still find self-catheterization difficult because of positioning problems. They may choose to use indwelling catheters. External urine collection devices for female clients are available but may be cumbersome.

Reliance on incontinence pads is discouraged for all clients because of the threat to skin integrity. The importance of adequate fluid intake must be stressed to clients. Some individuals limit fluid intake in an effort to lessen the chances of incontinence. This predisposes the client to constipation, urinary tract infection, and renal calculi.

Constipation

Once oral feedings are begun, a bowel management program should be instituted. The client will have decreased or absent sphincter tone. This, combined with an inability to detect the need to defecate, puts the client at risk for incontinence. Slowed bowel motility, as well as generalized immobility, contributes to constipation. A high-fiber diet with adequate fluid intake is important. Use of a suppository on a scheduled daily or every-other-day basis enables most clients to maintain bowel continence.

Self-Care Deficit

Explaining the rationale for nursing activities prepares the client and significant others to assume responsibility for care. Encourage the client and significant others to participate in hands-on care as much as possible. If the client will not be able to perform self-care, assist him or her to learn to direct care. Physical and occupational therapists can help the client adapt to wheelchair or other mobility aids. Most clients spend some time in a rehabilitation facility in order to learn to function independently. Some clients may require long-term care.

Risk for Impaired Coping

The psychosocial impact of a spinal cord injury is devastating. The client may be afraid of dying, yet express the feeling that he or she would be better off dead than being paralyzed. These types of statements are very difficult for significant others to cope with. Encourage the client to focus on reasons for living (e.g., seeing children or grandchildren grow up, or a loving partner). Consult a social worker or pastoral care worker who is familiar with spinal cord–injured clients. Support groups may also be helpful (see Table 46–7).

Dysreflexia

If you suspect autonomic dysreflexia, immediately take the client's blood pressure and continue to monitor it every 5 minutes. Remember that clients with spinal cord injury are typically hypotensive, so a finding of even mild hypertension may represent a dramatic increase from their baseline blood pressure.

Uncontrolled blood pressure may cause seizures, intracerebral hemorrhage, or death. Place the client in a Fowler's position to utilize the effect of orthostasis to control blood pressure. The goal of treatment is to identify the cause and relieve it without increasing the sympathetic nervous system response. Notify the physician immediately. If removal of the cause does not relieve hypertension, an antihypertensive agent may be ordered.

A rectal examination is performed to determine if an impaction is present. Apply anesthetic ointment to the rectum before disimpaction, because further rectal stimulation may exacerbate symptoms. Simultaneously monitor blood pressure and stop disimpaction if the blood pressure increases.

Evaluate the indwelling catheter for patency. If it is not patent or a catheter is not in place, obtain an order to insert one immediately. Monitor blood pressure during catheterization. If bowel or bladder distention is not present, examine the client for other causative mechanisms. It may be necessary to treat the hypertension if a cause cannot be quickly found and treated. If hypertension is treated with medications, remember that the blood pressure may decrease rapidly once the cause of the autonomic dysreflexia is corrected. Continue to carefully monitor blood pressure.

Once the acute episode is past, significant others and the nurse should devise a plan to prevent reoccurrence. The client should be taught how to direct caregivers in treating autonomic dysreflexia.

Airway Clearance

Clients with cervical injuries have difficulty clearing secretions. They no longer have adequate muscle strength to cough effectively. Initially, suctioning will be required to keep the airway clear. Once the client is stable, an assisted cough may be used to clear secretions. This involves the nurse or other caregiver gently pushing upward and inward on the client's chest while the client coughs as strongly as possible. It is similar to the Heimlich maneuver but not as forceful. Humidified air and oral or enteral fluids will help keep secretions thin and mobile.

Skin Integrity

Extreme care must be taken to protect the skin of the injured client, beginning with the initial emergency treatment. In the emergency department the nurse should remove anything between the client and the backboard. Clients have developed pressure ulcers from lying on keys or other objects in their pockets. If the client is on a Roto-Rest bed, make sure the client is not sliding as the bed turns. This could cause shearing of the skin. When permitted by the physician, turn the client frequently and assess bony prominences for redness. Ensure that the client's extremities do not get caught in side rails or wheelchair spokes. If a client is in traction or a halo brace, the pin sites should be assessed frequently. Keep the sites clean and dry and report any sign of infection.

Sexual Dysfunction

Paraplegic males usually have difficulty achieving and maintaining an erection. Quadriplegic males may develop an erection during any penile stimulation. This includes catheterization and can be embarrassing to the client. If this occurs the nurse should discontinue the procedure and continue at a later time if possible. It should be treated with a matter-of-fact attitude. Males with spinal cord injuries do not ejaculate in the normal manner. Consultation with a fertility specialist or urologist may provide some help for conception if desired.

Spinal cord injury does not impair female fertility. Clients who wish to become pregnant should seek an obstetrician familiar with spinal cord injuries. See Table 46–9 for contraception for females with spinal cord injuries.

Altered Role Performance

Interpersonal relationships are significantly stressed by spinal cord injury. Both short-term and long-term relationships may become stronger or disintegrate. Clients and significant others should be encouraged to draw support from all available sources. Friends, family, and members of one's religious affiliation can provide emotional and physical help.

Table 46–9. *Birth Control Issues for Clients with Spinal Cord Injury*

Method	Comments
Oral contraceptives	Contraindicated because of the risk of deep vein thrombosis
Diaphragm	May be difficult for a client with poor hand function to insert
Intrauterine device	Client may not feel IUD move out of position; client may not feel perforation of uterus
Norplant	No contraindications
Condom	No contraindications

Loss of income may be temporary or permanent. Financial concerns add to the burden of spinal cord injury. Not all insurance policies cover the extensive inpatient rehabilitation needed by spinal cord–injured clients. Uninsured clients may have a very difficult time finding a rehabilitation program that will accept them. Adaptive equipment is expensive and may not be covered by insurance. A social worker can help the client gain access to appropriate assistance.

Client Education

Education of the spinal cord–injured client is an ongoing process. It begins with a basic explanation of the anatomy and physiology of the spine. Treatment of spinal cord injury and prognosis are early learning needs.

As the client's condition stabilizes, teaching focuses on caring for the client. This can seem overwhelming to the client and caregiver. Break tasks down into simple steps. Focus on one body system at a time. For example, do not try to teach suctioning and bowel care at the same time.

Be aware that performing tasks such as catheterization or bowel care may interfere with feelings of intimacy between partners. Encourage partners to verbalize these feelings and make alternative arrangements for care if possible. Some clients prefer to hire an attendant rather than rely on significant others for personal care.

Both clients and caregivers should be involved in determining contingency plans. These include what to do in the event of a power failure, fire, or illness of the caregiver.

Spinal cord–injured clients experience the same basic health care needs as noninjured individuals. Encourage the client to establish a relationship with a primary practitioner who is familiar with spinal cord injury. This facilitates the client's adaptation to changes in his or her condition. Female clients may find that they do not fit in the wheelchair as pregnancy advances. A client who requires cardiac bypass may be unable to transfer or propel the wheelchair because use of his or her arms is impaired by the sternal incision. These and many other situations require creativity and flexibility on the part of the client, caregiver, and health professional.

Evaluation

Avoidance of preventable complications is one sign of a successful care plan. The client should have regular bowel and bladder function. Mobility is maximized based on the client's rehabilitation potential. The client and significant others should verbalize basic understanding of spinal cord injury and self-care.

akinesia: a—not + kinesis—movement

Degenerative Neuromuscular Disorders

Degenerative nervous system disorders involve the extrapyramidal tracts and basal ganglia in the brain. The extrapyramidal tracts are the efferent pathways outside the pyramidal system that connect the cerebral cortex with the spinal nerve pathways. Because these are motor pathways, movement rather than sensation is affected. The resulting symptoms can include rigidity, tremor, and abnormal movements.

PARKINSON'S DISEASE

Parkinson's disease is a chronic degenerative movement disorder that arises in the basal ganglia in the cerebrum. It usually begins in the fourth or fifth decade of life, with symptoms becoming progressively worse as the client ages. The disease is characterized by tremors, changes in posture and gait, rigidity, and slowness of movements. Approximately 1 million people in the United States are currently living with Parkinson's disease.

Pathophysiology

The substantia nigra is a group of cells located within the basal ganglia, which is situated deep within the brain. These cells are responsible for the production of dopamine, an inhibitory neurotransmitter. Dopamine facilitates the transmission of impulses from one neuron to another. Parkinson's disease is caused by widespread destruction of the cells of the substantia nigra, resulting in decreased dopamine production. Loss of dopamine function results in impairment of semiautomatic movements. Dopamine also plays a part in the fight-or-flight mechanism by activating epinephrine and norepinephrine.

Acetylcholine, an excitatory neurotransmitter, is secreted normally in individuals with Parkinson's disease. The normal counterbalance of acetylcholine and dopamine is interrupted in these clients, causing a relative excess of acetylcholine, which results in the tremor, muscle rigidity, and **akinesia** (loss of muscle movement) characteristic of Parkinson's disease.

Etiology

The etiology of Parkinson's disease is unknown. It was first described in 1817 by London surgeon James Parkinson. Although scientists now know that the symptoms are caused by death of dopamine-producing cells in the substantia nigra, they do not know what causes the cells to die. Parkinson's-like symptoms, referred to as parkinsonism, may be associated with use of certain drugs, such as phenothiazines. Parkinsonism was also linked to an outbreak of encephalitis in the 1920s.

Signs and Symptoms

The onset of symptoms in clients with Parkinson's disease is usually gradual and subtle. A substantial percentage of the dopamine-producing cells are nonfunctional before the client becomes symptomatic. Symptoms may be mistakenly attributed to aging or fatigue. In retrospect, clients and their significant others often identify a long period in which symptoms were present but not identified as symptoms of Parkinson's disease.

The primary symptoms of Parkinson's disease are muscular rigidity, **bradykinesia** (slow movement) or akinesia, changes in posture, and tremors. The brain is no longer able to direct the muscles to perform in the usual manner. This lack of communication between the brain and the muscles can have profound impact on the client's ability to ambulate safely, perform ADL and job functions, or enjoy leisure activities. The symptoms may also have a significant negative impact on the client's self-esteem.

The client may have difficulty in initiating movement; this may be particularly apparent when the client attempts to start walking, rise from a sitting position, or begin dressing. Because considerable effort is required to move the rigid muscles, the client performs voluntary movements very slowly.

The extensor muscles are more affected by Parkinson's disease than the flexor muscles. This impaired function of the extensor muscles results in the stooped posture typical of clients with Parkinson's disease (Fig. 46–16). Flexion of the hips, knees, and neck shifts the center of gravity forward. The gait is characterized by shuffling, short steps. This shuffling gait may increase in speed once the client finally gets walking, and the client may have difficulty stopping. The client maintains a broad base when making turns to try to compensate for imbalance. These changes place clients at high risk for falls. Slowness of movement and stiff muscles make it much harder for clients to catch themselves if they start to fall or to relax the muscles to minimize injury.

Tremors typically begin in the hand and then progress to the **ipsilateral** foot. In most clients the tremor then moves to the **contralateral** side. Many clients identify one side of the body as being more affected by the tremor than the other. Tremor of the hand has been described as a pill-rolling tremor; the thumb typically moves back and forth across the fingers and looks like the client is rolling a pill. Tremors typically lessen or disappear during movement and are more noticeable when the extremity is at rest or when trying to hold an object still (this is called a resting tremor). The tremors disappear when the client is asleep. The inability to hold an object still can make simple acts such as drinking a glass of water or reading a book nearly impossible. The signs and symptoms of Parkinson's disease tend to increase in severity when the client becomes fatigued.

Another type of tremor, a benign familial (or essential) tremor, may sometimes be mistaken for Parkinson's dis-

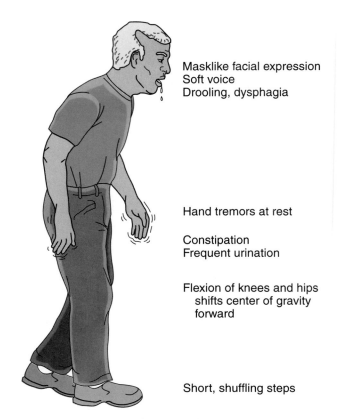

Masklike facial expression
Soft voice
Drooling, dysphagia

Hand tremors at rest

Constipation
Frequent urination

Flexion of knees and hips shifts center of gravity forward

Short, shuffling steps

Figure 46–16. Manifestations of Parkinson's disease.

ease. Treatment is different for each. See Table 46–10 for differentiation of these tremors. The secondary symptoms of Parkinson's disease include generalized weakness, muscle fatigue and cramping, and difficulty with fine motor activities. This fine motor dysfunction may make it difficult for the client to button a shirt or tie shoes. Handwriting typically deteriorates as the disease progresses. A soft, monotone voice and masklike facial expression may make the client appear to be lacking in emotional responses. It may be necessary to ask clients about their emotional status and help them develop ways of expressing their emotions. The normal blink response is diminished, so the client and his or her significant others must be educated about eye care to prevent corneal abrasions.

Dysfunction of the autonomic system may be manifested by diaphoresis, constipation, orthostatic hypotension, drooling, dysphagia, seborrhea, and frequent urination. Clients who experience seborrhea and diaphoresis need frequent attention to personal hygiene. Drooling and dysphagia may make the client reluctant to appear in public. Slowness in initiating walking, balance problems, and frequent urination place the client at risk for urinary incon-

---

bradykinesia: brady—slow + kinesis—movement
ipsilateral: ipsi—same + lateral—side
contralateral: contra—opposite + lateral—side

Table 46–10. **Symptoms of Parkinson's Disease vs. Essential Tremor**

	Parkinson's Disease	Benign Familial Tremor
Resting tremor	Yes	No
Intention tremor (with movement)	No	Yes
Pill-rolling tremor	Yes	No
Head/voice tremor	No	Yes
Relieved with beta-blocking medication (propranolol)	No	Yes
Relieved with anti-Parkinson's medications	Yes	No

tinence, which may also increase the client's reluctance to leave home.

Late in the disease, mental function may become slowed and the client may become demented. This is compounded by the side effects of many anti-Parkinson's drugs. Death is usually from complications of immobility.

Complications

The most typical acute complications of Parkinson's disease are related to the client's difficulties with mobility and balance. These clients are very prone to falls, which may result in injuries ranging from bruises to fractures to head or spinal cord injuries. Constipation is common due to decreased activity, diminished ability to take in food and fluids, and the side effects of anticholinergic medications.

Clients are encouraged to increase the fiber and roughage in their diet. If constipation is not alleviated by dietary modifications, the client may need to use stool softeners. The client should be counseled not to rely on laxatives or enemas.

Muscular rigidity and bradykinesia contribute to joint immobility, which decreases a client's ability to ambulate and care for himself or herself. Position changes may be painful for clients. A turning sheet and adequate personnel are necessary when turning a client in bed to prevent stress on the joints. Tremors interfere with ADL, consume immense amounts of energy, and may prevent the client from working or performing leisure activities. Swallowing may become so impaired that enteral (tube) feeding is required. Depression is a common complication at any stage of Parkinson's disease and may compromise communication, ability to learn, and performance of ADL. Clients may require counseling or antidepressants.

Diagnostic Tests

No specific tests diagnose Parkinson's disease. The diagnosis is based on the history given by the client and a thorough physical examination.

Medical Treatment

There is no cure for Parkinson's disease. Treatment is aimed at controlling symptoms and maximizing the client's functional level. Drugs used to control symptoms are listed in Table 46–11.

Many clients with Parkinson's disease experience fluctuations in motor function related to their drug therapy.

Table 46–11. **Medications Used to Treat Parkinson's Disease**

Medication	Use	Side effects/Comments
Anticholinergic (trihexyphenidyl [Artane])	Block action of acetylcholine to control tremor, salivation.	Urine retention, dry mouth, constipation, blurring of memory, dizziness, confusion.
Antiviral (amantadine [Symmetrel])	Dopamine agonist that facilitates the production and secretion of dopamine.	Leg edema, hypotension, dizziness, confusion.
Monoamine oxidase B inhibitor (selegiline [Eldepryl])	Blocks the metabolism of central dopamine, increasing dopamine in CNS.	Nausea, dizziness, confusion; may have the potential to slow the progression of Parkinson's disease.
Dopamine agonist (levodopa [L-Dopa])	Levodopa is converted into dopamine in the brain by the amino acid decarboxylase. Reduces tremor, rigidity, and bradykinesia.	May cause nausea, vomiting, and dyskinesias: dystonia (repetitive involuntary contraction of muscles), athetosis (twisting, writhing movement of arms and hands), and chorea (involuntary muscle twitching; may resemble a dance). The breakdown products of protein metabolism compete with levodopa for transport from the intestine to the brain. Clients should take levodopa 15–30 min before meals and minimize their protein intake during the times they need to be most active.
Peripheral decarboxylase inhibitor (carbidopa) (Sinemet is levodopa/carbidopa combination)	Carbidopa prevents peripheral breakdown of levodopa so more is available in the CNS.	

This is referred to as the on-off phenomenon. Clients may experience a decreased response to levodopa, or off period, particularly as the dose is wearing off. As the disease progresses, clients may notice that the off periods become less predictable and occur more rapidly. The client may have a delayed or absent response to the next dose of levodopa, resulting in the client being stuck in the off stage and being significantly disabled for that time period. Fluctuations in motor function may be accompanied by other symptoms such as pain, diaphoresis, anxiety attacks, hallucinations, or mood swings. These symptoms significantly increase the disability associated with the episodes.

Clients who are taking maximum doses of medication for Parkinson's symptoms may benefit from a "drug holiday." During a drug holiday, clients are taken off all drugs for a period of time, then restarted on lower doses. Hospitalization may be necessary during this time to maintain client safety.

Surgical Treatment

Pallidotomy is an option for clients whose rigidity, tremor, and bradykinesia are uncontrollable by medical management. During this stereotactic procedure a destructive lesion is placed in the basal ganglia. The surgery is only performed on one side at a time. The client remains awake during the surgery to make sure that the lesion is being placed in the appropriate location. These clients need a great deal of education and support before and during the surgery. Some centers are experimenting with implanting fetal tissue or adrenal gland tissue in the brain to produce dopamine.

Nursing Process: The Client with Parkinson's Disease

Assessment

The client is assessed for symptoms of Parkinson's disease and their effect on level of functioning. Ability to move, walk, and perform ADL is assessed. Risk for injury related to immobility or falls should be determined. Nutritional status and condition of skin are assessed. Presence of confusion and side effects of medications are identified. Psychosocial assessment includes the client's and caregiver's response to the disease, coping strategies, and support systems.

Nursing Diagnosis

The client with Parkinson's disease is at risk for many problems. Typical diagnoses include the following:

- Impaired physical mobility related to muscle stiffness and tremor
- Self-care deficit related to reduced mobility
- Altered nutrition related to dysphagia and reduced mobility

- Altered thought processes related to effects of disease and medication
- Caregiver role strain related to demands of caring for client
- Risk for injury related to falls

Planning and Implementation

IMPAIRED PHYSICAL MOBILITY. Clients frequently plan their daily activities based on anticipated response to their medications. This allows them to be as active as possible within the restrictions of the medication schedule. The client is encouraged to determine his or her own best schedule for activities that require mobility. For clients in skilled nursing facilities, leisure activities are planned around the client's most active times.

Physical and occupational therapy sessions can help maintain mobility, provide assistive devices, and provide diversional activities. The nurse provides assistance with range-of-motion exercises. The client who has difficulty initiating walking can be taught to pick her or his foot up as if attempting to step over something to take the first step. It may also help to take several steps in place before starting to walk.

SELF-CARE DEFICIT. The most common setting for treatment of the client with Parkinson's disease is the home. The client is encouraged to participate in ADL as much as possible. The occupational therapist can assist with devices and strategies for maintaining independence. Clients have usually developed their own coping strategies, such as wearing clothing without buttons or shoes with adherent fasteners. As self-care abilities further decline, the nurse provides more assistance with ADL.

As the client ages so do the significant others who are providing care. The point may be reached at which the caregiver is no longer able to meet the increasing needs of the client. The decision to place the client in a skilled nursing facility is an extremely difficult and emotional one. Every effort should be made to retain as much of the client's usual routine as possible during hospitalization or admission to a skilled nursing facility.

ALTERED NUTRITION. The nurse helps open packages and prepares the meal so the client can feed himself or herself if at all possible. If the client has a severe tremor a spoon may be safer than a fork for self-feeding. Finger foods may also be helpful. A cup with a lid and spout can help minimize spilling. Clients in the advanced stages of Parkinson's disease are at high risk for aspiration due to difficulty swallowing. Thickening agents in liquids and assisting the client to a chair or high Fowler's position for meals may help prevent aspiration. Meals that are high in fiber help prevent constipation. Small, frequent meals may be less overwhelming to the client who must eat slowly.

ALTERED THOUGHT PROCESSES. Memory impairment is one of the most distressing symptoms that clients with

Parkinson's disease experience. Many clients state that memory impairment and loss of social outlets are more troublesome than the physical impairments. The nurse can assist the client to devise coping methods, such as written daily schedules, calendars, and reminders to take medications. If the client becomes confused, frequent reorientation may be helpful.

CAREGIVER ROLE STRAIN. The significant others and caregivers of the client with Parkinson's disease should be included in the plan of care. These individuals should be encouraged to utilize all community, personal, and governmental support systems available. Caregivers may need to be reminded that if they neglect their own health, both physical and mental, it will have a negative impact on the client as well. Some caregivers may only need an hour or two away on an occasional basis. Others may require a more extended break. Options for relief from caregiving range from having a friend or neighbor visit to employing a home health aide or utilizing adult day care on a part-time or full-time basis. Some skilled care facilities offer respite care, in which the client is admitted for a short time. This may be a viable option for a caregiver who must be hospitalized for his or her own health care.

RISK FOR INJURY. The client is at risk for injury from falls related to problems with mobility. The client's call light should be within reach at all times. The bed should be kept in the low position, with side rails raised. Restraints should be avoided, but alarm systems are available that alert the nurse that the client is getting up. The environment should be kept free from clutter, throw rugs, or other items that may cause a client to trip. The nurse assists with ambulation. Walkers and other assistive devices may be helpful.

> ### CRITICAL THINKING: Ms. Simpson
>
> Ms. Simpson is a 47-year-old Caucasian female. She has had Parkinson's disease for the last 5 years, and the symptoms are becoming progressively worse. She is now admitted for a urinary tract infection.
>
> 1. What problems do you foresee when caring for Ms. Simpson?
> 2. What safety measures should you implement?
>
> *Answers at end of chapter.*

HUNTINGTON'S DISEASE

Huntington's disease is a progressive, hereditary, degenerative, incurable neurological disorder. It was first described in 1872 by George Huntington, a general practitioner from New York. The uncontrolled movements associated with Huntington's disease caused some sufferers in the seventeenth century to be accused of, and exe-

cuted for, witchcraft. Many of the cases around the world can be traced back to specific individuals.

Pathophysiology and Etiology

Huntington's disease is inherited in the autosomal dominant manner, meaning that each offspring of an affected parent has a 50 percent chance of inheriting the disorder. It is uncertain what caused the mutation of the gene responsible for Huntington's disease. Structurally, the disease is characterized by degeneration of the corpus striatum, caudate nucleus and other deep nuclei of the brain, and portions of the cerebral cortex.

Signs and Symptoms

Signs and symptoms develop slowly and become progressively more apparent. Cognitive signs may be noticed before movement problems. Clients who are not aware of their hereditary risk for Huntington's disease may be incorrectly diagnosed as being mentally ill or alcoholic.

The client may display personality changes and inappropriate behavior. The client may be euphoric or irritable and may rapidly alternate between moods. Paranoia is common, and behavior may become violent as **dementia** (mental impairment) worsens. The client eventually becomes so demented that he or she is incontinent and totally dependent on others for care. These symptoms are difficult for caregivers, whether family members or professionals, to cope with. They are particularly devastating for offspring, who may or may not know whether they have inherited the disease.

Physical symptoms also develop slowly. Huntington's disease is characterized by involuntary, irregular, jerky, dancelike movements. Initially these symptoms may take the form of mild fidgeting and facial grimacing. In the early stages of the disease the client may try to cover the movements by incorporating them into a voluntary movement such as crossing the arms or scratching. The involuntary movements usually start in the arms, face, and neck and progressively involve the remainder of the body. Clients display hesitant speech, eye blinking, irregular trunk movements, an abnormal tilt of the head, and constant motion (Fig. 46–17). The gait is wide based, and the client may appear to be dancing. Emotional upset, stress, or trying to perform a voluntary task can significantly increase the severity and rate of the abnormal movements. The movements typically diminish or disappear during sleep. Dysphagia may significantly impair the client's nutritional status.

Depression and suicide are common in the earlier stages of the disease. As the disease progresses, the client becomes more and more dependent. Aspiration resulting in respiratory failure is the primary cause of death for individuals suffering from Huntington's disease. Life span following diagnosis is about 10 to 20 years.

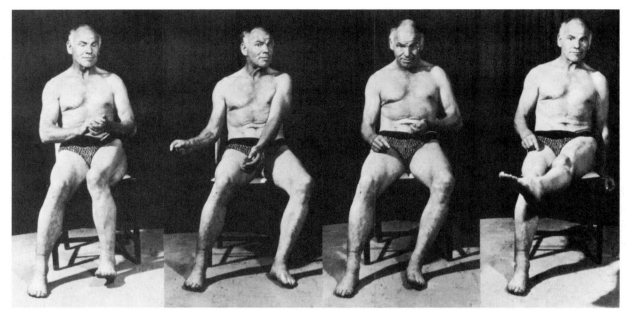

Figure 46–17. 47-year-old client with Huntington's disease. Note constant fidgety movement. (From Spillane, JD: An Atlas of Clinical Neurology. Oxford University Press, New York, 1968, p 219, by permission of Oxford University Press.)

Diagnostic Tests

Huntington's disease has typically been diagnosed based on the clinical examination and a family history of the disease. MRI or CT may be helpful. Genetic testing is available for prenatal use and to determine if an individual has Huntington's disease before he or she becomes symptomatic. This is a dramatic breakthrough because Hunington's disease does not become symptomatic until the client is in his or her thirties or forties, when he or she may already have children who may be affected.

Medical Treatment

Because there is no cure, treatment of Huntington's disease focuses on minimizing symptoms and preventing complications. Antipsychotic drugs are frequently used to treat both the involuntary movements and behavioral outbursts.

Nursing Management

Clients with Huntington's disease are typically cared for on an outpatient basis. When a client with Huntington's disease is admitted to an inpatient facility it is important to obtain as much information as possible about that person's response to medication, daily routine, and emotional and cognitive functioning from the caregivers. For example, knowing that a certain client is intensely afraid of bathtubs but willingly takes showers can prevent unnecessary struggles and outbursts. Providing some objects from home may make the new environment seem less threatening. The caregivers may relate that the client has better cognitive functioning at a particular time of day. As the dementia progresses, the client will respond less to attempts to reason with him or her. Giving directions in a calm but firm tone may help the client cooperate with activities. The environment should be modified to keep the client safe. Keep in mind that forceful, involuntary movements of the client's extremities can happen at any time. These movements should never be misinterpreted as an attempt to harm caregivers.

Difficulty swallowing typically begins toward the middle of the disease course. Clients exhibit trouble swallowing liquids in particular. At this stage it may still be possible to teach the client to hold the chin down to the chest while swallowing, which lessens the chance of aspiration. Clients should sit straight upright while eating. Adaptive devices may prolong the client's ability to eat independently. Soft foods that are easily manipulated in the mouth are most suitable. These clients may have difficulty taking in adequate calories to maintain a normal body weight, even if a caregiver assists with feeding them. One of the many ethical issues faced by these clients and their significant others is whether artificial feeding should be used, and if so, for how long. Early in the course of the disease clients and their significant others should be encouraged to discuss end-of-life decisions.

ALZHEIMER'S DISEASE

Alzheimer's disease (also called dementia of the Alzheimer's type, or DAT) is the most common of several types of dementia. Dementia is "a loss of intellectual function (thinking, remembering, and reasoning) so severe that it interferes with an individual's daily functioning and eventually results in death."[1]

Alois Alzheimer, a German neurologist, first described the disease in 1907. He described pathological changes, now referred to as neurofibrillary tangles and neuritic plaques, that he discovered while performing an autopsy. Alzheimer's disease is a progressively degenerative disease that is inevitably fatal. The incidence of Alzheimer's disease is more common in women than men and doubles for every 5 years the individual lives beyond the age of 65 years.

Etiology and Pathophysiology

Many different etiologies have been theorized for Alzheimer's disease, including a genetic cause. Chromosome 21 is the location for the gene sequence that is associated with Alzheimer's disease. Chromosome 21 is also the location of the genetic abnormality responsible for Down syndrome. Clients over the age of 40 who have Down syndrome will usually develop Alzheimer's disease. The exact correlation between the two disorders is still being studied.

Although the exact cause of Alzheimer's disease is unknown, the structural changes associated with it have been well documented. An abnormality exists within the protein of the cell membrane of a neuron. As the axon terminals and dendrite branches disintegrate, they collect in neuritic plaques. Within the normal brain is a precise arrangement of filaments and tubules, responsible for cell integrity. Individuals with Alzheimer's disease develop neurofibrillary tangles instead of the normal orderly arrangement. Instead of remaining a small area of abnormality, these neuritic plaques and neurofibrillary tangles spread via axons to other areas of the brain.

Advancement of neurofibrillary tangles and neuritic plaques typically affect the hippocampus first, resulting in short-term memory dysfunction. As the tangles and plaques spread to the temporal lobe, the memory impairment becomes more severe. It may be at this point that the client accesses the health care system. Personality changes and incontinence are inevitable results of Alzheimer's disease. These symptoms can be attributed to the spread of plaques and tangles to the frontal lobes of the brain.

It is believed that the younger the client is at the time of onset, the faster the neurofibrillary tangles and neuritic plaques spread. Therefore these clients tend to deteriorate faster, require complete care earlier, and have a shorter life span.

One area of the brain that is left relatively untouched by tangles and plaques is the subcortical area. This structure is responsible for our subconscious urge to survive. The needs for basic requirements such as shelter, food and water, security, and reproduction are controlled by the subcortical area, as are emotional responses to situations. The client with Alzheimer's disease may experience hunger, but no longer know how to meet that basic need. Left to their own devices these individuals would starve.

Signs and Symptoms

The signs and symptoms of Alzheimer's disease are typically broken down into three stages. The *early stage* lasts from 2 to 4 years and is characterized by increasing forgetfulness. At this stage the client may attempt to cope by using lists and reminders. Interest in day-to-day activities, acquaintances, and surroundings tends to diminish. The client is reluctant to take on tasks because of uncertainty in how to perform them. If the client is still working his or her performance deteriorates and may result in being terminated from the job.

The *middle stage* is the longest in duration, lasting 2 to 12 years. Progressive memory loss is demonstrated by difficulty doing simple calculations or answering questions. Clients may become irritable, particularly when asked to perform a task that they know they should be able to perform but cannot. It may help the client to break the task down to manageable steps. Depression is common. Aphasia and the resulting inability to make himself understood may exacerbate the client's irritability. It is during the middle stage, as cognitive function significantly deteriorates, that the client becomes more physically active. The normal sleep-wake cycle is disrupted, and the client tends to wander aimlessly, particularly at night. The client may become lost in familiar surroundings, which compounds the anxiety that typically develops during this stage. Hallucinations and seizures may occur. Management of day-to-day activities such as feeding a pet or paying bills becomes overwhelming. Personal hygiene deteriorates, as does appropriate social behavior. Clients may make up stories to cover for deficits, saying that possessions they misplaced were stolen. Some clients hoard food or money.

The *third stage* of Alzheimer's disease is characterized by progression to complete dependency. The client loses the ability to converse or control bowel or bladder function. Constant supervision is required if the client is still mobile to protect from wandering and avoid injury. Emotional control and ability to recognize significant others are lost. This lack of recognition is particularly devastating for family members. Eventually the client is unable to move independently, swallow, or express his or her needs. Death occurs from complications of immobility.

The duration of the final stage of Alzheimer's disease, characterized by complete dependence, depends in part on the physical stamina and general health of the individual. The healthier the client, the longer the body will continue to function. Another factor is the decisions that have been made regarding artificial feeding and respiratory support. Few significant others, or health care practitioners, advocate intubation and mechanical ventilation for clients with Alzheimer's disease. The issue of enteral feedings, however, is an emotional one with few easy answers. The use of enteral feedings can prolong the client's life, despite the absence of cognitive functioning. As with clients suffering from Huntington's disease, every effort should be made to determine the client's wishes before cognitive impairment makes that impossible. See Table 46–12 for a comparison of the symptoms of Parkinson's, Huntington's, and Alzheimer's diseases.

Diagnostic Tests

The only absolute method of confirming a diagnosis of Alzheimer's is by pathological examination at autopsy. In actuality, the disease is diagnosed on the basis of clinical examination, history, and elimination of other possible causes of the symptoms. MRI may reveal the presence of the classic neurofibrillary tangles and neuritic plaques. Positron emission tomography (PET) and single photon emission computed tomography (SPECT) scans show areas of neuronal inactivity. Newer tests are being evaluated that hold promise for better diagnosis.

Medical Treatment

There is no known cure for Alzheimer's disease. Treatment has traditionally focused on minimizing the effects of the disease and maintaining independence as long as possible. Two drugs are currently available for the treatment of the disease itself. Tacrine (Cognex) was the first drug released expressly for the treatment of Alzheimer's disease. Cognex is thought to inhibit the breakdown of the neurotransmitter acetylcholine. Increased levels of acetylcholine in the brain allow better functioning of the remaining neurons. Cognex appears most effective for those clients who exhibit mild to moderate symptoms of Alzheimer's disease. A minimum of 19 weeks may be required to notice any effects of the drug. Use of Cognex diminishes the amount of medical care and social service interventions required and delays admission to skilled nursing facilities. This delay in institutionalization can result in significant positive impact on quality of life, as well as thousands of dollars in savings. Donepezil (Aricept) also inhibits the breakdown of acetylcholine in the brain, but it has fewer side effects than Cognex.

Antidepressants, antipsychotics, and antianxiety drugs may be used as a last resort to control symptoms of depression and behavioral disturbances, but they do not treat the dementia. Clients should be carefully monitored for drug interactions and side effects.

Nursing Process: The Client with Dementia

Assessment

The nurse assesses mental status, including memory, orientation, and judgment (see Chapter 45). The client's functional level is assessed to determine the level of self-care he or she is able to engage in. The abilities of the family or caregiver to provide the care needed are also assessed, so that appropriate referrals can be made. Availability and use of resources are determined. Nutritional status and usual food preferences are assessed to aid in planning for adequate nutritional intake.

Nursing Diagnosis

Clients with dementia are at risk for numerous problems. Priority diagnoses include risk for injury, altered nutrition, altered thought processes, incontinence, and caregiver role strain.

Planning and Implementation

Goals include helping the client maintain the ability to care for himself or herself for as long as possible. Maintenance of safety and nutrition are priorities. Incontinence should be minimized and skin protected. Goals should include not only the client but the caregiver as well. If the caregiver does not have adequate support, the burden of caring for the client may become overwhelming.

RISK FOR INJURY. Many individuals who have a loved one with dementia wish to keep that individual at home as long as possible. These caregivers need a great deal of education and support. Although every effort should be made to retain the client's dignity, devices designed to protect small children may be effectively used in the home. Baby gates at stairways and baby latches on doors and outlets provide relatively unobtrusive protection. Because they may misinterpret the environment, clients may find mirrors frighten-

Table 46–12. *Symptoms of Parkinson's Disease, Huntington's Disease, and Alzheimer's Disease*

	Parkinson's Disease	Huntington's Disease	Alzheimer's Disease
Tremors	Present	Absent	Absent
Bradykinesia/akinesia	Present	Absent	Absent
Muscle rigidity	Present	Absent	Absent
Memory dysfunction	Late	Late	Early
Cognitive dysfunction	Late	Present	Early
Inability to perform ADL	Progressive	Progressive	Progressive
Involuntary movements	Absent	Present	Absent
Depression	Present	Present	Present

ing. Forgetfulness and impaired judgment make safety a major concern for Alzheimer's clients who live at home. Clients may strongly resist efforts to keep them from cooking or driving. It may be necessary to remove car keys from the client's access. If the client lives alone, he or she may resist changes in living arrangements.

The client with dementia is typically admitted to a skilled nursing facility when the significant other can no longer handle care at home. Clients may wander, making them prone to injury. Doors of units should be equipped with alarms indicating when they have been opened. A Medic Alert bracelet can be worn to identify the client in case he or she wanders and becomes lost.

NUTRITION. Maintaining adequate nutrition intake for a client with limited attention span is a nursing challenge. Because these clients have difficulty making choices, one food at a time should be offered. Frequent high-calorie meals and snacks that can be eaten with the fingers may help increase intake.

ALTERED THOUGHT PROCESSES. To facilitate communication, the nurse should gently touch the client to get his or her attention before speaking. Gestures, simple phrases, and a quiet setting may also help. The client must be allowed adequate time for the information to be processed before a response is expected.

Difficult behavior may be caused by inability to express needs or fears. The client may feel the urge to urinate but can no longer communicate this need or accomplish the process independently. Because understanding the environment is difficult, the nurse tries to maintain a predictable routine. Scheduled voiding may minimize incontinence. Clients feel safer and may cope better in a stable environment.

Clients often rummage through drawers, closets, or boxes. Unfortunately, these clients do not recognize the difference between their own possessions and those of others, which becomes more problematic if they are in a nursing facility. These clients may not know what they are looking for, but they do feel that they need to find something. Giving the client a box of safe, familiar items, such as empty thread spools, may occupy the client repeatedly.

INCONTINENCE. Regular toileting for both bowel and bladder can help prevent episodes of incontinence. As incontinence becomes more frequent, adult briefs should be used. An indwelling catheter should be avoided because of the risk for injury and infection. Briefs should be changed regularly to prevent skin breakdown.

CAREGIVER ROLE STRAIN. Dementia often takes at least as much of a toll on caregivers as it does on the sufferer. Fear of the diagnosis may keep people from seeking medical care. Some clients consider suicide due to fear of losing their dignity and becoming a burden on their significant others. As the disease progresses, the client gradually loses awareness of the neurological deterioration. Occasional lucid moments can be very difficult for client and caregiver as they realize what has been lost.

Caregivers should be encouraged to share their perspectives and coping strategies with others in similar situations. Support, both informal and formal, is vital to caregiver coping. Caregivers of clients with Alzheimer's disease have unique concerns and needs. The nurse can help caregivers find Alzheimer's support groups and resources (see Table 46–7).

HOME HEALTH HINTS

To assess a client's neurological status at home:

- Note whether the client's clothes are matched and properly fastened. Is the client clean and well groomed?
- Observe the client during bathing, grooming, or dressing to assess motor function and coordination.
- Assess energy level by noting if the client makes frequent requests to sit or lie down.
- Observe the client's gait for steadiness.

To help the client perform ADLs easier at home:

- Ask permission to move furniture and small rugs in order to provide a clear path for ambulation.
- Position frequently used items such as a comb, glass of water, eyeglasses, books, tissues, and phone where they are easily accessible.
- Recommend shoes with Velcro closures.
- Use chairs with armrests—the client can use the armrests to push against to stand.
- Keep the client cleaner at meals with a clip-on bib such as those used at the dentist's office. Attach clips from suspenders to a piece of elastic and place around the back of the client's neck. Attach a clean napkin or washcloth for each meal.

To help the client with Alzheimer's disease who has perceptual deficits:

- Have things used together the same color (e.g., toothbrush and toothpaste).
- Contrast colors in the environment to help clients function independently—slipper color should be different than the floor, a dark-colored placemat can be used under light dishes, the first and last steps of a stairway can be painted a contrasting color.
- Use a bath or shower seat, handheld shower head, and soothing music to help the client feel safe and oriented to the task while bathing.
- Cover doorknobs with a piece of cloth to keep the client from wandering away.

Evaluation

If the plan of care is successful, the client with dementia will remain safe and without injury, in an environment that is as comfortable and nonrestrictive as possible. If nutrition is adequate, the client's weight will remain stable. The client's needs will be anticipated so that communication frustrations will be kept to a minimum. Incontinence will be managed without skin breakdown. Clients and caregivers should be able to identify resources and obtain relief from caregiver activities when needed.

Review Questions

1. Which of the following problems predisposed Jennie to develop meningitis?
   a. A muscle injury in her back
   b. A migraine headache
   c. A sore throat for 3 days
   d. Vision changes

2. Mr. Delmar has receptive aphasia. This means that he has difficulty:
   a. Swallowing
   b. Speaking
   c. Hearing
   d. Understanding language

3. David complains of seeing flashing lights. You know he has a history of seizures. Which of the following actions do you take first?
   a. Help him lie down in a safe place.
   b. Record the events of the seizure.
   c. Take him to the emergency department.
   d. Assess his eyes.

4. Teresa is admitted following a traumatic brain injury. Which of the following actions do you take to help prevent increased ICP?
   a. Cluster care so she can have long periods of rest.
   b. Keep the head of her bed elevated at 30 degrees.
   c. Suction frequently to keep her airway clear.
   d. Do not give her anything by mouth.

5. Intracranial hemorrhage can be caused by which of the following etiologies?
   a. Hypertension
   b. Trauma
   c. Ruptured aneurysm
   d. All of the above

6. Jason is admitted following a T4 spinal injury. When taking his morning vital signs you note that he appears restless and his blood pressure is elevated. Which of the following actions is correct?
   a. Recheck his blood pressure in an hour.
   b. No action is necessary.
   c. Check for a full bladder.
   d. Encourage him to express his anxiety.

7. The symptoms of Parkinson's disease are caused by depletion of which neurotransmitter?
   a. Dopamine
   b. Acetylcholine
   c. Serotonin
   d. Norepinephrine

8. The symptoms of Alzheimer's disease are caused by depletion of which neurotransmitter?
   a. Dopamine
   b. Acetylcholine
   c. Serotonin
   d. Norepinephrine

9. Ellie has Alzheimer's disease and is losing weight because she does not remember how to eat. Which of the following interventions is appropriate?
   a. Request an order for intravenous nutrition.
   b. Remind her that it is important to eat a variety of foods.
   c. Give her frequent small meals with finger foods.
   d. Do not interfere; she will eat when she is hungry.

10. Which disease is characterized by involuntary twisting movements?
    a. Parkinson's disease
    b. Huntington's disease
    c. Alzheimer's disease
    d. Multiple sclerosis

11. Frances is confused and wanders. Which intervention will best maintain safety?
    a. Use a vest restraint to keep her in her chair.
    b. Allow her to wander in a safe, locked environment.
    c. Reorient her and remind her not to leave the floor.
    d. Keep her TV on to distract her.

 ANSWERS TO CRITICAL THINKING

CRITICAL THINKING: Mr. Chung

1. CT scan and lumbar puncture.
2. Short, simple sentences, because he may be very anxious or disoriented. Further education can be provided when he is feeling better.
3. Because meningococcal meningitis is contagious, he should be placed in isolation. Gloves, gowns, and masks should be used. The nurse should explain the need for these practices to Mr. Chung and his visitors.
4. Tepid baths, a quiet dark environment, minimal stimulation. If ordered, acetaminophen and analgesics.
5. The health service at his college should be notified of his diagnosis. Close contacts may require prophylactic treatment. If Mr. Chung lives at home rather than at college, his family should be advised to see their family practitioner and begin prophylactic treatment.

CRITICAL THINKING: *Mrs. Washington*

1. Uncontrolled hypertension.
2. Left.
3. Mrs. Washington is disoriented. Her room should be as close to the nurse's station as possible. Reorient her to her surroundings and condition frequently. Keep side rails up when Mrs. Washington is alone.

   Mrs. Washington is also hemiparetic. Obtain a commode because Mrs. Washington will probably not be able to walk to the bathroom. Place the call light and telephone on her right side. Assist Mrs. Washington with positioning to prevent injury to hemiparetic limbs.
4. The relationship of uncontrolled hypertension to intracranial hemorrhage; options for inpatient, outpatient, or in-home therapy; memory strategies to prevent missed medication doses (e.g., weekly pill box, keeping medications with breakfast food or an alarm clock or watch).

CRITICAL THINKING: *Mr. Esposito*

1. Impaired speech, right-sided weakness, rapid decrease in consciousness.
2. Intubation equipment, mannitol, IV access. NPO status and results of lab work in the event of emergency surgery. The whereabouts of Mr. Esposito's next of kin.
3. Who are Mr. Esposito's support people? Was this drinking episode an isolated incident or a chronic problem?

CRITICAL THINKING: *Ms. Simpson*

1. Urinary tract infection is often accompanied by urinary urgency. Ms. Simpson may have difficulty getting to the bathroom quickly and safely.
2. Keep a bedside commode nearby if the bathroom is not close. Assist Ms. Simpson to the bathroom or commode at regular intervals to prevent urgency. Remind her to ask for help if she needs to get up. Make sure that her call light is within reach.

REFERENCE

1. Alzheimer's Association. Http://www.alz.org/dinfo/factsheet/ADFS.html, 1998.

BIBLIOGRAPHY

Abudi, S, Bar-Tal, Y, Ziv, L, and Fish, M: Parkinson's disease symptoms—patients' perceptions. J Adv Nurs 25(1):54, 1997.
Ackley, BJ, and Ladwig, GB: Nursing Diagnosis Handbook: A Guide to Planning Care. Mosby, St Louis, 1997.

Adams, RD, Victor, M, and Ropper, AH: Principles of Neurology, ed 6. McGraw-Hill, New York, 1997.
Albanese, A, Cassetta, E, Caretta, D, et al: Acute challenge with apomorphine in Huntington's disease: A double-blind study. Clin Neuropharmacol 18(5):427, 1995.
Berkow, R (ed): The Merck Manual of Diagnosis and Therapy, ed 16. Merck, Rahway, NJ, 1992.
Black, JM, and Matassarin-Jacobs, E (eds): Medical-Surgical Nursing: Clinical Management for Continuity of Care, ed 5. WB Saunders, Philadelphia, 1997.
Bunch, B (ed): Disease, vol 4. Grolier Educational, Danbury, Conn, 1997.
Carroll, DL: Living with Parkinson's: A Guide for the Patient and Caregiver. Harper Perennial, New York, 1992.
Cohen, D, and Eisdorfer, C: The Loss of Self. New American Library, New York, 1986.
Cutler, NR, and Sramek, JJ: Understanding Alzheimer's Disease. University Press of Mississippi, Jackson, Miss, 1996.
Delieu, J, and Keady, J: The biology of Alzheimer's disease: 1. Br J Nurs 5(3):162, 1996.
Delieu, J, and Keady, J: The biology of Alzheimer's disease: 2. Br J Nurs 5(4):216, 1996.
Ditunno, JF, Graziani, V, and Tessler, A: Neurological assessment in spinal cord injury. Advanced Neurology 72:325, 1997.
Gresham, GE, Duncan, PW, Stason, WB, et al: Post-Stroke Rehabilitation: Assessment, Referral, and Patient Management. Clinical Practice Guideline, No. 16. AHCPR Pub. No. 95-0662. U.S. Department of Health and Human Services, Public Health Service, Agency for Health Care Policy and Research, 1995.
Hall, JK: Caring for corpses or killing patients. Nurs Manage 25(10):81, 1994.
Henke, CJ, and Burchmore, MJ: The economic impact of Tacrine in the treatment of Alzheimer's disease. Clin Ther 19(2):330, 1997.
Hickey, JV: The Clinical Practice of Neurological and Neurosurgical Nursing, ed 4. JB Lippincott, Philadelphia, 1997.
Hinkle, JL: New developments in managing transient ischemic attack and acute stroke. AACN Clin Issues 8(2):205, 1997.
Hodgson, H: Alzheimer's: Finding the Words. Chronimed, Minneapolis, 1995.
Hughes, AJ: Drug treatment of Parkinson's disease in the 1990s. Achievements and future possibilities. Drugs 53(2):195, 1997.
Kulisevsky, J, Avila, A, Barbanoj, M, et al: Levodopa does not aggravate postural tremor in Parkinson's disease. Clin Neuropharmacol 18(5):435, 1995.
Lile, J: Alzheimer's drug update: Learn what drugs look promising. Nursing 27(2):32111, 1997.
McGoon, DC: The Parkinson's Handbook. WW Norton, New York, 1990.
Mistretta, EF, and Kee, CC: Caring for Alzheimer's residents in dedicated units. Developing and using expertise. J Gerontol Nurs 23(2):41, 1997.
Mittelman, MS, Ferris, SH, Shulman, E, et al: Family intervention to delay nursing home placement of patients with Alzheimer disease. JAMA 276(21):1725, 1996.
Moreau, D (ed): Nursing 96 Drug Handbook. Springhouse, Springhouse, Pa, 1996.
National Institute of Neurological Disorders and Stroke: A systems approach to immediate evaluation and management of hyperacute stroke: Experience at eight centers and implications for community practice and patient care. Stroke 28(8):1530, 1997.
van Vugt, JP, Siesling, S, Vergerr, M, Vander Velde, EA, Roos, RA: J Neurol Neurosurg Psychiatry 63:35–39, 1997.
World Health Organization: Dementia in later life: Research and action. Report of the WHO Scientific Group on Senile Dementia. WHO Technical Report Series 730, WHO, Geneva, Switzerland, 1986.
Wooten, C: The top 10 ways to detect deteriorating central neurological status. J Trauma Nurs 3(1):25, 1996.
Wynbrandt, J, and Ludman, MD: The Encyclopedia of Genetic Disorders and Birth Defects. Facts on File, New York, 1991.

47

Nursing Care of Clients with Peripheral Nervous System Disorders

Marsha A. Miles and Deborah L. Roush

Learning Objectives

Upon completion of this chapter, the student will be able to:

1. Identify the disorders caused by disruption of the peripheral nervous system.
2. Describe the pathophysiology, major signs and symptoms, and complications of selected peripheral nervous system disorders.
3. Discuss medical and surgical treatment of selected peripheral nervous system disorders.
4. Use the nursing process to plan care for the client with a peripheral nervous system disorder.

Key Words

anticholinesterase (AN-ti-KOH-lin-**ESS**-ter-ays)
atrophy (**AT**-ruh-fee)
degeneration (de-jen-er-**AY**-shun)
demyelination (dee-MY-uh-lin-**AY**-shun)
exacerbation (egg-sass-sir-**BAY**-shun)
fasciculation (fah-SIK-yoo-**LAY**-shun)
neuralgia (new-**RAL**-jee-ah)
neuropathies (new-**RAH**-puh-thees)
plasmapheresis (PLAS-mah-fer-**EE**-sis)
polyneuropathy (PAH-lee-new-**RAH**-puh-thee)
ptosis (**TOH**-sis)
remyelination (ree-MY-uh-lin-**AY**-shun)
sclerosis (skle-**ROH**-sis)

Peripheral Nervous System Disorders

The peripheral nervous system (PNS) consists of all nervous system structures outside of the central nervous system (CNS). A variety of disorders affect the PNS. Some of these disorders become chronic and cause **degeneration** of body systems. Other disorders are of a temporary nature. Two common types of PNS disorders will be discussed in this chapter. Neuromuscular disorders compose one group of disorders. The second group includes cranial nerve disorders. Both types of disorders present a challenge to the nurse caring for the patient and family.

NEUROMUSCULAR DISORDERS

This group of neurological conditions is chronic and degenerative in nature. Neuromuscular disorders involve a disruption of the transmission of impulses between neurons and the muscles that they stimulate (Fig. 47–1). This breakdown in transmission results in muscle weakness, including the muscles used for breathing (diaphragm, intercostals). Due to the weakness of respiratory muscles experienced by these clients, deadly complications of the respiratory system develop, including pneumonia and respiratory failure. Common neuromuscular disorders include multiple **sclerosis** (MS), myasthenia gravis (MG), amyotrophic lateral sclerosis (ALS), and Guillain-Barré syndrome (GBS). An additional neuropathic disorder is discussed in Cultural Considerations Box 47–1.

Multiple Sclerosis

Etiology

Multiple sclerosis is an autoimmune process. Viral infections, heredity, and other factors are suspected of contributing to the development of MS. However, the cause of

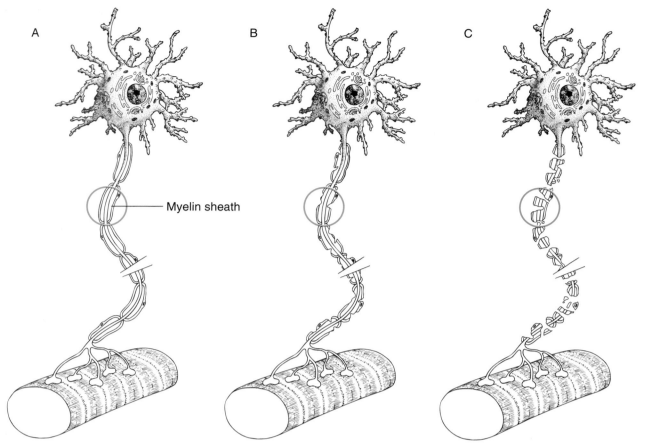

A

B

C

— Myelin sheath

Figure 47–1. The myelin sheath breaks down in multiple sclerosis, interrupting transmission of nerve impulses. *(A)* Normal myelin sheath. *(B)* Myelin beginning to break down. *(C)* Total myelin disruption. (Modified from Scanlon, VC, Sanders, T: Workbook for Essentials of Anatomy and Physiology, ed 2. FA Davis, Philadelphia, 1995, p 109, with permission.)

MS is not known. This disease affects 36 to 80 per 100,000 persons in the United States. Onset of the disease usually occurs between 15 and 50 years of age. Women are affected more than men.

CULTURAL CONSIDERATIONS BOX 47-1

Navajo neuropathy is unique to the Navajo Indian population. Characteristics include poor weight gain, short stature, sexual infantilism, serious systemic infections, and liver derangement. Manifestations include weakness, hypotonia, areflexia, loss of sensation in the extremities, corneal ulcerations, acral mutilation, and painless fractures.[1] Nerve biopsies show a nearly complete absence of myelinated fibers, which is different from other neuropathies that present as a gradual demyelination process. Individuals who survive have many complications and are generally ventilator dependent. None have been known to survive past the age of 24.

Pathophysiology

Myelin is responsible for the smooth transmission of nerve impulses. Muscles contract when nerve impulses stimulate the muscle tissue. If the myelin sheath is damaged, nerve impulses cannot be transmitted to the muscle and contraction of the muscle will not occur. In multiple sclerosis, the myelin sheath begins to break down (degenerate) due to activation of the body's immune system. The nerve becomes inflamed and edematous. Nerve impulses to the muscles slow down. As the disease becomes worse, sclerosis from scar tissue damages the nerve. Nerve impulses are completely blocked, causing permanent loss of muscle function in that area of the body.

Signs and Symptoms

The client with MS will present with muscle weakness, tingling sensations, and numbness. These symptoms may begin slowly over weeks to months or suddenly and dramatically. MS affects many systems of the body. Table 47–1 lists other problems experienced by clients with this neurological condition. A variety of factors can trigger the onset of symptoms or can aggravate the condition.

Table 47–1. **Problems Associated with Multiple Sclerosis**

Weakness/paralysis of limbs, trunk or head	Impaired hearing
Dipoplia (double vision)	Nystagmus
Slurred speech	Ataxia
Spasticity of muscles	Dysarthria
Numbness and tingling	Dysphagia
Patchy blindness (scotomas)	Constipation
Blurred vision	Spastic (uninhibited) bladder
Vertigo	Flaccid (hypotonic) bladder
Tinnitus	Sexual dysfunction
	Anger, depression, euphoria

These factors include extreme heat and cold, fatigue, infection, and physical and emotional problems. Periods of **exacerbation** and remission of symptoms lead clients with MS to be uncertain about when the disease will flare up and what system of the body will be affected. Intense fatigue is a common complaint among clients. Therefore immobility can become a problem. Accidents are common due to muscular weakness of extremities and trunk. Pneumonia can occur from immobility and weakness of the diaphragm and intercostal muscles. Death, usually due to respiratory infections, occurs 20 to 35 years after diagnosis.

Diagnostic Tests

Diagnosis is based on the history and signs and symptoms experienced by the client. MS cannot be diagnosed by a specific test. Analysis of cerebrospinal fluid (CSF) may show an increase in oligoclonal immunoglobulin G (IgG). Magnetic resonance imaging (MRI) may be helpful in diagnosis because sclerotic plaques can be detected.

Medical Treatment

Multiple sclerosis has no cure. Treatment is supportive and symptomatic. Steroids are given to decrease inflammation and edema at the neuron, which decreases symptoms experienced by the client. Immunosuppressant drugs such as azathioprine (Imuran) and cyclophosphamide (Cytoxan) may be given to depress the immune system. Anticonvulsants such as phenytoin (Dilantin) and carbamazepine (Tegretol) help relieve pain. Valium (Diazepam) and physical therapy assist in controlling muscle spasms. Bladder problems are treated with several different medications such as bethanechol (Urecholine), neostigmine (Prostigmin), propantheline (Pro-Banthine), and oxybutynin (Ditropan). Rehabilitation after an acute episode includes physical, speech, and occupational therapy. Rehabilitation therapy assists the client and family in adapting the home environment. Instruction in the use of assistive devices (braces, canes, wheelchairs, splints) by physical and occupational therapists allows the client increased mobility and independence. Clients who develop speech difficulties benefit from speech therapy.

Nursing Process

ASSESSMENT. When assessing a client with MS, special attention should be directed toward what symptoms the client is experiencing. Factors that triggered the onset of symptoms need to be identified. Determining specific areas of muscle weakness, sensation, and potential visual difficulties will dictate what precautions are needed to prevent injuries. Assessing respiratory rate and depth will reveal any potential respiratory problems. Vital signs and laboratory tests can indicate the presence of infection. Frequent skin assessments are important due to risk of skin breakdown from immobility. The client's ability to swallow while eating needs to be carefully assessed during meals because aspiration is a great risk.

NURSING DIAGNOSIS. Priority nursing diagnoses include impaired physical mobility related to muscle weakness and ineffective airway clearance related to impaired ability to cough. Other nursing diagnoses include self-care deficit, alteration in sensory perception, and risk for impaired skin integrity.

PLANNING AND IMPLEMENTATION. The nurse assists the client in activities of daily living (ADL) and other activities to conserve energy. Active range-of-motion exercises should be done at least two times a day to prevent contractures and decrease muscle atrophy. Providing assistive devices for activities helps decrease fatigue and encourages independence, comfort, and safety. If the client is bedridden, position changes every 2 hours prevent skin breakdown and pooling of pulmonary secretions. Assisting and encouraging coughing and deep breathing exercises at least every 4 hours while awake maintains an open airway and prevents respiratory complications. Client should be positioned upright while eating to prevent aspiration. Physical therapy helps relieve spasticity and increases muscle coordination. (See also Home Health Hints at the end of the chapter.)

CLIENT EDUCATION. The nurse instructs the client to avoid factors that can cause an exacerbation of symptoms. The client needs to include rest periods throughout the day to conserve energy. Eating well-balanced and nutritious meals needs to be emphasized. The client should be encouraged to perform exercises to prevent contractures. Skin care and assessment need to be taught to the client and family members. Any infection, especially respiratory, should be reported immediately to a physician.

EVALUATION. Strength and mobility should be maintained or increased. The client should be able to demonstrate use of assistive devices to increase mobility and decrease potential for injury. Breath sounds should be clear with absence of respiratory infection.

NURSING CARE PLAN BOX 47–2 FOR THE CLIENT WITH MULTIPLE SCLEROSIS

Impaired physical mobility related to muscle weakness

Outcomes
Client will identify measures to help maintain activity level. Client will perform exercises that help maintain current activity level.

Evaluation of Outcomes
Can client identify measures that will help maintain activity level? Does client perform exercises that help maintain activity level?

Interventions	*Rationale*	*Evaluation*
• Determine current level of activity.	Provides information to formulate plan of care.	What is client's present level of activity?
• Identify factors that affect ability to be active.	Provides opportunity to seek answers for problems.	Is client able to identify factors that affect mobility?
• Encourage client to perform self-care to maximum ability.	Promotes sense of control and independence for client.	Does client perform self-care activities? Is assistance required?
• Consult physical or occupational therapist to provide assistive devices for walking (canes, braces, walker, and wheelchair).	Walking improves safety of client. Assistive devices decrease fatigue and promote independence, comfort, and safety.	Does client use assistive devices safely during activities?
• Reposition frequently when client is immobile.	Prevents skin breakdown and stasis of pulmonary secretions.	Is client free of skin breakdown and pulmonary congestion?
• Provide active and passive range-of-motion exercises on a regular basis.	Prevents contractures and disuse atrophy.	Does client have any contractures or atrophy?
• Administer medications as ordered (Valium, baclofen, steroids, immunosuppressants).	Valium and baclofen reduce spasticity. Steroids decrease edema. Immunosuppressants slow progression of disease.	Is client free of muscle spasms? Is progression of the disease slowing down for client?

Ineffective airway clearance related to muscle weakness, impaired cough and gag reflex

Outcomes
Client will maintain a patent airway. Client will be free of signs and symptoms of respiratory distress.

Evaluation of Outcomes
Is client's airway patent? Is client free of signs and symptoms of respiratory distress?

Interventions	*Rationale*	*Evaluation*
• Monitor respiratory rate and depth and oxygen saturation.	Increasing respiratory distress indicates progressing muscle weakness that may require mechanical ventilation.	Is client's respiratory rate within normal limits and respiratory effort regular and easy?
• Observe client for breathlessness while speaking.	Inability to speak without breathlessness indicates declining respiratory function.	Is client able to finish sentences without needing to take a breath?
• Elevate head of bed.	Improves lung expansion and decreases work of breathing. Improves cough efforts and decreases risk for aspiration.	Does elevation of head of bed help relieve dyspnea and prevent aspiration?
• Evaluate cough, swallow, and gag reflexes frequently. Notify physician if absent.	Frequent evaluation of reflexes is needed to prevent aspiration, respiratory infections, and respiratory failure.	Is client able to cough effectively? Is gag reflex intact? Does client eat meals and drink fluids without aspirating?
• Suction secretions as needed, noting color and amount of secretions.	Muscle weakness may result in inability to clear airway.	Does client require suctioning to clear airway?

continued

NURSING CARE PLAN BOX 47–2 (continued)

Activity intolerance related to muscle weakness and fatigue

Outcomes
Client will maintain or improve current activity level. Client will participate in rehabilitation program.

Evaluation of Outcomes
Has client maintained or improved current activity level? Is client able to participate in rehabilitation program?

Interventions	Rationale	Evaluation
• Note presence of fatigue.	Fatigue interferes with ability to participate in ADL and other activities.	Does client complain of or demonstrate fatigue with activities?
• Assist client with self-care activities.	Muscle weakness may cause difficulty in performing activities independently.	Are client's self-care needs met? Is assistance required?
• Encourage client to perform activities to maximum of ability.	Promotes independence and sense of control.	Does client perform some activities independently?
• Plan activities with a balance of frequent rest periods.	Decreases fatigue.	Do rest periods after activities reduce fatigue?
• Encourage use of assistive devices for activities.	Enhances independence, safety, and control. Decreases fatigue.	Are assistive devices helpful for performing activities?
• Consult with physical and occupational therapists. Encourage client to participate in exercise program.	Helps develop individualized exercise program and identify assistive devices needed.	Does client participate in exercise program?

See also Nursing Care Plan Box 47–2 for the Client with Multiple Sclerosis.

LEARNING TIP

Myelin facilitates impulse transmission to the muscle. If myelin is interrupted, the impulse cannot get to the muscle efficiently.

Myasthenia Gravis

Etiology

Myasthenia gravis is an autoimmune process. No specific cause has been found for MG. However, current thought is that a virus may initiate the disease. Prevention of MG is not possible at this time. Incidence of the disease is estimated from 43 to 84 persons per million. Peak age of onset in women is 20 to 30 years. MG occurs slightly more often in women than men.

Pathophysiology

Myasthenia gravis is a disease of the neuromuscular junction (Fig. 47–2). At the neuromuscular junction, the neuron releases the chemical neurotransmitter acetylcholine (ACh), which crosses the synaptic cleft. Receptors on the muscle tissue take up ACh, and contraction of the muscle results. In MG, the body's immune system is activated. Antibodies produced by the immune system attack and destroy ACh receptors at the neuromuscular junction. Acetylcholine cannot stimulate muscle contraction because the number of ACh receptors has been reduced, resulting in loss of voluntary muscle strength.

Signs and Symptoms

Myasthenia gravis results in progressive extreme muscle weakness. Muscles are strongest in the morning, when the person is rested. Activity causes the muscles to fatigue easily, but rest allows the muscles to regain strength. Activities affected by MG include eye and eyelid movements, chewing, swallowing, speaking, and breathing, as well as skeletal muscle function. Clients often present with drooping of eyelids (**ptosis**). Facial expressions will be masklike. After long conversations, the voice will fade. Falls occur due to weakness of the arm and leg muscles. Clients with MG experience periods of exacerbation and remission of symptoms, as do clients with multiple sclerosis. Exacerbations can be caused by emotional stress, pregnancy, menses, secondary illness, trauma, extremes in temperature, electrolyte imbalance, surgery, and drugs that block actions at the neuromuscular junction.

Complications

Major complications associated with MG result from weakness of muscles that assist with swallowing and

A

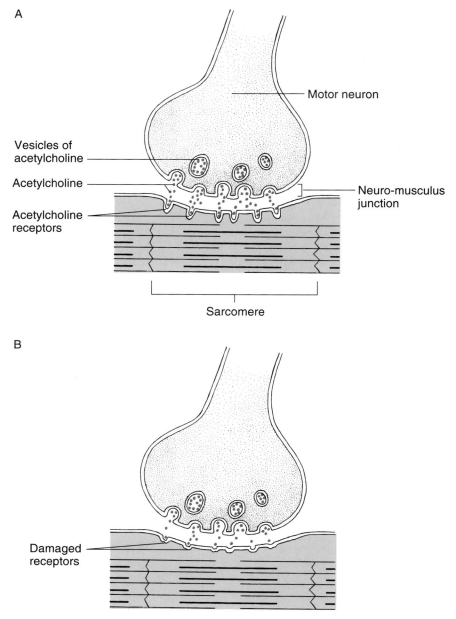

Motor neuron

Vesicles of
acetylcholine

Acetylcholine

Acetylcholine
receptors

Neuro-musculus
junction

Sarcomere

B

Damaged
receptors

Figure 47–2. Myasthenia gravis. *(A)* Normal neuromuscular junction. *(B)* Note damaged acetylcholine receptor sites in myasthenia gravis. (Modified from Scanlon, VC, Sanders, T: Workbook for Essentials of Anatomy and Physiology, ed 2. FA Davis, Philadelphia, 1995, p 97, with permission.)

breathing. Aspiration, respiratory infections, and respiratory failure are the leading causes of death. Sudden onset of muscle weakness in clients with MG resulting from not enough medication is called a *myasthenic crisis.* Overmedication with **anticholinesterase** drugs will cause a *cholinergic crisis* (Table 47–2). Both crises require immediate medical attention.

Diagnostic Tests

Diagnosis of myasthenia gravis is based on history of symptoms and physical examination of the client. A simple test involves the client looking upward for 2 to 3 minutes. Increased droop of the eyelids (ptosis) will occur if MG is present. After a brief rest, the eyelids can be opened without difficulty. Another test involves an intravenous injection of Tensilon (an anticholinesterase drug). If muscle strength improves dramatically, MG is diagnosed. However, improvement is only temporary. If the client's symp-

anticholinesterase: anti—against + cholinesterase—chemical that breaks down acetylcholine

Table 47–2. *Comparison of Myasthenic Crisis and Cholinergic Crisis*

Myasthenic Crisis	Cholinergic Crisis
Cause	*Cause*
Too little medication	Too much medication
Signs and Symptoms	*Signs and Symptoms*
Ptosis	Increasing muscle weakness
Difficulty swallowing	Dyspnea
Difficulty speaking	Salivation
Dyspnea	Nausea or vomiting
	Abdominal cramping
	Sweating
	Increased bronchial secretions
	Miosis (contraction of pupils)

toms become worse after Tensilon is given, the condition known as cholinergic crisis exists. An increased number of anti-ACh receptor antibodies in the blood are present in 90 percent of patients with MG. Electromyography (EMG) may be done to rule out other conditions.

Medical Treatment

As with multiple sclerosis, no cure has been found for MG. Treatment options include the use of drugs and **plasmapheresis.** Removal of the thymus gland (thymectomy) can decrease production of ACh receptor antibodies and decrease symptoms in most clients. Medications used to treat MG include the anticholinesterase drugs neostigmine (Prostigmin) and pyridostigmine (Mestinon). These drugs improve symptoms of MG by destroying the acetylcholinesterase that breaks down ACh. Remember that ACh causes muscles to contract. If ACh is allowed more time to attach to muscle tissue receptors, the muscle will contract and strength will be increased. Steroids such as prednisone and immunosuppressants are used to suppress the body's immune response. Plasmapheresis (similar to dialysis) can be used to remove antibodies from the client's blood.

Nursing Process

ASSESSMENT. The nurse should ask the client about any progressive muscle weakness after activities, what body parts are affected, and the severity of weakness. Strength of all face and limb muscles along with swallowing, speech, and gag and cough reflexes should be assessed. Respiratory rate and depth are monitored. Results of arterial blood gases (ABGs) and pulmonary function tests should be reviewed to assess respiratory function.

NURSING DIAGNOSIS. Priority nursing diagnoses include risk for ineffective airway clearance related to muscle weakness and impaired cough and gag reflex and activity intolerance related to muscle weakness. Other important diagnoses to consider in the care of clients with MG are impaired verbal communication related to muscle fatigue, altered nutrition: less than body requirements related to dysphagia, and sensory or perceptual visual alterations.

PLANNING AND IMPLEMENTATION. The nurse assists the client in maintaining an open airway and addresses activity intolerance using a variety of interventions. Turning and position changes every 2 hours prevent pooling of respiratory secretions. Coughing and deep breathing exercises every 2 to 4 hours promote clearance of secretions. Suction should be available at the bedside. Positioning the client upright at mealtimes minimizes the risk for aspiration. Correct scheduling of drugs should be done so that peak action occurs at times when increased muscle strength is needed for activities such as meals and physical therapy. Frequent assessments of respiratory status allow for early detection of complications. Plan activities for morning when muscle strength is greatest. Encouraging frequent rest periods and assisting with ADL conserves energy. The nurse must be able to distinguish a myasthenic from a cholinergic crisis to determine what immediate actions need to be taken. Physical therapy assists the client and family in adapting lifestyle and home environment to increase the client's independence and conservation of energy.

CLIENT EDUCATION. The client is instructed that nutritious, well-balanced meals provide caloric intake to maintain strength and resistance to infections. Clients with MG should choose foods that are easy to chew and swallow; semisolid foods are easier to chew and swallow than solid or liquids. Clients should be instructed to schedule activities at times when medication is at peak strength so that muscle strength will be increased. Balancing activities with periods of rest helps conserve energy. Avoidance of persons with infections and exposure to cold will minimize risk for respiratory infections, which can exacerbate symptoms and increase risk for ineffective airway clearance. Clients need to be familiar with signs and symptoms of crisis conditions (see Table 47–2) because both crises constitute medical emergencies and require immediate medical attention. Support groups can provide encouragement and assistance to clients and their families.

EVALUATION. The client will demonstrate no signs and symptoms of respiratory infection. Breath sounds will be clear, and respiratory effort will be regular and easy. Client will demonstrate sufficient muscle strength to complete ADL without difficulty.

LEARNING TIP

Rest promotes an increase in ACh, which results in an increase in muscle strength.

---

plasmapheresis: plasma—liquid of blood + apheresis—removal

CRITICAL THINKING: Jamie

Jamie is admitted with complaints of muscle weakness.

1. What history can help differentiate between MS and MG?
2. What assessment can be done to differentiate between MS and MG?

Answers at end of chapter.

Amyotrophic Lateral Sclerosis

Pathophysiology and Etiology

Amyotrophic lateral sclerosis (also called Lou Gehrig's disease) is a progressive, degenerative condition that affects motor neurons. Within the brain and spinal cord, motor neurons begin to degenerate and form scar tissue. Transmission of nerve impulses is blocked. Without stimulation, **atrophy** of muscle tissue occurs. Muscle strength and coordination decrease. As the disease progresses, more muscle groups, including muscles controlling breathing and swallowing, become involved. However, the ability to think and reason is not affected. ALS may have a genetic predisposition in some cases. Symptoms usually do not appear until adulthood. A specific cause has not been discovered.

Signs and Symptoms

Symptoms are vague early in the course of ALS. Primary symptoms include progressive muscle weakness and decreased coordination of arms, legs, and trunk. Atrophy of muscles and twitching (**fasciculations**) also occur. Muscle spasms can cause pain. Difficulty with chewing and swallowing place the client at a risk for choking and aspiration as the disease progresses. Inappropriate emotional outbursts of laughing and crying may occur. Speech becomes increasingly difficult. Bladder and bowel functions remain intact, yet problems such as constipation, urinary urgency, hesitancy, or frequency may occur. Late in the disease, communication becomes limited to moving of eyes and blinking of eyelids in response to questions. Pulmonary function becomes severely compromised to the point of requiring mechanical assistance (ventilator). Other complications that may occur include extreme malnutrition, falls, pulmonary emboli, and congestive heart failure. ALS eventually leads to death from respiratory complications (atelectasis, respiratory failure, and pneumonia). Death usually occurs 3 to 10 years after diagnosis.

Diagnostic Tests

Diagnosis is made from clinical symptoms. Other tests may be done to rule out other conditions (CSF analysis, EEG, nerve biopsy, EMG). Blood enzymes may be increased due to muscle atrophy.

Medical Treatment

Goals of treatment are aimed at improving function as long as possible and emotionally supporting the client and family through the process. Baclofen (Lioresal) and diazepam (Valium) may be given to relieve spasticity. Quinine is used for muscle cramps. Nonpharmacological measures such as physical therapy, massage, position changes, and diversional activities may be instituted for pain control. Tube feedings help provide adequate nutrition. Prevention of infections, such as pneumonia and urinary tract infection (UTI), is vital. Skin care and frequent assessments minimize the incidence of pressure sores. Rehabilitation therapy, including physical, occupational, and speech therapy, allows the client to maximize function and control. Therapy also decreases the occurrence of complications such as aspiration, falls, and contractures. Support groups and counseling provide emotional support for the client and family.

Nursing Process

ASSESSMENT. The nurse assesses the client for fatigue, muscle weakness, cramping, and twitching. Sensation should be intact. Swallowing difficulties should be identified. Respiratory rate and effort, and pulse oximetry if ordered, are monitored to detect decreasing pulmonary function. Skin integrity must be assessed daily. Vital signs and laboratory tests are monitored for infection.

NURSING DIAGNOSIS. Priority diagnoses include ineffective airway clearance related to muscle weakness, impaired cough and gag reflex, and impaired physical mobility related to muscle weakness. Risk for impaired skin integrity and impaired communication may also be problems.

PLANNING AND IMPLEMENTATION. Suction should be available at the bedside in case the client is unable to clear secretions. The nurse or family member stays with the client during meals in case problems with swallowing occur. Semisolid foods should be offered instead of solids or liquids, because these are easier to chew and swallow. Frequent (every 2 hours) position changes promote removal of pulmonary secretions and help prevent skin breakdown. Range-of-motion exercises promote circulation to extremities and prevent contractures. Asking questions that require a yes or no answer or using a picture board can improve communication for the client who has difficulty speaking. A nonhurried, calm, and caring approach while providing care will help decrease anxiety and provide emotional support to the client and family.

CLIENT EDUCATION. Information about ALS and its prognosis should be given to the client and family. Referral to support groups can provide emotional support as the client and family deal with the reality of eventual death. Rehabilitation using assistive devices and exercises will help prevent complications. Teaching family members how to per-

---

atrophy: a—without + trophy—nourishment

form physical therapy and other health care activities allows the client to spend as much time as possible at home. Teach the client to avoid exposure to persons with infections, because an infection can be deadly to the client with a debilitating disease.

EVALUATION. If the care plan has been effective, the client will maintain a patent airway and breath sounds will be clear. No evidence of infection will be present. The client will be free of complications from immobility (pressure sores, contractures). The client will be able to communicate needs effectively.

LEARNING TIP

The individual with ALS has an intact mind—it is the body that is deteriorating.

CRITICAL THINKING: Mr. Miller

Mr. Miller has been having difficulty swallowing. He is diagnosed with ALS.

1. What are the priority nursing diagnoses for him?
2. How can the client and his family be supported in coping with this disease?

Answers at end of chapter.

Guillain-Barré Syndrome

Etiology

Guillain-Barré syndrome is also called acute inflammatory **polyneuropathy.** This term is more descriptive of the actual disease process. Guillain-Barré syndrome is an inflammatory disorder characterized by abrupt onset of symmetrical paresis (weakness) that progresses to paralysis. An autoimmune response to some type of viral infection or vaccination is the most widely accepted theory about the cause of Guillain-Barré syndrome. Usually the viral illness occurs within 2 weeks of the onset of symptoms. Incidence is 1 to 2 per 100,000 people, with men and women being equally affected. Average age at onset is 30 to 50 years old.

Pathophysiology

The myelin sheath of the spinal and cranial nerves is destroyed by a diffuse inflammatory reaction. The peripheral nerves are infiltrated by lymphocytes, which leads to edema and inflammation. Segmental **demyelination** causes axonal atrophy, resulting in slowed or blocked nerve conduction. Typically, the demyelination begins in the most distal nerves and ascends in a symmetrical fashion. **Remyelination,** which is a much slower process, occurs in a descending pattern and is accompanied by a resolution of symptoms.

There are four recognized variants of Guillain-Barré syndrome. The most common form is ascending Guillain-Barré. It is characterized by progressive weakness and numbness that begins in the legs and ascends up the body. The numbness tends to be mild, but the muscle weakness usually progresses to paralysis. The paralysis may ascend all the way to the cranial nerves or stop anywhere between the legs and head. Deep tendon reflexes are either depressed or absent. In approximately 50 percent of clients with ascending Guillain-Barré, respiratory function is compromised.

Descending Guillain-Barré is less common. It affects the cranial nerves that originate in the brain stem first. These clients present with difficulty swallowing and speaking. The weakness progresses downward toward the legs. Respiratory compromise is rapid. Numbness is more problematic in the hands than in the feet, and the reflexes are diminished or absent.

Miller Fisher syndrome, a variant of Guillain-Barré syndrome, is rare. Typically, there is no respiratory compromise or sensory loss. The classic symptoms are profound ataxia, absence of reflexes, and paralysis of the extraocular muscles. Some people believe that the fourth form, pure motor Guillain-Barré, is actually a milder version of ascending Guillain-Barré syndrome. The symptoms are the same, except for the lack of numbness or paresthesias.

Signs and Symptoms

Guillain-Barré syndrome is divided into three stages. The first stage starts with the onset of symptoms and lasts until the progression of symptoms stops. This stage can last from 24 hours to 3 weeks and is characterized by abrupt and rapid onset of muscle weakness and paralysis, with little or no muscle atrophy. Many clients give a history of a recent viral illness or vaccination, supporting the theory that the cause is autoimmune in nature. The degree of respiratory involvement correlates to the type of Guillain-Barré syndrome and the level of paralysis. Clients with ascending Guillain-Barré may gradually notice a reduced ability to take deep breaths or carry on conversations and may feel short of breath. These clients are terrified that they will not be able to breathe. Clients with descending Guillain-Barré may require intubation on an emergent basis.

The autonomic nervous system is frequently affected by Guillain-Barré syndrome. Clients may experience labile blood pressure, cardiac dysrhythmias, urinary retention, paralytic ileus, or syndrome of inappropriate antidiuretic hormone (SIADH). Client complaints of discomfort range from annoying numbness and cramping to severe pain. The discomfort is exacerbated by the client's inability to move voluntarily.

The second stage is the plateau stage, when symptoms are most severe but progression has stopped. It may last from 2 to 14 days. Clients may become discouraged if no improvement is evident.

Axonal regeneration and remyelination occur during the recovery phase. This stage lasts from 6 to 24 months. Symptoms slowly improve.

Complications

Complications that can occur include respiratory failure, infection, and depression. Fatigue and paralysis of the respiratory muscles lead to insufficient respiratory effort. Some clients with impending respiratory failure will attempt to convince the staff that they are not in distress and do not need to be intubated. Discussion of the possible need for intubation early in the client's course is important. Constant monitoring of respiratory parameters and continuous pulse oximetry will provide information indicating the need for immediate intervention.

Clients with Guillain-Barré syndrome are prone to pneumonia and urinary tract infections. Maintaining infection control practices and maximizing the client's nutritional status help decrease the likelihood of infections occurring. Immobility leads to such problems as skin breakdown, pulmonary embolus, deep vein thrombosis, and muscle atrophy. Clients with Guillain-Barré have little time to adjust to their illness and deterioration. They fear that they will not recover function. Calm, supportive reassurance is important.

Diagnostic Tests

A lumbar puncture is performed to obtain CSF. The CSF analysis shows a normal cell count with an elevated protein level. Electromyogram and nerve conduction velocity tests are done to evaluate nerve function.

Medical Treatment

During the first stage clients are partially or completely dependent for all needs. They are often frightened and anxious. In an effort to reduce inflammation, steroids are often administered. Plasmapheresis is used to remove the client's plasma and replace it with albumin. This procedure is thought to lessen the body's immune response. To be most effective, plasmapheresis should begin 7 to 14 days from the onset of symptoms.

During the plateau phase clients may become very discouraged because they are not getting any better. Clients may become fearful and very demanding of attention from significant others and staff. Emotional support is very important during this phase.

Axonal regeneration and remyelination occur during the recovery phase. Intensive rehabilitation helps the client regain function during this phase.

Nursing Process

ASSESSMENT. In the acute phase, assessment of the client is extremely important. The nurse needs to monitor progression of paralysis, assess respiratory function, and monitor ABGs and pulse oximetry. Gag, corneal, and swallowing reflexes should be a part of the routine assessment so pro-

tective interventions can be implemented if necessary. Frequent skin assessments are important due to the risk of skin breakdown from immobility. Abnormal vital signs and complete blood count (CBC) may indicate presence of infection.

NURSING DIAGNOSIS. A priority nursing diagnosis for clients with Guillain-Barré syndrome is risk for impaired gas exchange related to respiratory muscle paralysis. Other related nursing diagnoses include risk for aspiration, pain, and impaired verbal communication.

PLANNING AND IMPLEMENTATION. The goal of therapy is to support body systems until the client recovers. Serial assessments of vital capacity and ABGs will reveal deterioration in respiratory function. Positioning the client in a semi-Fowler's position with the head of the bed elevated at least 30 degrees will make respiratory effort easier and prevent aspiration. Suction must be available at the bedside. Meticulous care must be taken when suctioning or doing any other invasive procedure to prevent infection. Position changes every 2 hours promotes drainage of pulmonary secretions and minimizes the possibility of skin breakdown. Physical therapy, range-of-motion exercises, and proper positioning of extremities help maintain joint and muscle function and minimize the occurrence of other complications of immobility. Pain management includes administration of narcotics and nonpharmacological methods such as position changes, massage, and diversional activities. Nutritional needs may be provided via tube feedings or parenteral nutrition if the client is unable to swallow. Communication boards provide a means for the client to indicate needs to staff. Because recovery can be prolonged, diversional activities such as visits from family and friends, listening to music or relaxation tapes, and watching TV or videos can help alleviate boredom, loneliness, and depression. As the client begins to regain function, the nurse needs to encourage participation in therapy and point out any returning function to the client and family.

CLIENT EDUCATION. All procedures should be explained to the client and family. The client and family need to understand the reasons for continuous respiratory monitoring. Clients may deny any respiratory difficulty due to fear of intubation and mechanical ventilation. Informing the client about the possibility of respiratory support and the measures taken to alleviate discomfort will help decrease anxiety and encourage client cooperation. Information about the disease, treatments, and recovery should be given, because recovery may take months or years. Educating family members about how to perform specific patient care activities will encourage participation and prepare the client and family for discharge.

EVALUATION. If the plan has been effective, the client will not experience any complications due to the disease process.

LEARNING TIP

Guillain-Barré syndrome: muscle weakness **A**scends, then **D**escends.

CRANIAL NERVE DISORDERS

Cranial nerves are the peripheral nerves of the brain. There are 12 pairs of cranial nerves. Areas that the cranial nerves innervate include the head, neck, and special sensory structures. Cranial nerve problems are classified as peripheral **neuropathies.** Disorders may affect the sensory, motor, or both branches of a single nerve. Causes of cranial nerve disorders include tumors, infections, inflammation, trauma, and unknown causes. Two common cranial nerve problems are trigeminal **neuralgia** (tic douloureux) and Bell's palsy.

Trigeminal Neuralgia

Pathophysiology and Etiology

Trigeminal neuralgia involves the fifth cranial nerve (trigeminal). This cranial nerve has three branches that include both sensory and motor functions. The branches innervate areas of the face, including the forehead, nose, cheek, and jaw. Trigeminal neuralgia affects only the sensory portion of the nerve. Irritation or chronic compression of the nerve is suspected as the event that initiates onset of symptoms. The incident rate per year is 4.3 per 100,000 persons. This condition is seen more often in women and usually begins around 50 to 60 years of age.

Signs and Symptoms

Intense recurring episodes of pain, described as sudden, jabbing, burning, or knifelike, characterize this condition. Episodes of pain begin and end suddenly, lasting a few seconds to minutes. Attacks can occur in clusters up to hundreds of times daily. However, some clients experience only a few attacks per year. Pain is felt in the skin on one side of the face. Slight touching, cold breezes, talking, or chewing can trigger attacks of pain. The areas of the face where pain is triggered are referred to as trigger zones. Areas affected include the lips, upper or lower gums, cheeks, forehead, or side of nose (Fig. 47–3). Sleep provides a period of relief from the pain. Therefore persons with trigeminal neuralgia may sleep most of the time to avoid painful attacks. They may also refrain from activities such as talking, face washing, teeth brushing, shaving, and eating to prevent pain. Frequent blinking and tearing of the eye on the affected side also occurs.

---

neuropathies: neuro—nerve + pathies—disease
neuralgia: neur—nerve + algia—pain

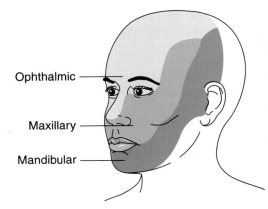

Figure 47–3. Areas innervated by the three main branches of the trigeminal nerve (CN V) are affected in trigeminal neuralgia.

Diagnostic Tests

History of symptoms and direct observation of an attack confirm diagnosis. Radiological studies, including computed tomography (CT) scan and MRI, may be used to rule out other causes of the pain.

Medical Treatment

Initial management includes the use of the anticonvulsants phenytoin (Dilantin) and carbamazepine (Tegretol) to reduce transmission of nerve impulses. Most persons experience relief with medications. These drugs cause bone marrow suppression, so routine complete blood counts are necessary. However, medications do not offer a permanent solution because they lose their effectiveness after a period of time. Another treatment option is nerve blocks using local anesthetics. This option offers 8 to 16 months of relief. If medications and nerve blocks do not provide relief, surgical options are available. Surgery is done to identify and remove the cause of irritation and inflammation of the nerve. Radiofrequency ablation is used to destroy some of the nerve branches resulting in anesthesia of the area.

Nursing Process

ASSESSMENT. The nurse assesses attacks using the WHAT'S UP? format, being sure to include factors that trigger pain. The effect of the pain on the client's life is assessed, including nutritional status, general and oral hygiene, behavior, and emotional state.

NURSING DIAGNOSIS. The priority diagnosis is pain related to inflammation or compression of the trigeminal nerve. Other important diagnoses include altered nutrition: less than body requirements and anxiety.

PLANNING AND IMPLEMENTATION. The nurse should administer analgesics as needed for pain. Alternative pain relief measures such as biofeedback and use of diversional activities may be used in addition to drugs or if drugs do not work. Evaluation of effectiveness of pain relief measures is important. The client's environment needs to be monitored and kept free of potential triggers. The room should be free of drafts and kept at an even, moderate temperature. A private room is preferable. Care must be taken to avoid touching the client's face. Hygiene measures should include the use of lukewarm water, soft cloths, and solutions not requiring rinsing when cleansing the face. A soft-bristled toothbrush or a warm mouthwash can provide adequate oral hygiene. However, the client must be given control over when and how care is provided. Hygiene may be avoided when an attack occurs. Small, frequent meals that are high in protein and calories and easy to chew help meet nutritional needs.

CLIENT EDUCATION. The nurse can instruct the client to chew on the unaffected side and to avoid food and drinks of extreme temperatures. The importance of meticulous oral hygiene should be emphasized. Men need to use electric razors when shaving the face. If corneal sensation is lost, goggles and sunglasses should be used as needed to protect the affected eye. An eye patch may be needed at night to prevent injury during sleep. Protecting the face from cold or windy weather helps prevent attacks.

EVALUATION. The client will express adequate pain relief with a decrease in or absence of attacks. Caloric intake will be adequate to meet nutritional needs. The client will verbalize understanding of the use of measures to prevent recurrent attacks.

Bell's Palsy

Pathophysiology and Etiology

In Bell's palsy, cranial nerve VII (facial) becomes inflamed and edematous, or compression of the blood vessel feeding the nerve occurs causing interruption of nerve impulses. Loss of motor control occurs on one side of the face. Contracture of facial muscles may occur if recovery is slow. The etiology is unknown.

Signs and Symptoms

Onset of symptoms occurs over a 48-hour period. Pain behind the ear may precede the onset of facial paralysis. The client may be unable to close the eyelid, wrinkle the forehead, smile, raise the eyebrow, or close lips effectively. The mouth is pulled toward the unaffected side (Fig. 47–4). Drooling of saliva also occurs. The affected eye has constant tearing. Sense of taste is lost over the anterior two thirds of the tongue. Speech difficulties are present.

Diagnostic Tests

History of the onset of symptoms is used to diagnose Bell's palsy. Observation of the client confirms the diagnosis. An EMG may be done. The possibility of a stroke is ruled out.

Medical Treatment

Prevention of complications is the goal of treatment because 80 percent of clients should have complete recovery

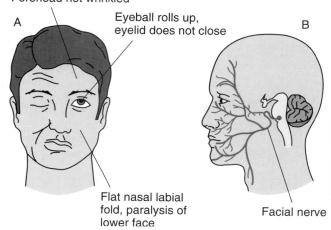

Forehead not wrinkled

Eyeball rolls up, eyelid does not close

Flat nasal labial fold, paralysis of lower face

Facial nerve

Figure 47–4. Bell's palsy. *(A)* Note weakness of affected side of face. *(B)* Distribution of facial nerve. (Modified from Lewis, SM, Collier, IC, and Heitkemper, MM: Medical-Surgical Nursing: Assessment and Management of Clinical Problems, ed 4. Mosby, St Louis, p 1795, with permission.)

of function within weeks to months. However, recovery may take up to a year. Prednisone may be given over 7 to 10 days to decrease edema. Analgesics are given for pain control. Moist heat with gentle massage to face and ear also eases pain. Use of a facial sling will aid in eating and support facial muscles.

Nursing Process

ASSESSMENT. The nurse should assess facial muscles for signs of weakness. Evaluation for other signs and symptoms of Bell's palsy should be done and carefully documented.

NURSING DIAGNOSIS. Priority diagnoses include pain related to inflammation of CN VII (facial), altered nutrition: less than body requirements related to inability to chew, and risk for trauma to eye related to inability to blink. An additional diagnosis would be body image disturbance.

PLANNING AND IMPLEMENTATION. Administration of analgesics, moist heat, and massage can help relieve pain. Eyedrops or eye ointment as ordered by the physician and a patch are used to protect the eye. Facial exercises several times a day will prevent muscle atrophy. Use of a facial sling aids in eating meals and prevents atrophy. A nutri-

HOME HEALTH HINTS

- If the client has difficulty speaking (dysarthria), try using magnetic alphabet letters. Ask questions that require a yes or no answer. The client can respond with the letter y or n.

- Bedside commode lids can be kept up with patches of Velcro attached to the seat and the frame.

tious, well-balanced diet in a consistency the client can tolerate is important.

CLIENT EDUCATION. The client needs to be instructed to chew on the unaffected side. Meticulous oral care needs to be emphasized. Protection of the eye using ointment and a patch needs to be included in client and family education. Clients need to demonstrate facial exercises and the use of a facial sling before discharge. Support from family and friends should be encouraged.

EVALUATION. The client will express adequate pain control. Caloric intake will meet nutritional needs as evidenced by maintenance of weight and normal laboratory values. The affected eye will remain free of injury.

LEARNING TIP

Trigeminal (CN V) neuralgia is a sensory disorder; Bell's palsy (CN VII) is a motor disorder.

Review Questions

1. Tegretol may be given to a client with MS for what purpose?
   a. Decrease inflammation
   b. Depress the immune system
   c. Help relieve pain
   d. Control bladder spasms

2. What medication is used to differentiate between myasthenic crisis and cholinergic crisis?
   a. Prostigmin
   b. Tensilon
   c. Acetylcholine
   d. Prednisone

3. Karesa comes to the clinic complaining of a burning pain on her right cheek. What assessment will help differentiate between trigeminal neuralgia and Bell's palsy?
   a. Tearing of the eye
   b. Application of cold compresses
   c. Asymmetry of facial expressions
   d. Pupillary response

4. What is the primary focus of nursing assessment for a client with ALS?
   a. Skin assessment
   b. Bowel function assessment
   c. Bladder function assessment
   d. Respiratory assessment

5. In planning care for a client with trigeminal neuralgia, what should be your priority nursing diagnosis?
   a. Pain related to inflammation of CN V
   b. Alteration in nutrition: less than body requirements
   c. Pain related to muscle spasms
   d. Ineffective coping related to facial deformity

6. In caring for a client admitted with a diagnosis of lain-Barré syndrome, the nurse should continuous monitor the client for which of the following?
   a. Increasing pain
   b. Urinary retention
   c. Respiratory distress
   d. Blurred vision

ANSWERS TO CRITICAL THINKING

CRITICAL THINKING: Jamie

1. Muscle weakness caused by myasthenia gravis improves with rest.
2. Have client look upward for 2 to 3 minutes. If ptosis occurs, let client close eyes for several minutes. If client can open eyelids and look upward, myasthenia gravis is confirmed.

CRITICAL THINKING: Mr. Miller

1. Ineffective airway clearance related to muscle weakness and risk for aspiration related to muscle weakness. If a client's respiratory system is compromised by a disease, nursing care should be focused on maintaining pulmonary function in order to preserve life.
2. Compassionate care for the client and providing information about the disease and its prognosis to the client and family establishes an honest and supportive environment. Support groups provide resources and emotional support.

REFERENCE

1. Singleton, R, et al: Neuropathy in Navajo children: Clinical and epidemiologic features. Neurology 40(2):363, 1990.

BIBLIOGRAPHY

Doenges, ME, et al: Nursing Care Plans: Guidelines for Planning and Documenting Patient Care, ed 3. FA Davis, Philadelphia, 1993.

Hanak, M: Rehabilitation Nursing for the Neurological Patient. Springer, New York, 1992.

Hoeman, SP: Rehabilitation in Nursing: Process and Application, ed 2. Mosby, St Louis, 1996.

Kuhn, MA: Pharmacotherapeutics: A Nursing Process Approach, ed 3. FA Davis, Philadelphia, 1994.

Lewis, SM, et al: Medical-Surgical Nursing: Assessment and Management of Clinical Problems, ed 4. Mosby, St Louis, 1996.

Miller, CM: The lived experience of relapsing multiple sclerosis: A phenomenological study. J Neurosci Nurs 29:5, 1997.

Pagana, KD, and Pagana, TJ: Mosby's Diagnostic and Laboratory Test Reference. Mosby, St Louis, 1995.

Thomas, CL (ed): Taber's Cyclopedic Medical dictionary, ed 18. FA Davis, Philadelphia, 1997.

Understanding the Sensory System

Sensory System Function, Assessment, and Therapeutic Measures— Vision and Hearing

Debra Aucoin-Ratcliff, Lazette Nowicki, and Valerie C. Scanlon

Learning Objectives

Upon completion of this chapter, the student will be able to:

1. Describe the basic anatomy and physiology of the eye and ear.
2. Describe techniques used in assessment of the eye and ear.
3. Explain the purpose of common diagnostic tests for the client with sensory-perceptual alterations.
4. Discuss nursing responsibilities for preparing clients for diagnostic tests related to sensory-perceptual alterations.
5. Describe care of healthy eyes, including safety and preventive measures.
6. Describe care of healthy ears, including safety and preventive measures.

Key Words

accommodation (uh-KOM-uh-**DAY**-shun)
arcus senilus (**AR**kus se-**NILL**-us)
cochlear implant (KOK-lee-er **IM**-plant)
consensual response (KON-**SEN**-shoo-uhl ree-**SPONS**)
electroretinography (ee-LEK-troh-RET-in-**AHG**-ruh-fee)
esotropia (ESS-oh-**TROH**-pee-ah)
exotropia (EKS-oh-**TROH**-pee-ah)
hearing aid (**HEER**-ing AYD)
nystagmus (nis-**TAG**-muss)
ophthalmologist (AHF-thal-**MAH**-luh-jist)
ophthalmoscope (ahf-**THAL**-muh-skohp)
optician (ahp-**TISH**-uhn)
optometrist (ahp-**TOM**-uh-trist)
otalgia (oh-**TAL**-jee-ah)
otorrhea (OH-toh-**REE**-ah)

ototoxic (OH-toh-**TOK**-sik)
ptosis (**TOH**-sis)
Rinne test (**RIN**-nee TEST)
Romberg's test (**RAHM**-bergs TEST)
Snellen's chart (**SNEL**-ens CHART)
tropia (**TROH**-pee-ah)
Weber test (**VAY**-ber TEST)

Our eyes and ears provide us with a myriad of stimuli and sensory input. It is difficult to imagine what it would be like not to see or hear the world around us. Nurses have an important role in assessing vision and hearing. Clients depend on health care personnel to assist them in maintaining these primary senses.

Vision

NORMAL ANATOMY AND PHYSIOLOGY OF THE EYE

The eye contains the receptors for vision and a refracting system that focuses light rays on these receptors in the retina.

External Structures

The eyelids are the protective covers for the front of the eyeball; on the border of each lid are eyelashes that help keep dust out of the eyes. The eyelids are lined with a thin transparent membrane called the conjunctiva, which is also folded over the white of the eye.

Associated with each eyeball is a lacrimal gland located within the bony socket at the upper, outer corner of the eyeball. Small ducts take tears to the front of the eyeball, and blinking helps spread the tears over the surface. Tears contain lysozyme, an enzyme that inhibits the growth of most bacteria on the surface of the eye. The lacrimal canals at the medial corner of each eye collect tears, which then drain into the lacrimal sac to the nasolacrimal duct to the nasal cavities.

Structure of the Eyeball

Most of the eyeball is within the orbit, the bony socket that provides protection from trauma. The six extrinsic muscles that move the eyeball are attached to the orbit and to the outer surface of the eyeball. There are four rectus muscles that move the eyeball side to side or up and down and two oblique muscles that rotate the eye. The cranial nerves that innervate these muscles are the oculomotor, trochlear, and abducens (third, fourth, and sixth cranial).

The wall of the eyeball has three layers: the outer sclera, the middle choroid (uvea), and the inner retina. The sclera is made of fibrous connective tissue that is visible as the white of the eye. The most anterior portion is the transparent cornea (Fig. 48–1), which has no capillaries and is the first part of the eye that refracts light rays.

The choroid layer contains blood vessels and a dark-blue pigment that prevents glare within the eyeball by absorbing light. The anterior of the choroid is modified into the ciliary body and the iris. The ciliary body (or muscle) is a circular muscle that surrounds the edge of the lens and is connected to the lens by suspensory ligaments. The lens is made of a transparent, elastic protein, and like the cornea,

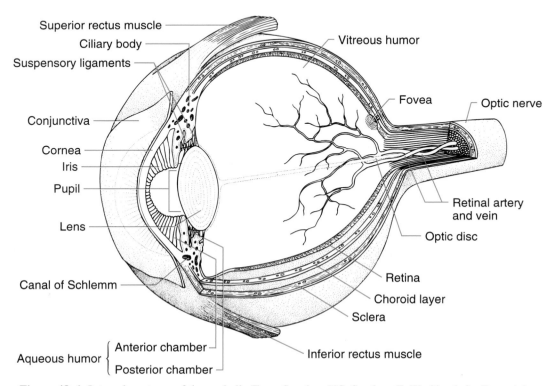

Figure 48–1. Internal anatomy of the eyeball. (From Scanlon, VC, Sanders, T: Workbook for Essentials of Anatomy and Physiology, ed 2. FA Davis, Philadelphia, 1995, p 138, with permission.) See Plate 15.

has no capillaries. The shape of the lens is changed by the ciliary muscle, which permits the focusing of light from objects at varying distances.

In front of the lens is the circular iris, which is made of two sets of smooth muscle fibers that change the diameter of the pupil, the central opening. Contraction of the radial fibers is a sympathetic response and dilates the pupil. Contraction of the circular fibers is a parasympathetic response (mediated by the oculomotor nerves) and constricts the pupil. Pupillary constriction is a reflex that protects the retina from intense light or that permits more acute near vision.

The retina lines the posterior two thirds of the eyeball and contains the rods and cones, the receptors for vision. Rods detect only the presence of light, whereas cones detect the different wavelengths of light as colors. The fovea centralis is a small depression in the macula lutea of the retina, directly behind the center of the lens, and contains only cones. It is therefore the area of most acute color vision. Rods are proportionally more abundant toward the periphery of the retina, and for this reason night vision is best at the sides of the visual field.

Neurons called ganglion neurons transmit the impulses generated by the rods and cones. These neurons all converge at the optic disc and pass through the wall of the eyeball as the optic nerve. The optic disc may also be called the blind spot because no rods or cones are present.

Cavities of the Eyeball

There are two cavities within the eye, posterior and anterior. The larger posterior cavity is between the lens and retina and contains vitreous humor. This semisolid substance helps keep the retina in place.

The anterior cavity is between the cornea and the front of the lens and contains aqueous humor, the tissue fluid of the eyeball that nourishes the lens and cornea. Aqueous humor is formed by capillaries in the ciliary body, flows anteriorly through the pupil, and is reabsorbed by the canal of Schlemm (scleral venous sinus) at the junction of the iris and the cornea. The rate of reabsorption normally equals the rate of production.

Physiology of Vision

Vision involves the focusing of light rays on the retina and the transmission of the subsequent nerve impulses to the visual areas of the cerebral cortex.

The refractive structures of the eye are, in order, the cornea, aqueous humor, lens, and vitreous humor. The lens is the only adjustable part of this focusing system. When the eye is focused on a distant object, the ciliary muscle is relaxed and the lens is elongated and thin. When the eye is focused on a near object, the ciliary muscle contracts and forms a smaller circle, and the elastic lens recoils and bulges in the middle and has greater refractive power.

When light rays strike the retina, they stimulate chemical reactions in the rods and cones. The receptors contain a light-absorbing molecule called retinal (a derivative of vitamin A) bonded to a protein called an opsin. In the rods, for example, light stimulates the breakdown of rhodopsin into scotopsin and retinal; this generates a nerve impulse. Rhodopsin is then resynthesized in a slower reaction. The cones also contain retinal, and similar reactions take place. The opsins of the cones are specialized to respond to a portion of the visible light spectrum; there are red-absorbing, blue-absorbing, and green-absorbing cones. The chemical reactions within the cones also generate electrical nerve impulses.

The impulses from the rods and cones are transmitted to the ganglion neurons, which converge at the optic disc and become the optic nerve. The optic nerves from both eyes converge at the optic chiasma, just in front of the pituitary gland. Here, the medial fibers of each optic nerve cross to the other side. This crossing permits each visual area to receive impulses from both eyes, which is important for binocular vision.

The visual areas are in the occipital lobes of the cerebral cortex. It is here that the upside-down retinal images are righted, and the slightly different pictures from the two eyes are integrated into one image; this is binocular vision, which also provides depth perception.

AGING AND THE EYE

The most common changes in the aging eye are those in the lens. Over a long period of time the lens may become partially or totally opaque. The lens also loses its elasticity with age; most people become far-sighted as they get older and by age 40 begin to need correction with glasses. Peripheral vision losses may occur. Depth perception decreases and glare is more difficult to adjust to, which can affect safety. Color vision fades with poorer discrimination of blue, green, and violet colors. Red, yellow, and orange colors are seen best.

NURSING ASSESSMENT OF THE EYE AND VISUAL STATUS

As with most examinations, nursing assessment of the eye begins with the collection of subjective data, then moves to observation and testing, and finally a more invasive physical examination is performed. LPN/LVNs generally do not conduct invasive examinations on the eye, but rather assist the advanced practitioner in conducting this portion of data collection.

Subjective Data

The nurse interviews clients and collects data about family history that may affect vision, particularly glaucoma, diabetes, blindness, and cataracts. Because many eye disorders are genetically transmitted, this information alerts the nurse to possible alterations in eye health. Clients should be asked about their general health and the presence of diseases such as diabetes and hypertension. The nurse determines the types of medication the client is taking to assess for any ocular (eye) effects. Last, the nurse asks the client about any changes in visual acuity or symptoms of abnormality (Table 48–1).

Objective Data

Visual Acuity

Objective data collection begins by assessing the client's visual acuity. Visual acuity is measured in a variety of ways but usually starts with the use of the **Snellen's chart,** E chart, or handheld visual acuity chart (Rosenbaum card) to test near and far vision. The Snellen's chart is imprinted with alphabetical letters graduating in size from the smallest on the bottom to the largest on the top (Fig. 48–2). The examiner measures out 20 feet and marks the distance on the floor. The examiner then asks the client to cover one eye with a 3 × 5 card or eye cover and then read out loud an indicated line of letters. The lowest line on the chart that the client is able to read accurately is used to indicate visual acuity for that eye. Normal vision is 20/20, which means the client can read at 20 feet what the normal eye can read at 20 feet. Visual impairment occurs at 20/70 and legal blindness at 20/200 or less with correction. An example of findings is the client who identifies all of the letters correctly on the line marked 30; he or she would have a visual acuity of 20/30. This means that the client can see at 20 feet what the average individual can see at 30 feet. The examination is conducted on both eyes separately, then together, and documented as follows: oculus dexter (OD)

20/30, oculus sinister (OS) 20/20, oculus uterque (OU) 20/20. In addition to identifying the eye tested, the examiner conducts the examination with and without the client's corrective lenses, if applicable. When corrective lenses are used, documentation reflects this as OD 20/100 without correction, OD 20/20 with correction. The E chart is used for clients who are illiterate. The client is asked to indicate the direction of the E-shaped figure. The handheld visual acuity chart is used to indicate visual acuity by having the client hold the card approximately 14 inches from the eyes. The test is conducted and documented in the same way as the Snellen's and E chart examinations.

VISUAL FIELDS BY CONFRONTATION. The examiner also tests peripheral vision, which is the ability of the eye to see objects peripherally while the eye is fixed or kept in one position. This is also known as testing visual fields by confrontation. To do this, the examiner compares his or her own ability to see peripheral objects with that of the client. This test should be done with an examiner who has normal peripheral vision. The examiner stands 2 feet in front of the client and instructs the client to cover one eye. The examiner covers his or her own corresponding eye (e.g., if the client's right eye is covered, the examiner's left eye is covered). The examiner uses the arm opposite the covered eye, extends it to the space midway between the client and the examiner, and brings it toward the eye from three directions: superior, inferior, and temporal (middle). The examiner wiggles the finger while moving the arm. The examiner asks the client to look straight ahead and indicate at what point he or she is able to see the examiner's finger. One eye is tested and then the other. The client has full visual fields if the point at which the client sees the finger matches that of the examiner. The examiner documents the

Table 48–1. **Subjective Nursing Assessment Data Questions**

To elicit information about the family history	Do you have any family members with a history of diabetes? Hypertension? Cataracts? Glaucoma? Blindness? Diabetes mellitus? Do any family members wear glasses or contact lenses? Is their vision corrected with the lens?
To find out about the client's general health	How would you describe your general health? What health problems do you currently have? How are they treated? What health problems have you had in the past? Have you ever had trauma to your eyes? What medications do you take? How often do you have eye examinations? When was the last time you had an eye examination?
To elicit information about visual acuity	Do you wear glasses or contact lenses? Have you had any changes in vision such as difficulty seeing distances, difficulty seeing close up, difficulty seeing at night? Do you see things double? Do you have clouded vision? Do you see halos around lights? Does it look like you are looking through a veil or web? Is there sensitivity to light? Is there pain? Itching? Tearing? Burning? Do you have headaches? If so, what are the precipitating events?

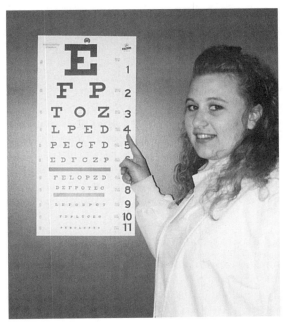

Figure 48–2. Snellen's chart examination.

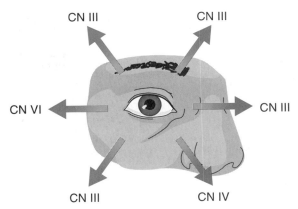

Figure 48–3. Six cardinal fields of gaze.

results as "visual fields equal to examiner," "full visual fields," or if abnormal "visual fields unequal to examiner in . . ." (identify position, e.g., left superior).

Muscle Balance and Eye Movement

The examiner tests extraocular muscle balance and cranial nerve function by instructing the client to look straight ahead and follow the examiner's finger movement without moving his or her head. As with the confrontation test, the client and examiner face each other either standing or sitting. The examiner moves his or her finger in the six cardinal fields of gaze, coming back to the point of origin between each field of gaze (Fig. 48–3). If the client's eyes are able to follow the examiner's finger in all fields of gaze without **nystagmus,** the client is assessed to have adequate extraocular muscle strength and innervation. Nystagmus is an involuntary, cyclical, rapid movement of the eyes in response to vertical, horizontal, or rotary movement.

The corneal light reflex test is used to assess muscle balance. This test is conducted by shining a penlight toward the cornea while the client is staring at an object straight ahead. The light reflection should be at exactly the same place on both pupils. If the eyes lack symmetry, muscle weakness could be present.

The cover test is used in conjunction with an abnormal corneal light reflex test to evaluate muscle balance. The client is asked to look straight ahead at a far object. The ex-

aminer covers one of the client's eyes with a 3 × 5 card. The uncovered eye should have a steady gaze; if it moves there may be muscle weakness. Next, the cover is quickly removed and the action of this eye is observed. If this eye moves to fixate on the light instead of staring straight ahead, it indicates a drifting of the eye when it was covered, which is a sign of muscle weakness. This deviation of the eye away from the visual axis is known as **tropia.** Deviation of the eye toward the nose is known as **esotropia,** movement laterally is known as **exotropia,** and downward deviation is hypotropia.

Pupillary Reflexes

The pupils are observed. They should be round, symmetrical, and reactive to light. To test pupillary response to light, both consensual and direct examinations should be completed. A slightly darkened room works best. The client is asked to look straight ahead, and the size of the pupil is noted. A penlight is shone toward the pupil from a lateral position, and the movement of the pupil is observed. The pupil should quickly constrict. The size of the pupil is noted when it constricts. This is known as direct response.

To conduct a consensual pupil examination, observe the eye just tested for reaction while shining the penlight into the other eye. The observed pupil should constrict. This is known as **consensual response.** Repeat the procedure for the opposite eye.

The examiner now proceeds to test for **accommodation.** Accommodation is the ability of the pupil to respond to near and far distances. The client is told to focus on an object far away. The size and shape of the pupils are observed. The examiner continues to observe the pupils as the client focuses on a near object (the examiner's penlight or finger) held approximately five inches from the client's face. Normally, the client's eyes should turn inward and the pupils should constrict. These responses, convergence and constriction, are called accommodation (Gerontological Issues Box 48–1). Examiners use the acronym PERRLA to indicate *p*upils *e*qual, *r*ound, *r*eact to *l*ight, *a*ccommoda-

---

esotropia: eso—inward + tropia—movement of the eye
exotropia: exo—out + tropia—movement of the eye

Safety Concerns for Older Adults Experiencing Changes in Eye and Ear Function

Because visual accommodation is decreased with aging, there is an increased potential for falls. An older person has difficulty visually accommodating the move from a well-lit building into evening darkness or stepping out of a dark area into the sunlight.

The increased time required to accommodate to near and far along with dark and light is often the reason that older adults do not drive at night. Usually they will complain that the lights of oncoming traffic blinds them or that their eyes do not focus properly.

Deafness or decreased hearing acuity is one of the main reasons that many older adults withdraw from social activities. The loss of high-pitched hearing causes the older adult to hear distracting background noises more clearly than conversation. Older adults who are deaf may require adaptive equipment in their home for safety. The use of a hearing aid can increase hearing for elderly individuals who do not have nerve damage deafness. The use of flashing lights instead of buzzers or alarms increases the safety of an older adult who is not able to hear a smoke detector or fire alarm.

tion. If accommodation is not tested along with the other tests, the examiner may use the acronym PERRL.

Inspection and Palpation of External Structures

The extraocular structures are inspected beginning with the eyebrows. The presence of eyebrows, symmetry, hair texture, size, and extension of the brow is noted. The examiner inspects and palpates the orbital area for edema, lesions, puffiness, and tenderness. Then the eyelids are inspected for symmetry, presence of eyelashes, eyelash position, tremors, flakiness, redness, and swelling. The client is asked to open and close the eyelids. When open, the eyelid should cover the iris margin but not the pupil. The distance between the upper and lower eyelid, known as the palpebral fissure, is inspected; it should be equal in both eyes. If the palpebral fissure is nonsymmetrical, observe for **ptosis,** a drooping of the eyelid, which is commonly seen in stroke clients. Next, the medial canthus of the lower lid is gently palpated and observed for exudate. The eyelids are palpated for nodules while the eye is palpated for firmness over the closed eyelid.

The lower eyelid is pulled down and the client is asked to look upward. The conjunctiva and sclera are inspected for color, discharge, and pterygium (thickening of the conjunctiva). To inspect the upper eyelid, the upper lid is everted over a cotton-tipped applicator. The client blinks to

return the eyelid to its resting position when the inspection is complete.

The external eyes are inspected for color and symmetry of the irides, clarity of the cornea, and depth and clarity of the anterior chamber. Shining a light obliquely across the cornea assesses the clearness of the cornea. The cornea should be transparent without cloudiness. In individuals over 40, there may be bilateral opaque whitening of the outer rim of the cornea known as **arcus senilus.** It is caused from lipid deposits and is considered normal. It does not affect vision. The anterior chamber (the area between the cornea and the iris) of the eye is inspected using oblique light. The anterior chamber should be clear when the light shines on it.

Internal Eye Examination

Examination of the internal eye is done by the advanced practitioner. The LPN/LVN may be required to explain the procedure to the client and to assist the practitioner in the examination. To perform the internal eye examination, specialized equipment must be used. It is useful, but not always necessary, to have the pupil dilated for the internal eye examination. Having a dark room allows the pupil to dilate, as does the application of anticholinergic mydriatic eyedrops.

The instrument used to examine the internal eye is called an **opthalmoscope.** The opthalmoscope magnifies the structures of the eye so the examiner can visualize the retina, optic nerve, blood vessels, and macula. The device is handheld and has a light source that is directed into the client's internal eye. The client should be instructed to hold the head still with the eyes focused on a distant object. The client should be notified that the bright light might be uncomfortable. The ophthalmologist may examine the eye using a stationary device called a slit-lamp microscope rather than the handheld opthalmoscope. The client is seated and rests the chin on a support. This examination allows the examiner to visualize the internal eye by use of a microscope and light source directed into the eye.

INTRAOCULAR PRESSURE. Estimation of intraocular pressure is measured by using one of several types of tonometer. Generally, the procedure is performed with the client lying down, and anesthetic drops may be instilled. One type of tonometer testing uses a puff of air to make an indentation in the cornea to measure intraocular pressure. Readings obtained above the normal range may indicate glaucoma.

Diagnostic Tests

Culture

If there is exudate from any portion of the eye or surrounding structure, a culture may be ordered. Results of the culture determine if antiinfective treatment is necessary.

Fluorescein Angiography

Fluorescein angiography is a procedure used to monitor, diagnose, and treat eye diseases. The client is assessed for dye allergies before the procedure. Then the pupil is dilated and fluorescence dye is injected into the client's venous system. The dye travels to the retinal arteriovenous circulation, and the eye is examined via a slit-lamp microscope. The blood vessels in the eye are extremely visible with the addition of the dye.

Electroretinography

Electoretinography is useful in diagnosing diseases of the rods and cones of the eye. The procedure evaluates differences in the electrical potential between the cornea and retina in response to light wavelengths and intensity. The test is conducted by placing contact lenses with electrodes directly on the eye.

Ultrasonography

Ultrasound is useful as an examination tool when the internal eye cannot be visualized directly due to obstructions such as corneal opacities or bloody vitreous. The eye is anesthetized with instillation of anesthetic drops and a transducer probe is placed on the eye to perform the ultrasound. Clients should be instructed to keep the eye and head still during the procedure.

Radiological Tests

Several radiological examinations are used to assess eye health. X-ray films are used to view bone structure and tumors. Computerized tomography (CT) and magnetic resonance imaging (MRI) are used to visualize ocular structures and abnormalities of the eye and surrounding tissues.

THERAPEUTIC MEASURES

Nurses have an important role in educating individuals, families, and the community about the care of healthy eyes. Nurses often have the opportunity to screen and educate people about the prevention of disease and impairment.

Regular Eye Examinations

Regular eye examinations should be encouraged. Individuals who are not known to have visual deficits and do not have diseases associated with visual loss such as diabetes should have their eyes examined at regular intervals throughout their life. Screening tests are usually done during an annual physical examination to detect gross visual deficits. Clients who wear corrective lenses or have disease processes that place them at risk for visual loss should have their eyes examined by an eye care provider at least yearly.

Eye care providers include the ophthalmologist and optometrist. An **ophthalmologist** is a physician who specializes in the comprehensive care of the eyes and visual system, including diagnosing and treating eye diseases. An **optometrist** is a health care provider who specializes in visual examinations, diagnosis, and treatment of visual problems, such as prescribing lenses. The optometrist is not a physician but is identified as a Doctor of Optometry. An **optician** is a person trained to grind and fit lenses according to prescriptions written by the ophthalmologist or optometrist.

Eye Hygiene

Individuals should be careful to keep debris out of their eyes to prevent scratching of the eye's delicate surfaces. When a foreign object gets into the eye, such as dirt or an eyelash, the individual should be taught not to rub the eye but allow tears to wash the object out. This can be done by pulling the eyelid down over the eye for a brief time. When wiping the eyes, the nurse should wipe from the inner canthus to the outer canthus.

Nutrition for Eye Health

Adequate nutrition is important for the whole body as well as the eye. Nutrition-related eye disorders are common in underdeveloped countries and include disorders related to inadequate vitamin A (corneal damage, night blindness) and vitamin B (optic neuritis). It is also thought that a combination of the antioxidants A, C, and E may reduce the risk of macular degeneration.[1]

Eye Safety and Prevention

Many people in the United States suffer eye injuries each year. Common household activities are responsible for the majority of injuries. Activities such as microwave cooking, lawn care, and shooting rubber bands and BB guns all contribute to eye injury. Many of these injuries could be prevented with education and implementation of safety measures (Table 48–2).

Eye Irrigation

It is sometimes necessary to irrigate foreign bodies or chemical substances out of the eye. The nurse prepares the client by explaining the procedure. Usually an isotonic solution is used to irrigate the eye. Refer to Table 48–3 and Figure 48–4.

Medication Administration

A variety of drugs are available for eye application. Most of the drugs are applied as drops, ointments, or irrigations. The nurse must know the usual dosage and strength, desired action, side effects, and contraindications of the med-

Table 48–2. **Eye Safety and Prevention**

To Protect From:	Use These Eye Safety Measures:
Foreign objects	Wear safety goggles.
	Avoid mowing over rocks or sticks.
	Always wear safety goggles when using lawn edging yard devices.
Chemical splashes	Use splash shields when working with chemicals such as cleaning solution or body fluids.
	Close eyes to avoid getting hair spray in them.
Contact lens abrasions/infections	Follow manufacturer's or eye care professional's directions for length of use and cleaning procedures. Do not overwear lenses.[2]
Ultraviolet light (UV)	Wear UV-protected sunglasses when outdoors.
	Instruct clients to wear sunglasses with side shields after administration of mydriatics.
	Wear hats to shield sun.
Visual deficits in adult with corrective lenses	Update prescription of glasses yearly. Glasses should fit properly, be clean, and be free of scratches.
Eye strain from computer usage	The position of the bottom of the monitor should be 20° below the line of sight and should be positioned 13 to 18 inches from the eyes.[3]
	The light in the room should prevent glare.
	Increase the font size on the screen if letters appear too small.
	If dry eyes are a problem while using a computer, adjust the monitor to a lower level so the eyes do not have to open as wide, which increases evaporation.
Eye injury from sports	Wear protective eyewear with polycarbonate lenses.
	Wear facemasks or helmets in any high-contact or high-impact sports.

ication being administered to prevent harm to the client. Systemic adverse reactions can occur and medical diseases can be exacerbated from the administration of eye medications. The elderly are especially susceptible to this because they have more chronic diseases, as well as long-term use of ophthalmic agents. These agents can interact with other medications the client is taking. The nurse needs to observe clients for possible reactions.

Table 48–3. **Eye Irrigation**

1. Explain the procedure to the client.
2. Wash hands.
3. Gather equipment. For low-volume irrigation, a prefilled squeezable bottle is used. For large-volume irrigation, an intravenous bag of isotonic solution such as normal saline or lactated Ringer's is used. Attach IV tubing to the bag and flush the line.
4. Apply anesthetic drops, if ordered.
5. Place a basin by the side of the client's head and pad the area with towels to absorb irrigant.
6. Apply gloves.
7. The eye may be irrigated by holding the distal end of the IV tubing at the inner canthus of the eye, or a Morgan lens (Fig. 48–4) may be attached. The lens is placed directly on the anesthetized eye and the tubing is connected to the IV bag tubing. Proceed with irrigation using a slow, steady stream of irrigant. Generally, use of the lens is more comfortable for clients because the eyelids do not need to be held open.
8. Assess client's tolerance to the procedure.
9. Remove Morgan lens.
10. Document assessment, type and amount of irrigant, and client's tolerance to procedure.

Chapter 49 discusses specific ophthalmic medications and their uses. Tables 48–4 and 48–5 identify the steps in the application of eyedrops and eye ointments, respectively. Figure 48–5 demonstrates application of eyedrops and eye ointments. It is important to administer eye medications correctly to help reduce the chances of systemic absorption and reactions. Whenever eye medications, especially eyedrops, are administered, the punctum (tear duct) of the eye should have pressure applied to it by either the nurse wearing gloves or the client if able for at least 1 minute. This reduces systemic absorption of the medication via the punctum. Some eye medications can have serious cardiac or respiratory effects, and clients have had life-threatening reactions to them. The nurse should educate the client on the proper instillation of eye medications to reduce these reactions.

LEARNING TIP

Elderly clients, when putting in their own eyedrops, may not feel the drops go in. Teaching clients to refrigerate the drops, if not contraindicated, for 15 minutes to 30 minutes before instillation helps them feel if the drops go into the eye or on the face.

Eye Patching

After treating an injured or infected eye, the physician may order the eye to be patched. The nurse applies ointment or drops if ordered, requests that the client keep

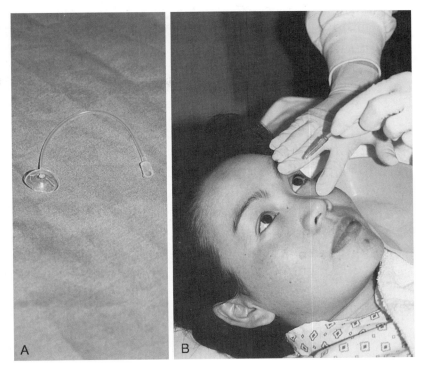

Figure 48–4. *(A)* Morgan lens. *(B)* Irrigation of eye.

the eyelid shut, and then places a disposable, cotton gauze eye patch over the depression of the eye socket. If the client has a deep eye socket, the nurse may need to place two pads over the socket to assist the eyelids in remaining closed. The purpose of eye patching is to protect

the eye from further damage by keeping the lids closed. Sometimes an additional metal shield is placed over the soft pads to protect the eye from external injury. The patch is taped in place and the client instructed to rest the eyes. The nurse should suggest quiet activities to the client such as listening to music or an audiotaped book or sleeping. Watching TV or reading is not recommended because the patched eye will follow the movement of the unpatched eye.

Table 48–4. *Administration of Eyedrops*

1. Explain procedure to the client.
2. Check medication for dosage, strength, side effects, contraindications, and expiration date.
3. Wash hands and apply gloves.
4. Instruct client to tilt head backward and look up toward the ceiling.
5. Gently pull the lower lid down and out. This forms a pocket to catch the eyedrop.
6. Approach the client's eye from the side with the dropper and instill the prescribed amount of medication into the pocket (Fig. 48–5). Be careful to avoid touching the client's eye or surrounding structure with the tip of the dropper. It is helpful for the nurse, and the client who is self-administering eyedrops, to use the forehead as a stabilizing area for the hand administering the drop.[4,5]
7. Release the lower eyelid.
8. Gently apply pressure to the punctum (over the tear duct) for 1 minute to prevent the medication from being drained. The nurse or client can do this. A tissue held against the punctum can be used.
9. Wipe any excess medication off of the eyelids or cheek.
10. Remove gloves.
11. Document medication administration and client tolerance to procedure.

Table 48–5. *Administration of Eye Ointments*

1. Explain procedure to the client.
2. Check medication for dosage, strength, side effects, contraindications, and expiration date.
3. Wash hands and apply gloves.
4. Instruct client to tilt head backward and look up toward the ceiling.
5. Gently pull the lower lid down. This forms a pocket into which the ointment is placed.
6. Express the ointment directly into the exposed palpebral conjunctiva in the direction of inner to outer canthus (Fig. 48–5). Be careful to avoid touching the client's eye or surrounding structure with the tip of the ointment tube.
7. Release the lower eyelid over the ointment.
8. Instruct the client to gently close the eyes.
9. Remove gloves.
10. Instruct client that vision may be blurred while the ointment is in the eye.
11. Document medication administration and client tolerance to procedure.

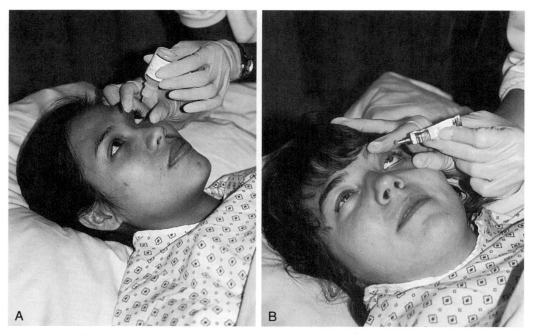

Figure 48–5. *(A)* Application of eyedrops. *(B)* Application of eye ointments.

Ear

NORMAL ANATOMY AND PHYSIOLOGY OF THE EAR

The ear consists of three areas: the outer ear, the middle ear, and the inner ear (Fig. 48–6). The inner ear contains the receptors for the senses of hearing and equilibrium.

Outer Ear

The outer ear consists of the auricle (or pinna) and the ear canal. The auricle is made of cartilage covered with skin. The ear canal is a tunnel into the temporal bone that curves slightly forward and downward. The canal is lined with skin that contains ceruminous glands. Cerumen, or earwax, is the secretion that keeps the eardrum pliable and, because it is sticky, traps dust.

Middle Ear

The middle ear is an air-filled cavity in the temporal bone. The eardrum (or tympanic membrane) is stretched across the end of the ear canal and vibrates when sound waves strike it. These vibrations are transmitted to the three auditory bones, the malleus, incus, and stapes. The stapes then transmits vibrations to the fluid-filled inner ear at the oval window.

The eustachian tube (or auditory tube) extends from the middle ear to the nasopharynx and permits air to enter or leave the middle ear cavity. The air pressure in the middle ear must be the same as the external atmospheric pressure in order for the ear drum to vibrate properly. Swallowing or yawning opens the eustachian tubes and permits equalization of these pressures.

Inner Ear

The inner ear is a cavity in the temporal bone called the bony labyrinth, lined with membrane called the membranous labyrinth. The fluid between bone and membrane is called perilymph, and that within the membrane is called endolymph. These membranous structures are the cochlea, concerned with hearing, and the utricle, saccule, and semicircular canals, all concerned with equilibrium.

The cochlea is shaped like a snail shell and partitioned internally into three fluid-filled canals. The medial canal is the cochlear duct, which contains the receptors for hearing in the organ of Corti (spiral organ). The receptors are called hair cells (their projections are stereocilia), which contain endings of the cochlear branch of the eighth cranial nerve. A membrane called the tectorial membrane hangs over the hair cells.

The process of hearing involves the transmission of vibrations and the generation of nerve impulses. When sound waves enter the ear canal, vibrations are transmitted by the following structures: eardrum, malleus, incus, stapes, oval window of the inner ear, perilymph and endolymph within the cochlea, and hair cells of the organ of Corti. When the hair cells bend, they generate impulses that are carried by the eighth cranial nerve to the brain. The auditory areas, for both hearing and interpretation, are in the temporal lobes of the cerebral cortex.

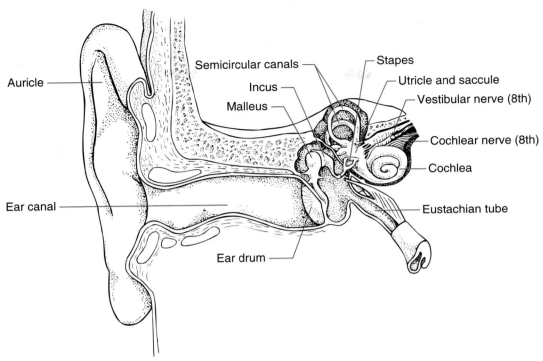

Figure 48–6. The ear in frontal section through the right temporal bone. (From Scanlon VC, Sanders, T: Workbook for Essentials of Anatomy and Physiology, ed 2. FA Davis, Philadelphia, 1995, p 140, with permission.) See Plate 15.

The utricle and saccule are membranous sacs between the cochlea and semicircular canals. Each contains a patch of hair cells embedded in a gelatinous structure that contains otoliths, small crystals of calcium carbonate. The hair cells bend in response to the pull of gravity on the otoliths as the position of the head changes. The impulses generated are carried by the vestibular branch of the eighth cranial nerve to the cerebellum, midbrain, and temporal lobes of the cerebrum. The cerebellum and midbrain use this information to maintain equilibrium at a subconscious level; the cerebrum provides a conscious awareness of the position of the head.

The three semicircular canals are fluid-filled membranous ovals oriented in three planes. At the base of each is an enlarged portion called the ampulla, which contains hair cells (the crista) that are affected by movement. As the body moves forward, for example, the hair cells at first bend backward. The bending of the hair cells generates impulses carried by the vestibular branch of the eighth cranial nerve to the cerebellum, midbrain, and temporal lobes of the cerebrum. These impulses are interpreted as starting or stopping, turning, or changing speeds, and this information is used to maintain equilibrium while a person is moving.

AGING AND THE EAR

In the ear, cumulative damage to the hair cells in the organ of Corti usually becomes apparent sometime after the age of 60. Hair cells that have been damaged by a lifetime of noise cannot be replaced. Sounds in high-pitched ranges are usually those lost first (presbycusis), while hearing may still be adequate for lower-pitched ranges. The high-pitched sounds f, s, k, and sh are usually lost first. It becomes more difficult to filter out background noises, so noisy environments make it difficult to hear conversations.

LEARNING TIP

Presbycusis is the loss of hearing high-pitched sounds (pitch = cycles per second; loudness = decibels). Because the ability to hear pitch is lost rather than loudness, it is not helpful to talk louder to a client with this type of hearing loss. In fact talking louder can make it more difficult to discriminate sounds. It is important to know the type of hearing loss a client has.

NURSING ASSESSMENT OF THE EAR AND HEARING STATUS

A nursing assessment of the ear includes the client's health history and physical examination. A complete nursing assessment is conducted on admission. The nurse provides privacy and makes the client as comfortable as possible before beginning the nursing assessment. A quiet environment is helpful for an accurate assessment of hearing. During the initial assessment, the nurse observes the client's behavior, as well as noting any information the client shares with the nurse.

Subjective Data

To understand the client's ear disorder, the nurse performs a focused health history. The nurse uses knowledge of pathophysiology to guide questions in an appropriate and complete manner. Assessment of symptoms includes asking questions for WHAT'S UP: where it is, how it feels, aggravating and alleviating factors, timing, severity, useful data for associated symptoms, and perception by the client of the problem.

Health History

Obtaining the client's self-appraisal of his or her hearing or related symptoms is completed during the health history.[6] The nurse also gathers information about medications, surgeries, treatments, allergies, and habits. The health history helps the nurse formulate the nursing care plan.

Symptoms and complaints related to the ear include decreased or loss of hearing, **otorrhea** (discharge), **otalgia** (ear pain), itching, fullness, tinnitus (ringing, buzzing, or roaring in the ears), or vertigo (dizziness). If any of these symptoms or complaints is positive, the nurse can explore the symptoms in more detail using the WHAT'S UP acronym. The nurse records all the information accurately and completely.

Other information about the client's past medical history, including asking about previous ear problems and use of hearing aids or assistive hearing devices, is obtained. The nurse also asks about any surgeries, allergies, recent upper respiratory infections, history of infections, injury to the ear, hospitalizations, swimming habits, exposure to pressure changes (flying or diving), medical diseases, and exposure to any loud noises. Positive findings should be assessed using the WHAT'S UP acronym and results recorded.

Information about current and past medications should be obtained. Many medications are potentially toxic to the ear and can cause hearing loss or decreased hearing. The nurse should pay particular attention to any exposure to medications that are potentially **ototoxic** such as certain antibiotics or diuretics (see Chapter 49).

Family history related to ear disorders includes any hearing problems or hearing loss and Ménière's disease. Significant findings are recorded, including the relationship of the family member with the problem to the client.

The nurse also gathers information about the client's care of his or her ears. It is important to assess what preventive measures the client practices and what the client's learning needs are concerning care and protection of the ears. The nurse determines how the client cleans his or her ears, any exposure to loud noises during recreational activities or during work activities, any changes in ability to hear, and any exposure to ototoxic medications. The nurse should determine if the client has had his or her hearing evaluated and if there is a history of ear problems. The nurse instructs the client in ways to care for the ears and maintain ear health (Table 48–6).

Objective Data

Physical assessment of the ear begins by observing the behaviors of the client. The nurse notes how the client communicates. The nurse observes how the client talks, noting any slurred speech or words. Certain behaviors can be early indicators of hearing loss as listed in Table 48–7. Examination of the ear includes inspection, palpation, testing auditory acuity, and, for the advanced practitioner, otoscopic examination.

Inspection and Palpation of the External Ear

Inspection of the external ear begins with examining the auricle. A penlight or otoscope may be used to improve visualization of the external ear. The external ear should be inspected for size, symmetry, configuration, and angle of attachment. The nurse notes any obvious deformities or scars. The skin should be smooth and without breaks, particularly behind the ear in the crevice. The color should be uniform, without signs of inflammation. To inspect the external ear canal, the nurse tips the adult client's head to the side and uses a penlight or otoscope to inspect the canal. The nurse notes any drainage or cerumen (wax), including the color, odor, and clarity of the drainage. The skin should be smooth and without inflammation, edema, or breaks. There should be no lesions, foreign bodies, erythema, or edema observed within the external ear canal. Inspection of the external ear canal should be completed before obtaining an infrared ear temperature because the presence of cerumen can alter the accuracy of the reading.[7]

Next, the auricles are palpated and any tophi, lesions, or masses are noted. Tophi are small, hard nodules in the helix (external ear margin) that are deposits of uric acid crystals that may also occur in gout. The auricle should be nontender when it is palpated; tenderness can indicate an external ear infection. A downward protrusion of the helix, called Darwin's tubercle, is a normal finding. The mastoid process should be smooth and hard when palpated. The mastoid process can be of different sizes but should not be tender or swollen.

Auditory Acuity Testing

Auditory function can be grossly evaluated using three different assessment tests. The whisper voice test is one test to check hearing function in each ear. The client occludes one ear with a finger and the nurse stands 1 to 2 feet away on the opposite side. The nurse whispers two-syllable words toward the unoccluded ear. The client restates the whispered words. The nurse should be by the client's side to prevent the client from lip-reading. The nurse's voice can be increased from a soft, medium, or loud whisper to a soft, medium, or loud voice. The process is repeated on the other ear. The client is asked if hearing is better in one ear than in the other

---

otorrhea: oto—related to the ear + rhea—to flow
otalgia: ot—related to the ear + algia—signifying pain
ototoxic: oto—related to the ear + toxic—poison

Table 48-6. *Prevention of Ear Problems*

Activity	Client Education	Rationale
Care of External Ear	Wash external ear with soap and water only. Do not routinely remove wax from the ear canal.	Keeps external ear clean. The ear is generally self-cleaning. Wax is normally removed during showering. Wax serves as a protective mechanism to lubricate and trap foreign material.
Preventing Ear Trauma	Avoid inserting any objects or solutions into the ear. Avoid swimming in polluted areas. Avoid flying when the ear or upper respiratory system is congested.	Prevents traumatizing the ear and tympanic membrane or exposing the ear to infection. Prevents barotrauma due to pressure changes.
Prevent Damage from Noise Pollution	Avoid exposure to excessive occupational noise levels.	Normal speech is 50 decibels; heavy traffic is 70 decibels. Above 80 decibels is uncomfortable. If there is ringing in the ear, damage may be occurring. Occupational noise is the primary cause of hearing loss.
	Avoid other causes of excessive noise such as use of firearms and high-intensity music. Use protective earplugs or earmuffs if exposure to noise cannot be avoided.	Hearing loss can occur due to exposure to loud noises. Protects ears from hearing loss by decreasing exposure to loud noises.
Early Detection of Hearing Loss	Instruct adults to have hearing checked every 2 to 3 years. Monitor side effects of ototoxic drugs. Instruct client to report any dizziness, decreased hearing acuity, or tinnitus when taking ototoxic medications. Caution elderly clients who use aspirin that it is ototoxic. Instruct client to report to physician any prolonged symptoms of ear pain, swelling, drainage, or plugged feeling. Instruct client to blow nose with both nostrils open during upper respiratory infections (colds).	Degenerative changes occur in the ear with aging. To prevent side effects of medications from causing hearing loss. Elderly clients may have hearing loss and not be able to hear the tinnitus. Many medical problems can be prevented with prompt treatment. Prevents infected secretions from moving up the eustachian tubes into the middle ear.

ear. The client should be able to hear a soft whisper equally well in both ears. Findings of one ear hearing better than the other or inability to hear a soft whisper can be indicative of hearing impairment. Results of the test are documented.

Table 48-7. *Behaviors Indicating Hearing Loss*

Adults with hearing loss may display any or all of the following behaviors:
- Turns up the volume on the television or radio
- Frequently asks, "What did you say?"
- Leans forward or turns head to one side during conversations to hear better
- Cups hand around ear during conversation
- Complains of people talking softly or mumbling
- Speaks in an unusually quiet or loud voice
- Answers questions inappropriately or not at all
- Has difficulty hearing high-frequency consonants
- Avoids group activities
- Loss of sense of humor
- Face looks strained or serious during conversations
- Appears to ignore people or aloof, does not participate
- Irritable or sensitive in interpersonal relations
- Complains of ringing, buzzing, or roaring noise in the ears

A second acuity test is the **Rinne test.** This test is performed with a tuning fork and is useful for differentiating between conductive and sensorineural hearing loss. To perform the test, the nurse strikes the tuning fork and places it on the client's mastoid process (Fig. 48-7). The nurse verifies that the client is able to hear the tuning fork and then instructs the client to tell the nurse immediately when the sound is no longer heard. When the client indicates that the sound is not heard, the nurse places the vibrating tuning fork 2 inches in front of the ear (see Fig. 48-7). The nurse asks the client if he or she hears the tuning fork and then to indicate when the sound is no longer heard. Normally, air conduction (AC) is heard twice as long as bone conduction (BC). The client reports this by hearing the tuning fork when placed in front of the ear (AC) after no longer hearing the tuning fork placed on the mastoid process (BC). Normal results are recorded as AC > BC (air conduction is greater than bone conduction). The test is repeated on the other ear and findings recorded. Abnormal findings can indicate conduction or sensorineural problems. See Table 48-8 for a summary of possible findings.

The **Weber test** is a third test to assess hearing acuity. The Weber test is also performed using a tuning fork. The

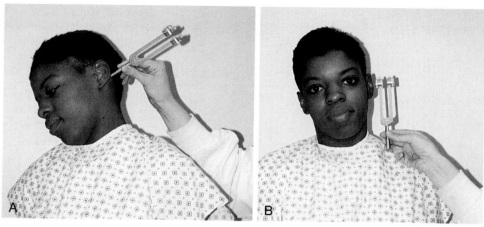

Figure 48–7. Rinne test.

nurse places the vibrating tuning fork on the center of the client's forehead or head (Fig. 48–8). The nurse verifies that the client can hear the tuning fork. Then, with a positive answer, the nurse asks the client if he or she hears the sound better in the left ear, better in the right ear, or the same in both ears. It is important to give the client three choices from which to choose. Normally, the client hears the sound the same in both ears. Table 48–8 identifies abnormal findings.

Balance Testing

When the client complains of dizziness, nystagmus, or problems with equilibrium, the nurse can perform simple tests to assess vestibular function. The first test is simply to observe the client's gait by having the client walk away from the examiner and then walk back to the examiner. The nurse notes the client's balance, posture, and movement of arms and legs. The client should be able to walk with an upright position with no difficulties in balance or movement.

The **Romberg's test,** or falling test, is another simple test to assess vestibular function. The nurse instructs the client to stand with feet together, first with eyes open and then with eyes closed. Normally, the client has no difficulty maintaining a standing position with only minimal swaying. If the client has difficulty maintaining balance or loses balance (a positive Romberg's test), it can indicate an inner ear problem. If a fall appears likely, the nurse should be prepared to support the client to prevent injury.

Otoscopic Examination

An otoscope is an instrument consisting of a handle, a light source, a magnifying lens, and an optional speculum for inserting in the ear. Some otoscopes have a pneumatic device for injecting air into the canal to test the eardrum's mobility and integrity. The otoscope is used to visualize the external ear, ear canal, and tympanic membrane. Otoscopic examination is completed to identify specific disorders or infections, remove wax, or remove foreign bodies. Examination of the ear canal should be completed during insertion and removal of the speculum. The ear canal should be smooth and empty. There should be no redness, scaliness, swelling, drainage, nodules, foreign objects, or excessive wax. The internal otoscopic examination is conducted to examine the eardrum and is done by the experienced practitioner. The eardrum should appear slightly conical, shiny, and smooth and be a pearly gray color.

Diagnostic Tests

Audiometric Testing

Audiometric testing is used as a screening tool to determine the type and degree of hearing loss. An audiologist conducts the hearing tests in a soundproof booth. The audiometer produces a stimulus that consists of a musical tone, pure tone, or speech. To test air conduction, the client is placed in the booth, wears earphones, and signals the au-

Table 48–8. **Auditory Acuity Tuning Fork Tests**

Test	Expected Results	Conductive Hearing Loss	Sensorineural Hearing Loss
Rinne Test	Air conduction heard longer than bone conduction	Bone conduction heard longer than air conduction in affected ear	Air conduction heard longer than bone conduction in affected ear (may be less than 2:1 ratio).
Weber Test	Tone heard in center of the head; no lateralization	Sound heard louder in affected ear	Sound heard louder in better ear

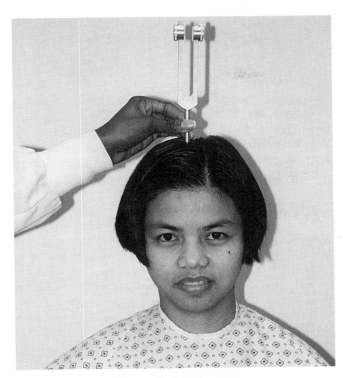

Figure 48–8. Weber test.

Table 48–9. *Common Noise Levels*

Human hearing threshold	**0–25 dB**
Quiet room	30–40 dB
Conversational speech	60 dB
Heavy traffic	70 dB
Telephone	70 dB
Alarm clock	80 dB
Vacuum cleaner	80 dB
Unsafe noise levels begin	**90 dB**
Circular saw	100 dB
Rock music	120 dB
Jet planes	120–130 dB
Pain threshold	**130 dB**
Firearms	140 dB

diologist when and if the tone is heard. Each ear is tested separately as the client is exposed to sounds of varying frequency or pitch (hertz) and intensity (decibels). By varying the levels of the sound, a hearing level is established (Table 48–9). The use of earphones measures air conduction, level of speech hearing, and understanding of speech. During bone conduction testing, a vibrator is placed on the mastoid process and the earphones are removed. Testing proceeds as with air conduction.

A client with normal hearing should have the same air conduction as bone conduction hearing levels. Alterations in testing air and bone conduction hearing can provide information about the location and type of hearing loss.

Tympanometry

Tympanometry is a test used to measure compliance of the tympanic membrane and differentiate problems in the middle ear. Varying amounts of pressure are applied to the tympanic membrane, and the results create a distinctive response recorded on a graph called a tympanogram. The test is useful in determining the amount of negative pressure within the middle ear. The client is informed that the tympanometry may cause transient vertigo. The client should report any nausea or dizziness experienced during the test.

Caloric Test

The caloric test is used to test the function of the eighth cranial nerve. It is used to assess vestibular reflexes of the inner ear that control balance. The test is performed first on one ear and then the other. Warm (44.5°C or 112°F) or cold (30°C or 86°F) water is instilled into the ear canal. This stimulates the endolymph of the semicircular canals, which stimulates movement of the head. A normal response is nystagmus. The client may also experience dizziness. No nystagmus is seen if the client has a disease of the labyrinth such as Ménière's disease. The test is contraindicated if the client has a perforated tympanic membrane. Otoscopic examination should be completed before this test to assess for excessive cerumen or perforated tympanic membrane.

Electronystagmogram

The electronystagmogram is used to diagnose the causes of unilateral hearing loss of unknown origin, vertigo, or ringing in the ears. It is similar to the caloric test. The test is usually completed in a darkened room. Five electrodes are taped to the client's clean face at certain positions around the eye. The electrodes measure nystagmus in response to vestibular stimulation. Measurements are taken at rest, looking at different objects, eyes open and closed, in different positions, with water of different temperatures, and air. Usually tranquilizers, alcohol, stimulants, and antivertigo agents are held for 1 to 5 days before the test. The client should also avoid tobacco and caffeine on the day of the test. The test is contraindicated in clients who have pacemakers. The client may experience nausea, vertigo, or weakness following the test.

Computed Tomography

Computed tomography (CT) produces x-rays similar to those used in conventional radiography. A special scanner system produces cross-sectional images of anatomical structures without superimposing tissues on each other. CT is useful for visualizing the temporal and mastoid bones, the middle and inner ears, and the eustachian tube. The client should remove hairpins and jewelry from the area of visualization.

Magnetic Resonance Imaging

Magnetic resonance imaging (MRI) produces cross-sectional images of the human anatomy through exposure to magnetic energy sources without using radiation. It is useful in differentiating between healthy and diseased tissue.

The MRI allows the membranous organs, nerve, and blood vessels of the temporal bone to be examined. The test is contraindicated in clients with implanted heart valves, surgical and aneurysm clips, and internal orthopedic screws and rods. The client should remove dental bridges and appliances, credit cards, keys, hairclips, shoes, belts, jewelry or clothing with metal fasteners, wigs, and hairpieces before entering the magnetic resonance room.

Laboratory Tests

CULTURE. Culture of drainage from the ear canal or surgical incision is important in diagnosis and treatment of acute infections. Identifying the organism responsible for the infection allows the appropriate antibiotic to be used. Often with chronic infections, the culture is less helpful because gram-negative bacilli cover up the original pathogen. Drainage from the external ear is collected using a sterile cotton-tipped or polyester-tipped swab. Samples should be taken to the laboratory immediately.

PATHOLOGICAL EXAMINATION. Pathological examination of tissue obtained during surgery is completed to rule out a malignancy and identify any unusual problems. A cholesteatoma (cyst of epithelial cells and cholesterol found in the middle ear) is usually documented by a pathological examination.

CRITICAL THINKING: Mr. Frank

Mr. Frank's wife expressed concern about his changing behavior over the last 6 months. She reports that Mr. Frank no longer enjoys talking to neighbors or visiting with friends in their church group, is irritable, has lost his sense of humor, and does not always answer her questions appropriately.

1. What do you suspect is wrong with Mr. Frank?
2. What examination techniques or tests might you use to assess Mr. Frank's signs and symptoms?
3. What would the expected findings be?

Answers at end of chapter.

THERAPEUTIC MEASURES

Medications

The medications most often used to treat ear disorders include antiinfectives, antiinflammatories, antihistamines, decongestants, ceruminolytics, and diuretics. Antiinfectives can be administered systemically or as a topical solution. Ear medications are generally in a liquid form for ease in administration as drops. Table 48–10 and Figure 48–9 guide the nurse in administering eardrops. Antiinflammatories, antihistamines, and decongestants are used with acute infections to reduce nasal and middle ear congestion. Ceruminolytics are used to soften cerumen and re-

move it from the ear canal. Diuretics are used with some inner ear disorders to reduce pressure caused by fluids.

Health Maintenance

Health maintenance focuses on care and health promotion of the ears. Routine cleaning and care of the ears should be taught to all clients. Client education should include prevention of trauma, prevention of hearing loss, and early detection of hearing loss. All clients can benefit from this type of education as found in Table 48–6.

Assistive Devices

Hearing aids are instruments that amplify sounds (see Fig. 49–10). Certain hearing aids may be designed to amplify sounds and attenuate certain portions of the sound signal. A microphone receives the sounds and converts them to electrical signals. These signals are amplified, and a receiver then converts the signal to sound. A small battery serves as the energy source. There are four types of commonly used hearing aids:

1. The in-the-ear aid fits into the ear. It is small and unobtrusive to the wearer and others.
2. The behind-the-ear or postauricular aid is the most common type. This type fits behind the ear and is comfortable to wear.
3. The all-in-one eyeglass aid combines eyeglasses with a hearing aid and is the least commonly used type.
4. The body-worn aid has a fitted ear mold inserted into the external ear and is connected to a receiver. The receiver is wired to a transmitter, which is worn around the neck. The wearer is not able to hide the receiver and wires.

To care for a hearing aid, the nurse should ensure that it is turned off and the battery is removed when it is not in use. This saves the battery and expense for the client, who may be on a fixed income. When turning the hearing aid on, it should be turned up just until it squeals and then turned down until the client indicates it is at the appropriate level for hearing. To clean the hearing aid, the ear mold

Table 48–10. *Administration of Eardrops*

1. Wash hands.
2. Ensure medication is at room temperature.
3. Position client sitting up with head tilted toward unaffected side or side lying on unaffected side.
4. Pull auricle down and back on children and pull auricle up and back for adults.
5. Instill prescribed number of drops, being careful not to touch the tip of the dropper to prevent contamination.
6. Have client remain in position for 2 to 3 minutes.
7. A small cotton plug may be inserted to prevent medication from running out of ear.

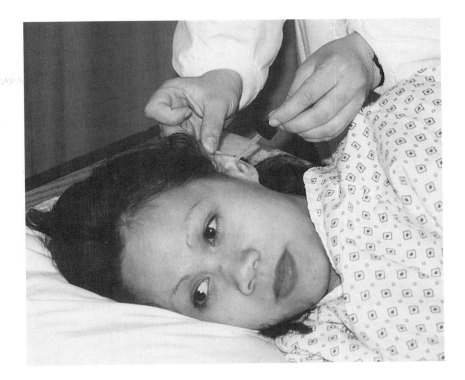

Figure 48–9. Eardrop administration.

portion is washed with either a dry cloth or a damp, soapy cloth and then rinsed with a damp cloth at least weekly. A brush may come with the hearing aid for cleaning, or a cotton-tipped swab can be used to clean the small tip that fits into the ear.

A person who is profoundly deaf and has lost all hearing may use a **cochlear implant.** All cochlear implants feature a microelectronic processor for converting the sound into electrical signals, a transmission system to relay signals to the implanted parts, and a long, slender electrode placed in the cochlea to deliver the electrical stimuli directly to the fiber of the auditory nerve. The electrode is surgically placed. Clients commonly have difficulty understanding and learning speech, even with the cochlear implant.

Diet

The client with an ear problem usually does not have any diet modifications. However, the client with Ménière's disease may benefit from a lower-sodium diet.

Review Questions

1. Which one of the following is the first part of the eye that refracts light rays?
   a. Aqueous humor
   b. Cornea
   c. Vitreous humor
   d. Lens

2. Which of the following are the receptors for color vision?
   a. Optic discs
   b. Rods and cones
   c. Elastic lens
   d. Rhodopsins

3. Which one of the following describes what 20/30 vision indicates for the client?
   a. The client is legally blind.
   b. The client's vision is better than the average person's vision.
   c. The client reads at 20 feet what normal vision reads at 30 feet.
   d. The client reads at 30 feet what normal vision reads at 20 feet.

4. Which of the following should the nurse do to reduce systemic absorption of eyedrops?
   a. Instruct the patient to keep eyes closed for 30 seconds after administration
   b. Apply pressure to punctum of the eye for 1 minute after application
   c. Keep eyedrops in the refrigerator before applying
   d. Have the client look up for 1 minute after application

5. Which one of the following methods can the nurse use to assess visual fields?
   a. Inspection with an ophthalmoscope
   b. Use of a tonometer
   c. Testing vision with a Snellen's chart
   d. Comparing client's visual fields with own

6. Which one of the following indicates where the receptors for hearing and equilibrium are located?
   a. Eardrum
   b. Inner ear
   c. Middle ear
   d. Outer ear

7. Which one of the following tests assesses auditory acuity?
   a. Caloric test
   b. Romberg's test
   c. Rinne test
   d. Tympanometry

8. Which one of the following behaviors is indicative of hearing loss?
   a. Client turns down the volume on the television
   b. Irritable or sensitive in interpersonal relations
   c. Answers questions appropriately
   d. Complains of people talking too loudly

9. Which one of the following is the most important nursing intervention during the Romberg's Test?
   a. Ensure client safety
   b. Whisper softly into each ear
   c. Ensure a quiet environment
   d. Remove all cerumen from ear canal

ANSWERS TO CRITICAL THINKING: Mr. Frank

1. He is exhibiting behaviors of hearing loss.
2. Ear inspection; whisper voice test; Rinne test; Weber test.
3. Inspection of ear—cerumen impaction may be found. Whisper voice test—not heard in affected ear. Rinne test—bone conduction heard longer than air conduction in affected ear. Weber—sound heard louder in affected ear.

REFERENCES

1. Eichenbaum, J: Vitamins for cataracts and macular degeneration. J Ophthalmic Nurs Technol 15:2, 1996.
2. Rakow, P: Identifying and managing complications in soft lens wearers. J Ophthalmic Nurs Technol 16:2, 1997.
3. McHugh, M, and Schaller, P: Ergonomic nursing workstation design to prevent cumulative trauma disorders. Comput Nurs 15:5, 1997.
4. Morlet, MB, and Kelly, M: Improving drop administration by patients. J Ophthalmic Nurs Technol 15:2, 1996.
5. Kelly, M: Medications and the visually impaired elderly. Geriatr Nurs 17:2, 1996.
6. Chen, H: Hearing in the elderly: Relation of hearing loss, loneliness and self-esteem. J Gerontol Nurs 20:22, 1994.
7. Hasel, K: Effect of cerumen on infrared ear temperature measurement. J Gerontol Nurs 21:6, 1995.

BIBLIOGRAPHY

Diamond, J: Systemic adverse effects of topical ophthalmic agents. Implications for older patients. Drugs Aging 11(5):352, 1997.
Fischbach, FT: A Manual of Laboratory and Diagnostic Tests. JB Lippincott, Philadelphia, 1996.
Hayes, D, and Chen, J: Bone-conduction amplification with completely-in-the-canal hearing aids. J Am Acad Audiol 9(1):59, 1998.
Heath, H: Sensory function in older people. Community Nurse 3(11):13, 1997.
Horowitz, A: The relationship between vision impairment and the assessment of disruptive behaviors among nursing home residents. Gerontologist 37(5):620, 1997.
Jaffe, M, and McVan, B: Davis's Laboratory and Diagnostic Test Handbook. FA Davis, Philadelphia, 1997.
Jupiter, T, and Spivey, V: Perception of hearing loss and hearing handicap on hearing aid use by nursing home residents. Geriatr Nurs 18(5):201, 1997.
Larson, P, Hazen, S, and Martin, J: Assessment and management of sensory loss in elderly patients. AORN J 65(2):432, 1997.
Lusk, SL: Noise exposures. Effects on hearing and prevention of noise induced hearing loss. AAOHN J 45(8):397, 1997.
Lusk, SL, Ronis, DL, and Hogan, MM: Test of the health promotion model as a causal model of construction workers' use of hearing protection. Res Nurs Health 20(3):183, 1997.
McConnell, E: Handling your patient's hearing aid. Nursing 26(7):22, 1996.
McConnell, E: Communicating with a hearing-impaired patient. Nursing 28(1):32, 1998.
Noble, W, Sinclair, S, and Byrne, D: Improvement in aided sound localization with open earmolds: Observations in people with high-frequency hearing loss. J Am Acad Audiol 9(1):25, 1998.
Resnick, H, Fries, B, and Verbrugge, L: Windows to their world: The effect of sensory impairments on social engagement and activity time in nursing home residents. J Gerontol B Psychol Sci Sco Sci 52(3):S135, 1997.
Shaw, L: Protocol for detection and follow-up of hearing loss. Clin Nurse Spec 11(6):240, 1997.
Thobaben, M, and Langlois, A: Patients with hearing impairments: Implications for home healthcare professionals. Home Healthc Nurse 14(4):290, 1996.
West, G: Detecting and treating eye problems in later life. Community Nurse 3(5):24, 1997

49

Nursing Care of Clients with Sensory Disorders— Vision and Hearing

Lazette Nowicki and Debra Aucoin-Ratcliff

Learning Objectives

Upon completion of this chapter, the student will be able to:

1. Describe pathophysiology, etiology, signs and symptoms, diagnostic tests, medical treatment, and nursing care for eye infections.
2. Describe pathophysiology, etiology, signs and symptoms, diagnostic tests, medical treatment, and nursing care for refractive errors of vision and blindness.
3. Describe pathophysiology, etiology, signs and symptoms, diagnostic tests, medical treatment, and nursing care for diabetic retinopathy.
4. Describe pathophysiology, etiology, signs and symptoms, diagnostic tests, medical treatment, and nursing care for retinal detachment, glaucoma, cataracts, and macular degeneration.
5. Identify medications contraindicated for clients with closed-angle glaucoma.
6. Describe emergency care for the client with eye trauma.
7. Explain nursing care and teaching for clients with sensory-perceptual alterations or having eye surgery.
8. Describe drug categories for ophthalmic medications.
9. Describe pathophysiology, etiology, signs and symptoms, diagnostic tests, medical treatment, and nursing care for external ear disorders.
10. Describe pathophysiology, etiology, signs and symptoms, diagnostic tests, medical treatment, and nursing care for middle ear, tympanic membrane, and mastoid disorders.
11. Describe pathophysiology, etiology, signs and symptoms, diagnostic tests, medical treatment, and nursing care for inner ear disorders.
12. Describe nursing care for the client with hearing impairment.
13. Identify ototoxic drugs.

Key Words

acute angle-closure glaucoma (ah-**KEWT ANG**-uhl **KLOH**-zhur glaw-**KOH**-mah)

astigmatism (uh-**STIG**-mah-TIZM)
blepharitis (BLEF-uh-**RIGH**-tis)
blindness (**BLYND**-ness)
carbuncle (**KAR**-bung-kull)
cataract (**KAT**-uh-rakt)
chalazion (kah-**LAY**-zee-on)
conductive hearing loss (kon-**DUK**-tiv **HEER**-ing LOSS)
conjunctivitis (kon-JUNK-ti-**VIGH**-tis)
enucleation (ee-NEW-klee-**AY**-shun)
external otitis (eks-**TER**-nuhl oh-**TIGH**-tis)
furuncle (**FYOOR**-ung-kull)
hordeolum (hor-**DEE**-oh-lum)
hyperopia (HIGH-per-**OH**-pee-ah)
macular degeneration (**MAK**-yoo-lar de-jen-er-**AY**-shun)
Ménière's disease (MAY-nee-**AIRZ** di-**ZEEZ**)
miotics (my-**AH**-tiks)
myopia (my-**OH**-pee-ah)
myringoplasty (mir-**IN**-goh-PLASS-tee)
myringotomy (MIR-in-**GOT**-uh-mee)
otosclerosis (OH-toh-skle-**ROH**-sis)
photophobia (FOH-toh-**FOH**-bee-ah)
presbycusis (PRESS-bee-**KYOO**-sis)
presbyopia (PREZ-bee-**OH**-pee-ah)
primary open-angle glaucoma (**PRY**-mer-ee **OH**-pen **ANG**-uhl glaw-**KOH**-mah)
retinopathy (ret-i-**NAH**-puh-thee)
sensorineural hearing loss (SEN-suh-ree-**NEW**-ruhl **HEER**-ing LOSS)
stapedectomy (stuh-puh-**DEK**-tuh-mee)

Nurses interact with clients who have sensory disorders in all phases of sensory loss, including prevention, detection, and treatment. Early detection and treatment of sensory injuries or diseases can reduce the impact that these disorders may have in an individual's life. Any disturbance in vision or hearing disrupts a person's role performance, safety, and activities of daily living (ADL). Treatment for sensory disturbances as simple as glasses for refractive errors or hearing aids may interfere with an individual's self-concept and body image. Nurses play an important role in recognizing symptoms of visual and hearing disorders and in assisting the individual to follow treatment, prevent recurrence, and learn new adaptive skills.

Vision

INFECTIONS AND INFLAMMATION

Infections and inflammation of the eye and surrounding structures can be bacterial or viral in origin. The eye may become aggravated by allergens, chemical substances, or mechanical irritation leading to infection by microorganisms. Mechanical irritation may be caused by sunburn or bacterial infection. Inflammation results from allergies to environmental substances or by irritation of chemical irritants found in perfumes, makeup, sprays, or plants. Viral agents that cause infection include herpes simplex virus, cytomegalovirus, and human adenovirus. Bacterial agents that infect the eye include staphylococcus and streptococcus. The most common type of acute infection is conjunctivitis, which accounts for over two thirds of all acute infections[1] (Cultural Considerations Box 49–1).

Conjunctivitis

Pathophysiology and Etiology

Conjunctivitis is the inflammation of the conjunctiva and is caused by either a virus or bacteria. Viral conjunctivitis is more commonly seen and is highly contagious. It is usually transmitted via contaminated eye secretions that are touched by a hand and then spread to an eye when the hand rubs or touches the eye. The virus is hardy and may live on dry surfaces for 2 weeks or more. This infection lasts 2 to 4 weeks. Bacterial conjunctivitis (commonly called pinkeye) is usually due to staphylococcal or streptococcal bacteria. Conjunctivitis can also be caused from the organisms *Haemophilus influenzae, Chlamydia trachomatis,* and *Neisseria gonorrhoeae.* Conjunctivitis is commonly transmitted among family members and child daycare groups. Interestingly, conjunctivitis may also be caused from the use of nonprescription decongestant eyedrops containing vasoconstrictors.[2] When the eyedrop is discontinued, a pharmacologically induced rebound phenomenon may occur. The eye vessels dilate and may become ischemic. This condition eventually subsides.

CULTURAL CONSIDERATIONS BOX 49–1

Vision

Onchocerciasis, commonly called river blindness, is a filarial (worm) infection in which larvae infect almost all ocular tissues. Blindness typically follows infestation of the choroid, retina, and optic nerve. The disease is spread by blood-sucking insects such as flies, gnats, or mosquitoes that ingest the larvae from blood and then inject another host. This infection affects over 18 million people and is predominant in Africa, South America, and Central America. Of the 18 million infected, 1 to 2 million are either blind or visually impaired. The use of the medication ivermectin has revolutionized the treatment of this disease. Ivermectin is administered annually to the infected individual for 10 years or longer.[22]

Trachoma, a form of conjunctivitis, is a common, chronic disease that affects approximately 600 million people worldwide. It is primarily seen among low-income persons in the Mediterranean, Africa, Brazil, and the Far East.[1] Trachoma is caused by a viral strain of *Chlamydia trachomatis* that is highly contagious. Following the acute conjunctivitis phase, the eyelids shrink as a result of scarring. The shrinking tends to pull the eyelashes inward (entropion), which may scratch the cornea. In addition, granulations form on the inner eyelids. This painful condition may eventually lead to corneal ulceration and blindness. Trachoma is medically treated with topical and oral erythromycin or tetracycline.

Signs and Symptoms

The symptoms of conjunctivitis include conjunctival redness and crusting exudate on the lids and corners of the eyes. Individuals may complain that their eyes itch and are painful. The eyes may tear excessively in response to the irritation.

Diagnostic Tests

Conjunctivitis is primarily diagnosed by symptoms; however, exudate cultures may be collected to determine the exact microorganism responsible for the infection.

Medical Treatment

Bacterial conjunctivitis is treated with antibiotic eyedrops or ointments (Table 49–1). Eyedrops are generally preferred by adults because they do not impair vision. Ointments are commonly used when the eye is resting (at night) or with children, who may squeeze their eyes shut and cry when ocular medications are applied, thus expelling the

---

conjunctivitis: conjunctive—joining membrane + itis—inflammation

Table 49–1. **Ophthalmic Medications**

Drug Type	Uses	Nursing Considerations
Diagnostic Aids		
Fluorescein sodium	Staining of eye. Lesions or foreign objects pick up bright yellow-orange stain so abnormality can be detected.	Stain needs to be irrigated out of eye when examination is complete. Stain is colorfast, so caution should be used when irrigating.
Topical anesthetics	Provides local anesthesia to area, making examination painless. Also used to reduce pain of injury.	Corneal anesthesia is achieved within 1 minute and lasts about 15 minutes. The eye must be protected because the blink reflex is temporarily lost. The lid should be kept closed to keep eye moist when examination and treatment are completed.
Anti-infectives		
Antibacterials	Combat eye infections of bacterial origin.	Clients must be asked about previous allergic reaction to any ophthalmic or systemic medications.
Antivirals	Combat eye infections of viral origin.	To minimize systemic absorption of anti-infectives, apply pressure on tear duct up to 5 minutes after medication is applied.
Antifungals	Combat eye infections of fungal origin.	
Anti-inflammatories		
Steroidal Nonsteroidal	Used to reduce inflammation of the conjunctiva, cornea, or eyelids, due to infection, edema, allergic reaction, or burns.	To minimize systemic absorption of anti-inflammatories, apply pressure on tear duct up to 5 minutes after medication is applied. Long-term use of corticosteroids can contribute to cataract formation.
Lubricants	Used to moisten the eyes in healthy and ill persons. Lubricants maintain the moisture on the eyeball, which contributes to maintenance of the epithelial surface.	Lubricants come in liquid and ointment forms. For clients who have ointments placed in the eye during surgery to prevent eye dryness, client teaching should be done, informing clients that vision will be distorted in the presence of ophthalmic ointments.
Miotics	Used to lower the intraocular pressure by stimulating pupillary and ciliary sphincter muscles. This assists in improving blood flow to the retina and flow of aqueous humor.	There are two types of miotics, which work differently to reduce ocular pressure—cholinergics and cholinesterase inhibitors. Miotic side effects include headache, eye pain, and brow pain. Systemic absorption can cause nausea, vomiting, diarrhea, respiratory attacks in asthmatics, and respiratory difficulty. Pilocarpine, a miotic, causes miosis (contraction of the pupil). Expect to see a smaller than normal pupil with little if any reaction to light.
Carbonic Anhydrase Inhibitors	Used to decrease aqueous humor formation and decrease intraocular pressure. Used primarily for treatment of glaucoma when other miotics have not been successful.	Side effects include lethargy, anorexia, depression, nausea, and vomiting. Do not administer to persons allergic to sulfonamides. Carbonic anhydrase inhibitors may also cause photosensitivity. Use of the medication may cause dry eyes and dry oral membranes. Encourage client to maintain eye and oral hygiene.
Osmotics	Used to reduce intraocular pressure in emergency situations such as acute open-angle glaucoma or used preoperatively and postoperatively to decrease vitreous humor volume, thereby reducing intraocular pressure.	Disorientation, especially in elderly, may be caused by change in electrolytes secondary to use of osmotics. Monitor for headache, nausea, vomiting, and confusion.
Anticholinergic Mydriatics	Used to dilate the pupils for examination or surgical procedures.	If pupils are dilated, they can no longer protect the eye from bright light. Instruct client to wear dark glasses until the effects of the drug have worn off.
Cycloplegics	Used to paralyze the muscles of accommodation for examination or surgical procedures.	Contraindicated in clients with glaucoma because of increase in intraocular pressure with use. Side effects include tachycardia, dry mouth, and symptoms of atropine toxicity.

mydriatics (handwritten annotation)

medication. Viral conjunctivitis is treated by supportive measures, which seek to keep the client comfortable until the infection resolves on its own. Treatment includes eyewashes or eye irrigations, which cleanse the conjunctiva and relieve the inflammation and pain. With either type of conjunctivitis, hand washing is the best means of preventing the spread of the disease. During home care, eyes should be cleansed gently to remove exudate and the cleansing tissues disposed of using Standard Precautions. The tissue should be used on only one eye and then disposed of to avoid cross-contamination. If washcloths are used, they should be laundered after use on one eye and not shared with other people.

Blepharitis

Pathophysiology and Etiology

Blepharitis is inflammation of the eyelids and is most often seen as a chronic inflammatory process involving the eyelid margins. There are thought to be several different etiologies for this disorder, including staphylococcal infection, seborrhea (dandruff), rosacea (a chronic disease of the skin usually affecting middle-aged and older adults), a dry eye, and abnormalities of the meibomian glands and their lipid secretions.

Signs and Symptoms

Blepharitis is characterized by reddened upper and lower eyelids with scales attached to the base of the lashes. The eyelids may appear edematous and sore. Eyelids chronically infected with staphylococcus may become thickened and the eyelashes may be less dense.

Diagnostic Tests

This disorder is diagnosed primarily by symptoms. Generally, obtaining cultures of the eyelids is controversial because most healthy individuals test positive for staphylococcus.

Medical Treatment

Treatment focuses on keeping the eyelids clean by washing them daily with either cotton-tipped applicators soaked with 50 percent strength baby shampoo or sterile eyelid cleanser solutions. Lifelong daily cleansing is important to prevent infection development. If infection occurs, antistaphylococcal antibiotic ointment is applied to the lid margins one to four times a day after the eyelids have been cleansed. The most commonly used antistaphylococcal antibiotics are bacitracin and erythromycin. The treatment may take several months to effectively eradicate this disorder.

Complications

Oftentimes, blepharitis causes some degree of conjunctivitis. If not kept under control, conjunctivitis and blepharitis can lead to the development of more serious eye disorders such as keratitis (inflammation of the cornea).

Hordeolum and Chalazion

Pathophysiology and Etiology

Another type of eyelid infection is a **hordeolum.** An external hordeolum (sty) is a small staphylococcal abscess in the sebaceous gland at the base of the eyelash (either Zeis' glands or glands of Moll). Use of cosmetics on the eyes may be a contributing factor to hordeolum formation. A second type of abscess may form in the connective tissue of the eyelids, specifically, in the meibomian glands. It is larger than an external hordeolum and is called a **chalazion** or internal hordeolum.

Signs and Symptoms

A sty may appear on the palpebral (eyelid) border. It is a small, raised, reddened area. Stys do not cause discomfort; however, the chalazion often puts pressure on the cornea and is more uncomfortable.

Medical Treatment

Hordeolums usually form and rupture spontaneously within a few days and require no treatment. Chalazions may require surgical incision and drainage (I & D) if they do not drain spontaneously. If either type of abscess persists, administration of oral antistaphylococcal antibiotics may be prescribed along with application of hot soaks to assist in the healing process.

Keratitis

Pathophysiology and Etiology

Keratitis is inflammation of the cornea and may be acute, chronic, superficial, or deep. The depth of keratitis refers to the layers of the cornea that may be affected. Keratitis may be associated with bacterial conjunctivitis, a viral infection such as herpes simplex, a corneal ulcer, or diseases such as tuberculosis and syphilis. Children may develop keratitis as a response to vitamin A deficiency, allergic reactions, or viral diseases such as mumps or measles. Herpes simplex keratitis is the most common corneal infection in developed countries; bacterial and fungal infections are more prevalent throughout the rest of the world.[3] People who have dry eyes, wear contact lenses, have poor contact lens hygiene, have decreased corneal sensation, or are immunosuppressed are at increased risk of keratitis.[3] Overnight wearing of soft contact lenses and wearing of disposable contact lenses increase the risk even more. *Pseudomonas aeruginosa* is the pathogen most commonly associated with infection following overnight wear of soft contact lenses. If this infection occurs, the client may be advised to dispose of the contaminated lenses and be treated with antibiotics.

Signs and Symptoms

The cornea has many pain receptors, so any inflammation of the cornea will be painful. This pain increases with movement of the lid over the cornea. Other symptoms of keratitis include decreased vision, **photophobia** (sensitivity to light), tearing, and blepharospasm (spasm of the eyelids). Oftentimes the conjunctiva also appear reddened. In advanced cases, the cornea may appear opaque (cloudy).

Diagnostic Tests

Assessment of keratitis or corneal ulcer is made by use of a slit lamp or a handheld light. The cornea is examined by shining the light source obliquely across the cornea. Oblique illumination allows visualization of opacity in the cornea. Fluorescein stain may also be used to outline the area of involvement. When the stained area is viewed with a blue light, the disruption of the corneal surface is clear. If the client is having pain from blepharospasm, the examiner may instill a topical ophthalmic anesthetic such as proparacaine.

Medical Treatment

Medical treatment includes topical antibiotics, cycloplegic agents, which keep the iris and ciliary body at rest, and warm compresses. If the keratitis is caused by herpes simplex, antiviral medications such as idoxurindine are used rather than antibiotics. If the cornea is severely damaged, corneal transplant may be required. The eye may be patched to decrease the amount of eyelid movement over the cornea during healing.

Complications

Corneal infections are usually serious and are often sight threatening. The corneal tissue may become thin and susceptible to perforation. Untreated, keratitis can cause permanent scarring of the cornea. Significant scarring of the cornea over the pupil results in permanent loss of vision.

Human Immunodeficiency Virus

Pathophysiology and Etiology

Infectious and noninfectious ocular conditions occur in 75 percent of persons with human immunodeficiency virus (HIV).[4] Keratitis, caused by herpes simplex or herpes zoster, is an opportunistic infection that develops because the client with acquired immunodeficiency syndrome (AIDS) is immunosuppressed. Kaposi's sarcoma, non-Hodgkin's lymphoma, and HIV retinopathy are noninfectious conditions. Cytomegalovirus (CMV) retinopathy is a sight-threatening infectious disease involving the retina. It usually begins in one eye and progresses to the other.

Medical Treatment

Pharmacological treatment for CMV includes gancyclovir and trisodium phosphonoformate, both of which require monitoring for bone marrow toxicity.[5] Other treatments include radiation and injection of chemotherapeutic agents into the lesion.

Pediculosis

Pathophysiology and Etiology

Eyelids may be infected with *Phthirus pubis,* the crab louse, which attaches nits (eggs) to the base of the eyelashes.

Medical Treatment

Application of an ointment such as petroleum jelly usually is enough to smother the lice, which prevents reproduction. If necessary, 1 percent lindane cream may be ordered for one application. Contact with the eyes should be avoided because the drug is harmful to ocular tissues.

Nursing Process—Inflammation and Infection of the Eye

Assessment

Assessment of symptoms for any eye problem includes asking the client for subjective data using the WHAT'S UP acronym:

Where is it? What part of the eye is affected? Eyelid, conjunctiva, cornea?

How does it feel? Pressure? Itchy? Painful? No pain? Irritated? Spasm?

Aggravating and alleviating factors. Worse when rubbing eyes, blinking? Photosensitivity?

Timing. Was there exposure to a pathogen? Previous infection or irritation? Length of time symptoms have persisted?

Severity. Is there visual impairment? Does pain affect ADL?

Useful data for associated symptoms. Is client infected with lice? Immunosuppression? Do other members of the family or peer group have symptoms? Are decongestant eyedrops used? Is there exudate? Are the eyelids stuck together on awakening? Does client wear contact lenses, soft contact lenses overnight, disposable contact lenses? Does client have dry eyes? Infection with tuberculosis, syphilis, HIV? What is typical eye hygiene?

Perception by the client of the problem. What does client think is wrong?

Objective assessment data collected by the nurse include the condition of conjunctiva, the condition of eyelids and eyelashes, the presence of exudate, whether tearing is occurring, any visible abscess on palpebral border, a palpable

---

photophobia: photo—light + phobia—fear of

abscess in eyelid, opacity of the cornea, and visual acuity testing comparing unaffected and affected eyes.

Nursing Diagnosis

The major nursing diagnoses for inflammation and infection of the eye include but are not limited to the following:

- Pain related to inflammation or infection of the eye or surrounding tissues
- Sensory-perceptual alteration (visual) related to blepharospasm, photophobia, diminished visual acuity (corneal opacity, eye patching), visual distortions (exudate, ophthalmic ointment)
- Risk for injury related to visual impairment
- Risk for infection related to poor eye hygiene, use of contact lenses
- Knowledge deficit related to disease process, prevention, and treatment

Planning

The client and family are included in the planning phase. Planning focuses on helping clients return to their preillness state and preventing any further eye disorders. Client goals include the following:

- States pain is decreased or acceptable on a scale of 1 (low) to 10 (severe)
- Vision returns to preillness state
- Does not become injured as a result of impairment
- Does not develop infection
- Explains disease process, prevention, and treatment measures
- Demonstrates treatment regimen correctly, such as administration of eyedrops

Nursing Interventions

Nursing care focuses on relieving the client's pain, promoting safety, maintaining eye function, educating the client about the disorder, application of medication if ordered, eye hygiene, and preventive eye care.

The client should be assessed for pain using objective and subjective cues. Use of dark glasses, rubbing the eye, squinting, and avoiding light are nonverbal indicators of pain that should also be assessed. Eye pain is generally treated with topical anesthetic drops or ointments, antibiotics, and antiinflammatory agents. Warm or cool packs may also assist in soothing the eye. Patching of the effected eye also helps reduce pain by decreasing the movement of the eye across the eyelid. For severe pain, analgesics may also be prescribed. The nurse and client should also explore methods of pain reduction such as guided imagery, relaxation techniques, music, or distraction.

Visual impairment of any type raises safety concerns for the client. The nurse must promote safety by assessing any visual impairment that may be present. Inflamed eyes often do not focus well and may have exudate, tearing, or ointment present, which interfere with vision. Clients with one eye patched should be advised that depth perception is al-tered and they should not drive. They must be taught to be cautious and careful when ambulating and reaching for things.

Interventions to maintain eye function must be implemented. If the client is to rest the eye, reading and television should be discouraged because they require use of the eyes. Quiet activity, which can be carried out with the eyes closed, is best. Listening to music, radio, or an audiorecorded book may provide distraction and rest for the eye. Contact lenses should be avoided when the eye or surrounding structure is inflamed. When the eye has healed and infection is gone, contact wear can usually be resumed. Contact lenses must be sterilized before use to prevent reinfection of the eye. Soft contact lenses that cannot be sterilized need to be discarded.

The nurse is responsible for educating the client in prevention, care of the affected eye, medication administration, safety issues, and outcomes. Clients should demonstrate the administration of ointments or drops after teaching has occurred. The client and family are taught how to prevent spreading the infection if it is contagious. The nurse also teaches the client how to maintain good eye hygiene to prevent further complications.

Evaluation

The goals for the client are met if the following occur:

- Pain is reduced to a lower acceptable rating
- Vision improves or returns to preillness level
- Injury does not occur as a result of visual impairment
- Infection does not occur as a result of poor eye hygiene or contact lens wear
- Explains disease process, prevention, or treatment regimen accurately
- Prescribed treatment is stated or demonstrated correctly (e.g., administering eyedrops or ointments)

REFRACTIVE ERRORS

Pathophysiology and Etiology

Refraction refers to the bending of light rays as they enter the eye. Emmetropia, or normal vision, means that light rays are bent to focus images precisely on the macula of the retina. An emmetrope is a person with normal vision. **Ametropia** is a term used to describe any refractive error. When an image is not clearly focused on the retina, refractive error is present. Refractive errors account for the largest number of impairments in vision. Ametropia occurs when parallel light rays entering the eye are not refracted to focus on the retina. There are four common ametropic disorders: **myopia, hyperopia, astigmatism,** and **presbyopia.**

---

ametropia: ametro—disproportionate + opia—concerning vision
presbyopia: presby—old age + opia—concerning vision

Hyperopia, also known as farsightedness, is caused by light rays focusing behind the retina (see Fig. 49–1). People who are hyperopic see images that are far away more clearly than images that are close. Physiologically, the globe or eyeball is too short from the front to the back, causing the light rays to focus beyond the retina. Hyperopia is often associated with primary angle-closure glaucoma and aging.[6] Hyperopia can be corrected with convex lenses.

Myopia, commonly referred to as nearsightedness, is caused by light rays focusing in front of the retina (Fig. 49–1). The eyeball is elongated and thus the light rays do not reach the retina. Persons with myopia hold things close to their eyes to see them well. Distance vision is blurred. Myopia can be corrected with concave lenses.

Astigmatism results from unequal curvatures in the shape of the cornea. When parallel light rays enter the eye, the irregular cornea causes the light rays to be refracted to focus on two different points. This can result in either myopic or hyperopic astigmatism. The person with astigmatism has blurred vision with distortion. The corneal irregularities can be caused by injury, inflammation, corneal surgery, or an inherited autosomal dominant trait.

Presbyopia is a condition in which the crystalline lenses lose their elasticity, resulting in a decrease in ability to focus on close objects. The loss of elasticity causes light rays to focus beyond the retina, resulting in hyperopia. This condition usually is associated with aging and generally occurs after age 40. If an individual has preexisting hyperopia, the onset of presbyopia may occur earlier than 40 years. Likewise, if an individual has myopia, presbyopia may correct the myopia by projecting the light rays directly on the retina. Because accommodation for close vision is accomplished by lens contraction, people with presbyopia exhibit the inability to see objects at close range. They often compensate for blurred close vision by holding objects to be viewed further away. Complaints of eyestrain and mild frontal headache are common. These symptoms are relieved with eye rest and corrective lenses.

Signs and Symptoms

Individuals with refractive errors often complain of difficulty reading or seeing objects. Often the eyestrain that occurs as one attempts to improve visual acuity causes headache. The nurse may observe myopic individuals holding reading material close to the eyes. Hyperopic individuals may hold reading materials far away from their eyes.

Diagnostic Tests

A refractive error may be roughly estimated by use of a Snellen's chart or by comparing the individual's vision at different distances and comparing it with that of the examiner. To obtain a more definitive refractive error measurement, a retinoscopic examination is necessary. Before this examination, a cycloplegic drug is often instilled (see Table 49–1). A cycloplegic drug dilates the pupil and temporarily paralyzes the ciliary muscle, thus preventing accommodation. During the examination, an ophthalmologist or optometrist examines the internal and external eye and uses trial lenses via a retinoscope to assess the type of lens best suited to correct the refractive error. If convex-shaped trial lenses correct the focusing power of the eyes,

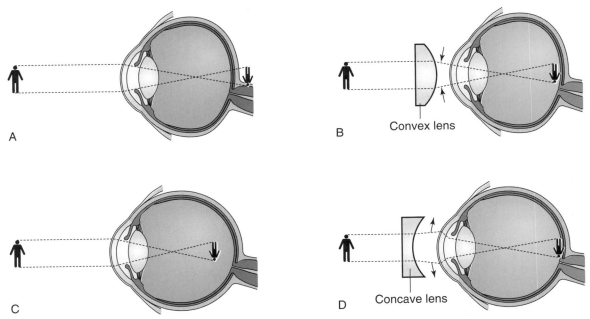

Figure 49–1. Refractive disorders. *(A)* Hyperopia. *(B)* Corrected hyperopia. *(C)* Myopia. *(D)* Corrected myopia.

the client is determined to be hyperopic. If concave-shaped trial lenses correct the focusing power, the client is said to be myopic. The amount of focusing power needed in the trial lens to correct the visual defect indicates the degree of refractive error. Left and right eyes of the same person may not have the same degree of refractive error. If a cycloplegic agent has been used, clients need to be told that blurred vision will be present and sunglasses need to be worn until the agent wears off. In addition, the client should be instructed that driving and reading is not possible until the effect of the cycloplegic drug is diminished.

Medical and Surgical Treatment

Refractive errors are commonly treated with corrective lenses, either eyeglasses or contact lenses. The lenses bend the parallel light rays so that they converge on the macula portion of the retina. Incisional radial keratotomy and photorefractive keratectomy (PRK) are surgical procedures that have been shown to be somewhat successful at correcting refractive error. With incisional radial keratotomy, surgical incisions are made on the cornea to reshape it. PRK utilizes laser technology (Table 49–2) to accomplish the same goal, reshaping of the cornea. The cornea is made flatter for individuals with myopia and more cone shaped for those with hyperopia.[7]

LEARNING TIP

To remember the normal type of vision a person has, use this saying: "You are what you say." For example, If you say "you are farsighted," this means that you have clear vision of far away images but difficulty seeing images that are nearer. If you say "you are nearsighted," this means that you have clear vision of near images but difficulty seeing images that are farther away.

Complications

Complications of corrective lens use are primarily related to safety. Eyeglasses can be broken. Eyeglass lenses can be made with special polymers that do not break as easily as

Table 49–2. Laser Treatment

Laser is an acronym for light amplification by stimulated emission of radiation. Lasers are devices that amplify light and produce synchronized light waves. Lasers are based on the principle that atoms, molecules, and ions can be excited by absorption of thermal, electrical, or light energy. After this energy is absorbed, the atoms, molecules, or ions give off a beam of synchronized light waves. By using this extremely intense, highly directional, pure-colored light, lasers can be used for a variety of purposes such as making incisions, removing tissue, or stopping bleeding.

---

traditional glass. It is a myth that if corrective lenses are not worn, vision becomes worse. Complications of contact lens use include corneal abrasions, infections, and keratitis. Incisional radial keratotomy and PRK both have surgical risks and are not always successful. Some individuals report a worsening of their vision after this surgery.

BLINDNESS

Blindness is described in many terms often reflective of the degree of visual impairment an individual has. Generally, blindness is the complete or almost complete absence of the sense of sight. Terms such as *profound blindness, partially sighted,* and *blind* may all have different meanings. Some people consider the terms *blind* and *partially sighted* to be negative and prefer the term *visually impaired* to describe their condition.

Pathophysiology and Etiology

Few people are born blind. Blindness is caused by a variety of factors, including trauma, complications from various diseases such as hypertension and diabetes, conditions such as cataracts and glaucoma, and in children malnutrition, infectious diseases, and parasitic infestations. Blindness is caused by any obstacle to the rays of light on their way to the optic nerve or by disease of the optic nerve or tract of the part of the brain connected with vision. It may be permanent or transient, complete or partial, or occur only in darkness (night blindness). In the United States, it is estimated that 10 million people are blind, even when wearing their glasses.[8] There are blind people in every age-group, but about half of the blind people in the United States are older adults.[8]

Signs and Symptoms

Aside from a general loss of vision, clients may describe their visual image as blurred, distorted, or absent in specific areas of the visual field. Objects may appear dark or absent around the peripheral field in glaucoma or retinitis pigmentosa. Retinitis pigmentosa causes this visual disturbance because the pigmented layer of the retina has degenerated. The center of the visual field may appear dark for individuals with diabetic retinopathy or macular degeneration. Half of the visual field may be impaired in clients with hemianopia. This results from a defect in the optic pathways in the brain and is often seen with stroke. Clients may report that the visual field appears blurry or hazy in corneal visual problems, cataracts, diabetic retinopathy, or refractive errors (Fig. 49–2).

Diagnostic Tests

Diagnostic tests are usually done to determine the exact cause of the blindness. A visual field examination is used

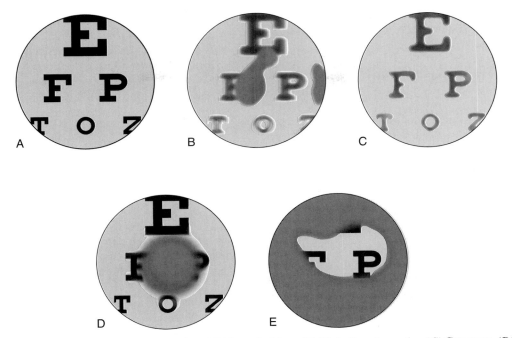

Figure 49–2. Visual field abnormalities. *(A)* Normal vision. *(B)* Diabetic retinopathy. *(C)* Cataracts. *(D)* Macular degeneration. *(E)* Advanced glaucoma.

to detect gaps in the visual field. Tonometry is performed to measure the intraocular pressure (Fig. 49–3). A slit lamp examination allows the examiner to microscopically examine the surface of the eye, the cornea, and the anterior segment of the eye. Retinal angiography is used to follow blood flow through the retinal vessels and to detect vascular changes. Ultrasonography may be used to visualize changes in the posterior eye that cannot be directly exam-

ined because of other pathology such as a cloudy cornea, bloody vitreous, or an opaque lens.

Medical Treatment

Medical treatment for blindness centers on treating the underlying condition and prevention of further impairment. Depending on the cause of the blindness, treatment may include

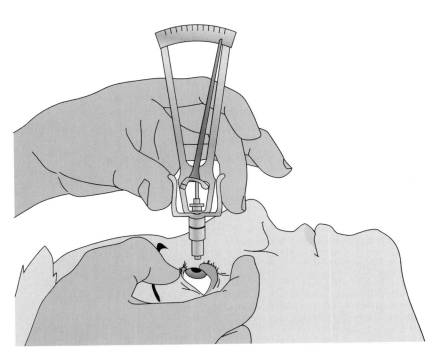

Figure 49–3. Tonometry to measure intraocular eye pressure.

medication prescription, surgical intervention, corrective eyewear prescription, and referral to supportive services.

Nursing Process for Visual Impairment

Assessment

Collection of subjective data for assessment of visual impairment can be made using the WHAT'S UP acronym:

Where is it? What part of the visual field is affected? If there is vision, what are the characteristics of what can be seen? Blurry? Hazy? Dark? Halos around lights?

How does it feel? Is there associated pain with the visual impairment? Headaches? How do you feel? Fearful? Anxious? Depressed? Helpless? Hopeless? Accepting?

Aggravating and alleviating factors. Is it worse when reading? Is it worse when watching TV? Does it affect the client only at night? Is vision better at distances or close up?

Timing. When did the symptoms start? Do they come and go? Is the impairment progressively getting worse? Was onset sudden?

Severity. Does the impairment affect the client's activities of daily living? If so, how severely? Does the client need assistance to cook, dress, bathe, read mail, pay bills, access health care, obtain transportation, maintain a household, shop?

Useful data for associated symptoms. Does the client have diabetes, hypertension, a family history of retinitis pigmentosa, a history of eye infection, or eye trauma? Has the client recently traveled out of the country?

Perception of the problem by the client. What does the client think is wrong? How severe does the client perceive the impairment to be?

Collection of objective data includes the nurse's observations of the client. Is there squinting? Rubbing of eyes? Is the client using compensatory measures—magnifying glass, sits close to television, uses large-print reading materials, avoids reading, uses eyeglasses? Nurses must also be aware of psychosocial data because a blind person may be withdrawn, be socially isolated, have low self-esteem, have poor coping mechanisms, or have poor interpersonal skills as a result of the visual impairment.

Nursing Diagnosis

The major nursing diagnoses for visual impairment include but are not limited to the following:

- Sensory-perceptual alteration (visual)
- Self-care deficit (specify area) related to visual impairment
- Risk for injury related to visual impairment
- Risk for impaired home maintenance management related to lack of assistance, lack of rehabilitation, or other factors

- Altered family processes related to change in role secondary to visual impairment
- Altered role performance related to visual impairment, lack of rehabilitation
- Knowledge deficit related to disease process, prevention, and treatment
- Diversional activity deficit related to transition from sighted to visually impaired
- Fear related to blindness
- Anxiety related to sensory-perceptual changes (visual)

See also Nursing Care Plan Box 49–2 for the Client with Visual Loss.

Planning

A client's level of independence must be included in the planning phase. If clients have minimal visual impairment or have attended rehabilitation, they may be able to function independently. If a client has recently become visually impaired, he or she may be completely dependent until learning alternative ways of coping with this impairment. Planning focuses on meeting self-care needs, keeping the client safe from injury, supporting the grieving process, and helping the client acquire knowledge of agencies, services, and devices that allow maintenance of independence. Families must be included in the planning phase because they need to understand and be supportive of the self-image and role performance changes that may occur.

Client goals include the following:

- Maintains ability to complete activities of daily living with minimal assistance
- Remains free of injury
- Demonstrates ability to access agencies and services for visually impaired
- Maintains healthy relationships among family members
- Maintains positive self-esteem
- Verbalizes understanding of disease process, prevention, and treatment
- Participates in diversional activities
- Verbalizes lessened fear or anxiety about perceptual changes

Nursing Interventions

Nursing care begins by understanding how to interact with the visually impaired client (Table 49–3). The nurse includes client teaching in the plan of care. The goal of the teaching is to promote independence and safety for the client while in the hospital and in the home. Several organizations exist whose mission is to enhance the independence of visually impaired persons. Referring clients to these resources enhances their ability to maintain independence (see References).

Evaluation

Evaluation of the nursing care plan is based on client attainment of goals. The goals for the visually impaired client are met if the client

NURSING CARE PLAN BOX 49-2 FOR THE CLIENT WITH VISUAL LOSS

Sensory-perceptual alteration: visual

Client Outcomes

Client will attain optimal level of sensory stimulation. Client will become aware of visual impairment and ways to compensate. Client will demonstrate ability to perform activities of daily living, with assistance if necessary.

Evaluation of Outcomes

Client perceives maximum visual sensory input. Client is able to compensate for sensory impairment by using other senses and resources. Client is able to perform activities of daily living as independently as possible.

Interventions	Rationale	Evaluation
• Assess visual acuity using a standard Snellen's vision chart. If the individual is unable to read letters, use directional arrows or pictures.	Determines client's ability to see.	Does client have 20/20 vision? Is there an impairment? If so, how severe is it?
• Assess visual fields using the cover test or confrontation test.	Identifies deficits in visual fields.	Are the visual fields of the client equal to the examiner's? Is there a deficit? Is it bilateral or unilateral?
• Structure the environment to compensate for the visual loss by adding color and contrast (e.g., chairs and carpeting should be in contrasting colors, bright tape or paint on stairs, medicine bottles color coded with colored dot stickers).	Makes the environment easier to visualize and interpret and assists in depth perception and identifying medications.	Does the environment have clearly delineated walkways, sitting areas, and doorways? Are areas with changes in elevation clearly identified using contrasting tape or paint? Is there a way for the client to safely administer his or her own medications?
• Structure the environment to compensate for visual loss by use of large-print directional signs and arrows, well-lit areas, nonglare surfaces, consistent placement of objects, traffic areas free of clutter.	Large directional signs will assist the individual in maintaining orientation. Shiny floors or areas with bright window glass can impair vision. Traffic areas free of clutter will assist in preventing injury.	Can the visually impaired individual identify locations such as bathroom, dining room, and office areas? Is the individual able to ambulate freely without safety hazards?
• Provide for optimal care of assistive appliances such as eyeglasses, including maintenance of proper prescription, fit, and cleaning.	Improperly fitting or dirty eyeglasses may impair vision even further. Older adults should have their eyeglass prescription checked yearly.	Do eyeglasses fit properly? Are the lenses clean? Is the prescription current?
• Introduce other assistive devices such as handheld magnifying glasses, table-side magnifiers, television magnifiers, large-print items, and phone dial covers with large numbers.	Clients may not be aware of assistive devices, which may help them adapt to visual loss and continue previous activities such as watching TV or reading letters and magazines.	Is client aware of assistive devices that allow participation in previously enjoyed activities such as TV or reading? Is the visually impaired client able to pay bills? Read mail? Communicate on the telephone?
• Allow client to verbalize feelings and grieving about visual loss.	Losing a primary sense such as vision can be devastating for clients. Opportunity to ventilate feelings will assist in processing the loss.	Is the client able to verbalize feelings about the visual impairment and its loss?
• Identify coping strategies that have been successful for the client in the past.	By identifying successful coping strategies, the nurse assists the client in dealing with the stress of visual loss. A positive approach for nurses to use focuses on the individual's capabilities rather than deficits.	Is client able to identify successful coping strategies and use them to deal with the stress of visual impairment?
• Refer to specialized clinician such as ophthalmologist or occupational therapist or to specialized resources such as American Federation for the Blind or Prevent Blindness America (see References).	Specialized clinicians can provide detailed examination and treatment for the disorder. Specialized resource groups have networks in place to assist individuals in coping with the loss and assisting them with maximizing abilities.	Does client know who to call for detailed examination and treatment of problems? Does the client know that there are specialized clinicians and resource groups to help with the visual impairment? Does the client know how to access these specialists?

Table 49–3. **Interacting with the Visually Impaired Client**

- People entering a room and at each contact with the client should identify themselves.
- Post a sign on the door or over the bed that identifies the client's visual status so that others can interact appropriately.
- Remember that the individual is not having hearing problems, so use a normal tone of voice and do not yell.
- Ask visually impaired clients what their needs are; do not assume they need help with everything.
- Do not hesitate to use the words "blind" and "see."
- Talk directly to the impaired client, not through a companion.
- At mealtime, explain the location of items on the tray by comparing their position to the numbers on a clock (e.g., milk is at 2 o'clock, peas are at 7 o'clock).
- Explain any activity going on in the room or within the client's auditory range.
- Explain procedures before beginning them. Speak to the client before touching him or her.
- When walking, allow client to grasp assistant's arm and walk a half step behind. Be aware of obstacles on either side when walking.
- When seating a client, place the client's hand on the arm of the chair.
- Tell client when leaving the room or area so the client does not continue conversation in an empty room, which may cause embarrassment.
- When orienting client to the hospital room, explain the location of items the client may need such as the water pitcher, call light, bed controls, urinal, tissues. Attempt to keep these items in the same place at all times.
- If client has a Seeing Eye dog, do not play with the dog, pet it, or feed it without consulting the client—the dog is working! Make sure the client's dog is near the bed, on a mat provided especially for the dog, preferably on the side of the bed that is less likely to be used by staff. Instruct staff and visitors about the Seeing Eye dog.

- Demonstrates ability to complete activities of daily living with increasing independence
- Remains free of injury
- Demonstrates ability to assess agencies and services for visually impaired
- Maintains healthy relationships among family members
- Maintains positive self-esteem
- Verbalizes understanding of disease process, prevention, and treatment
- Participates in diversional activities
- Verbalizes lessened fear or anxiety about perceptual changes

DIABETIC RETINOPATHY

Pathophysiology and Etiology

Retinopathy is a disorder in which there are vascular changes in the retinal blood vessels. The most common incidence of retinopathy is found in diabetics. It is estimated that half of the approximately 14 million diabetics in the United States have at least early signs of retinopathy.[6] The pathological changes that occur with diabetic retinopathy are related to excess glucose, changes in the retinal capillary walls, formation of microaneurysms, and constriction of retinal blood vessels. Three stages of diabetic retinopathy have been identified: background retinopathy, preproliferative retinopathy, and proliferative retinopathy.

Background retinopathy is the earliest stage, in which microaneurysms form on the retinal capillary walls. These microaneurysms may leak blood into the central retina or macula. If the leakage causes edema, the client may notice a decrease in color discrimination and visual acuity.

The second stage, preproliferative retinopathy, is characterized by swollen and irregularly dilated veins, which results in sluggish or blocked blood flow. Clients generally are not aware of this stage because there are no symptoms.

Proliferative retinopathy, the third stage, is characterized by the formation of new blood vessels growing into the retinal and optic disc area as an attempt to increase the blood supply to the retina. The newly formed blood vessels are fragile and often leak blood into the vitreous and retina. In addition to leaking, the newer vessels may grow into the vitreous, which causes a traction effect, pulling the vitreous away from the retina and subsequently pulling the retina away from the choroid. This condition is called retinal detachment and is discussed later in this chapter.

Signs and Symptoms

Individuals may experience a reduction in central visual acuity or color vision due to macular edema (see Fig. 49–2). Many clients with diabetic retinopathy do not have any symptoms until the proliferative stage, at which point vision is lost. Visual loss at the last stage usually cannot be restored.

Diagnostic Tests

Diabetic retinopathy, as well as the other retinopathies, can be diagnosed only on examination of the internal eye. The examination is conducted with an ophthalmoscope following dilation of the pupil using a cycloplegic agent. The examination may be enhanced by use of retinoangiography. In the initial stages, vessels may appear swollen and tortuous (twisted).

Medical Treatment

Treatment of diabetic retinopathy focuses on stopping the leakage of blood and fluid into the vitreous and retina. The leaking microaneurysms are sealed by use of laser photocoagulation (see Table 49–2). If blood has already leaked into the vitreous, a vitrectomy is performed. During a vitrectomy, the vitreous humor is drained out of the eye

---

retinopathy: retino—having to do with the retina + pathy—illness, disease, or suffering

chamber and replaced with saline or silicon oil. The replacement fluid is necessary to support the structures of the eyeball until healing can occur. Further treatment may be needed if the client has sustained retinal detachment.

Complications

Early treatment for diabetic retinopathy is highly successful in preventing further visual loss; however, visual loss cannot be reversed. For this reason it is very important for diabetic clients to have a comprehensive eye examination through dilated pupils at least once each year or as directed by their physician. Careful control of diabetes during the first 5 years following diagnosis has been shown to reduce the frequency and delay the onset of diabetic retinopathy.[9]

Nursing Process for Retinopathy

Assessment

Nursing assessment for diabetic retinopathy focuses on risk factors associated with the incidence of the disease. The client may not have any symptoms. If diabetic clients do have changes in perceptions of visual acuity or color discrimination, they should be immediately referred to the physician.

Nursing Diagnosis

Nursing diagnoses for diabetic retinopathy include but are not limited to the following:

- Risk for (or actual) impaired home maintenance management
- Risk for (or actual) impaired medical regimen management
- Sensory-perceptual alteration: visual

Planning

The planning phase of the nursing process focuses on prevention of visual loss by early detection and treatment. If the client has entered phase three and is already visually impaired, the nursing care plan for the visually impaired client is used. Additionally, planning includes a method for monitoring blood glucose and for drawing up and administering the correct amount of insulin for the visually impaired diabetic client. Specialty devices are available that can be preset to draw up amounts of insulin for the visually impaired diabetic. Family members may have to assist the client.

Nursing Interventions

Nursing interventions for diabetic retinopathy focus on preventive eye care. Clients are taught the importance of yearly comprehensive eye examinations. Assisting clients to keep their diabetes under control also helps reduce the onset of this condition. If the diabetic client has experienced visual loss, nursing interventions focus on assisting the individual with home and health maintenance.

Evaluation

Client goals are met if the client is able to

- Manage home maintenance
- Manage medication regimen
- Prevent further visual impairment via preventive care (e.g., manage blood sugars within normal limits)

RETINAL DETACHMENT

Pathophysiology and Etiology

Retinal detachment is a separation of the retina from the choroid layer of the eye. There are three types of retinal detachment. Rhegmatogenous retinal detachment is caused by a hole or tear in the retina that allows fluid to flow between the two layers. The tears are related to degenerative changes in the retina or vitreous. This type of retinal detachment can also be precipitated by moderate trauma, such as stooping or lifting weights, or by direct trauma to the eye. The incidence of rhegmatogenous detachment increases with age. Nonrhegmatogenous tractional detachment occurs when fibrous tissue in the vitreous humor attaches to the sensory retina and, as it contracts, pulls the retina away from its normal position. This type of detachment is seen in patients with sickle cell disease or diabetes mellitus. The third type of detachment is called exudative detachment. This type of detachment occurs when fluid or exudate accumulates in the subretinal space and separates the layers. Exudative detachment occurs most often in conditions such as advanced hypertension, preeclampsia, or eclampsia and from intraocular tumors.

Signs and Symptoms

Clients experiencing a retinal detachment report a sudden change in vision. Initially, as the retina is pulled "flashing lights" are reported, and then "floaters" are seen. The flashing lights are caused by vitreous traction on the retina, and the floaters are caused by the hemorrhage of vitreous fluid or blood. When the retina detaches, the client describes it as "looking through a veil" or "cobwebs," and finally "like a curtain being lowered over the field of vision" with darkness resulting. There is no pain because the retina does not contain sensory nerves. On visual examination, the client generally has a loss of peripheral vision when the visual fields are tested and a loss of acuity in the affected eye.

Diagnostic Tests

Indirect ophthalmoscopy is used by the physician to examine the interior of the eye. This examination allows the examiner to visualize the retina, which may be pale, opaque, and in folds with retinal detachment. The examiner is able to diagnose the type of detachment based on this examination. If there are lesions in the eye, the slit lamp examination allows the examiner to magnify the lesions.

Medical Treatment

Prompt medical treatment must be sought to prevent loss of vision. One of several procedures may be performed. The goal of each procedure is to reattach the retina to prevent blindness. Laser reattachment, electrodiathermy, laser cryosurgery, scleral buckling, and pneumatic retinopexy are the procedures that may be utilized.

Laser reattachment involves focusing a laser beam (see Table 49–2) on the detached area of the retina and causing a controlled burn, which reattaches the layers together by forming an adhesion. This procedure is used only when a small area of the retina is involved.

Cryosurgery involves the placement of a supercooled probe on the sclera. The probe causes injury to the tissue causing an adhesion, a principle similar to the laser procedure.

Electrodiathermy, the least used procedure, involves placement of an electrode needle into the sclera to allow fluid that has accumulated to drain. The retina later adheres to the choroid layer.

Scleral buckling is a surgical procedure that involves placing a silicon implant in conjunction with a beltlike device around the sclera to bring the choroid in contact with the retina (Fig. 49–4). Cryosurgery or laser is used concomitantly to assist in forming adhesion of the retina and choroid layers.

Pneumatic retinopexy is a procedure that can be conducted in the physician's office and is very time consuming for the client. This procedure involves injecting air or gas into the chamber to hold the retina in place. The client must be extremely compliant with the treatment regimen, reclining for about 16 hours before the procedure to allow the retina to fall back toward the choroid. Because air rises, the client must maintain a position that keeps the air bubble against the detached area for up to 8 hours a day for 3 weeks.

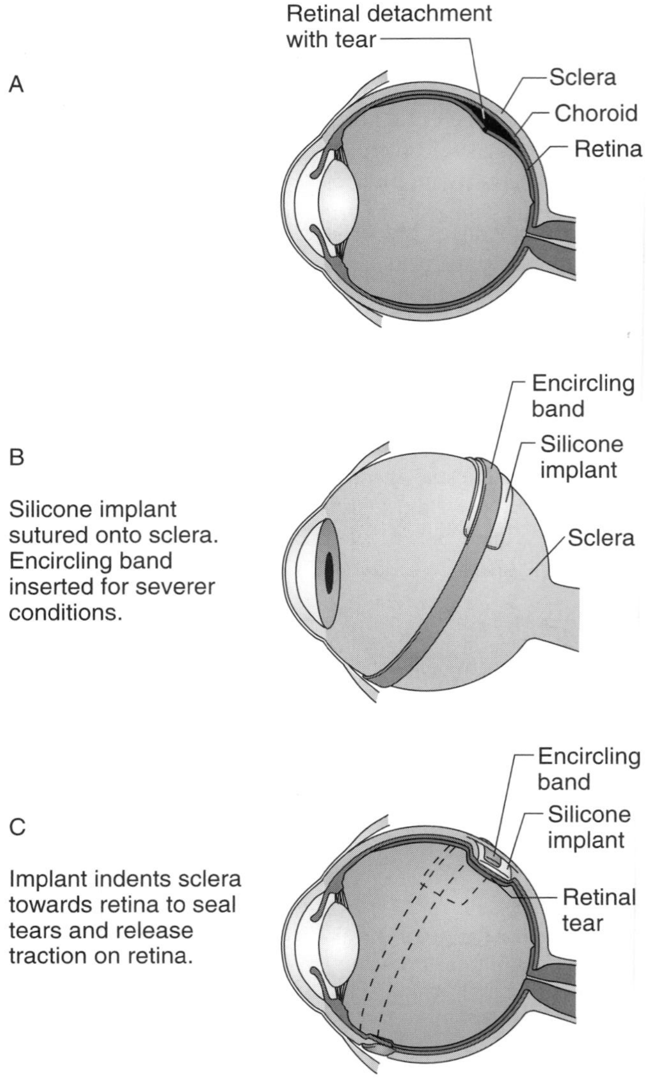

Complications

With any of the retinal reattachment procedures there is risk of increased intraocular pressure (IOP) and recurrent detachment. The client is also at risk of future breaks in the retina.

Nursing Process for Retinal Detachment

Nursing process for clients with retinal detachment can be found in the section on nursing process for clients undergoing eye surgery. Assessment data specific to retinal detachment follows.

Assessment

Subjective data collected include client observation of the loss of peripheral vision, any change in visual acuity, and

A

Silicone implant sutured onto sclera. Encircling band inserted for severer conditions.

B

Implant indents sclera towards retina to seal tears and release traction on retina.

C

Figure 49–4. Scleral buckling repair for retinal detachment.

the presence of floaters, flashing lights, or cobweb or veil-like visual impairments. There should be an absence of pain.

Objective data collected include the client's visual acuity, visual fields, ability to perform ADL, and level of anxiety.

CRITICAL THINKING: Mr. Samuel

Mr. Samuel, 65, is working in the yard when a branch strikes his right eye. He sees flashes of light and then a short time later a dark shadow out of the right eye.

1. What should Mr. Samuel do?
2. After having a scleral buckling procedure, Mr. Samuel reports nausea. What should the nurse do?

Answers at end of chapter.

GLAUCOMA

Glaucoma is a group of diseases characterized by abnormal pressure within the eyeball. This pressure causes damage to the cells of the optic nerve, the structure responsible for transmitting visual information from the eye to the brain. The damage is silent, progressive, and irreversible until the end stages when loss of peripheral vision occurs, followed by reductions in central vision and eventually blindness (see Fig. 49–2). Once glaucoma occurs, the client will always have it and must follow treatment to maintain stable intraocular eye pressures.

Pathophysiology

The most common form of glaucoma, called primary, consists of two types: **primary open-angle glaucoma** (POAG) and **acute angle-closure glaucoma** (AACG). Secondary glaucoma may be caused by infections, tumors, or injuries. A third form, congenital glaucoma, is primarily due to developmental abnormalities.

AACG occurs in people who have an anatomically narrowed angle at the junction where the iris meets the cornea (Fig. 49–5). When nearby eye structures such as the iris protrude into the anterior chamber, the angle is occluded, which blocks the flow of aqueous fluid. This is considered a medical emergency and results in partial or total blindness if not treated. POAG occurs when the drainage system of the eye, the trabecular meshwork and Schlemm's canal, degenerate and subsequently block the flow of aqueous humor (see Fig. 49–5).

Etiology and Prevention

The incidence of AACG is highest among Asians, women over 45, and nearsighted individuals; the incidence of POAG increases with those over 40 years of age (over 50 for European-Americans, over 35 for African-Americans),

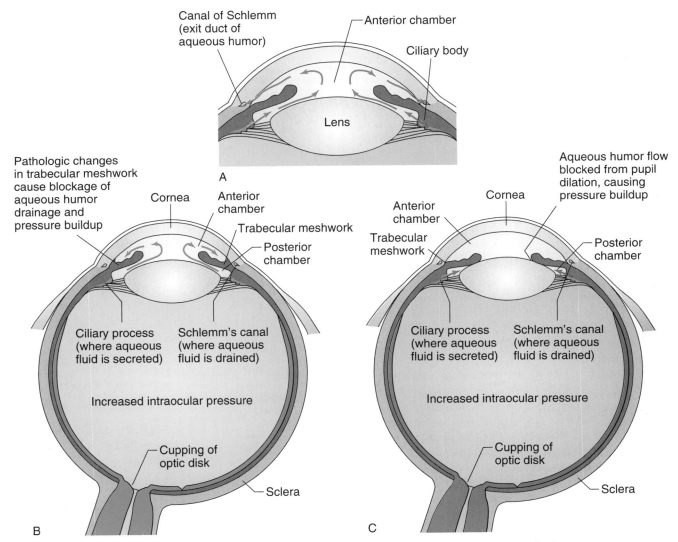

Figure 49–5. (*A*) Normal flow of aqueous humor. (*B*) Open-angle glaucoma. (*C*) Closed-angle glaucoma.

diabetes, and family history of glaucoma and is four to five times more prevalent in African-Americans than European-Americans.[10,11] Those in high-risk groups should have yearly eye examinations for glaucoma detection.

Signs and Symptoms

An ophthalmic emergency, AACG typically has a unilateral, rapid onset. The client may complain of severe pain over the affected eye, blurred vision, rainbows around lights, eye redness, a steamy-appearing cornea, photophobia, and tearing. Nausea and vomiting may occur from the increased IOP.

POAG develops bilaterally. The onset is usually gradual and painless, so the client may not experience noticeable symptoms or after time may experience mild aching in the eyes, headache, halos around lights, or frequent visual changes that are not corrected with eyeglasses.

Diagnostic Tests

Tonometry is utilized to detect increased IOP (normal IOP: 12 to 20 mm Hg) but is not adequate to detect glaucoma alone (see Fig. 49–3). The eye must be examined through dilated pupils to adequately diagnose the disease. The visual field examination may demonstrate a loss of peripheral vision. In AACG, IOP may exceed 50 mm Hg.

Medical Treatment

The first-line treatment for glaucoma focuses on opening the aqueous flow by administering **miotics** such as pilocarpine (Pilocar) to constrict the pupil. When the pupil is constricted, the iris pulls away from the drainage canal so that the aqueous fluid can flow freely. A second type of medication may be given to slow the production of aqueous fluid such as acetazolamide (Diamox) or beta blockers such as timolol (Timoptic). Slowing the aqueous fluid production helps decrease IOP. Additionally, the physician may order steroid eyedrops to reduce inflammation. The client experiencing an acute attack of angle-closure glaucoma is given these medications and mannitol, an osmotic diuretic, to rapidly reduce IOP, as well as analgesics and complete bed rest.

Clients with glaucoma are required to administer lifelong eyedrop medications twice or more daily. In the absence of symptoms, compliance is often an issue. Other factors that contribute to noncompliance include age of the client, inability to afford the medication, and lack of understanding of the disease process.[12] Clients need to carry Medic Alert identification indicating they have glaucoma and what their medications are. This can help prevent administration of contraindicated medications in emergency situations.

Certain medications, regardless of their route, are contraindicated in narrow-angle glaucoma and can result in blindness if given to a client with narrow-angle glaucoma.

These medications include any anticholinergics such as atropine and antihistamines such as diphenhydramine (Benadryl) or hydroxyzine (Vistaril) because they are mydriatics. Before a medication is given, it should be determined that it is not contraindicated in glaucoma to prevent blindness from occurring.

LEARNING TIP

- Mydriatic medications are contraindicated in closed-angle (narrow-angle) glaucoma because they can cause acute glaucoma by dilating the pupil and pushing the iris back to block flow of aqueous humor, which further increases IOP.
- Miotic medications constrict the pupil and so may be given to clients with closed-angle glaucoma.
- To remember what miotic medications and mydriatic medications do, so that the appropriate medication is given and contraindicated ones are never given, remember the following:

| D = dilate | = my**d**riatic | = do not give |
| No D = constricts | = miotic | = okay to give |

Surgical Management

When medication is no longer able to control the aqueous humor flow, surgical intervention may become necessary. Surgery focuses on creating an area for the aqueous humor to flow freely, thus preventing increased IOP. The most common surgical procedures for treating glaucoma are laser iridectomy and laser trabeculoplasty (Fig. 49–6). Laser iridectomy is a noninvasive procedure utilizing a laser to remove a portion of the iris, thus allowing aqueous fluid to flow through the area. Prophylactic iridectomy may be performed on the other eye to prevent AACG.[13] Laser trabeculoplasty is also noninvasive and involves utilizing a laser beam to create openings in the trabecular meshwork.

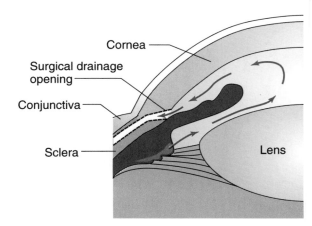

Figure 49–6. Flow of aqueous humor after surgery (*arrows*).

Nursing Process for Glaucoma

Assessment

The client should be assessed for loss of both central and peripheral vision, discomfort, understanding of disease and compliance with treatment regimen, and ability to conduct activities of daily living.

Nursing Diagnosis

- Sensory-perceptual alteration: visual, related to disease process
- Knowledge deficit related to medical regimen, disease process
- Self-care deficit related to decreased vision
- Anxiety related to partial or total visual loss
- Altered home maintenance related to decreased vision
- Pain related to increased intraocular pressure
- Risk for injury related to decreased vision

Planning

Planning for nursing interventions needs to take into account the client's level of understanding of disease process and medical regimen. Planning must also include the client's ability to comply with the time-consuming medication regimen. The goal of nursing care for the glaucoma client is to prevent further visual loss and to promote comfort if the client is experiencing pain such as in acute glaucoma. The client who needs surgical intervention has additional goals, which are included in the section on nursing process for the client having eye surgery.

Nursing Interventions

The client is taught how to administer medications. The nurse watches a return demonstration to ensure that eyedrops are administered properly. If the client is unable to see the label on the eyedrop bottle, consider large-print labels or audiotaped directions. For clients with multiple medications, the nurse may want to consider the use of large, different-colored dot stickers that are placed on the medication bottle and a corresponding direction card with a matching colored dot.[12] If the client has trouble with a steady hand when administering eyedrops, the nurse

should teach the client to rest his or her hand on the forehead to steady the hand.

Clients are taught the need for having regular eye examinations through dilated pupils. Family members should also be advised that they are at increased risk of developing glaucoma and should have regular eye examinations.

Analgesics are given as needed for acute glaucoma. The client is also assisted with self-care and home maintenance referrals as needed. The nurse listens to clients' concerns about losing their sight.

Other interventions that may be implemented if the client is experiencing severe visual loss or having surgery are in the nursing process sections for impaired vision and the client having eye surgery, respectively.

Evaluation

Client goals are met if the client

- Has no further loss of vision
- Is able to verbalize understanding of condition and treatment
- Is able to care for self with assistance if needed
- Expresses concerns and anxieties
- Is able to manage home maintenance with assistance if needed
- Demonstrates correct instillation of eye medications
- Maintains an acceptable level of comfort
- Does not suffer injury as a result of the visual impairment

CATARACTS

Pathophysiology and Etiology

A **cataract** is an opacity in the lens of the eye that may cause a loss of visual acuity (see Fig. 49–2). Vision is diminished because the light rays are unable to get to the retina through the clouded lens (Fig. 49–7).

The most common cause of cataract formation is aging. These cataracts are called senile cataracts. Other causes include intraocular infections, trauma, and congenital defects. Factors that may contribute to cataract formation in-

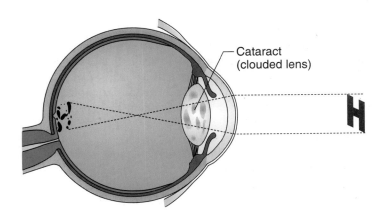

Figure 49–7. Cataract vision pathology.

clude ultraviolet radiation, diabetes, use of steroids, drugs, and nutritional deficiencies.

Signs and Symptoms

Cataracts are painless. Symptoms of cataract formation may include halos around lights, difficulty reading fine print or seeing in bright light, increased sensitivity to glare such as when driving at night, double or hazy vision, and decreased color vision.

Diagnostic Tests

Cataract formation is diagnosed through an eye examination. Visual acuity is tested for near and far vision. The direct ophthalmoscope and slit lamp are used to examine the lens and other internal structures.

Surgical Treatment

The only treatment for cataract formation is surgical removal. There are several types of cataract surgery. If the no-stitch operation is done, there are no restrictions in activities postoperatively with vision being fine in about 2 days. Cataract surgery is painless.

After the lens is removed there are several treatment options to correct the visual deficit that occurs when the eye is aphakic (absence of lens) and cannot accommodate or refract light properly. One treatment option is to provide the client with eyeglasses or contact lenses that help correct the visual deficit. A more common option is to replace the lens with a synthetic intraocular lens.

Complications

Complications of cataract surgery are rare but include inflammation, increased IOP, macular edema, retinal detachment, vitreous loss, hyphema, endophthalmitis, and expulsive hemorrhage.

Nursing Process

Preoperative and postoperative nursing care is the primary nursing responsibility for the client with cataracts. The client is assessed for visual deficits to assist the nurse in planning care. The client may have cataracts in both eyes and have severe visual impairment or may be able to adequately cope with slightly diminished sight in one eye. The client should also be assessed for knowledge deficits about the disease process, surgical intervention, postoperative care, and medical regimen.

The majority of clients undergoing cataract surgery have same-day surgery and go home. The nurse must evaluate the home situation, the ability of the client or family member to follow the medical regimen, and transportation to and from the hospital for the client.

NURSING PROCESS FOR CLIENTS HAVING EYE SURGERY

Assessment

Subjective data can be collected using the WHAT'S UP acronym:

Where is the visual disturbance—centrally? Peripherally? Throughout the entire visual field? Unilateral? Bilateral?

How does it feel? Painful? Absence of pain?

Aggravating or alleviating factors. Worse in bright light, at night? Better when resting eyes, with head of bed elevated?

Timing. Sudden onset? Gradual onset?

Severity. Does it affect ADL? Does it affect closeup work?

Useful data for associated symptoms. Does the client suffer from hypertension? Diabetes? Has there been trauma? Vascular disease? What is the level of anxiety? Is the client over 50?

Perception of the problem by the client. Will the visual disturbance impair ADL? Ability to carry out medical regimen? Ability to manage home maintenance?

Objective data may include visual acuity and peripheral field measurements. Visual acuity should be tested with and without corrective lenses. Eye tearing, redness, or swelling is noted.

Nursing Diagnosis

Nursing diagnoses for the client undergoing eye surgery may include but are not limited to the following:

- Sensory-perceptual alteration related to trauma or disease of the eye
- Knowledge deficit related to preoperative and postoperative eye care
- Risk for infection related to surgical procedure
- Risk for injury related to altered visual acuity
- Anxiety related to visual alteration
- Fear or anxiety related to surgery

Planning

The client goals are to remain free of injury, to prevent further visual impairment by rapid diagnosis and treatment, and to have minimal anxiety surrounding the visual alteration, treatment, and recovery.

Nursing Interventions

A key nursing intervention involves client teaching about the disease process, surgical intervention, preoperative and postoperative activity restrictions, use of dark glasses to decrease the discomfort of photophobia, use of correct technique for administration of eye medications, reporting for medical follow-up as instructed, keeping eye patched or pressure dressing on if ordered, and how to protect the eye from further injury. Clients are advised to avoid activities that would increase intraocular pressure such as vomiting, coughing, sneezing, straining, or bending over. They should not drive a car. They are told to return to the hospital if they experience worsening pain, increase in watery or bloody discharge, or sudden loss of vision, because hemorrhaging may be occurring.

Nurses also must focus on reducing anxiety by allowing clients the opportunity to discuss their feelings about the visual loss, by answering questions honestly, and by explaining any restrictions in activity. To help prevent injury, clients should be aware that their depth perception may be affected, which can result in falls. Client should walk carefully and clearly mark stairs. To prevent spills and slippery floors, beverages can be poured ahead of the surgery and stored in the refrigerator in single-serving glasses.

Evaluation

The client goals have been met

- If the client is able to regain visual loss as a result of corrective treatment
- If injury is prevented
- If anxiety is lessened

MACULAR DEGENERATION

Pathophysiology and Etiology

Age-related **macular degeneration** (ARMD) is the leading cause of visual impairment in Americans over the age of 50. It involves a deterioration in the macular area of the retina, the area on the retina where light rays converge for sharp, central vision needed for reading and seeing small objects, as well as color vision. There are two types of ARMD: dry (atrophic) and wet (exudative). In the dry form, photoreceptors in the macula fail to function and are not replaced due to advancing age. This accounts for 70 to 90 percent of the cases.[14] In the wet form, retinal tissue degenerates, allowing vitreous fluid or blood into the subretinal space. New blood vessels are formed and compromise the macular tissue, causing subretinal edema. Eventually fibrous scar tissue is formed, severely limiting central vision.

People at risk of developing macular degeneration include those over age 60, those with a family history of macular degeneration, diabetics, smokers, those frequently exposed to ultraviolet light, and light-skinned people.

Signs and Symptoms

Macular degeneration of the dry type is characterized by slow, progressive loss of central and near vision (see Fig. 49–2). Although individuals usually have the condition in both eyes, each eye may be affected in different degrees. Macular degeneration of the wet type has the same loss of central and near vision, but the onset is sudden. The loss can occur in one or both eyes. This visual loss is described as blurred vision, distortion of straight lines, and a dark or empty spot in the central area of vision. For some clients there may be a decreased ability to distinguish colors.

Diagnostic Tests

Examination of the client begins with visual acuity for near and far vision and an examination of the internal eye structures with an ophthalmoscope. The examiner uses an Amsler grid (Fig. 49–8) to detect central vision distortion and a color vision test to evaluate color differences. Clients are given an Amsler grid to take home and look at on a regular basis to monitor their vision changes. If any of the grid lines look crooked or disappear, the client should contact the physician. Intravenous fluorescein (dye) angiography to look at the retina may also be utilized to evaluate blood vessel leakage or abnormalities in the eye.

Medical Treatment

Unfortunately, there is no treatment for the dry type of ARMD. Most clients with the dry type do not lose peripheral vision or become totally blind, but most are classified as legally blind (less than 20/200 vision with correction). Special low-vision lenses can enhance remaining vision. If the wet type of ARMD is diagnosed early, argon laser photocoagulation can seal the leaking blood vessels, slowing the rate of vision loss. With either type of ARMD, the client has significant visual loss and needs to adapt her or his patterns of daily living.

Current research is exploring cell transplant in an attempt to provide a cure in the future. Studies are focusing on transplanting retinal-pigmented epithelial cells that grow and function normally.

Complications

If the client receives argon laser photocoagulation, there is a small, permanent blind spot at the point of laser contact with the macula.

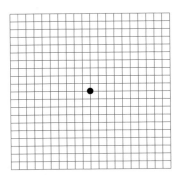

Figure 49–8. Amsler grid.

Nursing Process

See the nursing process section for the visually impaired.

TRAUMA

Emergencies and trauma of the eye must be assessed immediately so that proper treatment can be initiated. Injuries to the eye include foreign bodies, burns, abrasions, lacerations, and penetrating wounds. The nurse must know which conditions require immediate treatment to prevent permanent visual loss and which situations allow for referral. Treatment for chemical burns and sudden, painless loss of vision should be initiated within minutes to preserve vision.

Pathophysiology and Etiology

Foreign bodies are the most common cause of corneal injury. Dust particles or propellants may lodge in the conjunctiva or cornea. Clients naturally rub their eyes to dislodge the object, which further irritates the cornea. Burns occur from chemical, ultraviolet, and direct heat sources. Depending on the agent causing the burn, it may be superficial or deep. Abrasions and lacerations usually occur as a result of something dragging across the eye, such as a fingernail or clothing.

Penetrating wounds are the most serious eye injury. Eye structures may be damaged permanently with complete blindness resulting. A penetrating wound also puts the client at great risk of infection.

Signs and Symptoms

Foreign bodies produce pain when the eyeball or eyelid moves, causing the foreign body to drag over the opposing surface. Usually the eye tears excessively in an attempt to irrigate the noxious substance out of the eye.

Injuries that irritate or penetrate layers of the cornea range from mild to severe pain. With corneal abrasions, the pain sensation may be delayed for several hours. Other symptoms that may be seen with abrasions, lacerations, and foreign bodies include conjunctival redness, photosensitivity, decreased visual acuity, erythema, and pruritis.

Acute pain and burning are characteristic symptoms of a burn to the eye. Chemical burns must be treated immediately with an eyewash or irrigation to remove the caustic substance from the eye.

Penetrating wounds may result in a variety of symptoms depending on the area of the eye involved and the extent of the damage. If the nerve has been damaged, the client may have no pain.

Diagnostic Tests

With any eye trauma or injury, visual acuity must be tested. It is important to establish baseline acuity to evaluate ef-

fectiveness of treatment, although many clients resist acuity testing due to discomfort. Testing includes examination by slit lamp and direct ophthalmoscope. Fluorescein staining is used to evaluate abrasions.

Medical Treatment

Foreign bodies are treated with a saline flush to irrigate the object out of the eye or to a point where it can be removed with a swab. Topical antibiotic ointment is prescribed to prevent infection.

Most chemical burns are treated with a 15- to 20-minute irrigation of either tap water at the work site or sterile solution in the health care facility. Topical antibiotic ointments are usually prescribed. Burns from heat or UV radiation are not irrigated.

Abrasions and lacerations are generally treated with antiinfective ointments or drops after cleansing the eye with a saline solution.

An eye specialist treats penetrating wounds. At initial injury, both eyes should be covered to prevent ocular movement. If there is a protruding object, it should be stabilized but not removed until the physician can assess the client. The nature and extent of the penetrating wound determine the necessary treatment.

Complications

If the eye cannot be saved via medical treatment, it may be necessary to surgically remove the eye. This procedure is called **enucleation** (entire eyeball removal).

Nursing Process

Assessment and Intervention

FOREIGN BODIES. The nurse should inspect the eye for foreign bodies, which may be visible on the eyeball. The lids should be everted to examine the surface. The nurse will assist with the irrigation of the eye.

BURNS. The nurse assesses the type of burn the client has because treatment options vary. The nurse should begin immediate irrigation of the eyes once it has been established that a chemical burn has taken place. The nurse may assist in applying medication and patching the eye if indicated.

ABRASIONS AND LACERATIONS. The nurse assesses the eye for visible lacerations and records the client's history. The nurse assists in cleaning the eye, applying medication, and patching the eye if indicated.

PENETRATING WOUNDS. The nurse attempts to keep the client calm and relaxed to minimize eye movement and in-

---

enucleation: e—removed from + nuclear—center

creased IOP. If a protruding object is present, the nurse should stabilize the object with tape or other supports.

Nursing Diagnosis

Nursing diagnoses for the client with eye trauma include

- Knowledge deficit related to medical regimen
- Sensory-perceptual alteration related to trauma or disease of the eye
- Risk for infection
- Anxiety related to visual sensory deficit
- Pain: acute, related to inflammatory process and injury

Planning

Planning for the eye trauma client must take into account the ability of the client to carry out the medical regimen, to verbalize concerns about the visual alteration, and to verbalize comfort levels.

Evaluation

Client goals have been met if

- Client is able to verbalize care of the eye
- Vision is retained
- Client remains free of infection

- Client is able to verbalize a reduction in anxiety
- Pain level is within an acceptable range for the client

Hearing

HEARING LOSS

Hearing loss is the most common disability in the United States and can be acquired or congenital. Hearing impairment ranges from difficulty understanding words or hearing certain sounds to total deafness. Hearing impairment can affect communication, social activities, and work activities. Hearing impairment can diminish the individual's quality of life. Nurses have a responsibility to communicate with the hearing impaired and provide necessary information regarding health care.

Conductive Hearing Loss

Conductive hearing loss is any interference with the conduction of sound impulses through the external auditory canal, the eardrum, or the middle ear (Fig. 49–9). The inner ear is not involved in a pure conductive hearing loss. Conductive hearing loss can be caused by anything that interferes with the ability of the sound wave to reach the inner ear. Conductive hearing loss is a mechanical problem.

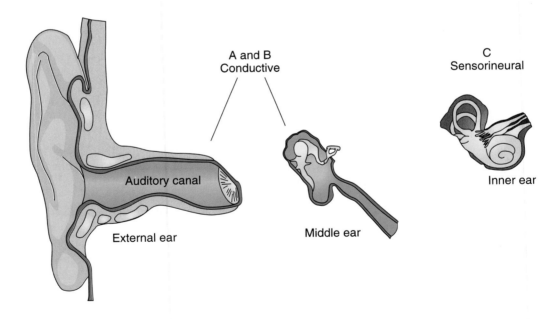

A and B
Conductive

C
Sensorineural

Auditory canal

Inner ear

External ear

Middle ear

A. External Ear
   impacted cerumen
   foreign body
   external otitis
   perforated eardrum

B. Middle Ear
   otitis media
   dislocation of
      ossicles
   otosclerosis

C. Inner Ear
   noise trauma
   drug toxicity
   presbycusis
   congenital defect
   syphilis
   Meniere's disease

Figure 49–9. Types of hearing losses and their causes.

Causes of conductive hearing loss include cerumen, foreign bodies, infection, perforation of the tympanic membrane, trauma, fluid in the middle ear, cysts, tumor, and otosclerosis. Many causes of conductive hearing loss such as infection, foreign bodies, and impacted cerumen can be corrected. Hearing devices may improve hearing for conditions that cannot be corrected such as scarred tympanic membrane or otosclerosis. Hearing devices are most effective with conductive hearing loss when no inner ear and nerve damage are present.

Sensorineural Hearing Loss

Sensory hearing loss originates in the cochlea and involves the hair cells and nerve endings. Neural hearing loss originates in the nerve or brainstem. **Sensorineural hearing loss** results from disease or trauma to the sensory or neural components of the inner ear (see Fig. 49–9). Some of the causes of nerve deafness are complications of infections (such as measles, mumps, and meningitis), ototoxic drugs (Table 49–4), trauma, noise, neuromas, arteriosclerosis, and the aging process.

Presbycusis is hearing loss caused by the aging process that results from degeneration of the organ of Corti. This degenerative process usually begins in the fifth decade of life. The individual develops an inability to decipher high-frequency sounds (consonants s, z, t, f, g). This interferes with the individual's ability to understand what has been said, especially in noisy environments. The aging individual commonly has more difficulty understanding higher-pitched female voices than lower-pitched male voices.

Other Types of Hearing Loss

Mixed hearing loss occurs when an individual has both conductive and sensorineural hearing loss. This can be caused by a combination of any of the disorders previously mentioned. Central hearing loss occurs when the central nervous system cannot interpret normal auditory signals. This condition occurs with such disorders as cerebrovascular accidents and tumors. Functional hearing loss is a hearing loss for which no organic cause or lesion can be found. It is also called psychogenic hearing loss and is precipitated by emotional stress.

Medical and Surgical Management

Medical management consists of improving the client's hearing. The majority of persons with ear disorders have some degree of hearing loss. With any permanent hearing loss, the use of a hearing aid should always be considered. A hearing aid is designed to amplify sound or attenuate certain portions of the sound signal and amplify other sounds. There are four types of hearing aids available (Fig. 49–10). The in-the-ear aid is a small device that fits either in the ear canal or in the canal and outside of the canal. The in-the-ear aid is unobtrusive and may be preferred by the individual. The behind-the-ear aid is worn postauricular and is the most common type of hearing aid used today. The all-in-one eyeglass aid is attached to glasses and is positioned behind the ear. The final type of hearing aid is the body-worn aid. This device is worn around the neck or connected to clothing. The client should have a trial period before making a final decision to purchase the hearing aid.

Surgical intervention may be available for clients whose hearing is not improved with hearing aids. Cochlear implants are surgically placed electrical devices that receive sound and transmit the resulting electrical signal to electrodes implanted in the cochlear of the ear. The signal stimulates the cochlea, allowing the client to hear. The cochlear implants are able to restore up to one half of the client's hearing.

Nursing Management

Nursing management includes identifying those clients at risk for hearing impairment. Clients with renal or hepatic disease, using two or more ototoxic drugs, or previously having used ototoxic drugs are at risk for developing hearing impairment. The nurse monitors for signs of vertigo,

Table 49–4. **Ototoxic Drugs**

Aminoglycosides (Antibiotic)
Streptomycin
Gentamycin
Amikacin
Tobramycin
Neomycin
Netilmicin
Kanamycin

Other Antibiotics
Vancomycin
Erythromycin
Minocycline

Diuretics
Furosemide
Bumetanide
Hydrochlorothiazide

Other Drugs
Salicylates
Indomethacin
Quinidine
Cisplatin
Methotrexate

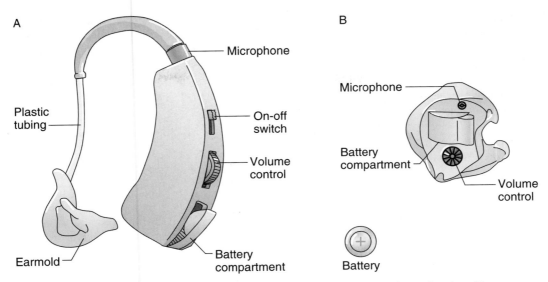

Figure 49–10. Hearing aids. *(A)* Behind-the-ear hearing aid. *(B)* In-the-ear hearing aid.

horizontal nystagmus, nausea, vomiting, and spinning or rocking sensation while sitting still.[15]

Nursing management for the client with hearing impairment focuses on enhancing communication and quality of life (Nursing Care Plan Box 49–3 for the Client with Hearing Loss). Social isolation may be more pronounced for the hearing impaired than it is for the visually impaired. Families should be included in discussions about therapeutic hearing devices and their care, enhancing communication, and limiting isolation.

Nursing Process—Hearing Impaired

Assessment

The nurse should ask family members as well as the client questions related to the client's hearing status. Assessment of symptoms for the client with hearing impairment includes gathering subjective data using the WHAT'S UP acronym:

Where is it? Are both ears affected? Is one side worse than the other?

How does it feel? Are certain words unclear, or entire conversations? Are high-frequency sounds (consonants s, t, z, f, g, and female voices) unclear or difficult to understand? Is there any pain associated with the hearing loss? Any tinnitus or vertigo?

Aggravating and alleviating factors. Is hearing worse in large groups or when there is a lot of background noise? Is hearing improved in a quiet environment or when speaking only to an individual? Is it easier to understand someone when seeing the person's lips move? Does the client own or use any assistive hearing devices? Are they effective? What type does the client use?

Timing. When did the hearing loss start? Was it gradual or sudden? Is the hearing loss associated with any illness or traumatic event? Is it associated with any recent flying? Any history of ototoxic drug use?

Severity. Does it cause communication impairment? How much? Does it affect ADL? Does it affect or limit usual social activities? Have family or friends commented on decreased hearing? Does client avoid communication or social activities because of difficulty hearing? Is client having difficulties hearing telephone voices, radio, television, or movies?

Useful data for associated symptoms. Is there any fever, nausea, vomiting, or dizziness? Is there any history of occupational or environmental exposure to loud noises? What are the usual ear self-care habits? Any history of impacted cerumen? Has client ever had cerumen removed from ears?

Perception of problem by the client. What does the client feel is wrong? Does the client think that he or she has a hearing problem? How does the client feel about hearing assistive devices? How does the client perceive the hearing loss, and how is it influencing his or her life?

Objective data focus on obtaining a gross screening of hearing function. Assessment should start with engaging in normal conversation with the client. Observe the client for any difficulty understanding conversation or interview questions. Clarity of the client's speech is also determined during the interview. Physical assessment includes the whisper voice, Rinne, and Weber tests. Test results provide an estimate of conductive or sensorineural hearing loss. The client should be assessed for the underlying cause of the problem to determine if it is an external, middle, or inner ear problem. Examination of the external ear may reveal an external ear problem. The experienced practitioner

NURSING CARE PLAN BOX 49–3 FOR THE CLIENT WITH HEARING LOSS

Sensory-perceptual alteration: hearing

Client Outcomes
Client will attain optimal level of sensory stimulation. Client will become aware of auditory impairment and ways to compensate. Client will demonstrate ability to perform activities of daily living, with assistance if necessary.

Evaluation of Outcomes
Client perceives maximum auditory sensory input. Client is able to compensate for sensory impairment by using other senses and resources. Client is able to perform activities of daily living as independently as possible.

Interventions	Rationale	Evaluation
• Begin assessment of hearing by inspecting the ear canals for mechanical obstruction. If cerumen is found to be present, the use of a softening product is recommended to assist in wax removal. If the canal is clear, continue assessment of hearing by use of a tuning fork, loud ticking clock, or verbal cues to determine auditory ability at various distances.	Hearing loss may occur due to the buildup of cerumen in the auditory canal. Determination of hearing ability will assist the nurse in developing interventions appropriate to the hearing level of the client.	Is ear canal free of mechanical obstruction? Is the client able to hear verbal input? If not, how severe is the impairment?
• Enhance hearing by giving auditory cues in quiet surroundings.	Background noise such as television, radio, or large numbers of people make hearing more difficult.	Are auditory cues being delivered in an environment free of extraneous background noises? Are auditory cues being understood by the client?
• Enhance understanding of auditory cues by getting the client's attention before speaking, speak slowly with careful enunciation of words, add hand gestures, speak face to face with the impaired person, and adjust pitch downward without increasing volume.	Hearing is enhanced when additional cues assist the impaired individual in understanding the message. Use of hand gestures to point, lip-reading, facial expression, and lower pitch all assist communication.	Are instructions given in step-by-step format with written cues?
• Structure the environment to compensate for the hearing loss by adding visual indicators to telephone ringer, doorbell, smoke detectors, and other emergency sounds.	Assists in communication.	Is client able to receive input in ways other than auditory?
• Provide for optimal care of assistive appliances such as hearing aids by making sure that cerumen has been cleaned from the device, that batteries are charged, and that the appliance is placed correctly in the ear.	Appliances that are not functioning properly will not assist the client in hearing.	Is client's hearing aid in place correctly? Is there cerumen blocking sound conduction? Do the batteries work?
• Introduce other assistive devices such as hearing amplifiers, telephone amplifiers, telephones with extra-loud bells, written communication, and sign language.	Clients may not be aware of assistive devices, which may help them adapt to hearing loss and continue previous activities such as talking on the telephone or listening to television.	Is client aware of assistive devices that will allow him or her to continue to verbally communicate with others? Is the client able to use the devices to compensate for the auditory impairment?
• Allow client to verbalize feelings and grieving about hearing loss.	Losing a primary sense such as hearing can be devastating for clients. Opportunity to ventilate feelings will assist in processing the loss.	Is client able to verbalize feelings about the auditory impairment and its loss?

continued

NURSING CARE PLAN BOX 49–3 *(continued)*

Interventions	Rationale	Evaluation
• Identify coping strategies that have been successful for the client in the past.	By identifying successful coping strategies, the nurse assists the client in dealing with the stress of hearing loss. A positive approach for nurses to use focuses on the individual's capabilities rather than deficits.	Is client able to identify successful coping strategies and use them to deal with the stress of hearing impairment?
• Refer to specialized clinician such as audiologist or occupational therapist or to specialized resources such as National Association of the Deaf or American Speech, Language and Hearing Association (see Reference).	Specialized clinicians can provide detailed examination and treatment for the disorder. Specialized resource groups have networks in place to assist individuals in coping with the loss and assisting them with maximizing abilities.	Does client know who to call for detailed examination and treatment of problems? Does client know that there are specialized clinicians and resource groups to help with the hearing impairment? Does client know how to access these specialists?

may examine the ear canal for impacted cerumen or a tympanic membrane problem. Any assistive hearing devices should be noted and inspected for proper functioning. The results of the examination are documented and communicated with other health team members.

Nursing Diagnosis

The major nursing diagnoses for the client with hearing impairment may include but are not limited to the following:

- Sensory-perceptual alterations (auditory) related to noise exposure, age, trauma, or ear disorder
- Impaired verbal communication related to impaired hearing
- Social isolation related to impaired hearing and decreased communication skills
- Body image disturbance related to impaired hearing and use of assistive hearing devices
- Ineffective individual coping related to difficult communication
- Knowledge deficit related to care of hearing aid

Planning

Planning focuses on helping the client optimize hearing, promoting communication, and promoting adjustment to impaired hearing. The client's goals are to

- Establish effective method of communication
- Maintain usual social activities
- Verbalize acceptance of altered appearance when using assistive device
- Develop coping responses to the emotional reaction of the hearing impairment
- Demonstrate care of hearing aid

Nursing Interventions

Nursing interventions focus on establishing and maintaining effective communication. Communicating with the

hearing impaired requires the nurse to be sensitive to the client's needs. Reducing or eliminating background noise provides a quiet environment. The nurse should allow extra time and maintain eye contact with clients. The client should be faced while speaking because many hearing-impaired individuals supplement hearing with lip-reading. The nurse should speak at a normal rate and volume, avoiding overarticulating or shouting, and keep hands away from the mouth when talking. If the client hears better out of one ear, the nurse speaks toward that ear. A paper and pencil should be available so the client may write responses or questions. Using gestures enhances communication. The client is informed of topics to be discussed and when a change of topic occurs. The nurse monitors the client's understanding by having the client repeat important information. While communicating, the nurse should avoid the appearance of frustration. Table 49–5 has additional information on communicating with the hearing impaired.

The client is encouraged to maintain usual social activities. The nurse assesses what the client's normal activities are and assists with participation in the activities by arranging transportation, scheduling activities, and involving other persons.

The client's feelings are discussed regarding the use of assistive devices. If the client has a hearing aid or is getting one for the first time, the nurse should ensure that the client is able to operate and care for it (Table 49–6). The nurse should check to see that hearing aid batteries are working and the volume is set at a minimal level to reduce humming. Ways to minimize the appearance of the assistive device are explored. Women may use a different hairstyle to cover the device. The nurse should stress the positive results of using the assistive device.

The client is asked to identify prior coping methods and discuss strategies to improve hearing. The nurse helps the client identify additional coping strategies to deal with the decreased hearing.

Table 49–5. *Communicating with the Hearing Impaired*

1. Get the person's attention before beginning to speak.
2. Face and stand close to the person being spoken to and maintain eye contact.
3. Avoid standing in the glare of bright sunlight or other bright lights.
4. Speak clearly, at a normal rate and volume. Do not shout or overarticulate.
5. Inform the listener of topics to be discussed and when a change of topic occurs. Stick to a topic for a while and avoid quick shifts.
6. Use short sentences and assess for understanding. If the listener does not understand after the message is repeated, rephrase the message. If the listener has difficulty with high-pitched sounds, lower the voice pitch.
7. Allow extra time for the listener to respond and do not rush the listener.
8. Ensure an optimum environment by reducing background noises by turning off television and radio, closing the door, or moving to a quieter area.
9. Encourage nonverbal communication such as touch or gestures as appropriate.
10. If the listener uses a hearing device, ensure that it is operational and in place before beginning to communicate. Give the person time to adjust the hearing device before speaking.
11. Do not smile, chew gum, or cover the mouth when talking.
12. Use active listening with attentive body posture, pleasant facial expressions, and a calm, unhurried manner.
13. Do not avoid conversation with a person who has hearing loss.
14. Use written communication if unable to communicate verbally.

Evaluation

The client's goals are met if the following occur:

- Client communicates effectively
- Client engages in usual social activities
- Client verbalizes acceptance of assistive hearing device

Table 49–6. *Care of Hearing Aids*

1. Insert hearing aid over a soft surface such as a pillow to prevent damage if the hearing aid is dropped during insertion.
2. Remove hearing aid before showering or bathing. Do not immerse in water.
3. Turn the hearing aid off when not in use.
4. Do not expose the hearing aid to extreme heat or cold.
5. Clean the hearing aid daily with a dry, soft cloth.
6. Turn off the hearing aid and turn the volume down before inserting. Turn hearing aid on and increase volume once it is inserted.
7. Minimize whistling noise by ensuring that the volume is not too high, the aid fits securely, and the aid is free from wax.
8. Check battery or lower the volume if sound is not clear or intermittent. Buzzing noise may indicate that the battery door is not completely closed.
9. Do not expose the hearing aid to medicinal or hair sprays. Apply sprays before inserting hearing aid.

- Client copes with emotional reaction of hearing impairment
- Client demonstrates care of hearing aid

EXTERNAL EAR

Infections

Pathophysiology and Etiology

Infections are the most common disorder of the external ear, with **external otitis** being the most common infection. Exposure to moisture, contamination, or local trauma provides an ideal environment for pathological growth in the external ear, which results in external otitis. It may be caused by bacterial or fungal pathogens. Staphylococci are the most common organisms, but other gram-negative or gram-positive bacteria can cause problems.[6] *Pneumocystis* infections have been seen in HIV-positive patients. A diffuse bacterial external otitis that occurs when water is left in the ear after swimming is known as swimmer's ear. External otitis occurs more often in the summer months than in the winter months. However, swimmer's ear can be seen year round in clients who swim indoors.

A localized infection called ear canal **furuncle** or abscess results when a hair follicle becomes infected. A **carbuncle** forms when several hair follicles are involved forming the abscess. Most furuncles and carbuncles erupt and drain spontaneously. Ostomycosis is an infection caused by fungal growth and is typically seen after topical corticosteroid or antibiotic use. Ostomycosis occurs more commonly in hot weather. An infection of the auricle is called perichondritis, which can result in necrosis of cartilage.

Signs and Symptoms

The most common sign of infection of the external ear is pain. An early indication of infection is pain with gentle pulling on the pinna. The client may also experience pain when moving the jaw or when the otoscope is inserted into the ear canal. Pruritis (itching) is also a common symptom and can be an early sign of infection. Signs of inflammation are present on the external ear. The ear canal may become swollen or occluded, and as a result hearing may be diminished. Redness, swelling, and drainage can be observed during otoscopic examination. If drainage is present, it usually starts out clear and becomes purulent as the disease progresses. The client may also be febrile.

Diagnostic Tests

Laboratory tests such as a complete blood count (CBC) and cultures of discharge may be completed to diagnose infections. The white blood cell (WBC) count may be elevated. Culture and sensitivity tests isolate the specific infective organism, as well as antibiotics to treat the infection. Rinne and Weber tests can indicate conductive hearing impairment.

Impacted Cerumen

Pathophysiology and Etiology

Normally, the ear is self-cleaning. However, cerumen may become impacted, blocking the ear canal. People with large amounts of hair in the ear canal or who work in dusty or dirty areas are prone to cerumen impaction. Improper cleaning can also result in cerumen impaction. The older adult is at risk to develop impacted cerumen. This occurs because the amount of cerumen secreted is decreased and because of increased amounts of keratin. These two factors cause the cerumen to be drier, harder, and more easily impacted.[16] Clients with hearing aids tend to have problems with impacted cerumen. Clients with bony growths secondary to osteophyte or osteoma are at risk for cerumen impaction.

Signs and Symptoms

The client may experience hearing loss, a feeling of fullness, or blocked ear if cerumen has become impacted. Otoscopic examination reveals cerumen blocking the ear canal.

Diagnostic Studies

Audiometric testing reveals conductive hearing loss in the affected ear. Hearing acuity can be decreased by 45 decibels due to impacted cerumen.[16] Whisper voice, Rinne, and Weber tests also indicate conductive hearing loss (see Chapter 48).

Masses

Pathophysiology and Etiology

Benign masses of the external ear are usually cysts resulting from sebaceous glands. Other benign masses are lipomas, warts, keloids, and infectious polyps. Infectious polyps usually arise from the middle ear and enter the external ear through a hole in the tympanic membrane. Actinic keratosis is a precancerous lesion that can be found on the auricle and may be seen in the elderly. Malignant tumors such as basal cell carcinoma on the pinna and squamous cell in the ear canal may develop. These tumors can spread to surrounding tissue and bones if not treated.

Signs and Symptoms

Changes in the appearance of the skin can occur with benign or malignant masses. Usually impaired conductive or sensorineural hearing occurs with masses. Pain is another symptom and is usually described as deep pain radiating inward on the affected side. Ear drainage may be present. As the condition progresses, facial paralysis occurs. Visualization of the mass may be observed during otoscopic examination.

Diagnostic Studies

A biopsy may be obtained to determine if the mass is benign or malignant. Imaging studies are also used to diagnose tumors. Audiometric studies reveal any hearing impairment.

Trauma

Pathophysiology and Etiology

Injuries to the external ear are commonly caused by a blow to the head, automobile accidents, burns, foreign bodies lodged in the ear canal, and cold temperatures. Foreign bodies in the ear canal are common among children, with small toys being the most common object. Cotton ball pieces and insects are the most common foreign bodies found in adults.

Signs and Symptoms

Lacerations, contusions, hematomas, abrasions, erythema, and blistering are signs seen with thermal or physical trauma. Repeated trauma to the ear can cause hypertrophy, also known as cauliflower ear. This is common among boxers. Conductive hearing loss can occur if the ear canal is partially or totally blocked. Clients who have contusions or hematomas commonly complain of numbness, pain, and paresthesia of the auricle. The client may or may not have symptoms associated with foreign bodies. Symptoms indicative of foreign bodies include decreased hearing, itching, pain, and infection. Examination of the ear canal with a penlight usually reveals the foreign body. Care should be taken during otoscopic examination not to push the foreign body further into the ear canal.

Diagnostic Studies

Imaging studies may be needed to determine the extent of the trauma. Audiometric, whisper voice, Rinne, and Weber testing may demonstrate conductive hearing loss.

Complications of External Ear Disorders

Complications can result from delayed treatment, no treatment, or spreading of the external ear disorder. If not treated, infections can spread, causing cellulitis, abscesses, middle ear infection, and septicemia. Metastasis can occur if malignant tumors are not treated. Infection, trauma, and malignant tumors may cause temporary or permanent hearing loss, disfigurement, discoloration, and scarring. Prompt identification and treatment of external ear disorders can prevent many complications.

Medical and Surgical Management of External Ear Disorders

External ear infections are treated with topical antibiotics in the form of drops or ointment. Systemic antibiotics are used for severe infections that are localized or have spread to surrounding tissues. Topical or systemic steroids may be used to treat inflammation. The ear is thoroughly cleaned before starting any topical treatment. If the external ear canal has drainage or is swollen shut, a wick may be inserted. The wick serves to aid in removing drainage or to aid in administering medication into the ear canal. Cerumen may be removed with installations, a blunt ear curette, or a wire ear curette. Installation is not used with history of perforated tympanic membrane (eardrum). External ear disorders are usually painful, and analgesics are used to control pain.

Debridement, surgical repair, or application of a protective covering may be done when trauma occurs to the external ear. Surgical management consists of incision and drainage of abscesses. Excision of cysts or cutaneous carcinomas may also be required.

Nursing Process—External Ear Disorders

Assessment

Subjective data are obtained in a client history. Data include any reports of pain, fullness, previous cerumen impaction, itching, or hearing loss, as well as onset, duration, and severity of symptoms. Additional data include client's occupation, previous ear problems, use of a hearing aid, and typical ear hygiene. Inspection and palpation are primarily used to obtain objective data. The nurse observes for redness, swelling, drainage, furuncles, carbuncles, lesions, abrasions, lacerations, growths, cerumen, scaliness, or crusting. The client may report pain when the ear is palpated. Basic hearing acuity tests are conducted to evaluate hearing loss (see Chapter 48).

Nursing Diagnosis

The major nursing diagnoses for external ear disorders may include but are not limited to the following:

- Pain related to inflammation or trauma
- Sensory-perceptual alterations (auditory) related to blockage of external ear
- Risk for injury related to self-cleaning of external ear
- Knowledge deficit related to lack of information on preventive ear care

Planning

Planning focuses on helping the client return to his or her preillness state and preventing any further ear disorders. The client's goals are as follows:

- States pain is decreased by a lower rating on a scale of 1 (low) to 10 (severe)
- Hearing returns to preillness state
- Explains or demonstrates prescribed treatment
- Explains or demonstrates procedures to maintain wellness of the external ear

Nursing Interventions

Nursing care focuses on relieving the client's pain, promoting hearing, maintaining ear function, and educating the client about the disease and preventive ear care. The client should be assessed for nonverbal signs of ear pain. External ear pain is relieved by pharmacological and nonpharmacological interventions. The nurse and client should identify the optimum analgesic schedule and administer the medications to promote comfort. Nonpharmacological methods such as relaxation, massage, music, guided imagery, or distraction techniques can also be used to relieve pain. The nurse can also apply warmth to the area to promote comfort. Liquid or soft foods may be offered if the client experiences pain when chewing.

Interventions to restore hearing and relieve blockage of the ear canal are important. Topical antibiotics and antiinflammatory medications should be administered using aseptic technique. If the client has a wick inserted into the ear canal, the nurse monitors for drainage. Experienced practitioners or physicians remove cerumen (Table 49–7).

The nurse should instruct the client how to complete the prescribed treatment and maintain ear health (Table 49–8). Client teaching includes how to administer eardrops or ointments. The client should keep the ear clean and dry. During an infection, cotton with petroleum jelly or earplugs should be used to avoid getting water in the ears.

Evaluation

The goals for the client are met if the following occur:

- Pain is reduced to a lower rating on a scale of 1 to 10
- Hearing improves or returns to preillness level
- States or demonstrates prescribed treatment (e.g., administering eardrops or ointments)
- Explains or demonstrates measures to maintain wellness of the external ear

Table 49–7. **Removing Cerumen**

Instillations and irrigations should not be used on any person with a history of perforated tympanic membrane. Commercial ceruminolytics or common products such as baby oil, mineral oil, and virgin olive oil can be used to soften impacted cerumen and aid in the removal of the impacted wax. The client should instill several drops of the solution at bedtime and then place a cotton plug in the ear to hold the solution in place. Excess oil and drainage are removed in the morning. Ear wax is usually softened for 3 to 4 days before an irrigation is attempted. Clients prone to cerumen buildup should be taught how to safely remove earwax. A few drops of half-strength peroxide may be instilled into the ear canal during the day and three drops of glycerin instilled at bedtime. This can be repeated each week to minimize wax buildup.

The ear can be irrigated with an ear irrigation syringe or a Water Pik. The irrigation solution, usually water, should be warmed to body temperature. The client is draped with a protective plastic drape, and a basin is placed below the ear to catch the irrigating solution. The client sits with the ear toward the nurse and the head tilted toward the opposite ear (Fig. 49–11). The external ear is pulled upward and backward for the adult. A low-pressure stream of water is directed toward the top of the ear canal. Care is taken not to obstruct the canal with the syringe so that the irrigation solution can backflow out of the canal. The nurse must ensure that only the tip of the syringe is in the ear canal to prevent perforation of the eardrum.

Table 49–8. *Ear Care*

1. Cleanse the external ear with a wet washcloth. Gently cleanse the helix.
2. Never insert anything into the ear canal, including hairpins, cotton-tipped applicators, matchsticks, safety pins, toothpicks, paper clips, and fingers.
3. An individual with a history of ear infections, perforated tympanic membrane, or swimmer's ear should prevent moisture from entering the ear canal. Avoid swimming in contaminated water. Moisture or water in the ear canal can be prevented by using special earplugs or by using a piece of cotton rolled into a cylinder and covered with petroleum jelly.
4. Avoid home remedies for ear care.
5. An individual with an upper respiratory infection should gently blow the nose with both nares open to prevent infection being forced up the eustachian tubes.

MIDDLE EAR, TYMPANIC MEMBRANE, AND MASTOID DISORDERS

Infections

Pathophysiology and Etiology

Otitis media is the most common disease of the middle ear. *Otitis media* is a general term for inflammation of the middle ear, mastoid, and eustachian tube. Inflammation of the nasopharynx causes most cases of otitis media. As inflammation occurs the nasopharynx mucosa becomes edematous and discharge is produced. When fluid, pus, or air builds up in the middle ear, the eustachian tube becomes blocked, and this impairs middle ear ventilation. There are several types of otitis media in which inflammation can occur alone, with infective drainage, or with noninfective drainage. The first type of otitis media is otitis media without effusion. This is an inflammation of the middle ear mucosa without drainage. The second type of otitis media oc-

curs when there is a bacterial infection of the middle ear mucosa. This is called acute otitis media, suppurative otitis media, or purulent otitis media. The infected fluid becomes trapped in the middle ear. If the infection continues longer than 3 months, chronic otitis media results. The third type of otitis media is otitis media with effusion. Other names include serous otitis media, nonsuppurative otitis media, and glue ear. With this type of otitis media, noninfective fluid accumulates within the middle ear.[6]

Signs and Symptoms

Acute otitis media commonly follows an upper respiratory infection. A fever, earache, and feeling of fullness in the affected ear are common symptoms. As purulent drainage forms, there is pain and conductive hearing loss. Nausea and vomiting may also be present. Purulent drainage may be evident in the external ear canal if the tympanic membrane ruptures. Mastoid tenderness indicates that the infection may have spread to the mastoid area. Otoscopic examination reveals a reddened, bulging tympanic membrane.

Symptoms of otitis media with effusion may go undetected in adults because there are no signs of infection. The client may complain of fullness, bubbling, or crackling in the ear. The client may have a slight conductive hearing loss or allergies or be a mouth breather. Otoscopic examination can reveal a bulging tympanic membrane with a fluid level, but the eardrum is not reddened.

Diagnostic Studies

Laboratory studies may indicate an elevated WBC count. Ear cultures may be obtained on any drainage to identify the specific infective organism. Conductive hearing loss is usually present on audiometric studies and Rinne, Weber, and whisper tests. Imaging studies may be done to diagnose infection.

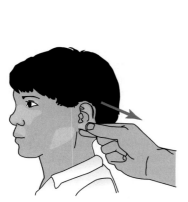

A Pull ear back and down to straighten ear canal

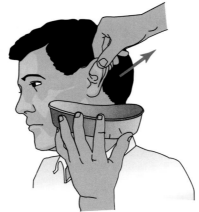

B Pull ear up and back to straighten ear canal

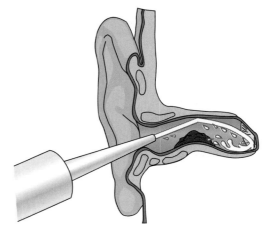

C Irrigation – Fluid is aimed off top of ear canal wall behind impacted cerumen

Figure 49–11. Ear irrigation. *(A)* Child. *(B)* Adult.

Complications

A perforation may occur with an acute or chronic infection. Buildup of fluid and pressure in the middle ear can cause a spontaneous perforation of the tympanic membrane. The client usually experiences pain before the rupture and relief of pain after the rupture. The fluid in the middle ear moves through the perforation into the ear canal, relieving the pressure and pain. A tympanic membrane perforation causes hearing loss. The location and size of the perforation determine the extent of hearing loss. Damage to the ossicles can also occur with perforation.

Repeated infections in the middle ear or mastoid can cause a cholesteatoma. A cholesteatoma is an epithelial cystlike sac that fills with debris such as degenerated skin and sebaceous material. The cholesteatoma starts in the external ear canal and spreads to the middle ear through a perforation in the tympanic membrane. Damage occurs in the middle ear structures due to pressure necrosis. The cholesteatoma causes conductive hearing loss. As the disease progresses, facial paralysis and vertigo may occur.

Tympanosclerosis is another complication of repeated middle ear infections. Tympanosclerosis consists of deposits of collagen and calcium on the tympanic membrane. The condition can slowly progress over time to the area around the middle ear ossicles. These deposits appear as chalky white plaques on the tympanic membrane and contribute to conductive hearing loss.

Mastoiditis can occur if acute otitis media is not treated. The infection spreads to the mastoid area, causing pain. Since the use of antibiotics, acute mastoiditis is relatively uncommon. Chronic mastoiditis is still seen with repeated middle ear infections.

Medical and Surgical Treatment

Medical treatment consists of treating the infections with antibiotics. Amoxicillin, penicillin V, erythromycin, cefaclor, and co-trimoxazole are commonly used. Analgesics such as aspirin, acetaminophen, or codeine or eardrops control the pain.

Surgical intervention includes several techniques. Paracentesis may be performed with a needle and syringe. The tympanic membrane is punctured with the needle and the fluid is drained from the middle ear. A **myringotomy** may also be performed. During this procedure, an incision is made on the tympanic membrane and fluid is allowed to drain out or is suctioned out of the middle ear. Various types of transtympanic tubes may be inserted to keep the incision open. The transtympanic tube keeps the incision in the tympanic membrane open, equalizes pressure, and prevents further fluid formation and buildup. The transtympanic tubes are left in place until the infection is cured. Most tubes spontaneously extrude in 3 to 12 months and rarely have to be removed.

Reconstructive repair of a perforated tympanic membrane is called a **myringoplasty.** One technique involves placing Gelfoam over the perforation. Then a graft from the temporal muscle behind the ear or tissue from the external ear is placed over the perforation and Gelfoam. The Gelfoam is absorbed and the graft repairs the perforation.

A mastoidectomy involves incision, drainage, and surgical removal of the mastoid process if the infection has spread to the mastoid area.

Otosclerosis

Pathophysiology and Etiology

Otosclerosis, or hardening of the ear, results from the formation of new bone along the stapes. With the new bone growth, the stapes becomes immobile and causes conductive hearing loss. The formation of the new bone growth begins in adolescence or early adulthood and progresses slowly. Hearing loss is most apparent after the fourth decade. Otosclerosis is more common in women than in men. The disease usually affects both ears. Although the exact cause of otosclerosis is not known, most clients have a family history of the disease. It is therefore thought to be a hereditary disease.

Signs and Symptoms

The primary symptom of otosclerosis is progressive hearing loss. The client usually experiences bilateral conductive hearing loss, particularly with soft, low tones. Usually medical assistance is sought when the hearing loss interferes with the client's ability to hear conversations. The client may also experience tinnitus. Otoscopic examination reveals a pinkish-orange tympanic membrane due to vascular and bony changes in the middle ear.

Diagnostic Studies

Audiometric testing indicates the type and extent of the hearing loss. Imaging studies indicate the location and the extent of the excessive bone growth. Whisper voice test and normal conversation show decreased hearing. The client hears best with bone conduction in the Rinne test, whereas lateralization to the most affected ear occurs with the Weber test.

Medical and Surgical Management

There is no cure for otosclerosis, but hearing aids may be used to improve hearing for the client. The hearing aid is most effective for conductive hearing loss when there is no sensorineural involvement.

Although total restoration of hearing is not possible, reconstruction of necrotic ossicles is done to restore some of the client's hearing. Various methods are used to reposition and replace some or all of the ossicles. Unfortunately, the surgeries are not always successful over the long term. Os-

---

myringoplasty: myringo—tympanic membrane + plasty—surgical repair

otosclerosis: oto—ear + sclerosis—hardening

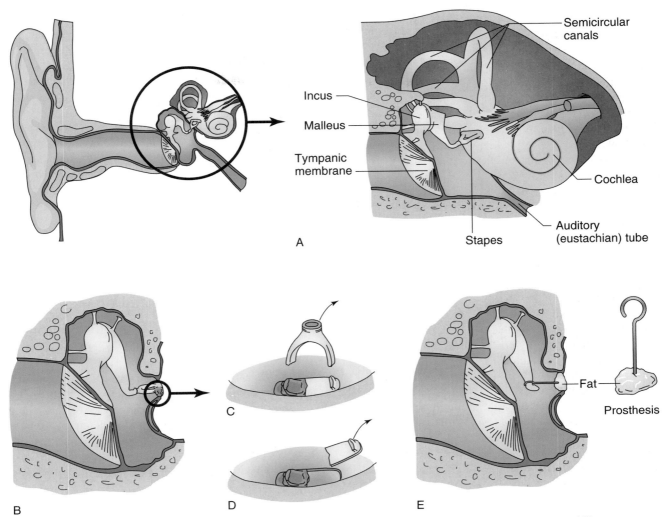

Figure 49–12. Stapedectomy. *(A)* Normal anatomy. *(B)* Sclerotic process at the foot of the stapes. *(C)* Stapes that is broken away surgically. *(D)* The footplate is removed. *(E)* Prosthesis implanted.

siculoplasty is the reconstruction of the ossicles. Prostheses made of plastic, ceramic, or human bone are used to replace the necrotic ossicles. Total or partial ossicular replacement prosthesis may be used. The **stapedectomy** is the treatment of choice for otosclerosis (Fig. 49–12). Either part or all of the stapes is removed and replaced with a prosthesis. The prosthesis is placed between the incus and the oval window. Advances in surgical treatment include the use of lasers for improved visualization, less trauma, and greater precision during surgery.[17] The goal is to restore vibration from the tympanic membrane to the oval window and allow sound transmission. Many clients experience improved hearing immediately, others not until swelling subsides. Complications of ossiculoplasty and stapedectomy include extrusion of the prosthesis, infection, hearing loss, dizziness, and facial nerve damage. Some clients may have the surgery repeated if complications develop.[18]

stapedectomy: stapes—stirrup + ectomy—excision of

Nursing Management

The operative ear is placed upward when lying in bed. An earplug may be used to help keep the area aseptic due to proximity of the brain. Activity orders may vary. The client may be dizzy and experience nausea. Antiemetics should be given promptly to prevent vomiting. The client's safety should be ensured if dizziness occurs. To prevent dislodgment or damage to the prosthesis, the client is instructed not to cough, sneeze, blow his or her nose, vomit, fly in an airplane, lift heavy objects, or shower. If the client develops a cold, the physician should be contacted.

 CRITICAL THINKING: Mrs. Smith

Mrs. Smith is an 83-year-old woman who is scheduled to be discharged from the hospital following a stapedectomy. She lives alone at home and is able to care for herself.

1. How would you communicate with Mrs. Smith to ensure that she understands the discharge instructions?
2. What teaching methods would you use to enhance communication?
3. What ear care instructions would you give her?

Answers at end of chapter.

Trauma

Etiology and Physiology

Trauma such as a blasting force, a blunt injury to the side of the head, or sudden changes in atmospheric pressure can cause the tympanic membrane to perforate and middle ear ossicles to fracture. Blast injuries cause injury from the direct pressure on the ear. Blunt injury to the head can cause temporal skull fractures and trauma to both the middle and inner ear. Barotrauma caused by sudden changes in atmospheric pressure in the ears can occur during scuba diving and airplane takeoffs and landings. Pressure changes can occur during normal atmospheric conditions such as nose blowing, heavy lifting, and sneezing.[19] During these rapid changes of pressure, the eustachian tube does not ventilate due to occlusion or dysfunction and a negative pressure develops in the middle ear. The resulting pressure can cause the tympanic membrane to rupture or cause damage to the middle and inner ear.

Signs and Symptoms

Pain and hearing loss are the most common symptoms associated with trauma. Other signs and symptoms of barotrauma include fullness of the ears, vertigo, nausea, disorientation, edema of the affected area, and hemorrhage in the external or middle ear. In severe cases of barotrauma when scuba diving, these symptoms can cause drowning or cerebral air embolism from an overly rapid ascent. Otoscopic examination may reveal a retracted, reddened, and edematous tympanic membrane.

Diagnostic Studies

Audiometric studies are completed to determine the hearing loss. Imaging studies may be done to determine the extent of middle and inner ear damage. Conductive or sensorineural hearing loss may be evident, depending on the extent and location of the damage.

Nursing Process—Middle Ear, Tympanic Membrane, and Mastoid Disorders

Assessment

Assessment of symptoms includes asking the client for subjective data using the WHAT'S UP acronym:

Where is it? Are both ears affected? Is it deep within the head?

How does it feel? Pressure? Fullness? Painful—sharp, dull, continuous, intermittent, throbbing, localized? No pain?

Aggravating and alleviating factors. Worse with change of position? Worse with movement? Relief after drainage? Relief with change of position? Relief with heat or analgesics?

Timing. When did it start? Any recent upper respiratory infections, airline travel, scuba diving, trauma, or weight lifting? Was it a gradual or sudden onset? Length of time symptoms have persisted? Has there been a change in symptoms?

Severity. Does it cause hearing impairment? How much? Does it affect ADL?

Useful data for associated symptoms. Is there any fever, drainage from the ear canal, nausea, vomiting, dizziness? Is there a family history of otosclerosis? Any previous ear problems or ear surgeries? Any occupational or recreational risk factors such as scuba diving, weight lifting, or frequent airline travel?

Perception by the client of the problem. What does the client think is wrong? Has problem occurred before? If so, how was it the same and what was different?

The external ear should be inspected and palpated to obtain objective data. Pain with palpation is indicative of external ear problems, not middle ear problems. Pain over the mastoid area can indicate a mastoid problem.

The middle ear and mastoid cavity cannot be visualized directly. The tympanic membrane is the only middle ear structure that can be directly visualized by the experienced practitioner with an otoscope.

Objective assessment should also include vital signs, noting any elevation in temperature. Hearing acuity should be screened by the experienced practitioner using the whisper voice, Rinne, and Weber tests. Any drainage from the ear should be noted and described.

Nursing Diagnosis

Nursing diagnoses for middle ear disorders may include but are not limited to the following:

- Risk for infection related to broken skin, pressure necrosis, chronic disease, or surgical procedure
- Sensory-perceptual alteration (auditory) related to blockage, infection, drainage, or fixation of the ear bones in the middle ear
- Pain related to fluid accumulation, inflammation, or infection
- Fear related to hearing loss and lack of information
- Knowledge deficit related to lack of exposure to information

Planning

The client and family are included in planning care. Planning focuses on improving hearing, controlling infection, and improving the quality of life. The client's goals include but are not limited to the following:

- Exhibits no signs of infection (no drainage from ear, no tenderness over mastoid, negative culture, afebrile)
- Hearing improves or stabilizes
- States pain is decreased or absent as evidenced by a lower rating on scale of 1 to 10
- States methods for preventing problems in the middle ear, tympanic membrane, and mastoid process
- States rationale and desired outcome of any impending surgery

Nursing Interventions

The family should be included in teaching sessions. The client is instructed about medications. The client is instructed to complete all therapy as directed by the physician. The nurse ensures that the client knows how to administer eardrops and ear ointment. Care of the ears to prevent infection is discussed. The client is taught to avoid getting water in the ears.

If medical or surgical management is necessary to improve the client's hearing, the client is instructed on this treatment. Methods to improve communication with the hearing impaired are used by the nurse (see Nursing Care Plan Box 49–3).

The nurse monitors pain using a pain scale and provides measures to promote comfort. Nonpharmacological measures for pain reduction may include heat, distraction, and relaxation techniques. If analgesics are used, the optimal schedule for pain control is identified.

The client is instructed on methods to maintain ear health. The nurse informs the client how to prevent ear damage from trauma, noise exposure, and environmental or occupational conditions. To equalize ear pressure, the client should yawn or jaw thrust (opening mouth wide and moving jaw). Preventing the spread of upper respiratory infections up the eustachian tube is accomplished by telling the client not to blow the nose by pinching off a nare. If the client's pain worsens, hearing decreases, or drainage from ear is present, the client is told to seek further medical attention.

The nurse assesses the client's knowledge regarding any surgical procedures. The nurse instructs the client as needed (Table 49–9).

Evaluation

The goals for the client are met if the following occur:

- Does not have ear drainage, pain over mastoid; has negative culture and remains afebrile

Table 49–9. **Preoperative and Postoperative Nursing Interventions for the Client Having Ear Surgery**

Preoperative Care

Nursing care for the client undergoing ear surgery begins as soon as the decision to have surgery is made. The nurse collects data, determines if the client understands the events, assesses the client's mental readiness, and obtains baseline physiological data.

1. Assess understanding of the surgery and explain whether local or general anesthesia will be used.
2. Help alleviate the client's fear by encouraging the client to ask questions. Ensure that all questions are answered before the surgery.
3. Explain the type of pain, any packing or dressings that may be in place postoperatively, and any other restrictions postoperatively that may be needed.
4. Establish baseline vital signs and document findings.
5. Ensure that the operative permit is signed.
6. Determine current medications the client is taking and document in the client's record.
7. Assess if the client understands that surgery does not always correct impaired hearing.
8. Leave any hearing devices in place as long as possible before the surgery.[18]

Postoperative Care

Postoperatively, the nurse is responsible for assessing the client's physiological status. The nurse is also responsible for ensuring that the client and family members understand discharge instructions.

1. Some degree of pain can be expected, even with minor procedures. Explain how and when to take pain medication when the client is discharged.
2. Monitor postoperative vital signs and return to presurgical baseline.
3. Tell clients that if an occlusive dressing is in place, hearing may be decreased until the dressing is removed.
4. Instruct clients with tubes to avoid getting water in the ear. A shower cap or earplugs may be used.
5. Instruct the client to seek medical attention if excessive bleeding or drainage occurs. If a cotton plug is to be left in place, instruct the client to change it daily.
6. Teach the client unless contraindicated to blow the nose very gently one side at a time for the first week after surgery. Instruct the client to sneeze or cough with the mouth open for 1 week after surgery.
7. Avoid airplane flights for 1 week after surgery. For sensations of ear pressure, hold nose, close mouth, and swallow to equalize pressure.
8. The client should avoid strenuous work for several weeks. The client may return to work in a few days, depending on the type of surgery done and the type of work the client does.
9. Tell client to take prescribed medication and antibiotics as ordered.
10. Have client arrange for follow-up appointment by calling physician's office.

- Responds appropriately to auditory cues indicating improvement of hearing
- States that no pain is present or pain is decreased
- Verbalizes care of ears, methods to prevent further infection; describes signs requiring medical attention
- Verbalizes rationale and outcome for any upcoming surgery

INNER EAR

Labyrinthitis

Pathophysiology and Etiology

Labyrinthitis is an inflammation or infection of the inner ear and can be caused by either viral or bacterial pathogens. The bacteria or virus enters the inner ear from the middle ear, meninges, or bloodstream. Serous labyrinthitis is a type of acute labyrinthitis that sometimes follows drug intoxication or overindulgence in alcohol. It can also be caused by an allergy. Diffuse suppurative labyrinthitis occurs when acute or chronic otitis media spreads into the inner ear or after middle ear or mastoid surgery. Destruction of soft tissue structures from the infection can cause permanent hearing loss.

Signs and Symptoms

Vertigo, tinnitus, and sensorineural hearing loss are the most common symptoms. Vertigo, or dizziness, occurs when the vestibular structures are involved. Tinnitus, or ringing in the ear, occurs when the infection is located in the cochlea. Sensorineural hearing loss can be caused by infections in the cochlea or vestibular structures. Nystagmus on the affected side may occur. Other signs and symptoms include pain, fever, ataxia, nausea, vomiting, and beginning nerve deafness.

Diagnostic Tests

Laboratory tests such as a complete blood count may be completed to diagnose infection. Thorough hearing evaluation by an audiologist may reveal mild to complete hearing loss. Rinne and Weber tests can indicate conductive or sensorineural hearing loss.

Medical Management

Antibiotics are used to treat bacterial inner ear infections. Viral infections usually run their course in about 1 week. Mild sedation may help the client relax. Although there is no specific medicine to relieve dizziness, antihistamines can be used if they prove helpful on an individual basis. Clients may be placed on bed rest.

Nursing Management

Nursing management includes helping the client manage symptoms, self-care, and educating the client about safety issues while on bed rest and sedatives. The client should avoid turning the head quickly to help alleviate the vertigo. The nurse also needs to assist the client with anxiety that may be present due to frustration surrounding hearing loss or loss of work.

Neoplastic Disorders

Pathophysiology and Etiology

Inner ear tumors can be benign or malignant. Acoustic neuroma, a tumor of the eighth cranial nerve, is the most common benign tumor. It is slow growing, occurs at any age, and usually occurs unilaterally. As it spreads, it compresses the nerve and adjacent structures. Malignant tumors arising from the inner ear are rare. Squamous and basal carcinoma arise from the epidermal lining of the inner ear.

Signs and Symptoms

Early symptoms of an acoustic neuroma include progressive unilateral sensorineural hearing loss of high-pitched sounds, unilateral tinnitus, and intermittent vertigo. Headache, pain, and balance disorders may also be present. Symptoms progress as the tumor spreads to other structures. Most malignant tumors grow quickly. The symptoms vary depending on the area of the ear that is involved.

Diagnostic Tests

Neurological, audiometric, and vestibular testing are used to diagnose the neuromas. Auditory brainstem evoked response (ABR) and electronystagmography (ENG) are completed. Examination of the cerebrospinal fluid shows increased protein. Computed tomography (CT) and magnetic resonance imaging (MRI) are used to determine size and location of the tumor.

Medical and Surgical Treatment

The preferred method of treatment involves surgical removal of the tumor. The labyrinth is destroyed, with a resulting permanent hearing loss. Steroids and radiation may be used to decrease the size of the tumor or for inoperable tumors.

Nursing Management

Nursing management focuses on preparing the client for surgery, adjusting to the diagnosis, and the resulting hearing loss.

Ménière's Disease

Pathophysiology and Etiology

Ménière's disease is a balance disorder. Its cause is unknown. With the disease, there is a dilation of the membranous labyrinth resulting from a disturbance in the fluid physiology of the endolymphatic system. The exact etiology is unknown but is thought to stem from hypersecretion, hypoabsorption, deficit membrane permeability, allergy, virus, hormonal imbalance, or mental stress. The disease usually develops between 40 and 60 years of age. The symptoms range from vague to severe and debilitating.

Signs and Symptoms

A triad of symptoms of vertigo, hearing loss, and tinnitus characterizes Ménière's disease. Recurring episodic bouts of the incapacitating triad of symptoms and nausea and vomiting occur with Ménière's disease. The attacks may occur suddenly, or the client may experience warning signs such as headache or fullness in the ears. During an acute episode, the client experiences vertigo that lasts 2 to 4 hours. The vertigo is usually accompanied by nausea and vomiting, followed by dizziness and unsteadiness. The client is uncoordinated and has gait changes when walking. Hearing loss is often described as a fluctuating fullness in the ears. Tinnitus is present. Irritability, depression, and withdrawal are common behavioral changes. The vital signs usually remain normal. It takes several weeks for symptoms to resolve, and hearing loss in the affected ear remains. The client then enters a stage of remission until the next attack. The acute episodes occur two to three times per year. Eventually, the client has complete remission with some degree of permanent hearing loss.

Diagnostic Tests

Diagnostic tests include audiometric studies, neurological testing, and x-rays of the internal ear. Audiometric studies identify the type and magnitude of the hearing loss. Neurological testing and radiographical studies are done to rule out other pathology. A caloric stimulation test may demonstrate a difference in eye movement.

Medical and Surgical Treatment

Medical treatment consists of symptomatic treatment for acute attacks and prophylactic treatment between attacks. Tranquilizers and vagal blockers may be needed during acute attacks. Salt-restricted diet, diuretics, antihistamines, and vasodilators are used during prophylactic treatment. The client should avoid alcohol, caffeine, and tobacco use. The client may be placed on bed rest during acute attacks. Most clients respond to medical protocol but continue to have acute attacks. The goal of medical treatment is to preserve hearing and reduce symptoms.

Surgical treatment is used only when medical management has failed. When involvement is unilateral, a labyrinthectomy is performed.[20] This causes complete loss of hearing in that ear. Another surgical intervention establishes a shunt from the inner ear to the subarachnoid space. This procedure helps drain the fluid and prevent future hearing loss. Another surgical treatment is intratympanic gentamycin injection, which is usually done in the physician's office.[21]

Nursing Management

Nursing management focuses on managing the client's symptoms and providing safety during the acute attacks. The nurse administers medication, monitors fluid and nutritional status, and ensures safety. Due to the unpredictability of Ménière's disease, the nursing care focuses on emotional support for the client during periods of remission. The nurse provides emotional support and resources to help the client cope with the unpredictable nature of the disease and the physical impairments associated with the disease.

Nursing Process for Inner Ear Disorders

Assessment

Assessment of symptoms for the client with inner ear disorders includes asking the client for subjective data using the WHAT'S UP acronym:

Where is it? Are both ears affected?

How does it feel? Pressure? Fullness? Vertigo? Tinnitus? Painful—sharp, dull continuous, intermittent, throbbing, localized? No pain?

Aggravating and alleviating factors. Worse with change of position? Worse with movement? Relief with medications? Current medications? Any allergies?

Timing. When did it start? Was it a gradual or sudden onset? Length of time symptoms have persisted? Do symptoms progress in a set timing pattern? Do the symptoms occur together or separate? Has there been a change in symptoms?

Severity. Does it cause hearing impairment? How much? Does it affect ADL, nutritional intake, work, or leisure?

Useful data for associated symptoms. Any fever, nausea, vomiting, or dizziness? Any previous ear problems or ear surgeries? Headache?

Perception by the client of the problem. What does the client think is wrong? Has client had this problem before? If so, what was the same and what was different?

Objective data include assessment of gross hearing. The whisper voice, Rinne, and Weber tests and a physical examination can be performed. The client should be assessed for any nutritional deficiencies, including dehydration, weight loss, or weight gain. Any musculoskeletal abnormalities such as unsteady gait are also noted. The client's vital signs are taken to determine if symptoms are associated with an infection. Laboratory data and diagnostic data are examined for abnormal findings.

Nursing Diagnosis

The major nursing diagnoses for internal ear disorders may include but are not limited to the following:

- Anxiety related to unpredictability of sudden and severe acute attacks
- Fear related to potential permanent hearing loss
- Altered role performance related to impaired equilibrium
- Social isolation related to hearing loss and experiencing an attack in public

- Grieving related to hearing loss
- Risk for injury related to impaired equilibrium
- Fluid volume deficit related to nausea and vomiting
- Nutrition, altered: less than body requirements related to nausea and vomiting
- Knowledge deficit related to lack of information of diagnosis and treatment

Planning

Planning focuses on helping the client maintain normal lifestyle, remain free of injuries, cope with the illness or hearing loss, and maintain adequate nutrition and hydration. The client's goals are as follows:

- Signs of anxiety are decreased
- Is not injured from falling
- Identify ways of increasing meaningful relationships and diversional activities
- Experience adequate nutrition and hydration

Nursing Interventions

Nursing care focuses on relieving anxiety, protecting the client from injuries, maintaining and developing relationships, and providing adequate nutrition. The nurse encourages the client to explore concerns about hearing loss and the unpredictability of acute attacks. The client's understanding about the disorder should be explored, with the nurse providing additional information as needed. Medication regimen to help control symptoms should be explained. The nurse explains methods to minimize symptoms during acute episodes, such as decreasing movement.

Nursing measures to prevent injury include assessing the client for any pattern of dizziness and environmental hazards. The nurse instructs the client to seek assistance before ambulating. Antivertiginous drugs are administered, and the client is taught the medication regimen. Environmental hazards such as throw rugs, electrical cords in walkways, and poor lighting should be removed by the family.

The nurse can assist the client in maintaining relationships and activities that were present before the disorder. The nurse can provide information about disease processes to ensure that the client is informed about the disease. Diversional activities are planned.

Evaluation

The goals for the client are met if the following occur:

- Signs of anxiety are decreased
- Client remains free from injury
- Client verbalizes satisfaction with relationships
- Client maintains weight within normal range

Review Questions

1. Which one of the following infections is described by the term *pinkeye?*

   a. Keratitis
   b. Bacterial conjunctivitis
   c. Viral conjunctivitis
   d. Blepharitis

2. Which one of the following symptoms is common with macular degeneration?
   a. Loss of peripheral vision
   b. Sudden darkness
   c. Dull ache in the eyes
   d. Loss of central vision

3. Which one of the following clients needs specific positioning orders postoperatively?
   a. 4-year-old child after removal of congenital cataract
   b. 30-year-old woman after a scleral buckling
   c. 52-year-old man after trabeculectomy
   d. 82-year-old man after corneal transplant

4. Which one of the following is the most common assessment finding associated with retinal detachment?
   a. Blurred vision
   b. Flashes of light
   c. Loss of central vision
   d. Halos around lights

5. Which one of the following is the most common assessment finding with an external ear infection?
   a. Pain
   b. Fullness in ears
   c. Fever
   d. Dizziness

6. When caring for a client with impacted cerumen, which one of the following would be an expected finding?
   a. Positive Romberg's test
   b. Greenish drainage
   c. Rinne test results BC > AC
   d. Reddened auricle

7. Which one of the following should a client experiencing vertigo be instructed to do to relieve the vertigo?
   a. Avoid all medications
   b. Avoid rapid movement of the head
   c. Avoid raising hands above the head
   d. Avoid eating until the vertigo passes

8. Which one of the following is the primary goal for a client with Ménière's disease?
   a. Prevent fluid volume deficit
   b. Prevent injury
   c. Decrease pain
   d. Preserve hearing

ANSWERS TO CRITICAL THINKING

CRITICAL THINKING: Mr. Samuel

1. Seek assistance. Patch both eyes. Have someone take him to medical care immediately.

2. The nurse should ensure that an antiemetic is ordered postoperatively on the client's return to the unit. When client reports nausea, the antiemetic should be given promptly.

CRITICAL THINKING: Mrs. Smith

1. Gain her attention, face and stand in client's visual field, avoid glare, speak clearly, inform her of topics to be discussed, assess for understanding, allow extra time, reduce background noises, use nonverbal communication, and do not cover mouth when talking.
2. Use active listening. Use written communication to enhance spoken words. Use demonstration and return demonstration. Allow questions. Do not hurry. Provide information in short segments. Reassess understanding at each session.
3. Place operative ear upward when lying in bed. Use ear plug as ordered. Do not cough, sneeze, blow nose, vomit, fly in an airplane, lift heavy objects, or shower. If cold develops, call physician. Be careful if dizzy when up.

REFERENCES

1. Phipps, WJ, et al: Medical-Surgical Nursing. Mosby, St Louis, 1995.
2. Soparkar, CN, et al: Acute and chronic conjunctivitis due to over-the-counter ophthalmic decongestants. Arch Ophthalmol 115:34, 1997.
3. Baum, J: Infections of the eye. Clin Infect Dis 21:479, 1995.
4. Greenwood, J, and Graham, E: The ocular complications of HIV and AIDS. Int J STD AIDS 8:358, 1997.
5. Schultz, PJ: Vision. In Harkness, GA, and Dischner, JR (eds): Medical Surgical Nursing: Total Patient Care. Mosby, St Louis, 1996.
6. Beare, PG, and Myers, JL: Principles and Practice of Adult Health Nursing. Mosby, St Louis, 1994, p 1413.
7. Birt, L: Making sense of photorefractive keratectomy. Nurs Times 91:30, 1995.
8. American Foundation for the Blind at www.afb.org/afb.
9. National Foundation for the Blind at http://www.nfb.org/aboutnfb.htm.
10. Bryson, MK: Caring for patients with glaucoma. Nursing 25:56, 1995.
11. Prevent Blindness America: http://www.prevent-blindness.org/about_eyes/faq_glaucoma.html.
12. Cooper, J: Improving compliance with glaucoma eye-drop treatment. Nurs Times 92(32):36, 1996.
13. Meissner, JE: Caring for patients with glaucoma. Nursing 25(1):56, 1995.
14. Vaughan, DG, Asbury, T, and Riordan-Eva, P: General Ophthalmology, ed 14. Norwalk, Conn, 1995, Appleton & Lange.
15. Epstein, S: What you should know about ototoxic medications. Self help for Hard of Hearing People Journal (on-line). Available: http://www.pub.utdallas/edu/~dybala/theaudpa/blah/shhh/ototoxic.htm.
16. Meador, JA: Cerumen impaction in the elderly. J Gerontol Nurs 21:43, 1995.
17. Lundy, LB: Otosclerosis update. Otolaryngol Clin North Am 29:257, 1996.
18. Somers, TS, et al: Revision stapes surgery. J Laryngol Otol 111:233, 1997.
19. Kozuka, M, et al: Inner ear disorders due to pressure change. Clin Otolaryngol 22:106, 1997.
20. Pereira, KD, and Kerr, AG: Disability after labyrinthectomy. J Laryngol Otol 110:216, 1996.
21. Murofushi, T, Halmagyi, GM, and Yavor, RA: Intratympanic gentamicin in Ménière's disease: Results of therapy. Am J Otolaryngol 18:52, 1997.
22. Malatt, AE, and Taylor, HR: Onchocerciasis. Infect Dis Clin North Am 6:963, 1992.

BIBLIOGRAPHY

Anders, N, et al: Combined phacoemulsification and filtering surgery with the "no-stitch" technique. Arch Ophthalmol 115(10):1245, 1997.

Andersson, G, Green, M, and Melin, L: Behavioural hearing tactics: A controlled trial of a short treatment programme. Behav Res Ther 35(6):523, 1997.

Brady, L, et al: Radiation therapy for macular degeneration: Technical considerations and preliminary results. Int J Radiat Oncol Biol Phys 39(4):945, 1997.

Cataract Management Guideline Panel: Management of Cataract in Adults. Clinical Practice Guideline. Quick Reference Guide for Clinicians, Number 4. AHCPR Pub No 93-0543. US Department of Health and Human Services, Public Health Service, Agency for Health Care Policy and Research, Rockville, Md, 1993.

Elfervig, L: Age-related macular degeneration. Insight 22(3):88, 1997.

Gandham, S: New topical medications in the treatment of glaucoma. J Ophthalmic Nurs Technol 16(6):290, 1997.

Gates, G, and Rees, T: Hear ye? Hear ye! Successful auditory aging. West J Med 167(4):247, 1997.

Georpopoulos, G, et al: Risk factors in ocular hypertension. Eur J Ophthalmol 7(4):357, 1997.

Kalina, R: Seeing into the future. Vision and aging. West J Med 167(4):253, 1997.

Kearney, K: Emergency! Retinal detachment. Am J Nurs 97(8):50, 1997.

Sandler, R: Glaucoma. Am J Nurs 95(3):34, 1995.

Schumacher, D, and Carruth, J: Long-term use of hearing aids in patients with presbycusis. Clin Otolaryngol 22(5):430, 1997.

Sunness, J: Age-related macular degeneration: How science is improving clinical care. Geriatrics 53(2):70, 1998.

Understanding the Integumentary System

50

Integumentary Function, Assessment, and Therapeutic Measures

Rita Bolek Trofino and Valerie C. Scanlon

Learning Objectives

Upon completion of this chapter, the student will be able to:

1. Identify the structures and accessory structures of the integumentary system.
2. Describe the functions of the integumentary system.
3. List the effects of aging on the integumentary system.
4. Describe nursing assessment of the integumentary system, including health history and physical assessment.
5. Explain common laboratory and diagnostic tests utilized when assessing integumentary disorders.
6. Describe common therapeutic measures for clients with integumentary disorders.

Key Words

alopecia (AL-oh-**PEE**-she-ah)
ecchymosis (eck-uh-**MOH**-sis)
erythema (ER-i-**THEE**-mah)
petechei (pe-**TEE**-kee-ee)
turgor (**TER**-ger)

Review of Normal Anatomy and Physiology

The skin, its accessory structures, and the subcutaneous tissue make up the integumentary system, the covering of the body that separates the living internal environment from the external environment. The skin itself is considered an organ and consists of two layers, the outer epidermis and the inner dermis (Fig. 50–1).

EPIDERMIS

The epidermis is made of stratified squamous epithelial tissue and is avascular, meaning that it has no capillaries within it. Its nourishment comes from the dermis beneath it. The epidermis is thickest on the palms of the hands and soles of the feet. The innermost layer of the epidermis is called the stratum germinativum, and it is here that mitosis takes place to produce new epidermal cells. The rate of mitosis is fairly constant, but it may be increased by chronic pressure on the skin (as in callus formation). The new cells produced contain the protein keratin. As they are pushed to the surface of the skin, they die and become the stratum corneum, the outermost of the epidermal layers.

The stratum corneum is many layers of dead cells; all that remains is their keratin. An unbroken stratum corneum is an effective barrier against pathogens and most chemicals, although even microscopic breaks are sufficient to permit their entry. Keratin is relatively waterproof, so it prevents the loss of water, that is, dehydration, and also prevents the entry of excess water by way of the body surface. As dead cells are worn off the surface of the skin (which also contributes to the removal of pathogens) they are continuously replaced by cells from within. Loss of large portions of the stratum corneum, as with extensive third-degree burns, greatly increases the risk for infection and dehydration.

Melanocytes are cells in the lower epidermis that produce the protein melanin; the amount of melanin is a genetic characteristic and gives color to skin and hair. When

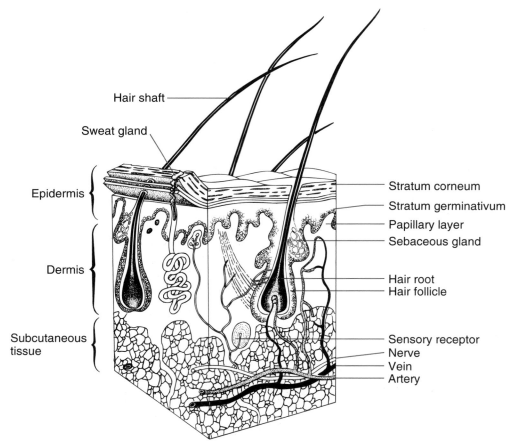

Figure 50–1. Structure of the skin and subcutaneous tissue. (Modified from Scanlon, VC, Sanders, T: Workbook for Essentials of Anatomy and Physiology, ed 2. FA Davis, Philadelphia, 1995, p 60, with permission.) See Plate 16.

the skin is exposed to ultraviolet rays (part of sunlight), production of melanin increases and it is incorporated into the epidermal cells before they die, making the cells darker. Melanin is a pigment barrier to prevent further exposure of living skin (the stratum germinativum within) to ultraviolet rays. Ultraviolet rays are considered mutagenic, that is, capable of damaging the DNA within cells and causing mutations that may result in malignant cells.

Also in the epidermis (and dermis) are Langerhans cells, a type of macrophage that presents foreign antigens to helper T cells. This is the first step in the destruction of pathogens that have penetrated the epidermis.

DERMIS

The dermis is also known as the "true skin." It is made of fibrous connective tissue; the cells present are called fibroblasts. Fibroblasts produce the protein fibers collagen and elastin. Collagen fibers are very strong and form the bulk of the dermis; elastin fibers are capable of recoil and make the dermis somewhat stretchable. Within the dermis are the hair and nail follicles, glands, nerve endings, and blood vessels. The capillaries in the papillary layer of the dermis are important to nourish the stratum

germinativum, which has no capillaries of its own. The papillary layer is responsible for the unique pattern of fingerprints.

APPENDAGES

Hair

Hair develops in epidermal structures called follicles. At the base of a follicle is the hair root, a group of cells that undergoes mitosis to produce the hair shaft. The cells quickly die after producing keratin and incorporating melanin. Hair growth is about 5 inches per year, with periods of growth and rest. Human hair with significant functions includes the eyelashes and eyebrows, which keep dust and sweat out of the eyes, and nostril hair, which blocks the entry of dust into the nasal cavities. Hair on the head provides thermal insulation (sparse body hair does not). If the shape of the hair shaft is flat, the hair is wavy; if round, the hair is straight.

Nails

Nail follicles are found at the ends of the fingers and toes, and growth of nails is similar to growth of hair. Mitosis in the nail root is a continuous process to produce new cells, which contain keratin. As these cells die, they form the visible nail. Nails protect the ends of the digits from mechanical injury and are useful for picking up small objects. Nail growth varies and is about 1.0 to 1.5 mm per week. Fingernails grow faster than toenails.

Receptors

The sensory receptors in the dermis are those for the cutaneous senses. Free nerve endings are the receptors for pain; encapsulated nerve endings are specific for touch, pressure, heat, or cold. The sensitivity of an area of skin is determined by the number of receptors present.

Sebaceous Glands

The ducts of sebaceous glands open into hair follicles or directly to the skin surface. Their secretion is sebum, a lipid substance that prevents drying of skin and hair. Skin that is dry tends to crack or fissure more easily, and even these small breaks in the epidermis are potential portals of entry for pathogens.

Modified sebaceous glands called ceruminous glands are found in the dermis of the ear canals. Their secretion is called cerumen or ear wax. Cerumen prevents drying of the outer surface of the ear drum. Excess cerumen, however, may become impacted against the eardrum, prevent it from vibrating properly, and diminish the acuity of hearing.

Sudoriferous (Sweat) Glands

Sudoriferous glands are also known as sweat glands. There are two kinds of sudoriferous glands: apocrine and eccrine. Apocrine glands are really modified scent glands most numerous in the axillae and genital area; they are activated by stress and emotions. Odor is produced when sweat mixes with bacteria on the skin.

Eccrine glands are found throughout the dermis but are most numerous on the face, palms, and soles. They are activated by high temperatures or by exercise and secrete sweat onto the skin surface. The sweat is evaporated by excess body heat, which is a very effective cooling mechanism, although it does have the potential to lead to dehydration if water is not replaced by drinking.

Blood Vessels

The blood vessels in the dermis serve the usual function of tissue nourishment, but the arterioles are also involved in the maintenance of body temperature. Blood carries the heat produced by active organs and distributes it throughout the body. In a warm environment, dilation of blood vessels in the dermis increases blood flow and loss of heat to air or clothing (if cooler than the body). Constriction of blood vessels in a cold environment decreases blood flow to the skin and conserves body heat.

Stressful situations also bring about vasoconstriction in the dermis, which allows blood to circulate to more vital organs such as the heart, liver, brain, or muscles.

Other functions of the skin are the formation of vitamin D from cholesterol when the skin is exposed to the UV rays of the sun and the excretion of small amounts of urea and sodium chloride in sweat.

SUBCUTANEOUS TISSUE

The subcutaneous tissue, between the dermis and the muscles, is made of areolar connective tissue and adipose tissue. Although an unbroken stratum corneum is an excellent barrier to pathogens, even small breaks provide portals of entry. In the subcutaneous tissue are numerous white blood cells to destroy any pathogens that have entered by way of broken skin. Subcutaneous adipose tissue cushions some bones and provides some insulation from cold, but its most important function is energy storage. Excess nutrients are changed to fat and stored as potential energy for times when food intake may decrease.

AGING AND THE INTEGUMENTARY SYSTEM

The effects of age on the integumentary system are often quite visible. Cell division in the epidermis slows, fibroblasts in the dermis die and are not replaced, and both skin layers become thinner and more fragile. Both the collagen and elastin fibers in the dermis deteriorate, causing wrinkles. Sebaceous glands and sweat glands decrease their activity. The skin becomes dry, and temperature regulation in hot weather becomes more difficult. There is often less fat in the subcutaneous layer, which may make an elderly person more sensitive to cold temperatures. Hair follicles become inactive and the hair thins. Melanocytes die and the hair that remains becomes gray.

Nursing Assessment

HEALTH HISTORY

Skin problems are a fairly common complaint for the client entering the health system. Many factors can influence the integumentary system. A skin problem may be the only problem the client has, or it may be one manifestation of an underlying systemic condition, or psychological stress. Most important, the skin visibly communicates the client's health. Therefore the questions that the nurse poses to the client are important in determining if the skin problem is a disease entity of its own or a sign of a more systemic disorder. Table 50–1 provides examples of general questions the nurse can ask the client to elicit further information.

If the nurse needs to further assess a particular problem area, the WHAT'S UP? line of questioning may be used.

Do you (or anyone in your family) have a history of dryness, rashes, pruritis, skin diseases, proriasis, eczyma, dermatitis, asthma, hay fever, hives, or allergies?

Have you noticed any changes in the skin, such as a sore that does not heal, rashes, or lumps?

Have you had any recent trauma to your skin?

Do you have a tendency to sunburn easily? Do you use some type of sunblock?

Do you frequent tanning salons or utilize sun lamps or tanning pills?

How often do you bathe or shower? What kind of soap do you use?

Do you wear a wig or hairpiece?

Have you noticed a change in the growth or loss of your hair?

Have you experienced recent trauma or changes in your nails? Do you wear artificial nails?

Do you, any members of your immediate family, or your co-workers have recent skin complaints?

What medications do you take every day (prescription or nonprescription)? What is the dosage and frequency of your medications?

What medications did you take most recently? When did you take your last dose?

What is your occupation?

Do you enjoy any recreational activities, such as sports or gardening?

Have you traveled recently?

Is there anything in your current environment, at home or work, that may be causing any skin problems (e.g., animals, plants, chemicals, infections, or new detergents or soaps)?

Is there anything that touches your skin that causes a rash?

For example, if the client has a rash, the nurse may respond with the following questions:

Where is it? Is that the only area where you have a rash?

How does it feel? Does it itch? Burn?

Aggravating and alleviating factors. Does scratching aggravate it? Does anything else aggravate it, such as soaps and detergents? What relieves it?

Timing. How long have you had this problem? Does it recur?

Severity. How bad is the discomfort on a scale of 0 to 10, with 0 being comfortable and 10 being unable to touch the area?

Useful other data. Do you have other symptoms besides the rash, such as itching, discharge, tingling, or loss of sensation?

Patient's perception. What do you think is causing your rash?

PHYSICAL ASSESSMENT

Assessment of the skin involves not only the entire skin area, but also the hair, nails, scalp, and mucous membranes. The main techniques utilized in the physical assessment of the skin are inspection and palpation. For this assessment, the nurse ensures that the client is disrobed but adequately draped in a well-lighted and warm environment. A hand magnifying glass or penlight may be utilized to see small details and further illuminate the area.

Normally the skin is intact, with no abrasions, and appears smooth, dry, well hydrated, and warm. Skin **turgor** is firm and elastic. The skin surface is flexible and soft. Skin color ranges from light to ruddy pink or olive in white-skinned clients and light brown to deep brown in dark-skinned clients.

The nurse needs to be aware of normal developmental changes when performing an assessment. The skin of the neonate is very thin and friable. During adolescence, the skin becomes thicker, with active sebaceous, eccrine, and apocrine glands. Body hair also changes during adolescence due to hormonal influences. With older clients, the skin loses some of its elasticity and moisture. There is decreased activity of sebaceous and sweat glands. The older client's skin is thinner, more fragile, and more wrinkled.

Inspection

The nurse inspects each area of the skin, including nails, hair, scalp, and mucous membranes, for color, moisture, lesions, edema, intactness, vascular markings, and cleanliness. This examination should be done in an orderly sequence, such as hair, scalp, nails, buccal mucosa, and then the general skin surface from head to toe. (See Gerontological Issues Box 50–1.)

Color

Skin color can be influenced by many factors, including the temperature of the client, oxygenation, and blood flow. Because skin color genetically can differ from very light to very dark, this can make skin assessment a little more difficult for the novice practitioner.

Common alterations noted can include pallor, **erythema** (redness), jaundice, cyanosis, or brown color. Pallor, a paleness or decrease in color, can be caused by vasoconstriction or decreased blood flow or decreased hemoglobin levels from anemia. Pallor is best assessed on the face, conjunctivae, nail beds, and lips. Erythema, or red discoloration, may indicate circulatory changes and can be caused by vasodilation or increased blood flow to the skin from fever or inflammation. Erythema is best assessed on the face or area of trauma.

Jaundice, or a yellow-orange discoloration, may occur due to liver diseases. The best place to inspect for jaundice is in the sclera. Cyanosis, or bluish discoloration, may indicate a cardiac or pulmonary problem. The best places to inspect for cyanosis are the lips, nail beds, conjunctivae, and palms. A brown color may be caused by increased melanin production that could be indicative of chronic exposure to sunlight or pregnancy. This is best assessed on the face, areola, nipples, and areas exposed to the sun. A brownish color may also be the result of chronic peripheral vascular

GERONTOLOGICAL ISSUES BOX 50-1

In acute care settings, priorities are determined by medical diagnoses and often center around cardiovascular, respiratory, nutrition, comfort, or other immediate concerns. The feet may be forgotten in the rush to care for the client and plan a timely discharge.

Feet are also viewed by some as dirty; washing the feet may be seen as a lowly job. It may be assumed that people take care of their own feet. However, many older people are unable to bend down or bring the feet up high enough to see or care for them.

For these reasons it is especially important for the nurse to assess and care for the feet, both in institutional settings and at home. General guidelines for assessment include the following:
- Inspect feet for redness or pressure ulcers over bony prominences
- Inspect feet for dryness or cracking
- Inspect between toes for cracking, wounds, or excess moisture
- Inspect and palpate for callouses
- Palpate dorsalis pedis and posterior tibial pulses for circulatory status

- Assess client's sensation using a wisp of cotton or light touch

Hints to promote healthy feet:
- Soak the client's feet briefly in warm water and wash using a gentle soap. Test the water to be sure it is not too warm, especially for the client with reduced sensation.
- Thoroughly dry the feet, including between the toes. Water left to evaporate can cause drying and cracking.
- Use a pumice stone to help remove dry dead skin over heels or calluses. Work gently, rubbing the stone in one direction only and removing only a small amount of dead skin at any one time.
- Use a cream or lotion that does not contain alcohol to moisturize the feet. Apply it with a gentle massage while moving the client's feet through range-of-motion exercises. To prevent falls, never apply lotion before the client steps into the tub or shower.
- Use gauze or a commercially made pad to decrease pressure and friction in areas between toes that cross or other areas where breakdown is likely.
- Encourage the client to wear cotton socks and shoes or slippers to avoid injury to the feet and prevent falls.

disease and may be especially noted on the lower extremities.

Lesions

A lesion is any change or injury to tissue. Assessment of skin lesions helps determine the skin disorder. Lesions are described as primary or secondary lesions. Primary lesions are the initial reaction to the disease process. Secondary lesions are the changes that take place in the primary lesion due to trauma, scratching, infection, or various stages of a disease. Lesions are further described according to type and appearance (Fig. 50–2).

When assessing and documenting skin lesions, the nurse notes the color or colors of the lesion, the size (usually in centimeters), location(s), distribution, and configuration. Configuration refers to the pattern of the lesions, as shown in Figure 50–3. Gently stretching the skin over the rash area will make it stand out more for further assessment.

In general, healthy clients with naturally dark skin have a reddish undertone, with pinkish buccal mucosa, tongue, nails, and lips. If a dark-skinned client is pale, the mucous membranes will have an ash-gray color, lips and nail beds will appear paler, and the skin will appear yellow-brown to ash-gray. Erythema will present as a purplish-grayish color. Cyanosis will present as a gray cast to the skin. The nail beds, palms, and soles may have a bluish cast. Jaun-

dice can be noted in the oral mucosa, particularly the hard palate and the sclera closest to the cornea.

Moisture/Dryness

The assessment of moisture provides clues to the client's level of hydration. The nurse observes the skin areas for dryness and moisture. The skin is assessed for scales and flakes. Moisture may be found in skin fold areas. The skin should normally be smooth and dry. Flaking and scaling of the skin are indicative of dry skin.

Edema

Edema occurs due to a buildup of fluid in the tissues. Edema can cause the skin to become stretched, dry, and shiny. The location, distribution, and color of edematous areas are determined and documented. *Dependent edema* is edema that occurs in the part of the body that is at the lowest point, typically noted in the feet and ankles, or in the sacrum if the client is lying down.

Vascular Markings

Vascular markings may be classified as normal and abnormal. Two common abnormal vascular changes are **petechiae** and **ecchymosis.** Petechiae are small purplish hemorrhagic spots, smaller than 0.5 mm in diameter. In the darker-skinned client, petechiae are usually not visible on the skin but can be visualized in the conjunctivae and oral mucosa. An ecchymosis is a bruise in which the color changes from blue-black to greenish-brown or yellow with time.

---

ecchymosis: ek—out + chymos—juice + osis—condition

PRIMARY LESIONS

Macule:
Flat, nonpalpable change in skin color, with different sizes, shapes, color; usually smaller than 1 cm. (e.g. rubella, scarlet fever)
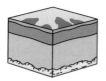

Papule:
Palpable solid raised lesion that is less than 1 cm. in diameter (e.g. ringworm, rosea, psoriasis, eczema)
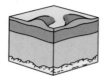

Nodule:
Solid elevated lesion that is larger and deeper than a papule (e.g. wart)
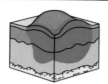

Vesicle:
Small raised area of the skin that contains serous fluid, less than 0.5 cm. in diameter (e.g. poison ivy, shingles, chicken pox)
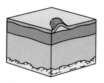

Bulla:
A vesicle or blister larger than 1 cm. (e.g. burns; scarlet fever-on palms and soles)
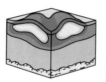

Pustule:
Small elevation of skin or vesicle or bulla that contains pus (e.g. impetigo, scabies, acne)
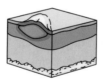

Wheal:
Round, transient elevation of the skin caused by dermal edema and surrounding capillary dilatation (e.g. hives, insect bites)
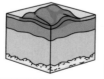

Plaque:
A patch or solid, raised lesion on the skin or mucous membrane that is greater than 1 cm. in diameter
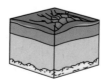

Cyst:
A closed sac or pouch tumor which consists of semisolid, solid, or liquid material
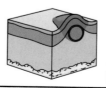

SECONDARY LESIONS

Scales:
Dry exfoliation of dead epidermis that may develop as a result of inflammatory changes (e.g. very dry skin, cradle cap)
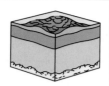

Crusts:
A scab formed by dry serum, pus, or blood (e.g. infected dermatitis's impetigo)
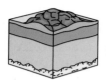

Excoriations:
Traumatized abrasions of the epidermis or linear scratch marks
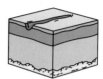

Fissure:
A slit or cracklike sore usually due to continuous inflammation and drying
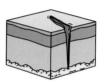

Ulcer:
An open sore or lesion that extends to the dermis (e.g. pressure sores)
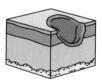

Lichenification:
Thickening and hardening of skin from continued irritation
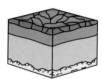

Scar:
A mark left in the skin due to fibrotic changes following healing of a wound or sore
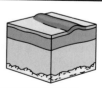

Figure 50–2. Description of skin lesions.

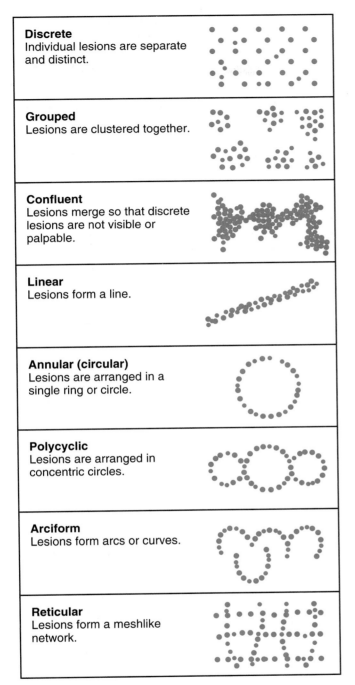

Discrete
Individual lesions are separate and distinct.

Grouped
Lesions are clustered together.

Confluent
Lesions merge so that discrete lesions are not visible or palpable.

Linear
Lesions form a line.

Annular (circular)
Lesions are arranged in a single ring or circle.

Polycyclic
Lesions are arranged in concentric circles.

Arciform
Lesions form arcs or curves.

Reticular
Lesions form a meshlike network.

Figure 50–3. To assess configuration, observe the relationship of the lesions to each other. Then characterize the configuration by one of the patterns illustrated in the chart. (Modified from Morton, PG: Health Assessment in Nursing, ed 2. Springhouse, Springhouse, Pa, p 169, with permission.)

General Integrity and Cleanliness

The nurse assesses the intactness of the skin. Elderly clients have thin, fragile skin that may have breaks in skin integrity. General cleanliness and odors are noted.

Palpation

Palpation is utilized in conjunction with inspection. The nurse utilizes the dorsum (back) of the hand to palpate temperature, because this part of the hand is most sensitive to changes in temperature. The fingertips are used to gently palpate over the skin to determine size, contour (flat, raised, depressed), and consistency (soft or indurated) of lesions. If the lesion is moist or draining, gloves should be worn to protect the client and nurse from the spread of infectious organisms. The degree of pain or discomfort associated with light palpation of lesions is documented.

The nurse assesses turgor and texture of the skin. Skin turgor is a measure of the amount of skin elasticity. To assess for turgor, the skin on the back of the forearm or over the sternum is pinched between the thumb and forefinger and then released. Normally, the skin will lift easily and then quickly return to its normal state. Poor skin turgor is indicated by "tenting" of the skin, with more gradual return to its normal state. Poor skin turgor may indicate dehydration. Normal aging of skin will produce some loss of skin elasticity; the preferred place to check skin turgor in the elderly is over the sternum.

If edema is suspected, the nurse palpates those areas to assess for tenderness, mobility, and consistency. When pressure from the nurse's fingers leaves an indentation, this is called pitting edema. Pitting edema is classified by its depth. The nurse presses the edematous area (against bone, if possible) with the thumb for 5 seconds and then releases. One way to measure edema is to measure depth of the pitting in millimeters: for example, 1+ edema = 1 mm depth or trace edema; 2+ edema = 2 mm depth of indentation or a small amount; 3+ is moderate edema; and 4+ is a large amount.

Hair distribution over the entire body is palpated. Assess for hair color, quantity, thickness, and texture. Note any areas of **alopecia** (hair loss). Determine any recent changes in color and growth pattern. Note cleanliness, itching, redness, scaling, flakes, and tenderness. If lesions or lice are suspected, utilize disposable gloves to avoid spread of infection.

Terminal hair is the hair on the scalp, axillae, and pubic areas. *Vellus hairs* are the soft, tiny hairs covering the body. Normally body hair has uniform distribution. Male and female pubic hair distribution is noted. Scalp hair can normally be thick, thin, coarse, smooth, shiny, curly, or straight. Scalp hair distribution and cleanliness are described.

Nails can reflect the client's general health. Fingers and nails are assessed for color, shape, texture, thickness, and abnormalities. The nails of elderly clients may have a yellowish-gray color, thickening, and ridges. Brown or black pigmentation between the nail and nail base is normal in dark-skinned clients. Normally, for all clients, the nail will appear pink, smooth, hard, and slightly convex (160-degree angle), with a firm base. Abnormal findings include clubbing (see Chapter 26), which may indicate hypoxia, and spoon nails (concave nails, also called koilonchia), which can indicate anemia. The nurse palpates for nail consistency and observes for redness, swelling, or tenderness

Table 50–2. **Abnormalities of the Nails**

Nail Abnormality	Description	Causes
Beau's lines	Transverse depressions in the nails	Systemic illnesses or nail injury
Splinter hemorrhages	Red or brown streaks in the nailbed	Minor trauma, subacute bacterial endocarditis, or trichinosis
Paronychia	Inflammation of the skin at the base of the nail	Local infection or trauma

Table 50–3. **Steps in Culturing a Wound**

1. Use sterile saline to remove excess drainage and debris from the wound. Purulent material may have different bacteria than those actually causing the infection.
2. Using a sterile calcium aginate swab in a rotating motion, swab wound and wound edges 10 times in a diagonal pattern across the entire surface of the wound.
3. Do not swab over eschar.

around the nail area. See Table 50–2 for other nail abnormalities.

Describe any abnormal skin conditions in detail. Include findings such as color of lesion, pain, swelling, redness, location, extent of lesion, and eruption patterns.

Diagnostic Tests

LABORATORY TESTS

Cultures

Skin cultures are done to determine the presence of fungus, bacteria, and viruses. When a fungal infection is suspected, the nurse gently scrapes scales from the lesion into a Petri dish or other indicated container. The specimen is then treated with a 10 percent potassium hydroxide (KOH) solution to make the fungi more prominent. The specimen can remain at room temperature until sent to the laboratory.

LEARNING TIP

When scraping scales, position the client so that the skin lesion is vertical. Place the slide against the skin below the lesion.

If a viral culture is ordered, the fluid is expressed (gently squeezed) from an intact vesicle, collected with a cotton swab, and placed in a special viral culture tube. If the lesion has crusts, they are removed or punctured before swabbing. The viral culture tube must be kept in ice and sent to the laboratory as soon as possible.

Wound cultures are also collected with a swab or wound culture kit. The wound should first be cleansed with normal saline. The red area of the wound is then swabbed, *not* the wound drainage itself. See Table 50–3 for specific instructions.

SKIN BIOPSY

A skin biopsy is indicated for deeper infections, to establish an accurate diagnosis, or for the assessment of the current treatment. A biopsy is an excision of a small piece of tissue for microscopic assessment. Three common types of skin biopsies are punch, shave, and incisional.

A punch biopsy utilizes a small round cutting instrument, called a punch, to cut a cylinder-shaped plug of tissue for a full-thickness specimen. An incisional biopsy is performed with a scalpel to make a deep incision, and, as such, almost always requires a suture closure. A shave biopsy removes just the area that is risen above the rest of the skin. For all of these biopsies, the nurse explains the procedure, calms and comforts the client, assists in preparing a sterile field, and assists in dressing the site following the procedure. The most uncomfortable part is usually the injection of the local anesthetic agent. Explaining the procedure and providing appropriate calming techniques can make the procedure less traumatic to the client.

OTHER DIAGNOSTIC TESTS

Wood's Light Examination

Wood's light examination is the use of ultraviolet rays to detect fluorescent materials in the skin and hair present in certain diseases such as tinea capitis. This examination is performed with a handheld black light in a darkened room.

Skin Testing

Patch and scratch tests are performed when allergic contact dermatitis is suspected. These tests are usually done by a dermatologist to uninvolved skin, such as the upper back and upper arms. Any hair in the area must first be shaved.

For the scratch test, the skin is superficially scratched or pricked with an allergen for an immediate reaction. If a reaction such as a wheal occurs, the test is positive for that allergen. Resuscitation equipment should be in the immediate vicinity in the event of a severe allergic (anaphylactic) reaction.

With the patch test, a delayed hypersensitivity reaction develops in 48 to 96 hours. The allergens are applied under occlusive tape patches. For this test, the skin should be free of oils. Alcohol promotes patch adhesion. The test site must remain dry and free from moisture. The patch is removed in 2 days. Any reaction is noted, with a final reading in 2 to 5 days.

Therapeutic Measures

OPEN WET DRESSINGS

Wet compresses may be ordered for acute, weeping, crusted, inflammatory, or ulcerative lesions. The purpose of these dressings is to decrease inflammation, cleanse and dry the wound, and continue drainage of infected areas. They may be ordered either sterile or unsterile depending on the risk for infection. The solutions commonly consist of room to cool temperature tap water or normal saline, aluminum acetate solution (Burow's solution), or magnesium sulfate.

The dressing is saturated with the solution before it is applied. Wet dressings are usually applied every 3 to 4 hours for 15 to 30 minutes. To prevent chilling, more than one third of the body should not be treated at one time. The client should be kept warm during this treatment. Wet dressings should not be prescribed for more than 72 hours, because the skin may become too dry or macerated. If cool compresses are used, they should be reapplied every 5 to 10 minutes, because they become too warm from body heat. If warm compresses are utilized, the skin is monitored closely to prevent burns.

Balneotherapy

Balneotherapy (therapeutic bath) is useful in applying medications to large areas of the skin. It is also useful for debridement, or removing old crusts, for removing old medications, and to relieve itching and inflammation. The temperature of the water should be kept at a comfortable level, avoiding hot baths. The bath should last for 15 to 30 minutes, while maintaining its warmth. The tub is filled half full. A bath mat should be used, because certain treatment baths may make the tub slippery. The room should be kept warm to minimize changes in temperature. The client is advised to wear loose clothing after the bath.

Water and saline are utilized for weeping, oozing, and erythematous lesions. Colloidal baths (such as oatmeal or Aveeno) are utilized for widely distributed lesions, for drying, and for the relief of itching. Medicated tar baths, such as Almar-Tar or Bainetar, are used for chronic eczema problems and psoriasis. Any loose skin crusts can be removed after the bath. The room should be well ventilated, because tars are volatile.

To increase hydration after the bath, a lubricating agent is applied to wet skin, if emollient action is prescribed. Bath oils, such as Alpha-Keri, Avenol, and Lubath, are utilized for lubrication and itching.

TOPICAL MEDICATIONS

Many types of topical medications are used to treat skin conditions. These include lotions, ointments and creams, powders, gels, pastes, and intralesional therapy. Systemic medications may also be given for more serious conditions.

Lotions tend to cool the skin through water evaporation. They may also have a protective effect and be antipruritic (treat itching). Lotions are usually applied with cotton gauze, gloves, or a soft brush.

Ointments and creams have a varied base (greasy, nongreasy, penetrating), depending on the drug applied. These medications can protect the skin, provide lubrication, and prevent water loss. These agents are utilized with localized or chronic skin conditions. Ointments and creams can cause some reduction in blood flow to the skin. They are applied with a gloved hand or wooden tongue depressor.

Powders usually have a zinc oxide, talc, or cornstarch base. They act as a hygroscopic agent, to absorb moisture and reduce friction. Powders are usually applied with a shaker top.

LEARNING TIP

Avoid applying too much powder in skin fold areas. Dermatitis can occur with too much powder in these areas. Products with a cornstarch base can provide a good medium for growth of microorganisms.

Gels, or semisolid emulsions, become liquid with topical application. They are usually greaseless and do not stain. Many topical steroids are prescribed in this manner.

Pastes are semisolid substances comprised of ointments and powders. They are utilized with inflammatory disorders. Mineral oil can facilitate removal of these agents.

Topical corticosteroids are used to reduce or relieve pain and itching by decreasing inflammation. Steroids should be used sparingly and according to package directions. Overuse of topical steroids can cause thinning of the skin. Caution is needed when used on the face to prevent glaucoma, cataracts, and perioral dermatitis.

Interlesional therapy has an anti-inflammatory action. This procedure utilizes a tuberculin syringe, most often of a sterile suspension of a corticosteroid, injected just below the lesion. Local atrophy may occur if the injection is made into subcutaneous tissue. Common conditions that are treated with the therapy include psoriasis and keloids.

 CRITICAL THINKING: Mr. Evans

Mr. Evans comes to the doctor's office with atrophic skin (thin, shiny, pink, with visible vessels) at the area of psoriasis where he is applying his corticosteroid ointment. He states that he has been generously applying a thick layer four times a day. What might be the cause of this condition?

Answer at end of chapter.

NURSING CARE PLAN BOX 50–2
FOR THE CLIENT WITH AN OCCLUSIVE DRESSING

Impaired skin integrity related to open lesions

Client Outcome
Improved skin integrity as evidenced by reduction in size of lesion.

Evaluation of Outcome
Is there a decrease in wound size?

Interventions	Rationale	Evaluation
• Assess areas of lesions for changes three times a day or as ordered. • Assess the lesions for presence or absence of dead tissue and exudate. • Cleanse the wound as prescribed (see text for specific bathing instructions). Lightly pat dry. • Apply the prescribed topical agent (see text for specifics) to moist skin. Apply sparingly or as directed. • Apply plastic film, cut to size. Cover with an appropriate dressing to seal the edges. • Remove dressing for 12 out of 24 hours.	Areas of redness, swelling, pain, and drainage may indicate infection. Indicates areas of healing and infection. Helps provide a healthy granulation area for healing. Various agents have specific properties (control bacterial growth, prevent itching, have a protective effect, provide lubrication, relieve pain, or decrease inflammation). Enhances absorption of medication and helps retain moisture. Continued use may cause skin atrophy, folliculitis, erythema, and systemic absorption of medication.	Are the lesions free of redness, swelling, pain, and drainage? Are the lesions free of exudate and dead tissue? Is the wound clean and free of debris, crusts, and exudate? Does the area exhibit signs of healing (e.g., decrease in size and numbers of lesions, free from infection, less itching)? Is the topical adherent to the skin? Are there signs of healthy granulation tissue? Is the skin pink? Are there less open areas? Is the dressing removed for at least 12 hours?

Knowledge deficit related to care of the dressing

Client Outcomes
Client and caregiver will be able to verbalize understanding of self-care, demonstrate dressing procedure, and state available resources for help following discharge.

Evaluation of Outcomes
Are client and caregiver able to verbalize self-care actions and rationale? Are client and caregiver able to correctly demonstrate dressing changes and care of skin? Is the client able to state how to obtain help following discharge?

Interventions	Rationale	Evaluation

• Assess client's and caregiver's baseline knowledge of self-care.
• Instruct client and caregiver in the following (see text for specifics):
  • Removal of old dressing
  • Cleansing of lesions
  • Application of topical agent
  • Application of plastic film
  • Application of dressing to seal the edges
  • Knowledge of signs and symptoms of infection
	Determines extent of teaching that is necessary.
	The client and caregiver need to be competent with wound care before discharge.
		Do the client and caregiver exhibit knowledge of self-care?
		Are the client and caregiver able to verbalize understanding of self-care and demonstrate all wound care before discharge?

continued

NURSING CARE PLAN BOX 50–2 *(continued)*

Body image disturbance related to presence of lesion or wound

Client Outcomes
Client verbalizes acceptance of condition. Client is willing to participate in care of lesion or wound.

Evaluation of Outcomes
Does client verbalize acceptance of condition? Does client participate in care of lesions?

Interventions	*Rationale*	*Evaluation*
• Assess client's feelings regarding condition.	Provides a baseline for care. If client denies condition, he or she may not comply with care.	Does client state willingness to follow care instructions?
• Care for the client with an accepting attitude.	Client will be aware of nuances in nurse's behavior.	Does the client allow the nurse to partake in the care of the lesion or wound?
• Allow opportunities for client to verbalize concerns about condition.	Verbalizations allow client to begin to accept and problem solve.	Does the client verbalize feelings appropriately?
• Provide referrals to support groups and counselors as appropriate.	Client may benefit from talking to others with similar condition or to another professional for objective evaluation.	Is the client receptive to appropriate referrals?
• Assist client in concealing the lesion or wound in a safe and appropriate manner.	Long sleeves and long pants may help conceal lesions, protect lesions, and prevent further skin damage.	Is the client accepting of appearance of lesions? Are lesions or wounds visible?

Bathing/hygiene self-care deficit, related to presence of lesions or wound and discomfort

Client Outcomes
Client verbalizes importance of good hygiene. Client is willing to participate in bathing/hygiene.

Evaluation of Outcomes
Does client verbalize importance of good hygiene? Is client clean?

Interventions	*Rationale*	*Evaluation*
• Assess client's level of hygiene.	Provides a baseline for care.	Is the client's level of hygiene at an acceptable level?
• Instruct client in appropriate bathing/hygiene: • Avoid strong detergents and soaps, utilize gentle emollient soaps or prescribed soaps • Gently stroke areas of lesions • Pat dry; no friction • Maintain a little moisture on skin • Maintain comfortable environmental temperature • Have temperature of bath at a comfortable level to client, but not too hot	The client needs to be able to properly cleanse lesions to prevent infection. Avoidance of friction and strong soaps prevents further trauma to skin. Client will not shiver in comfortable temperatures.	Is the client able to verbalize understanding, as well as demonstrate good bathing techniques? Are the lesions free of infection?

Dressings

Dressings may be used to enhance absorption of topical medications, encourage retention of moisture, prevent evaporation of medication, and reduce pain and itching. Occlusive dressings (for sealing the wound) are commonly used for skin disorders. An airtight plastic film is applied directly over the topical agent. Corticosteroids are also available as a special plastic surgical tape and can be cut to size. (See Nursing Care Plan Box 50–2 for the Client with an Occlusive Dressing.) Proper application of a plastic wrap dressing includes washing the area, lightly patting dry, applying the medication to moist skin, covering the medicated area with plastic wrap, and covering with a dressing to seal the edges. Plastic wrap dressings should be utilized for no more than 10 to 12 hours a day.

LEARNING TIP

Continued use of occlusive dressings may cause skin atrophy, folliculitis, maceration, erythema, and systemic absorption of the medication. To prevent some of these complications, the dressing is removed for 12 out of every 24 hours.

Other dressings commonly used with topical treatments for skin conditions include gauze or cotton cloth held in place with small, stretchable tubular material (Surgitube, Tubegauze) for fingers, toes, and extremities; disposable polyethylene gloves sealed at the wrist; cotton socks or plastic bags for the feet; cotton cloth held in place with tubular material for the extremities; disposable diapers or cotton diapers for the groin and perineal areas; cotton cloth held in place with dress shields for the axillae; cotton or light flannel pajamas for the trunk; a shower cap for the scalp; and a face mask made from gauze and stretchable dressings with holes cut out for eyes, nose, mouth, and ears. The client's physician can specify the type of dressing and particular materials needed for this dressing.

OTHER DRESSINGS

A variety of other types of dressing materials are available for wound and skin care. Transparent dressings (Op-Site, Tegaderm) can be used over skin tears or intravenous insertion sites. Hydrocolloid dressings can help protect areas exposed to pressure and treat pressure ulcers in early stages. Gels, pastes, and granules can be used to fill in deep wounds to aid healing. See Chapter 51 for additional dressings used specifically for pressure ulcers.

Wound Healing

Wounds can heal by first intention, second intention, and third intention. The edges of the wound are approximated with staples or sutures with first-intention healing. This usually results in minimal scarring. With healing by second intention, the wound is usually left open and allowed to heal by granulation. Scarring is usually extensive with prolonged healing. With healing by third intention, an infected wound is left open until there is no evidence of infection, and the wound is then surgically closed.

Review Questions

1. The protein in epidermal cells that makes the skin relatively waterproof is:
   a. Collagen
   b. Keratin
   c. Melanin
   d. Elastin

2. Which of the following skin lesions is typically seen in chickenpox?
   a. Macule
   b. Papule
   c. Vesicle
   d. Wheal

3. Which of the following terms describes a slit or crack-like sore?
   a. Scales
   b. Excoriations
   c. Ulcer
   d. Fissure

4. Which of the following actions by the nurse is appropriate when applying an occlusive dressing on a client?
   a. Remove the dressing for 12 out of 24 hours
   b. Apply a thick layer of the topical agent
   c. Apply aluminum foil
   d. Dry the client vigorously after the bath

5. Why should wet dressings be applied only to one third of the body at one time?
   a. So the rest of the body can be observed for reaction to the dressing
   b. To prevent chilling the client
   c. To prevent absorption of too much water causing fluid overload
   d. To enable the client to be more mobile

6. Which of the following terms describes a small, flat, red lesion?
   a. Macule
   b. Papule
   c. Bulla
   d. Crust

ANSWERS TO CRITICAL THINKING

CRITICAL THINKING: Mr. Evans

He may be sensitive or allergic to the medication. Most likely, he is applying too much, too often. This ointment is applied as a thin layer, and usually only twice daily.

BIBLIOGRAPHY

Alvarez, O, Rozint, J, and Wiseman, D: Moist environment for healing: Matching the dressing to the wound. Wounds 1(1):35, 1989.

Barkauskas, V, et al: Health and Physical Assessment. Mosby, St Louis, 1994.

De Witt, S: Nursing assessment of the skin and dermatologic lesions. Nurs Clin North Am 25(1):235, 1990.

Flory, C: Perfecting the art: Skin assessment. RN 55(6):22, 1992.

Gaskin, FC: Detection of cyanosis in the person with dark skin. J Natl Black Nurses Assoc 1(1):52, 1986.

Hill, M: The skin: Anatomy and physiology. Dermatol Nurs 2(1):13, 1990.

Ignatavicius, DD, et al: Medical-Surgical Nursing, ed 2. WB Saunders, Philadelphia, 1995.

Mairis, E: Four senses for a full skin assessment: Observation and assessment of the skin. Prof Nurse 7(6):376, 1992.

McConnel, E: Clinical do's and don'ts: Assessing the skin. Nursing 22(4):86, 1992.

Potter, PA, and Perry, AG: Fundamentals of Nursing, ed 4. Mosby, St Louis, 1997.

Reeves, JR, and Maibach, H: Clinical Dermatology Illustrated, ed 3. FA Davis, Philadelphia, 1998.

Watson, J, and Jaffe, MS: Nurse's Manual of Laboratory and Diagnostic Tests, ed 2. FA Davis, Philadelphia, 1995.

51

Nursing Care of Clients with Skin Disorders

Rita Bolek Trofino

Learning Objectives

Upon completion of this chapter, the student will be able to:

1. Describe the pathophysiology, etiology, signs and symptoms, and treatment of pressure ulcers.
2. Use the nursing process to plan care for the client with a pressure ulcer.
3. Describe the pathophysiology, etiology, signs and symptoms, and treatment of inflammatory skin disorders.
4. Use the nursing process to plan care for the client with dermatitis and psoriasis.
5. Describe pathophysiology, etiology, signs and symptoms, and treatment of infectious skin disorders.
6. Use the nursing process to plan care for the client with infectious skin disorders.
7. Describe the pathophysiology, etiology, signs and symptoms, and treatment of parasitic skin disorders.
8. Describe the pathophysiology, etiology, signs and symptoms, and treatment of pemphigus vulgaris.
9. Describe the pathophysiology, etiology, and signs and symptoms of a burn injury.
10. Use the nursing process to plan care for the client with a burn injury.
11. Describe the pathophysiology, etiology, and signs and symptoms of skin lesions.
12. Discuss nursing care of clients with skin lesions.
13. Describe types of skin grafts.
14. Discuss nursing care of clients undergoing plastic surgery.

Key Words

blanch (BLANCH)
cellulitis (sell-yoo-**LYE**-tis)
comedone (**KOH**-me-doh)
dermatitis (DER-mah-**TIGH**-tis)
dermatophytosis (DER-mah-toh-fye-**TOH**-sis)
eczema (**EK**-zuh-mah)
epithelialization (ep-i-THEE-lee-al-eye-**ZAY**-shun)

eschar (**ESS**-kar)
escharotomy (ess-kar-**AHT**-oh-mee)
lichenified (lye-**KEN**-i-fyed)
onychomycosis (ON-i-koh-my-**KOH**-sis)
pediculosis (pe-DIK-yoo-**LOH**-sis)
pemphigus (**PEM**-fi-gus)
pruritus (proo-**RYE**-tus)
psoriasis (suh-**RYE**-ah-sis)
purulent (**PURE**-u-lent)
pyoderma (PYE-oh-**DER**-mah)
seborrhea (SEB-oh-**REE**-ah)
serosanguineous (SEER-oh-**SANG**-gwin-ee-us)

Skin disorders cover a wide array of diseases and conditions. Disorders can be generalized or localized, acute, chronic, or traumatic. This chapter will discuss the more common skin disorders encountered by nurses.

Pressure Ulcers

PATHOPHYSIOLOGY AND ETIOLOGY

Pressure ulcers are often referred to by clients with old terms such as bed sores, decubitus ulcers, or pressure sores. Essentially a pressure ulcer is a sore caused by prolonged pressure against the skin. This may occur from a prolonged period of time in one position, causing the weight of the body to compress the capillaries against a bed or chair, especially over bony prominences. Other causes may be a tight splint or cast, traction, or other device. Pressure ulcers are the result of tissue anoxia and begin to develop within 20 to 40 minutes of unrelieved pressure on the skin. Those at risk are immobile clients, those with decreased circulation, and those with impaired sensory perception or neurological function.

Mechanical forces (pressure, friction, and shear) lead to the formation of pressure ulcers. The pressure level that closes capillaries in healthy people is 25 to 32 mm Hg. When pressure applied to the skin is greater than the pressure in the capillary bed, it can impair cellular metabolism. It decreases the blood supply to the tissues and eventually causes tissue ischemia. This reduction in blood flow causes **blanching** of the skin. The longer the pressure occurs, the greater the risk of skin breakdown and the development of a pressure ulcer.

Friction is the rubbing of the skin surface with an external mechanical force. This is also referred to as "sheet burns." This can happen when the client is dragged or pulled across the bed linens instead of being lifted.

Shearing occurs when the client slides down in bed while in a high Fowler's position or when being pulled or repositioned without being lifted off of the sheets. With shearing, the skin and subcutaneous tissue remain stationary, and the fat, muscle, and bone shift in the direction of body movement. As a result, there is damage deep within the tissues.

Any client experiencing prolonged pressure is at risk for a pressure ulcer. Elderly clients have increased risk because of normal aging changes of the skin. Because thin clients have little padding when pressure is present, they have the greatest pressure applied to their capillaries. Obesity also is a contributing factor, because adipose tissue is poorly vascularized and is therefore more likely to develop ischemic changes. Impaired peripheral circulation also makes the skin more susceptible to ischemic damage.

PREVENTION

There are many interventions for the prevention of pressure ulcers. The condition of the skin should be documented daily to be aware of developing problems. The skin should be gently cleansed daily with tepid water and mild soap to prevent drying. To reduce friction the skin is patted dry rather than rubbed dry. After bathing, daily lifelong lubrication of the skin with moisturizers is important to prevent dryness. Skin-to-skin surfaces, such as under the breasts, skin folds, and between the toes, should be thoroughly patted dry to prevent prolonged exposure to moisture. Moisture barriers should be used when incontinence is a problem. The skin should be promptly cleaned and dried after soiling occurs to prevent breakdown. Bony prominences or reddened skin areas should never be massaged; research has shown that blood vessels are damaged by massage when ischemia is present or when they lie over a bone.

Pressure on the skin should be avoided. If possible, teach clients to shift their weight every 15 minutes when lying or sitting. When the client is immobile, the highest level of mobility should be maintained, as well as frequent active or passive range of motion and turning according to a written repositioning schedule. If the client is on bed rest, he or she should be turned and repositioned at least every 2 hours, but preferably more often because ischemia development begins after 20 to 40 minutes of pressure application. When positioning clients on their side, they should be placed at a 30-degree angle or less and not directly on their trochanter because this area is especially sensitive to pressure and can quickly break down. If clients are placed on the trochanter, they usually become restless and squirm around to get off the trochanter. If the client is seated in a chair, repositioning every hour is important. A mobility program specific to the client must be developed.

The client's heels should not rest on the bed surface. They should be elevated off the bed with pillows placed lengthwise under the calf or with heel elevators. Care should be taken so pressure is not applied on the calf from the pillows. The client's elbows, sacrum, scapula, ears, and occipital area should also be protected from pressure.

Donut-shaped cushions should never be used. They create a circle of pressure that cuts off the circulation to the surrounding tissue, promoting ischemia rather than preventing it. Skin contact surfaces are padded, especially bony prominences, so they do not press against each other. Appropriate pressure-relieving or pressure-reducing mattresses and chair cushions are provided for immobile clients. To avoid friction, a sheet should be used to lift and move the client; a trapeze to assist the client to move herself or himself should be provided. Malnutrition and dehydration should be prevented by ensuring an adequate intake of protein, calories, and fluid; 2500 mL of fluid should be provided each day if not contraindicated by other medical problems. See Gerontological Issues Box 51–1 for additional preventive measures.

SIGNS AND SYMPTOMS

The most common sites for pressure ulcers are the sacrum, heels, elbows, lateral malleoli, greater trochanters, and ischial tuberosities. Most clients experience pain at the ulcer site. A report of pain requires continual assessment and treatment.

Pressure ulcers may be described according to a three-color system.

- Black wounds indicate necrosis.
- Yellow wounds have exudate and are infected.
- Red wounds are pink or red and are in the healing stage.

A wound may contain a mixture of these colors. Necrotic wounds are the worst, because they have dead tissue. Beefy red wounds are desired because they are healing wounds. It is important to consider treating the worst color present first or healing will be delayed. For example, if a wound is both yellow and black, the dead tissue must be removed first before the infection can be effectively treated. This color system is a helpful system for clients and families to use to describe wounds to the home care nurse, because colors are easily recognized and understood by most people.

COMPLICATIONS

Wound infection is a common complication. New ulcers can also appear, and the present ulcer can progress to a deeper wound. Wounds that do not heal or take prolonged time to heal also occur and may cause pain.

DIAGNOSTIC TESTS

All pressure ulcers are considered to be colonized with bacteria. This means that bacteria are present, but the wound is not necessarily infected. Swab cultures and culture and sensitivity tests may be done to identify the causative organism in suspected infection sites (see Chapter 50 for instructions for obtaining a culture). Results need to be interpreted to distinguish between true wound infection and bacterial colonization. If the wound is healing by second intention, it becomes colonized by bacterial flora on the skin and from the environment. If, however, the wound is extensive, bacterial growth may exceed the local tissue defenses and a true wound infection results.

If the wound does not demonstrate any healing, or if an ischemic ulcer is suspected, noninvasive and invasive arterial blood studies are recommended. Also, quantitative wound biopsies may also be performed for very large, extensive wounds.

MEDICAL TREATMENT

Treatment varies according to the size, depth, and stage of the pressure ulcer, as well as special needs of the client and health care provider preference. All pressure must be removed from the affected area for healing to occur. Cleanliness must be maintained. Basic treatment includes debridement, cleansing, and dressing of the wound to provide a moist and healing environment.

LEARNING TIP

The epidermis skates on moisture, so the wound must be kept moist to heal.

Debridement

Debridement can be nonsurgical or surgical. Nonsurgical methods include mechanical, enzymatic, and autolytic de-

---

GERONTOLOGICAL ISSUES BOX 51–1

Interventions to Prevent Skin Breakdown

- Avoid the use of soap and water on dry skin areas. Use a moisture barrier cream or ointment on dry skin areas *before* bathing to protect the skin from the drying effects of water.
- Use perineal cleansing products to cleanse urine and feces residue from the perineum and anal areas. These products are specially designed to break down and facilitate the complete removal of urine and feces without irritating the skin.
- Use moisturizing creams that have no alcohol or perfume that can irritate the skin.
- Avoid areas of skin pressure, especially over bony areas, by assisting the older adult to change positions on a regular schedule.
- Assess skin for areas of redness. If redness (stage I breakdown) occurs, the positioning schedule should be more frequent.
- Use pillows and pads to help maintain alignment with position changes. Use specialized mattresses and chair cushions designed to decrease pressure.
- Encourage the older adult to be out of bed and active throughout the day. Remember to assess skin and reposition frequently even when out of bed, because areas of pressure occur whether the client is in or out of bed.

bridement. Surgical debridement is utilized only if the client has sepsis or cellulitis or to remove extensive **eschar.** Eschar is a black, hard scab or dry crust that forms from necrotic tissue. It may hide the true depth of the wound and must be removed before the wound will heal.

Mechanical debridement can utilize scissors and forceps to selectively debride nonviable tissue. Dextranomer beads, another method of mechanical debridement, may also be sprinkled over the wound to absorb exudate and all other products of tissue breakdown, as well as surface bacteria. Whirlpool baths and wet-to-dry saline gauze dressings may also be utilized for mechanical debridement. The wet gauze is placed directly on the wound and allowed to dry completely. The nurse then pulls off this adherent gauze, removing tissue with it. This results in nonselective debridement, because viable tissue may also be removed in this process. These methods are painful; the client should be premedicated for pain and assessed frequently.

Enzymatic debridement involves the application of a topical debriding agent. These agents vary as to application methods, so careful reading of instructions is necessary. Most of these debriding agents are proteolytic enzymes that selectively digest necrotic tissue.

Autolytic debridement is the use of a synthetic dressing, or moisture-retentive dressing over the ulcer. The eschar is then self-digested via the action of the enzymes that are present in the fluid environment of the wound. This method is not utilized for infected wounds.

Surgical debridement is the removal of devitalized tissue, or thick, adherent eschar, utilizing a scalpel, scissors, or other sharp instrument. Depending on the amount of debridement to be done, this may be performed in the operating room, the treatment room, or the client's room. Following surgical debridement, grafting may be necessary to close the wound. This becomes necessary if it is a full-thickness ulcer, if there is loss of joint function, or for cosmetic purposes. The client is assessed continually for pain during the procedure, especially if there is a donor site for grafting.

Wound Cleansing

The ulcer should be thoroughly cleansed via whirlpool, handheld shower head, or an irrigating system with a pressure between 4 and 15 psi (such as a 30 mL syringe with an 18-gauge needle). If an irrigating system is used, 250 mL of normal saline or tap water for home wound care should be used to thoroughly cleanse any wound. If the wound is red, gentle irrigation with a needleless 30 to 60 mL syringe should be used to prevent wound trauma and bleeding. When bleeding occurs, wound healing has been impaired. However, if the wound has been diagnosed as being infected, pressure flushing with a 30 to 60 mL syringe and an 18-gauge needle is needed to help remove bacteria.

LEARNING TIP

Dilution is the solution to wound pollution!

Once the wound is cleansed and debrided, a dressing is applied. The wound heals more rapidly in a moist environment, with minimal bacterial colonization, and a healing temperature. This takes 12 hours to occur after the wound is covered with an occlusive dressing. If a dressing is frequently removed, the wound may not reach its healing temperature and healing may be impaired. When possible, the dressing should be left in place for extended periods. Infected wounds are not covered with occlusive dressings; draining wounds may require frequent dressing changes.

Wound Dressings

Dressings vary according to size, location, depth, stage of ulcer, and physician preference. Commonly used dressing materials include hydrogel dressings, polyurethane films, hydrocolloid wafers, biological dressings, alginates, and cotton gauze. These materials provide an optimal healing environment. Hypoallergenic tape should be used to secure dressings if tape is necessary. Protective paste may be applied to protect nonaffected tissue from topical agents. In all cases, pressure should be kept off of the wound. No treatment will be effective if pressure continues to damage the tissue.

NURSING PROCESS

Assessment

The nurse provides ongoing assessment of the status of the pressure ulcer, as well as underlying causes and impediments to healing. Clients should be monitored for risk factors such as prolonged immobility, incontinence, and inadequate hydration and nutrition.

Use transparency film or a disposable ruler to measure and document the diameter of the ulcer. Depth can be measured with a cotton-tipped applicator. Also, gently probe a cotton-tipped applicator under the skin edges to detect tunnelling and measure lateral tissue destruction.

There are several different staging systems for pressure sores based on the depth of tissue destroyed. In general, the staging systems are categorized from I to IV. See Figure 51–1 for photos of ulcers at each stage.

- Stage I: The skin is still intact, but the area is red and does not blanch. There may also be warmth, hardness, and discoloration of the skin.

---

eschar: eschara—scab

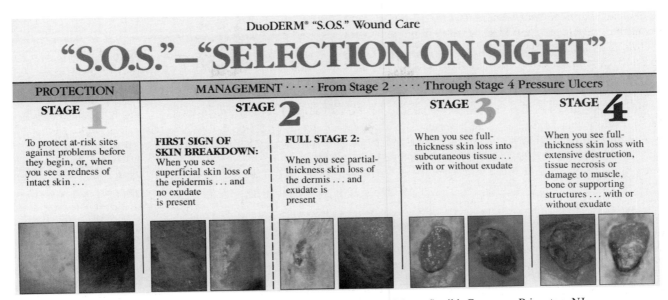

Figure 51–1. Pressure ulcers. (Courtesy of ConvaTec, a Bristol-Myers Squibb Company, Princeton, NJ, with permission.)

- Stage II: There is partial-thickness skin loss of epidermis, dermis, or both. The ulcer may appear as an abrasion, a shallow crater, or a blister.
- Stage III: There is full-thickness skin loss, which extends to the subcutaneous tissue, but not fascia. The ulcer looks like a deep crater.
- Stage IV: There is full-thickness skin loss with damage to the muscle, bone, or support structures such as tendons.

Wound exudate should be assessed. Two common types of wound exudate are **serosanguineous** and **purulent.** Serosanguineous exudate is fluid consisting of serum and blood. It is blood-tinged, amber-colored fluid. Purulent fluid is a fluid that contains pus. It can vary in color with different odors, which are suggestive of different wound colonizations. Creamy yellow pus may indicate *Staphylococcus.* Beige pus that has a fishy odor may suggest *Proteus.* Green-blue pus with a fruity odor may indicate *Pseudomonas.* Brown pus with a fecal odor may suggest *Bacteroides.*

The nurse should gently palpate the wound with a gloved hand to assess the texture of granulations. If the granulations are healthy, they will have a slightly spongy texture.

Nursing Diagnosis

Possible nursing diagnoses include impaired skin integrity related to immobility or pressure on skin surface; high risk for infection, related to open wound; pain, related to ulcer and treatments; and ineffective individual coping, related to chronic condition of ulcer.

Nursing Care

See Nursing Care Plan Box 51–2 for the Client with a Pressure Ulcer.

Inflammatory Skin Disorders

DERMATITIS

Pathophysiology and Etiology

Dermatitis is the inflammation of the skin and is characterized by itching, redness, and skin lesions, with varying borders and distribution patterns. Dermatitis can be caused by exposure to allergens or irritants, heredity, or emotional stress. Many times the cause is not known. When the cause is not known, the term **eczema** or *nonspecific eczematous dermatitis* may be used. The terms *eczema* and *dermatitis* are often used interchangeably. There are three common types of dermatitis: contact dermatitis, atopic dermatitis, and seborrheic dermatitis. All types tend to be chronic and respond well to treatment, but are prone to occur again. See Table 51–1 for common types of dermatitis.

Prevention

The client should prevent irritation to the skin by avoiding irritants, allergens, excessive heat, and dryness and controlling perspiration. Baths should be short, and water should not be overly hot. Deodorant soaps should be

---

serosanguineous: serum—whey + sanguineous—bloody
purulent: purulentus—pus
dermatitis: dermatos—skin + itis—inflammation

NURSING CARE PLAN BOX 51–2 FOR THE CLIENT WITH A PRESSURE ULCER

Impaired skin integrity related to pressure on skin surface

Client Outcomes

Skin integrity is improved as evidenced by decrease in wound size, no further development of other pressure ulcers.

Evaluation of Outcomes

Is there a decrease in wound size? Are there any new pressure ulcers?

Interventions	Rationale	Evaluation
• Assess the status of the pressure ulcer according to stage, color, exudate, texture, size, and depth.	Provides baseline data on which care is based.	What stage is the ulcer in? Are there any other outstanding characteristics?
• Assess the cause of pressure (e.g., immobility, friction, shearing).	Allows for correction and also prevents further trauma.	What is the cause of this ulcer?
• Cleanse wound gently with warm water; rinse; pat dry gently with gauze.	Reduces the number of bacteria. Drying prevents maceration of skin. Gentle handling prevents further trauma.	Is the wound clean and dry?
• Debride the wound as prescribed (method depends on client's condition and the goals of care).	Debridement removes drainage and wound debris. Permits granulation of tissue.	Does the wound look clean and free of debris?
• Dress the wound appropriately for the prescribed topical agent.	Protects the underlying wound and helps promote healing.	Is the dressing applied appropriately?
• Position the client off the ulcer.	Prevents further pressure and trauma on the ulcer.	Is the client positioned off the ulcer?
• If a leg ulcer, provide for frequent rest periods with leg elevation; if immobile, reposition every 2 hours.	Prevents further tissue breakdown.	Is the leg elevated? Is the client repositioned every 2 hours?

Risk for infection related to open wound

Client Outcomes

The client will not experience further wound infection or systemic sepsis. (Total elimination of bacteria is impossible due to the nature of the condition.)

Evaluation of Outcomes

Is the client free from signs and symptoms of further infection? Is the client free from systemic infection?

Intervention	Rationale	Evaluation
• Assess the ulcer at every dressing change or at least every 24 hours. Note color and appearance of skin; diameter and depth of ulcer; areas of tenderness, swelling, redness, and heat; and drainage.	Allows for early recognition of infection and response to treatment.	Are signs of infection present?
• Monitor temperature at least every 12 hours.	Elevated body temperature is one sign of infection.	Is the client afebrile?
• Provide meticulous wound care (see under Impaired Skin Integrity).	Helps decrease the level of contamination. Prevents further infection.	Is the wound showing signs of healing?
• Use thorough hand-washing techniques. Use sterile gloves for dressing changes.	Prevents cross-contamination.	Does the nurse take proper wound precautions?

continued

NURSING CARE PLAN BOX 51–2 *(continued)*

Pain related to ulcer and treatments

Client Outcomes
Client will be as comfortable and as pain free as possible as evidenced by statement of increased comfort, statement of decreased pain, and ability to sleep at night.

Evaluation of Outcomes
Does the client express comfort? Does the client express a decrease in pain? Is the client able to sleep?

Interventions	*Rationale*	*Evaluation*
• Assess the level of pain through verbalizations, facial expressions, and positioning of the body.	Monitors level of pain and response to therapy.	At what level is the pain? Is it better or worse with treatment?
• Offer analgesics as prescribed.	Analgesics help relieve pain.	Do the analgesics relieve the pain?
• Decrease anxiety with relaxation techniques (e.g., distraction, music).	Relaxation can lessen pain intensity.	Is the client less anxious? Does the client verbalize less pain?
• Maintain a comfortable environment: cover; provide for privacy; position in good alignment and comfortably; and maintain a comfortable room temperature.	This relaxes the client and lessens the intensity of the discomfort.	Does the client express an increase in comfort?

Ineffective individual coping related to chronic condition of the ulcer

Client Outcome
The client will better cope with the chronic ulcer as evidenced by changing the dressing or assisting in the dressing change as much as physically possible.

Evaluation of Outcome
Is the client helping in wound care as much as possible?

Interventions	*Rationale*	*Evaluation*
• Explain all care to the client.	Understanding will encourage further independence.	Is the client able to verbalize the plan of care?
• Determine extent of the client's mobility.	Provides important data in how much control the client will have over care.	Is the client able to see and reach the wound?
• Involve the client in the care as much as possible (e.g., bathing self or partial bathing; assisting in wound care as much as possible).	Gives the client more control and boosts self-esteem.	Can the client wash self totally? How much of the wound care is the client able to accomplish?
• Encourage involvement with a therapist or support group.	Provides emotional support and helps the client to better cope with the situation.	Does the client see a therapist? Does the client attend support groups?

avoided; mild superfatted soaps are recommended instead. Dry skin is lubricated with creams, oils, or ointments as appropriate. Itching and scratching are prevented as much as possible.

Signs and Symptoms

Itching and rash or lesions are the main clinical manifestations of dermatitis. The lesions vary depending on the type and location of dermatitis. Rashes and lesions can be dry, flaky scales, yellow crusts, red, fissures, macules, papules, and vesicles (these are described in Chapter 50, Table 50–2). Scratching can make any of these lesions worse.

LEARNING TIP
Itching and scratching can occur during sleep, causing the rash to worsen. Place mitts on baby's hands or have the adult or older child wear cotton gloves at night.

Table 51-1. **Common Types of Dermatitis**

Type	Description
Contact	Acute or chronic condition; due to contact with irritant or allergen
Irritant contact	Caused by direct contact with an irritating substance, such as soap, detergent, strong medication, astringent, cosmetic, or industrial chemical
Allergic contact	From contact with an allergen, such as perfume, tanning lotion, medication, hair dye, poison ivy, poison oak; contact results in cell-mediated immune response
Atopic	Chronic inherited condition; may be associated with respiratory allergies or asthma; can vary between bright red maculas, papules, oozing, **lichenified,** and hyperpigmented
Seborrheic	Chronic, inflammatory disease usually accompanied by scaling, itching, and inflammation; **seborrhea** is excessive production of sebaceous secretions; found in areas with abundant sebaceous glands (scalp, face, axilla, genitocrural areas) and where there are folds of skin; can appear as dry, moist, or greasy scales, yellow or pink-yellow crusts, redness, and dry flakiness; can be associated with emotional stress; may be genetic predisposition

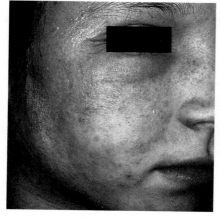

Allergic contact dermatitis from the poison oak plant. See Plate 20.

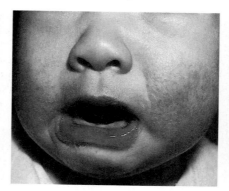

Atopic dermatitis as typical "chapped cheeks" in infant. See Plate 20.

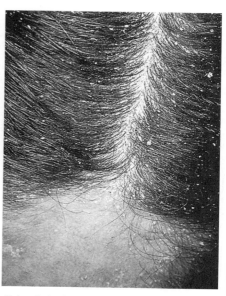

Seborrheic dermatitis as seen in dandruff, or excessive scaling of the scalp. See Plate 20.

(From Reeves J, Maibach H. Clinical Dermatology Illustrated, 2nd ed, 1998. Reproduced with permission: MacLennan & Petty, Sydney.)

Complications

The lesion or rash will worsen with continued irritation, exposure to offending agents, or scratching. Infections of the skin are common due to the many open areas and breaks in the skin, as well as the client's reluctance to properly wash the affected area due to pain from the lesions. Many infections can also become systemic.

Diagnostic Tests

Diagnosis is usually based on history, symptoms, and clinical findings. If infection is suspected, cultures of the lesions may be ordered to identify the infecting agent.

Medical Treatment

Treatment varies according to symptoms. Basic treatment objectives may be to control itching; alleviate discomfort and pain; decrease inflammation; control or prevent crust formation and oozing; prevent infection; prevent further damage to the skin; and heal the skin as much as possible.

Itching and discomfort can be somewhat relieved by antihistamines, analgesics, and antipruritic medications as ordered. Colloidal oatmeal preparations added to baths can also help relieve some of the **pruritus.**

Steroids may be used to suppress inflammation. They may be administered as a topical, intralesional, or systemic agent. The specific type and vehicle used depends on the type of lesion, the body area involved, and the extent of the

---

pruritus: prur—itch + itis—condition

lichenified: leichen—scaly growth on rocks and bark of trees + facere—to make

seborrhea: sebum—tallow + rhoia—flow

lesion. Topical administration is preferred if possible, because systemic preparations can cause systemic side effects, including adrenal suppression.

Tub baths and wet dressings help control oozing and prevent further crust formation. These interventions serve to loosen exudates, scales, and other wound debris, providing a clean area for topical application of medication. Skin is protected by lightly patting dry, avoiding friction, avoiding hot water, and using a sunscreen agent when outdoors.

Nursing Process

Assessment

The nurse can use the WHAT'S UP format to assess the rash:

- Where is it? Location and distribution are determined.
- How does it feel? Is it itchy? Painful?
- Aggravating and alleviating factors. What aggravates or alleviates the rash? Allergies to foods, drugs, medications, soaps, or other allergens are identified. Has the client been exposed to allergens?
- Timing. When did it start? Has it occurred before?
- Severity. How severe is it? Are lesions open or infected?
- Useful data. What useful other data are available? Are there related signs and symptoms?
- Perception. What is the client's perception of the problem? Is there a family or personal history of rash? What does the client think it is?

(Also refer to Table 50–1 for specific questions to ask.) The nurse also needs to observe the rash or lesions for character, distribution, description (see Table 50–2), skin tenderness, signs of scratching, and other associated problems.

Nursing Diagnosis

Possible nursing diagnoses include impaired skin integrity related to rash or lesions; alteration in comfort related to pain and itching; body image disturbance related to visible rash or lesions; and knowledge deficit related to disease and treatment.

Planning

The goals of treatment are to keep the skin intact or improve integrity, prevent infection, and maintain comfort. The client will have improved body image as evidenced by a statement of acceptance of the condition and ability to socialize with others. The client will verbalize understanding of the condition and demonstrate ability to perform self-care measures.

Implementation

SKIN INTEGRITY. The nurse cleanses the area as ordered by the physician, taking care not to further irritate the skin. Moist compresses, dressings, or tepid tub baths may be ordered to help relieve inflammation, debride lesions, and soften crusts and scales. The skin is patted rather than rubbed dry, to prevent further trauma. Topical agents are applied as directed to help suppress inflammation. If lesions are generalized, protein can be lost through oozing of serum. Clients are encouraged to eat a high-protein diet to promote healing and replace lost protein.

COMFORT. Medications to reduce inflammation and itching are administered as ordered. Administration at bedtime will help promote comfortable sleep. Many antihistamines also have a sedative effect. Cool moist compresses or tepid baths with soothing agents added as ordered can help relieve itching and discomfort. Gloves or mitts, especially at night, help prevent scratching. The client is also encouraged to keep fingernails short to prevent scratching. Application of slight pressure with a clean cloth may help relieve itching. Relaxation exercises or referral to a support group may help the client cope with distressing symptoms.

BODY IMAGE. The client is allowed to verbalize concerns. Referral to a support group, if available, will provide support from others in similar circumstances. The nurse displays an accepting attitude while caring for skin lesions. The client will be quick to pick up the nurse's reaction to the lesions, especially if it is negative. The client is encouraged to participate in skin care, to allow more control over the situation. Long sleeves or other appropriate covers may make the lesions less noticeable and the client more comfortable.

KNOWLEDGE DEFICIT. The client is instructed in application of topical agents and dressings. Overuse of medications can further traumatize skin, so application of a very thin layer is advised. The client is also instructed in how to recognize changes, improvement, or flare-ups of the disorder and what symptoms to report to the health care provider. Because most skin conditions are cared for at home, it is important for the client to have the skills needed to monitor the condition and institute treatment appropriately. The client is advised to avoid overexposure to sun, to prevent skin damage. Sunscreen agents should be used when outdoors. A humidifier in the home helps maintain hydration of skin and control itching during dry weather, especially in winter. It is important for the client to know if the condition is chronic and how to prevent flare-ups if possible.

Evaluation

If medical and nursing care have been effective, the lesions will be controlled or in remission, the client will state that itching and other discomforts are controlled, the client will be able to socialize without undue difficulty, and the client will be able to describe and demonstrate self-care measures.

PSORIASIS

Pathophysiology and Etiology

Psoriasis is a chronic inflammatory skin disorder in which the epidermal cells proliferate abnormally fast. Usually, epidermal cells take about 27 days to shed. With psoriasis, the cells shed every 4 to 5 days. The abnormal keratin forms loosely adherent scales with dermal inflammation.

Psoriasis is characterized by exacerbations and remissions. The cause is not known; however, there often may be a positive family history. The onset can be at any age, with 27 years the average age. The condition can be severe if the onset is in childhood. Many factors can influence the suppression and outbreak of lesions, but this varies from individual to individual. Sun and humidity may suppress lesions. Aggravating factors include streptococcal pharyngitis, emotional upset, stress, hormonal changes, and certain drugs (e.g., antimalarials, lithium, beta blockers).

Prevention

Because the exact etiology is not known, measures to prevent exacerbation of symptoms are specific to the client's circumstances. General preventive measures include avoidance of upper respiratory infections, especially streptococcal infections; avoidance of or coping with emotional stress; avoidance of skin trauma, including sunburns; and medications that may precipitate a flare-up.

Signs and Symptoms

Signs and symptoms vary according to the client and the particular type of psoriasis. Lesions are red papules that join to form plaques with distinct borders (Fig. 51–2). Silvery scales develop on untreated lesions. Areas most often affected are the elbows and knees, scalp, umbilicus, and genitals. Other signs and symptoms include nail involvement, intergluteal pinking, itching, and dry or brittle hair.

Complications

Because of the nature of the disease, with its lesions and itching, secondary infections can occur. Psoriatic arthritis may develop after the psoriasis has developed, with nail changes and destructive arthritis of large joints, the spine, and interphalangeal joints (Fig. 51–3). If the psoriasis becomes severe and widespread, fever, chills, increased cardiac output, and benign lymphadenopathy can result.

Diagnostic Tests

Testing depends on the severity of the psoriasis. Normally, this disease is diagnosed by physical assessment alone. Diagnostic tests may be performed to rule out concurrent disease or secondary infections.

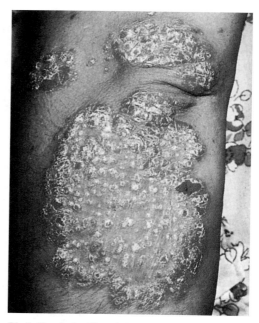

Figure 51–2. Psoriasis. Note bright red scaly plaque with silvery scale. (From Reeves J, Maibach H. Clinical Dermatology Illustrated, 2nd ed, 1998. Reproduced with permission: MacLennan & Petty, Sydney.) See Plate 21.

Medical Treatment

Treatment varies according to the type and extent of the disease, as well as physical preference. Psoriasis is a chronic disease with remissions and exacerbations. Basic treatment objectives are to decrease the rapid epidermal proliferation, decrease inflammation, and decrease the itching and scaling. Generally the client is instructed to bathe daily in a tub bath, using a soft brush to assist in the removal of scales.

Topical therapy includes steroids, salicylic acid, keratolytics, coal tar, anthralin, ultraviolet (UV) light, and, in severe cases, antimetabolite chemotherapy agents. Topical corticosteroids may be used for their anti-inflammatory effect. Occlusive dressings (see Chapter 50) are commonly used to enhance penetration of medications. Keratolytic ointments or gels enhance the effects of salicylic acid to loosen or remove scales.

Tar preparations are usually prescribed along with the corticosteroids for conditions that warrant it. The tar acts as an antimitotic, or slows the epidermal cell division. Occlusive dressings are not used with tars. Anthralin is a substance extracted from coal tar. It also suppresses mitotic activity. The anthralin may be mixed with salicylic acid in a stiff paste. The client must be closely observed, because the anthralin is a strong irritant and can cause chemical burns. It is usually applied for no longer than 2 hours. Both coal tar and anthralin are commonly used in combination

---

psoriasis: psora—itch + itis—inflammation

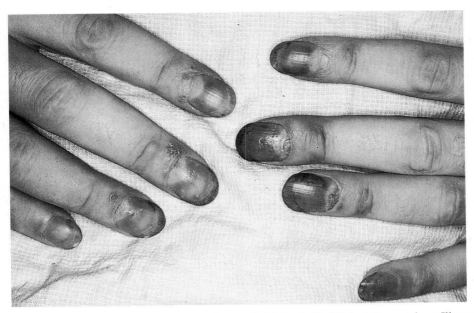

Figure 51–3. Acute psoriatic arthritis. (From Reeves J, Maibach H. Clinical Dermatology Illustrated, 2nd ed, 1998. Reproduced with permission: MacLennan & Petty, Sydney.) See Plate 21.

with UV light and are usually administered in inpatient settings or specialized outpatient clinics.

Ultraviolet light may be designated as UVB, shorter wavelength, or UVA, longer wavelengths. UVA is from an artificial source, such as special mercury vapor lamps or special cabinets. The amount of exposure depends on the client's condition, pigmentation, and susceptibility to burning. The client must wear eye guards during treatments. Oral psoralen tablets (a photosensitizing agent) followed by exposure to UVA is called PUVA therapy. PUVA therapy temporarily inhibits DNA synthesis, which is antimitotic. Because psoralen is a photosensitizing agent, the client must not only wear dark glasses during the treatment period, but also for the entire day of any treatments. The long-term safety of PUVA therapy is still unknown. Possible side effects include increased skin carcinomas, premature skin aging, and actinic keratosis (premalignant lesions of the skin). The client should be observed closely for redness, tenderness, edema, and eye changes. Therefore initial and follow-up eye examinations, skin biopsies, urinalysis, and blood tests may be ordered.

Antimebolites are reserved for the most severe cases, as a last resort. Methotrexate is the most common agent given. Because of its hepatoxicity, it is contraindicated in clients with liver disease, alcoholism, renal disease, and bone marrow suppression. Before therapy, a liver biopsy and routine blood work are completed.

 CRITICAL THINKING: Mrs. Long

Mrs. Long arrives at the health clinic to complain that the prescribed shampoo she is using for her scalp is not working. She states that she washes her hair thoroughly with the medicated shampoo and immediately rinses completely. She wants to know why her scalp shows no signs of improvement.
Answers at end of chapter.

Nursing Process

Nursing care for the client with psoriasis is the same as nursing care for the client with dermatitis. The only addition would be to encourage frequent periods of rest to enhance the antimitotic effects of the therapeutic agents.

Infectious Skin Disorders

A variety of infections can infect the skin. The most common disorders are discussed in this section. See Table 51–2 for a summary of additional skin infections.

HERPES SIMPLEX

Pathophysiology and Etiology

Herpes simplex virus (HSV) is a common viral infection that tends to recur repeatedly. There are two types: type 1 virus (HSV1), which occurs above the waist and causes the fever blister or cold sore (Fig. 51–4); and type 2 virus (HSV2), which occurs below the waist and causes genital herpes.

The primary infection occurs through direct contact, respiratory droplet, or fluid exposure from another infected person. Following this, the virus lies dormant in nerve gan-

Table 51-2. **Infectious Skin Disorders**

Type	Description	Complications	Treatment/Nursing Care
Impetigo contagiosa	Common contagious, infectious, inflammatory skin disorders usually caused by streptococcus or *Staphylococcus aureus;* sources of infection include swimming pools, pets, dirty fingernails, beauty and barber shops, and contaminated clothing, towels, sheets; may occur secondary to scrapes, cuts, insect bites, burns, dermatitis, poison ivy. Primary skin infection can appear on exposed areas of the body (extremities, hands, face, neck) or skin-fold areas (axillae). Rash appears as oozing, thin-roofed vesicle that rapidly grows and develops a honey-colored crust; crusts are easily removed, and new crusts appear; lesions heal in 1 to 2 weeks if allowed to dry.	Glomerulonephritis due to a particular strain of streptococcus infection. Lesions may spread from one skin area to another. Lesions may persist if not permitted to dry. Secondary **pyoderma,** or acute inflammatory purulent dermatitis, may occur if lesions are unresponsive to treatment.	Systemic antibiotics are administered as prescribed. Topical antibiotics are utilized after crust removal. Gentle washing with a mild soap, or soaking with warm, moist compresses, aids in crust removal, removes debris, and provides a clean bed for topical therapy. Appropriate antipyretics are prescribed as necessary. Keep fingernails short and clean. Glove or mitt hands as necessary to prevent scratching. Client must remain home until all lesions are healed. Teach proper disposal or washing of any material that comes in contact with lesions. Appropriate hygienic practices must be adhered to in preventing skin-to-skin or person-to-person spread. Observe client for 6 to 7 weeks for signs/symptoms of glomerulonephritris.

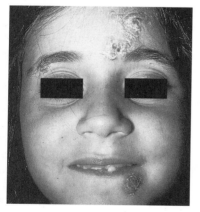

Impetigo on the face. Note honey-colored crusts on red erosions. See Plate 21.

continued

glia near the spinal column, where the immune system cannot destroy it. The client is asymptomatic at this time.

Recurrence of the infection can happen spontaneously or be triggered by fever, sunburn, stress, illness, menses, fatigue, or injury. The secondary lesion may appear as isolated or groups of small vesicles or pustules on an erythematous base. Crusts eventually form, and the lesions heal in about 1 week. The lesions are contagious for 2 to 4 days before dry crusts form.

Prevention

This disease can recur spontaneously. Avoidance of certain stressors such as sunburn, injury, and fatigue may delay a recurrence. The use of sunscreens, especially on the lips, may be helpful. Avoidance of contact with a known in-

pyoderma: pyo—pus + derma—skin

Table 51–2. (continued)

Type	Description	Complications	Treatment/Nursing Care
Furuncles and carbuncles	A furuncle is a small, tender boil that occurs deep in one or more hair follicles and spreads to surrounding dermis; may be single or multiple; usually caused by *Staphylococcus;* usually occurs on body areas prone to excessive perspiration, friction, and irritation (e.g., buttocks, axillae); can recur; the boil eventually comes to a soft yellow, black, or white head; there is localized pain, tenderness, and surrounding cellulitis; lymphadenopathy may be present. A carbuncle is an extension of a furuncle; an abscess of skin and subcutaneous tissue; deeper than furuncle; caused by *Staphylococcus;* usually appears where skin is thick, fibrous, and inelastic (e.g., back of neck, upper back, and buttocks); associated symptoms may include fevers, pain, leukocytosis, prostration. Both tend to occur in debilitated clients, and more often in diabetics.	Furuncles may progress to carbuncles. Carbuncles may progress to infection of bloodstream. Further spread of infection can occur to self and others. Occasionally, scarring may occur.	Prevent trauma; avoid squeezing or irritation. Cleanse surrounding skin with antibacterial soap, followed by application of antibacterial ointment. Surgical incision and drainage may be performed. Cover draining lesion with dressing. Follow Standard Precautions. Double bag all soiled dressings and dispose of properly. Systemic antibiotic therapy (based on sensitivity studies) is instituted for carbuncles or spreading furuncles. Analgesia and antipyretics are ordered as necessary. Bed rest is advised with carbuncles or furuncles on perineal or anal regions. Cover mattress and pillows with plastic and wipe daily with a disinfectant. Wash all linens, towels, and clothing after each use. Properly discard razor blades after each use. Strict hand washing is maintained to prevent cross-contamination.

(From Reeves J, Maibach H. Clinical Dermatology Illustrated, 2nd ed, 1998. Reproduced with permission: MacLennan & Petty, Sydney.)

fected lesion during the blistering phase can prevent the primary lesions. Clients should also be taught to avoid sharing contaminated items such as toothbrushes and drinking glasses.

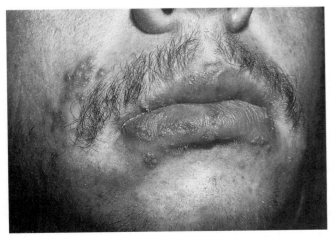

Figure 51–4. Herpes simplex around mouth. (From Reeves J, Maibach H. Clinical Dermatology Illustrated, 2nd ed, 1998. Reproduced with permission: MacLennan & Petty, Sydney.) See Plate 22.

Signs and Symptoms

Some clients may have a prodromal phase of burning or tingling at the site for a few hours before eruption. The area becomes erythematous and swollen. Vesicles and pustules erupt in 1 to 2 days. There may also be redness with no blistering. Lesions can burn, itch, and be painful. The attacks vary in frequency, but diminish with age. The client is contagious until scabs are formed.

Complications

If herpes simplex is present in the vagina at childbirth, the newborn may be infected (meningoencephalitis or a panvisceral infection may occur). If the person touches the affected area and then rubs the eyes, the eyes can become severely infected.

Diagnostic Tests

Cultures of the lesions provide a definitive diagnosis. Most lesions are diagnosed on the basis of history, signs, and symptoms.

Medical Treatment

There is no complete cure. Recurrences will happen. Topical acyclovir (Zovirax) ointment is the drug of choice for primary lesions, to suppress the multiplication of vesicles. It will not benefit secondary lesions. Oral acyclovir may be recommended for severe or frequent attacks (six or more attacks per year) or for clients who are immunosuppressed. Various lotions, creams, and ointments may be prescribed to accelerate drying and healing of lesions (e.g., camphor, phenol, alcohol). Antibiotics may be indicated for secondary infections.

Nursing Care

Educating the client about the disease and recurrences is very important. The client should be instructed about when the infection is contagious and how to prevent spreading the virus from one part of the body to another or to other individuals.

HERPES ZOSTER (SHINGLES)

Pathophysiology and Etiology

Herpes zoster, or shingles, is an acute inflammatory and infectious disorder that produces a painful vesicular eruption on bright red edematous plaques, along the distribution of nerves from one or more posterior ganglia. This eruption follows the course of the nerve and is almost always unilateral (one sided) (Fig. 51–5).

Herpes zoster is caused by the varicella-zoster virus. This virus appears identical to the one that causes chickenpox. It is thought that herpes zoster is a reactivation of this latent varicella virus. The incubation period is 7 to 21 days. The vesicles appear in 3 to 4 days. Eruption usually occurs posteriorly and progresses anteriorly and peripherally along the dermatome. The total duration of the disease can vary from 10 days to 5 weeks.

This disease occurs most frequently in the elderly who have a diminished resistance, in the immunosuppressed client, and in the client with a malignancy or an injury to the spinal or cranial nerve.

Prevention

Avoidance of the person with this disease during the contagious phase (a few days before eruption until vesicles dry or scab) is the best prevention.

Signs and Symptoms

In addition to the vesicles and plaques, there may be irritation, itching, fever, malaise, and, depending on the location of lesions, visceral involvement. Lesions may be very painful; the likelihood of pain increases with age.

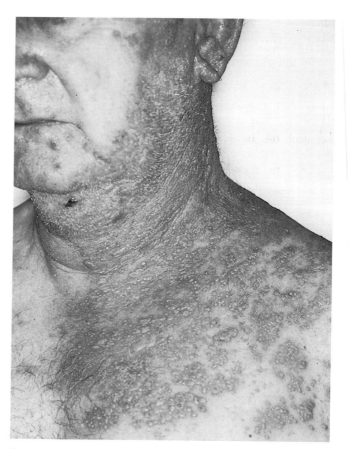

Figure 51–5. Herpes zoster (shingles). (From Reeves J, Maibach H. Clinical Dermatology Illustrated, 2nd ed, 1998. Reproduced with permission: MacLennan & Petty, Sydney.) See Plate 22.

Complications

Postherpetic neuralgia, persistent dermatomal pain, and hyperesthesia are common in the elderly and can last for weeks to months after the lesions have healed. The incidence and severity of these complications increases with age.

Ophthalmic herpes zoster, involvement of the fifth cranial nerve, can be a very serious complication. Consultation with an ophthalmologist is imperative. Other complications can occur with facial and acoustic nerve involvement. These complications can include hearing loss, tinnitus, facial paralysis, and vertigo. Full-thickness skin necrosis and scarring can occur if lesions do not heal properly, or systemic infection can occur from scratching, causing the virus to enter the bloodstream.

Diagnostic Tests

Diagnosis is usually confirmed by the clinical picture of the client and associated signs and symptoms. Cultures may be ordered if secondary bacterial infections are suspected.

Medical Treatment

Treatment is aimed at controlling the outbreak, reducing pain and discomfort, and preventing complications. Acyclovir (Zovirax), either IV, oral, or topically, may be prescribed in the early stages of the initial infection, for a severe outbreak, and if the client is immunosuppressed or debilitated. Acyclovir does not cure, but it may help control the initial outbreak. Analgesics are prescribed for pain and discomfort. Corticosteroids may be administered to prevent postherpetic neuralgia and reduce pain. Topical steroids should not be applied if a secondary infection is present, because they suppress the immune system. Antihistamines are administered to control itching. Antibiotics are prescribed for secondary bacterial infections.

Nursing Care

Appropriate precautions during the contagious stage are necessary to prevent spread. Cool compresses two or three times a day help cleanse and dry lesions, as well as lessen itching. Hyperesthesia may be somewhat relieved with stockings, wraps, or a tight T-shirt that provides continuous firm pressure. Any appropriate measures to increase comfort should be initiated.

FUNGAL INFECTIONS

Pathophysiology and Etiology

Dermatophytosis, or a fungal infection of the skin, occurs when there is an impairment of the skin integrity in a warm moist environment. This infection occurs through direct contact with infected humans or animals or an object. *Tinea* is the term used to describe fungal skin infections; the name used after tinea indicates the body area affected. For example, tinea capitis is a fungal infection of the scalp. Common fungal infections and treatments are described in Table 51–3.

CELLULITIS

Pathophysiology and Etiology

Cellulitis in the inflammation of skin cells or cellular or connective tissue, due to a generalized infection, usually with *Staphylococcus* or *Streptococcus*. It can occur as a result of skin trauma or the secondary bacterial infection of an open wound, such as a pressure sore, or it may be unrelated to skin trauma.

dermatophytosis: derma—skin + phyton—plant + osis—condition

cellulitis: cell + itis—inflammation

Prevention

Good hygiene and prevention of cross-contamination are very important. If there is an open wound, preventing infection and promoting healing are important.

Signs and Symptoms

The initial sign of cellulitis is a localized area of inflammation that may become more generalized if not treated properly. Common clinical manifestations include warmth, redness, edema, pain, tenderness, fever, and lymphadenopathy. It may be seen in any areas of an open wound, with skin trauma, and in the lower legs. The infection can worsen rapidly if not treated properly.

Diagnostic Tests

Culture and sensitivity of any pustules or drainage are necessary to identify the infecting organism. Blood cultures may also be indicated to rule out bacteremia.

Medical Treatment

Appropriate Standard Precautions are used. Topical and systemic antibiotics are prescribed according to results of laboratory tests. Debridement of nonviable tissue is necessary when there is an open wound. Systemic antibiotics are indicated if fever and lymphadenopathy are present.

Nursing Care

The nurse assesses for history of recent skin trauma. The affected extremity can be measured to determine degree of edema and to monitor for improvement. Temperature and other signs of worsening or systemic infection are monitored for and reported. The affected extremity should be elevated to decrease edema. Analgesics and application of warm compresses as ordered may increase comfort. Antibiotics are administered as ordered. Use of Standard Precautions, including frequent, thorough hand washing, is a must to prevent spread of infection. The client should be taught infection control measures, especially if home dressing changes are ordered.

ACNE VULGARIS

Pathophysiology and Etiology

Acne vulgaris is a common skin disorder of the sebaceous glands and their hair follicles that usually occurs to the face, chest, upper back, and shoulders. The etiology is multifocal. The most common cause is hormonal changes.

The sebaceous glands are under endocrine control, especially the androgens. Stimulation of androgens (e.g., during adolescence or the menstrual cycle) in turn stimulates

text continues on page 1110

Table 51–3. **Fungal Infections**

Type	Description	Treatment/Nursing Care
Tinea pedis (athlete's foot)	Common fungal infection, most frequently seen in those with warm, moist, sweaty feet; occlusive shoes; or friction/trauma to the feet. Three types: chronic plantar scaling, acute vesicular, and interdigital. Chronic plantar scaling will have slight redness and mild to severe scaling; fold lines on sole appear to have white powder due to scaling; may be toenail involvement; itching is usually not present. Acute vesicular appears as a sudden eruption of small, painful, itchy vesicles; may also accompany chronic plantar scaling. Interdigital is more common; there is erosion, scaling, and fissuring in toe webs; area is painful, burning, and itchy, and there is usually an offensive odor.	Chronic plantar scaling may be treated with kerolytics and topical antifungal agents; these agents help in relieving symptoms and improve appearance; they are not curative. Acute vesicular is treated with soaks or baths two or three times a day for 2 to 3 days to dry up blisters; astringent paint is applied to debrided areas; topical corticosteroids help relieve itching. Interdigital may be treated with combined antifungal and antibacterial therapies or antifungals alone; soak feet twice daily and dry well. Teach client prevention measures: keep feet dry; dry carefully between toes; apply foot powder to absorb perspiration; wear cotton socks to absorb perspiration; if weather permits, use perforated shoes or sandals; avoid plastic or rubber-soled shoes; wear water shoes in public showers and near swimming pools. Apply topical agents properly: apply antifungals thinly; treat for time specified, even after apparent clearing.

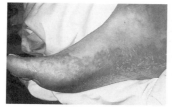 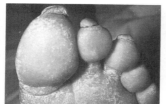 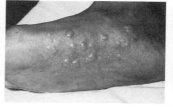 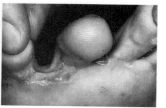

Tinea pedis—chronic plantar scaling. See Plate 23.

Tinea pedis with toenail involvement. See Plate 23.

Acute vesicular tinea pedis. See Plate 23.

Interdigital tinea pedis is itchy and malodorous. See Plate 23.

Type	Description	Treatment/Nursing Care
Tinea capitas (ringworm of scalp)	Contagious; commonly causes hair loss in children. Appears as scattered round, red, scaly patches; small papules or pustules may be evident at edges of patches; hair is brittle at site, breaks off, and temporary areas of baldness result; may be mild itching; kerion inflammation may occur after weeks.	Teach prevention measures: never share combs, brushes, pillowcases, or headgear. Systemic antifungals are prescribed due to high relapse rate with topical agents; review side effects with client. Oral corticosteroids are indicated for kerion inflammation to help prevent alopecia; review side effects with client. Instruct family on contagious aspect of disease; assess other family members and pets for organism.

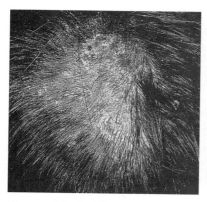 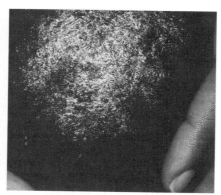

Tinea capitis. See Plate 24.

Tinea capitis—kerion inflammation. See Plate 24.

continued

Table 51–3. (continued)

Type	Description	Treatment/Nursing Care
Tinea corporis (tinea circinata; ringworm of body)	Erythematous macule that progresses to rings of vesicles or scale with a clear center that appears alone or in clusters; usually occurs on exposed areas of body; can be moderately to intensely itchy. Infected pet is common source of infection.	Teach prevention measures: keep skin areas, especially folds, dry; use clean towel and washcloth daily; wear cotton clothing, especially on hot, humid days. Topical antifungals are prescribed for small, localized lesions. Oral antifungals are indicated for severe, widespread, resistant, or follicular cases. Topical corticosteroids are prescribed for itching.

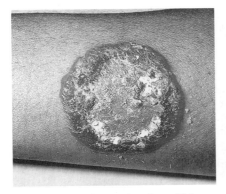

Tinea corporis—singular. This woman worked in a school where many children had scalp ringworm. See Plate 25.

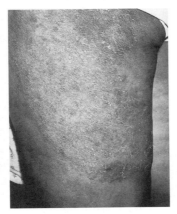

Tinea corporis—clusters and plaques. See Plate 25.

Type	Description	Treatment/Nursing Care
Tinea cruris (jock itch)	Ringworm of groin that may extend to inner thighs and buttocks area; may occur with tinea pedis; often in obese people who are athletic. Lesion first appears as a small red scaly patch and then progresses to a sharply demarcated plaque with elevated scaly or vesicular borders; itching can range from absent to severe.	Teach client prevention measures: avoid heat, moisture, and friction. Topical antifungals are prescribed; apply in a thin layer to rash and a few centimeters beyond border. Oral antifungals may be indicated for widespread cases or those resistant to topical therapy. Topical corticosteroids may be prescribed for itching.

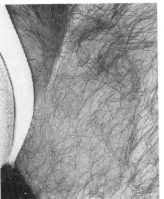

Tinea cruris. The inner thigh is the typical location for tinea cruris, or "jock itch." The border is pronounced and scaly. See Plate 25.

continued

Table 51–3. (continued)

Type	Description	Treatment/Nursing Care
Tinea unguium	Ringworm of the nails; also referred to as **onychomycosis.** Chronic fungal infection of nails, usually the toenails; a lifelong disease. There is yellow thickening of nail plate; it is friable and lusterless; eventually crumbly debris accumulates under free edge of the nail and causes nail plate to become separated; over time, the nail may become thickened, painful, and destroyed.	Systemic antifungals are rarely given for toenail involvement, but may be prescribed for fingernail involvement (review side effects). Nail may have to be surgically removed (nail avulsion). Explain high relapse rate to client. Keep nails neatly trimmed and buffed flat; gently scrape out any nail debris.

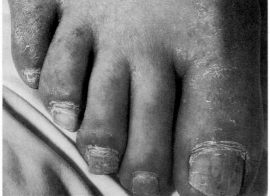

Onychomycosis (tinea unguium). See Plate 26.

(From Reeves J, Maibach H. Clinical Dermatology Illustrated, 2nd ed, 1998. Reproduced with permission: MacLennan & Petty, Sydney.)

the sebaceous glands to increase sebum production. This, along with gradual obstruction of the pilosebaceous ducts with accumulated debris, ruptures the sebaceous glands, which causes an inflammatory reaction that may lead to papules, pustules, nodules, and cysts. Acne occurs when the ducts through which this sebum flows become plugged.

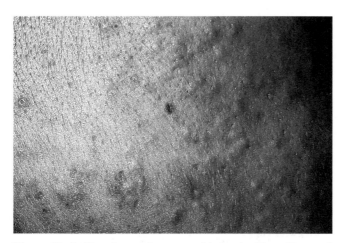

Figure 51–6. Closed comedones, or whiteheads. (From Reeves J, Maibach H. Clinical Dermatology Illustrated, 2nd ed, 1998. Reproduced with permission: MacLennan & Petty, Sydney.) See Plate 26.

Other factors that influence occurrence and severity of acne include genetic factors, stress, and external irritants such as strong soaps or cosmetics. It is not related to diet, chocolate, sexual activity, or uncleanliness.

Prevention

Acne vulgaris will occur regardless of interventions; however, certain interventions can lessen the severity or prevent complications. Avoidance of "picking" pimples will prevent further inflammation and scarring. The client should also avoid excessive washing, irritants, and abrasives.

Signs and Symptoms

The initial lesions are **comedones.** Closed comedones, or whiteheads (Fig. 51–6), are small white papules with tiny follicular openings. This may eventually become an open comedone, or blackhead (Fig. 51–7). The color is not due to dirt, but to lipids and melanin pigment. Scarring occurs due to significant skin inflammation, not due to picking, although picking can worsen inflammation and lead to

onychomycosis: onyx—nail + mykes—fungus + osis—condition

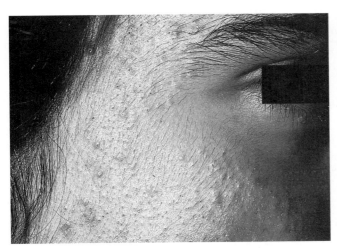

Figure 51–7. Open comedones, or blackheads. (From Reeves J, Maibach H. Clinical Dermatology Illustrated, 2nd ed, 1998. Reproduced with permission: MacLennan & Petty, Sydney.) See Plate 26.

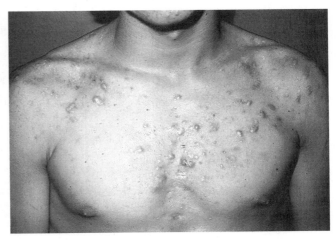

Figure 51–8. Nodular acne vulgaris. (From Reeves J, Maibach H. Clinical Dermatology Illustrated, 2nd ed, 1998. Reproduced with permission: MacLennan & Petty, Sydney.) See Plate 26.

further scarring. The resulting inflammation can lead to papules, pustules, nodules (Fig. 51–8), cysts, or abscesses.

Medical Treatment

Medical treatment prevents new lesions and helps control current lesions. Effective topical agents include benzoyl peroxide, an antibacterial that may help prevent pore plugging (e.g., Desquam-X; Benzagel); antibiotics to kill bacteria in follicles (erythromycin, tetracycline); and vitamin A acid (Retin-A, tretinoin) to loosen pore plugs and prevent occurrence of new comedones. Topical agents may be used alone or in combination. It may take 3 to 6 weeks before improvement is seen.

Systemic antibiotics (long term, low dose) and isotretinoin (Retin-A) may be prescribed for severe cases; however, the client must be closely monitored for side effects. Estrogen therapy (oral contraceptives) may also be prescribed for young women; however, the risks often outweigh the benefits. Systemic corticosteroids may occasionally be prescribed for severe nodular acne. Clients are observed closely for side effects.

Other medical treatments include comedo extraction, intralesional injections of corticosteroids, cryosurgery (freezing with liquid nitrogen), mild peeling (UV light, carbon dioxide, liquid nitrogen, mild acid), dermabrasion (deep chemical peel), excision of scars, and injection of fibrin or collagen below the scars. These treatments depend on the severity, age, condition, and physician and client preference.

Nursing Care

The nurse should review all medication instructions. Antibiotics should be used as directed to avoid development

of antibiotic-resistant strains. The client should be encouraged to gently wash his or her face twice daily, especially before topical application, using a mild soap. All topical agents should be applied to acne-prone areas, not just where the acne is. These agents must be applied to dry skin. Medications should not be applied near eyes, nasolabial folds, and corners of the mouth, due to potential irritation.

LEARNING TIP

Topical benzoyl peroxide may bleach colored fabrics.

If the client is ordered a combination of topical agents, unless contraindicated, the tretinoin is used at night and the others in the morning or afternoon, Tretinoin could be neutralized if mixed directly with other agents. The client must be careful with sun or sunlamp exposure while using tretinoin. Also, the client should be reminded that it may be necessary to continue treatment even when the skin clears.

Above all, try to dispel misconceptions on the cause of the acne and give appropriate health education. Advise the client to keep hands away from the face and especially not to squeeze pimples. Keep hair clean and off of the face. Avoid cosmetics, lotions, and shaving creams on the face.

Parasitic Skin Disorders

PEDICULOSIS

Pathophysiology and Etiology

Pediculosis is an infestation by human lice. There are three basic types: pediculosis capitis (head lice), pediculosis cor-

pediculosis: pediculus—louse + osis—condition

poris (body lice), and pediculosis pubis (pubic or crab lice). Generally, the lice bite the skin and feed on human blood, leaving their eggs and excrement, which can cause very intense itching. The lice are oval in shape and are approximately 2 mm in length.

With pediculosis capitis, the female louse lays eggs (nits) close to the scalp, where the nits become firmly attached to hair shafts (Fig. 51–9). The most common areas of infestation are the back of the scalp and behind the ears. The nits are about 1 mm in length and appear silvery white and glistening. Transmission is by direct contact or contact with infested objects, such as combs, brushes, wigs, hats, and bedding. It is most common in children and people with long hair.

Pediculosis corporis is caused by body lice that lay eggs in the seams of clothing and then pierce the skin. Areas of the skin usually involved are the neck, trunk, and thighs.

Pediculosis pubis is caused by crab lice. It is generally localized in the genital region, but it can also be seen on hairs of the chest, axillae, eyelashes, and beard. The lice are about 2 mm in length and appear crablike (Fig. 51–10). It is chiefly transmitted through sexual contact, or to a lesser degree by infested bed linen.

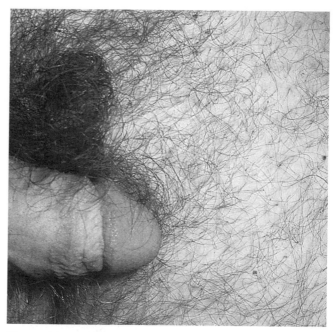

Figure 51–10. Pubic lice infestation is usually very itchy and shows only scattered excoriations. (From Reeves J, Maibach H. *Clinical Dermatology Illustrated*, 2nd ed, 1998. Reproduced with permission: MacLennan & Petty, Sydney.) See Plate 27.

Prevention

Obvious prevention is avoidance of contact with an infected person or object. Brushes, combs, hats, and other personal items should not be shared. Good personal hygiene and routine clothes washing are other preventive measures; however, even someone with meticulous hygiene can develop this infection if there is contact with the organism.

Signs and Symptoms

Pediculosis capitis can result in no itching or intense itching and scratching, especially at the back of the head. Nits may be noticeably attached to hair. A papular rash may be seen (Fig. 51–11).

Pediculosis corporis may appear as minute hemorrhagic points. Excoriations may be noted on the back, shoulders, abdomen, and extremities. It may also cause intense itching.

Pediculosis pubis results in mild to severe itching, especially at night. Black or reddish-brown dots may be noted at the base of hairs or in underclothing. Gray-blue macules may also be noted on the trunk, thighs, and axillae; this is the result of the insects' saliva mixing with bilirubin.

Complications

Secondary bacterial infections can occur with pediculosis capitis, resulting in impetigo, furuncles, pustules, crusts, and matted hair. Secondary lesions that can occur with pediculosis corporis include parallel linear scratches,

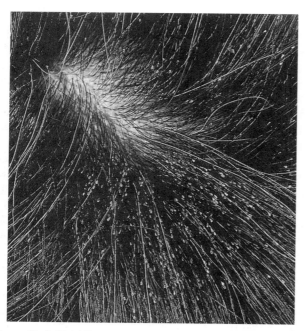

Figure 51–9. Head lice—nits are attached to hairs. (From Reeves J, Maibach H. *Clinical Dermatology Illustrated*, 2nd ed, 1998. Reproduced with permission: MacLennan & Petty, Sydney.) See Plate 27.

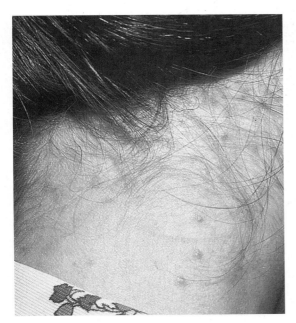

Figure 51–11. Head lice—bite papules at nape of neck. (From Reeves J, Maibach H. Clinical Dermatology Illustrated, 2nd ed, 1998. Reproduced with permission: MacLennan & Petty, Sydney.) See Plate 27.

hyperemia, eczema, and hyperpigmentation. Most important, body lice may be vectors for rickettsiae disease. Complications with pediculosis pubis include dermatitis and the coexistence of other sexually transmitted diseases.

Diagnostic Tests

Diagnosis is through history and physical assessment. The client may also be tested for sexually transmitted diseases if pediculosis pubis is present.

Medical Treatment

Medical treatment is aimed at killing the parasites and mechanically removing nits. Pediculosides containing pyrethrum or permethrin are the most commonly recommended compounds. These agents should kill the lice and nits, although some lice develop pesticide resistance, making mechanical removal necessary. Permethrin (Nix) remains active for about a week, killing the adult lice immediately, and the nits when they hatch days later. Pyrethrins (RID, A-200 Pyrinate) must be reapplied in 1 week to kill newly hatched lice.

Complications are treated, as appropriate, with antipruritics, topical corticosteroids, and systemic antibiotics. Physostigmine ophthalmic ointment is applied to affected eyebrows and eyelashes. Other medications should not be applied to eyebrows or eyelashes.

Nursing Care

The nurse reassures the client and family that head lice can happen to anyone, and this is not a sign of uncleanliness. These infections are treated on an outpatient basis, so patient education is very important. Package instructions should be followed for correct usage of all medications.

The nurse instructs the client to bathe with soap and water and to disinfect combs and brushes in hot, medicated soapy water. A fine-toothed comb dipped in vinegar can be used to remove nits from hairy areas. Nits can be removed from eyebrows and eyelashes with a cotton-tipped applicator after treatment. Clothing, linens, and towels should be laundered in hot water and detergent; unwashable clothing should be dry-cleaned or sealed in a plastic bag for 10 days. Treatment should be started immediately to prevent rapid spread. Family members and close contacts (sexual contact with pediculosis pubis) should be examined for infestation and should put on clean clothing.

Shampoos and lotions kill nits, but they do not remove them. To loosen nits from the scalp, the hair may be soaked in a solution of equal parts vinegar and water and a shower cap worn for 15 minutes. The hair is then combed with a fine-toothed comb and thoroughly rinsed or shampooed to mechanically remove the nits. Children may return to school after adequate medical treatment, even if nits are still present (the nits are dead).

LEARNING TIP

It is not possible to dry-clean or wash all infected items such as mattresses and upholstered furniture. Adult lice can live away from humans for only 3 to 4 days. Therefore simply vacuum the upholstered furniture. The lice will die in 3 to 4 days without human contact anyway.

SCABIES

Pathophysiology and Etiology

Scabies is a contagious skin disease caused by the mite *Sarcoptes scabiei*. It is caused by intimate or prolonged skin contact, or prolonged contact with infected clothing, bedding, or animals (dogs, cats, small animals). The parasite burrows into the superficial layer of the skin (Fig. 51–12). These burrows appear as short, wavy, brownish-black lines. The client is asymptomatic while the organism multiplies, but it is most contagious at this time. Symptoms do not occur for almost 4 weeks from time of contact.

Prevention

All persons (and animals) in intimate contact with an infected client should be treated at the same time to eliminate the mites. The mites survive less than 24 hours without human contact. Therefore bed linen, clothes, and towels

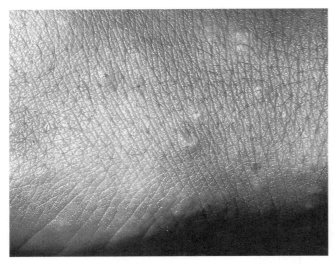

Figure 51–12. Scabies—the J-shaped white lesion in the center of the photograph is a burrow that contains an organism. (From Reeves J, Maibach H. Clinical Dermatology Illustrated, 2nd ed, 1998. Reproduced with permission: MacLennan & Petty, Sydney.) See Plate 28.

should be washed, but furnishings need not be cleaned. Clean clothing and linens should be applied.

Signs and Symptoms

The major complaints are itching and rash. Itching can be intense, especially at night. The itching occurs 1 month after infestation and may persist for days to weeks after treatment. The rash may appear as small, scattered erythematous papules, concentrated in fingerwebs (Fig. 51–13), axillae, wrist folds, umbilicus, groin, and genitals. Male clients may exhibit excoriated papules on the penis and groin area.

Complications

Hypersensitivity reactions to the mite can result in crusted lesions, vesicles, pustules, excoriations, and bacterial superinfections.

Diagnostic Tests

Diagnosis is confirmed by a superficial shaving of a lesion and microscopic evaluation for adult mite, eggs, or feces (Fig. 51–14).

Medical Treatment

Topical scabicides are used for chemical disinfection. Usually the cream or lotion is applied in a thin layer to the entire body from neck to feet (including genitals, umbilicus, and skin-fold areas), is left on overnight (8 to 12 hours), and is washed off in the morning; however, package in-

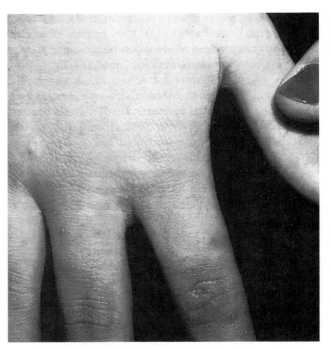

Figure 51–13. Scabies—fingerweb involvement is common. (From Reeves J, Maibach H. Clinical Dermatology Illustrated, 2nd ed, 1998. Reproduced with permission: MacLennan & Petty, Sydney.) See Plate 28.

structions should be referred to for each medication. One or two applications is usually curative, depending on the agent prescribed. Antipruritics and corticosteroids may be prescribed for itching.

Nursing Care

The client needs to take a warm soapy bath or shower to remove scales and skin debris. Advise the client to apply the topical medication as ordered; not repeatedly use scabicides because it can increase itching and cause further skin irritation; follow medication directions; treat family members and close contacts simultaneously to eliminate mites; wear clean clothing; and use clean linens. Remind the client that itching may continue for up to 2 weeks after treatment, until the allergic reaction subsides (dead mites remain in the epidermis until exfoliated). Infected animals should be treated by a veterinarian.

Pemphigus

PATHOPHYSIOLOGY AND ETIOLOGY

Pemphigus is an acute or chronic serious skin disease characterized by the appearance of bullae (blisters) of vari-

---

pemphigus: pemphix—blister

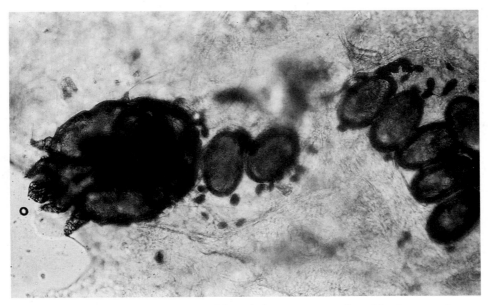

Figure 51–14. Scabies—adult mite, eggs, and feces in burrow are seen in a skin shave specimen under the microscope. (From Reeves J, Maibach H. Clinical Dermatology Illustrated, 2nd ed, 1998. Reproduced with permission: MacLennan & Petty, Sydney.) See Plate 28.

ous sizes on normal skin and mucous membranes. The etiology is unknown, but it is probably due to an autoimmune disorder. It usually occurs in clients from middle to older age.

Successive crops of bullae suddenly appear on normal skin or mucous membranes. The bullae are fragile and flaccid. They enlarge, rupture, and form painful, raw, eroded, partial-thickness wounds that bleed, ooze, and form crusts. Pemphigus usually originates in the oral mucosa and then spreads to the trunk. Large areas of the body become involved.

SIGNS AND SYMPTOMS

Besides the appearance of the blisters, the client experiences pain, burning, and itching. The lesions have a foul smell. Involvement of the oral mucosa can interfere with chewing, swallowing, and talking. The client is in constant misery.

COMPLICATIONS

The major complication is a bacterial superinfection or a secondary infection. There is a high morbidity and mortality rate associated with this disease.

DIAGNOSTIC TESTS

A positive Nikolsky's sign is a characteristic finding; this occurs when there is sloughing or blistering of normal skin

when minimal pressure is applied. A biopsy of a blister will reveal acantholysis, or separation of epidermal cells from one another.

MEDICAL TREATMENT

Treatment is aimed at controlling the disease, healing the skin, and preventing complications. Corticosteroids in large doses and cytotoxic agents are prescribed to control the disease and bring about remission. Medicated mouthwashes may be prescribed for mouth lesions. Analgesics and antipruritics are prescribed according to the client's specific signs and symptoms. Because of fluid, blood, and protein losses through the partial-thickness injury, a high-protein, high-calorie diet is recommended along with appropriate fluid replacement therapy.

NURSING CARE

The client is educated on the effects and side effects of medications. Fluid balance is monitored with regular intake and output, body weight, and blood pressure measurement. The client is encouraged to maintain adequate fluid intake. Administer tepid wet dressings or baths to lessen secondary infection, cleanse the area, decrease odor, and increase the comfort level of the client. Potassium permanganate baths may decrease infection and clean and deodorize the area. Always thoroughly dissolve potassium permanganate crystals in a small container before adding to tub water. Undissolved crystals may further damage and burn the skin. Dry the client thoroughly after the bath. Do not use tape on the client because this may cause further blistering. Talcum powder may be indicated to keep the client from sticking to linens and bedclothes. Maintain meticulous oral hygiene. Offer cool drinks often to lessen discomfort. Provide appropriate psychosocial support due to the length of illness, chronic nature of the condition, and physical appearance of lesions.

Burns

Many people are hospitalized each year for burns. Burns not only affect the skin, but can affect every major body system. Smoke inhalation and wound infections complicate care of the client who has been burned.

PATHOPHYSIOLOGY AND SIGNS AND SYMPTOMS

Burns are wounds caused by an energy transfer from a heat source to the body, heating the tissue enough to cause damage. Locally, the heat denatures cellular protein and interrupts the blood supply. The three zones of tissue damage are described in Figure 51–15.

The amount of skin damage is related to (1) the temperature of the burning agent; (2) the burning agent itself; (3) the duration of exposure; (4) the conductivity of tissue; and (5) the thickness of the involved dermal structures. Alterations in normal skin functioning due to a major burn injury include loss of protective functions, impaired temperature regulation, increased risk for infection, changes in sensory function, loss of fluids, impaired skin regeneration, and impaired secretory and excretory functions.

Systemic Responses

The alterations in the functional capacity of the skin affect virtually all major body systems. Following a major burn, increased capillary permeability leads to the leakage of plasma and proteins into the tissue, resulting in the formation of edema and loss of intravascular volume. There is also an evaporative water loss through burn tissue that can be 4 to 15 times that which is normal. The increase in metabolism leads to further water loss through the respiratory system.

Cardiac function is affected. There is an initial decrease in cardiac output, which is further compromised by the circulating plasma volume loss. Severe hematological changes occur in major burns due to tissue damage and vascular changes. Plasma moves into the interstitial space due to increased capillary permeability. In the first 48

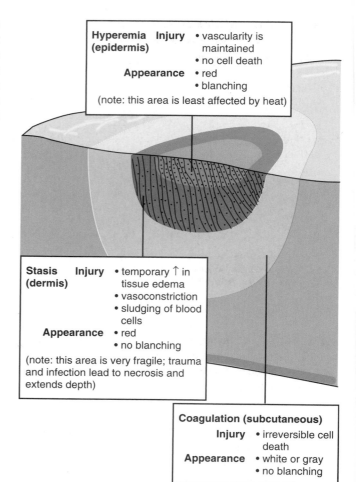

Figure 51–15. Three zones of tissue damage. (Modified from Ruppert, SD, Kernick, JG, and Dolan, JT: Dolan's Critical Care Nursing. FA Davis, Philadelphia, 1996, p 942, with permission.)

hours after a burn, fluid shifts lead to hypovolemia and, if untreated, hypovolemic shock. Loss of intravascular fluid causes an increase in hematocrit, and there is red blood cell destruction. The intense heat decreases platelet function and half-life. Leukocyte and platelet aggregation may progress to thrombosis.

The metabolic demands are very high. A high metabolic rate proportional to the severity of the burn is usually maintained until wound closure. This hypermetabolism is further compromised by associated injuries, surgical interventions, and the stress response. Severe catabolism also begins early and is associated with a negative nitrogen balance, weight loss, and decreased wound healing. Elevated catecholamine levels are triggered by the stress response. This, along with elevated glucagon levels, can stimulate hyperglycemia.

Gastrointestinal problems that can develop with a major burn include gastric dilation, Curling's ulcer, paralytic ileus, and superior mesenteric artery syndrome. Most of

Table 51–4. **Classification of Burn Depth**

Classification	Formerly	Areas Involved	Appearance	Sensitivity	Healing Time
Partial-thickness (superficial)	1°–2°	Epidermis Papillae of dermis	Bright red to pink. Blanches to touch. Serum-filled blisters. Glistening, moist.	Sensitive to air, temperature, and touch.	7–10 days
Partial-thickness (deep)	2°	Epidermis, ½ to ⅞ of dermis Appendage usually present	Blisters may be present. Pink to light red to white. Soft and pliable. Blanching present.	Pressure may be painful from exposed nerve endings.	14–21 days. May need grafting to decrease scarring.
Full-thickness	3°–4°	Epidermis Dermis Tissue Muscle Bone	Snowy white, gray, or brown. Texture is firm and leathery. Inelastic.	No pain as nerve endings are destroyed, unless surrounded by areas of partial-thickness burns.	Needs grafting to complete healing.

Source: Trofino, RB: Nursing management of the patient with burns. In Ruppert, SD, Kernick, JG, and Dolan, JT (eds): Dolan's Critical Care Nursing. FA Davis, Philadelphia, 1996, p 943.

these problems occur in response to fluid shifting, dehydration, narcotic analgesics, immobility, depressed gastric motility, and the stress response.

Acute renal insufficiency can occur as a result of hypovolemia and decreased cardiac output. Fluid loss and inadequate fluid replacement can lead to decreased renal plasma flow and glomerular filtration rate. With an electrical burn injury, renal damage can occur from direct electrical current or the formation of myoglobin casts (due to the muscle destruction), which can cause acute tubular necrosis.

Pulmonary effects are mostly related to smoke inhalation. However, hyperventilation is usually proportional to the severity of the burn. There is increased oxygen consumption due to the hypermetabolic state, fear, anxiety, and pain.

Immunologically, with the skin destroyed, the body loses its first line of defense against infection. Major burns

also cause a depression of the immunoglobulins IgA, IgG, and IgM.

Classification of Burn Injuries

The severity of a burn injury is influenced by the depth of destruction, percentage of injury, cause of the burn, age of the client, concomitant injuries, past medical history (e.g., heart disease, diabetes), and location of the burn wound. Table 51–4 describes classification of burn depth (Figs. 51–16, 51–17, and 51–18).

The size of the burn wound is determined by an estimation of the extent of the burn injury. A common method is the rule of nines. This method divides the body into segments whose areas are either 9 percent or multiples of 9 percent of the total body surface, with the perineum counted as 1 percent. This formula may be easy, but it is not accurate in assessing children. A more accurate method

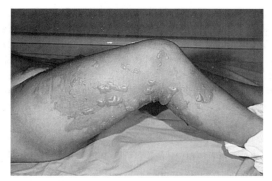

Figure 51–16. Partial-thickness burn. (From Trofino, RB: Nursing Care of the Burn-Injured Patient. FA Davis, Philadelphia, 1991, plate 1, with permission.)

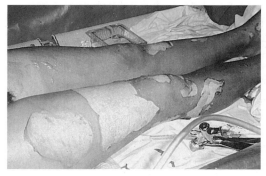

Figure 51–17. Deep partial-thickness burn. (From Trofino, RB: Nursing Care of the Burn-Injured Patient. FA Davis, Philadelphia, 1991, plate 2, with permission.)

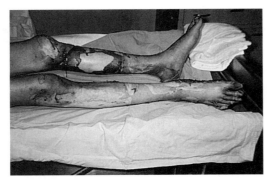

Figure 51–18. Full-thickness burn. (From Trofino, RB: Nursing Care of the Burn-Injured Patient. FA Davis, Philadelphia, 1991, plate 3, with permission.)

utilizes a table with a relative anatomical scale or diagram that estimates total burned area by ages and by smaller anatomical areas of the body. Figure 51–19 provides an example of each method.

ETIOLOGY

Burn injuries occur due to many causes. The most common causes include flame, contact, chemical, electrical, and radiation (Table 51–5).

COMPLICATIONS

A major complication that can occur with a flame burn in an enclosed space is inhalation injury. Infection is another common complication with a major burn. The incidence of infection increases with the size of the burn wound, because the first line of defense against microorganisms is the skin.

Neurovascular compromise can also occur with a major burn. Eschar formation creates pressure and contributes to decreasing blood flow to areas distal to the burned area. Other systemic complications are reviewed under Systemic Responses, earlier in this chapter.

DIAGNOSTIC TESTS

Burns are diagnosed through clinical manifestations. Various diagnostic tests are performed for systemic reactions, infection, and other complications. Common tests include complete blood count (CBC) and differential; blood urea nitrogen (BUN); serum glucose and electrolytes; arterial blood gases; blood protein and albumin; urine cultures; urinalysis; clotting studies; cervical spine series; electrocardiogram; wound cultures; and, if suspected inhalation injury, bronchoscopy and carboxyhemoglobin levels.

MEDICAL TREATMENT

Medical treatment varies according to the severity of the burn and the stage the client is in. The treatment of the client is managed over three overlapping stages (Table 51–6).

Emergent Stage

At the time of injury, the burning process must be stopped. The clothes are removed and the wound is cooled with tepid water and covered with clean sheets to decrease shivering and contamination. The burn wound itself takes a lower priority to the ABCs (airway, breathing, circulation) of trauma resuscitation. The client should be stabilized in terms of fractures, hemorrhage, spine immobilization, and other injuries. Inhalation injury is suspected if the client sustained a burn from a fire in an enclosed space or was exposed to smoldering materials, if the face and neck were burned, if there are vocal changes, and if the client is coughing up carbon particles. Intravenous fluids are given to prevent and treat hypovolemic shock. The client is treated for pain with appropriate IV narcotic analgesia. Patient-controlled analgesia (PCA) is very effective.

An accurate history of the injury is obtained in order to determine severity, probable complications, and any associated trauma. The client's past medical history is also obtained. Admission to the facility and burn care treatment are explained to the client and family.

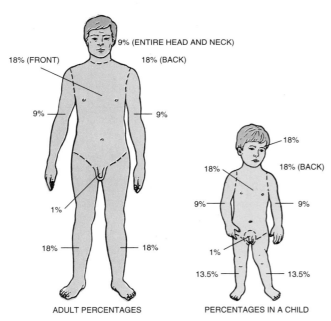

Figure 51–19. Estimation of extent of burn injury. (From Thomas, C.L. (ed):Taber's Cyclopedic Medical Dictionary, ed 18. FA Davis, Philadelphia, 1997, p 1700, Beth Anne Willert, M.S., Dictionary Illustrator.)

Table 51–5. *Common Causes of Burns*

Flame	House fire is a common cause.
	Usually associated with an inhalation injury.
	Flash injury occurs from a sudden ignition or explosion.
Contact	Hot tar, hot metals, hot grease will produce a full-thickness injury on contact.
Scald	A burn from hot liquid.
	Common in children less than 5 years and adults older than 65 years.
	With an immersion scald, there are usually no splash marks; usually involves lower regions of body.
Chemical	Usually occurs in an industrial setting.
	Extent and depth of injury are directly proportional to concentration and quantity of agent, duration of contact, and chemical activity and penetrability of agent.
Electrical	One of the most serious types of burn injury; can be full-thickness with possible loss of limbs, as well as cause internal injuries.
	Entry wound is usually ischemic, charred, and depressed.
	Exit wound may have an explosive appearance.
	Extent of injury depends on voltage, resistance of body, type of current, amperage, pathway of current, and duration of contact.
	Bones offer greatest resistance to the current; can have much damage.
	Tissue fluid, blood, and nerves offer least resistance; therefore the current travels this path.
Radiation	Can occur in an industrial setting, due to treatment of diseases, or from ultraviolet light (sun or tanning salons).
	Severity depends on type of radiation, duration of exposure, depth of penetration, distance from source, and the absorbed dose.

Acute Stage

If the client is in a facility with a special burn unit, multidisciplinary care from a burn team will be provided during the acute stage. Management goals include wound closure with no infection; minimal scarring; maximal function; maintenance of comfort as much as possible; adequate nutritional support; and maintenance of fluid, electrolyte, and acid-base balance. The client continues to be medicated for pain as needed, especially before painful treatments. Nutritional support is maintained via a small Silastic nasogastric feeding tube.

The wound is cleansed and debrided daily to promote healing, prevent infection, and provide a clean bed for grafting. Wound cleansing is achieved by tubbing with a Hubbard tank, showering utilizing a shower trolley or shower chair, and bedside care.

Debridement, or the removal of nonviable tissue (eschar), can be mechanical, chemical, surgical, or a combination of these methods. Mechanical debridement can involve the use of scissors and forceps to manually excise loose nonviable tissue, or the use of wet-to-moist or wet-to-dry mesh gauze. Chemical debridement involves the use of a proteolytic enzymatic debriding agent that digests necrotic tissue. Surgical debridement is the excision of full-thickness and deep partial-thickness burns. This method is followed by an application of a skin graft.

If the client has a circumferential burn (one that surrounds an extremity or area), there is an increase in tissue

pressure secondary to tissue edema. The burn then acts like a tourniquet, impeding arterial and venous flow. Common sites for these burns are the extremities, trunk, and chest. If this occurs to the chest and trunk, respiratory insufficiency can occur due to restricted chest expansion. An **escharotomy** is immediately necessary to relieve this pressure. An escharotomy is a linear excision through the eschar to the superficial fat that allows for expansion of the skin and return of blood flow (Fig. 51–20).

Once the area is cleaned, the burn dressing and topical treatment are prescribed. The type of dressing and topical agent chosen are dependent on the area involved, extent and depth of injury, and physician preference. Several common topical agents are listed in Table 51–7.

Dressings may be open, closed, biological, synthetic, or a combination. The open method is the use of a topical agent without any dressing. The closed method involves

Table 51–6. *Stages of Burn Care*

Stage	Duration
I (emergent)	From onset of injury to completion of fluid resuscitation
II (acute)	From start of diuresis to near completion of wound closure
III (rehabilitation)	From wound closure to return of optimal level of physical and psychosocial function

Source: Trofino, RB: Nursing management of the patient with burns. In Ruppert, SD, Kernick, JG, and Dolan, JT (eds): Dolan's Critical Care Nursing. FA Davis, Philadelphia, 1996, p 948.

escharotomy: eschara—scab + otomy—incision

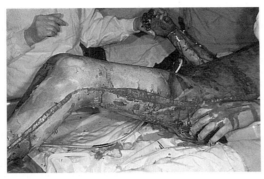

Figure 51–20. Escharotomy. (From Trofino, RB: Nursing Care of the Burn-Injured Patient. FA Davis, Philadelphia, 1991, plate 16, with permission.)

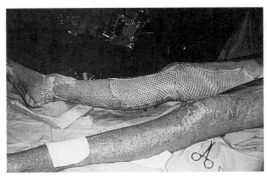

Figure 51–21. Meshed graft. (From Trofino, RB: Nursing Care of the Burn-Injured Patient. FA Davis, Philadelphia, 1991, plate 17, with permission.)

the use of an occlusive dressing over the wound. General principles to follow with dressings include the following: limit the bulk of the dressing to facilitate range of motion; never wrap skin-to-skin surfaces (e.g., wrap fingers or toes separately; place a "donut" gauze dressing around the ear); base dressings on the size of wounds, absorption, protection, and debridement; wrap extremities distal to proximal to promote venous return; and elevate affected extremities.

Biological dressings refer to tissue from living or deceased humans (cadaver skin) or deceased animals (e.g., pigskin). These dressings may be used as a donor site dressing, to manage a partial-thickness burn, and to cover the clean, excised wound before autografting. The biological dressings assist with wound healing and stimulate **epithelialization.**

Synthetic dressings are utilized in the management of partial-thickness burns and donor sites. These dressings are more readily available, less costly, and easier to store than biological dressings. They are made from a variety of materials and come in many different sizes and shapes. Most of these dressings contain no antimicrobial agents.

Biological and synthetic dressings are utilized as temporary wound coverings over clean partial- and full-thickness injuries. These skin substitutes help maintain the wound surface until healing occurs, a donor site becomes available, or the wound is ready for autografting.

Skin Grafts

An autograft is a skin graft from the client's unburned skin to be placed on the clean excised burn. The two common types of autografts are the split-thickness skin graft (STSG), which includes the epidermis and part of the dermis, and the full-thickness skin graft (FTSG), which includes the epidermis and entire dermal layer.

An STSG (0.006 to 0.016 inch) may be applied as a sheet graft or a meshed graft. A sheet graft is used for cosmetic effect, such as for a face, neck, upper chest, breast, or hand burn. It is placed on the area as a full sheet. A meshed

graft is passed through a mesher that produces tiny splits in the skin, similar to a fishnet, with openings in the shape of diamonds (Fig. 51–21), to permit the skin to expand 1.5 to 9 times its original size. The meshing allows for coverage of a large burn area with a small piece of skin by stretching it and securing it with sutures or staples. A mesh graft is especially useful when there are extensive burns resulting in few available donor sites. Graft "take," or vascularization, is complete in about 3 to 5 days.

Full-thickness skin grafts (0.035 to 0.040 inch) can be sheet grafts or pedicle flaps. FTSGs are used over areas of muscle mass, soft tissue loss, hands, feet, and eyelids. They are not used for extensive wounds, because the donor sites usually require an STSG for closure, or closure from the wound edges. A pedicle graft or flap includes the skin flap and subcutaneous tissue that is attached by its pedicle to a blood supply—artery and vein; it is then attached to the area in need of grafting. Once the distal part of the graft takes, it remains in place, and the flap is divided with the remainder returning to the original site. Pedicle flaps are not as popular as free skin flaps, because they require more than one surgery and take longer for the graft site and donor site to heal. Table 51–8 provides a comparison of split-thickness and full-thickness grafts.

Donor sites are considered a partial-thickness wound. Donor sites usually heal in 10 to 14 days, but this is dependent on thickness and method of grafting. Treatment for the donor site varies with the individual client, the area of the body, and physician preference. Considerations for care include promoting comfort and preventing trauma and infection. An outer dressing, used to apply pressure for hemostasis, remains in place for 1 to 2 days. For dry exposure healing, a bed cradle may be used to promote circulation and avoid pressure on the site. A heat lamp (60 to 100 watts) may be employed to assist in drying, but it must be kept at least 2 feet away from the site. Loose, separating

epithelialization: epi—over + thele—nipple + ation—condition

Table 51–7. **Common Topical Antibiotic Agents**

Agent	Dressings	Advantages	Disadvantages
Silver sulfadiazine 1% cream *Silvadene* *H2o soluble*	Buttered on. With light dressings once or twice a day.	Broad spectrum. Low toxicity. Painless, easy to apply and remove. Can be used with or without dressings.	Intermediate penetration of eschar; leukopenia.
Mafenide acetate (Sulfamylon)	Buttered on. Open exposure method. Applied 3–4 times daily.	Broad spectrum. Rapid, deep penetration of eschar. Rapid excretion.	Pain on application. Pulmonary toxicity. Metabolic acidosis. Inhibits wound healing. Hypersensitivity.
Silver nitrate solution 0.5%	Wet dressings. Change bid. Resoak every 2 hr.	Broad spectrum. Nonallergenic. Low toxicity. Inexpensive. Does not interfere with healing.	Poor penetration of eschar. Ineffective on established wound infections. Can cause an electrolyte imbalance. Discoloration of wound and environment makes assessment difficult.
Bacitracin	Buttered on. Reapply every 4–6 hr.	No pain. Clear, odorless. Useful for face burns. Softens eschar.	Poor penetration of eschar. Not effective in reducing sepsis in large burns. Occasional allergic sensitivity.
Gentamicin	Apply gently 3–4 times daily.	Broad spectrum. May be covered or left open to air.	Ototoxic. Nephrotoxic. Pain on application.
Nitrofurazone	Apply thin layer directly to wounds or impregnate into gauze. Change dressings twice daily.	Bactericidal. Broad spectrum.	Painful application. May lead to overgrowth of fungus and pseudomonas.

Source: Trofino, RB: Nursing management of the patient with burns. In Ruppert, SD, Kernick, JG, and Dolan, JT (eds): Dolan's Critical Care Nursing. FA Davis, Philadelphia, 1996, p 951.

gauze is trimmed to avoid accidental trauma. The donor site is very painful. Appropriate pain medications are provided, along with nonpharmacological measures (e.g., back rub, distraction).

With any type of graft, the client must keep the graft site immobilized until the graft takes, to prevent movement or slippage of the grafted skin. Dressings may be bulky to assist in immobilization. These dressings must not be disturbed. The involved area requires frequent circulatory checks (color, warmth, sensation, pulses, and capillary refill). Any involved extremities must be elevated to maintain circulation. Table 51–9 describes factors affecting graft viability. A good take of a graft involves adherence of the graft to the wound with no evidence of necrosis or infection.

Rehabilitation Phase

The therapy started during the acute phase continues in the rehabilitation phase. There is wound closure, and the goal is to return the client to an optimal level of physical and psychosocial function. This may take months to years to

Table 51–8. **Comparison of Split-Thickness and Full-Thickness Skin Grafts**

	Split-Thickness	Full-Thickness
Layers	Epidermis Partial layer of dermis	Epidermis Entire dermal layer
Advantages	Donor site may be reused Healing of donor site is more rapid, results in good "take"	Allows more elasticity over joints Can reconstruct cosmetic defects Soft, pliable Gives full appearance Provides good color-match Less hyperpigmentation May allow hair growth
Disadvantages	Prone to chronic breakdown Likely to hypertrophy More likely to contract	Donor site takes longer to heal Requires split-thickness graft to heal or closure from wound edges

Source: Konop, D: General local treatment. In Trofino, RB (ed): Nursing Care of the Burn-Injured Patient. FA Davis, Philadelphia, 1991, p 61.

Table 51–9. **Factors Affecting Graft Viability**

Factors Inhibiting Graft "Take"	Factors Promoting Graft "Take"
Infection	Adequate hemostasis
Necrotic skin (tissue)	Anatomic location of graft
Anatomic location of graft	Smooth contour
Perineum	Nonjoints
Axilla	Graft secured well
Buttocks	Immobilization of graft area
Poor-quality donor skin	Good nutritional status
Poor nutritional status	
Bleeding	
Mechanical trauma	
Shock	

Source: Konop, D: General local treatment. In Trofino, RB (ed): Nursing Care of the Burn-Injured Patient. FA Davis, Philadelphia, 1991, p 62.

accomplish. Reconstructive surgery can be ongoing for many years.

Two things to keep in mind when caring for the client with a major burn are that the most comfortable position (flexion) is the position of contracture, and that the burn wound will shorten until it meets an opposing force. To avoid contractures (Fig. 51–22), a specific exercise program is begun 24 to 48 hours after injury, along with the use of splinting devices to maintain proper positioning and stretching. Hypertrophic scarring, or a proliferation of scar tissue, can be minimized or prevented through the use of a pressure garment (Fig. 51–23).

The burn affects the client's psychosocial status in many ways. The magnitude of these effects are related to the age of the client, location of the burn (e.g., face, hands), recovery from injury, cause of the injury (especially if related to negligence or a deliberate act), and ability to continue at preburn level of normal daily activities, disruption of role, family involvement, and general personality and health. Treatment involves the client and significant others. Support groups, counselors, and psychiatrists should be utilized appropriately.

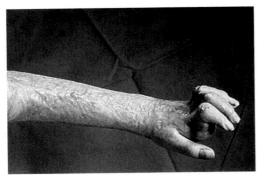

Figure 51–22. Burn deformity: contracture. (From Trofino, RB: Nursing Care of the Burn-Injured Patient. FA Davis, Philadelphia, 1991, plate 36, with permission.)

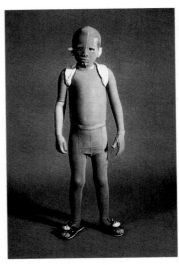

Figure 51–23. Full-body pressure garment. (From Trofino, RB: Nursing Care of the Burn-Injured Patient. FA Davis, Philadelphia, 1991, plate 39, with permission.)

NURSING PROCESS

Assessment

A major burn is very painful and frightening to the client and very frightening to the family. Elicit information from the client, family, and rescuers. If the injury occurred in an enclosed space with flames or smoldering materials, inhalation injury is suspected. If an electrical injury, determine voltage, duration of contact, host susceptibility (wet or dry skin), entry and exit sites, and associated falls. With chemical burns, determine type of agent and duration of exposure.

General information to assess with all burns (in addition to normally assessed data, such as past medical history, known allergies, current medications) include extent, depth, and type of burn; duration of contact with the burning agent; amount and location of pain; and associated injuries. Determine the immediate first aid treatment provided at the scene. Elicit psychosocial information: other people injured; additional losses (home, pets); whether the client was at fault; and how this injury affects the client role.

Nursing Diagnosis

Possible nursing diagnoses for a client with a major burn include impairment of skin integrity; impaired gas exchange; fluid volume deficit; pain; alteration in peripheral perfusion; risk for sepsis; alteration in nutrition; impairment of activity; and ineffective coping.

Nursing Care

See Nursing Care Plan Box 51–3 for the Client with a Burn Injury.

text continues on page 1127

NURSING CARE PLAN BOX 51-3 FOR THE CLIENT WITH A BURN INJURY

Impaired skin integrity related to thermal injury

Client Outcomes

Skin integrity is improved as evidenced by healing of burned areas with no infection present, healing of the burning process.

Evaluation of Outcomes

Is the burned area healed? Is it free from infection? Did the burning process stop?

Interventions	*Rationale*	*Evaluation*
Assess the burning process. If heat is felt on the wound, cool with tepid tap water or sterile water. If a chemical burn, immediately lavage with copious amounts of water for 20 minutes (do not neutralize the chemical, because this takes too much time and the resulting reaction may generate heat and cause further skin injury).	Depth of injury increases with length of exposure to burning agent.	Is heat felt over the wounds?
Assist RN or MD to assess the burn area for extent (percentage) and depth (partial-thickness, full-thickness) of injury.	Provides a basis for triage of care. Important also for calculating resuscitation fluid therapy.	What is the estimation of percentage of burn injury? What is the depth of injury?
Remove clothing and jewelry.	These items can retain heat and thermal agent, therefore increasing the depth of injury. Jewelry can be constrictive when edema develops.	Are clothing and jewelry removed?
Do not apply ice.	Ice causes vasoconstriction, further increasing wound damage. Ice also causes a decrease in core body temperature, which may promote shock.	Is the water tepid? Has the use of ice been avoided?
Cover the client with a clean sheet or blanket.	Prevents excessive heat loss. Decreases pain from air exposure. Protects the client from environmental contamination.	Is the client covered?
Obtain history of the burning agent.	Provides information related to depth, duration of contact, and resistance of tissues. If fire scenario, provides clues to possible inhalation injury.	What caused this thermal injury? How long was the client in contact with the agent?
Initiate copious tepid water lavage for 20 minutes for all chemical burns, along with simultaneous removal of contaminated clothing. Brush off dry chemicals before lavage. Use heavy rubber gloves or thick gauze for removal of clothing.	Dilution and removal of chemical agent will halt the burning process. Lavage dissipates heat. Gloves and gauze are necessary to protect health care workers from injury.	Has the lavage been initiated? Were there any injuries to health care workers?
Cleanse wound via tubbing or showers.	Promotes healing and helps decrease infection.	Is the burn wound clean and free of wound debris?
Assist RN or MD with debriding the wound via surgical, chemical, or mechanical means. Apply topical agent as prescribed.	Promotes healing and healthy granulation bed. Most agents prevent infection and promote healing.	Is there any eschar? Is the wound free of wound debris? Is the agent applied as directed?

continued

NURSING CARE PLAN BOX 51-3 *(continued)*		
Interventions	*Rationale*	*Evaluation*
Apply dressing as prescribed. Use common practices: 1. Do not wrap skin surface to skin surface (e.g., wrap fingers and toes separately; "donut" bandage around ears). 2. Limit the bulk of dressings. 3. Wrap extremities distal to proximal.	Dressing types vary and are influenced by area, extent, and depth of injury, as well as by topical agent used. The dressing protects the burn area and promotes healing. Wrapping separately prevents webbing and contractures. Mobility is enhanced with a less bulky dressing. Circulation is increased when extremities are wrapped distal to proximal.	Is the dressing applied appropriately?

Impaired gas exchange related to upper airway edema, carbon monoxide poisoning, edema of alveolar capillary membranes

Client Outcomes
Gas exchange will be improved as evidenced by patent airway, CO level less than 10%, clear lung sounds, PaO_2 80–100 mm Hg, $PaCO_2$ 35–45 mm Hg, responsive and aware.

Evaluation of Outcomes
Are blood levels improved: CO, PaO_2, $PaCO_2$? Do the lungs sound clear on auscultation? Is the client aware of surroundings? Are there no signs of respiratory distress (e.g., retractions, nasal flaring, use of accessory muscles)?

Interventions	*Rationale*	*Evaluation*
Assess respiratory status: auscultate breath sounds every 15 minutes or as necessary; note any adventitious breath sounds; observe for chest excursion: monitor ability to cough.	Detects changes in pulmonary function to alter therapy.	What is the client's respiratory status? Are any adventitious lung sounds noted?
Monitor arterial blood gases and CO level.	Assesses level of oxygenation. Helps guide oxygen therapy.	What are the client's blood gas levels? Are they abnormal?
Monitor for nasal flaring, retractions, wheezing, and stridor.	Stridor may signal upper airway involvement; nasal flaring, retractions, and wheezing may indicate lower airway involvement.	Does the client exhibit nasal flaring, retractions, wheezing, and stridor?
Administer humidified 100% oxygen by tight-fitting face mask for the breathing client.	Provides oxygen for adequate gas exchange.	Is the oxygen administered appropriately? Are the blood gases improving?
Elevate head of bed (if no cervical spine injuries or no history of multiple trauma).	Decreases swelling of face and neck.	Is the head of the bed elevated? Is there any change in facial or neck swelling?
Provide appropriate pulmonary care: turn, cough, deep breathe every 2–4 hours. Incentive spirometer every 2–4 hours, suction frequently as needed.	Mobilizes secretions and promotes lung expansion.	Is the client on scheduled activities for vigorous pulmonary care?
Obtain sputum cultures. Note amount, color, and consistency of pulmonary secretions.	Carbonaceous sputum is diagnostic for smoke inhalation injury. Infection will change color, amount, and consistency of sputum. Assists in selection of appropriate antibiotic.	Is the client coughing up any sputum? Has the character of the sputum been documented?
Administer bronchodilators and antibiotics as prescribed.	Bronchodilators decrease bronchospasms and edema; antibiotics fight infection.	Are medications given appropriately?

continued

NURSING CARE PLAN BOX 51–3 *(continued)*

Fluid volume deficit related to evaporative losses from wound, capillary leak, and decreased fluid intake

Client Outcomes
The client will maintain adequate circulating volume as evidenced by urine output of 50 mL/hr (in the adult), blood pressure within normal limits, heart rate at about 100 beats per minute (adult), and stabilized body weight.

Evaluation of Outcomes
Is the urine output maintained at least at 50 mL/hr? Are the blood pressure and heart rate within normal limits? Is the client's weight stable?

Interventions	Rationale	Evaluation
Obtain admission weight and monitor weight daily.	Helps measure fluid loss or gain.	Is the client's weight documented? Is it stable?
Record intake and output (I & O) hourly.	Serves as a guide for fluid loss and replacement.	What is the client's I & O?
Assess for signs and symptoms of hypovolemia (hypotension, tachycardia, tachypnea, extreme thirst, restlessness, disorientation).	Fluid volume loss is multifocal (e.g., through increased capillary permeability, insensible loss).	Does the client exhibit any signs or symptoms of hypovolemia?
Monitor electrolytes, CBC.	Serves as guide for electrolyte replacement and blood product replacement.	What are the client's lab values? Are they within normal limits?
Administer IV fluids as ordered. Insert a large-bore catheter.	Fluid replacement begins immediately. Large vessels are needed for rapid delivery of fluids.	Is the client's fluid replacement adequate? Is the catheter patent?
Insert indwelling urinary catheter.	Fluid replacement is titrated based on urine output.	Is the catheter patent?
Monitor urine for amount, specific gravity, and hemochromogens.	Specific gravity can predict volume replacement; hemochromogens can cause renal-tubular damage.	What are the client's urine values?
Administer osmotic diuretics as ordered; monitor response to therapy.	Decreased urinary output can be caused by decreased renal flow (due to myoglobin in urine).	What is the urinary output? Has it changed due to therapy?
Assess gastrointestinal function for absence of bowel sounds. Maintain nasogastric tube.	Splanchnic constriction due to hypovolemia can cause a paralytic ileus.	Are the client's bowel sounds normal? Is the nasogastric tube patent?

Pain related to burns or graft donor sites

Client Outcomes
The client will experience pain control as evidenced by verbalizations of pain tolerance, nonverbal cues: less thrashing; better rest or sleep; body positioning.

Evaluation of Outcomes
Does the client verbalize better pain control? How many hours of rest/sleep does the client have in 24 hours? Does the client state she or he feels rested?

Interventions	Rationale	Evaluation
Assess level of pain: nature, location, intensity, and duration at various times (during procedures, at rest). Rate pain on visual analogue scale.	Provides a baseline to monitor response to therapy.	Is the client's individual response to pain documented?

continued

NURSING CARE PLAN BOX 51–3 (continued)

Interventions	Rationale	Evaluation
Observe for varied responses to pain: increase in blood pressure, pulse, respiration; increased restlessness and irritability; increased muscle tension; facial grimaces; guarding.	Responses to pain are variable. These parameters change in response to pain.	What are the client's responses to pain? Do responses change with treatment?
Acknowledge the presence of pain. Explain causes of pain.	Encourages understanding.	Is the client more trusting of the treatments?
Administer narcotics IV. Utilize patient-controlled analgesia (PCA) as appropriate.	IV administration is necessary due to edema and poor tissue perfusion. Narcotics are necessary for severe burn pain. PCA allows client more control.	Is the client being medicated for pain appropriately?
Offer diversional activities (e.g., music, TV, books, games, relaxation techniques).	Helps the client focus on something other than pain.	Does the client utilize diversional activities? Do they help?
Properly position client. Elevate burned extremities.	Increases comfort. Elevation decreases edema and pain.	Is the client positioned as comfortably as possible? Are extremities elevated?
Maintain comfortable environment (e.g., bed cradle; comfortable environmental temperature, 86–91.4°F; quiet environment).	Pressure from bed linens may cause discomfort; with loss of integument, the body cannot self-regulate temperature.	Does the client verbalize comfort of environment?

Alteration in peripheral perfusion related to circumferential burns, blood loss, decreased cardiac output

Client Outcomes
The client will maintain adequate tissue perfusion as evidenced by presence of peripheral pulses; minimal edema; adequate circulation, sensation, and motion; and warm extremities.

Evaluation of Outcomes
Are peripheral pulses present? Are extremities warm, with adequate sensation, motion, and circulation? Is edema decreased?

Interventions	Rationale	Evaluation
Elevate the burned extremity above the level of the heart.	Enhances venous return and decreases edema formation.	Are all burned extremities elevated above heart level? Is edema decreasing?
Assess pulses on burned extremities every 15 minutes.	Assesses need for escharotomy.	Are pulses documented every 15 minutes?
Use Doppler as necessary. Assess capillary refill, sensation, color, swelling, and motion.	Assesses peripheral perfusion.	Is the extremity warm, with adequate color, sensation, motion, and capillary refill?
Assess for numbness, tingling, and increased pain in the burned extremity.	Can be indicative of increased pressure from edema.	Does the client complain of numbness, tingling, or pain?
Measure circumference of burned extremities.	Monitors edema formation.	Is there a change in measurements of circumference?
Apply burn dressing loosely.	Prevents constriction and allows for expansion as edema forms.	Is the dressing too tight?
Assist with muscle compartment pressures.	Helps determine need for escharotomy (if pressure greater than 25 mm Hg).	What is the client's pressure?
Assist with escharotomy as necessary.	If indicated, removal of eschar allows for edema expansion and permits peripheral perfusion.	Does the client require an escharotomy? Is the edema relieved?

continued

NURSING CARE PLAN BOX 51–3 *(continued)*

Risk for sepsis related to wound infection

Client Outcomes
The client will not develop a wound infection.

Evaluation of Outcomes
Is there healthy granulation tissue on unhealed areas with less than 10^5 colonies of bacteria (wound culture)? Are the donor sites free of infection? Have the skin grafts taken? Is there absence of clinical manifestation of infection (temperature 98.6°F; normal WBC)?

Interventions	Rationale	Evaluation
Use sterile technique with wound care.	The unhealed burn wound is a culture medium for bacterial growth.	Is sterile technique used for all wound care?
Maintain protective isolation with good hand-washing technique.	Prevents the spread of bacteria from client to client or nurse to client.	Do all persons in contact with client maintain proper precautions?
Administer immunosupportive medications as prescribed: tetanus and gamma globulin.	Immunoglobulins are depressed at time of severe burn injury.	Does the client require these medications?
Perform wound care as prescribed, which may include the following: inspect and debride wounds daily; culture wound three times a week or at sign of infection; shave hair at least 1 inch around burn areas (excluding eyebrows); inspect invasive line sites for inflammation (especially if line is through a burn area).	Provides quick identification of bacterial wound invasion and decreases incidence of infection. Presence of hair increases medium for bacterial growth.	What does the wound look like? Is it debrided? What are the culture results? Is there any hair near burn or line sites?
Continually assess for signs and symptoms of sepsis: temperature elevation; change in sensorium; changes in vital signs and bowel sounds; decreased output; positive blood/wound cultures.	The burn client may experience several septic episodes until the wound is healed.	Does the client exhibit any signs or symptoms of sepsis?
Administer systemic antibiotics and topical agents as prescribed.	Useful in eliminating or controlling infection. Systemic antibiotics are prescribed based on results of wound cultures.	Does the client require systemic antibiotics? Are they working? Are topical agents applied appropriately? Is the wound healing?

Skin Lesions

Skin lesions can be either benign (noncancerous) or malignant. Benign lesions are described in Table 51–10. Malignant lesions are discussed below. See also Cultural Considerations Box 51–4.

MALIGNANT SKIN LESIONS

Pathophysiology and Etiology

The most common skin malignancies include basal cell carcinoma, squamous cell carcinoma, and malignant melanoma. The major causative factor is overexposure to ultraviolet rays, most commonly sunlight. Other factors include being fair skinned and blue eyed; genetic tendencies; history of x-ray therapy; exposure to certain chemical agents (e.g., arsenic, paraffins, coal tar); burn scars; chronic osteomyelitis; and immunosuppressive therapy.

Basal cell carcinoma (Fig. 51–24) arises from the basal cell layer of the epidermis. It is the most common type of skin cancer. This tumor is mainly seen on sun-exposed areas of the body. The lesion appears as a small "pearly" or translucent papule with a rolled, waxy edge, depressed center, telangiactasia (lesion formed by dilation of vessels), crusting, and ulceration. Metastasis is rare.

Squamous cell carcinoma arises from the epidermis. This tumor can occur on sun-exposed areas of the skin and mucous membranes and is mainly seen on the lower lip, neck, tongue, head, and dorsa of the hands. It can occur on normal skin or a preexisting lesion (actinic kerotosis). The lesion appears as a single, crusted, scaled, eroded papule, nodule, or plaque (Fig. 51–25). A neglected lesion will appear more rough, scaly, and darker colored (Fig. 51–26).

The lesion is fragile and prone to oozing and bleeding. This is a truly invasive carcinoma. Metastasis is related to histological type, the depth of invasion, and the size of the lesion.

text continues on page 1130

Table 51–10. **Benign Skin Lesions**

Type	Description	Treatment
Cyst	A saclike growth with a definite wall that may contain liquid, semifluid, or solid material. An epidermal cyst is a saclike growth of the upper portion of a hair follicle. It is due to blockage of the pilosebaceous follicle. It is a soft hemispherical module, usually with an overlying comedo, that is usually seen on the face, neck, or upper trunk. It is usually asymptomatic. A pilar cyst, or sebaceous cyst, is a saclike growth of the middle portion of the hair follicle that contains hair and cuticle-like material. It is a hard, hemispherical nodule without a surmounted pore that is usually seen on the scalp.	If bothersome, it may be surgically excised. If excision is done, the entire cyst wall is removed to prevent recurrence.
Seborrheic keratosis	A benign skin lesion that is pigmented light tan to dark brown patches. The plaques or papules have a "stuck on" appearance due to the proliferation of epidermal cells and keratin piled on the skin surface. Etiology is unknown, but it tends to occur in middle-aged to older clients, most commonly on the trunk, scalp, face, and extremities.	Treatment is cosmetic only, or if lesion becomes irritated from friction. Liquid nitrogen cryotherapy or light curettage is performed if necessary for removal.

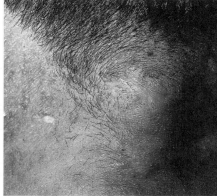

Epidermal cyst at nape of neck. See Plate 29.

Keloid	A benign growth of fibrous tissue (scar formation) at the site of trauma or surgical incision; occurs in various sizes. Growth of tissue is out of proportion to what is needed for normal healing. The benign wartlike lesion or nodule extends beyond the original injury and occurs mainly in middle-aged and elderly clients and darker-skinned clients.	Treatment varies, is not always successful, and is difficult; a larger scar may ensue. Treatments include surgical excision, intralesional steroid therapy, low-dose radiation, and pressure garments worn over the area, or a combination of these therapies.

continued

Table 51–10. (continued)

Type	Description	Treatment
Pigmented nevi	A benign, flesh-colored to dark brown macule or papule located randomly over the entire skin surface of the body. Can be inherited or acquired and occurs mostly in light-skinned clients. Usually begin to appear between 1 to 4 years of age, increasing in number into adulthood. Some contain a few hairs. There are many variations. Rate of transformation to a malignant melanoma is higher in congenital moles and larger lesions. Clinical signs to observe for in differentiating between a mole and a melanoma include change in color or size; inflammation of surrounding skin; irregular borders; spreading borders; variegated colors, especially a bluish pigmentation; bleeding; and oozing, crusting, and itching. Usually nevi over 1 cm should be carefully examined.	Treatment is indicated for any of the previously listed indications of melanoma; unsightly nevi (cosmetic); repeated irritation (rubbing from belt, bra); trauma; large moles; and client conviction of a change in the mole. Surgical removal can include excision (preferred) or surgical shave. All excised moles should be examined histologically.

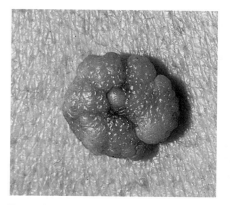

Dermal mole. See Plate 29.

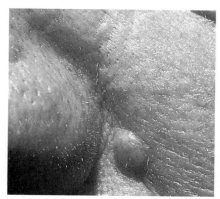

Nonpigmented dermal mole. See Plate 29.

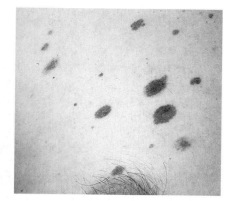

Dysplastic nevi. See Plate 29.

Type	Description	Treatment
Warts	Small, common, benign growths of the skin resulting from the hypertrophy of the papillae and epidermis. Caused by a virus. Common warts, often seen on hands and fingers, appear as raised, flesh-colored papules that have a rough surface. These warts may crack, fissure, bleed, and be painful to lateral pinching and direct, firm pressure. Plantar warts occur on the sole of the foot. They may appear granular, pitted, or protuberant, with a callous of surrounding normal skin. Incubation period can be several weeks to months. Virus is spread by direct contact into areas of broken skin or to other nails by nail cuticle biting.	If no pain or discomfort, no treatment may be indicated. Client should be cautioned not to spread lesions by picking or biting them. Treatment is indicated for symptomatic warts and for cosmetic purposes. General treatments include kerolytic agents (e.g., salicylic acid plasters) to soften and reduce keratin; cryotherapy (liquid nitrogen); and light electrodesiccation and curettage (requires local anesthesia). Treatment of choice is usually cryotherapy, because local anesthesia is not necessary and it leaves little scarring.

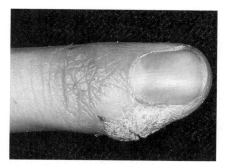

Wart near nail. See Plate 30.

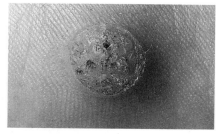

Plantar wart. This wart was painful during walking. Pressure caused irritation of surrounding skin. See Plate 30.

continued

Table 51–10. (continued)

Type	Description	Treatment
Hemangiomas (angiomas)	Benign vascular tumors of dilated blood vessels that can have varied clinical manifestations. Nevus flammeus involves mature capillaries on the face and neck. It is a congenital neoplasm that appears as a pink-red to bluish-purple macular patch. Port-wine stains or port-wine angiomas appear as violet-red macular patches, usually singular lesions, growing proportionately as the child grows. These lesions can persist indefinitely. Cherry hemangiomas are commonly seen in the elderly client. They appear as small round papules that can vary in color from red to purple.	Nevus flammeus is usually treated for cosmetic reasons. Port-wine stains, if large enough, may require surgical excision with skin grafting. Laser therapy may also be utilized. Noninvasive treatment is the use of cosmetics to camouflage the affected area. Treatment for cherry hemangiomas is usually not prescribed, except for cosmetic purposes.

(From Reeves J, Maibach H. Clinical Dermatology Illustrated, 2nd ed, 1998. Reproduced with permission: MacLennan & Petty, Sydney.)

Malignant melanoma, as the name implies, is a malignant growth of pigment cells (melanocytes). It is highly metastatic, with a higher mortality rate than basal or squamous cell carcinoma. This tumor can occur anywhere on the body, especially where there are moles. There are three general types: lentigo maligna, superficial spreading, and nodular.

Lentigo maligna melanoma (Fig. 51–27) appears as a slow-growing dark macule on exposed skin surfaces (especially the face) of elderly clients. The lesion has irregular borders and brown, tan, and black coloring. Prognosis is good if treated in the early stage.

Superficial spreading melanoma (Fig. 51–28) is the most common melanoma. It can occur anywhere on the body, usually to middle-aged clients. The lesion appears as a slightly elevated plaque with an irregular border. The coloring of the lesion varies in combinations of black, brown, and pink. The fragile surface may bleed or ooze. Eventually the plaque develops into a nodule. The cure rate is excellent when it is in the plaque phase; prognosis is poor with the nodular phase.

CULTURAL CONSIDERATIONS
BOX 51–4

Some African-American men have facial hair that is kinky, curls back on itself, and penetrates the skin, which can result in pustules and small keloids. Many use depilatories or electric razors to prevent nicking the skin, which can also cause keloids.

Darker-skinned people have an increased incidence of birth marks and mongolian spots compared with lighter-skinned people. Mongolian spots disappear over time. The nurse must be cautious and not mistake these spots for bruising indicating injury or abuse.

Darker-skinned people have a tendency toward an overgrowth of connective tissue components concerned with the protection against infection and repair after injury. Keloid formation is one example of this tendency toward overgrowth of connective tissue. Lymphoma and systemic lupus erythematosus may occur due to this overgrowth of connective tissue.

For people with light skin such as Germans, Polish, and Irish, prolonged exposure to the sun may increase the incidence of skin cancer. The nurse needs to teach clients to protect themselves from sun exposure to reduce their risk of skin cancer. Nevi (freckles and skin discolorations) occur more often in lighter-skinned individuals. They are most common in European-Americans, followed by Asians, and then darker skinned African-Americans.

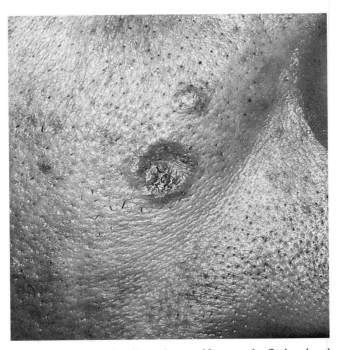

Figure 51–24. Basal cell carcinoma. Note pearly flesh-colored papule with depressed center and rolled edge. (From Reeves J, Maibach H. Clinical Dermatology Illustrated, 2nd ed, 1998. Reproduced with permission: MacLennan & Petty, Sydney.) See Plate 30.

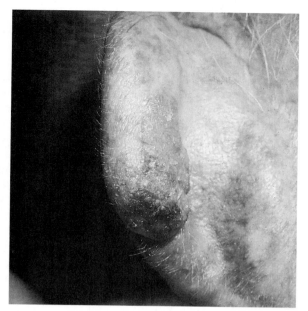

Figure 51–25. Squamous cell carcinoma. Surface is fragile and bleeds easily. (From Reeves J, Maibach H. Clinical Dermatology Illustrated, 2nd ed, 1998. Reproduced with permission: MacLennan & Petty, Sydney.) See Plate 31.

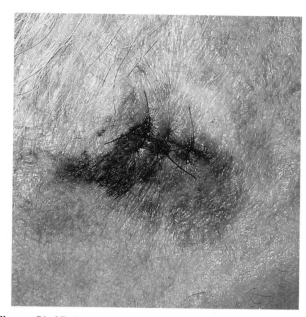

Figure 51–27. Lentigo maligna. (From Reeves J, Maibach H. Clinical Dermatology Illustrated, 2nd ed, 1998. Reproduced with permission: MacLennan & Petty, Sydney.) See Plate 31.

Nodular melanoma (Fig. 51–29) occurs suddenly as a spherical papule or nodule on the skin or in a mole. Coloration in blue-black, blue-gray, or reddish-blue color that may have a rim of inflammation. The lesion is fragile and bleeds easily. Metastasis occurs rapidly. This type of melanoma has the least favorable prognosis. Early treatment is imperative.

Prevention

Most types of skin cancer can be prevented by limiting or avoiding direct exposure to ultraviolet rays (sun, tanning booths). If exposure to the sun is necessary, exposure should be avoided during its highest intensity (10 A.M. to 2 P.M.). The client should use a protective sunscreen, with sun protection factor (SPF) of 15 or more. The client should also wear sun-protective clothing, such as hats and

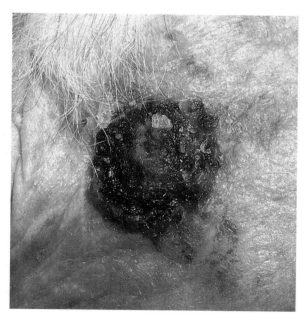

Figure 51–26. Squamous cell carcinoma that has been neglected. (From Reeves J, Maibach H. Clinical Dermatology Illustrated, 2nd ed, 1998. Reproduced with permission: MacLennan & Petty, Sydney.) See Plate 31.

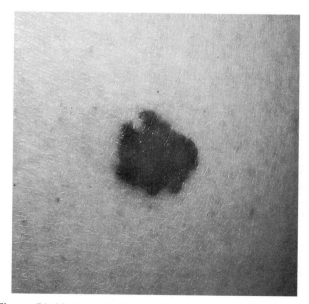

Figure 51–28. Superficial spreading melanoma. Note irregular border and variegated pigment. (From Reeves J, Maibach H. Clinical Dermatology Illustrated, 2nd ed, 1998. Reproduced with permission: MacLennan & Petty, Sydney.) See Plate 32.

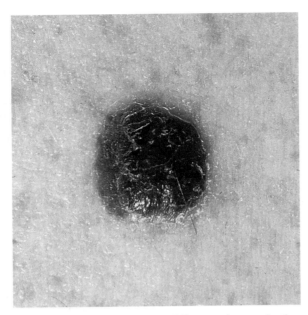

Figure 51–29. Nodular melanoma. Microscopic examination revealed that it arose from a mole. (From Reeves J, Maibach H. Clinical Dermatology Illustrated, 2nd ed, 1998. Reproduced with permission: MacLennan & Petty, Sydney.) See Plate 32.

long sleeves. The client should seek medical advice if there is a change in color, shape, sensation, or character of a lesion or mole.

Diagnostic Tests

A preliminary diagnosis can be based on the appearance of the lesion. A definite diagnosis is made by biopsy. Other tests are performed based on the results of the pathological examination.

Medical Treatment

Medical treatment depends on the type, thickness, and location of the lesion, the stage of the disease, and the age and general health of the client. Generally, lesions are excised with a 1 to 2 cm margin. Regional node dissection varies; it may be advised if the nodes in the area drain to one group. Grafting may be necessary for closure or repair. Chemotherapy may be utilized for metastasis. Radiation therapy may be recommended for elderly clients with a deeply invasive tumor or those who are poor surgical risks. Other therapies that also may be used include cryosurgery and curettage and electrodesiccation.

Nursing Care

The nurse performs a complete skin assessment. Lesions are palpated to determine texture. All lesions should be described as to size, location, color, surface characteristics, pain, discomfort, itching, and bleeding.

Nursing care of the client with cancer is documented in Chapter 10. Specific nursing care related to cryosurgrey includes preparing the client for the procedure: Minor discomfort can be expected with little or no local anesthesia, swelling, local tenderness, and hemorrhagic blister formation 1 to 2 days after the procedure. After the procedure, the area is cleansed as ordered and prescribed ointments are applied. Specific nursing care for curettage and electrodesiccation include preparing the client for the procedure: After local anesthesia, a dermal curette is used to scrape away the lesion followed by electrodesiccation of the remaining wound; the wound heals by secondary intention, usually with minimal scarring; and after the procedure the wound is cleansed and dressed as prescribed.

Dermatological Surgery

Plastic or reconstructive surgery is performed to correct certain defects, scars, and malformations, as well as restore function or prevent further loss of function. This type of surgery is usually an elective procedure; it may be prescribed by the physician or it may be the wish of the client in hopes of improving his or her body image. Common types of plastic surgical procedures are listed in Table 51–11.

HOME HEALTH HINTS

- A wound-measuring device that will not be misplaced is your hand. Measure your hand, such as the nailbed of the particular finger or a joint of a finger. Use these as a guide to determine wound measurements.
- Sanitary pads make great cushions for bony prominences. You can also place them in a cotton sock for better molding purposes.
- A handheld shower head is useful in debriding some leg ulcers. Do not use it if it is too painful.
- To relieve itchy skin (pruritis), oatmeal baths are sometimes prescribed. An inexpensive way to do this is to place a half cup of quick-cooking oatmeal in a cotton sock. Put is under the faucet as you fill the tub and ring out the sock.
- Instruct clients to prevent red, dried, cracked skin on hands by doing the following: wear gloves outside in the cold or windy weather to prevent chapping; avoid overheating the house; use a humidifier to keep the air moist; apply hand lotion two or three times a day and after each hand washing; use soaps with added oil and avoid those with deodorants; use sunscreen of at least SPF 15; and stop smoking (smoking reduces blood flow to the skin).

Table 51-11. **Common Plastic Surgical Procedures**

Operation	Description	Purpose	Possible Complications	Postoperative Nursing Treatment Considerations
Rhinoplasty (nose)	Removal of excessive nasal cartilage, tissue, or bone; reshaping of nose.	Correct congenital or acquired septal defects; improve cosmetic shape of nose.	Hemorrhage, hematoma; temporary ecchymosis and edema; infection, septal perforation.	Monitor dressing and packings for bright-red bleeding; monitor vital signs and level of consciousness; maintain semi-Fowler's position to minimize edema.
Blepharoplasty (eyelid)	Incisions on upper and lower lids with excision of fat and skin and primary closure.	Removal of bags under eyes and wrinkles and bulges.	Corneal injury; hematoma; ectropion; rarely visual loss and wound infection.	Eye dressings; antibiotic ointment around eyes and lids; discoloration and swelling usually subsides in about 10 days; maintain semi-Fowler's position to minimize edema.
Rhytidoplasty (face-lift)	Incision anterior to ear with removal of excessive skin and tissue; the subcutaneous tissue and fascia are folded and stretched.	Removal of excessive wrinkling or sagging skin.	Hemorrhage; hematoma, ecchymosis, and edema (temporary); wound infection, facial nerve damage.	Surgical improvement lasts from 5–10 years; antibiotic ointment to suture line; maintain semi-Fowler's position to minimize edema.
Otoplasty (ear)	Incision of ear for correction of defect.	Correct congenital defects; correct deformities; improve cosmetic shape of ear.	Hemorrhage; hematoma; edema; wound infection.	Ear dressing for about 1 week; protect ear at times of sleep for about 3 weeks.
Breast augmentation	Skin incision to insert breast implant.	Improve cosmetic shape and size of breasts.	Hemorrhage; hematoma, wound infection.	Dressing to site; antibiotic ointment to suture line. Drains may by in place—note color and amount of drainage.
Breast reduction	Skin incision to excise excess breast tissue and skin.	Improve cosmetic shape and size of breasts; comfort measure.	Hemorrhage; hematoma, wound infection; wound dehiscence; necrosis of areola and nipple area.	Dressing to site; antibiotic ointment to suture line. Drains may be in place—note color and amount of drainage.

Review Questions

1. Mechanical forces that can lead to formation of a pressure ulcer include:
   a. Pressure
   b. Friction
   c. Shear
   d. All of the above

2. Which of the following actions by the nurse is appropriate when caring for the client with dermatitis?
   a. Bathe in hot oatmeal baths
   b. Dry vigorously to prevent moisture buildup
   c. Apply gloves to hands at night
   d. Apply a thick layer of prescribed topical agent

3. Psoriasis is an inflammatory skin disorder that is characterized by which underlying condition?
   a. Epidermal proliferation
   b. Excessive subcutaneous fat
   c. A herpes infection
   d. Excessive melanin production

4. Which of the following is appropriate instruction for the parent of a child with impetigo contagiosa, to help prevent spread of infection? Send back to school:
   a. One week after treatment is started.
   b. After the lesions scab.
   c. When all lesions are healed.
   d. After spread of lesions has stopped.

5. In general, which of the following actions is most important in preventing infectious skin disorders?
   a. Use of isolation precautions
   b. Careful hand washing

c. Use of antibacterial soap

d. Sterilizing all contaminated objects.

6. Which of the following is appropriate patient education about treating scabies?

a. Dry-clean all linens, towels, clothes

b. Throw away infested mattresses

c. Wash linens, towels, clothes

d. Remove infested pets

7. Jan Smith, 42 years old, is admitted to the emergency department with flame burns to her entire chest, back, and upper extremities. Using the rule of nines you would estimate the percentage of burns to be:

a. 36%

b. 45%

c. 54%

d. 64%

8. Which of the following actions is appropriate initial treatment of a chemical burn?

a. Neutralize the chemical

b. Lavage with water

c. Apply the prescribed topical agent

d. Wrap the client in sterile sheets

9. Which of the following is the most common cause of malignant skin lesions?

a. Overexposure to ultraviolet rays

b. Genetic predisposition

c. Fair skin, blue eyes, red hair

d. Numerous moles on body

ANSWERS TO CRITICAL THINKING

CRITICAL THINKING: Mrs. Long

The nurse should ask Mrs. Long if she read the package instructions. She would find that for medicated scalp shampoos to work properly, they must remain on the scalp for several minutes. Package instruction should be carefully checked for each product, because they vary from product to product.

BIBLIOGRAPHY

Arnold, H, Odum, R, and James, W: Diseases of the Skin: Clinical Dermatology, ed 2. WB Saunders, Philadelphia, 1990.

Arturson, MG: The pathophysiology of severe thermal injury. J Burn Care Rehabil 6:129, 1985.

Barkauskas, V, et al: Health and Physical Assessment. Mosby, St Louis, 1994.

Bergstrom, N, Bennett, MA, Carlson, CE, et al: Treatment of Pressure Ulcers. Clinical Practice Guideline, No. 15. AHCPR Publication No. 95-0652. US Department of Health and Human Services, Public Health Service, Agency for Health Care Policy and Research, Rockville, Md, December 1994.

Bohon, L, and Rijswijk, L: Wound dressings: Meeting clinical and biological needs. Dermatol Nurs 3(3):146, 1991.

Cuzzell, JZ: Choosing a wound dressing: A systematic approach. AACN Clin Issues Crit Care Nus 1(3):566, 1990.

De Witt, S: Nursing assessment of the skin and dermatologic lesions. Nurs Clin North Am 25(1):235, 1990.

Doctor, JN, et al: Health outcome for burn survivors. J Burn Care Rehabil 18:490, 1997.

Grizzard, D: Understanding of the pathophysiology of psoriasis: A nursing perspective. Dermatol Nurs 3(5):305, 1991.

Hansbourgh, JF: The promises of excisional therapy of burn wounds: Have they been achieved? J Intensive Care Med 9:1, 1994.

Krasner, D: Resolving the dressing dilemma: Selecting wound dressings by category. Ostomy Wound Manage 35:62, 1991.

Lawrence, JC: Dressings and wound infection. Am J Surg 167:215, 1994.

Lazarus, GS, et al: Definitions and guidelines for assessment of wounds and evaluation of healing. Arch Dermatol 130:489, 1994.

Lookingbill, DB, and Marks, JG, Jr: Principles of Dermatology, ed 2. WB Saunders, Philadelphia, 1993.

Murray, M, and Blaylock, B: Maintaining effective pressure ulcer prevention programs. Medsurg Nurs 3(2):85, 1994.

Nicol, N: Current considerations and management of atopic dermatitis. Dermatol Nurs 2(3):129, 1990.

Polednak, A: Connective tissue responses in Negroes in relation to disease. Am J Phys Anthropol 41:49, 1974.

Porth, CM: Pathophysiology: Concepts of Altered Health States. JB Lippincott, Philadelphia, 1994.

Reeves, JR, and Maibach, H: Clinical Dermatology Illustrated, ed 3. FA Davis, Philadelphia, 1998.

Rudy, S: Skin cancer incidence and risk. Dermatol Nurs 2(3):129, 1990.

Ruppert, SD, et al: Dolan's Critical Care Nursing, ed 2. FA Davis, Philadelphia, 1998.

Somma, S, and Glassman, D: Malignant melanoma. Dermatol Nurs 3(2):93, 1991.

Trofino, RBT: Nursing Care of the Burn-Injured Patient. FA Davis, Philadelphia, 1991.

Vargo, N: Basal and squamous cell carcinomas: An overview. Semin Oncol Nurs 7(1):13, 1991.

Understanding the Immune System

52

Immune System Function, Assessment, and Therapeutic Measures

Sharon M. Nowak and Valerie C. Scanlon

Learning Objectives

Upon completion of this chapter, the student will be able to:

1. Define immunity.
2. Define antigens and describe their function.
3. Describe what role lymphocytes have in the immune system.
4. Explain the difference between T cells and B cells.
5. Explain how antibodies function in an immune response.
6. Describe cell-mediated immunity.
7. Describe humoral immunity.
8. Describe an antibody response.
9. Differentiate between the various types of immunity.
10. List two effects that aging has on the immune system.
11. Explain how past surgeries may affect current immune system function.
12. Explain how past or current medications may affect immune system function.
13. State the purpose of biopsies.
14. List three structures that may be biopsied related to the immune system.
15. Identify screening blood tests for the immune system and state their importance.
16. Identify the common specific blood tests used for immune system dysfunction and state their importance.

Key Words

active immunity (**AK**-tiv im-**YOO**-ni-tee)
anaphylactic (AN-uh-fi-**LAK**-tik)
antibody (**AN**-ti-bod-ee)
antigen (**AN**-ti-jen)
cell-mediated immunity (SELL **ME**-dee-ay-ted im-**YOO**-ni-tee)
humoral immunity (**HYOO**-mohr-uhl im-**YOO**-ni-tee)
lymphocyte (**LIM**-foh-site)
neutrophil (**NEW**-troh-fil)
passive immunity (**PASS**-iv im-**YOO**-ni-tee)
white blood cells (WIGHT BLUHD SELLS)

Normal Immune Anatomy and Physiology

Immunity may be defined as the ability to destroy pathogens or other foreign material and to prevent further cases of certain infectious diseases. When we think of immunity we most often think of microorganisms such as bacteria, viruses, and fungi, and these are indeed foreign to the body. Malignant cells, however, are also foreign in that they have mutated from the normal state, and they too are usually destroyed before they can establish themselves as cancer. Transplanted organs are unfortunately also perceived as foreign, and rejection of a transplanted organ is an immune response. Occasionally the immune system mistakenly reacts to part of the body itself; this is an autoimmune disease.

The immune system consists of lymphoid organs, **lymphocytes** and other **white blood cells,** and many chemicals they produce that are involved in activation of our own cells for the destruction of foreign **antigens** (Fig. 52–1).

ANTIGENS

Antigens are chemical markers that identify cells or molecules. The antigens of pathogens or foreign tissue are recognized as foreign and may be destroyed in one of several ways. Antigens that are not cellular include bacterial toxins, plant pollens or proteins that trigger allergies, and the protein products of viral activity within cells. Human cells (except red blood cells [RBCs]) have their own "self" antigens, thousands of markers that identify the cell as belonging in the body. These are the major histocompatibility complex (MHC) antigens, also called human leukocyte antigens (HLAs), and are genetically determined. The MHC antigens of identical twins will be identical. These MHC antigens serve as a comparison for cells of the immune system; foreign antigens will not "match" them and may therefore be recognized as foreign and destroyed.

LYMPHOCYTES

There are three types of lymphocytes: natural killer (NK) cells, T cells, and B cells, each with very different functions.

Natural Killer Cells

Natural killer cells are found in the blood, bone marrow, lymph nodes, and spleen and are able to destroy many kinds of pathogens and tumor cells. How NK cells recognize foreign antigens is not known with certainty, but they may respond to the absence of MHC antigens on foreign cells. It is believed that NK cells destroy foreign cells by rupturing their membranes or by some other form of direct contact. The action of NK cells is considered a nonspecific resistance mechanism because it is effective against a great variety of foreign antigens.

T Cells and B Cells

The lymphocytes called T cells and B cells are involved in specific immune responses; that is, each cell is genetically programmed to respond to one kind of foreign antigen. It is estimated that the human immune system can respond to hundreds of millions of different foreign antigens.

In the fetus, both T cells and B cells develop in the bone marrow. T cells then migrate to the thymus, where the thymic hormones bring about their maturation. From the thymus, T cells migrate to the lymph nodes and nodules throughout the body and to the spleen. B cells mature in the bone marrow and migrate directly to lymphatic tissue. When activated during an immune response, some B cells will become plasma cells that produce antibodies to a specific foreign antigen.

ANTIBODIES

Antibodies may also be called immunoglobulins (Ig) or gamma globulins and are proteins produced by plasma cells

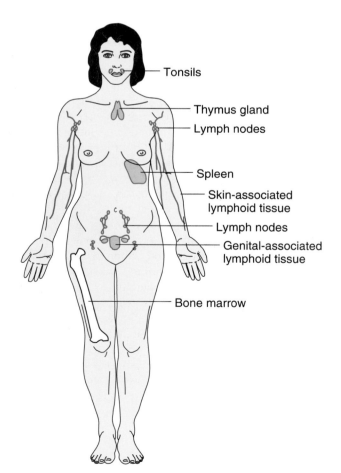

- Tonsils
- Thymus gland
- Lymph nodes
- Spleen
- Skin-associated lymphoid tissue
- Lymph nodes
- Genital-associated lymphoid tissue
- Bone marrow

Figure 52–1. Immune system organs.

lymphocytes: lympha—lymph + kytos—cell
antigens: anti—against + gennan—to produce

Table 52–1. **Classes of Antibodies**

Name	Location	Function
IgG	Blood, extracellular fluid	Crosses the placenta to provide passive immunity for newborns
IgA	External secretions: tears, saliva, etc.	Provides long-term immunity following a vaccine or illness recovery
		Provides passive immunity for breast-fed infants
IgM	Blood	Found in secretions of all mucous membranes
		Produced first by the maturing immune system of the infant
IgD	B cells	Produced first during an infection (IgG production follows)
IgE	Mast cells or basophils	Are antigen-specific receptors on B lymphocytes
		Important in allergic reactions; mast cells release histamine

in response to foreign antigens. Antibodies do not themselves destroy foreign antigens, but rather become attached to such antigens to "label" them for destruction. Each **antibody** is specific for only one antigen, and the B cells (to become plasma cells) of an individual are capable of producing millions of different antibodies. There are five classes of human antibodies, designated by letter names: IgG, IgM, IgA, IgE, and IgD. Their functions are summarized in Table 52–1.

MECHANISMS OF IMMUNITY

The two mechanisms of **immunity** are **cell-mediated immunity,** which involves T cells, and **humoral immunity,** which involves both T cells and B cells. Although the mechanisms are different, invasion by a pathogen often triggers both.

The first step in the destruction of a foreign antigen is the recognition of it as foreign. B cells in lymphatic tissue are able to recognize the foreign antigens for which they are genetically programmed and become activated B cells. Their activation is greatly enhanced if the foreign antigen is presented to them by antigen-processing cells called dendritic cells. T cells called helper T cells (CD4) also recognize the foreign antigen and provide a further stimulation to B cells, causing them to divide (proliferate) and become more specialized (differentiate). Helper T cells are assisted in their recognition of foreign antigens by macrophages or other antigen-processing cells, which present the foreign antigen as well as their own MHC antigens to the T cell, providing a comparison. The macrophages also provide chemical stimulation to the T cells, which then begin to divide and become more specialized.

Cell-Mediated Immunity

This mechanism of immunity does not involve the production of antibodies, but it is effective against intracellular pathogens (such as viruses), fungi, malignant cells, and grafts of foreign tissue. The first step is the recognition of the foreign antigen by helper T cells, assisted by macrophages. The activated T cells divide many times and become specialized in one of several ways.

Cytotoxic, or killer, T cells (CD8) are able to lyse cells such as cancer cells or those infected by viruses or other intracellular parasites. They also release chemicals that activate phagocytes such as macrophages and **neutrophils.**

Memory T cells will remember the specific foreign antigen and very quickly activate an immune response should it reappear. Suppressor T cells are believed to inhibit the proliferation of both T cells and B cells, which limits the immune response to just what is needed and no more.

Humoral Immunity

Humoral immunity may also be called antibody-mediated immunity, and does indeed involve antibody production. Again the first step is the recognition of the antigen as foreign, this time by B cells. Helper T cells that recognize the antigen further stimulate the B cells to proliferate and differentiate. Some B cells will become plasma cells that produce antibodies specific for this particular antigen. Other B cells will become memory B cells that will remember this antigen and initiate a very rapid response should it return.

Although B cells are stationary, the antibodies produced by plasma cells circulate throughout the body. The antibodies bond to the antigen, forming an antigen-antibody complex. This is termed *opsonization,* which means that the antigen is now "labeled" for phagocytosis by macrophages or neutrophils. The antigen-antibody complex also stimulates the process of complement fixation.

Complement is a group of about 20 plasma proteins that circulate in the blood until activated by an antigen-antibody complex. The activation of complement may result in the formation of an enzyme complex that punches a hole in a cellular antigen to bring about its death. Other complement proteins bind to foreign antigens and serve as further "labels" to attract macrophages.

Antibody Responses

The first exposure to a foreign antigen stimulates antibody production, but the antibodies are produced so slowly and

---

immunity: immunis—safe

neutrophils: neuter—neither + philein—to love

Primary and secondary antibody responses

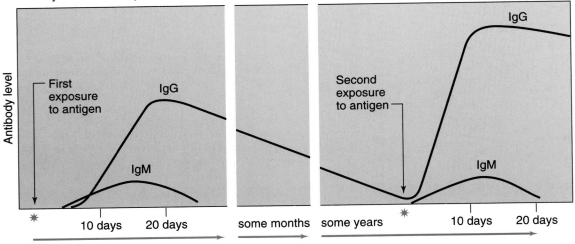

Figure 52–2. Antibody responses to a first and then subsequent exposure to a pathogen. (From Scanlon, V, and Sanders, T: Understanding Human Structure and Function. FA Davis, Philadelphia, 1997, p 258, with permission.)

in such small amounts that this production may be too late to prevent the disease. With recovery from the disease, however, the person has antibodies and memory cells that are specific for that pathogen. On a second exposure, the memory cells initiate rapid production of large amounts of antibody, often enough to prevent a second case of the illness (Fig. 52–2). This is the basis for the protection given by vaccines. A vaccine contains an antigen that is not pathogenic (e.g., bacterial capsules in the case of the pneumococcal vaccine). The vaccine stimulates the formation of antibodies and memory cells.

Antibodies may also neutralize viruses, that is, attach to a virus and render it unable to enter a cell. Outside living cells, viruses cannot reproduce, and those coated with antibodies will be phagocytized by macrophages. Another aspect of our defenses against viruses is interferon, a chemical produced by cells infected with viruses. Although it does not help the infected cell, interferon protects surrounding cells by enabling them to resist viral reproduction by limiting or slowing growth of the virus.

Antibodies are also involved in allergies, in which the immune system responds to an antigen that is actually harmless, such as plant pollen. IgE antibodies bond to mast cells, which break down and release histamine and other chemicals that contribute to inflammation. **Anaphylactic shock** is a massive allergic reaction characterized by loss of plasma from capillaries (an effect of histamine) and a sudden drop in intravascular blood volume and blood pressure.

Types of Immunity

Two categories of immunity are **passive immunity** and **active immunity.** In passive immunity, antibodies are not

produced by the individual, but are obtained from another source. Naturally acquired passive immunity includes placental transmission of antibodies from mother to fetus and transmission of antibodies in breast milk. Artificially acquired passive immunity involves injection of preformed antibodies; this may help prevent disease after exposure to a pathogen such as the hepatitis A virus. Passive immunity is always temporary, in that antibodies from another source eventually break down.

Active immunity means that the individual produces his or her own antibodies. Naturally acquired active immunity means that a person has recovered from a disease and now has antibodies and memory cells specific for that pathogen. Artificially acquired active immunity is the result of a vaccine that has stimulated production of antibodies and memory cells. The duration of active immunity depends on the particular disease or vaccine; some confer lifelong immunity, but others do not.

Aging and the Immune System

The efficiency of the immune system decreases with age. Elderly people are more susceptible to infections, especially secondary infections such as developing pneumonia following the flu (Gerontological Issues Box 52–1). Autoimmune disorders are also more common among older people; the immune system mistakenly perceives the

anaphylactic: ana—up + phylaxis—protection

body's own tissues as foreign and initiates their destruction. The incidence of cancer is also higher; malignant cells that might once have been quickly destroyed by the immune system remain alive and proliferate.

Immune System Assessment

NURSING ASSESSMENT

A thorough assessment of the immunologically compromised client is the first step in the nursing process. It gives substance to the nursing care plan, which guides nursing practice. Because disorders of the immune system can affect every system in the body, it is vitally important that a thorough head-to-toe assessment and history is performed.

Subjective Data

Demographic Data

The client's age, gender, race, and ethnic background data are important because some disease processes tend to be associated with a particular gender, race, or age-group. For instance, systemic lupus erythematosus (SLE) tends to affect women eight times more frequently than men. Inquiring about the client's place of birth may give insight to ethnic ties that are not initially evident in the interview. Also locations where the client lives and has lived may shed light on the client's current problem.

History

Inquiry into medication, food, and environmental allergies such as dust, pollen, and insects should include the client's allergies, as well as those that are present in the family history. Many times if there is a family history of a severe reaction (anaphylaxis) to penicillin, a physician does not order penicillin for the client. There may be a familial tendency to react negatively to penicillin or other substances,

so a previous exposure resulting in sensitization to a substance may not be necessary before a severe reaction occurs. Some reactions can be fatal within minutes without immediate medical treatment.

As with allergies, inquiring about past and present medical conditions or disease processes should also include a family history, as well as the client's history. Numerous conditions, such as allergic rhinitis, SLE, ankylosing spondylitis, multiple sclerosis, myasthenia gravis, diabetes mellitus, and asthma, are thought to be either familial or have a genetic predisposition in certain races or cultures (Cultural Considerations Box 52–2).

The client's previous surgeries may play an important bearing on the client's current condition. If the client has had his or her thymus gland removed (thymectomy), T cell production may be altered, which affects the cell-mediated immune response. If the client has had his or her spleen removed (splenectomy), lymphocyte and plasma cell production may be altered, which affects humoral immune response.

Further questioning about previous blood transfusions, radiation exposure (therapeutic or accidental), and current medications (prescription and over-the-counter drugs) provides further data that may be associated with the current problem. For example, corticosteroids and immunosuppressants alter the immune response. Other medications such as some anti-infectives or antineoplastics depress the bone marrow, resulting in decreased production of the cells made in the bone marrow. Bone marrow depression of white blood cells can alter cell-mediated and humoral immune responses.

A client's lifestyle may influence immune system function and should be assessed. Are there exposures to caustic chemicals or fumes at work? If so, they may lead to systemic or topical immune reactions or bone marrow depression. Is the client exposed to or allergic to latex? Anaphylactic reactions can be caused by exposure to latex, which is found in gloves and other medical products that health care workers and their clients touch. The nurse should be aware of this potentially life-threatening reaction and know the agency's latex allergy protocol. These clients should wear a Medic Alert bracelet and carry an anaphylactic epinephrine kit. Does the client use illicit drugs or have multiple sexual partners or partners of the same gender? These behaviors place the client at risk for contracting the human immunodeficiency virus (HIV). Does the client eat a balanced diet or use vitamins? Knowing the client's diet habits and supplemental vitamins gives insight into the potential reserve of the immune system for fighting infection.

The client's life stressors, coping behaviors, and support systems are explored. Stress (environmental, physical, and psychological) can depress the immune system's function. Coping behaviors are essential in keeping stress within manageable limits to maintain an optimal functioning immune system. Support systems play an important role in coping with stress and should be encouraged and nurtured by nurses.

Current Problem

Use the WHAT'S UP format to collect data about the current immune system problem. For immune disorders, the client is asked the following questions:

- **W**here is it? What part of the body is affected?
- **H**ow does it feel? Painful? No pain?
- **A**ggravating and alleviating factors?
- **T**iming. Was there exposure to a pathogen? Did you have a previous infection? Did you have chemotherapy or radiation therapy? Length of time symptoms have persisted?
- **S**everity. Does it affect activities of daily living (ADL)? Work? Roles?
- **U**seful data for associated symptoms. Immunosuppression? Family history? Allergies?
- **P**erception of the client of the problem. What do you think is wrong?

When investigating the client's current problem the following are examples of common signs and symptoms that may be found with immune disorders: fever, fatigue, joint pain, swollen glands, weight loss, and skin rash.

CRITICAL THINKING: Laura

Laura is scheduled for a lymph node biopsy and is seen in preadmission testing before surgery. As the LPN/LVN prepares to draw blood specimens, he learns that Laura is allergic to latex.

1. Why is this client information important?
2. What should the LPN/LVN do next?

3. What precautions should the LPN/LVN use to draw the blood specimen?

Answers at end of chapter.

Objective Data

Physical Assessment

The physical assessment begins by observing the client's general appearance and expressions. The nurse observes for generalized edema, color, posture, gait, facial expressions, or lack of expression. While talking with the client, alertness and orientation to person, place, and time are assessed. Clients with various immune disorders, such as SLE or acquired immunodeficiency syndrome (AIDS), may exhibit mentation changes, especially in advanced stages.

A client may be febrile and have no other signs or symptoms of infection such as redness, pain, swelling, and warmth when the immune system is compromised. This may be the first and only sign that a problem exists and should be promptly reported. An elevation in respirations and pulse may accompany this febrile state. The client may be hypertensive or hypotensive, depending on the affected organ and stage of the disease process.

LEARNING TIP

A normally functioning immune system is required to trigger an inflammatory response that produces the signs of inflammation or infection: fever, redness, pain, swelling, and warmth. If the immune system is suppressed or functioning abnormally, this normal inflammatory response may not occur. Thus the client may exhibit only a low-grade fever with none of the other signs of inflammation or infection: redness, pain, swelling, and warmth.

The nurse must recognize clients with suppressed immune systems so that low-grade fevers are reported to the physician for prompt treatment. This may be the only sign of a life-threatening infection that is developing. The infection can become life threatening due to the suppressed immune system, which may not be able to fight it off.

The client's skin, bone joints, and nailbeds should be carefully examined. Any cyanosis or erythema (redness) is noted. Rashes need to be examined for size, shape, location, texture, drainage, and pruritis (itching). Painless, small purple lesions are Kaposi's sarcoma (Fig. 52–3). This sarcoma is frequently associated with AIDS. Bone joints, especially of the hands, should be inspected for swollen, painful nodules that are associated with rheuma-

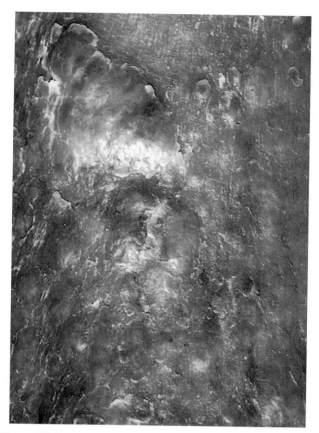

Figure 52–3. Kaposi's sarcoma of the skin. (From Wells, J: Clinical Immunology Illustrated. Adis International, Philadelphia, 1986, p 96, with permission.)

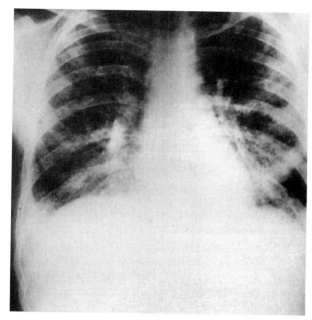

Figure 52–4. *Pneumocystis carinii* pneumonia. (From Wells, J: Clinical Immunology Illustrated. Adis International, Philadelphia, 1986, p 96, with permission.)

toid arthritis. Any swelling, tenderness, or limited range of motion in them is noted. Nails are assessed. If they separate from the nail bed, it is called onycholysis and can be associated with thyroiditis.

Vision and hearing changes can be associated with an immunological disorder. Eye movements are assessed by using the six cardinal positions test for muscle weakness (see Chapter 48). The conjunctiva should be deep pink and moist. If the client is anemic, it is pale. Edema around the eyes (periorbital edema) may indicate hypothyroidism or renal disease. Darkened areas under the eyes are called shiners and are common in clients experiencing allergic rhinitis.

Adventitious lung sounds, such as wheezing, may indicate asthma or an allergic response. Crackles are frequently associated with an upper respiratory infection. Crackles heard with a dry cough and labored tachypnea are a sign of *Pneumocystis carinii* pneumonia, a common opportunistic lung infection of clients afflicted with AIDS (Fig. 52–4). A pleural or pericardial friction rub may be a sign of rheumatoid arthritis or SLE.

Lymph nodes should be inspected and then gently palpated (Fig. 52–5). Normally, lymph nodes are not palpable. If on palpation a lymph node is enlarged, the following characteristics need to be noted: location, size, shape, tenderness, temperature, consistency, mobility, symmetry, and any pulsation. Generally, when lymph nodes are tender and enlarged, there is inflammation present. Nodes that are nontender, hard, fixed, and enlarged are frequently associated with cancer.

The spleen may be enlarged and palpable in the left upper quadrant of the abdomen with disorders in which there is an overproduction or excessive destruction of red blood cells. The advanced practitioner usually palpates the spleen.

Gastrointestinal signs and symptoms such as nausea, vomiting, and diarrhea are noted. They may also have an immunological disorder basis. The renal system may also show impairment due to an immunological disorder. This may be exhibited through a change in urinary output, flank pain, edema, weight gain, or elevated renal function studies.

A general neurological assessment of muscle strength and coordination, changes, or abnormalities is noted. Changes may be an indication of an immunologically based disorder such as multiple sclerosis or myasthenia gravis.

DIAGNOSTIC TESTS

Blood Tests

Initially, screening tests are performed. Table 52–2 describes the most common screening blood tests for clients with allergic, autoimmune, or immune disorders. If the screening tests detect an abnormality, further specific tests may be ordered to precisely identify the disorders. Table

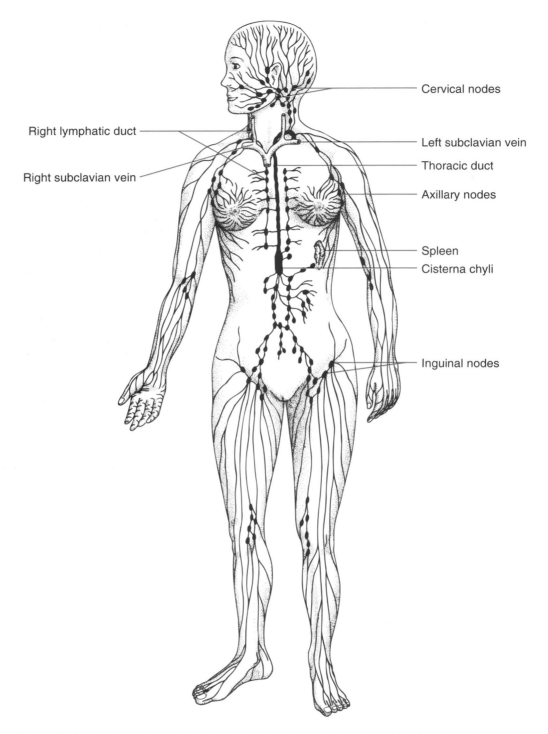

Figure 52–5. Lymph vessels and major lymph nodes. (From Scanlon, V, and Sanders, T: Understanding Human Structure and Function. FA Davis, Philadelphia, 1997, p 250, with permission.)

52–3 examines the more common of these specific immune tests.

Radiographic Tests

A routine chest x-ray may be performed to examine the lung fields and the thymus gland, which lies behind the sternum. Magnetic resonance imaging (MRI) or computed tomography (CT) may also be performed to identify size and density of structures, as well as new abnormal growths.

Biopsies

Biopsies of organs or structures possibly affected by an immune disorder aid in confirming a diagnosis, determining a

Table 52–2. **Common Screening Tests for Allergic, Immune, and Autoimmune Disorders**

Test	Explanation of Normal Values	Explanation of Abnormal Values
Red Blood Cell Count	Number of red blood cells per mm of blood	Decreased in anemias, multiple myeloma; may be low in rheumatoid arthritis
Total White Blood Cell Count (WBC)	Number of white blood cells per mm of blood	Increased in acute infection, inflammation, and leukemias Decreased in chronic infections, cancer, bone marrow failure and immunosuppression (AIDS), chronic cortisol therapy, antibiotic therapy, chemotherapy, myelosuppression
WBC Differential	Percentage of type of white blood cells in 1 mm of blood	
Neutrophils		Increased in acute bacterial infections Decreased in acute viral infections, chemotherapy, radiation therapy, aplastic anemia, and neoplastic invasion of bone marrow
Lymphocytes		Increased in leukemias, pertussis, TB, and viral infections Decreased in acute bacterial infections, AIDS
Eosinophils		Increased in allergic reactions and parasitic infestations Decreased in corticosteroid therapy, bone marrow failure, and immunosuppression
Basophils		Increased in allergic reactions Decreased in bone marrow failure and immunosuppression
Serum IgG Levels	Amount of IgG in milligrams per deciliter of blood and percentage of IgG of total immunoglobulins Normal: 70–75%	Increased in infection, AIDS, and autoimmune disorders Decreased in lymphocytic leukemia and agammaglobulinemia
Serum IgA Levels	Amount of IgA in milligrams per deciliter of blood and percentage of IgA of total immunoglobulins Normal: 10–15%	Increased in chronic infections, autoimmune disorders Decreased in immunosuppression, lymphocytic leukemias, and agammaglobulinemia
Serum IgM Levels	Amount of IgM in milligrams per deciliter of blood and percentage of IgM of total immunoglobulins Normal: 10%	Increased in autoimmune disorders, systemic lupus erythematosus Decreased in immunosuppression and chronic lymphocytic leukemia
Serum IgE Levels	Amount of IgE in milligrams per deciliter of blood and percentage of IgE of total immunoglobulins Normal: 0.002%	Increased in asthma and allergic conditions Decreased in immunosuppression
Complement Assay	Measures the amount of each of the components in the complement system	Increased in thyroiditis, rheumatoid arthritis, ulcerative colitis Decreased in systemic lupus erythematosus, acute poststreptococcal glomerulonephritis, acute serum sickness, multiple myeloma, and hereditary angioedema
Sedimentation Rate	Measures the red blood cell descent (in mm) in test tube after being in normal saline for 1 hour	Increased in inflammatory, infectious, necrotic, and cancerous conditions due to the increased protein content in plasma
C-reactive Protein Test	An abnormal protein found in plasma during acute inflammatory processes; more sensitive than sedimentation rate	Increased in rheumatoid arthritis, cancer, systemic lupus erythematosus Aspirin and steroids suppress

prognosis, or evaluating a treatment. These may include lymph node biopsies, organ biopsies, or bone marrow aspirations. These procedures require a consent to be signed by the client. They may be performed as inpatient, outpatient, or physician's office procedures. The specific biopsy being performed determines any required client preparation or postprocedure care.

Skin Tests

Skin testing may be utilized to test for *Candida,* tetanus, or tuberculosis (PPD). Clients who have allergic rhinitis or drug and food allergies may also have skin testing performed to determine the specific allergen they are sensitive to. This information allows the client to either avoid the al-

Table 52–3. **Common Specific Tests Performed for Allergic, Immune, and Autoimmune Disorders**

Test	Explanation of Test	Explanation of Abnormal Values
Rheumatoid Factor (RF)	An abnormal protein found in serum when IgM reacts with an abnormal IgG; found in 80% of clients with rheumatoid arthritis, as well as other autoimmune disorders	Increased in rheumatoid arthritis, systemic lupus erythematosus, leukemia, tuberculosis, older age, scleroderma, infectious mononucleosis
Antinuclear Antibodies (ANA)	Measures antibodies that attack the cell's nuclei	Most commonly present in systemic lupus erythematosus, leukemia, scleroderma, rheumatoid arthritis, and myasthenia gravis; many medications influence these levels
Lupus Erythematosus Test (LE Prep)	Nonspecific test for lupus ANA is a more sensitive test for lupus	Increased in lupus erythematosus, rheumatoid arthritis, scleroderma; many medications influence levels
Western Blot	Tests for antibodies to HIV; technical and labor-intensive test, therefore not used as a screening test; used as a confirmation test; positives are difficult to determine	Positive when antibodies for HIV are present
Murex SUDS	Tests for antibodies to HIV-1; manual, qualitative test; visually read in 10 minutes; used as a screening test	Positive when antibodies for HIV are present
ELISA (Enzyme-Linked Immunosorbent Assay)	Tests for antibodies to HIV; inexpensive and easily performed, therefore a good screening test for HIV; high incidence of false-positive results due to the test's nonspecificity	Positive when antibodies for HIV are present, as well as numerous other viruses
p24 Antigen Testing	Tests for the formation of the p24 antigen, which occurs before the production of antibodies, therefore testing can occur during the window between infection and seroconversion (antibody production); p24 antigen is present for only a short time and is replaced with the antibodies	Positive when p24 antigen produced by HIV is present
Polymerase Chain Reaction Testing	Detects nonreplicating viral genomes; requires only 1–2 mL of blood; very costly and time consuming, therefore not a screening test	Positive when the human immunodeficiency virus is present
CD4+ T cells	Measures the actual number and percentage of CD4+ T cells in a specimen	Increased in allergy-proven clients Decreased in cancer, AIDS, and immunosuppression
CD8+ T cells	Measures the actual number and percentage of CD8+ T cells in a specimen	Increased in viral infections Decreased in systemic lupus erythematosus

lergen or have immunotherapy (allergy shots) to desensitize the immune system to the specific offending allergen.

Therapeutic Measures

ALLERGIES

A Medic Alert bracelet or some sort of readily available identification of an allergy should be worn by the client. The nurse should always be aware of client allergies. Allergies should be noted before giving any medications or foods.

If the antigen is environmental, such as bee or wasp stings, obtaining and carrying an epinephrine pen may be vital. Epinephrine is the drug of choice for an anaphylactic reaction. Time plays a crucial role when this type of reaction occurs. The client must seek immediate medical care

and begin treatment until help is available by administering the epinephrine.

An anaphylaxis kit is prescribed for clients with allergies to insect stings. The kit contains injectable epinephrine, oral chewable antihistamine tablets, a tourniquet, and instructions for use. The client must carry the kit at all times when insect stings are possible. The client is taught how to use the kit and how to give the subcutaneous epinephrine injection. The tourniquet is applied to the extremity that was stung to slow blood flow carrying the allergen to reduce its spread in the body. The tourniquet is released every 15 minutes to allow some blood flow in the extremity.

IMMUNOTHERAPY

To help desensitize a client with anaphylactic reactions to allergens, immunotherapy involves injecting small amounts of an extract of the allergen. Over time the strength of the allergen injection is increased until the desired hyposensitivity is reached. The subcutaneous injections are given once or twice a week initially, then every few weeks indefinitely for years. It is important that the client does not miss a dose. If this happens, the allergen strength may need to be reduced. This therapy is helpful for insect sting allergies.

When the nurse is administering the injection, it is important to understand that an anaphylactic reaction can occur. A physician and emergency equipment should be readily available. The client should be observed following the injection for about 20 to 30 minutes to detect a reaction. The client should be taught that a reaction could occur up to 24 hours after the injection.

MEDICATIONS

Medications are one of the primary treatment options for immune disorders. General categories of these medications include epinephrine, corticosteroids, antihistamines, histamine H_2 blockers, decongestants, mast-cell stabilizing drugs, antivirals, antibiotics, immunosuppressants, interferon, and hormone therapy. The use of these medications is discussed in Chapter 53.

SURGICAL MANAGEMENT

In some cases, splenectomy is necessary to control symptoms of an immunological disorder.

NEW THERAPIES

Monoclonal antibodies can be produced against a variety of antigens. A monoclonal antibody is made by cloning one specific antibody and then growing unlimited amounts of it in tissue cultures. Many uses are being found for these antibodies such as in dealing with transplant rejections. Further study will lead to expanding knowledge on these antibodies.

Recombinant DNA technology combines genes from one organism with genes from another organism. This therapy is used for replacing an abnormal or missing gene to produce a normal gene. The normal gene can then be injected into the client in an attempt to cure the disorder as the client's body reproduces the normal genes. T lymphocyte–directed gene transfer for severe combined immune deficiency has been performed successfully. Studies continue in this area for possible uses of gene therapy.

Review Questions

1. In the embryo, both B cell and T cells are produced in which one of the following parts of the body?
   a. Liver
   b. Thymus
   c. Bone marrow
   d. Kidney

2. A vaccine provides which one of the following types of immunity?
   a. Naturally acquired passive immunity
   b. Artificially acquired passive immunity
   c. Naturally acquired active immunity
   d. Artificially acquired active immunity

3. The immune system usually does not destroy the individual's own cells because of the presence of which one of the following cell characteristics?
   a. DNA genes in the nucleus
   b. MHC antigens on the cell membrane
   c. DNA genes on the cell membrane
   d. ABO antigens in the nucleus

4. In humoral immunity, which one of the following cells produce antibodies?
   a. T cells
   b. NK cells
   c. Plasma cells
   d. Macrophages

5. Which of the following cells are responsible for initiating a stronger and quicker response to subsequent exposures to an antigen?
   a. Memory cells
   b. Natural killer T cells
   c. Plasma cells
   d. B cells

6. Whenever a person suffers from a deficiency in the immune system, the person is at risk for which one of the following complications?
   a. Experiencing a fatal allergic reaction
   b. Suffering an overwhelming infection
   c. Death from asphyxiation
   d. Having an excessive inflammatory reaction

7. Which one of the following general client data may be useful in assessing potential immune system dysfunction?
   a. Weight
   b. Occupation
   c. Size of family
   d. Home layout

8. Which one of the following past surgeries may be useful in assessing potential immune system dysfunction?
   a. Splenectomy
   b. Thyroidectomy
   c. Pneumonectomy
   d. Parathyroidectomy

9. Lymph nodes that are enlarged and tender are usually indicative of which of the following problems?
   a. Cancer
   b. Degeneration
   c. Inflammation
   d. Arthritis

10. Which of the following is a confirmation test used to test for HIV antibodies?
    a. Murex SUDS
    b. Enzyme-linked immunosorbent assay
    c. Western blot
    d. P24 antigen testing

ANSWERS TO CRITICAL THINKING: Laura

1. The client can have an anaphylactic reaction if exposed to latex, which may result in death for some clients.
2. The LPN/LVN should follow the agency's latex allergy protocol, enter this information into the client medical record, notify surgery scheduling so latex precaution protocols can be planned for surgery, and have the client's physician informed.
3. Follow the agency's protocol, wear nonlatex gloves, and use nonlatex equipment to draw the specimens.

REFERENCE

1. Still, O, and Hodgins, D: Navajo Native Americans. In Purnell, L, and Paulanka, B (eds): Transcultrual Health Care: A Culturally Competent Approach. FA Davis, Philadelphia, 1997.

BIBLIOGRAPHY

Banov, C: Latex hypersensitivity: A worldwide crisis. J Investig Allergol Clin Immunol 7(5):322, 1997.

Evangelisto, M: Latex allergy: The downside of Standard Precautions. Todays Surg Nurse 19(5):28, 1997.

Fuchs, T, et al: Natural latex, grass pollen and weed pollen share IgE epitopes. J Allergy Clin Immunol 100(3):356, 1997.

Hammer, AL, et al: Latex allergy: Implementation of an agency program. Gastroenterol Nurs 20(5):156, 1997.

Jaffe, M, and McVan, B: Nurse's Manual of Laboratory and Diagnostic Tests. FA Davis, Philadelphia, 1997.

Lundberg, M, et al: Latex allergy from glove powder—an unintended risk with the switch from talc to cornstarch? Allergy 52(12):1222, 1997.

Onodera, M, et al: Successful peripheral T-lymphocyte-directed gene transfer for a patient with severe combined immune deficiency caused by adenosine deaminase deficiency. Blood 91(1):30, 1998.

Oppenheimer-Marks, N, et al: Interleukin 15 is produced by endothelial cells and increases the transendothelial migration of T cells in vitro and in the SCID mouse-human rheumatoid arthritis model in vivo. J Clin Invest 15:101(6):1261, 1998.

Post-White, J: The immune system. Semin Oncol Nurs 12(2):89, 1996.

Price, SA, and Wilson, LM: Pathophysiology: Clinical Concepts of Disease Processes, ed 5. Mosby, St Louis, 1997.

Reddy, S: Latex allergy. Am Fam Physician 57(1):93, 1998.

Smart, BA, et al: The molecular basis and treatment of primary immunodeficiency disorders. Curr Opin Pediatr 9(6):570, 1997.

Stevens, CD: Clinical Immunology and Serology: A Laboratory Perspective. FA Davis, Philadelphia, 1996.

Thompson, G: Ways of avoiding latex allergy. Community Nurse 3(2):33, 1997.

van Halteren, HK, et al: Discontinuation of yellow jacket venom immunotherapy: Follow-up of 75 patients by means of deliberate sting challenge. J Allergy Clin Immunol 100(6 pt 1):767, 1997.

Nursing Care of Clients with Immune Disorders

Sharon M. Nowak

Learning Objectives

Upon completion of this chapter, the student will be able to:

1. Describe the immunological mechanism for each of the four types of hypersensitivity.

2. Describe the pathophysiology, etiology, complications, diagnostic tests, medical treatment, nursing management, and education of each hypersensitivity disorder.

3. Describe the difference between urticaria and angioedema.

4. List the factors that alter or influence the self-recognition portion of the immune system.

5. Describe the pathophysiology, etiology, complications, diagnostic tests, medical treatment, nursing management, and education of each autoimmune disorder.

6. Describe the pathophysiology, etiology, and nursing management of DiGeorge's syndrome and hypogammaglobulinemia.

7. Describe the pathophysiology, etiology, complications, diagnostic tests, medical treatment, nursing management, and prevention of HIV/AIDS.

Key Words

acquired immunodeficiency syndrome (AIDS) (uh-**KWHY**-erd IM-yoo-noh-de-**FISH**-en-see **SIN**-drohm)

anaphylaxis (an-uh-fi-**LAK**-sis)

angioedema (AN-gee-o-eh-**DEE**-ma)

ankylosing spondylitis (ANG-ki-**LOH**-sing SPON-da-**LIGHT**-is)

histamine (**HISS**-ta-mean)

human immunodeficiency virus (**HYOO**-man im-YOO-noh-dee-**FISH**-en-see **VIGH**-rus)

Kaposi's sarcoma (Ka-**POE**-sees sar-**CO**-mah)

Pneumocystis carinii pneumonia (new-moh-**SIS**-tis ca-**RIN**-ee-eye new-**MOH**-nee-ah)

urticaria (UR-ti-**KAIR**-ee-ah)

Immune Disorders

Disorders of the immune system can be divided into three categories. The first is hypersensitivity reactions, which include conditions such as anaphylaxis, hemolytic transfusion reactions, measles, and transplant rejections. Autoimmune disorders (e.g., rheumatoid arthritis, ulcerative colitis, and multiple sclerosis) are the second category. The third category includes the immune deficiencies, such as hypogammaglobulinemia and acquired immunodeficiency syndrome (AIDS).

HYPERSENSITIVITY REACTIONS

The immune system usually is an adaptive or protective system of the body. However, there are times when this system causes injury to the body due to its exaggerated response. One of these occasions is when a hypersensitivity reaction occurs.

In the past these reactions were classified as either immediate or delayed hypersensitivity. Gell and Coombs have developed a more precise classification system, which is used today.[1] This four-division system classifies hypersensitivity reactions according to the way the tissue is injured.

Type I

A type I reaction is also called an anaphylactic-type reaction. It is an immediately occurring reaction when exposure to a specific antigen occurs. This reaction can be life threatening. The client must have had previous exposure (sensitization) to the antigen. During this exposure, immunoglobulin E (IgE) antibodies are made and attach to mast cells throughout the body. When a subsequent exposure occurs, the antigen causes IgE to trigger mast cells to release their contents. One of the substances released is **histamine,** which causes vasodilation, changes in vascular permeability, an increase in mucus production, and contraction of various smooth muscles.

If the second antigen exposure is localized, the reaction is small and remains local. However, if the exposure is systemic, the reaction is massive and widespread. Respiratory allergies, such as allergic rhinitis and allergic asthma, with associated disorders of atopic dermatitis, tend to be reactions of a larger scale. **Anaphylaxis, urticaria,** and **angioedema** are the severest forms of type I reactions (Fig. 53–1).

A type I reaction occurs when the client has a positive reaction to a scratch test. A scratch test is done to identify specific allergens to which a client is reactive. Tiny amounts of a variety of common allergens are scratched onto the skin, which is then observed for indications of a reaction: redness, edema, and pruritus. If these indicators occur, it is considered to be a local reaction.

Allergic Rhinitis

Allergic rhinitis is the most common form of allergy. If symptoms occur throughout the year, it is called perennial allergic rhinitis. If the symptoms occur seasonally, it is called hay fever. The causative antigens are environmental and airborne.

PATHOPHYSIOLOGY. Allergic rhinitis is the result of an antigen-antibody reaction. Ciliary action decreases and mucus secretions increase. Vasodilation and local tissue edema occur.

SIGNS AND SYMPTOMS. Signs and symptoms vary in intensity and include sneezing, nasal itching, profuse watery rhinorrhea (runny nose), and itchy red eyes. The nasal mucosa is pale, cyanotic, and edematous. Frequently there are dark circles under the eyes called allergic shiners. They are due to venous congestion in the maxillary sinuses.

COMPLICATIONS. Allergic rhinitis may be minor and self-limiting for most clients. Repeated occurrences of allergic rhinitis can lead to infection of the sinuses (sinusitis), nasal polyps, asthma, or chronic bronchitis

DIAGNOSTIC TESTS. Diagnosis is generally made from a detailed history and interview and visual inspection of the nasal passages. Sometimes, skin testing may also be performed to identify the specific offending allergens to allow avoidance of the allergen. However, it is expensive and does not always identify the allergen.

MEDICAL TREATMENT. Initial treatment involves eliminating the offending environmental stimuli. Antihistamines and nasal decongestants may be prescribed for symptomatic relief. If the symptoms are severe, corticosteroids via inhalation or nasal spray may also be given. Immunotherapy, previously referred to as allergy shots, is reserved for clients with severe or debilitating symptoms. Immunotherapy involves receiving weekly subcutaneous injections of tiny amounts of the offending antigen. Once a tolerance to a particular dose is reached, the amount of antigen is slightly increased. This therapy continues until the client no longer exhibits symptoms when exposed to the environmental antigen.

NURSING MANAGEMENT. Client and significant other education is an important nursing function. Monitoring the client's symptoms and compliance with the treatment plan is also a nursing responsibility. Skin testing and immunotherapy injections, given in the allergist's office, may also be performed by the nurse.

Education. The nurse may need to be creative in helping the client find ways to avoid the antigen. It may mean wearing a mask when mowing the lawn or working outdoors. Heating ducts may need to be cleaned and heat registers covered with filters. Frequent home vacuuming and dusting should also be recommended. The nurse needs to assess the client's knowledge of prescribed medications and their correct usage.

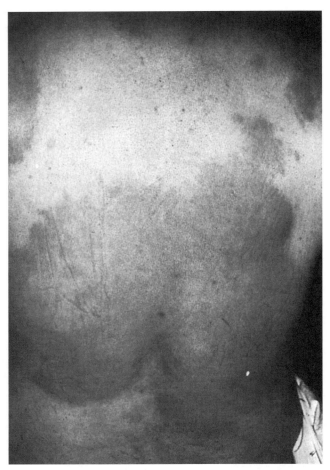

Figure 53–1. Urticaria. Large wheals in client allergic to penicillin. (From Reeves J, Maibach H. Clinical Dermatology Illustrated, 2nd ed, 1998. Reproduced with permission: MacLennan & Petty, Sydney.)

anaphylaxis: ana—up + phylaxis—protection
angioedema: angeion—vessel + oidema—swelling

Atopic Dermatitis

PATHOPHYSIOLOGY. Atopic dermatitis is an inflammatory skin response. The skin lesions are not typical for a type I hypersensitivity reaction, and there usually is not a specific antigen identified as the cause. However, it is believed that the pathophysiology of atopic dermatitis is a type I hypersensitivity reaction, mediated by IgE antibodies, because it is commonly found in clients with allergic rhinitis or allergic asthma.

SIGNS AND SYMPTOMS. Initially, there is pruritus, edema, and extremely dry skin. This is followed by eruptions of tiny blister lesions, which eventually break open, crust over, and scale off. There is decreased sweating in these areas with the skin eventually thickening in the areas of dermatitis.

COMPLICATIONS. With open skin lesions, there is always a risk for infection. Staphylococci are found on the dermal layer of the skin, so these bacteria tend to be the most frequent source of secondary infections of the affected area of skin.

DIAGNOSTIC TESTS. There are no tests to confirm this diagnosis. A detailed history and physical examination are used to diagnose it. Of course, if there is an infection, a culture and sensitivity may be ordered to determine the infecting organism and appropriate treatment.

MEDICAL TREATMENT. Treatment is symptomatic in nature. Lubricants, especially oil-in-water lubricants such as Alpha-Keri oil, tend to be the most effective. Topical corticosteroids may be ordered for their anti-inflammatory properties. If the lesions become infected, topical or systemic antibiotics may need to be prescribed.

NURSING MANAGEMENT. The nurse needs to assess the lesions for signs of infection: redness, warmth, swelling, and purulent drainage. Following assessment, the primary function of nursing care is client education.

Education. The client needs to be instructed on the signs and symptoms of infection. Assessment of the client's knowledge base regarding medications and over-the-counter preparations as prescribed in the treatment plan is also needed. The client is told that humidification during the winter months is a necessity, cotton clothing may minimize irritation, and cool soaks decrease pruritus.

Anaphylaxis

PATHOPHYSIOLOGY. Anaphylaxis is a severe systemic type I hypersensitivity reaction. IgE antibodies produced from previous antigen sensitization are attached to mast cells throughout the body. In this reaction, the antigen is introduced at a systemic level, which causes widespread release of histamine and other chemical mediators contained within the mast cells.

ETIOLOGY. There are numerous causes of anaphylaxis. See Table 53–1 for potential causes.

SIGNS AND SYMPTOMS. There are sudden and severe types of signs and symptoms with anaphylaxis. Generalized smooth muscle spasms occur. The bronchi spasm, creating stridor, wheezing, dyspnea, and laryngeal edema, which can lead to respiratory arrest. Cramping, diarrhea, nausea, and vomiting also result from these spasms.

Capillary permeability increases, allowing fluid to shift from the vessels to the interstitium. This causes hypotension, tachycardia, and an increase in respiratory symptoms. The blood volume within the vessels decreases while the blood vessels dilate, resulting in a further decrease in circulating blood volume. The dilation also causes diffuse erythema (redness) and warmth of the skin. Neurological changes include apprehension, drowsiness, profound restlessness, headache, and possible seizures.

COMPLICATIONS. The most profound complications of an anaphylactic reaction are respiratory and cardiac arrest. Fast treatment is necessary to prevent death.

DIAGNOSTIC TESTS. There is no time for tests to be performed during an anaphylactic reaction other than tests to guide symptom treatment such as arterial blood gases or electrocardiogram (ECG) monitoring. This diagnosis is based on physical assessment and a history, if obtainable,

Table 53–1. **Substances That Commonly Trigger Anaphylactic Reactions**

Antibiotics	*Foods*
Penicillins	Beans
Sulfonamides	Chocolate
Tetracyclines	Eggs
Cephalosporins	Fruits (e.g., strawberries)
Amphotericin B	Grains (e.g., wheat)
Aminoglycosides	Nuts
	Shellfish
Medical Products	
Latex rubber	*Pollens*
	Grass
Diagnostic Agents	Ragweed
Contrast dyes	
	Proteins
Anesthetics/Antiarrhythmics	Horse serum
Lidocaine	Rabbit serum
Procaine	
	Venoms
Other Medications	Bees, wasps, hornets
Barbiturates	Fire ants
Dilantin	Snakes
Protamine	
Salicylates	*Hormones*
Valium	Insulin
	Vasopressin
Food Additives	Estradiol
Bisulfites	Adrenocorticotropic hormone
MSG	

from the client or significant other. After the client's recovery, allergen testing may be considered.

MEDICAL TREATMENT. Intravenous access is a priority, with administration of intravenous epinephrine. Vasopressor drugs may be used to increase blood pressure. Oxygen therapy is started. If respiratory symptoms are severe, a tracheostomy or intubation may be necessary with mechanical ventilation. Antihistamines and corticosteroids may also be given either orally or intravenously.

NURSING MANAGEMENT. Early recognition of anaphylaxis is important. Staying with the client while calling for immediate help minimizes the client's anxiety and allows close monitoring of vital signs and symptoms. Maintaining a patent airway is vital. Anticipation of emergency medication and equipment needs by the nurse facilitates rapid treatment.

Education. The nurse must educate the client who is prone to anaphylactic reactions the importance of avoiding the offending antigen. Medic Alert identification must be worn by the client. If the antigen is environmental, such as bee or wasp stings, obtaining a prescription and providing instruction on the use of an anaphylaxis kit or an epinephrine pen is vital (see Chapter 52).

Urticaria

PATHOPHYSIOLOGY. Urticaria (hives) is a type I hypersensitivity reaction. It is caused by the antigen-stimulated reaction of IgE antibodies causing the release of mast cell contents, especially histamine.

ETIOLOGY. There are numerous etiologies of urticaria. In addition to medications and foods, cold, local heat, pressure, and stress can also cause urticaria. Many times clients with an underlying chronic condition such as systemic lupus erythematosus, lymphomas, hyperthyroidism, or cancer are susceptible to urticaria.

SIGNS AND SYMPTOMS. Urticaria are raised, pruritic, nontender, erythematous wheals on the skin. They tend to be concentrated on the trunk and proximal extremities.

DIAGNOSTIC TESTS. Diagnosis is made on the basis of physical examination and client history.

MEDICAL TREATMENT. Treatment depends on the degree of symptoms. In the most severe cases, epinephrine may be given to quickly resolve the urticaria. Corticosteroids may be prescribed orally, topically, or intravenously. Antihistamines and histamine H_2 blockers, such as cimetidine and ranitidine, may aid in resolution by blocking the release of histamine.

NURSING MANAGEMENT. Nursing management includes monitoring the client's symptoms, administering prescribed medications, and evaluating the client's response to medications. In severe cases, maintaining a patent airway

is a priority. Cool soaks and diversionary activities may help with pruritus.

Education. Instructing the client on the use and side effects of prescribed medications is the nurse's responsibility. The nurse may need to be very creative in investigating ways with the client to avoid the causative agent of the urticaria. Some clients benefit from instruction on stress management and relaxation techniques.

Angioedema

PATHOPHYSIOLOGY AND ETIOLOGY. Angioedema is a form of urticaria. The pathophysiology and etiology of angioedema are the same as for urticaria.

SIGNS AND SYMPTOMS. Angioedema is painless, minimally pruritic, with dermal erythematous and subcutaneous eruptions. There is also skin and mucous membrane edema. The eruptions may last longer than with urticaria.

DIAGNOSTIC TESTS. A comprehensive history and physical examination confirms the diagnosis. Skin testing may be performed to determine the specific antigen.

MEDICAL TREATMENT. The most basic treatment involves avoidance of the antigen. Symptomatic relief may be obtained through the use of antihistamines and corticosteroids. For long-term treatment, immunotherapy for allergen desensitization may be indicated.

NURSING MANAGEMENT. Assessment of the client's symptoms is needed, as well as the administration and then evaluation of the client's response to medications. If the reaction is severe, maintenance of a patent airway is a priority.

Education. Assessing the client's baseline knowledge of the condition and medications is necessary. Further education may be indicated. The client and nurse may need to find creative ways for the client to either avoid or minimize future exposure to the causative antigen.

Type II

A type II hypersensitivity reaction is the destruction of a cell or substance that has an antigen attached to its cell membrane, which is sensed by either immunoglobulin G (IgG) or immunoglobulin M (IgM), as being a foreign antigen. When an antigen marker is sensed as foreign, an antibody attaches to the antigen on the cell membrane causing lysis of the cell or accelerated phagocytosis (engulfing and ingestion). When a cell is foreign, such as a bacterium, this process is beneficial. However, sometimes antigens on a red blood cell (RBC) can be sensed as foreign for the different blood types, which results in the RBC being destroyed.

Hemolytic Transfusion Reaction

PATHOPHYSIOLOGY. A hemolytic transfusion reaction is a type II hypersensitivity reaction in which RBCs with antigens foreign to the individual are rapidly lysed. The rapid RBC lysis results in a massive amount of cellular debris that occludes the blood vessels throughout the body. This leads to ischemia and necrosis of tissue and organs and can be life threatening.

ETIOLOGY. Occasionally, antibodies form after a bacterial or viral infection. However, prior sensitization is usually from a previous blood transfusion or past pregnancy. If maternal and fetal blood Rh factors (red blood cell surface antigens) are different, the mother becomes sensitized by the fetal Rh type, which can affect future fetuses. For example, an Rh-negative pregnant woman becomes sensitized by an Rh-positive fetus. As a result, the blood cells of future Rh-positive fetuses may be destroyed by the maternal antibodies that cross the placenta.

SIGNS AND SYMPTOMS. There is usually a rather sudden onset of low back or chest pain, hypotension, fever rising more than 1.8°F (1°C), chills, tachycardia, tachypnea, wheezing, dyspnea, urticaria, and anxiety. The client may also complain of a headache and nausea.

COMPLICATIONS. Clients that survive severe reactions are at risk for developing shock and acute renal failure due to the massive occlusion of blood vessels.

DIAGNOSTIC TESTS. The direct Coombs' test confirms this diagnosis. In the laboratory, a small amount of the client's RBCs are washed to remove any unattached antibodies. Antihuman globulin is added to see if agglutination (clumping) of the RBCs results. If agglutination occurs, an immune reaction such as a hemolytic transfusion reaction is taking place.

MEDICAL TREATMENT. The medical treatment depends on the severity of the reaction and what tissue and organs are specifically affected by the reaction. Antihistamines, corticosteroids, or even epinephrine may be given. Diuretics may be given to assist the kidneys with excretion if they become occluded with cellular debris.

NURSING MANAGEMENT. Prevention of hemolytic reaction is crucial. Following strict guidelines for blood transfusions helps ensure the client's safety. When blood is released from the blood bank, two health care workers double-check specified data. On the unit, transfusion guidelines may include double-checking at the bedside the client's name and identification number on the chart, bag of blood, and client's identification bracelet, as well as checking the client's blood type in the chart, on the unit of blood, and paperwork with the unit of blood. This double-checking is usually performed by two licensed nursing staff members, one of whom is a registered nurse, at the client's bedside.

Agency policy is followed for taking vital signs during a blood transfusion. Usually, baseline vital signs are taken before the beginning of the blood transfusion, then every 15 minutes for 30 minutes, then every half hour or hourly, and again when the transfusion is completed. It takes only a small amount of blood to trigger a hemolytic transfusion reaction, so it is critical that the nurse stays with the client at the bedside during the first 15 minutes of any blood transfusion. This enables the nurse to detect symptoms of a blood transfusion reaction early and act quickly to help minimize cell destruction.

LEARNING TIP

Every unit of blood, even if of the same blood type, is unique and can trigger a blood transfusion reaction. Careful monitoring with every transfusion is necessary.

If symptoms of a reaction are noted, agency policy is followed and the blood is immediately stopped. The vein is kept patent with a normal saline infusion. The physician and blood bank are immediately notified. A nurse remains with the client for reassurance and monitoring of symptoms and vital signs. If a blood incompatibility is suspected, the unused blood and blood tubing is returned to the blood bank for testing. A series of blood and urine specimens are collected and sent to the laboratory for analysis. The physician's orders are followed to treat the client's symptoms and stabilize him or her.

Education. Once clients have had a hemolytic transfusion reaction it is important to inform them and their significant others of this. They should also inform their health care providers that this reaction occurred. A number of very specific blood tests can be performed to test for less common antibodies if the client is ever typed for a blood transfusion again. These tests are costly and time consuming, so they are not routinely performed unless there is a history of a reaction. Autologous (self) blood donation may be an option for clients having elective surgery to help avoid a transfusion reaction.

Type III

A type III hypersensitivity reaction involves immune complexes formed by antigens and antibodies, usually of the IgG type. The client is sensitized with an initial exposure. Then on a subsequent exposure the reaction occurs. The reaction is localized and evolves over several hours, with symptoms ranging from a red, edematous skin phase, to hemorrhage and necrosis. The process involves the formation of antigen-antibody complexes within the blood vessels, as the antigen is absorbed through the vessel wall. Neutrophils are attracted to the area and release enzymes that ultimately lead to blood vessel damage.

Serum Sickness

PATHOPHYSIOLOGY. Serum sickness is a type III hypersensitivity immune reaction in which antigen-antibody complexes are formed and cause symptoms of inflammation.

ETIOLOGY. In the past, serum sickness occurred after inoculation of equine (horse) antiserum for diseases such as tetanus and diphtheria. With the refinement of these vaccines, serum sickness does not usually occur from them. Today serum sickness is seen occasionally after administration of penicillin and sulfonamide.

SIGNS AND SYMPTOMS. The signs and symptoms usually occur 7 to 10 days after the exposure. The most predominant manifestation is severe urticaria and angioedema. The client may experience a fever, malaise, muscle soreness, arthralgia, splenomegaly, and occasionally nausea, vomiting, and diarrhea. Lymphadenopathy may occur, especially at the lymph nodes closest to the antigen entry site.

COMPLICATIONS. Serum sickness is usually a brief and self-limiting condition, although at times it can become chronic. Systemic complications may arise, such as renal failure.

DIAGNOSTIC TESTS. Frequently there is a slight elevation in the white blood cell count and the sedimentation rate, and a complement assay decreases.

MEDICAL TREATMENT. Antipyretics may be given for the fever and analgesics for the arthralgia. Antihistamines and epinephrine may be prescribed for the urticaria and angioedema. If the symptoms continue to persist, corticosteroids may be ordered.

NURSING MANAGEMENT. Nursing care focuses on assessing symptoms, evaluating the effectiveness of prescribed medications, and client education regarding the therapeutic regimen and measures to prevent further exposure to the antigen. The nurse may also play an important part in identification of the causative agent, through the history taking process or recollection of recent exposures by the client.

Education. Knowledge of the disease and offending agent is important for the client. This knowledge may help clients prevent a reoccurrence of the condition.

Type IV

A type IV hypersensitivity reaction, also called a delayed reaction, occurs when a sensitized T lymphocyte comes in contact with the particular antigen to which it is sensitized. The resulting necrosis is due to the actions of the macrophages and the various T lymphocytes involved in the cell-mediated immune response.

Contact Dermatitis

PATHOPHYSIOLOGY. When a substance or chemical comes in contact with the skin, it is absorbed into the skin and binds with special skin proteins called haptens. With the first contact, there is no reaction or symptoms, but within 7

to 10 days T memory cells are formed. Therefore on subsequent exposures the T memory cells quickly become activated T cells, which secrete the chemicals that cause symptoms.

ETIOLOGY. Poison ivy and poison oak are the most common irritants causing this reaction. Latex rubber has also been found to be a cause for contact dermatitis. It has also been known to trigger type I anaphylactic reactions.

SIGNS AND SYMPTOMS. Within a number of hours from the exposure, the area of contact becomes reddened and pruritic, with fragile vesicles.

DIAGNOSTIC TESTS. Diagnosis is usually made by assessment of the skin and lesions, as well as a detailed client history.

MEDICAL TREATMENT. Treatment consists of controlling symptoms. Oral or topical antihistamines and topical drying agents may be used. If the symptoms are severe, corticosteroids may be prescribed.

NURSING MANAGEMENT. To aid in the relief of symptoms, tepid baking soda baths may help dry the vesicle and minimize the pruritus. The nurse may administer and evaluate the effectiveness of medications.

Education. The client is instructed to immediately wash with a brown soap called Fels-Naptha or if unavailable any soap when contact with the offending agent is suspected. The best advice is to avoid contact with the agent. The client should also be instructed not to scratch the skin to prevent the spread of the dermatitis, as well as infection development.

Transplant Rejection

ETIOLOGY AND PATHOPHYSIOLOGY. Any form of transplanted living tissue is sensed as foreign material by the immune system. Lymphocytes become sensitized during an induction phase immediately after the tissue is transplanted. The sensitized lymphocytes invade the transplanted tissue and destroy it via the release of chemicals and macrophage activity.

SIGNS AND SYMPTOMS. Various signs and symptoms occur depending on the transplanted tissue or organ that is involved and the severity of the reaction. Signs and symptoms reflect failure of the organ or tissue such as renal failure for a rejected kidney.

COMPLICATIONS. A total failure and loss of the transplanted tissue or organ can occur, or the tissue or organ can be damaged from immunological reactions and not function at full capacity. The greatest cause of death following a transplant is from infection. Immunosuppression therapy, which is necessary to prevent tissue rejection following the transplant, is a major contributory factor for severe infection development. Because the immune system is suppressed, it is unable to effectively fight infections.

DIAGNOSTIC TESTS. Biopsy, scans, blood tests, arteriogram, and ultrasound are some tests that may be performed to aid in diagnosing a transplant rejection.

MEDICAL TREATMENT. Depending on the type of transplant, the body's immunological system is prepared before surgery with medications, transfusions, or radiation to minimize the risk of rejection.

NURSING MANAGEMENT. Nursing care depends greatly on the type of transplant performed. Initially, the client is in an intensive care unit under close observation and support. Observing for signs of rejection is a priority throughout the client's hospitalization.

Another consideration for nursing is the psychological support of the client and family. Many clients wait on a transplant list a long time before a donor match is found. Once a matching donor is found there is usually great elation. Yet if a donor's death made the transplant possible, the client and family may be simultaneously feeling a profound sadness for the donor's family. They need time to verbalize these feelings and understand that they are normal and diminish with time. Also, a fear of rejection is always present that must be discussed.

Education. Rejection can take place weeks, months, or years following a transplant (with decreasing risk). The client and family need to be educated about specific signs and symptoms of rejection. Also, because infection is a major complication due to long-term immunosuppressive medications, the client and family need to know signs and symptoms of infection and when to notify the physician of problems. Steroid use may mask the symptoms of infection, so small indicators such as a low-grade fever should be promptly reported. Education regarding prescribed medications is a must because long-term success of a transplant is dependent on compliance with immunosuppressive medication therapy. Avoidance of people with colds or infections is also important to reduce the client's infection risk.

AUTOIMMUNE DISORDERS

In autoimmune disorders, the immune system no longer recognizes the body's normal cells as self and not foreign. Instead, the antigens on these normal body cells are recognized as foreign material, and an immune response to destroy them is launched.

A number of factors either cause or influence this breakdown of self-recognition, including viral infections, drugs, and cross-reactive antibodies. Some microbes stimulate the production of antibodies, but are so closely related to normal cell antigens that the antibodies also attack some normal cells. Hormones have also been found to influence this breakdown of self-recognition.

Table 53–2 lists additional autoimmune disorders and chapters in which they are discussed.

Table 53–2. **Immune Disorders**

Idiopathic thrombocytopenic purpura	Refer to Chapter 24.
Multiple sclerosis	Refer to Chapter 47.
Myasthenia gravis	Refer to Chapter 47.
Rheumatoid arthritis	Refer to Chapter 44.
Systemic lupus erythematosus	Refer to Chapter 44.
Ulcerative colitis	Refer to Chapter 31.

Pernicious Anemia

Pathophysiology

Antibodies against the gastric parietal cells and intrinsic factor lead to destruction of these cells and decrease secretion and function of intrinsic factor. Because intrinsic factor is needed for vitamin B_{12} to be absorbed in the small bowel, a vitamin B_{12} deficiency ensues and production of RBCs is decreased.

Etiology

There tends to be a familial tendency toward pernicious anemia in relation to immune causes. Non–immune-related causes of pernicious anemia include any type of gastric or small bowel resections coupled with no or inadequate vitamin B_{12} or intrinsic factor replacement.

Signs and Symptoms

The client experiences increasing weakness, loss of appetite, glossitis, and pallor. Irritability, confusion, and numbness or tingling in the extremities (peripheral neuropathy) occur because the nervous system is affected.

Complications

Clients with pernicious anemia have a greater risk of developing gastric carcinoma.

Diagnostic Tests

On microscopic examination of the client's RBCs, macrocytic (enlarged cells) anemia is diagnosed. Macrocytic anemia and low vitamin B_{12} levels are indicators of pernicious anemia and folic acid deficiency. To further determine if the diagnosis is pernicious anemia or folic acid deficiency, the Schilling test can be performed. For the Schilling test, radioactive vitamin B_{12} is administered to the client. The client's urine is then collected for 24 hours (48 hours for clients with renal disease) and the amount of radioactive vitamin B_{12} excreted in the urine is measured. If intrinsic factor is decreased, gastric absorption of vitamin B_{12} is also decreased, resulting in pernicious anemia and more vitamin B_{12} being excreted in the urine. Gastric secretion analysis is done to measure levels of hydrochloric acid (HCl) because low or absent HCl may be indicative of pernicious anemia.

Medical Treatment

Treatment with corticosteroids may rectify the problem if it is immunologically based. Otherwise, weekly and then monthly intramuscular injections of vitamin B_{12} must be taken for life to prevent pernicious anemia.

Nursing Management

Nursing measures are aimed at caring for the anemic client. Care related to fatigue and safety are important. Care with ambulation, frequent rest periods, and providing assistance with activities of daily living (ADL) as indicated by the client's activity tolerance are helpful for the client with anemia.

EDUCATION. The client and family need education regarding medication therapy. If vitamin B_{12} injections are prescribed, they must understand that this is a lifelong need to prevent the return of symptoms. Clients should not miss injections or follow-up appointments.

Idiopathic Autoimmune Hemolytic Anemia

Pathophysiology

Autoantibodies, for no known reason, are produced that attach to RBCs and cause them to either lyse or agglutinate (clump). When lysis occurs, fragments of the destroyed RBCs circulate in the blood. If agglutination occurs, occlusions in the small blood vessels result from the clumping and then tissue ischemia follows.

Signs and Symptoms

Clinical manifestations vary from mild fatigue and pallor to severe hypotension, dyspnea, palpitations, and jaundice.

Diagnostic Tests

The RBC count, hemoglobin (Hgb), and hematocrit (Hct) are low, and microscopic examination reveals fragmented RBCs. Lactic dehydrogenase (LDH) is elevated due to RBC destruction and tissue ischemia.

Medical Treatment

Supportive measures such as supplemental oxygen may be initiated. Folic acid may be prescribed to increase production of RBCs. The use of immunosuppressive medications and corticosteroids may be useful in obtaining remission. In more severe cases, blood transfusions and erythrocytapheresis (a process whereby abnormal RBCs are removed and replaced with normal RBCs) may be instituted. A splenectomy may be performed in an attempt to stop the destruction of RBCs for severe cases.

Nursing Management

The client's signs and symptoms should be monitored and reported as necessary. Frequent rest periods should be planned into the client's daily routine to prevent fatigue. Blood products are administered as ordered to replace RBCs. The client and family are instructed on the medical regimen and their understanding is verified.

Hashimoto's Thyroiditis

Pathophysiology

Autoantibodies for thyroid-stimulating hormone (TSH) form in Hashimoto's thyroiditis. However, instead of inactivating TSH, the autoantibodies bind with the hormone receptors on the thyroid gland and stimulate the thyroid gland to secrete thyroid hormones. The thyroid gland enlarges due to this overstimulation (hyperthyroidism). It becomes infiltrated with lymphocytes and phagocytes, causing inflammation and further enlargement. Then different autoantibodies appear that destroy thyroid cells, which slows secretion activity, causing hypothyroidism.

Etiology

The exact cause is unknown, although it occurs in females eight times more often than in males.[2] It is also more common in people 30 to 50 years old and clients with Down syndrome and Turner's syndrome.

Signs and Symptoms

Initially, the manifestations are those of hyperthyroidism, such as restlessness, tremors, chest pain, increased appetite, diarrhea, moist skin, heat intolerance, and weight loss. These manifestations may go unrecognized and progress quickly into hypothyroidism. At this point, an enlarged thyroid gland (goiter) may be seen. Clinical manifestations may include fatigue, bradycardia, hypotension, dyspnea, anorexia, constipation, dry skin, weight gain, sensitivity to cold, facial puffiness, and a slowing of mental processes.

Diagnostic Tests

Immunofluorescent assay, a test that detects antigens on cells using an antibody with a fluorescent tag, detects antithyroid antibodies. Serum thyroid-stimulating hormone levels are elevated, while T3 and T4 levels are low.

Medical Treatment

Thyroid hormone replacement therapy of thyroxine is the primary means of treatment. Lifelong thyroid hormone therapy is needed.

Nursing Management

If the client has a goiter, a soft diet may be necessary for comfort. Frequent rest periods are necessary, as well as slowly increasing client activity. Antiembolic stockings may help prevent venous stasis during the low-energy, decreased-activity phase. Daily weights and monitoring intake and output when cardiac status is compromised are important to detect abnormalities such as fluid retention.

Because weight gain and facial puffiness alter clients' self-image, they need an opportunity to verbalize their feelings to help them adjust to this disease process.

EDUCATION. Clients taking thyroid hormone replacement therapy should avoid foods high in iodine. The diet should also consist of high bulk and fiber to combat constipation. During the hyperthyroidism phase, a diet high in protein and carbohydrates encourages weight gain. Education regarding prescribed medications is also needed.

Ankylosing Spondylitis

Pathophysiology

Ankylosing spondylitis, also called rheumatoid spondylitis, is a chronic progressive inflammatory disease of the sacroiliac, costovertebral, and large peripheral joints. The inflammatory process begins in the lower region of the back and progresses upward. A specific histocompatibility antigen (antigen that identifies self), human leukocyte antigen (HLA) B27, is formed that stimulates an immune response.

Etiology

There is strong evidence that there is a familial tendency, but no other specific causes are known. It tends to afflict men more than women.

Signs and Symptoms

There is an insidious onset of lower back stiffness and pain, which is worse in the morning. As the disease progresses, the pain worsens and there are spasms of the back muscles. The normal curvature of the lower back (lordosis) flattens, and the curvature of the upper back increases (kyphosis). Clients may also experience fatigue, anorexia, and weight loss.

Complications

Due to thoracic structural changes that occur, carditis, pericarditis, and pulmonary fibrosis may develop occasionally.

Diagnostic Tests

A culmination of findings, such as a positive family history, radiographic x-rays of the joints, a positive HLA-B27 blood test, and negative Rh, confirms a diagnosis of ankylosing spondylitis. There are no specific immunological tests to diagnose ankylosing spondylitis.

Medical Treatment

Because there is no cure for ankylosing spondylitis, treatment consists of measures to minimize the symptoms. Analgesics for pain relief, anti-inflammatory agents to decrease joint inflammation, and physical therapy to maintain muscle strength and joint range of motion are used. Surgery can be done to replace fused joints. For kyphosis, cervical or lumbar osteotomy can be performed.

Nursing Management

Nursing care focuses on client education and administration and evaluation of prescribed medications.

EDUCATION. The client and family need knowledge of the disease process. Proper posture and range-of-motion exercises may be taught by physical therapy and need to be reinforced by nursing staff. The client should also be instructed not to stay in any one position for any length of time. The client should sleep on a mattress that is firm without a pillow to help reduce pain and stiffness.

IMMUNE DEFICIENCIES

Immune deficiencies occur when one or more components of the immune system are either completely absent or deficient in quantities sufficient to elicit or sustain an adequate immune response to combat an infectious agent.

DiGeorge's Syndrome

Pathophysiology and Etiology

DiGeorge's syndrome is also called congenital thymic hypoplasia. There is a partial or complete absence of the thymus gland and parathyroid gland. It is in this gland that T lymphocytes mature and differentiate, so there is either a complete absence or reduced number of T lymphocytes. This leaves the client with impaired immunity. Hypocalcemia develops from the absent parathyroid gland.

This syndrome has been associated with fetal alcohol syndrome. It occurs from abnormal fetal development resulting in a complete or partial absence of the thymus gland.

Signs and Symptoms

The symptoms of DiGeorge's syndrome are noticed shortly after an infant's birth. These infants usually have low-set ears, notched ear pinnae, an undersized jaw, a fish-shaped mouth, and wide-set eyes with eyelids that slant downward. Frequently, there are great blood vessel anomalies such as tetralogy of Fallot. If the thymus is partially absent, the infant may have a spontaneous return of cell-mediated immunity, but later in life may develop a severe T cell deficiency. With an absence of severely impaired cell-mediated immune response, the infant is extremely prone to recurrent infections. Hypocalcemia tetany can develop.

Diagnosis

DiGeorge's syndrome diagnosis is difficult to make initially unless the infant has facial anomalies. Immunoglobu-

---

ankylosing spondylitis: ankyle—stiff joint + osis—condition + spondylos—vertebrae

lin assays are useless in the infant because the maternal antibodies are present for months. Chest x-ray may reveal an absent thymus gland. Blood tests for T lymphocytes are abnormally low.

Medical Treatment

A fetal thymic transplant can restore T lymphocytes. Hypocalcemia is treated with calcium administration.

Nursing Management

The infant is monitored for hypocalcemia. Emotional support for the infant's parents and significant others is provided. Education on signs and symptoms of infection and hypocalcemia is a priority for the parents. The infant's parents are also taught that a low-phosphorus diet aids in maintaining calcium levels. Measures to minimize the risk of infection are discussed, such as avoidance of crowds, good hygiene, and adequate nutrition and hydration.

Hypogammaglobulinemia

Pathophysiology and Etiology

This condition is either a hereditary congenital disorder or acquired after childhood from unknown causes. It is characterized by the absence or deficiency of one or more of the five classes of immunoglobulins (IgG, IgM, IgA, IgD, and IgE) from defective B cell function. The lack of normal function of these antibodies makes the client prone to infections. The congenital form of this disorder affects males. Clients usually live a normal life span.

Signs and Symptoms

The infant is usually asymptomatic until 6 months of age when the maternal immunoglobulins are gone. At this time, the infant begins having many recurrent infections, especially from staphylococcus and streptococcus organisms.

Diagnosis

Until the infant is 9 months old, diagnosis is extremely difficult. At 9 months of age, immunoelectrophoresis, which measures the level of each immunoglobulin, can be performed.

Medical Treatment

Treatment is aimed at minimizing infections while increasing the immune system through injections of immunoglobulin. These injections mainly contain IgG, so fresh frozen plasma is given to replace IgM. IgA cannot be replaced, increasing the risk for frequent pulmonary infections.

Nursing Management

The infant is monitored for infections. The family is educated on signs and symptoms of a variety of infections and the importance in seeking medical help immediately. The infant should not be around crowds. Good nutrition, hydration, and hygiene are important in preventing infections. Any break in the skin must be cleansed immediately and monitored for infection development. Genetic counseling may be recommended for parents.

Acquired Immunodeficiency Syndrome

Over 29.5 million adults and 1.1 million children have been infected with **human immunodeficiency virus (HIV)** since the HIV/AIDS epidemic began.[3] Women are increasingly becoming affected with HIV. It is estimated that 12.1 million women are infected with HIV.[2] Over 8 million children have lost their mothers to AIDS.[2] By the year 2000, about 60 million adults will be infected with HIV.[2]

Transmission

Acquired immunodeficiency syndrome is the final phase of infection with the human immunodeficiency viruses, of which there are two, HIV-1 and HIV-2. HIV has been isolated in urine, semen, vaginal secretions, blood, saliva, and tears. HIV is contracted from an infected person's blood coming into contact with the recipient's blood via a break in the recipient's skin or mucous membranes. The virus is acquired through vaginal, anal, or oral sexual intercourse, contaminated blood transfusions and needles, and transfer of HIV from mother to fetus or infant during pregnancy, birth, or breast feeding. Unsafe sexual practices and intravenous drug use presents the greatest risk for HIV development. If the mother, before and during delivery, and then the infant for 6 weeks after delivery, are given zidovudine, it greatly reduces the transmission of HIV to the infant.[4] After delivery, infants must have long-term monitoring. Health care workers who follow Standard Precautions are not at increased risk.[2]

Pathophysiology

AIDS is caused by a virus, HIV. This virus mainly infects immune system cells, specifically T4 lymphocytes, also referred to as CD4+. As these cells are destroyed by the virus and become fewer in number, infections and cancers can take over as the immune system is not able to detect and destroy them.

HIV first attaches itself to CD4 receptors, a protein found on the surface of many cells, including T lymphocytes, monocytes, macrophages, and some nerve cells (Fig. 53–2). The viral particle is taken into the cell and its covering destroyed to expose the viral genome (chromosomes). HIV is a retrovirus that uses an enzyme called reverse transcriptase to produce viral DNA from viral RNA. This is integrated into the host cell's DNA and causes the cell to create more virus. The cell eventually ruptures and releases more HIV into the lymph and then circulatory systems.

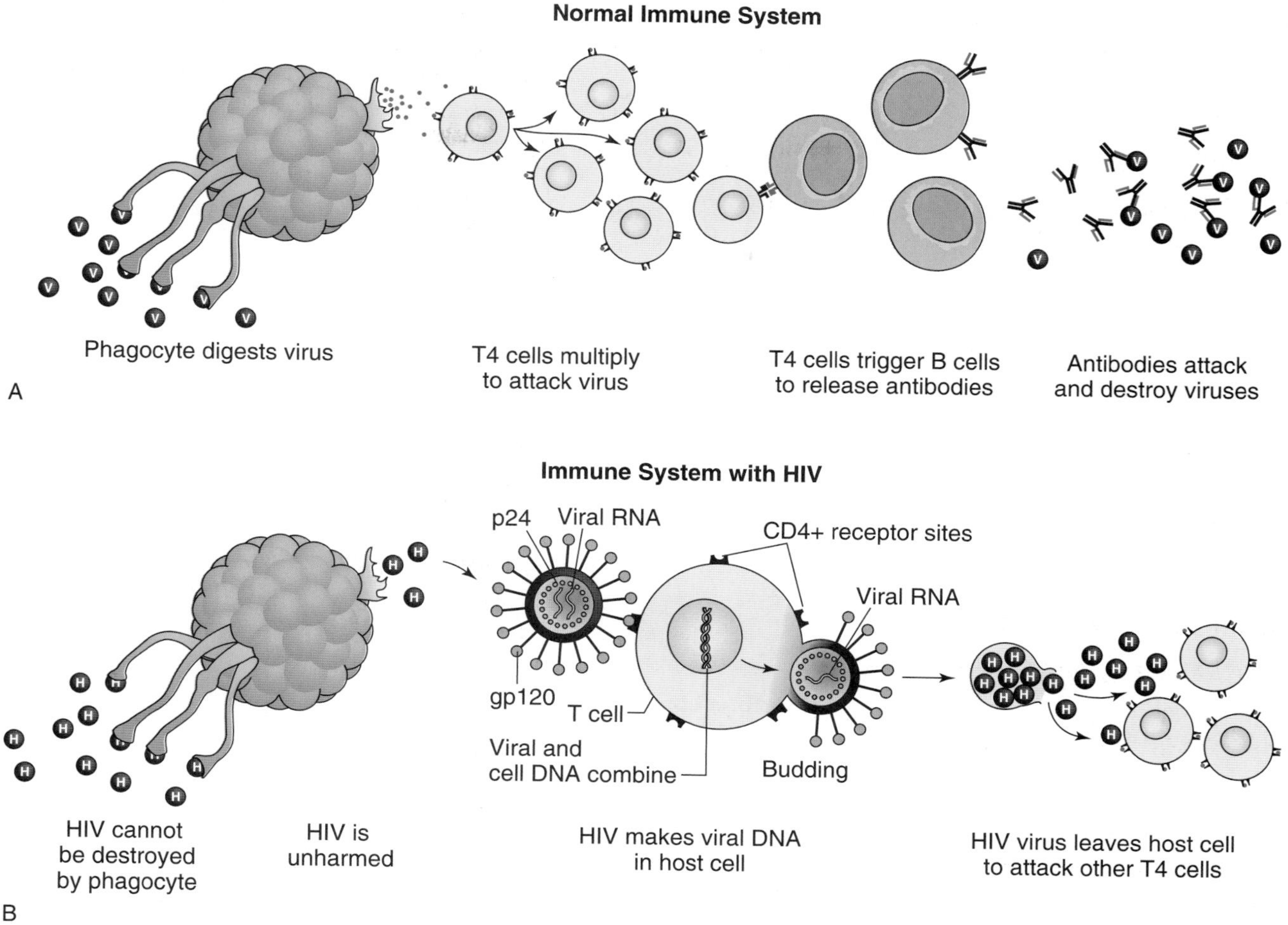

Normal Immune System

| Phagocyte digests virus | T4 cells multiply to attack virus | T4 cells trigger B cells to release antibodies | Antibodies attack and destroy viruses |

A

Immune System with HIV

| HIV cannot be destroyed by phagocyte | HIV is unharmed | HIV makes viral DNA in host cell | HIV virus leaves host cell to attack other T4 cells |

B

Figure 53–2. *(A)* Normal immune system. *(B)* Human immunodeficiency virus (HIV) contains several proteins, gp 120 protein around it and viral RNA and p24 protein inside. The gp 120 proteins attach to CD4+ receptors of T lymphocytes; HIV enters the cell and makes viral DNA; and the enslaved host cell produces new viruses that bud, which destroys the host cell's membrane, causing cellular death and allowing the virus to leave to attack other T4 cells.

Following exposure to HIV, incubation occurs over a period of several weeks (Fig. 53–3). There are usually no symptoms while the virus replicates. Then an acute infection, seroconversion illness, develops with general symptoms such as fever, rash, joint pain, lymphadenopathy, or malaise. These symptoms do not often require medical care, so testing for HIV is not usually done during this phase. HIV antibodies are now present at this time. The person is said to have seroconverted, or is HIV-positive, when these antibodies have been produced.

After the exposure and incubation phase, there is a latent period when there are no symptoms. This latent period may last 5 to 10 years. A decrease in CD4+ T lymphocytes continues and is the only sign of the infection. The virus remains in the lymph nodes, liver, and spleen and continues viral replication, which is undetected by blood testing.

After enough CD4+ T lymphocytes and other white blood cells are destroyed to impair immune function, symptoms are seen. This phase may last about 3 years before AIDS is diagnosed. The AIDS diagnosis is made when there are opportunistic infections present. These infections are opportunistic because a person with a normal immune system would be able to destroy them. However, with an impaired immune system the organisms and conditions have the opportunity to survive. Common opportunistic organisms include *Candida albicans* (yeast), *Pneumocystic carinii* (fungus), and **Kaposi's sarcoma** (skin cancer).

Signs and Symptoms

Initially after HIV infection, the client may have no symptoms or exhibit symptoms of mononucleosis (Epstein-Barr virus infection), such as extreme fatigue, headache, fever, generalized lymphadenopathy (enlarged lymph nodes in

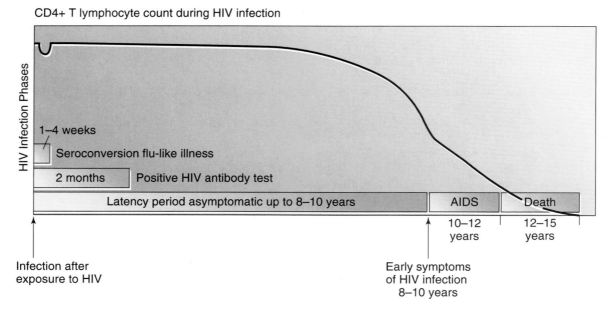

Figure 53–3. Typical time phases of HIV infection, AIDS development, and CD4+ T lymphocyte counts.

two different sites other than inguinal nodes), diarrhea, or a sore throat. These symptoms generally develop 6 to 12 weeks after HIV exposure and may last a few days to weeks.

After an extended asymptomatic phase, the syndrome progresses to a symptomatic stage when the virus has impaired the immune system. During this time, the client may exhibit weight loss, fatigue, night sweats, persistent diarrhea, oral and vaginal candidiasis ulcers, low-grade fever, peripheral neuropathy, shingles (varicella zoster virus reactivation), or dementia. These symptoms last up to 3 years.

In the final stage of HIV infection, AIDS disease is diagnosed. Opportunistic diseases and infections with their specific symptoms occur (Table 53–3).

Complications

HIV wasting syndrome occurs in most clients with the disease. This syndrome is defined by the occurrence of the two following criteria:

- Involuntary baseline body weight loss of more than 10 percent
- Chronic weakness or fever for more than 30 days or chronic diarrhea of two loose stools daily for more than 30 days

Several causes contribute to this syndrome, such as decreased appetite, increased metabolic rate, altered metabolism, malabsorption, gastrointestinal (GI) infections, diarrhea, dysphagia, medication side effects, and cognitive impairment. It is a very challenging condition that is one of the AIDS diagnostic conditions. The significant weight loss results in impaired function of all body systems due to

malnourishment. The weight loss is progressive and is accompanied by a loss of muscle mass, which is a significant cause of death. Careful intervention, planning, and education of the client when HIV is first diagnosed are necessary to help maintain body weight.

Table 53–3. ***Conditions and Opportunistic Infections Indicating AIDS***

Candidiasis infections of mouth, trachea, bronchi, lungs
Candidiasis of esophagus
Cervical cancer, invasive
Coccidioides immitis: extrapulmonary infections or disseminated
Cryptococcus neoformans: infections outside lung
Cryptosporidium: chronic GI tract infections
Cytomegalovirus infections other than liver, spleen, lymph nodes
Cytomegalovirus retinitis with loss of vision
Herpes simplex: chronic
Histoplasma capsulatum
Encephalopathy, HIV related
Isosporiasis, chronic intestinal
Kaposi's sarcoma
Lymphoma: Burkitt's
Lymphoma: immunoblastic
Lymphoma: primary brain
Mycobacterium avium complex or *M. kansasii*
Mycobacterium tuberculosis
Mycobacterium, any variety of species
Pneumocystis carinii pneumonia
Pneumonia, recurrent
Progressive multifocal leukoencephalopathy
Salmonella, recurrent
Toxoplasmosis
Wasting syndrome of HIV

Source: CDC: MMWR 41(RR-17):2, 1992.

Opportunistic infections are a primary complication of HIV infection and indicate the onset of AIDS from an impaired immune system. Kaposi's sarcoma is a skin cancer that can invade organs and has no cure (see Fig. 52–3). It appears as purple-red lesions on fair-skinned clients and dark brown in dark-skinned clients.

Pneumocystis carinii pneumonia is caused by a fungus that produces shortness of breath, cough, and fatigue. Chest x-ray shows infiltrates (see Fig. 52–4). The pneumonia may be resolved by treatment with oxygen, and oral trimethoprim-sulfamethoxazole (Bactrim) or pentamidine inhalation usually in an intensive care setting.

Dementia can occur from HIV infecting the brain. It impairs memory and concentration and causes depression, personality changes, hallucinations, and slower responses. Coma may result. Client safety is an important consideration for the nurse and caregiver.

Diagnosis

Testing for HIV infection may include one or more of the following categories: antibody detection, antigen detection, detection of the viral nucleic acid, or culturing of the virus. Antibody detection tests are the most commonly used screening tests. They are relatively inexpensive and quick to perform. The enzyme-linked immunosorbent assay (ELISA) is used (see Table 52–3). When the test result is positive after being repeated, the Western blot test is done for confirmation. To detect the HIV antigen (p24), a p24 antigen test is performed. This test is fairly accurate during the "window" of negativity, when the client has not seroconverted and has negative results with the antibody detection tests. The polymerase chain reaction (PCR) test is used to identify the presence of the viral nucleic acid. It is an expensive and time-consuming test, as is viral culturing.

The typical HIV diagnostic tests and testing pattern include the following:

1. ELISA test is done to detect antibodies to HIV antigen on test plates.
2. If positive, the ELISA test is repeated.
3. If the ELISA test is again positive, another test, often the Western blot, is done for confirmation.
4. If all test results are positive, the client is HIV-antibody positive.
5. Other tests can be used, especially if initial test results are not conclusive.

The CD4+ T cell count and beta-2 microglobulin levels (immune activity indicator) are used to monitor the disease's progression. CD4+ T cell counts decline as the disease progresses. Viral load studies monitor the speed of the disease's progress. The Centers for Disease Control and Prevention (CDC) defines AIDS in those with HIV infection by a CD4+ T lymphocytes count of less than 200/μL, [4] or the presence of one of the specified clinical conditions (see Table 53–3).[5] These conditions are primarily opportunistic infections.

Infants of HIV-positive mothers are tested at birth, 1, 3, and 6 months of age for HIV antibodies. A positive ELISA test at 15 or 18 months of age in children indicates HIV infection.

Medical Treatment

Because there is no cure for HIV/AIDS, treatment focuses on delaying or preventing its progression and development of opportunistic diseases. Treatment with medication is often recommended when the CD4+ T cell count falls under 500/μL.

The medications used to treat HIV infection are antiretrovirals. Two main kinds of antiretrovirals are used: nucleoside analogues and protease inhibitors. Nucleoside analogues inhibit reverse transcriptase, which is needed for HIV replication in the cells. Protease inhibitors are newer, potent medications that act on the virus by inhibiting enzyme action at a different time in the reproduction cycle. Some examples of these medications are listed in Table 53–4. Research for new medications to treat HIV is ongoing and includes non-nucleoside reverse-transcriptase inhibitors.

The HIV virus can become resistant to some of the commonly used medications over time, when used as single-drug therapy. Therefore early, aggressive treatment with multiple-drug therapy, aimed at reducing the viral load to an undetectable amount, is the most effective line of treat-

Table 53–4. *Antiretroviral Medications Used in Treating AIDS*

Nucleoside Analogues
Zidovudine (AZT, Retrovir)
Zalcitabine (ddC, HIVID)
Didanosine (ddl, Videx)
Lamivudine (3TC, Epivir)
Stavudine (d4T, Zerit)

Protease inhibitors
Saquinavir (Invirase)
Ritonavir (Norvir)
Indinavir (Crixivan)

Experimental Medications
Delavirdine (Rescriptor)
Nevirapine (Viramune)
Nelfinavir (Viracept)
HIV/AIDS vaccines

Table 53–5. **Prophylactic Treatment Used to Prevent AIDS Complications**

Complication	Treatment
HIV wasting	Client education: eat three high-calorie, high-protein meals and snacks daily; drink liquids before meals; eat low-residue diet for diarrhea control; control odors; develop easy meal plan—favorite foods, meal programs, frozen dinners; cold food controls nausea; use antiemetics; rest; listen to music; numb painful oral sores with ice, popsicles, or topical analgesic; avoid spicy foods; use artificial saliva for dry mouth; use nutritional supplements; referral for food stamps or free meal programs as needed; exercise to increase muscle mass; take prescribed medications designed to treat HIV wasting
Influenza	Annual influenza vaccine
Pneumococcal pneumonia	Pneumococcal vaccine when HIV infection diagnosed
Hepatitis B virus	Hepatitis B virus vaccine when HIV infection diagnosed
Tuberculosis	Test with PPD; treat as indicated with INH for 12 months; if active TB, multidrug treatment needed
Herpes simplex	Acyclovir therapy
Pneumocystis carinii *pneumonia*	Oral trimethoprim-sulfamethoxazole (Bactrim) or pentamidine inhalation

ment. Many drugs have side effects. If side effects occur, the drug may be changed to another one or interventions to help control the side effects may be used. The client should always report side effects.

To increase life expectancy and treatment cost-effectiveness, it is also recommended that clients should be prophylactically treated for opportunistic infections, especially hepatitis B virus, herpes simplex virus, and *Pneumocystis carinii* pneumonia (Table 53–5). Other opportunistic infections are treated with appropriate medications.

Nursing Management

Nursing care is individualized to the client's presenting symptoms and may include many different nursing diagnoses (Nursing Care Plan Box 53–1). Emotional and spiritual support for the client and the family, caregivers, and significant others is an important intervention that is provided throughout the disease process (Ethical Considerations Box 53–2). Nonjudgmental care should be provided. The nurse should be knowledgeable about the transmission of AIDS so that clients are not made to feel isolated. The Americans with Disability Act (ADA) makes discrimination toward clients with AIDS illegal, which the nurse should understand as the client's advocate.

Extensive teaching is necessary to assist clients in understanding this chronic, life-threatening disease that alters everything in their lives. Teaching must be done about all aspects of client care. Compliance is necessary to help prolong the time span before AIDS occurs. Financial resources may need to be addressed, because treatment can be expensive and an inability to work may occur.

For the client exhibiting diarrhea due to a variety of opportunistic causes (except *Salmonella*), an antimotility agent may be prescribed. To maintain nutritional status,

a high-calorie, high-protein, low-residue diet may be needed. Sitz baths may be soothing, and thorough cleansing of the rectal area after each stool is imperative. Ointments may be applied to protect and soothe if the anal area is excoriated.

In AIDS clients who smoke, there is an increased incidence of oral thrush (candidiasis). Therefore clients should be encouraged to quit smoking. Candidiasis, medications, and peripheral and central nervous system disease tend to decrease the senses of taste and smell. This predisposes the client with AIDS to nutritional deficiencies. Medicated oral swish and swallow medications, topical anesthetic sprays, and flavor enhancers may promote an increased food intake.

As the disease progresses, the client may require more care from caregivers and home health nurses. The home health nurse, in addition to providing physical care, establishes a therapeutic relationship with clients with AIDS and their significant others. When the client is terminal, comfort care and emotional support for the family are essential. Hospice care may be used at this time.

Prevention

Prevention is the best management of the HIV/AIDS epidemic. Education regarding the disease and transmission should begin with the older school-age child either at home or in school, and include the general population as well as older adults (Gerontological Issues Box 53–3).

STANDARD PRECAUTION USE. All those at risk of coming in contact with blood and body fluids and substances must follow CDC Standard Precautions to reduce their risk of HIV exposure. Health care workers are a primary category of workers that should use these precautions to protect themselves and other clients.

NURSING CARE PLAN BOX 53–1
FOR THE CLIENT WITH ACQUIRED IMMUNODEFICIENCY SYNDROME (AIDS)*

Risk for ineffective individual coping related to terminal disease and progressive debility

Outcome
Client will show use of effective coping skills.

Evaluation of Outcome
Does client show the use of effective coping skills?

Interventions	Rationale	Evaluation
• Establish and maintain an open and trusting therapeutic relationship.	Effective communication is based on trust—assurance of confidentiality is essential.	Does the client talk about concerns with the nurse?
• Allow grieving to take place (keeping a journal has been effective for some clients who have AIDS).	AIDS brings about losses of health, strength, employment, and in many cases friends and threatens one's sense of security and reasonableness of life. Healthy grieving is a natural coping response.	Is grief being expressed? Is client finishing things that matter to him or her?
• Encourage the client to express feelings and concerns. Contact a counselor, chaplain, or AIDS support worker if the client so desires.	Talking about feelings and concerns helps defuse anger, clarify needs, and relieve tension.	How are family members, friends, and support persons interacting with the client? How is he or she responding to family members, friends, and support persons?
• Provide the client with desired information or refer to others who can supply the information.	Knowledge dispels unreasonable fears and helps the client prepare adequately to cope with stressors.	Does the client evidence enough understanding of his or her disease to be able to cope effectively?
• Ask the client if he or she would like information about a support group and arrange such.	Social support can help the client cope.	Does the client show satisfaction with his or her coping resources?

Pain related to neuropathies, cancer growth, yeast and fungal overgrowth, dyspnea with pneumonia, decreased mobility, anxiety, and diagnostic procedures

Outcome
The client will express pain relief and will rest and move well.

Evaluation of Outcome
Does client express satisfaction with pain relief?

Interventions	Rationale	Evaluation
• Assess the pain.	Assessment of the characteristics of the pain assists the nurse in providing appropriate relief measures.	Can the client describe the pain characteristics?
• Offer pain relief measures appropriate to the type and location of the pain (both alternative measures, such as heat, ice, massage, and change of position, and medicine may be offered).	Not all types of pain respond well to the same treatment.	Does the client express satisfactory relief of pain? Does the client move and rest without evidence of pain?
• Document results of pain relief measures.	Documentation alerts other caregivers about what works and does not work, thus providing effective pain relief sooner.	Has client given sufficient information to document results?

*Written by Linda Hopper Cook

continued

NURSING CARE PLAN BOX 53–1 (continued)

Interventions	Rationale	Evaluation
• Notify the appropriate team member of a need for a change in the pain relief measures.	Changes in condition may require that pain relief measures change to provide effective relief.	How effective were the various relief measures (on a scale of 0 to 10 with 0 signifying no pain and 10 signifying the worst imaginable pain)?

Risk for infection, nosocomial related to weakened immune system, skin breakdown, intravenous therapy, and possible invasive procedures

Outcomes
Client will remain free of nosocomial infections. Client will describe measures to maintain skin integrity and avoid infections.

Evaluation of Outcomes
Is client free of nosocomial infections? Can client explain and demonstrate skin maintenance techniques?

Interventions	Rationale	Evaluation
• Assess the client's risk factors, such as skin condition, laboratory results, portals of entry for infections, and presence of any infections.	Status of these assessment factors determines plan for care.	Does the client have intact skin or nonreddened, nonpurulent sites of interrupted integrity?
• Caregivers should use Standard Precautions and strict aseptic technique for *all* clients and procedures.	Transmission of microorganisms can occur in both directions.	Do all caregivers use Standard Precautions?
• Instruct visitors about techniques to avoid transmission of infection, such as hand washing and not visiting when they have an infection. The nurse with an infection, especially a respiratory infection, should not care for a client with AIDS.	The immune system is damaged by HIV. Ability to combat infections is severely compromised. A minor infection for most people may kill a person who has AIDS.	Do those with infections avoid contact with the client until their infection is resolved? Do the laboratory tests indicate that the client is so immunocompromised that reverse isolation may be necessary?
• Promote skin integrity by frequent turning, optimal mobilization, protective mattress and chair pads, application of emollient to dry areas, and prompt treatment of any injuries.	The skin is the body's first line of defense.	Does the client's skin remain intact and infection free?
• Teach strategies for skin care and avoidance of infection to the client.	Self-care offers a measure of control in a frequently uncontrollable situation.	Does the client satisfactorily explain or demonstrate good skin care and knowledge of how to avoid infection?

Risk for injury related to impaired mobility, weakness, fatigue, possible electrolyte imbalances, neurological impairment, and sedative effects of pain medications

Outcomes
Care and mobility needs will be met without injury.

Evaluation of Outcomes
Does client remain free from injury?

continued

NURSING CARE PLAN BOX 53–1 *(continued)*

Interventions	Rationale	Evaluation
• Assess the client's abilities and disabilities.	Particular disabilities may increase the danger to the client.	Does client have deficits?
• Look for potential hazards in the environment (hospital or home) and eliminate as many hazards as possible.	Awareness of hazards is necessary to decrease occurrence of accidents and injuries.	Are there any hazards in the environment presently?
• Instruct the client about how to avoid hazards (if cognitively and physically able to comply).	Clients can help avoidance of injury if they understand hazards.	Is the client effectively avoiding hazards, or is the client a danger to self?
• Encourage self-care as much as is feasible without tiring the client.	Self-care promotes feelings of self-efficacy and can combat depression.	Does the client evidence satisfaction with his or her self-care efforts?
• Assist with care activities as needed.	Varying levels of assistance with care are necessary due to the debilitating nature of the disease.	Are client's care and mobility needs being met satisfactorily without injury?
• Institute safety measures as required, such as close observation, frequent reorientation, two staff members for ambulation, use of side rails, a bed motion alarm, or a room near nurse's station.	Protection of the client against inadvertent removal of tubes or equipment, falls, and other injuries may require extraordinary measures due to neurological damage.	Are safety measures effective for client? Does the client respond negatively to the protective measures? Can these be modified to be less offensive?

SAFER SEX TO REDUCE RISKS. Abstaining from sexual intercourse is the best way to prevent exposure to HIV. A mutually monogamous sexual relationship is considered safe if the partners are not or will not become infected with HIV. Alternative methods of sexual activities can be used that prevent exposure to blood and secretions, such as masturbation or massage. The benefits of limiting sexual partners should be explained. For sexual intercourse, the use of male or female condoms and safer sex techniques should be discussed, especially with young adults. Condoms should be

- New for each intercourse act
- Latex or polyurethane because other kinds have large pores that allow HIV to pass
- Current and not past expiration date
- Used with water-soluble lubricants only, not oil-based lubricants
- Withdrawn from the partner while penile erection is still present to avoid semen leakage

Dental dams of latex or plastic wrap can be used for oral protection.

REDUCING RISK FROM DRUG USE. Recreational and illegal drug use can contribute to HIV infection. The best prevention is to avoid drug use. Drug equipment should not be shared, especially needles. Sexual activity should not occur when judgment is impaired from drug use, because protective measures may not be used.

Education

For the client infected with HIV, education regarding the signs and symptoms of progression to AIDS and the need for immediate medical treatment is necessary. Clients with AIDS need education on ways that they may reduce the possibility or frequency of developing opportunistic infections. This may include avoiding areas containing birds and bird droppings to prevent *Cryptococcus neoformans*

ETHICAL CONSIDERATIONS BOX 53–2

Caring for a Client with AIDS

Edward, 28, is hospitalized in a large research hospital in California. He is in the terminal stages of AIDS, with widespread metastatic cancer and lung infections. He wants to see his parents before he dies. However, when he left his middle-class home on a ranch in Oklahoma in the middle of the Bible Belt to attend college, his parents had no knowledge of his homosexual lifestyle. They have not seen him since that time, and still have no knowledge that he is homosexual.

Edward does not want his parents to know about his homosexuality or AIDS. He feels that their rigid religious beliefs may make them disown him and cause a scene in the hospital. Before they come to visit him at the hospital, he asks the LPN/LVN assigned to care for him to answer any of his parents' questions about his illness by telling them he has leukemia or pneumonia, or another rare disease that they would not know anything about. After the third day of visiting their severely ill son, Edward's parents directly ask the LPN/LVN, "Does our son have AIDS?"

How should the LPN/LVN respond? Does the LPN/LVN's obligation to confidentiality outweigh the obligation to veracity? Are there any other alternative solutions to this dilemma?

GERONTOLOGICAL ISSUES BOX 53-3

HIV, AIDS, and Older Adults

It is a myth that older adults are not at risk for HIV infection and transmission. Societal biases support this myth.

Issues and Behaviors That Place Older Adults at Risk

- Risk of HIV infection is increased for anyone who had a blood transfusion before 1985. Hip replacements and open heart surgeries often require transfusion of donated blood.
- Older adults are sexually active and retain this ability and desire despite myths to the contrary.
- Previously monogamous men and women may enter into sexual relationships with others after the death of a spouse. This behavior increases the potential of HIV infection. Monogamous long-term homosexual or heterosexual relationships did not require the partners to use items to protect against HIV transmission because of the safety of monogamy. Older adults' sexual practices may have to be altered. They may need to learn about new products to decrease the potential of HIV and sexually transmitted disease infection.
- Older adults may resist using condoms because of the association with them as birth control rather than as a barrier to the spread of infection.
- The lifestyle of intravenous drug users puts them at risk for an early death. Older people can be intravenous drug users and at high risk for HIV infection.
- There is a lack of screening and screening information available to older adults. Because older adults are not candidates to donate blood, the potential to be identified as infected when donating blood is not an option.
- HIV infection symptoms can be interpreted as normal aging or as part of a chronic disease process. The effects of HIV on the brain that cause dementia can be misdiagnosed as Alzheimer's disease. This misdiagnosis keeps the individual from making treatment choices for HIV/AIDS.

HOME HEALTH HINTS

- Instruct clients in ways to reduce allergens in the home: (a) keep the bedroom clear of articles that collect dust or mold, such as knickknacks, stuffed animals, books, wall hangings, plants (real or artificial), and aquariums; (b) dust with a wet cloth to pick up dust, not just move it around; and (c) cover the mattress and box spring with vinyl covers.
- Teach clients with AIDS and their family members how to properly clean and disinfect the home. The recommended disinfectant is household bleach in a 1:10 dilution mixture. Use it to (a) clean toilet seats and bathroom fixtures, (b) clean inside the refrigerator to avoid growth of mold, and (c) wash clothing separately that is soiled with blood, urine, feces, or semen.
- Clients with AIDS do not require separate sets of dishes or silverware. Dishes are washed normally in hot soapy water and rinsed thoroughly after use.
- Teach the family of AIDS clients signs and symptoms to report to the physician and nurse immediately: fever, increased dyspnea, pain, change in sputum production, upper respiratory tract infection, pneumonia, respiratory distress syndrome, diarrhea 5 times per day or more for 5 days, uncontrolled weight loss greater than 10 pounds in the last month, persistent headaches, falling, seizures, mental status changes including memory loss and personality changes, rashes and skin changes, difficulty swallowing, and problems with urination.
- Many of the infections people with AIDS develop are similar to other illnesses and may be mistaken if potential exposure to HIV is not considered. AIDS dementia, for example, may look like Alzheimer's disease when it shows up in an elderly sick person.

infection. Fitting water faucets with 1 μm filters, frequent hand washing (especially after gardening or changing a baby's diaper), avoiding public pools, avoiding unfiltered tap water and ice, and avoiding oral-anal sexual practices help prevent cryptosporidium infections.

CRITICAL THINKING: Zoe

Zoe, 22, is diagnosed as HIV-positive. She is tearful and asks many questions.

1. How would you answer her questions:
   a. "Am I going to die?"
   b. "How is AIDS diagnosed?"
   c. "Can my boyfriend get it?"

2. Years later Zoe's CD4+ lymphocyte count is 200/μL. Why is she started on the following medications?
   a. Bactrim
   b. Acyclovir
3. Zoe is malnourished. What interventions can you use to promote nutrition?
   Answers at end of chapter.

Review Questions

1. Ronald has been sneezing and has had itchy watery eyes throughout the summer. He's diagnosed with allergic rhinitis. Which one of the following other signs and symptoms may Ron exhibit?
   a. Sore throat

b. Urticaria
c. Allergic shiners
d. Otitis media

2. Ron's treatment may include which of the following?
   a. Epinephrine
   b. Gold salts
   c. Anticholinergic medication
   d. Avoiding environmental stimuli

3. The nurse is admitting Mrs. Romerez to a medical unit. When asked if she has any allergies she responds, "Yes, to erythromycin and some kind of dye." What should be the nurse's next question to Mrs. Romerez?
   a. "How old were you when you took these medications?"
   b. "What happens when you take these medications?"
   c. "Under what circumstances were you given these medications?"
   d. "What type of doctor prescribed these to you?"

4. Brad is receiving preoperative medications, which include Zantac, Reglan, and Ancef 2 g intravenous piggyback. He states an allergy to penicillin. Fifteen minutes after the Ancef is started, Brad reports an uneasy feeling as well as feeling very warm. Brad is probably experiencing which of the following?
   a. Urticaria
   b. Anaphylaxis
   c. Angioedema
   d. Contact dermatitis

5. Jane, 55, is admitted with a 2-month history of fatigue, shortness of breath, pallor, and dizziness. She is diagnosed with idiopathic autoimmune hemolytic anemia. Which of the following may be the cause of this disease?
   a. Spleen malfunction
   b. Liver malfunction
   c. Bone marrow suppression
   d. Unknown

6. Clients who have pernicious anemia are at greater risk for developing which of the following?
   a. Heart disease
   b. Ulcers
   c. Stomach cancer
   d. Goiters

7. In planning nursing care for a client with ankylosing spondylitis, which of the following should be included?
   a. Avoid any exercise or massage
   b. Use interferon injections
   c. Avoid one position for prolonged periods
   d. Use topical steroids

8. Whenever people suffer from a deficiency of a component of the immune system, they are in danger of which one of the following?

a. Suffering an overwhelming infection
b. Experiencing a fatal allergic reaction
c. Dying from asphyxiation
d. Having a delayed anaphylactic reaction

9. An autoimmune disease occurs when which one of the following occurs with the body's immune cells?
   a. Produce too many antibodies
   b. Grow and multiply too rapidly
   c. Are not produced in sufficient amounts
   d. Are unable to distinguish between "self" and "not self"

10. Mr. Vida is experiencing an outbreak of chronic urticaria. Which of the following will assist him to control the symptoms of this disease?
    a. Managing daily stress
    b. Avoiding tub baths
    c. Drinking decaffeinated tea
    d. Taking one aspirin every morning

11. If an initial HIV test returns positive, which one of the following is recommended?
    a. The same test is repeated.
    b. Antibiotics are started.
    c. A different HIV test is performed.
    d. Rest and isolation are initiated.

12. Which of the following is one of the most common opportunistic infections that a client with AIDS may develop?
    a. Toxoplasmosis
    b. Cryptococcis
    c. Cryptosporidiosis
    d. *Pneumocystis carinii* pneumonia

13. Which one of the following cells of the immune system is most involved in the development of AIDS?
    a. Neutrophils
    b. T4 lymphocytes
    c. B lymphocytes
    d. Phagocytes

ANSWERS TO CRITICAL THINKING: Zoe

1. a. There currently is no cure for HIV/AIDS. However, medications are available that slow the disease's progression. AIDS onset typically occurs 10 years after HIV infection and may be fatal within 3 years. Research continues on finding improved treatments and a cure.
   b. AIDS is diagnosed when CD4+ T lymphocyte counts are below $200/\mu L$ or 1 of 25 clinical conditions as defined by the CDC is present.
   c. Zoe's boyfriend could become infected through exposure to her blood or vaginal secretions. She must learn about preventive measures and discuss them with him.

2. a. Bactrim is given prophylactically to prevent *Pneumocystis carinii* pneumonia when the CD4+ T cell count goes below 200/μL.
   b. Acyclovir is given prophylactically to prevent herpes simplex virus.
3. Client education; eat three high-calorie, high-protein meals and snacks daily; drink liquids before meals; eat a low-residue diet for diarrhea control; develop an easy meal plan; use antiemetics; numb painful oral sores; avoid spicy foods; refer for food stamps or free meal programs; and exercise.

REFERENCES

1. Stevens, CD: Clinical Immunology and Serology: A Laboratory Perspective. FA Davis, Philadelphia, 1996.
2. Thomas, CL (ed): Taber's Cyclopedic Medical Dictionary, ed 17. FA Davis, Philadelphia, 1997.
3. CDC AIDS Information: International Projections/Statistics, http://www.cdc.gov/nchstp/hiv_aids/stats/internat.htm.
4. CDC: MMWR 47 (RR-02): January 30, 1998—Preview, http://www.cdc.gov/epo/mmwr/preview/rr4702.html.
5. CDC: MMWR 41(RR-17):2, 1992.

RESOURCES

CDC National AIDS Hotline: http://www.cdc.gov/nchstp/hiv_aids/hiv-info/nah.htm. English: 1-800-342-AIDS; Spanish: 1-800-344-7432; TTY service for the deaf: 1-800-243-7889.
CDC National AIDS Clearinghouse Electronic Access to HIV/AIDS Information: http://www.caps.uof.edu/capsweb/aidslist.html.

BIBLIOGRAPHY

Agency for Health Care Policy and Research, Public Health Service, US Department of Health and Human Services: Evaluation and management of early HIV infection. AHCPR Pub No 94-0572. US Government Printing Office, Rockville, Md, 1994.
Augustus, LJ: Nutritional care for patients with HIV. Am J Nurs 97(10):62, 1997.
Behrens, DR: Allergies, immune, and autoimmune disorders. In White, L, and Duncan, G (eds): Medical-Surgical Nursing: An Integrated Approach. Delmar, Albany, NY, 1998.
Bright, DC: Pharmacologic management of cytomegalovirus retinitis: Review of current and future therapeutic modalities. J Optometrist Assoc 68(1):11, 1997.
Coleman, RM, Lombard, MF, and Sicard, RE: Fundamental Immunology, ed 3. Wm C Brown, Chicago, 1993.
Crossley, ML: "Survivors" and "victims": Long-term HIV positive individuals and the ethos of self-empowerment. Soc Sci Med 45(12):1863, 1997.
Decker, CF, and Masur, J: Pneumonia in AIDS patients in the critical care unit. Crit Care Clin 14(1):135, 1998.
Freedberg, KA, et al: The cost-effectiveness of preventing AIDS-related opportunistic infections. JAMA 279(2):130, 1998.
Gibb, L, Ellershaw, J, and Williams, MD: Caring for patients with HIV disease: The experience of a generic hospice. AIDS Care 9(5):601, 1997.
Harley, JB, and Scofield, RH: The spectrum of ankylosing spondylitis. Hosp Pract 30(7):37, 1996.
Heald, AE, and Schiffman, SS: Taste and smell. Neglected senses that contribute to the malnutrition of AIDS. N C Med J 58(2):100, 1997.
Holzemer, WL, Henry, SB, and Reilly, CA: Assessing and managing pain in AIDS care: The patient perspective. J Assoc Nurses AIDS Care 9(1):22, 1998.
Lewis, JS II, et al: Protease inhibitors: A therapeutic breakthrough for the treatment of patients with human immunodeficiency virus. Clin Ther 19(2):187, 1997.
Lisanti, P, and Zwolski, K: Understanding the devastation of AIDS. Am J Nurs 97(7):27, 1997.
McMahon, E, and Weinstein, E (eds): Immunological Disorders. Springhouse, Springhouse, Pa, 1995.
Melton, ST, Kirkwood, CK, and Ghaemi, SN: Pharmacotherapy of HIV dementia. Ann Pharmacother 31(4):457, 1997.
Mueller, MR: Social barriers to recognizing HIV/AIDS in older adults. J Gerontol Nurs 23(11):17, 1997.
Neal, LJ: The rehabilitation nurse in the home care setting: Care of the client with HIV or AIDS. Rehabil Nurse 22(5):239, 1997.
Nokes, KM, et al: Development of an HIV educational needs assessment tool. J Assoc Nurses AIDS Care 8(6):46, 1997.
Ostrow, MJ, et al: Determinants of complementary therapy use in HIV-infected individuals receiving antiretroviral or antiopportunistic agents. J Acquir Immune Defic Syndr 15(2):115, 1997.
Pearlin, LI, Aneshensil, CS, and LeBlanc, AJ: The forms and mechanisms of stress proliferation: The case of AIDS caregivers. J Health Soc Behav 38(3):223, 1997.
Post-White, J: The immune system. Semin Oncol Nurs 12(2):82, 1996.
Price, SA, and Wilson, LM: Pathophysiology: Clinical Concepts of Disease Process, ed 5. Mosby, St Louis, 1997.
Roitt, IM: Essential Immunology, ed 9. Blackwell Scientific, London, 1997.
Simms, J: Latex allergy client. Can Nurse 91(2):27, 1995.
Smith, KV, and Russell, J: Ethical issues experience by HIV-infected African-American women. Nurs Ethics 4(5):394, 1997.
Smith, MY, et al: Zidovudine adherence in persons with AIDS. The relation of patient beliefs about medication to self-termination of therapy. J Gen Intern Med 12(4):216, 1997.
Spector, SA, et al: Plasma cytomegalovirus (CMV) DNA load predicts CMV disease and survival in AIDS patients. J Clin Invest 101(2):497, 1998.
Thomson, CM: The potential risks of latex. Br J Theatre Nurs 6(5):12, 1996.
Ungvarski, P: Waging war on HIV wasting. RN 96(2):26, 1996.
Walsek, C, Zafonte, M, and Bowers, JM: Nutritional issues and HIV/AIDS: Assessment and treatment strategies. J Assoc Nurses AIDS Care 8(6):71, 1997.
Wilson, IB, and Cleary, PD: Clinical predictors of declines in physical functioning in persons with AIDS: Results of a longitudinal study. J Acquir Immune Defic Syndr 16(5):343, 1997.
Yu, LM, Easterbrook, PJ, and Marshall, T: Relationship between CD4 count and CD4% in HIV-infected people. Int J Epidemiol 26(6):1367, 1997.

Plate 17

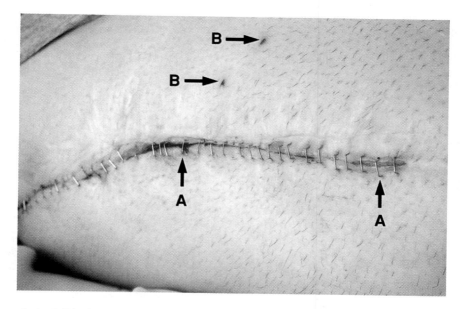

A stapled incision. *(A)* Note wound edges not approximated at arrows. *(B)* Arrows indicate puncture sites where drains were inserted.
(See Fig. 11–9, p. 207.)

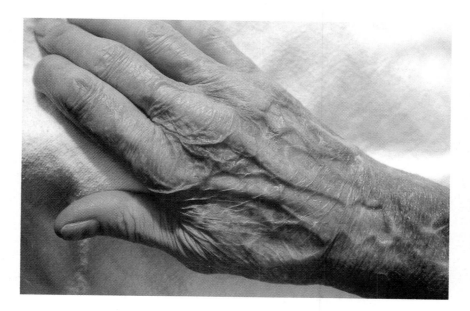

Thin, fragile skin of older client.
(See Fig. 13–3, p. 236.)

Plate 18

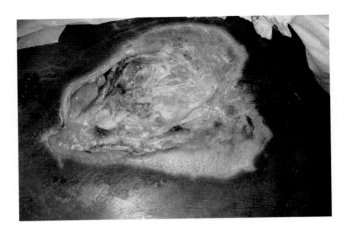

Pressure ulcer. (From Goldsmith: Adult and
Pediatric Dermatology: A Color Guide to
Diagnosis and Treatment. FA Davis,
Philadelphia, p. 445, with permission.)
(See Fig. 13–4, p. 236.)

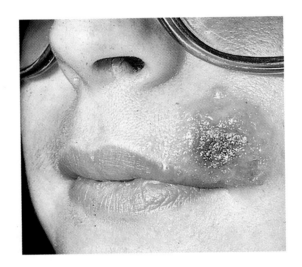

Herpes simplex. (From Reeves J, Maibach H.
Clinical Dermatology Illustrated, 2nd ed, 1998.
Reproduced with permission: MacLennan &
Petty, Sydney.)
(See Fig. 30–1, p. 577.)

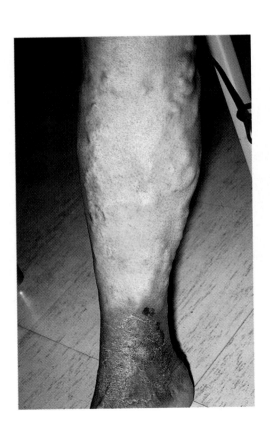

Varicose veins and chronic stasis dermatitis of the
ankle. (From Reeves J, Maibach H. Clinical
Dermatology Illustrated, 2nd ed, 1998.
Reproduced with permission: MacLennan &
Petty, Sydney.)
(See Fig. 18–5, p. 345.)

Plate 19

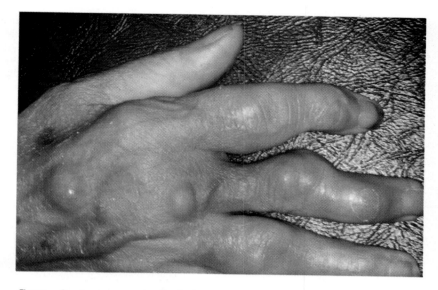

Gout: subcutaneous nontender lesions near joints. (From Goldsmith, LA, et al:
Adult and Pediatric Dermatology. FA Davis, Philadelphia, 1997, p. 405, with permission.)
(See Fig. 44–4, p. 892.)

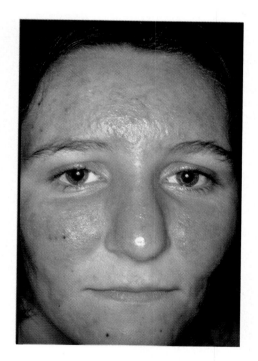

Lupus erythematosus: red papules and plaques in butterfly pattern on face.
(From Goldsmith, LA, et al: Adult and Pediatric Dermatology. FA Davis, Philadelphia, 1997,
p. 230, with permission.)
(See Fig. 44–5, p. 894.)

Plate 20

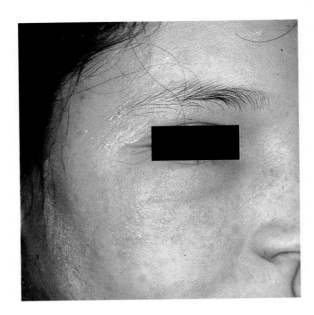

Allergic contact dermatitis from the poison oak plant.
(From Reeves J, Maibach H. Clinical Dermatology
Illustrated, 2nd ed, 1998. Reproduced with permission:
MacLennan & Petty, Sydney.)
(See first figure in Table 51–1, p. 1100.)

Seborrheic dermatitis as seen in dandruff, or excessive
scaling of the scalp. (From Reeves J, Maibach H. Clinical
Dermatology Illustrated, 2nd ed, 1998. Reproduced with
permission: MacLennan & Petty, Sydney.)
(See third figure in Table 51–1, p. 1100.)

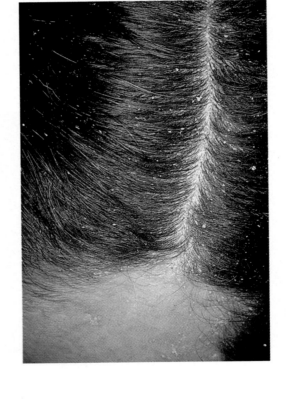

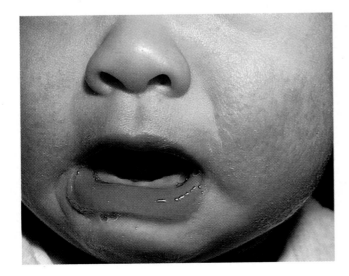

Atopic dermatitis as typical "chapped cheeks" in infant.
(From Reeves J, Maibach H. Clinical Dermatology
Illustrated, 2nd ed, 1998. Reproduced with permission:
MacLennan & Petty, Sydney.)
(See second figure in Table 51–1, p. 1100.)

Plate 21

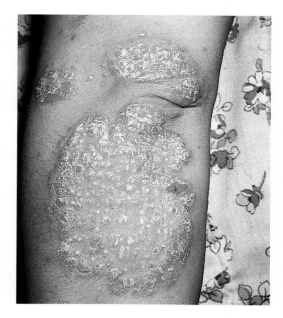

Psoriasis. Note bright red scaly plaque with
silvery scale. (From Reeves J, Maibach H. Clinical
Dermatology Illustrated, 2nd ed, 1998.
Reproduced with permission: MacLennan &
Petty, Sydney.)
(See Fig. 51–2, p. 1102.)

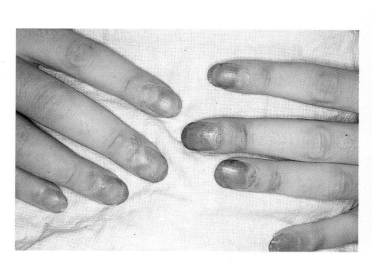

Acute psoriatic arthritis. (From Reeves J, Maibach H. Clinical
Dermatology Illustrated, 2nd ed, 1998. Reproduced with
permission: MacLennan & Petty, Sydney.)
(See Fig. 51–3, p. 1103.)

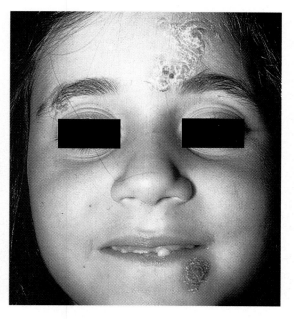

Impetigo on the face. Note honey-color crusts on
red erosions. (From Reeves J, Maibach H. Clinical
Dermatology Illustrated, 2nd ed, 1998. Reproduced
with permission: MacLennan & Petty, Sydney.)
(See figure in Table 51–2, p. 1104.)

Plate 22

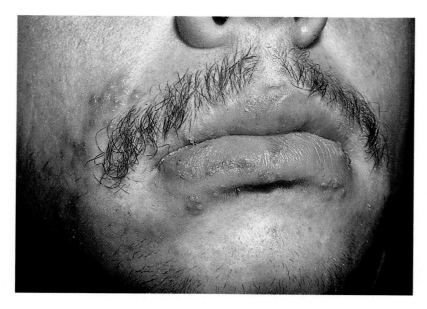

Herpes simplex around mouth. (From Reeves J, Maibach H. Clinical Dermatology Illustrated, 2nd ed, 1998. Reproduced with permission: MacLennan & Petty, Sydney.)
(See Fig. 51–4, p. 1105.)

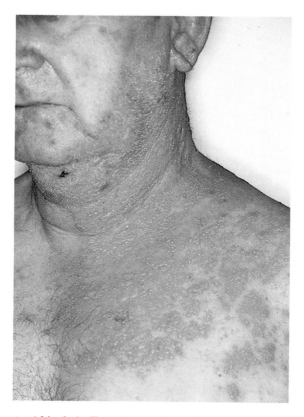

Herpes zoster (shingles). (From Reeves J, Maibach H. Clinical Dermatology Illustrated, 2nd ed, 1998. Reproduced with permission: MacLennan & Petty, Sydney.)
(See Fig. 51–5, p. 1106.)

Plate 23

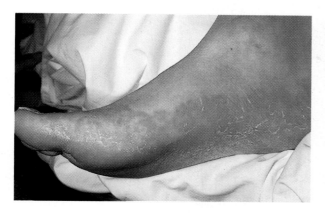

Tinea pedis—chronic plantar scaling. (From Reeves J, Maibach H. Clinical Dermatology Illustrated, 2nd ed, 1998. Reproduced with permission: MacLennan & Petty, Sydney.)
(See first figure in Table 51–3, p. 1108.)

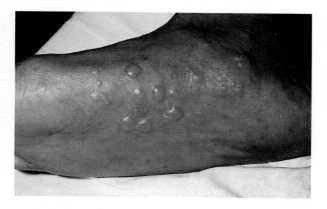

Acute vesicular tinea pedis. (From Reeves J, Maibach H. Clinical Dermatology Illustrated, 2nd ed, 1998. Reproduced with permission: MacLennan & Petty, Sydney.)
(See third figure in Table 51–3, p. 1108.)

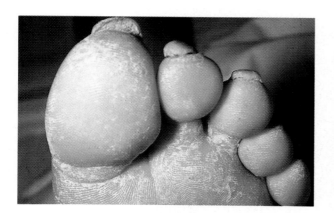

Tinea pedis with toenail involvement. (From Reeves J, Maibach H. Clinical Dermatology Illustrated, 2nd ed, 1998. Reproduced with permission: MacLennan & Petty, Sydney.)
(See second figure in Table 51–3, p. 1108.)

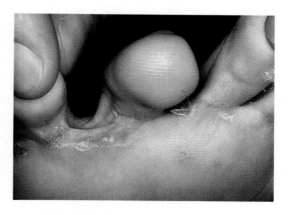

Interdigital tinea pedis is itchy and malodorous. (From Reeves J, Maibach H. Clinical Dermatology Illustrated, 2nd ed, 1998. Reproduced with permission: MacLennan & Petty, Sydney.)
(See fourth figure in Table 51–3, p. 1108.)

Plate 24

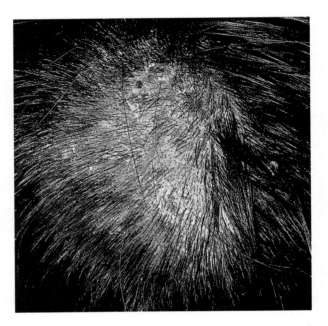

Tinea capitis. (From Reeves J, Maibach H. Clinical Dermatology
Illustrated, 2nd ed, 1998. Reproduced with permission:
MacLennan & Petty, Sydney.)
(See fifth figure in Table 51–3, p. 1108.)

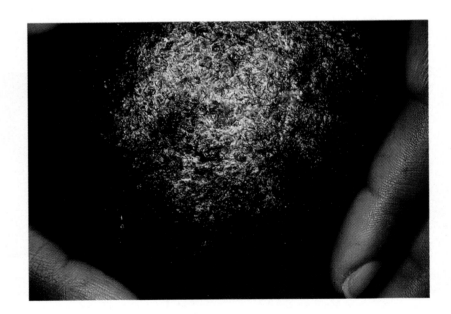

Tinea capitis—kerion inflammation. (From Reeves J, Maibach H. Clinical
Dermatology Illustrated, 2nd ed, 1998. Reproduced with permission:
MacLennan & Petty, Sydney.)
(See sixth figure in Table 51–3, p. 1108.)

Plate 25

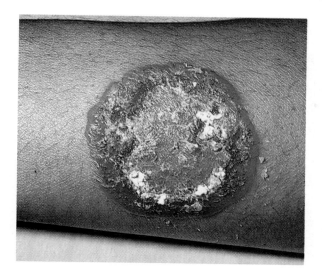

Tinea corporis—singular. This woman worked in a school where many children had scalp ringworm. (From Reeves J, Maibach H. Clinical Dermatology Illustrated, 2nd ed, 1998. Reproduced with permission: MacLennan & Petty, Sydney.) (See first figure in Table 51–3, p. 1109.)

Tinea cruris. The inner thigh is the typical location for tinea cruris, or "jock itch." The border is pronounced and scaly. (From Reeves J, Maibach H. Clinical Dermatology Illustrated, 2nd ed, 1998. Reproduced with permission: MacLennan & Petty, Sydney.) (See third figure in Table 51–3, p. 1109.)

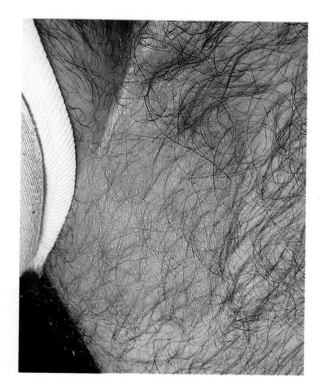

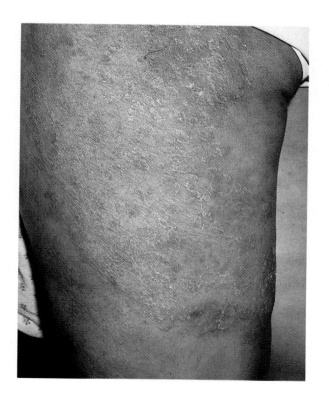

Tinea corporis—clusters and plaques. (From Reeves J, Maibach H. Clinical Dermatology Illustrated, 2nd ed, 1998. Reproduced with permission: MacLennan & Petty, Sydney.) (See second figure in Table 51–3, p. 1109.)

Plate 26

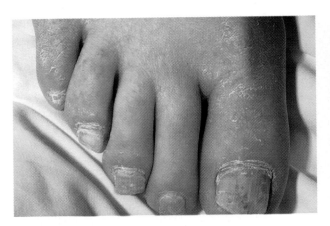

Onychomycosis (tinea unguium). (From Reeves J, Maibach H. Clinical Dermatology Illustrated, 2nd ed, 1998. Reproduced with permission: MacLennan & Petty, Sydney.) (See figure in Table 51–3, p. 1110.)

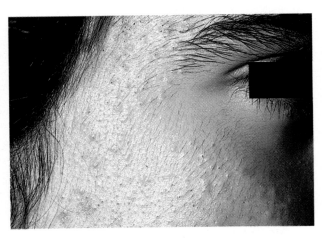

Open comedones, or blackheads. (From Reeves J, Maibach H. Clinical Dermatology Illustrated, 2nd ed, 1998. Reproduced with permission: MacLennan & Petty, Sydney.) (See Fig. 51–7, p. 1111.)

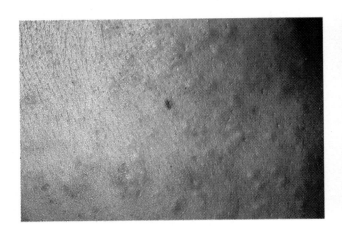

Closed comedones, or whiteheads. (From Reeves J, Maibach H. Clinical Dermatology Illustrated, 2nd ed, 1998. Reproduced with permission: MacLennan & Petty, Sydney.) (See Fig. 51–6, p. 1110.)

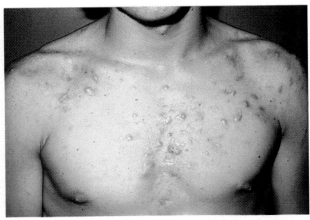

Nodular acne vulgaris. (From Reeves J, Maibach H. Clinical Dermatology Illustrated, 2nd ed, 1998. Reproduced with permission: MacLennan & Petty, Sydney.) (See Fig. 51–8, p. 1111.)

Plate 27

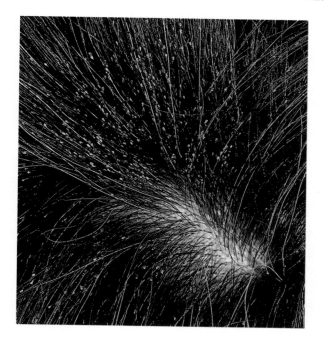

Head lice—nits are attached to hairs. (From Reeves J, Maibach H. Clinical Dermatology Illustrated, 2nd ed, 1998. Reproduced with permission: MacLennan & Petty, Sydney.)
(See Fig. 51–9, p. 1112.)

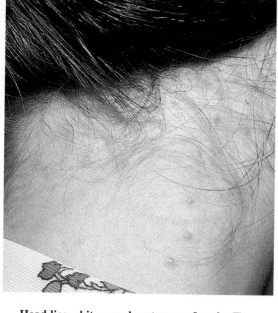

Head lice—bite papules at nape of neck. (From Reeves J, Maibach H. Clinical Dermatology Illustrated, 2nd ed, 1998. Reproduced with permission: MacLennan & Petty, Sydney.)
(See Fig. 51–11, p. 1113.)

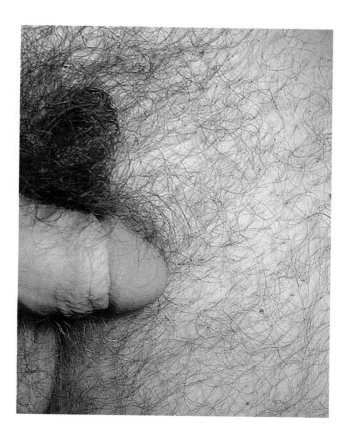

Pubic lice infestation is usually very itchy and shows only scattered excoriations. (From Reeves J, Maibach H. Clinical Dermatology Illustrated, 2nd ed, 1998. Reproduced with permission: MacLennan & Petty, Sydney.)
(See Fig. 51–10, p. 1112.)

Plate 28

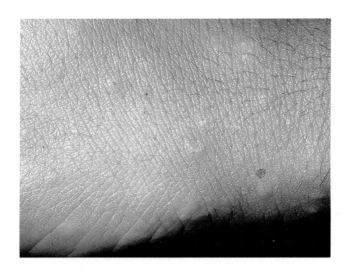

Scabies—the J-shaped white lesion in the center of the photograph is a burrow that contains an organism. (From Reeves J, Maibach H. Clinical Dermatology Illustrated, 2nd ed, 1998. Reproduced with permission: MacLennan & Petty, Sydney.) (See Fig. 51–12, p. 1114.)

Scabies—adult mite, eggs, and feces in burrow are seen in skin shaved specimen under the microscope. (From Reeves J, Maibach H. Clinical Dermatology Illustrated, 2nd ed, 1998. Reproduced with permission: MacLennan & Petty, Sydney.) (See Fig. 51–14, p. 1115.)

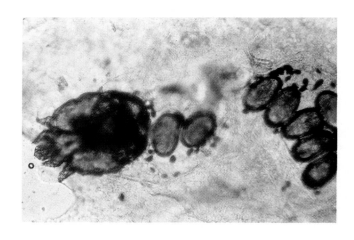

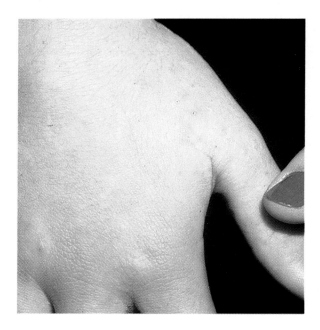

Scabies—fingerweb involvement is common. (From Reeves J, Maibach H. Clinical Dermatology Illustrated, 2nd ed, 1998. Reproduced with permission: MacLennan & Petty, Sydney.) (See Fig. 51–13, p. 1114.)

Plate 29

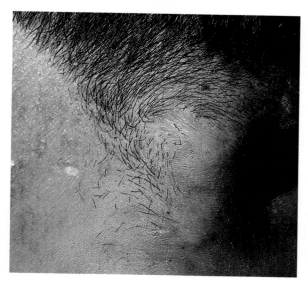

Epidermal cyst at nape of neck. (From Reeves J,
Maibach H. Clinical Dermatology Illustrated, 2nd ed,
1998. Reproduced with permission:
MacLennan & Petty, Sydney.)
(See figure in Table 51–10, p. 1128.)

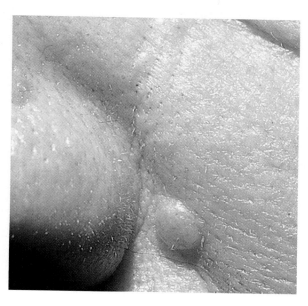

Nonpigmented dermal mole. (From Reeves J,
Maibach H. Clinical Dermatology Illustrated, 2nd ed,
1998. Reproduced with permission:
MacLennan & Petty, Sydney.)
(See second figure in Table 51–10, p. 1129.)

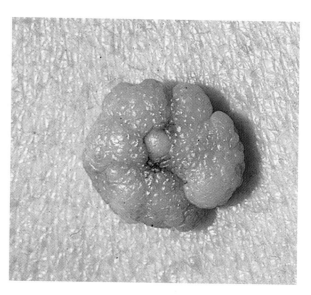

Dermal mole. (From Reeves J, Maibach H. Clinical
Dermatology Illustrated, 2nd ed, 1998. Reproduced
with permission: MacLennan & Petty, Sydney.)
(See first figure in Table 51–10, p. 1129.)

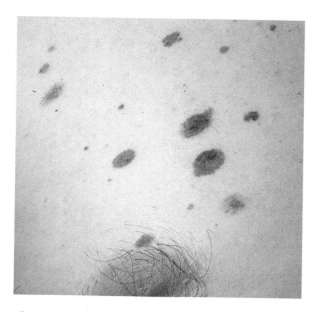

Dysplastic nevi. (From Reeves J, Maibach H. Clinical
Dermatology Illustrated, 2nd ed, 1998. Reproduced
with permission: MacLennan & Petty, Sydney.)
(See third figure in Table 51–10, p. 1129.)

Plate 30

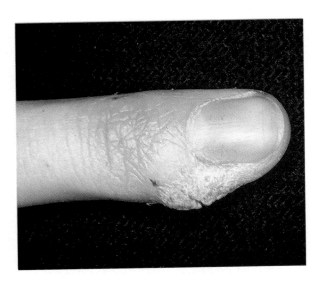

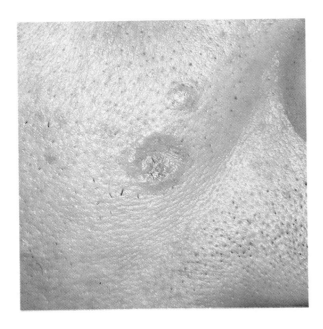

Wart near nail. (From Reeves J, Maibach H. Clinical Dermatology Illustrated, 2nd ed, 1998. Reproduced with permission: MacLennan & Petty, Sydney.) (See fourth figure in Table 51–10, p. 1129.)

Basal cell carcinoma. Note pearly flesh-colored papule with depressed center and rolled edge. (From Reeves J, Maibach H. Clinical Dermatology Illustrated, 2nd ed, 1998. Reproduced with permission: MacLennan & Petty, Sydney.) (See Fig. 51–24, p. 1130.)

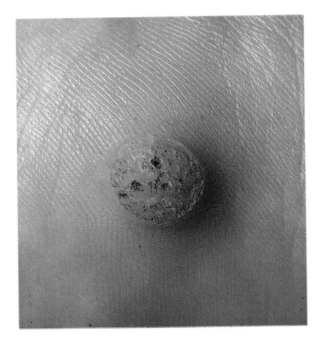

Plantar wart. This wart was painful during walking. Pressure caused irritation of surrounding skin. (From Reeves J, Maibach H. Clinical Dermatology Illustrated, 2nd ed, 1998. Reproduced with permission: MacLennan & Petty, Sydney.) (See fifth figure in Table 51–10, p. 1129.)

Plate 31

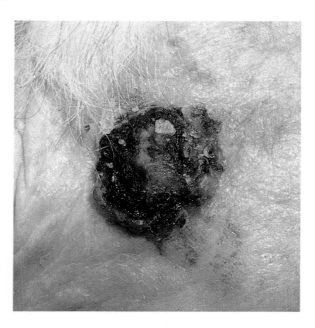

Squamous cell carcinoma that has been neglected. (From Reeves J, Maibach H. Clinical Dermatology Illustrated, 2nd ed, 1998. Reproduced with permission: MacLennan & Petty, Sydney.) (See Fig. 51–26, p. 1131.)

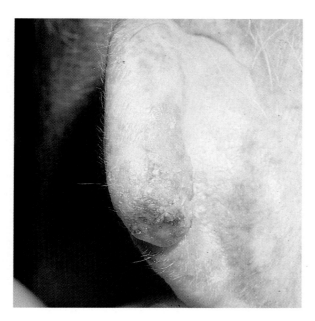

Squamous cell carcinoma. Surface is fragile and bleeds easily. (From Reeves J, Maibach H. Clinical Dermatology Illustrated, 2nd ed, 1998. Reproduced with permission: MacLennan & Petty, Sydney.) (See Fig. 51–25, p. 1131.)

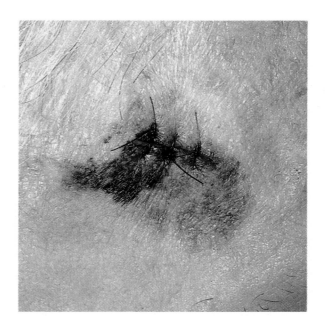

Lentigo maligna. (From Reeves J, Maibach H. Clinical Dermatology Illustrated, 2nd ed, 1998. Reproduced with permission: MacLennan & Petty, Sydney.) (See Fig. 51–27, p. 1131.)

Plate 32

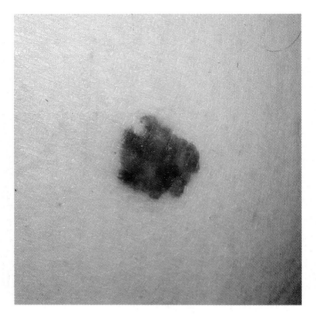

**Superficial spreading melanoma. Note irregular
border and variegated pigment. (From Reeves J,
Maibach H. Clinical Dermatology Illustrated, 2nd ed,
1998. Reproduced with permission:
MacLennan & Petty, Sydney.)
(See Fig. 51–28, p. 1131.)**

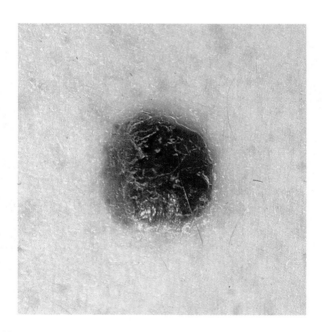

**Nodular melanoma. Microscopic examination revealed that it
arose from a mole. (From Reeves J, Maibach H. Clinical
Dermatology Illustrated, 2nd ed, 1998. Reproduced with
permission: MacLennan & Petty, Sydney.)
(See Fig. 51–29, p. 1132.)**

Understanding Emergency Care

Nursing Care of Clients with Emergent Conditions

54

Kate Schmitz

Learning Objectives

Upon completion of this chapter, the student will be able to:

1. Identify common signs and symptoms of shock.
2. Differentiate anaphylactic shock from hemorrhagic shock.
3. List the components of the primary survey.
4. Describe interventions for the multisystem trauma victim.
5. Define partial-thickness and full-thickness burns.
6. Identify symptoms of inhalation injury.
7. Describe stages of hypothermia.
8. Describe stages of hyperthermia.
9. Describe priorities of care for poison overdose.
10. Identify the nurse's role in psychiatric emergencies.

Key Words

abrasion (a-**BRAY**-shun)
amputation (am-pew-**TAY**-shun)
anaphylactic shock (an-uh-fi-**LAK**-tik SHAHK)
asphyxia (as-**FIX**-ee-a)
capillary permeability (**KAP**-i-lar-ee PER-me-a-**BILL**-i-tee)
capillary refill (**KAP**-i-lar-ee **RE**-fill)
cardiogenic shock (kar-dee-o-**JEN**-ick SHAHK)
distributive shock (dis-**TRIB**-u-tive SHAHK)
full-thickness burn (full **THICK**-ness BERN)
gastric lavage (**GAS**-trik la-**VA**-ge)
heatstroke (**HEET**-strohk)
hypoproteinemia (HIGH-poh-pro-teen-**EE**-mee-ah)
hypovolemic shock (HIGH-poh-voh-**LEEM**-ik SHAHK)
laceration (la-sir-**A**-shun)
obstructive shock (ub-**STRUK**-tive SHAHK)
partial-thickness burn (**PAR**-shul THICK-ness BERN)
rule of nines (ROOL of NINES)
shock (SHAHK)
tetanus (**TET**-uh-nus)

Essential for successful emergency nursing is the ability to recognize life-threatening conditions, conduct quick and complete client assessments, and provide appropriate interventions for optimal client outcome. A variety of emergency situations and resulting client injuries that may be encountered by the LPN/LVN are presented. Chapter content includes a framework to conduct initial assessment, implement interventions, and contribute to identifying nursing diagnoses and their interventions.

Shock

Shock is a condition of acute peripheral circulatory failure, causing inadequate and progressively failing tissue perfusion that can result in cellular death. During initial phases of shock, compensatory adjustments allow the body to adapt to the circulatory changes. Eventually, these compensatory mechanisms fail and decreased cellular perfusion occurs, causing cellular death. Because measuring shock at the cellular level as it occurs is difficult, clinical assessment is based on the effect of shock on the major organ systems.

There are four types of shock: hypovolemic, cardiogenic, obstructive, and distributive. **Hypovolemic shock** is due to a decrease in circulating blood volume. It is often caused by hemorrhage. Shock can also result from decreased volume of plasma as is seen in burn victims or in severely dehydrated clients. **Cardiogenic shock** is caused by inadequate contractility of the cardiac muscle. This results in decreased cardiac output and causes ineffective tissue perfusion. Causes of cardiogenic shock are myocardial infarction, myocardial contusion, dysrhythmias, and heart failure. **Obstructive shock** results from inadequate circulating blood volume due to an obstruction or compression of the great veins, aorta, pulmonary arteries, or the heart itself. Cardiac tamponade can compress the heart during filling, which leads to a decrease in stroke volume. A tension pneumothorax can displace the inferior vena cava and obstruct venous return to the right atrium, causing inadequate stroke volume. **Distributive shock** results from poor distribution of blood flow. Vascular tone is lost because of the release of vasodilating substances (anaphylactic or septic shock) or the loss of autonomic nervous innervation (spinal or neurogenic shock). The end result is profound vasodilation in the circulatory system and a decrease in systemic vascular resistance. This reduces venous return, causing decreased cardiac output and decreased blood pressure, resulting in shock.

NURSING PROCESS

Assessment

When assessing a client at risk for shock, the nurse must be aware of important signs and symptoms that are common to all types of shock. Client assessment requires the nurse to look (inspect), listen (auscultate), and feel (palpate) for vital signs, level of consciousness, skin color, and capillary refill. Common signs and symptoms of shock are listed in Table 54-1.

Normally, the rate of respirations is between 12 and 20 breaths per minute. Rapid, shallow respirations are frequently associated with shock because the body is trying to compensate and maintain an adequate supply of oxygen. The nurse must ensure that the airway is kept patent at all times.

It is important to note the level of consciousness of a client early in the course of evaluation and monitor for any subsequent changes. Progressive deterioration in the level of consciousness indicates an urgent need for intervention.

The pulse indicates the strength of the heart's contractions. A rapid, thready, weak pulse indicates shock from blood loss. Because the pulse is an immediate indicator of the client's condition, it should be taken frequently during any emergency condition.

LEARNING TIP

The term *thready* is used when referring to a weak pulse because when blood flow is reduced the pulse feels thin like a thread instead of full and bounding.

Changes in blood pressure may indicate changes in blood volume. These blood pressure changes can occur rapidly but usually not as swiftly as pulse changes occur.

Table 54–1. **Common Signs and Symptoms of Shock**

- Restlessness and anxiety
- Weak, rapid, thready pulse
- Cold and clammy skin
- Pale skin color
- Shallow, rapid, labored breathing
- Gradual and steadily falling blood pressure
- Alteration in consciousness in severe shock state
- Thirst

Initially for a short time, the blood pressure rises to compensate for the reduced blood volume. However, severe states of shock can cause the blood pressure to fall dramatically. This indicates insufficient pressure in the arterial system to supply blood to all the body organs.

Changes in skin temperature can result from shock. Cool, clammy skin is indicative of the sympathetic nervous system, the system activated for "fight or flight," being activated in response to the severe blood loss. Peripheral blood vessels constrict to shunt additional blood to vital organs. The vasoconstriction results in cool or cold skin. Clammy or diaphoretic skin is caused by sympathetic stimulation that attempts to cool the body, which it believes is working hard to "fight," and vasoconstriction because it is blood that makes the body warm. Skin color depends on the presence of circulating blood in the vessels of the skin. Pale, white, or ashen skin is indicative of insufficient circulation. In clients with deeply pigmented skin, color changes may be apparent in the nail beds, sclera of the eye, or mucous membranes in the mouth.

Capillary refill is checked on nailbeds to evaluate arterial circulation to an extremity. The nailbed is compressed to produce blanching and then released. Normally, the release of the pressure should result in a return of blood flow and nail color in less than 3 seconds. Clients in shock may have delayed or completely absent capillary refill.

Nursing Diagnosis

- Decreased cardiac output related to hypovolemia
- Altered cerebral tissue perfusion related to hypovolemia

Planning

The client's goal is to maintain vital signs and level of consciousness within normal limits.

Interventions

Clients who exhibit signs or symptoms of shock must be treated as soon as the evaluation of shock is made. It is important to help identify the probable cause of shock with data collection so the appropriate treatment is given.

Guiding principles for the nurse treating clients in shock are listed in Table 54-2. Administering supplemental oxy-

Table 54–2. **Guiding Principles for Treating Shock**

- Maintain an open airway and give oxygen as ordered.
- Control external bleeding by direct pressure.
- Elevate the lower extremities 10 to 12 inches.
- If possible, keep the client supine.
- Accurately record vital signs.
- Do not give the client anything to eat or drink.
- Administer IV fluids as ordered.

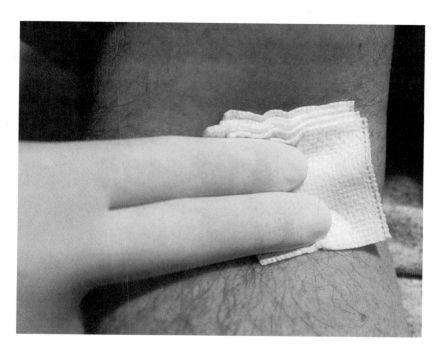

Figure 54–1. Application of pressure.

gen to the client in shock increases tissue oxygenation. External bleeding is controlled by applying direct pressure to stop the flow of blood and allow normal coagulation to occur (Fig. 54–1). If bleeding continues after a dressing is in place, additional manual pressure may be indicated. If additional dressings are needed, they are applied over the initial dressing. Elevation of a bleeding extremity helps stop venous bleeding and should be combined with direct pressure. When direct pressure and elevation do not control hemorrhage, pressure-point control should be attempted (Fig. 54–2). The chosen artery must be proximal to the injury site and overlie a bony structure against which the artery can be compressed to reduce blood flow to the injured site.

The client is protected from becoming cold by application of a blanket. The client should not be overheated because this causes peripheral blood vessels to dilate, which then takes blood away from vital organs. If possible, the client is kept calm and in a supine position. The lower extremities are elevated to promote venous return to the heart. Vital signs are continually taken, recorded, and reported to the physician if changes occur for treatment. The client is not given anything by mouth because the possibility of surgery exists. The physician orders IV fluids to increase circulating volume, which the LPN/LVN monitors.

Tourniquets are used only as a last resort in the control of bleeding. Their use is rarely necessary and generally not beneficial or effective. Absolute indications for the use of tourniquets are very few because they often produce more problems than benefits. Tourniquets can cause damage to nerves and blood vessels when they are improperly applied. If a tourniquet must be used, it should be applied in a very specific manner and, if possible, under physician direction. A wide bandage should always be used for a tourniquet. A wire, rope, belt, or any other material that is narrow or cuts into the skin should never be used. A tourniquet is never placed below the knee or elbow because nerves lie closer to the skin and are more susceptible to damage from compression. A blood pressure cuff can serve as a very effective tourniquet by applying the cuff proximal to the bleeding point and inflating it to stop the bleeding (Fig. 54–3). A tourniquet should never be covered with a bandage because it may be forgotten if it is not visible. The time of tourniquet application must always be documented, and it usually should be periodically released for a brief time.

The application of a pneumatic antishock garment (PASG) for the treatment of shock remains controversial,

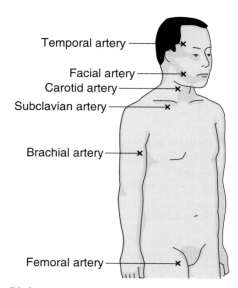

Temporal artery

Facial artery

Carotid artery

Subclavian artery

Brachial artery

Femoral artery

Figure 54–2. Arterial pressure points for control of bleeding.

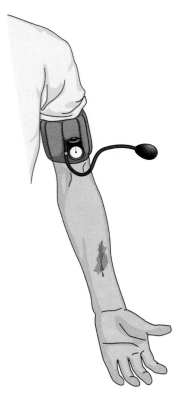

Figure 54–3. Use of a blood pressure cuff to apply pressure to an area of bleeding.

and some experts in emergency medicine recommend that it never be used. However, the PASG may have already been applied by prehospital personnel before the nurse encounters the client in shock. Possible indications of PASG are hypotension from hypovolemia due to abdominal or pelvic trauma. It is also used for splint of pelvic and extremity fractures. The inflated PASG causes an increase in tissue pressure and subsequent increase in total peripheral resistance. Its purpose is to improve blood flow to the brain, heart, and lungs. Once the blood pressure is stabilized by fluid replacement, the PASG is carefully discontinued with deflation. Deflation of the PASG should take place only in the emergency department or operating room under the supervision of a physician. The blood pressure must be carefully monitored during the deflation process.

Evaluation

Criteria for evaluating the outcome in the treatment of shock include a rising blood pressure, a bounding pulse, and warm, dry skin. The restless client becomes calmer. If signs of shock persist without desirable outcome criteria, the physician must be notified. Persistent shock can lead to irreversible shock and death.

Irreversible shock occurs when attempts to increase cardiac output and tissue perfusion fail. The body's compensatory mechanisms are no longer helpful, and medical interventions to alleviate shock are unsuccessful. The body's major organs can no longer function efficiently because organ tissue lacks adequate nutrition and perfusion. A backup of waste products causes acidosis. Severely decreased cardiac output and acidosis with multisystem organ failure leads to cardiac arrest and death.

Anaphylaxis

Anaphylaxis is a potentially life-threatening allergic reaction. Anaphylactic shock occurs when an individual has been previously sensitized to a foreign substance and reacts violently to a subsequent dose or contact with the substance. If the first exposure does not cause an allergic reaction, the nurse should not be misled by a client who reports prior contact with a suspected substance without incident. Every exposure after sensitization tends to produce a progresssively more severe reaction.

Clinical symptoms of an allergic reaction are listed in Table 54–3. Symptoms occur from a massive release of chemical mediators from mast cells and basophils throughout the body. Chemical mediators lead to vasodilation and capillary leaking that results in hypotension. Anaphylactic reactions may occur quickly and can result in a life-threatening condition.

PATHOPHYSIOLOGY

Anaphylactic shock is a form of distributive shock. There is no loss of blood, but there is excessive vasodilation. Bronchi constrict and air movement into the lungs becomes increasingly difficult. Increased fluid and mucus are secreted into the bronchial passages. Fluid in the air passages and constricted bronchi cause the development of wheezing. The body is rapidly deprived of needed oxygen by this respiratory system reaction. Signs of severe anaphylaxis include profound hypotension, decreased level of consciousness, and respiratory distress with stridor and cyanosis.

Nursing Diagnosis

- Breathing patterns ineffective related to airway compromise
- Decreased cardiac output related to vasodilation

Table 54–3. ***Clinical Symptoms of Allergic Reaction***

- Generalized itching and burning
- Urticaria (hives)
- Swelling about the lips and tongue
- Dyspnea
- Bronchospasm and wheezing
- Chest tightness and cough
- Anxiety
- Hypotension

Planning

The client's goal is to maintain vital signs and level of consciousness within normal limits.

Interventions

Nursing care quickly begins with monitoring the respiratory and cardiovascular status of the client. If possible, the offending antigen or allergen is identified and removed if still present, such as an insect stinger. When acute anaphylaxis occurs, airway compromise is an immediate threat to life. Symptoms of anaphylaxis must be treated quickly. The client is given oxygen for respiratory distress. Epinephrine is the drug of choice for treatment. Its effects decrease edematous tissue, dilate bronchial smooth muscle, and increase blood pressure by vasoconstriction. The standard adult dose of epinephrine is 0.2 mg to 0.5 mg of a 1:1000 solution given subcutaneously. Injections can be repeated every 10 to 15 minutes until the desired effect is achieved or significant side effects occur. Antihistamines are used as adjuncts in the therapy of anaphylaxis for control of rash and pruritis. Steroids may be given to prevent reexacerbation of symptoms.

Evaluation

When treatment is effective for anaphylactic shock, the client should show immediate reversal of shock symptoms. Breathing is easy, and blood pressure and pulse return to normal range. Breath sounds remain clear, and hives and pruritis subside.

Trauma

Trauma is the third-leading cause of death for all ages combined in the United States and the leading cause of death for persons between the ages of 1 and 44.[1] Injuries result in the death of more persons between the ages of 25 and 34 than in any other age group. The leading cause of death from 6 years to 33 years of age is motor vehicle crashes.

MECHANISM OF INJURY

When assessing the victim of trauma, it is important to determine the mechanism of injury (Gerontological Issues Box 54–1). This refers to the mechanisms whereby energy is transferred from the environment to the person. Injuries sustained from motor vehicle crashes, falls, gunshots, or any other moving source result from the mechanical energy that is loaded onto the victim and the body's response to that energy.

Injuries resulting from the transfer of mechanical energy are either penetrating or blunt. Penetrating, or open, injuries disrupt the skin; in blunt, or closed, injuries the skin surface is intact. The energy associated with blunt trauma

---

GERONTOLOGICAL ISSUES BOX 54–1

Injuries and Older Adults

Older adults are at a high risk for falls that put them at risk for bruises, abrasions, cuts, and fractures. Nurses who initially assess older adults with injuries requiring treatment must ask questions and perform assessments that would identify if the client is a victim of abuse or neglect.

Injuries Due to Falls versus Battery or Assault

Any unexplained bruises, burns, abrasions, cuts, fractures, evidence of old injuries or bruises, burns, and cuts that are in different stages of healing suggest abuse. The pattern of an injury can also suggest abuse—for example, cigarette burns in areas covered with clothing; bruises or friction burns in a ring around the neck, ankles, or wrists; welts, burns, or bruises in the outline of a hand or belt buckle; multiple similar injuries in an area, such as whip marks across the buttocks or back of the legs; defensive injury pattern of bruising; and trauma to the hands and forearms.

Injuries related to falls have a predictable injury pattern related to the history and report of the fall. If an older adult falls there would be bruising of the hands and knees as the person attempted to break the fall. Additional bruising or injuries to the front of the body, arms, and head could be caused by hitting furniture or other items during the fall. Skin tears on the arms are common with a fall. Often, a friend or family member sees the older adult starting to fall and tries to steady the person by grabbing the area, tearing the skin. Ask questions to be sure that the report of the fall incident is consistent with the presenting injuries.

Any form of abuse or suspicion of abuse needs to be reported to the state agency that investigates reports of suspected abuse. It is not the nurse's responsibility to prove that there has been abuse or neglect, only to report incidents or cases of possible abuse.

---

is more widespread around the impact point but can be absorbed by the underlying structures. Most injuries associated with motor vehicle crashes, motorcycle crashes, and falls are blunt. Penetrating trauma may be caused by a stick, a piece of glass, a bullet, or a knife.

The mechanism of injury from firearms is related to the energy created and dissipated by the bullet into the surrounding tissues. The localized crush of tissue in the missile's path causes tissue injury. The wounding forces of a missile depend on the projectile mass, type of tissue struck, striking velocity, and range. Entrance wounds are round or oval and may be surrounded by an abrasion rim. Powder burns are usually present if the firearm was discharged at close range. Exit wounds are usually larger than entrance wounds because the skin may "explode" as the bullet exits the body. This often produces a star-burst or stellate wound.

Penetrating injury can cause thoracic trauma in the absence of visible chest wounds. A bullet may enter the abdomen and travel upward through the diaphragm and into the thorax. All victims of gunshot wounds to the abdomen should be evaluated for thoracic injury. Victims of thoracic gunshot wounds should be evaluated for abdominal injury.

SURFACE TRAUMA

In a closed wound, the skin does not break. Damage occurs to tissues and blood vessels. Types of closed wounds include contusion (bruising), ecchymosis (discoloration), and hematoma (collection of blood under the skin).

In open wounds, the skin is broken. These wounds are susceptible to external hemorrhage and wound contamination. Types of open wounds are abrasions, lacerations, puncture wounds, avulsions, amputations, and impaled objects.

Abrasions are a scratching of the surface of the skin. The epidermis and part of the dermis are lost. Abrasions have little bleeding involved but can be extremely painful from involved nerve endings. Dirt may be ground into the wound and can pose an infection threat when large areas of skin are involved.

Lacerations are open wounds resulting from snagging or tearing of tissue. Skin tissue may be partly or completely torn away. Lacerations can cause significant bleeding if blood vessels or arteries are involved.

Puncture wounds result from sharp, narrow objects such as knives, nails, or high-velocity bullets. They can often be deceptive because the entrance wound may be small with little or no bleeding. It is difficult to estimate the extent of damage to underlying organs. Puncture wounds are usually not a bleeding problem unless they are located in the chest or abdomen.

Avulsions are full-thickness skin loss in which wound edges cannot be approximated. This type of injury is frequently seen with machine operators or lawn mower and power tool accidents.

Amputations occur when there is a tearing away or crushing of limbs from the body. There are three general types of amputation: complete, in which the body part is completely severed; partial, in which more than 50 percent of the body part is severed; and degloving, in which the skin and adipose tissue are torn away but underlying tissue is left intact. Complete amputations usually have less bleeding because blood vessels spasm and retract into the tissue. In partial or degloving amputations, lacerated arteries continue to bleed.

NURSING PROCESS OF SURFACE TRAUMA

Nursing Diagnosis

- Alteration in skin integrity related to tissue trauma
- Risk for fluid volume deficit related to hemorrhage
- Risk for infection related to tissue trauma

Planning

The client's goal is to maintain vital signs within normal limits, remain free of infection, and restore skin integrity.

Interventions

The management of closed soft tissue wounds includes ice and elevation of the affected part to decrease swelling of the injured tissue. The management of open wounds includes application of pressure to control bleeding. Open wounds are irrigated with sterile saline to thoroughly remove dirt and debris and clean exposed tissue to prevent infection. Saline irrigation is performed by using a gentle but firm stream of 100 mL of saline per centimeter of laceration. Potential injuries that could cause shock are identified and treated accordingly. Tetanus prophylaxis is administered to clients, if indicated by the last date of their tetanus booster.

If the client has sustained an amputation, bleeding is controlled with direct pressure and elevation. A tourniquet is applied only as a last resort. If a tourniquet is necessary, a blood pressure cuff is used to help control bleeding. A dressing is applied to the amputated extremity (referred to as the stump) with an elastic bandage for pressure. A degloving injury occurs when the mechanism of injury causes the skin of an extremity to be peeled away, exposing underlying bone and tissue. If there is a degloving injury, saline-soaked gauze is applied to the area to keep the tissue moist. Ice is never applied to a degloving injury because it may cause tissue necrosis.

Amputated parts should be sent to the hospital for possible reattachment. At the hospital, the amputated part is rinsed with a saline solution and wrapped in sterile gauze. It is placed in a plastic bag and sealed. The sealed plastic bag containing the amputated body part is placed in slushy ice water. The open end of the amputated limb is covered with sterile saline–moistened gauze and a dry dressing.

When caring for a client who has sustained an impaled-object injury, it is imperative that the object not be removed until the client is seen by a physician. Removing an impaled object may cause additional trauma during its extraction. A bulky dressing is applied to stabilize the object. The impaled object is removed only if it is causing airway obstruction. No pressure should be exerted on the object. Dressings are packed around the object and taped securely to reduce motion. Impaled objects are never cut off, broken off, or shortened unless transportation to the emergency department is otherwise impossible.

Evaluation

When treatment is effective for fluid volume deficit, vital signs remain normal, and for impaired skin integrity and risk for infection, the client's wound heals without development of infection.

SURFACE TRAUMA COMPLICATIONS

Tetanus is a serious disease caused by the bacillus *Clostridium tetani*. The bacillus organism enters the body through an open wound. Tetanus causes convulsions, muscle spasms, stiffness of the jaw, coma, and death. Immunization with tetanus toxoid should be initiated at 2 months of age and included in a series of pediatric immunizations. Additional booster vaccinations are recommended every 10 years. Tetanus prophylaxis is given after trauma when the wound is contaminated with dirt and the client has not had a booster for 5 years.

MULTISYSTEM TRAUMA

The victim of trauma may receive injury to an isolated organ system or multiple body systems. To recognize life-threatening conditions and determine priorities of care, the nurse must use a systematic process for the initial assessment of the trauma client. Experts in trauma care endorse the use of the primary survey when assessing the victim of major trauma. The primary survey has five components to guide the nurse in finding the most life-threatening injuries first. As each component is used for assessment, any life-threatening injuries are determined and interventions are implemented to correct them immediately. Priority is always given to the airway, breathing, and circulation. The components of the primary survey are listed in Table 54–4.

Primary Survey

A = Airway

The airway is the most important component of the primary survey. The airway is inspected while keeping the cervical spine stabilized. Partial or total airway obstruction may threaten the patency of the upper airway. The nurse should look for causes of airway obstruction, including loose teeth or foreign objects, bleeding, and vomitus.

Interventions include opening the airway, maintaining cervical spine immobilization, and removing obstructions. The jaw-thrust or chin-lift maneuver is used to open the airway. The neck is not hyperextended, flexed, or rotated until spinal injury is ruled out because any movement may cause cervical spine injury. If any life-threatening conditions compromising airway status are found, action must

be taken to correct the problem before assessment continues.

B = Breathing

After the patency of the airway is ensured, spontaneous breathing and respiratory rate and depth are noted. If breathing is absent, interventions are conducted before proceeding. The client is ventilated with a bag-valve-mask. Endotracheal intubation is always the preferred method of maintaining an airway because it ensures airway patency and eliminates the possibility of aspiration. After the airway is secure, spontaneous breathing is assessed by noting if the chest rises and falls and breath sounds are auscultated without passive ventilation being provided. The color of the skin is also noted to determine the oxygenation status.

C = Circulation

Pulses are palpated for quality and rate. The skin is inspected for color and temperature. Obvious signs of external bleeding are noted. Any life-threatening conditions that may compromise circulation are assessed and intervention provided before proceeding with further assessment. Examples of conditions that may compromise circulation include uncontrolled external bleeding, shock due to hemorrhage, or massive burns. Large-gauge IV cannulas (16, 18 gauge) are initiated for fluid resuscitation. If the client does not have a pulse, cardiopulmonary resuscitation must be initiated. If a pulse can be palpated, all vital signs are taken and recorded.

D = Disability

After assessing airway, breathing, and circulation, a brief neurological assessment is conducted to determine the degree of disability (D) as measured by the client's level of consciousness. The client's level of consciousness is determined by assessing responses to verbal or painful stimuli. Level of consciousness may range from being alert and talking to unresponsive. If the client appears unresponsive, a painful stimulus is applied such as rubbing the sternum, pressing a pen against the base of the nail, or applying periorbital pressure. The client is observed for any response to the pain, and the response is recorded.

E = Expose

To continue the assessment process and identify further injuries, the client must be exposed. Clothing is removed and, if necessary, cut off in order to perform an adequate head-to-toe assessment. History taking is initiated and not only includes details of the accident, but any available information regarding the client's medical history.

After the primary survey is done, a head-to-toe assessment is conducted on the entire body. Major body areas that may sustain trauma resulting in serious injury include the head and spine, chest, abdomen, and musculoskeletal system.

Table 54–4. Components of the Primary Survey

A—Airway
B—Breathing
C—Circulation
D—Disability (neurological status)
E—Expose the client

HEAD TRAUMA

Sharp blows to the head can cause shifting of intracranial contents and lead to brain tissue contusion. The pathophysiology of head trauma can be divided into two phases. The initial injury occurs at the time of the accident and cannot be reversed. The second phase of head injury involves the sequelae of the primary injury. Space-occupying lesions such as intracerebral bleeding or edema cause increased intracranial pressure (ICP). Management of head trauma is directed at decreasing volume and consequently decreasing ICP. Nursing care includes accurate identification of changes in neurological status and interventions to prevent further injury.

NURSING PROCESS OF HEAD TRAUMA

Assessment

The mechanism of injury is determined to identify the extent of injury. The level of consciousness is assessed. The Glasgow Coma Scale is a tool that is used to objectively rate a client's level of consciousness.[2] It has become the most popular tool used to assess level of consciousness after head trauma (Fig. 54–4). The highest score that a client can obtain is 15, which indicates that the client is alert and only needs observation. The lowest possible score is 3, which indicates coma and the need for immediate intervention. Morbidity and mortality sharply increase for clients with scores of eight and below. Early and late signs and symptoms of increased ICP are listed in Table 54–5. Pupil size and reaction are noted and monitored. A dilated or nonreactive pupil indicates increased ICP and requires immediate physician notification and intervention to reduce ICP.

Nursing Diagnosis

- Tissue perfusion, altered cerebral, related to cerebral edema

Planning

The client's goal is to remain alert and oriented.

Interventions

Oxygen is administered to the client who has sustained head trauma. If the client has an altered level of consciousness or deteriorating respiratory effort, endotracheal intubation is performed. Oxygen delivery and ventilation improve cerebral tissue oxygenation and perfusion. Intravenous access is established to maintain hemodynamic stability and access for medications. Mannitol IV, an osmotic diuretic, may be ordered to decrease cerebral edema. Computed tomography (CT) and magnetic resonance imaging (MRI) scans with x-rays direct definitive treatment for the client.

Evaluation

Criteria for evaluating a positive outcome in the treatment of head trauma include a client's Glasgow Coma Score of 14 to 15. The goal is met if the client is alert, oriented, and able to follow verbal commands; vital signs are within nor-

GLASGOW COMA SCALE	
Areas of Response	**Points**
Eye Opening	
Eyes open spontaneously	4
Eyes open in response to voice	3
Eyes open in response to pain	2
No eye opening response	1
Best Verbal Response	
Oriented (e.g., to person, place, time)	5
Confused, speaks but is disoriented	4
Inappropriate, but comprehensible words	3
Incomprehensible sounds but no words are spoken	2
None	1
Best Motor Response	
Obeys command to move	6
Localizes painful stimulus	5
Withdraws from painful stimulus	4
Flexion, abnormal decorticate posturing	3
Extension, abnormal decerebrate posturing	2
No movement or posturing	1
Total Possible Points	**3–15**
Major Head Injury	**≤8**
Moderate Head Injury	**9–12**
Minor Head Injury	**13–15**

Figure 54–4. The Glasgow Coma Scale is used to determine level of consciousness.

Table 54–5. **Signs and Symptoms of Increased Intracranial Pressure**

Early Signs and Symptoms of Increased ICP
Headache
Nausea and vomiting
Amnesia
Altered level of consciousness
Changes in speech
Drowsiness

Late Signs and Symptoms of Increased ICP
Dilated nonreactive pupils
Unresponsiveness
Abnormal posturing
Widening pulse pressure
Decreased pulse rate
Changes in respiratory pattern

mal limits; and pupils are equal in size, shape, and reactivity to light.

SPINE TRAUMA

The cervical spine is vulnerable to injury when trauma occurs. Clients who have sustained multiple injuries should be suspected of having spinal cord injury, especially when signs of head trauma are present. All trauma clients should be treated for spinal cord injury until it is proven otherwise. This involves stabilization of the neck and back by using cervical collars and backboards (Fig. 54–5).

NURSING PROCESS OF SPINE TRAUMA

Assessment

Spinal cord injury at the level of C5 and above interferes with diaphragmatic function and affects respiratory effort, which must be carefully assessed.

Spinal nerves are located in the spinal cord and transmit motor impulses to the body. The thoracic nerves innervate the thorax, abdomen, buttocks, and portions of the upper arm. The lumbar nerves innervate the groin region and lower extremities. The sacral nerves supply the perianal muscles, which control voluntary contraction of the external bladder sphincter and the external anal sphincter. The higher the traumatic lesion on the spinal column, the greater the loss of muscle and sensory function (Table 54–6). The client's ability to move each extremity is noted and recorded.

Nursing Diagnosis

- Ineffective breathing pattern related to neck injury
- Ineffective airway clearance related to neck injury
- Impaired mobility related to neck injury

Table 54–6. *Assessment of Motor Function*

If the Client Is Unable to:	The Lesion Is above the Level of:
Extend and flex arms	C5 to C7
Extend and flex legs	L2 to L4
Flex foot, extend toes	L4 to L5
Tighten anus	S3 to S5

Planning

The client's goal is to maintain arterial blood gases within normal limits and maintain or increase mobility.

Interventions

During initial treatment of a client with probable neck trauma, it is imperative that the neck remain immobilized. A cervical collar and backboard must be in place. If the cervical spinal cord has been traumatized, the effectiveness of breathing may be altered. If signs of respiratory distress are present, oxygen is administered to improve tissue oxygenation. Adjunct airway equipment, including an endotracheal tube, must be readily available.

Evaluation

Outcome criteria for effectively treating cervical spine trauma include a regular rate, rhythm, and pattern of breathing; maintaining clear lung sounds by protecting the airway from aspiration; and maintaining mobility.

CHEST TRAUMA

Chest trauma can present significant problems because of the organ systems involved. Damage to the heart and lungs can result in life-threatening injuries. Immediately life-

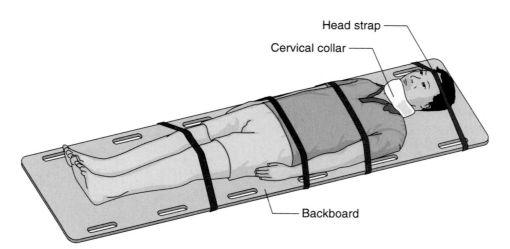

Figure 54–5. Immobilization of client suspected of having spinal cord injury using backboard and cervical collar.

threatening injuries include pericardial tamponade, massive hemothorax, tension pneumothorax, and flail chest. Potentially life-threatening injuries include pulmonary contusion, aortic disruption, diaphragmatic hernia, tracheobronchial disruption, and myocardial contusion.

Chest trauma can result in laceration of lung tissue and cause a change in the negative intrapleural pressure. Air or blood leaking into the intrapleural space collapses the lung, resulting in a hemothorax and ineffective ventilation. Deep penetrating wounds to the chest can cause a tension pneumothorax in which a flap of skin acts as a one-way valve allowing air to enter the wound during inhalation and trapping it inside the pleural space during exhalation. Air that is forced into the pleural cavity without being able to escape causes increased pressure, which compresses the lung and displaces the heart and great vessels toward the unaffected side. The trachea shifts from the midline and impairs ventilation. Blood flow to and from the heart is greatly reduced, causing a decrease in cardiac output. An uncorrected tension pneumothorax is fatal.

Chest trauma can cause injury to the heart and great vessels and reduce the amount of circulating blood volume. The heart may be bruised (myocardial contusion) or may sustain direct trauma. Blood can rapidly accumulate in the pericardial sac around the heart, causing pericardial tamponade. Increased pressure causes the heart to become compressed, resulting in a significant decrease in cardiac output. The client with cardiac tamponade exhibits hypotension, tachycardia, and neck vein distention and requires immediate intervention.

NURSING PROCESS OF CHEST TRAUMA

Assessment

The mechanism of injury is determined to identify the extent of injury. Clients with major chest injuries can have dramatic symptoms. They may exhibit classic signs of shock with cyanosis, dyspnea, and restlessness. The client's breathing pattern and effectiveness of respirations are assessed. The rise and fall of the chest is observed, as well as symmetrical chest movement. Multiple rib fractures may cause a paradoxical movement resulting in lung injury. Distended neck veins may indicate increased intrathoracic pressure because of a tension pneumothorax or pericardial tamponade. If the trachea is shifted to one side, a tension pneumothorax or massive hemothorax may be present. Any bruising on the skin is noted. Seat belts and restraint systems can cause significant bruising in high-impact crashes. Penetrating chest wounds may compromise ventilation.

Nursing Diagnosis

- Ineffective breathing pattern related to unstable chest wall segment or lung collapse
- Fluid volume deficit related to hemorrhage

- Decreased cardiac output related to compression of heart and great vessels

Planning

The client's goal is to maintain arterial blood gases and vital signs within normal limits.

Interventions

Clients with major chest injuries require immediate treatment. Supplemental oxygen is administered to promote tissue oxygenation. The nurse should be prepared to assist with chest tube insertion to relieve a tension pneumothorax or hemothorax. IV fluids are initiated to increase circulating volume. The client's vital signs are continuously monitored to detect signs of shock. Respiratory status is observed to detect ineffective ventilation.

Clients with unstable vital signs need immediate surgical intervention in the operating room. Clients with stable vital signs undergo radiographic studies to determine the extent of cardiac or pulmonary injury.

Evaluation

Outcome criteria for evaluating the client with chest trauma include maintenance of a patent airway and effective breathing pattern. Respirations are of normal rate and depth with equal chest expansion. Dyspnea and cyanosis are absent. Vital signs are within normal limits. Urinary output is 30 to 50 mL per hour. Skin color is normal, and skin is warm and dry. Jugular vein distention is absent and the trachea is midline.

ABDOMINAL TRAUMA

The abdominal cavity contains solid and hollow organs. The organs of the abdomen are vulnerable to injury because there is limited bony protection. Extensive hemorrhage can result from injuries to the abdomen. The spleen and liver have a rich blood supply and are frequently injured in severe blunt abdominal trauma. Rapid loss of large blood volumes can occur. A full bladder can rise into the abdominal cavity. If a distended bladder ruptures, urine is likely to leak into the abdomen. Abdominal organs can be bruised or rupture from blunt trauma. Penetrating trauma can cause lacerations to abdominal organs.

NURSING PROCESS OF ABDOMINAL TRAUMA

Assessment

Vital signs are taken to detect tachycardia and hypotension from shock. The shape of the abdomen is observed to detect distention from intra-abdominal hemorrhage. Skin color and any bruising across the abdomen are noted. Open wounds and penetrating trauma are noted. The abdomen is auscultated for bowel sounds. The perineum is inspected and observed for blood from the urethra.

Nursing Diagnosis

- Fluid volume deficit related to abdominal organ injury
- Altered urinary elimination related to urethral or renal trauma

Planning

The client's goal is to maintain vital signs and urinary output within normal limits.

Interventions

Abdominal organs may be injured as a result of severe blunt or penetrating trauma. If hypotension is present, intra-abdominal hemorrhage may exist. IV fluids are administered to restore circulating volume. An indwelling urinary catheter may be ordered. Catheterization is contraindicated if blood is present at the urethra. A nasogastric tube may be inserted to decompress the stomach. Abdominal wounds are covered with a sterile dressing. If abdominal organs are exposed, they are covered with a sterile saline–soaked dressing to prevent tissue necrosis.

Evaluation

Expected outcome criteria for clients with abdominal trauma include effective circulating volume as evidenced by vital signs within normal limits. Skin or mucous membrane color is pink, and skin is warm and dry to touch. Urine output is 30 to 50 mL per hour. Hematuria is absent.

ORTHOPEDIC TRAUMA

Fractured bones can result in blood loss, compromised circulation, and immobility. Unstable pelvic fractures can cause injury to the genitourinary system or a disruption to the veins in the pelvis. Large bone fractures can cause significant blood loss. For example, a fractured femur can cause up to 1500 mL of blood loss. A fractured tibia or humerus can cause up to 750 mL of blood loss. Multiple fractures with other injuries can result in hemorrhagic shock. Joint dislocations can cause neurovascular compromise by the bones applying pressure to the nerve and blood vessel. Delayed fracture reduction (realignment or setting) can lead to avascular necrosis, which leads to dead tissue and bone.

NURSING PROCESS OF ORTHOPEDIC TRAUMA

Assessment

Vital signs are assessed to detect abnormalities. The injured extremity is inspected, and skin color and capillary refill are noted. Skin integrity and any protruding bone or deformity are observed. If a joint is dislocated, the distal pulses are palpated to assess circulation to the area. Motor function is assessed to determine abnormality in movement or sensation of the injured extremity.

Nursing Diagnosis

- Fluid volume deficit related to hemorrhage
- Impaired physical mobility related to bone injury

Planning

The client's goal is to maintain vital signs within normal limits and mobility at baseline level.

Interventions

The nurse prepares to splint and immobilize the affected extremity if there is a deformity. Splinting the extremity prevents further damage to surrounding tissue by broken bone ends. It also provides comfort for the client. A piece of cardboard or a pillow can be used as a splint until the client is evaluated by a physician. Jewelry is removed before applying the splint. The joints above and below the deformity are immobilized. Pulses and **capillary refill** are assessed after splint application to determine circulatory status. The extremity is elevated and ice applied to reduce edema. Dislocated joints are splinted in the position they are found. If distal circulation is compromised, medical treatment, by a physician only, is immediately required to relocate the joint. If the client exhibits symptoms of hypovolemic shock, IV fluids are administered as ordered. IV fluids are used to increase circulatory volume.

LEARNING TIP

Splint it where it lies, to prevent further damage.

Evaluation

Outcome criteria for clients with orthopedic trauma include effective circulating volume as evidenced by strong, palpable pulses and normal blood pressure. Skin color is normal, and skin is warm and dry to touch. Capillary refill is less than 3 seconds. Motor function of the affected extremity is normal.

Burns

Burn injuries are acutely painful events that may be dramatic in appearance. Burn victims often face devastating problems, not only from the initial event but from subsequent hospitalizations, long-term rehabilitation, and psychosocial impact. Nursing care depends on the extent and depth of the burn injury and the presence of any associated factors such as smoke inhalation, blunt trauma, or fractures. The client's age may contribute to potential mortality. Infants less than 2 years of age and elderly clients over 60 years of age have less reserve available to survive a major burn.

The skin protects the body by preventing bacterial or viral invasion, enhancing temperature regulation, and conserving body fluids and electrolytes. These functions are impaired with a burn injury and can cause physiological alterations that can be multisystem in scope. The more extensive the burn injury, the greater the potential for complications and mortality.

TYPES OF BURNS

Burns can be thermal, chemical, or electrical. The most common burns are thermal burns, caused by steam, scalds, fire injuries, or contact with hot substances. Chemical burns are caused by acids or alkalis. Alkali burns are usually more serious than acid burns because alkali penetrate deeper and burn longer. The concentration of the chemical agent and the duration of exposure determine the extent and depth of damage. Electrical burns can be caused by low-voltage (alternating) current or high-voltage (alternating or direct) current. Radiation burns are similar to thermal burns and can occur from overexposure to ultraviolet light (sunburn) or heat of an atomic explosion. Nuclear radiation burns vary in severity depending on the distance between the victim and heat of the atomic explosion.

BURN PATHOPHYSIOLOGY

Three factors influence the extent of the burn injury: the intensity of the energy source, the duration of exposure to the energy source, and the conductance of the tissue exposed. Increased intensity with increased exposure causes increased amounts of tissue damage. Initially, there is decreased blood flow to the local burn area followed by vasodilation and increased **capillary permeability.** Vasodilation and increased capillary permeability occur as a result of histamine release from thermally injured cells. This causes fluid and electrolytes to leak from cells into the interstitial space. These responses cause intravascular fluid loss and can place the client at risk for hypovolemic shock. Fluid can also be lost directly through the burn wound. As fluid evaporates, body temperature decreases. Hypothermia can occur in the client with extensive thermal burn injuries. **Hypoproteinemia** results from capillary permeability, allowing fluid to leak and cause edema in the nonburned tissue. The severity of the burn injury is determined by the extent of the burn (percentage of body surface area burned), the depth of the burn wounds, age of the client, past medical history, and area of the body burned.

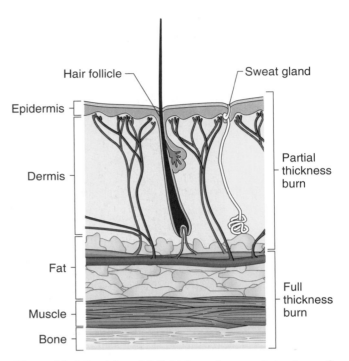

Figure 54–6. Partial- and full-thickness burns and structures affected.

BURN CLASSIFICATION

Burns are classified as either **partial-thickness burns** or **full-thickness burns** based on the surface appearance of the wound (Fig. 54–6). Partial-thickness burns can be either superficial or deep. Superficial partial-thickness burns involve only the first two or three layers of the epidermis of the skin. These wounds appear red and moist and cause local pain. Common examples of this type of burn include sunburns and minor steam burns. This type of burn generally heals in 2 to 7 days.

Deep partial-thickness burns involve the entire epidermal layer and part of the dermis. These burns appear red or mottled and are more painful. The epidermis is blistered or broken (Fig. 54–7). Deep partial-thickness burns can become full-thickness injuries if they become infected or if there is further trauma to the site.

Full-thickness burns involve all the layers of the skin and the subcutaneous tissue. The burn appears pale white or charred, red or brown, and leathery. Nerve endings have been destroyed, so the severely burned area may be without feeling and is usually painless. However, the surrounding less severely burned areas may remain extremely painful and sensitive to circulating air movement.

The extent of the burn is the percent of total body surface area (TBSA) burned. The most common method of estimating the burn area is called the **rule of nines,** which di-

---

hypoproteinemia: hypo—under + protos—first + haima—blood

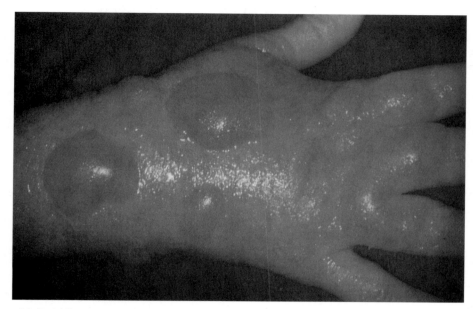

Figure 54–7. A blistered partial-thickness thermal burn. (From Goldsmith, Lazarus, and Tarp: Adult and Pediatric Dermatology: A Color Guide to Diagnosis and Treatment. FA Davis, Philadelphia, 1997, p 318, with permission.)

vides the total body surface into areas consisting of 9 percent or multiples of 9 percent (Fig. 54–8).

NURSING PROCESS FOR BURNS

Assessment

The assessment of the burn client begins with the ABCs of the primary survey. The history should include the mechanism and time of the injury and a description of the surrounding environment. Information is obtained regarding the presence of noxious chemicals, the possibility of smoke inhalation, or any related trauma. The greatest threat to life in a major burn is smoke or heat inhalation injury. Continuous assessment of respiratory status is essential. Burns of the face, sooty mucous membranes, singed nasal hairs, a hoarse voice, and restlessness are signs of potential lung injury.

Nursing Diagnosis

- Fluid volume deficit related to abnormal fluid loss secondary to increased capillary permeability
- Pain related to major burn
- Risk for infection related to impaired skin integrity

See Nursing Care Plan Box 54–2.

Planning

The client's goals are to maintain vital signs within normal limits, have pain relieved, remain free of infection, and restore skin integrity.

Interventions

The first responsibility when caring for a burned person is to stop any further burning from occurring. The victim is removed from the burning area. If the victim's clothing is on fire, the victim is placed on the ground and rolled in a blanket. All jewelry is removed as soon as possible because swelling begins soon after injury. The burned area is covered with a dry sterile dressing or clean linen. If the TBSA appears to be less than 10 percent, cool saline-moistened sterile dressings may be applied within the first 10 minutes to help relieve pain and reduce the heat content of the tissue. Generally, wet dressings should not be used if the TBSA is greater than 10 percent because they provide an open pathway for bacteria and cause hypothermia. Ointments, lotions, butter, and antiseptics are never used on the burn area because they may promote infection, hold in heat, and cause more pain to the victim. Blisters should not be broken because they provide a protective covering to underlying tissue. Cold packs and ice are never placed over the burn area because they can cause further tissue damage.

Burns of the face swell rapidly and can compromise the airway. The head of the stretcher is elevated 30 degrees to minimize edema. Oxygen is administered to the client with potential pulmonary injury. Because abnormal fluid losses occur in burn injuries, an IV infusion should be initiated. The client's weight and extent of the burn determines fluid resuscitation needs.

The client is kept warm because the burn victim cannot maintain body heat. Narcotics are administered for pain. Partial-thickness burn wounds that involve a small area can be cleansed with a sterile saline solution. Silver sulfadiazine (Silvadene) cream is applied in a ⅛-inch layer and

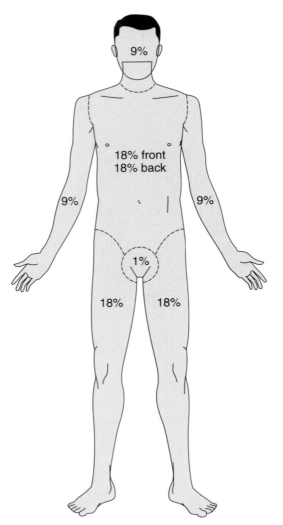

Figure 54–8. The rule of nines: used to assess the body surface extent of burns using 9 percent and multiples of 9 percent.

covered with bulky, fluffed dressings. Silvadene facilitates germicidal activity and is soothing to the burn. Major full-thickness wounds are covered with dry, sterile dressings or linen. Clients who have sustained major full-thickness burns are transferred to the burn unit.

Evaluation

When treatment is effective for fluid volume deficit, vital signs remain normal. The goal for pain is met if the client reports satisfactory relief. The goal for impaired skin integrity and risk for infection is met if the client's wounds heal without development of infection.

CHEMICAL BURNS

Chemical burns differ from thermal burns in that the burning process continues until the agent is inactivated, neutralized, or diluted with water. The degree of damage by a chemical agent is dependent on the concentration and quantity of the agent, its mechanism of action, and the duration of contact. Most chemical burns are caused by strong acids or alkalis that get on the skin or clothing. Fumes of strong chemicals can cause pulmonary burns. Eyes can also be exposed to chemical burns.

To stop the burning process of most chemical burns, all saturated clothing is removed and the burn is copiously irrigated with water. A forceful stream of water is not used on the client because the extreme water pressure may add injury to the burned skin. Strong alkalis may cause more severe burns than strong acids because they penetrate more deeply into the tissues. Dry chemicals such as lime must be brushed off before flushing with water because they may be activated by contact with water and cause more damage to the skin. Because residual amounts of chemicals can be retained in the creases of clothes, all clothing and shoes must be removed.

Many times the eyes are involved in chemical burns and can have serious damage. The eye must be flooded with water. In the prehospital area, flush the eye by supporting the client's head under a faucet of running water. Be careful not to wash the chemicals into the uninjured eye. The eyelids must be held open while irrigating the eye. Use a gentle stream of water and flood the eye for at least 5 minutes for an acid chemical burn and 10 to 20 minutes for an alkali burn. After flushing the eye, the client should immediately seek medical care for evaluation of the injury and further irrigation in the emergency department. Nothing but water is put in the eye because other substances may cause further injury.

ELECTRICAL BURNS

Electrical burns frequently are much more serious than their surface appearance. As the electrical current passes through the body, it damages the inner tissues, leaving little evidence of a burn on the skin surface. The type and voltage of the circuit, resistance, pathway of transmission through the body, and duration of contact are taken into consideration to determine the amount of damage sustained.

The energy from a high-voltage electrical current passing through the body may disrupt the normal electrical rhythm of the heart and cause cardiac arrest. The electrical current may cause violent muscle contractions that could result in fractures or dislocations. From the point of entry, the electrical current follows the path of least resistance, causing one or more tracks of damage.

Lightning strikes contain massive amounts of energy (up to 50 million volts) and can cause temperatures in excess of 50,000°F. Although there is much greater energy from a lightning injury, its duration is usually only a fraction of a second and rarely causes deep tissue injury. A victim may suffer a direct lightning strike or a flashover when lightning strikes nearby. The major types of injuries that

NURSING CARE PLAN BOX 54–2 FOR THE CLIENT WITH BURNS

Fluid volume deficit related to abnormal fluid loss secondary to increased capillary permeability

Client Outcome
Client has adequate fluid volume as evidenced by normal vital signs.

Evaluation of Outcome
Are blood pressure, pulse, and respiratory rate within normal limits? Is urinary output adequate?

Interventions	Rationale	Evaluation
Monitor vital signs and report abnormalities.	Changes in heart rate and blood pressure can be readily detected.	Is pulse rate less than 100? Is blood pressure within normal limits?
Give intravenous fluids as ordered.	Adequate fluid volume can be achieved by infusing intravenous fluids.	Is client's urinary output 30–50 mL/hr?

Potential for ineffective airway clearance related to edema from burn injury

Client Outcome
Client has airway clearance as evidenced by absence of respiratory distress and hoarse voice.

Evaluation of Outcome
Is respiratory rate within normal limits? Is pulse oximetry reading above 90%? Can the client talk without a hoarse voice?

Interventions	Rationale	Evaluation
Assess for burns to the face or soot around the mouth and nose.	Burns to the face swell rapidly and can compromise airway. Evidence of soot can be a sign of smoke inhalation and pulmonary injury.	Is respiratory rate between 10 and 20? Is pulse oximetry reading above 90%?
Elevate the head of the bed 30 degrees.	Elevation can minimize edema by dependent gravity.	Can client talk without a hoarse voice?

Pain related to major burn

Client Outcome
Client states pain is relieved.

Evaluation of Outcome
Does client state pain is relieved?

Interventions	Rationale	Evaluation
Administer narcotics as ordered.	Burns cause damage or exposure of the nerve endings.	Does client state pain is relieved?
Cover burned areas with sterile dressings or linen.	Air movement over exposed nerve endings increases pain.	Does client report comfort?

Body image disturbance related to burns

Client Outcome
Client can verbalize feelings about the burn experience and body appearance.

continued

NURSING CARE PLAN BOX 54–2 *(continued)*

Evaluation of Outcome
Does the client talk about the burn experience and altered body appearance?

Interventions	Rationale	Evaluation
Demonstrate acceptance of client's experience and appearance. Encourage client to verbalize feelings about the burns.	Changes in physical appearance can alter client's self-perception.	Does the client verbalize feelings to staff and family members?

Potential for infection related to altered skin integrity

Client Outcome
Client will show no signs of infection as evidenced by vital signs, absence of purulent wound drainage, and lab results.

Evaluation of Outcome
Is the client afebrile? Is the white blood cell (WBC) count less than 10,000? Is the burn wound absent of purulent drainage?

Interventions	Rationale	Evaluation
Wear gown, gloves, and mask when caring for client. Do frequent hand washing. Monitor client's temperature and lab results.	The client's first line of defense (the skin) can no longer provide protection from bacterial or viral invasion. Abnormal readings are detected and can be reported to physician.	Is the burn wound absent of purulent wound drainage? Is WBC count less than 10,000? Is client's core temperature normal?

---

result from lightning are cardiac arrest, neurological injuries, blunt trauma, and superficial burns. Surface burns from lightning have a spidery, feathery, branching appearance.

Clients with minor injuries are usually conscious. They may have briefly lost consciousness and are frequently confused. Moderately injured persons show more obvious altered mentation and may be combative or comatose. The most common cause of death in lightning injuries is cardiopulmonary arrest. Severe lightning strikes may cause paralysis to the medullary respiratory center, causing respiratory arrest before cardiac arrest. For this reason, when assessing the client who sustained a lightning strike, the cardiopulmonary status must be assessed immediately.

 CRITICAL THINKING: Mr. Smith

Mr. Smith is a 28-year-old man who was welding close to a natural gas line. The flame of the welder caused an explosion of the gas line, throwing Mr. Smith 50 feet. He landed on his back. He is brought to the emergency department by rescue squad. Mr. Smith is awake, alert, and oriented. He has soot around his mouth and nose. He sustained deep partial-thickness burns to his neck, upper chest, and both forearms. He is complaining of pain from his burns and also thoracic back and hip pain. His pulse rate is 100. His blood pressure is 160/90. Respiratory rate is 20.

1. What is the first priority of care for Mr. Smith?
2. What can soot around the mouth and nose indicate?
3. What symptoms should the nurse look for during assessment?
4. Are Mr. Smith's vital signs within normal limits?
5. Would wet dressings or dry dressings be preferable for large areas of deep partial-thickness burns?
6. Mr. Smith is wearing a gold chain necklace and a wedding ring. Should they be removed immediately, or should the nurse wait until Mr. Smith's wife arrives to take them? Why?
7. Mr. Smith continues to complain of hip and back pain. In reviewing his mechanism of injury, what other injuries could Mr. Smith have?
8. After 30 minutes in the emergency department, Mr. Smith is transferred to the burn unit. He is still alert and able to talk, but his voice sounds raspy. Is airway clearance still a priority when assessing Mr. Smith?

Answers at end of chapter.

Hypothermia

Body temperature is maintained within a narrow range on either side of 98.6°F (36°C) to allow chemical reactions in the body to work most efficiently. When the body is exposed to freezing temperatures, mechanisms that maintain body temperature may become overwhelmed and cold exposure results. Cold exposure may cause injury to individual body parts or the entire body. When the body temperature falls, hypothermia occurs.

Body heat is lost to the environment through conduction, convection, radiation, and evaporation. Heat loss is inversely proportional to body size and body fat. Fat insulates because it has less blood flow and consequently has less ability to vasodilate and lose heat. Therefore large people conserve heat better than small people, obese people better than thin people, and adults better than children.

NURSING PROCESS

Assessment of Stages of Hypothermia

Hypothermia occurs when the core body temperature falls below 95°F (35°C). As core temperature falls below 95°F, the body is less able to regulate its temperature and generate body heat, causing progressive loss of body heat to occur (Table 54-7).

Table 54-7. **Hypothermia Related to Exposure to Cold Environment**

Defining Characteristics
- Core body temperature below 95°F (35°C)
- Skin cold to touch
- Uncoordination, slurred speech
- At core body temperature below 91.4°F (33°C):
    Cardiac dysrhythmias
    Cyanosis
- At core body temperature below 89.6°F (32°C):
    Shivering replaced by muscle rigidity
    Hypotension
    Dilated pupils
- At core body temperature below 82.4°F (28°C):
    Absent deep tendon reflexes
    Hypoventilation (3 to 4 breaths/min)
    Ventricular fibrillation possible
- At core body temperature below 80.6°F (27°C):
    Coma
    Flaccid muscles
    Fixed, dilated pupils
    Ventricular fibrillation to cardiac standstill
    Apnea

Outcome Criteria
- Core body temperature is greater than 95°F (35°C).
- Client is alert and oriented.
- Cardiac dysrhythmias are absent.
- Acid-base balance is normal.
- Pupils react normally.

In cases of mild hypothermia (core temperature between 90°F and 95°F) the client is usually alert and shivering. Clients may appear clumsy, apathetic, or irritable. Metabolism initially increases to generate heat. Hypoglycemia can occur because glucose and glycogen stores are depleted by long-term shivering. Symptoms of mild hypothermia include shivering, hypoglycemia, and increased respiratory rate, heart rate, and cardiac output.

More severe hypothermia occurs between 85°F and 90°F (29°C and 32°C). Shivering stops and muscle activity decreases. Initially, fine muscle coordination ceases. As core body temperature continues to drop, all muscle activity stops and all muscles become rigid. The client becomes lethargic and less interested in combating the cold environment. Metabolism begins to decrease. Level of consciousness begins to markedly decrease at 89.6°F (32°C), and clients become lethargic or disoriented and begin to hallucinate. The pupils become dilated. As the core body temperature falls to 82°F (28°C), there is a decrease in vital signs. The client hypoventilates, taking only 3 or 4 breaths per minute, or becomes apneic. The pulse becomes slower and weaker. Cardiac dysrhythmias may occur. The profoundly hypothermic client has a core temperature of less than 80°F (27°C) and usually appears dead without obtainable vital signs. Determination of death can be made only after aggressive core rewarming to at least 90°F (32°C) occurs without return of a cardiac rhythm.

Nursing Diagnosis

- Hypothermia related to cold exposure

See Nursing Care Plan Box 54–3.

Planning

The client's goal is to maintain a body temperature within normal limits.

Interventions

Initial treatment of the hypothermic client consists of stabilizing the vital functions and preventing further heat loss. The client is removed from the cold environment. All wet clothing is removed to prevent further heat loss. The client is wrapped in warm, dry blankets. Active core rewarming interventions include administering warm, humidified oxygen and placing the client on a thermal heating blanket. Core body temperature is constantly monitored using a rectal probe. If available, warm IV fluids should be administered. Aggressive measures for the critically hypothermic client may include heated gastric lavage, heated peritoneal dialysis, or cardiopulmonary bypass. During aggressive resuscitation emergency, cardiac drugs are given sparingly because as the body warms, peripheral vasodilation occurs. Drugs that remain in the periphery are suddenly released, leading to a bolus effect that may cause fatal dysrhythmias.

NURSING CARE PLAN BOX 54–3 FOR THE CLIENT WITH HYPOTHERMIA		
Hypothermia related to exposure to cold environment		

Client Outcome
Client's body temperature and vital signs are within normal limits.

Evaluation of Outcome
Is client's body temperature greater than 95°F (35°C)? Is client alert and oriented? Is cardiac rhythm normal?

Interventions	*Rationale*	*Evaluation*
Monitor client's core body temperature. Assess skin temperature. Monitor pulse and electrocardiogram rhythm. Monitor client's level of consciousness.	Abnormal body temperature can be detected and treated. Cardiac dysrhythmias may occur at temperatures below 91.4°F (33°C). Level of consciousness becomes markedly decreased at temperatures of 89.6°F (32°C).	Is body temperature greater than 95°F (35°C)? Is skin cold to touch? Are pulse rate and electrocardiogram rhythm normal? Is the client alert?
Institute rewarming by applying a thermal blanket.	Rapid, active rewarming is necessary to return body temperature to desirable range.	Is body core temperature rising to normal range?

Evaluation

Desired outcome criteria for the client with hypothermia include a core body temperature greater than 95°F (35°C). The client is alert and oriented. Cardiac dysrhythmias are absent, and pulse and blood pressure are within normal limits.

Frostbite

The extremities are vulnerable to cold injury. Frostnip occurs when exposed parts of the body become very cold but not frozen. This condition is usually not painful. The skin becomes pale and blanched. Contact with a warm object such as someone's hand may be all that is needed to rewarm the part. During rewarming, tingling and redness of the affected part occur.

Frostbite occurs when body parts become frozen. The affected tissues feel hard and frozen. Most frostbitten parts are a white, yellow-white, or blue-white color. Similar to a burn, the depth of damage to the skin can vary. When rewarmed, the skin appears deep red, hot, and dry to touch. After thawing, damaged cells die and gangrene can occur. The severity of a cold injury is determined by the duration of the exposure, the temperature to which the body part was exposed, and the wind velocity during exposure. Shunting of blood away from the extremities occurs to maintain core body temperature. This increases the risk of cold injury to the extremities.

Interventions for frostbite include protecting the affected area from further trauma. The frostbitten part is never rubbed with anything because this causes further tissue damage. The injured part is loosely covered with a dry, sterile dressing. The client is not allowed to stand or walk on a frostbitten foot. The affected extremity is elevated to minimize edema to promote blood flow.

Hyperthermia

When heat exposure causes the body's normal regulatory mechanisms to become overwhelmed, the body is no longer able to tolerate the excessive heat. The body's heat-dissipation mechanisms fail, causing heat-related emergencies to occur. Usually, the body's heat-regulating mechanisms work very well and people are able to tolerate significant temperature changes quite well. However, when these mechanisms become overwhelmed, the consequences can be disastrous and irreversible at a rapid rate.

The body absorbs heat from a warm environment by radiation (heat emission), convection (heat transfer by atmospheric motion), and conduction (heat transfer by conductive medium). The body's most efficient mechanisms to decrease body heat are sweating and dilation of skin blood vessels. When blood vessels dilate, blood is brought to the skin surface to increase the rate of radiation of heat from the body. People at greatest risk for heat illnesses include children, the elderly, and clients with cardiac disease. Certain drugs may make a person more susceptible to heat illness.

Thermoregulation by the hypothalamus balances heat production and heat loss. Hyperthermia results when thermoregulation breaks down because of excess heat generation, inability to dissipate heat, overwhelming environmental conditions, or a combination of these factors. It is important to note that two different mechanisms are involved in fever and heat illness. In fever, the thermal set point is elevated because the body is trying to fight off an infection from an invading organism. Salicylates are used to inhibit these reactions, causing a reduction of the thermal set point and relieving hyperthermia caused by fever. In heat illness, the thermal set point remains normal and hyperthermia occurs because of inability to dissipate heat. Normal defense mechanisms that protect the set point are overwhelmed. Antipyretics are of no use in this setting and in fact may contribute to complications of clotting problems and liver damage.

LEARNING TIP

The older adult is vulnerable to temperature extremes. In times of extreme temperatures such as temperatures over 100°F, the elderly who live alone should have someone designated to check on them and ensure that they are not experiencing hyperthermia. They should be taken to a cooler environment if they do not have air conditioning available in their residence.

STAGES OF HYPERTHERMIA

Assessment

As heat illness progresses, circulatory blood volume decreases, causing dehydration. The more severe the dehydration, the faster the physiological compensation will be exhausted. Fluid intake is crucial in the prevention of heat illness. Illness from heat exposure can take three forms: heat cramps, heat exhaustion, and heatstroke (Table 54–8).

Table 54–8. **Hyperthermia Related to Exposure to Hot Environment**

Defining Characteristics
Early signs:
• Core body temperature 100.4°F to 102.2°F (38°C to 39°C)
• Diaphoresis
• Cool, clammy skin
• Dizziness
• Pulse rate > 100
Late signs:
• Increasing body core temperature of 106°F (41°C) or more
• Hot, dry, flushed skin
• Altered mental status
• Coma or seizures possible
• Hypotension

Outcome Criteria
• Core body temperature is less than 101°F (38.3°C).
• Client is alert and oriented.
• Skin is warm and dry to touch.

Heat Cramps

Heat cramps, a mild form of heat illness, are painful muscle spasms that occur after strenuous exercise. Sweat produced during vigorous exercise in a warm environment causes a change in the body's salt balance, resulting in cellular loss of essential electrolytes. Large amounts of water can be lost as a result of excessive sweating, causing stressed muscles to go into spasm. Heat cramps usually occur in the leg or abdominal muscles.

When heat cramps occur, the client should be removed from the hot environment. Tight clothing should be loosened. The client should sit or lie down until the cramps subside. The client is given water or a diluted (half-strength) balanced electrolyte solution to drink. Solutions high in salt concentration or salt tablets are not given because the client has an adequate amount of circulating electrolytes, but needs water. With adequate rest and fluid replacement, the body adjusts the distribution of electrolytes and the cramps disappear.

Heat Exhaustion

Heat exhaustion occurs when the body loses so much water and electrolytes through heavy sweating that hypovolemia occurs. Heat exhaustion is largely a manifestation of the strain placed on the cardiovascular system attempting to maintain normothermia. Cerebral function is unimpaired, although the client may exhibit minor irritability and poor judgment. The ability to sweat remains. The skin is usually cold and clammy and the face gray. Sodium and water loss cause the client to become dehydrated. The body temperature is usually normal or slightly elevated from 100.4°F to 102.2°F (38°C to 39°C). The client may complain of feeling dizzy, weak, or faint, with nausea or headache. Vomiting and diarrhea may also be present.

The client is removed from the hot environment. Tight clothing is loosened. If the client is fully alert, oral fluids of water or diluted balanced salt solution are administered. Fluids by mouth are not given if the client is not fully alert. If symptoms do not clear promptly, the client needs to be given IV fluids.

Heatstroke

If symptoms of heat exhaustion are not treated, **heatstroke** can develop. Central nervous system disruption with altered mental status is a key diagnostic pattern in heatstroke. Some clients show confusion, irrational behavior, or psychosis and others may present in a coma or with seizures. The sweating mechanism has been overwhelmed, so many heatstroke victims have hot, dry, flushed skin. The body temperature rises rapidly to 106°F (41°C) or more. As the core body temperature rises, the level of consciousness decreases. If heatstroke is not treated, it always results in death.

Nursing Diagnosis

- Hyperthermia related to exposure to hot environment
- Fluid volume deficit related to hypovolemia

Planning

The client's goal is to maintain a body temperature within normal limits.

Interventions

Emergency treatment of heatstroke consists of reducing the body temperature and rapidly cooling the victim. The client should be undressed and allowed to cool. Evaporative cooling is the most efficient method of cooling. Tepid water is used as a mist spray over the client with a strong continual breeze from electric fans to enhance evaporation. If the client is hypotensive, give IVs as ordered to increase circulating volume.

Clients suffering from heatstroke are admitted to the intensive care unit because late complications can appear suddenly and require immediate management. Relatively common occurrences include seizures, cerebral ischemia, renal failure, late cardiac decompensation, and gastrointestinal bleeding. Long-term prognosis is variable, depending on prior state of health, length of time under heat stress, and adequate oxygenation.

Evaluation

Desired outcome criteria for the hyperthermic client include a core body temperature that is below 101°F (38.3°C). The client is alert and oriented. The skin is warm and dry to touch. The pulse is bounding, and the blood pressure is within normal limits.

Poisoning and Drug Overdose

Poisons are introduced into the body by ingestion, inhalation, injection, absorption, or venom bites. Poisons act by changing cellular metabolism, causing damage to structures or disturbances of function. Many toxins and poisons alter the client's mental status, making it difficult to obtain an accurate history.

NURSING PROCESS

Assessment

The primary nursing responsibility is to recognize that a poisoning has occurred and then attempt to determine the nature of the poison. The method of exposure is established so that removal or interruption of the toxin can be initiated. Objects at the scene such as empty bottles, scattered pills,

chemicals, damaged plants, or any suspicious material should be sent with the client to the hospital to help establish poison or drug identification. The client's physical appearance may give a clue to the type of poison or overdose taken. Intravenous needle tracks, burns, erythema, flushed skin, or bite marks may help identify the poison or toxic exposure. Poison control centers have access to information concerning virtually all substances that could possibly be poisonous, any available antidotes, and appropriate emergency treatment. In general, the most important treatment for poisons involves dilution and physical removal of the agent.

Drugs represent the majority of ingested poisons, but approximately one third of poisonings are caused by cleaners, soaps, insecticides, acids, or alkalis. Many household plants are poisonous if they are accidentally ingested. Some plants cause local irritation of the skin and others can affect the circulatory system, the gastrointestinal tract, or the central nervous system.

Nursing Diagnosis

- Risk for injury related to absorption of poisoning agent

Planning

The client's goal is to be free of injury.

Interventions for Ingested Poisons

Emergency treatment for the client after ingesting poisons includes rapid removal of the poison from the gastrointestinal tract and diluting the remainder. Syrup of ipecac can be used to induce vomiting if the client is fully alert. The usual dose of syrup of ipecac is 15 mL for children between the ages of 1 and 5 years and 30 mL for older children and adults. Several glasses of water should be given to the client after administering syrup of ipecac. Vomiting usually occurs within 30 minutes. The dose may be repeated once if vomiting does not occur after 30 minutes. Contraindications to forced vomiting include a semiconscious client, corrosive poisons, or ingestion of a petroleum product. If clients are not fully alert, aspiration may occur because they may not be able to protect their airway. If the poison is a corrosive material, serious burns may occur to the gastrointestinal tract if vomiting occurs. Petroleum products cause a serious chemical pneumonia if they are aspirated into the lungs or if their vapors are inhaled during forced vomiting.

Gastric lavage may be indicated if the client has altered level of consciousness. A large gastric tube is inserted orally into the client's stomach. Water is instilled via the tube in 50 to 60 mL doses and withdrawn to evacuate any remaining poison in the stomach. A total of 2 L of water is required or more until gastric return is clear of any pill fragments or substance. Activated charcoal with sorbitol can be administered before pulling the tube. Activated charcoal is given because it binds most drugs and helps prevent systemic absorption. Sorbitol hastens gastrointestinal transit.

Evaluation

The goal for risk for injury is met if the client remains free from injury.

INHALED POISONS

Inhaled poisons include natural gas, certain pesticides, carbon monoxide, chlorine, and other gases. Carbon monoxide is odorless and can produce profound hypoxia by combining with the hemoglobin molecule in the red blood cell. It competes with oxygen for hemoglobin. Carboxyhemoglobin levels are done on the client to direct appropriate therapy. Chlorine is very irritating and can produce airway obstruction and pulmonary edema.

When an inhalation injury occurs, the client must be moved into fresh air and away from the toxin. Supplemental oxygen is given as ordered. Clients exposed to prolonged inhalation of a poison may experience lung damage. Respiratory status must be closely monitored to detect complications.

INJECTED POISONS

Injected poisons pose compelling problems because they are difficult to remove or dilute. Usually they are the result of drug overdose, but they can also result from the bites and stings of insects or animals. Local swelling and tissue destruction may occur at the injection site. All jewelry is removed because swelling may occur. A cold pack is applied to decrease local pain and swelling about the injection site. The identity of the injected drug or toxin must be identified to establish the course of side effects that occur. It is also important to determine if antivenom is available.

INSECTS

Insect stings or bites can have serious consequences for certain people. Potentially dangerous stings or bites are associated with bees, wasps, yellow jackets, hornets, certain ants, scorpions, and some spiders. Symptoms usually occur at the site of injury, producing sudden pain, swelling, heat, and redness about the affected area. There is no specific treatment for these injuries, but ice applied to the site can make them less irritating. Cellulitis can occur hours later and may require medical treatment. A small percentage of people are allergic to the insect venom and suffer anaphy-

laxis. If anaphylaxis occurs after an insect sting, the client requires immediate treatment.

When a client has sustained a bee or wasp sting, examine the area for the stinger. If the stinger remains in the wound, attempt to remove it by gently scraping it off the skin. Do not use tweezers or forceps to remove the stinger, because squeezing the stinger can inject more venom into the client. Ice application placed over the injury site may help slow the rate of absorption of toxin.

Many spider bites do not produce serious complications. However, two species of spiders—black widow and the brown recluse—are able to inflict serious and sometimes life-threatening bites. Black widow spiders are glossy black and have a distinctive, bright red-orange marking in the shape of an hourglass on the abdomen. They are found in dry, dim places around buildings, in woodpiles, and among debris. Their venom is neurotoxic and causes systemic symptoms, including cramps, dyspnea, dizziness, sweating, nausea, vomiting, and skin rashes. Death is not common, and symptoms generally subside in 48 hours. Antivenom is available.

The brown recluse spider is dull brown and has a dark violin-shaped mark on its back. It tends to live in dark areas, under rocks, in woodpiles, and in old abandoned buildings. It is found in the southern and central United States. The venom of the brown recluse causes severe local tissue damage. The area becomes red, swollen, and tender and develops a pale, mottled, cyanotic center. A large ulcer can develop over the next several days if not treated promptly. Antivenom is available.

SNAKE BITES

A small percentage of snake bites are caused by poisonous snakes. There are four poisonous snakes in the United States: the rattlesnake, the copperhead, the cottonmouth moccasin, and the coral snake. The most prevalent venomous snakes are the pit vipers, which include rattlesnakes, copperheads, and cottonmouth moccasins. Envenomation is the deposit of venom into the wound. Hollow fangs in the roof of the snake's mouth inject the poison from two sacs located at the back of the head. The poisonous snake bite has a characteristic appearance of two small puncture wounds with surrounding discoloration, swelling, and pain.

Envenomation by a pit viper produces burning pain at the site of the injury. Local tissue destruction starts from the moment of envenomation. Signs of swelling and discoloration occur within 5 to 10 minutes after the bite. Interventions used to decrease the circulation of venom throughout the client's system include keeping the client calm and immobilizing the affected part. Venous tourniquets placed above and below the fang marks help limit the spread of the venom through the veins of the extremity. Constricting bands can be used to stop venous blood flow.

The tourniquets should not stop arterial flow. The client's pulse should be palpable below the tourniquets after they are applied. The site of the bite is cleaned with soap and water. The client is kept calm until antivenom can be given. Medical treatment of the client with a poisonous snake bite should be directed by an experienced toxicologist.

TICK BITES

Tick bites occur during warm weather when people are outside, especially in wooded areas. The bite itself is painless. The tick attaches itself to the skin and sucks blood. The saliva of the tick is injected into the skin, causing infections to spread. It usually takes at least 18 hours for the infection to be transmitted from the tick to the person.

When the tick is found, it should be removed carefully and slowly. Tweezers should be used to pull the tick straight out of the skin. The tick is never handled with fingers. The nurse never applies gasoline or vaseline to the tick or tries to burn it with a lighted match.

Tick bites can spread infectious diseases. Two diseases commonly spread by tick bites are Rocky Mountain spotted fever and Lyme disease. Rocky Mountain spotted fever occurs 7 to 10 days after a bite from an infected tick and causes symptoms of nausea, vomiting, headache, weakness, paralysis, or even cardiorespiratory collapse. Symptoms of Lyme disease from an infected tick develop about 3 days after the tick bite. A red rash develops and spreads to several parts of the body with joint swelling. Clients are treated with antibiotics.

Psychiatric Emergencies

A psychiatric emergency exists when people no longer possess the coping skills necessary to maintain their usual level of functioning. Clients' moods, thoughts, or actions are so disordered that they have the potential to produce danger, harm, or death to themselves or to others if the situation is not quickly controlled. As a result, a behavioral or mental status change occurs. Frequently the change is sudden, but it can be insidious in onset. If acute psychiatric episodes are not managed, they can result in life-threatening suicidal, violent, or psychologically damaging behavior. A crisis is characterized by escalating levels of tension and anxiety with resulting cognitive, emotional, and behavioral disorganization.

NURSING PROCESS

Assessment

Causes of psychiatric emergency symptoms are varied and require thorough assessment of the client's history, physi-

cal examination, and mental status. Information from the client's past medical history may produce possible organic causes that may be contributing to the client's presenting symptoms. Endocrine dysfunction, electrolyte abnormalities, and head trauma are examples of medical conditions that may cause changes in mental status. A medication history is obtained to determine compliance with medication regimens and any recent changes in medications. A mental status examination consists of assessing the cognitive and psychological status of a client. The major components of the mental status examination include behavior and general appearance, affect and mood, mental content and thought processes, judgment and insight, perception, and cognitive ability. The nurse observes if the client is having problems concentrating on information that is being given. The more serious the disruption in cognitive abilities, the more significant the mental derangement.

Common emotional or behavioral manifestations of psychiatric crises include emotional responses to stressful events, anxiety, depression, psychosis, and mania. A crisis occurs when people enter a sudden state of emotional turmoil. They are unable to resolve the situation with their own resources and need assistance.

Anxiety may range in severity from mild to panic. Panic evolves into complete disorganization and loss of control. The client in panic is terrified and needs external controls to avoid harm.

Depression is an affective disorder most commonly characterized by physical ailments and somatizations. An assessment of the persons's suicide risk is important. Antidepressants are used to diminish symptoms of depression.

Psychotic clients experience impaired reality testing. Their disorderly thought processes are often characterized by hallucination, delusions, ideas of reference, thought broadcasting, and thought insertion. Psychotic thinking and abnormal speech patterns interfere with the client's attempt to communicate rationally.

Manic behavior is most commonly the result of manic-depressive illness. It is characterized by abnormally increased expansiveness in a person's feeling, thinking, and doing. Manic persons are often insulting toward others and express sexual desires with frequent use of obscenities. Manic persons are also at high risk for injuring themselves or others.

Nursing Diagnosis

- Anxiety related to situational stress
- Risk for injury related to impaired judgment
- Fear, related to alteration in thought content

Planning

The client's goals are to reduce anxiety, remain free from injury, and reduce fear.

Interventions

During crisis intervention, there are strategies designed to reduce the negative impact of a distressing event. It is important to establish an atmosphere of trust for clients so they feel free to discuss problems. The nurse acknowledges the client's physical and emotional complaints by using active listening. The environment is made safe, and external sources of stimulation are reduced. When speaking to the client, the nurse speaks directly and truthfully to the client and never promises unachievable things. Trusted supportive members of the client's family are involved to calm the person and encourage cooperation. Bystanders or adversive family members that could create further complications are restricted. The client is prepared for each new development as the circumstances evolve. The nurse does not threaten, challenge, or argue with the disturbed client. Misconceptions are corrected, but not in an argumentative manner. The nurse is firm but not threatening and shows respect for the client by never laughing or joking. It is important not to "play along" with distorted thinking because it can make matters much worse.

Intervention for all psychotic persons consists of reducing the fear and potential harm to self or others. Sometimes physical restraint is necessary, as ordered, to prevent harm or injury to the client or others. Restraint equipment is not shown to the client until sufficient help is available to use it. The client's behavior is documented on the chart, as well as written physician orders for the use of physical restraints.

Antipsychotic medications are administered as ordered, and their response is monitored. Haloperidol (Haldol) is used when rapid tranquilization of a client is required. It has strong antipsychotic properties and a rapid onset. The nurse should assist in coordinating necessary support services for the client's aftercare.

Evaluation

The client's goals are met if the client reports reduced anxiety and fear and remains free from injury.

Near-Drowning

Drowning is death from **asphyxia** after submersion in water. Near-drowning is submersion with at least temporary survival of the victim. Life-threatening complications of submersion are respiratory failure and ischemic neurological injury from hypoxia and acidosis.

When submersion occurs, conscious victims take in several deep breaths in an attempt to store oxygen. Victims hold their breath until reflex inspiratory efforts override breath holding. As water is aspirated, laryngospasm occurs, producing severe hypoxia. In wet drownings, fluid is inhaled or aspirated into the lungs after the vocal cords re-

lax. In dry drownings, no fluid has been inhaled or aspirated because of prolonged laryngospasm. Most successfully resuscitated victims experience dry drownings.

If a person survives submersion, acute respiratory failure may follow. Fluid in the alveoli and interstitial spaces causes poor perfusion and hypoxemia. The incidence of serious pulmonary complications is high in this group. Symptoms of impaired gas exchange may be delayed as long as 24 hours after the incident. Contaminants in the water can irritate the pulmonary system and cause additional complications. Cardiovascular complications can occur secondary to hypoxia and metabolic acidosis, resulting in dysrhythmias.

NURSING PROCESS

Assessment

Vital signs are assessed to detect abnormal readings. Respiratory rate and pattern are observed. Any dyspnea or signs of airway obstruction are noted. The skin color or cyanosis is noted. The client's level of consciousness may be altered due to anoxia.

Nursing Diagnosis

* Altered tissue perfusion related to severe anoxia

Planning

The client's goal is to maintain level of consciousness and vital signs within normal range.

Interventions

When submersion occurs, avoid initial attempts to drain fluid from the lungs or stomach. Resuscitative efforts should always start with ventilation. Supplemental oxygen is administered to increase tissue oxygenation. Adjunct airway equipment should be available. The nurse prepares the client for endotracheal intubation and insertion of a nasogastric tube to decompress the stomach.

Aggressive resuscitative efforts should be used on victims of cold water drowning where submersion time has been 1 hour or less. Rapid hypothermia may serve as a protective function. Hypothermia can decrease the metabolic needs of the brain and contribute to neurological recovery after prolonged submersion.

Evaluation

Factors that influence the outcome of near-drowning victims include the temperature of the water, length of time of submersion, cleanliness of the water, and age of the victim. The younger the client, the better the chance for survival. Expected outcome criteria to evaluate the near-drowning client include effective ventilation. Respiratory rate and pattern of breathing will be normal. The client is alert. Skin color is normal, and skin is warm and dry to touch. Palpable pulses and blood pressure are normal.

Disaster Response

When a disaster strikes a community, several area agencies are activated to coordinate search, rescue, transportation, and treatment of multiple victims. Involved agencies include emergency medical system (EMS) providers, fire agencies, law enforcement, and hospitals. Each agency must evaluate its available resources to determine the ability of handling a major incident. Resources include manpower, equipment, and communication capabilities. Preparedness is the key to successful disaster management.

Disaster is defined as any event that overwhelms existing manpower, facilities, equipment, and capabilities of a responding agency or institution. Its available resources are insufficient to manage the number of casualties or the nature of the emergency. Disaster response involves a massive effort of multiple coordinating agencies working together.

The development and implementation of a well-researched and well-prepared plan is important for disaster management. Each agency should develop internal plans, as well as work with other agencies to develop community plans. Drills are conducted regularly to evaluate and rework plans. Nurses should be familiar with their agency's disaster plans and policies.

Review Questions

1. Signs and symptoms of profound shock include which one of the following?
   a. Sacral edema
   b. Jugular vein distention
   c. Palpable, bounding pulse
   d. Decreasing blood pressure

2. Which one of the following is the purpose of checking capillary refill?
   a. To evaluate arterial blood flow in an extremity
   b. To assess venous blood flow in an extremity
   c. To measure oxygen saturation of the blood
   d. To assess peripheral edema

3. Which one of the following is usually used to control bleeding?
   a. Application of a tourniquet
   b. Application of pressure
   c. Pressure point massage
   d. Antishock garment application

4. Which one of the following is an immediate threat to life during acute anaphylaxis?
   a. Airway obstruction
   b. Generalized itching
   c. Hypotension
   d. Rapid pulse

5. Which one of the following is the most important component of the primary survey?
   a. Airway
   b. Breathing
   c. Circulation
   d. Level of consciousness

6. Which one of the following may result from an extensive thermal burn injury?
   a. Fluid volume excess
   b. Hyperthermia
   c. Hypothermia
   d. Hemorrhage

7. Treatment for heat exhaustion includes which one of the following?
   a. Restrict oral fluids
   b. Cool Environment
   c. Aspirin
   d. Apply tight clothing

8. Treatment for a semiconscious client who has ingested 50 tablets of Xanax includes which one of the following?
   a. Tracheostomy
   b. Activated charcoal
   c. Forced vomiting
   d. Elevating the lower extremities

9. During crisis intervention with a psychotic client with distorted thinking, which one of the following interventions is helpful to gain the client's trust?
   a. "Play along"
   b. Make promises
   c. Avoid eye contact
   d. Show respect

▼ **ANSWERS TO CRITICAL THINKING: Mr. Smith**

1. The airway is the first priority because edema from inhalation burns can occlude the airway.
2. Soot around the mouth and nose are signs of inhalation burns. Assess the respiratory status of the client.
3. Assessment should include respiratory rate and pattern. Assess the client's ability to speak without a hoarse voice. Abnormal breathing sounds such as wheezing indicate partial upper airway occlusion.
4. The vital signs are within normal limits.
5. Deep partial-thickness burns should be covered with dry dressings. Because the skin can no longer protect the client, wet dressings provide a medium for bacterial invasion. Wet dressings can

also cause a decrease in temperature because the skin can no longer help with thermoregulation.

6. Jewelry should always be immediately removed before edema formation begins.

7. Mr. Smith was involved in an explosive incident and thrown 50 feet. He could have sustained fractures of the pelvis or back. He is also suspect for internal organ injuries from blunt trauma.

8. Mr. Smith's respiratory status should continue to be closely monitored because edema can still pose a problem for airway occlusion. Mr. Smith is developing a hoarse voice, and that can be a precursor to airway occlusion from edema formation.

REFERENCES

1. National Center for Health Statistics: Advance report of final mortality statistics. Monthly Vital Statistics Report 43:1, 1994.

2. Teasdale, G and Jennett, B: Assessment of coma and impaired consciousness: A practical scale. Lancet 2(7872):81, 1974.

BIBLIOGRAPHY

Cardona, VD, et al (eds): Trauma Nursing: From Resuscitation through Rehabilitation, ed 2. WB Saunders, Philadelphia, 1994.

Emergency Nurses Association: Emergency Nursing Core Curriculum, ed 4. WB Saunders, Philadelphia, 1994.

Emergency Nurses Association: Trauma Nursing Core Course Provider Manual. Mosby, St Louis, 1995.

Kitt, S, et al (eds): Emergency Nursing: A Physiologic and Clinical Perspective, ed 2. WB Saunders, Philadelphia, 1995.

Mattox KL (ed): Complications of Trauma. Churchill Livingstone, New York, 1994.

Mozingo, DW, Cioffi, WG, and Pruitt, BA: Burns. In Bongard, F, and Sue, D (eds): Current Critical Care Diagnosis and Management. Appleton & Lange, Norwalk, Conn, 1994.

Porth, CM: Pathophysiology: Concepts of Altered Health States, ed 4. JB Lippincott, Philadelphia, 1994.

Saunders, M: Mosby's Paramedic Textbook. Mosby, St Louis, 1994.

Understanding Mental Health Care

Nursing Care of Clients with Mental Health Disorders

55

Kathy Neeb

Learning Objectives

Upon completion of this chapter, the student will be able to:

1. Define mental health and mental illness.
2. Identify the components of a mental health status assessment.
3. Define DSM-IV and other methods for diagnosing mental illness.
4. Identify common defense mechanisms.
5. Describe a therapeutic milieu.
6. Identify classifications, uses, actions, side effects, and nursing considerations for selected classifications of psychoactive medications.
7. Describe methods for psychoanalysis, behavior modification, rational-emotive therapy, humanistic/person-centered therapy, counseling, electroconvulsive therapy, group therapy, and relaxation therapy.
8. Identify the nurse's role in therapy.
9. Define and identify symptoms, treatment modalities, and nursing care for anxiety disorders, mood disorders, somatoform disorders, schizophrenia, substance abuse disorders, and codependency.

Key Words

abuse (uh-**BYOOS**)
addiction (uh-**DIK**-shun)
affect (**AF**-feckt)
anxiety (ang-**ZIGH**-uh-tee)
behavior modification (be-**HAYV**-yer MAH-di-fi-**KAY**-shun)
biofeedback (BYE-oh-**FEED**-bak)
bipolar (bye-**POH**-ler)
codependence (KO-de-**PEN**-dense)
cognitive (**KAHG**-ni-tiv)
compulsion (kum-**PUHL**-shun)
conversion disorder (kon-**VER**-zhun dis-**OR**-der)
coping (**KOH**-ping)
counseling (**KOWN**-sel-ing)
delirium tremens (dee-**LIR**-ee-uhm **TREE**-menz)

delusions (dee-**LOO**-zhuns)
dependence (di-**PEN**-dens)
displacement (dis-**PLAYSS**-ment)
dysfunctional (dis-**FUNCK**-shun-uhl)
electroconvulsive therapy (ee-**LEK**-troh kun-**VUL**-siv **THER**-uh-pee)
eustress (**YOO**-stress)
hallucinations (huh-LOO-si-**NAY**-shuns)
illusions (i-**LOO**-zhuns)
imagery (**IM**-ij-ree)
mania (**MAY**-nee-ah)
mental health (**MEN**-tuhl HELLTH)
mental illness (**MEN**-tuhl **ILL**-ness)
milieu (me-**LYU**)
obsession (ub-**SESH**-un)
orientation (OR-ee-en-**TAY**-shun)
paranoia (PAR-uh-**NOY**-uh)
phobia (**FOH**-bee-ah)
psychoanalysis (SIGH-koh-uh-**NAL**-i-sis)
psychopharmacology (SIGH-koh-FAR-meh-**KAHL**-uh-jee)
psychosomatic (SIGH-koh-soh-**MAT**-ik)
somatoform (soh-**MAT**-uh-form)
stress (STRESS)
stressor (**STRESS**-er)
tolerance (**TALL**-ler-ens)
withdrawal (with-**DRAW**-ul)

Normal Function

The study of mental illness is fairly new to the health care field. There are differing opinions within the mental health community as to what **mental health** and **mental illness** are. *Mental health* has been defined in many ways. These definitions include the ability to

- Be flexible
- Be successful
- Form close relationships
- Make appropriate judgments
- Solve problems
- Cope with daily **stress**
- Have a positive sense of self

Mental illness is defined as

- Impairment of ability to think
- Impairment of ability to feel
- Impairment of ability to make sound judgments
- Difficulty or inability to cope with reality
- Difficulty or inability to form strong personal relationships

It is important to remember that mental health and mental illness exist on a continuum. It is natural for individuals' emotions to ebb and flow from day to day in response to the degree of stress that is experienced. Individuals who remain mentally healthy are able to keep their stress in perspective. Others are not able to do so, and over a period of time, they may develop physical or emotional illnesses as a result of the constant stress in their life. Visualize the seesaw that children play on. Mental health and mental illness are like a seesaw. When children of approximately equal weight get on each end of the seesaw, they can balance each other and keep the seesaw even. Mentally healthy people keep themselves in a state of emotional balance. Sometimes, one child weighs just a little more than the other and the seesaw tips just a *little* to one side or the other. Mentally healthy people can cope with this fluctuation. Sometimes, another child gets on or one child greatly outweighs the other and the seesaw gets out of balance *completely;* one end goes way up while the other goes way down, and it stays there until someone alters the balance. Ultimately, it must be the client who finds his or her own balance. When people's moods get way down or way up, they are not in emotional homeostasis.

The discussion surrounding the etiology (causes) of mental illness continues to revolve around the "nature versus nurture" or "organic versus inorganic or functional" arguments. The connections between physical and emotional health are so closely intertwined that it is sometimes hard to decide if emotional causes trigger physical responses or vice versa. Nurses must have a basic understanding of both the "nature" and the "nurture" schools of thought on the causes of alterations in mental health.

Explanations of mental illness include concepts from the psychoanalytic (or psychological) theory and the psychobiological (or biological) theory. When pertinent, other theories (behavioral, environmental, etc.) will also be presented. Most mental illnesses have no absolute etiology. Some etiological theories have stronger positive correlations to illnesses than others. When it is appropriate, this chapter will give the most popular or most widely accepted view of an etiology.

Many professionals in the field of psychology believe that social and cultural environments have a great influence on the way people develop and process life experiences. Some psychoanalysts believe that some cultural traditions and beliefs cause disturbances in personal relationships, which can lead to forms of emotional disturbances. It is part of the nurse's role to take time to learn about the traits that are common among people and those traits that are different. It is important to have an understanding of people's customs and beliefs to avoid unrealistic expectations of clients. See Cultural Considerations Box 55–1 for more detailed information about culture and mental health issues.

Spirituality and religion are extremely important to some clients and unimportant or nonexistent to others. A person's success at recuperating from physical or emotional illness may be deeply tied to his or her spirituality. It is necessary for the nurse to be comfortable talking to the client about spiritual needs while being careful not to impose personal values on the client. Nurses who are not comfortable in these situations should offer to call the chaplain in the facility or the spiritual leader of the client's choice. It is important to keep the lines of communication open. People learn by sharing with each other. It is much better to ask a person about something than to make an assumption about it.

Nursing Assessment

During the data collection/assessment part of the nursing process, the mental status examination is performed. This is a series of questions and activities that check eight areas: appearance and behavior, level of awareness and reality **orientation,** thinking/content of thought, memory, speech and ability to communicate, mood and **affect,** judgment, and perception. These examinations are of varying names, lengths, and formats, but they all assess the client's mental capabilities. See Table 55–1 for a sample mental status examination.

After data have been collected, the licensed practical nurse/licensed vocational nurse (LPN/LVN) collaborates with the registered nurse (RN) to develop nursing diagnoses. Table 55–2 lists nursing diagnoses commonly used when caring for clients experiencing mental health problems.

CULTURAL CONSIDERATIONS BOX 55-1

Among many Haitians and some African-Americans, conjure (practicing magic) and root doctors are believed to know more about mental illness than Western-educated physicians. Some depressive and obsessive behaviors are viewed as culture-bound syndromes. These behaviors are expected of some Haitians, and those affected fulfill some expected roles in the society. Some of these illnesses are viewed as having no cure.[1] Thus, the nurse may need to include folk healers when working with African-Americans and clients of Haitian descent.

Smoking, alcoholism, and deaths from suicide or violence are prevalent problems in the American culture. Violent deaths account for high mortality rates among adolescents and young adults of African-American, Cuban, Mexican-American, and Puerto Rican origin.[2] Programs geared to these target populations should be personalized to include adolescents and their families. Given their strong family values, an important approach is to begin early in church groups or family settings.

Hispanics require lower doses of antidepressants and experience greater side effects than whites. Thus, careful observations need to be undertaken when observing for side effects of medications in clients of Mexican heritage.

One of the few drugs found to have a higher rate of side effects in individuals of Ashkenazi ancestry is clozopine, used to treat schizophrenia. Twenty percent of Jewish clients taking this drug developed agranulocytosis compared with about 1 percent of non-Jewish patients. Thus, the nurse may need to suggest testing for agranulocytosis when Jewish clients are prescribed clozopine.

Asian clients require lower dosages and have side effects at lower dosages than whites for a variety of psychoactive drugs (lithium, haloperidol) even when matched with body weight. Asians commonly believe that Western drugs are too strong for them and take less than prescribed. Most Asians are more sensitive to alcohol, resulting in facial flushing, palpitations, and tachycardia.

Many Vietnamese people believe that mental illness results from offending a deity and that such a condition brings disgrace to the family and must be concealed. A shaman may be enlisted to help. Additional therapy is sought only with the greatest discretion and often after a dangerous delay. Unmistakable emotional disturbance is usually attributed to possession by malicious spirits, the bad luck of familial inheritance, or, for Buddhists, to bad karma accumulated by misdeeds in past lives.[3] Additionally, the term *psychiatrist* has no direct translation in Vietnamese and may be interpreted to mean nerve physician or specialist who treats crazy people. The nervous system sometimes is seen as the source of mental problems, neurosis being thought of as "weakness of the nerves" and psychosis as "turmoil of the nerves."[4]

Poles usually look for a physical basis of disease before considering a mental disorder. If mental health problems exist, home visits are preferred to clinic visits, and talk therapies without suitable psychosocial strategies are not maintained unless interventions are action oriented.[5] In addition, Poles look to other family members and the community to assess appropriateness of treatments. Polish-Americans often seek self-help groups such as Alcoholics Anonymous before seeing a health care provider. A family physician is preferred over a specialist.[6]

Mental illness among the Navajo is perceived as resulting from placing a curse on an individual. In these instances, a healer who deals with dreams or a crystal gazer is consulted. Individuals may wear turquoise to ward off evil; however, an individual who wears too much turquoise is sometimes thought to be an evil person and someone to avoid. In some tribes, mental illness may mean that the affected person has special powers.[7] Additionally, many Native-Americans metabolize alcohol at a faster rate than European-Americans, resulting in them having a lowered tolerance for alcohol.

Mental illness in the Korean culture is viewed as a stigma. Hwabyung, a traditional Korean illness, occurs from the suppression of sadness, depression, worry, anger, fright, and fear. These emotions are commonly related to conflicts with close relatives or significant others. Symptoms include physical complaints such as headaches, poor appetite, insomnia, and lack of energy. Most people accept the symptoms as inevitable.[8]

Newer immigrants from Ireland have a higher incidence of mental illness than the rest of the population. Undocumented Irish immigrants in the United States report more stressors and mental health problems than their legal counterparts.[9] Because many Irish people have difficulty expressing emotions, health care providers may need to encourage Irish-Americans to express their concerns.

Mental illness is strongly stigmatized among Iranians and is thought to be genetic. Should a family member have mental illness, it is likely to be called a "neurological disorder" so as not to stigmatize the family, which may result in daughters having a lesser chance of marrying. Psychotherapeutic help may be avoided because of stigma or because it is perceived as irrelevant. People prefer a medicine that might cure them. There is a tendency to pay more attention to somatic symptoms when under emotional stress, and Iranians consider psychopharmacology most effective, with a high rate of compliance.

Because of the stigma attached to seeking professional psychiatric help, many Hindus do not access the health care system. Instead, family and friends seem to be the best help, and a general belief is that time is the best healer. Physical and mental illnesses are considered God's will, or karma, and are associated with a fatalistic attitude.[10]

Among Greeks, mental illness is accompanied by social stigma for the afflicted individual as well as the relatives. The shame originates in the notion that mental illness is hereditary, and afflicted individuals are viewed as having lifelong conditions that pollute the bloodline.[11]

Because of social stigma attached to mental illness and retardation, the Arab family may keep their family from pub-

continued

lic view.[12] However, when Arab clients suffer from mental distress, they seek medical care. They are likely to have complaints such as abdominal pain, lassitude, anorexia, or shortness of breath. Arabs have an increased tendency to experience elevated blood levels and adverse affects when customary dosages of antidepressants are prescribed. Patients often expect and insist on somatic treatment, at least vitamins and tonics.

African-Americans may be at a greater risk for being misdiagnosed with a psychiatric disorder than whites. African-Americans with psychiatric disorders are more likely to have hallucinations, delusions, somatization, and hostility even when controlled for socioeconomic class. Maintaining direct eye contact with some African-Americans may be misinterpreted as an aggressive behavior. Thus, nurses must take these nonverbal behaviors into consideration when working with the client with an emotional or mental concern. Additionally, African-Americans are more susceptible to tricyclic antidepressants and thus experience more toxic side effects.[13]

Diagnostic Tests

The diagnostic tool that is used most widely by psychiatrists and psychologists is the Diagnostic and Statistical Manual of Mental Disorders—IV, or DSM-IV. The DSM-IV uses a system for grouping illnesses into categories of clinical disorders. This is a very complex diagnostic tool that nurses do not need to memorize but should be aware of.

Physicians also use other diagnostic criteria to diagnose mental illness. Sometimes they test for other illnesses in an effort to rule out physical illness. The physician may choose to refer the client to a psychiatrist or psychologist for further testing and diagnosis.

There are also batteries of psychological tests that can be administered and interpreted by psychiatrists or psychologists. Age, hand tremors, vision, language barriers, educational background, and the interpretation of the psychiatrist or psychologist are some factors that could either positively or negatively influence the results of these tests.

Tests that may be performed to either confirm or rule out a diagnosis of a mental illness include the following:

- Blood work (to rule out electrolyte imbalances, dehydration, drug toxicity, etc.)
- Computed tomography (CT) scans (to rule out tumors, lesions, or other physical problems)
- Positron emission tomography (PET) scans (to identify how the parts of the brain are functioning by showing chemical activity or metabolism)

Coping and Defense Mechanisms

"Oh, just learn to cope with it." "Get a grip." "Don't make a mountain out of a molehill." These are pieces of advice that people may have heard or given at some point. But what do they mean? What is **coping?** *Coping* is the way one adapts psychologically, physically, and behaviorally to a **stressor.** Individuals have different methods of coping or dealing with their stressors. Culture, religion, individual belief systems, and personal choice seem to be major reasons for these differences in people's responses to stress. It is not the value of a behavior that we assess as nurses; it is the desired outcome that is important. What is an effective coping skill? How do nurses observe and measure it?

CRITICAL THINKING: Grieving

A man is noted wailing loudly and continuously after the death of his wife. It is disturbing the other clients on the wing, and one of the nurses comments, "He is a real nut case. Get him out of here."

What is an appropriate response to this nurse and client?

Answers at end of chapter.

Effective coping skills offer healthy choices for dealing with stressors. Hospitalization is stressful for clients and families. Many things are unknown and unfamiliar. The client may not understand the illness or the implications of the treatment plan. It is common for clients to use mechanisms to help them cope during hospitalization. The process of effective coping is sometimes called adaptation. Allowing the client to practice new coping techniques will give him or her confidence and will decrease the stress that can accompany change.

Often, the dividing line between effective and ineffective coping is the frequency of its use. For instance, a little worry or **anxiety** can be positive (Fig. 55–1). Generally, when there is a little tension, people are more alert and ready to respond. The fight or flight mechanism can actually help one adapt to a new situation. However, too much worry begins to cloud the consciousness and interfere with the ability to make appropriate choices and to recall the new

Table 55–1. **Sample Mental Status Examination**

Area of Assessment	Type of Assessment	Normal Parameters	Alterations from Normal
Appearance and Behavior	Objective and subjective observations about dress, hygiene, posture, and appearance and about the client's actions and reactions to health care personnel.	Clean, combed, hair. Clothing intact and appropriate to weather or situation. Teeth/dentures in good repair. Posture erect. Cooperates with health care personnel.	Displays either unusual apathy or concern about appearance. Displays uncooperative, hostile, or suspicious behaviors toward health care personnel.
Level of Awareness and Orientation	Subjective and objective assessment of the client's degree of alertness (wakefulness) and the degree of client's knowledge of self.	Awareness is measured on a continuum that ranges from unconsciousness to mania. "Normal alertness" is the desired behavior. Facilities may provide a standard guideline for helping with this assessment, but subjective observations can be documented as well, if the client is not able to stay awake for even short intervals or if the client is overly active and has difficulty staying in one place for any period of time.	Outcome is not considered within accepted normal limits if the client is difficult to arouse and keep awake or if the client has difficulty feeling calm. Abnormal results of orientation are the client's inability to correctly answer questions pertaining to the self or to commonly known social information, such as who is the president.
Thinking/Content of Thought	Subjective assessment of what the client is thinking and the process the client uses in his or her thinking.	Formal testing may be done by the psychologist or psychiatrist to determine the client's general thought content and pattern. Nurses may contribute to the assessment of thought by documenting statements the client makes regarding daily care and routines.	Behaviors including flight of ideas, loose associations, phobias, delusions, and obsessions may become apparent.
Memory	Subjective assessment of the mind's ability to recall recent and remote (long-term) information.	Recent memory: Recall of events that are immediately past or within 2 weeks before the assessment, such as a recent news event. One measurement technique is to verbally list five items. After 1 minute, client can recall four or five of those items. Continue with assessment and at 5 minutes, client should be able to recall three or four of the items. Remote memory: Recall of events of the past beyond 2 weeks before assessment. Clients may be asked where they were born, where they went to grade school, etc.	Inability to accurately perform recent or remote (long-term) recall exercises within parameters. May indicate symptom of delirium or dementia.

continued

Table 55–1. (continued)

Area of Assessment	Type of Assessment	Normal Parameters	Alterations from Normal
Speech and Ability to Communicate	Objective and subjective assessment of aspects of how client uses verbal and non-verbal communication.	Client can coherently produce words appropriate to age, education, and life experience. Rate of speech reflects other psychomotor activity (e.g., faster if client is agitated). Volume is not too soft or too loud. Stuttering, repetition of words, and words that the client makes up (neologisms) are also assessed.	Limited speech production. Rate of speech is inconsistent with other psychomotor activity. Volume is not appropriate to situation (speaks in very loud volume even when asked to speak more quietly). Presence of stuttering, word repetition, or neologisms may indicate physical or psychological illness.
Mood and Affect	Subjective and objective assessment of the client's stated feelings and emotions. Affect measures the outward expression of those feelings.	Mood is the stated emotional condition of the client and should fluctuate to reflect situations as they occur. Facial expression, body language (affect) should match (be congruent with) the stated mood. Affect should change to fluctuate with the changes in mood.	Mood and affect do not match (e.g., facial expression does not appear sad while client is expressing sad feelings).
Judgment	Subjective assessment of a client's ability to make appropriate decisions about his or her situation or to understand concepts.	Give client a proverb or situation to solve, such as "You can't teach an old dog new tricks." Client should be able to give some sort of acceptable interpretation, such as "old habits are hard to break" or "it is hard to learn something new." Another example is to ask the client what he or she would do if a small child was lost in the store. An appropriate response might be "call the manager" or "try to calm the child."	Client cannot interpret the sayings in some acceptable manner. Client cannot complete problem-solving questions appropriately. The client might answer very literally, "dogs can't learn anything when they get old" or might say, "I would go through the child's pockets looking for phone numbers."
Perception	Assesses the way a person experiences reality. Assessment is based on the client's statements about his or her environment and the behaviors expressed in association with those statements. Nurses and health team members must document this often subjective information in very objective terms.	All five senses are monitored for interaction with the client's reality. Client's insight into his or her condition is also assessed.	Presence of hallucinations and illusions (schizophrenia). Individuals who are not within normal boundaries of judgment or insight will not be able to state understanding of the origin of the illness and the behaviors that are associated with it.

adaptive tools one has learned. One of the most helpful roles a nurse can perform is to listen to the client's thoughts and feelings about the stressor and then provide information that will reinforce the client's positive feelings.

Ineffective coping is another story. When conscious techniques are not successful, humans often unconsciously fall into habits that give the illusion of coping. These habits are called defense mechanisms (or coping or mental mechanisms). Defense mechanisms are mental pressure valves. The purpose of defense mechanisms is to reduce or eliminate anxiety. They give the impression that they are helping alleviate the stress level. When used in very small doses, defense mechanisms can be helpful. When they are overused, they become ineffective and can lead to a break-

Table 55–2. *Nursing Diagnoses Commonly Used for Clients with Mental Health Problems*

Altered thought processes
Altered role performance
Anxiety (mild to panic)
Body image disturbance
Dysfunctional grieving
Impaired social interaction
Ineffective individual coping
Personal identity disturbance
Powerlessness
Risk for violence (toward self or others)
Self-care deficit
Self-esteem disturbance
Sensory-perceptual alteration
Sexual dysfunction
Sleep pattern disturbance
Social isolation

down of the personality. People are not born with these behaviors; they are learned as responses to stress. Many times, they develop by the age of 10 years old. They appear to be conscious, but they are, for the most part, unconscious mechanisms.

Some commonly used defense mechanisms are listed in Table 55–3.

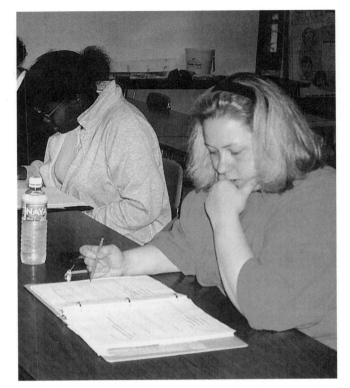

Figure 55–1. A little worry or anxiety can be positive, such as that experienced by these students studying for a test.

CRITICAL THINKING: Mrs. Beison

Mrs. Beison, a 44-year-old mother of three teenagers, is diagnosed with breast cancer. She is refusing treatment because she does not believe she has cancer. She says if anything is really wrong, her vitamins will take care of it.

What coping mechanism is Mrs. Beison using? Is it effective or ineffective? Why? How can you help?

Answers at end of chapter.

Therapeutic Measures

People who have alterations in their mental health have special treatment needs. When emotional health is threatened, many other daily activities can be altered as well. **Cognitive** ability (the ability to think rationally and to process those thoughts) can be decreased. Emotional responses can be decreased or even absent in some conditions. This can be extremely frightening and can lead to a

worsening of the mental disorder, or even the development of another disorder. Some therapies are described next.

MILIEU

One area over which nurses have some control is the therapeutic environment. In mental health, this therapeutic environment is called the **milieu** or therapeutic milieu (Fig. 55–2). It is believed that environment has an effect on behavior.

The milieu is the area that will provide safety and help during the client's stay. A nurse can keep the area calm and quiet and arrange for roommate changes if needed. As the client progresses, the milieu will be changed to allow the client to take on more responsibility.

PSYCHOPHARMACOLOGY

Psychopharmacology is the use of medications to treat psychological disorders. Since the introduction of the phenothiazine class of drugs in the 1950s, the number of medications available for treating mental health disorders has increased greatly. The reason for using medications is twofold: First, the medications control symptoms, helping the client feel more comfortable emotionally. Second, the client is generally more receptive and able to focus on other types of therapy if medications are effective. Classi-

---

psychopharmacology: psycho—soul or mind + pharmaco—drug or medicine + ology—study of

Table 55–3. **Defense Mechanisms**

Mechanism	Description	Examples
Denial	Usually the first defense learned and used. Unconscious refusal to see reality. Is *not* conscious lying.	The alcoholic states, "I can quit any time I want to."
Repression (Stuffing)	An unconscious "burying" or "forgetting" mechanism. Excludes or withholds from our consciousness events or situations that are unbearable.	A step deeper than "denial." A client may "forget" about an appointment he or she does not want to keep.
Rationalizing	Using a logical-sounding excuse to cover up true thoughts and feelings. Is the most frequently used defense mechanism.	1. "I did not make a medication error; I followed the doctor's order." 2. "I failed the test because the teacher wrote bad questions."
Compensation	Making up for something we perceive as an inadequacy by developing some other desirable trait.	1. The small boy who wants to be a basketball center instead becomes an honor roll student. 2. The physically unattractive person who wants to model will instead become a famous designer.
Reaction Formation (Overcompensation)	Similar to compensation, except the person will usually develop the exact opposite trait.	1. The small boy who wants to be a basketball center may become a political voice to decrease the emphasis of sports in the elementary grades. 2. The physically unattractive person who wants to be a model may speak out for eliminating beauty pageants.
Regression	Emotionally returning to an earlier time in life when client experienced far less stress. Commonly seen in clients while hospitalized. Note: Everyone will not go back to the same developmental age. This is highly individualized.	1. Children who are toilet trained beginning to wet themselves. 2. Adults who may start crying and have a "temper tantrum."
Projection (Scapegoating)	Blaming others. A mental or verbal "finger-pointing" at another for client's own problem. **Memory tool:** Think of a projector at the movie theater. It "points" the images of the film onto the screen just as a person using this defense mechanism "points" blame on another person or situation.	1. "I didn't get the promotion because you don't like me." 2. "I'm overweight because you make me nervous."
Displacement (Transference)	The "kick the dog syndrome." Transferring anger and hostility to another person or object that is perceived to be less powerful than yourself.	Parent loses job without notice; goes home and verbally abuses spouse, who unjustly punishes child, who slaps the dog.
Restitution (Undoing)	Make amends for a behavior one thinks is unacceptable. Makes an attempt at reducing guilt.	1. Giving a treat to a child who is being punished for a wrongdoing. 2. The person who sees someone lose a wallet with a large amount of cash does not return the wallet, but puts extra in the collection plate at the next church service.
Conversion Reaction	Anxiety is channeled into physical symptoms. Note: Often, the symptoms disappear soon after the threat is over.	Nausea develops the night before a major exam, causing the person to miss the exam. Nausea may disappear soon after the scheduled test is finished.
Avoidance	Unconsciously staying away from events or situations that might open feelings of aggression or anxiety.	"I can't go to the class reunion tonight. I'm just so tired, I have to sleep."

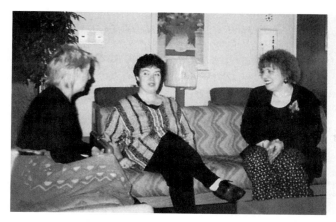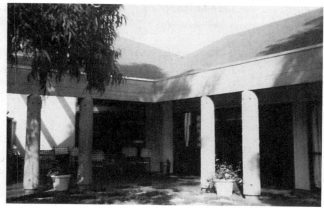

Figure 55–2. The therapeutic milieu is important in treating the client. (From Fortinash, KM, and Holoday-Worret, PA: Psychiatric-Mental Health Nursing. Mosby, St Louis, 1996, p 311, with permission of Grossmont Hospital/Sharp Health Care, San Diego.)

fications of psychoactive drugs are provided in Table 55–4. See also Nutrition Notes Box 55–2 for the impact of nutrition on the effects of some drugs.

PSYCHOTHERAPIES

Psychotherapy is the term used to describe the form of treatment chosen by the psychologist or psychiatrist. The goals of psychotherapy are to

1. Decrease the client's emotional discomfort
2. Increase the client's social functioning
3. Increase the ability of the client to behave or perform in a manner appropriate to the situation

Several specific types of therapy that are typically used are described next.

Psychoanalysis

Psychoanalysis is the form of therapy that was born from the theory of Sigmund Freud. In psychoanalysis, the focus is on the cause of the problem, which is believed to be buried somewhere in the unconscious. In psychoanalysis, the therapist uses questioning and memory probing techniques to take the client into the past in an effort to determine where the problem began.

Behavior Modification

Behavior modification is a treatment method that is a result of the studies of behavioral theorists such as Skinner and Pavlov. It is a common treatment modality used in long-term care facilities and facilities that treat clients with alterations in mental health.

Behavior can be changed, according to behavior modification theory, by either positive or negative reinforcement.

Positive reinforcement is the act of rewarding the client with something pleasant when the desired behavior has been performed. For instance, if Mrs. Powell has the habit of using foul language in an attempt to have a need met, it might be assumed that the desired behavior change would be to come to a staff member and ask quietly for what she needs. Mrs. Powell loves to be outside but is not allowed out except at supervised times. A suitable positive reinforcement for her might be to allow 15 more minutes outdoors when she remembers to come ask for her needs quietly.

Negative reinforcement is the act of responding to the undesired behavior by taking away a privilege or adding a responsibility. Negative reinforcement can be misinterpreted as punishment. It is necessary to be very careful when performing behavior modification to avoid an infraction of the Patient's Bill of Rights. A signed consent from the client is advised when using this form of therapy. Parents who "ground" their children for unacceptable behavior are using negative reinforcement; requiring the child to perform extra household tasks for a stated period of time is reinforcing the fact that the behavior has consequences. The child may not repeat the undesired behavior after negative reinforcement has been used.

The client must understand the consequences of the behavior to be changed and the purpose for the type of consequence that is chosen. If the person is not capable of understanding the situation or is not able to remember the consequences due to some other problem, behavior modification could be considered a questionable alternative to other kinds of treatment.

Cognitive Therapies

Rational-Emotive Therapy

Dr. Albert Ellis and other cognitive therapists believe that people teach themselves to be ill because of the way they

---

psychoanalysis: psycho—soul or mind + analysis—dissolving

Table 55–4. **Medications Used for Alterations in Mental Health**

Classification and Common Trade Names	Uses	Side Effects	Nursing Considerations	Client Teaching
Antipsychotics Thorazine (chlorpromazine), Haldol (haloperidol), Stelazine (trifluoperazine), Prolixin (fluphenazine), Clozaril (clozapine), Risperdal (risperidone)	Treatment of schizophrenia and other psychotic behavior that is violent or potentially violent	Blood dyscrasias, photosensitivity Darkening of the skin Extrapyramidal side effects (EPSEs): parkinsonism, akathisia, dystonia, tardive dyskinesia	Observe for any signs of EPSEs. Monitor blood work for any kind of abnormality. Discontinue slowly. Antacids will decrease absorption of antipsychotics.	These are very strong medications. Wear a large-rimmed hat, cover all exposed skin, and use a sunscreen when in the sun, especially if using Thorazine. Avoid alcohol, sleeping pills, and other medications. Do not alter dose before discussing it with the doctor. Take medication 1–2 hours before going to bed. Take antacids 1–2 hours after oral doses of antipsychotics.
Antianxiety Drugs Xanax (alprazolam), BuSpar (buspirone), Valium (diazepam), Ativan (lorazepam)	Decrease the effects of stress or mild depression without causing sedation	Can cause physical and psychological dependence, drowsiness, lethargy, fainting, transient hypotension, nausea, and vomiting; if discontinued abruptly, severe side effects, including nausea, hypotension, and fatal grand mal seizures	Administer intramuscular (IM) dosages deeply, slowly, and into large muscle masses. Z-track method of IM administration is preferred.	Teach the client and family that it is not safe to drive or use alcohol while using this classification of medication.
Antidepressants Elavil (amitriptyline), Triavil (perphenazine/amitriptyline), Tofranil (imipramine), Pamelor (nortriptyline), Paxil (paroxetine), Prozac (fluoxetine), Zoloft (sertraline), Xanax (alprazolam), Asendin (amoxapine), Ludiomil (maprotiline), Parnate (tranylcypromine), Nardil (phenelzine), Marplan (isocarboxazid)	Treatment of depression	Dependence, sedation, dry mouth, agitation, hypotension, vertigo, blood dyscrasias	Encourage clients to continue taking the medication during this time, because they may not feel any change in their mood for up to 3 weeks after starting medication.	Reinforce the teaching that these medications may take 2–3 weeks to reach a therapeutic level and provide the desired effect for the client.

continued

think about their situations. Cognitive (or cognitive/behavioral) therapy stresses ways of rethinking situations. The therapist confronts the client with certain behaviors and then works out ways of thinking about them differently.

Feeling sad about an unpleasant experience (such as the death of a loved one) is acceptable and normal, but long-term depression about the death is an extreme emotion and therefore considered to be unhealthy. In this situation, the client might be helped to see the death as a sad loss, but extreme, long-term depression would be viewed as an inappropriate response.

Cognitive therapies are gaining in popularity because they are usually significantly more short term than psychoanalysis and therefore less costly to the client. It is com-

Table 55–4. (continued)

Classification and Common Trade Names	Uses	Side Effects	Nursing Considerations	Client Teaching
Stimulants Acutrim, Dexatrim (phenylpropanolamine), Dexedrine (dextroamphetamine), Ritalin (methylphenidate)	Promotes alertness, diminishes appetite, combats narcolepsy, local anesthesia	Rapid or irregular heart rates, hypertension, hyperactivity, hand tremor, rapid speech, confusion, depression, seizures, suicidal thoughts, psychological dependence	Physical or psychological dependence, especially with long-term use. Diabetic clients should be informed that amphetamines can cause changes in their insulin requirements. Can also cause changes in judgment; people should use extreme caution when driving or operating equipment, and should avoid these activities if possible.	Diabetic clients should monitor insulin carefully and inform the doctor of any changes. Use extreme caution when driving or operating equipment, and avoid these activities if possible. Do not stop medication without consulting doctor. Use plain water to rinse mouth or use hard, sugarless candy to relieve dry mouth.
Antiparkinsonism Agents Cogentin (benztropine), Artane (trihexyphenidyl), Akineton (biperiden)	Decrease the effects of drug-induced and non-drug-induced symptoms of parkinsonism	Blurred vision, dry mouth, dizziness, drowsiness, confusion, tachycardia, urinary retention, constipation, changes in blood pressure, and melanoma	They should be avoided in children under 12 years old. Monitor blood pressure carefully (at least every 4 hours when beginning the course of treatment).	Use hard, sugarless candy to combat the effects of dry mouth. Increase dietary roughage to maintain bowel functioning. May cause drowsiness, so should not drive or operate equipment until the response to medication is established.

monly performed in groups. The clients are given "homework" that is specific to their needs. Clients practice their assignments between sessions.

Person-Centered/Humanistic Therapy

Abraham Maslow and Carl Rogers are two theorists who are often credited with the concept of person-centered or humanistic therapy. In this form of treatment, all caregivers focus on the whole person and work in the "present." It is not important in humanistic treatment to understand the cause of the problem or what happened in the person's past; what is important is the here and now. With this therapy the client will learn to see himself or herself as a person who has value and who is respected by others.

Nursing is very strongly centered in person-centered ideals. Three qualities are essential for caregivers: empathy, which is the ability to identify with the client's feelings without actually experiencing them with the client; unconditional positive regard (respect); and genuineness or honesty. Although nurses may not be active participants in the actual therapy sessions with clients, it is important to maintain these three qualities in all therapeutic relationships.

Counseling

Counseling is the provision of help or guidance by a health care professional. The area of counseling is licensed and regulated differently not only state by state, but sometimes municipality by municipality. Nurses prepared at an LPN/LVN level or at an RN level can, in some areas and with special training, practice some forms of counseling.

Nurses may be asked or required to accompany their clients to counseling sessions or even to facilitate a group discussion. The nurse must remember that these are confidential sessions, even if they are group oriented. Clients are there to work; others are there by invitation for special reasons.

Group Therapy

Groups are formed for many reasons; they can be ongoing or short term, depending on the needs of the clients or the type of disorder. For example, Alcoholics Anonymous (AA) and similar 12-step groups are well-established, ongoing groups formed around treatment of a specific problem (Fig. 55–3). Family counseling sessions may occur with individual therapists with a specialty in the problem area for that family. Marriage counseling may be done in a

Monoamine Oxidase Inhibitors

Several antidepressant drugs (isocarboxazid, phenelzine, tranylcypromine) are monoamine oxidase inhibitors (MAOIs). These drugs counteract depression by preventing the breakdown of dopamine and tyramine, an intermediate product in the conversion of tyrosine to epinephrine. The increased concentration of these chemicals in the central nervous system elevates the client's mood.

When a client taking MAOIs consumes foods high in tyramine, the drug prevents the normal breakdown of tyramine, leading to excessive epinephrine. Hypertension results, sometimes severe enough to cause intracranial hemorrhage. Some other drugs (furazolidone, isoniazid, procarbazine) produce similar reactions with tyramine-containing foods.

All food groups except breads and cereals have some items with sufficient tyramine to create problems for clients taking MAOIs. Example of common foods to be avoided are bananas, aged cheese, yogurt, bologna, salami, pepperoni, summer sausages, chocolate, beer, and wine.

Lithium Carbonate

The antimanic drug lithium carbonate is absorbed, distributed, and excreted along with sodium. Fluctuations in sodium intake will affect the metabolism of lithium. Thus, decreased sodium intake with decreased fluid intake may lead to retention of lithium and overmedication. Increased sodium intake from food or medications and increased fluid intake may hasten excretion of lithium, resulting in increased symptoms of mania.

group with other couples. Many times, peer counselors are used.

Therapists and counselors are tools. They do not heal the client; the client heals himself or herself. Clients must take the suggestions given by the therapist, try them, and see what works for them. Nurses can help by reinforcing the good work clients do in learning to stay healthy.

Electroconvulsive Therapy

Electroconvulsive therapy (ECT), sometimes called electroshock therapy (EST), is another form of treatment that is used in special situations. Some experts believe ECT works because it breaks up thought patterns in the brain, helping people to forget painful past experiences. It is very frightening to some people. Many changes have been made in this form of therapy since the 1940s to make it safer for the client.

Clients are generally given a sedative before the treatment. Nurses carefully monitor blood pressure and pulse before and after the treatment. The amount of electrical energy used is individualized to the client. A treatment usually lasts only a few seconds, and if the nurse is slow to look, he or she might miss seeing any kind of convulsion. Often, only a toe or a finger twitches slightly.

Side effects of ECT can be unpleasant. The client may feel confused and forgetful immediately after the treatment. This can be from a combination of the ECT itself and the medication that was used before the treatment. If there has been a strong seizure, the client may have some muscle soreness. Clients are secured with restraints during the treatment so movement is minimal.

Electroconvulsive therapy is not used indiscriminately. It is used when other therapies have not been helpful, and it is usually reserved for severe or long-term depression and certain types of schizophrenia.

The nurse's responsibilities include careful monitoring of vital signs and accurate documentation relating to the client's subjective and objective responses to the treatment. The client should receive nothing by mouth (NPO) for at least 4 hours before a treatment. Reminding the client to empty his or her bladder and to remove dentures, contact lenses, hair pins, and so on is also important. Because of the possibility of confusion and forgetfulness, it is common to restrict activity for 24 hours after a treatment. It is recommended that the nurse stay with the client until he or she is oriented and able to care for himself or herself. Ensuring that the person is kept safe after therapy is a major concern.

Relaxation Therapy

A variety of relaxation techniques can be taught to help clients control their responses to stress. Relaxation exercises such as deep, rhythmic breathing can increase oxygenation and provide distraction from stressors. Breathing exercises may be coupled with progressive muscle relaxation exercises. For this technique, clients are taught to start at the head and neck and systematically tense and then relax muscle groups as they progress toward the lower extremities. Soft music may enhance the ability to fully relax.

Imagery is the use of the imagination to promote relaxation. For this technique, the client is taught to imagine a pleasurable experience from his or her past, such as lying on a beach or soaking in a warm bath. Use of all senses is encouraged—for a beach image, the client might see the beach, feel the warm sun, smell the salt air, and hear the waves crashing against the shore.

Biofeedback uses computerized or other instruments to provide feedback about the client's degree of relaxation. Heart rate, skin temperature, and muscle tension might be measured; the client is taught by a specialist to control these variables with a variety of relaxation techniques.

Relaxation techniques may be used individually, but they are often used in combination with each other for maximum effect.

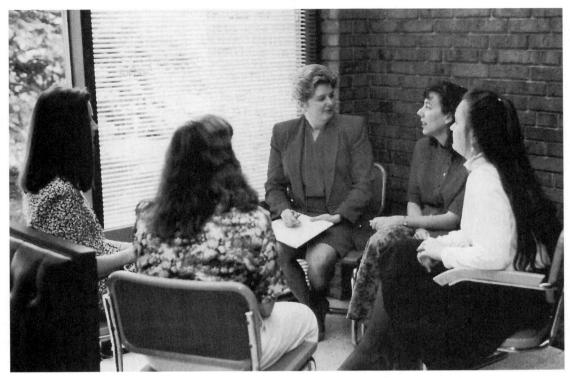

Figure 55–3. Group therapy may be helpful for some conditions. (From Fortinash, KM, and Holoday-Worret, PA: Psychiatric-Mental Health Nursing. Mosby, St Louis, 1996, p 366, with permission.)

Mental Health Disorders

ANXIETY DISORDERS

Stress is everywhere in our society. Stress produces anxiety. Most often, stress is associated with negative situations, but the good things that happen to us, such as weddings and job promotions, also produce stress. The stress from positive experiences is called **eustress.** It can produce just as much anxiety as the negative stressors. A *stressor* is any person or situation that produces an anxiety response. Stress and stressors are different for each person; therefore, it is important that nurses ask clients what their personal stress producers are.

Anxiety is the uncomfortable feeling of dread that occurs in response to extreme or prolonged periods of stress. It is commonly ranked as mild, moderate, severe, or panic. It is believed that a mild amount of anxiety is a normal part of being human and that mild anxiety is necessary to change and develop new ways of coping with stress.

Anxiety may also be influenced by one's culture. It may be acceptable for some people to acknowledge and discuss stress, but others may believe that one does not discuss personal problems with others. This cultural behavior can be a challenge for the nurse during an assessment.

Anxiety is usually referred to as either free-floating anxiety or signal anxiety. Free-floating anxiety is described as a general feeling of impending doom. The person cannot pinpoint the cause, but might say something like "I just know something bad is going to happen if I go on vacation." Signal anxiety, on the other hand, is an uncomfortable response to a known stressor ("Finals are only a week away and I've got that nausea again.") Both types of anxiety are involved in the various anxiety disorders.

Etiological Theories

Psychoanalytical theory says that anxiety is a conflict between the id (the "all for me" part of the personality) and the superego (the conscience), which was repressed in early development but which emerges again in adulthood.

Biological theory looks at this situation differently. Biological theories consider the sympathoadrenal (fight or flight) responses to stress and observe that the blood vessels constrict because epinephrine and norepinephrine have been released. Blood pressure rises. If the body adapts to the stress, hormone levels adjust to compensate for the epinephrine-norepinephrine release, and body functions return to homeostasis. If the body does not adapt to the stress, the immune system is challenged, lymph nodes swell, and risk for physical illness increases.

The LPN/LVN will usually observe mental illness in conjunction with medical-surgical illness. It is important

---

eustress: eu—normal or good + stress

for nurses to recognize the relationship between physical and emotional responses to stress. Some examples of medical conditions and the effects of the body's adaptation response to stress are shown in Table 55–5.

Differential Diagnosis

Because there are so many symptoms associated with anxiety disorders, it is important for people to have a complete physical examination before diagnosing an anxiety disorder. More than one condition may occur at the same time.

Types of Anxiety Disorders

Phobia

Phobia is the most common of the anxiety disorders. Phobia is defined as an irrational fear of a specific object or situation. The person is very aware of the fear and even the fact that it is irrational, but the fear continues.

Psychoanalytical view implies that it really is not the object that is the source of the fear, but rather the fear is a result of a defense mechanism called **displacement.** For example, the person with a phobia of snakes may have seen a frightening movie in which someone died from a snakebite. The stated object of the phobia would be interpreted as a symbol for the underlying cause of the fear.

Panic Disorder

Panic is a state of extreme fear that cannot be controlled. It is also referred to as panic attack, and people may not consider it to be a serious disorder.

Panic episodes present quickly. Clients must exhibit several episodes at a time in order to be given the diagnosis of panic disorder. Some of the symptoms associated with panic disorder are

- Fear (usually of dying, losing control of self, or "going crazy")
- Dissociation (a feeling that it is happening to someone else or not happening at all)
- Nausea
- Diaphoresis
- Chest pain
- Increased pulse
- Shaking

Generalized Anxiety Disorder

In generalized anxiety disorder (GAD), the anxiety itself (also referred to as excessive worry or severe stress) is the expressed symptom. Symptoms that may be present in GAD include the following:

- Restlessness or feeling "on edge"
- Shaking

Table 55–5. **Adaptation Responses to Stress**

Stress-related Medical Condition	Body's Adaptation to the Stress	Outcome of Stress on the Body
Lowered Immunity	Interferes with effectiveness of the body's antibodies; possibly related to interactions among the hypothalamus, pituitary gland, adrenal glands, and the immune system	Increased susceptibility to colds and other viruses and illnesses
Burnout	Associated with stress-related depression	Emotional detachment
Migraine, Cluster, and Tension Headaches	Tightening skeletal muscles, dilating of cranial arteries	Nausea, vomiting, tight feeling in or around head and shoulders, tinnitus, inability to tolerate light, weakness of a limb
Stress (Peptic) Ulcers	Stress contributes to the formation of ulcers by stimulating the vagus nerve and ultimately leading to hypersecretion of hydrochloric acid	Nausea, vomiting, gastrointestinal bleeding, perforation of intestinal walls
Hypertension	Role of stress not positively known; thought to contribute to hypertension by negatively interacting with the kidneys, autonomic nervous system, and endocrine system	Resistance to blood flow through the cardiovascular system, causing pressure on the arteries; can lead to stroke, heart attack, and kidney failure
Coronary Artery Disease	Stressor increases the amount of epinephrine and norepinephrine	Coronary vessels dilate, pulse and respirations increase
Cancer	Stress lowers immune response	Lowered immunity may allow for overcolonization of opportunistic cancer cells
Asthma	Autonomic nervous system stimulates mucus, increases blood flow, and constricts bronchial tubes; may be associated with other stress-related conditions such as allergy and viral infection	Wheezing, coughing, dyspnea, apprehension; may lead to respiratory infections, respiratory failure, or pneumothorax

- Palpitations
- Dry mouth
- Nausea, vomiting
- Easy frightening
- Hot flashes
- Chills
- Polyuria
- Difficulty swallowing

Obsessive-Compulsive Disorder

Obsessive-compulsive disorder (OCD) is a different type of anxiety disorder. It consists of two parts: **obsession** (repetitive thought, urge, or emotion) and **compulsion** (repetitive act that may appear purposeful). An example of obsessive-compulsive disorder is the need to check that the doors are locked numerous times before one is able to sleep or leave the house. In reality, this need to repetitively check the locks may prevent the person from sleeping or leaving at all. Behaviors become very ritualistic. The person with OCD is unable to stop the thought or the action. Performing the thought or the action is the mechanism that reduces the anxiety.

Posttraumatic Stress Disorder

Posttraumatic stress disorder (PTSD) develops in response to some unexpected emotional or physical trauma that could not be controlled. People who have fought in wars, who have been raped, or who have survived violent storms or violent acts (such as the Oklahoma Federal Building bombing in 1995) are examples of people who are susceptible to suffering from this disorder.

A term that is associated with PTSD is *survivor guilt.* This is the feeling of guilt expressed by those who survived. A survivor of an airline crash may say "Why me? Why did I make it? I should have died too!"

Symptoms may appear immediately or may be repressed until years later. Symptoms include the following:

- "Flashbacks" in which the person may relive and act out the traumatic event
- Social **withdrawal**
- Feelings of low self-esteem
- Changes in relationships with significant others
- Difficulty forming new relationships
- Irritability and outbursts of anger seemingly for no obvious reason
- Depression
- Chemical dependency

Medical Treatment for Clients with Anxiety Disorders

Treatment is individualized for the client and may include one or more of the following: psychopharmacology, individual psychotherapy, group therapy, systematic desensi-tization, hypnosis, imagery, relaxation exercises, and biofeedback.

Psychopharmacology usually involves the antianxiety classification of medications. The benzodiazepines such as diazepam (Valium) and alprazolam (Xanax) are commonly used and are effective in most cases. Use of antianxiety drugs is short term whenever possible because of the strong potential for dependency. Individuals who have anxiety disorders and who are chemically dependent are managed with other medications that have calming qualities but do not have the same high potential for **addiction** as the antianxiety drugs. Hydroxyzine hydrochloride (Atarax), clonidine (Catapres), and sertraline (Zoloft) are common alternatives in this situation.[14]

Nursing Interventions for Clients with Anxiety Disorders

1. Maintain a calm milieu.
2. Maintain open communication.

Encourage the client to verbalize all thoughts and feelings. Honesty in dealing with clients will help them learn to trust others and will enhance their self-esteem. Observe nonverbal communication.

3. Observe for signs of suicidal thoughts.
4. Report and document any changes in behavior.

Any change can be significant to that client's care. Positive or negative alterations in the way a client responds to the nurse, to the treatment plan, or to other people and situations should be reported.

5. Encourage activities.

Activities that are enjoyable and nonstressful will provide diversion and will give staff an opportunity to provide positive feedback about the progress the client is making. The client should not be put in a situation of competition.

CRITICAL THINKING: Tommy

Tommy has come to your clinic with numerous cracks on his hands. They are bleeding and very sore. Tommy tells you that he just has to wash his hands all of the time. His mother says he will wash for 2 to 3 hours at a time, and he will not stop when she tells him to. The doctor has diagnosed Tommy with obsessive-compulsive disorder and has explained the illness to Tommy and his mother. When the doctor leaves the room, Tommy's mother begins to cry. "What did he just say? What am I supposed to do? What did I do wrong that Tommy got this illness?" How do you respond?

Answers at end of chapter.

MOOD DISORDERS

Mood disorders (also called affective disorders) are disorders in which people experience extreme changes in mood (emotions) and affect (the outward expression of the mood). Sadness becomes depression when it lasts a very long time (generally two years or more) or when it begins to interfere with normal day-to-day functioning (Fig. 55–4). People of all age groups and all ethnic and socioeconomic groups develop mood disorders.

Etiological Theories

Psychoanalytical theory indicates that people who have suffered loss in their life are at risk for developing depressions. Depression is also associated with unresolved anger and has been explained as "anger turned inward." In other words, people who cannot or do not deal appropriately with situations that anger them tend to repress the anger (turn it inside) and become depressed.

Cognitive theorists believe that the way people perceive events and situations may lead to depression. Instead of thinking about failing an exam as being unfortunate and disappointing, some people with tendencies toward depression will exaggerate the emotion and turn the situation into something much deeper, such as thoughts of "I'm stupid" or "I'll never get anywhere."

Biological theories offer genetic links and neurochemical interactions as two etiologies. Serotonin and norepinephrine have an effect on mood; if these neurochemicals are elevated, mood is elevated, and if they are low, mood will be low. Biological theorists also believe that there is a connection between these neurochemicals and female hormones.

Differential Diagnosis

Symptoms of depression may occur as a result of other disorders, such as schizophrenia or drug side effects or overuse. Symptoms can mimic heart failure, nutritional deficiencies, fluid and electrolyte imbalances, infections, or diabetes.

Types of Mood Disorders

Major (Unipolar) Depression

People who develop major depression exhibit a vast array of symptoms. Some behavioral and physical symptoms of major depression include the following:

- Sad mood
- Loss of pleasure in things that are usually pleasurable
- **Hallucinations** or **delusions** (possible, but uncommon)
- Weight loss or gain resulting from changes in appetite
- Sleep pattern disturbances
- Increased fatigue
- Increased agitation
- Increase or decrease in normal activity
- Lowered pleasure for life, including sexual activity
- Decreased ability to think, remember, or concentrate
- Suicidal thoughts

Bipolar Depression

Approximately 2 million Americans suffer from **bipolar** depression. Bipolar depression (or manic-depressive illness or bipolar disorder) is a type of depression with both extreme **mania** (extreme elation or agitation) and extreme depression. The mania is part of the depression. Think of a color you like. Now think of all the shades of that color

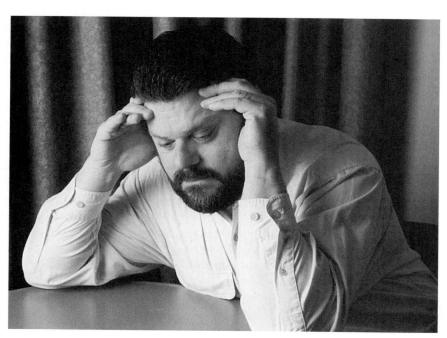

Figure 55–4. Depression interferes with normal day-to-day functioning.

from the very palest shade to the brightest shade (like the color cards that you can get in paint stores). Both extremes of color are very different, but both are still part of the same color. This is one way to remember that mania and depression are just opposite poles of the same illness. It takes only one episode of mania to be diagnosed with bipolar disorder, but it is more common to see the client alternating, or cycling, from one "pole" to the other. Individuals can cycle slowly (over weeks or months or even years), or they can be "quick cyclers" who can change moods several times in an hour.

Common signs of mania include the following:

- Excessive high moods
- Sustained period of behavior that is different from usual
- Increased energy, activity, restlessness, racing thoughts, and rapid talking
- Decreased need for sleep
- Unrealistic beliefs in one's abilities and powers
- Extreme irritability and distractibility
- Uncharacteristically poor judgment
- Increased sexual drive
- Abuse of drugs, particularly cocaine, alcohol, and sleeping medications
- Obnoxious, provocative, or intrusive behavior
- Denial that anything is wrong

Common signs of depression include the following:

- Persistent sad, anxious, or empty mood
- Feelings of guilt, worthlessness, hopelessness, or pessimism
- Loss of interest or pleasure in usual activities, including sex
- Decreased energy—a feeling of fatigue or being slowed down
- Difficulty concentrating, remembering, and making decisions
- Restlessness or irritability
- Sleep disturbances
- Loss of appetite and weight loss or gain
- Thoughts of death or suicide; suicide attempts

Medical Treatment for Clients with Mood Disorders

With treatment, it is estimated that approximately 80 percent of people with serious depression can be helped in a matter of a few weeks. Some common medical treatments for depression are

- Lithium
- Antidepressants
- Psychotherapy
- Electroconvulsive therapy

---

psychosomatic: psyche—soul or mind + soma—body

Lithium is the drug of choice in most instances for the treatment of bipolar depression. Antidepressants such as Elavil (amitriptyline), Prozac (fluoxetine hydrochloride), and Desyrel (trazodone hydrochloride) and antianxiety drugs such as Ativan (lorazepam) may also be used.

Psychotherapy for the client and family may be helpful in understanding the illness and learning problem solving and other new adaptive coping behaviors. For young children, play therapy is the most common and effective form of therapy.

Electroconvulsive therapy is an option when other therapy is not effective.

Nursing Interventions for Clients with Mood Disorders

1. Be patient!
2. Monitor lithium levels. Normal range of lithium is 1.0 to 1.5 mEq/L while loading and 0.6 to 1.2 mEq/L when on maintenance.
3. Be honest in communicating thoughts and feelings with the client.
4. Be consistent in communication and in all areas of implementation of the care plan.
5. Provide appropriate activities. Activity needs to be planned carefully and should be age appropriate. Activity that includes small groups can be helpful for building esteem. Activities that can be done alone will be helpful when it is necessary to decrease stimulation.
6. Maintain nutrition. Physical health is important for mental health. The dietitian may be consulted for assistance.
7. Use therapeutic communication and active listening. This is not a time for false reassurance. Do *not* use phrases such as "Cheer up!" or "It could be worse!" Making an observation such as "I like the way you look in that blue outfit. Is it new?" may go farther in helping the person improve self-esteem than "Cheer up!" (See Gerontological Issues Box 55–3 for interventions for older adults who are suicidal.)

SOMATOFORM/PSYCHOSOMATIC DISORDERS

The **somatoform** (or **psychosomatic**) disorders are conditions in which physical symptoms occur with no known organic cause. It is believed that the physical symptoms are connected to a psychological conflict. Because the client is not able to control the symptoms, they are considered to be caused from some unconscious mechanism.

Etiological Theories

Psychoanalytical theorists believe that the somatoform disorders are rooted in unconscious mechanisms that develop

GERONTOLOGICAL ISSUES BOX 55–3

Suicide and the Older Adult

Older adults are not immune to suicidal thoughts. White males over the age of 75 have an especially high suicide rate.

Comments by any older adult referring to hopelessness or desire to die must be explored to assess suicide risk. The following comments could be a reflection of suicide potential in an older adult who is depressed:

"Living is harder than dying could ever be."

"I am a used-up old man who is a burden for everyone."

"I am useless. I can't do anything anymore."

"I don't know why God won't take me."

To adequately assess suicide potential, the nurse must ask questions that establish whether the older adult has

- Thought about ending his or her life
- Attempted to end his or her life in the past
- Developed a plan to end his or her life
- Set the plan into action (i.e., bought a gun, has a full bottle of pills in the bed stand)

Any older adult who has a plan to end his or her life and has the ability or resources to do so must be immediately referred for psychological evaluation.

Crisis Intervention for an Older Adult Who Is Suicidal

- Remove any items that the older adult could use to inflict an injury or end his or her life.

- Make arrangements for direct supervision and observation that are reliable, considering personnel and family resources. Often, hospital admission is the most appropriate intervention for a person at a very high risk for suicide.
- Help the older adult talk about the crisis or life event that has devastated his or her desire to live. For example, encourage reminiscence about the client's spouse, or allow the older person to express the frustration of being unable to physically meet the daily demands of life.
- Develop a "do no harm" or suicide contract with the older adult. Outline a short-term, structured plan to keep the older adult safe. Focus on decreasing social isolation by requiring personal social contacts (e.g., stay at daughter's home for a weekend; go to the senior center for lunch; call a specific person who is willing and wants to listen to feelings and concerns; exercise; take a walk outside; volunteer services at a nursing home, hospital, or school).

Older adults often need assistance to develop or enhance skills required to cope with life events. Self-care and personal independence in care choices need to be encouraged. Developing an understanding and a manner of avoiding personal thinking patterns and behaviors that increase depression are important skills to learn as part of managing depression.

to deny, repress, and displace anxiety. Biologically, there is research into the possibility of a genetic predisposition to somatic difficulties.

Types of Somatoform Disorders

There are five separate illnesses within the category of somatoform disorders and two additional illnesses that are closely related. These include conversion disorder, hypochondriasis, dysmorphophobia/body dismorphic disorder, somatization disorder, and somatoform pain disorder. This chapter will give a brief explanation of conversion disorder.

Conversion Disorder

Conversion disorder is an illness that emerges from overuse of the conversion reaction defense mechanism (refer to Table 55–3). In conversion disorder, there is a loss or decrease in physical functioning that seems to have a neurological connection. Paralysis and blindness are two common examples of this disorder. Age of onset is usually adolescence and young adulthood, but it can occur later in life as well.

The symptoms, although not supportive of organic disease, are very real to the client. It should not be conveyed

to the client that the nurse thinks the person is "faking" the illness; this is not true. Clients are truly experiencing the symptoms.

The belief about this disorder is that the symptom is allowing the person to avoid some situation that is unacceptable to him or her. The symptom helps the client relieve the anxiety. This is called primary gain. Secondary gain results from the extra benefits one may acquire as a result of staying ill, such as extra emotional support, sympathy, love, or financial benefits.

Medical Treatment for Clients with Somatoform Disorders

Hospitalized clients will usually be admitted to a medical unit rather than a psychiatric unit. Treatment will be individualized for the client. Hypnosis and relaxation techniques are used with many clients. Methods of stress management are taught. Behavior modification may be effective for some clients. Clients may resist accepting the fact that their problem is psychological or emotional in nature and may feel insulted and become resistant to treatment.

Medications are used sparingly. When they are ordered for a client, the classifications of choice are usually antidepressants, antianxiety drugs, or both.

Nursing Management for Clients with Somatoform Disorders

1. *Skillful communication.* Honesty and gaining trust will encourage the client to verbalize thoughts and feelings about the physical and emotional aspects of this disorder. An example of a way to be honest about the situation would be for the nurse to say, "Ms. P., your doctor can find no physical or life-threatening conditions at this time. We will continue to observe and examine you. We will make every attempt to help you improve."
2. *Therapy.* Keeping the client focused on other topics may help in the recovery.
3. *Support.* The nurse caring for the client with a somatoform disorder must pay attention to the person but must not reinforce the symptom. A thorough head-to-toe assessment should always be done. The client will see the nurse's concern for his or her health, but the nurse will not be focusing on the area of dysfunction or reinforcing the problem. All findings are documented objectively.

SCHIZOPHRENIA

Schizophrenia is becoming more widely viewed as a group of illnesses rather than a single condition. People with schizophrenia seem very distractible. It is difficult for them to focus on one topic for any length of time.

Schizophrenia most often strikes adolescents and young adults. The National Institute of Mental Health estimates that nearly 3 million Americans will develop schizophrenia during the course of their lives.

The term *schizophrenia* (which means "split mind") was first used by a Swiss psychiatrist, Eugene Bleuler.[15] Schizophrenia is a serious psychiatric disorder. People who have schizophrenia have a "split" between their thoughts and their feelings and between their reality and society's reality. The person may have splits concerning gender identity. People who have schizophrenia may not be able to differentiate between what is "theirs" and what is "everybody else's" in relation to social functioning. Poor self-esteem is an issue for clients with schizophrenia. People with schizophrenia are generally highly intelligent. Schizophrenia is *not* the same thing as multiple personality disorder.

Schizophrenia has an insidious onset. This means that it is "sneaky." The early symptoms of quietness and withdrawal in an adolescent person may be shrugged off as normal adolescent behavior. It may be a school nurse or counselor who begins to notice these changes. Grades may begin to suffer. The adolescent may have a change in personality or a change in the way he or she relates to other people. It is easy to misinterpret these new behaviors as part of the adolescent experience.

Eugene Bleuler used a system of "four A's" to define schizophrenia. The four A's are associative disturbance, affect, autism, and ambivalence.

Associative Disturbance

In associative disturbance (also referred to as associative looseness), the client typically exhibits three main behaviors: (1) making up words (neologisms); (2) rambling from topic to topic; and (3) using revolving words and syllables that may be associated with a specific word but that are out of context with the conversation. Making up words that rhyme with other words is another behavior that is sometimes observed.

Affect

Affect, as discussed earlier, is the outward expression of emotion. People with schizophrenia generally have what is called a "flat" or "blunted" affect. This means that they rarely show signs of any emotion.

In schizophrenia there may also be inappropriate or incongruent affect. The outward expression of the mood does not match the stated feeling (e.g., clients laughing when they state they feel sad or depressed). Exaggerations of affect are also present in some clients.

Autism

Autism associated with schizophrenia is an emotional detachment. People who display autistic behavior are preoccupied with the self and show little concern for any reality outside their own world (Fig. 55–5).

Ambivalence

Ambivalence means to have opposite feelings about a person or situation at the same time. An example of this is the love/hate relationships sometimes seen in jobs or marriages. (Caution: not all people who have love/hate relationships are schizophrenic.)

In addition to the four A's, clients with schizophrenia display other common symptoms such as delusions, hallucinations, and **illusions.** *Delusions* are fixed, false beliefs that cannot be changed by logic. Clients resist any factual proof that their beliefs do not exist. Typically, clients exhibit delusions of grandeur, persecutory delusions, or guilt. *Hallucinations* are false sensory perceptions. They can affect any of the five senses. *Illusions* are mistaken perceptions of reality.

Hallucinations and illusions are easily confused. Anyone who has ever watched a magician or seen certain pictures in cloud formations has witnessed an illusion. In illusion, *something* is there; it is just perceived incorrectly. The card did not magically appear; it was set up to appear when the magician wanted it to. In hallucination, there is nothing to misinterpret. The person who sees a lamb in a certain cloud formation is experiencing an illusion; the person who sees a lamb in the sky and there are no clouds is experiencing a hallucination.

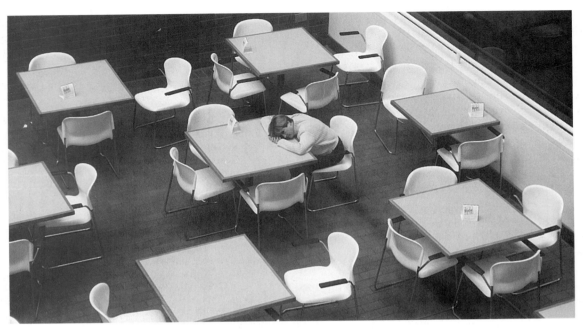

Figure 55–5. The client with schizophrenia may withdraw.

Etiological Theories

There are psychoanalytical and biological theories of the causes of schizophrenia. The symptoms of schizophrenia are highly debated on both sides of the nature versus nurture theory.

The psychoanalytical, or nurture, theories revert to the anal stage of freudian theory. The inability to meet the challenge of oral gratification leaves people in the adolescent and young adult years unable to handle their developing sexuality, according to Freud. Lack of nurturing mother-child relationships can also lead to personalities that are cool or aloof (or indifferent) in their relationships. Freud would also attribute the disruption of effective communication to failure to reach oral gratification.

Schizophrenia and its relationship to genetics has been examined in twins studies, family studies, and adoption studies for approximately 75 years. Studies of identical twins (the psychobiological, or nature, theory) show that if one twin has schizophrenia, the other has approximately a 50 percent chance of developing it also. In fraternal twins, that percentage drops to approximately 10 percent. It is believed that the more genes twins or family members have in common, the greater the chance for the second twin developing schizophrenia. Clients with schizophrenia generally have elevated amounts of dopamine or a brain that overreacts to the amount of dopamine that is present.

Types of Schizophrenia

There are several categories of schizophrenia. This chapter will discuss only the most common one of those categories: paranoid schizophrenia. *Paranoid schizophrenia* is defined as schizophrenia in which the person exhibits unusual suspiciousness and fear. The main symptom of paranoid schizophrenia is suspiciousness. People who have paranoid schizophrenia may also be hostile and aggressive in their behavior.

Clients with this type of schizophrenia tend to have delusions of persecution and grandeur. In persecutory delusions, clients state that they feel tormented and followed by people. These people could be staff, relatives, or the announcer on the radio or television. In delusions of grandeur, the client may state that he or she is God or the president of the United States.

Hallucinations almost always go along with the delusions. The hallucinations can affect any of the five senses but are most commonly auditory or visual. Clients with paranoid schizophrenia will speak about "the voices." These voices are frightening and derogatory to the client and are responsible for many of the actions performed by people with paranoid schizophrenia. Clients will experience increased fear, anxiety, and suicidal ideation as a result of the voices. The nurse caring for a client with paranoid schizophrenia may see or hear the client arguing with what at first appears to be himself or herself. Actually, the client is arguing with the voices. Describing the voices is difficult, but imagine that you are in a room with six televisions on different stations at the same time. This example comes close to what some clients have described as the voices.

Medical Treatment for Clients with Schizophrenia

Medications, ECT, and psychotherapy are indicated for clients with schizophrenia.

Among the classifications of medications that will be prescribed for certain clients are the antipsychotics, which block dopamine action in the brain. Decreased dopamine action creates extrapyramidal side effects. Anticholinergic medications such as Cogentin (benztropine) or Artane (trihexphenidyl) are used to combat the extrapyramidal side effects of the antipsychotics by helping return balance between dopamine, acetylcholine, and other neurotransmitters. New antipsychotic medications such as Clozaril (clozapine) and Risperdal (risperidone) are being developed specifically for use in schizophrenia.

Psychotherapy may include individual, group, and family therapy. Electroconvulsive therapy is used in some severe cases or in cases that are difficult to treat; ECT is usually not used until other methods of therapy have been attempted.

Nursing Interventions for Clients with Schizophrenia

1. *Never reinforce hallucinations, delusions, or illusions.* It is necessary to keep the client in reality as the nurse knows it. Some examples of responses to clients who are hallucinating are listed in Table 55–6.
2. *Never whisper or laugh when the client cannot hear the whole conversation.* Face the client when having a conversation, even a personal conversation. Turning away may be interpreted as rejection.
3. *Avoid placing the client in situations of competition or embarrassment.*
4. *Develop trust.* It is crucial for a trusting relationship to exist between the nurse and the client. Promises must be kept. The nurse should be honest and consistent in all areas of the client's treatment plan. The client is allowed to vent thoughts and feelings, when

appropriate to the time and place. Whenever possible, the same nurse should be assigned to the same clients to ensure the best possible continuity of care.
5. *Provide a therapeutic milieu.* Structure the treatment setting in a way that promotes healthy behaviors and minimizes anxiety. Providing written instructions or information boards can help promote reality and self-responsible behavior.
6. *Keep communication simple.* Be brief and clear with all directions. State what is acceptable; give the rationale and consequences at the same time. Stating information in positive rather than negative terms will also be helpful; for example, "Eat your food calmly" rather than "Do not throw your food!"

SUBSTANCE ABUSE DISORDERS

Alcoholism and chemical dependency are serious conditions in American society. People start using alcohol and drugs for many reasons, but often it is to feel accepted by a peer group or to feel comfortable in a social situation. People mistake the temporary high as a stimulant. In reality, alcohol is a depressant. Nurses must understand that any chemical can be potentially dangerous.

Physical **dependence** on a substance, **tolerance** (the ability to endure the effects of a drug or the need for higher amounts of the drug to produce the high), and **withdrawal** (unpleasant physical, psychological, or cognitive effects that result from decreasing or stopping the use of the chemical after regular use) are characteristics of addiction. The general definitions of substance **abuse** and substance dependence apply to any substance. *Substance dependence* (Fig. 55–6) is a condition in which a person has had several (usually three) of the following symptoms for 1 month or longer:

Table 55–6. **Suggested Interventions for Clients with Schizophrenia Who Are Hallucinating**

Suggested Action	Rationale
1. "Mr. R., I don't see any snakes. It is time for lunch. I will walk to the dining room with you."	1. Lets the client know you heard him, but brings him immediately into the reality of time of day and need to go to the dining room.
2. "I see a crack in the wall, Mr. R. It is harmless; you are safe. Susan is here to take you down to occupational therapy now."	2. This is in response to a probable illusion. It lets the client know that you see something. It validates his fear, but it tells him what you see and then moves him into the here and now.
3. "I know that your thoughts seem very real to you, Ms. C., but they do not seem logical to me. I would like for you to come to your room and get dressed now, please."	3. Again, you are validating the client's concern without exploring and focusing on the delusion.
4. "Ms. C, it appears to me that you are listening to someone. Are you hearing voices other than mine?"	4. This is a method of validating your impression of what you see. This is as far as you will go into exploring what she may be hearing.
5. "Thank you, Ms. C. I want to help you focus away from the other voices. I am real; they are not. Please come with me to the reading room."	5. Responds to her in the present and reinforces her response to you. Attempts to redirect her thinking.

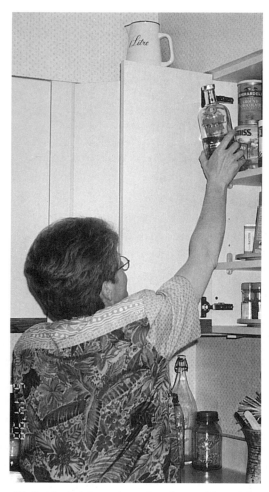

Figure 55–6. Alcohol dependence interferes with social and professional activities.

- The client needs more of the substance and at more frequent intervals to achieve the "high," or the effect of the substance.
- The client spends much time obtaining the substance.
- The client gives up important social or professional functions in order to use the substance.
- The client has tried at least once to quit but still obsesses about the substance.
- Misuse or withdrawal symptoms interfere with job, family, or social activities.
- The client uses the substance regardless of the problems it causes.
- Tolerance increases greatly (by approximately 50 percent).
- The client uses the substance to avoid withdrawal symptoms.

Substance abuse is defined differently than dependence and is often diagnosed by a rating system similar to the following one:

- *Mild*—The person meets three of the above criteria, but social functioning is only minimally affected.

- *Moderate*—Symptoms are somewhere between mild and severe.
- *Severe*—The client meets more than three of the above criteria, and social obligations are impaired.
- *Partial remission*—No substance use for over 6 months, some symptoms have occurred.
- *Full remission*—No substance use for over 6 months, no symptoms have occurred.

Not all clients who have a substance abuse disorder go through all stages, and not everyone will go through them in the same order.

Nurses need to develop an interest in chemical dependency for several reasons. First, many medical-surgical clients are chemically dependent. This affects their healing and the effect of their medications. Second, as part of the human experience, the nurse's chance of being in a close personal relationship with a person who is chemically dependent is great. Third, and maybe most important, nurses are part of a profession that is statistically a high user and abuser of drugs and alcohol. (See Ethical Considerations Box 55–4.) Studies indicate that 10 to 20 percent of all nurses in the United States will be chemically dependent at some point in their lifetime.[16]

Substance abuse is not a one-person illness; it affects personal and professional relationships with people who are associated with the user. The term **dysfunctional** is often used to refer to the relationships within an alcoholic family or work environment. Dishonesty and inability to discuss the situation are strong components of the disease. Many times, people who live or work in the dysfunctional group begin to cover up for the user's behaviors and lack of responsibility. Family members or significant others will take sides, begin to be dishonest with each other, and erode the bond within that group. Eventually, this leads to a condition called **codependence,** which is as serious as the use and abuse of the substance. In codependence, the significant others in the family group begin to lose their own sense of identity and purpose and exist solely for the abuser. Their actions take away the opportunity for the user to take responsibility for his or her own actions.

Why do some people become addicted or dependent and others do not? Can it be the chemical or is it the person? Some theorists believe in the existence of an addictive personality, which may begin to explain addictions to food, sex, and gambling, as well as alcohol, chemicals, and other dependencies.

Etiological Theories

Psychoanalytical theories state that people who develop addictions to alcohol or other substances are people who failed to successfully pass through the "oral" stage of development.

---

dysfunctional: dys—bad or difficult + functional—performance

ETHICAL CONSIDERATIONS BOX 55-4

Nurses Who Abuse Drugs

Ellen and Julie are LPNs who work in a busy medical unit in a large hospital. They were close friends in nursing school and have been working the night shift together for 3 years. Recently, Ellen went through a difficult and painful divorce, and Julie has noticed that Ellen's personality has changed. Ellen, usually serious, and almost compulsive in the completion of her work, has taken on a very lackadaisical attitude, laughs or giggles at inappropriate times, and frequently calls in sick. She also displays hostility toward the hospital administration and seems very irritated when corrected. Julie has observed Ellen taking increasingly large doses of "nerve medication" and fears that her friend is becoming a drug abuser.

One evening, Ellen arrives at work with glassy eyes and slurred speech. She asks Julie to watch her patients for her while she takes a little nap to "sleep it off." Julie asks Ellen if she is becoming a drug abuser, and after some initial denial, Ellen admits that she has been taking increasingly large doses of medication in order to continue functioning from day to day. Ellen pleads with Julie not to tell the head nurse or anyone else about the drug problem. Because of their friendship, Julie consents to cover for Ellen this night.

The next night, Ellen again comes to work with obvious signs of drug intoxication. She again asks Julie to cover for her, swearing that this would be the absolute last time it would happen. Ellen falls asleep while listening to the taped report for the change of shifts. What should Julie do?

The substance-abusing nurse is one of the most common situations that nurses may encounter during their careers. It is estimated that about 40,000 nurses who work in the United States are alcoholics, and drug addiction among nurses is reported to be 30 to 100 times greater than among the general population. Nurses have easy access to drugs because they are usually responsible for obtaining and maintaining the supply of controlled drugs in a hospital. Other factors that contribute to the increased drug abuse among nurses include job stress, short staffing, double shifts, unrealistic expectations, frustration and anxiety, personal problems, and lack of autonomy in practice.

Professional and emotional conflicts are felt by the drug-abusing nurse's colleagues, who must use their professional training as promoters of health to try to understand a nurse's abuse of drugs. Underlying the ethical dilemma is the right of the patient to safe and competent treatment versus the nurse's right to self-determination (freedom to abuse drugs). According to the nurses' code of ethics, nurses have a major obligation to protect the public from practitioners who are unsafe, which far outweighs the nurse's right to self-determination.

In this particular situation, Julie does have an obligation to do something about Ellen's drug problem. Covering for Ellen will not solve the problem. The first thing to do is to get a second opinion about Ellen's drug problem and then to confront her. She can also file a report through the institution's chain of command to the unit manager and head nurse, and finally the director of nursing. If the institution hierarchy will not take any action, the nurse should submit the report to the state board of nursing. This report should be well documented and signed, and it should include a request for confidentiality if the nurse submitting the report does not want to be known. To allow Ellen to practice while under the influence of drugs puts Julie in a very serious legal position. If Ellen were to do something wrong and harm a patient, and Julie knew that Ellen was under the influence of drugs, Julie could be held liable under the law.

Biological theories include numerous studies that imply that there is some sort of genetic metabolic disorder. Many of these studies were done on twins born to an alcoholic parent or parents who were separated from the parents at birth or shortly after birth. The number of twins who were born of alcoholic parents but raised by nonalcoholic parents and yet developed alcoholism is consistently high.

Cognitive-behavioral theorists suggest the way in which a person perceives being high may influence the act of becoming high. It can be a very innocent beginning: obtaining relief from the medications given by the doctor can, according to cognitive theory, leave people perceiving that the use of these drugs is a "miracle cure." It becomes appealing to want that kind of relief again, and very soon a pattern is formed and other substances may be involved.

Differential Diagnosis

Commonly, the alcoholic client is admitted to the medical unit with primary medical diagnoses including dehydra-tion, hyperemesis, or respiratory infections. Data collected by the nurse, laboratory test results, client need for frequent pain medication, or symptoms of withdrawal may lead the nurse or physician to pursue the possibility of chemical dependency.

Types

Alcohol Abuse and Dependence

Use and abuse of alcohol is present in all walks of life, in all economic levels, and in both genders. Sometimes a very fine line exists between a person who is a social drinker and a person who has an abuse condition. One factor used to make that differentiation is the degree of need or compulsion to drink. There is a high incidence of alcohol use and abuse among the elderly, teenagers, and even younger children. Alcoholism either directly or indirectly decreases a person's life expectancy by an average of 10 to 12 years.

Denial is a common defense mechanism used by people who are substance abusers. The alcohol-dependent person will often use statements such as "I can quit anytime I want to" or "I just need a little bump to loosen me up."

Typical symptoms of alcohol dependence include the following:

- Impaired social function and relationships
- Inability to cut down or stop using; daily use is common
- Binges usually lasting 2 days or more
- Blackouts (amnesia while intoxicated)
- Vomiting
- Dehydration
- Disorientation
- Increased vulnerability to infections, accidents, and other injury

Sometimes clients who are actively using drugs or alcohol when admitted to an inpatient setting, or who are cut off from their alcohol abruptly, experience a condition called **delirium tremens** (DTs). In DTs, hyperexcitability in the sensory activity of the individual can cause visual hallucinations, tremors, and possibly tonic-clonic seizures. Elevated blood pressure and pulse and cardiac dysrhythmias may also occur. This condition occurs within hours or days after the client has stopped drinking and can last a week or more; hospitalization is necessary.

TREATMENTS FOR ALCOHOL ABUSE AND DEPENDENCE. Perhaps the single most effective treatment for alcoholism is involvement in Alcoholics Anonymous (AA). Treatment for and recovery from alcohol dependency and abuse is a slow process. With very few exceptions, an alcoholic who is recovering cannot ever have another drink, or he or she will risk the chance of returning to previous abusive patterns.

Rationale-emotive therapy (RET) is being used as well. RET advocates believe that with homework and practice, a person can learn to think differently about the event that led to the drinking. When the person changes the belief system about the activating event and the drinking, the consequences of drinking will be less powerful. AA and RET are group activities.

Psychoanalysis may also be used. Psychoanalysis provides one-on-one therapy. Family therapy is important in reinstating honesty in communications.

Medications are used cautiously. It is not always wise to substitute the alcohol with another chemical. If, however, the anxiety level prohibits participation in therapy, or if a depressive disorder accompanies the abuse, medications may be prescribed. Antidepressant or antianxiety drugs are most often prescribed. Disulfiram (Antabuse) is a medication that is sometimes prescribed for the person who abuses alcohol. The client taking Antabuse who ingests alcohol develops a severe reaction, causing chest pain, nausea, vomiting, confusion, and other symptoms. This reaction discourages the client from using alcohol. Nurses need to be aware that the person on Antabuse can also be adversely affected if he or she uses products that contain alcohol, such as cologne, mouthwash, aftershave, or cough syrup.

Use of benzodiazepines (Valium, Ativan) can help prevent symptoms of DTs during acute withdrawal.

Milieu can be varied as well. Therapy may range from in-house hospitalizations of 2 weeks or more to independent attempts to help oneself by attending AA. It is not uncommon for clients to seek treatment more than once. This is not to be interpreted as a weakness in the individual or the treatment program. It is only a sign that the person is learning more about the disorder and the need to help himself or herself.

NURSING CARE FOR CLIENTS WITH ALCOHOL ABUSE AND DEPENDENCE

1. *Be honest.* Effective therapeutic communication is essential. Nurses need to be in touch with their own thoughts and feelings about addictions.
2. *Provide group support.* Many chemical dependency units provide group support meetings.
3. *Be aware of the use of defense mechanisms.* The client should be confronted if rationalization or denial behaviors are noted.
4. *Use positive reinforcement.* Positive reinforcement for successes is important when helping a person with an addiction. Every step is a big one in this field; every step taken is a new one.
5. *Provide a safe environment.* Clients who are chemically addicted may become suicidal or display other bizarre behavior, especially during DTs. Maintaining a safe milieu and calm demeanor will help the client through this difficult time. Also, the fact that a client is hospitalized does not guarantee that he or she does not have access to the chemical or even use it in the presence of the nurse. The nurse must be constantly alert. Suspicions should be expressed honestly and nonjudgmentally to the client. All findings and behaviors that may be potential safety issues for the client are reported and documented.
6. *Practice tough love.* This concept encourages the client to be responsible for his or her own healing. "Doing for" clients may be tempting, but it is not in the client's best interest most of the time. Nurses need to toughen up the caretaking side of their personality when working with people who are alcohol or drug dependent. Praising the client's attempts at self-responsible behavior and using therapeutic communication skills to constructively confront behaviors that are inconsistent with the plan of care are two examples a nurse can use to begin practicing this skill.

Drug Abuse and Dependence

Many substances can be addictive to humans. Caffeine and nicotine are two that are very readily available. Coffee, tea, soda, and cigarettes are everywhere in our society and yet are very addicting. Many experts believe that the single most difficult addiction to overcome is the addiction to nicotine.

Illegal substances such as marijuana, cocaine, crack, and PCP and prescription medications for pain and mental health treatment are also among potentially addictive substances.

It is becoming popular among the youth in the United States to use inhalants such as lighter fluid, paint, paint thinners, and gasoline to get high. These are highly toxic, potentially lethal, and usually available in the house or garage.

SIGNS AND SYMPTOMS OF DRUG ABUSE AND DEPENDENCE. The signs and symptoms of drug abuse and dependence can be very similar to those of people who are alcohol abusers. Signs and symptoms that may also be seen in people who abuse other drugs are

- Red, watery eyes
- Runny nose
- Hostile behavior
- **Paranoia**
- Needle tracks on arms or legs

TREATMENTS FOR CLIENTS WITH DRUG ABUSE AND DEPENDENCE

1. Narcotics anonymous
2. Group therapy
3. Psychotherapy
4. Methadone programs

Methadone acts as a sort of "stepdown" for drug addicts. Methadone can be legally prescribed and dispensed. It, too, is potentially addicting, and its critics believe it is only a substitute. It is typically given once a day. Psychotherapy is also provided for clients in methadone programs.

NURSING INTERVENTIONS FOR CLIENTS WITH DRUG ABUSE AND DEPENDENCE. Nursing care for people who are drug dependent is essentially the same as for those who are alcohol dependent. It is very important to remember that nurses and doctors do not "fix" the client who is chemically dependent. The desire to be chemically free must come from the individual who is addicted.

Caring for clients with mental health disorders is challenging and rewarding. Nurses learn that there are very few absolutes in the area of mental health nursing. There are many guidelines about the illnesses, but caring for the clients who have the illnesses is as individualized as the clients themselves. It is also important to remember to care for the whole person. The mind and body work together, so nurses must be sure to take care of the physical, emotional, cognitive, and behavioral parts of our clients.

CRITICAL THINKING: Maria

You are one of the team of school nurses in your local high school. You notice that Maria, a 17-year-old student, is behaving oddly. She has always been

HOME HEALTH HINTS

- Listen to what your client says and how he or she says it. Listen to what is said by other persons in the home who are familiar with the client.
- Look for signs of any chemical use, misuse, or abuse by the client or any caregiver. Count pills and take note of alcohol containers in refrigerators, on counters, or in trash cans.
- Be observant of the health status of the client's caregiver(s), with particular attention to signs of exhaustion, depression, or anger. Discuss this with your supervisor.
- Familiarize yourself with the mental health services and professionals in your community. Learn about criteria for admission, cost, and modalities of treatment.

rather loud and even has been referred to as "obnoxious" by several of her peers. Lately, you have observed her sitting alone, as if waiting for someone, but when you approach her, she barely greets you and then leaves. What are your concerns about Maria? What are some of the possibilities that might be affecting her? How will you approach her more effectively the next time you see her?

Answers at end of chapter.

Review Questions

1. When assessing mental health, which client behavior would cause the nurse to be concerned or ask further questions?
   a. Client is always happy and smiling.
   b. Client can verbalize emotions.
   c. Client is able to cope with bad news.
   d. Client maintains some close, personal relationships.

2. The mental status examination is done in which part of the nursing process?
   a. Assessment
   b. Plan
   c. Implementation
   d. Evaluation

3. A person who always sounds like he or she is making excuses is displaying which defense mechanism?
   a. Denial
   b. Fantasy
   c. Rationalization
   d. Transference

4. The alcoholic who says, "I don't have a problem; I can quit any time I want to; I just don't want to," is displaying which of the following defense mechanisms?
   a. Denial
   b. Fantasy
   c. Dissociation
   d. Transference

5. A therapeutic environment (milieu) is *best* defined as an environment that is
   a. Able to provide for all of the client's needs
   b. Locked and supervised
   c. Structured to decrease stress and encourage learning new behavior
   d. Designed to be homelike for persons who are hospitalized for life

6. Which of the following does *not* state a goal of psychotherapy?
   a. Decrease emotional pain/discomfort
   b. Increase social functioning
   c. Increase ability to behave appropriately
   d. Allow client to avoid/deny uncomfortable situations

7. Which of the following is *false* regarding ECT/EST?
   a. It is used to treat depression and schizophrenia.
   b. It is used to stop convulsive seizures.
   c. Fatigue and disorientation are immediate side effects.
   d. Memory will gradually return.

8. Psychopharmacology is used for which of the following purposes?
   a. As a cure for mental illness and substance abuse
   b. Only when necessary to control violent behavior
   c. To alter the pain receptors in the brain
   d. To decrease symptoms and facilitate other therapies

9. Mrs. Henderson has been started on Thorazine. Which of the following side effects will you include in your teaching?
   a. Photosensitivity
   b. Weight loss
   c. Elevated blood pressure
   d. Hypoglycemia

10. Avoiding such foods as bananas, cheese, and yogurt should be stressed to clients who are taking which drug?
    a. Prozac
    b. Lithium
    c. Parnate
    d. Elavil

11. If an extrapyramidal side effect such as tardive dyskinesia occurs, the treatment of choice is to
    a. Administer anticholinergic drugs as ordered
    b. Discontinue the drugs per order
    c. Increase the dose per order
    d. Administer antianxiety drugs per order

12. Your significant other is a veteran of the Gulf War. It is very difficult for him or her to drive through a parking ramp because "there are people hiding behind the pillars! They have guns! Be careful!" This person is most likely experiencing
    a. Auditory hallucinations
    b. Flashbacks
    c. Delusions of grandeur
    d. Free-floating anxiety

13. Mrs. T. cannot leave her home without checking the coffee pot numerous times. This makes her late to many functions, and she misses engagements on occasion because of it. Mrs. T. probably is suffering from which kind of anxiety disorder?
    a. Generalized anxiety disorder
    b. Phobia
    c. Posttraumatic stress disorder
    d. Obsessive-compulsive disorder

14. Which of the following descriptions best represents somatoform disorders?
    a. Physical symptoms with organic causes
    b. Physical symptoms that are confirmed with MRI
    c. Physical symptoms with hallucinations
    d. Physical symptoms with no organic cause

ANSWERS TO CRITICAL THINKING

CRITICAL THINKING: Grieving

Different people cope in different ways. This may be a healthy way to cope in this gentleman's culture. Gently guide the grieving husband to a room where he can express his emotions without disturbing others. Ask if he would like you to contact someone to come in to support him.

CRITICAL THINKING: Mrs. Beison

Mrs. Beison is using denial to cope with her cancer diagnosis. Although at times denial can be an effective coping mechanism, if Mrs. Beison continues to deny her disease and refuse treatment, her life will be in danger. The nurse can help Mrs. Beison verbalize her fears about cancer and cancer treatment and can provide accurate information to help her make wise choices. If necessary, a psychiatric evaluation can be requested.

CRITICAL THINKING: Tommy

You can reassure Tommy's mother that his OCD is not her fault. Tommy can learn to control his illness with medications and therapy. The family must be part of the therapy, for both Tommy's sake and the family's sake. Positive communication between Tommy and his family is encouraged. Tommy's mother can also be encouraged to attend a support group herself.

CRITICAL THINKING: Maria

A number of options may explain Maria's behavior, including depression, drug use, schizophrenia, anorexia, or bulimia. Next time you see Maria you might try constructively confronting her behavior by saying something like "Maria, you used to be much more outgoing. We always were friendly and now you leave when I'm near. That change in you concerns me. I'm here if you want to talk." Or, "Maria, I see your behavior is changing. You are loud one moment and very quiet the next. That is unusual for you. What is happening?"

REFERENCES

1. Gustafson, M: Western voodoo: Providing mental health care to Haitian refugees. J Psychosoc Nurs 27(12):22, 1989.
2. Council on Scientific Affairs, American Medical Association: Hispanic health in the United States. JAMA 265(2):248, 1991.
3. Muecke, MA: In search of healers—Southeast Asian refugees in the American health care system. West J Med 139(6):835, 1983.
4. Nowak, T: Vietnamese-Americans. In Purnell, L, and Paulanka, B (eds): Transcultural Health Care: A Culturally Competent Approach. FA Davis, Philadelphia, 1998.
5. McGoldrick, M, Pearce, J, and Giordano, J: Ethnicity and Family Therapy. Guilford, New York, 1982.
6. Fandetti, V, and Gelfand, DE: Attitudes toward symptoms and services in the ethnic family and neighborhoods. Am J Orthopsychiatry 48(3):477, 1977.
7. Still, O, and Hodgins, D: Navajo Indians. In Purnell, L, and Paulanka, B (eds): Transcultural Health Care: A Culturally Competent Approach. FA Davis, Philadelphia, 1998.
8. Pang, KY: Hwabyung: The construction of a Korean popular illness among Korean elderly immigrant women in the United States. Cult Med Psychiatry 14:495, 1990.
9. Aroian, KJ: Mental health risks and problems encountered by illegal immigrants. Issues in Mental Health 14:379, 1993.
10. Jambanathan, J: Hindu-Americans. In Purnell, L, and Paulanka, B (eds): Transcultural Health Care: A Culturally Competent Approach. FA Davis, Philadelphia, 1998.
11. Mavreas, V, Bebbington, P, and Der, G: Acculturation and psychiatric disorder: A study of Greek Cypriot immigrants. Psychol Med 20:941, 1990.
12. AbuGharbieh, P: Arab-Americans. In Purnell, L, and Paulanka, B (eds): Transcultural Health Care: A Culturally Competent Approach. FA Davis, Philadelphia, 1998.
13. Campinha Bacote, J: African-Americans. In Purnell, L, and Paulanka, B, (eds): Transcultural Health Care: A Culturally Competent Approach. FA Davis, Philadelphia, 1998.
14. Shives, L: Basic Concepts of Psychiatric Mental Health Nursing, ed 3. JB Lippincott, Philadelphia, 1994.
15. Bleuler, E: Dementia Praecox (Emil Kraepelin) or the Group of Schizophrenias. International Press, New York, 1911, p 26.
16. Skinner, K: The hazards of chemical dependency among nurses. JPN 8, December 1993.

BIBLIOGRAPHY

Aiken, LR: Psychological Testing and Assessment, ed 7. Allyn and Bacon, Boston, 1991.

Alcohol, Drug Abuse and Mental Health Administration. DHHS Pub No (ADM) 90-1609, Bethesda, Md, 1990.

Bailey, DS, and Bailey, DR: Therapeutic Approaches to the Care of the Mentally Ill, ed 3. FA Davis, Philadelphia, 1993.

Diagnostic and Statistical Manual of Mental Disorders—IV. American Psychiatric Association, Washington, DC, 1994.

Ellis, A: A Guide to Rational Living. Thinking Allowed Productions, Oakland, Calif, 1988.

Helpful Facts about Depressive Illness. DHHS-NIH Pub. No. 94-3875, Bethesda, Md, 1994.

Kalman, N, and Waughfield, C: Mental Health Concepts, ed 3. Delmar, New York, 1993.

McEnany, G: Managing Mood Disorders. RN 53(9):28, 1990.

McGue, M, and Gottesman, II: Genetic linkage in schizophrenia: Perspectives from a genetic epidemiology. Schizophr Bull 15:453, 1989.

Merikangas, K: The genetic epidemiology of alcoholism. Psychol Med 20:11, 1990.

Townsend, MC: Nursing Diagnoses in Psychiatric Nursing. FA Davis, Philadelphia, 1997.

Weiten, W: Psychology Themes and Variations—Briefer Version, ed 3. Brooks/Cole, Pacific Grove, Calif, 1997.

List of NANDA-Approved Nursing Diagnoses

Activity intolerance
Activity intolerance, risk for
Adaptive capacity: intracranial, decreased
Adjustment, impaired
Airway clearance, ineffective
Anxiety
Anxiety, death
Aspiration, risk for
Autonomic dysreflexia, risk for
Bed mobility, impaired
Body image disturbance
Body temperature, altered, risk for
Breastfeeding, effective
Breastfeeding, ineffective
Breastfeeding, interrupted
Breathing pattern, ineffective
Cardiac output, decreased
Caregiver role strain
Caregiver role strain, risk for
Communication, impaired verbal
Community coping, ineffective
Community coping, potential for enhanced
Confusion, acute
Confusion, chronic
Constipation
Constipation, colonic
Constipation, perceived
Constipation, risk for
Coping, defensive
Coping, individual, ineffective
Decisional conflict (specify)
Denial, ineffective
Dentition, altered
Development, altered, risk for
Diarrhea
Disuse syndrome, risk for
Diversional activity deficit
Dysreflexia
Energy field disturbance
Environmental interpretation syndrome, impaired
Failure to thrive, adult
Family coping: ineffective, compromised
Family coping: ineffective, disabling
Family coping: potential for growth

Family process, altered: alcoholism
Family processes, altered
Fatigue
Fear
Fluid volume deficit
Fluid volume deficit, risk for
Fluid volume excess
Fluid volume imbalance, risk for
Gas exchange, impaired
Grieving, anticipatory
Grieving, dysfunctional
Growth, altered, risk for
Growth and development, altered
Health maintenance, altered
Health-seeking behaviors (specify)
Home maintenance management, impaired
Hopelessness
Hyperthermia
Hypothermia
Incontinence, bowel
Incontinence, functional
Incontinence, reflex
Incontinence, stress
Incontinence, total
Incontinence, urge
Incontinence, urinary urge, risk for
Infant behavior, disorganized
Infant behavior, disorganized, risk for
Infant behavior, organized, potential for enhanced
Infant feeding pattern, ineffective
Infection, risk for
Injury, risk for
Knowledge deficit (specify)
Latex allergy
Latex allergy, risk for
Loneliness, risk for
Memory, impaired
Nausea
Noncompliance (specify)
Nutrition: altered, less than body requirements
Nutrition: altered, more than body requirements
Nutrition, altered, risk for more than body requirements
Oral mucous membrane, altered
Pain

Pain, chronic
Parental role conflict
Parent/infant/child attachment, altered, risk for
Parenting, altered
Parenting, altered, risk for
Perioperative positioning injury, risk for
Peripheral neurovascular dysfunction, risk for
Personal identity disturbance
Physical mobility, impaired
Poisoning, risk for
Post-trauma response
Post-trauma syndrome, risk for
Powerlessness
Protection, altered
Rape-trauma syndrome
Rape-trauma syndrome: compound reaction
Rape-trauma syndrome: silent reaction
Relocation stress syndrome
Role performance, altered
Self-care deficit, bathing/hygiene
Self-care deficit, dressing/grooming
Self-care deficit, feeding
Self-care deficit, toileting
Self-esteem, chronic low
Self-esteem disturbance
Self-esteem, situational low
Self-mutilation, risk for
Sensory/perceptual alterations (specify): visual, auditory, kinesthetic, gustatory, tactile, olfactory
Sexual dysfunction
Sexuality patterns, altered
Skin integrity, impaired
Skin integrity, impaired, risk for

Sleep deprivation
Sleep pattern disturbance
Social interaction, impaired
Social isolation
Sorrow, chronic
Spiritual distress
Spiritual distress, risk for
Spiritual well-being, potential for enhanced
Spontaneous ventilation, inability to sustain
Suffocation, risk for
Surgical recovery, delayed
Swallowing, impaired
Therapeutic regimen: community, ineffective management of
Therapeutic regimen: families, ineffective management of
Therapeutic regimen: individuals, ineffective management of
Therapeutic regimen (individuals), ineffective management of
Thermoregulation, ineffective
Thought processes, altered
Tissue integrity, impaired
Tissue perfusion, altered (specify): cerebral, cardiopulmonary, renal, gastrointestinal, peripheral
Trauma, risk for
Unilateral neglect
Urinary elimination, altered
Urinary retention
Ventilatory weaning response, dysfunctional
Violence, risk for, directed at self/others
Walking, impaired
Wheelchair mobility, impaired
Wheelchair transfer ability, impaired

Normal Reference Laboratory Values

Blood, Plasma, or Serum Values

	Reference Range	
Determination	Conventional	SI
Aldolase	1.3–8.2 U/L	22–137 nmol · sec^{-1}/L
Ammonia	12–55 μmol/L	12–55 μmol/L
Amylase	4–25 units/ml	4–25 arb. unit
Ascorbic acid	0.4–1.5 mg/100 ml	23–85 μmol/L
Bilirubin	Direct: up to 0.4 mg/100 ml	Up to 7 μmol/L
	Total: up to 1.0 mg/100 ml	Up to 17 μmol/L
Blood volume	8.5–9.0% of body weight in kg	80–85 ml/kg
Calcium	8.5–10.5 mg/100 ml (slightly higher in children)	2.1–2.6 mmol/L
Carbamazepine	4.0–12.0 μg/ml	17–51 μmol/L
Carbon dioxide content	24–30 mEq/L	24–30 mmol/L
Chloride	100–106 mEq/L	100–106 mmol/L
CK isoenzymes	5% MB or less	
Creatine kinase (CK)	Female: 10–79 U/L	167–1317 nmol · sec^{-1}/L
	Male: 17–148 U/L	283–2467 nmol · sec^{-1}/L
Creatinine	0.6–1.5 mg/100 ml	53–133 μmol/L
Ethanol	0 mg/100 ml	0 mmol/L
Glucose	Fasting: 70–110 mg/100 ml	3.9–5.6 mmol/L
Iron	50–150 μg/100 ml (higher in males)	9.0–26.9 μmol/L
Iron-binding capacity	250–410 μg/100 ml	44.8–73.4 μmol/L
Lactic dehydrogenase	45–90 U/L	750–1500 nmol · sec^{-1}/L
Lipase	2 units/ml or less	Up to 2 arb. unit
Lipids		
Cholesterol	120–220 mg/100 ml	3.10–5.69 mmol/L
Very low density lipoprotein	13–32 mg/dL	
Low density lipoprotein	38–40 mg/dL	
High density lipoprotein	20–48 mg/dL	
Triglycerides	40–150 mg/100 ml	0.4–1.5 g/L
Lithium	0.5–1.5 mEq/L	0.5–1.5 mmol/L
Magnesium	1.5–2.0 mEq/L	0.8–1.3 mmol/L
Osmolality	280–296 mOsm/kg water	280–296 mmol/kg
Oxygen saturation (arterial)	96–100%	0.96–1.00
PCO_2	35–45 mm Hg	4.7–6.0 kPa
pH	7.35–7.45	Same
PO_2	75–100 mm Hg (dependent on age) while breathing room air Above 500 mm Hg while on 100% O_2	10.0–13.3 kPa
Phenobarbital	15–50 μg/ml	65–215 μmol/L
Phenytoin (Dilantin)	5–20 μg/ml	20–80 μmol/L
Phosphatase (acid)	Male—Total: 0.13–0.63 sigma U/ml	36–175 nmol · sec^{-1}/L
	Female—Total: 0.01–0.56 sigma U/ml	2.8–156 nmol · sec^{-1}/L
	Prostatic: 0–0.5 Fishman–Lerner U/100 ml	
Phosphatase (alkaline)	13–39 U/L, infants and adolescents up to 104 U/L	217–650 nmol · sec^{-1}/L, up to 1.26 μmol · sec^{-1}/L
Phosphorus (inorganic)	3.0–4.5 mg/100 ml (infants in first year up to 6.0 mg/100 ml)	1.0–1.5 mmol/L
Potassium	3.5–5.0 mEq/L	3.5–5.0 mmol/L

continued

Blood, Plasma, or Serum Values (continued)

Determination	Reference Range	
	Conventional	SI
Protein: Total	6.0–8.4 g/100 ml	60–84 g/L
Albumin	3.5–5.0 g/100 ml	35–50 g/L
Globulin	2.3–3.5 g/100 ml	23–35 g/L
Salicylate:	0	
Therapeutic	20–25 mg/100 ml;	1.4–1.8 mmol/L
	25–30 mg/100 ml to age 10 yr 3 hr post dose	1.8–2.2 mmol/L
Sodium	135–145 mEq/L	135–145 mmol/L
Transaminase, aspartate amino-transferase	7–27 U/L	117–450 nmol · sec^{-1}/L
Transaminase, alanine aminotransferase	1–21 U/L	17–350 nmol · sec^{-1}/L
Urea nitrogen (BUN)	8–25 mg/100 ml	2.9–8.9 mmol/L
Uric acid	3.0–7.0 mg/100 ml	0.18–0.42 mmol/L

Urine Values

Determination	Reference Range	
	Conventional	SI
Acetone plus acetoacetate (quantitative)	0	0 mg/L
Amylase	24–76 units/ml	24–76 arb. unit
Calcium	300 mg/day or less	7.5 mmol/day or less
Catecholamines	Epinephrine: under 20 μg/day	<109 nmol/day
	Norepinephrine: under 100 μg/day	<590 nmol/day
Creatine	Under 100 mg/day or less than 6% of creatine. In pregnancy: up to 12%. In children under 1 yr: may equal creatinine. In older children: up to 30% of creatinine.	<0.75 mmol/day
Creatinine	15–25 mg/kg of body weight/day	0.13–0.22 mmol · kg^{-1}/day
Cystine or cysteine	0	0
Hemoglobin and myoglobin	0	
pH	5–7	5–7
Phosphorus (inorganic)	Varies with intake; average, 1 g/day	32 mmol/day
Protein:		
Quantitative	<150 mg/24 hr	<0.15 g/day
Steroids:		
17-Ketosteroids (per day)	Age　Male　Female	
	10　1–4 mg　1–4 mg	3–14 μmol　　3–14 μmol
	20　6–21　　4–16	21–73　　　14–56
	30　8–26　　4–14	28–90　　　14–49
	50　5–18　　3–9	17–62　　　10–31
	70　2–10　　1–7	7–35　　　　3–24
17-Hydroxysteroids	3–8 mg/day (women lower than men)	8–22 μmol/day as tetrahydrocortisol
Sugar:		
Quantitative glucose	0	0 mmol/L
Urobilinogen	Up to 1.0 Ehrlich U	To 1.0 arb. unit

Hematologic Values

Determination	Reference Range	
	Conventional	SI
Coagulation screening tests:		
Bleeding time (Simplate)	3–9.5 min	180–570 sec
Prothrombin time	Less than 2-sec deviation from control	Less than 2-sec deviation from control
Partial thromboplastin time (activated)	25–38 sec	25–38 sec
Whole-blood clot lysis	No clot lysis in 24 hr	0/day
"Complete" blood count:		
Hematocrit	Male: 45–52%	Male: 0.45–0.52
	Female: 37–48%	Female: 0.37–0.48
Hemoglobin	Male: 13–18 g/100 ml	Male: 8.1–11.2 mmol/L
	Female: 12–16 g/100 ml	Female: 7.4–9.9 mmol/L
Leukocyte count	4300–10,800/mm^3	4.3–10.8 $\times 10^9$/L
Erythrocyte count	4.2–5.9 million/mm^3	4.2–5.9 $\times 10^{12}$/L
Mean corpuscular volume (MCV)	86–98 μm^3/cell	86–98 fl
Mean corpuscular hemoglobin (MCH)	27–32 pg/RBC	1.7–2.0 pg/cell
Mean corpuscular hemoglobin concentration (MCHC)	32–36%	0.32–0.36
Platelet count	150,000–350,000/mm^3	150–350 $\times 10^9$/L

Miscellaneous Values

Determination	Reference Range	
	Conventional	SI
Carcinoembryonic antigen (CEA)	0–2.5 ng/ml	0–2.5 μg/L
Digoxin	1.2 ± 0.4 ng/ml	1.54 ± 0.5 nmol/L
	1.5 ± 0.4 ng/ml	1.92 ± 0.5 nmol/L
Gastric analysis	Basal:	
	Females: 2.0 ± 1.8 mEq/hr	0.6 ± 0.5 μmol/sec
	Males: 3.0 ± 2.0 mEq/hr	0.8 ± 0.6 μmol/sec
	Maximal (after histalog or gastrin):	
	Females: 16 ± 5 mEq/hr	4.4 ± 1.4 μmol/sec
	Males: 23 ± 5 mEq/hr	6.4 ± 1.4 μmol/sec
Gastrin-I	0–200 pg/ml	0–95 pmol/L
Immunologic tests:		
Alpha-fetoprotein	Undetectable in normal adults	
Alpha-1-antitrypsin	85–213 mg/100 ml	0.85–2.13 g/L
Rheumatoid factor	<60 IU/ml	
Antinuclear antibodies	Negative at a 1:8 dilution of serum	

Reference range values may differ from one institution to another. These data from Scully, Robert E. (ed.): Case Records of the Massachusetts General Hospital, *N Engl J Med* 314:39–49, 1986.

Answers to Chapter Review Questions

C

Chapter 1:	1. a	2. c	3. c	4. d	5. b	6. b	7. a						
Chapter 2:	1. c	2. a	3. c	4. a	5. b	6. d							
Chapter 3:	1. b	2. d	3. b	4. a	5. c	6. a	7. c	8. d	9. b	10. d			
Chapter 4:	1. b	2. a	3. a	4. d	5. a	6. b	7. c						
Chapter 5:	1. b	2. c	3. a	4. d	5. a	6. a	7. d	8. b					
Chapter 6:	1. b	2. c	3. a	4. d	5. b	6. c	7. b	8. b					
Chapter 7:	1. c	2. c	3. b	4. c	5. a	6. d	7. b	8. a	9. c				
Chapter 8:	1. c	2. d	3. d	4. b	5. a	6. c	7. c	8. b					
Chapter 9:	1. b	2. b	3. a	4. c	5. c	6. d	7. d						
Chapter 10:	1. b	2. d	3. a	4. b	5. d	6. b	7. a	8. c	9. b	10. c	11. d	12. b	
Chapter 11:	1. a	2. c	3. a	4. b	5. d	6. c	7. b	8. a	9. c	10. b	11. c	12. a	13. b	14. d
Chapter 12:	1. a	2. b	3. d	4. a	5. b								
Chapter 13:	1. d	2. b	3. a	4. c	5. c	6. d	7. a						
Chapter 14:	1. c	2. b	3. d	4. a	5. b	6. c	7. d						
Chapter 15:	1. a	2. c	3. b	4. d	5. b	6. c	7. d	8. a	9. b	10. d	11. a	12. b	
Chapter 16:	1. d	2. b	3. d	4. b	5. c	6. a	7. a						
Chapter 17:	1. c	2. a	3. d	4. a	5. b	6. b	7. c						
Chapter 18:	1. b	2. b	3. b	4. a	5. c	6. d	7. c						
Chapter 19:	1. d	2. b	3. b	4. c	5. d	6. c	7. b						
Chapter 20:	1. d	2. d	3. a	4. d	5. b	6. c	7. c						
Chapter 21:	1. b	2. a	3. d	4. a	5. d								
Chapter 22:	1. b	2. a	3. a	4. a	5. b	6. b	7. c	8. a	9. d	10. d			
Chapter 23:	1. b	2. c	3. c	4. d	5. b	6. c	7. a	8. c					
Chapter 24:	1. b	2. c	3. c	4. d	5. a	6. d	7. a	8. b					
Chapter 25:	1. c	2. a	3. b	4. d	5. a								
Chapter 26:	1. a	2. d	3. c	4. b	5. d	6. a	7. c	8. c					
Chapter 27:	1. d	2. b	3. a	4. a	5. c								
Chapter 28:	1. c	2. b	3. b	4. d	5. d	6. a	7. c	8. b	9. a				
Chapter 29:	1. a	2. d	3. d	4. d	5. b	6. a	7. a						
Chapter 30:	1. b	2. b	3. c	4. d	5. d	6. c	7. c	8. a					
Chapter 31:	1. c	2. a	3. c	4. c	5. b	6. a	7. b	8. a	9. d	10. d			
Chapter 32:	1. a	2. b	3. b	4. c	5. a								
Chapter 33:	1. d	2. a	3. b	4. c	5. a	6. b	7. d	8. a					
Chapter 34:	1. b	2. c	3. b	4. b	5. c	6. c	7. b	8. d					
Chapter 35:	1. a	2. c	3. d	4. b	5. c	6. c	7. a	8. a					
Chapter 36:	1. a	2. b	3. d	4. c	5. a	6. b	7. b	8. a					
Chapter 37:	1. b	2. c	3. a	4. a	5. d	6. a	7. b	8. c					
Chapter 38:	1. b	2. a	3. d	4. a	5. a	6. c	7. d	8. b					
Chapter 39:	1. c	2. d	3. b	4. c	5. b	6. c							
Chapter 40:	1. a	2. a	3. e	4. d	5. b	6. c	7. c	8. c	9. c	10. d			
Chapter 41:	1. c	2. b	3. c	4. b									
Chapter 42:	1. c	2. a	3. d	4. d	5. b	6. a	7. c	8. c	9. b				
Chapter 43:	1. d	2. c	3. a	4. b	5. d	6. c	7. d						
Chapter 44:	1. b	2. b	3. a	4. d	5. a	6. d	7. d	8. b	9. c	10. b	11. a	12. c

Chapter 45:	1. b	2. c	3. b	4. d	5. a	6. d	7. c	8. c	9. b	10. a			
Chapter 46:	1. c	2. d	3. a	4. b	5. d	6. c	7. a	8. b	9. c	10. b	11. b		
Chapter 47:	1. c	2. b	3. c	4. d	5. a	6. c							
Chapter 48:	1. b	2. b	3. c	4. b	5. d	6. b	7. c	8. b	9. a				
Chapter 49:	1. b	2. d	3. b	4. d	5. a	6. c	7. b	8. b					
Chapter 50:	1. b	2. c	3. d	4. a	5. b	6. a							
Chapter 51:	1. d	2. c	3. a	4. c	5. b	6. c	7. c	8. b	9. a				
Chapter 52:	1. c	2. d	3. b	4. c	5. a	6. b	7. b	8. a	9. c	10. c			
Chapter 53:	1. c	2. d	3. b	4. b	5. d	6. c	7. c	8. a	9. d	10. a	11. a	12. d	13. b
Chapter 54:	1. d	2. a	3. b	4. a	5. a	6. c	7. b	8. b	9. d				
Chapter 55:	1. a	2. a	3. c	4. a	5. c	6. d	7. b	8. d	9. a	10. c	11. a	12. b	13. d

Chapter 55 also has: 14. d

Medical Abbreviations

ABG	arterial blood gas	hor. som., h.s.	bedtime
a.c.	before a meal	IM	intramuscular
AD	advance directive	IUD	intrauterine device
ad lib.	freely; as desired	IV	intravenous
ALT	alanine aminotransferase	IVP	intravenous pyelogram
AM	morning	J	joule
A-P	anterior-posterior	kg	kilogram
AST	aspartate aminotransferase	KUB	kidney, ureter, and bladder
AV	atrioventricular	L	liter
b.i.d.	twice a day	lb	pound
BM	bowel movement	lmp	last menstrual period
BP	blood pressure	mEq	milliequivalent
BUN	blood urea nitrogen	mg	milligram
c̄	with	ml	milliliter
cap.	a capsule	mm	millimeter
CBC	complete blood count	MRI	magnetic resonance imaging
cc	cubic centimeter	MS	mitral stenosis; multiple sclerosis
cm	centimeter	μEq	microequivalent
CNS	central nervous system	μg	microgram
CSF	cerebrospinal fluid	n.p.o.	nothing by mouth
CV	cardiovascular	NSAID	nonsteroidal anti-inflammatory drug
D and C	dilatation and curettage	NSR	normal sinus rhythm
dc	discontinue	OB	obstetrics
DNR	do not resuscitate	OC	oral contraceptive
DOA	dead on arrival	O.D.	right eye
dr.	dram	O.S.	left eye
Dx	diagnosis	OU	both eyes open
ECF	extracellular fluid	oz	ounce
ECG	electrocardiogram	p̄	after
ECT	electroconvulsive therapy	p.c.	after meals
EEG	electroencephalogram	PCO_2	carbon dioxide pressure
EMG	electromyogram	PERRLA	pupils equal, regular, react to light and accommodation
EMS	emergency medical service		
ENT	ear, nose, and throat	pH	hydrogen ion concentration
EOM	extraocular muscles	PM	afternoon/evening
ER	Emergency Room	PMI	point of maximal impulse
ESR	erythrocyte sedimentation rate	post.	posterior
F	Fahrenheit	p.r.	through the rectum
g, gm	gram	p.r.n.	as needed
GERD	gastroesophageal reflux disease	q.h.	every hour
GI	gastrointestinal	q.2h.	every 2 hours
gr	grain	q.3h.	every 3 hours
Gtt, gtt	drops	q.i.d.	four times a day
GYN	gynecology	q.s.	as much as is needed
h, hr	hour	RBC	red blood cell; red blood count
hgb	hemoglobin	s̄	without

SA	sinoatrial	URI	upper respiratory infection
SC, sc, s.c.	subcutaneous(ly)	USP	United States Pharmacopeia
SOB	shortness of breath	UTI	urinary tract infection
s.o.s.	if necessary	WBC	white blood cell; white blood count
s.q.	subcutaneous(ly)	WF/BF	white female/black female
stat.	immediately	WM/BM	white male/black male
STD	sexually transmitted disease	wt.	weight
T	temperature		
tab.	medicated tablet		
temp.	temperature		
t.i.d.	three times a day		
top.	topically		

Adapted from Thomas, CL: Taber's Cyclopedic Medical Dictionary, 18th ed. FA Davis, Philadelphia, 1997, pp 2224–2226, with permission.

Prefixes, Suffixes, and Combining Forms

a-, an-. Without; away from; not.

ab-, abs-. From; away from; absent.

abdomin-, abdomino-. Abdomen.

-ad. Toward; in the direction of.

aden-, adeno-. Gland.

adip-, adipo-. Fat.

-aemia. Blood.

aer-, aero-. Air.

-algesia, -algia. Suffering; pain.

andro-. Man; male; masculine.

angi-, angio-. Blood or lymph vessels.

aniso-. Unequal; asymmetrical; dissimilar.

ankyl-, ankylo-. Crooked; bent; fusion or growing together of parts.

ante-. Before.

antero-. Anterior; front; before.

ant-, anti-. Against.

arteri-, arterio-. Artery.

arthr-, arthro-. Joint.

-ase. Enzyme.

-asis, esis, -iasis, -isis, -sis. Condition; pathological state.

aut-, auto-. Self.

axo-. Axis; axon.

bacteri-, bacterio-. Bacteria; bacterium.

bi-, bis-. Two; double; twice.

bili-. Bile.

bio-. Life.

blast-, -blast. Germ; bud; embryonic state of development.

blephar-, blepharo-. Eyelid.

brady-. Slow.

bronch-, bronchi-, broncho-. Airway.

cardi-, cardio-. Heart.

cat-, cata-, cath-, kat-, kata-. Down; downward; destructive; against; according to.

cent-. Hundred.

cephal-, cephalo-. Head.

cervic-, cervico-. Head; the neck of an organ.

chrom-, chromo-. Color.

-cide. Causing death.

contra-. Against; opposite.

crani-, cranio-. Skull; cranium.

cry-, cryo-. Cold.

cyan-, cyano-. Blue.

cyst-, cysto-, -cyst. Cyst; urinary bladder.

cyt-, cyto-, -cyte. Cell.

derm-, derma-, dermato-, dermo-. Skin.

di-. Double; twice; two; apart from.

dors-, dorsi-, dorso-. Back.

-dynia. Pain.

dys-. Difficult; bad; painful.

ec-, ecto-. Out; on the outside.

-ectomy. Excision.

ef-, es-, ex-, exo-. Out.

electr-, electro-. Electricity.

-emesis. Vomiting.

-emia. Blood.

en-. In; into.

end-, endo-. Within.

ent-, ento-. Within; inside.

enter-, entero-. Intestine.

ep-, epi-. Upon; over; at; in addition to; after.

erythr-, erythro-. Red.

eury-. Broad.

ex-. Out; away from; completely.

exo-. Out; outside of; without.

extra-. Outside of; in addition; beyond.

-facient. Causing; making happen.

-ferous. Producing.

ferri-, ferro-. Iron.

fluo-. Flow.

fore-. Before; in front of.

-form. Form.

-fuge. To expel; to drive away; fleeing.

gaster-, gastero-, gastr-, gastro-. Stomach.

gen-. Producing; forming.

-gen, -gene, -genesis, -genetic, -genic. Producing; forming.

glosso-. Tongue.

gluc-, gluco-, glyc-, glyco-. Sugar; glycerol or similar substance.

gyn-, gyne-, gyneco-, gyno-. Woman; female.

hem-, hema-, hemato-, hemo-. Blood.

hemi-. Half.

hepat-, hepato-. Liver.

heter-, hetero-. Other; different.

histo-. Tissue.

homo-. Same; likeness.

hydra-, hydro, hydr-. Water.

hyp-, hyph-, hypo-. Less than; below; under.

hyper-. Above; excessive; beyond.

hyster-, hystero-. Uterus.

-ia. Condition, esp. an abnormal state.

-iasis. SEE: *-asis.*

-iatric. Medicine; medical profession; physicians.

in-. In; inside; within; intensive action; negative.

infra-. Below; under; beneath; inferior to; after.

inter-. Between; in the midst.

intra-, intro-. Within; in; into.

ipsi-. Same.

irid-, irido-. Iris.

-ism. Condition; theory.

iso-. Equal.

-itis. Inflammation of.

kera-, kerato-. Horny substance; cornea.

kolp-, kolpo, colp-, colpo-. Vagina.

kypho-. Humped.

leuk-, leuko-. White; colorless; rel. to a leukocyte.

lip-, lipo-. Fat.

-lite, -lith, lith-, litho-. Stone; calculus.

-logia, -logy. Science of; study of.

lumbo-. Loins.

-lysis. 1. Setting free; disintegration. **2.** In medicine, reduction of; relief from.

macr-, macro-. Large; long.

mal-. Ill; bad; poor.

med-, medi-, medio-. Middle.

mega-, megal-, megalo-. Large; of great size.

-megalia, -megaly. Enlargement of a body part.

melan-, melano-. Black.

mening-, meningo-. Meninges.

-meter. Measure.

metr-, metra-, metro-. Uterus.

micr-, micro-. Small.

mon-, mono-. Single; one.

muc-, muci-, muco-, myxa-, myxo-. Mucus.

multi-. Many; much.

musculo-, my-, myo-. Muscle.

my-, myo-. SEE *musculo-.*

myel-, myelo-. Spinal cord; bone marrow.

naso-. Nose.

necr-, necro-. Death; necrosis.

neo-. New; recent.

nephr-, nephra-, nephro-. Kidney.

neur-, neuri-, neuro-. Nerve; nervous system.

non-. No.

normo-. Normal; usual.

oculo-. Eye.

-ode, -oid. Form; shape; resemblance.

-odynia, odyno-. Pain.

olig-, oligo-. Few; small.

-ology. Science of; study of.

-oma. Tumor.

onco-. Tumor; swelling; mass.

oo-, ovi-, ovo-. Egg; ovum.

oophor-, oophoro-, oophoron-. Ovary.

ophthalm-, ophthalmo-. Eye.

-opia. Vision.

optico-, opto-. Eye; vision.

orchi-, orchid-, orchido-. Testicle.

orth-, ortho-. Straight; correct; normal; in proper order.

os-. Mouth; bone.

-osis. Condition; status, process; abnormal increase.

oste-, osteo-. Bone.

ot-, oto-. Ear.

-otomy. Cutting.

-ous. 1. Possessing; full of; **2.** Pertaining to.

pan-. All; entire.

para-, -para. 1. Prefix; near; alongside of; departure from normal. **2.** Suffix: Bearing offspring.

path-, patho-, -path, -pathic, -pathy. Disease; suffering.

ped-, pedi-, pedo-. Foot.

-penia. Decrease from normal; deficiency.

peri-. Around; about.

perineo-. Perineum.

phaco-. Lens of the eye.

phag-, phago-. Eating; ingestion; devouring.

-phil, -philia, -philic. Love for; tendency toward; craving for.

phlebo-. Vein.

-phobia. Abnormal fear or aversion.

photo-. Light.

phren-, phreno-, -phrenia. Mind; diaphgram.

-phylaxis. Protection.

-plasia. Growth; cellular proliferation.

plasm-, -plasm. 1. Prefix: Living substance or tissue. **2.** Suffix: To mold.

-plastic. Molded; indicates restoration of lost or badly formed features.

-plegia. Paralysis; stroke.

pneo-. Breath; breathing.

pneum-, pneuma-, pneumato-. Air; gas; respiration.

-poiesis, -poietic. Production; formation.

poly-. Much; many.

post-. After.

pre-. Before; in front of.

presby-. Old age.

pro-. Before; in behalf of.

proct-, procto-. Anus; rectum.

pseud-, pseudo-. False.

psych-, psycho-. Mind; mental processes.

pulmo-. Lung.

py-, pyo-. Pus.

pyro-. Heat; fire.

ren-, reno-. Kidneys.

retro-. Backward; back; behind.

rheo-, -(r)rhea. Current; stream; to flow; to discharge.

rhino-. Nose.

-(r)rhage, -(r)rhagia. Rupture; profuse fluid discharge.

-(r)rhaphy. A suturing or stitching.

salping-, salpingo-. Auditory tube; fallopian tube.

sclero-. Hard; relating to the sclera.

-scopy. Examination.

semi-. Half.

sero-. Serum.

somat-, somato-. Body.

sperma-, spermat-, spermato-. Sperm; spermatozoa.

steno-. Narrow; short.

-stomosis, -stomy. SEE: *-ostomosis.*

sub-. Under; beneath; in small quantity; less than normal.

super-. Above; beyond; superior.

supra-. Above; beyond; on top.

tachy-. Swift; rapid.

tel-, tele-. 1. End. 2. Distant; far.

tendo-, teno-. Tendon.

thorac-, thoraci-, thoraco-. Chest; chest wall.

thrombo-. Blood clot; thrombus.

thyro-. Thyroid gland; oblong; shield.

-tomy. Cutting operation; excision.

top-, topo-. Place; locale.

tox-, toxi-, toxico-, toxo-, -toxic. Toxin; poison; toxic.

tracheo-. Trachea; windpipe.

trans-. Across; over; beyond; through.

-tropin. Stimulation of a target organ by a substance, esp. a hormone.

tympano-. Eardrum; tympanum.

ultra-. Beyond; excess.

-uria. Urine.

uter-, utero-. Uterus.

vaso-. Vessel (e.g., blood vessel).

veno-. Vein.

ventro-, ventr-, ventri-. Abdomen; anterior surface of the body.

vertebro-. Vertebra; vertebrae.

vesico-. Bladder; vesicle.

Adapted from Thomas, CL: Taber's Cyclopedic Medical Dictionary, 18th ed. FA Davis, Philadelphia, 1997, pp 2214–2218, with permission.

GLOSSARY

Abrasion: (a-**BRAY**-shun) A scraping away of skin or mucus membrane as a result of injury or by mechanical means. (Ch. 54)

Abuse: (uh-**BYOOS**) Misuse; excessive or improper use. (Ch. 55)

Acidosis: (ass-I-**DOH**-sis) An actual or relative increase in the acidity of blood caused by an accumulation of acid or a loss of base. (Ch. 5, 8)

Accommodation: (uh-KOM-uh-**DAY**-shun) A reflex action of the eye for focusing. (Ch. 48)

Acoustic neuroma: (uh-**KOO**-stik new-**ROH**-mah) A benign tumor of the vestibular, or acoustic, nerve. (Ch. 49)

Acquired immunodeficiency syndrome (AIDS): (uh-**KWHY**-erd IM-yoo-noh-de-**FISH**-en-see **SIN**-drohm) Suppression or deficiency of the cellular immune response, acquired by exposure to human immunodeficiency virus (HIV). (Ch. 53)

Active immunity: (**AK**-tiv im-**YOO**-ni-tee) Acquired immunity attributable to the presence of antibodies or of immune lymphoid cells formed in response to antigenic stimulus. (Ch. 7, 52)

Activities of daily living (ADL): (ack-**TIV**-i-tees of **DAY**-lee **LIV**-ing) Those activities and behaviors that are performed in the care and maintenance of self (e.g., bathing, dressing, eating). (Ch. 13)

Acute angle-closure glaucoma: (ah-**KEWT ANG**-uhl **KLOH**-zhur glaw-**KOH**-mah) A form of adult primary glaucoma in which the chamber angle is narrowed or completely closed because of forward displacement of the final roll and root of the iris against the cornea. (Ch. 49)

Acute pulmonary hypertension: (ah-**KEWT PULL**-muh-NER-ee HIGH-per-**TEN**-shun) Sudden obstruction of the pulmonary artery causes excessive buildup of pressure in the pulmonary arteries. (Ch. 8)

Addiction: (uh-**DIK**-shun) Psychological dependence characterized by drug seeking and craving for an opioid or other substance for effects other than the intended purpose of the substance. (Ch. 9, 55)

Adjunct: (**ADD**-junkt) An addition to the principal procedure or course of therapy. (Ch. 11)

Adjuvant: (ad-**JOO**-vant) Something that assists something else, such as a second form of treatment added to treat a disease. (Ch. 9, 28)

Administrative laws: (ad-MIN-i-**STRAY**-tiv LAWZ) Establishes the licensing authority of the state to create, license, and regulate the practice of nursing. (Ch. 1)

Adnexa: (ad-**NECK**-sah) Appendages or accessory organs. (Ch. 39)

Adventitious: (ad-ven-**TI**-shus) Abnormal or extra; often refers to extra breath sounds, such as wheezes or crackles. (Ch. 26)

Affect: (**AF**-feckt) Emotional tone. (Ch. 36, 55)

Agenesis: (ay-**JEN**-uh-sis) Failure of an organ or part to develop or grow. (Ch. 40)

Agonist: (**AG**-on-ist) A type of opioid that binds to opioid receptors in the central nervous system to relieve pain. (Ch. 9)

Akinesia: (a-ki-**NEE**-zee-ah) Absence or loss of the power of voluntary movement. (Ch. 46)

Alkalosis: (al-ka-**LOH**-sis) An actual or relative decrease in the acidity of blood caused by loss of acid or accumulation of base. (Ch. 5)

Alopecia: (AL-oh-**PEE**-she-ah) The loss of hair from the body and the scalp. (Ch. 10, 50)

Alternative therapy: (all-**TURN**-a-tive **THAIR**-a-pee) A therapy that is not taught widely in medical schools or is not generally available inside hospitals. (Ch. 4)

Amenorrhea: (ay-MEN-uh-**REE**-ah) The absence or suppression of menstruation. Amenorrhea is normal before puberty, after menopause, and during pregnancy and lactation. (Ch. 37, 40)

Ametropia: (AM-e-**TROH**-pee-ah) An ocular disorder in which parallel rays fail to come to a focus on the retina. (Ch. 49)

Amputation: (am-pew-**TAY**-shun) The removal of a limb or other appendage or outgrowth of the body. (Ch. 54)

Amsler grid: (**AMZ**-ler GRID) A grid of lines used in testing for macular degeneration of the eye. (Ch. 49)

Anaerobic: (AN-air-**ROH**-bik) Able to live without oxygen. (Ch. 8)

Analgesic: (AN-uhl-**JEE**-zik) A drug that relieves pain. (Ch. 9)

Anaphylactic shock: (AN-uh-fi-**LAK**-tik SHOCK) Systemic reaction that produces life-threatening changes in the circulation and bronchioles. (Ch. 52, 54)

Anaphylaxis: (AN-uh-fi-**LAK**-sis) A sudden severe allergic reaction. (Ch. 8, 53)

Anastomose: (uh-NAS-tuh-**MOS**) To surgically connect two parts. (Ch. 22)

Anemia: (uh-**NEE**-mee-yah) A condition in which there is reduced delivery of oxygen to the tissues as a result of reduced numbers of red cells or hemoglobin. (Ch. 10, 24)

Anergy: (**A**-ner-jee) Diminished ability of the immune system to react to an antigen. (Ch. 28)

Anesthesia: (AN-es-**THEE**-zee-uh) Lack of feeling or sensation; artificially induced loss of ability to feel pain. (Ch. 11)

Anesthesiologist: (an-es-**THEE**-zee-uhl-la-just) A physician who specializes in anesthesiology. (Ch. 11)

Aneurysm: (**AN**-yur-izm) A sac formed by the localized dilation of the wall of an artery, a vein, or the heart. (Ch. 18)

Angina pectoris: (an-**JIGH**-nah **PEK**-tuh-riss) Severe pain and constriction around the heart caused by insufficient supply of blood to the heart. (Ch. 18)

Angioedema: (AN-gee-o-eh-**DEE**-ma) A localized edematous reaction of the deep dermis or subcutaneous or submucosal tissues appearing as giant wheals. (Ch. 53)

Anion: (**AN**-eye-on) Electrolyte that carries a negative electrical charge. (Ch. 5)

Anisocoria: (an-i-soh-**KOH**-ree-ah) Inequality in size of the pupils of the eyes. (Ch. 45)

Ankylosing spondylitis: (ANG-ki-**LOH**-sing SPON-da-**LIGHT**-is) Inflammatory disease of the spine causing stiffness and pain. (Ch. 53)

Annuloplasty: (**AN**-yoo-loh-PLAS-tee) Plastic repair of a cardiac valve. (Ch. 19, 22)

Anorexia: (AN-oh-**REK**-see-ah) Absence or loss of appetite for food. Seen in depression, with illness, and as a side effect of some medications. (Ch. 30)

Anorexia nervosa: (AN-oh-**REK**-see-ah ner-**VOH**-sah) Refusal to maintain body weight over a minimal normal weight for age and height. (Ch. 30)

Antagonist: (an-**TAG**-on-ist) Medication used to counteract the effects of an opioid (e.g., naloxone). (Ch. 9)

Anteflexion: (AN-tee-**FLECK**-shun) The abnormal bending forward of part of an organ. (Ch. 40)

Anteversion: (AN-tee-**VER**-zhun) A tipping forward of an organ as a whole, without bending. (Ch. 40)

Antiarrhythmics: (an-ti-a-**RITH**-micks) Medications used to treat irregular heart rhythms. (Ch. 8)

Antibodies: (**AN**-ti-bod-es) An immunoglobin molecule having a specific amino acid sequence that gives each antibody the ability to adhere to and interact only with the antigen that induced the synthesis. (Ch. 7, 52)

Anticholinesterase: (AN-ti-KOH-lin-**ESS**-ter-ays) A substance that breaks down acetylcholinesterase. (Ch. 47)

Antidiuretic: (AN-ti-DYE-yoo-**RET**-ik) Lessening urine excretion. (Ch. 5)

Antigen: (**AN**-ti-jen) A protein marker on the surface of cells that identifies the type of cell. (Ch. 7, 52)

Antitussive: (an-tee-**TUSS**-iv) An agent that prevents or relieves cough. (Ch. 28)

Anuria: (AN-**YOO**-ree-ah) Complete suppression of urine formation by the kidney. (Ch. 35)

Anxiety: (ang-**ZIGH**-uh-tee) The uncomfortable feeling of apprehension or dread that occurs in response to a known or unknown threat. (Ch. 55)

Aphakic: (ah-**FAY**-kik) Absence of the lens of the eye, occurring congenitally or as a result of trauma or surgery. (Ch. 49)

Aphasia: (ah-**FAY**-zee-ah) Defect or loss of the power of expression by speech, writing, or signs, or of comprehension of spoken or written language, caused by disease or injury of the brain centers, such as stroke syndrome. (Ch. 45)

Aphthous stomatitis: (**AF**-thus STOH-mah-**TIGH**-tis) Small, white, painful ulcers (also known as canker sores) that appear on the inner cheeks, lips, gums, tongue, palate, and pharynx. They tend to recur. (Ch. 30)

Apnea: (ap-**NEE**-ah) Temporary absence of breathing. (Ch. 26)

Appendicitis: (uh-PEN-di-**SIGH**-tis) Inflammation of the vermiform appendix. (Ch. 31)

Arcus senilus: (**AR**-kus se-**NILL**-us) A benign white or gray opaque ring in the corneal margin of the eye. (Ch. 48)

Arrhythmia: (uh-**RITH**-mee-yah) Irregular rhythm, especially heartbeat. (Ch. 13)

Arteriosclerosis: (ar-TIR-ee-oh-skle-**ROH**-sis) Term applied to a number of pathological conditions in which there is gradual thickening, hardening, and loss of elasticity of the walls of the arteries. (Ch. 15, 18)

Arthritis: (are-**THRYE**-tis) Inflammation of a joint. (Ch. 43)

Arthrocentesis: (AR-throw-cen-**TEE**-sis) Surgical puncture of a joint cavity for aspiration of fluid. (Ch. 44)

Arthroplasty: (**AR**-throw-PLAS-te) Repair of a joint. Also called joint replacement. (Ch. 44)

Arthroscopy: (are-**THROW**-scop-ee) Examination of the interior of a joint with an arthroscope. (Ch. 43)

Articular: (ar-**TIK**-yoo-lar) Pertaining to a joint. (Ch. 43)

Ascites: (a-**SIGH**-teez) Abnormal accumulation of fluid in the peritoneal cavity. (Ch. 33)

Asepsis: (ah-**SEP**-sis) A condition free from germs, infection, and any form of life. (Ch. 7)

Aseptic: (ah-**SEP**-tik) Free of pathogenic organisms; asepsis. (Ch. 11)

Asphyxia: (as-**FIX**-ee-a) A condition in which there is a deficiency of oxygen in the blood and an increase in carbon dioxide in the blood and tissues. (Ch. 54)

Aspiration: (ASS-pi-**RAY**-shun) Accidental drawing in of foreign substances into the throat or lungs during inspiration. (Ch. 13)

Assessment: (ah-**SESS**-ment) An appraisal or evaluation of a client's condition. (Ch. 2)

Asterixis: (AS-ter-**ICK**-sis) Hand flapping tremor and involuntary movements of tongue and feet; may be present in hepatic encephalopathy. (Ch. 35)

Astigmatism: (uh-**STIG**-mah-**TIZM**) An error of refraction in which a ray of light is not sharply focused on the retina but is spread over a more or less diffuse area. (Ch. 49)

Ataxia: (ah-**TAK**-see-ah) Failure of muscular coordination; irregularity of muscular action. (Ch. 46)

Atelectasis: (AT-e-**LEK**-tah-sis) Collapsed or airless condition of the lung or portion of lung, caused by obstruction or hypoventilation. (Ch. 11, 22, 28)

Atherosclerosis: (ATH-er-oh-skle-**ROH**-sis) A form of arteriosclerosis characterized by accumulation of plaque, blood, and blood products lining the wall of the artery, causing partial or complete blockage of an artery. (Ch. 15, 18)

Atherosclerosis obliterans: (ATH-er-oh-skle-**ROH**-sis uh-**BLI**-ter-anz) A term used to describe the chronic arterial occlusion that is a slow, progressive disease attributed to the atherosclerotic process. (Ch. 18)

Atrial depolarization: (**AY**-tree-uhl DE-poh-lahr-i-**ZAY**-shun) Electrical activation of the atria. (Ch. 20)

Atrial kick: (**AY**-tree-uhl KIK) The contraction of the atria just before ventricular stimulation and contraction. Atrial kick contributes 15% to 30% of additional blood volume for greater cardiac output. (Ch. 19)

Atrial systole: (**AY**-tree-uhl **SIS**-tuh-lee) The contraction of the atria. (Ch. 20)

Atrioventricular node: (**AY**-tree-oh-ven-trick-yoo-lar nodh) Located in lower right atrium; receives an impulse from the SA node and relays it to the ventricles. (Ch. 20)

Atrophy: (**AT**-ruh-fee) Without nourishment; wasting. (Ch. 47)

Atypical: (ay-**TIP**-i-kuhl) Deviating from normal. (Ch. 28)

Augmentation: (AWG-men-**TAY**-shun) The act or process of increasing in size, quantity, degree or severity. (Ch. 40)

Auscultation: (AWS-kul-**TAY**-shun) Process of listening for sounds within the body, usually sounds of thoracic or abdominal viscera, to detect an abnormality. (Ch. 2)

Autocratic leadership: (AW-tu-**KRAT**-ik **LEE**-der-ship) A leadership style in which the leader has a high degree of control. (Ch. 1)

Autoimmune: (AW-toh-im-**YOON**) A condition in which the body does not recognize itself and the immune system attacks normal cells. (Ch. 37, 52, 53)

Autologous vaccine: (aw-**TAHL**-ah-gus **VACK**-seen) A vaccine derived from one's own tissues or fluids. (Ch. 42)

Avascular necrosis: (a-**VAS**-kue-lar ne-**KROW**-sis) Disruption of blood supply causing tissue death. (Ch. 44)

Bacteremia: (back-ter-**EE**-mee-ah) Bacteria in the blood. (Ch. 7)

Bacteria: (back-**TEAR**-e-ah) One-celled organism that can reproduce but needs a host for food and supportive environment. Bacteria can be harmless, normal flora, or disease-producing pathogens. (Ch. 7)

Bactericidal: (back-ter-i-**SIGH**-del) Destructive to, or destroying of, bacteria. (Ch. 7)

Bacteriostatic: (back-te-re-o-**STAT**-ik) Inhibiting or retarding bacterial growth. (Ch. 7)

Balanitis: (BAL-uh-**NIGH**-tis) Inflammation of the skin covering the glans penis. (Ch. 40)

Baroreceptor: (BA-roh-ree-**SEP**-tur) Sensory nerve endings found in the heart, vena cave, aortic arch, and carotid sinus that are stimulated by changes in pressure. (Ch. 5)

Barotrauma: (BAR-oh-**TRAW**-mah) Injury caused by pressure differences between the external environment and the inside of a bodily structure. (Ch. 49)

Barrel chest: (**BA**-ruhl CHEST) Increased anterior-posterior diameter of the chest caused by air trapping; often seen in clients with emphysema. (Ch. 26)

Basal cell secretion test: (**BAY**-zuhl SELL see-**KREE**-shun TEST) Part of a gastric analysis; measures the amount of gastric acid produced in 1 hour. (Ch. 29)

Behavior modification: (be-**HAYV**-yer MAH-di-fi-**KAY**-shun) A treatment method that uses positive reinforcement, aversive conditioning, and other methods to change behavior. (Ch. 55)

Belief: (bee-**LEEF**) Something accepted as true. Does not have to be proven. (Ch. 3)

Beneficence: (buh-**NEF**-i-sens) To provide good care; to do good for clients. One of the oldest requirements for health care providers. (Ch. 1)

Benign: (bee-**NIGHN**) Not progressive; for example, a tumor that is not cancerous. (Ch. 10)

Beta-hemolytic streptococci: (**BAY**-tuh-HEE-moh-**LIT**-ick STREP-tah-**KOCK**-sigh) Gram-positive bacteria that when grown on blood-agar plates completely hemolyze the blood and produce a clear zone around the bacteria colony. Group A beta-hemolytic streptococci cause disease in humans. (Ch. 17)

Bigeminy: (bye-**JEM**-i-nee) Occurring every second beat, as in bigeminal premature ventricular contractions. (Ch. 20)

Bilateral salpingo-oophorectomy: (by-**LAT**-er-uhl sal-PINJ-oh-ah-fuh-**RECK**-tuh-mee) Surgical removal of both fallopian tubes and ovaries. (Ch. 40)

Bimanual: (by-**MAN**-yoo-uhl) With both hands. (Ch. 39)

Biofeedback: (BYE-oh-**FEED**-bak) A form of therapy that uses provision of visual or auditory evidence to a person of the status of an autonomic body function such as heart rate, blood pressure, or respiratory rate. (Ch. 55)

Biopsy: (**BY**-ahp-see) A sample of tissue removed for examination. (Ch. 10)

Bipolar: (bye-**POH**-ler) Having two poles or pertaining to both poles. Bipolar disorder is characterized by episodes of manic and depressive behavior. (Ch. 55)

Blanch: (BLANCH) To lose color. (Ch. 51)

Bleb: (BLEB) An irregularly shaped elevation of the skin, such as a blister. May also occur in lung tissue. (Ch. 28)

Blepharitis: (BLEF-uh-**RIGH**-tis) Inflammation of the glands and lash follicles along the margin of the eyelids. (Ch. 49)

Blepharospasm: (BLEF-uh-roh-**SPAZM**) Spasm of the orbicular muscle of the eyelid. (Ch. 49)

Blindness: (**BLYND**-ness) Lack or loss of ability to see. (Ch. 49)

Bolus: (**BOH**-lus) A dose of intravenous medication injected all at once. (Ch. 6)

Bone: (BOWN) The hard, rigid form of connective tissue constituting most of the skeleton of vertebrates, composed chiefly of calcium salts. (Ch. 43)

Bowel sounds: (BOW'L SOWNDS) Gurgling and clicking sounds heard over the abdomen caused by air and fluid movement from peristaltic action. Normal bowel sounds occur every 5 to 15 seconds at a rate of 5 to 35 sounds per minute. Absent—no bowel sounds heard after 5 minutes of listening in each quadrant. Hyperactive—bowel sounds that are rapid, high-pitched, and loud. Hypoactive—bowel sounds that occur at a rate of one every minute or longer. (Ch. 29)

Bradycardia: (BRAY-dee-**KAR**-dee-yah) A slow heartbeat characterized by a pulse rate below 60 beats per minute. (Ch. 15, 20)

Bradykinesia: (BRAY-dee-kin-**EE**-zee-ah) Abnormal slowness of movement; sluggishness. (Ch. 46)

Bronchiectasis: (BRONG-key-**EK**-tah-sis) Chronic dilation of a bronchus or bronchi, usually associated with secondary infection and excessive sputum production. (Ch. 28)

Bronchitis: (brong-**KIGH**-tis) Inflammation of the mucous membrane of the bronchial airways; may be viral or bacterial. (Ch. 28)

Bronchodilator: (BRONG-koh-**DYE**-lay-ter) A drug that expands the bronchial tubes by relaxing bronchial smooth muscle. (Ch. 28)

Bronchospasm: (**BRONG**-koh-spazm) Spasm of the bronchial smooth muscle resulting in narrowing of the airways; associated with asthma and bronchitis. (Ch. 8, 28)

Bruit: (BROUT) A humming heard when auscultating a blood vessel that is caused by turbulent blood flow through the vessel. (Ch. 15)

Bulimia nervosa: (buh-**LEE**-mee-ah ner-**VOH**-sah) Recurrent episodes of binge eating and self-induced vomiting. (Ch. 30)

Bulimic: (buh-**LEE**-mick) The condition of having bulimia nervosa. (Ch. 30)

Bulla: (**BUHL**-ah) A large blister or skin lesion filled with fluid. May also occur in lung tissue. (Ch. 28)

Bundle of His: (**BUN**-duhl of HISS) A bundle of fibers of the impulse-conducting system of the heart. Originates in the AV node. (Ch. 20)

Bursae: (**BURR**-sah) A small fluid-filled sac or saclike cavity situated in tissues such as joints where friction would otherwise occur. (Ch. 43)

Calculi: (**KAL**-kyoo-lye) An abnormal concentration, usually composed of mineral salts, occurring within the body, chiefly in the hollow organs or their passages. Called also stones, as in kidney stones and gallstones. (Ch. 35)

Cancer: (**KAN**-sir) A general name for over 100 diseases in which abnormal cells grow out of control; a malignant tumor. (Ch. 10)

Candidiasis: (**KAN**-di-di-ah-sis) Infection of the skin or mucous membrane with any species of *Candida* (yeast-like fungi). (Ch. 7)

Cannula: (**KAN**-yoo-lah) A flexible tube that can be inserted into the body guided by a stiff, pointed rod. For example, an intravenous cannula is guided by a metal needle. (Ch. 6)

Capillary permeability: (**KAP**-i-lar-ee per-me-a-**BILL**-i-tee) The ability of substances to diffuse through capillary walls into tissue spaces. (Ch. 54)

Capillary refill: (**KAP**-i-lar-ee **RE**-fill) Indicator of peripheral circulation. (Ch. 54)

Caput medusae: (**KAP**-ut mi-**DOO**-see) Dilated veins around the umbilicus, associated with cirrhosis of the liver. (Ch. 32, 33)

Carbuncle: (**KAR**-bung-kull) A necrotizing infection of skin and subcutaneous tissue composed of a cluster of boils. (Ch. 49)

Carcinoembryonic antigens (CEA): (**KAR**-sin-oh-EM-bree-ah-nik **AN**-ti-jens) A class of antigens normally present in the fetus; CEA is elevated in many cancers. (Ch. 29)

Carcinogen: (kar-**SIN**-oh-jen) Specific agents known to promote the cancer process. (Ch. 10)

Cardiac output: (**KAR**-dee-yak **OWT**-put) A measure of the pumping ability of the heart; amount of blood pumped by the heart per minute. (Ch. 8, 16)

Cardiac tamponade: (**KAR**-dee-yak TAM-pon-**AYD**) The life-threatening compression of the heart by the fluid accumulating in the pericardial sac surrounding the heart. (Ch. 17)

Cardiogenic shock: (kar-dee-o-**JEN**-ick SHOCK) Occurs when the heart muscle is unhealthy and contractility is impaired. (Ch. 54)

Cardiomegaly: (KAR-dee-oh-**MEG**-ah-lee) Enlargement of the heart. (Ch. 17)

Cardiomyopathy: (KAR-dee-oh-my-**AH**-pah-thee) A group of diseases that affect the myocardium's structure or function. (Ch. 17)

Cardioplegia: (KAR-dee-oh-**PLEE**-jee-ah) Arrest of myocardial contraction, as by use of chemical compounds or cold temperatures in cardiac surgery. (Ch. 22)

Cardioversion: (KAR-do-oh-**VER**-zhun) An elective procedure in which a synchronized shock is delivered to attempt to restore the heart to a normal sinus rhythm. (Ch. 20)

Caring: (**KARE**-ring) The fostering of trust, respect, well-being, and growth by a caregiver with an individual, family, or the community. (Ch. 1)

Carrier: (**CARE**-ee-er) A person who harbors a specific pathogenic organism in the absence of discernible symptoms or signs of the disease and who is capable of spreading the organism to others. (Ch. 7)

Cataract: (**KAT**-uh-rakt) Opacity of the lens of the eye. (Ch. 13, 49)

Cation: (**KAT**-eye-on) Electrolytes that carry a positive electrical charge. (Ch. 5)

Cautery: (**CAW**-tur-ee) A device used to destroy tissue by electricity, freezing, heat, or corrosive chemicals. (Ch. 40)

Ceiling effect: (**SEE**-ling e-**FEKT**) The dose of medication at which the maximum therapeutic effect is achieved. Increasing the dose beyond the therapeutic dose will *not* result in increased relief and may result in undesirable side effects. (Ch. 9)

Cell-mediated immunity: (SELL **ME**-dee-ay-ted im-**YOO**-ni-tee) Production of lymphocytes by thymus in response to antigen exposure. (Ch. 52)

Cellulitis: (sell-yoo-**LYE**-tis) Inflammation of cellular or connective tissue. (Ch. 51)

Central hearing loss: (**SEN**-truhl **HEER**-ing LOSS) Occurs when there is a pathologic condition above the junction of the acoustic nerve and the brain stem. (Ch. 49)

Cerebrovascular: (SER-ee-broh-**VAS**-kyoo-lur) Pertaining to the blood vessels of the cerebrum or brain. (Ch. 45)

Chalazion: (kah-**LAY**-zee-on) A small eyelid mass resulting from chronic inflammation of a meibomian gland. (Ch. 49)

Chancre: (**SHANK**-er) A hard, syphilitic primary ulcer, the first sign of syphilis, appearing approximately 2 to 3 weeks after infection. (Ch. 42)

Chemotherapy: (KEE-moh-**THER**-uh-pee) The treatment of disease with medication; often refers to cancer therapy. (Ch. 10)

Cholecystitis: (KOH-lee-sis-**TIGH**-tis) Inflammation of the gallbladder. (Ch. 33)

Cholecystokinin: (KOH-lee-sis-toh-**KYE**-nin) A hormone secreted by the small intestine that stimulates contraction of the gallbladder. (Ch. 32)

Choledocholithiasis: (koh-LED-oh-koh-li-**THIGH**-ah-sis) Gallstones in the common bile duct. (Ch. 33)

Choledochoscopy: (KOH-LED-oh-**KOS**-koh-pee) An endoscopic test of the gallbladder and common bile duct. (Ch. 33)

Cholelithiasis: (KOH-lee-li-**THIGH**-ah-sis) Gallstones in the gallbladder. (Ch. 33)

Cholesteatoma: (KOH-lee-STEE-ah-**TOH**-mah) A cyst-like mass with a lining of stratified squamous epithelium, filled with desquamating debris frequently including cholesterol, which occurs in the meninges, central nervous system, and bones of the skull, but most commonly in the middle ear and mastoid region. (Ch. 49)

Chorea: (kaw-**REE**-ah) A nervous condition marked by involuntary muscular twitching of the limbs or facial muscles. (Ch. 17)

Circumcise: (**SIR**-kuhm-size) Surgical removal of the foreskin covering the head of the penis. (Ch. 39)

Cirrhosis: (si-**ROH**-sis) Chronic disease of the liver, associated with fat infiltration and development of fibrotic tissue. (Ch. 33)

Civil law: (**SIV**-il LAW) Provides the rules by which individuals seek to protect their personal and property rights. (Ch. 1)

Claudication: (KLAW-di-**KAY**-shun) A severe pain in the calf muscle from inadequate blood supply. (Ch. 15)

Clubbing: (**KLUB**-ing) A condition in which the ends of the fingers and toes appear bulbous and shiny, most often the result of lung disease. (Ch. 15)

Cochlear implant: (**KOK**-lee-er **IM**-plant) A device consisting of a microphone, signal processor, external transmitter, and implanted receiver to aid hearing. (Ch. 48, 49)

Code of ethics: (KOHD of **ETH**-icks) A traditional compilation of ideal behaviors of a professional group. (Ch. 1)

Codependence: (KO-de-**PEN**-dense) A situation in which the significant others in a family group begin to lose their own sense of identity and purpose and exist solely for the abuser. (Ch. 55)

Cognitive: (**KAHG**-ni-tiv). The ability to think rationally and to process thoughts. (Ch. 55)

Colectomy: (koh-**LEK**-tuh-me) Excision of the colon or a portion of it. (Ch. 31)

Colic: (**KAH**-lick) Spasm of a hollow organ or duct, causing pain. (Ch. 33)

Colitis: (koh-**LYE**-tis) Inflammation of the colon. (Ch. 31)

Collateral circulation: (koh-**LA**-ter-al SIR-kew-**LAY**-shun) Small branches off of larger blood vessels that will increase in size and capacity next to a main vessel that is obstructed. (Ch. 18)

Colonoscopy: (KOH-lun-**AHS**-kuh-pee) Examination of the upper portion of the rectum with a colonoscope. (Ch. 29)

Colostomy: (koh-**LAH**-stuh-me) An artificial opening (stoma) created in the large intestine and brought to the surface of the abdomen for evacuating the bowels. (Ch. 31)

Colporrhaphy: (kohl-**POOR**-ah-fee) Surgical repair of the vagina. (Ch. 40)

Colposcopy: (kul-**POS**-koh-pee) Examination of the vulva, vagina, and cervix by means of a magnifying lens and a bright light. (Ch. 39)

Comedone: (**KOH**-me-doh) Skin lesion that occurs in acne vulgaris. (Ch. 51)

Commissurotomy: (KOM-i-shur-**AHT**-oh-mee) Surgical incision of any commissure as in cardiac valves to increase the size of the orifice. (Ch. 19, 22)

Compliance: (kom-**PLIGH**-ens) The ability to alter size or shape in response to an outside force; the ability of the lungs to distend. (Ch. 28)

Compulsion: (kum-**PUHL**-shun) A recurrent, unwanted, and distressing urge to perform an act. (Ch. 55)

Compulsive: (kum-**PUHL**-siv) Repetitive act that may appear purposeful. (Ch. 55)

Conductive hearing loss: (kon-**DUK**-tiv **HEER**-ing LOSS) Impaired transmission of sound waves through the external ear canal to the bones of the middle ear. (Ch. 49)

Condylomata acuminata: (KON-di-**LOH**-ma-tah ah-KYOOM-in-**AH**-tah) Warts in the genital region caused by the human papillomavirus (HPV); a contagious sexually transmitted disease. (Ch. 41)

Condylomatous: (KON-di-**LOH**-ma-tus) Pertaining to a condyloma. (Ch. 41)

Confidentiality: (KON-fi-den-she-**AL**-i-tee) Maintaining privacy of client information. Client and client's care can be discussed only in the professional setting. (Ch. 1)

Conization: (KOH-ni-**ZAY**-shun) The removal of a cone of tissue, as in partial excision of the cervix uteri. (Ch. 39)

Conjunctivitis: (kon-JUNK-ti-**VIGH**-tis) Inflammation of the conjunctiva of the eye. (Ch. 42, 49)

Consensual response: (KON-**SEN**-shoo-uhl ree-**SPONS**) Reaction of both pupils when one eye is exposed to greater intensity of light than the other. (Ch. 48)

Constipation: (KON-sti-**PAY**-shun) A condition of sluggish or difficult bowel action/evacuation. (Ch. 13, 31)

Contraceptive: (KON-truh-**SEP**-tiv) Any process, device, or method that prevents conception. (Ch. 40)

Contracture: (kon-**TRACK**-chur) Abnormal accumulation of fibrosis connective tissue in skin, muscle or joint capsule that prevents normal mobility at that site. (Ch. 13, 45, 46)

Contralateral: (KON-truh-**LAT**-er-uhl) Originating in or affecting the opposite side of the body. (Ch. 46)

Conversion disorder: (kon-**VER**-zhun dis-**OR**-der) An illness that emerges from overuse of the conversion reaction defense mechanism, in which there is impaired physical functioning that appears to be neurological, but no organic disease can be identified. (Ch. 55)

Coping: (**KOH**-ping) The process of contending with the stresses of daily life in an effort to overcome or work through them. (Ch. 55)

Corneal light reflex test: (**KOR**-nee-uhl LIGHT **REE**-fleks TEST) Testing of the corneal reflex action of the eye. Absence of the corneal reflex indicates deep coma or injury of one of the nerves carrying the reflex arc. (Ch. 48)

Corneal transplant: (**KOR**-nee-uhl **TRANS**-plant) Transplantation of a donor cornea into the eye of the recipient. (Ch. 49)

Coronary artery disease: (**KOR**-uh-na-ree **AR**-tuh-ree di-**ZEEZ**) Narrowing of the coronary arteries sufficient to prevent adequate blood supply to the myocardium. (Ch. 18)

Counseling: (**KOWN**-sel-ing) The provision of help or guidance by a health care professional. (Ch. 55)

Craniectomy: (KRAY-nee-**EK**-tuh-me) Excision of a segment of the skull. (Ch. 46)

Cranioplasty: (KRAY-nee-oh-plas-tee) Any plastic repair operation on the skull. (Ch. 46)

Craniotomy: (KRAY-nee-**AHT**-oh-mee) Any incision through the cranium. (Ch. 46)

Crepitation: (crep-i-**TAY**-shun) A dry, crackling sound or sensation, such as that produced by the grating of the ends of a fractured bone. (Ch. 43)

Crepitus: (**KREP**-i-tuss) Crepitation. (Ch. 26)

Criminal law: (**KRIM**-i-nuhl LAW) Regulates behaviors for citizens within a country. (Ch. 1)

Critical thinking: (**KRIT**-i-kuhl **THING**-king) Use of knowledge and skills to make the best decisions possible in client care situations. (Ch. 2)

Cryotherapy: (KRY-oh-**THER**-uh-pee) The therapeutic use of cold. (Ch. 40)

Cryptorchidism: (kript-**OR**-ki-dizm) A birth condition in which one or both of the testicles have not descended into the scrotum. (Ch. 41)

Culdocentesis: (KUL-doh-sen-**TEE**-sis) The procedure for obtaining material from the posterior vaginal cul-de-sac by aspiration or surgical incision through the vaginal wall, performed for therapeutic or diagnostic reasons. (Ch. 40)

Culdoscopy: (kul-**DOS**-koh-pee) Direct visual examination of the female viscera through an endoscope introduced into the pelvic cavity through the posterior vaginal fornix. (Ch. 39)

Culdotomy: (KUL-**DOT**-uh-mee) Incision or needle puncture of the cul-de-sac of Douglas through the vagina. (Ch. 40)

Cultural awareness: (**KUL**-chur-uhl a-**WARE**-ness) Being aware of history and ancestry and having an appreciation of and attention to the crafts, arts, music, foods, and clothing of various cultures. (Ch. 3)

Cultural competence: (**KUL**-chur-uhl **KOM**-pe-tens) Having an awareness of one's own culture and not letting it have an undue influence over another person's culture. Having the knowledge and skills about a culture that are required to provide care. (Ch. 3)

Cultural diversity: (KUL-chur-uhl di-**VER**-si-tee) Representing two or more cultures; the differences among cultures. For example, the United States includes people from many different countries. (Ch. 3)

Cultural sensitivity: (KUL-chur-uhl SEN-si-**TIV**-i-tee) Being aware of and sensitive to cultural differences. Avoiding behavior or language that may be offensive to another person's cultural beliefs. (Ch. 3)

Curet: (kyoo-**RET**) A loop, ring, or spoon-shaped instrument, attached to a handle and having sharp or blunt edges; used to scrape tissue from a surface. (Ch. 39)

Custom: (**KUS**-tum) A custom is the usual way of acting in a given circumstance or something that an individual or group does out of habit. For example, many people have turkey on Thanksgiving. (Ch. 3)

Cyanosis: (SIGH-uh-**NOH**-sis) Slightly bluish, grayish, or dark purple discoloration of the skin caused by the presence of abnormal amounts of reduced hemoglobin in the blood. (Ch. 8, 21, 26)

Cycloplegic: (sigh-kloh-**PLEE**-jik) Pertaining to paralysis of the ciliary muscle of the eye. (Ch. 49)

Cystic: (**SIS**-tik) Pertaining to cysts or the urinary bladder. (Ch. 39)

Cystitis: (sis-**TIGH**-tis) Inflammation of the urinary bladder. (Ch. 35)

Cystocele: (**SIS**-toh-seel) A bladder hernia that protrudes into the vagina. (Ch. 40)

Cystoscopy: (sis-**TAHS**-koh-pee) A diagnostic procedure using an instrument (cystoscope) via the urethra to view the bladder. (Ch. 34)

Cytotoxic: (SIGH-toh-**TOCK**-sick) Destructive to cells. (Ch. 10, 42)

Data: (**DAY**-tuh) A group of facts or statistics. (Ch. 2)

Data, objective: (ob-**JEK**-tiv) Factual data obtained through physical assessment and diagnostic tests; objective data are observable or knowable through the five senses. (Ch. 2)

Data, subjective: (sub-**JEK**-tiv) Information that is provided verbally by the client. (Ch. 2)

Debridement: (day-breed-**MENT**) The removal of foreign material and contaminated and devitalized tissues from or adjacent to a traumatic or infected area until surrounding healthy tissue is exposed. (Ch. 11)

Decerebrate: (dee-**SER**-e-brayt) Posture of an individual with absence of cerebral function. (Ch. 45)

Decorticate: (dee-**KOR**-ti-kayt) Posture of an individual with a lesion at or above the upper brain stem. (Ch. 45)

Defibrillate: (dee-**FIB**-ri-layt) Stopping fibrillation of the heart by using an electrical device that applies countershock to the heart through electrodes placed on the chest wall. (Ch. 20)

Degeneration: (de-jen-er-**AY**-shun) Deterioration. (Ch. 47)

Dehiscence: (dee-**HISS**-ents) A splitting open (i.e., rupture) of an incision. (Ch. 11)

Dehydration: (DEE-high-**DRAY**-shun) A condition resulting from excessive loss of body fluid that occurs when fluid output exceeds intake. (Ch. 5)

Delirium tremens: (dee-**LIR**-ee-uhm **TREE**-menz) An acute alcohol withdrawal syndrome marked by acute, transient disturbance of consciousness. (Ch. 55)

Delusions: (dee-**LOO**-zhuns) False beliefs that are firmly maintained in spite of incontrovertible proof to the contrary. (Ch. 55)

Dementia: (dee-**MEN**-cha) A broad term that refers to cognitive deficit, including memory impairment. (Ch. 13, 46)

Democratic leadership: (DEM-ah-**KRAT**-ik **LEE**-dership) A leadership style in which the leader has a moderate degree of control. (Ch. 1)

Demyelination: (dee-MY-uh-lin-**AY**-shun) Loss of myelin from neurons. (Ch. 47)

Dependence: (di-**PEN**-dens) A state of reliance on something. Psychological craving for a drug that may or may not be accompanied by a physiological need. (Ch. 55)

Depression: (dee-**press**-shun) A mental disorder marked by altered mood with loss of interest. (Ch. 13)

Dermatitis: (DER-mah-**TIGH**-tis) Inflammation of the skin. (Ch. 51)

Dermatophytosis: (DER-mah-toh-fye-**TOH**-sis) A fungal infection of the skin. (Ch. 51)

Dermoid: (**DER**-moyd) Resembling the skin. (Ch. 40)

Developmental stage: (dee-vell-up-**MEN**-tal STAYJ) An age-defined period with specific psychological tasks that need to be accomplished to maintain ego as proposed by Erik Erikson, a psychoanalyst. (Ch. 12)

Diabetes mellitus: (DYE-ah-**BEE**-tis mel-**LYE**-tus) A chronic disease characterized by impaired production or use of insulin and high blood glucose levels. (Ch. 38)

Diagnosis-related groups: (DYE-ag-**NOH**-sis ree-**LAY**-ted GROOPS) A system designed to standardize prospective payment for medical care for specific medical diagnoses. (Ch. 1, 4)

Diarrhea: (DYE-uh-**REE**-ah) Frequent passage of loose, fluid, or unformed stools. (Ch. 31)

Diastolic blood pressure: (dye-ah-**STAH**-lik BLUHD **PRE**-shure) The amount of pressure exerted on the wall of the arteries when the ventricles are at rest. The bottom number in a blood pressure reading. (Ch. 16)

Diffusion: (di-**FEW**-zhun) The tendency of molecules of a substance (gaseous, liquid, or solid) to move from a region of high concentration to one of lower concentration. (Ch. 5)

Dilation and curettage: (DIL-**AY**-shun and kyoor-e-**TAHZH**) A surgical procedure that expands the cervical canal of the uterus (dilation) so that the surface lining of the uterine wall can be scraped (curettage). (Ch. 40)

Displacement: (dis-**PLAYSS**-ment) Transference of emotion from the original idea with which it was associated to a different idea, allowing the client to avoid acknowledging the original source. (Ch. 55)

Disseminated intravascular coagulation: (dis-**SEM**-i-NAY-ted IN-trah-**VAS**-kyoo-lar koh-AG-yoo-**LAY**-shun) A pathological form of coagulation that is diffuse rather than localized, as would be the case in normal coagulation. Clotting factors are consumed to such an extent that generalized bleeding may occur. (Ch. 24, 40)

Distributive justice: (dis-**TRIB**-yoo-tiv **JUS**-tiss) The right of individuals to be treated equally regardless of race, sex, marital status, sexual preference, medical diagnosis, social standing, economic level, or religious belief. (Ch. 1)

Diverticulitis: (DYE-ver-tik-yoo-**LYE**-tis) Inflammation of a diverticulum (a sac or pouch in the walls of a canal or organ, usually the colon), especially inflammation involving diverticula of the colon. (Ch. 31)

Diverticulosis: (DYE-ver-tik-yoo-**LOH**-sis) The presence of diverticula in the absence of inflammation. (Ch. 31)

Dressler's syndrome: (**DRESS**-lers **SIN**-drohm) Post–myocardial infarction syndrome; pericarditis. (Ch. 17)

Dumping syndrome: (**DUHM**-ping **SIN**-drohm) The rapid entry of food into the jejunum without proper mixing of the food with digestive juices causing dizziness, tachycardia, fainting, sweating, nausea, diarrhea, a feeling of fullness, and abdominal cramping. Occurs in some clients after gastric surgery. (Ch. 30)

Dysarthria: (dis-**AR**-three-ah) Imperfect articulation of speech caused by disturbances of muscular control resulting from central or peripheral nervous system damage. (Ch. 45)

Dysfunctional: (dis-**FUNCK**-shun-uhl) Family or work environment that does not function effectively, sometimes because of other problems of members. (Ch. 55)

Dysmenorrhea: (DIS-men-oh-**REE**-ah) Pain in association with menstruation. (Ch. 40)

Dyspareunia: (DIS-puh-**ROO**-nee-ah) Occurrence of pain in the labia, vagina, or pelvis during or after sexual intercourse. (Ch. 40)

Dysphagia: (dis-**FAYJ**-ee-ah) Inability to swallow or difficulty swallowing. (Ch. 27, 37, 45)

Dysplasia: (dis-**PLAY**-zee-ah) Abnormal development of tissue. (Ch. 40)

Dyspnea: (**DISP**-nee-ah) Subjective sense of labored breathing that occurs because of insufficient oxygenation. (Ch. 26)

Dysreflexia: (DIS-re-**FLEK**-see-ah) State in which an individual with a spinal cord injury at or above T7 experiences an uninhibited sympathetic response to a noxious stumulus. (Ch. 46)

Dysrhythmia: (dis-**RITH**-mee-yah) Abnormal, disordered, or disturbed cardiac rhythm. (Ch. 5, 8, 15, 20)

Dysuria: (dis-**YOO**-ree-ah) Difficult or painful urination. (Ch. 34, 35, 41)

Ecchymoses: (eck-uh-**MOH**-sis) A bruise of varying size, the color of which may be blue-black, changing to greenish yellow or yellow with time. (Ch. 23, 24, 50)

Ectasia: (ek-**TAY**-zee-ah) Replacement of normal tissue with fibrous tissue. (Ch. 40)

Ectopic: (eck-**TOP**-ick) Ectopic hormones are secreted from sites other than the gland where they would normally be found. (Ch. 28, 37, 39)

Eczema: (**EK**-zuh-mah) Acute or chronic inflammatory conditions of the skin. (Ch. 51)

Edema: (uh-**DEE**-muh) Collection of excess fluid in body tissues. (Ch. 13)

Ejaculation: (ee-JAK-yoo-**LAY**-shun) The release of semen from the male urethra. (Ch. 39)

Electrocautery: (ee-**LECK**-troh-**CAW**-tur-ee) Cauterization using platinum wires heated to red or white heat by an electric current, either direct or alternating. (Ch. 42)

Electrocardiogram: (ee-**LECK**-troh-**KAR**-dee-oh-GRAM) A recording of the electrical activity of the heart. (Ch. 20)

Electrocoagulated: (ee-**LECK**-troh-coh-**AG**-yoo-LAY-ted) Coagulation of tissue by means of a high-frequency electric current. (Ch. 42)

Electroconvulsive therapy (ECT): (ee-**LEK**-troh-kun-**VUL**-siv **THER**-uh-pee) A type of somatic therapy in which an electric current is used to produce convulsions to treat such conditions as depression. (Ch. 55)

Electroencephalogram: (ee-**LEK**-troh-en-**SEFF**-uh-loh-gram) A record produced by electroencephalography; tracing of the electrical impulses of the brain. (Ch. 45)

Electrolyte: (ee-**LEK**-troh-lite) A substance that when dissolved in water can conduct electricity. (Ch. 5)

Electroretinography: (ee-LEK-troh-RET-in-**AHG**-ruh-fee) Measurement of the electrical response of the retina to light stimulation. (Ch. 48)

Emboli: (**EM**-boh-li) Solid, liquid, or gaseous masses of undissolved matter traveling with the fluid current in a blood or lymphatic vessel. (Ch. 17)

Embolism: (**EM**-boh-lizm) Foreign substance or blood clot that travels through the circulatory system until it obstructs a vessel. (Ch. 18, 28)

Emmetrope: (**EM**-e-trohp) A person who has no refractive error of vision. (Ch. 49)

Emmetropia: (**EM**-e-**TROH**-pee-ah) The ideal optical condition. (Ch. 49)

Empathy: (**EM**-puh-thee) Objective awareness of and insight into the feelings, emotions, and behavior of another person. (Ch. 1)

Emphysema: (**EM**-fi-**SEE**-mah) Distention of interstitial tissue by gas or air; chronic pulmonary disease marked by terminal bronchiole and alveolar destruction and air trapping. (Ch. 28)

Empyema: (**EM**-pigh-**EE**-mah) Pus in a body cavity, especially the pleural space. (Ch. 28)

Encephalitis: (EN-seff-uh-**LYE**-tis) Inflammation of the brain. (Ch. 46)

Encephalopathy: (en-SEFF-uh-**LAHP**-ah-thee) Dysfunction of the brain. (Ch. 22, 46)

Endarterectomy: (end-AR-tur-**ECK**-tuh-mee) Excision of thickened atheromatous areas of the innermost coat of an artery. (Ch. 22, 46)

Endogenous: (en-**DAH**-jen-us) Produced or originating from within a cell or organism. (Ch. 38, 40)

Endometritis: (EN-doh-me-**TRY**-tis) Inflammation of the endometrium of the uterus. (Ch.42)

Endorphins: (en-**DOR**-fins) Naturally occurring opioids in the body, many times more potent than analgesic medications. (Ch. 9)

Endoscope: (**EN**-doh-skohp) A device consisting of a tube and optical system for observing the inside of a hollow organ or cavity. Can be flexible or rigid. (Ch. 29)

Enkephalins: (en-**KEF**-e-lins) One type of endorphin. (Ch. 9)

Enteritis: (en-ter-**EYE**-tis) Inflammation of the intestines, particularly of the mucosa and submucosa of the small intestine. (Ch. 31, 42)

Enucleation: (ee-NEW-klee-**AY**-shun) Removal of an organ or other mass intact from its supporting tissues, as of the eyeball from the orbit. (Ch. 49)

Epidemiological: (EP-i-DEE-me-ah-**LAHJ**-i-kuhl) The study of the distribution and determinants of health-related states and events in populations and the application of this study to the control of health problems. (Ch. 42)

Epididymitis: (EP-i-DID-i-**MY**-tis) Inflammation or infection of the epididymis. (Ch. 41)

Epidural: (EP-i-**DUHR**-uhl) Situated on or outside the dura mater. (Ch. 46)

Epinephrine: (EP-i-**NEFF**-rin) A hormone secreted by the adrenal medulla in response to stimulation of the sympathetic nervous system. (Ch. 8)

Epistaxis: (EP-iss-**TAX**-iss) Nosebleed. (Ch. 27)

Epithelialization: (ep-i-THEE-lee-al-eye-**ZAY**-shun) The growth of skin over a wound. (Ch. 51)

Equianalgesic: (EE-kwee-AN-uhl-**JEE**-zik) Drugs having equal pain killing effect. The same degree of pain relief may require different doses when different medications are given or medications are given by different routes. (Ch. 9)

Erectile dysfunction: (e-**RECK**-tile dis-**FUNCK**-shun) Inability to have an erection sufficient for sexual intercourse. (Ch. 41)

Erection: (e-**REK**-shun) Enlargement and hardening of the penis caused by engorgement of blood. (Ch. 39)

Erythema: (ER-i-**THEE**-mah) Diffuse redness over the skin. (Ch. 50)

Eschar: (**ESS**-kar) Hard scab or dry crust that results from necrotic tissue. (Ch. 51)

Escharotomy: (ess-kar-**AHT**-oh-mee) Removal of a slough or scab formed on the skin and underlying tissue of severely burned skin. (Ch. 51)

Esophagogastroduodenoscopy: (e-SOFF-uh-go-GAS-troh-DOO-od-e-**NOS**-kuh-pee) An endoscopic procedure that allows the physician view the esophagus, stomach, and duodenum. (Ch. 32)

Esophagoscopy: (ee-soff-ah-**GAHS**-kuh-pee) Examination of the esophagus using an endoscope. (Ch. 29)

Esotropia: (ESS-oh-**TROH**-pee-ah) Strabismus in which there is deviation of the visual axis of one eye toward that of the other eye, resulting in diplopia. Also called cross-eyed. (Ch. 48)

Ethical rights: (**ETH**-i-kuhl RIGHTS) Rights that are based on a moral or ethical principle. (Ch. 1)

Ethnic: (**ETH**-nick) Pertaining to a religious, racial, national, or cultural group. For example, individuals may identify with the Jewish, Catholic, or Islamic religions. (Ch. 3)

Ethnocentrism: (ETH-noh-**SEN**-trizm) The tendency to think that one's own ways of thinking, believing, and acting are the only right ones. People who are different are seen as strange or bizarre. For example, one who believes that his or her religious beliefs are the only right beliefs and other religions are wrong. (Ch. 3)

Euthyroid: (yoo-**THY**-royd) Normal thyroid function. (Ch. 37)

Evaluation: (e-VAL-yoo-**AY**-shun) The judgment of anything. (Ch. 2)

Evisceration: (e-**VIS**-sir-a-shun) Extrusion of viscera outside the body, especially through a surgical excision. (Ch. 11)

Exacerbation: (egg-sass-sir-**BAY**-shun) Aggravation of symptoms. (Ch. 47)

Exophthalmos: (ECKS-off-**THAL**-mus) Abnormal protrusion of the eyeball. (Ch. 36, 37)

Exotropia: (EKS-oh-**TROH**-pee-ah) Abnormal turning outward of one or both eyes; divergent strabismus. (Ch. 48)

Expectorant: (ek-**SPEK**-tuh-rant) Agent that promotes removal of pulmonary secretions. (Ch. 28)

Expectorate: (eck-**SPECK**-tuh-RAYT) The act or process of coughing up materials from the air passageways leading to the lungs. (Ch. 13)

External otitis: (eks-**TER**-nuhl oh-**TIGH**-tis) Inflammation of the external ear. (Ch. 49)

Extracellular: (EX-trah-**SELL**-yoo-ler) Outside the cell. (Ch. 5)

Extracorporeal shock wave lithotripsy (ESWL): (ECKS-trah-koar-**POR**-ee-uhl SHAHK WAYV LITH-oh-**TRIP**-see) Noninvasive treatment using shock waves to break up gallstones or kidney stones. (Ch. 33)

Extrinsic factors: (eks-**TRIN**-sik **FAK**-ters) External variables. (Ch. 13)

Exudate: (**EKS**-yoo-dayt) Accumulated fluid in a cavity; oozing of pus or serum; often the result of inflammation. (Ch. 27, 28)

Fasciculation: (fah-SIK-yoo-**LAY**-shun) Twitching. (Ch. 47)

Fasciotomy: (fash-e-**OTT**-oh-me) Incision of a fascia. (Ch. 44)

Fetor hepaticus: (**FEE**-tor he-**PAT**-i-kus) Foul breath associated with liver disease. (Ch. 33)

Fibrinolytic: (FIGH-brin-oh-**LIT**-ik) A complicated system of biochemical reactions for lysis of clots in the vascular system. (Ch. 40)

Fibrocystic: (FIGH-broh-**SIS**-tik) Consisting of fibrocysts, which are fibrous tumors that have undergone cystic degeneration or accumulated fluid. (Ch. 40)

Fidelity: (fi-**DEL**-i-tee) The obligation to be faithful to commitments made to self and others. (Ch. 1)

Filtration: (fill-**TRAY**-shun) The process of removing particles from a solution by allowing the liquid portion to pass through a membrane or other partial barrier. (Ch. 5)

Fissure: (**FISH**-er) A narrow slit or cleft, especially one of the deeper or more constant furrows separating the gyri of the brain. (Ch. 31)

Fistula: (**FIST**-yoo-lah) Any abnormal, tubelike passage within body tissue, usually between two internal organs, or leading from an internal organ to the body surface. (Ch. 31)

Flaccid: (**FLA**-sid) Weak, lax, soft muscles. (Ch. 46)

Fluoroscope: (**FLAW**-or-oh-skohp) A device consisting of a fluorescent screen suitably mounted, either separately or in conjunction with an x-ray tube, by means of which the shadows of objects interposed between the tube and the screen are made visible. (Ch. 29)

Fluoroscopy: (fluh-**RAHS**-kuh-pee) The use of a fluoroscope for medical diagnosis or for testing various materials by roentgen rays. (Ch. 20)

Full-thickness burn: (full-**THICK**-ness BERN) Burn in which all of the epithelializing elements and those lining the sweat glands, hair follicles, and sebaceous glands are destroyed. (Ch. 54)

Functional hearing loss: (**FUNK**-shun-uhl **HEER**-ing loss) Affecting the function but not the structure. (Ch. 49)

Fungi: (**FUNG**-guy) A general term for a group of eukaryotic organisms (mushrooms, yeasts, molds, etc.). (Ch. 7)

Furuncle: (**FYOOR**-ung-kull) An acute circumscribed inflammation of the subcutaneous layers of the skin or of a gland or hair follicle. (Ch. 49)

Gamete: (**GAM**-eet) A mature male or female reproductive cell; the spermatozoon or ovum. (Ch. 40)

Gastrectomy: (gas-**TREK**-tuh-mee) Any surgery that involves partial removal of the stomach. (Ch. 30)

Gastrectomy, total: (gas-**TREK**-tuh-mee, **TOE**-tal) Total surgical removal of the stomach. (Ch. 30)

Gastric acid stimulation test: (**GAS**-trik **ASS**-id STIM-yoo-**LAY**-shun TEST) A test that measures the amount of gastric acid for 1 hour after subcutaneous injection of a drug that stimulates gastric acid secretion. (Ch. 29)

Gastric analysis: (**GAS**-trik ah-**NAL**-i-sis) A test performed to measure secretions of hydrochloric acid and pepsin in the stomach. (Ch. 29)

Gastric lavage: (**GAS**-trik la-**VA**-ge) Washing out of the stomach; used to empty the stomach when the contents are irritating. (Ch. 54)

Gastritis, acute: (gas-**TRY**-tis) The inflammation of the stomach mucosa. Also known as heartburn or indigestion. (Ch. 30)

Gastritis, chronic: (gas-**TRY**-tis) Gastritis that is recurrent. Classified as type A (asymptomatic) or type B (symptomatic). (Ch. 30)

Gastroduodenostomy: (**GAS**-troh-DOO-oh-den-**AHS**-toh-mee) Excision of the pylorus of the stomach with anastomosis of the upper portion of the stomach to the duodenum. (Ch. 30)

Gastroepiploic: (**GAS**-troh-EP-i-**PLOH**-ick) Pertaining to the stomach and greater omentum. (Ch. 22)

Gastrojejunostomy: (**GAS**-troh-JAY-joo-**NAHS**-toh-mee) Subtotal excision of the stomach with closure of the proximal end of the duodenum and side-to-side anastomosis of the jejunum to the remaining portion of the stomach. (Ch. 30)

Gastroparesis: (**GAS**-troh-puh-**REE**-sis) Paralysis of the stomach, resulting in poor emptying. (Ch. 38)

Gastroplasty: (**GAS**-troh-PLAS-tee) Plastic surgery of the stomach. Used to decrease the size of the stomach to treat morbid obesity. (Ch. 30)

Gastroscopy: (gas-**TRAHS**-kuh-pee) Examination of the stomach and abdominal cavity by use of a gastroscope. (Ch. 29)

Gastrostomy: (gas-**TRAHS**-toh-mee) Surgical creation of a gastric fistula through the abdominal wall. (Ch. 29)

Gavage: (gah-**VAZH**) Feeding with a stomach tube or with a tube passed through the nares, pharynx, and esophagus into the stomach. The food is in liquid or semiliquid form at room temperature. (Ch. 29)

Generalization: (JEN-er-al-i-**ZAY**-shun) An assumption about a group or an individual item or person that leads to seeking additional information to determine if the generalization fits the individual. Whereas generalizations are true for the group, they may not be true for the individual. (Ch. 3)

Glaucoma: (glaw-**KOH**-mah) A group of eye diseases characterized by increased intraocular pressure. (Ch. 13)

Glomerulonephritis: (gloh-MER-yoo-loh-ne-**FRY**-tis) A form of nephritis in which the lesions involve primarily the glomeruli. (Ch. 35)

Glossitis: (glah-**SIGH**-tis) An inflammation of the tongue. (Ch. 24)

Glycosuria: (GLY-kos-**YOO**-ree-ah) Abnormal amount of glucose in the urine, often associated with diabetes mellitus. (Ch. 38)

Goiter: (**GOY**-ter) Abnormal enlargement of the thyroid gland. (Ch. 37)

Guaiac: (**GWY**-ak) A resin obtained from trees used in testing for occult blood in feces. (Ch. 29)

Gummas: (**GUM**-ahs) A soft granulomatous tumor of the tissues characteristic of the tertiary stage of syphilis. (Ch. 42)

Gynecomastia: (JIN-e-koh-**MASS**-tee-ah) Excessive breast tissue on a male. (Ch. 39)

Hallucinations: (huh-LOO-si-**NAY**-shuns) False perceptions having no relation to reality and not accounted for by any exterior stimuli. (Ch. 55)

Health: (**HELLTH**) A condition in which all functions of the body and mind are normally active. (Ch. 1, 12)

Health care delivery systems: (HELLTH KAIR dee-**LIV**-er-ee **SIS**-tems) Groups of health care services that attempt to cover all or most health care needs across a broad continuum and across the life span. (Ch. 4)

Health-illness continuum: (HELLTH ill-ness kon-**TIN**-u-m) A continuum represents an individual's life span with health on one end and illness on the other end. The person then moves back and forth along the continuum throughout life toward health or illness. (Ch. 1)

Hearing aid: (**HEER**-ing AYD) An instrument to amplify sounds for those with hearing loss. (Ch. 48)

Heatstroke: (**HEET**-strohk) An acute and dangerous reaction to heat exposure, characterized by high body temperature, usually above 105°F. (Ch. 54)

***Helicobacter pylori*:** (**HE**-lick-co-back-tur **PIE**-lori) Bacterium that causes some peptic ulcers. (Ch. 30)

Hemangioma: (hee-MAN-jee-**OH**-mah) A benign vascular tumor. (Ch. 51)

Hematochezia: (HEM-uh-toh-**KEE**-zee-uh) Blood in the feces. (Ch. 31)

Hematoma: (HEE-muh-**TOH**-mah) A localized collection of extravasated blood, usually clotted, in an organ, space, or tissue. (Ch. 11, 35)

Hematuria: (HEM-uh-**TYOOR**-ee-ah) Blood in the urine. (Ch. 34, 41)

Hemiparesis: (hem-ee-puh-**REE**-sis) Weakness affecting one side of the body. (Ch. 45, 46)

Hemipelvectomy: (hem-ee-pell-**VEC**-toe-me) The surgical removal of half of the pelvis and the leg. (Ch. 44)

Hemiplegia: (hem-ee-**PLEE**-jee-ah) Paralysis of only one side of the body. (Ch. 46)

Hemodialysis: (HEE-moh-dye-**AL**-i-sis) A method for replacing the function of the kidneys by circulating blood through tubes made of semipermeable membranes. (Ch. 35)

Hemodynamic: (he-mo-di-**NAM**-ik) The stability of the body systems as maintained by adequate blood circulation. (Ch. 18)

Hemolysis: (he-**MAHL**-e-sis) The destruction of the membrane of red blood cells with the liberation of hemoglobin, which diffuses into the surrounding fluid. (Ch. 22, 24)

Hemophilia: (HEE-moh-**FILL**-ee-ah) A hereditary blood disease marked by greatly prolonged coagulation time, with consequent failure of the blood to clot and abnormal bleeding. (Ch. 24)

Hemoptysis: (hee-**MOP**-ti-sis) Coughing up of blood from respiratory tract. (Ch. 28)

Hemorrhoids: (**HEM**-uh-royds) A mass of dilated, tortuous veins in the anorectum involving the venous plexuses of that area. (Ch. 31)

Hemothorax: (HEE-moh-**THAW**-raks) Blood in the pleural space; may be associated with trauma, tuberculosis, or pneumonia. (Ch. 28)

Hepatitis: (HEP-uh-**TIGH**-tis) Inflammation of the liver, most often viral. (Ch. 33)

Hepatorenal syndrome: (hep-**PAT**-oh-REE-nuhl **SIN**-drohm) A deadly kidney failure that sometimes accompanies liver disease. (Ch. 33)

Hepatosplenomegaly: (he-PA-toh-SPLE-noh-**MEG**-ah-lee) Enlargement of the liver and spleen. (Ch. 42)

Hernia: (**HER**-nee-uh) The protrusion or projection of an organ or a part of an organ through the wall of the cavity that normally contains it. (Ch. 31)

Herpetic: (her-**PET**-ick) Pertaining to herpes. (Ch. 42)

Hiatal hernia: (high-**AY**-tuhl **HER**-nee-ah) A condition in which part of the stomach protrudes through and above the diaphragm. (Ch. 30)

High-density lipoprotein (HDL): (HIGH **DEN**-si-tee LIP-oh-**PROH**-teen) Plasma lipids bound to albumin consisting of lipoproteins. It has been found that those with high levels of HDL have less chance of having coronary artery disease. (Ch. 18)

Histamine: (**HISS**-ta-mean) A substance produced in the body that increases gastric secretion, increases capillary permeability, contracts the bronchial smooth muscle. Plays a role in allergic reaction. (Ch. 53)

Histoplasmosis: (HISS-toh-plaz-**MOH**-sis) A systemic fungal respiratory disease due to *Histoplasma capsulatum* (causative agent). (Ch. 7)

Homans' sign: (**HOH**-manz SIGHN) An assessment for venous thrombosis in which calf pain with dorsiflexion occurs if thrombosis is present. (Ch. 15)

Homeostasis: (HOH-mee-oh-**STAY**-sis) Maintaining a constant balance, especially whenever a change occurs. (Ch. 5, 13)

Hordeolum: (hor-**DEE**-oh-lum) Sty. (Ch. 49)

Human immunodeficiency virus (HIV): (**HYOO**-man im-YOO-noh-dee-**FISH**-en-see **VIGH**-rus) A retrovirus that causes acquired immunodeficiency syndrome (AIDS). (Ch. 53)

Humoral: (**HYOO**-mohr-uhl) Pertaining to body fluids or substances contained in them. (Ch. 7)

Hydrocele: (**HIGH**-droh-seel) A collection of fluid in the scrotal sack. (Ch. 41)

Hydrocephalus: (HIGH-droh-**SEF**-uh-luhs) A condition caused by enlargement of the cranium caused by abnormal accumulation of cerebrospinal fluid within the cerebral ventricular system. (Ch. 46)

Hydronephrosis: (HIGH-droh-ne-**FROH**-sis) Abnormal dilation of kidneys caused by obstruction of urine flow. (Ch. 35, 41)

Hydrostatic: (HIGH-droh-**STAT**-ik) Pertaining to the pressure of liquids in equilibrium and to the pressure exerted by liquids. (Ch. 5)

Hypercalcemia: (HIGH-per-kal-**SEE**-mee-ah) An excessive amount of calcium in the blood. (Ch. 5)

Hypercoagulability: (HIGH-per-koh-AG-yoo-lah-**BILL**-i-tee) The increased ability of the blood to clot. (Ch. 17)

Hypercoagulation: (HIGH-per-koh-AG-yoo-**LAY**-shun) Increased blood clotting. (Ch. 40)

Hyperglycemia: (HIGH-per-gligh-**SEE**-mee-ah) Excess glucose in the blood. (Ch. 38)

Hyperkalemia: (HIGH-per-kuh-**LEE**-mee-ah) An excessive amount of potassium in the blood. (Ch. 20)

Hyperlipidemia: (HIGH-per-LIP-i-**DEE**-mee-ah) Excessive quantity of fat in the blood. (Ch. 18)

Hypermagnesemia: (HIGH-per-MAG-nuh-**ZEE**-mee-ah) Excess magnesium in the blood. (Ch. 5)

Hypermenorrhea: (HIGH-per-MEN-oh-**REE**-ah) An abnormal increase in the duration or amount of menstrual flow. (Ch. 40)

Hypernatremia: (HIGH-per-nuh-**TREE**-mee-ah) Excess sodium in the blood. (Ch. 5)

Hyperopia: (HIGH-per-**OH**-pee-ah) Farsightedness. (Ch. 49)

Hyperplasia: (HIGH-per-**PLAY**-zee-ah) Excessive increase in the number of normal cells. (Ch. 37, 41)

Hypertension: (HIGH-per-**TEN**-shun) Abnormally elevated blood pressure. (Ch. 16)

Hypertensive crisis: (HIGH-per-**TEN**-siv **CRY**-sis) Arbitrarily defined as severe elevation in diastolic blood pressure above 120 to 130 mm Hg. (Ch. 16)

Hypertonic: (HIGH-per-**TAHN**-ik) Exerts greater osmotic pressure than blood. (Ch. 5, 6)

Hypertrophy: (high-**PER**-truh-fee) An increase in the size of an organ or structure, or of the body, owing to growth rather than tumor formation. (Ch. 16, 40)

Hyperuricemia: (HIGH-per-yoor-a-**SEE**-me-ah) An excess of uric acid or urates in the blood. (Ch. 44)

Hyperventilation: (HIGH-per-VEN-ti-**LAY**-shun) Increased ventilation that results in a lowered carbon dioxide (CO_2) level (hypocapnia). (Ch. 5)

Hypervolemia: (HIGH-per-voh-**LEE**-mee-ah) An abnormal increase in the volume of circulating blood. (Ch. 5)

Hypocalcemia: (HIGH-poh-kal-**SEE**-mee-ah) Reduced amount of calcium in the blood. (Ch. 5)

Hypoglycemia: (HIGH-poh-gligh-**SEE**-mee-ah) Below-normal amount of glucose in the blood. (Ch. 38)

Hypokalemia: (HIGH-poh-kuh-**LEE**-mee-ah) Reduced amount of potassium in the blood. (Ch. 5)

Hypomagnesemia: (HIGH-poh-MAG-nuh-**ZEE**-mee-ah) Reduced amount of magnesium in the blood. (Ch. 5, 20)

Hypomenorrhea: (HIGH-poh-MEN-oh-**REE**-ah) A deficient amount of menstrual flow, but with regular periods. (Ch. 40)

Hyponatremia: (HIGH-poh-nuh-**TREE**-mee-ah) Reduced amount of sodium in the blood. (Ch. 5)

Hypophysectomy: (HIGH-pah-fi-**SECK**-tuh-mee) Surgical removal of the pituitary gland. (Ch. 37)

Hypoplasia: (HIGH-poh-**PLAY**-zee-ah) Underdevelopment of a tissue organ or body. (Ch. 40)

Hypoproteinemia: (HIGH-poh-pro-teen-**EE**-mee-ah) A decrease in the amount of protein in the blood. (Ch. 54)

Hypospadias: (HIGH-poh-**SPAY**-dee-ahz) A congenital male defect in which the opening of the urethra is on the underside of the penis, instead of the tip. (Ch. 39)

Hypostatic: (HIGH-poh-**STA**-tik) Hypostatic pneumonia occurs from congestion in the lungs associated with lack of activity. (Ch. 28)

Hypotension: (HIGH-poh-**TEN**-shun) Abnormally low blood pressure below 90 mm Hg systolic. (Ch. 8)

Hypothermia: (HIGH-poh-**THER**-mee-ah) Low body temperature. (Ch. 11, 22)

Hypotonic: (HIGH-poh-**TAHN**-ik) Pertaining to defective muscular tone or tension; having a lower concentration of solute than intracellular or extracellular fluid. (Ch. 5, 6)

Hypovolemia: (HIGH-poh-voh-**LEE**-mee-ah) The most common form of dehydration resulting from the loss of fluid from the body; results in decreased blood volume. (Ch. 5)

Hypovolemic: (HIGH-poh-voh-**LEEM**-ick) Low volume of blood in the circulatory system. (Ch. 8, 37)

Hypovolemic shock: (HIGH-poh-voh-**LEEM**-ick SHAHK) Shock that occurs when blood or plasma is lost in such quantities that the remaining blood cannot fill the circulatory system despite constriction of the blood vessels. (Ch. 54)

Hypoxemia: (HIGH-pock-**SEE**-mee-ah) Deficient oxygenation of the blood. (Ch. 22)

Hypoxia: (high-**POCK**-see-ah) Diminished availability of oxygen to the body tissues. (Ch. 22)

Hysterectomy: (HISS-tuh-**RECK**-tuh-mee) Surgical removal of the uterus through the abdominal wall or vagina. (Ch. 40)

Hysterosalpingogram: (**HIS**-tur-oh-SAL-pinj-oh-gram) Radiograph of the uterus and fallopian tubes. (Ch. 39)

Hysteroscopy: (HIS-tur-**AHS**-koh-pee) Endoscopic direct visual examination of the canal of the uterine cervix and the cavity of the uterus. (Ch. 39)

Hysterotomy: (HISS-tuh-**RAH**-tuh-mee) Incision of the uterus. (Ch.40)

Icterus: (**ICK**-ter-us) Yellowing of the skin and the sclera of the eye. (Ch. 32)

Idiopathic thrombocytopenic purpura: (ID-ee-oh-**PATH**-ik THROM-boh-SIGH-toh-**PEE**-nik **PUR**-pew-rah) The total number of circulating platelets is greatly diminished, even though platelet production in the bone marrow is normal, resulting in slowed blood clotting. (Ch. 24)

Ileostomy: (ILL-ee-**AH**-stuh-me) An artificial opening (stoma) created in the small intestine (ileum) and brought to the surface of the abdomen for the purpose of evacuating feces. (Ch. 31)

Illness: (**Ill**-ness) The state of being sick. (Ch. 1, 12)

Illusions: (i-**LOO**-zhuns) Mistaken perceptions of reality. (Ch. 55)

Imagery: (**IM**-ij-ree) The use of the imagination to promote relaxation. (Ch. 55)

Immunocompromised: (IM-yoo-noh-**KAHM**-prah-mized) Having an immune system that is not capable of reacting to a pathogen or tissue damage. (Ch. 28)

Impaction: (im-**PAK**-shun) An immovable accumulation of feces in the bowels. (Ch. 29, 31)

Imperforate: (im-**PER**-foh-rate) Without an opening. (Ch. 40)

Incisional radial keratotomy: (in-**SIZ**-zhun-uhl **RAY**-dee-uhl ker-ah-**TAH**-tu-mee) Excision of a portion of the cornea. (Ch. 49)

Increased intraocular pressure: (**IN**-creesed in-trah-**OK**-yoo-lur **PRESS**-ure) Increase in the fluid (aqueous humor) pressure compromising blood flow to the optic nerve and retina. (Ch. 49)

Induction: (in-**DUCK**-shun) The process or act of causing to occur. (Ch. 11)

Induration: (IN-dyoo-**RAY**-shun) Area of hardened tissue. (Ch. 28)

Infarction: (in-**FARK**-shun) An area of tissue in an organ or part that undergoes necrosis following cessation of blood supply. (Ch. 18)

Infective endocarditis: (in-**FECK**-tive EN-doh-kar-**DYE**-tis) Inflammation of the heart lining caused by microorganisms. (Ch. 17)

Initiation: (i-NI-she-**AY**-shun) The onset of a process, such as the uncontrolled growth of cells in cancer. (Ch. 10)

Inspection: (in-**SPEK**-shun) Use of observation skills to systematically gather data that can be seen. (Ch. 2)

Insufficiency: (IN-suh-**FISH**-en-see) The condition of being inadequate for a given purpose, such as heart valves that do not close properly. (Ch. 19)

Insufflation: (in-suff-**LAY**-shun) Used to inflate the abdomen during laparoscopic or endoscopic procedures to enhance visualization of structures. (Ch. 39, 40)

Interferons: (IN-ter-**FEER**-ons) Any of a group of glycoproteins with antiviral activity. (Ch. 42)

Intermittent claudication: (IN-ter-**MIT**-ent KLAW-di-**KAY**-shun) A symptom associated with arterial occlusive disease. It refers to pain in the calf of a lower extremity, usually brought on by activity or exercise, and ceases with rest. (Ch. 18)

International normalized ratio: (IN-ter-**NASH**-uh-nul **NOR**-muh-lized **RAY**-she-oh) The World Health Organization's standardization for reporting the prothrombin time assay test when the thromboplastin reagent developed by the first International Reference Preparation is used. The reagent was developed to prevent variability in prothrombin time testing results and provide uniformity in monitoring therapeutic levels for coagulation during oral anticoagulation therapy. (Ch. 17)

Interstitial: (IN-ter-**STISH**-uhl) Fluid between tissues. (Ch. 5)

Intervention: (in-ter-**VEN**-shun) One or more actions taken in order to modify an effect. (Ch. 2)

Intracellular: (IN-trah-**SELL**-yoo-ler) Fluids located within the blood cell. (Ch. 5)

Intracranial: (IN-trah-**KRAY**-nee-uhl) Within the cranium or skull. (Ch. 5)

Intraocular pressure: (**IN**-trah-**OK**-yoo-lur **PRESH**-uhr) Pressure within the eye. (Ch. 48)

Intraoperative: (**IN**-trah-**AHP**-er-uh-tiv) Occurring during a surgical procedure. (Ch. 11)

Intrarenal failure: (In-tra-**REE**-nuhl **FAYL** yur) Renal failure caused by a problem within the kidney. (Ch. 35)

Intravascular: (In-trah-**VAS**-kyoo-lar) Fluids located within the blood vessels. (Ch. 5)

Intravenous: (IN-trah-**VEE**-nus) Within or into a vein. (Ch. 6)

Intrinsic factors: (in-**TRIN**-sik **FAK**-ters) Internal variables. (Ch. 13)

Intussusception: (IN-tuh-suh-**SEP**-shun) The slipping of one part of an intestine into another adjacent to it. (Ch. 31)

In vitro fertilization: (in **VEE**-troh FER-ti-li-**ZAY**-shun) Fertilization in a test tube. (Ch. 40)

Ipsilateral: (IP-si-**LAT**-er-uhl) On the same side; affecting the same side of the body. (Ch. 46)

Ischemia: (iss-**KEY**-me-ah) Condition of inadequate blood supply. (Ch. 8, 15)

Isoelectric line: (EYE-so-e-**LEK**-trick LINE) The period when the electrical tracing is at zero and is neither positive nor negative. (Ch. 20)

Isolated systolic hypertension: (**EYE**-suh-lay-ted sis-**TAH**-lik HIGH-per-**TEN**-shun) The systolic pressure is 160 mm Hg or more, but the diastolic pressure is below 95 mm Hg. (Ch. 16)

Isotonic: (EYE-so-**TAHN**-ik) A fluid that has the same osmolarity as the blood. (Ch. 5, 6)

Jaundice: (**JAWN**-diss) Yellowing of the skin and the sclera of the eye. (Ch. 32)

Joint: (JOYNT) An articulation. The point of juncture between two bones. (Ch. 43)

Kaposi's sarcoma: (ka-**POE**-sees sar-**CO**-mah) A vascular malignancy that is often first apparent in the skin or mucous membranes but may involve the viscera. (Ch. 53)

Keratitis: (KER-uh-**TIGH**-tis) Inflammation of the cornea, which is usually associated with decreased visual acuity. (Ch. 49)

Ketoacidosis: (KEE-toh-ass-i-**DOH**-sis) A condition in which fat breakdown produces ketones, which cause an acidic state in the body; may be associated with weight loss or diabetes mellitus. (Ch. 38)

Kussmaul's: (**KOOS**-mahlz) Term describing deep respirations of an individual with ketoacidosis. (Ch. 38)

Labyrinthitis: (LAB-i-rin-**THIGH**-tis) An inflammation of the labyrinth; otitis internal. (Ch. 49)

Laceration: (la-sir-**A**-shun) A wound or irregular tear of the flesh. (Ch. 54)

Lactic acid: (**LAK**-tik **ASS**-id) By-product of anaerobic metabolism. (Ch. 8)

Laissez-faire leadership: (LAS-ay-**FAIR LEE**-der-ship) A leadership style in which the leader exerts no control over the group he or she is leading. (Ch. 1)

Laminectomy: (LAM-i-**NEK**-toh-mee) The excision of a vertebral posterior arch, usually to remove a lesion or herniated disk. (Ch. 46)

Lanugo: (la-**NU**-go) Downy hair covering the body. (Ch. 30)

Laparoscopy: (LAP-uh-roh-**SKOP**-ee) Exploration of the abdomen with an endoscope. (Ch. 33)

Laparotomy: (LAP-uh-**RAH**-tuh-mee) The surgical opening of the abdomen; an abdominal operation. (Ch. 40)

Laryngeal edema: (lah-**RIN**-jee-uhl uh-**DEE**-muh) Sudden swelling of the larynx occurring with severe allergic reactions. (Ch. 8)

Laryngectomy: (lar-in-**JEK**-tah-mee) Surgical removal of the larynx. (Ch. 27)

Laser ablation: (**LAY**-zer uh-**BLAY**-shun) Therapeutic destruction of a growth or part of a growth by laser treatment. (Ch. 40)

Lavage: (lah-**VAZH**) Washing out of a cavity. (Ch. 29)

Law: (LAW) The further formalization of moral considerations. (Ch. 1)

Leadership: (**LEE**-der-ship) Involves decision making, communicating, motivating, and guiding others. (Ch. 1)

Leiomyoma: (LYE-oh-my-**OH**-ma) A myoma consisting principally of smooth muscle tissue. (Ch. 40)

Leukemia: (loo-**KEE**-mee-ah) A malignancy of the blood-forming cells in the bone marrow. (Ch. 24)

Leukocytes: (**LOO**-ko-sites). White blood corpuscles. (Ch. 7)

Leukocytosis: (LOO-koh-sigh-**TOH**-sis) An increase in the number of leukocytes in the blood, generally caused by presence of infection and usually transient. (Ch. 22)

Leukopenia: (LOO-koh-**PEE**-nee-yah) Abnormal decrease of white blood cells, usually below 5000/mm³. (Ch. 10)

Liability: (LYE-uh-**BIL**-i-tee) The level of responsibility that society places on individuals for their actions. (Ch. 1)

Libido: (li-**BEE**-doh) Sexual drive, conscious or unconscious. (Ch. 39)

Lichenified: (lye-**KEN**-i-fyed) Thickened or hardened from continued irritation. (Ch. 51)

Lifestyle modifications: (**LYEF**-style MAH-di-fi-**KAY**-shuns) Nonpharmacologic management of primary hypertension; may include weight reduction, dietary sodium and alcohol restriction, and regular aerobic exercise. (Ch. 16)

Limitation of liability: (lim-i-**TAY**-shun OF LYE-uh-**BIL**-i-tee) Steps that health care professionals can take to limit their liability. (Ch. 1)

Lobectomy: (loh-**BEK**-tuh-mee) Surgical removal of a lobe of any organ or gland. (Ch. 28)

Lower gastrointestinal series (lower GI): (**LOH**-er GAS-troh-in-**TES**-ti-nuhl **SEER**-ees) The use of barium sulfate as an enema to facilitate x-ray and fluoroscopic examination of the colon. (Ch. 29)

Lymphadenopathy: (lim-FAD-e-**NAH**-puh-thee) Any disorder of the lymph nodes. (Ch. 42)

Lymphangitis: (lim-FAN-je-**EYE**-tis) Inflammation of lymphatic channels or vessels. (Ch. 18)

Lymphedema: (LIMPF-uh-**DEE**-mah) An abnormal accumulation of tissue fluid (potential lymph) in the interstitial space. (Ch. 23)

Lymphocytes: (**LIM**-foh-sites) Cells present in the blood and lymphatic tissue that provide the main means of immunity for the body; white blood cells. (Ch. 52)

Lymphoma: (lim-**FOH**-mah) A usually malignant lymphoid neoplasm. (Ch. 25)

Macular degeneration: (**MACK**-you-lar dee-JEN-uh-**RAY**-shun) Age-related breakdown of the macular area of the retina of the eye. (Ch. 13, 49)

Malignant: (muh-**LIG**-nunt) Growing, resisting treatment; used to describe a tumor of cancerous cells. (Ch. 10)

Malpractice: (mal-**PRAK**-tiss) A breach of duty arising out of the relationship that exists between the client and the health care worker. (Ch. 1)

Mammography: (mah-**MOG**-rah-fee) Use of radiography of the breast to diagnose breast cancer. (Ch. 39)

Mammoplasty: (**MAM**-oh-PLAS-tee) Plastic surgery of the breast. (Ch. 40)

Mania: (**MAY**-nee-ah) Mental disorder characterized by excessive excitement. (Ch. 55)

Marsupialization: (mar-SOO-pee-al-i-**ZAY**-shun) Process of raising the borders of an evacuated tumor sac to the edges of the abdominal wound and stitching them there to form a pouch. (Ch. 40)

Mastalgia: (mass-**TAL**-jee-ah) Pain in the breast. (Ch. 40)

Mastectomy: (mass-**TECK**-tuh-mee) Excision of the breast. (Ch. 40)

Mastitis: (mass-**TIGH**-tis) Inflammation of the breast. (Ch. 40)

Mastoiditis: (MASS-toy-**DYE**-tis) Inflammation of the air cells of the mastoid process. (Ch. 49)

Mastopexy: (**MAS**-toh-PEKS-ee) Correction of a pendulous breast by surgical fixation and plastic surgery. (Ch. 40)

Mediastinum: (ME-dee-ah-**STYE**-num) A septum or cavity between two principal portions of an organ. (Ch. 22)

Megacolon: (**MEG**-ah-KOH-lun) Extremely dilated colon. (Ch. 31)

Melena: (muh-**LEE**-nah) Black, tarry feces caused by action of intestinal secretions on free blood. (Ch. 31)

Menarche: (me-**NAR**-kee) The initial menstrual period, normally occurring between the ninth and seventeenth year. (Ch. 39)

Meniere's disease: (MAY-nee-**AIRZ** di-**ZEEZ**) A recurrent and usually progressive group of symptoms including progressive deafness, ringing in the ears, dizziness, and a sensation of fullness or pressure in the ears. (Ch. 49)

Meningitis: (men-in-**JIGH**-tis) Inflammation of the membranes of the spinal cord and brain. (Ch. 46)

Menometrorrhagia, metromenorrhagia: (MEN-oh-MET-roh-**RAY**-jee-ah) (MET-roh-MEN-oh-**RAY**-jee-ah) Excessively long and heavy menstrual flow. (Ch. 40)

Menopause: (**MEN**-oh-pawz) The period that marks the permanent cessation of menstrual activity, usually occurring between the ages of 35 and 58. (Ch. 39)

Menorrhagia: (MEN-oh-**RAY**-jee-ah) Passing more than 80 mL of blood per menses. (Ch. 40)

Mental health: (**MEN**-tuhl HELLTH) State of being adjusted to life; able to be flexible, successful, maintain close relationships, solve problems, make appropriate judgments, and cope with daily stresses. (Ch. 55)

Mental illness: (**MEN**-tuhl ILL-ness) Any illness that affects the mind or behavior. (Ch. 55)

Metastasis: (muh-**TASS**-tuh-sis) Movement of bacteria or body cells (especially cancer cells) from one part of the body to another. (Ch. 10, 40)

Milieu: (me-**LYU**) Environment. (Ch. 55)

Miotic: (my-**AH**-tik) An agent that causes the pupil to contract. (Ch. 49)

Mixed hearing loss: (MIXD **HEER**-ing LOSS) A functional and conductive hearing loss. (Ch. 49)

Morality: (muh-**RAL**-i-tee) A social barometer that dictates what is good or bad in a society. (Ch. 1)

Motility: (moh-**TIL**-i-tee) The power to move spontaneously. (Ch. 40)

Mucolytic: (MYOO-koh-**LIT**-ik) Agent that liquefies sputum. (Ch. 28)

Mucopurulent cervicitis: (MYOO-koh-**PYOOR**-uh-lent SIR-vi-**SIGH**-tis) Inflammation of the cervix producing mucus and purulent discharge. (Ch. 40, 42)

Mucositis: (MYOO-koh-**SIGH**-tis) Inflammation of a mucous membrane. (Ch. 10)

Multifocal: (MUHL-tee-**FOH**-kuhl) Many foci or sites. (Ch. 20)

Murmur: (**MUR**-mur) An abnormal sound heard on auscultation of the heart and adjacent large blood vessels. (Ch. 15, 19)

Muscle: (**MUSS**-uhl) A bundle of long slender cells or fibers that have the power to contract and hence to produce movement. (Ch. 43)

Mutation: (myoo-**TAY**-shun) A change in a gene potentially capable of being transmitted to an offspring. (Ch. 10)

Myalgia: (my-**AL**-jee-ah) Muscle pain or tenderness. (Ch. 27)

Myectomy: (my-**ECK**-tuh-mee) Surgical removal of a hypertrophied muscle. (Ch. 17)

Myelogram: (**MY**-e-loh-gram) The film produced by radiography of the spinal cord after injection of a contrast medium into the subarachnoid space. (Ch. 45)

Myocardial infarction: (MY-oh-**KAR**-dee-yuhl in-FARK-shun) Death of cells of an area of the heart muscle, myocardium, as a result of oxygen deprivation, which in turn is caused by obstruction of the blood supply. Commonly referred to as a heart attack. (Ch. 18)

Myocarditis: (MY-oh-kar-**DYE**-tis) The inflammatory process that causes nodules to form in the myocardial tissue; the nodules become scar tissue over time. Inflammation of the heart muscle. (Ch. 8, 17)

Myomectomy: (my-oh-**MECK**-tuh-mee) Removal of a portion of muscle or muscular tissue. (Ch. 40)

Myopia: (my-**OH**-pee-ah) The error of refraction in which rays of light entering the eye parallel to the optic axis are brought to a focus in front of the retina; nearsightedness. (Ch. 49)

Myringoplasty: (mir-**IN**-goh-PLASS-tee) Surgical reconstruction of the tympanic membrane. (Ch. 49)

Myringotomy: (MIR-in-**GOT**-uh-mee) Incision of the tympanic membrane, usually performed to relieve pressure and allow for drainage of either serous or purulent fluid in the middle ear behind the tympanic membrane. (Ch. 49)

Myxedema: (MICK-suh-**DEE**-mah) Condition resulting from hypofunction of the thyroid gland. (Ch. 37)

Negligence: (**NEG**-li-jense) An unintentional tort. (Ch. 1)

Neoplasia: (NEE-oh-**PLAY**-zee-ah) The development of new abnormal tissue. (Ch. 40)

Neoplasm: (**NEE**-oh-PLAZ-uhm) New abnormal tissue growth, as in a tumor. (Ch. 10)

Nephrectomy: (ne-**FREK**-tuh-mee) Surgical removal of a kidney. (Ch. 35)

Nephrogenic: (NEFF-roh-**JEN**-ick) Caused by the kidneys. (Ch. 37)

Nephrolithotomy: (NEFF-roh-li-**THOT**-uh-mee) Incision of a kidney for removal of kidney stones. (Ch. 35)

Nephropathy: (ne-**FROP**-uh-thee) Any disease of the kidney. (Ch. 35, 38)

Nephrosclerosis: (NEFF-roh-skle-**ROH**-sis) Hardening of the kidney associated with hypertension and disease of the renal arterioles. (Ch. 35)

Nephrostomy: (ne-**FRAHS**-toh-mee) Creation of a permanent opening into the renal pelvis. (Ch. 35)

Nephrotoxin: (NEFF-roh-**TOK**-sin) A toxin having a specific destructive effect on kidney tissue. (Ch. 22, 35)

Neuralgia: (new-**RAL**-jee-ah) Nerve pain. (Ch. 47)

Neurogenic: (NEW-roh-**JEN**-ik) Originating in the nervous system. (Ch. 8)

Neuromuscular junction: (NOOR-o-**MUS**-ku-lar **JUNC**-tion). Point at which nerve and muscle meet. (Ch. 47)

Neuropathic pain: (NEW-roh-**PATH**-ik PAYN) Pain resulting from peripheral nerve injury. (Ch. 9)

Neuropathy: (new-**RAH**-puh-thee) A general term denoting functional disturbances and pathologic changes in the peripheral nervous system. (Ch. 45, 47)

Neutropenia: (noo-tro-**PE**-ne-ah) Abnormally small number of neutrophil cells in the blood. (Ch. 7)

Neutrophils: (**NEW**-troh-fils) Granular leukocytes (white blood cells) having a nucleus with three to five lobes connected by threads of chromatin and cytoplasm containing very fine granules. (Ch. 52)

Nit: (NIT) Egg of a louse or other parasitic insect. (Ch. 49)

Nociceptive: (NOH-see-SEP-tiv) Pain sensitive. (Ch. 9)

Nocturia: (nock-**TYOO**-ree-ah) Excessive urination at night. (Ch. 12, 13, 37, 38, 41)

Nodal or junctional rhythm: (**NOHD**-uhl or **JUNGK**-shun-uhl **RITH**-uhm) A cardiac rhythm with its origin at the atrioventricular (AV) node. (Ch. 20)

Nonmaleficence: (NON-muh-**LEF**-i-sens) The requirement that health care providers do no harm to their clients, either intentionally or unintentionally. (Ch. 1)

Nonpathogenic: (non-path-o-**JEN**-ic) Inability to produce a disease. (Ch. 7)

Norepinephrine: (NOR-ep-i-**NEFF**-rin) A hormone produced by the adrenal medulla, similar in chemical and pharmacological properties to epinephrine, but chiefly a vasoconstrictor with little effect on cardiac output. (Ch. 8)

Normotensive: (nor-moh-**TEN**-siv) Normal blood pressure. (Ch. 16)

Nosocomial infection: (no-zoh-**KOH**-mee-uhl in-**FECK**-shun) Infection acquired in a health care agency. (Ch. 7)

Nuchal rigidity: (**NEW**-kuhl re-**JID**-i-tee) Rigidity of the nape, or back, of the neck. (Ch. 46)

Nursing diagnosis: (**NUR**-sing DYE-ag-**NOH**-sis) A standardized label placed on a client's problem to make it understandable to all nurses. (Ch. 2)

Nursing process: (**NUR**-sing **PRAH**-sess) An orderly, logical approach to administering nursing care so that the client's needs for such care are met comprehensively and effectively. (Ch. 2)

Nystagmus: (nis-**TAG**-muss) Involuntary, rapid, rhythmic eye movement. (Ch. 45, 48)

Obesity: (oh-**BEE**-si-tee) Abnormal amount of fat on the body from 20% to 30% over average weight for age, sex, and height. (Ch. 30)

Obsession: (ub-**SESH**-un) Repetitive thought, urge, or emotion. (Ch. 55)

Obstipation: (OB-sti-**PAY**-shun) Intractable constipation. (Ch. 31)

Obstructive shock: (ub-**STRUCK**-tive SHAHK) Shock caused by indirect pump failure. (Ch. 54)

Occult blood test: (ah-**KULT** BLUHD TEST) A chemical test or microscopic examination for blood, especially in feces, that is not apparent on visual inspection. (Ch. 29)

Oligomenorrhea: (AH-li-goh-MEN-uh-**REE**-ah) Scanty or infrequent menstrual flow. (Ch. 40)

Oligura: (AH-li-**GYOO**-ree-ah) Diminished urination. (Ch. 8, 35)

Onchocerciasis: (ONG-koh-sir-**KIGH**-uh-sis) Infection with worms of the genus *Onchocerca*. (Ch. 49)

Oncologist: (on-**KAH**-luh-jist) A specialist in oncology (the study of tumors). (Ch. 10)

Oncology: (on-**KAH**-luh-jee) The study of cancer and cancer treatment. (Ch. 10)

Oncovirus: (**ONK**-oh-**VIGH**-russ) Viruses linked to cancer in humans. (Ch. 10)

Onychomycosis: (ON-i-koh-my-**KOH**-sis) Disease of the nails caused by fungus. (Ch. 51)

Ophthalmia neonatorum: (ahf-**THAL**-mee-ah NEE-oh-nuh-**TOR**-uhm) Conjunctivitis in the newborn resulting from exposure to infectious or chemical agents. (Ch. 40, 42)

Ophthalmologist: (AHF-thal-**MAH**-luh-jist) A physician who specializes in the treament of disorders of the eye. (Ch. 48)

Ophthalmoscope: (ahf-**THAL**-muh-skohp) An instrument used for examining the interior of the eye, especially the retina. (Ch. 48)

Opioid: (O-pe-**OYD**) A narcotic drug with morphine-like effects. True opioids are derived from opium. (Ch. 9)

Optician: (ahp-**TISH**-uhn) One who specializes in filling prescriptions for corrective lenses for eyeglasses and contact lenses. (Ch. 48)

Optimum level of functioning: (**OP**-teh-mum **LEV**-uhl of **FUNK**-shun-ing) Highest level of client activity considering the client's condition. (Ch. 13)

Option rights: (**OP**-shun RIGHTS) Rights that are based on a fundamental belief in the dignity and freedom of human beings. (Ch. 1)

Optometrist: (ahp-**TOM**-uh-trist) A doctor of optometry who diagnoses and treats conditions and diseases of the eye per state laws. (Ch. 48)

Orchiectomy: (or-ki-**EK**-toh-mee) Removal of one or both testicles; a treatment for prostate cancer. (Ch. 41)

Orgasm: (**OR**-gazm) Pleasurable physical release sensation related to physical, sexual, and psychological stimulation. (Ch. 39, 41)

Orientation: (OR-ee-en-**TAY**-shun) The ability to comprehend and to adjust oneself in an environment with regard to time, location, and identity of persons. (Ch. 55)

Osmolality: (ahs-moh-**LAL**-i-tee) Osmotic concentration; ionic concentration of the dissolved substances per unit of solvent. (Ch. 37)

Osmosis: (ahs-**MOH**-sis) The passage of solvent through a semipermeable membrane that separates solutions of difference concentrations. (Ch. 5)

Ossiculoplasty: (ah-SIK-yoo-loh-**PLASS**-tee) Surgical reconstruction of the middle ear to improve hearing caused by conductive hearing loss. (Ch. 49)

Osteomyelitis: (AHS-tee-oh-my-**LIGHT**-tis) Inflammation of bone, especially the marrow, caused by a pathogenic organism. (Ch. 44)

Osteoporosis: (AHS-tee-oh-por-**OH**-sis) A condition in which there is a reduction in the mass of bone per unit volume. (Ch. 5, 13, 40)

Osteosarcoma: (AHS-tee-oh-sar-**KOH**-mah) A malignant sarcoma of a bone. (Ch. 44)

Otalgia: (oh-**TAL**-jee-ah) Pain in the ear. (Ch. 48)

Otomycosis: (OH-toh-my-**KOH**-sis) An infection of the external auditory meatus of the ear caused by a fungus infestation. (Ch. 49)

Otorrhea: (Oh-toh-**REE**-ah) Inflammation of the ear with purulent discharge. (Ch. 48)

Otosclerosis: (OH-toh-skle-**ROH**-sis) A condition characterized by chronic, progressive deafness, especially for low tones. (Ch. 49)

Ototoxic: (OH-toh-**TOK**-sik) Having a detrimental effect on the eighth cranial nerve or the organs of hearing. (Ch. 48)

Pain: (PAYN) An unpleasant sensory and emotional experience associated with actual or potential tissue damage, or described in terms of such damage. Whatever the client says it is whenever the client says it occurs. (Ch. 9)

Palliation: (PAL-ee-**AY**-shun) The relief of symptoms without cure. (Ch. 10)

Palpation: (pal-**PAY**-shun) Use of the fingers or hands to feel something. (Ch. 2)

Palpebral fissure: (**PAL**-puh-burhl **FISH**-er) Fissure of the eyelid. (Ch. 48)

Pancarditis: (PAN-kar-**DYE**-tis) Inflammation of all the structures of the heart. (Ch. 17)

Pancreatectomy: (PAN-kree-uh-**TECK**-tuh-mee) Removal of all or part of the pancreas. (Ch. 33)

Pancreatitis: (PAN-kree-uh-**TIGH**-tis) Inflammation of the pancreas. (Ch. 22)

Pancytopenia: (PAN-sigh-toh-**PEE**-nee-ah) Abnormal depression of all the cellular elements of the blood. (Ch. 24)

Panhysterectomy: (PAN-hiss-tuh-**RECK**-tuh-mee) Excision of the entire uterus, including the cervix uteri. (Ch. 40)

Panmyelosis: (PAN-my-e-**LOH**-sis) Increased level of all bone marrow components, red blood cells, white blood cells, and platelets. (Ch. 24)

Paradoxical respirations: (PAR-uh-**DOK**-si-kuhl RES-pi-**RAY**-shuns) Chest movement on respiration that is opposite to that expected. (Ch. 28)

Paranoia: (PAR-uh-**NOY**-uh) Behavior that is marked by delusions of persecution or delusional jealousy. (Ch. 55)

Paraparesis: (PAR-ah-pah-**RE**-sis) Partial paralysis of the lower extremities. (Ch. 46)

Paraphimosis: (PAR-uh-figh-**MOH**-sis) Uncircumcised foreskin that has swollen and stuck behind the head of the penis. (Ch. 41)

Paraplegia: (PAR-ah-**PLEE**-jah) Paralysis of the lower body, including both legs, resulting from a spinal cord lesion. (Ch. 46)

Paresis: (puh-**REE**-sis) Weakness; incomplete paralysis. (Ch. 45)

Paresthesia: (PAR-es-**THEE**-zee-ah) A heightened sensation, such as burning, prickling, or tingling. (Ch. 22, 45, 46)

Partial-thickness burn: (**PAR**-shul **THICK**-ness BERN) Burn in which the epithelializing elements remain intact. (Ch. 54)

Passive immunity: (**PASS**-iv im-**YOO**-ni-tee) Reinforcement of the immune system with immune serum for such conditions as tetanus, diptheria, and venomous snake bite. (Ch. 7, 52)

Paternalism: (puh-**TER**-nuhl-izm) A unilateral and sometimes unreasonable decision by health care providers that implies they know what is best, regardless of the client's wishes. (Ch. 1)

Pathogen: (**PATH**-o-jen) A microorganism or substance capable of producing a disease. (Ch. 7)

Pathological fracture: (PATH-uh-**LAH**-jik-uhl **FRAHK**-chur) Fracture resulting from weakening of the bone structure by pathological processes such as neoplasia or osteomalacia. (Ch. 24, 25)

Patient-controlled analgesia (PCA): (**PAY**-shent kon-**TROHLD** an-uhl-**JEE**-zee-ah) An apparatus that delivers an intravenous analgesic to relieve pain, which is controlled by the client. (Ch. 9)

Pedicle: (**PED**-i-kuhl) The stem that attaches a new growth. (Ch. 40)

Pediculosis: (pe-DIK-yoo-**LOH**-sis) Infestation with lice. (Ch. 51)

Pemphigus: (**PEM**-fi-gus) Acute or chronic serious skin disease characterized by the appearance of bullae (blisters) of various sizes on normal skin and mucous membranes. (Ch. 51)

Peptic ulcer disease: (**PEP**-tick **UL**-sir di-**ZEEZ**) A condition in which the lining of the esophagus, stomach, or duodenum is eroded. (Ch. 30)

Perception: (per-**SEP**-shun) A unique impression of events by an individual. These impressions are strongly influenced by personality, cultural orientation, attitudes, and life experiences. (Ch. 13)

Percussion: (per-**KUSH**-un) A tapping technique used by physicians and advanced practice nurses to determine the consistency of underlying tissues. (Ch. 2)

Percutaneous: (PER-kyoo-**TAY**-nee-us) Through the skin; may refer to an injection, a medication application, or a biopsy. (Ch. 34)

Perfusion: (per-**FEW**-zhun) Supplying an organ or tissue with blood. (Ch. 8)

Pericardial effusion: (PER-ee-**KAR**-dee-uhl ee-**FYOO**-zhun) A buildup of fluid in the pericardial space. (Ch. 17)

Pericardial friction rub: (PER-ee-**KAR**-dee-uhl **FRICK**-shun RUB) Friction sound heard over the fourth left intercostal space near the sternum; a classic sign of pericarditis. (Ch. 15, 17)

Pericardial tamponade: (PER-ee-**KAR**-dee-uhl TAM-pon-**AYD**) Compression of the heart by an abnormal filling of the pericardial sac with blood. (Ch. 8)

Pericardiectomy: (PER-ee-kar-dee-**ECK**-tuh-mee) Excision of part or all of the pericardium. (Ch. 17)

Pericardiocentesis: (PER-ee-**KAR**-dee-oh-sen-**TEE**-sis) Surgical perforation of the pericardium. (Ch. 17, 22)

Pericardiotomy: (PER-ee-KAR-dee-**AH**-tah-mee) Incision of the pericardium. (Ch. 22)

Pericarditis: (PER-ee-kar-**DYE**-tis) Inflammation of the pericardium. (Ch. 17, 22)

Perichondritis: (PER-ee-kon-**DRY**-tis) Inflammation of the perichondrium. (Ch. 49)

Perimenopausal: (PER-ee-MEN-oh-**PAWS**-uhl) The phase before the onset of menopause, during which the woman with regular menses changes, perhaps abruptly, to a pattern of irregular cycles and increased periods of amenorrhea. (Ch. 40)

Perinatal: (PAIR-ee-**NAY**-tuhl) Concerning the period beginning after the 28th week of pregnancy and ending 28 days after birth. (Ch. 42)

Perioperative: (PER-ee-**AHP**-er-uh-tiv) Occurring in the period immediately before, during, and after surgery. (Ch. 11)

Peripheral arterial disease: (puh-**RIFF**-uh-ruhl ar-**TIR**-ee-uhl di-**ZEEZ**) Disease of the peripheral arteries that interferes with adequate flow of blood. (Ch. 18)

Peripheral parenteral nutrition: (puh-**RIFF**-uh-ruhl par-**EN**-te-ruhl new-**TRISH**-un) Nutrition by intravenous injection. (Ch. 29)

Peripheral vascular resistance: (puh-**RIFF**-uh-ruhl **VAS**-kyoo-lar ree-**ZIS**-tense) Opposition to blood flow through the vessels. (Ch. 16, 21)

Peristomal: (PER-i-**STOH**-muhl) Area around a stoma. (Ch. 31)

Peritoneal dialysis: (PER-i-toh-**NEE**-uhl dye-**AL**-i-sis) The employment of the peritoneum surrounding the abdominal cavity as a dialyzing membrane for the purpose of removing waste products or toxins accumulated as a result of renal failure. (Ch. 35)

Peritonitis: (per-i-toh-**NIGH**-tis) Inflammation of the peritoneum. (Ch. 31)

Persistent vegetative state: (per-**SISS**-tent **VEJ**-uh-tay-tiv STAYT) A person showing no evidence of cortical functioning but having the sustained capacity for spontaneous breathing and heartbeat. (Ch. 46)

Petechiae: (pe-**TEE**-kee-ee, puh-**TEE**-kee-eye) Small, purplish, hemorrhagic spots on the skin that appear in certain illnesses and bleeding disorders. (Ch. 17, 23, 24, 40, 50)

Peyronie's disease: (pay-roh-**NEZ**) Hardening of the corpora cavernosa of the penis, causing distortion and curvature of the penis. (Ch. 41)

Phagocytes: (**FAY**-go-sites). Cells that have the ability to ingest and destroy particulate substances such as bacteria, protozoa, and cell debris. (Ch. 7)

Phagocytosis: (fay-go-sigh-**TOH**-sis) Ingestion and digestion of bacteria and particles by phagocytes. (Ch. 7)

Pheochromocytoma: (**FEE**-oh-KROH-moh-sigh-**TOH**-mah) Rare tumor of the adrenal system that secretes catecholamines. (Ch. 37)

Phimosis: (figh-**MOH**-sis) Uncircumcised foreskin that cannot be moved down from the head of the penis. (Ch. 41)

Phlebotomy: (fle-**BAH**-tuh-mee) Entry into a vein for the removal or withdrawal of blood. (Ch. 24)

Phobia: (**FOH**-bee-ah) A persistent, irrational, intense fear of a specific object, activity, or situation. (Ch. 55)

Photophobia: (FOH-toh-**FOH**-bee-ah) Abnormal visual intolerance to light. (Ch. 46, 49)

Photorefractive keratoectomy: (FOH-toh-ree-**FRAK**-tiv KER-ah-toh-**EK**-tuh-mee) Use of a laser to reshape the cornea to correct refractive errors of light rays entering the eye. (Ch. 49)

Phthirus pubis: (**THIR**-us **PEW**-biss) Crab lice. Infects primarily the pubic region but may also be found in armpits, beard, eyebrows, and eyelashes. (Ch. 49)

Physical dependence: (**FIZ**-ik-uhl dee-**PEN**-dens) A pharmacologic phenomenon characterized by signs and symptoms of withdrawal when medication is withdrawn. (Ch. 9)

Plaque: (PLAK) A deposit of fatty material on the lining of an artery. (Ch. 16, 18)

Plasmapharesis: (PLAS-mah-fer-**EE**-sis) Removal of blood to separate cells from plasma. (Ch. 47)

Pleurodesis: (PLOO-roh-**DEE**-sis) Creation of adhesions between the parietal and visceral pleura to treat recurrent pneumothorax. (Ch. 28)

***Pneumocystis carinii* pneumonia:** (new-mo-**SIS**-tis ca-**RIN**-ee-eye new-**MOH**-nee-ya) An acute pneumonia caused by *Pneumosyctis carinii,* a fungus. It occurs in immunodeficient adults and is a defining opportunistic infection of AIDS. (Ch. 53)

Pneumonectomy: (NEW-moh-**NEK**-tuh-mee) Surgical removal of all or part of a lung. (Ch. 28)

Pneumothorax: (NEW-moh-**THAW**-raks) Air in the pleural space. (Ch. 28)

Poikilothermy: (POY-ki-loh-**THER**-mee) The absence of sufficient arterial blood flow, causing the extremity to become the temperature of the environment. (Ch. 15, 18)

Point of maximal impulse: (POYNT of **MAKS**-i-muhl **IM**-puls) The area of the chest where the greatest force can be felt with the palm of the hand when the heart contracts or beats. Usually at the fourth to fifth intercostal space in the midclavicular line. (Ch. 15)

Polycythemia: (PAH-lee-sigh-**THEE**-mee-ah) Excessive red cells in the blood. (Ch. 18, 24, 28)

Polydipsia: (PAH-lee-**DIP**-see-ah) Excessive thirst. (Ch. 37)

Polymenorrhea: (PAH-lee-MEN-uh-**REE**-uh) Menstrual periods occurring with abnormal frequency. (Ch. 40)

Polymyositis: (PAH-lee-my-oh-**SIGH**-tis) A rare, inflammatory disease of the skeletal muscle tissue characterized by symmetric weakness of proximal muscles of the limbs, neck, and pharynx. (Ch. 44)

Polyneuropathy: (PAH-lee-new-**RAH**-puh-thee) A disease involving multiple nerves. (Ch. 47)

Polyphagia: (PAH-lee-**FAY**-jee-ah) Excessive eating. (Ch. 38)

Polyuria: (PAH-lee-**YOOR**-ee-ah) Excessive urination. (Ch. 35, 37)

Portal hypertension: (**POR**-tuhl HIGH-per-**TEN**-shun) Persistent blood pressure elevation in the portal circulation of the abdomen. (Ch. 33)

Postcoital: (post-**KOH**-i-tal) Following sexual intercourse. (Ch. 40)

Postictal: (pohst-**IK**-tuhl) Occurring after a sudden attack, such as an epileptic seizure. (Ch. 46)

Postoperative: (post-**AHP**-er-uh-tiv) Following a surgical operation. (Ch. 11)

Postrenal failure: (post-**REE**-nuhl **FAYL**-yur) Inability of the kidney to maintain normal function resulting from the obstruction of urine flow out of the kidneys. (Ch. 35)

Preload: (**PREE**-lohd) End-diastolic stretch of cardiac muscle fibers; equals end-diastolic volume. (Ch. 15, 21)

Preoperative: (pre-**AHP**-er-uh-tiv) Preceding an operation. (Ch. 11)

Prerenal failure: (**PREE**-**REE**-nuhl **FAYL**-yur) Inability of the kidney to maintain normal function resulting from poor systemic perfusion and decreased renal blood flow. (Ch. 35)

Presbycusis: (PRESS-bee-**KYOO**-sis) Progressive, bilaterally symmetrical perceptive hearing loss occurring with age; usually occurs after age 50 and is caused by structural changes in the organs of hearing. (Ch. 49)

Presbyopia: (PREZ-bee-**OH**-pee-ah) Diminution of accommodation of the lens of the eye occurring normally with aging, and usually resulting in hyperopia, or farsightedness. (Ch. 49)

Pressure ulcer: (**PRESS**-sure **ULL**-sir) An open sore or lesion of the skin that develops because of prolonged pressure against an area. (Ch. 13)

Priapism: (**PRY**-uh-pizm) Erection that lasts too long. (Ch. 41)

Primary care: (**PRY**-mer-ee KAIR) A type of health care that includes health promotion, preventive care and continuing care for common health problems, and health teaching. It may also include a family focus. (Ch. 4)

Primary hypertension: (**PRY**-mer-ee HIGH-per-**TEN**-shun) Abnormally elevated blood pressure of unknown cause. Also called essential hypertension. (Ch. 16)

Primary open-angle glaucoma: (**PRY**-mer-ee **OH**-pen **ANG**-guhl glaw-**KOH**-mah) Most common type of glaucoma. Optic disc cup is enlarged. Affects both eyes. Intraocular pressure may be normal. (Ch. 49)

Proctitis: (prock-**TIGH**-tis) Inflammation of the rectum and anus. (Ch. 42)

Proctosigmoidoscopy: (PROK-toh-SIG-moy-**DAHS**-kuh-pee) Visual examination of the rectum and sigmoid colon by use of a sigmoidoscope. (Ch. 29)

Prodrome: (**PROH**-drohm) A symptom indicating the onset of a disease. (Ch. 46)

Promotion: (proh-**MOH**-shun) Encouragement, such as when a carcinogen encourages development of a tumor. (Ch. 10)

Prostaglandins: (PRAHS-tah-**GLAND**-ins) Chemical neurotransmitters usually associated with pain at the site of an injury, periphery. (Ch. 9)

Prostatectomy: (PRAHS-tuh-**TEK**-tuh-mee) Removal of the prostate gland. (Ch. 41)

Prostatitis: (PRAHS-tuh-**TIGH**-tis) Inflammation or infection of the prostate gland. (Ch. 41)

Protozoa: (pro-tow-**ZOH**-ah) Single-celled parasitic organisms that can move and live mainly in the soil. (Ch. 7)

Pruritis: (proo-**RYE**-tis) Severe itching. (Ch. 51)

Pseudoaddiction: (soo-doh-ad-**DICK**-shun) Syndrome in which behaviors similar to addiction appear as a result of inadequate pain control and clients fear not receiving adequate pain medications. (Ch. 9)

Psoriasis: (suh-**RYE**-ah-sis) Chronic inflammatory skin disorder in which epidermal cells proliferate abnormally fast. (Ch. 51)

Psychoanalysis: (SIGH-koh-uh-**NAL**-i-sis) Form of therapy based on the theories of Sigmund Freud, regarding the dynamics of the unconscious. (Ch. 55)

Psychogenic: (SIGH-koh-**JEN**-ick) Of mental origin. (Ch. 37)

Psychological dependence: (SY-ko-**LOJ**-ick-al dee-**PEN**-dens) Obsession of obtaining drugs for use other than medicinal; addiction. (Ch. 9)

Psychopharmacology: (SIGH-koh-FAR-meh-**KAHL**-uh-jee) The study of the action of drugs on psychological functions and mental states. (Ch. 55)

Psychosomatic: (SIGH-koh-soh-**MAT**-ik) Having bodily symptoms of psychological, emotional, or mental origin; illness traceable to an emotional cause. (Ch. 55)

Ptosis: (**TOH**-sis) Drooping of eyelid. (Ch. 47, 48)

Puerperal: (pyoo-**ER**-per-uhl) Concerning the puerperium, or period of 42 days after childbirth. (Ch. 42)

Pulse deficit: (PULS **DEF**-i-sit) A condition in which the number of pulse beats counted at the radial artery is less than those counted in the same period of time at the apical heart rate. (Ch. 15)

Purpura: (**PUR**-pur-uh) Hemorrhage into the skin, mucous membranes, internal organs, and other tissues. (Ch. 23)

Purulent: (**PURE**-u-lent) Fluid that contains pus. (Ch. 11, 51)

Pyelogram: (**PIE**-loh-**GRAM**) A diagnostic procedure involving x-ray of the kidneys; may be done after injection of a dye into the bloodstream or directly into the kidneys. (Ch. 34)

Pyelonephritis: (**PYE**-e-loh-ne-**FRY**-tis) Inflammation of the kidney and renal pelvis. (Ch. 35)

Pyoderma: (**PYE**-oh-**DER**-mah) Any acute, inflammatory, purulent bacterial dermatitis. (Ch. 51)

Quadriparesis: (kwod-ri-par-**E**-sis) Weakness involving all four limbs caused by spinal cord injury. (Ch. 46)

Quadriplegia: (**KWA**-dri-**PLEE**-jah) Paralysis of all four limbs caused by spinal cord injury. (Ch. 46)

Radiation therapy: (RAY-dee-**AY**-shun **THER**-uh-pee) Cancer treatment with ionizing radiation. (Ch. 10)

Radiculopathy: (ra-DIK-yoo-**LAH**-puh-thee) Disease of the nerve roots. (Ch. 45)

Range of motion (ROM): (RANJE of **MOH**-shun) The range of movement of a body joint. (Ch. 13)

Raynaud's disease: (ra-**NOHZ** di-**ZEEZ**) A primary or idiopathic vasospastic disorder characterized by bilateral and symmetrical pallor and cyanosis of the fingers. (Ch. 18)

Reality orientation: (ree-**AL**-i-tee OR-ee-en-**TAY**-shun) A process to orient a person to facts such as names, dates, and time, through the use of verbal and nonverbal repeating messages. (Ch. 13)

Rectocele: (**RECK**-toh-seel) Protrusion or herniation of the posterior vaginal wall with the anterior wall of the rectum through the vagina. (Ch. 40)

Reflux: (**REE**-fluks) Backward flow; may refer to backflow of blood through a cardiac valve or backflow of urine from the bladder toward the kidneys. (Ch. 41)

Regurgitation: (ree-GUR-ji-**TAY**-shun) A backward flowing, as in the backflow of blood through a defective heart valve. (Ch. 19)

Remission: (ree-**MISH**-uhn) Diminution or abatement of the symptoms of disease. (Ch. 10)

Remyelination: (ree-MY-uh-lin-**AY**-shun) Replacement of myelin or neurons. (Ch. 47)

Replantation: (re-plan-**TAY**-shun) The replacement of an organ or other structure, such as a digit, limb, or tooth, to the site from which it was previously lost or removed. (Ch. 44)

Respiratory excursion: (**RES**-pi-rah-TOR-ee eks-**KUR**-zhun) Downward movement of diaphragm with inspiration. (Ch. 26)

Respondeat superior: (ress-**POND**-ee-et sue-**PEER**-ee-or) An institution that employs a worker may be liable for the acts or omissions of its employees. (Ch. 1)

Retinal detachment: (**RET**-i-nuhl de-**TACH**-ment) Complete or partial separation of the retina from the choroid, the middle coat of the eyeball. (Ch. 49)

Retinopathy: (ret-i-**NAH**-puh-thee) Disease of the retina of the eye. (Ch. 49)

Retroflexion: (RET-roh-**FLECK**-shun) A bending or flexing backward. (Ch. 40)

Retrograde: (**RET**-roh-grayd) Moving backward; degenerating from a better to a worse state. (Ch. 40, 41)

Retrograde cholangiopancreatography: (**RET**-roh-grayd koh-LAN-jee-oh-PAN-kree-ah-**TOG**-rah-fee) An endoscopic procedure that permits the physician to visualize the liver, gallbladder, and pancreas using an endoscope, dye, and x-rays. (Ch. 32)

Retroversion: (RET-roh-**VER**-zhun) A turning, or a state of being turned back; the tipping of an entire organ. (Ch. 40)

Rheumatic fever: (roo-**MAT**-ick **FEE**-ver) A hypersensitivity reaction to antigens of group A beta-hemolytic streptococci. (Ch. 17)

Rheumatic heart disease: (roo-**MAT**-ick HART di-**ZEEZ**) Severe damage to the heart from complications of rheumatic fever. (Ch. 17)

Rhinitis: (rye-**NIGH**-tis) Inflammation of the nasal mucosa, usually associated with congestion, itching, sneezing, and nasal discharge. (Ch. 27)

Rhinoplasty: (**RYE**-noh-plass-tee) Plastic surgery of the nose. (Ch. 27)

Rickettsia: (ra-**KET**-see-ah) A genus of bacteria of the tribe *Rickettsiae* that multiply only in host cells. (Ch. 7)

Rinne test: (**RIN**-nee TEST) A test of hearing made with tuning forks. (Ch. 48)

Romberg's test: (**RAHM**-bergs TEST) A test to determine if a person has the ability to maintain body balance when the eyes are shut and the feet are close together. (Ch. 48)

Rule of nines: (ROOL of NINES) A formula for estimating percentage of body surface areas, particularly helpful in judging the portion of skin that has been burned. (Ch. 54)

Sacral radiculopathy: (**SAY**-krul ra-DICK-yoo-**LAH**-puh-thee) Pathology of sacral nerve roots. (Ch. 42)

Salpingitis: (SAL-pin-**JIGH**-tis) Inflammation of a fallopian tube. (Ch. 42, 43)

Scleroderma: (SKLER-ah-**DER**-ma) A chronic manifestation of progressive systemic sclerosis in which the skin is taut, firm, and edematous, limiting movement. (Ch. 44)

Sclerosis: (skle-**ROH**-sis) A hardening or induration of an organ or tissue, especially from excessive growth of fibrous tissue. (Ch. 47)

Seborrhea: (SEB-oh-**REE**-ah) Disease of the sebaceous glands marked by increase in the amount and often alteration of the quality of sebaceous secretions. (Ch. 51)

Secondary hypertension: (**SEK**-un-DAR-ee HIGH-per-**TEN**-shun) High blood pressure that is a symptom of a specific cause, such as a kidney abnormality. (Ch. 16)

Semipermeable: (SEM-ee-**PER**-mee-uh-buhl) Partly permeable; said of a membrane that will allow fluids but not the dissolved substance to pass through it. (Ch. 5)

Sensorineural hearing loss: (SEN-suh-ree-**NEW**-ruhl HEER-ing LOSS) Hearing loss caused by impairment of a sensory nerve. (Ch. 49)

Sensory deprivation: (SEN-suh-ree DEP-ri-**VAY**-shun) No or minimal stimulation of the senses that creates the potential for maladaptive coping. (Ch. 13)

Sensory overload: (SEN-suh-ree OH-ver-lohd) Excessive stimulation of the senses that creates the potential for maladaptive coping. (Ch. 13)

Sepsis: (SEP-sis) Systematic infection caused by microorganisms in the bloodstream. (Ch. 7, 8)

Septa: (SEP-tuh) Wall dividing two cavities. (Ch. 15, 40)

Serologic: (SEAR-uh-**LAJ**-ick) Study of substances present in blood serum. (Ch. 42)

Serosanguineous: (SEER-oh-**SANG**-gwin-ee-us) Fluid consisting of serum and blood. (Ch. 11, 51)

Serotonin: (SER-ah-**TOH**-nin) A chemical neurotransmitter important in sleep-wake cycles. Reduced serotonin levels are associated with depression. (Ch. 9)

Shock: (SHAHK) A clinical syndrome in which the peripheral blood flow is inadequate to return sufficient blood to the heart for normal function, particularly transport of oxygen to all organs and tissues. (Ch. 54)

Sinoatrial node: (SIGH-noh-**AY**-tree-al NOHD) Node at the junction of the superior vena cava and right atrium, regarded as the starting point of the heartbeat. (Ch. 20)

Snellen's chart: (SNEL-ens CHART) A chart imprinted with lines of black letters graduating in size from smallest on the bottom to largest on top; used for testing visual acuity. (Ch. 48)

Somatoform: (soh-**MAT**-uh-form) Denoting psychogenic symptoms resembling those of physical disease; psychosomatic. (Ch. 55)

Spider angioma: (SPY-der an-jee-**OH**-mah) Thin reddish-purple vein lines close to the skin surface. (Ch. 32)

Splenectomy: (sple-**NEK**-tuh-mee) Excision of the spleen. (Ch. 25)

Splenomegaly: (SPLEE-noh-**MEG**-ah-lee) Enlargement of the spleen. (Ch. 25)

Standard of best interest: (**STAND**-erd of BEST **IN**-ter-est) A type of decision made about clients' health care when they are unable to make an informed decision about their own care. (Ch. 1)

Standard Precautions: (**STAN**-derd pre-**KAW**-shuns) Guidelines recommended by the Centers for Disease Control and Prevention to reduce the risk of the spread of infection. (Ch. 7)

Stapedectomy: (stuh-puh-**DEK**-tuh-mee) Excision of the stapes in order to improve hearing, especially in cases of otosclerosis. (Ch. 49)

Staphylococcus: (STAFF-il-oh-**KOCK**-uss) A genus of gram-positive bacteria; they are constantly present on the skin and in the upper respiratory tract and are the most common cause of localized suppurating infections. (Ch. 7)

Status asthmaticus: (**STAT**-us az-**MAT**-i-kus) Prolonged period of unrelieved asthma symptoms. (Ch. 28)

Steatorrhea: (STEE-ah-toh-**REE**-ah) Fat in the stools; may be associated with pancreatic disease. (Ch. 29, 30, 31, 33)

Stenosis: (ste-**NOH**-sis) The constriction or narrowing of a passage or orifice, such as a cardiac valve. (Ch. 18, 19)

Stent: (STENT) Any mold or device used to hold tissue in place or to provide a support, graft, or anastomosis while healing is taking place. (Ch. 35)

Stereotype: (**STER**-ee-oh-TIGHP) An opinion or belief about an individual or group that may not be true. (Ch. 3)

Sternotomy: (stir-**NAH**-tuh-mee) The operation of cutting through the sternum. (Ch. 22)

Stoma: (**STOH**-mah) A mouth, small opening, or pore. (Ch. 31)

Stomatitis: (STOH-mah-**TIGH**-tis) Inflammation of the mouth. (Ch. 10, 30)

Streptococcus: (STREP-toh-**KOCK**-uss) A bacterial organism of the genus *Streptococcus*. (Ch. 7)

Stress: (STRESS) The physical (gravity, mechanical, pathogenic, injury) and psychological (fear, anxiety, crisis, joy) forces that are experienced by individuals. (Ch. 55)

Stressor: (**STRESS**-er) Any person or situation that produces an anxiety response. (Ch. 55)

Striae: (**STRIGH**-ee) A line or band of elevated or depressed tissue; may differ in color or texture from surrounding tissue. (Ch.32)

Sty: (STY) A localized circumscribed inflammatory swelling of one or more of the sebaceous glands of the eyelid. (Ch. 49)

Subarachnoid: (SUB-uh-**RAK**-noyd) Below or under the arachnoid membrane and the pia mater of the covering of the brain and spinal cord. (Ch. 45)

Subdural: (sub-**DUHR**-uhl) Beneath the dura mater. (Ch. 46)

Suffering: (**SUFF**-er-ing) A state of severe distress associated with events that threaten the intactness of the person. Emotional pain associated with real or potential tissue damage. (Ch. 9)

Summons: (**SUM**-muns) A notice of suit. (Ch. 1)

Suprapubic: (SOO-pruh-**PEW**-bik) Bone of the groin (or region) located above the pubic arch. (Ch. 41)

Surgeon: (**SURGE**-on) A medical practitioner who specializes in surgery. (Ch. 11)

Swimmer's ear: (**SWIM**-mers EAR) A type of external otitis seen in persons who swim for a considerable amount of time or fail to completely dry their ear canals after swimming. (Ch. 49)

Sympathectomy: (sim-pa-**THEK**-to-me) Excision of a portion of the sympathetic division of the autonomic nervous system. (Ch. 18)

Synovitis: (sin-oh-**VIGH**-tis) Inflammation of the synovial membrane that may be the result of an aseptic wound, a subcutaneous injury, irritation, or exposure to cold and dampness. (Ch. 43, 44)

Systolic blood pressure: (sis-**TAH**-lik BLUHD **PRESS**-ur) Maximal pressure exerted on the arteries during contraction of the left ventricle of the heart. The top number of a blood pressure reading. (Ch. 16)

Tachycardia: (TAK-ee-**KAR**-dee-yah) An abnormal rapidity of heart action, usually defined as a heart rate greater than 100 beats per minute in adults. (Ch. 8)

Tachydysrhythmia: (TACK-ee-dis-**RITH**-mee-yah) An abnormal heart rhythm with rate greater than 100 beats per minute in an adult. (Ch. 22)

Tachypnea: (TAK-ip-**NEE**-ah) Abnormally rapid respiratory rate. (Ch. 8, 28)

Tamponade: (TAM-pon-**AYD**) Compression of a part. (Ch. 41)

Tension pneumothorax: (**TEN**-shun NEW-moh-**THAW**-raks) Abnormal accumulation of air with buildup of pressure in the pleural space. (Ch. 8)

Teratoma: (ter-uh-**TOH**-muh) A congenital tumor containing one or more of the three primary embryonic germ layers. (Ch. 40)

Tetanus: (**TET**-uh-nus) A highly fatal disease caused by the bacillus *Clostridium tetani* and characterized by muscle spasm and convulsions. (Ch. 54)

Tetany: (**TET**-uh-nee) Muscle spasms, numbness, and tingling caused by changes in pH and low serum calcium. (Ch. 37)

Thoracentesis: (THOR-uh-sen-**TEE**-sis) Insertion of a large-bore needle into the pleural space to remove fluid. (Ch. 26)

Thoracotomy: (THAW-rah-**KAH**-tah-mee) Surgical incision into the chest wall. (Ch. 28)

Thrill: (THRILL) Abnormal vessel that has a bulging or narrowed wall; a vibration is felt. (Ch. 15)

Thrombi: (**THROM**-bye) Blood clots. (Ch. 8)

Thromboangitis obliterans: (THROM-boh-an-je-**EYE**-tis uh-**BLI**-ter-ans) Chronic inflammatory vascular occlusive disease mainly of peripheral extremity vessels; commonly in men who smoke cigarettes, Buerger's disease. (Ch. 18)

Thrombocytopenia: (THROM-boh-SIGH-toh-**PEE**-nee-uh) Abnormal decrease in the number of blood platelets. (Ch. 10, 23, 24)

Thrombolytic: (throm-bo-**LIT**-ik) Agent that dissolves or splits up a thrombus, an aggregation of blood factors. (Ch. 46)

Thrombophlebitis: (THROM-boh-fle-**BYE**-tis) The formation of a clot and inflammation within a vein. (Ch. 17, 40)

Thrombosis: (throm-**BOH**-sis) Formation, development, or presence of a thrombus, an aggregation of blood factors. (Ch. 18)

Tidaling: (**TIGH**-dah-ling) Rise and fall; may refer to water in water-seal chamber of a chest drainage system. (Ch. 26)

Titration: (tigh-**TRAY**-shun) Adjustment of medication up or down to meet client needs. (Ch. 9)

Tolerance: (**TALL**-er-ens) The response of the body to medication that requires increased medication administration to achieve the same effect. Often refers to opioids. (Ch. 9, 55)

Tonometer: (tuh-**NAHM**-uh-tur) An instrument for measuring tension or pressure, especially intraocular pressure. (Ch. 48)

Tophi: (**TOH**-fye) A chalky deposit of sodium urate occurring in gout and most often forming around the joints in cartilage, bone, and bursae. (Ch. 48)

Torts: (TORTS) Lawsuits involving civil wrongs. (Ch. 1)

Tortuous: (**TOR**-choo-us). Twisted and enlarged veins. (Ch. 18)

Toxemia: (tock-**SEE**-me-ah) Spread of poisonous products of bacteria throughout the body. (Ch. 8)

Tracheostomy: (TRAY-key-**AHS**-tuh-me) A surgical opening in the neck into the trachea to provide an airway when the trachea is obstructed. (Ch. 26)

Tracheotomy: (TRAY-key-**AH**-tuh-me) An opening in the neck into the trachea. (Ch. 26)

Trachoma: (truh-**KOH**-mah) Chronic contagious form of conjuctivitis caused by *Chlamydia trachomatis;* may cause blindness. (Ch. 49)

Traditional: (tra-**DISH**-un-al) Relating to practices and customs handed down through the generations, often by word of mouth. (Ch. 3)

Transcellular: (trans-**SELL**-yoo-lar) Across cell membranes. (Ch. 5)

Transdermal: (trans-**DER**-mal) Entering through the dermis, or skin, as in administration of a drug applied to the skin in ointment or patch form. (Ch. 9)

Transillumination: (TRANS-i-loo-mi-**NAY**-shun) The passage of strong light through a body structure to permit inspection of an observer on the opposite side. (Ch. 39)

Transjugular intrahepatic portosystemic shunt (TIPS): (trans-**JUG**-yoo-lar intra-hep-**PAT**-ik POR-toh-sis-**TEM**-ik SHUNT) Shunt that sidetracks venous blood around the liver to the vena cava for treatment of ascites. (Ch. 33)

Transmural myocardial infarction: (trans-**MYOOR**-uhl MY-oh-**KAR**-dee-uhl in-**FARK**-shun) Death of tissue through the full thickness of the heart wall caused by sudden blockage of a coronary artery. (Ch. 8)

Trauma: (**TRAW**-mah) Physical injury caused by an external force. (Ch. 8)

Trendelenburg: (tren-**DELL**-en-berg) A position in which the client's head is low and the body and legs are on an elevated and inclined plane. (Ch. 8)

Trigeminy: (try-**JEM**-i-nee) Occurring every third beat, as in trigeminal premature ventricular contractions. (Ch. 20)

Tropia: (**TROH**-pee-ah) A manifest deviation of an eye from the normal position when both eyes are open and uncovered. (Ch. 48)

T-tube: (**TEE**-toob) A T-shaped tube in the bile duct that allows drainage of bile following gallbladder surgery. (Ch. 33)

Tumor: (**TOO**-mur) An abnormal growth of cells or tissues; tumors may be benign or malignant. (Ch. 10)

Turbid: (**TER**-bid) Cloudy. (Ch. 46)

Turgor: (**TER**-ger) The resistance of the skin to being grasped between the fingers. Dehydration causes poor skin turgor. (Ch. 50)

Tympanosclerosis: (tim-PAN-oh-skle-**ROH**-sis) A condition characterized by the presence of masses of hard, dense connective tissue around the auditory ossicle in the middle ear. (Ch. 49)

Unifocal: (YOO-ni-**FOH**-kuhl) Coming or originating from one site or focus. (Ch. 20)

Upper gastrointestinal series (upper GI, UGI): (**UH**-per GAS-troh-in-**TES**-ti-nuhl **SEER**-ees) X-ray and fluoroscopic examinations of the stomach and duodenum after the ingestion of a contrast medium. (Ch. 29)

Uremia: (yoo-**REE**-mee-ah) An excess in the blood of urea, creatinine, and other nitrogenous end products of protein and amino acid metabolism. (Ch. 34, 35)

Urethritis: (YOO-ree-**THRIGH**-tis) Inflammation of the urethra. (Ch. 35, 42)

Urethroplasty: (yoo-REE-throh-**PLAS**-tee) Plastic repair of the urethra. (Ch. 35)

Urinary incontinence: (**YOOR**-i-NAR-ee in-**KON**-ti-nents) Inability to control urine excretion creating accidental urinary leakage. (Ch. 13)

Urodynamic: (YOO-roh-dye-**NAM**-ik) The study of the holding or storage of urine in the bladder, the facility with which it empties, and the rate of movement of urine out of the bladder during urination. (Ch. 41)

Urosepsis: (YOO-roh-**SEP**-sis) Septicemia resulting from urinary tract infection. (Ch. 35, 41)

Urticaria: (UR-ti-**KAIR**-ee-ah) Hives signifying an allergic reaction. (Ch. 8, 53)

Vaginosis: (VAJ-i-**NOH**-sis) Inflammation of the vagina caused by *Gardnerella vaginalis*. (Ch. 40)

Values: (**VAL**-use) Ideals or concepts that give meaning to an individual's life. (Ch. 1, 3)

Valvuloplasty: (**VAL**-vyoo-loh-PLAS-tee) Plastic or restorative surgery on a valve, especially a cardiac valve. (Ch. 19)

Varices: (**VAR**-i-seez) Dilated veins. (Ch. 33)

Varicocele: (**VAR**-i-koh-seel) Varicose veins of the scrotum; can lead to infertility. (Ch. 39, 41)

Varicose veins: (**VAR**-i-kohs VAINS) Swollen, distended, and knotted veins, usually in the subcutaneous tissue of the leg. (Ch. 18)

Varicosities: (**VAR**-i-kos-i-tez) Varicose veins; varicose condition. (Ch. 18)

Vasculitis: (VAS-kue-**LIGH**-tis) Inflammation of a vessel. (Ch. 44)

Vasectomy: (va-**SEK**-tuh-mee) Surgically cutting and sealing the vas deferens to prevent sperm from getting outside the body. Used as a birth control method for men. (Ch. 41)

Vasovagal reflex: (VAY-zoh-**VAY**-gull **REE**-fleks) Reflex stimulation of vagus nerve resulting in slowed heart rate and decreased cardiac output. (Ch. 40)

Venipuncture: (**VEE**-nuh-PUNK-shur) Puncture of a vein for the purpose of drawing blood or instilling fluid or medication into the bloodstream. (Ch. 6)

Venous stasis ulcers: (**VEE**-nus **STAY**-sis **UL**-sers) Poorly healing ulcers that result from inadequate venous drainage. (Ch. 18)

Ventricular diastole: (ven-**TRICK**-yoo-lar dye-AS-tuh-lee) The period of relaxation of the two ventricles. (Ch. 20)

Ventricular escape rhythm: (ven-**TRICK**-yoo-lar es-**KAYP RITH**-uhm) The naturally occurring rhythm of the ventricles when the rest of the cardiac conduction system fails. (Ch. 20)

Ventricular repolarization: (ven-**TRICK**-yoo-lar RE-pol-lahr-i-**ZAY**-shun) Reestablishment of the polarized state of the muscle after contraction. (Ch. 20)

Ventricular systole: (ven-**TRICK**-yoo-lar **SIS**-tuh-lee) The contraction of the two ventricles. (Ch. 20)

Ventricular tachycardia: (ven-**TRICK**-yoo-lar TACK-ee-**KAR**-dee-yah) A series of at least three beats arising from a ventricular focus at a rate greater than 100 beats per minute. (Ch. 20)

Veracity: (vuh-**RAS**-i-tee) The principle of "truthfulness." (Ch. 1)

Verrucous: (ve-**ROO**-kus) Wartlike, with raised portions. (Ch. 42)

Vertebrae: (**VER**-te-bray) Any of the 33 bony segments of the spinal column: 7 cervical, 12 thoracic, 5 lumbar, 5 sacral, and 4 coccygeal vertebrae. (Ch. 43)

Vesicant: (**VESS**-i-kant) Agent that causes blistering of tissue. (Ch. 10)

Vesicular: (ve-**SICK**-yoo-ler) Pertaining to vesicles or small blisters. (Ch. 42)

Virus: (**VI**-russ) The smallest organism identified by use of electron microscopy; intracellular parasites that may cause disease. (Ch. 7)

Viscosity: (vis-**KAH**-si-tee) Thickness, as of the blood. (Ch. 16)

Volvulus: (**VOL**-view-lus) A twisting of the bowel on itself, causing obstruction. (Ch. 31)

Weber test: (**VAY**-ber TEST) A test for unilateral deafness. (Ch. 48)

Welfare rights: (**WELL**-fare RIGHTS) Also called legal rights; rights that are based on a legal entitlement to some good or benefit. (Ch. 1)

Whisper voice test: (**WISS**-per VOYSS TEST) A simple hearing acuity test in which the client blocks one ear canal and the tester quietly whispers a statement and asks the client to repeat it. (Ch. 48)

White blood cells: (WIGHT BLUHD SELLS) Leukocytes; the body's primary defense against infection. (Ch. 52)

Withdrawal: (with-**DRAW**-ul) Symptoms caused by cessation of administration of a drug, especially a narcotic or alcohol, to which the individual has become either physiologically or psychologically addicted. (Ch. 55)

Worldview: (**WERLD**-vyoo) The way individuals look on the world to form values and beliefs about life and the world around them. (Ch. 3)

Xerostomia: (ZEE-roh-**STOH**-mee-ah) Dry mouth caused by reduction in secretions. (Ch. 10)

Zygote: (**ZYE**-goht) The cell produced by the union of two gametes; the fertilized ovum. (Ch. 40)

Index